KT-872-260

Oxfo[illegible]
End[illegible]ogy and Diabetes

WITHDRAWN

WILLIAM HARVEY LIBRARY
GETEC
GEORGE ELIOT HOSPITAL NHS TRUST
COLLEGE STREET, NUNEATON CV10 7DJ

William Harvey Library
T13061

Oxford University Press makes no representation, express or implied, that the drug dosages in this book are correct. Readers must therefore always check the product information and clinical procedures with the most up-to-date published product information and data sheets provided by the manufacturers and the most recent codes of conduct and safety regulations. The authors and publishers do not accept responsibility or legal liability for any error in the text or for the misuse or misapplication of material in this work. Except where otherwise stated, drug dosages and recommendations are for the non-pregnant adult who is not breast-feeding.

VOLUME 1

Oxford Textbook of Endocrinology and Diabetes

SECOND EDITION

Edited By

John A.H. Wass

Paul M. Stewart

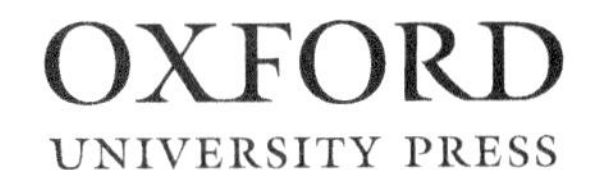

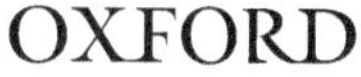

UNIVERSITY PRESS

Great Clarendon Street, Oxford, OX2 6DP,
United Kingdom

Oxford University Press is a department of the University of Oxford.
It furthers the University's objective of excellence in research, scholarship,
and education by publishing worldwide. Oxford is a registered trade mark of
Oxford University Press in the UK and in certain other countries

© Oxford University Press 2011

The moral rights of the authors have been asserted

First published 2002
Second published 2011
First published in paperback 2016

Impression: 1

All rights reserved. No part of this publication may be reproduced, stored in
a retrieval system, or transmitted, in any form or by any means, without the
prior permission in writing of Oxford University Press, or as expressly permitted
by law, by licence or under terms agreed with the appropriate reprographics
rights organization. Enquiries concerning reproduction outside the scope of the
above should be sent to the Rights Department, Oxford University Press, at the
address above

You must not circulate this work in any other form
and you must impose this same condition on any acquirer

Published in the United States of America by Oxford University Press
198 Madison Avenue, New York, NY 10016, United States of America

British Library Cataloguing in Publication Data
Data available

Library of Congress Cataloging in Publication Data
Data available

ISBN 978–0–19–923529–2 (Hbk)
ISBN 978–0–19–879192–8 (Pbk, volume 1)
ISBN 978–0–19–879193–5 (Pbk, volume 2)
ISBN 978–0–19–876649–0 (Pbk, set)

Printed in Great Britain by
Ashford Colour Press Ltd, Gosport, Hampshire

Links to third party websites are provided by Oxford in good faith and
for information only. Oxford disclaims any responsibility for the materials
contained in any third party website referenced in this work.

Brief contents

Contents

PART 3
The thyroid

PART 5 The adrenal gland and endocrine hypertension

PART 6 Neuroendocrine tumours and genetic disorders

PART 7 Growth and development during childhood

Contributors

Amanda I. Adler, Institute of Metabolic Science, Wolfson Diabetes & Endocrine Clinic, Addenbrooke's Hospital, Cambridge, UK

Tomas Ahern, Department of Endocrinology, St Columcille's Hospital, Loughlinstown, Co Dublin, Ireland

S. Faisal Ahmed, University of Glasgow, Royal Hospital For Sick Children, Glasgow, UK

Thankamma Ajithkumar, Department of Clinical Oncology, Norfolk and Norwich University Hospital, Norwich, UK

Kyriaki S. Alatzoglou, Developmental Endocrinology Research Group, Clinical and Molecular Genetics Unit, Institute of Child Health, London, UK

Sir K. George M. M. Alberti, Type 2 Diabetes Group, Division of Medicine, Imperial College London, London, UK, and Diabetes UK, London, UK

K. J. Allen, The Royal Childrens Hospital, Melbourne, Australia

Stephanie A. Amiel, Guy's, King's and St Thomas' School of Medicine, King's College London, London, UK

Nobuyuki Amino, Kuma Hospital, Center for Excellence in Thyroid Care, Kobe, Japan

Stig Andersen, Aalborg Hospital, Aarhus University Hospital, Aalborg, Denmark

Bo Angelin, Department of Endocrinology, Metabolism and Diabetes, Department of Medicine and Molecular Nutrition Unit, Center for Biosciences, Novum, Karolinska Institute at Karolinska University Hospital Huddinge, Stockholm, Sweden

Alessandro Antonelli, Metabolism Unit, Department of Internal Medicine, University of Pisa

Aurora Aragon-Alonso, Department of Endocrinology, University Hospitals Birmingham NHS Foundation Trust, Queen Elizabeth Hospital, Edgbaston, UK

Laleh Ardeshirpour, Department of Pediatrics, Yale University School of Medicine, New Haven, Connecticut, USA

Wiebke Arlt, Centre for Endocrinology, Diabetes and Metabolism (CEDAM), College of Medical and Dental Sciences, School of Clinical and Experimental Medicine, University of Birmingham, Edgbaston, UK

Robert Arnott, Univeristy of Birmingham, Birmingham, UK

Anna Aulinas, Department of Endocrinology/Medicine and Centro de Investigación Biomédica en Red de Enfermedades Raras (CIBER-ER, Unidad 747), Hospital Sant Pau, Universitat Autònoma de Barcelona, Barcelona, Spain

John Ayuk, Department of Endocrinology, Queen Elizabeth Hospital Birmingham and School of Clinical and Experimental Medicine, University of Birmingham, Birmingham, UK

Usha Ayyagari, Oxford Centre for Diabetes, Endocrinology and Metabolism, University of Oxford, Churchill Hospital, Oxford, UK, and National Institute for Health Research, Oxford Biomedical Research Centre, Oxford, UK

Ricardo Azziz, Center for Androgen Related Disorders, Cedars-Sinai Medical Center, and Department of Obstetrics and Gynecology and Department of Medicine, The David Geffen School of Medicine at UCLA, Los Angeles, USA

Michael N. Badminton, Department of Infection, Immunity and Biochemistry, School of Medicine, Cardiff University, Heath Park, Cardiff, Wales, UK

Cliff J. Bailey, Aston Pharmacy School, School of Life and Health Sciences, Aston University, Birmingham, UK

Stephen C. Bain, Institute of Life Science, School of Medicine, Swansea University, Swansea, Wales, UK

H.W. Gordon Baker, Department of Obstetrics and Gynaecology, University of Melbourne, The Royal Women's Hospital, Parkville, Australia

Sabapathy P. Balasubramanianh, Academic Unit of Surgical Oncology, University of Sheffield, Sheffield, UK

Adam Balen, Department of Reproductive Medicine, Leeds General Infirmary, Leeds, UK

Stephen G. Ball, The Medical School, Newcastle University, and Newcastle Hospitals NHS Trust, Newcastle, UK

Anthony H. Barnett, School of Clinical and Experimental Medicine, College of Medical and Dental Sciences, University of Birmingham, Birmingham, UK, and Department of Diabetes and Endocrinology, Heart of England NHS Foundation Trust, Birmingham, UK

Christopher L. R. Barratt, Reproductive and Developmental Biology, Maternal and Child Health Science Laboratories, Centre for Oncology and Molecular Medicine, Ninewells Hospital, University of Dundee, Dundee, Scotland, UK

Luigi Bartalena, Department of Clinical Medicine, Division of Endocrinology, University of Insubria, Varese, Italy

Duncan Bassett, Molecular Endocrinology Group, Division of Medicine, MRC Clinical Sciences Centre, Imperial College London, Hammersmith Hospital, London, UK

Paolo Beck-Peccoz, Department of Medical Sciences, University of Milan, Fondazione Policlinico IRCCS, Milano, Italy

Hermann M. Behre, Center for Reproductive Medicine and Andrology, University Hospital Halle, Martin Luther University, Halle, Germany

Srikanth Bellary, Department of Diabetes and Endocrinology, Heart of England NHS Foundation Trust, Birmingham, UK, and School of Clinical and Experimental Medicine, College of Medical and Dental Sciences, University of Birmingham, Birmingham, UK

Finn N. Bennedbæk, Department of Internal Medicine and Endocrinology, Herlev Hospital, University of Copenhagen, Copenhagen, Denmark

Sarah L. Berga, Department of Gynecology and Obstetrics, Emory University School of Medicine, Atlanta, USA

Ignacio Bernabeu, Endocrinology Section, Hospital Clinico Universitario de Santiago de Compostela, Santiago de Compostela, A Coruña, Spain

Xavier Bertagna, Service des Maladies Endocriniennes et Métaboliques, Hôpital Cochin, Département Endocrinologie, Métabolisme et Cancer, Institut Cochin, and Université Paris Descartes, Paris, France

Jérôme Bertherat, Service des Maladies Endocriniennes et Métaboliques, Hôpital Cochin, Département Endocrinologie, Métabolisme et Cancer, Institut Cochin, and Université Paris Descartes, Paris, France

Rudi Beschorner, Department of Neuroradiology, University of Tuebingen, Tuebingen, Germany

Rachel Besser, Monogenic Research Group, Peninsula Clinical Research Facility, Peninsula Medical School/Royal Devon and Exeter NHS Foundation Trust, Exeter, UK

John Betteridge, University College London Hospitals, London, UK

John S. Bevan, Aberdeen Royal Infirmary, and Department of Endocrinology, University of Aberdeen, Aberdeen, Scotland, UK

John P. Bilezikian, Department of Medicine, College of Physicians and Surgeons, Columbia University, New York, New York, USA

Stephen R. Bloom, Department of Investigative Medicine, Imperial College London, London, UK

Claire Bournaud, Université Claude-Bernard Lyon-1, and Hospices Civils de Lyon, Service d'Endocrinologie-Diabétologie-Maladies Métaboliques, Groupement Hospitalier Sud, Pierre-Bénite, France

G. Brabant, Department of Endocrinology, The Christie, Manchester, UK

Michael Brada, Neuro-oncology Unit, The Institute of Cancer Research and the Royal Marsden NHS Foundation Trust, Sutton, Surrey, UK, and Fulham Road, London, UK

Edward M. Brown, Division of Endocrinology, Diabetes and Hypertension, Department of Medicine, Brigham and Women's Hospital, Boston, Massachusetts, USA

Morris J. Brown, Clinical Pharmacology Unit, Addenbrooke's Hospital, Cambridge, UK

Iain E. Buchan, University of Manchester, Manchester, UK

Henry G. Burger, Prince Henry's Institute of Medical Research, Monash Medical Centre, Clayton, Australia

Gary Butler, Department of Paediatric and Adolescent Medicine and Endocrinology, University College London Hospital and Great Ormond Street Hospital for Children, London, UK, and UCL Institute of Child Health, London, UK

J. V. Byrne, Department of Neuroradiology, The John Radcliffe Hospital, Oxford, UK

Ernesto Canalis, Saint Francis Hospital and Medical Center, Hartford, Connecticut, USA

Martyn E. Caplin, Neuroendocrine Tumour Unit, Centre for Gastroenterology, Royal Free Hospital, London, UK

Cesare Carani, Department of Medicine, Endocrinology and Metabolism, Faculty of Medicine, University of Modena and Reggio, Emilia, Italy, and Nuovo Ospedale Civile S. Agostino-Estense, Modena, Italy

Jean-Claude Carel, Endocrinologie Diabétologie Pédiatrique, INSERM U690, Université Paris 7 Denis Diderot, Hôpital Robert Debré, Paris, France

Marian Carey, Leicester Royal Infirmary, Leicester, UK

Thomas O. Carpenter, Department of Pediatrics, Yale University School of Medicine, New Haven, Connecticut, USA

Felipe F. Casanueva, Department of Medicine, Santiago de Compostela University, Complejo Hospitalario Universitario de Santiago (CHUS), and CIBER de Fisiopatologia Obesidad y Nutricion, Instituto Salud Carlos III, Santiago de Compostela, Spain

Sophie Catteau-Jonard, Department of Endocrine Gynaecology and Reproductive Medicine, Hôpital Jeanne de Flandre, Centre Hospitalier de Lille, France

Filomena Cetani, Department of Endocrinology, University of Pisa, Pisa, Italy

Pierre Chatelain, Université Claude Bernard, Groupe Hospitalier EST, Hôpital Mère–Enfant de Lyon, Service d'Endocrinologie and Diabétologie Infantiles, Bron, France

V. Krishna Chatterjee, Department of Medicine, Addenbrooke's Hospital, University of Cambridge, Cambridge, UK

Moira S. Cheung, Molecular Endocrinology Group, Division of Medicine, MRC Clinical Sciences Centre, Imperial College London, Hammersmith Hospital, London, UK

Shern L. Chew, Department of Endocrinology, St Bartholomew's Hospital, London, UK

Luca Chiovato, Department of Endocrinology, University of Pisa, Pisa, Italy

Pratik Choudhary, Diabetes Research Group, Guy's, King's and St Thomas' School of Medicine, King's College London, London, UK

Adrian J. L. Clark, Centre for Endocrinology, Barts and the London School of Medicine and Dentistry, London, UK

Orlo Clark, UCSF Mt. Zion Medical Center, University of California San Francisco, San Fransisco, USA

P. E. Clayton, Endocrine Science Research Group, Division of Investigative Science, Imperial College London, London, UK

Karine Clément, INSERM, U872 Nutriomic team 7, Centre de Recherche des Cordeliers, Paris, France

Cristina Colom, Department of Internal Medicine, Centre d'Atenció Integral Hospital Dos de Maig, Consorci Sanitari Integral, Barcelona, Spain

John M. C. Connell, Faculty of Medicine, University of Glasgow, Glasgow, UK

Gerard S. Conway, Department of Endocrinology, Institute for Women's Health, UCLH NHS Foundation Trust, London, UK

Andrew Cotterill, Departments of Paediatric Endocrinology, Mater Hospitals, and Department of Paediatrics and Child Health, University of Queensland, Brisbane, Queensland, Australia

Christopher T. Cowell, Institute of Endocrinology, Diabetes and Metabolism, The Children 's Hospital at Westmead, Sydney, Australia

David Cowley, Departments of Paediatric Biochemistry, Mater Hospitals, and Department of Pathology University of Queensland, Brisbane, Queensland, Australia

George Creatsas, Second Department of Obstetrics and Gynecology, Aretaieion Hospital, Athens University School of Medicine, Athens, Greece

David E. Cummings, Division of Metabolism, Endocrinology and Nutrition, Department of Medicine, University of Washington, Seattle, Washington, USA, and Diabetes Endocrinology Research Center, University of Washington, Seattle, Washington, USA, and Diabetes and Obesity Center of Excellence, University of Washington, Seattle, Washington, USA

Janine A. Danks, School of Medical Sciences, RMIT University, Bundoora, Australia

Mehul T. Dattani, Developmental Endocrinology Research Group, Clinical and Molecular Genetics Unit, UCL Institute of Child Health, London, UK

Melanie C. Davies, Reproductive Medicine Unit, Institute for Women's Health, UCLH NHS Foundation Trust, London, UK

Melanie J. Davies, Vascular Medicine Research Group, Department of Cardiovascular Sciences, University of Leicester, Leicester, UK, and Department of Diabetes and Endocrinology, University Hospitals of Leicester NHS Trust, Leicester, UK

Terry F. Davies, Division of Endocrinology and Metabolism, Department of Medicine, Mount Sinai School of Medicine, and the James J. Peters VA Medical Center, New York, New York, USA

Julian R. E. Davis, Endocrine Sciences Research Group, Manchester Academic Health Science Centre, University of Manchester, Manchester, UK

W. W. de Herder, Department of Medicine, Erasmus Univerisity Medical Centre, Rotterdam, The Netherlands

Leonard John Deftos, University of California San Diego, and San Diego VA Medical Center, San Diego, USA

Didier Dewailly, Department of Endocrine Gynaecology and Reproductive Medicine, Hôpital Jeanne de Flandre, Centre Hospitalier de Lille, France

Waljit S. Dhillo, Department of Investigative Medicine, Hammersmith Hospital, Imperial College, London, UK

Kevin Docherty, School of Medical Sciences, University of Aberdeen, Institute of Medical Sciences, Aberdeen, UK

Ines Donangelo, Pituitary Center, Cedars-Sinai Medical Center, UCLA David Geffen School of Medicine at University of California Los Angeles, Los Angeles, USA

Franco Dondero, Department of Medical Pathophysiology, University of Rome, Rome, Italy

Jacqueline Doyle, Clinical Psychologist, Institute for Women's Health, UCLH NHS Foundation Trust, London, UK

W. M. Drake, The Christie, Manchester, UK

Ian F. Dunn, Department of Neurosurgery, Brigham and Women's Hospital, Harvard Medical School, Boston, Massachusetts, USA

Pamela Dyson, Oxford Centre for Diabetes, Endocrinology and Metabolism, University of Oxford, Churchill Hospital, Oxford, UK

Richard Eastell, Academic Unit of Bone Metabolism, Metabolic Bone Centre, Northern General Hospital, Sheffield, UK

Jakob Eberhard, Department of Oncology, Lund University Hospital, Lund, Sweden

Alison Edelman, Department of Obstetrics and Gynaecology, Oregon Health & Science University, Portland, USA

Michael Edmonds, Diabetic Foot Clinic, King's Diabetes Centre, King's College Hospital, London, UK

Thomas Edouard, Department of Paediatric Endocrinology, Hôpital des Enfants, Toulouse, France

George H. Elder, Department of Infection, Immunity and Biochemistry, School of Medicine, Cardiff University, Heath Park, Cardiff, Wales, UK

Rossella Elisei, Department of Endocrinology and Metabolism, University of Pisa, Pisa, Italy

Charis Eng, Genomic Medicine Institute; Center for Personalized Genetic Healthcare, Cleveland Clinic; and Department of Genetics, Case Western Reserve University School of Medicine, Cleveland, USA

Mikael Englund, Cellartis AB, Dundee, Scotland, UK

Ulrike Ernemann, Department of Neuroradiology, University of Tuebingen, Tuebingen, Germany

Poupak Fallahi, Department of Internal Medicine, University of Pisa, Pisa, Italy

I. Sadaf Farooqi, Metabolic Research Laboratories, Institute of Metabolic Science, Addenbrooke's Hospital, Cambridge, UK

Alan P. Farwell, Division of Endocrinology, Diabetes, and Nutrition, Boston University School of Medicine, Boston, Massachusetts, USA

R. A. Feelders, Department of Medicine, Section of Endocrinology, Erasmus University Medical Centre, Rotterdam, The Netherlands

Clodoveo Ferri, Postgraduate School of Clinical Immunology, University of Pisa, Pisa, Italy

Leon Fogelfeld, John H. Stroger Jr Hospital of Cook County, Section of Endocrinology, Chicago, USA

John V. Forrester, Section of Immunology and Infection, Division of Applied Medicine, School of Medicine and Dentistry, Institute of Medical Sciencess, University of Aberdeen, Aberdeen, UK

A. V. M. Foster, Diabetic Foot Clinic, King's Diabetes Centre, King's College Hospital, London, UK

Jayne A. Franklyn, The Medical School, University of Birmingham, Birmingham, UK

Karin Frank-Raue, Endokrinologische Gemeinschaftspraxis, Heidelberg, Germany

E. Marie Freel, Faculty of Medicine, University of Glasgow, Glasgow, UK

Dagmar Führer, Department of Internal Medicine, Division of Endocrinology and Nephrology, University of Leipzig, Leipzig, Germany

John W. Funder, Prince Henry's Institute of Medical Research, Monash Medical Centre, Clayton, Australia

John S. Fuqua, Section of Pediatric Endocrinology and Diabetology, Indiana University School of Medicine, Riley Hospital for Children, Indianapolis, USA

Cécile Gallo, Department of Endocring Gynaecology and Reproductive Medicine, Hôpital Jeanne de Flandre, Centre Hospitalier de Lille, Lille, France

Loredana Gandini, Department of Medical Pathophysiology, University of Rome, Rome, Italy

James Gibney, Department of Endocrinology and Diabetes, Adelaide and Meath Hospital, Tallaght, Dublin, Ireland

Neil J. L. Gittoes, Department of Endocrinology, Queen Elizabeth Hospital Birmingham and School of Clinical and Experimental Medicine, University of Birmingham, Birmingham, UK

Linda C. Giudice, Department of Obstetrics and Gynaecology, Stanford University School of Medicine, Stanford, USA

Andrea Giustina, Department of Medical and Surgical Sciences, University of Brescia, Italy

Aleksander Giwercman, Reproductive Medicine Centre, Malmö University Hospital, Malmö, Sweden

Helen Gleeson, Department of Paediatric Endocrinology, Royal Manchester Children's Hospital, Manchester, UK

Apostolos I. Gogakos, Molecular Endocrinology Group, Division of Medicine, MRC Clinical Sciences Centre, Imperial College London, Hammersmith Hospital, London, UK

David Goltzman, Calcium Research Laboratory, Royal Victoria Hospital, Montreal, Quebec, Canada

Louis J. G. Gooren, Division of Andrology, Free University Hospital Amsterdam, Amsterdam, The Netherlands

Stephen C. L. Gough, Centre for Endocrinology, Diabetes and Metabolism, School of Clinical and Experimental Medicine, College of Medical and Dental Sciences, Institute of Biomedical Research, University of Birmingham, Birmingham, UK

Antonio R. M. Granata, School of Endocrinology and Metabolic Disorders, Faculty of Medicine, University of Modena and Reggio, Emilia, Italy

Peter J. Grant, Division of Cardiovascular and Diabetes Research, Faculty of Medicine and Health, University of Leeds, Leeds, UK

Niels Grarup, Steno Diabetes Center and Hagedorn Research Institute, Gentofte, Denmark

Ristan Greer, Departments of Paediatric Endocrinology, Mater Hospitals, and Department of Paediatrics and Child Health, University of Queensland, Brisbane, Queensland, Australia

Simon Griffin, MRC Epidemiology Unit, Institute of Metabolic Science, Addenbrooke's Hospital, Cambridge, UK

Steven K. Grinspoon, MGH Program in Nutritional Metabolism and Neuroendocrine Unit, Harvard Medical School, Boston, Massachusetts, USA

Lionel Groussin, Service des Maladies Endocriniennes et Métaboliques, Hôpital Cochin, Département Endocrinologie, Métabolisme et Cancer, Institut Cochin, and Université Paris Descartes, Paris, France

Peter Guest, Queen Elizabeth Medical Centre, Queen Elizabeth Hospital, University Hospital Birmingham NHS Foundation Trust, Birmingham, UK

Catherine M. Guly, Aberdeen Royal Infirmary, Aberdeen, UK

Mark Gurnell, Metabolic Research Laboratories, Institute of Metabolic Science, Addenbrooke's Hospital, University of Cambridge, Cambridge, UK

Bjorn I. Gustafsson, Department of Cancer Research and Molecular Medicine, Norwegian University of Science and Technology, Trondheim, Norway

Andrew P. Hall, Sleep Disorders Service, Division of Anaesthesia, Critical Care and Pain Management, University Hospitals of Leicester NHS Trust, Leicester, UK

Saira Hameed, Department of Investigative Medicine, Imperial College London, London, UK

Maggie Sinclair Hammersley, Oxford Radcliffe Hospitals NHS Trust, Oxford, UK

David J. Handelsman, ANZAC Research Institute, and Department of Andrology, Concord Hospital, Sydney, Australia

Torben Hansen, Steno Diabetes Center and Hagedorn Research Institute, Gentofte, Denmark

Barney J. Harrison, Royal Hallamshire Hospital, Sheffield, UK

Andrew Hattersley, Peninsula Clinical Research Facility, Peninsula Medical School, and Royal Devon and Exeter NHS Foundation Trust, Exeter, UK

Laszlo Hegedüs, Department of Endocrinology and Metabolism, Odense University Hospital, University of Southern Denmark, Odense, Denmark

Simon R. Heller, Department of Human Metabolism, University of Sheffield Medical School, Sheffield, UK

Geoffrey N. Hendy, Calcium Research Laboratory, Royal Victoria Hospital, Montreal, Canada

David E. Henley, Department of Endocrinology and Diabetes, Sir Charles Gairdner Hospital, Perth, Australia

Jacqueline K. Hewitt, Department of Endocrinology and Diabetes, Royal Children's Hospital, Parkville, Australia

Raimund Hirschberg, Los Angeles Biomedical Research Institute at Harbor-UCLA Medical Center, Torrance, USA

Ken K. Y. Ho, Pituitary Research Unit, Garvan Institute of Medical Research and Department of Endocrinology, St Vincent's Hospital, Darlinghurst, Sydney, Australia

Humphrey Hodgson, Neuroendocrine Tumour Unit, Centre for Gastroenterology, Royal Free Hospital, London, UK

Jürgen Honegger, Department of Neurosurgery, University of Tuebingen, Tuebingen, Germany

Eva Horvath, Department of Laboratory Medicine, St Michael's Hospital, University of Toronto, Toronto, Canada

Roman Hovorka, Institute of Metabolic Science, University of Cambridge, Cambridge, UK

Trevor A. Howlett, Leicester Royal Infirmary, University Hospitals of Leicester NHS Trust, Leicester, UK

Claire Hughes, Centre for Endocrinology, Barts and the London School of Medicine and Dentistry, London, UK

Ilpo Huhtaniemi, Department of Surgery and Cancer, Imperial College London, London, UK

Andrei Iagaru, Division of Nuclear Medicine and Molecular Imaging, Stanford University Hospital and Clinics, Stanford, USA

Misa Imaizumi, Department of Clinical Studies, Radiation Effects Research Foundation, Nagasaki, Japan

Khalida Ismail, Department of Psychological Medicine, Institute of Psychiatry, King's College London, London, UK

James E. Jackson, Department of Imaging, Imperial College School of Medicine, Hammersmith Hospital, London

Jesper Johannesen, Department of Paediatrics, Glostrup University Hospital, Glostrup, Denmark

Stephen Johnston, Breast Unit, Royal Marsden Hospital, London, UK

A. Kamischke, European Academy of Andrology, Department of Gynaecology and Obstetrics, University Ratzeburger, Lübeck, Germany

Beth Kaplan, Division of Endocrinology, Diabetes, and Nutrition, Boston University School of Medicine, Boston, USA

Janaka Karalliedde, Vascular Cell Biology and Inflammation Research Group, Cardiovascular Division, School of Medicine, King's College London, London, UK

Niki Karavitaki, Department of Endocrinology, Oxford Centre for Diabetes, Endocrinology and Metabolism, Churchill Hospital, Oxford, UK

Joey M. Kaye, Department of Endocrinology and Diabetes, Sir Charles Gairdner Hospital, Perth, Australia

Mark T. Kearney, Division of Cardiovascular and Diabetes Research, Faculty of Medicine and Health, University of Leeds, Leeds, UK

Kamlesh Khunti, Department of Health Sciences, University of Leicester, Leicester UK

Mark Kidd, Yale University School of Medicine, New Haven, Connecticut, USA

Abbas E. Kitabchi, Division of Endocrinology, Diabetes and Metabolism, University of Tennessee Health Science Center, Memphis, Tennessee, USA

Joanna Klubo-Gwiezdzinska, Division of Endocrinology, Washington Hospital Center, Washington, DC, USA

Ulrich A. Knuth, Endokrinologikum Hamburg, Hamburg, Germany

Josef Köhrle, Institut für Experimentelle Endokrinologie und Endokrinologisches Forschungs-Centrum der Charité EnForCé, Charité Universitätsmedizin Berlin, Berlin, Germany

Márta Korbonits, Centre for Endocrinology, William Harvey Research Institute, Barts and The London School of Medicine and Dentistry, London, UK

Kalman Kovacs, Department of Laboratory Medicine, St Michael's Hospital, University of Toronto, Toronto, Canada

Gerasimos E. Krassas, Department of Endocrinology, Diabetes and Metabolism, Panagia General Hospital, Thessaloniki, Greece

Jelena Kravarusic, Division of Endocrinology, Metabolism & Molecular Medicine, Feinberg School of Medicine, Northwestern University, Chicago, USA

Nils Krone, Institute of Biomedical Research, Division of Medical Sciences, University of Birmingham, Birmingham, UK

Sumihisa Kubota, Department of Internal Medicine, Kuma Hospital, Center for Excellence in Thyroid Care, Kobe, Japan

Annie W. C. Kung, The University of Hong Kong, Queen Mary Hospital, Hong Kong, China

L.D. Kuvera, Centre for Endocrine and Diabetes Sciences, Cardiff University School of Medicine, University Hospital of Wales, Cardiff, UK

Robert Lachmann, Charles Dent Metabolic Unit, National Hospital for Neurology and Neurosurgery, London, UK

Steven W. J. Lamberts, Department of Internal Medicine, Erasmus Medical Centre, Rotterdam, The Netherlands

Michael Lassmann, Klinik und Poliklinik für Nuklearmedizin, Julius-Maximilians-Universität Würzburg, Würzburg, Germany

Francesco Latrofa, Department of Endocrinology and Metabolism, University of Pisa, Pisa, Italy

Peter Laurberg, Department of Endocrinology, Aalborg Hospital, Aarhus University Hospital, Aalborg Hospital Science and Innovation Centre, Aalborg, Denmark

Edward R. Laws Jr, Department of Neurosurgery, Brigham and Women's Hospital, Harvard Medical School, Boston, Massachusetts, USA

John H. Lazarus, Centre of Endocrine and Diabetes Sciences, Cardiff University School of Medicine, and Department of Medicine, University of Wales College of Medicine, Cardiff, UK

Sophie Leboulleux, Department of Nuclear Medicine and Endocrine Oncology, Institut Gustave-Roussy, Villejuif, France

Harold E. Lebowitz, Division of Endocrinology, State University of New York Health Science Center, Brooklyn, USA

William L. Ledger, University of Sheffield, Academic Unit of Reproduction and Development, Royal Hallamshire Hospital, Sheffield, UK

Juliane Léger, Department of Pediatric Endocrinology and Diabetology, INSERM CIC-EC05 U676, and Centre de Référence des Maladies Endocriniennes de la Croissance, Robert Debré Hospital and University Paris 7 Denis Diderot, Paris, France

Richard S. Legro, Department of Obstetrics and Gynecology, Pennsylvania State University, College of Medicine, Hershey, Pennsylvania, USA

Andrea Lenzi, Department of Medical Pathophysiology, University of Rome, Rome, Italy

Ronen Levi, Nephrology, Hadassah Hospital, Jerusalem, Israel

Michael A. Levine, Division of Endocrinology and Diabetes, Children's Hospital of Philadelphia and Department of Pediatrics, University of Pennsylvania School of Medicine, Philadelphia, USA

Rossella Libè, Service des Maladies Endocriniennes et Métaboliques, Hôpital Cochin, Département Endocrinologie, Métabolisme et Cancer, Institut Cochin, and Université Paris Descartes, Paris, France

Uri A. Liberman, Department of Physiology and Pharmacology, Sackler School of Medicine, Tel Aviv University, Tel Aviv, Israel

Steven A. Lietman, Department of Orthopaedic Surgery and Department of Biomedical Research, Cleveland Clinic Lerner Research Institute, Cleveland, USA

Stafford L. Lightman, Henry Wellcome Laboratories for Integrative Neuroscience & Endocrinology, University of Bristol, Bristol, United Kingdom

Siew Lim, CSIRO Human Nutrition, Discipline of Physiology, The University of Adelaide, Australia

Francesco Lombardo, Department of Medical Pathophysiology, University of Rome, Rome, Italy

David Lowe, The London Clinic, London, UK

C. Marc Luetjens, Covance Laboratories GmbH, Münster, Germany

Markus Luster, Klinik und Poliklinik für Nuklearmedizin, Uniklinik Ulm, Ulm, Germany

Isla S. Mackenzie, Hypertension Research Centre, University of Dundee and Ninewells Hospital, Dundee, UK

Jane R. MacKinnon, Department of Opthalmology, Aberdeen Royal Infirmary, Aberdeen, UK

Eamonn R. Maher, Department of Medical and Molecular Genetics, School of Clinical and Experimental Medicine, University of Birmingham College of Medical and Dental Sciences, Birmingham, UK

Monica Marazuela, Endocrinology Section, Hospital de la Princesa, Madrid, Spain

Claudio Marcocci, Department of Endocrinology and Metabolism, University of Pisa, Pisa, Italy

Stefano Mariotti, Endocrinology Unit, Department of Medical Sciences, University of Cagliari, Monserrato, Cagliari, Italy

Niamh M. Martin, Endocrine Unit, Department of Investigative Medicine, Imperial College London, London, UK

George Mastorakos, Endocrine Unit, Second Department of Obstetrics and Gynecology, Aretaieion Hospital, Athens University School of Medicine, Athens, Greece

David Matthews, Oxford Centre for Diabetes, Endocrinology and Metabolism, University of Oxford, Churchill Hospital, Oxford, UK, and National Institute for Health Research, Oxford Biomedical Research Centre, Oxford, UK

Krystyna A. Matyka, Clinical Sciences Research Institute, University of Warwick Medical School, Coventry, UK

Gherardo Mazziotti, Department of Medical and Surgical Sciences, University of Brescia, Italy

Christopher J. McCabe, Department of Endocrinology, Queen Elizabeth Hospital Birmingham and School of Clinical and Experimental Medicine, University of Birmingham, Birmingham, UK

David R. McCance, Regional Centre for Endocrinology and Diabetes, Royal Victoria Hospital, Belfast, Northern Ireland, UK

I. Ross McDougall, Division of Nuclear Medicine and Molecular Imaging, Stanford University Hospital and Clinics, Stanford, California, USA

Paul G. McNally, Department of Diabetes and Endocrinology, Leicester Royal Infirmary, Leicester, UK

Karim Meeran, Department of Investigative Medicine, Imperial College London, London, UK

Puja Mehta, Department of Endocrinology and Metabolic Medicine, Hammersmith Hospital, Imperial College London, London, UK

Shlomo Melmed, Pituitary Center, Cedars-Sinai Medical Center, UCLA, and David Geffen School of Medicine at University of California Los Angeles, Los Angeles, California, USA

Francesca Menconi, Division of Endocrinology and Metabolism, Department of Medicine, Mount Sinai School of Medicine, and the James J. Peters VA Medical Center, New York, New York, USA

Dieter Meschede, Praxis für Humangenetik, Köln, Germany

Dieter Mesotten, Intensive Care Medicine Research Group, Department of Acute Medical Sciences, Faculty of Medicine, University Hospital Gasthuisberg, Catholic University of Leuven, Belgium

Louise A. Metherell, Centre for Endocrinology, Barts and the London School of Medicine and Dentistry, London, UK

Paula Midgley, Centre for Reproductive Health, University of Edinburgh, Edinburgh, UK

Dan Mihailescu, Section of Endocrinology, Diabetes and Metabolism, University of Illinois at Chicago, Chicago, USA

Irvin M. Modlin, Yale University School of Medicine, New Haven, Connecticut, USA

Mark E. Molitch, Division of Endocrinology, Metabolism and Molecular Medicine, Northwestern University, Feinberg School of Medicine, Chicago, USA

Michael Monteiro, Brighton and Sussex Medical School; and Gatwick Park Spire Hospital, Brighton and Sussex University Hospitals NHS Trust, Horley, UK

Mauricio Moreno, MD Anderson Cancer Center, Houston, TX, USA

Primus E. Mullis, Paediatric Endocrinology/Diabetology and Metabolism, University Children's Hospital, Inselspital, Bern, Switzerland

Robert D. Murray, Department of Endocrinology, Leeds Teaching Hospitals NHS Trust, Leeds, UK

Shigenobu Nagataki, Nagasaki University, Nagasaki, Japan

C. Nelson-Piercy, St Thomas' Hospital, London, UK

John P. New, Salford Royal NHS Foundation Trust Hope Hospital, Salford, UK

John W. Newcomer, Washington University School of Medicine, St Louis, Missouri, USA

John Newell-Price, Academic Unit of Diabetes and Endocrinology, University of Sheffield, Sheffield, UK

Eberhard Nieschlag, Institute of Reproductive Medicine, University of Münster, Münster, Germany

G. M. K. Nijher, Department of Investigative Medicine, Hammersmith Hospital, Imperial College London, London, UK

Errol R. Norwitz, Yale University School of Medicine, and Department of Obstetrics, Gynecology and Reproductive Sciences, Yale-New Haven Hospital, New Haven, Connecticut, USA

Ebenezer Nyenwe, University of Tennessee Health Science Center, Memphis, Tennessee, USA

John O'Grady, King's College Hospital NHS Foundation Trust, London, UK

Ciara O'Hanlon Brown, Department of Oncology, Imperial College, London, UK

Stephen O'Rahilly, Cambridge Metabolic Research Laboratories, Institute of Metabolic Science, Addenbrooke's Hospital, Cambridge, UK

Donal O'Shea, St Vincent's University Hospital, Dublin; Department of Endocrinology, St Columcille's Hospital, Loughlinstown; and University College Dublin, Dublin, Ireland

Yolanda C. Oertel, FNA Service, Pathology Department, Washington Hospital Center, Cancer Insitute, Washington, DC, USA

Wilma Oostdijk, Department of Paediatrics, Leiden University Medical Center, Leiden, The Netherlands

Jacques Orgiazzi, Université Claude-Bernard Lyon-1, and Hospices Civils de Lyon, Service d'Endocrinologie-Diabétologie-Maladies Métaboliques, Groupement Hospitalier Sud, Pierre-Bénite, France

Furio Pacini, Department of Endocrinology and Metabolism, University of Pisa, Pisa, Italy

Socrates E. Papapoulos, Department of Endocrinology and Metabolic Diseases, Leiden University Medical Centre, Leiden, The Netherlands

Paolo Parini, Division of Clinical Chemistry, Department of Laboratory Medicine and Molecular Nutrition Unit, Center for Biosciences, Novum, Karolinska Institute at Karolinska University Hospital Huddinge, Stockholm, Sweden

Jong Chan Park, Division of Nephrology & Hypertension, Harbor-UCLA Medical Center, Torrance, CA, USA

L. Patel, University of Manchester, Department of Paediatric Endocrinology, Royal Manchester Children's Hospital, Manchester, UK

Mark Peakman, Peter Gorer Department of Immunobiology, Guy's, King's and St Thomas' School of Medicine, King's College London, London, UK

Elizabeth N. Pearce, Division of Endocrinology, Diabetes, and Nutrition, Boston University School of Medicine, Boston, Massachusetts, USA

Inge Bülow Pedersen, Department of Endocrinology and Medicine, Aalborg Hospital, Århus University Hospital, Aalborg, Denmark

Oluf Pedersen, Steno Diabetes Center and Hagedorn Research Institute, Gentofte, Denmark

R. P. Peeters, Department of Endocrinology, Thyroid Laboratory, Erasums Medical Center, Rotterdam, The Netherlands

Nancy D. Perrier, Department of Surgical Oncology, The University of Texas M. D. Anderson Cancer Center, Houston, USA

Luca Persani, Department of Medical Sciences, University of Milan, Istituto Auxologico Italiano IRCCS, Milano, Italy

Frank Petrak, LWL-Klinik Dortmund, Universitätsklinik der Ruhr-Universität Bochum, Dortmund, Germany

John Pickup, Diabetes Research Group, King's College London School of Medicine, Guy's Hospital, London, UK

Aldo Pinchera, Department of Endocrinology and Metabolism, University of Pisa, Pisa, Italy

E. Premawardhana, Centre for Endocrine and Diabetes Sciences, Cardiff University School of Medicine, University Hospital of Wales, Cardiff, UK

Jackie Price, Public Health Sciences Section, Centre for Population Health Sciences, The University of Edinburgh Medical School, Edinburgh, UK

R. L. Prince, Department of Medicine, Sir Charles Gairdner Hospital, Nedlands, USA

Margit G. Proescholdt, Psychiatric Hospital, Division of Substance Use Disorders, University of Basel, Switzerland

A. Ramachandran, India Diabetes Research Foundation, Chennai, India, and Dr A Ramachandran's Diabetes Hospitals, Chennai, India

R. Ramachandran, Department of Investigative Medicine, Hammersmith Hospital, Imperial College, London, UK

Andrea Rapkin, Department of Obstetrics and Gynecology, David Geffen School of Medicine at UCLA, Los Angeles, USA

Friedhelm Raue, Endokrinologische Gemeinschaftspraxis, Heidelberg, Germany

David W. Ray, Endocrine Sciences Research Group, University of Manchester, Manchester, UK

Samantha J. Richardson, School of Medical Sciences, RMIT University, Bundoora, Australia

Felix G. Riepe, Department of Paediatrics, Division of Paediatric Endocrinology, Christian-Albrechts-Universität Kiel, Kiel, Germany

Paul Riley, Molecular Medicine Unit, Institute of Child Health, University College London, London, UK

Vincenzo Rochira, Nuovo, Ospedale Civilie S. Agostino Estense, Unità di Endocrinologia, Modena, Italy

Martina Rodie, University of Glasgow, Royal Hospital For Sick Children, Glasgow, UK

Alan D. Rogol, Department of Pediatrics, Section of Pediatric Endocrinology and Diabetology, University of Virginia; Indiana University School of Medicine, Charlottesville, Virginia, USA; and Riley Hospital for Children, Indianapolis, Indiana, USA

Claus Rolf, Klinik Norderney, Norderney, Germany

Stefano Romeo, School of Clinical Medicine, University of Cambridge, Cambridge, UK

Stefan Rossner, Karolinska Institutet, Stockholm, Sweden

R. Santen, Division of Endocrinology, Department of Medicine, University of Virginia, Charlottesville, USA

Ferruccio Santini, Department of Endocrinology and Metabolism, University of Pisa, Pisa, Italy

David A. Savage, Genetic Epidemiology Research Group, Centre for Clinical and Population Sciences, Queen's University Belfast, Belfast, Northern Ireland, UK

David B. Savage, Univeristy of Cambridge Metabolic Research Laboratories, Institute of Metabolic Science, Addenbrooke's Hospital, Cambridge, UK

Martin O. Savage, Centre for Endocrinology, William Harvey Research Institute, Barts and The London School of Medicine and Dentistry, London, UK

Philip Savage, Imperial College London, London, UK

Clark Sawin, Veterans Health Administration, Washington DC, USA†

W. A. Scherbaum, Department of Endocrinology, University Hospital Düsseldorf, Düsseldorf, Germany

Martin Jean Schlumberger, Department of Nuclear Medicine and Endocrine Oncology, Institut Gustave-Roussy, Villejuif, France

Arthur B. Schneider, Section of Endocrinology, Diabetes and Metabolism, University of Illinois at Chicago, Chicago, USA

Matthias Schott, Department of Endocrinology, University Hospital Düsseldorf, Düsseldorf, Germany

Wolfgang Schulze, Department of Andrology, University of Hamburg, Hamburg, Germany

Michael J. Seckl, Imperial College London, London, UK

Robert K. Semple, University of Cambridge Metabolic Research Laboratories, Institute of Metabolic Science, Addenbrooke's Hospital, Cambridge, UK

Markku Seppälä, Department of Obstetrics and Gynaecology, University of Helsinki Biomedicum, Helsinki, Finland

M. Guftar Shaikh, Royal Hospital for Sick Children, Glasgow, UK

James A. M. Shaw, Institute of Cellular Medicine (Diabetes)/North East England Stem Cell Institute, Newcastle University, and Newcastle Diabetes Centre and Freeman Hospital, Newcastle upon Tyne, UK

Amna Sheri, Breast Unit, Royal Marsden Hospital, London, UK

Mark Sherlock, Department of Endocrinology, University Hospitals Birmingham NHS Foundation Trust, Queen Elizabeth Hospital, Edgbaston, UK

Angela Shore, Institute of Biomedical and Clinical Science, Peninsula Medical School, University of Exeter, Hevitree, UK

Martin Silink, University of Sydney, Australia, and The Children's Hospital at Westmead, Sydney, Australia

Justin Silver, Nephrology and Hypertension Services, Hadassah Hospital, Jerusalem, Israel

Shonni J. Silverberg, Department of Medicine, College of Physicians and Surgeons, Columbia University, New York, New York, USA

Matthew J. Simmonds, Oxford Centre for Diabetes, Endocrinology and Metabolism, Churchill Hospital, University of Oxford, Oxford, UK

C. Snehalatha, India Diabetes Research Foundation, Chennai, India, and Biochemistry Department, Dr A Ramachandran's Diabetes Hospitals, Chennai, India

Eugène Sobngwi, Department of Internal Medicine and Specialties, Faculty of Medicine and Biomedical Sciences, University of Yaoundé 1; National Obesity Centre, Yaoundé Central Hospital, Yaoundé, Cameroon; and Institute of Health and Society, Newcastle Biomedicine, Newcastle University, Newcastle upon Tyne, UK

Parthi Srinivasan, Institute of Liver Studies, King's College Hospital, London, UK

Rajaventhan Srirajaskanthan, Neuroendocrine Tumour Unit, Centre for Gastroenterology, Royal Free Hospital, London, UK

Olof Ståhl, Department of Oncology, Lund University Hospital, Lund, Sweden

Takara L. Stanley, Harvard Medical School, Boston, MA, USA

Paul Stewart, Department of Endocrinology, Queen Elizabeth Hospital, University of Birmingham, Birmingham, UK

Jim Stockigt, Monash University, and Epworth and Alfred Hospitals, Melbourne, Australia

Helen L. Storr, Centre for Endocrinology, William Harvey Research Institute, Barts and The London School of Medicine and Dentistry, London, UK

Constantine A. Stratakis, Program in Developmental Endocrinology and Genetics, National Institute of Child Health and Human Development, National Institutes of Health, Bethesda, Maryland, USA

Noboru Takamura, Department of Radiation Epidemiology, Nagasaki University Graduate School of Biomedical Sciences, Nagasaki, Japan

Maïthé Tauber, Departement Lipoprotéines et Médiateurs Lipidiques, Hôpital Purpan, Toulouse, and Unité d'Endocrinologie Pédiatrique, Maladies Osseuses, Génétique et Gynécologie Médicale, Hôpital des Enfants, Toulouse, France

Helena J. Teede, Prince Henry's Institute of Medical Research, Monash Medical Centre, Clayton, Australia

Massimo Terzolo, Department of Clinical and Biological Sciences, San Luigi Faculty of Medicine, Orbassano, Italy

† It is with regret that we report the death of Dr Clark Sawin.

Solomon Tesfaye, Royal Hallamshire Hospital, Sheffield, UK, and University of Sheffield, Sheffield, UK

Rajesh V. Thakker, Academic Endocrine Unit, Nuffield Department of Clinical Medicine, University of Oxford, and Oxford Centre for Diabetes, Endocrinology and Metabolism, Churchill Hospital, Oxford, UK

George Tharakan, Section of Investigative Medicine, Department of Medicine, Hammersmith Hospital, London, UK

Gilbert R. Thompson, Imperial College School of Medicine, Hammersmith Hospital, Imperial College London, London, UK

Jeannie F. Todd, Department of Endocrinology and Metabolic Medicine, Hammersmith Hospital, Imperial College London, London, UK

Anthony Toft, Endocrine Clinic, Royal Infirmary, Edinburgh, UK

Yaron Tomer, Division of Endocrinology and Metabolism, Department of Medicine, Mount Sinai School of Medicine, and the James J Peters VA Medical Center, New York, New York, USA

Massimo Tonacchera, Department of Endocrinology, University of Pisa, Pisa, Italy

Andrew A. Toogood, Department of Endocrinology, University Hospitals Birmingham NHS Foundation Trust, Queen Elizabeth Hospital, Edgbaston, UK

Christos Toumpanakis, Neuroendocrine Tumour Unit, Centre for Gastroenterology, Royal Free Hospital, London, UK

Herman J. Tournaye, Centre for Reproductive Medicine, Dutch-speaking Free University Brussels, Brussels, Belgium

Peter J. Trainer, The Christie, Manchester, UK

Frank Tüttelman, Institute of Human Genetics, University of Münster, Münster, Germany

Nigel Unwin, Institute of Health and Society, Newcastle Biomedicine, Newcastle University, Newcastle upon Tyne, UK

Greet Van den Berghe, Intensive Care Medicine Research Group, Department of Acute Medical Sciences, Faculty of Medicine, University Hospital Gasthuisberg, Catholic University of Leuven, Belgium, and Department of Intensive Care Medicine, Katholieke Universiteit Leuven, Leuven, Belgium

A. J. van der Lely, Department of Medicine, Section of Endocrinology, Erasmus University Medical Centre, Rotterdam, The Netherlands

Elisabeth F. C. van Rossum, Department of Internal Medicine, Erasmus Medical Centre, Rotterdam, The Netherlands

A. S. Paul van Trotsenburg, Department of Pediatric Endocrinology, Acadmeic Medical Centre, University of Amsterdam, Amsterdam, The Netherlands

Guy Van Vliet, University of Montreal, and Endocrinology Service, Sainte-Justine Hospital, Montreal, Canada

Mark P. J. Vanderpump, Department of Endocrinology, Royal Free Hampstead NHS Trust, London, UK

Yoo-Mee Vanwijngaerden, Intensive Care Medicine Research Group, Department of Acute Medical Sciences, Faculty of Medicine, University Hospital Gasthuisberg, Catholic University of Leuven, Belgium

Hilke Vervenne, Department of Intensive Care Medicine, Katholieke Universiteit Leuven, Leuven, Belgium

Giancarlo Viberti, Cardiovascular Division, King's College London School of Medicine, Guy's Hospital Campus, King's College London, London, UK

Theo J. Visser, Department of Internal Medicine, Erasmus University Medical Center, Rotterdam, The Netherlands

Paolo Vitti, Department of Endocrinology and Metabolism, University of Pisa, Pisa, Italy

Robert Volpé, Department of Medicine, The Wellesley Hospital, Toronto, Canada[†]

Thomas Vulsma, Department of Pediatric Endocrinology, Acadmeic Medical Centre, University of Amsterdam, Amsterdam, The Netherlands

Mike Wallace, Department of Clinical Biochemistry, University of Glasgow, Glasgow, UK

Marc Walter, Psychiatric Hospital, Division of Substance Use Disorders, University of Basel, Switzerland

Garry L. Warne, Department of Endocrinology and Diabetes, Royal Children's Hospital, Parkville, Australia

Leonard Wartofsky, Department of Medicine, Washington Hospital Center, Washington, DC, USA

John A.H. Wass, Department of Endocrinology, Oxford Centre for Diabetes, Endocrinology, and Metabolism, Churchill Hospital, Oxford, UK

Jonathan Waxman, Department of Oncology, Imperial College London, London, UK

Susan M. Webb, Department of Endocrinology/Medicine, Centro de Investigación Biomédica en Red de Enfermedades Raras, and Hospital Sant Pau, Universitat Autònoma de Barcelona, Barcelona, Spain

Anthony P. Weetman, Faculty of Medicine, Dentistry, and Health, The University of Sheffield Medical School, Sheffield, UK

Gerhard F. Weinbauer, Covance Laboratories GmbH, Münster, Germany

Ram Weiss, Department of Human Nutrition and Metabolism, Braun School of Public Health, Hebrew University - Hadassah Faculty of Medicine, Jerusalem, Israel

Erika F. Werner, Department of Obstetrics, Gynecology and Reproductive Biology, Yale University School of Medicine, New Haven, Connecticut, USA

Michael P. Whyte, Center for Metabolic Bone Disease and Metabolic Research, Shriners Hospital for Children, and Division of Bone and Mineral Diseases, Departments of Medicine, Pediatrics, and Genetics, Washington University School of Medicine, St Louis, Missouri, USA

Wilmar M. Wiersinga, Department of Endocrinology and Metabolism, University of Amsterdam, Amsterdam, The Netherlands

Sarah Wild, Public Health Sciences Section, Centre for Population Health Sciences, The University of Edinburgh Medical School, Edinburgh, UK

Bryan Williams, University of Leicester School of Medicine, and Leicester Blood Pressure Clinic, University Hospitals of Leicester NHS Trust, Leicester, UK

Graham R. Williams, Molecular Endocrinology Group, Division of Medicine, MRC Clinical Sciences Centre, Imperial College London, Hammersmith Hospital, London, UK

Jan M. Wit, Department of Paediatrics, Leiden University Medical Center, Leiden, The Netherlands

Katie Wynne, Department of Investigative Medicine, Imperial College London, London, UK

Bulent O. Yildiz, Hacettepe University School of Medicine, Department of Internal Medicine, Endocrinology and Metabolism Unit, Ankara, Turkey

Hannele Yki-Järvinen, Department of Medicine, University of Helsinki, Helsinki, Finland

Mya Zapata, Department of Obstetrics and Gynecology, David Geffen School of Medicine at UCLA, Los Angeles, USA

Michael B. Zimmermann, The Human Nutrition Laboratory, Swiss Federal Institute of Technology (ETH) Zürich, Switzerland, and the Division of Human Nutrition, Wageningen University, Wageningen, The Netherlands

Paul Zimmet, Baker IDI Heart & Diabetes Institute, Melbourne, Australia

[†] It is with regret that we report the death of Dr Robert Volpé.

Abbreviations

1,25$(OH)_2$D	1,25-dihydroxvitamin D
21-OHD	21-hydroxylase deficiency
25(OH)D	25-hydroxyvitamin D
5-HIAA	5-hydroxyindoleacetic acid
5-HT	5-hydroxytryptamine
5-HTP	5-hydroxytryptophan
5α-DHT	5α-dihydrotestosterone
β_2M	β_2 microglobulin
βhCG	β-human chorionic gonadotropin
λ_s	sibling recurrence risk ratio
β-HSD	17β-hydroxysteroid dehydrogenase/isomerase
A4	androstenedione
ABCC8	adenosine triphosphate (ATP)-binding cassette, subfamily C, member 8
ACE	angiotensin-converting enzyme
ACOG	American College of Obstetricians and Gynecologists
ACS	acute coronary syndromes
ACTH	adrenocorticotropic hormone
ADA	American Diabetes Association
ADAM	A disintegrin and metalloprotease (proteins)
ADAMTS9	ADAM metallopeptidase with thrombospondin type 1 motif, 9
ADH	antidiuretic hormone
ADH	atypical ductal hyperplasia
ADH	autosomal dominant hypocalcaemia
ADHH	autosomal dominant hypocalcaemic hypercalciuria
ADP	adenosine diphosphate
AFC	antral follicle count
AFP	α-fetoprotein
AFS	American Fertility Society
AGA	American Gastroenterological Association
AGB	adjustable gastric banding
AGE	advanced glycation end product
AgRP	agouti-related protein
AH	autoimmune hypophysitis
AHC	adrenal hypoplasia congenital
AHH	acquired hypocalciuric hypercalcaemia
AHI	apnoea/hypopnea index
AHO	Albright's hereditary osteodystrophy
AIB1	activated in breast cancer 1
AID	autoimmune diseases
AIDS	acquired immune deficiency syndrome
AIS	androgen insensitivity syndrome
AITD	autoimmune thyroid diseases
ALL	acute lymphoblastic leukaemia
ALS	acid labile subunit
AMH	anti-müllerian hormone
AMPA	α-amino-5-hydroxy-3-methyl-4-isoxazole propionic acid
AMPK	adenosine monophosphate-activated protein kinase
ANOVA	analysis of variance
ANP	atrial natriuretic peptide
AO	acridine orange
AO	autoimmune oophoritis
APC	antigen presenting cell
APECED	autoimmune polyendocrinopathy, candidiasis, and ectodermal dystrophy syndrome
apoB	apolipoprotein B
APS	autoimmune polyendocrine syndrome
APS	autoimmune polyglandular syndrome
AR	androgen receptor
ARB	angiotensin-receptor blocker
ARC	arcuate nucleus
ARDS	adult respiratory distress syndrome
ARE	androgen response element
ART	assisted reproduction techniques
ASA	antisperm antibodies
ASRM	American Society for Reproductive Medicine
ATC	anaplastic thyroid cancer
ATD	antithyroid drug medication
ATP	adenosine triphosphate
AUC	area under (the) curve
AVP	arginine vasopressin
BA	bone age
BACH2	BTB and CNC homology 1, basic leucine zipper transcription factor 2 protein (human)
BAFF	B-cell activating factor belonging to the TNF family
BBS	Bardet–Biedl syndrome
BCL	B-cell lymphoma
BCR	B-cell receptor
BDNF	brain-derived neurotropic factor
BED	biologically effective dose
BMC	bone mineral content
BMD	bone mineral density

BMI	body mass index
BMP	bone morphogenetic protein
BMT	bone marrow transplantation
BNP	brain natriuretic peptide
BPA	bisphenol A
BPD	biliopancreatic diversion
BSA	body surface area
BSO	bilateral salpino-oophorectomy
BSPED	British Society of Paediatric Endocrinology and Diabetes
BTB	broad complex, tramtrack, bric-a-brac
BWS	Beckwith–Wiedemann syndrome
C12orf30	chromosome 12 open reading frame 30
C19	19 carbon
C1QTNF6	C1q and tumour necrosis factor related protein 6
CAH	congenital adrenal hyperplasia
CAIS	complete androgen insensitivity syndrome
CAMK1D	calcium/calmodulin-dependent protein kinase 1D
cAMP	cyclic AMP
CASA	computer-aided sperm analysis
CaSR	calcium-sensing receptor
CBAVD	congenital bilateral absence of the *vas deferens*
CBG	corticosteroid-binding globulin
CBT	cognitive behaviour therapy
CC	clomiphene citrate
CCK	cholecystokinin
CCR5	chemokine (C-C motif) receptor 5
CCSS	Childhood Cancer Survival Study
CD127low	surface marker
CDC123	cell division cycle 123 homolog (*Saccharomyces cerevisiae*)
CDG	congenital disorders of glycosylation
CDGP	constitutional delay of growth and puberty
CDKAL1	CDK5 regulatory subunit associated protein 1-like 1
CDK	cyclin-dependent kinase
CETP	cholesterol ester transfer protein
CF	cystic fibrosis
CFC	cardiofaciocutaneous
CFTR	cystic fibrosis transmembrane regulator
CgA	chromogranin A
CGM	continuous glucose monitoring
cGMP	cyclic guanosine monophosphate
CGMS	continuous glucose monitoring system
CGRP	calcitonin gene-related protein
CHI	congenital hyperinsulinism of infancy
CHM	complete molar pregnancies
CI	confidence interval
CIS	carcinoma *in situ*
CJD	Creutzfeldt–Jakob disease
CLAH	congenital lipoid adrenal hyperplasia
CLEC16A	C-type lectin domain family 16, member A
CMI	carbimazole
CMV	cytomegalovirus
CNC	cap 'n' collar; family of basic leucine zipper transcription factors
CNS	central nervous system
CO2	carbon dioxide
COC	combined oral contraceptive
COH	controlled ovarian hyperstimulation
COPE	Calendar of Premenstrual Experiences
CRE	cyclic AMP response element
CREB	cyclic AMP response element binding protein
CREM	cyclic AMP (cAMP) responsive element modulator (CREM)
CRF	chronic renal failure
CRH	corticotropin-releasing hormone
CRP	C-reactive protein
CRT	conformal radiotherapy
CS	Cushing's syndrome
CSF	cerebrospinal fluid
CSII	continuous subcutaneous insulin infusion
CSK	C-terminal Src kinase
CSW	central salt wasting
CT	computed tomography
cTECs	cortical thymic epithelial cells
CTGF	connective tissue growth factor
CTL	cytotoxic T lymphocyte
CTLA4	cytotoxic T-lymphocyte-associated protein 4 (human); cytotoxic T-lymphocyte antigen 4
CTL	cytotoxic T lymphocyte
CTSH	cathepsin H
CUAVD	congenital unilateral absence of the vas deferens
CVD	cardiovascular disease
D1–3	deiodinase 1–3
DAG	diacylglycerol
DALY	disability-adjusted life year
DAX1	dosage-sensitive sex reversal-adrenal hypoplasia gene 1
DCCT	Diabetes Control and Complications Trial
DDAVP	1-desamino-8-D-arginine vasopressin
DDE	dichlorodiphenyldichloroethylene
DDI	dipsogenic diabetes insipidus
DEND	developmental delay, epilepsy, and neonatal diabetes
DES	diethylstilbestrol
DET	double embryo transfer
DGGE	denaturing gradient gel electrophoresis
DHA	docosahexaenoic acid
DHEA	dehydroepiandrosterone
DHEAS	dehydroepiandrosterone sulfate
DHT	dihydrotestosterone
DIDMOAD	diabetes insipidus, diabetes mellitus, optic atrophy, and deafness
DIT	diiodotyrosine
DJB	duodenal–jejunal bypass
DKA	diabetic ketoacidosis
DMPA	depo-medroxyprogesterone acetate
DNA	deoxyribonucleic acid
DON	dysthyroid optic neuropathy
DPP4	dipeptidyl-peptidase 4; also known as adenosine deaminase complexing protein 2 or CD26 antigen
DSD	disorders of sex development
DSM-IV	*Diagnostic and Statistical Manual of Mental Disorders*, 4th edition
DTC	differentiated thyroid cancer
DTT	dithiothreitol
DUOX	dual oxidase
DVT	deep venous thrombosis
EAT	experimental autoimmune thyroiditis
ECG	electrocardiogram
ECL	enterochromaffin-like
ECM	extracellular matrix
EDTA	ethylenediaminetetraacetic acid
EEG	electroencephalogram
EGF	epidermal growth factor
EGFR	epidermal growth factor receptor
EIF2AK3	eukaryotic translation initiation factor 2-alpha kinase 3
eIFs	eukaryotic initiation factors
ELISA	enzyme-linked immunosorbent assay
EMEA	European Medicines Agency

EMH	estimated mature height
EMS	external masculinization score
EPA	eicosapentaenoic
EPO	erythropoietin
ER	oestrogen receptor
ERBB3	v-erb-b2 erythroblastic leukaemia viral oncogene homolog 3 (avian) [*Homo sapiens*]
ERK	elk-related tyrosine kinase
ESHRE	European Society of Human Reproduction and Embryology
ESPE/GRS	European Society of Paediatric Endocrinology and Growth Hormone Research Society
ESR	erythrocyte sedimentation rate
EUGOGO	European Group on Graves' Orbitopathy
EUS	endoscopic ultrasonography
FAI	free androgen index
FasL	Fas ligand
FDG	[^{18}F]2-fluoro-2-deoxy-D-glucose
FDH	familial dysalbuminaemic hyperthyroxinaemia
FEV$_1$	forced expiratory volume in 1 s
FFA	free fatty acids
FGF	fibroblast growth factor
FGFR3	fibroblast growth factor receptor-3
FHA	functional hypothalamic anovulation
FHH	familial hypocalciuric hypercalcaemia
FHPP	familial hypokalaemic periodic paralysis
FISH	fluorescence *in situ* hybridization
FNA	fine-needle aspiration
FNAB	fine-needle aspiration biopsy
FOXP3	forkhead box P3 protein, human
FPG	fasting plasma glucose
FSCRT	fractionated stereotactic conformal radiotherapy
FSH	follicle-stimulating hormone
FSRT	fractionated stereotactic radiotherapy
FSS	familial short stature
FTC	follicular thyroid cancer
FTO	fat mass and obesity associated
G6PD	glucose-6-phosphate dehydrogenase
GABA	γ-aminobutyric acid
GAD	glutamic acid decarboxylase; glutamate decarboxylase
GAD65	glutamic acid decarboxylase 2; glutamate decarboxylase 2
GAP	GTPase activating protein
GAT	gelatin agglutination test
GCK	glucokinase (hexokinase 4)
GCKR	glucokinase (hexokinase 4) regulator
GCM2	glial cells missing 2
GCMS	gas chromatography mass spectrometry
GCSF	granulocyte colony-stimulating factor
GDM	gestational diabetes
GFR	glomerular filtration rate
GGTP	γ-glutamyl transpeptidase
GH	growth hormone
GHBP	growth hormone-binding protein
GHD	growth hormone deficiency
GHI	growth hormone insensitivity
GHIS	growth hormone insensitivity syndrome
GHR	growth hormone receptor
GHRH	growth hormone-releasing hormone
GHRHR	growth hormone-releasing hormone receptor
GHRP	growth hormone-releasing peptides
GI	glycaemic index
GIP	gastric inhibitory polypeptide; glucose-dependent-insulinotropic polypeptide
GLIS3	GLI-similar family zinc finger protein 3
GLP-1	glucagon-like peptide-1
GLUT4	glucose transporter type 4
GnRH	gonadotropin-releasing hormone
GnRHa	gonadotropin-releasing hormone analogue
GoKinD	Genetics of Kidneys in Diabetes
GO-QOL	Graves' ophthalmopathy quality of life
GR	glucocorticoid receptor
GRE	glucocorticoid response element
GSD	glycogen storage disease
GST	glucagon stimulation test
GTD	gestational trophoblastic disease
GTN	gestational trophoblastic neoplasia
GTP	guanosine triphosphate
GTT	gestational trophoblast tumour
GTV	gross tumour volume
GV	growth velocity
HA	hyperandrogenism
HAART	highly active antiretroviral therapy
HADH	3-hydroxy-acyl-CoA dehydrogenase
HAIRAN	hyperandrogenism, insulin resistance and acanthosis nigricans
HbA$_{1c}$	glycated haemoglobin
HB-EGF	heparin-binding epidermal growth factor
HBGM	home blood glucose monitoring
HCB	hexachlorobenzene
HCDC	hydrocortisone day curve
hCG	human chorionic gonadotropin
HDI	hypothalamic diabetes insipidus
HDL	high density lipoprotein
HDR	hypoparathyroidism, deafness, and renal anomalies syndrome
HEPES	4-(2-hydroxyethyl)-1-piperazineethanesulfonic acid
hES	human embryonic stem cells
HES	hydroxyethyl starch
HFEA	Human Fertilization and Embryology Authority
HGH	human growth hormone
HH	hypogonadotropic hypogonadism
HHEX	haematopoietically expressed homoeo box
HHV	human herpesvirus
HI	hyperinsulinism of infancy
HI/HA	hyperinsulinism/hyperammonaemia
HIV	human immunodeficiency virus
HLA	human leucocyte antigen
HMG	3-hydroxy-3-methylglutaryl
HMG	high-mobility group
hMG	human menopausal gonadotropin
HMG CoA	hydroxymethylglutaryl CoA
HNF	hepatocyte nuclear factor
HOMA	homoeostatic model assessment
HONK	hyperosmolar nonketotic state
HOS	hypo-osmotic swelling
HPA	hypothalamic–pituitary–adrenal
HPLC	high-performance liquid chromatography
HPG	hypothalamic–pituitary–gonadal
HPT	hypothalamic–pituitary–thyroid
HPTP	hypothalamic–pituitary–thyroid–periphery
HPV	human papillomavirus
HR	hazard ratio
HRT	hormone replacement therapy
HSD3B2	3B-hydroxysteroid dehydrogenase 2
HSG	hysterosalpingography
HSP	heat shock proteins
HSV	herpes simplex virus

HT	Hashimoto's thyroiditis
HTLVI	human T-cell lymphotropic virus type I
HU	Hounsfield unit
HV	height velocity
IA-2	insulinoma-associated protein 2
IAA	insulin autoantibodies
ICAM-1	intercellular adhesion molecule 1
ICD-10	*International Classification of Diseases, 10th Revision*
ICM	inner cell mass
ICOS	inducible T-cell costimulator
ICSI	intracytoplasmic sperm injection
ICTP	C-telopeptide pyridinoline cross-links of type I collagen
IDD	iodine deficiency disorders
IDDM	insulin-dependent diabetes mellitus
IDE	insulin-degrading enzyme
IDL	intermediate density lipoprotein
IDM	infant diabetes mellitus
IDPP	Indian Diabetes Prevention Programme
IFCC	International Federation of Clinical Chemistry
IFG	impaired fasting glycaemia; impaired fasting glucose
IFIH1	interferon induced with helicase C domain 1
IFMA	immunofluorometric assays
IFN-α	interferon
Ig	Immunoglobulin
IGF	insulin-like growth factor
IGFBP	insulin -like growth factor binding protein
IGF-1	insulin-like growth factor 1
IGF-IR	insulin-like growth factor 1 receptor
IGHD	isolated growth hormone deficiency
IGRP	islet-specific glucose-6-phosphatase catalytic subunit related protein
IGT	impaired glucose tolerance
IHC	immunohistochemical
IHH	isolated hypogonadotropic hypogonadism
Ii	invariant chain
IL	interleukin
IM	intramuscular
IMRT	intensity-modulated radiotherapy
INR	international normalized ratio
INS	insulin
INSR	insulin receptor
IP_3	inositol 1,4,5-trisphosphate
IPEX	immunodysregulation polyendocrinopathy enteropathy X-linked (syndrome)
IPH	index of potential height
IQ	intelligence quotient
IRB	immune radio binding
IRD	inner ring deiodination
IRMA	immunoradiometric assays
IRS1	insulin receptor substrate 1
ISPAD	International Society for Pediatric and Adolescent Diabetes
ISS	idiopathic short stature
ISSCR	International Society for Stem Cell Research
ITT	insulin tolerance test
IUD	intrauterine device
IUGR	intrauterine growth restriction
IUI	intrauterine insemination
IV	intravenous
IVF	*in vitro* fertilization
IVF-ET	*in vitro* fertilization and embryo transfer
JAK	Janus tyrosine kinase
JAZF1	juxtaposed with another zinc finger gene 1 protein, human
JMML	juvenile myelomonocytic leukaemia
JNK	c-Jun N-terminal kinase
K_{ATP} channel	ATP-sensitive potassium channel
KS	Kallmann's syndrome
KTS	Wilms' tumor protein
LADA	latent autoimmune diabetes
LCAT	lecithin cholesterol acyl transferase
LC-NE	locus coeruleus-noradrenergic
LCR	locus control region
LDL	low-density lipoprotein
LDLR	LDL receptor
LGA	large-for-gestational-age
LGR5	leucine-rich repeat-containing G protein-coupled receptor 5
LH	luteinizing hormone
LHRH	luteinizing hormone-releasing hormone
LIF	leukaemia inhibitory factor
LOH	late-onset hypogonadism
LOH	loss of heterozygosity
LPD	luteal phase deficiency
LPL	lipoprotein lipase
LRP	LDL receptor-related protein
Lyp	lymphoid-specific tyrosine phosphatase
MAP	mitogen activated protein
MAPK	mitogen-activated protein kinase
MAR	mixed antiglobulin reaction test
MC4R	melanocortin 4 receptor
MCAD	medium chain acyl coenzyme A dehydrogenase deficiency
MCB	master cell bank
MCH	melanin-concentrating hormone
MCP-1	monocyte chemoattractant protein-1
M-CSF	macrophage colony-stimulating factor
MD	maturational delay
MDA5	melanoma differentiation-associated protein 5
mDC	myeloid dendritic cell
MDI	multiple daily injection
Med OOX	medical oophorectomy
MELAS	mitochondrial encephalopathy, lactic acidosis, stroke-like episodes syndrome
MEN	multiple endocrine neoplasia
MESA	microsurgical epididymal sperm aspiration
Met-rGH	recombinant methionyl growth hormone
MGD	mixed gonadal dysgenesis
MHC	major histocompatibility complex
MHT	menopausal hormone therapy
MIBG	metaiodobenzylguanidine
MIDD	maternally inherited diabetes and deafness
MIS	müllerian inhibitory substance
MIT	monoiodotyrosine
MLC	multileaf collimator
MMI	methimazole
MMP	matrix metalloproteinase
MODY	maturity-onset diabetes of the young
MP	molar pregnancy
MPA	medroxyprogesterone acetate
MPD	myeloproliferative disorders
MPH	mid-parental height
MPHD	multiple pituitary hormone deficiency
MPS	mucopolysaccharidosis
MR	mineralocorticoid receptor
MRI	magnetic resonance imaging
MRKH	Mayer–Rokitansky–Kuster–Hauser

MS	mass spectrometry
MSH	melanocyte-stimulating hormone
MSY	male-specific region of the Y chromosome
MTC	medullary thyroid carcinoma
mtDNA	mitochondrial DNA
mTECs	medullary thymic epithelial cells
MTNR1B	melatonin receptor 1B
MURCS	mullerian, renal, cervical spine syndrome
NAD	nicotinamide-adenine-dinucleotide
NAFLD	non-alcoholic fatty liver disease
NANC	nonadrenergic-noncholinergic
NASH	nonalcoholic steatohepatitis
NCAH	nonclassic congenital adrenal hyperplasia
NCFC	neuro-cardio-facial-cutaneous
NCGS	National Cooperative Growth Study
NCHS	National Center for Health Statistics
NDDG	National Diabetes Data Group
NDI	nephrogenic diabetes insipidus
NEFA	nonesterified fatty acid
NET	neuroendocrine tumour
NEUROD1	neurogenic differentiation 1
NF	neurofibromatosis
NF-AT	nuclear factor of activated T cells
NF-κB	Nuclear factor κ-B
NGT	normal glucose tolerance
NHANES	National Health and Nutrition Examination Survey
NHPT	neonatal primary hyperparathyroidism
NICE	National Institute for Health and Clinical Excellence
NICHD	National Institute of Child Health and Human Development
NICU	neonatal intensive care unit
NIDDM	noninsulin-dependent diabetes mellitus
nIHH	normosmic idiopathic hypogonadotropic hypogonadism
NIS	sodium-iodide symporter
NK	natural killer
NMDA	*N*-methyl-D-aspartate
NO	nitrogen oxide
NOD mice	non-obese diabetic mice; animal model
NOTCH2	notch 2 (notch homolog 2 (*Drosophila*))
NPY	neuropeptide Y
NS	Noonan's syndrome
NSAID	nonsteroidal anti-inflammatory drug
NSHPT	neonatal severe hyperparathyroidism
nsSNP	nonsynonymous single nucleotide polymorphism
NTG	nontoxic goitre
OA	oligo and/or anovulation
OGTT	oral glucose tolerance test
OHSS	ovarian hyperstimulation syndrome
ONH	optic nerve hypoplasia
OPN	osteopontin
OR	oestrogen receptor
ORD	outer ring deiodination
ORF	open reading frame
OSAS	obstructive sleep apnoea syndrome
P450scc	P450 cholesterol side chain cleavage enzyme
$Paco_2$	partial pressure of carbon dioxide
PAH	polycyclic aromatic hydrocarbons
PAI-1	plasminogen activator inhibitor 1
PAIS	Partial androgen insensitivity syndrome
PAS	periodic acid–Schiff
PAX4	paired box 4
PBB	polybrominated biphenyls
PBDE	polybrominated diphenyl ethers
PBR	peripheral-type benzodiazepine receptor
PCB	polychlorinated biphenyls
PCDF	polychlorinated dibenzofurans
PCO	polycystic ovary
PCoA	posterior communicating artery
PCOS	polycystic ovary syndrome
PCR	polymerase chain reaction
pDC	plasmacytoid dendritic cell
PDX1	pancreatic and duodenal homoeo box 1
PET	positron emission tomography
PFS	progression-free survival
PG	prostaglandin
PGD	preimplantation genetic diagnosis
PGHS	prostaglandin H synthase
PGS	preimplantation genetic screening
PHM	partial molar pregnancies
PHP	pseudohypoparathyroidism
PHPT	primary hyperparathyroidism
PICP	propeptide of type I procollagen
Pit-hGH	pituitary human growth hormone
PKA	protein kinase A
PKC	protein kinase C
PLAP	placental/germ alkaline phosphatase
PLTP	phospholipid transfer protein
PMDD	premenstrual dysphoric disorder
PMDS	persistent müllerian duct syndrome
PMS	premenstrual syndrome
PMTS	premenstrual tension syndrome
PNDM	permanent neonatal diabetes mellitus
PO	per oral
POF	premature ovarian failure
POMC	proopiomelanocortin
POP	persistent organohalogen pollutant
POR	P450 oxidoreductase
PP	Pancreatic polypeptide
PPAR	peroxisome proliferator-activated receptor
PPi	inorganic pyrophosphate
PPI	proton pump inhibitor
PPT	postpartum thyroiditis
PRKCθ	protein kinase C, theta
PRL	prolactin
PRLR	prolactin receptor
proTRH	protein precursor of thyrotropin-releasing hormone
PSA	prostate specific antigen
PSD	psychosocial deprivation
PSTT	placental site trophoblastic tumours
PSU	pilosebaceous unit
PTC	papillary thyroid cancer
PTF1A	pancreas-specific transcription factor 1a
PTH	parathyroid hormone
PTHrP	parathyroid hormone-related protein
PTPN	protein tyrosine phosphatase nonreceptor
PTU	propylthiouracil
PTV	planning target volume
PVN	paraventricular nucleus
PWS	Prader–Willi syndrome
QCT	quantitative computed tomography
RAD	relative absolute difference
RAIT	radioactive iodine therapy
RAIU	radioactive iodine uptake

RAS renin–angiotensin system
Rb retinoblastoma protein
RBM17 RNA binding motif protein 17
RCT randomized controlled trial
REM rapid eye movement
rhGH recombinant human growth hormone
rhTSH recombinant human thyroid-stimulating hormone
RIA radioimmunoassays
ROC receiver–operating characteristic (curve)
ROS reactive oxygen species
ROS resistant ovary syndrome
RPLND retroperitoneal lymph node dissection
RXR retinoid X receptor
RYGB Roux-en-Y gastric bypass
SAH subarachnoid haemorrhage
SAHA suberoylanilide hydroxamic acid
SARMs specific androgen receptor modulators
SC subcutaneous
SCGE single-cell gel electrophoresis
SCHAD short chain 3-hydroxy-acyl-CoA dehydrogenase
SCNT somatic cell nuclear transfer
SCO Sertoli cell-only
SCSA sperm chromatin structural assay
SD standard deviation
SDH succinate dehydrogenase
SDS sodium dodecyl sulfate
SDS standard deviation score
SEER surveillance epidemiology and end results database
SEMS self-expanding metallic stent
SERMs selective oestrogen receptor modulators
SET single embryo transfer
SF-1 steroidogenic factor-1
SGA small for gestational age
SHBG sex hormone-binding globulin
SHOX short stature homoeobox-containing gene
SIAD syndrome of inappropriate antidiuresis
SIGN Scottish Intercollegiate Guideline Network
SLC30A8 solute carrier family 30 (zinc transporter), member 8
SLE systemic lupus erythematosus
SMBG self-monitoring of blood glucose
SMR standardized mortality ratio
SMS somatostatin
SNP single nucleotide polymorphism
SNR signal-to-noise ratio
SNRI serotonin norepinephrine reuptake inhibitors
SOD septo-optic dysplasia
SPA sperm penetration assay
SPECT single photon emission computed tomography
SR-A scavenger receptor class A
SR-B1 scavenger receptor class B type 1
SRBD sleep-related breathing disorders
SRCs steroid receptor coactivator proteins
SRS Silver–Russell syndrome
SRS somatostatin receptor scintigraphy
SS short stature
SSCP single strand conformation polymorphism
SSKI saturated solution of potassium iodide
SSRI selective serotonin reuptake inhibitors
SST short Synacthen test
SST somatostatin
SSTR somatostatin receptor
StAR steroid acute regulatory protein
StAR steroidogenic acute regulatory protein
STAT signal transducers and activators of transcription
STC stanniocalcin
SUR1 sulphonylurea receptor 1
T_2 diiodothyronine
T_3 triiodothyronine
T_4 thyroxine/tetraiodothyronine
tagSNP tag single nucleotide polymorphism
TART testicular adrenal rest tumour
TAT tray agglutination test
TBCE tubulin chaperone E
TBG thyroxine-binding globulin
TBI traumatic brain injury
TBI TSH-binding inhibition
TBII TSH-binding inhibiting immunoglobulins
TCF7L2 transcription factor 7-like 2
TCR T-cell receptor
TDS testicular dysgenesis syndrome
TdT terminal deoxynucleotide transferase
TESA testicular sperm aspiration
TESE testicular sperm extraction
Tfh follicular helper T lymphocytes
TGCC testicular germ cell cancer
TGF transforming growth factor
Th T helper
TH Target height
Th17 subset of T helper cells (Th1) producing interleukin-17
THADA thyroid adenoma associated
THDPs thyroid hormone distributor proteins
TIC theca-interstitial cells
TIMP tissue inhibitors of metalloproteinase
TLP transthyretin-like protein
TLP TTR-like protein
TLR toll-like receptor
TNDM transient neonatal diabetes
TNF tumour necrosis factor
TNM classification of malignant tumours (tumour, node, metastases)
TPN total parenteral nutrition
TPO thyroid peroxidase
TPP thyrotoxic periodic paralysis
TRA tissue-restricted antigens
TRAb thyrotropin/thyroid-stimulating hormone-receptor antibodies
TRE T_3 response element
Treg T regulatory cell
TRH thyrotropin-releasing hormone
TRHDE TRH-degrading ectoenzyme
TRHR thyrotropin-releasing hormone receptor
tPA tissue plasminogen activator
TS Turner's syndrome
TSH thyroid-stimulating hormone
TSHR thyroid-stimulating hormone receptor
TSI thyroid-stimulating immunoglobulin/TSH-receptor stimulating immunoglobulin
TSPAN8 tetraspanin 8
TSPY testis-specific protein Y encoded
TTR transthyretin
TUNEL terminal deoxynucleotidyl transferase-mediated dUTP nick-end labelling
TW3 Tanner Whitehouse-3
UAER urinary albumin excretion rate
UBASH3A ubiquitin associated and SH3 domain containing protein A (human)

UDH usual ductal hyperplasia
UFC urine for free cortisol
UKPDS United Kingdom Prospective Diabetes Study
uPA urokinase plasminogen activator
UPD uniparental disomy
USI universal salt iodization
VAS visual analogue scale
VDDR vitamin D-dependent rickets
VDR vitamin D receptor
VDRE vitamin D response element
VEGF vascular endothelial growth factor
VHL von Hippel–Lindau disease
VIP vasoactive intestinal polypeptide
VLDL very-low-density lipoprotein
VMN ventromedial nucleus
VNTR variable number of tandem repeats
VO_2 max maximal oxygen uptake
VTE venothrombotic episodes
WAGR WAGR syndrome
WBS whole body scan
WCB working cell bank
WFS1 Wolfram syndrome 1 (wolframin)
WHI Women's Health Initiative
WHO World Health Organization
WT1 Wilms' tumour-related gene-1
ZnT8 zinc transporter 8
ZP zona pellucida

PART 1

Principles of international endocrine practice

1.1

A brief history of endocrinology

Robert Arnott

Introduction

This chapter traces the history of endocrinology, principally through the nineteenth and the beginning of the twentieth centuries, but also looks further back to antiquity and the early modern period when the function of the glandular system was beginning to be recognized and partly understood. It also takes us through to later in the twentieth century, when therapeutics were developed that could tackle endocrine disease, and at the significant discoveries and those scientists and clinicians who made them, placing them in context of what appears later in this volume.

As a modern biomedical discipline, endocrinology can trace its origins back to the end of the nineteenth and the beginnings of the twentieth centuries, especially to 1905, when Ernest Starling (1866–1927) first used the word 'hormone' (1). This is not, however, to ignore what was learned in antiquity and the early modern period. In fact, most of the organs and tissues that form the body's endocrine system were known in some way by the early seventeenth century, particularly the pituitary, adrenal glands, gonads, and the likely cause of goitres, although most of these discoveries are now seen as purely isolated and not linked until the larger picture of the physiology of the human body eventually emerged. It took, for example, another 200 years to discover the islets of Langerhans and the function of the thyroid, although the thyroid gland itself it, as well as the function of the thymus and the spleen, had been described by the German polymath Albrecht von Haller (1708–77) and the French physician Théophile de Bordeu (1722–76) who wrote in the mid-eighteenth century about the body's organs discharging secretions (or 'emanations') into the bloodstream.

Early experimentation to support the ideas of von Haller and de Bordeu, that secretions from the glands played an important part in the function of the human body, can also be traced to around this time. The effects of castration, both animal and human were understood by many, including the distinguished London anatomist and surgeon, John Hunter (1728–93), who was aware that the secondary sex characteristics of castrated cockerels could be maintained by implanting their testes at other places. Later on in the nineteenth century, Arnold Berthold (1803–61), working in Göttingen, not only confirmed Hunter's work but also developed an understanding that the testes controlled the sex characteristics through the bloodstream (2). It was, however, the Parisian scientist Claude Bernard (1813–78), who actually first observed internal secretions, by discovering in 1855 that glucose synthesized in the liver was secreted into the portal vein, differentiating it from bile (1). Endocrinology was now taking it first and faltering steps.

Other work in this period included that of Thomas Addison (1793–1860) of Guy's Hospital in London (3) who gave his name to Addison's disease, describing the function of the adrenal glands. In 1873, Sir William Gull (1816–90) also of Guy's Hospital, working on goitre and cretinism, already attributed to iodine deficiency, described the 'cretinous state', (4) which he also called myxoedema. This was supported by the work of the Swiss scientist Emil Theodor Kocher (1841–1917) (5) and the London laryngologist Sir Felix Semon (1848–1921), who described the medical conditions brought about by the absence or malfunction of the thyroid gland. Early treatments for myxoedema were at first a complete failure, but George R. Murray (1865–1939) working first in Newcastle-upon-Tyne successfully managed to inject an extract of sheep thyroid into a patient with the condition, and oral therapy with sheep thyroid proved to be equally effective, soon becoming the established treatment for hypothyroidism (1).

It was not until well into the nineteenth century that work on Addison's disease was resumed. George Oliver (1841–1915) and later Sir Edward Sharpey-Schäfer (1850–1935), both working at University College London, found that adrenal extract, later called adrenaline after its isolation by John Abel (1857–1938) and Albert Crawford (1869–1921), when injected into dogs, caused a rapid increase of the heart rate and blood pressure. Shortly afterwards adrenaline was synthesized, and became the very first secretion of a ductless gland to be characterized chemically. Proved ineffective in the treatment of Addison's disease, Sir William Osler (1849–1919) is reported to have revived at least one patient with orally administered adrenaline (1).

It was the Greek physician Aretaeus of Cappadocia (81 – c.AD 138), believed to have first described the destructive nature of diabetes (διαβήτης), the Greek word for a siphon, who linked the disease to excessive discharge of urine (6). Mellitus, the Latin word for sweet, was added later, because some early Roman physicians believed that the urine tasted of honey, taste being a standard diagnostic test at the time. In his *Therapeutics of Chronic Diseases* (II.ii.485–6), Aretaeus mentions 'in diabetes the flow of the humour from the affected part and the melting is the same, but the abnormal discharge of urine is linked to the kidneys and the bladder, as in dropsy. In diabetes, the thirst is greater; for the fluid being passed dries out the body. For the thirst there is need of a very powerful remedy, for this is one of the worst of all sufferings, for when a fluid is drunk, it stimulates the discharge of urine' [translation: author]. The leading Greek physician of his time, Galen of Pergamum (AD 129–216), wrongly believed, perhaps not unreasonably, that diabetes was a disease of the kidneys. From then until the twentieth century, diabetes was an indiscriminate killer. Until then, however, only occasionally did some observations point to the correct determination of its actual cause; the Leiden physician Johann Brunner (1653–1727) had observed in 1673 that a dog experienced polyuria and thirst after experimental removal of both its pancreas and spleen. Thomas Willis (1621–1675) wrote of the 'pissing evil' and that the urine of diabetes patients tasted very sweet.

Over 200 years later, two French scientists, Xavier Arnozan (1852–1928) and Louis Vallard (1850–1935), found that the ligation of the ducts of the pancreas led to atrophy of the acinar tissue, while the islets, described by the German pathologist Paul Langerhans (1847–88), now called the islets of Langerhans, remained largely intact (1). Later that century, the work of Joseph von Mering (1849–1908) and Édouard Hèdon (1863–1933) developed a deeper understanding that diabetes was associated with the pancreas. In 1893, Gustave-Édouard Languesse (1861–1927) demonstrated that the pancreatic secretions arose from the islets of Langerhans and introduced the term 'endocrine' into the medical language to distinguish their function from that of exocrine acinar cells (1). The medical world was now beginning to understand that the lack of a still unknown internal secretion from the islets led to diabetes.

Early work in the field of endocrinology substantially changed when it became firmly understood that the central nervous system no longer controlled most bodily functions, after the work of bioscientists such as Sharpey-Schäfer, who in 1895 successfully described almost the complete endocrine system (7). This led the way to the work of the physiologists Sir William Bayliss (1860–1924) and Starling, who in 1902 at University College London discovered secretin, a completely new class of body substances beyond internal secretions. Starling proposed in 1905 the use of the word hormone, (8) which was soon universally accepted, although many scientists continued not to understand their actual function.

Sir William Bayliss expanded on this work in his *Principles of General Physiology*, published in 1915 (9). Here he referred to cell processes, which were a reflection of the understanding up to that time of body metabolism and the role of enzymes. This significantly enhanced endocrinology as a new discipline, which was still in its infancy, born not only out of biochemistry and physiology, but more importantly out of an understanding of the needs of patients. On the agenda of research and applied clinical practice was now the quest to identify new hormones and how they worked. What Bayliss and Starling actually achieved was to map the physiology and pathology of the endocrine system and to identify new scientific techniques that would complete this work and bring these discoveries to the bedsides of the patients.

One of the great setbacks at the time for the development of endocrinology as a serious medical and research specialization was the belief by many in the theory of organotherapy (5). This was the view that the intravenous injection of, for example, human male sperm and eventually other secretions, could be used to rejuvenate and treat patients with endocrine disease. The first to put forward this theory was Charles Édouard Brown-Séquard (1817–94) in 1889, who based it on the belief that the lack of secretions in the body caused specific disease and that organotherapy was the answer. Although treated sceptically or with outright concept by many of his contemporaries at the time, the idea lingered on right into the twentieth century and created a great deal of confusion with serious research in the field of endocrinology, considerably delaying its advance (1).

Endocrinology comes of age

The pioneering years of the discovery of secretions led to a speeding up of research, firstly in Europe, but now in Canada and the USA, with a few of these pioneers, such as Kocher, winning the Nobel Prize (Kocher won it in 1909 for his work on the thyroid). Science and medicine began to recognize discoveries that led to the acceptance as endocrine glands of the parathyroids, the gonads and that, apart from the pituitary and the adrenal glands, some secreted more than one hormone. Equally, the effects of adrenaline began to be understood, particularly through the work of Walter Cannon (1871–1945), who described in 1911, how the hormone adrenaline was secreted by the adrenal medulla in response to fear or anger (10). Iodine was now proved essential to normal thyroid function and a thyroid hormone, controlling the body's general metabolism, later named thyroxine was synthesized by the Welsh chemist Sir Charles Harington (1897–1972) at University College London.

It was not until 1921 that insulin was extracted from the cells of the islets of Langerhans by a team from the University of Toronto, comprising Sir Frederick Banting (1892–1941), Charles Best (1899–1978), John Macleod (1876–1935) and James Collip (1892–1965) (11). They begun to prove that insulin, a peptide hormone, plays a decisive role in regulating carbohydrate metabolism and soon was to change remarkably the treatment of diabetes in which the team was engaged.

On a similar level, groups of scientists working in various parts of Europe and North America began to make important discoveries in the field, supporting clinical treatment. For example, the pituitary extract of Schäfer and Oliver was found to contain two hormones, vasopressin, an antidiuretic, and oxytocin, which stimulated uterine contractions and the ejection of milk in women (1). In the following 20 years, this particular lobe was also found to secrete several peptide and protein hormones and to play a crucial role in regulating somatic growth and lactation, using growth hormones and prolactin. The other hormones produced stimulated growth and secretions of the thyroid, the adrenal cortex, and the gonads. In males, similarly the same two hormones were found to promote spermatogenesis and stimulate the interstitial (Leydig) cells of the testes. Sir Walter Langdon Brown (1870–1946), working in Cambridge, was now able to fully describe the significant role to the endocrine system of the anterior pituitary gland (1, 12).

In other fields we witness adrenocortical extracts being obtained, with the active principal now called cortin. By the 1940s, cortin was found to influence carbohydrate and protein metabolism, thus protecting the body from forms of stress. This led eventually to the extraction and synthesis of cortisone, first used clinically in 1948, revolutionizing the treatment of adrenal insufficiency but also establishing the anti-inflammatory effects of glucocorticoids. This work resulted in a Nobel Prize to Kendall, Reichstein, and Hench. In this latter period, some equally important discoveries were now made, in fields such as the invention of a radioimmunoassay for insulin; the role of the gut as a diffuse gastro-enteropancreatic endocrine organ, now emerging as the largest endocrine organ (1).

Right through to the 1970s and beyond, there was a continuation of scientific research into the hormonal system, with a better understanding of release, transport, and modes of action, which were now much better described. Also the synthesis of hormones took steps forwards, particularly insulin and growth hormone, brought about by recombinant DNA, making a huge difference to people's lives. In 1953, working in Cambridge, Frederick Sanger (b.1918), analysed insulin; and the analysis of other peptides and proteins followed in its wake. In the same year, James Watson (b.1928) and Francis Crick (1918–2004) described the structure of DNA and the world of biomedical research entered it genetic age.

Endocrinology from laboratory to bedside: disease and treatment

Understood today, hypofunction, hyperfunction, and dysfunction are the three disturbances of the endocrine system. All the glands of the body can be affected by at least one of these disturbances and sometimes by all three, and those glands that secrete a variety of hormones may well exhibit quite complex combinations of all three. In the field of hypofunction, for example, iodine deficiency was confirmed quite early on as the major cause of goitre and cretinism and in 1956, Deborah Doniah (b.1912) and Ivan Roitt (b.1927) discovered that autoimmune disease was a cause of thyroiditis and later on the cause of other endocrine disease. As early at the beginning of the nineteenth century, some clinicians began to describe patients with multiple endocrine disorders (1).

Over the preceding centuries, the treatment of thyroid disease has been varied, such as natural pharmacopeia and surgery, and it was not until last century that we begin to see modern medicine being introduced into this field. Radiotherapy as a treatment for cancer of the pituitary gland was first used in 1907, just 12 years after Röntgen, and more reliable treatment of many deficiency states followed with the synthesis of insulin in 1922, sex hormones in the 1930s, cortisone in 1948, and recombinant peptides in the 1980s. The surgical transplantation of endocrine animal glands, even after the work on immunosuppressants and human grafting to treat thyroid, adrenal, parathyroid, gonadal deficiency, and diabetes, proved of no benefit to the patient. Some small-scale pancreatic transplantation continued, while clinicians now turned almost exclusively to replacement therapy.

The treatment of hyperfunction had traditionally required a combination of surgery, radiotherapy, and drug treatment. Surgery performed by specialists proved at the time to be the only effective treatment for toxic goitre until the mid-twentieth century, and continues to be important in the treatment of pituitary, islet cell, gonadal, parathyroid, and adrenal lesions. Radioiodine was first used therapeutically for thyroid disease in 1942. Drug treatment that blocked the secretion of hormones, or which antagonized their actions on the tissues, were developed somewhat later. Clinical endocrinology was also able to export its knowledge to other areas of medicine. For example, hormone treatment continued to be effective for rheumatoid arthritis and contraception; other therapies have played a role in the treatment of prostate and breast cancer (1).

Of course, clinical endocrinology's reputation did and does not lie in the laboratory, but in its ability to treat patients with endocrine disease. Some early endocrinologists saw its importance, but many were still unable to distinguish between endocrinology and organotherapy, even after the discovery in 1922 of insulin (11). Many in science and medicine could now, however, look confidently into the future and predict effective stimuli of hormone production, the extraction, analysis and synthesis of further hormones, replacement therapy, and finally the promotion and suppression of secretory cells.

By the year 1923, as Starling pointed out, (13) endocrinology was accepted as reputable and clinical journals and international societies were founded. By 1955, when radioiodine, antithyroid drugs, and corticosteroids became more generally available, life-saving treatment for a number of conditions became the norm. Steroids still remained at the centre of research until the 1960s, when they gave way to looking at amines, peptides, and molecular biology – the future of research in this field.

The pancreas: diabetes mellitus

Diabetes is by far the most common of all endocrine diseases. Until the nineteenth century, treatment was often worthless as there was absolutely no knowledge of the nature of the disease. Sometimes patients were put on diets that positively harmed them, although only by chance, some mildly obese diabetic people who lost weight by reducing the intake of food responded well to this form of treatment.

The metabolic disturbances that cause diabetes were not to be fully understood until 1922, with the discovery of the peptide insulin. It was this discovery by Banting, Best, Macleod, and Collip at the University of Toronto (11) that introduced insulin treatment of both types of diabetes, and insulin soon became to be produced commercially and in large quantities. People with diabetes could now receive proper life-saving treatment. It was hailed by medical science as a huge breakthrough, and Banting and Macleod received the Nobel Prize, although many thought that Best should also have been included. A serious breakdown in the personal relationship between Banting and Macleod over this issue did nothing to create a productive research atmosphere for the future.

Banting and his team found that regular injections, combined with strict diet, could correct the metabolic disorder. Over the years after the discovery, insulin was improved with many different preparations; in the mid-1950s this was supplemented with oral hypoglycaemic remedies, such as metformin, which stimulates the secretion of insulin in the pancreas. Unlike many other conditions, diabetes could also be treated with insulin taken from animals, mostly bovine and porcine.

Alongside these treatments, the causes of diabetes began to be better understood; all revealing a deficient (or in cases of type 1) non-production of insulin by the islets, its wholly defective utilization by the body's tissues and inactivation, by unknown factors or increased antagonistic diabetogenic factors. It was also now that the two forms of diabetes were identified and differentiated. As therapies improved and patients began to live longer, many of them were to develop the traditional and now well-known effects of diabetes, such as hypertension, neuropathy, renal lesions, and retinopathy. For the latter condition, ablation of the patient's pituitary gland was used in the 1950s, but the procedure was later abandoned. Renal failure was and still is treated by dialysis or transplantation, although it became clear that regular dialysis can be complicated by anaemia. As far back as the 1900s, a renal erythropoietic factor in diabetes has been suspected, but then ignored and later rediscovered.

Soon after the introduction of insulin treatment, one of the complications of diabetes therapeutics was inadequate therapy.

Although animal insulin was synthesized by Sanger in 1964, human insulin became fully available only a few years ago, when a recombinant preparation was manufactured commercially, although it was found to have little practical advantage over animal insulin. Islet cell transplantation and pancreatic grafting is still imperfect, although a great deal of research these days has gone into developing better and more user-friendly methods of administering insulin, such as the inhaler and the development of better and more effective hypoglycaemic drugs.

The thyroid gland (14)

Iodine deficiency was first properly understood scientifically as the principal cause of goitre in 1918 by the US pathologist David Marine (1888–1976), who is remembered for his clinical trial of the effect of administering iodine to a group of adolescent girls in Ohio between 1917 and 1922 and demonstrating that this greatly reduced the instance of goitre. Although in the nineteenth century some goitre had been treated with iodine, with great benefit to patients, mostly in the early stages, those who did so did not really know why. From 1885, thyroid extract was used as a treatment with similar results and surgical techniques were developed to treat the most serious of cases. However, total thyroidectomy was abandoned and bilateral partial resections introduced. Thyroid extract for the treatment of hypothyroidism was first introduced commercially in 1902; thyroxine being made available later during the period of the Second World War, when the first reliable preparations were made. It was not until the 1950s that it was synthesized.

Toxic goitre was first named 'hyperthyroidism' and described by Charles Mayo (1865–1939) in 1907 (15). Again, thyroidectomy was the most effective treatment, but the surgical mortality was higher than for simple goitre, although the work of the Australian surgeon Sir Thomas Dunhill (1876–1957) showed that it could be successful. Iodine treatment has been used for toxic goitre, but with much less success, and it was Henry Plummer (1874–1936) who discovered that, given as a preoperative treatment, iodine could lower the basal metabolic rate to normal and reduce the surgical mortality. This became the standard treatment for a number of years.

In 1942, radioiodine therapy was introduced and in 1943, antithyroid drugs were first administered, either standalone or preoperative. By the 1950s, all were being used successfully and the mortality rate was effectively reduced to zero. When thyrotrophin was first discovered in 1931, it was assumed by endocrinologists that thyrotoxicosis was due to pituitary malfunction. However in 1956, a pathological thyroid stimulator was discovered in the blood of thyrotoxic patients (1). In the field of research and treatment of thyroid disease, a number of world centres subsequently emerged, no less than that at the University of Birmingham under the leadership of Sir Raymond Hoffenberg (1923–2007).

The pituitary gland

In 1886, Pierre Marie (1853–1929), working in Paris with Jean-Martin Charcot (1825–93), described and gave the world the word acromegaly (Pierre Marie's disease). It was realised also that acromegaly and gigantism were associated with pituitary tumours, and at the end of the nineteenth century it was suggested that both were caused by excess of a pituitary growth factor (1). At the same time, hypopituitarism was described. It was realized that children exhibit dwarfism and sexual infantilism, while adults develop amenorrhoea or anaphrodisia. Later on, Harvey Cushing (1869–1939) in 1912 (16) described the close relationship between pituitary tumours and syndromes. Again, surgery was the default treatment and transcranial and transsphenoidal operations and radiotherapy were recommended to reduce pressure, relieve headaches and improve eyesight. Treatment of pituitary tumours continued to improve and many acromegalic patients were treated with very good results. Until 1932, when Cushing proposed a syndrome of pituitary basophilia (Cushing's disease), (17) a tumour-secreting growth hormone was the only known manifestation of hyperpituitarism (18). Later on, radioimmunoassay and radiography allowed many cases of the disease to be diagnosed and treated and the use of cortisone-replacement facilitated advances in pituitary surgery. Subsequent progress allowed surgeons to remove some of the tumours completely: in others advances in radiotherapy provided some additional avenues of treatment (1).

In 1914, Morris Simmons (1855–1925) described pituitary cachexia (or Simmons' disease), caused by infarction of the gland. When hypopituitarism is only partial, he noted that gonadal function usually failed first. Hypothyroidism could be treated with thyroid extract, but hypogonadism could not be treated until the sex hormones were first available in the late 1930s. In 1939, the pathologist Harold Sheehan (1900–88) found that postpartum haemorrhage was the most common cause of pituitary infarction (Sheenan's syndrome). This was followed by the development of cortisone treatment in the 1950s. The treatment of pituitary dwarfism with human growth hormone initially involved material derived from cadaveric pituitary glands and with it a significant risk of Creutzfeldt–Jakob disease. It was in the mid-1980s that a recombinant form was finally synthesized (1).

The gonads

Primary hypogonadism due to castration and the secondary form, due to pituitary tumours, had been recognized for a long time and other causes, including autoimmune disease, came later. In the early 1920s it was suggested that ligation of the vas deferens or the transplantation of the testicles of an ape would be the ultimate panacea in rejuvenation. However, no active testicular extract was found until slightly later, when androsterone was first used clinically, being replaced by testosterone in 1935. Similarly we see about this time the discovery of additional hormones and the development of a number of treatments, including oestrone, oestriol, progesterone; all were effective as replacement therapies for hypogonadism for example, but did not restore fertility (1).

Sir Edward Dodds (1899–1973) at the Middlesex Hospital in 1938 discovered stilboestrol and oestrogens soon became widely used for retarding the process of osteoporosis after the menopause in women; hormone replacement therapy or HRT was born, as was around the same time the start of the use of androgens to improve and enhance athletic performance. Of major social consequence was the discovery in 1957 by the US bioscientist Gregory Pincus (1903–67), of suppression of ovulation in women treated with oral synthetic oestrogens and progestogens. Within 10 years, 'the pill' had helped change social behaviour, particularly among the young. Similarly, treatment for breast and prostate cancer was transformed when it was understood that prostate cancer was stimulated by androgens, and hormone treatment proved to be effective.

References

1. Welbourne RB. Endocrine diseases. In: Bynum WF, Porter R, eds. *Companion Encyclopaedia of the History of Medicine*. London: Routledge, 1994: 484–511.
2. Jørgensen CB. *John Hunter, A. A. Berthold and the Origins of Endocrinology*. 1971: Odense, Editit Bibliotheca Universitatis Havniensis (Acta Historica Scienatrun Naturalium et Medicinalium 24).
3. Addison T. *On the Constitutional and Local Effects of Disease of the Suprarenal Capsules*. London: Samuel Highley, 1855.
4. Gull W. On a cretinoid state supervening in adult life in women. *Trans Clin Soc Lond*, 1973; **7**: 180–5.
5. Borrell M. Organotherapy, British physiology and the discovery of the internal secretions. *J Hist Biol*, 1976; **2**: 235–68.
6. Aretaeus The Cappadocian. *The Extant Works,* ed. and tr. Adams F. London: The Sydenham Society, 1856: 338–9.
7. Schäfer EA. Internal secretions. *Lancet*, 1895; **ii**: 321–4.
8. Starling EH. The Croonian Lectures on the chemical correlation of the functions of the body. *Lancet*, 1905; **ii**: 339–41.
9. Bayliss, WM. *Principles of General Physiology*. London: Longman, Green, 1915.
10. Cannon WB, de la Paz D. Emotional stimulation of adrenal secretion. *Am J Physiol*, 1911; **28**: 64–70.
11. Bliss M. *The Discovery of Insulin*. London: Macmillan, 1987.
12. Brown WL. Recent observations on the pituitary body. *Practitioner*, 1931; **127**: 614–25.
13. Starling EH. Harveian Oration on the 'wisdom of the body'. *Lancet*, 1923; **ii**: 865–70.
14. Merke F. *History and Iconography of Endemic Goitre and Cretinism*. Lancaster: MTP Press, 1984.
15. Mayo CH. Goiter with preliminary report of 300 operations. *JAMA*, 1907; **48**: 273–7.
16. Cushing H. *The Pituitary Body and its Disorders*. Philadelphia: Lippincott, 1912.
17. Cushing H. The basophil adenomas of the pituitary body and their clinical manifestations (pituitary basophilism). *Bull Johns Hopkins Hosp*, 1932; **50**: 137–95.
18. Cope O. The story of hyperparathyroidism at the Massachusetts General Hospital. *N Engl J Med*, 1961; **274**: 1174–82.

For additional reading on the history of endocrinology, see Medvei VC (1982), *A History of Endocrinology*. Lancaster: MTP Press; and McCann SM (1988), *Endocrinology, People and Ideas*, Bethesda: American Physiological Society.

1.2

Prevention in endocrinology

Peter Laurberg, Stig Andersen

Introduction

The basis of health care is that it is much better for the individual member of society to be healthy and well than to be ill or deceased (1). To assist the individual in staying alive and well the health care system provides a broad range of services aimed at cure or control of disease. These services are available when someone becomes ill.

A different approach to preservation of good health and longevity is the prevention of disease. Prevention may take many forms. This may vary from legislation on food declaration via public campaigns on the importance of physical exercise to neonatal screening programmes. The intervention may be directed at decreasing the risk for disease in healthy subjects (primary prevention). A common variation is prevention of the severe consequences of disease by early detection of subclinical disease by screening or case-finding (secondary prevention). Other variants are prevention of complications of disease (tertiary prevention) or prevention of recurrence of disease by secondary intervention.

Often the costs of classic clinical care and prevention are compared in a way suggesting that the primary advantage of prevention is that it saves money. This conclusion may be correct in some areas of prevention such as in iodine deficiency disorders. It is, however, far too simple when it comes to many other areas such as prevention of complications in elderly patients with diabetes mellitus (1). The major appeal of prevention is that it is a most effective and often also a cost-effective way of reducing the burden of disease.

Identification of risk factors

A major obstacle to prevention may be uncertainty of risk factors. For many years it was debated whether tight blood glucose control in patients with type 1 diabetes would prevent development of diabetic retinopathy and nephropathy and other late complications of diabetes. Tight blood glucose control involves a high degree of focus on the balance between insulin, meals, and physical activity, and it increases the risk of hypoglycaemia. Thus, tight control is not that attractive to patients. Results of large intervention studies were necessary to document the overall beneficial effects of keeping blood glucose near normal in diabetes. Now tight control of blood glucose is essential in diabetes care (2). The importance of carefully controlled studies to document the beneficial effects (and possible adverse effects) of preventive measures cannot be stressed too much. Often large-scale studies involving much public funding are necessary.

The relations of risk to exposure

Another problem may be lack of knowledge on dose–effect relationship. The relation between exposure to a risk factor (e.g. high blood glucose) and the risk for disease (e.g. retinopathy) may vary. In the case of diabetes it is assumed that absolute normalization of blood glucose (if possible) would reduce the diabetes related risk to zero. Hence there is a certain threshold level of safety above which the risk increases more or less linearly. Several other types of relation between exposure and risk may exist (Fig. 1.2.1). The risk may increase gradually over the whole range of exposure. Probably such a relation exists between external radiation to the thyroid gland during childhood and later development of thyroid cancer. It means that no absolute safety limit can be delineated (Fig. 1.2.1(b)). The relation may be more exponential with acceleration in risk with increasing exposure. Such a relation exists between low bone mineral density and risk of fracture (Fig. 1.2.1(c)).

A special case is where both low and high exposure is associated with an increase in risk of disease. This type of relation is well known from several studies of alcohol consumption and disease. Optimal health is found in those with a moderate consumption while both heavy users and abstainers have a lower life expectancy. In endocrinology a similar relation is found between thyroid disease and iodine intake (Fig. 1.2.1(d)). The serious consequences

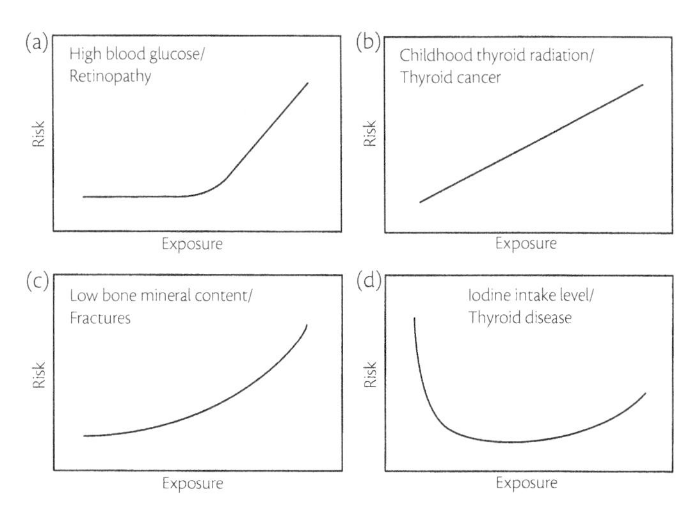

Fig. 1.2.1a–d Various types of relation between a risk factor (e.g. high blood glucose in diabetes) and the risk for disease (e.g. retinopathy). Examples are given for each type.

of extremes are found in severe iodine deficiency with cretinism, but a high iodine intake also correlates to an increase in disease frequency. Such a relation reinforces the need for monitoring to see that prevention of the consequences of one extreme should not lead to disease caused by the other extreme.

Preventive strategies

Population strategy of prevention

Several strategies of preventive medicine exist. In general, mass disease and mass exposure require a population strategy of prevention. A typical example of this is the widely applied iodine supplementation programmes where the iodine intake levels of populations are increased by the addition of iodine to salt. The risk of type 2 diabetes as part of the metabolic syndrome with overweight and sedate lifestyle is another mass problem clearly needing a population strategy of prevention, as well as more individual guidance. Some reasons for adoption of a population strategy of prevention are given in Box 1.2.1.

Effective population-based prevention depends on some kind of monitoring of disease frequency. This is necessary to evaluate whether a prevention programme should be initiated and to see if a running programme is effective.

The high-risk strategy of prevention

The high-risk strategy implies that individuals with a particularly high risk for disease are identified and prevention attempted. The power of this type of prevention is that the intervention is matched to the needs of the individual. This improves motivation and accommodates naturally into the organization of medical care. Resources can be directed at those in need, and if a small risk for side effects is part of the prevention this is much better balanced in high-risk/high-benefit subjects.

A weakness of the high-risk prevention strategy is that it tends to tackle the situations mentioned in Box 1.2.1 insufficiently. It means that an isolated high-risk strategy in some situations will fail if not combined with a population strategy of prevention. Type 2 diabetes is an example. Even considerable efforts to modify lifestyle by individual education of patients with type 2 diabetes might be insufficient or only temporarily effective if not combined with a population-directed programme to reinforce exercise and nonsmoking, and to modify diet and reduce overweight. The practical consequence of a lack of population prevention will be that modifications of lifestyle in patients with type 2 diabetes will be more or less hopeless and totally replaced by prescription of a series of medications to lower the blood glucose, treat hypertension, and regulate blood lipids. Both population and high-risk strategies are needed to obtain a proper balance between prevention by lifestyle modifications and prevention of diabetic complications by medication.

In some areas of endocrinology the high-risk strategy is optimal. In families where multiple endocrine neoplasia type 2 has been found, investigation of genomic DNA for mutation of the *RET* proto-oncogene may identify family members who should be offered thyroidectomy to prevent medullary thyroid carcinoma.

Screening

The high-risk strategy of prevention often involves screening to identify high-risk subjects. Screening implies an early detection of an asymptomatic condition which might develop to a symptomatic disease if not detected and treated. In the pure form of screening the full initiative for the investigation comes from the health system to which the subjects are urged to respond. The clinical policy guidelines for screening were set up by Wilson and Jungner (3) in a WHO report (Box 1.2.2). Rose (1) has given the following additional principles relating to examinations aimed at risk assessment.

Box 1.2.1 Need for a population strategy of prevention (adapted from Rose (1))

- When the underlying behavioural causes are socially conditioned: It is difficult to change eating, drinking, smoking and exercise habits out of proportion with the social environment. Individual guidance alone is then ineffective and a general change is needed.
- When a high disease rate is caused by population-wide distributional shifts in associated risk factors, and not by development of high risk in small groups: In many areas of the world even a 'healthy' food intake does not supply adequate iodine for prevention of thyroid disease.
- When most of the attributed cases arise around the middle of the exposure distribution and are individuals exposed to only a small excess risk. In many countries the majority of low energy bone fractures in elderly women occur in subjects with a bone mineral density that is not extreme for this age group.

Box 1.2.2 Policy guidelines for screening (from Wilson and Jungner (3))

- The condition sought should be an important health problem.
- There should be an accepted treatment for patients with recognized disease.
- Facilities for diagnosis and treatment should be available.
- There should be a recognizable latent or early symptomatic stage.
- There should be a suitable test or examination.
- The test should be acceptable to the population.
- The natural history of the condition, including development from latent to declared disease, should be adequately understood.
- There should be an agreed policy on whom to treat as patients.
- The cost of case-finding (including diagnosis and treatment of patients diagnosed) should be economically balanced in relation to possible expenditure in medical care as a whole.
- Case-finding should be a continuing process and not a 'once and for all' project.

There should be no screening without adequate resources for advice and long term care. Risk identification should be linked to professional care and follow-up, which may need to be maintained for years. Hence screening of selected groups for osteoporosis implies that a follow-up system of adequate capacity should be ready to care for subjects with low bone mineral density.

Selective screening and care are more cost-effective than mass screening. Screening of pregnant women for diabetes is more relevant than whole population screening. Gestational diabetes mellitus is more prevalent than undiagnosed diabetes in otherwise similar nonpregnant women, and not diagnosing the condition may have consequences for the outcome of pregnancy.

The purpose is to assess reversible risk—not risk factors. A single risk factor should be evaluated in concert with other risk factors to assess the overall reversible risk and the need for intervention. Blood pressure should be measured regularly in type 1 diabetics. Risk assessment and need for intervention should include measurements of urinary albumin excretion and be influenced by the higher risk of increased blood pressure in people with diabetes.

Other important aspects to take into consideration before a screening programme is initiated are the consequences of false-positive and false-negative results. The increase in techniques allowing early detection of disease or risk of disease has made both theoretical and practical aspects of screening an area of development (4). A form of screening is case-finding, where a patient seen for another reason is investigated. This overlaps with normal patient care.

Prevention integrates itself in many parts of endocrinology. Two areas will be mentioned where public programmes of classic prevention have been implemented worldwide: one is iodine deficiency disorders and the other is learning difficulties due to congenital hypothyroidism.

Type 1 and type 2 diabetes and osteoporosis have special relations with preventive medicine because they are large and expanding disorders where the major part of normal clinical care aims at prevention at one or another level. Finally it is interesting to evaluate with an endocrinologist eye the targets for public preventive campaigns in many countries, such as smoking, diet, and exercise.

Iodine deficiency disorders

Prevention of iodine deficiency disorders using a population strategy was introduced in the mid-western states of the USA and in Switzerland early in the twentieth century. At the beginning of the present century it had become the classic and most widespread preventive measure in endocrinology. Around two billion people in more than 100 countries live in areas where the natural supply of iodine through locally produced food and beverage is low enough to cause an increase in the incidence and prevalence of thyroid disorders (5).

Iodine is a component of thyroid hormones and severe iodine deficiency as found in areas with an average daily iodine intake below 25 μg may cause impaired thyroid hormone synthesis and secretion. Risk of such impairments also exists in moderate iodine deficiency, with an average daily iodine intake of 25–50 μg. Thyroid hormones are essential for normal brain development in the fetus and during the first years of life, and the most severe consequence of iodine deficiency is the complex of developmental brain disorders known as cretinism (6). In severely iodine deficient isolated areas this may affect up to 5–10% of the population and subtle brain damage with reduction in performance may be even more common. Abortion and stillbirths may be prevalent in areas with severe iodine deficiency.

The second main type of complication caused by iodine deficiency is related to thyroid growth. The thyroid gland possesses a number of mechanisms to compensate for variations in iodine supply. A low iodine supply is, among other things, accompanied by thyroid cell proliferation. When the iodine intake is permanently low this process tends to 'get out of control' with irreversible multiple foci of autonomous growth and function. In severe iodine deficiency nearly the entire population may be affected by goitre, but increases in the prevalence rate of goitre and of the incidence of hyperthyroidism due to autonomous thyroid nodules may be seen when the average iodine intake of adults is below approximately 100 μg per day. This inflicts considerable burden on affected patients and on the health economy.

Screening for iodine deficiency disorders

Screening for iodine deficiency is not individual oriented case-finding. Goitre may occur sporadically even in high iodine intake areas, and day-to-day variations in individual iodine intake and thereby iodine excretion in urine are large. Iodine deficiency in an area is usually evaluated by examination of the distribution of urinary iodine excretion, which reflects intake (up to 90%) and of the prevalence rate of goitre in a subpopulation.

The recommended daily iodine intake in adults is 150 μg/day with extra iodine intake during pregnancy and lactation (7). From individual variation in iodine excretion it has been calculated that examination of urinary iodine excretion should be performed in at least 100 people to give a reliable estimate of iodine intake in the group of population under study (8).

Prevention of iodine deficiency disorders

Iodine supplementation is the most effective way of eradicating iodine deficiency disorders. This is of urgent importance in areas with severe iodine deficiency to prevent iodine deficiency-induced brain damage in the fetus and infant. Worldwide programmes involving regional health authorities and governed by international organizations have made major progress in the field. Also the consequences of a more moderate iodine deficiency—high prevalence and incidence of non-toxic and multinodular toxic goitre in the elderly (9, 10)—should be prevented by an iodine supplementation programme.

The most widespread type of population iodine supplementation is by iodization of salt. Preferably all salt—both table salt and salt used by various food industries, bakeries etc.—should be fortified to obtain a universal increase in iodine intake irrespective of dietary habits. Where iodization of salt is not feasible, other principles have been used such as iodized bread or water, iodized vegetable oil or iodine tablets given as a bolus.

Precautions in the prevention of iodine deficiency

Iodine is a major substrate for thyroid hormone production. Individuals with autonomous thyroid nodules may develop hyperthyroidism when the iodine intake is increased. Since longstanding low iodine intake may lead to the development of such nodules an

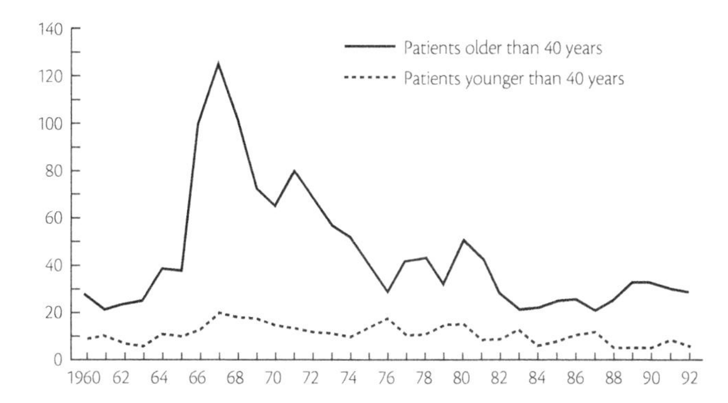

Fig. 1.2.2 New cases of hyperthyroidism reported from Tasmania before and after iodine supplementation of the population (initiated early 1966). Separate lines for patients younger and older than 40 years. Peaks in 1964, 1971, 1972, 1978, and 1980 coincided with rises in ambient iodine levels (11) Number of cases is not corrected for variations in size of population. (With permission from Stanbury JB, Ermans AE, Bourdoux P, Todd C, Oken E, Tonglet R, *et al.* Iodine-induced hyperthyroidism: occurrence and epidemiology. *Thyroid*, 1998; **8**: 83–100 (11).)

increase in the iodine intake level of the population may provoke a surge of hyperthyroidism. Figure 1.2.2 demonstrates the increase in cases of hyperthyroidism after iodine supplementation in Tasmania (11). The surge was self-limiting as should be expected, since the increase in iodine intake would prevent future development of autonomous thyroid nodules. Severe cases of hyperthyroidism with mortality have been seen where iodine supplementation has been too active.

Another concern is the long time effects of a high iodine intake. Figure 1.2.3 shows the difference in the prevalence rates of subclinical hyperthyroidism with low serum thyroid-stimulating hormone (TSH) and subclinical hypothyroidism with high serum TSH in elderly people from areas with longstanding mild to moderate iodine deficiency (Jutland, Denmark) and longstanding high iodine intake (Iceland). The autonomous nodules leading to hyperthyroidism with low TSH which was common in Denmark was prevented by the high iodine intake in Iceland. On the other hand subclinical hypothyroidism with elevated TSH was much more common when the iodine intake was high.

Excess iodine inhibits many processes in the thyroid gland, and it may worsen autoimmune thyroiditis, but the exact mechanism behind the increase in hypothyroidism with high iodine intake remains to be elucidated. The level of iodine intake that gives the lowest risk for thyroid disorders in a population is within a rather narrow interval around the recommended intake level of 150 μg/day in adults (7).

In many countries iodine intake of the population has varied unpredictably and unplanned due to variation in farming practices and the use of iodine-containing chemicals in the food industry. Ample supportive evidence exists that this has major consequences for the occurrence of thyroid disorders and that iodine intake of populations should be monitored. Also programmes of monitoring the effects and quality should be obligatory parts of iodine supplementation programmes. Detailed guidelines on the identification and eradication of iodine deficiency have been published by the World Health Organization (WHO)/UNICEF/International Council for the Control of Iodine Deficiency Disorders (ICCIDD) (7), and information is available via the ICCIDD website (www.iccidd.org).

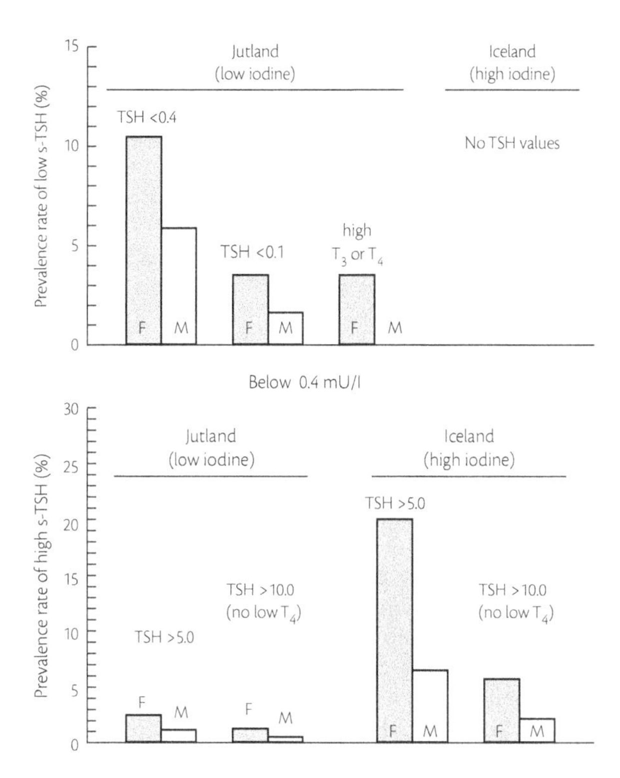

Fig. 1.2.3 Prevalence rates of subclinical hyper- and hypothyroidism in random population samples of 68-year-old subjects in Jutland, Denmark, with longstanding mild iodine deficiency, and in Iceland with longstanding high iodine intake. Subjects receiving thyroid medication were excluded. F: females; M: males. Young healthy subjects had serum thyroid-stimulating hormone (s-TSH) 0.4–4.0 mU/l. Note the high prevalence of various degree of hyperthyroidism with low TSH in the low iodine intake area versus the high prevalence of impaired thyroid function with high TSH in the high iodine intake area. (With permission from Laurberg P, Pedersen KM, Hreidarsson A, Sigfusson N, Iversen E, Knudsen PR. Iodine intake and the pattern of thyroid disorders: a comparative epidemiological study of thyroid abnormalities in the elderly in Iceland and in Jutland, Denmark. *J Clin Endocrinol Metab*, 1998; **83**: 765–9 (10).)

Congenital hypothyroidism

Another programme of prevention in endocrinology, which is well organized in many areas of the world, is screening for and early treatment of congenital hypothyroidism (12). Approximately 1 in 4000 newborns has permanent hypothyroidism. The major cause is dysgenesis of the thyroid gland but various selective defects in thyroid gland function are also found. Even if the placental crossing of thyroid hormones is limited, the fetus develops nearly normal due to thyroid hormones received from the mother. After birth, permanent brain malfunction with learning difficulties may develop if thyroid hormone substitution therapy is delayed until the condition is diagnosed from clinical findings. Before screening was introduced, the majority of cases were diagnosed too late and the average IQ in children with congenital hypothyroidism was reduced to 70–80%. If, on the other hand, the diagnosis is made and therapy started within the first month after birth the child develops normally.

Neonatal screening for congenital hypothyroidism was introduced in the 1970s when cheap and sensitive diagnostic methods had been developed. They were modified to enable measurements on eluates of blood spots collected for the screening of phenylketonuria. The organization of screening and subsequent follow-up varies, being adapted to local puerperal and neonatal care. TSH or TSH + thyroxine (T_4) in serum or blood is measured during the first week of life. Abnormal values are followed by retesting and clinical evaluation to allow rapid confirmation of the diagnosis and start of therapy.

Neonatal screening for congenital hypothyroidism clearly follows the guidelines for screening given in Box 1.2.2. Since the costs of lifelong caring for an individual with brain damage are very high in developed countries, it is an area of screening and prevention which is highly cost-effective.

Type 1 diabetes mellitus

Type 1 diabetes results from autoimmune destruction of the insulin-producing β cells in the pancreatic islets of Langerhans. Like other autoimmune disorders the pathogenic mechanisms are only partially known. Both genetic and environmental aetiological factors seem to be involved.

The idea to be able to prevent autoimmunity is very appealing and various ideas and principles have been tested in subjects with a high risk of developing type 1 diabetes. Unfortunately this has achieved limited success, and prevention of type 1 diabetes plays at present no practical role.

This is in sharp contrast to the clinical situation once the disease has developed. The goal of diabetic care is dual: one is to enable normal daily living and wellbeing. This may be problematic in some patients but is often not so difficult. Many patients feel quite comfortable if ketosis and hypoglycaemia are absent and with blood glucose giving a HbA_{1c} level of 9–10% (74.9–85.8 mmol/mol). This can often be achieved with one or two daily insulin injections, and moderate restrictions in the diet. The problems develop after years: nephropathy, retinopathy, neuropathy, accelerated atherosclerosis, etc. Hence the other goal of diabetes care is to prevent (tertiary prevention) diabetic complications. After years of uncertainty the results of the Diabetes Control and Complications Trial (DCCT) (13) finalized discussions on the importance of near normalization of blood glucose levels for the prevention of complications in type 1 diabetes.

Screening of diabetic patients for subclinical complications with measurements of urinary albumin, blood pressure, ophthalmoscopy, and foot examination is a well-established part of diabetes care. The aim is to prevent or delay disease progression by early intervention. Hence the majority of efforts in care of patients with type 1 diabetes as described elsewhere in this book aim at tertiary prevention.

Type 2 diabetes

Type 2 diabetes develops epidemically in many countries because of changes in lifestyle with a high fat intake, low levels of physical exercise and a high frequency of overweight. This is a prime target for both a population-based and a high-risk individual prevention. A type 2 diabetes risk assessment form has been developed for public use with guidance on lifestyle modifications, and recommendations on who should have blood glucose measured (14, 15).

Subclinical type 2 diabetes is common and screening of selected groups such as pregnant women is performed in many countries. Case-finding in overweight patients is the normal practice with the aim of preventing complications by intervention (16). Currently various studies are evaluating the effect of medications to prevent development of type 2 diabetes.

It is in general easy to treat patients to the level of having no diabetic symptoms. These patients have a high morbidity and mortality due to complications. The UK Prospective Diabetes Study (UKPDS) (17, 18) demonstrated the importance (and difficulty) of blood glucose normalization, with treatment of hypertension and regulation of blood lipids being particularly important as dealt with in detail in Part 13.

Osteoporosis

Although most health care efforts in type 2 diabetes are in essence prevention, this is even more so in osteoporosis. Osteoporosis has few if any clinical symptoms and signs, but it increases the risk for fractures (19). Hence it can be discussed whether osteoporosis is a disease or a risk factor.

The whole spectrum of preventive medicine as described previously in this chapter is applied in osteoporosis. Primary prevention is attempted using both a population and a high-risk strategy, and guidelines include both screening of selected groups and case-finding (19).

Osteoporosis is dealt with in detail in Part 4. The approach to identifying and treating osteoporosis covers both secondary prevention (of fractures) in patients diagnosed as having osteoporosis with low bone mineral density, and tertiary prevention (of more fractures) in patients who already have fractures due to osteoporosis. A tool to estimate absolute risk for fracture in a patient based on the presence of various risk factors is available (20). This allows discussing with the patient the change in risk induced by a certain change in lifestyle. A special area of current concern in this field is the role of widespread vitamin D deficiency for development of osteoporosis, and how this may be prevented (21).

Endocrinology and lifestyle modifications

Campaigns to reinforce physical exercise and nonsmoking and to modify diet and reduce overweight are common in many countries. Such lifestyle modifications are important for prevention of endocrine diseases.

Smoking is a risk factor for development of goitre, probably due to generation of thiocyanates, which inhibit thyroid iodine transport and hormone formation. Smoking increases the risk of development of Graves' disease and especially the development of orbitopathy, where a 10-fold increase in risk has been observed (22). Accordingly many patients with severe orbitopathy are heavy smokers. Even if controlled studies directly demonstrating a beneficial effect of stopping smoking are few, this should be encouraged because the consequences of Graves' orbitopathy are often severe and treatment is difficult. Cessation of smoking and avoidance of radioiodine therapy are the most important tertiary preventive measures in orbitopathy (22).

In diabetic people treated with insulin smoking alters subcutaneous blood flow and insulin absorption and thereby tends to induce more brittle diabetes. More importantly smoking increases the risk for diabetic micro- and macrovascular disease considerably. Smoking is an independent risk factor for osteoporosis.

Regular aerobic exercise improves glycaemic control in diabetes and prevents osteoporotic fractures, and weight reduction is probably the single most important factor in prevention of type 2 diabetes. Even if there are side effects such as the tendency to increase in weight after cessation of smoking and an increase in osteoporotic fractures with low body weight, the overall picture is that many endocrine disorders can be prevented by lifestyle modifications and that population-directed campaigns are important in this field of medicine.

References

1. Rose G. *The Strategy of Preventive Medicine.* Oxford: Oxford Medical Publications, 1992.
2. Bangstad HJ, Danne T, Deeb LC, Jarosz-Chobot P, Urakami T, Hanas R. International Society for Pediatric and Adolescent Diabetes (ISPAD). Insulin treatment. ISPAD clinical practice consensus guidelines 2006–2007. *Pediatr Diabetes*, 2007; **8**: 88–102.
3. Wilson JMG, Jungner G. *Principles and Practice of Screening for Disease.* Geneva: WHO, 1968.
4. Peckham C, Dezateux C, eds. Screening. *Br Med Bull*, 1998; **54**: 4.
5. Zimmermann MB, Jooste PL, Pandav CS. Iodine-deficiency disorders. *Lancet*, 2008; **372**: 1251–62.
6. Williams GR. Neurodevelopmental and neurophysiological actions of thyroid hormone. *J Neuroendocrinol*, 2008; **20**: 784–94.
7. WHO, UNICEF, ICCIDD. Elimination of Iodine Deficiency Disorders. A Manual for Health Workers. *EMRO Technical Publications Series*, No. **35**, 2008.
8. Andersen S, Karmisholt J, Pedersen KM, Laurberg P. Reliability of studies of iodine intake and recommendations for number of samples in groups and in individuals. *Br J Nutr*, 2008; **99**: 813–18.
9. Laurberg P, Pedersen KM, Vestergaard H, Sigurdsson G. High incidence of multinodular toxic goitre in the elderly population in a low iodine intake area vs. high incidence of Graves' disease in the young in a high iodine intake area: comparative surveys of thyrotoxicosis epidemiology in East-Jutland, Denmark and Iceland. *J Intern Med*1991; **229**: 415–20.
10. Laurberg P, Pedersen KM, Hreidarsson A, Sigfusson N, Iversen E, Knudsen PR. Iodine intake and the pattern of thyroid disorders: a comparative epidemiological study of thyroid abnormalities in the elderly in Iceland and in Jutland, Denmark. *J Clin Endocrinol Metab*, 1998; **83**: 765–69.
11. Stanbury JB, Ermans AE, Bourdoux P, Todd C, Oken E, Tonglet R, *et al.* Iodine-induced hyperthyroidism: occurrence and epidemiology. *Thyroid*, 1998; **8**: 83–100.
12. Grüters A, Krude H. Update on the management of congenital hypothyroidism. *Horm Res*, 2007; **5**: 107–111.
13. The Diabetes Control and Complications Trial Research Group. The effect of intensive treatment of diabetes on the development and progression of long-term complications in insulin-dependent diabetes mellitus. *N Engl J Med*, 1993; **329**: 977–86.
14. Lindstrom J, Tuomilehto J. The Diabetes Risk Score: A practical tool to predict type 2 diabetes risk. *Diabetes Care*, 2003; **26**: 725–31.
15. Alberti KG, Zimmet P, Shaw J. International Diabetes Federation: a consensus on Type 2 diabetes prevention. *Diabet Med*, 2007; **24**: 451–63.
16. IDF Clinical Guidelines Task Force. Global Guideline for Type 2 Diabetes: recommendations for standard, comprehensive, and minimal care. *Diabet Med*, 2006; **23**: 579–93.
17. UK Prospective Diabetes Study (UKPDS) Group. Intensive blood glucose control with sulphonylureas or insulin compared with conventional treatment and risk of complications in patients with type 2 diabetes (UKPDS 33). *Lancet*, 1998; **352**: 837–53.
18. UK Prospective Diabetes Study Group. Tight blood pressure control and risk of macrovascular and microvascular complications in type 2 diabetes: UKPDS 38. *BMJ*, 1998; **317**: 703–13.
19. Kanis JA, Burlet N, Cooper C, Delmas PD, Reginster JY, Borgstrom F, *et al.* European Society for Clinical and Economic Aspects of Osteoporosis and Osteoarthritis (ESCEO). European guidance for the diagnosis and management of osteoporosis in postmenopausal women. *Osteoporos Int*, 2008; **19**: 399–428.
20. Kanis JA, McCloskey EV, Johansson H, Strom O, Borgstrom F, Oden A, National Osteoporosis Guideline Group. Case finding for the management of osteoporosis with FRAX—assessment and intervention thresholds for the UK. *Osteoporos Int*, 2008; **10**: 1395–408.
21. Holick MF, Chen TC. Vitamin D deficiency: a worldwide problem with health consequences. *Am J Clin Nutr*, 2008; **87**: 1080S–6S.
22. Wiersinga WM. Preventing Graves' ophthalmopathy. *N Engl J Med* 1998; **338**: 121–2.

1.3

Endocrinology and evolution: lessons from comparative endocrinology

Janine A. Danks, Samantha J. Richardson

Introduction

Comparative endocrinology is the study of the endocrine glands and their hormones in different species of animals. It is undergoing a renaissance because of the new tools and techniques provided by genome sequencing and molecular biology. Until relatively recently, characterization and detection of hormones in lower vertebrates relied on biological assays and protein chemistry approaches, whereas now gene sequences can be readily revealed from whole genome sequencing. Gene expression and synthesis can be used to develop antibodies and other reagents for sensitive assays and revealing physiological experiments can be carried out.

Endocrinology traditionally used a range of animal species, including many lower vertebrates. Comparative endocrinology became a separate specialty only in the last 50 years when endocrinologists concentrated on rodents as their model animals. In 1933, Riddle demonstrated that an avian pituitary factor that promoted growth of the pigeon crop-sac was identical to a mammalian pituitary factor that earlier had been found to initiate and maintain milk secretion in mammals. Riddle called this avian factor prolactin and the response of the crop-sac provided a sensitive assay for the detection of human prolactin in pituitary extracts. Pigeon prolactin was the first pituitary hormone to be crystallized and purified in 1937 and led to the purification of mammalian prolactin. Prolactin has a number of roles in lower vertebrates, including a vital role as a hypercalcaemic factor in fish.

The first part of this chapter focuses on the calcium-regulating factors including parathyroid hormone (PTH), parathyroid hormone-related protein (PTHrP), and stanniocalcin (STC), and the second part will discuss comparative endocrinology of thyroid hormones and transthyretin (a thyroid hormone distributor in blood the cerebrospinal fluid).

Calcium regulation

Regulation of calcium levels within cells (Ca^{2+} = 0.1 μmol/l) and in extracellular compartments is fundamental in all vertebrate physiology. The regulation of calcium content in body fluids reflects a boundary between invertebrates and vertebrates. Marine invertebrates have plasma calcium levels of around 10 mmol/l, which is the same as the concentration in the surrounding environment. Primitive marine vertebrates (cyclostomes) have plasma calcium levels of 5 mmol/l in the same environment, and most cartilaginous and bony fish, regardless of their environment, have plasma calcium levels of around 2 mmol/l, similar to mammals. Most aquatic vertebrates are less dependent on a skeleton as a calcium source; instead the aquatic environment provides an inexhaustible supply of calcium ions.

Fish cannot use their skeleton as a rapidly accessible calcium store as it consists of acellular bone and so use their scales instead for this purpose. In contrast, terrestrial vertebrates have an internal skeleton that serves not only as physical support but also as a reservoir of calcium. They acquire calcium through their diet, and because this supply is episodic and uncertain, calcium needs to be labile so that it can be deposited or mobilized at any time. All vertebrates possess several factors with complex interrelated mechanisms for controlling circulating ionic calcium and these are essential for survival.

Calcium-regulating factors in lower vertebrates

The major difference in calcium control between lower and tetrapod vertebrates is the evolution of the parathyroid gland and its secretory product, PTH. An anatomically distinct parathyroid gland first appeared in amphibians but no comparable gland has been observed in fish. PTH is of paramount importance in calcium homoeostasis at all stages of tetrapod development, and interacts with calcitonin and 1,25-dihydroxyvitamin D_3. PTH elevates serum calcium by binding to receptors in bone to cause calcium release and by inhibiting calcium excretion via the kidney.

Parathyroid hormone

In spite of the absence of a parathyroid gland, there have been a number of reports of the presence of an immunoreactive PTH-like protein in fish, detected by antisera to mammalian PTH (1). These antisera were against the mid-molecule portion of the bovine PTH molecule and were used in both radioimmunoassay and immunohistochemistry. PTH-like immunoreactivity was demonstrated in brain and pituitary of goldfish and platyfish, the pituitary of eel and cod, and in the plasma of trout and goldfish. There were several problems with these studies including a lack of sufficient controls as well as poor characterization of the antibodies. Despite physiological studies by Parsons *et al.*(2) also predicting a rapidly acting hypercalcaemic factor in cod pituitary that was PTH-like in the N-terminus, the case for a fish PTH homologue remained unproven until 2003. A *PTH* gene has been identified from the *Fugu rubripes* genome database (3). Fugu PTH has low overall homology with human PTH (32%) and *Fugu* PTH (1-34) has only 56% identity with human PTH (1-34). However, Fugu PTH (1-34) was found to have *in vitro* biological activity resembling that of human PTH (1-34). A second Fugu PTH gene and protein were identified subsequently and this gene is not present in the human gene database, indicating that it is probably a gene duplication that took place in bony fish. There are two zebrafish *PTH* genes that provide weight to this argument.

Subsequent studies have identified two *PTH* genes in the elephant shark (*Callorhinchus milii*) genome (4). Cartilaginous fish are the oldest living group of jawed vertebrates and the elephant shark is one of the most ancient (approximately 450 million years old) (Fig. 1.3.1) Its genome has been termed the reference vertebrate genome, as initial studies have shown that the sequence and the gene order are more like human than other fish (e.g. Fugu or zebrafish) (5). These two elephant shark PTH proteins have different biological activity and the gene for elephant shark *PTH2* does not appear to exist in other fish or humans (4).

Parathyroid hormone-related protein

The earliest studies of PTH-like immunoreactivity in fish prompted studies in the early 1990s(6) that demonstrated the presence of immunoreactive PTHrP in a range of tissues including the pituitary as well as in the circulation of a marine bony fish. This molecule is highly homologous with the N-terminus of PTH and may be the factor predicted by Parsons *et al.* (2) in cod pituitary. PTHrP was first isolated from human tumours (1, 7, 8) and identified as the factor causing humoral hypercalcaemia of malignancy (HHM) through its actions on the classical PTH receptor (PTH1R) in bone and kidney.

Both PTH and PTHrP bind to this receptor with different affinities. PTH and PTHrP share sequence homology only at the N-terminal region of the molecule, notably in the 1-34 region, with eight of the first 13 amino acids being identical. The N-terminus in both PTH and PTHrP is required for binding to the common receptor, PTH1R. Subsequent studies indicated that PTHrP is synthesized in many normal adult and embryonic mammalian tissues, implying numerous potential functions, predominantly as an autocrine/paracrine factor (1).

The *PTHrP* and *PTH* genes

The *PTHrP* gene is more complex in structure than the *PTH* gene (Fig. 1.3.2). Genes for rat and chicken *PTHrP* consist of five exons which code for a protein of 139 or 141 amino acids (Fig. 1.3.2). The gene for human *PTHrP* has nine exons and codes for at least three isoforms of 139, 141, and 173 amino acids (1). This is contrasted with the *Fugu PTHrP* gene which has only three exons, reflecting the structure of the *PTH* gene. The *PTH* gene, composed of only three exons, is conserved among these species and generates a protein of 84 or 88 amino acids. The increasing complexity and number of proteins transcribed from the *PTHrP* gene from avian to human genes may be related to the increase in the number of roles of PTHrP through evolution. The increased roles for PTHrP implies that *PTHrP* may be the original gene and *PTH* may be the copy. This is supported by the highly conserved gene structure of *PTH*, and the single protein it codes for, and suggests its role(s) remain unchanged through evolution.

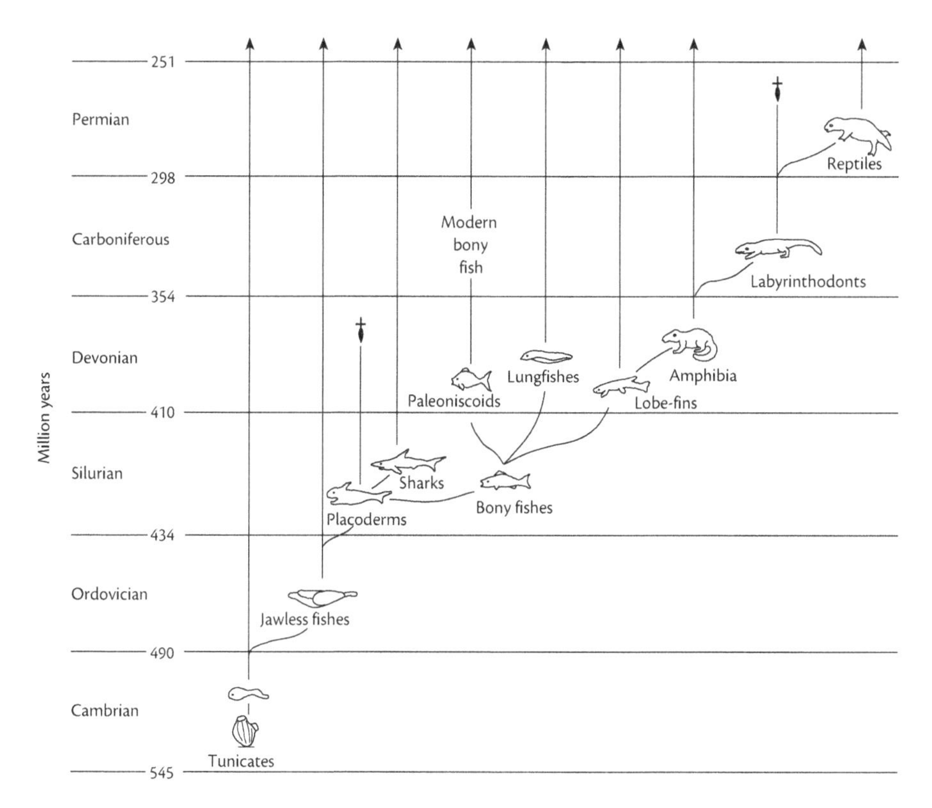

Fig. 1.3.1 Classification of chordates, including the tunicates and lower vertebrates, in relation to their phylogenetic origins and time in terms of palaeontological periods.

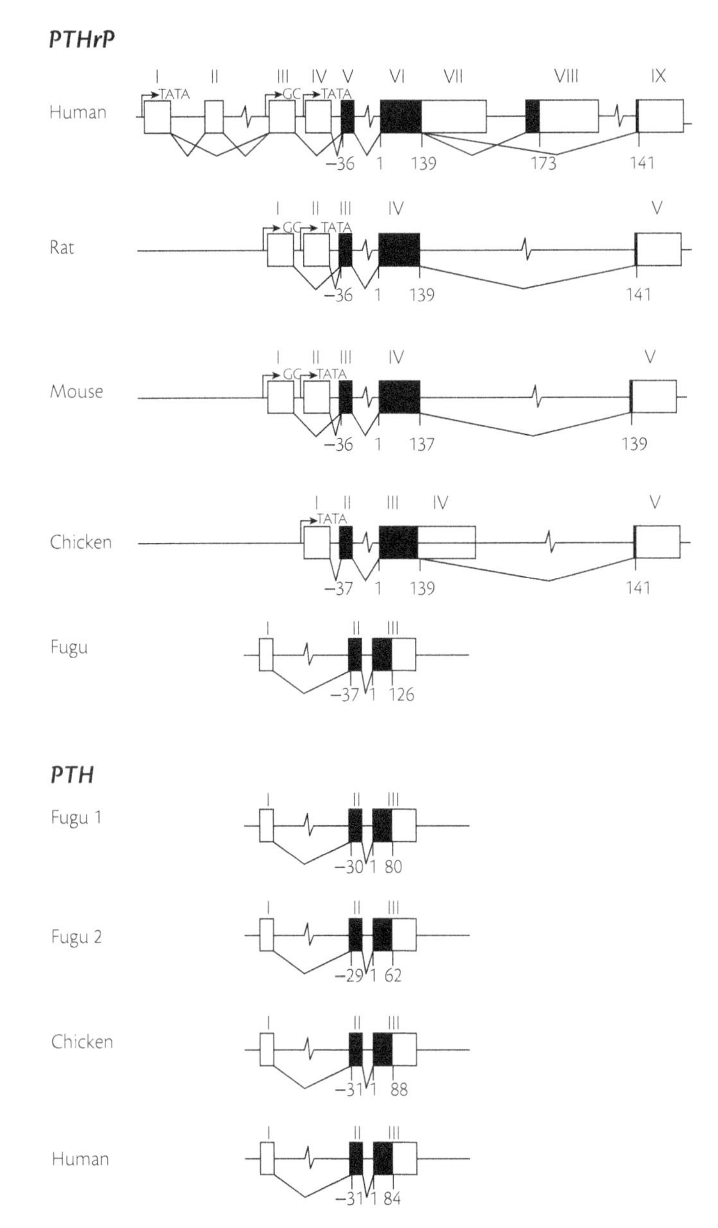

Fig. 1.3.2 A comparison of the gene structure of fugu, chicken, rat, and human parathyroid hormone-related protein (*PTHrP*), and fugu, chicken, and human parathyroid hormone (*PTH*).

Duplication of the *PTHrP* and *PTH* genes

The gene for human *PTHrP* is on chromosome 12 while the *PTH* gene is located on chromosome 11. The *PTH* and *PTHrP* genes are considered to be paralogous genes, that is, they have arisen following a duplication event involving a single ancestral gene and exist within a species (9). This is opposed to orthologous genes, which are found in different species and have diverged from their common ancestral gene as part of speciation and separate evolution. This divergence has been documented for other gene families that have members on both chromosomes 11 and 12, such as the insulin-like growth factors, the aromatic amino acid hydroxylases, lactate dehydrogenases, and the *Ras* gene family (Table 1.3.1). All these genes map to the same regions of these two chromosomes, suggesting that a single duplication event gave rise to all members of these gene families. Additionally, chromosome 12 appears to have a central position in the human genome (9) indicating that it might be a primordial chromosome retained within the human genome. Hence the genes on this chromosome may have a long evolutionary history.

The principles of tetraploidization and gene duplication

The duplication event that led to the two members of the parathyroid hormone family may well have been one of the two tetraploidization events that occurred between invertebrates and vertebrates (10).

A tetraploidization event means that every gene locus in the genome is duplicated. This is in contrast to regional duplication, where only some gene loci are duplicated. Regional duplication is thought to have given rise to the *IGF2* gene from *insulin* on chromosome 11 while the *IGF1* gene on chromosome 12 is believed to have arisen from a tetraploidization event (9) (Table 1.3.1).

Implications of gene duplication

The two tetraploidization events early in vertebrate evolution led to the expansion of the genome, thereby creating new genomic and phenotypic diversity resulting in the survival of the species. This 'safety net' is exemplified by knockout mice studies. These studies are based on the premise that 'nature is thrifty' and one gene is responsible for a defect. Frequently, knockout animals do not have the expected defect therefore, molecular biologists are now learning what evolutionary biologists have always known—that nature is extravagant and genes can sometimes fulfil multiple roles. Logically nature has to be extravagant to ensure survival of the species, and consequently, many diseases are going to be polygenic. Thus, several separate lines of knockout mice, each with a specific gene knocked out, will need to be bred together to get the expected defect originally thought to be caused by only one gene.

Timing of the duplication of *PTH* and *PTHrP* genes

The gene for PTHrP has been cloned from a number of mammals (human, rat, mouse, dog) and chicken and the level of homology is so great that its evolutionary development and variation can only be determined with the sequences from lower vertebrates, including fish and sharks. Certainly the gene structures have less exons and introns in the fish PTHrP whereas the PTH structure is maintained

Table 1.3.1 Paralogous genes in portions of human chromosomes 11 and 12

Chromosome 11	Chromosome 12
Lactate dehydrogenase A	Lactate dehydrogenase B
Lactate dehydrogenase C	
Hras	*Kras*
Parathyroid hormone	Parathyroid hormone-related protein
Glutathione S-transferase 3	Glutathione S-transferase 3-like
	Glutathione S-transferase 12
Tyrosine hydroxylase	Phenylalanine hydroxylase
Tryptophan hydroxylase	
Insulin	Insulin-like growth factor 1
Insulin-like growth factor 2	
Progesterone receptor	Vitamin D receptor
	Retinoic acid receptor G

from fish through to the human gene (Fig. 1.3.2). It appears likely that divergence between the two genes occurred prior to the evolution of cartilaginous fish. The presence of *PTHrP* and *PTH* genes in elephant shark indicates that clues to the evolutionary relationship of *PTH* and *PTHrP* and possible role(s) in calcium metabolism and other functions may be found in lampreys, a jawless fish.

Fish as a model vertebrate species

Numerically, fish constitute the major group of vertebrates, with estimates of total species varying from 25 000 to 35 000. They are highly successful with evolved physiologies ensuring survival in water of high or low ionic strength and, in some species, with the ability to adapt to both conditions. Today there are two major groups—the jawed bony fish and the jawed cartilaginous fish, including the sharks and rays (see Fig. 1.3.1). The surviving jawless fish, the lampreys and hagfishes, also have a cartilaginous skeleton. It seems likely that among the bony fish there has been a modification in calcium metabolism resulting in ossification of the internal skeleton. This development was essential for the future evolution of terrestrial vertebrates as it provided an internal calcium store. Thus the foundations were laid for the exploitation of internal calcium stores for maintaining calcium homoeostasis even if the environment has an abundant supply.

Originally, all fish were marine and logically they would have been more dependent on hypocalcaemic factors as they would need to maintain tissue calcium levels lower than the surrounding water. During evolution, as fish colonized the freshwater environment, hypercalcaemic agents would have been essential for survival. A hypercalcaemic agent, essential for the evolution of terrestrial vertebrates, may have developed from a factor already present in marine fish but fulfilling a different role. Both PTH and PTHrP could be such factors. Over the last 10 years we have demonstrated the presence of PTHrP in tissues of a range of lower vertebrates by immunohistochemistry and *in situ* hybridization with antisera and probes to human PTHrP (11). We examined tissues from both bony fish, including the lungfish (a 'living fossil' that is believed to be the link between fish and amphibians), and cartilaginous fish as well as jawless fish. PTHrP protein and messenger RNA (mRNA) localized to kidney, epidermis, vertebral elements, and muscle in all these animals, and this distribution reflects that reported in higher vertebrates. The conservation of PTHrP localization indicates that the function of PTHrP in these tissues is basic and fundamental. Futhermore, the successful use of antisera and probes to human PTHrP indicates that the *PTHrP* gene and the protein are highly conserved throughout vertebrate evolution, lending support to the hypothesis that its function is basic and essential for survival. PTHrP was localized to tissues that are unique to lower vertebrates, such as gills, saccus vasculosus and the rectal gland of sharks, all of which are involved in mineral ion regulation. The examination of PTHrP in these tissues could lead to the discovery of new roles for PTHrP. Using a polyclonal antiserum to human PTH (1-34) no PTH could be detected in the tissues of any of the lower vertebrates we examined, due to low homology between human and fish PTH.

PTHrP is an onco-fetal hormone in mammals and from the findings of our initial study in bony fish, we hypothesized that PTHrP could be a classic hormone in fish (6). Comparative endocrinology allows us to examine the normal physiological roles of PTHrP in simpler systems as there appears to be an elaboration of roles through evolution. The dissection of PTHrP roles in fish has been assisted by the isolation and cloning of zebrafish *PTH1R* and *PTH2R* genes (12).

Stanniocalcin

Calcium regulation in most marine fish should be more dependent on hypocalcaemic agents, such as STC, a hormone produced by the corpuscles of Stannius, an organ unique to some bony and cartilaginous fish. Since fish generally have abundant supplies of environmental calcium, STC prevents hypercalcaemia by targeting gill and gastrointestinal tract calcium transport (13). This factor was initially thought to be unique to those fish that had corpuscles of Stannius, but in 1995 human STC was isolated and cloned (14). Fish STC mRNA is expressed by specific tissues while mammalian STC mRNA is expressed in a wide range of tissues, including ovary, prostate, and thyroid. Human STC protein has been localized to the renal tubule cortex adjacent to the glomeruli and has been detected in the circulation. The isolation and analysis of the mouse *STC* gene found the protein was the same length as the human STC with very high level of amino acid sequence similarity (15).

The function of mammalian STC

Rodent STC is localized in the renal cortical brush-border membrane vesicle of rats and decreases calcium absorption and increases phosphate absorption in the duodenum of swine and rats, respectively. STC expression has been found in developing mouse chondrocytes and acts as a probable autocrine/paracrine factor (13, 15).

Mammalian STC may be a regulator of calcium and phosphate homoeostasis, and have an autocrine/paracrine role as well as an endocrine role in cellular growth and differentiation. This progression is also seen with PTHrP—from a classic hormone in lower vertebrates to predominantly autocrine/paracrine roles in mammals.

Stanniocalcin-2

A second mouse and human STC (STC2) was isolated and cloned in 1998 (15). *STC2* is expressed in a number of human tissues ranging from spleen to peripheral blood leucocytes, small intestine, and the ovaries and testes. It is also expressed in rat kidney, skeletal muscle, liver, and brain. The STC2 protein has significant similarity with fish STCs and mammalian STC1. The difference between the two mammalian STCs is the presence of 15 histidine residues in STC2, with four of them forming a cluster towards the end of the C-terminus of this protein (16). Clusters of histidine residues have been shown to interact with metal ions such as Co^{2+}, Ni^{2+}, Cu^{2+}, and Zn^{2+}. It has not been established whether the cluster of mammalian STC2 interacts with metal ions. A second fish STC was described in salmon corpuscles of Stannius in the same year (17). Salmon STC2 was less effective as an inhibitor of gill calcium transport in fish, supporting a non-calcaemic role for STC2. Additionally, salmon STC2 also appears to have fewer histidine residues than human, eel, or coho salmon STC1. This increase in the number of histidine residues in STC2 with the transition from fish to mammals may to be due to an alteration in, or an elaboration of, STC's roles through evolution.

Thyroid hormones

The first clear demonstration of the function of thyroid hormones was performed by Gudernatsch in 1912 (18), when he showed that diced horse thyroid gland prematurely turned tadpoles into 'mini-frogs'. Much of our understanding of the requirements and function of thyroid hormones in humans has come from studying the evolution of thyroid hormone distribution in vertebrates, both in the body and in the brain. Furthermore, insights into mechanisms of transthyretin amyloidosis through studying evolution of the transthyretin protein will be discussed.

Apart from the number of systemic calcium-regulating hormones that affect calcium and bone metabolism, other peripheral hormones including thyroid hormones play a significant role in bone remodelling. The thyroid hormones (thyroxine (T_4) and triiodothyronine (T_3)) are essential in humans for normal skeletal developmental, growth, and maintenance of adult bone mass (19). The thyroid hormones are involved in the regulation of development and metabolism, particularly of the brain. In humans, insufficient thyroid hormone levels during gestational development leads to cretinism and mental retardation, whereas in adults reduced levels can result in depression. A classic example of the potent effects of thyroid hormones in development is the metamorphosis of tadpoles into frogs, which is controlled by these hormones. The fine control of regulation of metabolism by the thyroid hormones requires the precise and accurate delivery of the thyroid hormone molecules to the target cells. Both the timing and the quantity of thyroid hormone delivered to the sites of action are crucial for normal development and metabolism to proceed. The delivery of thyroid hormone to target cells via the blood and the cerebrospinal fluid (CSF) is carried out by a group of proteins called thyroid hormone distributor proteins (THDPs). In humans, the THDPs are albumin, thyroxine-binding globulin, and transthyretin (TTR). This chapter will focus on the insights into thyroid hormone metabolism and human amyloid formation from TTR evolution. We will show that mammalian TTRs are the exception, not the rule.

Thyroid hormone distributor proteins ensure that the hormones get from the thyroid gland to target cells Thyroid hormones are synthesized in the thyroid gland then secreted into the blood, where they are distributed around the body bound to THDPs. More than 99% of thyroid hormone in blood is bound to the THDPs: albumin, TTR, and thyroxine-binding globulin (TBG).

The older literature and some current textbooks (e.g. see Alberts *et al.* (20)) state that thyroid hormones are bound to THDPs due to their low solubility in blood. This is incorrect, as the solubility of thyroid hormones at pH 7.4 is 2.3 μM and the concentration of free TH in blood is 24 pM, i.e. 1/100 000 the solubility limit (for review, see Schreiber and Richardson (21)).

Thyroid hormones are lipophilic molecules, which partition between the lipid phase and the aqueous phase with a ratio of 20 000:1 (22, 23). THDPs counteract the avid partitioning of thyroid hormones into cell membranes, maintain a pool of circulating thyroid hormones in the blood and ensure an even delivery of the hormones throughout the tissues (24). Thus, the plasma proteins that bind thyroid hormones have been called thyroid hormone *distributor* proteins. This clearly distinguishes the role of the thyroid hormone binding proteins in plasma from the other classes of thyroid hormone binding proteins. (The five classes of thyroid hormone binding proteins are: THDPs in the blood and cerebrospinal fluid; membrane-bound thyroid hormone transporters; thyroid hormone deiodinases; cytosolic thyroid hormone binding proteins; and thyroid hormone nuclear receptors).

From the bloodstream and CSF, thyroid hormones can dissociate from the THDPs and enter the cells. The two major modes of entry into the cells are via passive diffusion or via membrane-bound thyroid hormone transporter proteins. The thyroid hormones are then subject to activation or inactivation by the family of deiodinases. In humans, the major form of thyroid hormone circulating in the blood is T4 (the "transport form"), whereas the form of the hormone with highest affinity for the nuclear receptors is T3 (the "active form"). However, there is now a rapidly expanding literature of non-genomic effects of forms of thyroid hormones other than T3 (e.g. T4, rT3, T2). Deiodinases types 1, 2 and 3 can either active (e.g. T4 to T3) or inactivate (e.g. T4 to rT3; T3 to T2) THs within a cell. Thus, deiodinases confer a tissue-specific level of regulation of thyroid hormone activity.

Within the cell, thyroid hormones are bound by specific cytosolic proteins and are translocated into the nucleus where they are bound by the thyroid hormone nuclear receptors (TRs). T_3 has the highest affinity for TRs and is the usual ligand. TRs are coded for by two genes: *TRα* and *TRβ*. Each of these genes produces at least two splice variants, resulting in the four main products TRα1, TRα2, TRβ1 and TRβ2. However, TRα2 does not bind T_3. Together with co-modulator proteins, T3-TRs dimerize with retinoid X receptor (RXR) and bind to thyroid hormone response elements (TREs) and either positively or negatively regulate expression of specific genes.

TTR is responsible for much of the thyroid hormone distribution in the body and in the brain Thyroid hormones are distributed around the body via the bloodstream. In the blood about 75% thyroid hormone is bound to TBG, 15% is bound to TTR, and 10% is bound to albumin. A small fraction is also bound to lipoproteins. Albumin, TBG, and TTR are synthesized by the liver and secreted into the blood. Of these three THDPs, TBG is lowest in concentration but has highest affinity for T_4, albumin is highest in concentration but lowest affinity for T_4, whereas TTR has intermediate concentration and affinity for T_4. T_4 bound to albumin rapidly dissociates, T_4 bound to TBG acts as a reservoir for T_4 in the blood and TTR is responsible for the bulk of the delivery of T_4 to tissues. (For a greater discussion on concentrations, k_d values, capillary transit times, the free hormone hypothesis, and the free hormone transport hypothesis, see Richardson (25)).

The body is separated from the brain by a series of barriers, collectively known as 'the blood–brain barriers'. One of these barriers is the choroid plexus, which is located in the lateral, third, and fourth ventricles of the brain and forms the blood–CSF barrier. The only THDP synthesized by the brain is TTR, which is synthesized in the choroid plexus and is involved in the transport of T_4 from the blood into the CSF (22, 26–28). However, a small amount of albumin and TBG are present in the CSF due to the leakiness of the blood–brain barrier, and the main THDP in the CSF is TTR. Thus, TTR is responsible for the majority of thyroid hormone distribution in the CSF.

Evolution of TTR synthesis in the body and brain

TTR synthesis in the liver TTR is synthesized by the livers of all classes of vertebrates at some stage during their life cycle (Fig. 1.3.3 (29; for review, see Richardson (25)). In some animals this is during development only (e.g. fish, amphibians, reptiles, monotremes, and Australian polyprotodont marsupials) whereas in birds, diprotodont marsupial and eutherians ('placental mammals') TTR is synthesized in the liver throughout life. In general, animals that are homoeothermic ('warm blooded') synthesize TTR in their livers throughout life. Thyroid hormoness are known to be involved

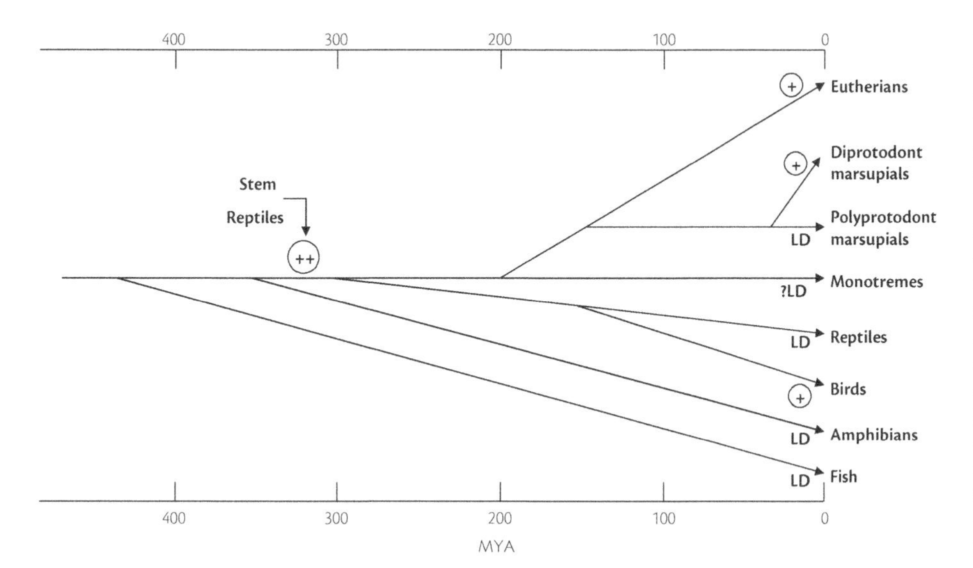

Fig. 1.3.3 Evolutionary/developmental tree for transthyretin (TTR) synthesis in choroid plexus and liver of vertebrates. The evolutionary tree based on the fossil record indicating onset of TTR synthesis in vertebrates. ++, onset of TTR synthesis in the choroid plexus, in juveniles and in adult of extant species; LD, hepatic TTR synthesis during development only; ?LD, possible onset of hepatic TTR synthesis during development only; +, hepatic TTR synthesis during development and in adult. MYA, millions of years ago. (From Richardson SJ, Monk JA, Shepherdley CA, Ebbesson LOE, Sin F, Power DM, *et al.* Developmentally regulated thyroid hormone distributor proteins in marsupials, a reptile and fishes. *Am J Physiol*, 2005; **288**: R1264–72.)

in the regulation of body temperature. Poikilothermic ('cold blooded') animals synthesize TTR in their livers only during specific stages of development that are regulated by thyroid hormones. From comparative endocrinology, we see that the function of TTR synthesized by the liver is related to an increased demand for thyroid hormone distribution: during thyroid hormone-regulated development and homoeothermy, which is governed largely by these hormones.

TTR synthesis in the brain TTR synthesis by the choroid plexus probably began with the stem reptiles about 320 million years ago (30). The stem reptiles are the common ancestors to the reptiles, birds and mammals (but not to amphibians and fish). Thus, TTR synthesis in the brain is a more recent event than TTR synthesis in the liver. The selection pressure for turning on the TTR gene in the choroid plexus could be the increase in brain volume, which occurred with the first traces of the cerebral cortex in the stem reptiles (31). This increase in lipid volume could have been the selection pressure requiring a protein to better distribute thyroid hormone around the brain via the CSF (see Schreiber and Richardson (20)). From comparative endocrinology, we see that the function of TTR synthesized by the brain is to counteract the partitioning of thyroid hormones into the increased lipid pool and to ensure their appropriate distribution throughout the CSF.

Evolution of TTR structure and function

The amino acid sequences of TTRs from more than 20 vertebrate species (including fish, amphibians, reptiles, birds, marsupials, and eutherians) have been determined. The amino acids in the central channel of the TTR homo-tetramer that are involved in ligand binding have been found tobe 100% conserved between species. A surprising finding, therefore, was that TTRs from lower vertebrates bind T_3 with higher affinity than T_4 (32). Only TTRs from mammals bind T_4 with higher affinity than T_3. Given that the amino acids in the thyroid hormone binding sites are identical in all TTRs sequenced to date, regions of the protein that changed during vertebrate evolution were sought and considered for influence of ligand binding. The region with the highest rate of evolution is the N-terminal region of the TTR subunit. This changed from longer and more hydrophobic in lower vertebrates to shorter and more hydrophilic in eutherian mammals. These structural characteristics correspond with ligand binding preferences: TTRs with longer and more hydrophobic N-termini bind T_3 with higher affinity than T_4, whereas TTRs with shorter and more hydrophilic N-terminal regions bind T_4 with higher affinity than T_3 (32). A series of chimeric TTRs were generated, where N-terminal regions were swapped or deleted. These studies confirmed the hypothesis that the N-terminal region of the TTR subunit confers ligand preference and affinity (33, 34). The mechanism for shortening the N-terminal region of the TTR subunit was found to be the stepwise shift in the position of the intron 1/exon 2 splice site in the 3′ direction (35). This is very unusual, as the thyroid hormone binding site in TTR does not determine which form of the thyroid hormone is bound.

TTR evolved from TTR-like protein, a 5-hydroxyisourate hydrolase There is a very high degree of amino acid identity across all vertebrate classes, suggesting that the *TTR* gene evolved prior to the divergence of the vertebrates from the invertebrates (36). Therefore, genomes of nonvertebrates were screened for open reading frames (ORFs) similar to *TTR* genes that could code for TTR-like proteins (TLPs). More than 100 ORFs coding for TLPs were identified, from all kingdoms (37). It was proposed that the *TTR* gene evolved as a duplication of the *TLP* gene. Five motifs were identified as defining TLPs and three motifs were identified as defining the set of TTRs + TLPs. These motifs mapped to structurally conserved and functionally important regions of the proteins. Transcription of these ORFs was shown in a bacterium, a plant, and an invertebrate animal, demonstrating their existence in nature. These TLPs had similar molecular weights and tetrameric structures to vertebrate TTRs. A subsequent study revealed the X-ray crystal structure of *Salmonella dublin* TLP to be extremely similar to that of vertebrate TTRs (Fig. 1.3.4) (38). Thus, the three-dimensional structure of TLP/TTR has not changed from bacteria to humans. The fact that the structure has been so highly conserved throughout evolution implies that this protein serves a very important function. Even within vertebrates, the structure of TTR is extremely highly conserved, similarly to histones. This remarkable degree of conservation of structure has been only revealed through comparative biochemistry.

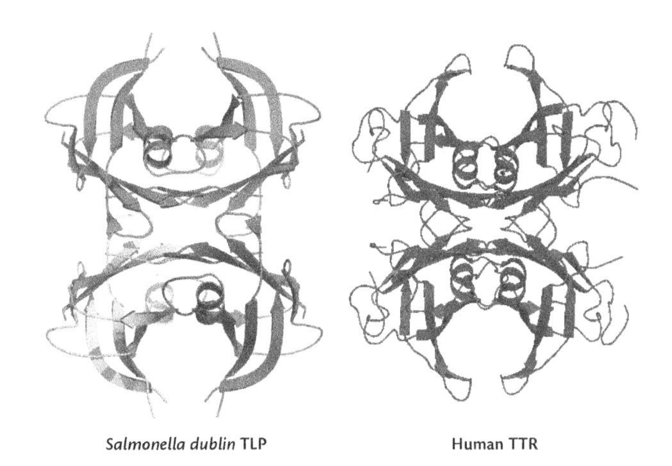

Fig. 1.3.4 Comparison of the X-ray crystal structures of *Salmonella dublin* transthyretin-like protein (TLP) and human transthyretin (TTR). (Adapted from Hennebry SC, Buckle AM, Law RH, Richardson SJ, Whisstock JC. The crystal structure of the transthyretin-like protein from *Salmonella dublin* reveals the structural basis for 5-hydroxyisourate hydrolase activity. *J Mol Biol*, 2006; **359**: 1389–99.)

TLPs do not bind thyroid hormones (39). TLPs from *Salmonella*, mouse, and zebrafish are enzymes involved in the oxidation of uric acid to allantoin. TLP is a 5-hydroxyisourate hydrolase, which hydrolyses 5-hydroxyisourate (5HIU) to 2-oxo-4-hydroxy-4-carboxy-5-ureidoimidazoline (38, 40, 41). A series of *Salmonella* TLPs with point mutations identified three conserved residues in the catalytic site that are essential for enzyme activity (38). Comparison between the thyroid hormone binding site in TTR and the equivalent region in *Salmonella* TLP revealed that the binding site was shallower and more positively charged in TLP compared with that of TTR, explaining why thyroid hormones cannot be bound by TLPs (38). TLP/TTR is a remarkable example of conservation of protein structure but evolution of its function: from a 5HIUase to distributor of T_3 to distributor of T_4.

Evolution of TTR structure sheds light on human amyloidosis The TTR tetramer is usually very stable. However, it can form amyloid fibrils naturally *in vivo*, and can be induced to form amyloid *in vitro* (42). There are two types of TTR amyloid. Senile systemic amyloidosis is an age-dependent disease and the TTR fibrils are formed from wild-type protein. At least 65% of people over 70 years have TTR senile systemic amyloidosis (see Calkins (43)). By contrast, familial amyloidotic polyneuropathy is a specific form of autosomal dominant hereditary polyneuropathy, which initially manifests as systemic deposition of amyloid in the peripheral nerves, but later effects many visceral organs.

There are at least 88 point mutations that have been documented in the 127 amino acids in the TTR subunit which result in familial amyloidotic polyneuropathy (see Connors *et al.* (44)). These mutations are evenly spread throughout the length of the TTR subunit—a sharp contrast to the evolutionary mutations, which are concentrated in the N-terminal regions of the subunit. TTR amyloidosis has not yet been described in a nonhuman species. Of the mutations in human TTR that result in amyloidosis, five are found in other species but do not result in amyloidosis: Val30Leu, Glu42Asp, Ile68Leu, Tyr69Ile, and Ala81Thr (Fig. 1.3.5) (see Richardson (25)). Of these, Leu30 is only found in sea bream TTR and Asp42 is only found in bullfrog TTR, both of which are evolutionarily quite distant from humans. However, the Ile68Leu substitution is found in 7 mammalian species studied to date. Further investigation of these TTRs and comparison to the mutated human Leu68 could give valuable insight as to why Leu is tolerated in position 68 without amyloidosis formation in other mammalian species, but leads to amyloid formation in humans. This could result in understanding a molecular basis of TTR amyloid formation in humans.

All five point mutations in human TTR that result in amyloidosis, that are the normal residue in that position in TTRs from other species, amyloidosis, but are result in cardiac amyloid deposition in humans. This is highly intriguing and requires further investigation.

Implications of the evolution of calcium regulation and thyroid hormone distributors for clinical endocrinology

In summary, there has always been considerable synergy between comparative and mammalian endocrinology with information from one field providing stimulus to the other. STC was originally identified in fish and subsequently found in mammals. Previous studies on fish STC provided information about the potential roles of human STC1 and the isolation of mammalian and fish STC2 will stimulate the search for its endocrine and physiological roles in both fish and mammals. In contrast, PTHrP and PTH were originally identified in mammals and then the search for fish genes began. There has been considerable interest in calcium-regulating factors from lower vertebrates because of the efficacy of salmon calcitonin in inhibiting bone resorption in mammals, including humans. Certainly a number of groups are interested in isolating fish PTH, or possibly PTHrP, as these fish factors or structural analogues, could be potential treatments for osteoporosis in humans.

The identification of a second STC in both fish and mammals reflects the principle Niall argued in 1982 (45)—that nature duplicates a gene rather than creating a new gene. Through this mechanism, when a gene for a hormone is duplicated, the copy is free to mutate and acquire new function(s) and receptors, leaving the first hormone carrying out its original role. This could also be the case with the duplication of PTH and PTHrP and calcitonin and calcitonin gene-related peptide. In his review, Ohno argued that for every gene present in invertebrates there could be up to four copies present in vertebrate genomes (10). He based his argument on the fact that there are 15 000 protein-coding genes in invertebrate genomes while he proposed that there should be 60 000 in vertebrate genomes as a result of two rounds of tetraploidization. He argued that there could be up to four oestrogen receptors in vertebrates, all of them not necessarily functional. Currently two oestrogen receptors have been isolated and cloned, and now we know that there are 30,00 genes in the human genome (http://www.ornl.gov/sci/techresources/Human_Genome/project/info.shtml) it may be a question of the gene is lost when it no longer has a function. But the one-to-four rule could apply to a number of other genes, including the PTH and calcitonin gene families. Prior to this, however, it is important to establish if there are members of these gene families present in an invertebrate genome. The sequencing of the *Caenorhabditis elegans* and *Ciona intestinalis* genomes have been completed and could be used for this purpose.

A number of other genes and hormones have been identified in fish but which have not yet been identified in mammals. One of these is somatolactin, a member of the growth hormone/prolactin family (46). Its relationship with two of the major vertebrate

```
                 <--- Presegment --->|Mature protein --->
                                     |---disordered----||β-strand|           |β-strand          |β-strand |  β-strand              |β-strand ||α-helix|
                                                          A                    B                  C           D                      E
Human            MASHRLLLLC LAGLVFVSEA GPT>        GTGESKC PLMVKVLDAV RGSPAINVAV HVFRKAADDT W>EPFASGKTS ESGELHGLTT EEEFVEGIYK VEIDTKSYWK ALGISPFHEH
                                                   S   A  P      Q I   NSS  M M   ITNP A   L G ST R AR GPEGPR RKA K  L    LHN A VH  YP   T S    QN
                                                                 G      T    L     L        D  D A II   KR  H      S    I        P       N    K
                                                                 N           A     V           S E P    Q                                  T
                                                                             G     C             V
Hedgehog         ******F*** ******M*** ***>         *Q*** ********** *****V**** K**K****E* * ********* ********** D*K****V** **L******* T********Y
Shrew            ***R****** *****L*T** ***>       ***Q*** ********** Q****V**** R**K****E* * ********* *F******** D*K*****I* **L***T*** ******S**Y
Pig              ***Y****** ********** **A        *A***** ********** *****V**G* K**K****G* * ****L**** *F******** D*K******* **L******* *********Y
Sheep            ***F****** ********** S*A        *A***** ********** *****A**G* K**K****E* * ********* D********* *DK****L** **L******* S********Y
Bovine           ***F**F*** ********** *SV        *A**P** ********** *****A**G* K**K****E* * ********* ********** *DK****L** **L******* S********F
Rabbit                                 **V        ***D*** ********** *****VD*S* ***K****E* * ********* KT******** S*K****V** **L******* *********Y
Rat              ***L**F*** ****I*A*** **G>       *A***** ********** *****VD*** K**K*T**GS * ********A ********** D*K*T**V*R **L******* *********Y
Mouse            ***L**F*** ********** **A>       *A***** ********** *****VD*** K**K*TSEGS *>********A ********** D*K****V*R **L******* T********F
Tammar Wallaby   **F*S***** ****A****T AAV>    H H EGEH*** ********** **R**V**D* K**K*TEEQ* * *L**A***N DN**I*E*** DDK*G**L** **F**I**** ***V*****Y
Grey Kangaroo    **F*S***** ****A****T AAV>    H H ESEH*** ********** **R**V**D* K**K*TEEQ* * *L**A***N DN**I*E*** DDK*G**L** **F**I**** ***V*****Y
Sugar Glider     **F*S***** ****L***** **V     A H *GED*** ********** **R**V**D* K**K*TEKQ* * *L******N DN**I*E**S DDK*G**L** **F**I**** ***V*****Y
Dunnart          **F*S***** ****L*L*** **V>    A H *AED*** ********S* *****V**D* K**K*TEEQ* * *L******N NN**I*E**S DDQ*G**L** **F**V**** TF*******Y
Grey Opossum     **F*S****G **S*L***D* A*V>    I H *AED*** ********** *****V**N* K**K*SEEQ* * ****T***N DY**I*E**N D*K*G**L** **F**F***N ***V*****Y
Chicken          **F*ST**VF ******L*** A*L>  V S H *SVD*** ********** *****A**** K**K****G* * QD**T***T *F**I*E*** **Q****V*R **F**S**** G**L*****Y
Crocodile        **F*SM**VF ******LT** A*L>  V S H *SID*** ********** *****A***I K**K*TS*GD * QE**A***T *F**V*E**S D*K******R **F**S**** ***L*****Y
Lizard           *G*SS***V* ***M*YLT** A*L>  V S H *SID*** ********** **R**TSI** K*SKMSEEGD * KE**N***N *F**I*E*** D*Q**Q*L** **F**S**** ***V*****Y
Bullfrog         **YYNT*A*L TIFIFSGAFH RAQ   G T H *EAD*** ********** **I**AKLP* K**KQNE*KS * DLIS**T** SD**I*N*A* **Q******* L*FA**RF*S K**LT****Y
Xenopus          ***FKSF**  **L*AI**** A*P>G H A S H *EAD*** ********** **I**A*LL* N****TNSGK * *QIT****T SD**I*N*** D*Q*T**V** I*FA**AF*G K**L*****Y
Sea Bream        *LQPLHC**L ASAVLCNTAP T**   D K H *GSDTR* *****I**** K*T**GS**L K*SQ*T**GG * TQI*T*V*D AT*EI*N*I* *QQ*PA*V*R **F***A**T NQ*ST****V
             -20        -10        -1+1 3-ε-δ-γ-β-α +4   10         20         30         40          50         60         70         80         90

                  |β-strand   |β-strand |  |β-strand
                    F           G          H
Human            AE>VVFTANDS GPRRYTIAAL LSPYSYSTTA VVTNPKE
                 SK    G     SRSC  VAT  MI C S  MS  I  S
                       S       H  M V      H        A
                                    S               Δ
Hedgehog         V* ******** *Q******** ********** L*SD***
Shrew            V* ******** *K******** ********** L*SD***
Pig              ** ******** *R*H****** ********** L*SS***GAL
Sheep            ** ******** *L*H****** ********** L*SS***
Bovine           ** ******** ***H****** ********** L*SS**A
Rabbit           ** ******** *H*S****** ***F****** **S**Q*
Rat              **>******** *H*H****** ********** **S**QN
Mouse            *D>******** *H*H****** ********** **S**QN
Tammar Wallaby   *D *******A *H*H****** *****F**** I*S**T*
Grey Kangaroo    *D *******A *H*H*****Q *****F**** I*S**T*
Sugar Glider     *D *******A *H*H*****Q *****F**** I*S**T*
Dunnart          *D *******A *H*H*****Q ***F*F**** **S***D
Grey Opossum     *D ***K***A *H*H****** ********** **S***D
Chicken          *D ******** *H*H****** ***F****** **SD*Q*
Crocodile        *D ******** *H*H****** ***F****** **SD*Q*
Lizard           *D ***S**** *H*H****** ***F****** **SD***
Bullfrog         VD *******A *H*H**T*V* *T***F**** **SDV**AHV
Xenopus          VD *******A *H*Q****V* *T***F*S** I*SE*HDDL
Sea bream        ** ***D*HPE *HGH**L*L* ***F**T*** **SSVH*
                        100        110        120        130
```

Bold in disordered region = N-terminal residue
Bold human mutation = found in another species
Italics = non-amyloidogenic mutation
> = position of intron
_ = residue in central channel
* = residue identical to that in human TTR
Δ = deletion of residue

Fig. 1.3.5 Human transthyretin (TTR) mutations compared with evolutionary mutations in vertebrate TTRs. TTR amino acid sequences and those derived from cDNA sequences from 19 species were aligned with that for human TTR. Secondary structural features for human TTR are indicated. Amino acids in other species identical to those in human TTR are indicated with asterisks. Point mutations detected in human TTRs are indicated below the human TTR sequence. (From Richardson SJ. Cell and molecular biology of transthyretin and thyroid hormones. *Int Rev Cytol*, 2007; **258**: 137–93.)

hormones should stimulate the search for it in the human genome and uncover its function in both lower and higher vertebrates. This will be another project where interaction between the two fields of endocrinology will prove fruitful.

Now that a number of whole genome sequencing projects, including the pufferfish (*Fugu rubripes*) and the human, are completed, and a number of other genomes are currently being sequenced (elephant shark, lamprey) more information about the genes for calcium-regulating factors as well as a number of other hormones will become accessible. When the complete sequences and genome structure are known, a shift in focus from gene to protein will be required, leaving comparative endocrinology to answer the following intriguing questions: what are the roles of these factors in lower vertebrates, compared with higher vertebrates, and how have evolutionary events modified these roles?

The evolution of the structure and function of TTR has given insights into the tissue-specific requirements of thyroid hormones, both during development and during evolution. TLPs exist in all kingdoms, whereas TTRs only exist in vertebrates. The highly conserved structure of TLP was very slightly modified to allow binding of thyroid hormones in the central channel. The N-terminal regions of each subunit were modified during evolution to change TTR from distributing T_3 to distributing T_4. This presumably resulted in an increased complexity of deiodinases at the tissue level. That certain amino acids in specific positions are tolerated in some species but result in amyloidosis in human TTR should be exploited to understand the mechanism of TTR amyloid formation in humans.

Large amounts of data are being generated by whole genome sequencing projects of a great range of vertebrates and invertebrates that are currently underway. There will be a number of exciting opportunities for collaboration between comparative and clinical endocrinology to learn more about the evolution of human endocrine conditions and possibly potential new treatments.

References

1. Ingleton PM, Danks JA. Distribution and functions of parathyroid hormone-related protein in vertebrate cells. *Int Rev Cytol*, 1996; **166**: 231–80.
2. Parsons JA, Gray D, Rafferty B, Zanelli JM. Evidence for a hypercalcaemic factor in the fish pituitary immunologically related to mammalian parathyroid hormone. In: Copp DH, Talmage RV, eds. *Endocrinology of Calcium Metabolism*. Amsterdam: Excerpta Medica, 1979: 111–14.
3. Danks JA, Ho PM, Notini AJ, Katsis F, Hoffmann P, Kemp BE, *et al.* Identification of a parathyroid hormone in the fish Fugu rubripes. *J Bone Miner Res*, 2003; **18**: 1326–31.
4. Liu Y, Ibrahim AS, Richardson SJ, Walker TI, Bell J, Ho PMW, *et al.* The parathyroid hormone gene family in a cartilaginous fish, the elephant shark (Callorhinchus milii) *J Bone Min Res.* doi 10.1002/jbmr. 178, 2008.
5. Yu WP, Rajasegaran V, Yew K, Loh W, Tay BH, Amemiya CT, *et al.* Elephant shark sequence reveals unique insights into the evolutionary history of vertebrate genes: a comparative analysis of the protocadherin cluster. *Proc Natl Acad Sci USA*, 2008; **105**: 3819–24.
6. Danks JA, Devlin AJ, Ho PM, Diefenbach-Jagger H, Power DM, Canario A, *et al.* Parathyroid hormone-related protein is a factor in normal fish pituitary. *Gen Comp Endocrinol*, 1993; **92**: 201–12.
7. Philbrick WM, Wysolmerski JJ, Galbraith S, Holt E, Orloff JJ, Yang KH, *et al.* Defining the roles of parathyroid hormone-related protein in normal physiology. *Physiol Rev*, 1996; **76**: 127–73.
8. Wysolmerski JJ, Stewart AF. The physiology of parathyroid hormone-related hormone: an emerging role as a developmental factor. *Annu Rev Physiol*, 1998; **60**: 431–60.
9. Lundin LG. Evolution of the vertebrate genome as reflected in paralogous chromosome regions in man and the house mouse. *Genomics*, 1993; **16**: 1–19.
10. Ohno S. The one-to-four rule and paralogues of sex-determining genes. *Cell Mol Life Sci*, 1999; **55**: 824–30.
11. Trivett MK, Officer RA, Clement JG, Walker TI, Joss JM, Ingleton PM, *et al.* Parathyroid hormone-related protein (PTHrP) in cartilaginous and bony fish tissues. *J Exp Zool*, 1999; **284**: 541–8.
12. Rubin DA, Hellman P, Zon LI, Lobb CJ, Bergwitz C, Jüppner H. A G-protein-coupled receptor from zebrafish is activated by human parathyroid hormone and not by human or teleost parathyroid hormone-related protein. *J Biol Chem*, 1999; **274**: 23035–42.
13. Yoshiko Y, Son A, Maeda S, Igarashi A, Takano S, Hu J, *et al.* Evidence for stanniocalcin gene expression in mammalian bone. *Endocrinology*, 1999; **140**: 1869–74.
14. Chang AC, Janosi J, Hulsbeek M, de Jong D, Jeffrey KJ, Noble JR, *et al.* A novel human cDNA highly homologous to the fish hormone stanniocalcin. *Mol Cell Endocrinol*, 1995; **112**: 241–7.
15. Chang AC-M, Dunham MA, Jeffrey KJ & Reddel RR. Molecular cloning and characterization of mouse stanniocalcin cDNA. *Molecular and Cellular Endocrinology*, 1996; **124**: 185–187.
16. Chang ACM, Reddel RR. Identification of a second stanniocalcin cDNA in mouse and human stanniocalcin 2. *Mol Cell Endocrinol*, 1998; **141**: 95–9.
17. Wagner GF, Jaworski EM, Haddad M. Stanniocalcin in the seawater salmon: structure, function, and regulation. *Am J Physiol*, 1998; **274**: R1177–85.
18. Gudernatsch JG Feeding experiments on tadpoles I. The influence of specific organs given as food on growth and differentiation: a contribution to the knowledge of organs with internal secretion. *Arch Entwicklungsmech Org*, 1912; **35**: 457–81.
19. Bassett JH, Williams GR. The molecular actions of thyroid hormones in bone. *Trends Endocrinol Metab*, 2003; **14**: 356–64.
20. Alberts B, Johnson J, Lewis J, Raff M, Roberts K, Walter P. *Molecular Biology of the Cell*, 4th edn. New York: Garland Science, 2002: P840.
21. Schreiber G, Richardson SJ. The evolution of gene expression, structure and function of transthyretin. *Comp Biochem Physiol*, 1997; **116B**: 137–60.
22. Dickson PW, Aldred AR, Menting JGT, Marley PD, Sawyer WH, Schreiber G. Thyroxine transport in choroid plexus. *J Biol Chem*, 1987; **262**: 13907–15.
23. Hillier AP. The binding of thyroid hormones to phospholipid membranes. *J Physiol*, 1970; **211**: 585–97.
24. Mendel CM, Weisiger RA, Jones AL, Cavalieri RR. Thyroid hormone-binding proteins in plasma facilitate uniform distribution of thyroxine within tissues: a perfused rat liver study. *Endocrinology*, 1987; **120**: 1742–9.
25. Richardson SJ. Cell and molecular biology of transthyretin and thyroid hormones. *Int Rev Cytol*, 2007; **258**: 137–93.
26. Southwell BR, Duan W, Alcorn D, Brack C, Richardson SJ, Köhrle J, *et al.* Thyroxine transport to the brain: role of protein synthesis by the choroid plexus. *Endocrinology*, 1993; **133**: 2116–26.
27. Schreiber G, Aldred AR, Jaworowski A, Nilsson C, Achen MG, Segal MB. Thyroxine transport from blood to brain via transthyretin synthesis in choroid plexus. *Am J Physiol*, 1990; **258**: R338–5.
28. Chanoine J-P, Alex S, Fang SL, Stone S, Leonard JL, Köhrle J, *et al.* Role of transthyretin in the transport of thyroxine from the blood to the choroid plexus, the cerebrospinal fluid, and the brain. *Endocrinology*, 1992; **130**: 933–8.
29. Richardson SJ, Monk JA, Shepherdley CA, Ebbesson LOE, Sin F, Power DM, *et al.* Developmentally regulated thyroid hormone distributor proteins in marsupials, a reptile and fishes. *Am J Physiol*, 2005; **288**: R1264–72.
30. Achen MG, Duan W, Pettersson TM, Harms PJ, Richardson SJ, Lawrence MC, *et al.* Transthyretin gene expression in choroid plexus first evolved in reptiles. *Am J Physiol*, 1993; **265**: R982–9.
31. Kent GC. *Comparative Anatomy of the Vertebrates.* St Louis: Time Mirror/Mosby College, 1987: 542.

32. Chang L, Munro SLA, Richardson SJ, Schreiber G. Evolution of thyroid hormone binding by transthyretins in birds and mammals. *Eur J Biochem*, 1999; **259**: 634–42.
33. Prapunpoj P, Richardson SJ, Schreiber G. Crocodile transthyretin: structure, function and evolution. *Am J Physiol*, 2002; **283**: R885–96.
34. Prapunpoj P, Leelawatwatana L, Schreiber G, Richardson SJ Change in structure of the N-terminal region of transthyretin produces change in affinity of transthyretin to T4 and T3. *FEBS J*, 2006; **273**: 4013–23.
35. Aldred AR, Prapunpoj P, Schreiber G. Evolution of shorter and more hydrophilic transthyretin N-termini by stepwise conversion of exon 2 into intron 1 sequences (shifting the 3′ splice site of intron 1). *Eur J Biochem*, 1997; **246**: 401–9.
36. Prapunpoj P, Yamauchi K, Nishiyama N, Richardson SJ, Schreiber G. Evolution of structure, ontogeny of gene expression and function of *Xenopus laevis* transthyretin. *Am J Physiol*, 2000 **279**: R2026–41.
37. Hennebry SC, Wright HM, Likic V, Richardson SJ. Structural and functional evolution of transthyretin and transthyretin-like proteins. *Proteins*, 2006; **64**: 1024–45.
38. Hennebry SC, Buckle AM, Law RH, Richardson SJ, Whisstock JC. The crystal structure of the transthyretin-like protein from *Salmonella dublin* reveals the structural basis for 5-hydroxyisourate hydrolase activity. *J Mol Biol*, 2006; **359**: 1389–99.
39. Eneqvist T, Lundberg E, Nilsson L, Abagyan R, Sauer-Eriksson AE. The transthyretin-related protein family. *Eur J Biochem*, 2003; **270**: 518–32.
40. Lee Y, Lee DH, Kho CW, Lee AY, Jang M, Cho S, *et al.* Transthyretin-related proteins function to facilitate the hydrolysis of 5-hydroxyisourate, the end product of the uricase reaction. *FEBS Letts*, 2005; **579**: 4769–74.
41. Ramazzina I, Folli C, Secchi A, Berni R, Percudani R. Completing the uric acid degradation pathway through phylogenetic comparison of whole genomes. *Nat Chem Biol*, 2006; **2**: 144–8.
42. Colon W, Kelly JW. Partial denaturation of transthyretin is sufficient for amyloid fibril formation in vitro. *Biochemistry*, 1992; **31**: 8654–60.
43. Calkins E. Amyloidosis. In: *Harrison's Principles of Internal Medicine*, 7th edn. Toyko: McGraw-Hill Kogakusha, 1974: 644–7.
44. Connors LH, Lim A, Prokaeva T, Roskens VA, Costello CE. Tabulation of transthyretin (TTR) variants 2003. *Amyloid*, 2003; **10**: 160–84.
45. Niall HD. The evolution of peptide hormones. *Annu Rev Physiol*, 1982; **44**: 615–24.
46. Rand-Weaver M, Noso T, Muramoto K, Kawauchi H. Isolation and characterization of somatolactin, a new protein related to growth hormone and prolactin from Atlantic cod (*Gadus morhua*) pituitary glands. *Biochemistry*, 1991; **30**: 1509–15.

Further reading

Ono S, Wolf U, Atkins NB. Evolution from fish to mammals by gene duplication. *Hereditas*, 1968; **59**: 169–87.

1.4

Hormones and receptors: fundamental considerations

John W. Funder

Background

The original endocrine physiologists viewed hormones as responses to homoeostatic challenge, any signal a call to arms; the word is thus derived from the classical Greek ωρμαειν—'to arouse'. In the twenty-first century a hormone is a molecule—small or large, protein or lipid—secreted in a regulated fashion from one organ and acting on another. The definition is firmly based on the anatomy of the seventeenth century, the histology of the nineteenth, and the physiology of the twentieth. It has been shaped by convention and clinical specialization: gut hormones are the marches between endocrinology and gastroenterology, and the adrenal medulla the territory of the cardiovascular physician. It has been refined by concepts of paracrine—where the secretion of one cell type in a tissue acts on another cell type in the same tissue—and autocrine, where a particular cell type both secretes and responds to a particular signal. Inherent in the concepts of paracrine and autocrine are that the signal is not secreted into blood or lymph, to be distributed more or less throughout the body, but is made locally to act locally. A very good example of a signalling system with both paracrine and autocrine activities is the neuronal synapse.

Inherent in the concept of the signal is that of a receptor: a signal without a receptor is the sound of one hand clapping. Inherent in the concept of a receptor are two functions: that of being able to discriminate between different signals, and to propagate the signal by activating cell membrane or intracellular signal transduction pathways. Discrimination by a receptor between different circulating potential signals is, in the first instance, a function of the likelihood of a particular signal being able to interact with the receptor, for a period of time sufficient to alter the confirmation of the receptor and thus to trigger propagation. This interaction is commonly referred to as binding, and thus the circulating hormone as a ligand (that which is bound). If the structures of ligand and receptors are such that the initial interaction is followed by formation of strong intermolecular bonds between the two, lessening the possibility of dissociation and the receptor returning to an unliganded state, the receptor is said to have high affinity for the ligand (and vice versa). If the binding is followed by propagation of the 'appropriate' signal the ligand is classified as an agonist, or active hormone; if a molecule occupies the binding site on the receptor but does not so alter its structure as to propagate a signal, it is classified as a hormone antagonist (and often, by extension, a receptor antagonist). In the past couple of decades, the concepts of 'agonist' and 'antagonist' have needed to be refined, as noted subsequently in this chapter.

Hormones and receptors: binding

In symbols, the reversible interaction between hormone and receptor can be simply written as follows;

$$[H]\cdot[R] \underset{}{\overset{K_1}{\rightleftharpoons}} [HR] \tag{1}$$

where [H] is the concentration of hormone, [R] the concentration of empty or unliganded receptor, and [HR] the concentration of occupied receptor, i.e. hormone-receptor complexes. The forward (to the right by convention) or association reaction is equally a function of hormone and receptor concentrations; the association rate constant $[K_1]$ is a reflection of the likeliness of apposition/goodness of fit of hormone and receptor, reflecting their structures plus extrinsic factors such as temperature, ionic strength of the milieu, and unstirred layers. The actual rate of the forward reaction is thus mulitfactorial, a function of the rate constant, the concentration of hormone, and the concentration of receptor, or

$$\text{forward rate (or on-rate)} = K_1\cdot[H]\cdot[R] \tag{2}$$

The dissociation of hormone receptor complexes [HR] is driven by one thing, and one thing only, the dissociation rate constant $[K_{-1}]$, a measure of the inherent probability of the two entities falling apart, under particular conditions of temperature, ionic strength, etc. The actual rate of dissociation is thus the product of K_{-1}, the dissociation rate constant, and the concentration of hormone-receptor complexes, or

$$\text{reverse rate (or off-rate)} = K_{-1}\cdot[HR] \tag{3}$$

At equilibrium, by definition, the rates of the forward and reverse reactions are equal, i.e. for every molecule of hormone that associates with a receptor molecule, a preformed hormone–receptor complex dissociates, or

$$K_1\cdot[H]\cdot[R] = K_{-1}\cdot[HR] \tag{4}$$

By simple rearrangement, this can be rewritten

$$\frac{K_{-1}}{K_1} = \frac{[H][R]}{[HR]} \tag{5}$$

The quotient of the two rates constants (K_{-1}/K_1) is termed the dissociation constant or Kd; its reverse (K_1/K_{-1}) is the less commonly used Ka or association constant of the reaction. The key outcome of all this relatively simple mathematics is to put a value on Kd, as a measure of affinity, or overall probability of the hormone–receptor complex being in existence, as follows.

$$Kd = \frac{K_{-1}}{K_1} = \frac{[H][R]}{[HR]} \quad (6)$$

If we where to choose a concentration of hormone which would half saturate the receptors, then [R] would equal [HR]. Under such circumstances the two terms can be cancelled in (6) above, and

$$Kd = [H] \quad (7)$$

where Kd equals [H], the hormone concentration at which half maximal receptor occupancy is achieved, and which has the dimensions of concentration, that is, molar.

From equations (1)–(7) there are a number of things that flow. First, in a simple binding system the dissociation of hormone from receptor is not accelerated by addition of excess hormone. What this does, when, for instance, 1000-fold nonradioactive hormone is added to a system containing tracer hormone–receptor complexes, is to operationally prevent (i.e. dilute 1000-fold) reassociation of tracer to receptor. Under such conditions then, the disappearance of tracer–receptor complexes over time thus provides an accurate estimate of the dissociation rate. There are receptors that oligomerize: in such circumstances binding of ligand can increase or decrease the affinity of the other binding sites for hormone, termed positive and negative cooperativity, respectively. Dissociation of bound tracer, for instance, is accelerated in systems displaying negative cooperativity.

Secondly, dissociation constants can only be derived from equilibrium studies, that is, those in which the rates of forward and backward reactions are equal. The association rate constant and dissociation rate constant are often very different, and are constant for a given set of physical circumstances; the actual rates of association and dissociation are determined by not just these constants, but also by the concentration of reactants, as noted above. Where this concept of equilibrium comes into play is in situations where binding is covalent, or essentially irreversible; under such circumstances Scatchard analysis, for example, is inappropriate for determining Kd. A practical case in point is triamcinolone acetonide (TA), a powerful synthetic glucocorticoid in clinical use, which (in contrast with dexamethasone or the physiological glucocorticoids) requires approximately 24 h to come into equilibrium in glucocorticoid receptor binding systems in vitro at 4 C; exposure for shorter time points will consistently underestimate the affinity of TA for the glucocorticoid receptor. Third, different binding systems respond differently to changes in physical conditions. Cortisol, for example, binds transcortin with an order of magnitude higher affinity at 4° C than at 37° C, across a number of species, and with clear differences in binding at physiologically relevant temperatures. In contrast, cortisol binding to glucocorticoid receptors is not particularly temperature dependent, but if anything is of a higher affinity at physiological than at lower temperatures.

Finally there is the inherent bias of endocrinology, that of seeing high-affinity binding as good ('binds well to the receptor ...'), and lower affinity binding as less good ('binds poorly ...'). The underpinnings of this bias is twofold, one theoretical and the other practical. Practically, particularly in often unstable broken cell preparations, the absence of high-affinity binding equates to experimental failure, a powerful driver of emotive language. Even if no experiment ever failed, however, an endocrinologist's bias is to regard high-affinity binding as good, for the following reason. The higher the affinity the lower the concentration of signal required to half-maximally occupy, and, other things being equal, activate the 'cognate' receptor. There are two consequences of this, one of which appears to be biologically sound, the other less so. The latter is a notion of economy; that it is better for an organ to make less rather than more signal, in that it poses less of a demand on precursors and metabolism. This is experientially not the case; every molecule of thyroglobulin, with a molecular weight in excess of 600 000 yields 4–16 molecules of thyroxine, at first sight an example of conspicuous biological extravagance. The other concept underlying the bias has more biological purchase, in that the higher the concentration required to activate cognate receptors, the more likely is the hormone to cross-react with other receptors, acting as an agonist or antagonist, and thus reducing the specificity of the signalling system. It is, of course, entirely possible that there have evolved circumstances in which such 'cross-reactivity' may reflect physiology, and that our bias is Ockham's razor cutting too close to the bone: on the whole, however, such a degree of cautious reductionism appears justified.

Hormones and neurotransmitters

In contrast with the previous discussion, if we take a broader biological view that low-affinity binding can be 'good'—when it enables rolling of platelets or leucocytes on endothelium, giving them time to 'sniff the wind' in terms of damage or inflammation. It is also not only advantageous, but functionally required, within the nervous system, where low-affinity binding of signal to receptor is a necessity for the time constants of neurotransmission.

When the electrical impulse underlying nerve conduction is translated into a chemical signal at a synapse or neuroeffector junction, minute quanta of neurotransmitter are released. Because the space into which the neurotransmitter is released is even more minute, the concentration of neurotransmitter becomes very high, so that receptors are rapidly occupied and activated. To achieve this, the 'on-rate' of neurotransmitter-receptor binding must be very rapid; and the off-rate (in contrast with hormone-receptor interactions) must also be very rapid, to enable the receptor to return to ground zero. Signal is rapidly cleared by reuptake, diffusion, and metabolism, so that quantal release of signal is followed essentially stochastically by a single response.

To achieve this rapid onset rapid offset binding and activation by neurotransmitters, receptors have to be low affinity, to allow the time constants that characterize neurotransmission. The nervous system does it by mass, 'brute-forcing' occupancy of low-affinity receptors, with a restricted spatial distribution of the mass of signal to allow the very high concentrations required, and very efficient mechanisms of rapidly reducing signal concentration. Reflecting this difference, hormones have time constants of minutes, hours, and days compared with the nervous system's milliseconds; the endocrine system sacrifices time to allow its signals to be distributed all over the body, to 'arouse' the diversity of cells that express receptors to which the particular signal can bind. Its signals are broadcast like radio, in contrast with the nervous system landline telephone network.

One striking anthropomorphic illustration of this difference may be worth a thousand words of theoretical justification. First, picture a hummingbird in the *National Geographic*, its wings still blurred despite shutter speeds of 1/500 or 1/1000 of a second. If acetylcholine had the same high affinity for its receptors at the neuromuscular junction as progesterone has for progesterone receptors, then a hummingbird could beat its wings twice a minute, aerodynamically challenging and clearly no evolutionary advantage. Even less of an evolutionary advantage accrues if progesterone receptors had the same affinity for progesterone as cholinergic receptors for acetylcholine. Unless the efficiency of steroidogenesis were vastly improved, the placenta would need to be considerably larger: to maintain plasma progesterone at the levels required, other things equal, it would need to be the size of a 0.4 m^3 (14 cubic foot) refrigerator. Other evolutionary considerations would be 9 months of somnolence that such levels of progesterone would almost certainly produce, difficult to reconcile with the additional 25 000 calories per day required to maintain the requisite levels of progesterone biosynthesis required.

Mineralocorticoid receptors: a case study

We have mercifully evolved otherwise, and evolution has exploited a range of interactions between signals and receptors in terms of growth, development, homoeostasis, and cognition. Sometimes we can second-guess nature, perhaps to our own disadvantage in terms of realizing our own physiology.

One example, within the author's area of experience, is that of the mineralocorticoid receptor. Mineralocorticoid hormones were defined in 1961 by Jean Crabbé as promoting unidirectional transepithelial sodium transport (1), a definition that has stood the test of time. The principal mineralocorticoid hormone, aldosterone, is secreted from the zona glomerulosa of the adrenal cortex in response to elevated plasma potassium concentrations, or increased levels of angiotensin II. In response to sodium deficiency, volume depletion or potassium loading, aldosterone incontestably acts via mineralocorticoid receptor in kidney and colon, salivary gland and sweat gland to retain sodium, *a la* Jean Crabbé and thus acting as a classic homoeostatic hormone. And yet ...

When human mineralocorticoid receptors were first cloned (2), the highest levels of mRNA were found in the hippocampus, not a classical site of aldosterone action, and recapitulating earlier binding studies on rat tissue extracts (3). Second, in both studies, mineralocorticoid receptors were shown to have equivalent affinity for the physiological glucocorticoids (cortisol, corticosterone) as for aldosterone, raising obvious questions of how aldosterone ever occupies epithelial mineralocorticoid receptors, given the orders of magnitude higher circulating concentrations of glucocorticoids.

The answer to this question appears to be the coexpression, in epithelial tissues, of the enzyme 11β-hydroxysteroid dehydrogenase (4, 5), which converts cortisol and corticosterone to their inactive 11-keto metabolites cortisone/11-dehydrocorticosterone. Aldosterone is not similarly metabolized, because its signature aldehyde group at C18 cyclizes with the hydroxyl at C11, forming a stable hemiacetal which is not susceptible to enzyme attack by 11β- hydroxysteroid dehydrogenase 2.

The enzyme is expressed at high abundance in aldosterone target cells (3–4 × 10^6 molecules/cell), and its operation—by metabolizing glucocorticoids (6) and probably by other mechanisms (7, 8)—appears sufficient to confer aldosterone selectivity on the epithelial mineralocorticoid receptor. When it is congenitally deficient, as in the autosomal recessive syndrome of apparent mineralocorticoid excess (9), cortisol activates epithelial mineralocorticoid receptors, leading to uncontrolled sodium retention and severe hypertension.

The enzyme 11β-hydroxysteroid dehydrogenase 2 is not found in nonepithelial tissues in which mineralocorticoid receptors are expressed at high (hippocampus) or modest (heart) abundance, and which thus aldosterone has prima facie little chance of occupying. An inescapable corollary of the last sentence is that such mineralocorticoid receptors are physiologically high-affinity glucocorticoid receptors.

Hormones and receptors evolutionary considerations

In the syndrome of glucocorticoid remediable aldosteronism (10), aldosterone is secreted primarily in response to adrenocorticotrophic hormone (ACTH), with aldosterone synthase activity expressed throughout the adrenal cortex. The underlying genetic defect is a chimeric gene in which the 5′ end of the gene for 11β-hydroxylase is fused with the 3′ end of the gene coding for aldosterone synthase. This can happen because the two parent genes lie next to one another, on chromosome 8, and because they are 94% identical in terms of nucleotide sequence. What the condition reflects is the product of an unequal crossing over at meiosis in an ancestral gamete, reflecting the relatively small misalignment required (gene proximity) and the possibility of realignment (sequence homology). In evolutionary terms, however, what the condition illustrates is the probability that the two genes (for 11β-hydroxylase and aldosterone synthase) share a relatively recent ancestor, and that their degree of identity and juxtaposition represent a relatively recent gene duplication event. Compare this with the gene coding for the mineralocorticoid receptor (chromosome 4) and the glucocorticoid receptor (chromosome 5).

Mineralocorticoid receptors and glucocorticoid receptors have one area of high (about 90%) sequence identity, the DNA-binding domain, and another of considerable homology, the ligand binding domain, with 57% identity: the majority of the two molecules, including major activation domains, have minimal (less than 15%) identity. It would thus appear that the mineralocorticoid receptor and glucocorticoid receptor are rather more evolutionary distant than are the enzymes 11β-hydroxylase and aldosterone synthase. Although classically mineralocorticoid and glucocorticoid receptors were thought to share a common immediate 'corticoid' receptor ancestor (11), more recently evidence has emerged for mineralocorticoid receptors being the first of the mineralocorticoid/glucocorticoid/androgen/progestin receptor subfamily to branch off (12).

In evolutionary terms aldosterone is thus a Johnny-come-lately, pressed into service as organisms became amphibious, to activate a pre-existing high-affinity glucocorticoid receptor (which we now term the mineralocorticoid receptor). Mineralocorticoid receptor selectivity in epithelial aldosterone target tissues is produced by coexpression of the enzyme 11β-hydroxsteroid dehydrogenase 2 at high abundance, and the integrity of a system for Na^+ retention out of seawater obtained by the expression of aldosterone synthase being yoked to surrogates of Na^+ deficiency (angiotensin II, K^+) rather than primarily to the brain hormone ACTH. To call aldosterone the cognate ligand for mineralocorticoid receptor—and the ascription 'mineralocorticoid receptor' itself—is thus understandable in terms of our historical knowledge of aldosterone, but it fails to recognize the previous, and current, physiological roles for mineralocorticoid receptors net of aldosterone. The rainbow trout, for instance, does not synthesize aldosterone. In an attempt to clone rainbow trout androgen receptors, an rtMR sequence was identified, related to rtGR but with much higher identity with mammalian mineralocorticoid receptors (13). Its physiologic role(s), like the pathophysiologic roles of mammalian nonepithelial mineralocorticoid receptors, await exploration.

A final fundamental consideration might thus be as follows. There are currently 49 members of the extended steroid/thyroid/retinoid/orphan receptor superfamily of ligand activated transcription factors in the human genome, evidence for enormous evolutionary scope and flexibility. One might thus be pardoned for asking why a 'specific' mineralocorticoid receptor did not evolve, responsive to a ligand with levels inversely related to Na^+ status, rather than the complicated system of highly reactive C18 aldehyde groups and epithelial 11β-hydroxsteroid dehydrogenase 2. This is in fact an impertinent question, bluntly put this way: what is the appropriate question to ask is where is the evolutionary gain in the system being how it is.

Receptor activation, receptor blockade

For aldosterone and mineralocorticoid receptors, the past decade has provided more questions than answers. Among the latter, for the hormone, is the acceptance that aldosterone can have both genomic and acute, nongenomic effects, and that most but probably not all such rapid effects are via the classic mineralocorticoid receptor. In addition, there is now general consensus that the syndrome of primary aldosteronism represents 10% of all 'essential hypertension', and that such patients show higher cardiovascular morbidity and mortality than age-, sex- and blood pressure-matched patients with essential hypertension. For the receptor, the RALES, EPHESUS, and 4E trials (14–16) have shown the beneficial effects of mineralocorticoid receptor blockade in heart failure and essential hypertension. The functions and roles of nonepithelial mineralocorticoid receptors, constitutively (90–99%) occupied by glucocorticoids, have hardly begun to be properly addressed. The mechanisms whereby the physiological glucocorticoids show bivalent activity when bound to mineralocorticoid receptors—normally antagonist, but agonist (in the sense of mimicking aldosterone) in the context of redox change (11β-hydroxysteriod dehydrogenase 2 blockade, reactive oxygen species generation (7, 8) similarly remain to be established.

In fact, the terms agonist and antagonist need to be seen for what they are—effector definitions, like that proposed for mineralocorticoids almost half a century ago by Jean Crabbé. For most hormone receptor systems, the last 20 years—and the past decade in particular—has seen the growing emergence of tissue selective agents, agonist in some organs, antagonist is others. While most microarray analyses have provided a formidable list of genes, expression of which is doubled or halved by a classical agonist, similar lists can be complied for classical antagonists. Some classical antagonists, e.g. spironolactone for epithelial mineralocorticoid receptors, demonstrate inverse agonist activity in experimental myocardial infarction (17). Aldosterone and cortisol aggravate the infarct area; spironolactone at low (EC50 3–5 nm) concentration reduces the infarct area, in the absence of any other steroid.

Spironolactone thus has its 'antagonist' effects in the context of cardiac damage not just by competing with agonist steroids for occupancy of mineralocorticoid receptors, but by inducing expression of protective genes and lowering that of proapoptotic genes. It does this at relatively low concentrations, evidence that not all mineralocorticoid receptors, or even a majority, need to be occupied for such an effect. Even before the advent of microarray, it was clear that the effects on enzyme induction, for example, in cultured cells could show distinct dose–response curves, evidence for maximal effects on some readouts at submaximal receptor occupancy. This has not been widely incorporated into consideration of the clinical roles of aldosterone and mineralocorticoid receptors. An example of the former is the demonstration that relatively mild elevations of aldosterone in primary aldosteronism, which would have minimal incremental effects on nonepithelial receptor occupancy, are accompanied by demonstrable cardiovascular damage (18), even in the absence of an elevated blood pressure (19), compared with age-, sex- and blood pressure- matched controls. An example of the latter would appear to be the otherwise curiously low dose (x = 26 mg/day) of spironolactone which, when added to standard care, produced a remarkable 30% improvement in survival, and 35% lower hospital admission rate, in the RALES trial (14).

ENV0I

Given the achievements of the human genome project, we are faced with a mass of information of daunting proportions. This brief chapter has attempted to raise questions, and thus help shape the mindsets of those who face the exciting but very challenging task of reconciling the enormity of information with the demands of clinical endocrinology, from individual patients through populations. For a chance of success, we need a degree of comfort with the underlying mathematics, the biology, and as best we can guess the historical record, the evolution.

References

1. Crabbe J. Stimulation of active sodium transport by the isolated toad bladder with aldosterone in *vitro*. *J Clin Investig*, 1961; **40**: 2103–10.
2. Arriza JL, Weinberger C, Cerelli G, Glaser TM, Handelin BL, Housman DE, *et al.* Cloning of human mineralocorticoid receptor complementary DNA: structural and functional kinship with the glucocortiod receptor. *Science*, 1987; **237**: 268–75.
3. Krozowski ZS, Funder JW. Renal mineralocorticoid receptors and hippocampal corticosterone-binding species have identical intrinsic steroid specificity. *Proc Natl Acad Sci USA*, 1983; **880**: 6036–60.
4. Funder JW, Pearce P, Smith R, Smith AL. Mineralocorticoid action: target-tissue specificity is enzyme, not receptor, mediated. *Science*, 1988; **242**: 583–5.
5. Edwards CR, Stewart PM, Burt D, Brett L, McIntyre MA, Sutanto WS, *et al.* Localisation of 11 beta-hydroxsteriod dehydrogenase–tissue specific protector of the mineralocorticoid receptor. *Lancet*, 1988; **2**: 986–9.
6. Funder JW, Myles K. Exclusion of corticosterone from epithelial mineralocorticoid receptors is insufficient for selectivity of aldosterone action: *in vivo* binding studies. *Endocrinology*, 1996; **137**: 5264–8.
7. Funder JW. Is aldosterone bad for the heart? *Trends Endocrinol Metab*, 2004; **15**: 139–42.
8. Feldman D, Funder JW, Eldelman IS. Subcellular mechanisms in the action of adrenal steroids. *Am J Med*, 1972; **53**: 545–60.
9. Wilson RC, Krozowski ZS, Li K, Obeyesekere VR, Razzaghy-Azar M, Harbison MD, *et al.* A mutation in the HSD11B2 gene in a family with apparent mineralocorticoid excess. *J Clin Endrocrinol Metab*, 1995; **80**: 2263–6.

10. Lifton RP, Dluhy RG, Powers M, Rich GM, Cook S, Ulick S, *et al.* A chimaeric 11 beta-hydroxylase/aldosterone synthase gene causes glucocortiod-remediable aldosteronism and human hypertension. *Nature*, 1992; **355**: 262–5.
11. Mangelsdorf DJ, Thummel C, Beato M, Herrlich P, Schutz G, Umesono K, *et al.* The nuclear receptor superfamily: the second decade. *Cell*, 1995; **83**: 835–9.
12. Hu X, Funder JW. The evolution of mineralocorticoid receptors. *Mol Endocrinol* 2006; **20**: 1471–8.
13. Colombe L, Fostier A, Bury N, Pakdel P, Gurgen YA. Mineralocorticoid receptor in the rainbow trout, *Oncorhynchus Mykiss*, cloning and characterization of its steroid binding domain. *Steroids*, 2000; **65**: 319–28.
14. Pitt B, Zannad F, Remme WJ, Cody R, Castaigne A, Perez A, *et al.* The effect of spironolactone on morbidity and mortality in patients with severe heart failure. *N Engl J Med*, 1999; **341**: 709–17.
15. Pitt B, Remme W, Zannad F, Neaton J, Martinez F, Roniker B, *et al.* Eplerenone, a selective aldosterone blocker, in patients with left ventricular dysfunction after myocardial infarction. *N Engl J Med*, 2003; **348**: 1309–21.
16. Pitt B, Reichek N, Willenbrock R, Zannad F, Phillips RA, Roniker B, *et al.* Effects of eplerenone, enalapril, and eplerenone/enalapril in patients with essential hypertension and left ventricular hypertrophy: the 4E-left ventricular hypertrophy study. *Circulation*, 2003; **108**: 1831–8.
17. Mihailidou AS, Loan Le Ty, Mardini M, Funder JW, Glucocorticoids activate cardial mineralcorticoid receptors during experimental myocardial infarction. *Hypertension*, 2009; **54**: 1211–12.
18. Milliez P, Girard X, Plouin P-F, Blacher J, Safar ME, Mourad J-J. Evidence for an increased rate of cardiovascular events in patients with primary aldosteronism. *J Am Coll Cardiol*, 2005; **45**: 1243–8.
19. Stowasser M, Sharman J, Leano R, Gordon RD, Ward G, Cowley D, *et al.* Evidence for abnormal left ventricular structure and function in normotensive individuals with familial hyperaldosteronism type 1. *J Clin Endocrinol Metab*, 2005; **90**: 5070–6.

1.5

Molecular aspects of hormonal regulation

Shern L. Chew

Introduction

The wide molecular effects of hormones have complicated the understanding of how hormones work on a cell. The old view was of a linear signalling pathway from the receptor to the nucleus, thereby stimulating gene transcription. This view is probably an oversimplification. Hormones can not only regulate most of the molecular machines of the cell, certainly the transcription machinery, but also others. These machines perform and coordinate functions such as RNA and protein biosynthesis, macromolecular transport, cell division or death, and intracellular signalling. Physiological studies have shown that hormonal regulation is specific, yet flexible, and has the ability to generate feedback loops. Advances in genetics, cellular, and molecular biology, and biochemistry have allowed much new, and sometimes confusing, data on the mechanisms underlying hormonal regulation. Many advances have been due to methods of identifying and verifying networks of interactions between proteins. One example is the yeast two-hybrid system, an *in vivo* genetic screening method for such interactions. Another example is the use of protein tagging (e.g. with histidine residues) which can allow rapid and high-yield protein purification for biochemical studies. This chapter will briefly review some of the mechanisms of hormonal regulation.

Gene expression

The control of the expression of a pattern or network of genes is an essential mechanism for the maintenance of stable, but specific, cellular state or differentiation. The hormonal milieu is often vital to the upkeep of specialized cellular functions, in both cultured cells and in tissues. Many hormones achieve these effects in a cell mainly by enhancing or silencing the transcription of specific genes (see Chapter 1.4 for details about transcription). The molecular details of several eukaryotic transcriptional enhancer systems have been elucidated (for a review, see Ogata *et al.* (1)).

The general principles are that transcriptional activation involves the formation of a multiprotein complex called an enhanceosome, which assembles at enhancer DNA sequence elements (Fig. 1.5.1). The enhanceosome complex attracts and engages the basal transcriptional machinery on several of its protein surfaces. The surface of the complex is made up of several peptide domains, either from different proteins, or from the multiple domains of one protein. The structure, shape, and domain components of this surface partly explain some of the specificity in transcriptional regulation. Only regulator protein domains that fit together can function together. Another principle is that the attraction between proteins within and between complexes is reciprocal. Thus, binding is cooperative: proteins that fit together help each other to bind to the activator complex. Transcription is stimulated in a synergistic (not additive) manner, once cooperative and specific binding has allowed a threshold of activator concentrations to be reached.

Proteins in the enhanceosome have several functions. Some are DNA sequence-specific transcriptional activators, which bind chromatin and hyperacetylate histones. This chemical modification results in the disruption of chromatin and histone structure around the DNA. The change in chromatin structure is required

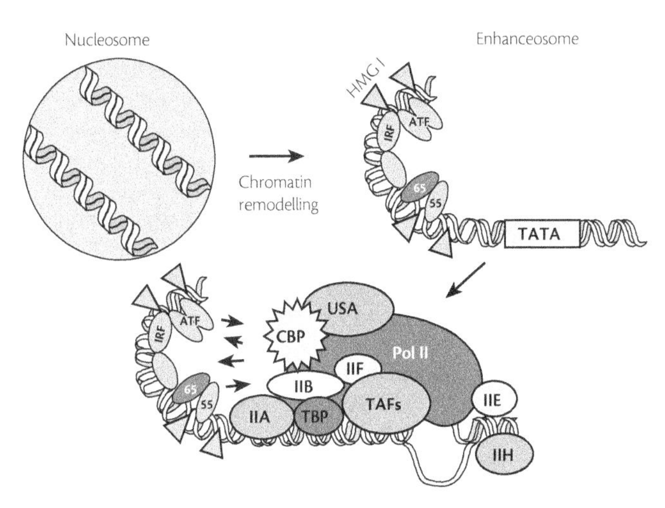

Fig. 1.5.1 The assembly of a higher order transcriptional complex. DNA is packed into a chromatin structure (nucleosome), but can be bound by several sequence specific activator proteins (ovals). These cooperate with structural proteins (triangles) which bend the DNA. The different proteins promote each other's binding, so that a stable enhanceosome is formed. The surface of the enhanceosome interacts with coactivators, such as CBP (star), and there is recruitment of pol II and other factors to the TATA box. The multiple, bidirectional arrows indicate that the interactions between the enhanceosome and the pol II apparatus is cooperative and leads to the stabilization and function of a higher order transcriptional complex. (Redrawn from Carey M. The enhanceosome and transcriptional synergy. *Cell*, 1998; **92**: 5–8.(2).)

for transcription to occur. Otherwise, the transcription complex fails to build properly and cannot progress along the DNA template to make pre-mRNA. Other proteins are architectural proteins, which bend the DNA to allow stabilization of the complex and further recruitment of activators. One example is the high-mobility group I(Y) protein (HMG I(Y)), which bends DNA to facilitate the binding of the transcriptional activator, nuclear factor kappa B (NF-κB). The interferon (IFN) β enhanceosome contains several other proteins, including members of the interferon regulatory factor family (IRF1, IRF3, IRF7) and activation transcription factor 2 (ATF2), and is capable of interactions with the basal transcriptional apparatus. Kinase-signalling pathways can modify the activator proteins in the enhanceosome and this phosphorylation stimulates cooperative binding and complex assembly. The enhanceosome now interacts with the basal RNA polymerase II transcriptional apparatus at the gene promoter. The multiple contacts between the surfaces of the enhanceosome complex and the basal transcription complex allow reciprocal strengthening of the stability of a higher order transcriptional complex. This is associated with the recruitment of more coactivator proteins (p300/CBP). The recruitment of p300/CBP (probably by interactions with IRF3) is associated with dramatic hyperacetylation of histones H3 and H4 at the site of the IFNβ promoter. Thus, specificity of transcription (i.e. localization of function at the IFNβ promoter) is achieved by the multiple stepwise interactions required to assemble the higher order transcriptional complex. Once the transcription complex is assembled, and the chromatin structure opened, transcription is activated in an exponential and synergistic manner in response to the external stimulus.

Hormones, such as glucocorticoids, may repress, as well as activate, gene expression. Some of the mechanisms of action of the glucocorticoid receptor (GR) have been elucidated by genetic technology in the mouse. In particular, these experiments have allowed the dissection of GR-mediated gene activation and repression (3). Mice have been made where the gene for the GR has been knocked out (GR null). The mice die after birth because of pulmonary atelectasis, but also show marked adrenal hyperplasia, high corticosterone levels, and reduced expression of gluconeogenic enzymes in the liver. Mice have also been engineered with a single mutation in the D-loop, which forms part of the DNA-binding domain of the GR. This mutation (GR dim) destabilizes the dimerization of the GR, thereby reducing cooperative binding between two GR monomers required for interactions with DNA. The GR dim mice show loss of functions that require dimerization and DNA binding. Conversely, functions that are mediated by interactions between GR monomers and other proteins are preserved. Comparison of the phenotypes of the two mutant mice, GR null and GR dim, and wild-type mice has allowed a functional classification of GR mechanisms (Table 1.5.1, based on Karin (4)). Examples of the positive transcriptional functions, requiring DNA binding by the GR, include transcription of liver genes such as tyrosine aminotransferase, and the viral MMTV genome. Transcriptional repression that requires DNA binding occurs in the proopiomelanocortin and prolactin genes. Finally, a set of functions not requiring DNA binding (and presumably due to interference with other transcription factors by protein–protein interactions) includes repression of the transcription of the osteogenic collagenase and gelatinase genes. The viability of the GR dim mice, in contrast to the lethality of the GR null mutant, reflects the importance of the transcriptional interference functions of the

Table 1.5.1 A functional classification of molecular mechanisms of glucocorticoid receptor function

Mechanism	Examples
Positive action via GRE	Tyrosine aminotransferase
	MMTV genome
	Metallothionein II_A
	Alanine aminotransferase
Negative action via GRE	Proopiomelanocortin
	α-subunit
	Prolactin
Interference with transcription factors (e.g. AP1)	Collagenase type I
	Gelatinase

GRE, glucocorticoid response element.

GR, particularly in adrenal and lung development. Additionally, these experiments opened avenues whereby treatments can be targeted to specific aspects of glucocorticoid function. Hopefully, drugs in development will retain the immunosuppressive effects of glucocorticoids (by interfering with the NF-κB signalling system), but without repressing transcription of osteogenic genes and thus avoiding glucocorticoid-associated osteopenia (5).

Post-transcriptional processing

After transcription, the newly made pre-mRNA must undergo several processing steps in order to be exported from the nucleus and made into protein in the cytoplasm. In humans and higher eukaryotes, substantial variations in the mRNA are introduced during these steps, such that one gene often encodes for several mRNA isoforms. Thus, the final pattern of cellular gene expression is very different from the genomic DNA sequence (6). Hormones can influence pre-mRNA processing mechanisms (7). Many examples have been reported where changes in the ratios of mRNA products from the same pre-mRNA gene transcript occur in response to changes in hormonal conditions (Table 1.5.2). Several processing steps may be involved, including pre-mRNA splicing (8), polyadenylation, and turnover (9). In some cases, the sequence elements on the pre-mRNA through which regulation is mediated and proteins acting as regulators have been identified (10).

Alternative pre-mRNA splicing significantly alters the patterns of gene expression in endocrine tissues such as the thyroid or testes (11). This results in diversity of protein expression, which is important to the specific functions of differentiated endocrine tissues. In the best studied example of the calcitonin/calcitonin gene-related protein (CGRP) pre-mRNA, regulatory pre-mRNA sequence elements have been mapped, and several RNA-binding proteins have been identified, which may function to control the tissue-specific splicing patterns.

Translational control

The expression of several endocrine genes can be regulated at the level of translation from mRNA into protein. This process occurs in the cytoplasm. Examples include insulin-like growth factor 2 (IGF2) and fibroblast growth factor 2 (FGF2), (12) which have alternative translation initiation sites. The use of the alternative

Table 1.5.2 Changes in mRNA isoforms in response to hormonal and other signals

Alternatively spliced mRNA	Stimulus
Insulin receptor	Dexamethasone
	Glucose
	Insulin
Cal/CGRP	Dexamethasone
Protein kinase C β	Insulin
IGFI	Growth hormone
FGF-R	Cytokines
TNFα	2-aminopurine
PTP1B	PDGF, EGF, basic FGF
TNFβ, β-globin	src
Hac1	UPR
hPMCA2	Calcium
CD44	TPA, PDGF, IGFI
	Concanavalin A
Fibronectin EIIIB (rat)	Insulin, via HRS
Fibronectin ED (human)	TGFβ1, vitamin D, retinoic acid
Kv3.1 channel	Basic FGF
Agrin	NGF
SRp20	Serum/cell cycle
Slo (K channel gene)	Hypophysectomy

CGRP, calcitonin gene-related protein; EGF, epidermal growth factor; FGF, fibroblast growth factor; HRS, hepatic serine-arginine protein 40 KD; IGF, insulin-like growth factor; NGF, nerve growth factor; PDGF, platelet-derived growth factor; TNF, tumour necrosis factor; TPA, tetradecanoyl phorbol acetate.

sites is regulated by the state of cellular growth and proliferation. IGF2 has two mRNAs. A minor 4.8 kb species is translated constitutively. A major 6.0 kb variant is generally sequestered and remains untranslated in a 100S ribonucleoprotein particle. In growing cells, however, the 6.0 kb variant is mobilized and translated by the mediation of a kinase signalling pathway. RNA-binding proteins and the signalling pathways have been identified which regulate IGF2 translation (13).

The general translational apparatus and the activity of the eukaryotic initiation factors (eIFs) may also be regulated by external signals, via phosphorylation pathways. One example is eIF4E, a component of the cap-binding complex. This complex binds the m^7G cap of mRNA to increase its interaction with the ribosome. Growth factors and hormones increase the state of eIF4E phosphorylation, and this may be associated with increases in the rate of translation of certain mRNA transcripts (14). A further level of complexity is added by the existence of a pathway for degrading mRNA in a mechanism that can be linked to the translational apparatus. This cotranslational degradation pathway involves small RNA molecules of 20–30 nucleotides in length. Such small RNA molecules are classed into two categories, small interfering RNAs and microRNAs. They are also involved in many aspects of post-transcriptional gene regulation (15).

Translation may also be regulated by localization of protein production to regions of the cell where the products are required at high concentrations. This may be accomplished by restriction of the relevant mRNA to a particular region, for example the transport of β-actin mRNA into cellular processes and growth cones. This transport process is regulated by signal transduction systems (16). While mRNA localization and regional translation has been known to be a mode of regulating embryo polarity and development, its role in other cells and tissues is beginning to emerge.

The cell cycle

The cell cycle coordinates cellular growth and division. The core of the cell cycle machinery consists of cyclins and cyclin-dependent kinases (CDKs) (17). Cyclins bind the CDKs and direct the phosphorylation activity of the CDKs to appropriate targets, for example, members of the retinoblastoma protein (Rb) family. Many hormones affect the cell cycle machinery. For example, growth factors promote progression of the cell cycle through G1 to the restriction point, at least in part, by signals to cyclin D. Conversely, inhibitory cytokines such as transforming growth factor β (TGFβ) negatively regulate the cell cycle via several pathways, including cyclin inhibitor proteins, the Smad proteins, or by interfering with MDM2 activation of Rb function (18).

One mechanism of control of the cell cycle is by the capacity of a cell to monitor its rate of cellular biosynthesis. In the budding yeast, *Saccharomyces cerevisiae*, the cyclin protein CLN3 (the homologue of human cyclin D) acts as a sensor of cellular biosynthesis. Once biosynthesis has exceeded a threshold, CLN3 stimulates the cell cycle, thereby triggering a cell division. Thus, a hormone with an effect on cellular biosynthesis may also potentially function to indirectly stimulate the cell cycle via a similar mechanism (19).

The cell cycle and hormonal systems may be linked in much more a complex relationship. There is recent evidence that a core protein of the cell cycle machinery, cyclin D1, can bind and activate the oestrogen receptor (ER), to enhance ER-mediated gene transcription (20). Like other steroid receptors, activation of the oestrogen receptor usually occurs when bound to the ligand, oestrogen. However, cyclin D1 activation of the ER is independent of ligand binding, nor is an interaction with a CDK needed. Furthermore, cyclin D1 acts as a bridge between the receptor and the steroid receptor coactivator proteins (SRCs). Binding between the ER and SRCs is normally regulated by the presence of ligand, so the control of the link between the receptor and its SRC partners can be subverted by cyclin D1. Thus, the activity of the ER has two inputs: by binding to its ligand, oestrogen; and via the cell cycle core protein, cyclin D1. These data show that there are intricate coordinations between the cell cycle machinery, cellular metabolism, and signalling and gene expression. The ultimate function of this coordination between cellular machines is not known.

Ageing and apoptosis

The process of ageing is associated with a decline in function of several hormonal systems in humans (see Chapter 10.1.1). Data from genetic studies in the worm, fruit fly and mouse suggest that the converse is also true (21): hormonal factors and signalling systems may play a role in the regulation of the ageing process (Table 1.5.3).

While ageing occurs at the level of the whole organism, apoptosis is a cellular process of programmed cell death. Some apoptosis is probably required in every tissue and organ. This may be to remove

Table 1.5.3 Genes involved in the regulation of ageing

Organism	Gene	Putative function
Caenorhabditis elegans	*age1*	Phosphatidylinositol 3-kinase
	daf2	Insulin receptor
Drosophila	*methuselah*	G-protein-linked transmembrane receptor
Mouse	*klotho*	Cell membrane signalling glucosidase

diseased cells, or to control the growth and morphology of a tissue. Apoptosis is generally tightly regulated. One example of the hormonal control of apoptosis is the effect of glucocorticoids on the involution of the thymus. This is due to the induction of apoptosis in thymocytes. There are several mechanisms for the proapoptotic effect of glucocorticoids. Glucocorticoids may exert effects at the level of gene transcription, by interfering with the function and formation of the AP1 and NF-κB transcription complexes. However, glucocorticoid stimulation also results in the sequestration of NF-κB in the cytoplasm, thereby preventing its action in the nucleus. This sequestration is due to the binding of NF-κB and masking of its nuclear localization signal by the inhibitory protein, IκB. Here, glucocorticoids function indirectly, by increasing transcription and levels of IκB family members (22). The outcome of these regulatory pathways is to influence the transcription of genes controlled by NF-κB, thereby inducing apoptosis.

Several cytokines and growth factors are cellular survival factors, reducing the likelihood of a cell undergoing apoptosis. In addition to pathways controlling expression of key genes (probably signal through the ras, raf, and mitogen activated protein (MAP) kinase pathway), signalling mechanisms that regulate the apoptosis machinery itself have been defined. In the case of cytokines and growth factors, an antiapoptotic signalling pathway involves phosphatidylinositol (3,4,5) kinase and the serine-threonine kinase, akt. Akt can directly phosphorylate and regulate the activity of a precursor of the apoptosis machinery, procaspase 9 (23).

Signalling networks, anchors, and scaffolds

Despite the many advances, a complete picture of the molecular mechanisms underlying hormonal regulation (encompassing all components: specificity, flexibility, and feedback) is still lacking for most systems. Study of proteins and complexes involved in signal transduction and action has shown that most signalling pathways are not linear. Instead, there are many interactions between different signalling pathways. This network of interactions is now beginning to be modelled and can, to some extent, predict and explain complex biological phenomena (24). These include persistent activation of downstream effector molecules, even when the original stimulus has been removed, and gate effects, where some levels of signals are transmitted, while other levels are not. Many of these signalling networks allow for complex positive and negative feedback controls. One example is the interaction of the phospholipase C and the ras pathways, which share protein kinase C activation in their chains (Fig. 1.5.2). Both pathways are activated at their apex by the epidermal growth factor receptor. The link via protein kinase C allows the establishment of a persistent activation of the outputs of the pathways after a threshold of stimulation is reached and then withdrawn. However, the effective modelling and prediction

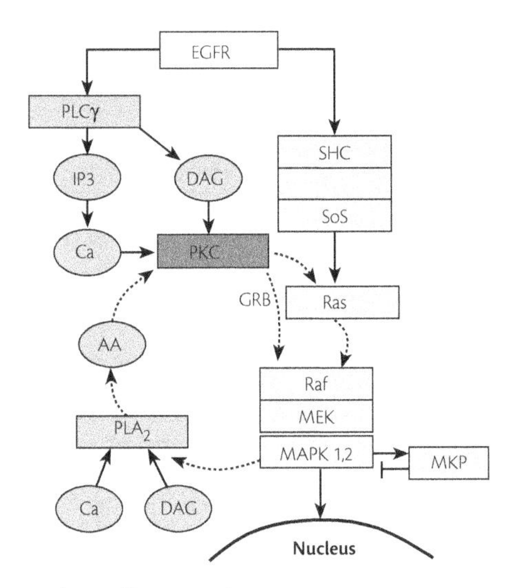

Fig. 1.5.2 A simple signalling network.
The epidermal growth factor receptor (EGFR) signals through two pathways (green and yellow). The pathways share protein kinase C (PKC; red) as a component. This leads to a positive feedback loop (red arrows). If a sufficiently strong signal from the EGFR is transmitted, then persistent activation of the MAP kinases may occur, even after the withdrawal of the stimulus. This drives the cell into a different, but stable, state. (Redrawn from. Bhalla US, Iyengar R. Emergent properties of networks of biological signaling pathways [see comments]. *Science*, 1999; **283**: 381–7 (25).)

of signalling networks will have to account for localization of signalling effectors to specific subcellular regions by anchor and scaffold proteins. Examples of such spatial restriction of signalling networks include the Smad network, and adds additional opportunities for specificity of function and regulation.

The molecular mechanisms of the response to a hormonal signal are increasingly well understood. These mechanisms involve networks of signalling effectors, which act to regulate nearly every major molecular machine of the cell. Furthermore, molecular machines do not function independently of each other. In some examples, interaction between types of cellular machines occurs via hormonal signalling intermediates. Specificity of action, once seen as simply the presence or absence of a receptor, must now be understood in terms of networks, localization of effectors, and the structural interactions between multidomain and multiprotein complexes.

References

1. Ogata K, Sato K, Tahirov TH. Eukaryotic transcriptional regulatory complexes: cooperativity from near and afar. *Curr Opin Struct Biol*, 2003; **13**: 40–8.
2. Carey M. The enhanceosome and transcriptional synergy. *Cell*, 1998; **92**: 5–8.
3. De BK, Haegeman G. Minireview: latest perspectives on antiinflammatory actions of glucocorticoids. *Mol Endocrinol*, 2009; **23**: 281–91.
4. Karin M. New twists in gene regulation by glucocorticoid receptor: is DNA binding dispensable? [comment]. *Cell*, 1998; **93**: 487–90.
5. Schacke H, Berger M, Rehwinkel H, Asadullah K. Selective glucocorticoid receptor agonists (SEGRAs): novel ligands with an improved therapeutic index. *Mol Cell Endocrinol*, 2007; **275**: 109–17.
6. Blencowe BJ. Alternative splicing: new insights from global analyses. *Cell*, 2006; **126**: 37–47.
7. Lonard DM, O'Malley BW. Nuclear receptor coregulators: judges, juries, and executioners of cellular regulation. *Mol Cell*, 2007; **27**: 691–700.

8. Auboeuf D, Batsche E, Dutertre M, Muchardt C, O'Malley BW. Coregulators: transducing signal from transcription to alternative splicing. *Trends Endocrinol Metab*, 2007; **18**: 122–29.
9. Misquitta CM, Chen T, Grover AK. Control of protein expression through mRNA stability in calcium signalling. *Cell Calcium*, 2006; **40**: 329–46.
10. Sen S, Talukdar I, Webster NJ. SRp20 and CUG-BP1 modulate insulin receptor exon 11 alternative splicing. *Mol Cell Biol*, 2009; **29**: 871–80.
11. Lou H, Gagel RF. Alternative ribonucleic acid processing in endocrine systems. *Endocr Rev*, 2001; **22**: 205–25.
12. Touriol C, Bornes S, Bonnal S, Audigier S, Prats H, Prats AC, *et al.* Generation of protein isoform diversity by alternative initiation of translation at non-AUG codons. *Biol Cell*, 2003; **95**: 169–78.
13. Gingras AC, Raught B, Sonenberg N. Regulation of translation initiation by FRAP/mTOR. *Genes Dev*, 2001; **15**: 807–26.
14. Day DA, Tuite MF. Post-transcriptional gene regulatory mechanisms in eukaryotes: an overview. *J Endocrinol*, 1998; **157**: 361–71.
15. Carthew RW, Sontheimer EJ. Origins and Mechanisms of miRNAs and siRNAs. *Cell*, 2009; **136**: 642–55.
16. Bassell GJ, Oleynikov Y, Singer RH. The travels of mRNAs through all cells large and small. *FASEB J*, 1999; **13**: 447–54.
17. Hahn WC, Weinberg RA. Rules for making human tumor cells. *N Engl J Med*, 2002; **347**: 1593–603.
18. Levav-Cohen Y, Haupt S, Haupt Y. Mdm2 in growth signaling and cancer. *Growth Factors*, 2005; **23**: 183–92.
19. Nasmyth K. Control of S phase. In: DePamphilis ML, ed. *DNA Replication in Eukaryotic Cells.* Cold Spring Harbor: Cold Spring Harbor Laboratory Press, 1996: 331–86.
20. Zwijsen RM, Buckle RS, Hijmans EM, Loomans CJ, Bernards R. Ligand-independent recruitment of steroid receptor coactivators to estrogen receptor by cyclin D1. *Genes Dev*, 1998; **12**: 3488–98.
21. Bishop NA, Guarente L. Genetic links between diet and lifespan: shared mechanisms from yeast to humans. *Nat Rev Genet*, 2007; **8**: 835–44.
22. Pascual G, Glass CK. Nuclear receptors versus inflammation: mechanisms of transrepression. *Trends Endocrinol Metab*, 2006; **17**: 321–7.
23. Manning BD, Cantley LC. AKT/PKB signaling: navigating downstream. *Cell*, 2007; **129**: 1261–74.
24. Papin JA, Hunter T, Palsson BO, Subramaniam S. Reconstruction of cellular signalling networks and analysis of their properties. *Nat Rev Mol Cell Biol*, 2005; **6**: 99–111.
25. Bhalla US, Iyengar R. Emergent properties of networks of biological signaling pathways [see comments]. *Science*, 1999; **283**: 381–7.

1.6

Endocrine autoimmunity

Matthew J. Simmonds, Stephen C.L. Gough

Introduction

Dysfunction within the endocrine system can lead to a variety of diseases with autoimmune attack against individual components being some of the most common. Endocrine autoimmunity encompasses a spectrum of disorders including, e.g., common disorders such as type 1 diabetes, Graves' disease, Hashimoto's thyroiditis, and rarer disorders including Addison's disease and the autoimmune polyendocrine syndromes type 1 (APS 1) and type 2 (APS 2) (see Table 1.6.1). Autoimmune attack within each of these diseases although aimed at different endocrine organs is caused by a breakdown in the immune system's ability to distinguish between self and nonself antigens, leading to an immune response targeted at self tissues. Investigating the mechanisms behind this breakdown is vital to understand what has gone wrong and to determine the pathways against which therapeutics can be targeted. Before discussing how self-tolerance fails, we first have to understand how the immune system achieves self-tolerance.

How the immune system screens the body for foreign antigens

The ability to be able to detect and destroy foreign molecules that have entered our bodies is essential for self-protection and survival. Antigens within the body have to be constantly monitored by the immune system to determine whether they are self, requiring no further action, or nonself, requiring activation by the immune system to ensure removal. This monitoring of endogenous and exogenous antigens occurs by two distinct routes.

Table 1.6.1 Prevalence and gender bias within the autoimmune endocrine diseases

Endocrine disorder	Population prevalence	Female to male ratio
Graves' disease	5–20/1000	5–10:1
Hashimoto's thyroiditis	4–15/1000	5–15:1
Type 1 diabetes	1–4/1000	1:1
Addison's disease	3–6/100 000	2.5:1
Autoimmune hypophysitis	Unknown, rare	8:1
APS 1	Rare	1:1
APS 2		2–3:1

APS, autoimmune polyglandular syndrome.

Internally or endogenously derived proteins, including those such as tumour or viral antigens, are presented to the immune system by human leucocyte antigen (HLA) class I molecules. Before presentation by the HLA class I molecules, ubiquitin is added to endogenous antigens to enable them to enter and be degraded by the cytosolic pathway. This involves the antigens entering the proteasome, which is composed of several proteases and generates specific HLA class I peptides. Peptides are then translocated from the cytosol into the rough endoplasmic reticulum by Tip-associated protein (TAP), which has the highest affinity for 8–10 amino acid peptides that are optimally bound by HLA class I molecules. The HLA class I α chain and associated β_2 microglobulin (β_2M) chain are synthesized along the rough endoplasmic reticulum. Calnexin associates with free HLA class I α chain to promote folding and β_2M binding. Calnexin is then released and the class I molecule associates with chaperone proteins calrecticulin, PDIA3, and tapasin. Tapasin binds to the TAP transporter bringing the newly synthesized HLA class I molecules into proximity with peptide, aiding peptide capture. Peptide binding further increases HLA class I stability, causing dissociation of calreticulin, tapasin and PDIA3 and exit from the rough endoplasmic reticulum before proceeding to the cell surface of the antigen-presenting cell (APC) for recognition by CD8$^+$ T lymphocytes and natural killer (NK) cells. If the peptide is recognized as nonself CD8$^+$ T cells become activated and functional effector cytotoxic T lymphocytes (CTLs) are produced, which possess lytic capabilities and play a role in CD8$^+$ T memory cell generation. Activated NK cells complement the CTL response by acting before T-cell expansion and differentiation of CD8$^+$ T cells and produce lymphokines, including interferons, which aid in the recruitment of additional cells to the site of inflammation and also produce cytokines and chemokines that aid cell destruction (see Fig. 1.6.1).

Extracellular or exogenous antigens, such as bacterial antigens, are handled by a separate pathway involving HLA class II presenting molecules. Exogenous antigens are internalized into the APC via endocytosis or phagocytosis and enter the endocytic pathway. The endocytic pathway consists of a series of compartments termed early endosome, late endosome, and lysosome, and as the antigen progresses through the compartments they become more acidic, leading to a series of proteolytic processes, resulting in the breakdown of the protein into 13–18 amino acid peptides, which HLA class II molecules preferentially bind. The HLA class II α and β chains association within the endoplasmic reticulum, where the peptide-binding domain is occupied by the invariant chain (Ii) to prevent endogenous peptide binding. The Ii also aids the HLA class

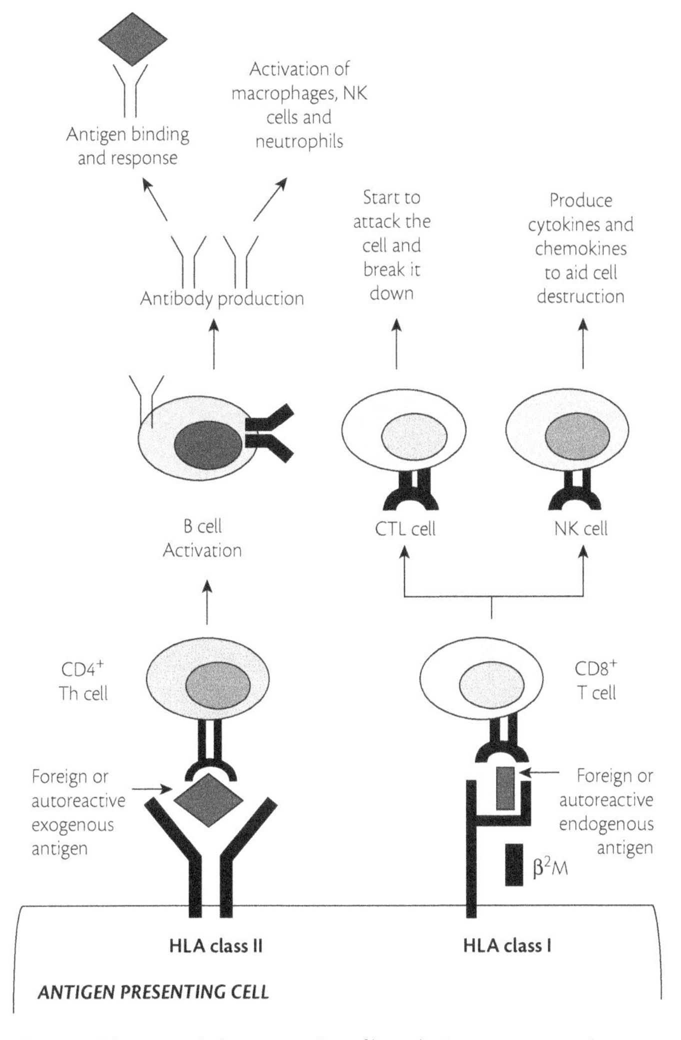

Fig. 1.6.1 Diagrammatical representation of how the immune response is triggered against foreign antigens or autoantigens. Antigens are presented to the immune system either by HLA class I molecules or HLA class II molecules depending on whether they are endogenously or exogenously derived, respectively. HLA class II molecules present antigens for recognition by $CD4^+$ T cells. If recognised as nonself (or the antigen is autoreactive), $CD4^+$ Th cells activate B cells. B cells produce antibodies (or if responding to an autoantigen autoantibodies), which aid in the removal of that specific antigen/autoantigen from the body and to the activation of other immune molecules including natural killer (NK) cells and neutrophils. HLA class I molecules present antigens for recognition by $CD8^+$ T cells. If the antigen/autoantigen is recognised as nonself cytotoxic T lymphocytes (CTLs) are produced, which aid in breaking down the cell containing the antigen/autoantigen and NK cells are also recruited to further aid cell destruction. β^2M, β^2 Microglobulin; Th cell, T helper cell.

II molecules to exit the endoplasmic reticulum, traverse the Golgi, and enter the endocytic pathway, where they encounter antigenic peptides. As the HLA class II molecules progress through the increasingly acidic compartments of the endocytic pathway, the Ii is degraded by proteolysis, leaving class II associated invariant chain peptide (CLIP) to occupy the binding domain. Removal of CLIP and exchange for antigenic peptide occurs by the HLA-DM accessory molecule, whose role is inhibited by HLA-DO. Once the HLA class II molecule has acquired peptide it is pulled out of the endocytic pathway and shuttled to the plasma membrane in transport vesicles before being displayed on the cell surface for recognition by $CD4^+$ T helper (Th) cells. If the $CD4^+$ Th cells determine that the antigen is non-self, two responses are generated, a T helper response 1 (Th1) which leads to macrophage activation, to kill the invading pathogen and a T helper response 2 (Th2) which leads to activation of B cells, which can produce antibodies. Antibodies are soluble copies of the antigen receptor that can bind to and eliminate the invading antigen and also bind to macrophages, neutrophils, and NK cells, stimulating these cells to attack the tissue directly (1) (See Fig. 1.6.1).

Correct functioning of the antigen presentation pathways is vital to enable foreign antigens to be quickly detected and removed, whilst protecting self. Although the need to produce a large repertoire of T and B cells to respond to a variety of invading pathogens is obvious, education of this T and B cell population is also vital to protect against autoimmunity, with systems in place in both the thymus for T cells and the bone marrow/lymph system for B cells to achieve this.

Thymic selection during T-cell generation

Random T-cell receptor (TCR) rearrangement is employed to enable the generation of a vast T cell population with varying antigen specificities. The downside of the random nature of the rearrangements inevitably leads to some of these T cells being self or autoreactive. Consequently, central tolerance mechanisms are employed during T cell development to ensure these cells do not enter the periphery (Fig. 1.6.2).

Progenitor double-negative $CD4^-/CD8^-$ T cells produced in the bone marrow progress to the thymus where random rearrangement of the TCR β and then TCR α chains (which compose the TCR) occurs, via recombination-activating gene 1 and gene 2 (*RAG1* and *RAG2*, respectively), to become double-positive $CD4^+/CD8^+$ T cells (1). As *RAG1* and *RAG2* function is random, once the TCR is expressed, the TCR needs to be checked to make sure that it can recognize self HLA molecules (HLA restricted) in a process referred to as positive selection. Positive selection occurs in the cortical region of the thymus, where cortical thymic epithelial cells (cTECs) expressing HLA class I and class II molecules present antigens for recognition by these $CD4^+/CD8^+$ T cells. T cells that bind to the peptide presenting HLA molecules receive a survival signal and progress to the next selection stage, whereas those that do not interact receive no survival signal and die via neglect (1). Once T cells have completed positive selection, they are then subjected to negative selection in the medullary thymic epithelial cells (mTECs) to remove any autoreactive T cells. Any cells that recognize HLA and self-antigens too strongly are either deleted by apoptosis or undergo TCR editing, where additional TCR rearrangements occur to try to prevent them expressing an autoreactive TCR, before being retested for autoreactivity (2). Only T cells that are HLA restricted and are not autoreactive are allowed to mature into $CD4^+$ Th or $CD8^+$ T cells.

Although central tolerance mechanisms attempt to remove many autoreactive T cells, inevitably some do progress into the periphery, highlighting the requirement for peripheral autoreactivity prevention mechanisms. Along with $CD4^+$ Th and $CD8^+$ T cell, an additional form of $CD4^+$ Th cells (which also express high levels of CD25 and foxp3) are generated known as T regulatory cells (Treg). These cells are mainly formed through interaction with cTECs (involved in positive selection) and are not believed to encounter mTECs (involved in negative selection) during their

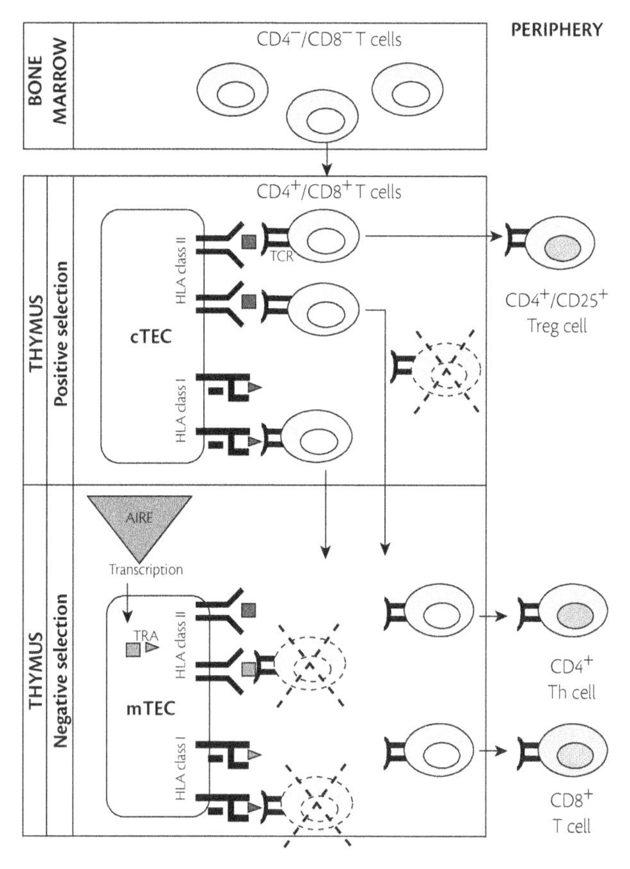

Fig. 1.6.2 Screening out autoreactive T cells during development
Double negative CD4⁻/CD8⁻ T cells released from the bone marrow enter the thymus and undergo random rearrangement of their T cell receptor (TCR) forming CD4⁺/CD8⁺ T cells. Before entering the periphery these T cells go through positive selection to check that these cells can bind to antigen being presented by self HLA class I or class II molecules on the surface of cortical thymic epithelial cells (cTECs). Only T cells that bind antigen are provided with survival signals and those that do not are deleted via apoptosis. T regulatory (Treg) cells, that monitor and prevent autoreactivity in the periphery, are also generated during this process and are released into the periphery without interacting with medullary thymic epithelial cells (mTECs). The remaining T cells undergo negative selection where the T cells are checked for autoreactivity and any showing signs of binding self-antigen too strongly are deleted. Expression of AIRE1 is also detected in mTECs which causes transcription of otherwise tissue restricted antigens (TRA) enabling the T cell population to be screened for autoreactivity against these. The remaining T cell population mature into either CD4⁺ T helper (Th) or CD8⁺ T cells.

generation. T regs represent approximately 6–7% of the mature CD4⁺ Th cell population and function by monitoring the periphery for autoreactive T cell activity and suppress the activation and expansion of autoreactive T cells, although the exact mechanisms by which they achieve this are still being elucidated (3).

Bone marrow/lymph node selection during B cell generation

In a similar manner to T cells, the majority of B cells formed during development are polyreactive and can recognize self and nonself, so also encounter a series of checkpoints to check their activity and/or autoreactive potential (see Fig. 1.6.3). Bone marrow hematopoietic stem cells give rise to progenitor B cells that do not possess a functional B-cell receptor (BCR). The BCR is composed of a immunoglobulin M (IgM) heavy and light chain together with a Igα and Igβ heterodimer (4). Random rearrangement of the BCR heavy and light chain is essential for BCR diversity and development. The heavy chain first undergoes rearrangement mediated by RAG1 and RAG2 and along with a surrogate light chain is presented on the progenitor B cell surface. It then interacts with bone marrow stromal cells to receive survival signals, enabling the cell to start dividing and progress into a precursor B cell. Rearrangement of the precursor B-cell light chain then occurs and together with the rearranged BCR heavy is expressed on the B cell surface as IgM. Further interaction between the precursor B cells and the stromal cells enables them to receive additional survival signals, triggering further proliferation and progression to become IgM expressing immature B cells that exit the bone marrow (1, 4).

Once released from the bone marrow immature B cells need antigen-induced activation for survival and to generate IgG that can be secreted from mature B cells. Immature B cells together with naïve T cells enter the lymph nodes and temporarily sequester into primary follicles and T-cell zones which are found between the follicles, respectively (1). Immature B cells internalize antigen present within the lymph nodes and present the antigen for recognition by antigen-specific naïve T cells at the primary follicle/T zone interface. On interaction, naïve T cells produce lymphokines, causing rapid proliferation and clonal expansion of that specific BCR, which then leads to the generation of a germinal centre consisting of a dark and light zone where two distinct phases of B-cell proliferation and differentiation occur. Within the dark zone activated immature B cells spontaneously undergo random rearrangement of their antibody genes and intense proliferation, giving rise to an immature B-cell-expressing membrane IgG. As B cell numbers increase, they move from the dark zone into the light zone. Due to the random nature of the heavy and light chain rearrangements many of the membrane IgGs produced are autoreactive or nonfunctioning, so are exposed to antigen to check binding ability and affinity. B cells with high affinity receptors for antigen make close contact with antigen displayed on the long extensions of the follicular dendritic cells, which act as an antigen reservoir for both foreign and self-antigens. Centrocytes bearing low-affinity IgG genes do not interact with the presented antigen and are destroyed via apoptosis. Centrocytes bearing IgG bind to antigen presented by the follicular dendritic cells, ingest and process the antigen, and display the antigen on their surface via HLA class II molecules. The B cell then presents the antigen to a T cell, which recognizes and binds to the presented antigen. This enables T-cell-dependent B cell activation to occur which induces the necessary stop signal to prevent apoptosis occurring within the B cell. This enables it to undergo differentiation into a large plasmablast, which migrates to the medulla of the lymph node where it will develop into a plasma cell and begin to secrete antibody molecules, or a small memory B cell which can remain in the lymph node or recirculate to other parts of the body ready to reactivate on reencountering that antigen. This process leads to the generation of a large and diverse repertoire of mature B cells that are not self-reactive and can be activated to produce high-affinity antibodies against foreign antigens.

Negative selection appears to occur at several stages during B cell maturation. Any developing B cell that binds self-antigen too

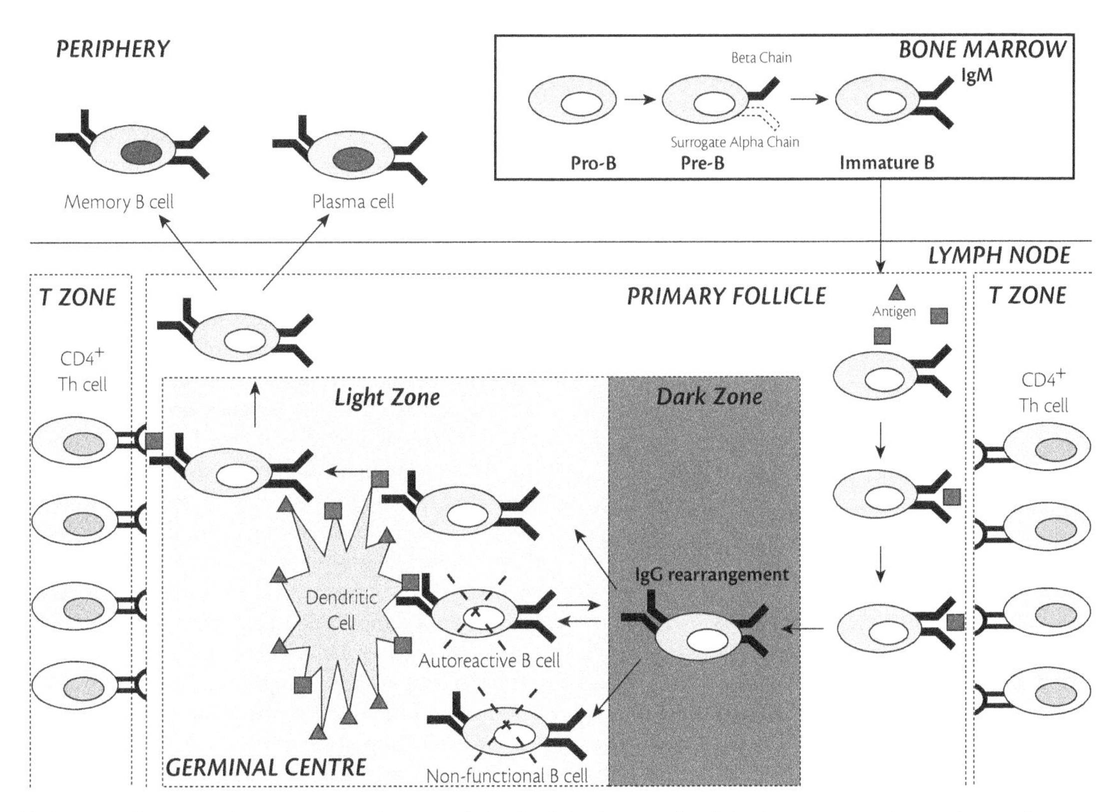

Fig. 1.6.3 Simplified version of negative selection processes that occur during B cell development. B cell development occurs in several stages. Rearrangement of the IgM B cell receptor occurs in the bone marrow before immature B cells are released into the periphery. To enable continued survival immature B cells enter the lymph node and need to take up antigen. Once they have taken up antigen, they interact with T cells (although interaction occurs through HLA class II molecules presenting antigen on the B cell surface and the T cell receptor for simplicity this is not shown) enabling them to start proliferating and form germinal centres. These proliferating B cells undergo IgG rearrangements before differentiating into mature plasma cell or memory B cells that express both IgM and IgG and can enter the periphery. Negative selection processes occur at several points to check that the randomly rearranged IgM and IgG are fully functional and are not autoreactive. In the light zone immature B cells with non-functional IgG rearrangements are apoptosed and those with autoreactive IgG receptors are either apoptosed or sent back to the dark zone for further rearrangements. Th, T helper; Ig, Immunoglobulin; Pro-B, Progenitor B; Pre-B, Precursor B.

strongly and is autoreactive is destroyed by either receptor editing (where BCR heavy chain undergoes further rearrangement to alter antigen specificity, making the cell less self-reactive), clonal deletion (where BCRs with high affinity for self-antigen are deleted by apoptosis) or clonal anergy (where autoreactive B cells are converted to a state that is no longer responsive to BCR engagement, due to constant receptor occupancy, making the B cell less able to compete for survival signal). Negative selection processes are, however, not complete and some autoreactive B cells do enter the periphery. A subset of regulatory B (Breg) cells that produce interleukin 10 (IL-10) have been identified in mice and have been proposed to play a role in down regulating peripheral B-cell autoreactivity by inhibiting their antigen-presentation abilities and proinflammatory cytokine production but to date identification of these Breg cells in humans is still awaited (5).

Immune system disruption leading to endocrine autoimmunity

Although mechanisms are in place to prevent autoimmunity, over 5% of the general population have autoimmune disease (AID), with the endocrine AIDs representing some of the most common AIDs, suggesting that a breakdown in these mechanisms can occur. Different endocrine diseases have differing population frequencies and vary with respect to the organ/s targeted (see Table 1.6.1). The generation of autoantibodies is common to all endocrine AIDs and tissue destruction is also found in several diseases, with GD being the major exception.

The first evidence that disruption of immune pathways is important in autoimmunity and could be caused by inherited genetic factors came from studies in families which showed clustering of AIDs in family members at a greater rate than would be expected in the general population. Twin studies showed further evidence of a genetic link with autoimmunity. In Graves' disease monozygotic twins, which share the same DNA, demonstrated concordance levels of about 30–40% compared with rates of 0–7% in dizygotic twins. The incomplete disease penetrance in monozygotic twins suggests that environmental factors also play a role. The relative contribution of genetic and environmental factors is difficult to estimate, with some studies suggesting that genetic factors may contribute up to 80% of the susceptibility. It has also been clearly established that with the exception of APS endocrine diseases are not simple monogenic disorders but are instead polygenic disorders caused by several different genetic effects. The co-existence of different endocrine AIDs and other nonendocrine AIDs (e.g. rheumatoid arthritis) has also been shown to run in individuals and families, suggesting that these diseases share a series of common AID pathways. However, as each of these diseases presents with autoimmunity against a different set of organs, it also suggests mechanisms unique to each disease. Taken together three distinct areas have been identified into which autoimmune endocrine mechanisms fall:

Factors that effect why a specific organ/s is prone to autoimmune attack

Variation in components of the immune system

External/environmental influences on the immune system

Factors that effect why a specific organ/s is prone to autoimmune attack

Autoantibody profiles vary disease by disease and even within a given disease autoantibodies can be detected against a variety of different molecules (Table 1.6.2). Variation in thymic expression of antigens and apoptotic clearance of autoantigens has been proposed to explain why certain antigens are targeted for autoimmune attack.

Thymic expression

Many of the molecules against which autoantibodies are raised are only expressed in a limited number of tissues. As a result of this limited expression of tissue-restricted antigens (TRAs) it was believed that they were not expressed by mTECs and, therefore, were not tolerated during negative selection of T cells. Investigation into the genetic causes of monogenic APS 1 determined that disease onset was caused by deletions within the autoimmune regulatory gene (*AIRE1*). APS 1 is characterized by autoimmune polyendocrinopathies, chronic mucocutaneous candidiasis and ectodermal dystrophies, suggesting a potential role for AIRE in controlling autoreactivity. This has been confirmed by findings in AIRE-deficient mice as they have been found to lack a subset of TRAs present in normal mice (6). This indicates that AIRE plays a key role in transcribing TRAs promiscuously in mTECs so that they can also form part of the repertoire of antigens that developing T cells are negatively selected against (see Fig. 1.6.2). *AIRE* expression is mainly restricted to mTECs and thymic dendritic cells and by mediating transcriptional regulation from multiple sites can transcribe up to 3000 genes including several thyroid, liver, and pancreas TRAs (6). Low levels of *AIRE* expression has also been detected in the periphery in the gonads, liver, central nervous system, and bone marrow and it has been proposed that the peripheral expression of self-antigens could complement *AIRE*'s role in the thymus and aid peripheral tolerance (7). Interestingly cTECs, which are involved in positive selection of $CD4^+$ Th cells and T regs do not express *AIRE* (6). A study on interindividual variation in thymic expression of several type 1 diabetes autoantigens, including insulin, glutamate decarboxylase 67 (GAD_{67}), and IA-2, demonstrated that there was up to a 50-fold variation in expression levels (8). An individual's own variation in TRA expression in the thymus could determine whether certain self-antigens are tolerated or not. *AIRE*, however, only acts on a limited set of antigens. Certain endocrine autoantigens including thyroid peroxidase and GAD_{65} are not under *AIRE* control, suggesting that other genes may also control thymic expression (6).

Whether influenced by *AIRE* or not, thymic expression does seem to be an important trigger for AID. This concept is eloquently highlighted by the role of the variable number of tandem repeats (VNTR) located in the 5′ region upstream from the insulin (*INS*) gene in type 1 diabetes. The *INS*-VNTR consists of tandem repeats of a 14–15 base-pair consensus sequence which clusters into sets of 30–60 repeats (class 1), 60–120 repeats (class II), and 120–170 repeats (class III). Homozygosity of class I alleles was found to be associated with type 1 diabetes, whereas presence of the class III allele offered protection from disease onset (9). When investigating

Table 1.6.2 Different autoantigens identified in each of the endocrine autoimmune diseases

Disease	Autoantigen	Percentage (%) prevalence of autoantibodies directed against autoantigen in disease versus control subjects	
		Disease cases	Control subjects
Type 1 diabetes	Islet cell antibody (antigen unknown)	70	1
	GAD_{65}	70–90	1–2
	GAD_{67}	10–20	1
	Insulin	40–70	1
	IA-2 and IA-2β proteins of protein tyrosine phosphatase	25–60	1
Graves' disease	TSHR	95–100	5
	TPO	90	10–30
	Tg	70	18–30
Hashimoto's thyroiditis	Tg	95–100	18–30
	TPO	95–100	10–30
Autoimmune hypoparathyroidism	Ca-SR	60	0
Addison's disease	Steroid 21-hydroxylase	70	1
	Steroid 17α-hydroxylase	5	1
APS 1 and APS 2	cytP450scc	9	1
APS 1 and APS 2	Organ specific antigens relating to disease component	Variable	

APS, autoimmune polyglandular syndrome; Ca-SR, calcium-sensing receptor; cytP450scc, cytochrome P450 side chain cleavage enzyme; GAD, glutamic acid decarboxylase; TPO, thyroid peroxidase; Tg, thyroglobulin; TSHR, thyroid-stimulating hormone receptor.

thymic *INS* expression transcriptional activity was found to be approximately 200–300% higher in *INS* transcripts encoded by the resistant class III alleles compared to levels of *INS* transcripts produced by the class I predisposing alleles (a). Mouse models which express low levels of insulin in the thymus presented with spontaneous peripheral reactivity to insulin, whereas mice with normal insulin levels did not, providing further support for this mechanism (10). Similarly the generation of autoantibodies to the thyroid-stimulating hormone receptor (TSHR) in Graves' disease has also been linked to differential expression of TSHR isoforms. After screening the *TSHR* for association with Graves' disease, a number of single nucleotide polymorphisms (SNPs) have been shown to be strongly associated with disease onset. Preliminary mRNA studies have shown differences in relative levels of full length TSHR (flTSHR) and two known TSHR isoforms, ST4 and ST5, in the thyroid between those with and without the associated SNPs. If differences between thyroid and thymic expression of these transcripts is demonstrated, as with INS in type 1 diabetes, this could have an effect on how these isoforms are tolerated during negative selection and/or their availability to be presented to the immune system in the periphery (11).

Apoptotic clearance of autoantigens

Apoptosis is a tightly controlled process that maintains homoeostasis in the immune system by deleting potentially autoreactive or nonfunctioning T and B cells, tumour cells, and virally-infected cells and by performing controlled destruction of dead or dying cells. Cells designated for apoptosis go through three phases, triggering, signalling, and execution. The triggering phase involves either engagement of death receptor machinery (including Fas (CD95) and Fas ligand (FasL) or tumour necrosis factor α (TNFα) and TNF-related apoptosis-inducing ligand (TRAIL)) or lack of survival signals triggered by growth factor deprivation, cellular stress, or cytotoxic drugs. Signalling is a multistep process achieved through a series of different accessory molecules including cytochrome c, mitogen-activated protein kinase (MAPK), c-Jun N-terminal kinase (JNK), and protein kinase A (PKA) and PKB, which enable activation of caspase 3, 7, and 8, key initiators of cellular destruction (12). These signalling pathways result in a programme of plasma membrane blebbing, cytoplasmic and organelle contraction and shrinkage, nuclear chromatin condensation, DNA and RNA degradation, and cytoskeletal rearrangements. To prevent proinflammatory cytokine release, apoptosed cells are removed by phagocytes, including macrophages and immature dendritic cells, which also present apoptosed antigens on their cell surface for recognition by the immune system. Apoptotic regulation can occur at several different levels including regulation of death receptor expression levels, expression of proapoptotic and antiapoptotic proteins, including the B-cell lymphoma (BCL) family, and changes in intracellular signalling (12).

Increased apoptosis or defects in phagocytosis of apoptotic cell debris, could lead to increased apoptotic debris that could accumulate and overwhelm the system providing an increased source of autoantigens which if presented to the immune system could trigger an immune response. Lack of or disrupted apoptosis has been proposed as a mechanism for triggering AID, in particular the thyroid autoimmune diseases' Graves' disease and Hashimoto's thyroiditis. Normal thyroid cells express low levels of death receptors and priming by cytokines is needed to trigger these receptors. Immunohistochemical staining of thyroid glands in Graves' disease suggests that Fas is upregulated and FasL downregulated by infiltrating immune cells (13). This suggests that thyroid cells are less resistant to Fas-mediated apoptosis and lose cytotoxic abilities against invading T cells. Interestingly, in Hashimoto's thyroiditis, which unlike Graves' disease displays autoimmune destruction of the thyroid gland, thyrocytes are committed to apoptosis by inappropriate Fas and TNFα mediated signalling. This suggests that on thyroid infiltration by immune cells, which precedes both diseases, there could be a battle in the thyroid gland between apoptosis and thyroid cell production/survival and which one wins could determine whether a person develops Hashimoto's thyroiditis or Graves' disease, respectively (14).

Variation in components of the immune system

Variation or disruption of antigen presentation and T- and B-cell recognition/activation is also key to autoimmune onset. Presentation of antigens by HLA class I and class II encoded molecules during central tolerance and in the periphery dictate how antigens are presented to CD4^{+} Th, CD8^{+} T and Treg cells. Variation within these molecules enables variation between different individual's immune systems to enable the human race to encounter new threats and survive. This variation occurs throughout the HLA molecules but tends to cluster within the antigen binding domains, suggesting that natural variations have not only protected us from diseases in the past but now may be aiding AID development.

HLA class II associations

The HLA region on chromosome 6 contains several important immune response genes and is split into three parts, the HLA class I, class II, and class III region. The HLA class II encoded DRB1, DQB1, and DQA1 molecules were the first to be investigated for association with AID, with association between these molecules being detected for most endocrine AIDs. Association of this region was first detected with type 1 diabetes, with the presence of aspartic acid at position β57 of the DQB1 chain shown to confer type 1 diabetes resistance, whereas presence of a neutral residue such as alanine or serine conferred susceptibility (15). Association was also reported at the DRB1 locus, with DRB1*04 and DRB1*03 shown to strongly predispose to type 1 diabetes. DRB1*04 has also been associated with Hashimoto's thyroiditis and DRB1*03 has been associated with Graves' disease, Hashimoto's thyroiditis and Addison's disease (16). These genes also form haplotypes encompassing DRB1-DQB1-DQA1, with the DR3 haplotype (containing DRB1*03) termed the 'autoimmunity haplotype' due to its association with so many AIDs, and the DR4 haplotype (containing DRB1*04) strongly associated with several endocrine AIDs. Strong linkage disequilibrium (in which variation in one gene is also linked with other variants in the same or neighbouring genes) between *DRB1-DQA1-DQB1* has made it difficult to determine which individual gene and, in turn, which molecule is the most important. A regression analysis performed in Graves' disease on the DRB1-DQB1-DQA1 haplotype revealed that *DQB1* was unable to explain association of this haplotype with Graves' disease and that the association was due to *DRB1* or *DQA1* (17). Further work in Graves' disease comparing the predisposing DRB1*03 allele against the protective DRB1*07 revealed that DRB1*03 contained a positively charged arginine at position β74, compared with DRB1*07, whch contained a noncharged glutamine (17). DRB1 position β74 has been shown to vary between the lower risk

DRB1*0403 and DRB1*0406 T1D alleles, which contains a negatively charged glutamic acid compared with the high risk non-charged polar alanine (16). Position β74 is also part of the shared epitope that is highly associated with RA and is composed of DRB1 positions β70–β74. DRB1-encoded position β74 spans several amino peptide binding domains which are important for antigen/autoantigen binding and TCR receptor docking and interaction, so any variations within this binding domain could be affecting how peptides are presented to the immune system and whether an immune response is mounted against them.

Several hypotheses have been put forward to explain how the DR and DQ molecules could be associated with autoimmunity (16).

Antigen-binding repertoire: variation in the binding grooves of DR/DQ could lead to preferential selection of only a specific limited set of self-peptides. This may allow autoreactive T cells to escape central tolerance and enter the periphery and/or may allow the generation of a Treg population that cannot recognize all self-antigens.

T-cell selection: polymorphic residues within TCR exposed surfaces of DR/DQ could select autoreactive T cells or fail to select a good Treg population.

Epitope stealing: preferential binding by a given allele in heterozygous DR/DQ subjects could cause epitope stealing and depending on whether this allele is predisposing, protective or neutral, peptide binding could be affecting whether an autoimmune response is mounted.

Cross-presentation of nonexogenous antigens: although the HLA class II molecules bind exogenous antigen and HLA class I molecules bind endogenous antigens crossover can occur where HLA class II bind endogenous antigen and vice versa. HLA class II binding of endogenous antigens could alter how they are displayed to the immune system and whether they are recognized as self or not.

HLA class I associations

Although originally investigation of the HLA region was limited to the HLA class II DR/DQ molecules, other parts of the HLA region also encode key parts of the immune system, none more than the HLA class I encoded A, B, and C molecules, which present endogenous antigen for recognition by $CD8^+$ T cells. Association of the HLA class I encoded HLA-B*27 with ankylosing spondylosis has been long established, but it was not until recent advances in statistical modelling for it to be possible to model the HLA class II effects and determine if HLA class I associations are still exerting a primary effect. Analysing over 1729 markers across the whole HLA region in several white Caucasian type 1 diabetes datasets revealed a secondary peak of association after accounting for HLA class II effects and demonstrated independent type 1 diabetes associations for the HLA-B locus and some evidence of association with HLA-A (18). In Graves' disease, when HLA-B and -C were screened for association and subjected to logistic regression to see if the effects were independent of HLA-DR/DQ, HLA-C and to a lesser extent HLA-B produced stronger association signals than that seen at the HLA class II region (19).

Several hypotheses have been suggested to try and explain these newly detected associations. Unlike HLA class II molecules, HLA class I molecules play a key role in presenting viruses to the immune system. There has been evidence to suggest that viruses could be one of the key environmental triggers for autoimmunity, with several different viruses proposed to play a role in endocrine AIDs (Table 1.6.3). Several different mechanisms have been proposed by which viruses could trigger disease including those listed below (16).

Molecular mimicry: where viral antigens are similar enough to self-antigens that when presented by HLA class I molecules they are still recognized as foreign but the immune response triggered can cross-react and attack self-antigens.

Superantigens: viruses could cause a strong, wide-ranging immune response that then cross-reacts with the host's cellular components and causes autoimmunity.

Increased expression of cell surface and soluble HLA class I: potentially enabling more viral antigens to be presented to the immune system, which could cause molecular mimicry or superantigen presentation.

NK-cell activation: NK-cell activation is controlled by a series of activating and inactivating signals, with signalling blocked by killer immunoglobulin-like receptors (KIR) which interact with HLA class I. HLA class I and KIR interaction can be affected by the peptide presented, so presented viral peptides could be altering this interaction and preventing the correct inhibitory signals being given to NK cells.

There are also some potential nonviral mechanisms proposed including conversion of the HLA class I molecules themselves into peptides which when presented by HLA class II could cause an autoimmune response to be triggered and cross presentation of exogenous antigen by HLA class I molecules with further studies needed to decipher the exact mechanism at play in endocrine autoimmunity.

T-cell signalling regulation by cytotoxic T-lymphocyte associated 4 (CTLA-4)

T-cell activation is a two-stage process whereby first, the T cell has to recognize and bind to peptides being displayed by a given HLA molecule and second, costimulatory signals are required from accessory molecules on the T cell surface to enable the signal to be transduced and the T cell to become activated. These signals are mediated and controlled by a balance between the T cell surface molecules CD28 and CTLA-4. CTLA-4 appears to downregulate T cell signalling whereas CD28 promotes T-cell signalling. CD28 is always expressed on T cells whereas CTLA-4 is normally up regulated during T-cell signalling but Tregs, unlike other T cells, consistently express CTLA-4 on their surface (20). CTLA-4 could function either by blocking positive signalling pathways or through initiating negative signalling pathways.

CTLA-4 has been proposed to block positive signalling through various mechanisms. CTLA-4 and CD28 both bind to CD80 (B7-1) and CD86 (B7-2) on the surface of APCs. CTLA-4 possess a 50–100-fold greater affinity for these molecules suggesting that CTLA-4 could either out compete CD28 for its ligands or could sequester available ligands, preventing CD28 binding and blocking CD28 positive signalling, causing T-cell anergy (20). It has also been suggested that CTLA-4 reduces lipid raft and microcluster formation that occurs after TCR ligation to increase adaptor molecules and local enzyme numbers essential for T-cell signalling, thereby preventing strong costimulation. More recently a reverse-stop signal model has also been suggested. T cells normally transit rapidly through the lymph node, scanning for APCs displaying antigens, 'sniffs' the antigen carefully and quickly moves on unless the antigen shows strong affinity for the TCR, preventing T cells slowing down for weakly bound antigen and weak TCR signalling (21). If a 'strong' antigen is detected, increased clustering of adhesion molecule lymphocyte function-associated antigen 1 (LFA1) on T cell surfaces occurs to reduce T cell speed to enable TCR/APC complex (also known as the immunological synapse) stabilization (22). This is known as inside out signalling as TCR binding to the HLA presented antigen, signals to within the cells to produce more LFA1 adhesion molecules which bind to intercell adhesion molecule 1 (ICAM-1) on the surface of the APC to further strength the interaction at the immunological synapse (21). Stable immunological synapse formation is key for TCR engagement and scanning of HLA presented peptide as there is minimal half-life between the HLA-TCR interaction necessary to produce a productive TCR signal. CTLA-4 controls LFA1 production thereby controlling T cell motility, which is proposed to reverse or override the TCR-induced upregulation of adhesion factors prematurely disrupting immunological synapse formation (22). Limiting TCR/APC contact time could result in more avid interactions still occurring but less reactive, low affinity antigens may be ignored, suggesting that not every antigen could be screened during central tolerance and that autoreactive T cells against low affinity peptides could escape central tolerance.

CTLA-4 is also believed to directly activate negative signals to prevent or dampen down TCR signalling by binding several protein tyrosine phosphatases including SHP2 and PP2A, which inhibit cell signalling proteins recruited to the TCR by dephosphorylation (23). CTLA-4 also inhibits JNK and elk-related tyrosine kinase (ERK) leading to reduced production of several transcription factors including nuclear factor κ-B (NF-κB), nuclear factor of activated T cells (NF-AT) and activator protein 1 (AP1). CTLA-4 can also up regulate the tryptophan degrading enzyme IDO (EC number 1.13.11.52), which can breakdown tryptophan in a manner that can inhibit T-cell activation (20).

Association of *CTLA-4* has been consistently reported with most AIDs, with fine mapping studies revealing that association was due to a small number of SNPs located within a 6.1 kb block (24). CTLA-4 exists in humans as both a full length version anchored to the T-cell membrane (flCTLA-4) and soluble form containing no transmembrane domain and, therefore, not anchored to the cell (sCTLA-4). Studies comparing flCTLA-4 and sCTLA-4 mRNA levels in serum and plasma samples demonstrated that possession of the susceptibility haplotype of these SNPs affected efficiency and splicing of sCTLA-4 producing less sCTLA-4 than the protective haplotype. Increased sCTLA-4 could be a marker of increased T cell activity, suggesting that possession of the susceptibility haplotype increased T cell function (24). These results could also indicate downregulation of Treg function. Other studies failed to detect sCTLA-4 in serum or replicate this effect suggesting the mechanism for action requires further confirmation.

Protein tyrosine phosphatase nonreceptor (PTPN) family

PTPN22 is another inhibitor of T-cell signalling, but acts further downstream than CTLA-4 on several molecules including lymphocyte-specific protein-tyrosine kinase (Lck), ζ-chain associated kinase (Zap-70), CD3ε/TCRζ-chains and valosin containing protein that all control T-cell signalling. The C1858T SNP within *PTPN22* has been consistently associated with several endocrine AIDs including type 1 diabetes, Graves' disease, and Hashimoto's thyroiditis and a series of other nonendocrine AIDs including rheumatoid arthritis (25). The C1858T variation encodes an amino acid change from arginine to tryptophan in the *PTPN22*-encoded LYP molecule at amino acid position 620 (R620W). The R620W variation is located within the first of four proline rich regions (P1) within LYP and interacts with the SH3 domain of Csk, an important intracellular tyrosine kinase. Csk suppresses the negative regulatory tyrosine in the c terminus of Lck (and Fyn) by dephosphorylation, leading to inhibition of Lck kinase activity which plays a role in T-cell signal transduction. Presence of LYP*620W severely impairs Lyp-Csk complexes and acts as a gain of function mutation by causing increased T-cell inhibition by dephosphorylating Lck and other signalling proteins more efficiently than LYP*620R (26).

Several mechanisms have been proposed to explain the LYP*620W gain of function. It has been suggested that stronger downstream inhibition of TCR signalling seen in those with LYP*W620 could effect autoreactive T-cell negative selection signals, particularly those with moderate autoreactive affinity, leading to a failure to delete these molecules prior to entry into the periphery (26). Presence of LYP*620W in Tregs may also inhibit their signalling pathways potentially preventing peripheral autoreactive T cell deletion (25). PTPN22 also interacts with other adaptor molecules including c-Cbl, a proto-oncogene which becomes phosphorylated after T cell stimulation and whose expression is reduced when LYP is overexpressed, and growth factor receptor bound protein 2 (Grb2), which like Csk has a SH3 domain binding site for LYP and is involved in negative regulation of the CD28 signalling pathway (27). Interestingly, interaction between CTLA-4 and LYP has been postulated. CTLA-4 and LYP both interact with Fyn, Lck and Zap70, with CTLA-4 believed to use LYP complexed with Grb2 to aid in downregulating T cell activation (27). LYP has also been proposed to play a role in lipid raft formation which CTLA-4 is believed to downregulate (25). *PTPN22* is also expressed in other cell types including B cells, NK cells, macrophages, and dendritic cells and could have an, as yet, unidentified role in controlling their signalling (26). Unsurprisingly, potential additional effects independent of R620W have also been detected in *PTPN22*, suggesting that there could be other variations in *PTPN22* leading to disease onset but due to a lack of replication between different studies further evidence is required to confirm these additional affects (26).

Between 60 and 70 of the over 100 PTPNs encoded within the human genome act as positive or negative regulators of T-cell activation (25), suggesting that further family members may too be playing a role in AID onset. *PTPN2* is one such family member. The *PTPN2* knockout mouse (lacking homologous *TCPTP*) exhibits defective T- and B-cell development and activation and when investigated within humans, variations within *PTPN2* were associated with type 1 diabetes, Graves' disease, and coeliac disease, with further work being performed to decipher the underlying disease mechanism (28).

Treg cell disruption

Disrupted Treg function is believed to be an important factor in preventing/controlling autoimmunity onset and specific mechanisms that control Treg function on top of CTLA-4 and PTPN22 have been identified. IL-2 mainly produced by activated T cells, promotes proliferation and enhances cytokine production. In Tregs IL-2 influences development and enhances Tregs ability to induce apoptosis of autoreactive T cells. IL-2 signals through the IL-2 receptor, which is composed of three subunits, an α chain (CD25 or IL-2 receptor α (IL-2Ra)) whose expression is restricted to T cells, in particular T regs, and a β (CD122) and γ chain (CD132) which are expressed on a variety of tissues and are involved in several cytokine signalling pathways. Screening of *IL-2Ra* and the surrounding region in type 1 diabetes showed strong evidence of association of two *IL-2Ra* SNPs with disease. Investigating individuals carrying two copies of the predisposing allele of either SNP had lower log concentrations of soluble IL-2Ra (sIl-2Ra), a marker of cell proliferation, than those carrying one or no copies, suggesting that reduced IL-2 signalling correlates with reduced T cell and, in particular, Treg function, which can in turn effect how the periphery is policed for autoreactive T cells (29).

B-cell regulation

Autoantibody production by B cells is key to autoimmune onset and can be either directed through binding to a receptor (such as TSHR autoantibodies in Graves' disease binding the TSHR) or through formation of immune complexes in tissues that locally activate the complement cascade (1). Hypermutation in the BCR during affinity maturation, failure to remove autoreactive B cells in the bone marrow/lymph nodes and periphery, and perturbations in signalling thresholds could all play a role in disease onset. Disruptions in several molecules that control B-cell signalling has been suggested, including B-cell activating factor (BAFF), whose expression in secondary lymphoid tissue is vital for providing prosurvival signals that enable transition from immature to mature B cell and sustaining long-term memory B cell survival (30). Inappropriate overexpression of BAFF can promote autoreactive B cells survival rather than deletion (1) with animals that express high levels of BAFF experiencing a number of autoimmune manifestations including high circulating antibody levels and immune complex formation in serum and kidneys. Variations within *Fc receptor like 3* (*FCRL3*), which encodes a member of the FC receptor-like family of proteins involved in regulating B cell signalling, have been detected in Graves' disease and other nonendocrine AIDs, including rheumatoid arthritis, which has been shown to disrupt gene expression and has been proposed to lead to unregulated B-cell activation.

Traditionally for many endocrine AIDs it has been viewed that B cells initiate autoimmunity and T cells progress disease. In the NOD mouse, a model for type 1 diabetes, for example, B cells are the first molecules to infiltrate the pancreas (31). The view of B cells as just producing autoantibodies and acting as bystanders in autoimmune disease such as type 1 diabetes, Graves' disease, and Hashimoto's thyroiditis, progression has been revised recently due to their ability to act as APCs to $CD4^{+}$ Th cells in low-antigen environments and their abilities to regulate inflammation through cytokine production. These features point to a larger and more active role for B cells in autoimmunity. It has also been suggested that T-cell-independent B-cell activation can also occur whereby antigens function as direct mitogenic stimuli causing antigen-specific B-cell activation through toll-like receptors (TLRs) or polysaccharides that directly engage the BCR (1). As TLR ligands, such as bacterial DNA and stimulatory CpG-oligodeoxyribonucleotides, are potent activators of B cells this could suggest another a way in which bacteria could be triggering autoimmunity.

External/environmental influences on the immune system

Although many of the mechanisms behind disease onset have so far focused on disruptions to specific molecules within the immune system, there are several 'external' factors that can also impact on the immune system, potentially triggering autoimmunity.

Sex differences in disease onset

Many AIDs have a strong female preponderance (see Table 1.6.1). Increased immune responsiveness in females, sex hormones, fetal microchimerism, and the presence of susceptibility loci on the sex chromosomes have all been put forward in an attempt to explain the female preponderance, although no single hypothesis has been confirmed. More recently, skewed X inactivation (XCI) has also been proposed as contributing to the female preponderance. During early development, females inherit one X chromosome from their father (XF) and one from their mother (XM). Males only inherit one X from their mother and a Y chromosome from their father. To enable dosage compensation to occur in females, one of the two X chromosomes present is randomly inactivated via methylation. Although XF:XM should be inactivated in a ratio of 50:50, skewed XCI can occur whereby more than 80% of one parent's X chromosome is inactivated. Evidence for higher rates of skewing have been detected in several Graves' disease datasets with 34–49% skewing seen in Graves' disease cases versus only 1–12% in control subjects (32). It has been proposed that in skewed XCI individuals, antigens on one X chromosome may fail to be expressed at a sufficiently high level in the thymus, preventing the immune system tolerating these antigens. When these antigens are presented to the immune system later in life they may, therefore, be recognized as foreign and an autoimmune response mounted, although further study is required to confirm these effects.

Environmental factors

Detecting the environmental contribution to disease is not easy because of the problems inherent in studying environmental impact during human development including the need for long-term follow-up and the reliance on patient recall. Even with these caveats in place, numerous potential environment factors have been suggested, including viruses (Table 1.6.3) and bacteria, chemicals, and stress (Table 1.6.4). These environmental factors are believed to impact upon the immune system in several different ways. First, fetal/maternal features such as birth weight, weight gain during pregnancy, and caesarean birth have all been proposed to contribute to onset of type 1 diabetes. Second, simply by the introduction of foreign particles into the body so that when the immune system tries to remove them autoimmunity is triggered as a side effect, as proposed for viruses or bacteria (Table 1.6.3 and HLA class I associations section). This is further supported by seasonal variation in the presentation of type 1 diabetes and Graves' disease. In the general population the majority of births occur within the spring or summer. This pattern is altered in type 1 diabetes and Graves' disease, with higher numbers born in the autumn or winter period, when an increased incidence of viral and bacterial infection occurs. Finally it can be affected by altering how the immune system functions. Stress and smoking are known to have immunosuppressive effects by stimulating the hypothalamo–pituitary–axis, which downregulates immune responsiveness. For example, an increase in the number of Graves' disease cases has

Table 1.6.3 Proposed viral triggers for endocrine autoimmune diseases

Virus	Symptoms caused by virus	Endocrine autoimmune disease/s affected
Adenovirus	Upper respiratory infections	GD
Coxsackie B virus	Gastrointestinal infections and in more extreme cases myocarditis and pericarditis	Type 1 diabetes
Hepatitis B	Liver inflammation	GD, HT
Hepatitis C	Liver inflammation	GD, type 1 diabetes
Human foamy virus	Asymptomatic	GD
Human T-cell leukaemia virus (HTLV)	T-cell leukaemia and T-cell lymphoma	GD
Parvovirus B19	Causes childhood exanthema	GD, HT, type 1 diabetes
Rotavirus	Infection of the gastrointestinal tract	Type 1 diabetes

GD, Graves' disease; HT, Hashimoto's thyroiditis.
Adapted from Gough, SCL Simmonds, MJ. The HLA region and autoimmune disease: Associations and mechanisms of action. *Curr Genomics*, 2007; **8**: 453–6 (16).

been noted during wartime and in type 1 diabetes both parental separation and bullying have been investigated as risk factors for disease onset. In type 1 diabetes there has been much debate concerning the benefits of breastfeeding over bottle feeding. It has been proposed that babies who are fed on cow's milk get more exposure to cow insulin leading to antibody formation. These antibodies could cross-react and attack an individual's own insulin-producing cells, whereas those who are breastfed would not get such early exposure to cow insulin. Although several studies have now been performed the data are inconclusive and further studies are required (33).

A lack of challenges to the immune system by foreign environmental factors has also been suggested as a potential cause of autoimmunity. The hygiene hypothesis suggests that changes in social behaviour combined with greater access to cleaning products could be contributing to the increased rates of AIDs. More sterile environments with a reduction in invading organisms could lead to autoimmune attack as our highly primed immune systems with less 'foreign' material to focus on could start to attack self-components.

Several large, long-term follow-up studies are currently being performed to evaluate the contribution of environmental factors, including investigating why different populations have variable disease rates, to see if changes in these differing populations' environments could provide further insights.

Summary

In summary, this chapter highlights some of the key mechanisms that are at play to prevent autoimmunity and describes how

Table 1.6.4 Proposed environmental triggers for endocrine autoimmune diseases subdivided by how they may trigger autoimmunity

	Proposed environmental factor	Endocrine autoimmune disease linked with environmental factor
Fetal/maternal environment		
	Maternal medicine during pregnancy	Type 1 diabetes
	Maternal age, excessive weight gain during pregnancy	Type 1 diabetes
	Birth by caesarean section	Type 1 diabetes
Introduction of foreign particles into the body		
	Chemicals – nitrates, nitrites, pesticides and industrial chemicals	GD, HT, type 1 diabetes
	Viruses and bacteria	GD, HT, type 1 diabetes
	Dietary factors – cereals, gluten	Type 1 diabetes
	Cow's milk	Type 1 diabetes
	Eczema	Type 1 diabetes
	Growing up in the city versus the country	Type 1 diabetes
	Iodine levels	GD, HT
Altering how the immune system functions		
	Vitamin D levels	Type 1 diabetes
	Smoking or passive smoking	GD, HT, type 1 diabetes
	Stressful life events	GD, HT, type 1 diabetes
	Excessive weight	Type 1 diabetes

GD, Graves' disease; HT, Hashimoto's thyroiditis.

disruptions within the immune system, both internally and externally can lead to the development of endocrine autoimmunity. As a result of advances in new genetic screening methodologies and long-term studies into environmental factors, our understanding of these mechanisms are constantly being updated and expanded on, with each new discovery helping to further identify the complex underlying pathologies involved in these diseases.

References

1. Monson NL. The natural history of B cells. *Curr Opin Neurol*, 2008; **21**(Suppl 1): S3–8.
2. Wagner DH Jr. Re-shaping the T cell repertoire: TCR editing and TCR revision for good and for bad. *Clin Immunol*, 2007; **123**: 1–6.
3. Torgerson TR. Regulatory T cells in human autoimmune diseases. *Springer Semin Immunopathol*, 2006; **28**: 63–76.
4. Wang LD, Clark MR. B-cell antigen-receptor signalling in lymphocyte development. *Immunology*, 2003; **110**: 411–20.
5. Jamin C, Morva A, Lemoine, S, Daridon, C, de Mendoza, AR, Youinou, P. Regulatory B lymphocytes in humans: a potential role in autoimmunity. *Arthritis Rheum*, 2008; **58**: 1900–6.
6. Kyewski B, Derbinski J. Self-representation in the thymus: an extended view. *Nat Rev Immunol*, 2004; **4**: 688–98.
7. Cheng MH, Shum AK, Anderson MS. What's new in the Aire?. *Trends Immunol*, 2007; **28**: 321–7.
8. Taubert R, Schwendemann J, Kyewski B. Highly variable expression of tissue-restricted self-antigens in human thymus: implications for self-tolerance and autoimmunity. *Eur J Immunol*, 2007; **37**: 838–48.
9. Bennett ST, Lucassen AM, Gough SC, Powell EE, Undlien DE, Pritchard LE, *et al.* Susceptibility to human type 1 diabetes at IDDM2 is determined by tandem repeat variation at the insulin gene minisatellite locus. *Nat Genet*, 1995; **9**: 284–92.
10. Chentoufi AA, Polychronakos C. Insulin expression levels in the thymus modulate insulin-specific autoreactive T-cell tolerance: the mechanism by which the IDDM2 locus may predispose to diabetes. *Diabetes*, 2002; **51**: 1383–90.
11. Brand OJ, Barrett J, Simmonds MJ, Newby PR, McCabe CJ, Bruce CK, *et al.* Association of the thyroid stimulating hormone receptor gene (TSHR) with Graves' disease (GD). *Hum Mol Genet*, 2009; **18**: 1704–13.
12. Eguchi K. Apoptosis in autoimmune diseases. *Intern Med*, 2001; **40**: 275–84.
13. Stassi G, Di Liberto D, Todaro M, Zeuner A, Ricci-Vitiani L, Stoppacciaro A, *et al.* Control of target cell survival in thyroid autoimmunity by T helper cytokines via regulation of apoptotic proteins. *Nat Immunol*, 2000; **1**: 483–8.
14. Stassi G, De Maria R. Autoimmune thyroid disease: new models of cell death in autoimmunity. *Nat Rev Immunol*, 2002; **2**: 195–204.
15. Todd JA, Bell JI, McDevitt HO. HLA-DQ beta gene contributes to susceptibility and resistance to insulin-dependent diabetes mellitus. *Nature*, 1987; **329**: 599–604.
16. Gough SCL, Simmonds MJ. The HLA region and autoimmune disease: Associations and mechanisms of action. *Curr Genomics*, 2007; **8**: 453–65.
17. Simmonds MJ, Howson JM, Heward JM, Cordell HJ, Foxall H, Carr-Smith J, *et al.* Regression mapping of association between the human leukocyte antigen region and Graves disease. *Am J Hum Genet*, 2005; **76**: 157–63.
18. Nejentsev S, Howson JM, Walker NM, Szeszko J, Field SF, Stevens HE, *et al.* Localization of type 1 diabetes susceptibility to the MHC class I genes HLA-B and HLA-A. *Nature*, 2007; **450**: 887–92.
19. Simmonds MJ, Howson JM, Heward JM, Carr-Smith J, Franklyn JA, Todd JA, *et al.* A novel and major association of HLA-C in Graves' disease that eclipses the classical HLA-DRB1 effect. *Hum Mol Genet*, 2007; **16**: 2149–53.
20. Gough SC, Walker LS, Sansom DM. CTLA4 gene polymorphism and autoimmunity. *Immunol Rev*, 2005; **204**, 102–15.
21. Mustelin T. Immunology. Restless T cells sniff and go. *Science*, 2006; **313**: 1902–3.
22. Schneider H, Downey J, Smith A, Zinselmeyer BH, Rush C, Brewer JM, *et al.* Reversal of the TCR stop signal by CTLA-4. *Science*, 2006; **313**: 1972–5.
23. Alegre ML, Frauwirth KA, Thompson CB. T-cell regulation by CD28 and CTLA-4. *Nat Rev Immunol*, 2001; **1**: 220–8.
24. Ueda H, Howson JM, Esposito L, Heward J, Snook H, Chamberlain G, *et al.* Association of the T-cell regulatory gene CTLA4 with susceptibility to autoimmune disease. *Nature*, 2003; **423**: 506–11.
25. Vang T, Miletic AV, Arimura Y, Tautz L, Rickert RC, Mustelin T. Protein tyrosine phosphatases in autoimmunity. *Annu Rev Immunol*, 2008; **26**: 29–55.
26. Bottini N, Vang T, Cucca F, Mustelin T. Role of PTPN22 in type 1 diabetes and other autoimmune diseases. *Semin Immunol*, 2006; **18**: 207–13.
27. Brand O, Gough S, Heward J. HLA, CTLA-4 and PTPN22:the shared genetic master-key to autoimmunity?. *Expert Rev Mol Med*, 2005; **7**: 1–15.
28. Wellcome Trust Case Control Consortium, Australo-Anglo-American Spondylitis Consortium. Genome-wide association study of 14,000 cases of seven common diseases and 3,000 shared controls. *Nature*, 2007; **447**: 661–78.
29. Lowe CE, Cooper JD, Brusko T, Walker NM, Smyth DJ, Bailey R, *et al.* Large-scale genetic fine mapping and genotype-phenotype associations implicate polymorphism in the IL2RA region in type 1 diabetes. *Nat Genet*, 2007; **39**: 1074–82.
30. Brink R. Regulation of B cell self-tolerance by BAFF. *Semin Immunol*, 2006; **18**: 276–83.
31. Silveira PA, Grey ST. B cells in the spotlight: innocent bystanders or major players in the pathogenesis of type 1 diabetes. *Trends Endocrinol Metab*, 2006; **17**: 128–35.
32. Invernizzi P. The X chromosome in female-predominant autoimmune diseases. *Ann NY Acad Sci*, 2007; **1110**: 57–64.
33. Peng H, Hagopian W. Environmental factors in the development of Type 1 diabetes. *Rev Endocr Metab Disord*, 2006; **7**: 149–62.

1.7

Measurement of hormones

Mike Wallace

Introduction

The role of accurate and reliable laboratory testing is particularly important for patients with potential endocrine disorders. The revolution which has taken place in the past 50 years in the methodology of hormone measurement is thus of considerable significance to this patient group. It is difficult to imagine that not too long ago common hormone measurements, such as thyroid function tests, took more than a week to produce. Now we live in a world where same day turnaround is the norm for the high throughput commonly requested tests. This is largely due to advances in the way hormones are measured and results delivered to the practising clinical endocrinologist.

Measuring hormones has always been a challenge as most circulate at extremely low concentrations, typically in the pico- (10^{-12}) or nanomolar (10^{-9}) range, and often in a milieu of closely related and potentially interfering compounds making great demands on method sensitivity and specificity. The most common procedures currently used are immuno- and immunometric assays but gas chromatography mass spectrometry (GCMS) and high-performance liquid chromatography (HPLC) also have a place. Liquid chromatography mass spectrometry (LC-MS/MS) is rapidly gaining acceptance for a limited number of hormone measurements.

It is not the aim of this chapter to provide precise detail on hormone measurement methodology but rather to overview general principles and applications of methods in current use. Attention is drawn to preanalytical and analytical problems which could have significant clinical consequences if not recognized.

Antibody-based methods

It was in late 1950s and early 1960s that it was first demonstrated that specific antibodies could be used to detect hormones and this discovery revolutionized clinical endocrinology. The first immunoassays were described by Yalow and Berson (1) and Ekins (2) for the measurement of insulin and thyroxine, respectively. Immunoassay is now the most widely applied technique for measuring hormones in biological samples. Nowadays, immunoassays are more likely to be developed within the diagnostics industry than by academic experts, with increasing emphasis on methods suitable for large, throughput automated platforms. Manual 'in house' or commercial kit procedures, however, remain prominent for the more specialist, lower throughput hormone measurements and are usually performed in specialized regional clinical laboratories.

The basic requirements for immunoassay are an antibody (or antibodies) to the analyte to be measured, a labelled form of the analyte (competitive immunoassay) or a labelled second antibody to the analyte (noncompetitive immunoassay). Procedures for separating antibody-bound tracer from unbound tracer and a means for detecting the tracer are also required. To facilitate separation, antibodies can be attached to solid surfaces, such as polystyrene reaction tubes or microtitre plates, plastic beads, or cellulose particles, thus allowing the unbound portion to be removed by a wash procedure. Commercial methods frequently use magnetized particles, which simplify separation on automated platforms.

Competitive immunoassay

Hormone immunoassays rely on high specific activity labels, such as radioisotopes, to reveal the products of the hormone–antibody reaction. The 'first generation' immunoassays—in common use from the 1960s to the mid-1980s—relied almost exclusively on the inclusion of a trace amount of radiolabelled hormone in a reaction mixture comprising the test sample (serum, urine, or saliva) and a limited amount of antibody (or other binding agent). The analytical principle governing these methods (termed RIA) involve 'competition' between labelled and unlabelled hormone molecules for the antibody present (Fig. 1.7.1). After incubation, the proportion of labelled analyte decreases as the concentration of the analyte being measured increases. Such assays are therefore often referred to as 'competitive' or 'displacement' assays. To avoid problems related to handling of radioactivity and the limited shelf-life of radiolabelled reagents these have now been largely, but not yet completely, superseded by labels employing fluorescent or chemiluminescent substances or enzymes.

One requirement for competitive immunoassay is that there should be no interference from circulating binding proteins which could participate in competition with the labelled analyte. Since many small-molecular-weight hormones, such as steroids, bind with high affinity to circulating binding proteins, the traditional approach was to separate them from the binding protein by extracting into an organic solvent such as diethyl ether. This has the added benefit of also removing water soluble, potentially cross-reacting, conjugated steroids. Unfortunately solvent extraction is a labour-intensive step that is difficult to automate. The introduction of simple, direct immunoassays for the measurements of steroids in unextracted serum or plasma was therefore a significant advance. In direct steroid immunoassays steroids are displaced from

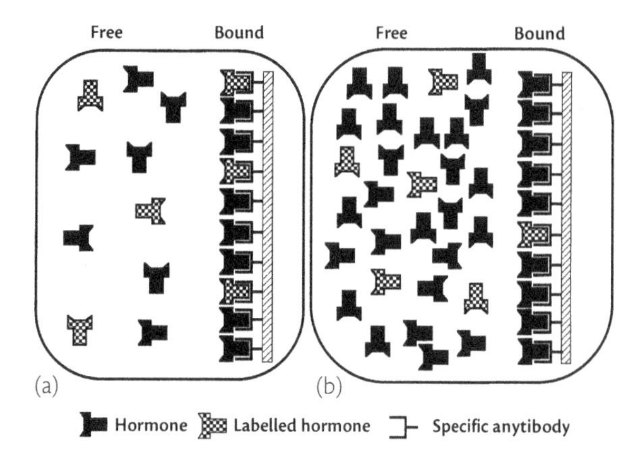

Fig. 1.7.1 The term 'competitive assay' derives from the perception that unlabelled hormone molecules (deriving from the test sample) 'compete' with labelled molecules for a limited number of specific hormone binding sites. When the concentration of unlabelled hormone molecules is low (a), the amount of labelled hormone bound is high, but falls with increase in unlabelled hormone concentration (b).

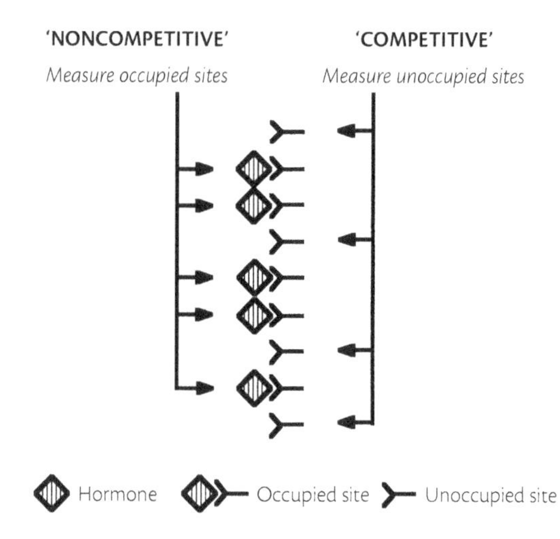

Fig. 1.7.2 'Competitive' binding assays' rely on measurement of unoccupied (antibody) binding sites either following or during exposure of specific binding agent (for example antibody) to the hormone-containing sample. 'Non-competitive' assays rely on measurement of occupied sites.

binding proteins by a chemical agent '*in situ*' and, ideally, these agents should not affect antibody-binding characteristics, but this is not always achieved (3). Although the advances in measuring steroid hormones directly have progressed the introduction of automated steroid measurements on large, fast throughput automated immunoassay platforms they do place great demand as illustrated later, on antiserum specificity as potentially cross-reacting steroid conjugates are not removed.

Noncompetitive immunoassays

In the late 1960s, methods relying on radiolabelled antibodies (termed immunoradiometric assays (IRMAs)) were first described (4, 5) As with competitive immunoassays as the labelled antibody procedure evolved a whole range of nonradioactive labels (enzymes, fluorofloures, chemiluminescent) were introduced. Since in these assays no competition occurs between labelled and unlabelled analyte for antibody-binding sites these immunometric assays have also been termed noncompetitive immunoassays or 'sandwich' assays. They rely on the detection of occupied antibody-binding sites to which the analyte has bound (Fig. 1.7.2). The amount of analyte bound to the first antibody is detected by the binding, and formation of a 'sandwich', with another antibody to which a label is attached. These assays are suitable for analytes of large molecular size (that is, of a molecular weight of approximately 1000 Da and above). For hormones of smaller molecular size (and thus incapable of binding simultaneously to two antibodies) the competitive approach continues to be generally employed.

Immunometric procedures require high concentrations of unlabelled antibody of known specificity. The full potential of the immunometric assay was, therefore, only realized with the introduction of *in vitro* monoclonal antibody procedures by Köhler and Milstein in 1975 (6). Further improvements were later made by the introduction of high activity labels for attachment to the second antibody in the 'sandwich' with remarkable improvement in sensitivity. In the 1970s, time-resolved fluorometric immunoassay methodology, now known as DELFIA (7, 8), was developed. Based on the use of lanthanide chelate fluorophors and labelled monoclonal antibodies, this was the first of many 'ultra-sensitive' nonisotopic immunoassay methodologies. The same approach has subsequently been adopted by many manufacturers using other high specific activity non-isotopic labels, as reviewed by Kricka (9). The use of such labels in immunoassays of noncompetitive design revolutionized the immunodiagnostic field towards the end of the twentieth century and underlies attempts to further improve assay sensitivities.

Very high sensitivity is clearly of particular importance in the case of certain hormones, for example, thyroid-stimulating hormone (TSH). Serum concentrations in hyperthyroid individuals not only fell below the limit of detection of the original radioimmunoassay methods used in the 1970s and 1980s, but were essentially indistinguishable from normal values. Ultrasensitive TSH methods (in combination with free thyroxine assays) are now widely used in the laboratory diagnosis of thyroid dysfunction. An equally important consequence of the development of ultrasensitive immunoassays has been a major reduction in assay performance times, resulting in the emergence of the automated immunoanalysers that now dominate the field. Total incubation times in the order of minutes are typical, replacing the hours or days characterizing first generation 'competitive' methodologies.

In summary, hormone immunoassay methods now in common use (and widely available as kits—usually incorporated in the menus provided by immunoanalyser manufacturers) are of both competitive single-site and noncompetitive two-site design. The former approach is generally adopted for the assay of hormones of small size (such as steroid and thyroid hormones), the latter for the assay of hormones of large molecular size (e.g. polypeptide and glycoprotein hormones). High specific activity nonisotopic labels, yielding higher sensitivities in assays of noncompetitive design, have largely replaced radioisotopic labels. Though their use does not significantly improve the sensitivities of competitive methods, the longer shelf lives of labelled reagents and other such practical benefits are also factors contributing to the general abandonment of radioisotopic labels by immunoassay kit manufacturers.

Free (nonprotein bound) immunoassays

In the case of those hormones (such as thyroid and steroid hormones) present in blood in free and protein-bound forms, it is widely accepted that the free hormone concentration measured under equilibrium conditions *in vitro* constitutes the determinant of the hormone's physiological activity. This concept, termed the 'free hormone hypothesis', derives primarily from observations that, in subjects in whom serum binding protein concentrations are 'abnormal', overall hormone effects correlate closely with the free hormone concentration. Despite doubts about the validity of the free hormone hypothesis (10, 11). Direct measurement of free thyroid and steroid hormones by equilibrium dialysis or centrifugal ultrafiltration is technically challenging and generally unavailable outside specialized research laboratories. Free hormone immunoassay methods have therefore been developed that rely on the basic physicochemical principle, which is that exposure of a small amount of antihormone antibody to a test serum sample results in occupancy of antibody-binding sites to an extent that reflects the ambient free hormone concentration in the sample (Fig. 1.7.3). Occupancy of binding sites can be determined in three different ways.

- The 'labelled hormone, back-titration' approach ('two-step' free hormone immunoassay) which relies on determination of unoccupied antibody-binding sites (the antibody being generally linked to a solid support) by their exposure to labelled hormone following removal of the test serum.
- The 'labelled hormone analogue' approach ('single-step' free hormone immunoassay), which obviates these sequential operations by the use of a labelled hormone analogue that must, in principle, be totally unreactive with serum proteins (though retaining the ability to react with antibody).
- The 'labelled antibody' approach (likewise a 'single-step' immunoassay), which also relies on the use of a hormone analogue. The analogue used in labelled antibody techniques, however, is coupled to a solid support, such attachment apparently contributing to a reduction of analogue binding to serum proteins. For this and other reasons, labelled antibody assay kits appear to conform more closely to the principles governing valid analogue-based free hormone immunoassays, and generally yield correct and clinically reliable results.

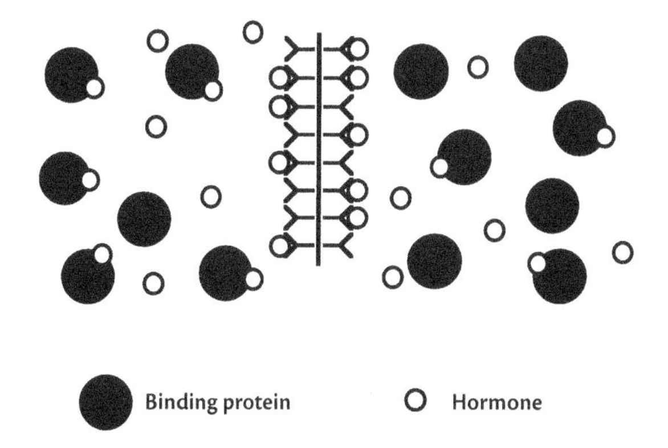

Fig. 1.7.3 When an antibody-coated probe is exposed to serum containing free and protein bound hormone, the fractional occupancy of antibody-binding sites reflects the ambient free hormone concentration, assuming the antibody binds only a small proportion (e.g. below 5%) of the total hormone in the sample. All free hormone immunoassays depend on measurement of the antibody fractional occupancy, either following, or during such exposure.

The main current application of free hormone immunoassay is for the measurement of free thyroxine. Undoubtedly reliable measurement of circulating 'free' thyroxine by immunoassay is a better diagnostic test than total thyroxine. Although a few commercial kits do exist for measuring free steroid concentrations, these have not received general acceptance. In contrast, in the case of testosterone, an index of the free hormone concentration is often calculated. For females the free androgen index (total testosterone/sex hormone-binding globulin × 100) (12) is generally used but this is not valid for males, in whim 'free' testosterone can be derived from measured circulating total testosterone, sex hormone-binding globulin, and albumin concentrations based on the binding constants of testosterone to these circulating proteins (13).

An alternative to measuring the circulating free hormone concentration is to measure the hormone in saliva. Saliva measurements have been developed for a number of steroids and have the potential to provide a convenient and noninvasive assessment of the serum 'free' steroid concentrations. Salivary concentrations of unconjugated steroids reflect those for free steroids in serum although concentrations may differ because of salivary gland metabolism. The use of salivary assays for both research and routine purposes has recently been reviewed in detail by Wood (14). Measuring salivary cortisol late evening is now an accepted and sensitive screening test for Cushing's. Salivary 17-hydroxyprogesterone and androstenedione assays are valued as noninvasive for home monitoring of hydrocortisone replacement in patients with the 21-hydroxylase deficiency variant of congenital adrenal hyperplasia. The diagnostic value of salivary oestradiol, progesterone, testosterone, dehydroepiandrosterone, and aldosterone testing is compromised by rapid fluctuations in salivary concentrations of these steroids.

Methods based on chromatographic separation followed by nonimmunological detection

Hormone analysis by gas chromatography and HPLC rely on chromatographic separation followed by a variety of detection procedures. As indicated in Table 1.7.1 these methods are usually restricted to measurement of nonprotein hormones such as steroids and related metabolites, vitamin D metabolites, catecholamines, and metabolites. Prior to chromatographic separation an initial purification step may be required: the simplest is extraction into an organic solvent(liquid/liquid extraction) but alternatively solid phase extraction (SPE) is becoming more popular. SPE can be used to effect sample extraction, concentration, and purification. The most commonly used hormone measurement procedure is reverse-phased SPE (polar liquid phase, nonpolar modified solid phase) which involves capture of the analyte from a liquid phase onto silica microparticles coated with sorbent packed into syringes or cartridges. One of the earliest descriptions of the use of SPE for hormone measurement is a method for purification of urinary steroids prior to gas chromatographic analysis described

Table 1.7.1 Procedures used to commonly measure hormone and hormone metabolites

Procedure	Sample type	Hormones measured
Immunoassay	Serum/plasma	Thyroid hormones
	Urine	Steroid hormones
	Saliva	Specific hormone-binding proteins
	Filter paper dried blood spots	Protein and peptide hormones
		Vitamin D metabolites
		Cortisol
		Cortisol, 17- hydroxyprogesterone
		Thyroid-stimulating hormone, 17-hydroxyprogesterone
High-performance liquid chromatography	Serum/plasma	Vitamin D metabolites
	Urine	Steroid hormones
		Catecholamines and metabolites
Gas chromatography mass spectrometry	Urine	Steroid metabolites
Tandem mass spectrometry (LC-MS/MS)	Serum/plasma	Vitamin D metabolites
	Urine	Testosterone
	Filter paper dried blood spots	Adrenal steroid profiles
		Cortisol
		17-hydroxyprogesterone

by Shackelton and Whitney in 1980 (15). Although it is not possible to automate liquid/liquid extraction procedures, recent advances in laboratory robotics allow automation of the solid phase extraction step off-line (16) or online, utilizing column-switching techniques, linked to either HPLC or LC-MS/MS (17).

Based on the knowledge of the chemical nature of both the hormone to be purified and any interferants, if present, the polarity of the organic solvent (for liquid/liquid extraction procedures) or type of solid phase and polarity of the eluting solvent (for SPE) can be selected to ensure adequate purification. The amount of purification and concentration required is governed, to some extent, by the efficiency of the next chromatographic stage and the sensitivity of the final detection stage.

In the chromatographic stage, in order to achieve separation a dynamic equilibrium distribution between compounds in a mobile phase such as a flowing gas or liquid and the stationary phase is established. As the analyte is propelled by the mobile phase over the stationary phase chromatographic separation is achieved with those compounds preferentially distributed in the mobile phase passing more quickly through the system than those preferentially distributed in the stationary phase. The stationary phase is contained in a fused silica (gas chromatography) or steel tube (HPLC) and a gas or liquid flow is maintained by the application of pressure. With careful optimization of the polarity of the stationary and/or the mobile phase very complex separations can be achieved.

Extraction and chromatographic separation will inevitably lead to loss of analyte necessitating the need for inclusion of an internal standard to correct for procedural losses. The internal standard should be indistinguishable from the analyte during the process of extraction and purification and the choice of internal standard is to some extent dictated by the quantification procedure. For example, for procedures employing mass spectrometry deuterated internal standards are ideal being chemically identical yet detectable by virtue of increased mass. This procedure generally compensates for any matrix related effects and is commonly termed isotope dilution mass spectrometry. When other types of detection systems such as light absorption, fluorescence, and electrochemical properties are used, an internal standard is usually selected which has similar chemical properties to the analyte but is not present in biological samples.

Gas chromatography mass spectrometry

GCMS has been established over several decades as an important procedure for measuring hormones. The combination of gas chromatography with mass spectrometry exploits the high-resolving power of gas chromatography to separate closely related molecules and the ability of mass spectrometry to provide precise data for identification and quantification of the separated substances. The two prerequisites are volatility and thermal stability of the compounds to be separated. This limits GCMS to measurement of compounds with a molecular weight of less than 800 Da such as steroids and thyroid hormones. Furthermore, derivatization is often required to increase volatility and thermo stability of the analyte.

During gas chromatography a liquid sample is evaporated at high temperature and the volatile constituents blown through a hollow flexible silica capillary column, to which is coated or bonded a liquid stationary phase. In most GCMS systems, the gas chromatography column passes through a vacuum seal delivering the separated molecules into the ion source of the mass spectrometer. Here, under vacuum, the molecules are bombarded with either electrons (electron impact ionization) or charged ions (chemical ionization) resulting in molecular instability and production of positively charged fragments. The mass spectrometer is able to use differences in the mass-to-charge ratio (m/z) of these ionized fragments to separate and detect each fragment. In essence the pattern of fragments provides a 'fingerprint' for the molecule under investigation allowing positive identification and quantification.

Unfortunately GCMS methods require laborious sample preparation limiting use for routine hormone measurements. Such methods have, however, provided a valuable tool for establishing reference methods for steroid and thyroid hormones where sample throughput is not an issue (18). GCMS has been more widely used in the specialized endocrine laboratory for profiling urinary steroid metabolites for both routine and research purposes by methods adapted from those first introduced by Shackleton in 1986 (19). The measurement of urinary steroid metabolites aids the diagnosis of a number of inherited disorders of the synthesis and metabolism of adrenal steroids, and steroid-producing tumours. (20) The procedure is particularly valuable in identifying the site of the enzyme defect in congenital adrenal hyperplasia. An example of a urinary steroid profile in a case of untreated late-onset congenital adrenal hyperplasia is shown in Fig. 1.7.4a. The full fragmentation pattern for each steroid metabolite permits absolute identification of the metabolite. An example of a fragmentation pattern for one of the abnormally elevated metabolites (11-oxo-pregnanetriol) is shown in Fig. 1.7.4b.

Tandem mass spectrometry

The relatively new procedure of tandem mass spectrometry is beginning to make a significant impact on hormone measurement. When linked to HPLC this procedure is commonly abbreviated to LC-MS/MS. As in the early days of immunoassay there is currently a flurry of LC-MS/MS method development activity within specialist endocrine laboratories. The revolution got going in the 1990s with the introduction of atmospheric pressure ionization (API) and electrospray ionization procedures allowing the first clinical applications which were in the areas of neonatal screening and therapeutic drug monitoring. Compared with GCMS sample preparation for LC-MS/MS is more straightforward and can be applied to thermo labile compounds. Instead of analytes being ionized in a gas phase they are ionized in liquid phase which is much more appropriate for biological samples. As with GCMS, mass spectrometry is used to identify, characterize, and quantitate but by utilizing two quadrupole mass filters, separated by a collision cell, far greater specificity is achieved (Fig. 1.7.5). The first quadrupole mass filter (QMF1) selects ions sharing identical mass-to-charge ratio (*m/z*), all other ions are filtered out. In the collision cell the selected ions are fragmented into characteristic product ions by collision with a

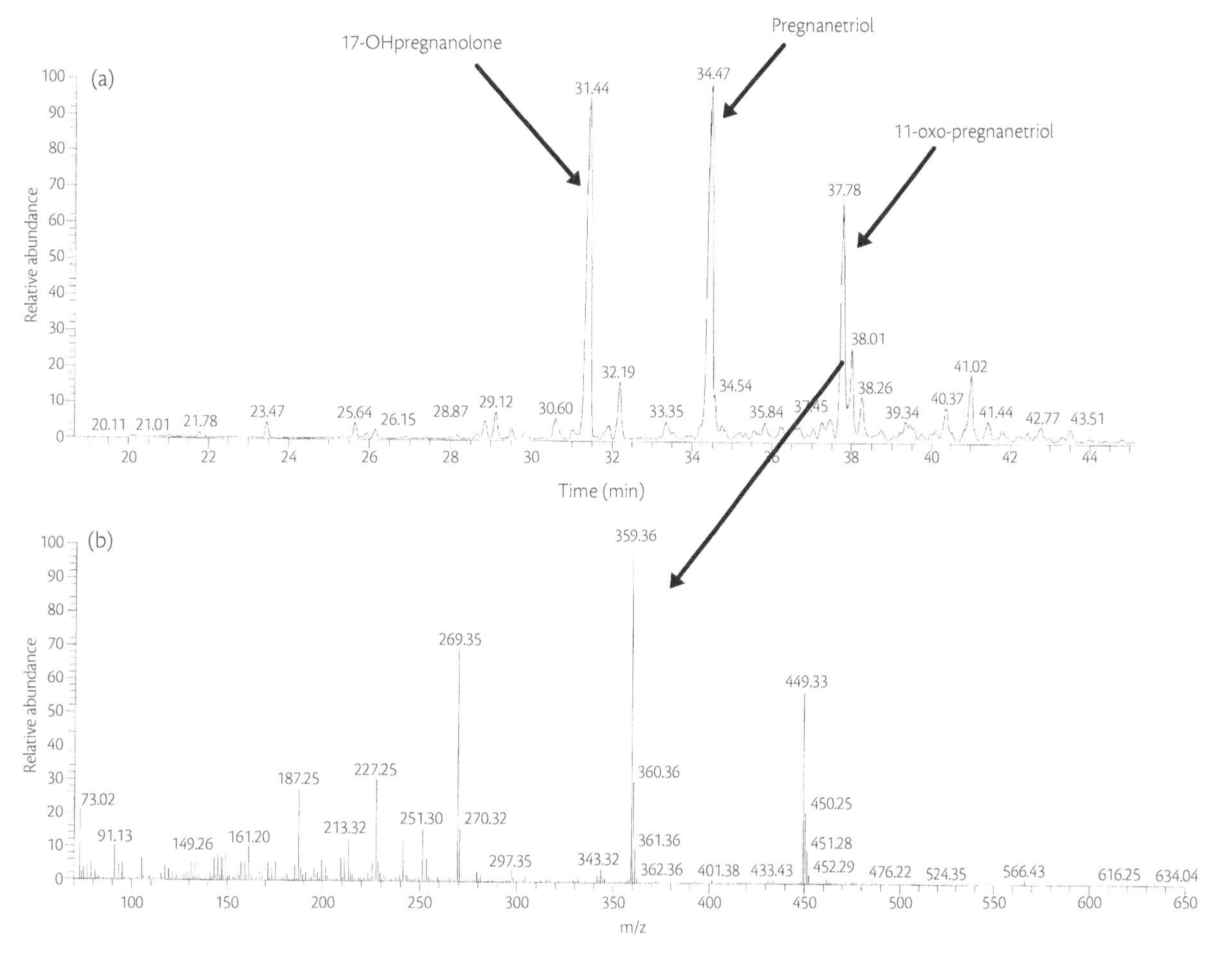

Fig. 1.7.4 Gas chromatography mass spectrometry. (a) Total ion chromatogram of a urinary steroid metabolite pattern from a patient with late-onset 21-hydroxylase deficiency variant of congenital adrenal hyperplasia. In this condition the most prominent steroid metabolites are 17-hydroxypregnanolone, pregnanetriol and 11-oxo-pregnanetriol. The x-axis shows the time in minutes at which the chromatographically separated steroid metabolites are detected and the y-axis the relative abundance (quantity of ions). (b) Complete pattern of ions produced by fragmentation of 11-oxopregnanetriol. The x-axis shows the *m/z* (mass to charge ratio) and the y-axis the relative abundance (quantity of ions).

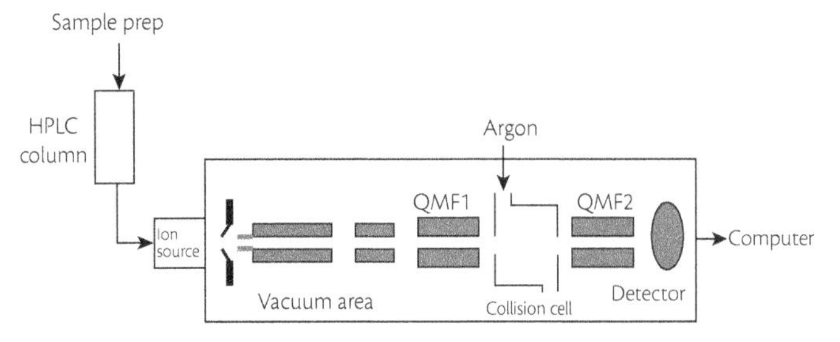

Fig. 1.7.5 Tandem mass spectrometry (MS/MS). After sample preparation components are separated by high performance liquid chromatography (HPLC). Molecular ions are produced and separated in the first quadrupole mass filter (QMF1) set to retain a predefined 'parent' ion. In the collision cell the parent ion is further fragmented by collision with an inert gas. One of the collision products, a 'daughter' ion, is retained by the quadrupole second mass filter (QMF2) and is focused towards the detector.

neutral gas (e.g. argon) and transmitted to the second quadrupole mass filter (QMF2). QMF2 is set to filter out all but the selected fragment ion. Thus, one defined 'daughter ion' from one defined 'parent ion' finally reaches the detector. The selection of masses by QMF1 and QMF2 can be changed within milli-seconds enabling a large number of different mass transitions to be monitored in parallel allowing multianalyte quantification. Illustrated in Fig. 1.7.6 are the output scans for a method developed for measurement of vitamin D metabolites by isotope dilution LC-MS/MS (16). After semiautomated SPE sample preparation analysis was performed using an automated LC-MS/MS system. The tandem mass spectrometer was used in positive ion mode with electrospray source and a stable isotope, hexadeuterated 25-hydroxyvitamin D_3, used as internal standard to correct for procedural losses. The multiple-reaction monitoring transitions (parent → daughter) selected for quantification of 25-hydroxyvitamin D_3, 25-hydroxyvitamin D_2, and hexadeuterated 25-hydroxyvitamin D_3 were *m/z* 401.35→159, 413.30→83, and 407.35→159, respectively. A more detailed account of principles of LC-MS/MS procedures and endocrine applications is provided in a two reviews by Vogeser and colleagues (21, 22).

Currently the methodology has been applied to steroids, vitamin D metabolites and catecholamines with greatest impact, so far, in the routine measurement of testosterone (23), vitamin D metabolites (16, 24) and urinary free cortisol (25). The ability to simultaneously measure a number of analytes is of value both for routine and research purposes. As previously illustrated (see Fig. 1.7.4) a number of vitamin D metabolites can be measured and likewise serum adrenal steroid profiles with simultaneous measurement of five, or more, steroids can be performed. A few further examples of methods developed to simultaneously measure hormones are test ostosterone;dihydrotestosterone (26), cortisol;cortisone (27), and plasma-free metanerphine;normetanephrine (28).

The main obstacles to the use of LC-MS/MS in the clinical laboratory are the high initial cost of instrumentation (£150 000–250 000) and the high level of expertise required to develop methods and run the equipment. To some extent the high initial cost can be offset by the low cost of reagent compared to diagnostic immunoassay kits and as LC-MS/MS becomes more widely used expertise in this area is rapidly increasingly within both specialist and routine clinical laboratories.

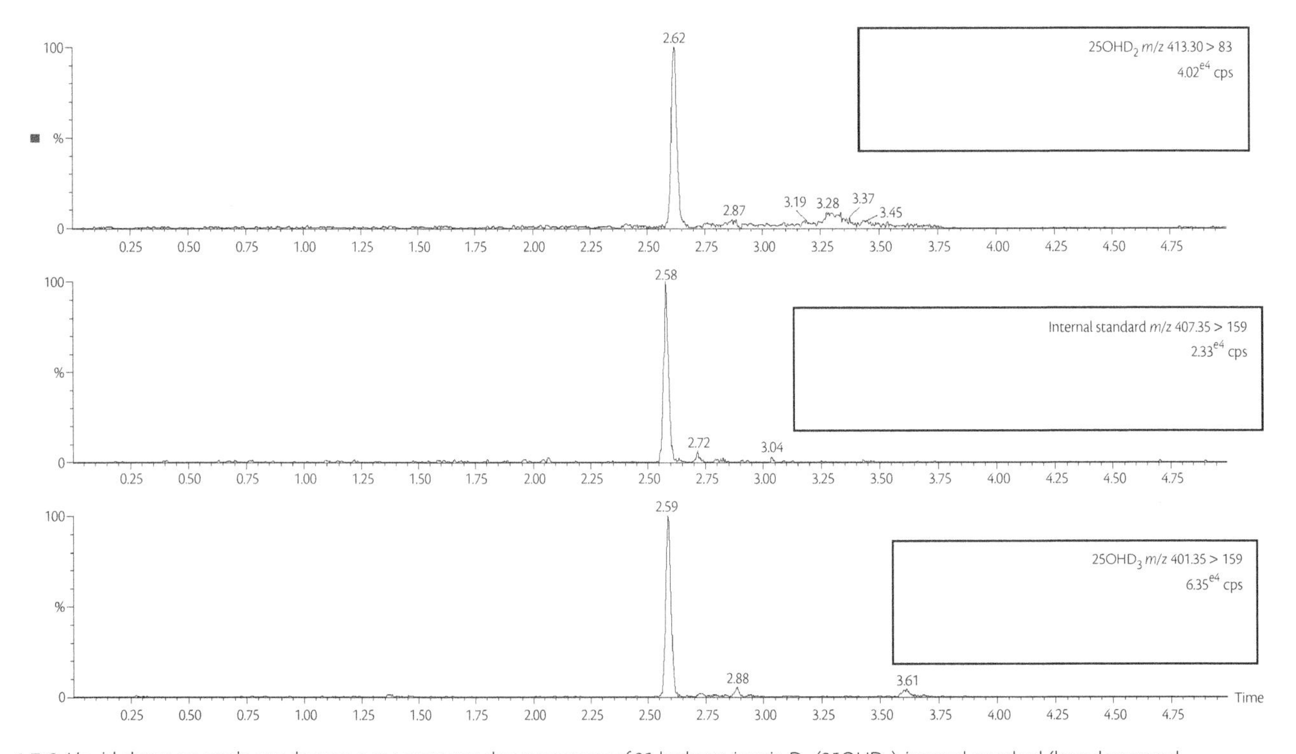

Fig. 1.7.6 Liquid chromatography-tandem mass spectrometry chromatograms of 25-hydroxyvitamin D_2 (25OHD$_2$), internal standard (hexadeuterated 25-hydroxyvitaminD$_3$) and 25-hydroxyvitamin D_3 (25OHD$_3$). The x-axis shows the time in minutes at which the chromatographically separated vitamin D metabolites are detected and the y-axis the relative abundance (quantity of ions). cps, counts per second.

Assay performance, interferences, and errors

Within the laboratory assay performance is assessed both internally and through external quality assessment schemes. It is important that each laboratory documents analytical accuracy, precision (both within and between batch) and reference ranges for all procedures. For procedures developed 'in house', or adapted from commercial procedures, more extensive evaluation on analytical and functional sensitivity and specificity are required. Comparison of results obtained by other methods and performance in external quality assessment schemes provide reassurance. Ideally methods should be compared to established reference methods but few are available in the endocrine field. Although this section focuses on analytical problems it is important to be aware that errors can also occur before and after the analytical process. Some of the causes of error from all three categories are summarized in Table 1.7.2.

The accuracy of hormone assays may be compromised by a variety of interfering substances. The interference may be positive or negative and may vary in magnitude depending on the concentration of interfering substance in the sample. Often samples circulated by external quality assessment schemes are selected to address such issues.

Immunoassays are prone to interference from endogenous binding proteins and drugs. This has been mentioned earlier in the case of steroid hormones and can also occur with other methods for hormone measurement. For instance growth hormone binding protein can interfere with the measurement of growth hormone to different extents in different immunoassays (29). In free thyroxine assays, drugs, including phenytoin, carbamazepine, and salicylate, compete with thyroid binding to serum-binding protein and may increase the free thyroxine concentration. The most common drug interference in cortisol immunoassays is with prednisolone, which cross-reacts, to varying degrees, with all cortisol antisera.

The presence of antibodies in a serum sample can cause numerous problems in immunoassay. The effect of the interference will depend on the type of assay used and the site where the antibody binds to the analyte. Interference may lead to either falsely elevated or decreased values (30). An example of a common interferant is macroprolactin. Prolactin mostly circulates in monomeric form with a molecular weight 23 KDa but in a few individuals a large antigen-antibody complex of molecular weight greater than 100 KDa, commonly called macroprolactin, is present which may be detected as prolactin in the assay. It is therefore good laboratory practice to further investigate samples giving unexpected elevated prolactin results for the presence of macroprolactin. This can he easily achieved by precipitating macroprolactin in the serum sample with a precipitation agent, such as polyethylene glycol, and remeasuring prolactin on the supernatant (31). Less common and more difficult to recognize is interference from endogenous antibodies. Heterophilic antibodies can be associated with autoimmune and other inflammatory diseases. Interference may occur in both competitive and noncompetitive assays, but the latter is more common. The same is true if specific human antianimal antibodies which are present in some individuals in response to prior immunizations. Monoclonal antibody-based immunometric assays are especially sensitive to the presence of heterophilic and antianimal antibodies, which interfere by linking the capture to the detection antibody, causing false-positive results. Commercial heterophilic, antibody-blocking reagents can be used to minimize the effect of this type of interference or, as described for macroprolactin, antibodies may be removed by polyethylene glycol precipitation.

A significant and potential extremely dangerous problem can also occur specifically in immunometric assays if an exceptionally high concentration of the hormone being measured is present which simultaneously binds both the capture and detecting antibodies. This prevents the formation of the required complexes with capture antibody, analyte, and detecting antibody producing an incorrect low result in a sample that actually contains extremely high concentrations of analyte. This type of interference is commonly known as the high-dose 'hook' effect. For immunoassay procedures a simple test to indicate the presence of interference is to measure the sample over a range of dilutions. Interference is likely if a nonlinear response is obtained.

One major advantage of LC-MS/MS over immunoassay is improved specificity and this has been demonstrated most vociferously in relation to the measurement of testosterone. Although many nonextraction immunoassay methods perform satisfactorily in males, measurement in females and children is fraught with problems. Interferences related to the presence of incompletely blocked binding proteins and conjugated interfering steroids can cause falsely elevated results. In 2003, Taieb *et al.* (32) reported on the measurement of female testosterone by using 10 direct commercially available immunoassays compared with an

Table 1.7.2 Errors related to laboratory testing

Preanalytical	Analytical	Postanalytical
Inappropriate patient preparation (fasting, posture, time of last medication, stress)	Poor analytical performance Incorrect assay standardization	Incorrect reference range
Dynamic function test performed incorrectly	Antibody interference in immunoassay	Incorrect interpretation Incorrect units
Incorrect name on sample	Drug interference	Computer error during processing of reports
Inadequate detail with request (e.g. clinical details age, sex, ethnicity, pregnancy, stage of menstrual cycle)	High dose 'hook' effect in immunometric assay Poor immunoassay specificity	
Wrong test requested	Ion suppression in LC-MS/MS	
Inappropriate sample type (serum, heparinized or EDTA plasma)		
Sample collected at inappropriate time of day		
Illegible handwriting on request form		

isotope-dilution GCMS reference method. They concluded that most nonextraction immunoassays showed a large positive bias. Such was the extent of the problem that it prompted a hard hitting editorial in *Clinical Chemistry*, 'Immunoassays for testosterone in women: better than a guess?' (33). Although the exact nature of the interference is unknown there is some evidence that implicates the adrenal steroid dehydroepiandrosterone sulfate, which circulates at extremely high concentrations (μmol/l) compared with testosterone (nmol/l). It is, however, probable that other conjugated steroids and also binding protein-related interferences play a part and that different direct immunoassays are affected to different degrees depending on the specificity of the antibody used. Recognizing this problem, the Endocrine Society in the USA commissioned a panel of experts to look into the issue, which has now published a position statement on the utility, limitations, and pitfalls in measuring testosterone (34). They concluded that 'direct' immunoassay procedures are too insensitive and inaccurate to measure testosterone in the plasma of women and children and recommend that assays after solvent extraction and chromatography, followed by mass spectrometry or immunoassay, are likely to furnish more reliable results. These findings have accelerated the progress of LC-MS/MS as the method of choice for measuring testosterone in the clinical laboratory.

Another area where LC-MS/MS has led to improved diagnostic accuracy is the measurement of 17-hydroxyprogesterone in neonates. Transient elevation of both unconjugated and conjugated Δ-5 adrenal steroids produced by the fetal zone of the adrenal cortex early in life, especially in neonates born prematurely, cause positive interference in most direct 17-hydroxyprogesteorne immunoassays but not in more specific LC-MS/MS procedures. There are, however, situations where poor immunoassay specificity may actually be advantageous. For instance to correctly assess vitamin D status it is important to measure both 25-hydroxyvitamin D_2 and 25-hydroxyvitamin D_3 in the same sample. It is claimed that a number of commercial immunoassays achieve or partially achieve this but there is at least one example of an extremely specific commercial immunoassay that only detects 25-hydroxyvitamin D_3 with the consequence that patients who are switched to vitamin D_2 are not correctly assessed (35). Of course the best solution, as described earlier, is to measure both metabolites simultaneously by LC-MS/MS. It is, however, worth mentioning that LC-MS/MS is not totally free from analytical problems. Ion suppression can affect the quantitative performance of a mass detector. This can be caused by the presence of nonvolatile compounds such as salts, ion-pairing agents, endogenous compounds, and drugs/metabolites. This problem can usually be minimized by modification of reagents or chromatographic conditions (36).

To end on a rather sobering thought, it is important for the clinician to realize that half of all errors in the diagnostic process are not related to methodology at all, but occur before the sample is analysed. In fact 20% of these preanalytical errors are related to sample collection (Table 1.7.2). Even in hospitals where there is a heightened awareness of these problems, there is a prevalence of 1% preanalytical errors. These effects can be of sufficient magnitude to alter the analysis enough to create situations for clinical errors. Most problems can be prevented by clear instructions and documented policies for sampling. Some issues are relatively straightforward such as collecting the sample into the correct blood tube at the correct time of day and ensuring that samples are transported to the laboratory fast enough and at the correct temperature. If in doubt contact your local laboratory for current protocols.

In addition samples can and do get mixed up and mislabelled. In some instances this is easily identifiable if a totally inappropriate result is obtained, for instance, a male testosterone concentration in a female patient, but often differences from previous results can be more subtle. It is important when unexpected results are obtained that the possibility of preanalytical, analytical error and postanalytical error is thoroughly investigated. The first step is often to repeat the test. This could be followed by arranging for the measurement to be performed by a different method or procedure. Whenever specimens with interfering substances are identified, other laboratory data and clinical information on the patient, especially any acute or chronic disease and medications should be obtained. This information may provide clues to the cause of the interference which can be investigated in more detail in the laboratory.

Since clinical endocrinology is so dependent on laboratory investigation it is important that a close working relationship is built up between the endocrine clinician and the clinical laboratory scientist. A climate of mutual respect and close collaboration should ensure that problems are recognized and attended to promptly and that procedures are developed that are fit for purpose.

References

1. Yalow RS, Berson SA. Assay of plasma insulin in human subjects by immunological methods. *Nature*, 1959; **194**: 1648–49.
2. Ekins RP. The estimation of thyroxine in human plasma by an electrophoretic technique. *Clin Chem Acta*, 1960; **5**: 453–9.
3. Ratcliffe WA. Direct (non-extraction) serum assays for steroids. In: Hunter WM, Corrie JET, eds. *Immunoassays for Clinical Chemistry 1983*. Ediburgh: Churchill Livingstone, 1983: 401–9.
4. Wide L, Bennich H, Johansson SGO. Diagnosis of allergy by an *in-vitro* test for allergen antibodies. *Lancet*, 1967; **2**: 1105–7.
5. Miles LEH, Hales CN. Labelled antibodies and immunological assay systems. *Nature*, 1968; **219**: 186–9.
6. Köhler G, Milstein C. Continuous cultures of fused cells secreting antibody of pre defined specificity. *Nature*, 1975; **256**: 495–7.
7. Marshall NJ, Dakubu S, Jackson T, Ekins RP. Pulsed light, time resolved fluoroimmunoassay. In: Albertini A, Ekins RP, eds. *Monoclonal Antibodies and Developments in Immunoassay*. Amsterdam: Elsevier, 1981: 101–8.
8. Soini E, Lövgren T. Time-resolved fluorescence of lanthanide probes and applications in biotechnology. *Anal Chem*, 1987; **18**: 105–54.
9. Kricka LJ. Trends in immunoassay technologies. *J Immunoassay*, 1993; **16**: 267–71.
10. Robbins J, Rall JE. Thyroid hormone transport in blood and extravascular fluids. In: Gray CH, James VHT, eds. *Hormones in Blood*. London: Academic Press, 1979: 575–688.
11. Tait JF, Burstein S. *In vivo* studies of steroid dynamics in man. In: Pincus V, Thimann KV, Astwood EB, eds. *The Hormones*. New York: Academic Press, Vol **V**, 1964: 441–57.
12. Nanjee MN, Wheeler MJ. Plasma free testosterone–is an index sufficient?. *Ann Clin Biochem*, 1985; **22**: 387–90.
13. Vermeulen A, Verdonck L, Kaufman JM. A critical evaluation of simple methods for the estimation of free testosterone in serum. *J Clin Endocrinol Metab*, 1999; **84**: 3666–72.
14. Wood P. Salivary steroid assays–research or routine?. *Ann Clin Biochem*, 2009; **486**: 183–96.
15. Shackleton CH, Whitney JO. Use of Sep-pak cartridges for urinary steroid extraction: evaluation of the method for use prior to gas chromatographic analysis. *Clin Chim Acta*, 1980; **107**: 231–43.

16. Knox S, Harris J, Calton L, Wallace AM. A simple automated solid-phase extraction procedure for measurement of 25-hydroxyvitamin D_3 and D_2 by liquid chromatography-tandem mass spectrometry. *Ann Clin Biochem*, 2009; **46**: 226–30.
17. Xu RN, Fan L, Rieser MJ, El-Shourbagy TA. Recent advances in high-throughput quantitative bioanalysis by LC-MS/MS. *J Pharm Biomed Anal*, 2007; **44**: 342–55.
18. Thienpont LM, Van Nieuwenhove B, Stöckl D, Reinauer H, De Leenheer AP. Determination of reference method values by isotope dilution-gas chromatography/mass spectrometry: a five years' experience of two EuropeanReference Laboratories. *Eur J Clin Chem Clin Biochem*, 1966; **34**: 853–60.
19. Shackleton CH. Profiling steroid hormones and urinary steroids. *J Chromatogr*, 1986; **379**: 91–156.
20. Shackleton CH. Mass spectrometry in the diagnosis of steroid-related disorders and in hypertension research. *J Steroid Biochem Mol Biol*, 1993; **45**: 127–4.
21. Vogeser M, Seger C. A decade of HPLC-MS/MS in the routine clinical laboratory - goals for further developments. *Clin Biochem*, 2008; **41**: 649–62.
22. Vogeser M, Parhofer KG. Liquid chromatography tandem-mass spectrometry (LC-MS/MS)–Technique and Applications in Endocrinology. *Exp Clin Endocrinol Diabetes*, 2007; **115**: 559–70.
23. Turpeinen U, Linko S, Itkonen O, Hämäläinen E. Determination of testosterone in serum by liquid chromatography-tandem mass spectrometry. *Scand J Clin Lab Invest*, 2007; **68**: 50–7.
24. Maunsell Z, Wright DJ, Rainbow SJ. Routine isotope-dilution liquid chromatography-tandem mass spectrometry assay for simultaneous measurement of the 25-hydroxymetabolites of vitamins D2 and D3. *Clin Chem*, 2005; **51**: 1683–90.
25. McCann SJ, Gillingwater S, Keevil BG. Measurement of urinary free cortisol using liquid chromatography-tandem mass spectrometry: comparison with the urine adapted ACS:180 serum cortisol chemiluminescent immunoassay and development of a new reference range. *Ann Clin Biochem*, 2005; **42**: 112–8.
26. Shiraishi S, Lee PW, Leung A, Goh VH, Swerdloff RS, Wang C. Simultaneous measurement of serum testosterone and dihydrotestosterone by liquid chromatography-tandem mass spectrometry. *Clin Chem*, 2008; **54**: 1855–63.
27. Vogeser M, Groetzner J, Küpper C, Briegel J. The serum cortisol:cortisone ratio in the postoperative acute-phase response. *Horm Res*, 2003; **59**: 293–6.
28. de Jong WH, Graham KS, van der Molen JC, Links TP, Morris MR, Ross HA, *et al.* Plasma free metanephrine measurement using automated online solid-phase extraction HPLC tandem mass spectrometry. *Clin Chem*, 2007; **53**: 1684–93.
29. Fisker S, Edrup L, Orsko. Influence of growth hormone binding protein estimation in different immunoassays. *Scand J Clin Lab Invest*, 1998; **58**: 373–81.
30. Jones AM, Honour JW. Unusual results from immunoassays and the role of the clinical endocrinologist. *Clin Endocrinol (Oxf)*, 2006; **64**: 234–44.
31. Sadideen H, Swaminathan R. Macroprolactin: what is it and what is its importance?. *Int J Clin Pract*, 2006; **60**: 457–61.
32. Taieb J, Mathian B, Millot F, Patricot MC, Mathieu E, Queyrel N, *et al.* Testosterone measured by 10 immunoassays and by isotope-dilution gas chromatography-mass spectrometry in sera from 116 men, women, and children. *Clin Chem*, 2003; **49**: 1381–95.
33. Herold DA, Fitzgerald RL. Immunoassays for testosterone in women: better than a guess?. *Clin Chem*, 2003; **49**: 1250–1.
34. Rosner W, Auchus RJ, Azziz R, Sluss PM, Raff H. Utility, limitations, and pitfalls in measuring testosterone: an Endocrine Society position statement. *J Clin Endocrinol Metab*, 2007; **92**: 405–13.
35. Cavalier E, Wallace AM, Knox S, Mistretta VI, Cormier C, Souberbielle JC. Serum vitamin D measurement may not reflect what you give to your patients. *J Bone Miner Res*, 2008; **23**: 1864–5.
36. Annesley TM. Ion suppression in mass spectrometry. *Clin Chem*, 2003; **49**: 1041–44.

1.8

Endocrine disruptors

George Creatsas, George Mastorakos

Introduction

During the past 50 years, there has been a huge increase in the number of chemical substances used worldwide as plasticizers, pesticides, detergents, paints, metal food cans, flame retardants, cosmetics, and chemical wastes, which exhibit the potential to interfere with the endocrine system of humans and animals. In addition, it has been found that many natural plant products have the same features (i.e. phyto-oestrogens). The public health risks related to these substances have raised reasonable concerns. Thus, the so-called endocrine disruptors have become the target of major scientific research.

Definition

According to the US Environmental Protection Agency '"an endocrine disruptor" is an exogenous agent that interferes with the synthesis, secretion, transport, binding, action, or elimination of natural hormones in the body that are responsible for the maintenance of homeostasis, reproduction, development and/or behavior' (1). Many endocrine disrupters are biologically active at extremely low doses. Their effects on humans, wildlife, and the environment have been the focus of attention of the international scientific community, since they mimic endogenous hormones and are supposed to cause adverse health effects such as infertility, abnormal prenatal development, precocious or delayed puberty, thyroid dysfunction, obesity, behavioural disorders, and cancer. The scientific research is focused on three general principles that characterize the endocrine disruptors. First, the timing of exposure (as well as the 'time window' of exposure) seems to be critical for the outcome, since prenatal or early postnatal exposure could cause permanent malfunction of certain systems and could affect the individual throughout life. Second, endocrine disruptor have different dose–responses and act through different cellular mechanisms. Third, endocrine disruptors may affect the offspring of the exposed individual, via genomic or epigenetic modifications (2).

Historical background

Endocrine disruptors have been known to exist since the 1930s, when the oestrogenic action of some chemicals, including bisphenol-A (BPA), was shown in laboratory animals. Later, in the 1950s, another chemical pesticide, dichloro-diphenyl-trichloroethane (DDT), was reported to have feminizing effects in roosters. During the 1970s, the use of diethylstilbestrol (DES), a synthetic oestrogen, for the prevention of abortions was common. Later, it was found that the children of those women treated with DES developed serious disorders such as vaginal carcinomas and infertility. The use of DES is now prohibited (3).

Mechanisms of action

Endocrine disruptors interfere with the endocrine system, affecting the hormonal action, the hormonal concentration, or the hormonal receptor concentration. Exogenous compounds might have agonistic or antagonistic action when binding at a hormone receptor. If the endocrine disruptor binds at the binding site of a specific receptor with high affinity and activates it (agonistic action), the result is the same as that caused by the endogenous hormone. This is the most common mechanism of action of endocrine disruptors. They usually interact with the oestrogen receptor (i.e. BPA, DES), the androgen receptor (i.e. vinclozolin) and the aryl hydrocarbon receptor (i.e. dioxins). Other substances bind on the hormone receptor, resulting in a competitive or noncompetitive antagonistic action. In a competitive antagonistic action an endogenous agonist and an exogenous antagonist compete for the same active binding site. On the other hand, in a noncompetitive antagonistic action the antagonistic exogenous compound binds on an area of the receptor, other than the active binding site. The competitive antagonistic action usually leads to total deactivation of the receptor, while the noncompetitive antagonistic action causes the receptor to react slower or less efficiently. Typical antagonists for the binding site are the herbicides linuron and vinclozolin and their metabolites.

In addition, chemicals can affect the endocrine system by inhibiting enzyme-dependent chemical reactions (i.e. the aromatization of testosterone to oestrogen) by inducing hormone metabolizing enzymes (i.e. cytochrome P450 group) or by antagonizing the binding sites of the transport proteins (a reduction in the transfer proteins causes the concentration of the free/active hormone to increase). Finally, an endocrine disruptor could affect the hormone receptor concentration by down-regulation or by increasing the degradation rate of the receptor (4).

Common categories of endocrine disruptors and exposure routes

The most common categories of endocrine disruptors (Table 1.8.1) as well as their exposure routes are described below.

Table 1.8.1 Effects of endocrine disruptors on humans

Substances	Effects
In utero exposure	
PCBs	Neuromuscular disorders, lower intelligence quota, hypothalamus–pituitary–testis axis dysregulation
Dioxins	Low birthweight, skin discoloration, bronchitis, developmental retardation
Phenols	Irregular menstrual cycles
Phyto-oestrogens, xenoestrogens, substances with oestrogenic bioactivity	Ambiguous genitalia, obesity later in life, sexual differentiation problems, hormone-dependent cancers
DES	Transplacental carcinogenesis (cervico-vaginal cancer in female offspring)
DDT, DDE	Low T_4 levels in infants
PCP	Alters thyroid hormone levels and thus causes neurodevelopmental deficits
Nitrofen (pesticide)	Lung hypoplasia
Phthalate esters	Morphological abnormalities of male reproductive tract
Disruption in pubertal timing	
Lead	Delayed pubertal onset
PCBs, phyto-oestrogens, pesticides, BPA	Precocious female reproductive tract development
DDE, DDT	Earlier menarche
Disruption in reproduction	
BPA	Oocyte meiotic disturbances (i.e. aneuploidy), PCOS
Phyto-oestrogen, genistein	Altered cyclicity, prolonged and abnormal cycles
Dioxins (TCDD)	Endometriosis
DES	Suppress lactation
DDE, PCBs	Reduction of duration of lactation
Endocrine disruptors and cancer development	
Oestrogen-mimicking compounds	Breast cancer, testicular cancer
PCBs, arsenic	Prostate cancer
Pesticides (i.e. atrazine)	Ovarian cancer
Endocrine disruptors and thyroid function	
BPA, PCBs, phyto-oestrogens	Hypo- or hyperthyroidism
Endocrine disruptors and obesity	
PCBs, pesticides, phthalates, BPA, metals	Weight gain
Endocrine disruptors and various functions	
BPA, phthalates, dioxins	Alterations in blood glucose homoeostasis

BPA, bisphenol-A; DDE, dichloro-diphenyl-dichloroethylene; DDT, dichloro-diphenyl-trichloroethane; DES, diethylstilbestrol; PCB, polychlorinated biphenyls; PCP, pentachlorophenol; TCDD, 2,3,7,8-tetrachlorodibenzo-p-dioxin.

Modified from Mastorakos G, Karoutsou EI, Mizamtsidi M, Creatsas G. The menace of endocrine disruptors on thyroid hormone physiology and their impact on intrauterine development. *Endocrine*, 2007; **31**: 219–37 (5).

Polychlorinated biphenyls

Polychlorinated biphenyls (PCBs) are synthetic organic chemicals that were used as coolants and lubricants in transformers, capacitors, and other electrical equipment. The use of these substances was stopped in 1977, when scientists recognized their negative health effects. Today, these compounds may be found in old microscope oil, old hydraulic oil, old fluorescent lighting fixtures, or electrical devices that contain old PCB capacitors. One route of human exposure includes the inhalation of PCBs released in the air when old electrical devices get hot during operation. Another exposure route is through the ingestion of contaminated food or through skin exposure. Infants could be exposed to PCBs through their mother's breast milk during nursing.

Phthalate esters

Phthalate esters are chemicals that are commonly used in plastics, in products such as wall coverings, vacuum pumps, tablecloths, floor tiles, furniture upholstery, shower curtains, garden hoses, swimming pool liners, rainwear, baby pants, squeeze toys and dolls, shoes, automobile upholstery and tops, packaging film and sheets, sheathing for wire and cable, medical tubing, and blood storage bags. They are also used as an additive in cosmetics. There is potential risk for exposure due to inhalation, however, there is minimal risk of exposure associated with drinking water due to the fact that it does not dissolve readily in water. Phthalates can enter the body during certain medical procedures. The greatest risks are run during blood transfusions, kidney dialysis, intravenous fluid administration and when a respirator for breathing support is used.

Phenols—bisphenol A

BPA is a light plastic with unique toughness, optical clarity, and high heat and electrical resistance. It is used widely in eyeglass lenses, medical equipment, water bottles, CDs and DVDs, cell phones, computers, household appliances, reusable food and drink containers, safety shields, sports equipment, industrial floorings, industrial protective coatings, can coatings, and electrical equipment. Although BPA is considered to be biodegradable, there is some risk of BPA leaching out of the lining of cans, which could potentially contaminate the foods and liquids inside (6).

Dioxins

Dioxins form a group of hundreds of chemicals that are highly persistent in the environment. The most toxic compound is 2,3,7,8-tetrachlorodibenzo-*p*-dioxin (TCDD). Dioxin is formed as an unintentional byproduct of many industrial processes involving chlorine, such as waste incineration, chemical and pesticide manufacturing, and pulp and paper bleaching. The major sources of environmental dioxin are the various kinds of waste-burning incinerator. Dioxin pollution is also associated with paper mills, where chlorine bleaching is used in various processes. Dioxin is also present in the human diet; as it is fat soluble, it bioaccumulates, climbing up the food chain (7).

Pesticides/herbicides

Pesticides and herbicides such as atrazine, DDT and trifuralin were used widely in the past. Atrazine is a white powder that is used to protect grasses and broadleaf weeds from pests. It dissolves in water and is taken up by plants growing in the soil. Atrazine may be inhaled as a dust and ingested through contaminated drinking water, but it is not absorbed through the skin.

DDT is extremely hydrophobic and signficantly absorbed by soils. Depending on conditions, its soil half-life can range from 22 days to 30 years. Routes of loss and degradation include run-off, volatilization, photolysis as well as aerobic and anaerobic biodegradation. When applied to aquatic ecosystems it is quickly absorbed by organisms and by the soil, or it evaporates, leaving little DDT dissolved in the water itself. Its breakdown products and metabolites, DDE and DDD, also persist for long periods and have similar chemical and physical properties.

Trifluralin is used as a herbicide for controlling the growth of grasses and some broadleaf weeds in a wide variety of vegetables and some fruit. It is usually directly incorporated into soils, although some trifluralin mixtures may be sprayed. Trifluralin may enter the aquatic environment via diffuse sources, resulting from its recommended use, e.g. in agricultural run-off bound mainly to soil particles. Industrial discharges, accidental spillages during transport, storage, and use are potential point sources of trifluralin contamination.

Phyto-oestrogens

Phyto-oestrogens are a diverse group of naturally occurring nonsteroidal plant compounds that, because of their structural similarity with oestradiol (17-β-oestradiol), have the ability to cause oestrogenic or/and antioestrogenic effects. These compounds in plants are an important part of their defence system, mainly against fungi. Foods with the highest relative phyto-oestrogen content are nuts and oilseeds, followed by soya products, cereals and breads, legumes, meat products, and other processed foods that may contain soya, vegetables, fruits, and alcoholic and nonalcoholic beverages.

Effects of endocrine disruptors on *in utero* development

The effects of *in utero* exposure to endocrine disruptors are a subject of scientific research. There is evidence suggesting that exposure at critical time points ('time window') during fetal development could cause a number of disorders, most of which are not reversible. Several chemicals or classes of chemicals can cause neurodevelopmental alterations by interfering with neuroendocrine function, including PCBs, dioxins, metals, pesticides, phyto-oestrogens, synthetic steroids, and triazine herbicides. It seems plausible that any compound which mimics or antagonizes the action of neurotransmitters, hormones, and growth factors in the developing brain, could cause adverse effects in the fetal neurodevelopment. The nature of the nervous system deficit, which could include cognitive dysfunction, altered neurological development, or sensory deficits, depends on the severity of the thyroid disturbance and the specific developmental period when exposure to the chemical occurred (Fig. 1.8.1) (8).

The almost classical case for endocrine disruption *in utero* which leads to adult disease in the offspring is that of previously described prenatal exposure to DES. Studies have confirmed the association between maternal treatment with the hormone and cervicovaginal cancer in daughters. This was the first demonstration of transplacental carcinogenesis in humans. In addition to a small number of genital tract cancers, the daughters of DES-exposed mothers also had functional and anatomical abnormalities of the uterus and fallopian tubes, and fertility was also compromised (9).

In addition, studies have found neuromuscular disorders and lower IQ in newborns, associated with *in utero* exposure to PCBs. Recent studies have demonstrated that exposure to DDE and its metabolites during fetal development is negatively associated with cord serum T_4 levels in infants, emphasizing the need to further investigate the adverse effects on thyroid hormones, growth, and neural development in children exposed in early life to high doses of DDT (5). An additional study revealed neuromuscular disorders in infants associated with *in utero* and lactational exposure to PCBs. Moreover, a lower IQ was reported in children 4–11 years of age, prenatally exposed to PCBs (5). Another chemical that belongs to the phenols group and is related to BPA, pentachlorophenol (PCP), has been found to alter thyroid hormones levels in newborns and consequently may lead to adverse neurodevelopmental defects. One study has demonstrated that the pesticide Nitrofen induces lung hypoplasia in rat fetuses when administered to the mother during gestation (5).

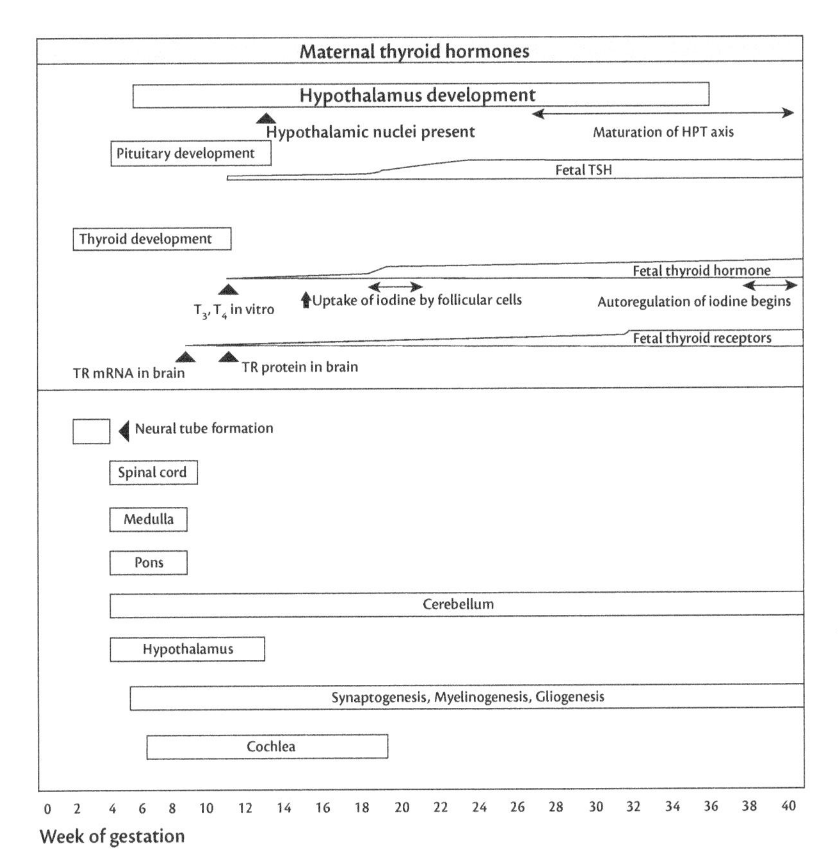

Fig. 1.8.1 Fetal development of the hypothalamus–pituitary–thyroid (HPT) axis components during gestation, with regard to the development of major thyroid hormone-dependent parts of the nervous system. It seems that exposure to endocrine disruptors at critical time points may induce irreversible disorders (5). TSH, thyroid stimulating hormone; TR, thyroid receptor.

A clinical study in Japan revealed that following contamination of rice oil with dioxins in 1968 in the city Yusho, significant adverse effects were observed in babies born to exposed women, including low birthweight, skin discoloration, bronchitis, and developmental retardation. Behavioural effects in the Yusho infants included hypoactivity and hypotony. Intrauterine exposure to dioxins causes a significant degree of thyroid dysfunction and affects development of newborns (5).

In addition, the maternal exposure to environmental pollutants during pregnancy and the high oestrogenic bioactivity in the serum of newborns strongly suggests that ambiguous genitalia are related to fetal exposure to endocrine disruptors (10). The literature states that perinatal exposure to BPA causes irregular cycles in mice, although there is not enough evidence of this in humans (11). Moreover, perinatal exposure to endocrine disruptors with oestrogenic activity is proposed to induce development of obesity later in life (12).

Phyto-oestrogens and xeno-oestrogens generally inhibit key steroidogenic enzymes, including 3β- and 17β- hydroxyl-steroid-dehydrogenase, aromatase, sulfatases, and sulfotransferases. There is also evidence that both phyto-oestrogens and xeno-oestrogens can modulate intracellular signalling pathways, thus inhibiting the synthesis and activity of steroidogenic enzymes. The ability of these compounds to modulate enzyme activity could be important in sexual differentiation and development as well as in the protection (or promotion) of hormone-dependent cancers (13).

In utero exposure to phthalate esters is associated with morphological abnormalities of the male reproductive tract, including decreased anogenital distance, cryptorchidism, hypospadias, diminished Leydig cell population, and decreased secretion of testicular testosterone. Testicular androgen signalling may also be impaired through suppression of the normal hypothalamus–pituitary–testis (HPTe) regulation of Leydig cell steroidogenesis. Disruption of the HPTe axis, resulting in low testicular testosterone levels, was demonstrated in the rat following exposure to a range of endocrine disruptors. Exposure to oestrogen-like DES impaired HPTe signalling in the rat, reducing plasma testosterone and increasing plasma follicle-stimulating hormone (FSH) levels. The HPTe axis was disrupted by PCB-169 exposure *in utero*, resulting in decreased spermatogenesis, Leydig cell number, and plasma testosterone levels in the rat. Atrazine, another herbicide that with antiandrogenic and oestrogenic properties, has been found to produce a number of adverse reproductive effects in the male rat. Atrazine was implicated in reduced secretion of testicular testosterone in males. Atrazine has a low affinity for androgen and oestrogen receptors, reduces androgen synthesis and enhances oestrogen production via the induction of aromatase. Both Leydig and Sertoli cells represent an intratesticular source of oestrogens via androgen aromatization (14).

Effects of endocrine disruptors on timing of puberty (female and male)

Recent studies have revealed the role of endocrine disruptors on the onset of puberty. Animal studies have demonstrated that both male and female pubertal timing is vulnerable to endocrine disruptors, particularly compounds that have oestrogenic or antiandrogenic effects (15). Endocrine disruptors can disturb the hypothalamic–pituitary–gonadal axis through negative feedback mechanisms as well as direct effects both centrally (hypothalamus and pituitary) and peripherally (ovary and testis). The effects may be seen after gestational, lactational, or juvenile exposure. Lead exposure has been shown to be associated with delayed pubertal onset, while phyto-oestrogen, PCBs, pesticides, and BPA exposure was related to precocious female development. On the other hand, transient neonatal androgen exposure resulted in reduced testis weight and testosterone production in rodents (16).

Another study revealed that exposure of adolescent girls in Canada to certain chemicals such as PCBs with potential oestrogenic features and lead may affect attainment of menarche. Lead was associated with a later median predicted age at menarche, when controlling for other toxicants, age, and socioeconomic status. However, at much higher or lower levels of lead and/or PCBs, different effects may occur (17).

Age at menarche is reduced in girls exposed to oestrogenic organochlorines, but the exact contribution of these substances to precocious menarche is unknown because of the numerous environmental variables influencing menarche. A study of women exposed to DDE through consumption of Great Lakes fish found a 1-year reduction in age at menarche for each increase of 15 mg/l serum DDE. Another study in Chinese textile workers showed that a 10 mg/l serum DDT increase was associated with 0.2-year reduction in menarcheal age (11).

Effects of endocrine disruptors on reproduction (female and male)

The impact of exposure to environmental contaminants on human fertility remains controversial. However, many studies have illuminated some aspects of the impact of endocrine disruptors on human reproduction. First, the ovarian effects of the exposure to endocrine disruptors will be discussed. Ten years ago, an observation that mice housed in damaged polycarbonate plastic cages had a high incidence of oocytes with meiotic disturbances led to investigations into the oocyte-damaging effect of the oestrogenic plasticizer BPA. It was determined that BPA was leaching into the water of animals in damaged cages, and when BPA purposely was added to the water in nondamaged cages similar oocyte meiotic disturbances were induced. Some of these meiotic disturbances resulted in aneuploidy. Experimental data from three different laboratories supported the conclusion that BPA exposure has a detrimental impact on the maturing oocyte. Besides BPA, other endocrine disruptors, such as DES, have been shown to cause meiotic disturbances.

Another common disturbance of ovarian function is the polycystic ovary syndrome (PCOS). An endocrine disruptor that has been associated with PCOS is BPA. BPA has been measured in serum and follicular fluid (1–2 ng/ml), as well as in fetal serum and term amniotic fluid, confirming passage through the placenta. There is a significant increase in serum BPA levels in women with PCOS. These results may partly prove the association of BPA with PCOS.

In addition, human cyclicity seems to be affected by endocrine disruptors. Experimental studies of exposure of neonatal mice to physiologically relevant concentrations of the phyto-oestrogen genistein causes prolonged and abnormal cycles in adult animals. In humans, altered cyclicity has been linked to adult exposures to persistent organic pollutants and contemporary pesticides. Studies examining the influence of organochlorine pesticide exposure on cyclicity and fecundity suggest that organochlorine exposure shortens the menstrual cycle, whereas women who are exposed to hormonally active pesticides (nonorganochlorine) have a 60–100% increased risk of long cycles, intermenstrual bleeding, and missed periods (18).

Second, endocrine disruptors cause structural changes in the human uterus. There are data implicating a role of endocrine disruptors in the development of uterine fibroids (leiomyomas). The consumption of phyto-oestrogens in a study conducted in Japanese women found that individuals consuming soya had a decreased incidence of hysterectomy. Considering that the principal diagnosis in women undergoing a hysterectomy is uterine fibroids, this study suggests a protective effect of modest phyto-oestrogen consumption (9).

The association between endometriosis and endocrine disruptors is still not clear. It has been shown that nonhuman primates exposed to the widespread environmental contaminant TCDD have a high rate of endometriosis. A recent evaluation of the cohort of women exposed to massive doses of dioxin after a chemical accident in Seveso, Italy, does not support these earlier findings in nonhuman primates (9). However, data linking organochlorine exposure and endometriosis in humans are equivocal, with some studies reporting significant correlations and others failing to find any significant relationship (11).

Finally, it seems that there is a correlation between exposure to endocrine disruptors and lactation. It is well known that exogenous oestrogens such as DES will effectively suppress lactation (9). Duration of lactation is reduced in women with elevated serum concentrations of PCBs and DDE. The effect of DDE and PCBs on duration of lactation is dose-dependent, with each additional part per million increase in serum concentration being associated with a 1-week reduction in lactation duration (11).

As far as the male reproductive system is concerned, there is a significant body of toxicological data based on laboratory and wildlife studies suggesting that exposure to certain endocrine disruptors is associated with reproductive toxicity, including abnormalities of the male reproductive tract (cryptorchidism, hypospadias), reduced semen quality, and impaired fertility in the adult. Endocrine disruption of spermatogenesis may occur by four mechanisms, including: (1) epigenetic changes to the genome; (2) apoptosis of germ cells; (3) dysregulation of androgenic signalling; and (4) disruption of Sertoli and other spermatogenesis supporting cells (14). The effects of some endocrine disruptors and their relation to male reproductive anomalies are presented in Table 1.8.2.

Effects of endocrine disruptors on cancer development

There is increasing concern about development of cancer after exposure to endocrine disruptors. Gestational and perinatal exposures to endocrine disruptors may have long-term effects on the endocrine system that can influence tumour development later in life. That a synthetic oestrogen such as DES could cause cancer in offspring should not be surprising, given that even elevated levels of natural oestrogens during gestation have been associated with an increase in breast cancer in the children later in life (18).

Developmental toxicants of the mammary gland may lead to an increase in the incidence of mammary tumours if they alter

Table 1.8.2 Effects of endocrine disruptors in male fertility

Compound	Outcome
Dibromochloropropane	Azoospermia and oligospermia
	Decreased motility and morphology
	Elevated FSH and LH
	Deficit of male births
Ethylene dibromide	Decreased sperm counts
Chlordecone (kepone)	Oligospermia, decreased sperm motility
Perchloroethylene	Dose-related morphological changes
Carbaryl	Impaired semen quality
Ethylene glycol ethers	Decreased sperm counts
	Decreased fertility
TCDD	Reduced serum testosterone, increased LH
	Deficit of male births
p-nitrophenol	Decreased sperm concentration
	Decreased percentage of motile sperm
	Increased serum LH

FSH, follicle-stimulating hormone; LH, luteinizing hormone; TCDD, 2,3,7,8-tetrachlorodibenzo-p-dioxin.

circulating or tissue-localized hormone levels, gland receptor expression patterns, hormone transport, or metabolism that results in altered response to endogenous hormones or growth factors. Many environmental chemicals with oestrogenic activity have been measured in the human breast and this could be associated to increased incidence of breast cancer. However, although animal models seem to support this point of view, studies are required to clarify the effects of endocrine disruptors on human mammary gland. The impact of multiple estrogen-mimicking compounds, as well as the dose to which the gland is more susceptible needs to be investigated. In addition, research is needed to determine whether the type of endocrine disruptor is an independent carcinogenic factor, or the exposure time and route are the most important factors in the development of neoplasia.

Studies conducted in the 1990s did not provide any significant evidence of association of PCBs exposure and breast cancer. In addition to these data, no association was found between DDT, its metabolite DDE and breast cancer, but further studies are needed. The role of phyto-oestrogens in the risk of developing breast cancer is controversial. Some studies have demonstrated that there may be an association with breast cancer, whereas others have found these compounds to have protective effects (19).

Although the initial thought that testicular cancer may be related to early life-stage exposure to environmental oestrogens and/or antiandrogens seemed logical, there is little evidence to support this notion. There is currently no compelling evidence that exposure to environmental oestrogenic or other hormonally active substances is contributing to the rise in testicular cancer incidence observed in Western countries over the past several decades; however, this question has not been extensively studied. Several factors have greatly hindered the understanding of environmental influences on the risk of testicular cancer: the rarity of this condition, the long lag time between the presumed sensitive period during fetal development and clinical appearance of the condition, and the lack of a good animal model to study the progression of the disease (20).

There is increasing evidence both from epidemiology studies and animal models that specific endocrine disruptors may influence the development or progression of prostate cancer. In large part, these effects appear to be linked to oestrogen signalling, either through interactions with endocrine disruptors or by influencing steroid metabolism and altering oestrogen levels in the body. In human studies, PCBs and inorganic arsenic exposure have been associated with an elevated risk of prostate cancer. However, this risk seems to exist only if the exposure took place during critical developmental 'time windows' (*in utero*, neonatal, puberty). Thus, infants and children may be considered as a highly susceptible population with regard to exposure to endocrine disruptors and the increased risk of prostate cancer on ageing (21).

Another cancer whose development is directly related to the action of some hormones is ovarian cancer. Pesticides with endocrine-disrupting activity remain in use in different countries. Scientific research to date suggests a link between atrazine and risk of ovarian cancer, and other environmental and occupational exposures may also be associated with ovarian cancer. It remains to be determined whether these risks can be modified by hormone use or genetic susceptibility (22).

Effects of endocrine disruptors on thyroid function

The existence of thyroid-disrupting chemicals has been confirmed through many animal and human studies. The disruption occurs at many different levels of thyroid hormone synthesis, binding, action, and metabolism. It has been demonstrated that the most common endocrine disruptors that affect thyroid function are BPA, pentachlorophenol, PCBs, and phyto-oestrogens. These compounds usually influence the hypothalamus–pituitary–thyroid axis, sodium-iodide symporter, thyroid-binding protein, the enzyme thyroperoxidase and many other sites. It seems possible that the endocrine disruptors that affect the thyroid could cause hypo- or hyperthyroidism, thyroid nodules and thyroid tumorigenesis. However, the limited data does not allow making reasonable conclusions about the effects of endocrine disruptors on thyroid function, and more scientific research is of crucial importance (5, 23).

Effects of endocrine disruptors on obesity development

The role of environmental chemicals in the development of obesity is an emerging area of research that is focusing on the identification of obesogens. Although until now data have been scant, some epidemiological and *in vitro* studies have suggested a link between environmental chemical exposure and obesity. Endocrine disruptors mimic natural lipophilic hormones that mediate their effects through members of the nuclear receptor transcription factors superfamily. Environmental estrogenic chemicals, such as BPA and nonylphenol, can promote adipocyte differentiation or proliferation of murine preadipocyte cell lines. Recently, studies have shown that chemicals including pesticides, organophosphates, polychlorinated biphenyls, polybrominated biphenyls, phthalates, BPA, heavy metals and solvents might cause weight gain possibly by interfering with weight homoeostasis via alterations in weight-controlling hormones, altered sensitivity to neurotransmitters, or altered activity of the sympathetic nervous system. However, more research is needed in this area (24).

Effects of endocrine disruptors on other body functions (autoimmunity, blood glucose homoeostasis)

It has been shown that endocrine disruptors might affect other systems such as the immune system and the endocrine pancreas. For example, some data suggest that EDs are involved in autoantibody production by B1 cells and could be an aetiologic factor in the development of autoimmune diseases. Other studies suggest that levels of BPA, phthalates, dioxins, and persistent organic pollutants are correlated with alterations of blood glucose homoeostasis in humans. However, these initial data about endocrine disruptor activity must be interpreted with caution (25, 26).

Conclusion

The impact of endocrine disruptors has been a matter of concern since the past 50 years. However, the results of the research remain controversial. This is because of the multitude of environmental effects on humans and because the genetic make-up of every individual is different, and the endocrine disruptor exposure duration and route may determine the outcome. In addition, the exact time point of the exposure is crucial. *In utero* exposure seems to cause irreversible outcomes. Moreover, experimental studies may not agree with studies in humans because exposure to endocrine disruptors varies and laboratory animals (rats, rodents, etc.) may also react differently. However, more experimental research is needed to clarify the possible mechanisms of action of endocrine disruptors.

References

1. U.S. Environmental Protection Agency. *Special Report on Environmental Endocrine Disruption: An Effects Assessment and Analysis.* EPA/630/R-96/012. Washington, DC: Office of Research and Development, 1997. Available at: http://www.epa.gov/raf/publications/pdfs/ENDOCRINE.PDF (accessed 14 December 2008).
2. Gore AC, Heindel JJ, Zoeller RT. Endocrine disruption for endocrinologists (and others). *Endocrinology*, 2006; **147**(Suppl 3): S1–3.
3. Solomon GM, Schettler T. Environment and health: 6. Endocrine disruption and potential human health implications. *CMAJ*, 2000; **163**: 1471–6.
4. Lintelmann J, Katayama A, Kurihara N, Shore L, Wenzel A. Endocrine disruptors in the environment. *Pure Appl Chem*, 2003; **75**: 631–81.
5. Mastorakos G, Karoutsou EI, Mizamtsidi M, Creatsas G. The menace of endocrine disruptors on thyroid hormone physiology and their impact on intrauterine development. *Endocrine*, 2007; **31**: 219–37.
6. Fall semester. PubH 5103: Exposure to environmental hazards. Endocrine disruptors. *Exposure Pathway, 2003*. Available at: http://enhs.umn.edu/current/5103/endocrine/pathwayofexposure.html (accessed 14 December 2008).
7. *Dioxin Homepage*. Available at: http://www.ejnet.org/dioxin/ (accessed 14 December 2008).
8. Tilson HA. Developmental neurotoxicology of endocrine disruptors and pesticides: identification of information gaps and research needs. *Environ Health Perspect*, 1998; **106**(Suppl 3): 807–11.
9. McLachlan JA, Simpson E, Martin M. Endocrine disrupters and female reproductive health. *Best Pract Res Clin Endocrinol Metab*, 2006; **20**: 63–75.
10. Paris F, Jeandel C, Servant N, Sultan C. Increased serum estrogenic bioactivity in three male newborns with ambiguous genitalia: a potential consequence of prenatal exposure to environmental endocrine disruptors. *Environ Res*, 2006; **100**: 39–43.
11. Crain DA, Janssen SJ, Edwards TM, Heindel J, Ho SM, Hunt P, *et al.* Female reproductive disorders: the roles of endocrine-disrupting compounds and developmental timing. *Fertil Steril*, 2008; **90**: 911–40.
12. Newbold RR, Padilla-Banks E, Snyder RJ, Jefferson WN. Perinatal exposure to environmental estrogens and the development of obesity. *Mol Nutr Food Res*, 2007; **51**: 912–17.
13. Whitehead S, Rice S. Endocrine-disrupting chemicals as modulators of sex steroid synthesis. *Best Pract Res Clinic Endocrin Metab*, 2006; **20**: 45–61.
14. Phillips KP, Tanphaichitr N. Human exposure to endocrine disrupters and semen quality. *J Toxicol Environ Health B Crit Rev*, 2008; **11**: 188–220.
15. Goldman JM, Laws SC, Balchak SK, Cooper RL, Kavlock RJ. Endocrine-disrupting chemicals: prepubertal exposures and effects on sexual maturation and thyroid activity in the female rat. A focus on the EDSTAC recommendations. *Crit Rev Toxicol Mar*, 2000; **30**: 135–96.
16. Jacobson-Dickman E, Lee MM. The influence of endocrine disruptors on pubertal timing. *Curr Opin Endocrinol Diabetes Obes*, 2009; **16**: 25–30.
17. Denham M, Schell LM, Deane G, Gallo MV, Ravenscroft J, DeCaprio AP. Relationship of lead, mercury, mirex, dichlorodiphenyldichloroethylene, hexachlorobenzene, and polychlorinated biphenyls to timing of menarche among Akwesasne Mohawk girls. *Pediatrics*, 2005; **115**: 127–34.
18. Soto A, Maffini M, Sonnenschein C. Neoplasia as development gone awry: the role of endocrine disruptors. *Int J Androl*, 2008; **31**: 288–93.
19. Salehi F, Turner MC, Phillips KP, Wigle DT, Krewski D, Aronson KJ. Review of the etiology of breast cancer with special attention to organochlorines as potential endocrine disruptors. *J Toxicol Environ Health B Crit Rev*, 2008; **11**: 276–300.
20. Garner M, Turner MC, Ghadirian P, Krewski D, Wade M. Testicular cancer and hormonally active agents. *J Toxicol Environ Health B Crit Rev*, 2008; **11**: 260–75.
21. Prins GS. Endocrine disruptors and prostate cancer risk. *Endocr Relat Cancer*, 2008; **15**: 649–56.
22. Salehi F, Dunfield L, Phillips K, Krewski D, Vanderhyden B. Risk factors for ovarian cancer: an overview with emphasis on hormonal factors. *J Toxic Environ Health, B Crit Rev*, 2008; **11**: 301–21.
23. Crofton KM. Thyroid disrupting chemicals: mechanisms and mixtures. *Int J Androl*, 2008; **31**: 209–23.
24. Grun F, Blumberg B. Environmental obesogens: organotins and endocrine disruption via nuclear receptor signaling. *Endocrinology*, 2006; **147**(Suppl 6): S50–5.
25. Ropero A, Alonso-Magdalena P, Garcia-Garcia E, Ripoll C, Fuentes E, Nadal A. Bisphenol-A disruption of the endocrine pancreas and blood glucose homeostasis. *Int J Androl*, 2008; **31**: 194–200.
26. Yurino H, Ishikawa S, Sato T, Akadegawa K, Ito T, Ueha S, *et al.* Endocrine disruptors (environmental estrogens) enhance autoantibody production by B1 cells. *Toxicol Sci*, 2004; **81**: 139–47.

1.9

Sports endocrinology: the use and abuse of performance-enhancing hormones and drugs

Leonard John Deftos and Mark Zeigler

Introduction

The endocrine system pervades all of sports, just as it pervades all of biology and medicine. The importance of endocrine glands and their hormonal products and effects in sports is axiomatic to the endocrinologist, and the actions in athletic activity of key hormones such as adrenaline are even known to much of the lay public. The other chapters in this textbook provided a systematic review of the effects of these hormones on organ systems, including those involved in sports as well as in health and disease. This chapter will only provide brief review of endocrine physiology that is relevant to sports. Such reviews can be readily found in other publications (1) as well as in the other chapters of this book. This chapter will instead focus on the role of hormones in the international sports arena, an arena that is populated by professional athletes, aspiring athletes, and the weekend warrior public of essentially all countries.

Unlike classic endocrinology, where primarily endogenous hormones play a role in both health and disease, exogenous hormones taken supraphysiologically as well as physiologically have a major role in contemporary sports endocrinology (2). Consequently, sports endocrinology often collides with the administrative, regulatory, and legal bodies that reside at its intersection with sports events (2, 3). While systematic research will inform the basis of much of this chapter, anecdotes taken from sport can also be provocative if not informative (3). For example, consider the role of thyroid hormone replacement in the athlete who has hypothyroidism, a situation recently manifest by a pitcher in major league baseball who had surgery for thyroid cancer. Without much research support, the temptation exists to try to enhance this athlete's performance by increasing his thyroid hormone dose before he is scheduled to pitch. At the other end of this particular spectrum is the athlete who chronically abuses androgens. Cases that also challenge the endocrinologist can fall in between these two extremes, such as glucose regulation for a diabetic footballer between games and during games and the cricketer who uses amphetamines intermittently.

While the use of hormones is at the centre of classic endocrinology, the medical periphery that is the ambit of some of sports endocrinology lurches beyond, into exercise pills and gene doping (1–4). It will become apparent that there is a paucity of controlled studies that demonstrate performance-enhancing effects of most of the agents abused by athletes (5). However, when all of the evidence is examined, exogenous androgens and perhaps growth hormone do seem to enhance athletic performance.

The central nervous system and pituitary hormones

The central nervous system–pituitary axis and its hypothalamic pathways, as the master regulatory system of endocrine function, play an important role in sports activity (6). The onset of such activity is accompanied by an acute increase in the secretion of adrenocorticotropin (ACTH) and growth hormone. The central nervous system origin of this secretory pattern seems to be mediated through the dorsomedial hypothalamus (7). In addition to the target organ action of each of these pituitary hormones, there is also an increase in cardiorespiratory function that accompanies central activation of the sympathetic axis (7, 8). The relationship of sports and exercise and the other pituitary hormones seem lesser and on a more chronic basis if at all.

Increased secretions of endorphins, oxytocin, vasopressin, and prolactin have been reported in sports activities, but the findings have been inconsistent (9, 10). The endorphins are postulated to counter the effects of stress during exercise, an action that might be shared with oxytocin and prolactin. But there is no good evidence that exercise-related euphoria, such as the runner's high, is associated with endogenous endorphins (11). Vasopressin acts to regulate fluid homoeostasis during exercise and sports activities, along with aldosterone and the natriuretic peptides. There is little evidence of the abuse of these hormones by athletes. However, electrolyte abnormalities can occur during sports activity. Interestingly, rather than hypernatraemia caused by excessive sweating, it is hyponatraemia induced by overhydration that is more likely to be problematic (12).

ACTH and the adrenal axis

The ACTH-adrenal axis is the major regulator of responses to perturbed homoeostasis. While there are distinct regulatory pathways and actions of adrenomedullary and adrenocortical hormones, there is both remote and recent evidence of a unitary sympathoadrenal system that involves circulating levels of ACTH, corticosteroids, and catecholamines of both adrenal and peripheral origin (8). These hormones are acutely increased during sports activities, where they exert their actions on organ systems and metabolic pathways that are invoked in exercise. As will be discussed later, forms of all of them, such as ephedrine and amphetamines, are abused by athletes.

Growth hormone

Growth hormone is well known to directly and indirectly regulate the growth and proliferation of most tissues. The exercise-related increase seen in growth hormone secretion produces the well-described metabolic effects of this hormone, which include gluconeogenesis and increased glucose metabolism, lipolysis, and increased fat metabolism, and proteolysis and increased protein metabolism. Skeletal muscle activity is nourished by these actions of growth hormone (13). In addition to these acute effects of growth hormone, there is a more chronic increase in muscle and bone mass, which is also mediated by the growth factors that are stimulated by growth hormone, notably insulin-like growth factor 1 (IGF-1) (14). In addition to growth hormone, there is evidence that IGF-1 itself is being used to enhance athletic performance, either alone, or in combination with growth hormone (13, 14).

The sports- and exercise-related actions of growth hormone have been best appreciated in growth hormone-deficient states. Exercise capacity and muscle strength are impaired in growth hormone deficiency, and physiological replacement therapy of growth hormone returns these parameters toward normal (15). Vigorous exercise regimens can magnify the growth hormone response to sports activity (16).

While administration of supraphysiological doses of growth hormone recapitulates the metabolic effects described above, there is little convincing evidence that these metabolic effects result in improved athletic performance. In fact, people with acromegaly increase their exercise capacity on successful treatment, which lowers growth hormone levels (17). Nevertheless, growth hormone abuse by athletes is widespread, and there is evidence that the administration of testosterone along with growth hormone does improve exercise performance and strength, especially in elderly subjects (5, 13). The growth hormone excess of acromegaly has only transient effects on sports activities. Andre the Giant (André René Roussimoff) was notoriously able to capitalize on these effects during a brief career as a wrestler. He chose not to be treated for his known pituitary tumour. However, he eventually succumbed to the complications of growth hormone excess that include hypertension, coronary artery disease, and diabetes mellitus (17). Malignancy is also a potential risk of growth hormone excess.

Gonadotropins

One of the most common athletic complications of pituitary function is the amenorrhoea seen in elite female athletes (18); in addition, delayed but normally progressing puberty can be seen in gymnasts (19). Since the gonadotropins do not seem to have a direct effect on exercise and sport but rather mediate their actions through their target hormones, these issues are discussed under gonadal steroids. But exercise-induced amenorrhoea is accompanied by decreases in gonadotropin-releasing hormone (GnRH) pulses from the hypothalamus and the consequent decrease in luteinizing hormone and follicle-stimulating hormone (18). A substantial number of such female athletes also have anorexia and bulimia. This can culminate in what has been termed the female athlete triad of osteoporosis, amenorrhoea, and eating disorders (18, 19).

Thyrotropin

The major effect of thyrotropin (thyroid-stimulating hormone (TSH)) in regulating the production and secretion of thyroid hormones by the thyroid gland is well known, and there is some recent evidence that TSH can have direct effects on its own (20). Although thyroid hormones are important in all metabolic pathways that underlie sports activity and exercise, most studies fail to show any remarkable changes in TSH and thyroid hormones during athletic activity, and they have has not found wide use of TSH as a drug of sports abuse (2, 3).

The calcaemic hormones and the skeletal system

The skeletal system plays an obviously important supporting role in athletic activity. However, the regulation of skeletal and calcium homoeostasis by the three calcaemic hormones—parathyroid hormone (PTH), calcitonin, and vitamin D—does not seem to manifest any substantial and acute changes during sports activities (21). The same holds true for calcium and magnesium concentrations. There are, however, some chronic changes of skeletal mass that correspond to the changes in muscle mass that can be readily appreciated in some sports, such as in the increased bone and muscle mass in the dominant arm of tennis players (22). But these changes are primarily mediated by the anabolic hormones, as discussed later. Exercise regimens, especially early in life, can results in an increase in peak bone mass, an effect that can be sustained by continuing exercise but diminishes with reduced exercise (22). Amenorrhoea, even when exercise related, can have the deleterious skeletal effect of reducing bone mass (18, 21).

Thyroid gland

The two thyroid hormones, thyroxine (T_4) and triiodothyronine (T_3), have actions on essentially every organ system in the body and notable muscle (20). While there are important sports-related actions by thyroid hormones on all organ systems, especially skeletal and cardiac muscle, these effects are not generally reflected by any consistent changes in circulating levels of the hormones during exercise. However, especially relevant to sports, peripheral muscle weakness and cardiac muscle dysfunction are seen in both hyperthyroidism and hypothyroidism. Since both conditions can be readily treated, the thyroid axis cannot be commonly blamed for impairing sports activity. Appropriate treatment of hyperthyroid and hypothyroidism maintains athletic performance. Abuse of thyroid hormone is more commonly seen in attempts to control weight and while this can occur in a sports context, it occurs more widely in the general population (2, 20).

The pancreatic hormones

The pancreatic hormones play a well-known role in glucose homoeostasis (23). Among the major pancreatic hormones, insulin and glucagon have sports-related significance. They served their well-known action in glucose metabolism of providing fuel, especially for muscles, during athletic activity. Insulin's general anabolic properties are important in maintaining the requisite integrity of exercise-related organ systems, especially muscle and bone. The anabolic activity of insulin provides the rationalization used by athletes to abuse insulin in their training regimens (1, 2). But, like most hormones, there is no convincing evidence that insulin enhances performance. Furthermore, insulin puts the abuser at great risk for hypoglycaemia. Of course, people with diabetes are expected to use insulin at all times, even during competitive sports activities (2).

The adrenal glands

The pleiotropic actions of cortisol are well- known. Equally well known is the fact that ACTH-stimulated cortisol levels increase during exercise and that there is a direct correlation between this increase and the intensity of the exercise (8). Along with the adrenergic axis, cortisol is a major participant in long-recognized and well-known fight or flight response. It is not then surprising that corticosteroids are among the most widely abused drugs in sport. This despite the fact that performance has not been shown to be improved by the administration of supraphysiological doses of cortisol (24). Furthermore, glucocorticoids used chronically decrease muscle mass and increase bone resorption, both of which are harmful, especially for athletes (6, 21, 24, 25). This abuse is complicated by the fact that there are legitimate uses of corticosteroids in sport, such as their intra-articular injection and use in asthmatic people. This widespread use results in a substantial incidence of adrenal gland suppression in athletes, best documented for cyclists.

The gonadal steroids

Sex steroids, also produced in lesser amounts in the adrenal cortex, have profound anabolic effects on most organ systems, especially bone and muscle. These effects are chronic, and exercise is not associated with a substantial increase in endogenous testosterone. (25). Nevertheless, androgens are among the most commonly abused drugs in sport. Athletes attempt to take advantage of their anabolic effects on the musculoskeletal system in order to enhance performance (1, 2). Early studies evaluated the relationship between performance parameters and physiological concentrations of testosterone and found no substantial relationship to muscle strength; however, later studies demonstrated a correlation with muscle strength and serum testosterone levels that exceed the normal range (26). In the male with hypogonadism, muscle mass is decreased and athletic ability impaired. In the male with precocious puberty and increased testosterone, muscle mass is increased. Both conditions can be ameliorated by appropriate treatment (2, 25, 26).

Conversely, impaired estrogen production in the exercising female is a major problem in sport for several reasons (18). Athletic-related amenorrhoea is seen in elite female athletes such as swimmers, runners, ballerinas, and gymnasts. Even eumenorrhoeic female athletes can have anovulatory cycles. Delayed puberty is common in this group of female athletes. (19) The low or absent oestrogens in such females leads to the failure to achieve peak bone mass and/or the development of osteoporosis, infertility, and abnormalities in lipid metabolism, which increase coronary heart disease risk. Oestrogen administration can be useful in reversing these abnormalities, but the reversal is often incomplete, especially as it relates to bone mass (18, 21).

Other endocrine organs

In addition to the classic endocrine organs, other organs secrete chemicals that have all of the characteristics of hormones. Most notable is erythropoietin (EPO) from the kidney. By increasing red blood cell mass, EPO helps to deliver oxygen, especially to active muscles (27). This regulatory pathway is abused by athletes in two ways, by the direct administration of EPO and by blood transfusion, called blood doping (2, 3). These forms of abuse are common among cyclists; here evidence for sustaining athletic activity is reasonably convincing despite the absence of controlled studies (3, 27).

Transgender issues

Sports activities have been classically divided according to gender in order to accommodate the seeming inherent performance advantages that males have over females (28). This gender difference can be largely attributed to the differences in muscle mass and circulating concentrations of testosterone found in males and females. Androgen administration to female to male transsexuals and androgen deprivation of male to female transsexuals can attenuate these differences in muscle mass (25, 26). For male to female transsexuals, anti-androgens are usually combined with oestrogens. Commonly used antiandrogens are cyproterone acetate and medroxyprogesterone. Finasteride, while an antiandrogen, is banned by the International Olympic Committee (IOC). Long-acting GnRH can also be used for male to female transsexuals. Testosterone is the common treatment for female to male transsexuals. These hormonal ministrations have the desired phenotypic results after about 1 year of treatment, but effects on athletic performance are more difficult to quantitate (28).

Chromosomal sex, specifically the determination of Barr bodies in buccal smears, had been commonly used to make the male to female distinction in athletes (2, 28). However, it has become increasingly appreciated that the male–female dichotomy for gender is an oversimplification and that there are many athletes, as well as nonathletes, who can be loosely categorized as intersex. Many sports organizations, most notably the IOC, but other international and national sports bodies as well, now allow sex-reassigned transsexuals to compete with members of their new sex if they meet certain criteria (28). In addition to hormonal administration, gonadectomy and legal recognition of newly assigned sex is required for athletic participation. It should be noted that sex steroid administration is generally prohibited otherwise for participants in competitive sports.

Performance-enhancing genetics and gene doping

In most instances, hormones are usually given as a pill or injection, and the hormones so delivered at a relatively short time of action (2). The identification and isolation of specific genes that encode

Box 1.9.1 Potential gene doping targets and agents

- Nervous system
- Endorphins and enkephalins—for pain and mood
- Oxytocin and vasopressin—for mood
- Cardiovascular
- Vascular endothelia growth factors—for vascularity
- Erythropoietin—for oxygen delivery
- Muscle
- Growth hormone—for muscle proliferation
- IGF-1—for growth and repair
- Myostatin—for muscle mass
- PPARδ—for muscle metabolism
- Mechano-growth factor—for repair
- Joints
- Interleukin 1 receptor agonist—for lubrication

peptides and proteins, including hormones, has led to the development of molecular methods that allow for the administration of these genes to experimental animals as well as patients (3). These genes can then express their product and provide a sustained amount to the recipient.

While this methodology can be effective in genetic treatment of disease, it could also be used to introduce to the recipient genes that encode for performance and enhancing agents–gene doping (2–4). Although there are other genetic procedures that can be used to enhance athletic performance, gene doping is the closest to realization. In fact, the World Anti-Doping Agency (WADA), formed in 1999, has identified gene doping as the nontherapeutic use of genes, genetic elements, and/or cells which have the capacity to enhance athletic performance (Box 1.9.1).

Although there has not been a confirmed episode of gene doping in sports, WADA has prohibited the technique for competing athletes worldwide. Many hormones with putative performance enhancing characteristics, such as growth hormone, are susceptible to such techniques that could be used in performance enhancement. As the medical use of gene therapy progresses, it is likely that unscrupulous athletes from all countries will appropriate the methodology for performance enhancement (2, 4).

Genetic variations that can confer extraordinary increases in bone and muscle mass are largely unknown (29). While the effects of increased bone mass on athletic ability is not well defined, the advantage that increased muscle mass can have in sport is well known (4). Some of the genes responsible for increased muscle mass, such as myostatin, have been identified. This opens the door to the use of gene doping to confer athletic advantage at local, regional, national, and international venues (30).

Exercise pills

The importance of exercise for athletic ability, as well as for the treatment of some diseases, is obvious. But the discipline necessary for regular exercise is often wanting. Agents have been recently identified that could serve as exercise mimetics by regulating the metabolic and contractile properties of muscle (29). These agents are based on the role for both the peroxisome-proliferator-activated receptor δ (PPARδ) and AMP-activated protein kinase in regulating muscle function. Both regulate the expression of oxidative genes in muscles and the metabolic phenotype of myofibres by causing a conversion from fast twitch type II myofibres to slow twitch type I myofibres fibres, which are able to perform sustained aerobic work, a conversion that is also caused by exercise. A PPAPδ agonist, named GW1516, given to exercising mice can increase the expression of oxidative genes in muscles and increase exercise endurance by about 70%. An activator of AMP-activated protein kinase, called AICAR (5-aminiimidizole-4-carboxamide-1-δ-ribofuranoside) given to sedentary mice can increase exercise endurance by about 40%. Pharmaceutical companies are developing agents like these in order to treat obesity in patients such as those with diabetes who are unable to exercise because of musculoskeletal or cardiovascular disease (29). Will they become the next generation of drugs for enhancing athletic ability?

The sports endocrine underground

The combination of sophistication and the naïveté about endocrinology that has been manifest in the international use, abuse, and detection of performance enhancing is surprising (1–4). The pharmacopoeia of agents, mostly hormones, that are used by athletes from all over the world to gain an unfair edge extend well beyond the scope of 'steroids' and include many if not most hormones. The method of abuse include oral, mucosal, dermal, and parenteral administration; the agents are taken in continuous, intermittent, and periodic regimens, many designed to avoid detection; and the regimens also use masking agents such as diuretics, α-reductase inhibitors, probenecid, urine dilution, and plasma expansion, and even contraptions to switch urine collections, such as intravaginal and intra-anal containers of substituted urine. The common use of urine rather than blood samples allows such switching to take place more readily. Furthermore, the common practices of 'stacking' (administration of multiple drugs) and 'pyramiding' (use of ascending and descending doses) are intended to elude detection as well as enhance performance. Random and unannounced testing, especially when performed unrelated to competition, may help to counter the deceit, but only a small percentage of the estimated cheaters are caught (3, 4).

Anabolic steroids are the biggest offenders (2, 31). Advances in steroid chemistry in the mid-1900s led to the development of many androgens, but toxicity and the limited legitimate market for these agents resulted in their commercial abandonment. Many of these abandoned agents, or agents relegated to veterinary use, became the basis of the illegitimate anabolic steroids use in sports. Legislation in this area has been complex and full of loopholes with many agents failing to be regulated or weakly regulated as dietary supplements (2, 32). And the internet has magnified this market by providing an international 24-h pharmacy. While there are attempts at regulation in many nations, WADA with its ever-expanding, frequently updated list of prohibited drugs, now dominates the regulation of these agents in sports, but enforcement remains elusive (33). The WADA list includes anabolic steroids, EPO, growth hormone, chorionic gonadotropin, LH, insulins, and corticotropins, Among the hormone modulators are aromatase inhibitors,

Box 1.9.2 Prohibited agents (modified from the 2009 WADA list)

Anabolic agents

- Anabolic androgenic steroids
  - Exogenous, including, oxandrolone, stanozolol, and tetrahydrogestrinone
  - Endogenous, including, dehydroepiandrosterone (DHEA) and testosterone
- Other anabolic agents, including, selective androgen-receptor modulators

Hormones

- Erythropoiesis-stimulating agents, erythropoietin, and darbepoietin
- Growth hormone, insulin-like growth factors, and mechano-growth factors
- Chorionic gonadotropin and luteinizing hormone
- Insulins
- Corticotropins

β_2 agonists, including formoterol and terbutaline

Hormone antagonists and modulators

- Aromatase inhibitors
- Selective oestrogen-receptor modulators including, raloxifene, tamoxifen, toremifene, and selective androgen-receptor modulators
- Other anti-oestrogenic substances, including clomifene, cyclofenil, fulvestrant

Glucocorticosteroids

β-blockers, including, atenolol, metoprolol, nadolol

Cannabinoids, including hashish and marijuana

Stimulants, including ephedrine, phenylephrine, and adrenaline

selective oestrogen receptor modulators and selective androgen receptor modulators, clomifene, adrenergic drugs, glucocorticoids, and cannabinoids. Box 1.9.2 lists the hormone and hormone-like agents prohibited by WADA. In addition, other prohibited agents include diuretics and masking agents such as probenecid, narcotics, alcohol in competition in certain sports, and PPARδ agonists. Prohibited methods include gene doping and enhancement of oxygen transfer with blood doping.

Endocrine testing in the context of sports endocrinology

Endocrine testing is at the core of clinical endocrinology. However, the methodology is often modified for testing in sports endocrinology. Here the task is more difficult, since immunoassays have to be designed that can distinguish exogenous, usually recombinant, recombinant molecules from endogenous hormones on the basis of the chemical and immunochemical signature that derives from their molecular size and glycosylation state (14). For example, because recombinant hormones are not glycosylated during the usual production processes, chemical methods, such as isoelectric focusing for recombinant EPO and darbepoetin, are needed to distinguish them from their glycosylated normal counterparts (2). Even so, agents such as these can be detected for only a few days in the blood, even though their effects can last for weeks. So the sophisticated abuser can stop taking the drug before an athletic event to allow for its decay and to diminish measurable levels in the blood. In addition, many monitoring programmes do not allow blood testing because of 'privacy' concerns.

Many endocrine tests are also performed by gas chromatography mass spectrometry and with use of liquid chromatography tandem mass spectrometry (2). Chromatography separates the analytes, and mass spectrometry identifies them by fragmentation patterns in comparison with known standards. These procedures are less widely applicable to proteins and peptides, for which immunochemically based methods are required. Even sensitive and specific immunoassays are limited in their application to illegal use of protein and peptide hormones. For example, insulin and its analogues, recombinant growth hormoneand EPO cannot be readily distinguished from their natural counterparts by standard immunoassays (2, 14). An additional example of testing complexity is illustrated by the procedures needed to distinguish natural testosterone from its pharmaceutical counterpart: gas chromatography-combustion-isotope ratio mass spectrometry can detect the 13C difference between the two. Similarly, the ratio of epitesterone to testosterone can be used to detect drug abuse because the pharmaceutical preparation of testosterone contains none (2).

Basic principles of endocrine regulation can also inform drug testing and deceit (3). Abusers learn about the half-lives of the various agents and the influence thereon of different routes of administration. The pseudosophisticated taking of clomifene has been used in an effort to stimulate suppressed levels of testosterone, resulting from endogenous administration (31). Furthermore, drug testing must conform to the rules of scientific reliability for the relevant jurisdiction (2).

There have been challenges in developing a test for recombinant growth hormone (14). The test used at the 2004 and 2008 Summer Olympics used an immunoassay to determine the difference between exogenous and endogenous growth hormone, but there have been difficulties in distributing testing kits to the WADA global network of accredited testing laboratories due to a limited supply of the distinguishing antibody. Even then, the test can only detect recombinant growth hormone use going back 1–2 days, severely limiting its effectiveness. Because the test was used almost exclusively at the Olympics, guilty athletes knew it was coming and simply stopped using recombinant growth hormone several days prior to the games. Indeed, through 2008, antidoping agencies had yet to announce a positive test for recombinant growth hormone.

'Designer' anabolic steroids create yet another challenge for the perpetually underfunded antidoping community (2, 31). Since the standard method for testing urine is performed using gas chromatography and high-resolution mass spectrometry, it can detect only some of the offending substances it is designed identify (2). Self-styled biochemists can render a known anabolic steroid virtually undetectable by tweaking a few molecules, or by re-engineering an old steroid that was created but never marketed (2). Victor Conte, the founder of BALCO and the architect of its underground doping programme, used what came to be known as tetrahydrogestrinone (THG), which had the unique characteristic of dissolving when the urine was heated for the purposes of gas chromatography. It was only after a used syringe of THG was mailed to the US Anti-Doping Agency that Dr Don Catlin and his UCLA laboratory were able to reverse-engineer THG and develop a method for detecting it in urine (2).

As a result of the above, in the USA the sport of baseball has belatedly begun to address drug abuse among its athletes. Even though years later than in other major sports, a drug policy was finally instituted in 2008. It took an exposé of drug use in baseball (4) to prompted Major League Baseball to begin an investigation of the problem. Some athletes, though, choose to beat the test instead of beating the tester (34). According to US Anti-Doping Agency statistics, nearly 10% of planned out-of-competition tests are 'missed,' either for innocent or more nefarious reasons (29). An athlete may have had a last-minute change in plans and neglected to update antidoping authorities. Or he or she may have purposely said they would be in one place when they were in another, creating a window to complete an anabolic steroid cycle or administer a dose of recombinant EPO. Several high-profile Russian track and field athletes were barred from the 2008 Summer Olympics after DNA testing allegedly proved their out-of-competition urine samples did not belong to them, suggesting a widespread conspiracy within the Russian track and antidoping federations. There also have been increasing reports of 'contraptions' designed to foil tests. An NFL player was caught in 2005 with 'The Whizzinator', a prosthetic penis attached to a jock strap with a compartment to store and heat 'clean' urine from freeze-dried packets. At the 2004 Summer Olympics, WADA officials accused members of Hungary's track and field team of using a crude device that stores a 'clean' urine sample in a small reservoir hidden in a body cavity. There have even been reports of athletes going so far as to use a catheter to fill their bladder with untainted urine shortly ahead of a drug test (31). All the while, presumably, their endocrine systems were dramatically being altered by an array of banned performance-enhancing substances (35).

Summary

There are hundreds of examples of athletes from essentially every country who have been caught abusing drugs and hormones (31). In addition to individual athletes, national programmes have been documented (East Germany) as well as suspected (China) of systematically providing their athletes with performance-enhancing drugs. This virtual epidemic is also illustrated by the recent identification of over 100 US baseball players who took performance-enhancing drugs. While recognizing that there are legitimate uses for physiological hormone replacement, endocrinologists have been naïve in failing to recognize the type of risk-to-benefit analysis that athletes apply in considering the pharmacological use of performance-enhancing agents. The abusing athletes consider the benefits to their performance while minimizing the risk, and some accept substantial risk for even the slightest edge. The practicing endocrinologist must be aware of this dissonance.

Acknowledgements

Supported by the Department of Veterans Affairs and the National Institutes of Health. Dr. Deftos is Distinguished Professor of Medicine at the University of California, San Diego, and Professor of Law at the California Western School of Law, San Diego California. Mr. Zeigler is on the staff of the San Diego Union Tribune.

Recent developments

The confrontation of medical science with the law and with sports culture continues. Jail sentences have been levied and several prominent athletes are being tried in court about lying to federal agents about illegal drug use. And sports legacies have been tarnished by admitted and even suspected use of performance enhancing drugs. Even related deaths have occurred. While some issues have been clarified others have been obscured. The selected illustrations that follow exemplify the continuing turmoil in this World.

Growth hormone and Testosterone

A recent study partially funded by WADA was conducted to determine the effect of growth hormone alone or with testosterone on body composition and measures of performance (36). The design was a randomized, placebo-controlled, blinded study of 8 weeks of treatment followed by a 6-week washout period of 96 recreationally trained athletes (63 men and 33 women) with a mean age of 27.9 years (SD, 5.7). Men were randomly assigned to receive placebo, growth hormone (2 mg/d subcutaneously), testosterone (250 mg/wk intramuscularly), or combined treatments. Women were randomly assigned to receive either placebo or growth hormone (2 mg/d).

Growth hormone significantly reduced fat mass, increased lean body mass through an increase in extracellular water, and increased body cell mass in men when coadministered with testosterone. Growth hormone significantly increased sprint capacity, by 3.9% in men and women combined and by 8.3% when coadministered with testosterone to men; other performance measures did not significantly change, and the increase in sprint capacity was not maintained 6 weeks after discontinuation of the drug.

The authors concluded that growth hormone supplementation influenced body composition and increased sprint capacity when administered alone and in combination with testosterone. But they noted that the athletic significance of the sprint capacity improvement was not clear. Furthermore, they pointed out that the study was limited to recreational, not elite, athletes and that a modest dose of growth hormone was used over a short period of time.

Growth hormone Testing

The United Kingdom Anti-Doping agency announced in early 2010 the first instance where human growth hormone blood testing resulted in an athletic sanction. A rugby player accepted a 2 year sanction from playing or coaching because of an out-of-completion positive test, a procedure that had been applied t the 2004 and 2008 Olympics without apparent impact. The athlete was subsequently found hanged (37). The improved blood test will now be applied to Minor League baseball players, but the U.S Major Leagues still resist.

Growth hormone and the Underground

The confusion that still reigns here has been recently displayed by the off label use of growth hormone in Canada and the United States (38). In Canada, human growth hormone can generally be prescribed for 'off-label' uses, whereas such uses are banned by U. S. Federal law (U.S. law limits distribution of human growth hormone to adults to three specific FDA-approved treatments: for

AIDS-related wasting, short bowel syndrome, and growth hormone deficiency). So while Canadian doctors can use human growth hormone to treat conditions for which the drug has not been explicitly approved, even bringing human growth hormone into the U.S. is illegal, and using human growth hormone to treat athletes without therapeutic-use exemptions violates sports doping rules. And while off-label prescribing of drugs is not uncommon in the U.S., federal law bans such use of human growth hormone. But in a seeming paradox, anabolic steroids, which are controlled substances, can be prescribed off-label. Legal complexities notwithstanding, human growth hormone use has been widely reported in athletics, including well-known international athletes. And interpreting the law has been confusing for many American and Canadian doctors.

Testosterone Administration

The safety and efficacy of testosterone treatment in older men who have limitations in mobility was studied in community-dwelling men, 65 years of age or older, with limitations in mobility and a low serum testosterone (39). The subjects were randomly assigned to receive placebo gel or testosterone gel, to be applied daily for 6 months. The testosterone group had significantly greater improvements in leg-press and chest-press strength and in stair climbing while carrying a load. But the application of a testosterone gel was associated with an increased risk of cardiovascular adverse events. So the risk/benefit analysis did not support testosterone use.

Transgender issues

Transgender disputes have invaded the usually sedate world of golf (40). A former police officer who had a male to female sex change operation challenged the female-at-birth requirements for competitors of the U. S. Ladies Professional Golf Association (LPGA). In a suit filed in San Francisco federal court claiming the LPGA violates a California civil rights law, the golfer is seeking to prevent the LPGA from holding tournaments in the state until its policy is changed to admit transgender players. She also sued three LPGA sponsors and the Long Drivers of America, which holds the annual women's long drive gold championship that she won in 2008 but was barred from competing in this year after organizers adopted the LPGA's gender rules. In double irony, a golfer was among the first athletes in America to be banned from professional golf tournaments, and he was not a good golfer (41).

References

1. Warren MP, Constantini NW, eds. *NW. Sports Endocrinology*. New York city: Humana Press, 2000.
2. Deftos LJ. Games of hormones: the para-endocrinology of sport. *Endocr Pract*, 2006; **12**: 472–4.
3. Wells DJ. Gene doping: the hype and the reality. *Br J Pharmacol*, 2008; **154**: 623–31.
4. Fainaru-Wada M, Williams L. *Game of Shadows*. New York, NY: Gotham Books, Penguin Group (USA), Inc., 2006.
5. Giannoulis MG, Sonksen PH, Umpleby M, Breen L, Pentecost C, Whyte M, *et al.* The effects of growth hormone and/or testosterone in healthy elderly men: a randomized controlled trial. *J Clin Endocrinol Metab*, 2006; **91**: 477–84.
6. Hackney AC, Viru A. Research methodology: endocrinologic measurements in exercise science and sports medicine. *J Athl Train*, 2008; **43**: 631–9.
7. Dampney RAL, Horiuchi J, McDowall LM. Hypothalamic mechanisms coordinating cardiorespiratory function during exercise and defensive behaviour. *Auton Neurosci*, 2008; **142**: 3–10.
8. Butler TH, Noakes TD, Soldin SJ, Verbalis JG. Acute changes in endocrine and fluid balance markers during high-intensity, steady-state, and prolonged endurance running: unexpected increases in oxytocin and brain natriuretic peptide during exercise. *Eur J Endocrinol*, 2008; **159**: 729–37.
9. Goldstein DS, Kopin IJ. Adrenomedullary, adrenocortical, and sympathoneural responses to stressors: a meta-analysis. *Endocr Regul*, 2008; **42**: 111–19.
10. Tworoger SS, Sorensen B, Chubak J, Irwin M, Stanczyk FZ, Ulrich CM, *et al.* Effect of a 12-month randomized clinical trial of exercise on serum prolactin concentrations in postmenopausal women. *Cancer Epidemiol Biomarkers Prev*, 2007; **16**: 895–9.
11. Meyer T, Schwartz L, and Kinderman W. Exercise and endogenous opiates. In: Warren MP, Constantini NW, eds, *NW. Sports Endocrinology*. New York city: Humana Press, 2000: 31–41.
12. Almond CSD, Shin AY, Fortescue EB, Mannix RC, Wypij D, Binstadt BA, *et al.* Hyponatremia among runners in the Boston Marathon. *N Engl J Med*, 2005; **352**: 1550–6.
13. Gibney J, Healy ML, Sonksen PH. The growth hormone/insulin-like growth factor-i axis in exercise and sport. *Endocr Rev*, 2007; **28**: 603–24.
14. Powrie JK, Bassett EE, Rosen T, Jørgensen JO, Napoli R, Sacca L, *et al.* Detection of growth hormone abuse in sport. *Growth Horm IGF Res*, 2007; **17**: 220–6.
15. Johansson G, Grimby G, Sunnerhagen KS, Bengtsson BA. Two years of growth hormone (GH) treatment increase isometric and isokinetic muscle strength in GH-deficient adults. *J Clin Endocrinol Metab*, 1997; **82**: 2877–84.
16. Ubertini G, Grossi A, Colabianchi D, Fiori R, Brufani C, Bizzarri C, *et al.* Young elite athletes of different sports disciplines present with an increase in pulsatile secretion of growth hormone compared with non-elite athletes and sedentary subjects. *J Endocrinol Invest*, 2008; **31**: 138–45.
17. Colao A, Cuolo A, Marzullo P, Nicolai E, Ferone D, Della Morte AM, *et al.* Is the acromegalic cardiomyopathy reversible? Effect of 5-year normalization of growth hormone and insulin-like growth factor I levels on cardiac performance. *J Clin Endocrinol Metab*, 2001; **86**: 1551–7.
18. Warren MP, Chua AT. Exercise-induced amenorrhea and bone health in the adolescent athlete. *Ann NY Acad Sci*, 2008; **1135**: 244–52.
19. Theodoropoulou A, Markou KB, Vagenakis GA, Benardot D, Leglise M, Kourounis G, *et al.* Delayed but normally progressed puberty is more pronounced in artistic compared with rhythmic elite gymnasts due to the intensity of training. *J Clin Endocrinol Metab*, 2005; **90**: 6022–7.
20. Bernet VJ, Wartofsky L. Thyroid function and exercise. In: Warren MP, Constantini NW, eds. *NW. Sports Endocrinology*. New York city: Humana Press, 2000: 97–118.
21. Grimston SK, Tanguay KE, Gundberg CM, Hanley DA. The calciotropic hormone response to changes in serum calcium during exercise in female long distance runners. *J Clin Endocr inol Metab*, 1993; **76**: 867–72.
22. Karlsson MK, Nordqvist A, Karlsson C. Physical activity increases bone mass during growth. *Food Nutr Res* 2008; **52**: doi: 10.3402/fnr.v52i0.1871.
23. Schneider S, Guleria PS. Diabetes and exercise. In: Warren MP, Constantini NW, eds. *NW. Sports Endocrinology*. New York city: Humana Press, 2000: 227–38.
24. Weise M, Drinkard B, Mehlinger SL, Holzer SM, Eisenhofer G, Charmandari E, *et al.* Stress dose of hydrocortisone is not beneficial in patients with classic congenital adrenal hyperplasia undergoing short-term, high-intensity exercise. *J Clin Endocrinol Metab*, 2004; **89**: 3679–84.
25. Kivlighan KT, Granger DA, Booth A. Gender differences in testosterone and cortisol response to competition. *Psychoneuroendocrinology*, 2005; **30**: 58–71.
26. Gooren LJ, Behre HM. Testosterone treatment of hypogonadal men participating in competitive sports. *Andrologia*, 2008; **40**: 195–9.

27. Nelson AE, Howet CJ, Nguyen TV, Seibel MJ, Baxter RC, Handelsman DJ, *et al.* Erythropoietin administration does not influence the GH-IGF axis or makers of bone turnover in recreational athletes. *Clin Endocrinol*, 2005; **63**: 305–9.
28. Gooren LJ. Olympic sports and transsexuals. *Asian J Androl*, 2008; **10**: 427–32.
29. Goodyear LJ. The exercise pill—too good to be true? *N Engl J Med*, 2008; **359**: 1842–4.
30. Gaffney GR, Parisotto R. Gene doping: a review of performance-enhancing genetics. *Pediatr Clin North Am*, 2007; **54**: 807–22.
31. Rosen DM. *Dope: A History of Performance Enhancement in Sports from the Nineteenth Century to Today*. Philadelphia, PA: Greenwood Publishing Group, 2008.
32. Butcher AR, Hong, CW. Doping. In: *Sport: Global Ethical Issues*. New Jersey: Rutledge: 2007.
33. WADA.Available at: http://en.wikipedia.org/wiki/World_Anti-Doping_Agency (accessed 26 October 2010).
34. Schneider AJ, Friedmann T. Gene doping in sports: the science and ethics of genetically modified athletes. *Adv Genet*, 2006; **51**: 1–110.
35. Wikipedia. List of doping cases in sport. Page last modified on 10 June 2010. Available at: http://www.wada-ama.org/en/World-Anti-Doping-Program/Sports-and-Anti-Doping-Organizations/International-Standards/Prohibited-List/ (accessed 26 October 2010).
36. Meinhardt U, Nelson AE, Hansen JL, Birzniece V, Clifford D, Leung KC, *et al.* The effects of growth hormone on body composition and physical performance in recreational athletes. *Ann Intern Med*, 2010; **152**: 568–57.
37. http://www.guardian.co.uk/sport/2010/sep/26/terry-newton-found-hanged-rugby. (accessed 26 October 2010).
38. Epstein D, Segura, M. The elusive Dr. Galea. Sports Illustrated. 2010. September 27, pp. 57–60.
39. Basaria S, Coviello AD, Travison TG, *et al.* Adverse events associated with testosterone administration. *N Engl J Med*, 2010; **363**: 109–22.
40. http://www.csmonitor.com/The-Culture/Sports/2010/1014/Lana-Lawless-Transgender-woman-sues-LPGA-for-right-to-tee-off. (accessed 26 September 2010).
41. http://deadspin.com/5396121/terrible-golfer-banned-for-using-drugs-to-enhance-his-terrible-performance. (accessed 27 September 2010).

PART 2

Pituitary and hypothalamic diseases

2.1

General concepts of hypothalamus-pituitary anatomy

Ignacio Bernabeu, Monica Marazuela, Felipe F. Casanueva

Introduction

The hypothalamus is the part of the diencephalon associated with visceral, autonomic, endocrine, affective, and emotional behaviour. It lies in the walls of the third ventricle, separated from the thalamus by the hypothalamic sulcus. The rostral boundary of the hypothalamus is roughly defined as a line through the optic chiasm, lamina terminalis, and anterior commissure, and an imaginary line extending from the posterior commissure to the caudal limit of the mamillary body represents the caudal boundary. Externally, the hypothalamus is bounded rostrally by the optic chiasm, laterally by the optic tract, and posteriorly by the mamillary bodies. Dorsolaterally, the hypothalamus extends to the medial edge of the internal capsule (Fig. 2.1.1) (1).

The complicated anatomy of this area of the central nervous system (CNS) is the reason why, for a long time, little was known about its anatomical organization and functional significance. Even though the anatomy of the hypothalamus is well established it does not form a well-circumscribed region. On the contrary, it is continuous with the surrounding parts of the CNS: rostrally, with the septal area of the telencephalon and anterior perforating substance; anterolaterally with the substantia innominata; and caudally with the central grey matter and the tegmentum of the mesencephalon. The ventral portion of the hypothalamus and the third ventricular recess form the infundibulum, which represents the most proximal part of the neurohypophysis. A bulging region posterior to the infundibulum is the tuber cinereum, and the zone that forms the floor of the third ventricle is called the *median eminence*. The median eminence represents the final point of convergence of pathways from the CNS on the peripheral endocrine system and it is supplied by primary capillaries of the hypophyseal portal vessels. The median eminence is the anatomical interface between the brain and the anterior pituitary. Ependymal cells lining the floor of the third ventricle have processes that traverse the width of the median eminence and terminate near the portal perivascular space; these cells, called tanycytes, provide a structural and functional link between the cerebrospinal fluid (CSF) and the perivascular space of the pituitary portal vessels.

The conspicuous landmarks of the ventral surface of the brain can be used to divide the hypothalamus into three parts: anterior (preoptic and supraoptic regions), middle (tuberal region), and caudal (mamillary region). Each half of the hypothalamus is also divided into a medial and lateral zone. The medial zone contains the so-called cell-rich areas with well-defined nuclei. The scattered cells of the lateral hypothalamic area have long overlapping dendrites, similar to the cells of the reticular formation. Some of these neurons send axons directly to the cerebral cortex and others project down into the brainstem and spinal cord.

Hypothalamic nuclei

Anterior group

Preoptic region

This region constitutes the periventricular grey of the most rostral part of the third ventricle. The preoptic periventricular nucleus surrounds the walls of the third ventricle and contains small cells poorly differentiated from the ependymal lining.

Supraoptic region

This region contains (midline to lateral) the paraventricular nucleus and its ventral expansion: the suprachiasmatic nucleus, the anterior hypothalamic nucleus, the lateral hypothalamic area, and the supraoptic nucleus. The paraventricular and supraoptic nuclei are prominent and highly vascularized. The cells of the paraventricular nucleus are densely packed and lie immediately beneath the ependyma of the third ventricle. They consist of several distinct cells groups, including a medial parvicellular group and a prominent magnocellular group. The supraoptic nucleus caps the optic chiasm and follows the optic tract laterally. This nucleus is composed mainly of uniformly large cells. Magnocellular components of both the supraoptic and paraventricular nuclei project fibres into the neural lobe of the hypophysis. Immunocytochemically,

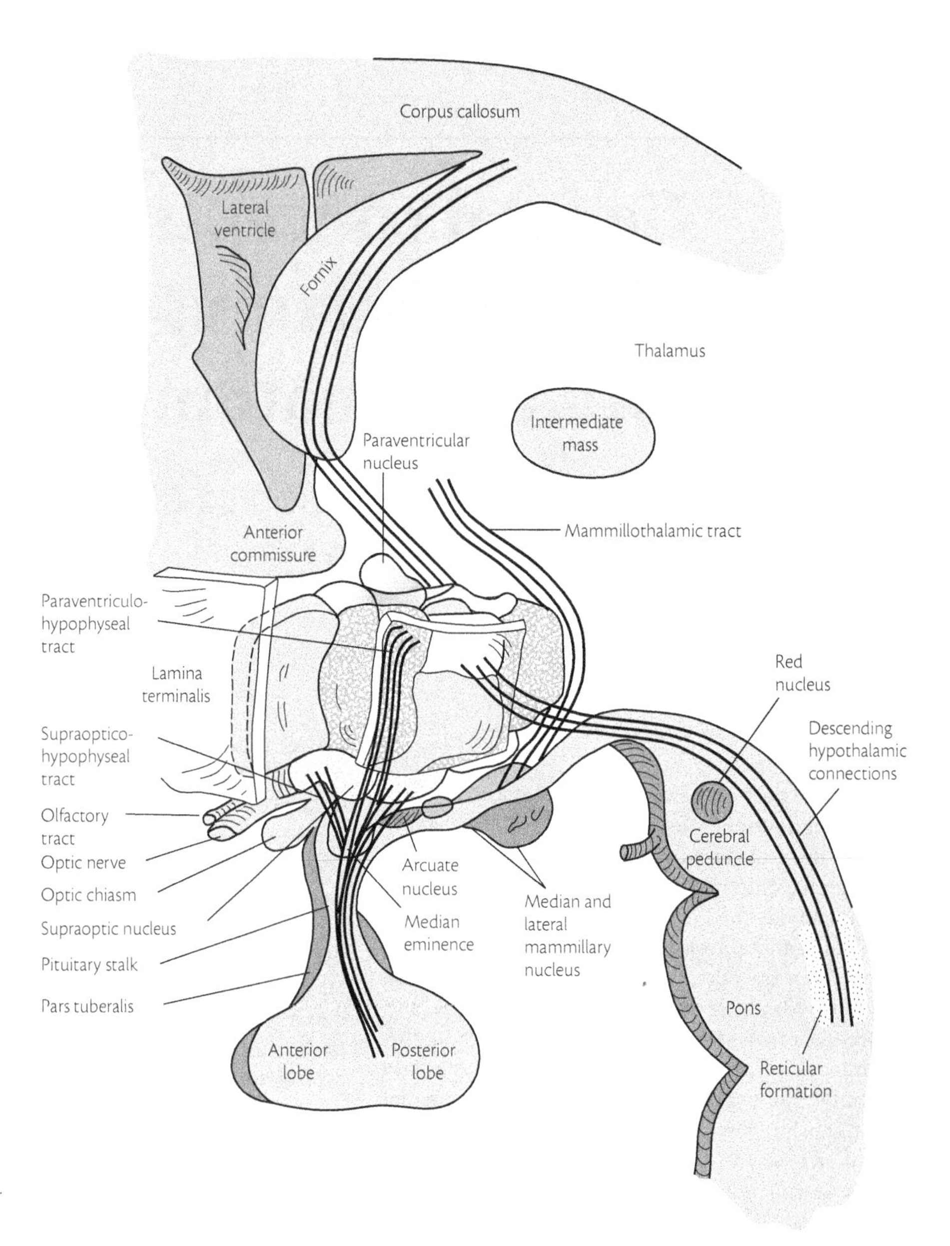

Fig. 2.1.1 The hypothalamic nuclei and hypothalamic-hypophyseal tracts in relation to the thalamus, ventricular system, and brainstem.

large cells in both nuclei contain either vasopressin (antidiuretic hormone (ADH)) or oxytocin, each of which is associated with a distinctive neurophysin. Regions of the paraventricular nucleus send axons to the brainstem and all levels of the spinal cord. The less differentiated central grey in the supraoptic region forms the anterior hypothalamic nucleus, which merges with the preoptic area. The suprachiasmatic nucleus constitutes a group of small round cells, dorsal to the optic chiasm. These neurons receive direct bilateral projections from the retina, and this connection provides the link between a cyclical environment and the internal clock.

Middle group (tuberal region)

The hypothalamus reaches its widest extent in the tuberal region, and the fornix separates the medial and the lateral hypothalamic areas. The medial portion contains three nuclei. The ventromedial nucleus occupies a strategic position in the hypothalamus and it has numerous afferent and efferent connections with many other regions of the CNS, including the brainstem. The dorsomedial nucleus is less distinct. Both nuclei are involved in autonomic function and emotional behaviour. The arcuate nucleus (infundibular nucleus) is situated in the most ventral part of the third ventricle and extends into the median eminence. This nucleus contains small cells that are in close contact with the ependymal lining. Axons from this nucleus form part of a diffuse projection system, the tuberoinfundibular tract, which terminates on the hypophyseal portal vessel system. This connection is of major importance to adenohypophyseal function.

Posterior group (mamillary region)

The posterior part of the hypothalamus consists of the posterior hypothalamic nucleus and the mamillary bodies. In humans, the mamillary body is a focal point for several prominent fibre bundles and it is formed by a large spherical medial mamillary nucleus containing small cells and surrounded by a capsule of heavily myelinated fibres. Lateral to this is the intermediate mamillary nucleus, with smaller cells, and even further laterally is a well-defined group of large cells, the lateral mamillary nucleus. The posterior hypothalamic nucleus is a large but poorly defined cell group that is continuous with the central grey matter of the mesencephalon. This nucleus consists of small and large cells. The latter are especially numerous in humans.

Rostrally and laterally, the hypothalamus is continuous with the basal olfactory region. Medially, this region extends dorsally, forming the so-called septal region, which is located beneath the rostral part of the lentiform nucleus and the head of the caudate nucleus. Beneath this region is a grey mass referred to as the substantia innominata, which contains clusters of large cholinergic neurons forming the basal nucleus of Meynert. Neurons in the basal nucleus constitute the major source of cholinergic innervation to the entire neocortex (2).

Major fibre systems

Due to its location at the base of the brain, access to the hypothalamus is limited in experimental investigations and thus it has been difficult to study the hypothalamic fibre connections. However, new tracing techniques have made this possible. The hypothalamus has extensive and complex connections with many regions in the forebrain, the brainstem and the spinal cord.

Afferent connections

Several afferent neural pathways provide the hypothalamus with input from the forebrain, limbic system, visual cortex, thalamus, and brain stem.

Medial forebrain bundle

This is a widespread, loosely arranged system arising from basal olfactory regions and monoaminergic cell groups in the brainstem, the periamygdaloid region, and the subiculum. In its parasagittal course, this bundle receives contributions from the substantia innominata and the amygdaloid complex.

Hippocampus-hypothalamic fibres (fornix)

This is a large fibre bundle that originates in the hippocampal formation and projects to the septal area, the anterior thalamus, and the hypothalamus. This bundle can be exposed by dissection of the lateral wall of the third ventricle and followed to the mamillary body where many of its fibres terminate. In the septal region, the fornix forms two distinct bundles: the precommisural fibres, which are distributed to the septal nuclei, the lateral preoptic region, and the dorsal hypothalamic area; and the postcommisural fibres of the fornix, which project to the medial mamillary nucleus, except for those that leave this bundle to terminate in the anterior thalamic nuclei.

Amygdalo-hypothalamic fibres

These fibres provides entry of emotional data from the amygdaloid nucleus into the hypothalamus. There are two different pathways: stria terminalis, which is the main pathway that connects the amygdaloid body and the medial hypothalamus, and the ventral-amygdalofugal fibres, which arise from the basolateral amygdaloid nucleus and extend to the lateral hypothalamic nucleus and medial forebrain bundle.

Brainstem reticular afferents

These fibres reach the hypothalamus through the mamillary peduncle of the lateral mamillary nucleu, and the ascending component of the dorsal longitudinal fasciculus from the central grey of the midbrain.

Cholinergic and monoaminergic pathways

The ascending cholinergic pathway, originating in the substantia nigra and ventral tegmental area, has widespread distribution in the forebrain, including the hypothalamus. The monoaminergic systems originating in the brainstem have a wide distribution in the forebrain and some of the projection systems, such as the mesolimbic dopamine pathway and the ventral ascending noradrenergic and the serotonergic pathways which pass through the lateral hypothalamic area. The ascending noradrenergic and the serotonergic systems distribute large number of fibres to the lateral and medial hypothalamus.

Retino-hypothalamic fibres

These fibres arise from ganglion cells of the retina and project bilaterally to the suprachiasmatic nuclei through the optic nerve and chiasm. These nuclei also receive inputs from the ventral and lateral geniculate nuclei and the paraventricular nuclei of the thalamus. This suprachiasmatic nucleus is well known as the pacemaker for circadian rhythms.

Cortico-hypothalamic fibres

The hypothalamus receives connections from the posterior orbital cortex, pyriform cortex, cingulated gyrus, and the entorhinal cortex. In each instance, the cortical projection is reinforced by a corresponding subcortical projection. Both the sense of taste and the sense of olfaction are directly involved in arousal mechanisms and phases of consummatory behaviour. Gustatory pathways to the hypothalamus are multisynaptic, whereas olfactory projections to the hypothalamus are relatively direct.

Efferent connections

These connections are partly reciprocal to the afferent systems. In addition, several efferent hypothalamic pathways have no counterpart among afferent systems. The medial forebrain bundle transmits impulses from the lateral hypothalamus to the hippocampal formation. The stria terminalis and the ventral pathway convey impulses from the hypothalamus to the amygdala. The dorsal longitudinal fasciculus carries descending fibres from the medial and periventricular hypothalamus to the midbrain and tegmentum. Mamillary efferent fibres arise mainly from the medial mamillary nucleus and quickly divide into two tracts: the mamillothalamic and the mamillotegmental tracts. The former projects to the anterior thalamic nuclei and the later terminates in the dorsal and ventral tegmental nuclei of the midbrain. It is not clear how the suprachiasmatic nucleus affects circadian rhythms, since its efferent projections are incomplete and do not reach the areas responsible for motor, autonomic or endocrine responses. Retrograde tracer injections in several hypothalamic areas have shown that suprachiasmatic nucleus subdivisions into core and shell areas differ with respect to afferents, local connections, and neuroactive substances. The paraventricular nucleus and the lateral and posterior hypothalamus send fibres to the dorsal motor nucleus of the vagus, the medial solitary nucleus, and the nucleus ambiguous. These hypothalamic nuclei also send fibres to the spinal cord, which terminate in the intermediolateral cell column at all levels, influencing autonomic functions.

Hypothalamus and adenohypophysis (tubero-hypophyseal tract)

The anatomical basis for the hypothalamic control of the anterior lobe of the pituitary is complex. Neurosecretory cells in the arcuatus (infundibular) nucleus, the ventromedial nucleus, and the neighbouring regions produce releasing and inhibiting factors that regulate the secretion of hormones from the anterior lobe of the pituitary. The hormones reach the anterior lobe by axoplasmic transport through the axons of the tubero-infundibular tract and are then discharged into capillary loops in the median eminence. The hormones are then transported by the hypophyseal portal veins to a second capillary network in the anterior lobe, where they influence the secretion of the various adenohypophyseal hormones, such as thyroid-stimulating hormone (TSH), adrenocorticotropin hormone (ACTH), follicle-stimulating hormone (FSH), luteinizing hormone growth hormone, and prolactin. This tract arises mainly from the arcuate nucleus and ends in the median eminence and the infundibular stem. Fibres of the tubero-infundibular tract convey releasing hormones to the anterior lobe of the pituitary. Dopamine was the first substance identified in the arcuate nucleus; in the hypophyseal portal system it inhibits the release of prolactin from the anterior pituitary. A short feedback loop suggests that pituitary prolactin inhibits dopamine release from the median eminence. The arcuate nucleus also contains a number of peptides similar to hormones in the anterior pituitary, such as ACTH, β-lipotropin, and β-endorphin. These peptides do not appear to coexist in neurons with dopamine (3, 4).

The pituitary

Embryology

The pituitary gland consists of an anterior lobe (adenohypophysis), a posterior lobe (neurohypophysis), and an intermediate zone. The adenohypophysis originates from the stomodeal ectoderm, which invaginates by the third week of gestation to form Rathke's pouch. In the sixth week of gestation it comes into contact with the infundibulum. A remnant of the pharyngo-hypophysis is occasionally encountered in adults, forming the pharyngeal pituitary in the midline of the nasopharynx, which contains the full spectrum of pituitary hormones.

The first type of cell to develop in the human fetal pituitary is the corticotroph at 6 weeks *in utero*, follows by somatotrophs (8 weeks), thyrotrophs and gonadotrophs (12 weeks), and lactotrophs (after 24 weeks). Pituitary development and differentiation involve the sequential expression of several transcription factors, among which POU1F1 (PIT1) and PROP1 are the most important. Mutations in genes encoding these transcription factors can not only produce combined pituitary hormone deficiency (mainly growth hormone, prolactin, TSH, FSH, and luteinizing hormone) but also pituitary hypoplasia or agenesis. Tpit is a transcription factor that is essential for preventing differentiation of corticotrophs into other pituitary cell types. Mutations in the gene encoding Tpit cause congenital isolated ACTH deficiency.

The posterior portion of Rathke's pouch gives rise to the intermediate lobe. This area normally contains microcystic remnants of Rathke's pouch, which rarely are clinically significant. The neurohypophysis develops from a neuroectodermal bud in the floor of the diencephalon at 4 weeks of gestation. The portal system starts to develop at 7 weeks but is not completed until 18–20 weeks of gestation. The body of the sphenoid bone and the sella turcica result from fusion of hypophyseal cartilage plates on either side of the developing pituitary. The sella is well formed at 7 weeks and matures by enchondral ossification.

Anatomy

The pituitary gland is centrally situated at the base of the brain, in the sella turcica, within the sphenoid bone. It is attached to the hypothalamus by both the pituitary stalk and a fine vascular network. The sphenoid bone forms a midline slope (the tuberculum sella) and a transverse indentation (the chiasmal sulcus). The optic canals lie anterolateral to the sulcus, whereas the optic tracts are posterolateral. The floor of the sella forms a portion of the roof of the sphenoidal air sinus, which permits easy surgical access. The sloping anterior sellar wall gives rise to posterolateral projections, the anterior clinoid processes. Posterior to the sella, the sphenoid bone continues as the dorsum sella, forming the posterior clinoid processes. The pituitary lacks leptomeninges. The sella turcica is lined by periosteal dura mater whereas the dura proper covers the lateral aspects of the cavernous sinuses and constitutes the sellar diaphragm. Leptomeninges circle the stalk, below the level of the sellar diaphragm and reflect upon themselves forming the infradiaphragmatic hypophyseal cistern. There are individual variations in this regard, with examples where the leptomeninges form a large diaphragmatic opening. If such an individual undergoes transsphenoidal surgery, it may result in persistent CSF rhinorrhoea due to violation of the subarachnoid space.

There are a number of important vascular structures in the vicinity of the sellar region. The cavernous sinuses are on either side of the sella, lateral and superior to the sphenoid sinuses. Venous drainage to the sinuses is through the superior ophthalmic vein, inferior, and middle cerebral veins and the spheno-parietal sinus. Both cavernous sinuses communicate anteriorly and posteriorly to the sella, forming a complex venous ring. The cavernous sinuses represent extradural cavities, which comprise important neurovascular structures, including the cavernous segments of the internal carotid arteries, and the cranial nerves III, IV, V, and VI. Several branches of the internal carotid artery originate within the cavernous sinus, including the meningohypophyseal trunk, the artery of the inferior cavernous sinus, and small capsular branches. The meningohypophyseal trunk gives rise to several vessels, including the inferior hypophyseal artery, which supplies the posterior lobe and the pituitary capsule.

Vascular supply: hypophyseal portal system

The hypophysis is supplied by two sets of arteries that arise from the internal carotid artery. The superior hypophyseal artery forms an arterial ring around the upper part of the hypophyseal stalk; the inferior hypophyseal artery forms a ring about the posterior lobe and gives branches to the lower infundibulum. A single superior hypophyseal artery leaves each carotid shortly after its entry into the cranial cavity and soon divides into posterior and anterior branches, each of which anastomoses with the corresponding branch from the opposite side, to form an arterial ring around the upper pituitary stalk. The posterior and anterior branches of the superior hypophyseal arteries are the source of the 'long stalk' and 'short stalk' arteries. Branches of the inferior hypophyseal arteries supply the posterior lobe and lower portion of the stalk, sending small branches to the periphery of the anterior lobe. Some arterioles

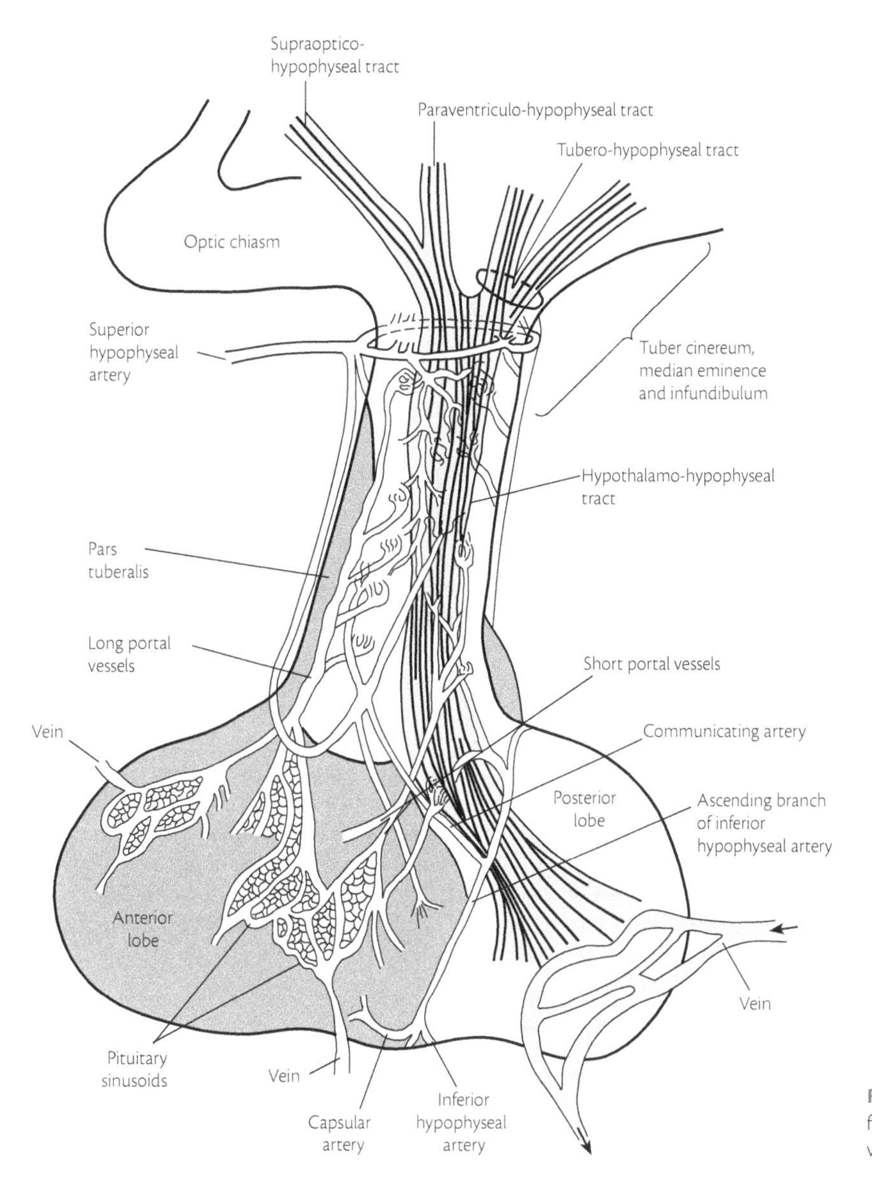

Fig. 2.1.2 Organization and functional significance of the vasculature of the pituitary gland.

and capillaries in the pituitary stalk and infundibulum give rise to unique vascular complexes named 'gomitoli', which consist of a central artery surrounded by a glomeruloid tangle of capillaries. The transition between the central artery and the capillaries consists of specialized arterioles with thick smooth muscle sphincters that regulate the blood flow (Fig. 2.1.2).

The hypophyseal portal system originates from the capillary plexus of the median eminence and superior stalk, which is derived from the terminal ramifications of the superior and inferior hypophyseal arteries. This capillary plexus in the median eminence and superior stalk drains into the long portal vessels but runs along the stalk to supply largely the anterior lobe, whereas the smaller capillary plexus in the lower stalk gives rise to the portal vessels. The portal system communicates with the capillary network in the anterior lobe that carries hypophyseotropic factors into the pituitary and delivers anterior lobe hormones to the periphery. The venous drainage of the pituitary is via collecting vessels that drain in the subhypophyseal sinus, cavernous sinus, and superior circular sinus. The majority of the anterior lobe circulation is venous and originates from the portal vessels. However, the blood supply of the posterior lobe is arterial and direct, which explains the predilection of metastatic carcinomas for the neural lobe.

Functional anatomy

The anterior lobe comprises about 80% of the gland and includes the pars distalis, pars intermedia, and pars tuberalis. Staining characteristics help divide the pars distalis into a central 'mucoid wedge' and two 'lateral wings'. On light microscopy the cells of the anterior lobe show variation in size, shape, and histochemical staining characteristics. They are organized in nests and cords, separated by a complex capillary network. This architectural pattern is altered in hyperplasia and adenomas (5, 6).

The pars distalis Large numbers of cells in the central zone are basophilic and stain with periodic acid-Schiff (PAS) method. These cells produce ACTH, luteinizing hormone, FSH, and TSH. Most of the cells in the lateral wings are acidophilic and produce growth hormone or less frequently prolactin. Somatotrophs or growth hormone-secreting cells are present in greatest density in the lateral wings comprising approximately 50% of all adenohypophyseal cells.

They are ovoid, medium size and with abundant acidophilic secretory granules. Pituitary somatotroph adenomas could be densely or sparsely granulated and the later is associated with aggressive tumours and worse response to therapy. Lactotrophs or prolactin-secreting cells comprise approximately 20% of anterior pituitary cells with wide variability related to age, sex, and parity in women. Lactotrophs are predominantly located in the posterior portions of the lateral wings. Histologically they are either acidophilic (densely granulated) or chromophobic (sparsely granulated). Densely granulated lactotrophs are thought to represent a storage phase, while sparsely granulated cells are associated with active secretion. A common feature of prolactin cells is their tendency to lie close to gonadotrophs, which is most likely due to a close physiological relationship. There are also mammosomatotroph cells producing prolactin and growth hormone. Prolactin cell adenomas could be densely or, more commonly, sparsely granulated.

Any space-occupying sellar or parasellar mass that compresses the pituitary stalk, impedes the principal hypothalamic prolactin-inhibitory factor delivery to the anterior lobe causing hyperprolactinaemia, a phenomenon termed 'stalk effect'. Corticotrophs or ACTH-producing cells, comprise 15–20% of adenohypophyseal cells and are most numerous in the mid and posterior portions of the mucoid wedge. Histologically, ACTH cells are medium to large polygonal cell. The strong PAS positivity is related to a carbohydrate moiety present in proopiomelanocortin (POMC), which is the precursor of ACTH. Perinuclear bundles of cytokeratin filaments are also typical of ACTH cells. In the context of glucocorticoid excess, ACTH cells accumulate type I microfilaments (Crooke's hyaline change). Thyrotrophs or TSH-secreting cells are located predominantly in the anterior part of the mucoid wedge, and represent approximately 5% of the adenohypophyseal cells. These are medium sized, elongated cells, which stain with basic dyes and are PAS positive. Gonadotrophs, or FSH and LH producing cells, represent about 10% of the pars distalis, are positive for basic dyes and PAS, and are evenly distributed throughout the anterior lobe. These cells have been shown to produce FSH and luteinizing hormone in isolation or by the same cell.

The pars intermedia (intermediate lobe) This is very poorly developed in humans, and is formed by epithelial-lined spaces containing colloid; the cells are ciliated, goblet, and endocrine.

The pars tuberalis (also named pars infundibularis) This is an extension of the anterior lobe along the pituitary stalk. It is formed by normal acini of pituitary cells distributed around surface portal vessels.

A different cell component in the anterior lobe is called follicular cell. These cells are derived from secretory cells and constitute follicles within the normal anterior pituitary. The folliculo-stellate cell is another unusual cell type that comprises less than 5% of the anterior lobe cells. These agranular cells are positive for S100 protein and their physiological role is unclear. These cells have been implicated in autocrine/paracrine regulation of anterior pituitary function, intrapituitary communication, and modulation of inflammatory responses.

Neurohypophysis

The posterior lobe or neurohypophysis is a ventral extension of the central nervous system, where the hypothalamic hormones oxytocin and vasopressin are released. The neurohypophysis is composed of unmyelinated axons that originate from the supraoptic and paraventricular nuclei and from cholinergic hypothalamic neurones, a prominent vascular network and specialized glial cells named pituicytes. These cells are reactive for glial fibrillary acidic protein, an intermediate filament characteristic of astrocytes, and are in close association with neurosecretory fibres; their morphology varies considerably, ranging from astrocytic to ependymal, and their role is yet unclear. The most important function of the neurohypophysis is the transfer of hormonal substances from neurosecretory granules to the intravascular space and its complex anatomy constitutes the basis for this process.

The framework of hypothalamo–pituitary functioning

The current paradigm accepts that the hypothalamus controls the pituitary by the release of activating and inhibitory factors called neurohormones, which are produced by neurons and secreted in the median eminence. These neurohormones travel from the median eminence to the pituitary target cells via the portal vessels. Acting on pituitary cells, they cause or stop the secretion of the pituitary hormones; some of these hormones act directly on different tissues and others activate target glands (Box 2.1.1). The system integrates information and amplifies the action, the neurohormones integrate environmental and neural information and this is translated by a few molecules in a very limited vascular space, the portal blood vessels. In its turn, the pituitary integrates information coming from the CNS and the general hormonal information

Box 2.1.1 Hormones with clinical relevance participating in the hypothalamo-adenohypophysis regulation

Hypothalamic hormones

- Gonadotropin-releasing hormone: 10 amino acids
- Corticotropin- releasing hormone: 41 amino acids
- Thyrotropin-releasing hormone: 3 amino acids
- Dopamine
- Growth hormone-releasing hormone: 44 amino acids
- Somatostatin: 14 amino acids

Pituitary hormones

- Luteinizing hormone: 204 amino acids
- Follicle-stimulating hormone: 204 amino acids
- Proopiomelanocortin (POMC)
- Adrenocorticotropin: 39 amino acids
- β-endorphin
- Melanocyte-stimulating hormone (MSH)
- Thyrotropin: 201 amino acids
- Prolactin: 199 amino acids
- Growth hormone: 191 amino acids

arriving from the rest of the body. This causes the pituitary hormones to be secreted in a meaningful concentration in to the general vascular space (7, 8).

Somatotroph axis

Growth hormone, also called somatotroph hormone, is mainly responsible for the physiological axial somatic growth and the general modulation of metabolism (Fig. 2.1.3). Growth hormone accounts for 10% of the net pituitary hormonal content. It is a single chain peptide molecule with several similarities to prolactin and placental lactogen, and is present in circulation and secreted in several isoforms. Growth hormone secretion occurs in pulses that occur every 3–4 h, the most pronounced discharge occurring during deep sleep or phases III–IV.

Somatotroph regulation

The somatotroph axis is based in three locations: hypothalamus, pituitary, and peripheral target tissues. The hypothalamic participation in the regulation of growth hormone secretion is exerted through two neurohormones, which reach the pituitary by the hypothalamo-pituitary portal vessels. One is growth hormone-releasing hormone (GHRH), which stimulates both synthesis and secretion of growth hormone, and the other is somatostatin, which inhibits the release, although not the synthesis, of growth hormone. In recent years it has been postulated that the endogenous ligand of the cloned growth hormone-secretagogue (GHS) receptor, i.e. ghrelin, may be implicated in the physiological regulation of growth hormone secretion, but this awaits definitive proof. Only after the full characterization of this third factor will it be possible to integrate it into a general framework of growth hormone regulation. Unlike other pituitary hormones, growth hormone does not have a target gland on which to operate, and its actions are exerted in a delocalized way over different peripheral tissues. Growth hormone exerts its action either directly or through the generation of insulin-like growth factor 1 (IGF-1) by the liver. Both growth hormone and IGF-1, by a feedback mechanism at hypothalamic and pituitary level, inhibit the further secretion of growth hormone. In contrast with other pituitary hormones, it is characteristic that growth hormone is powerfully regulated by peripheral signals such as thyroid and adrenal hormones, nutrients, and metabolites (see Fig. 2.1.3).

The biological action of GHRH is located in the first 28 amino acids, a fact being used to develop shorter analogues with diagnostic and therapeutic use. GHRH is abundant in splanchnic tissues, so circulating GHRH levels do not reflect the hypothalamic activity and are not usually measured for this purpose. Its determination has clinical utility only in ectopic tumours secreting GHRH causing acromegaly. The neurohormone somatostatin acting at the pituitary level inhibits the basal release of growth hormone as well as the growth hormone discharge elicited by all known stimuli. This action gave the name to somatostatin after its discovery, but later on other actions of the hormone became evident, such as inhibition of TSH, insulin, glucagon, and several other gastrointestinal hormones and functions. As somatostatin has abundant gastrointestinal distribution, it is not measured in the circulation in a clinical setting, because levels do not reflect hypothalamic activity. The significance of this widespread distribution and different actions, which are mediated by at least five types of receptors, are not clear. But the development of somatostatin analogues, with selective and powerful actions inhibiting GH and TSH secretion, have made possible their current use in clinical practice.

Except in tumoral hypersecretory states, GH secretion occurs in a pulsatile manner with eight to 12 pulses occurring in a 24-h period. Most of its daily output occurs during sleep (Fig. 2.1.4) especially in males. It is currently believed that growth hormone pulses are generated by the interplay of the two antagonist hormones GHRH and somatostatin, and it has been suggested that for growth hormone to be released, GHRH and somatostatin secretion by the hypothalamus should be out of phase, an attractive mechanistic view that lacks, at present, definitive proof. This scheme of regulation has also been used to explain the growth hormone discharge induced by stress, physical exercise, arginine infusion, or drugs such as clonidine or pyridostigmine, as well as insulin-induced hypoglycaemia. Artificial compounds such as growth hormone-releasing peptide-6 (GHRP-6), hexarelin, and others collectively called GHSs, have been used as stimulants of growth hormone secretion, and for cloning their receptor; interestingly the endogenous ligand of this receptor has been discovered and named ghrelin. The nutritional and metabolic control of growth hormone secretion is remarkable. In fact, insulin-mediated hypoglycaemia, as in the classic insulin tolerance test (ITT), not only leads to a reflex discharge of growth

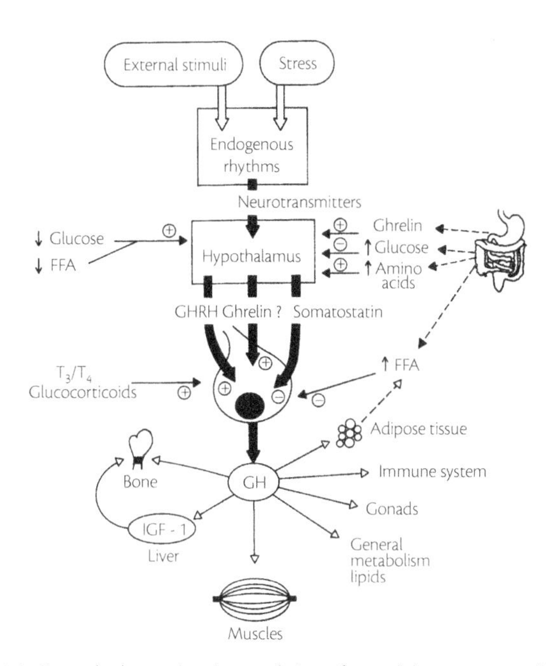

Fig. 2.1.3 General scheme showing regulation of growth hormone secretion. FFA, free fatty acids; GHRH, growth hormone-releasing hormone.

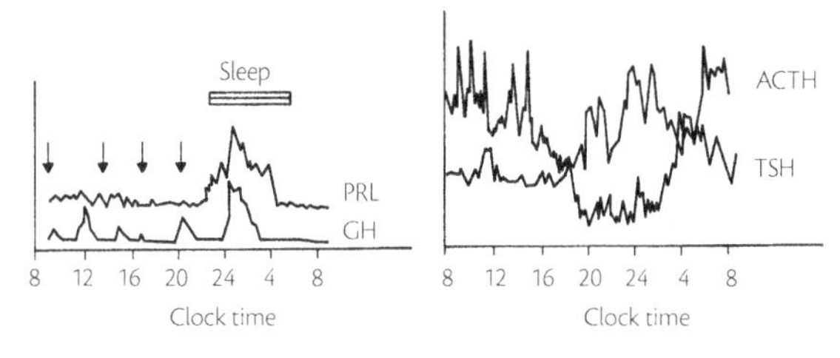

Fig. 2.1.4 Secretion of growth hormone (GH), prolactin (PRL), thyroid-stimulating hormone (TSH), and adrenocorticotropic hormone (ACTH), and their relationship to circadian rhythm and sleep. Values are depicted in arbitrary units, arrows indicate meal times.

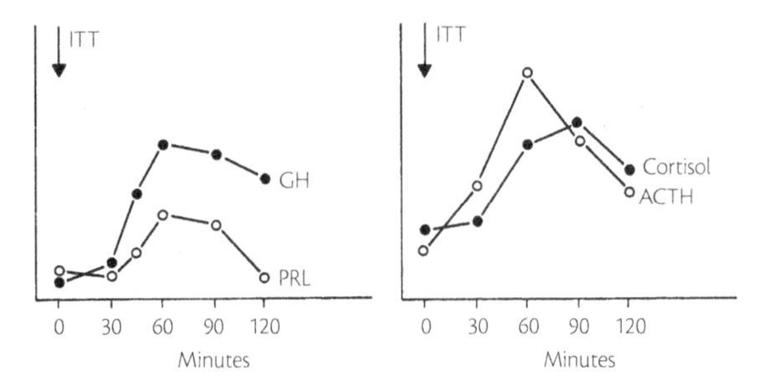

Fig. 2.1.5 Reflex discharge of growth hormone (GH), prolactin (PRL), and adrenocorticotropic hormone (ACTH) alters insulin-induced hypoglycaemia (ITT). The rise in cortisol is ACTH mediated. Arbitrary units.

hormone but also of prolactin, and ACTH/cortisol (Fig. 2.1.5). On the contrary, glucose administration inhibits growth hormone secretion, either basal or stimulated. A similar role is exerted by free fatty acids, the plasma reduction of which by pharmacological means enhances growth hormone secretion. On the contrary, their elevation by physiological or pharmacological means inhibits growth hormone secretion elicited by all stimuli so far known. Arginine and other amino acids stimulate the secretion of growth hormone by mechanisms that are still not well understood.

In summary, several physiological or pharmacological factors acting at hypothalamic level stimulate growth hormone secretion, namely deep sleep, hypoglycaemia, arginine, glucagon administration, physical exercise, clonidine, L-dopa, cholinergic agonists, and stress; others stimulate growth hormone, acting at the pituitary level, e.g. GHRH and free fatty acid reduction. On the contrary, growth hormone is reduced or inhibited by factors acting at the hypothalamic level, such as glucose load or cholinergic antagonists (atropine, pirenzepine) or at the pituitary level, such as somatostatin or free fatty acid rise.

Growth hormone actions

Growth hormone is rapidly cleared with a half-life between 10 and 20 min after its secretion into the circulation. Growth hormone circulates complexed to transporter proteins called growth hormone-binding proteins (GHBP), which are structurally equivalent to the extracellular region of the growth hormone receptor. The binding of growth hormone to the GHBP leads to a delayed clearance, but the physiological and pathological implications of such binding are at present controversial and it has not yet been ascertained whether variations in the growth hormone-GHBP complex may represent a new level of regulation in the somatotroph axis.

Acting at the liver, growth hormone generates IGF-1, which, either in free form or complexed to the several binding proteins, exerts widespread actions from which it is difficult to discern which are exerted by growth hormone and IGF-1. The main actions of growth hormone are the promotion of skeletal growth, mainly of long bones, and the regulation of several metabolic actions. In long bones growth hormone promotes growth by acting on the growing cartilage by a dual action, i.e. growth hormone initiates chondrocyte replication, which along with the maturative process, releases IGF-1 locally and expresses the IGF-1 receptor. This means that growth hormone initiates a local process, which is then propagated by the combined action of growth hormone and IGF-1. In the muscles, growth hormone acts as a trophic hormone, promotes the incorporation of amino acids and protein synthesis. On the contrary, at the adipose tissue level growth hormone promotes lipolysis and release of free fatty acids, exerting antagonistic actions on insulin.

With the availability of recombinant growth hormone, some previously unexpected actions of this hormone have been well defined. In this regard, growth hormone deficiency is clinically characterized by changes in body composition including increase in fat mass and reduction in lean mass, reduced muscular strength and exercise capability, as well as impaired psychological wellbeing, reduction in bone mineral density, alterations in lipoprotein and carbohydrate metabolism, and changes in renal and cardiac function. Growth hormone replacement reverses several of these adverse body composition changes. Recently, pegvisomant a bioengineered analogue of growth hormone, which blocks growth hormone receptor, has been developed. Pegvisomant inhibits IGF-1 synthesis and reverses most of the morbid consequences of growth hormone excess.

The reduction in growth hormone levels that occurs with progressive ageing may be in part responsible for the deleterious changes in body composition associated with ageing (see also Chapter 2.3.7).

Pituitary-adrenal axis

ACTH is a single chain peptide released by specific cell types of the pituitary, the corticotroph cells. The initial synthesis is of a larger peptide called POMC, which after proteolytic cleavage generates several peptides and hormones, among which are ACTH, and β-lipotropin. The main role of ACTH is to stimulate synthesis and secretion of the adrenal cortex hormones, mainly cortisol. ACTH is secreted in a pulsatile fashion, which is under positive hypothalamic control through a neurohormone called corticotropin-releasing hormone (CRH), which acting on specific pituitary receptors, increases ACTH secretion and *POMC* gene expression (Fig. 2.1.6). Direct evidence for a regulatory role of factors other than CRH is absent in human. Levels of ACTH and cortisol follow a circadian rhythm with higher values in the first hour of the

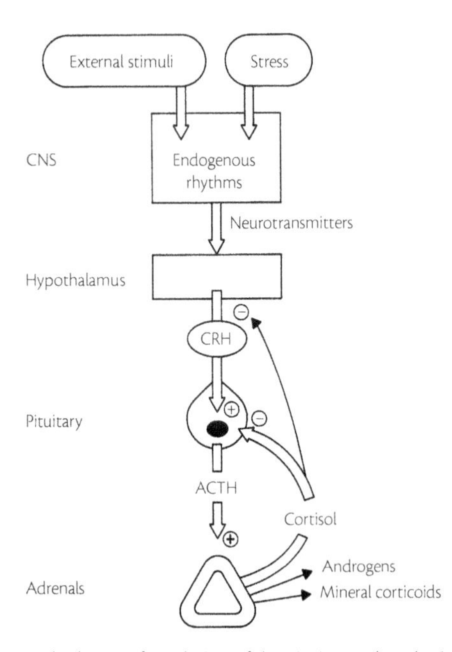

Fig. 2.1.6 General scheme of regulation of the pituitary-adrenal axis. CNS, central nervous system.

morning (06.00–08.00 h) that become progressively reduced, reaching the nadir (approximately 50% of morning levels) at around 20.00 h (see Fig. 2.1.4). This circadian rhythm is generated in the suprachiasmatic and paraventricular nucleus of the hypothalamus. Superimposed onto the circadian rhythm and at any time, a stressful situation, either physical or mental, may induce a large discharge of ACTH into the circulation with a similar increase in cortisol; this stress-mediated release is more robust if the stressful situation is unexpected. Apart from the above situations, the system is maintained under equilibrium by the feedback regulatory action of cortisol, which acting mainly on the pituitary and also on the hypothalamus, inhibiting or reducing ACTH release. A classic regulatory feedback is established between ACTH and cortisol, and the role of CRH is to determine the set point of the system, to modulate the circadian rhythm and, in case of stress, to start a stress response. The biological variable to be maintained is cortisol, and the other adrenal cortex hormones whose secretions are enhanced by ACTH, such as androgens, do not exert a regulatory feedback action at the pituitary. This explains why in situations of enzymatic defects that selectively lead to a reduced cortisol secretion, overstimulation exerted by ACTH normalizes cortisol levels at the expense of hypertrophy of the adrenal glands, thereby inducing different degrees of virilization due to androgen oversecretion. ACTH has no biological actions other than stimulating the adrenal cortex; therefore the clinical manifestations of its abnormal secretion will be those of either excess or reduced secretion of adrenal hormones, mainly cortisol. The system is exquisitely regulated and the simultaneous evaluation of ACTH and cortisol is valuable. On a theoretical basis, a deficit in cortisol secretion with elevated ACTH levels (also elevated melanocyte-stimulating hormone levels, and then skin hyperpigmentation) is indicative of an adrenal defect (Addison's disease), and the same cortisol deficit with normal or low ACTH levels (no pigmentation) suggests ACTH deficiency. However, in most cases dynamic or provocative tests are needed to firmly establish the diagnosis.

The negative feedback of cortisol on the ACTH secretion by corticotrophs may be imitated by synthetic glucocorticoids such as dexamethasone. As tumorous corticotrophs are more resistant to this feedback than normal ones, this fact has been exploited in the differential diagnosis of Cushing's syndrome. A low dexamethasone dose able to reduce ACTH secretion and then cortisol levels in healthy people will fail in the case of a pituitary adenoma secreting ACTH (Cushing's disease). A high dose of dexamethasone will usually overcome the resistance of the pituitary adenoma inhibiting ACTH and cortisol, but will not suppress the hypercortisolism of an adrenal adenoma, which is associated with low ACTH levels.

Pituitary-gonadal axis

The neurons secreting gonadotropin-releasing hormone (GnRH) into the arcuate nucleus of hypothalamus are modulated for many neurotransmitters and peptides from various brain regions and also by environmental and hormonal signals. GnRH neurons may have an intrinsic pulse-generating capacity and they secrete and release GnRH in a pulsatile manner. This GnRH pulsatility is essential for maintenance of normal gonadotropin pulsatile secretion and gonadal steroids synthesis, which in turn exert both stimulatory and inhibitory actions at the hypothalamic level.

Kisspeptins are a family of peptides that act through the specific G-protein-coupled receptor (KISS1) to markedly stimulate GnRH-induced gonadotropin secretion. Mutations in the gene coding for this receptor, result in idiopathic hypogonadotropic hypogonadism. Kisspeptin–KISS1 signalling has an important role in initiating GnRH secretion at puberty. Levels of gonadotropins are very low in children but are already pulsatile in prepuberty. In females, GnRH pulsatility controls the activation of the reproductive system as well as its deactivation. In prepuberty, very low plasma gonadotropin values increase progressively and the pulsatile pattern is mainly nocturnal. These changes are accentuated in puberty. In women the pulsatile pattern of gonadotropins is regarded as a reflection of the rhythm induced by GnRH secretion, with the difference that an external increase in the frequency or quantity of GnRH leads to receptor desensitization and to the paradoxical inhibition in the release of gonadotropins. This fact is used in the clinical setting for inducing a reversible chemical castration by the administration of large doses of exogenous GnRH.

The hypothalamic control of luteinizing hormone and FSH secretion is extremely sensitive to environmental conditions such as stressful situations and to changes in nutrition or energy homoeostasis (Fig. 2.1.7). It is assumed that stress activates the intrahypothalamic corticotropin-releasing hormone pathways, which would inhibit the GnRH neurons through opiate pathways. Mental or psychological stress, such as changing home, or problems at work, or alternatively a relevant reduction in the daily food intake leads to a reduction in GnRH secretion translated into a reduced and non-pulsatile secretion of luteinizing hormone and FSH in the circulation. In fact, in patients with malnutrition-mediated amenorrhoea, such as in anorexia nervosa, gonadotropins return to the prepubertal pattern.

In the follicular phase most of the luteinizing hormone pulses are followed by a release of oestrogens from the ovary, and in the mid and late luteal phase the luteinizing hormone pulses induce

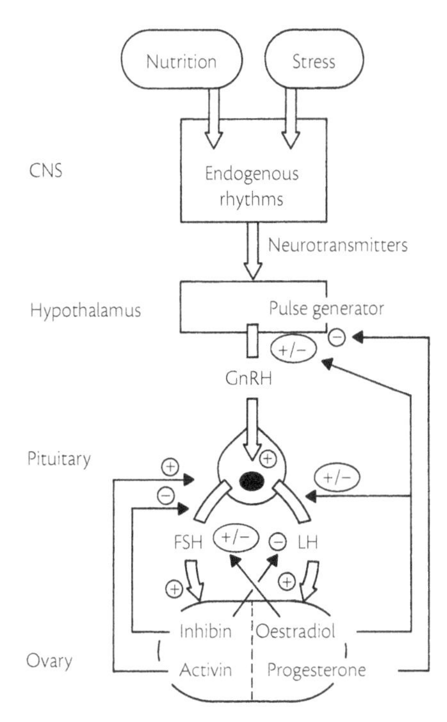

Fig. 2.1.7 General scheme showing regulation of the female pituitary–gonadal axis. CNS, central nervous system; FSH, follicle-stimulating hormone; GnRH, gonadotropin-releasing hormone; LH, luteinizing hormone.

a progesterone secretion. Oestradiol and progesterone exert an inhibitory action on the release of luteinizing hormone, acting at both hypothalamic and pituitary level; however, in the follicular phase associated with an enhanced release of oestradiol the inhibitory action suddenly changes to a stimulatory one, inducing a large discharge of luteinizing hormone, which is responsible for ovulation (see Fig. 2.1.7). The ovary exerts negative feedback on FSH secretion mostly through the secretion of the peptide hormone inhibin, which is synthesized in granulosa cells of the ovarian follicle and counterbalanced by activin. In the late follicular phase inhibin levels increase and, in combination with oestradiol, inhibit the synthesis and release of FSH, an inhibition that is overcome at the preovulatory gonadotrophin discharge. The regulation of the gonadal axis is equally complex but more static in males. No clear data regarding the regulation of GnRH by stress, or nutrition exist in males (Fig. 2.1.8). It is assumed that gonadotropin pulses in males follow the scarce pulses of hypothalamic GnRH and in fact are highly variable and of small amplitude. Unlike in females, the luteinizing hormone pulses are not translated into a peripheral pulse of testosterone, and no positive feedback on luteinizing hormone secretion has been reported, the system being operative on simple negative feedback. Sertoli cells in the male secrete activin and inhibin in order to regulate FSH secretion.

Pituitary-thyroid axis

The axis is regulated at three levels and the hypothalamic participation is exerted through the synthesis and release in the median eminence, and hence in the portal vessels, of thyrotropin-releasing hormone (TRH). Acting through specific receptors on thyrotroph cells, TRH induces the secretion of TSH, which in turn activates follicular cells in the thyroid gland to secrete into circulating blood the thyroid hormones triiodothyronine (T_3) and thyroxine (T_4). Thyroid hormones act on practically all tissues of the body, exerting multiple functions but mainly on general metabolic homoeostasis. Acting on the pituitary gland, they exert a negative feedback on thyrotrophs, inhibiting the release of TSH thereby closing the regulatory circuit (Fig. 2.1.9). They also act at hypothalamic level to reduce TRH secretion but this action is at best ancillary.

TSH secretion follows a circadian rhythm with elevation in the late hours of the evening (see Fig. 2.1.4). In addition to thyroid hormones, it is under the negative control of dopamine and somatostatin, and under the positive control of oestrogens. The physiological

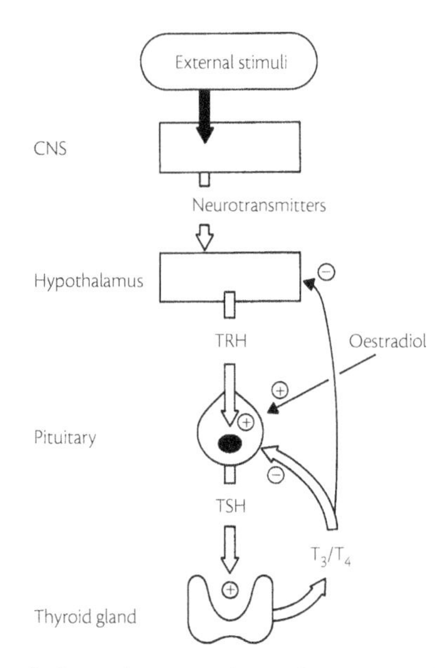

Fig. 2.1.9 General scheme showing regulation of the pituitary-thyroid axis. CNS, central nervous system; T_3/T_4 thyroid hormones; TRH, thyrotropin-releasing hormone; TSH, thyroid-stimulating hormone.

meaning and relevance of these regulations is controversial. The inhibitory action of somatostatin on TSH secretion is currently used employing somatostatin analogues in clinical practice to control pituitary tumours that secrete TSH. Between the two messages arriving at the pituitary thyrotroph cell, the stimulatory message of TRH and the inhibitory one of the thyroid hormones, the latter is more powerful. In fact, the administration of exogenous TRH to elicit a TSH discharge becomes dampened or blocked in situations of hyperthyroidism and is enhanced in hypothyroidism.

Lactotroph axis

The main action of prolactin is to initiate and maintain physiological lactation (Fig. 2.1.10). Released by lactotroph cells of the adenohypophysis, its molecular structure is similar to growth hormone and placental lactogen and they share a common phylogenetic origin. Similar to growth hormone, prolactin is a pituitary hormone acting on peripheral tissues without the intervention of a target gland.

The hypothalamic tubero-infundibular dopaminergic system is the main regulator of prolactin secretion. Among the pituitary

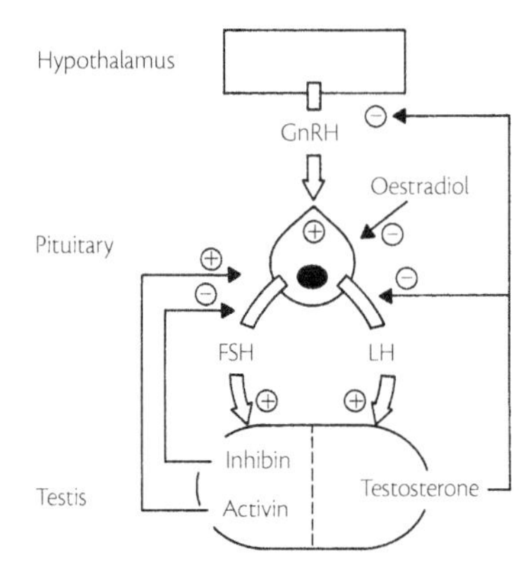

Fig. 2.1.8 General scheme showing regulation of the male pituitary-gonadal axis. FSH, follicle-stimulating hormone; GnRH, gonadotropin-releasing hormone; LH, luteinizing hormone.

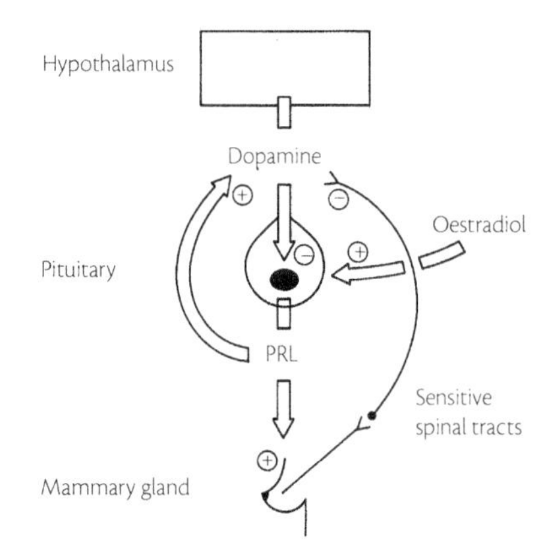

Fig. 2.1.10 General scheme showing regulation of the lactotroph axis. PRL, prolactin.

secreted hormones, prolactin is the only one with a negative hypothalamic control through dopamine. This fact confers some peculiarities to prolactin regulation and in cases of pituitary stalk section, prolactin secretion may be maintained, and when the hypothalamo-pituitary connection is impeded, all pituitary hormones are reduced except for prolactin. Dopamine reaches the lactotrophs through the hypothalamic-pituitary portal system and inhibits prolactin release. Dopamine is the only widely accepted physiological regulator of prolactin secretion. Hypothalamic stressors such as the insulin tolerance test (ITT) are able to release prolactin, and exogenous administration of TRH releases prolactin in addition to TSH, operating through specific lactotroph receptors. Both tests have been used for assessing the pituitary reserve of prolactin but they are not considered to be physiological regulators of its secretion.

Prolactin is secreted in a pulsatile fashion with a rhythm that shows an enhanced nocturnal secretion not associated with specific sleep stages (see Fig. 2.1.4). Nonspecific stress is able to release prolactin in some individuals, a fact that must be taken into account in clinical testing. Oestrogens have a marked effect on lactotroph cells, producing hyperplasia as well as enhanced prolactin secretion. The increment in pituitary volume in pregnant women may be in part due to the large oestrogenic production by the fetoplacental unit. Lactation and sexual intercourse increase prolactin secretion, and hypothyroidism in both genders is able to increase prolactin secretion through an unexplained mechanism; perhaps due to the hypersecretion of TRH by the thyroid hormone-deprived hypothalamus plus enhanced TRH receptor expression in lactotrophs.

Abnormally elevated levels of prolactin are capable of altering several endocrine axes in both sexes, inducing different degrees of hypogonadism. However the physiological role of this hormone is only accepted in pregnant or lactating women. Prolactin is viewed as the hormone that induces the maternal instinct. In mammary tissue primed with oestrogens and progesterone, prolactin induces the synthesis of milk proteins. After partum, the stimulation on the mammary nipple during lactation induces a nervous signal, which on reaching the hypothalamus inhibits dopamine secretion, releasing prolactin, which in turn stimulates milk production. Oxytocin, which is released simultaneously, ejects the accumulated milk.

Summary

The hypothalamus through specific neurohormones controls the release and action of several pituitary hormones that play a leading role in endocrine physiology. Hypothalamic hormones are not commonly measured in blood, but are injected for diagnostic testing. On the contrary, pituitary hormones and their target peripheral hormones are commonly measured in the clinical setting. Except ITT, the most provocative tests of pituitary secretion, such as the administration of GnRH, GHRH, and TRH, are less commonly used and have been replaced by the analysis of pituitary hormone basal value weighted against the peripheral hormone.

Further reading

1. Kovacs K, Scheithauer BW, Horvath E, Lloyd RV. The World Health Organization classification of adenohypophyseal neoplasms. *Cancer*, 1996; **78**: 502–10.
2. Nieuwenhijzen Kruseman AC. Structure and function of the hypothalamus and pituitary. In: Grossman A, ed. *Clinical Endocrinology*. 2nd edn. Oxford: Blackwell Science, 1998: 83–9.
3. Nieuwenhuys R. *Chemoarchitecture of the Brain*. Berlin: Springer-Verlag, 1985.
4. Clemmons D, Robinson I, Christen Y. IGFs: Local repair and survival factors throughout life span. 1st Edition; 2010, XIII, 157 p.
5. Casanueva FF, Molitch ME, Schlechte JA, Abs R, Bonert V, Bronstein MD, et al. Guidelines of the Pituitary Society of the diagnosis and management of prolactinomas. *Clin Endocrinol (Oxf)*, 2006; **65**(2):265–73.

References

1. Couce M, Dieguez C, Casanueva FF. Pituitary anatomy and physiology. In: Wass JAH, Shalet SM, eds. *Oxford Textbook of Endocrinology and Diabetes*. Oxford: Oxford University Press, 2002: 75–85.
2. Anderson E, Haymaker W. Breakthroughs in hypothalamic and pituitary research. *Prog Brain Res*, 1974; **41**: 1–60.
3. Carpenter MB. *Core Text of Neuroanatomy*. 4th edn. Baltimore: Williams and Wilkins, 1991; 297–324.
4. Heimer L. *The Human Brain and Spinal Cord. Functional Neuroanatomy and Dissection Guide*. NewYork: Springer-Verlag, 1983: 296–307.
5. Bevan JS, Scanlon MF. Regulation of the hypothalamus and pituitary. In: Grossman A, ed. *Clinical Endocrinology*. 2nd edn. Oxford: Blackwell Science, 1998: 90–112.
6. Leakk RK, Moore RY. Topographic organization of suprachiasmatic nucleus projecting neurons. *J Comp Neurol*, 2001; **433**: 312–34.
7. Casanueva FF. Enfermedades del hipotalamo y la adenhipofisis. In: Rozman C, ed. *Medicina Interna Textbook*. Vol. 11. 16th edn. Barcelona: Harcourt, 2008: 2028–54.
8. Sam S, Frohman LA. Normal physiology of hypothalamic pituitary regulation. *Endocrinol Metab Clin North Am*, 2008; **37**: 1–22.

2.2

The neurohypophysis

Stephen G. Ball

Neuroanatomy, molecular biology, and physiology of the neurohypophysis

The neurohypophysis is a complex neurohumoral system with a key role in body fluid homoeostasis and reproductive function. This chapter will concentrate on the physiology and pathophysiology of the two hormones made by the neurohypophysis, vasopressin and oxytocin, outlining the roles of both hormones together with the molecular, cellular, and anatomical basis of their regulation and function.

The neurohypophysis: neuroanatomy

The neurohypophysis consists of three parts: the hypothalamic nucleii (supraoptic and paraventricular) containing the cell bodies of the magnocellular, neurosecretory neurons that synthesize and secrete vasopressin and oxytocin; the supraoptico-hypophyseal tract, which includes the axons of these neurons; and the posterior pituitary, where the axons terminate on capillaries of the inferior hypophyseal artery (Fig. 2.2.1).

The supraoptic nucleus (SON) is situated along the proximal part of the optic tract. It consists largely of the cell bodies of discrete vasopressinergic and oxytocic magnocellular neurosecretory neurons projecting to the posterior pituitary along the supraoptico-hypophyseal tract. In humans, vasopressinergic neurons are found in the ventral SON, with oxytocic neurons situated dorsally. The paraventricular nucleus (PVN) also contains discrete vasopressinergic and oxytocic magnocellular neurons projecting to the posterior pituitary along the supraoptico-hypophyseal tract. In humans, magnocellular neurons of the PVN synthesizing vasopressin are found centrally in the nucleus, with oxytocic neurons in the periphery. The PVN contains additional smaller parvicellular neurons projecting to the median eminence and additional extrahypothalamic areas including the forebrain, brainstem, and spinal cord. Some of these parvicellular neurons are vasopressinergic. Some vasopressinergic parvicellular neurons terminate in the hypophyseal-portal bed of the pituitary. These neurons cosecrete corticotropin-releasing hormone, and have a role in the regulation of adrenocorticotropin (ACTH) release.

The posterior pituitary receives an arterial blood supply from the inferior hypophyseal artery and the artery of the trabecula (a branch of the superior hypophyseal artery). Both these vessels derive from the internal carotid artery and its branches. The SON and PVN receive an arterial supply from the suprahypophyseal, anterior communicating, anterior cerebral, posterior communicating, and posterior cerebral arteries, via the circle of Willis. Venous drainage of the neurohypophysis is via the dural, cavernous and inferior petrosal sinuses.

Molecular and cell biology

Mammalian vasopressin is a basic nonapeptide, with a disulfide bridge between the cysteine residues at positions 1 and 6 (Fig. 2.2.2). Most mammals have the amino acid arginine at position 8. In the pig family, arginine is substituted by lysine. Oxytocin differs from vasopressin by only two amino acids—isoleucine for phenylalanine at position 3, and leucine for arginine at position 8. Nonmammalian species have a variety of peptides very similar to vasopressin and oxytocin. The similarities between vasopressin and oxytocin, and the degree of conservation among similar peptides across the animal kingdom, probably reflects derivation from a common ancestral gene.

The vasopressin-neurophysin and oxytocin-neurophysin genes

The *VP* and *OT* genes lie in tandem array on chromosome 20, separated by 8 kb and 11 kb of DNA in humans and rats, respectively. Both genes are composed of three exons, and encode polypeptide precursors with a common modular structure: an N-terminal signal peptide, the specific vasopressin or oxytocin sequence, a hormone-specific mid-molecule peptide termed a neurophysin (Np), and a C-terminal peptide (Fig. 2.2.3). There is considerable homology between the Np sequences of the two genes, positions 10–74 being highly conserved at the amino acid level.

Hypothalamic-specific expression of *VP* and *OT* genes is conferred through selective repressor elements within both structural genes and the 5′ flanking sequences (1). Expression of the *VP* gene has been observed in extrahypothalamic tissues, such as adrenal gland, gonads, cerebellum, and probably the pituicytes of the posterior pituitary gland (2). Additional loci of control involved in *VP* expression in these tissues remain to be determined.

The regulation of *VP* gene expression is mediated through positive and negative regulatory elements in the proximal promoter. Several transcription factors bind to these elements; activating proteins 1 and 2 (AP1 and AP2) and cAMP-responsive element

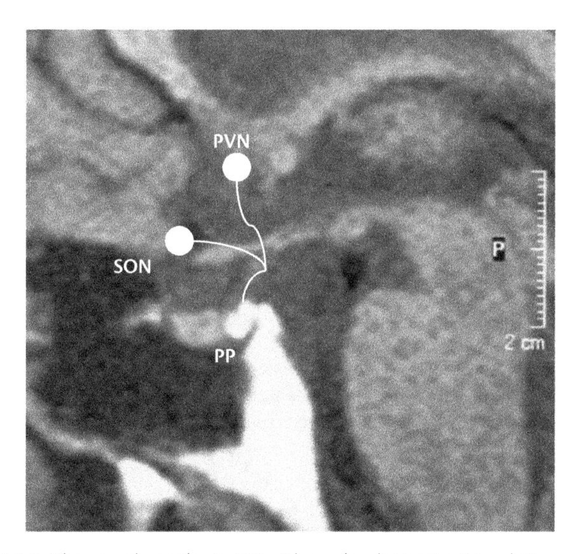

Fig. 2.2.1 The neurohypophysis. MRI with overlay demonstrating relative positions of the paraventricular nucleus (PVN), supraoptic nucleus (SON) connecting to the posterior pituitary (PP) via the supraoptico-hypophyseal tract.

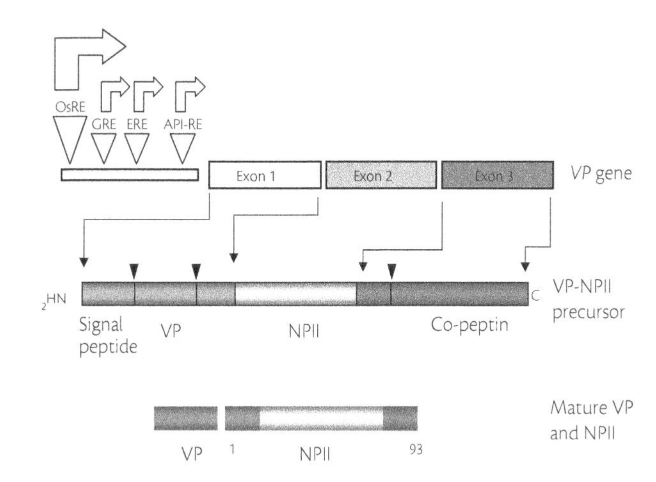

Fig. 2.2.3 Functional organization of the *VP* gene. The *VP* gene consists of three exons encoding a large precursor which is cleaved to produce the mature peptide through post-translational modification. The VP 5′-promoter contains a number of response element sites that interact with transcription factors regulating *VP* gene expression. Os-RE, GRE, ERE, and API-RE represent the response elements for osmoregulation: the glucocorticoid receptor, the oestrogen receptor, and AP1, respectively.

binding proteins (CREB) stimulate expression, while the glucocorticoid receptor negatively regulates expression (3, 4). The human, rat, and mouse *OT* promoters contain oestrogen-response elements and interleukin 6 (IL-6) response elements. However, the functional significance of these remain unclear (5).

VP gene expression can also be regulated at a post-transcriptional level. Water deprivation leads to an increase in length of the poly(A) tail of vasopressin mRNA, altering mRNA stability. Vasopressin mRNA processing may be further influenced through the interaction of a dendritic localization sequence, contained within the mRNA, with a multifunctional poly(A) binding protein (PABP). This RNA-protein interaction may play key role in RNA stabilization, initiation of translation, and translational silencing (6, 7).

Synthesis, release, and metabolism of neurohypophyseal hormones

Synthesis of vasopressin and oxytocin precursors occur separately in the cell bodies of specific magnocellular neurosecretory neurons of the SON and PVN. Generation of both mature hormones entails substantial post-translational modification of the large primary precursor. Following translation, the C-terminal domains are glycosylated and the precursors packaged in vesicles of the regulated secretory pathway which migrate along neuronal axons toward the nerve terminals of the neurohypophysis. Migration is microtubule dependent. During this process, the vasopressin and oxytocin precursors are cleaved by basic endopeptidases. The final products of processing, the mature hormone and the respective Nps, are stored as a complex in secretory granules within the nerve terminals of the posterior pituitary (8). An increase in the firing frequency of vasopressinergic and oxytocic neurons result in the opening of voltage-gated $Ca^{2?}$ channels in the nerve terminals which, through transient $Ca^{2?}$ influx, results in fusion of the neurosecretory granules with the nerve terminal membrane and release of their contents into the circulation. The hormone and its Np are cosecreted into the systemic circulation in equimolar quantities (9). Both Nps can bind both vasopressin and oxytocin *in vitro*. However, apart from acting as carrier proteins for vasopressin and oxytocin during axonal migration, Nps appear to serve no specific biological function.

The half-life of both vasopressin and oxytocin is short, that of vasopressin being 5–15 min (10). Both hormones circulate in the free form, unbound to plasma proteins. However, vasopressin does bind to specific receptors on platelets. Vasopressin concentrations in platelet-rich plasma are thus about fivefold higher than in platelet-depleted plasma (11). Both vasopressin and oxytocin are degraded by several endothelial and circulating endo- and aminopeptidases. A specific placental cysteine aminopeptidase degrades vasopressin and oxytocin rapidly during pregnancy and the immediate postpartum period.

Physiology of vasopressin

Regulation of vasopressin release

Neurophysiology of vasopressin release

Neurohypohyseal hormone release is modulated by sensory signals. In the case of vasopressin, the key sensory regulatory inputs reflect osmotic status and blood pressure/circulating volume. The relationships of the SON and PVN with the autonomic afferents and central nervous system nucleii responsible for osmo- and baroregulation are thus key to the physiological regulation of vasopressin. Functional osmoreceptors are situated in anterior circumventricular structures: the subfornicular organ, and the

	Amino acid position 1 2 3 4 5	6 7 8 9	Distribution
Arginine vasopressin: Cys-Tyr-Phe-Glu(NH_2)-Asp(NH_2)-Cys-Pro-Arg-Gly(NH_2)			Most mammals
Lysine vasopressin	Phe Glu(NH_2)	Lys	Pig family
Oxytocin	Ile Glu(NH_2)	Leu	Mammals, birds

Fig. 2.2.2 Amino acid sequences of vasopressin and oxytocin.

organum vasculosum of the lamina terminalis (OVLT) (12). Local fenestrations in the blood–brain barrier allow this neural tissue direct contact with the circulation. However, the presence of specific water channels (aquaporin 4) in both SON and PVN suggests that vasopressin neurons may have independent osmoreceptor function (13, 14). Moreover, vasopressin neurons of the SON and PVN express vasopressin receptors, highlighting the potential for autocontrol of vasopressin release through small branching neurites (15, 16). The act of drinking causes rapid suppression of vasopressin secretion. This response is mediated by oropharyngeal receptors. The afferent pathway(s) for this additional inhibitory influence on vasopressin release have not been identified.

Baroregulatory influences on vasopressin release derive from aortic arch, carotid sinus, cardiac atrial, and great vein afferents via cranial nerves IX and X. These project to the nucleus tractus solitarius (NTS) in the brainstem, from where further afferents project to the SON and PVN. Additional adrenergic afferents project to the SON and PVN from other brainstem nucleii, such as the locus coeruleus. Together, these act to integrate afferent inputs reflecting volume status. Interruption of ascending baroafferents increases plasma vasopressin concentrations, consistent with some degree of tonic inhibitory drive (17, 18).

Humoral regulation of vasopressin release

The renin–angiotensin system is intricately involved in the regulation of vasopressin production. Circulating angiotensin II stimulates vasopressin secretion through receptors in the subfornicular organ and activation of subfornicular organ afferents. In addition, angiotensin II stimulates vasopressin release via a direct effect on vasopressin magnocellular neurons, where type 2 angiotensin II receptors have been identified (19). In rat, atrial natriuretic peptide (ANP) inhibits both osmo- and barostimulated vasopressin release via subfornicular organ afferents (20). The related brain natriuretic peptide (BNP) also inhibits vasopressinergic neurons in the SON *in vitro*. However, there are no data to suggest that ANP is a key regulator of physiological vasopressin release in humans (21).

Osmoregulation of vasopressin release

Plasma osmolality is the most important determinant of vasopressin secretion. The osmoregulatory system for thirst and vasopressin secretion maintains plasma osmolality within the narrow limits of 284–295 mOsml/kg. The osmoregulation of vasopressin production and the physiological relationship between plasma osmolality and plasma vasopressin concentration is described by three characteristics: the linear relationship between plasma osmolality and plasma vasopressin concentration; the osmotic threshold or 'set point' for vasopressin release; and the sensitivity of the osmoregulatory mechanism.

Increases in plasma osmolality increase plasma vasopressin concentrations in a linear manner (Fig. 2.2.4). The abscissal intercept of this regression line, 284 mOsml/kg, indicates the mean 'osmotic threshold' for vasopressin release: the mean plasma osmolality above which plasma vasopressin starts to increase. Though there is no level of plasma osmolality below which vasopressin release is completely suppressed (22), such low levels of vasopressin have little antidiuretic effect. The concept of a threshold of vasopressin release thus remains a pragmatic means to characterize the physiology of osmoregulation; vasopressin release being increased from

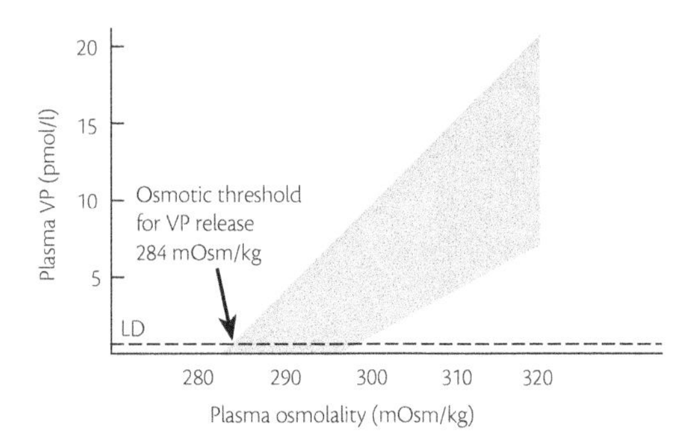

Fig. 2.2.4 Relationship between plasma osmolality and plasma vasopressin (VP) concentration during progressive hypertonicity induced by infusion of 855 mmol/l saline in a group of healthy adults. LD represents the limit of detection of the assay, 0.3 pmol/l.

a basal rate by activation of stimulatory osmoreceptor afferents, and decreased to minimal values by removal of this drive and the activation of synergistic inhibitory afferents. The slope of the regression line reflects the sensitivity of osmoregulated vasopressin release. There are considerable interindividual variations in both threshold and sensitivity of vasopressin release. Twin studies indicate a strong heritable component in this variation. However, over time, these parameters are remarkably reproducible within an individual (23).

There are several physiological situations where the tight relationship between plasma osmolality and vasopressin concentration is lost. The act of drinking results in rapid suppression of vasopressin release, independent of changes in osmolality. In addition, the rate of change of plasma osmolality can influence the vasopressin response; rapid increases in plasma osmolality result in exaggerated vasopressin release. The osmotic threshold for vasopressin release is lowered in normal pregnancy, and a similar though smaller change occurs in the luteal phase of the menstrual cycle. Plasma vasopressin concentrations increase with age, together with enhanced vasopressin responses to osmotic stimulation. In contrast, thirst appreciation is blunted and fluid intake reduced. These changes, together with age-related decreases in renal handling of water loads and generation of maximal urine concentration, form the basis for the predisposition of elderly people to both hyper- and hyponatraemia (24).

Baroregulation of vasopressin release

As a principal determinant of fluid homoeostasis, vasopressin is a key player in maintaining haemodynamic integrity. Significant reduction in circulating volume stimulates vasopressin release through the activation of mechanoreceptors in the cardiac atria and central veins. Hypotension stimulates vasopressin release through the activation of aortic arch and carotid sinus afferents. In contrast to osmoregulated vasopressin release, progressive reduction in blood pressure produces an exponential increase in plasma vasopressin. Falls in arterial blood pressure of 5–10% are necessary to increase circulating vasopressin concentrations in humans. Changes in circulating volume and blood pressure trigger an autonomic and endocrine cascade resulting in a coordinated physiological response. Baroregulated vasopressin responses can be modified by other neurohumoral influences triggered as part of this coordinated response: ANP inhibiting and noradrenaline augmenting baroregulated vasopressin release. Importantly, baroregulated vasopressin release can occur at low levels of plasma osmolality—levels that would normally act to suppress vasopressin production. This apparent 'hierarchy' of regulation is important when considering the integrated physiological response to volume depletion and the pathophysiology of hyponatraemia.

Other regulatory mechanisms of vasopressin release

Nausea and emesis are potent stimuli to vasopressin release, independent of osmotic and haemodynamic status. Manipulation of abdominal contents is another powerful stimulus to vasopressin release. Both contribute to the high plasma vasopressin values and consequent impairment of water load excretion observed after gastrointestinal surgery. Vasopressin release in response to these stimuli and others, such as neuroglycopenia, justify its classification as a stress response hormone.

Thirst

Thirsts, and the drinking response to thirst, are key components maintaining fluid homoeostasis. The basis of thirst and the regulation of water ingestion involve complex, integrated neural and neurohumoral pathways. Animal data place the osmoreceptors regulating thirst in the circumventricular AV3V region of the hypothalamus, anatomically distinct from those mediating vasopressin release (25). Rostral projections to higher centres remain largely unmapped. In rat, lesions in the ventral nucleus medianus can produce adipsia and hyperdipsia, indicating this to be one route through which afferent pathways reach the cerebral cortex.

There is a linear relationship between thirst, determined by visual analogue scale, and plasma osmolalities in the physiological range (Fig. 2.2.5). The mean osmotic threshold for thirst perception is 281 mOsml/kg, similar to that for vasopressin release. Thirst occurs when plasma osmolality rises above this threshold, the intensity varying in relation to the ambient plasma osmolality. The functional characteristics of osmoregulated thirst, just as vasopressin release, remain consistent within an individual on repeated testing, despite wide variations between individuals (23).

As with osmoregulated vasopressin release, there are also specific physiological situations in which the relationship between plasma osmolality and thirst breaks down. The act of drinking reduces osmostimulated thirst, just as it does vasopressin release. There is a fall in the osmotic threshold for thirst in the luteal phase of the menstrual cycle. In contrast, thirst appreciation and fluid intake are blunted in elderly people. Thirst can be stimulated by extracellular volume depletion through volume sensitive cardiac autonomic afferents. In addition, hypovolaemia and hypotension lead to the generation of circulating and intracerebral angiotensin II, a powerful dipsogen (Table 2.2.1).

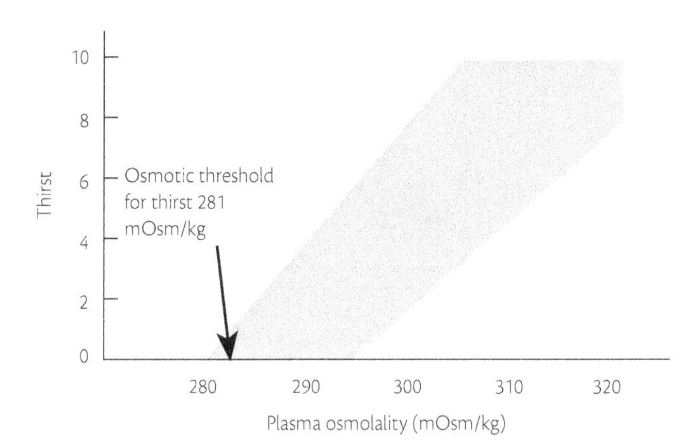

Fig. 2.2.5 Relationship between thirst and plasma osmolality during progressive hypertonicity induced by infusion of 855 mmol/l saline in a group of healthy adults.

Actions of vasopressin

Vasopressin receptors

There are three vasopressin receptor (V-R) subtypes, encoded by different genes (Table 2.2.2). All have seven transmembrane spanning domains, and all are G-protein coupled. They differ in tissue distribution, signal transduction mechanisms, and function. There is 70–80% human–rat subtype homology at the amino acid level (26, 27). The human *V2-R* gene has been mapped to Xq28. The murine *V2-R* gene maps to a syntenic X-chromosome locus. In contrast to many other hormone receptors, the V2-R is up-regulated by its ligand.

Renal effects of vasopressin

Although vasopressin has multiple actions, its principal physiological effect is in the regulation of water reabsorption in the distal nephron. The hairpin structure and electrolyte transport processes of the nephron allow the kidney to both concentrate and dilute urine in response to the prevailing circulating vasopressin concentration. Active transport of solute out of the thick ascending loop of Henle generates an osmolar gradient in the renal interstitium which increases from renal cortex to inner medulla, a gradient through which distal parts of the nephron pass *en route* to the collecting system. This is the basis of the renal countercurrent osmolar exchange mechanism. The presence of selective water channel proteins (aquaporins) in the wall of the distal nephron allows reabsorption of water from the duct lumen along an osmotic gradient, and excretion of concentrated urine.

Thirteen different mammalian aquaporins have been identified to date. Seven (AQP1-4, AQP6-8) can be found in the kidney (28). Aquaporins act as passive pores for small substrates and are divided

Table 2.2.1 Neurotransmitter and humoral regulators of vasopressin release

Enhancers of vasopressin release	Suppressors of vasopressin release
Catecholamines	Catecholamines
Dopamine	Dopamine? (central)
Noradrenaline (β1)	Noradrenaline (α1)
Acetyl choline	Amino acids
	N-methyl-D-aspartate agonists
Amino acids	Peptides
Glutamate	Atrial natriuretic peptide
Aspartate	Brain natriuretic peptide
Peptides	Opioids
Angiotensin II	Leu-encephalin
	β-endorphin
Others	
Nitric oxide	

Table 2.2.2 Vasopressin receptor subtypes

	Vasopressin receptor		
	V1a	**V1b**	**V2**
Expression	◆ Vascular smooth muscle ◆ Liver ◆ Platelets ◆ CNS	Pituitary corticotroph	Basolateral membrane of distal nephron
Amino acid structure	418 amino acids (human)	424 amino acids (human)	
Second messenger system	Gq/11mediated phospholipase C activation: Ca^{2+}, inositol triphosphate and diacylglycerol mobilization	As V1a	
Physiological effects	◆ Smooth muscle contraction ◆ Stimulation of glycogenolysis ◆ Enhanced platelet adhesion ◆ Neurotransmitter and neuromodulatory function	Enhanced adrenocorticotropic hormone release	Increased production and action of aquaporin-2

into two families: the water-only channels; and the aquaglyceroporins that can conduct other small molecules such as glycerol and urea. Specific structural arrangements within the primary, secondary, and tertiary structure convey the three functional characteristics of permeation, selectivity, and gating. The structure of aquaporins involves two tandem repeats, each formed from three transmembrane domains, together with two highly conserved loops containing the signature asparagine-proline-alanine (NPA) motif. All aquaporins form homotetramers in the cell membrane, providing four functionally independent pores with an additional central pore formed between the four monomers. Water can pass through all the four independent channels of water-permeable aquaporins, while the central pore may act as independent channel in some aquaporins (29, 30).

AQP1 is constitutively expressed in the apical and basolateral membranes of the proximal tubule and descending loop of Henle, where it facilitates isotonic fluid movement. Loss of function mutations of AQP1 in humans leads to defective renal water conservation (31). AQP3 and AQP4 are constitutively expressed on the basolateral membrane of collecting duct cells. They facilitate the movement of water from collecting duct cells into the interstitium. Expression of AQP3, but not AQP4 is modulated by vasopressin.

AQP2 is expressed on the luminal surface of collecting duct cells, and is responsible for water transport from the lumen of the nephron into collecting duct cells. Expression of AQP2 is vasopressin dependent; activation of the V2-R producing a biphasic increase in expression of the protein. Generation of intracellular cAMP by ligand activation of the V2-R triggers an intracellular phosphorylation cascade, ultimately resulting in the phosphorylation of nuclear CREB and expression of c-Fos. Activation of these transcription factors stimulates *AQP2* gene expression through CRE and AP1 elements in the AQP2 promoter (32). In addition, vasopressin stimulates an immediate increase in *AQP2* expression by accelerating trafficking of presynthesized protein from intracellular vesicles, and the assembly of functional water channels, composed of AQP2 tetramers, in luminal cell membranes (33).

Maximum diuresis occurs at plasma vasopressin concentrations of 0.5 pmol/l or less. As vasopressin levels rise, there is a sigmoid relationship between plasma vasopressin concentration and urine osmolality, with maximum urine concentration achieved at plasma vasopressin concentrations of 3–4 pmol/l (Fig 2.2.6).

Following persistent vasopressin secretion, antidiuresis may diminish. Down-regulation of both V2-R function and *AQP2* expression may be responsible for this escape phenomenon (34). Vasopressin has additional effects at other parts of the nephron; decreasing medullary blood flow, and stimulating an active urea transporter in the distal collecting duct. Vasopressin can also stimulate active sodium transport into the renal interstitium. These effects contribute to the generation and maintenance of a hypertonic medullary interstitium, thus increasing the osmotic gradient across collecting tubules, and augmenting the antidiuresis produced by the action of vasopressin on distal water channels.

Cardiovascular effects of vasopressin

Vasopressin is a potent pressor agent, its effects mediated via a specific membrane receptor (V1a-R). Systemic effects on arterial blood pressure are only apparent at high concentrations due to compensatory buffering haemodynamic mechanisms. Nevertheless, vasopressin is important in maintaining blood pressure in mild

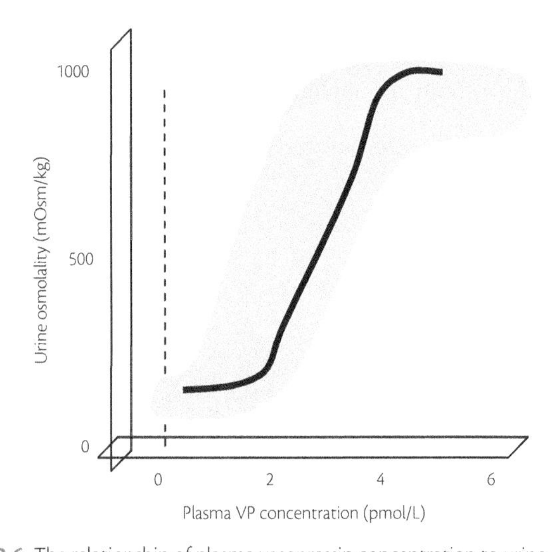

Fig. 2.2.6 The relationship of plasma vasopressin concentration to urine concentrating ability. There is a sigmoid relationship between plasma vasopressin concentration and urine osmolality, with maximum urine concentration occurring at plasma vasopressin concentrations of 4–6 pmol/l. There is a range of response in the normal population depicted by the grey area, within which an individual response is demonstrated.

volume depletion. The most striking vascular effects of vasopressin are in the regulation of regional blood flow. The sensitivity of vascular smooth muscle to the pressor effects of vasopressin vary according to the vascular bed; vasoconstriction of splanchnic, hepatic, and renal vessels occurring at vasopressin concentrations close to the physiological range. Furthermore, there are differential pressor responses within a given vascular bed; selective effects on intrarenal vessels resulting in redistribution of renal blood flow from medulla to cortex. Such effects suggest that baroregulated vasopressin release constitutes one of the key physiological mediators of the integrated haemodynamic response to volume depletion.

Effects of vasopressin on the pituitary

Vasopressin is an ACTH secretagogue, acting through pituitary corticotroph-specific V3-Rs. Though the effect is weak in isolation, vasopressin and corticotropin-releasing factor act synergistically. Vasopressin and corticotropin-releasing factor colocalize in neurohypophyseal parvicellular neurons projecting to the median eminence and the neurohypophyseal portal blood supply of the anterior pituitary. Levels of both vasopressin and corticotropin-releasing factor in these neurons are inversely related to glucocorticoid levels, clearly suggesting a role in feedback regulation.

Central nervous system and other miscellaneous effects of vasopressin

Vasopressinergic fibres and V-Rs are present in many areas of the brain, including the cerebral cortex and limbic system. These extensive neural networks are anatomically and functionally independent of the neurohypophysis (no neuronal connections being apparent, and the blood–brain barrier excluding the majority of circulating factors from these sites). In rodents, these central vasopressinergic systems have key roles in mediating complex social behaviour such as mating patterns. There are similar emerging data in humans, with association studies linking *V1a-R* gene sequence variation with autistic spectrum disorder, social phobia, and interpersonal behaviour patterns (35–37).

A number of other actions of vasopressin are listed in Table 2.2.3 (38–42).

Integrated physiology of vasopressin release and body fluid homoeostasis

The physiological regulation of water balance is intimately linked with that of circulating volume; common systems are involved in both processes. As sodium is the major cationic osmolyte, the interrelationships of sodium and water excretion with circulating volume regulation are key to appreciating the position of vasopressin in the physiology of fluid homoeostasis.

At plasma osmolalities of 285–295 mOsml/kg, osmolar balance can be maintained by vasopressin-dependent regulation of renal water loss. A rise in plasma osmolality within this range produces a progressive increase in plasma vasopressin to a concentration of 3–4 pmol/l, and antidiuresis. Further increases in plasma osmolality stimulate further vasopressin release, but this does not result in any further reduction of renal water excretion. Correction of plasma osmolality back to the range over which osmolar balance can be maintained by vasopressin requires thirst-stimulated drinking. As the osmolar threshold for thirst is similar to that for vasopressin release (284 mOsml/kg), the maintenance of water balance through a combination of osmoregulated vasopressin release and thirst is clearly a seamless, coordinated process of subtle complexity.

If excessive fluid volumes are consumed, greater than those demanded by thirst, plasma vasopressin levels are suppressed to below 0.3 pmol/l, resulting in maximum diuresis of up to 15–20 l/24 h. Ingestion of water in excess of this causes a reduction of plasma osmolality into the subnormal range, and hyponatraemia.

Vasopressin release is also regulated by other, nonosmotic stimuli. This complex regulation has a hierarchy, with significant physiological and pathophysiological sequelae. Hypovolaemia shifts the relationship of plasma osmolality with vasopressin concentration to the left. During moderate hypovolaemia, osmoregulation is maintained around a lower osmolar set point. As the degree of hypovolaemia progresses, baroregulated vasopressin release overrides the osmolar set point, and antidiuresis is maintained despite the potential for ensuing hyponatraemia. Coincident activation of the systemic and intracerebral renin–angiotensin systems stimulates drinking and augments vasopressin release, in addition to independent pressor and antinatriuretic effects. The homoeostatic response to hypovolaemia thus involves an integrated neurohumoral cascade, of which vasopressin is one component.

Table 2.2.3 Miscellaneous effects of vasopressin

Action	Receptor involved
Coagulation/clotting cascade	
Factor VII release from hepatocytes	V2
von Willebrand factor release from vascular endothelium	V2
Bone	
Maintenance of bone mineral density	V1a
Liver metabolism	
Glycogen phosphorylase A activation	V1a
Central nervous system	
Modulation of baroreceptor reflex	
Central temperature control	

Physiology of oxytocin

Oxytocin binds to specific G-protein coupled cell surface receptors (OT-Rs) on target cells to mediate a variety of effects concerned with reproductive function: the regulation of lactation, parturition, and reproductive behaviour. Recent data from animals lacking oxytocin because of targeted disruption of the oxytocin gene, have challenged this dogma, forcing a review of the physiological roles of the hormone (43).

Oxytocin and lactation

In the rat, the stimulation of sensory afferents in the nipple by the act of suckling trigger a reflex cascade leading to synchronized firing bursts of oxytocic magnocellular neurons, and pulsatile oxytocin release corresponding to this burst activity. The released oxytocin acts on OT-Rs on smooth muscle cells lining the milk ducts of the breast, initiating milk ejection. Oxytocin is essential for completion of this milk ejection reflex in rodent. Mice lacking oxytocin fail to transfer milk to their suckling young, and this deficit is corrected by injection of oxytocin. In contrast, women lacking posterior pituitary function can breastfeed normally, illustrating that oxytocin is not necessary for lactation in humans.

Pituitary lactotrophs express OT-R mRNA, and oxytocin released into the hypophyseal portal blood supply from the median eminence can stimulate prolactin release. However, the role of oxytocin in the physiology of prolactin release remains to be defined (5).

Oxytocin and Parturition

Oxytocin is the most powerful uterotonic agent identified. Furthermore, in many mammals there is both an increase in oxytocin secretion during parturition, and an increase in uterine responsiveness to oxytocin at term (5). These data suggest a key role for the hormone in the initiation and progression of labour. It is believed that falling progesterone concentrations toward the end of pregnancy lead to up-regulation of uterine myometrial OT-Rs, enhanced contractility, and increased sensitivity to circulating oxytocin. Stretching of the 'birth canal' during parturition leads to the stimulation of specific autonomic afferents, triggering increased burst firing of oxytocic magnocellular neurons and oxytocin release. A positive feedback loop is formed, with oxytocin both stimulating uterine contraction further and enhancing the production of local uterotonic mediators such as prostaglandins. It has been difficult to demonstrate increased circulating oxytocin levels in women during labour. This has been attributed to the difficulties of analysing pulsatile release, coupled with the short circulating half-life of the hormone due to the action of placental cysteine aminopeptidase. In mice lacking oxytocin, parturition is normal. Moreover, women with absent posterior pituitary function can have a normal labour. However, the importance of oxytocin in the birth process is highlighted by the effectiveness of oxytocin antagonists in the management of pre-term labour (44).

Recent data have highlighted an additional role of oxytocin in parturition. Maternal oxytocin produces a switch in fetal central nervous system (CNS) neurotransmission with enhanced inhibitory γ-aminobutyric acid (GABA)ergic signalling. This increases fetal neuronal resistance to hypoxaemic damage that may occur during delivery. These data suggest an adaptive mother–fetal signalling during parturition in which oxytocin is a major player (45).

Oxytocin and behaviour

OT-R expression is widespread in the CNS of many species. There is clear evidence that oxytocin has important influences on reproductive behaviour in rat; facilitating both lordosis and the development of maternal behaviour patterns (5). However, mice lacking oxytocin exhibit normal sexual and maternal behaviour, indicating these effects may be species-dependent. Central oxytotic transmission appears to reduce anxiety and hypothalamo-pituitary-adrenal stress responses in female rats (46). However, the same central oxytotic function may be required for normal adrenocorticotropin responses to stress. Together, these data suggest a complex role for oxytocin in the stress and other behavioural responses, with species and context-dependent differential effects (47, 48). Oxytocin release from both dendrites and nerve terminals of hypothalamic magnocellular neurons can be regulated by other neuropeptides, highlighting the potential for magnocellular oxytocin to integrate with central neurotransmission (49).

Integrated physiology of oxytocin

How are the proposed roles of oxytocin in reproductive function reconciled with both human and mouse data that highlight normal function in the absence of the hormone? First, there are interspecies differences in oxytocin-modulated processes that contribute important qualifications to the data. The mouse gravid uterus does not express OT-Rs, in contrast to human and rat. It is perhaps not surprising therefore, that parturition is normal in the oxytocin null-mouse. Similarly, in contrast to rat, maternal behaviour evolves gradually in mouse, and is not acquired rapidly in the postpartum period. Mouse may therefore not be a good model for the uterine and behavioural effects of oxytocin. Second, there is clearly variable redundancy in some of the physiological pathways in which oxytocin is involved. This redundancy may vary between species. The extrapolation of oxytocin's role in normal physiology from those responses found in its absence should thus be made with caution.

Clinical endocrinology of the neurohypophysis

There are no recognized clinical sequelae of oxytocin deficiency in humans. The pathophysiology of the neurohypophysis thus reflects the physiology of vasopressin and the regulation of water excretion. Defects in vasopressin production or action impact through disturbances in fluid and electrolyte balance. Another, less common, group of conditions reflect primary defects in thirst. In some cases, the two may coincide, reflecting the close anatomical and functional relationship of both processes.

Polyuric syndromes

Classification

Polyuria is defined by the excretion of urine in excess of 3 l/24 h (over 40 ml/kg per 24 h in adults and over 100 ml/kg per 24 h in infants). Diabetes insipidus is simply the excretion of large amounts of dilute urine. One of three mechanisms may be responsible:

- deficiency of vasopressin: termed hypothalamic diabetes insipidus (HDI)
- renal resistance to the antidiuretic action of vasopressin: termed nephrogenic diabetes insipidus (NDI)
- inappropriate, excessive water drinking: termed dipsogenic diabetes insipidus (DDI) or primary polydipsia

Box 2.2.1 gives a classification of diabetes insipidus based on aetiology.

Hypothalamic diabetes insipidus

HDI (also known as neurogenic, central, or cranial diabetes insipidus) is due to deficient osmoregulated vasopressin secretion. In most cases it is a partial defect, with patients having inappropriately low plasma vasopressin concentrations with respect to concomitant plasma osmolalities. Presentation with HDI implies destruction or loss of function of more than 80% of vasopressinergic magnocellular neurons. Though persistent polyuria can lead to dehydration, given free access to water, most patients can maintain water balance through an intact thirst mechanism. HDI is rare, with an estimated prevalence of 1:25 000, and equal gender distribution.

Aetiology

Most cases of HDI are acquired. Improvements in imaging and an appreciation of the varied presentation of inflammatory/autoimmune forms are responsible for fewer cases being designated idiopathic. Trauma, either as a result of head injury or surgery, can produce HDI through damage to the hypothalamus, pituitary stalk,

Box 2.2.1 Classification of polyuric syndromes

Hypothalamic diabetes insipidus

- Primary
  - Genetic
    - DIDMOAD (Wolfram) syndrome
    - Autosomal dominant
    - Autosomal recessive
  - Developmental syndromes
    - Septo-optic dysplasia
  - Idiopathic
- Secondary/acquired
  - Trauma
    - Head injury
    - Post surgery (transcranial, transsphenoidal)
  - Tumour
    - Craniopharyngioma, germ cell tumour, metastases, pituitary macroadenoma
  - Inflammatory
    - Granulomata
    - Sarcoidosis, histiocytosis
    - Infection
    - Meningitis, encephalitis
    - Infundibulo-neurohypophysitis
    - Guillain–Barré syndrome
    - Autoimmune (anti-vasopressin neuron antibodies)
  - Vascular
    - Aneurysm
    - Infarction
    - Sheehan's syndrome
    - Sickle cell disease
  - Pregnancy (associated with vasopressinase)

Nephrogenic diabetes insipidus

- Primary
  - Genetic
    - X-linked recessive (V2-R defect)
    - Autosomal recessive (AQP2 defect)
    - Autosomal dominant (AQP2 defect)
  - Idiopathic
- Secondary
  - Chronic renal disease
    - Polycystic kidneys
    - Obstructive uropathy
  - Metabolic disease
    - Hypercalcaemia
    - Hypokalaemia
  - Drug induced
    - Lithium
    - Demeclocycline
  - Osmotic diuretics
    - Glucose
    - Mannitol
  - Systemic disorders
    - Amyloidosis
    - Myelomatosis
  - Pregnancy

Dipsogenic diabetes insipidus

- Compulsive water drinking
- Associated with affective disorders
- Drug induced?
- Structural/organic hypothalamic disease
  - Sarcoid
  - Tumours involving hypothalamus
  - Head injury
  - Tuberculous meningitis

or posterior pituitary. Pituitary stalk trauma may lead to a triphasic disturbance in water balance; an immediate polyuria characteristic of HDI followed within days by a more prolonged period of antidiuresis suggestive of vasopressin excess. This second phase may last up to several weeks, and can be followed by reversion to HDI or recovery. Such a 'triple response' reflects initial magnocellular axonal damage; the subsequent unregulated release of large amounts of presynthesized vasopressin; and ultimately, either recovery or development of permanent HDI, as determined by the degree of initial neuropraxia/axonal shearing and damage. There is evidence that the polyuric phase may be associated with the presence of circulating inhibitors of vasopressin action, which may be partly processed vasopressin precursors (50). Not all phases of the response may be apparent. Recent data suggest acute HDI can occur in up to 22% of nonselected patients presenting with traumatic brain injury (TBI), persisting in some 7% of the total TBI cohort on long-term follow-up (51).

Although primary pituitary tumours rarely cause HDI, hypothalamic or pituitary metastases (for example, breast or bronchus) can present with HDI. In childhood, hypothalamic tumours, such as craniopharyngioma and germinoma/teratoma, are relatively common causes of HDI; together with developmental defects, such as septo-optic dysplasia (SOD), they account for up to 50% of cases in children (52). HDI can present in pregnancy, placental vasopressinase activity decompensating previously limited antidiuretic capacity through increased vasopressin degradation that cannot be matched by increased hormone release. This can revert to normal after delivery, though permanent HDI may ultimately develop if the natural history of the central defect is progressive.

Familial forms account for 5% of HDI. The Wolfram (WS) or DIDMOAD syndrome is a rare autosomal recessive, progressive neuro-degenerative disorder characterized by the association of HDI with *d*iabetes *m*ellitus, *o*ptic *a*trophy and bilateral sensorineural *d*eafness. The natural history, of sequential development of the features, can be distorted by factors influencing presentation. Diabetes mellitus and optic atrophy are generally present in the first or second decade. HDI and deafness follow in the second or third decade. Additional features may then follow. Renal outflow tract dilatation is common, while gonadal atrophy and progressive ataxia with brain stem dysfunction can occur. Wolfram syndrome is caused by loss of function mutations in the *WFSI* gene on Ch.4p16. The gene encodes an 890 amino acid glycoprotein (wolframin). Non-inactivating mutations in the same gene are associated with autosomal dominant sensorineural hearing loss, suggesting the possibility of a spectrum disorder. An additional locus for Wolfram syndrome has been identified at Ch.4q22-24, suggesting genetic heterogeneity (53–55).

Autosomal dominant familial HDI is caused by mutations in the *VP* gene on chromosome 20. While it typically presents in childhood, the age of presentation varies considerably, reflecting variation in the progressive loss of vasopressin secretion. A variety of different missense and nonsense mutations within exons 1 and 2 of the *VP* gene have been identified in affected kindreds. Mutant vasopressin precursors accumulate in the endoplasmic reticulum of magnocellular neurons, to which they are neurotoxic. This explains the progressive loss of vasopressin release in the condition, and its dominant inheritance (56, 57). Growth failure may be an early clinical feature (58). The inherited HDI of the Brattleboro (BB) rat is due to a frame shift in exon 2 of the *VP* gene, resulting in a vasopressin precursor with an altered C-terminus which also accumulates in the endoplasmic reticulum of vasopressinergic neurons. Interestingly, the HDI of the BB rat is inherited in a recessive manner, in contrast to the equivalent condition in humans.

Circulating antibodies to vasopressin-secreting neurons can be found in 30% of patients classified previously as having HDI with no identifiable cause, implying an autoimmune aetiology. Presence of antivasopressin neuron antibodies in patients with HDI is particularly associated with pituitary stalk thickening on MRI. However, antivasopressin neuron antibodies can also be found at low prevalence in patients with HDI secondary to histiocytosis X and following pituitary surgery, suggesting the specificity of the test or the autoantibody response is low (59).

Investigation

The strategy of investigation of HDI is to confirm the polyuric state, define its basis, and to explore possible primary aetiologies. After establishing significant polyuria of greater than 3 l/24 h in adults and excluding hyperglycaemia, hypokalaemia, hypercalcaemia, and significant renal insufficiency, attention should be focused on the vasopressin axis.

Direct measurement of plasma vasopressin in response to osmotic stimulation differentiates HDI from other causes of polyuria. However, access to reliable vasopressin assays is limited. Thus, a dynamic test using a surrogate endpoint of vasopressin release has been developed. This assesses the capacity to concentrate urine during the osmotic stress of controlled water deprivation: the water deprivation test. The period of water deprivation can be followed by evaluation of the antidiuretic response to exogenous vasopressin: the aim being to confirm renal sensitivity to vasopressin or establish renal resistance. A standard protocol is outlined in Box 2.2.2. HDI can be distinguished by urine osmolality less than 300 mOsml/kg, accompanied by plasma osmolality greater than 290 mOsml/kg after dehydration. Urine osmolality should rise above 750 mOsml/kg after desmopressin (DDAVP), indicating normal renal responsiveness. In contrast, failure to increase urine osmolality above 300 mOsml/kg after dehydration together with failure to respond to DDAVP is diagnostic of NDI. Patients with DDI should concentrate urine appropriately during dehydration, without significant rise in plasma osmolality.

Box 2.2.2 Protocol for water deprivation/desmopressin test

Preparation

- Free access to fluid given overnight prior to test
- Avoid caffeine and smoking
- 0750 h—weigh patient

Dehydration phase

- 0800—plasma and urine osmolality, and urine volume
- Restrict fluids up to 8 h
- Weigh patient at 2-h intervals
- Plasma and urine osmolality, and volume measurements 2 hourly
- Stop test if weight loss exceeds 5% of starting weight, or thirst is intolerable
- Supervise patient closely to avoid non-disclosed drinking

Desmopressin phase

- Inject intramuscularly 1 μg desmopressin
- Allow patient to eat and drink up to 1.5–2.0 times the volume of urine passed during dehydration phase
- Collect urine for osmolality and volume at 2000 h
- Plasma and urine osmolality, and volume measurements at 0900 h next day

In reality however, many patients have incomplete defects and manifest mild or moderate forms of diabetes insipidus. Moreover, prolonged polyuria of any type can impair urine concentrating ability through dissipation of the medullary interstitial concentration gradient, resulting in a partial functional NDI. The water deprivation test can be a poor discriminator in these circumstances. An accurate diagnosis of HDI can be made by direct measurement of plasma vasopressin during the controlled osmotic stress of a hypertonic 5% sodium chloride infusion (60). Patients with HDI have either undetectable vasopressin levels, or values falling to the right of the normogram relating plasma vasopressin to plasma osmolality. In NDI, plasma vasopressin is inappropriately high for the prevailing urine and plasma osmolality, indicating vasopressin resistance. In DDI, the relationship of plasma vasopressin to osmolality is normal. The test is not interpretable if the patient experiences nausea, a powerful non-osmotic stimulus of vasopressin release, during the test.

A pragmatic alternative to vasopressin measurements during hypertonic stress if there is diagnostic uncertainty following water deprivation is a controlled therapeutic trial of DDAVP: 10–20 μg of intranasal DDAVP per day for 2–4 weeks, with monitoring of plasma sodium every 2–3 days. Patients with DDI exhibit progressive dilutional hyponatraemia, whereas those with NDI remain unaffected. Patients with HDI experience improvement in polyuria and polydipsia, but remain normonatraemic.

Imaging of the hypothalamus, pituitary, and surrounding structures is essential in patients with HDI. MRI is the modality of choice. HDI is associated with the loss of the normal hyperintense signal of the posterior pituitary on T_1-weighted images. Signal intensity is correlated strongly with vasopressin content of the gland (61). As some hypothalamic germ cell tumours can be slow growing, imaging should be repeated at an interval of 6–18 months if the initial scan shows no demonstrable lesion. A negative scan at this stage should be taken as reassuring in the absence of a change in clinical features.

Treatment

Patients with a urine output of less than 4 l/24 h can be managed by advising adequate fluid intake. The treatment of choice for those with more severe symptoms is the synthetic, long-acting vasopressin analogue DDAVP; given as an intranasal spray (5–100 µg daily), parenterally (0.1–2.0 µg daily), or orally (100–1000 µg daily) in divided doses. There is wide individual variation in the dose required to control symptoms. DDAVP has twice the antidiuretic potency of vasopressin, but has minimal vasopressor activity. It is well tolerated. Dilutional hyponatraemia is the most serious potential adverse effect. This can be avoided by omitting treatment on a regular basis (perhaps weekly), to allow a short period of breakthrough polyuria and thirst.

Nephrogenic diabetes insipidus

NDI is due to renal resistance to the antidiuretic effects of vasopressin. Primary familial forms are rare. X-linked recessive familial NDI is caused by inherited mutations of the *V2-R* gene on chromosome Xq28. Over seventy different mutations have been described: affecting receptor expression, ligand binding, and G-protein coupling. Most lead to complete loss of function; only a few are associated with a mild phenotype (62).

An autosomal recessive form is observed in 10% of kindreds with familial NDI, with normal V2-R function. Affected individuals harbour mutations of the *AQP2* gene, leading to expression of dysfunctional water channels. Most mutations occur in the region coding for the transmembrane domain of the protein. Additional NDI kindreds harbour a mutation of the C-terminal intracellular tail of *AQP2*, leading to expression of a mutant protein that sequesters wild-type *AQP2* (expressed by the normal allele) in nonfunctioning mixed tetramers in a dominant-negative manner (63). This form of NDI is inherited as an autosomal dominant trait.

More commonly, NDI is due to a variety of acquired metabolic or drug effects. The final common pathway producing NDI in many of these is down-regulation of *AQP2* expression. NDI secondary to lithium toxicity can persist after drug withdrawal, and may not always be reversible.

Diagnosis of NDI is based on documenting inappropriately low urine osmolality with respect to circulating vasopressin levels, or lack of response to exogenous DDAVP. Secondary/acquired cases are managed by removing the underlying cause, and ensuring adequate hydration. Additional measures for persistent, severe symptoms rarely reduce urine volumes by more than 50%, though this may still be worthwhile. High dose DDAVP (4 µg IM twice daily) may produce a response in partial NDI, especially if the lesion is acquired. Thiazide diuretics (hydrochlorothiazide 25 mg/24 h), nonsteroidal anti-inflammatory drugs (ibuprofen 200 mg/24 h) and low-salt diets, singly or in combination, can also be effective. All probably work through reducing glomerular filtration rate, and interfering with the diluting capacity of the distal nephron.

Dipsogenic diabetes insipidus

DDI is a syndrome of excess fluid intake, and consequent polyuria. Though structural abnormalities may be the cause, more commonly it is a manifestation of primary hyperdipsia, psychiatric disease, or secondary to drug effects. DDI in the absence of other identifiable illness is compulsive water drinking. It is associated with abnormalities of thirst perception, including; a low osmotic threshold for thirst; an exaggerated thirst response to osmotic challenge; and an inability to suppress thirst at low osmolalities. The structural and/or functional basis for any of these abnormalities has not been identified. The association of DDI with affective disorders is well recognized. Up to 20% of patients with chronic schizophrenia have polydipsia. Although in some cases abnormal drinking is in response to beliefs founded in the primary thought disorder, complex abnormalities in both osmoregulated vasopressin release and osmoregulated thirst have been described. Whether these reflect long-term effects of drug therapy, or a primary defect in the central integration of thirst, is unclear.

Confirmation of the diagnosis of DDI is through direct or indirect demonstration of normal osmoregulated vasopressin release and antidiuretic action. As with many conditions, the treatment of DDI should address the underlying disorder. This can be difficult. Clozapine has been shown to reduce polydipsia in patients with refractory schizophrenia and a history of hyponatraemia. Whether this is due to an effect on central thirst mechanisms, or on suppressing disordered thought, remains to be clarified. Individuals with persistent DDI are at risk of hyponatraemia if treated with DDAVP, as fluid intake is maintained despite an obligate antidiuresis. In such cases a reduced fluid intake is the only rational treatment.

Syndrome of inappropriate antidiuresis

Pathophysiology

Hyponatraemia (serum sodium concentration less than 130 mmol/l) is common, occurring in about 15% of hospitalized patients (64). Hyponatraemia is not invariably associated with a low serum osmolality; high concentrations of other circulating osmolytes (for example, glucose), or a reduced plasma aqueous phase secondary to dyslipidaemia can result in hyponatraemia but normal plasma osmolality. Moreover, even when hyponatraemia is a true indicator of hypo-osmolality, it may reflect an appropriate physiological response. In order to maintain circulating volume in hypovolaemia, baroregulated vasopressin release proceeds despite plasma osmolalities well below the normal osmotic threshold. However, an individual with hypoosmolar plasma but a normal circulating volume, in whom the plasma vasopressin concentration is high for the prevailing osmolality, has a syndrome of inappropriate antidiuresis (SIAD) due to vasopressin excess. A variety of conditions are associated with SIAD, and to date four patterns of abnormal vasopressin secretion have been identified, as shown in Table 2.2.4 (65). Absolute plasma vasopressin concentrations may not be strikingly high; the key finding is that that they are inappropriate for the prevailing plasma osmolality. When this obligate antidiuresis is not accompanied by decreased water intake, haemodilution is inevitable.

Table 2.2.4 Classification of the syndrome of inappropriate antidiuresis (SIAD)

SIAD type	Characteristics
SIAD type A	Wide fluctuations in plasma vasopressin concentration, independent of plasma osmolality. Accounts for 35% of SIAD
SIAD type B	Osmotic threshold for vasopressin release subnormal Patients osmoregulate around subnormal plasma osmolar set point Accounts for 30% of SIAD
SIAD type C	Failure to suppress vasopressin release at low plasma osmolality, normal response to osmotic stimulation
SIAD type D	Normal osmoregulated vasopressin release, but unable to excrete a water load. Accounts for less than 10% of SIAD

Aetiology

Many conditions have been reported to cause SIAD (Box 2.2.3). SIAD is a nonmetastatic manifestation of small cell lung cancer and other malignancies. Some tumours are an ectopic source of vasopressin, and produce a type A syndrome. However, excessive posterior pituitary vasopressin secretion also occurs in association with malignancy. In fact the mechanism(s) of inappropriate vasopressin release in many cases of SIAD are not clear. The absence of an ectopic vasopressin source suggests a lesion in the neurohypophysis or its regulatory afferent pathways. The similarities between SIAD type B and the changes in vasopressin regulation in response to hypovolaemia and hypotension, suggest a single lesion in the baroregulatory afferent pathways. In contrast, the normal osmoregulated vasopressin release found in the type D syndrome suggests an increase in renal sensitivity to vasopressin, or the action of an as yet unidentified antidiuretic factor.

SIAD is a common mechanism of drug induced hyponatraemia. It can reflect direct stimulation of vasopressin release from the hypothalamus; indirect action on the hypothalamus via effects on higher centres; or aberrant resetting of the hypothalamic osmostat (66). Dopamine antagonists cause SIAD through stimulation of vasopressin release. Hyponatraemia is not restricted to one particular class of these agents, and has been reported with metoclopramide and newer antipsychotic compounds such as risperidone. Tricyclic antidepressants, monoamine oxidase inhibitors (MAOIs), and selective serotonin reuptake inhibitors (SSRIs)

Box 2.2.3 Causes of syndrome of inappropriate antidiuresis (SIAD)

Neoplastic disease
- Carcinoma (bronchus, duodenum, pancreas, prostate)
- Thymoma
- Mesothelioma
- Lymphoma, leukaemia
- Ewing's sarcoma
- Carcinoid
- Bronchial adenoma

Neurological disorders
- Head injury, neurosurgery
- Brain abscess or tumour
- Meningitis, encephalitis
- Guillain–Barré syndrome
- Cerebral haemorrhage
- Cavernous sinus thrombosis
- Hydrocephalus
- Cerebellar and cerebral atrophy
- Shy–Drager syndrome
- Peripheral neuropathy
- Seizures
- Subdural haematoma
- Alcohol withdrawal

Chest disorders
- Pneumonia
- Tuberculosis
- Empyema
- Cystic fibrosis
- Pneumothorax
- Aspergillosis

Drugs
- Chlorpropamide
- Opiates
- Vincristine, vinblastine, cisplatin
- Thiazides
- Dopamine antagonists
- Tricyclic antidepressants
- Monoamine oxidase inhibitors
- Serotonin selective reuptake inhibitors
- 3,4-MDMA ('Ecstasy')
- Anticonvulsants

Miscellaneous
- Idiopathic
- Psychosis
- Porphyria
- Abdominal surgery

potentiate stimulatory central α_1 adrenergic input to vasopressin-producing neurons. Opiates also stimulate inappropriate vasopressin release through enhancing central adrenergic drive. SIAD is commonly associated with antiseizure medication. The frequency of hyponatraemia in patients treated with carbamazepine ranges from 4.8–40%, though the majority of such cases are asymptomatic. Carbamazepine increases both the sensitivity of central osmoreceptors, and renal sensitivity to vasopressin.

Clinical features, diagnosis and differential diagnosis of SIAD

The major features in the diagnosis of SIAD are given in Box 2.2.4. The most frequent problem in clinical practice is distinguishing SIAD from chronic, mild hypovolaemia. In both conditions, urine osmolality tends to be higher than plasma osmolality. Plasma vasopressin will be detectable or elevated in both. Neither is therefore diagnostic of SIAD. The diagnosis hinges on confirming excretion of urine that is not maximally dilute in the context of a dilute plasma (i.e. urine concentration greater than 100mOsml/Kg). Renal sodium excretion should be above 20 mmol/l to make a diagnosis of SIAD. Below this value, volume depletion needs to be considered more likely. SIAD is often associated with urine sodium concentrations of 60 mmol/l or more. The hyponatraemia of chronic SIAD is not simply the result of haemodilution through reduced water excretion. SIAD is a volume-expanded state. Consistent with this, there is evidence of mild sodium loss as other regulators of volume homoeostasis attempt to minimize volume expansion (67).

Given the positive correlation between plasma vasopressin concentration and urinary excretion of AQP2, urine AQP2 excretion may be useful in the differentiation of SIAD from other causes of hyponatraemia (68). However, urinary AQP2 cannot differentiate clearly between hyponatraemic states associated with significant vasopressin production. SIAD and chronic hypovolaemia may generate similar plasma vasopressin concentrations and similar urine AQP2 levels and these two conditions are the most common differential diagnoses which we have difficulty in resolving. In addition, there are situations in which plasma vasopressin levels, urinary AQP2 excretion and renal concentrating ability are dissociated (e.g. following glucocorticoid replacement in hypopituitarism, central volume expansion, the newborn, the elderly). The clinical utility of the test thus remains to be clarified (69, 70).

The role of vasopressin production or action in producing hyponatraemia can be confirmed indirectly by assessing excretion of a standard water load over a fixed time: the water load test (Table 2.2.5). Normal subjects excrete 78–82% of the ingested water load in the 4h observation period. This is reduced to 30–40% in the presence of constitutive vasopressin production or action.

Box 2.2.4 Diagnosis of syndrome of inappropriate antidiuresis (SIAD)

- Hyponatraemia with appropriately low plasma osmolality
- Urine osmolality that is not maximally dilute in context of on-going hyponatraemia (i.e. urine osmolality >100mOsm/kg)
- Urine sodium concentration >20 mmol/l
- Absence of hypotension, hypovolaemia, and oedema-forming states
- Normal renal and adrenal function

Table 2.2.5 Protocol for water load test

Preparation	◆ Free access to fluid overnight prior to test ◆ Avoid caffeine and smoking ◆ 0730 h weigh patient ◆ Cannulate patient ◆ Rest patient 30 min
Water load phase	◆ 0800 h plasma and urine osmolality, plasma vasopressin ◆ Patient to drink 20 ml/kg water over 15 min ◆ Measure hourly urine output for 4 h ◆ Measure urine osmolality, plasma osmolality and plasma vasopressin hourly for 4 h
Recovery phase	◆ Plasma sodium 2 h after test completed ◆ Plasma sodium and osmolality 0900 h next day

The test is not essential to establish a diagnosis, although it can be helpful in planning management of chronic or recurrent hyponatraemia (60, 71).

Exercise-associated hyponatraemia

Extreme endurance exercise is a physiological stressor. The magnitude of the physiological stress will reflect a number of factors: duration of the event; and the effort entailed. Non-osmoregulated vasopressin release is a feature of extreme endurance exercise, leading to a state of antidiuresis. If endurance athletes maintain a fluid intake in excess of water loss, hyponatraemia is inevitable. Athletes developing hyponatraemia demonstrate weight gain over the course of the event, consistent with water intake in excess of water loss. Health professionals attending endurance events need to be aware of the problem of exercise associated hyponatraemia. Athletes should be advised to follow their thirst. In addition, athletes who collapse during the course, or at the end of the event, should not be routinely resuscitated with large volumes of hypotonic fluid in the absence of appropriate indications and without biochemical monitoring as this may contribute to worsening hyponatraemia (72, 73).

Nephrogenic syndrome of inappropriate antidiuresis

While loss of function mutations of the *V2-R* are the cause of X-linked nephrogenic diabetes insipidus, rare individuals express the reciprocal problem: constitutively activating mutations in the *V2-R* that lead to vasopressin-independent, but V2-R mediated, antidiuresis resulting in persistent hyponatraemia. This nephrogenic syndrome of inappropriate antidiuresis (NSIAD) can have a variable phenotype. Although initially described in male infants with persistent hyponatraemia, the condition is not limited to males and may manifest in adulthood (74, 75). This is consistent with in the condition being X-linked but with variable expression in heterozygous females. Some 10% of patients with apparent SIAD have undetectable vasopressin. It is likely that at least some of these cases may be due to activating mutations of the V2-R.

Central salt wasting

Central salt wasting (CSW) is an acquired primary natriuresis found in a variety of neurological situations and a rare cause of hypovolaemic hyponatraemia. The underlying mechanism(s) involve increased release of natriuretic peptides and/or reduced sympathetic drive. The natural history of the process is key in establishing the diagnosis: hyponatraemia is preceded by natriuresis and diuresis with ensuing clinical and biochemical features of hypovolaemia. Depending on the point in the natural history at which the clinician meets the patient, urea and creatinine are generally elevated and there may be postural hypotension, in contrast to SIAD. The simple observation of weight loss over the period in question can be helpful. CSW is a particular concern in the neurosurgical patient: when autoregulation of cerebral blood flow is disturbed and small reductions in circulating volume can lead directly to reduced cerebral perfusion with secondary ischaemic brain injury. While both SIAD and CSW are associated with urine sodium concentrations greater than 40 mmol/l, the natriuresis of CSW is much more profound than that of SIAD and precedes the development of hyponatraemia. The management of CSW is volume replacement with 0.9% saline, balancing net sodium loss together with the requirement for circulating volume support (76).

Treatment of hyponatraemia secondary to SIAD

The clinical impact of hyponatraemia secondary to SIAD reflects the combined effects of cerebral oedema and direct CNS dysfunction (Box 2.2.5). The clinical spectrum is wide. While values of serum sodium around 100 mmol/l are life-threatening, some patients with less marked hyponatraemia or in whom the problem has developed slowly commonly have mild symptoms or are asymptomatic due to CNS adaptation. CNS adaptation is limited: rapid changes in plasma sodium are accommodated less well than gradual changes, even if the scale of the change is relatively small. Moreover, this adaptation can complicate the management of hyponatraemia. Rapid correction of hyponatraemia following CNS adaptation can lead to significant changes in brain volume as the osmolar gradient across the blood-brain barrier alters. This may trigger CNS demyelination, a rare but serious complication of hyponatraemia and its treatment which develops within 1–4 days of rapid (>12 mmol/24 h) correction of plasma sodium. Other factors may play a role in susceptibility: concurrent hepatic dysfunction; potassium depletion; malnutrition; and it can occur even when sodium levels are corrected slowly Neurological manifestations include quadriplegia, ophthalmoplegia, pseudobulbar palsy and coma. Intervention to correct plasma sodium in SIAD must thus balance the morbidities of nonintervention with the risks of iatrogenic complications.

Box 2.2.5 Symptoms and signs of hyponatraemia secondary to SIAD

- Headache
- Nausea
- Vomiting
- Muscle cramps
- Lethargy
- Disorientation
- Seizure
- Coma
- Brain-stem herniation
- Death

Chronic asymptomatic hyponatraemia with plasma sodium concentrations greater than 125 mmol/l, may not require specific treatment. More severe degrees of hyponatraemia, particularly if symptomatic, require some form of intervention. Correction of the underlying cause(s) is appropriate if the clinical situation allows it (treatment of infection, removal of the causative drug). Such approaches may prevent worsening hyponatraemia and allow the body's own physiology to address the deficit in plasma sodium. Additional intervention should adhere to two key principles:

- correction should not risk morbidity and mortality (such as that from osmotic demyelination) in excess of that associated with the initial degree of hyponatraemia
- correction should be at sufficient pace to reverse life-threatening features of hyponatraemia as quickly as is feasible and safe

Initial intervention in hyponatraemia associated with SIAD

Fluid restriction of 0.5–1 l/day can be used safely when the clinical condition is not critical. The aim should be to have plasma sodium increase at a rate not exceeding 8–10 mmol/l per 24 h. Plasma sodium therefore needs to be measured regularly and all fluids need to be included in the restriction. Sodium intake should be maintained. It may be several days before sodium levels rise and it is important that a negative fluid balance is confirmed during this period. However, prolonged fluid restriction can be distressing and it is not always effective. The higher the baseline urine osmolality, the less likely fluid restriction is to work.

If the symptoms and signs of hyponatraemia due to SIAD are life-threatening, a more aggressive intervention may be required with hypertonic 3% sodium chloride. The aim of such an approach must be clear;

- reversal of life-threatening manifestations of hyponatraemia
- moderation of other nonlife-threatening manifestations of hyponatraemia

Clinical endpoints may be achieved through only a relatively small rise of 2–4 mmol/l in plasma sodium over 2–4 h. Importantly, normalization of plasma sodium is not the therapeutic target. Plasma sodium concentration should rise no more than 1–2 mmol/l per hour, with a total increment of no more than 8–10 mmol/l per 24 h. The volume of administered fluid required may be calculated through consideration of target plasma sodium, the sodium content of the administered fluid and the estimated deficit in plasma sodium based on body weight (64). If such an approach is used, it is imperative that the fluid regimen is reassessed at regular intervals, guided by careful clinical assessment and laboratory monitoring. However, the clinical utility of fixed replacement models in day-to-day practice is limited, especially if partial correction of plasma sodium to clinical endpoints is accepted and asymmetric increases biased toward more rapid changes in the first 1–4 hours of intervention are employed. An alternative approach is to use 100 ml boluses of 3% sodium chloride, with careful clinical and biochemical monitoring. Hypertonic fluid should be stopped when the defined clinical target or a sodium concentration of 125 mmol/l is reached, whichever is first. As before, the approach aims to reduce the neurological morbidity of hyponatraemia while minimizing the risk of precipitating osmotic demyelination (77).

Recurrent or persisting hyponatraemia associated with SIAD

If hyponatraemia persists or recurs after initial intervention, the underlying diagnosis should be reviewed and the basis for intervention reconsidered. If the diagnosis of SIAD remains intact, clinicians need to balance the merits of further incremental intervention with those of tolerating persisting hyponatraemia.

Demeclocycline produces a form of NDI and so increases renal water loss even in the presence of vasopressin. It is effective in treating hyponatraemia of SIAD at 600–1200 mg/day in divided doses. There is a lag time of some 3–4 days in onset of action. Treatment should be stopped if significant renal impairment develops. Lithium has similar effects and can be used as an alternative. However, the effects of lithium are less and the drug is associated with more adverse effects.

Urea increases renal free water excretion and decreases urinary sodium excretion. It can be used to treat the hyponatraemia of SIAD at doses of 30 g/day by mouth. It may be have clinical utility as an adjunctive therapy to allow reduction in water restriction and improvement in quality of life.

The nonpeptide V2-R antagonists (the vaptans) are a rational approach to the treatment of SIAD. They are aquaretic: increasing renal water excretion with no significant impact on renal electrolyte loss. Vaptans are either selective (V2-R specific) or nonselective (V2-and V1a antagonism). Both improve hyponatraemia associated with normal or increased plasma volume. Changes in plasma sodium can be seen within 4–6 hours. The drugs appear to be well tolerated. The developing role of vaptans in the management of SIAD needs to balance time course of action, tolerance, and long-term efficacy in specific clinical contexts (78, 79).

Hypodipsia

Adipsic and hypodipsic disorders are characterized by inadequate spontaneous fluid intake due to a primary defect in osmoregulated thirst. Patients are hypovolaemic and dehydrated, with elevated plasma sodium and urea. Despite this, they deny thirst and do not drink. If the defect is mild, the resultant hypernatraemia is often well tolerated. Severe disorders leading to marked electrolyte

Table 2.2.6 Classification of adipsic/hypodipsic syndromes

Classification	Osmoregulated thirst	Osmoregulated vasopressin release
Type A (essential hypernatraemia)	Osmotic threshold increased Normal sensitivity	Osmotic threshold increased, normal sensitivity Normal response to nonosmotic stimuli
Type B	Normal osmotic threshold Reduced sensitivity	Normal osmotic threshold, reduced sensitivity Normal response to nonosmotic stimuli
Type C	No thirst response to osmotic stimulation	Persistent low level vasopressin release, no response to osmotic stimulation or inhibition Normal response to nonosmotic stimulation
Type D		Normal

disturbances are tolerated poorly, and can lead to somnolence, seizures, coma and renal failure. Because of the close anatomical relationship of the osmregulatory centres for thirst and vasopressin release, adipsic syndromes are often associated with defects in osmoregulated vasopressin release and HDI, which can exacerbate electrolyte and water balance problems.

Aetiology

Four distinct patterns of osmoregulated thirst and associated vasopressin release are recognized (23). These are outlined in Table 2.2.6 and Figure 2.2.7. In addition, conditions producing adipsia/hypodipsia syndromes are outlined in Box 2.2.6.

The type A syndrome can be mistaken for HDI, as patients are hyperosmolar with a dilute urine. Formal assessment of thirst, by analogue scale during osmotic stimulation, confirms the diagnosis. Normal vasopressin responses to nonosmotic stimuli place the lesion responsible at the level of the osmoreceptor, rather than the vasopressin magnocellular neuron. The nature of the lesion remains unknown. Imaging is generally normal. Patients effectively osmoregulate around a higher osmolar set point, and are protected

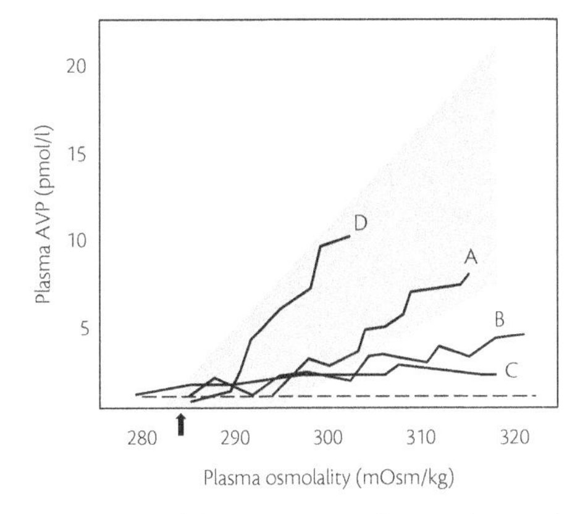

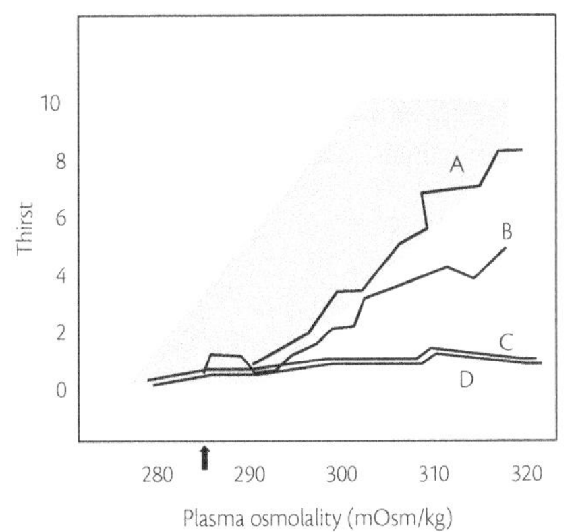

Fig. 2.2.7 Patterns of plasma vasopressin and thirst responses to hypertonic stress in patients with adipsic syndromes. Normal range responses to osmolar stimulation are shown by the shaded areas. The four types of adipsic syndrome are demonstrated. Patients with the type A syndrome osmoregulate around a higher osmolar set point. Those with the type B syndrome mount vasopressin and thirst responses but with reduced sensitivity to increases in plasma osmolality. Patients with the type C syndrome have much reduced or absent vasopressin and thirst responses to osmolar stimulation while those with the type D syndrome demonstrate normal vasopressin responses to osmolar stimulation but much reduced thirst responses.

Box 2.2.6 Causes of adipsic/hypodipsic syndromes

- Neoplastic (50%)
  - Primary
    - Craniopharyngioma
    - Pinealoma
    - Meningioma
  - Secondary
    - Pituitary tumour
    - Bronchial carcinoma
    - Breast carcinoma
- Vascular (15%)
  - Internal carotid ligation
  - Anterior communicating artery aneurysm
  - Intrahypothalamic haemorrhage
- Granulomatous (20%)
  - *Histiocytosis*
  - *Sarcoidosis*
- Miscellaneous (15%)
  - *Hydrocephalus*
  - *Ventricular cyst*
  - *Trauma*
  - *Toluene poisoning*

from extreme hypernatraemia, as are those with the type B syndrome. In contrast, type C adipsia is associated with complete lack of osmoregulated thirst and vasopressin release, consistent with complete destruction of osmoreceptors. Patients present with adipsic HDI. Specific precipitants include rupture and repair of anterior communicating artery aneurysm. One of the putative locations of the osmoreceptors mediating both thirst and vasopressin release, the OVLT, receives its blood supply from perforating branches of the anterior cerebral artery and anterior communicating artery. Some patients with the type C syndrome have persistent, constitutive low level vasopressin release. The resultant low level obligatory antidiuresis places such individuals at risk of dilutional hyponatraemia if large volumes of fluid are administered. Impaired osmoregulated thirst with normal osmoregulated vasopressin release (type D adipsia) is very rare.

Treatment

Because patients with type A and type B adipsia are protected from extreme hypernatraemia, treatment is to recommend an obligate fluid intake of about 2 l/24 h, with appropriate adjustment for climate and season. If fluid balance cannot be maintained during intercurrent illness, in-hospital management may be required. The adipsic HDI of the type C syndrome can be difficult to manage. Structural and vascular causes of the type C syndrome may lead to associated cognitive defects in short term memory and task organization, which can complicate any intervention. The principle of management is to define an acceptable urine output (1–2 l/24 h) with regular DDAVP, and to vary the daily fluid intake depending on day-to-day fluctuation from a target weight at which the patient is euvolaemic and normonatraemic:

Daily fluid intake in litre = 1–2 l (i.e. the targeted urine output as dictated by the DDAVP dose set and taking into account insensible loss) + (target weight - daily weight in kg).

This formula, together with weekly checks of plasma sodium to avoid the creeping development of hyper- and hyponatraemia, can result in stable fluid balance (80).

References

1. Ang H-L, Carter DA, Murphy D. Neuron-specific expression and physiological regulation of bovine vasopressin transgenes in mice. *EMBO J*, 1993; **12**: 2397–409.
2. Richter D, Mohr E, Schmale H. Molecular aspects of the vasopressin gene family: evolution, expression and regulation. In: Jard S, Jamison R, eds. *Vasopressin*. Montrouge, France: John Libbey, 1991: 3–10.
3. Waller SJ, Ratty A, Burbach JPH, Murphy D. Transgenic and transcriptional studies on neurosecretory cell gene expression. *Cell Mol Neurobiol*, 1998; **18**: 149–71.
4. Iwasaki Y, Oiso Y, Saito H, Majzoub JA. Positive and negative regulation of the rat vasopressin gene promoter. *Endocrinology*, 1997; **138**: 5266–74.
5. Russell JA, Leng G. Sex, parturition and motherhood without oxytocin? *J Endocrinol*, 1998; **157**: 343–59.
6. Carter DA, Murphy D. Rapid changes in poly (A) tail length of vasopressin and oxytocin m RNAs from common early components of neurohypophyseal peptide gene activation following physiological stimulation. *Neuroendocrinology*, 1991; **5**: 1–6.
7. Mohr E, Kachele I, Mullin C, Richter D. Rat vasopressin mRNA: a model system to characterize cis-acting elements and trans-acting factors in dendritic mRNA sorting. *Prog Brain Res*, 2002; **139**: 211–24.
8. Russell JT, Brownstein MJ, Gainer H. Biosynthesis of vasopressin, oxytocin and neurophysins: isolation and characterization of two common precursors (propressophysin and prooxyphysin). *Endocrinology*, 1980; **107**: 1880–91.
9. Sinding C, Robinson AG. A review of neurophysins. *Metabolism*, 1977; **26**: 1355–70.
10. Lauson HD. Metabolism of neurohypophysial hormones. In: Knobil E, Sawyer WH, eds. *Handbook of Physiology*, Section 7, Endocrinology, Washington DC: American Physiological Society, 1974: **4**: 287–393.
11. Bichet DG, Razi M, Lonergan M, Arthus MF, Papukna V, Kortas C. Human platelet fraction arginine–vasopressin: potential physiological role. *J Clin Invest*, 1987; **79**: 881–7.
12. McKinley MJ, Mathai ML, McAllen RM, McClear RC, Miselis RR, Pennington GL, *et al.* Vasopressin secretion: osmotic and hormonal regulation by the lamina terminalis. *J Neuroendocrinol*, 2004; **16**: 340–7.
13. Agre P, Brown D, Nielsen S. Aquaporin water channels: unanswered questions and unresolved controversies. *Curr Opin Cell Biol*, 1995; **7**: 472–83.
14. Oliet SH, Bourke CW. Mechanosensitive channels induce osmosensitivity in supraoptic neurons. *Nature*, 1993; **364**: 341–3.
15. Hurbin A, Boisin-Agasse L, Orcel H, Rabie A, Joux N, Desarmenien MG, *et al.* The V(1a) and V(1b), but not the V2, vasopressin receptor genes are expressed in the supraoptic nucleus of the rat hypothalamus, and the transcripts are essentially colocalized in the vasopressinergic magnocellular neurons. *Endocrinology*, 1998; **139**: 4701–7.
16. Ludwig M. Dendritic release of vasopressin and oxytocin. *J Neuroendocrinol*, 1998; **10**: 881–95.
17. Cunningham JT, Bruno SB, Grindstaff RR, Grindstaff RJ, Higgs KH, Mazzella D, *et al.* Cardiovascular regulation of supraoptic vasopressin neurons. *Prog Brain Res*, 2002; **139**: 257–73.
18. Ishikawa S, Schrier RW. Pathophysiological roles of arginine vasopressin and aquaporin-2 in impaired water excretion. *Clin Endocrinol*, 2003; **58**: 1–17.

19. Shelat SG, Reagan LP, King JL, Fluharty SJ, Flanagan-Cato LM. Analysis of angiotensin type 2 receptors in the vasopressinergic neurons and pituitary in the rat. *Regul Pept*, 1998; **73**: 103–12.
20. Samson WK. Atrial natriuretic factor inhibits dehydration and hemorrhage-induced vasopressin release. *Neuroendocrinology*, 1985; **40**: 277–9.
21. Wazna-Wesley JM, Meranda DL, Carey P, Shenker Y. Effect of atrial natriuretic hormone on vasopressin and thirst response to osmotic stimulation in human subjects. *J Lab Clin Med*, 1995; **125**: 734–42.
22. Baylis PH, Pippard C, Gill GV, Burd J. Development of a cytochemical assay for plasma vasopressin: application to studies on water loading normal man. *Clin Endocrinol*, 1986; **24**: 383–92.
23. McKenna K, Thompson C. Osmoregulation in clinical disorders of thirst and thirst appreciation. *Clin Endocrinol*, 1998; **49**: 139–52.
24. Baylis PH. Vasopressin and its neurophysin. In: DeGroot LJ, Jameson JL, eds. *Endocrinology*. 4th edn. Philadelphia: WB Saunders, 2001: 1: 363–76.
25. Zimmerman EA, Ma L-Y, Nilaver G. Anatomical basis of thirst and vasopressin secretion. *Kidney Int*, 1987; **32** (Suppl 21): 514–19.
26. Zing HH. Vasopressin and oxytocin receptors. *Bailliére's Clin Endocrinol Metab*, 1996; **10**: 75–96.
27. Laycock JF, Hanoune J. From vasopressin receptor to water channel: intracellular traffic, constraint and by-pass. *J Endocrinol*, 1998; **159**: 361–72.
28. King LS, Yasui M. Aquaporins and disease: lessons from mice to humans. *Trends Endocrinol Metab*, 2002; **13**: 355–60.
29. Agre P, King LS, Yasui M, Guggino WB, Ottersen OP, Fujiyoshi Y, *et al.* Aquaporin water channels- from atomic structure to clinical medicine. *J Physiol*, 2002; **542**: 3–16.
30. Nielsen S, Kwon T-H, Frokiaer J, Agre P. Regulation and dysregulation of aquaporins in water balance disorders. *J Intern Med*, 2007; **261**: 53–64.
31. King LS, Choi M, Fernandez PC, Cartron JP, Agre P. Defective urinary-concentrating ability due to a complete deficiency of aquaporin-1. *N Engl J Med*, 2001; **345**: 175–9.
32. Yasui M, Zelenin SM, Celsi G, Aperia A. Adenylate cyclase-coupled vasopressin receptor activates AQP2 promoter via a dual effect on CRE and AP1 elements. *Am J Physiol*, 1997; **272**: F443–50.
33. Martin P-Y, Schrier RW. Role of aquaporin-2 water channels in urinary concentration and dilution defects. *Kidney Int*, 1998; **53** (Suppl 65): 557–62.
34. Ishikawa S, Saito K, Kasono K. Pathological role of aquaporin-2 in impaired water excretion and hyponatraemia. *J Neuroendocrinol*, 2004; **16**: 293–6.
35. Young LJ, Nilsen R, Waymire KG, MacGregor GR, Insel TR. Increased affiliative response to vasopressin in mice expressing the V1a receptor from a monogamous vole. *Nature*, 1999; **400**: 766–8.
36. Bielsky IF, Hu S-B, Szegda KL, Westphal H, Young LJ. Profound impairment in social recognition and reduction in anxiety-like behaviour in vasopressin V1a receptor knockout mice. *Neuropsychopharmacology*, 2004; **29**: 483–93.
37. Walum H, Westberg L, Henningsson S, Neiderhiser JM, Reiss D, Igl W, *et al.* Genetic variation in the vasopressin receptor 1a gene (*AVPR1A*) associates with pair-bonding behavior in humans. *Proc Natl Acad Sci U S A*, 2008; **105**: 14153–6.
38. Mannucci PM, Ruggeri ZM, Pareti FI, Capitanio A. DDAVP: a new pharmacological approach to the management of haemophilia and von Willebrand disease. *Lancet*, 1977; **1**: 869–72.
39. Hashemi S, Tackaberry ES, Palmer DS, Rock G, Ganz PR. DDAVP induced release of von Willebrand factor from endothelial cells *in vitro*: the effect of plasma and red cells. *Biochim Biophys Acta*, 1990; **1052**: 63–70.
40. Pivonello R, Colao A, Di Somma C, Facciolli G, Klain M, Faggiano A, *et al.* Impairment of bone status in patients with central diabetes insipidus. *J Clin Endocrinol*, 1998; **83**: 2275–80.
41. Spruce BA, McCulloch AJ, Burd J, Orskov H, Heaton A, Baylis PH, *et al.* The effect of vasopressin infusion on glucose metabolism in man. *Clin Endocrinol*, 1985; **22**: 463–8.
42. Nakayama Y, Takano Y, Eguchi K, Migita K, Saito R, Tsujimoto G, *et al.* Modulation of the arterial baroreceptor reflex by the vasopressin receptor in the area prostrema of the hypertensive rat. *Neurosci Letters*, 1997; **226**: 179–82.
43. Nishimori K, Young LJ, Guo Q, Wang Z, Insel TR, Matzuk MM. Oxytocin is required for nursing but is not essential for parturition or reproductive behaviour. *Proc Natl Acad Sci U S A*, 1996; **93**: 11699–704.
44. Goodwin TM, Valenzuela GJ, Silver H, Creasy G. Dose ranging study of the oxytocin antagonist atosiban in the treatment of preterm labor. Atosiban Study Group. *Obstet Gynaecol*, 1996; **88**: 331–6.
45. Tyzio R, Cossart R, Khalilov I, Minlebaev M, Hübner CA, Represa A, *et al.* Maternal oxytocin triggers a transient inhibitory switch in GABA signaling in the fetal brain during delivery. *Science*, 2006; **15**: 1788–92.
46. Windle RJ, Gamble LE, Kershaw YM, Wood SA, Lightman SL, Ingram CD. Gonadal steroid modulation of stress-induced hypothalamo-pituitary-adrenal activity and anxiety behavior: role of central oxytocin. *Endocrinology*, 2006; **147**: 2423–31.
47. Hammock EAD, Young LJ. Oxytocin, vasopressin and pair bonding: implications for autism. *Philos Trans R Soc Lond B Biol Sci*, 2006; **29**: 2187–98.
48. Neumann ID, Torner LN, Veenema AH. Oxytocin actions within the supraoptic and paraventricular nuclei: differential effects on peripheral and intranuclear vasopressin release. *Am J Physiol*, 2006; **291**: R29–36.
49. Sabatier N. α-melanocyte-stimulating hormone and oxytocin: a peptide signaling cascade in the hypothalamus. *J Neuroendocrinol*, 2006; **18**: 9703–10.
50. Seckl JR, Dunger DB, Bevan JS, Nakasu Y, Chowdrey C, Burke CW, *et al.* Vasopressin antagonist in early postoperative diabetes insipidus. *Lancet*, 1990; **355**: 1353–6.
51. Aghar A, Thornton E, O'Kelly P, Tormey W, Phillips J, Thompson CJ. Posterior pituitary dysfunction after traumatic brain injury. *J Clin Endocrinol Metab*, 2004; **89**: 5987–92.
52. Baylis PH, Cheetham T. Diabetes insipidus. *Arch Dis Child*, 1998; **79**: 84–9.
53. Barrett TG, Bundey S. Wolfram (DIDMOAD) syndrome. *J Med Genet*, 1997; **34**: 838–41.
54. Domenecch E, Gomez-Zaera M, Nunes V. WFS1 mutations in spanish patients with diabetes mellitus and deafness. *Eur J Hum Genet*, 2002; **10**: 421–6.
55. Cryns K, Sivakumaran TA, Van den Ouweland JMW, Pennings RJ, Cremers CW, Flothmann K, *et al.* Mutational spectrum of the WFS1 gene in wolfram syndrome, non-syndromic hearing impairment, diabetes mellitus and psychiatric disease. *Hum Mutat*, 2003; **22**: 275–87.
56. Ito M, Jameson JL, Ito M. Molecular basis of autosomal dominant neurohypophyseal diabetes insipidus. Cellular toxicity caused by the accumulation of mutant vasopressin precursors within the endoplasmic reticulum. *J Clin Invest*, 1997; **99**: 1897–905.
57. Siggaard C, Ritig S, Corydon TJ, Andreasen PH, Jensen TG, Andresen BS, *et al.* Clinical and molecular evidence of the abnormal processing and trafficking of the vasopressin preprohormone in a large kindred with familial neurohypophyseal diabetes insipidus due to a signal peptide mutation. *J Clin Endocrinol Metab*, 1999; **84**: 2933–41.
58. Nijenhuis M, van den Akker ELT, Zalm R, Franken AAM, Abbes AP, Engel H, *et al.* Familial neurohypophyseal diabetes insipidus in a large dutch kindred: effect of the onset of diabetes on growth in children and cell biological defects of the mutant vasopressin prohormone. *J Clin Endocrinol Metab*, 2001; **86**: 3410–20.
59. Pivoello R, De Bellis A, Faggiano A, Di Salle F, Petretta M, Di Somma C, *et al.* Central diabetes insipidus and autoimmunity: relationship between the occurrence of antibodies to arginine vasopressin-secreting cells and clinical, immunological, and radiological features in a large cohort of patients with central diabetes insipidus of known and unknown etiology. *J Clin Endocrinol Metab*, 2003; **88**: 1629–36.

60. Ball SG, Barber T, Baylis PH. Tests of posterior pituitary function. *J Endocrinol Invest*, 2003; **26** (Suppl): 15–24.
61. Kurokowa H, Fujisawa I, Nakano Y, Kimura H, Akagi K, Ikeda K, *et al.* Posterior lobe of the pituitary gland: correlation between signal intensity on T1-weighted images and vasopressin concentration. *Radiology*, 1998; **207**: 79–83.
62. Barbieris C, Mouillac B, Durroux T. Structural basis of vasopressin/oxytocin receptor function. *J Endocrinol*, 1998; **156**: 223–9.
63. Mulders SM, Bichet DG, Rijss JP, Kamsteeg EJ, Arthus MF, *et al.* An aquaporin-2 water channel mutant which causes autosomal dominant nephrogenic diabetes insipidus is retained in the golgi complex. *J Clin Invest*, 1998; **102**: 57–66.
64. Adrogue HJ, Madias NE. Hyponatraemia. *N Engl J Med*, 2000; **342**: 1581–9.
65. Verbalis JG. Hyponatremia. In: Baylis PH, ed. Water and Salt Homeostasis in Health and Disease. London: Bailliére Tindall, 1989: 499–530.
66. Ball SG, Baylis PH. Mechanisms of drug induced hyponatraemia. *Adverse Drug React Bull*, 1998; **192**: 734–7.
67. Verbalis JG. Pathogenesis of hyponatremia in an experimental model of the syndrome of inappropriate antidiuresis. *Am J Physiol*, 1994; **267**: R1617–25.
68. Ishikawa S-E, Saito T, Fugagawa A, Higashiyama M, Nakamura T, Kusaka I, *et al.* Close association of urnary excretion of aquaporin-2 with appropriate and inappropriate arginine vasopressin-dependent antidiuresis in hyponatraemia in elderly subjects. *J Clin Endocrinol Metab*, 2001; **86**: 1665–71.
69. Saito T, Higashiyama M, Nakamura T, Kusaka I, Nagasaka S, Saito T, *et al.* Urinary excretion of the aquaporin-2 water channel exaggerated in pathological states of impaired water excretion. *Clin Endocrinol*, 2001; **55**: 217–21.
70. Pedersen RS, Bentzen H, Bech JN, Pedersen EB. Effect of water deprivation and hypertonic saline infusion on urinary AQP2 excretion in healthy humans. *Am J Physiol*, 2001; **280**: F860–7.
71. Ball SG. Vasopressin and disorders of water balance: the physiology and pathophysiology of vasopressin. *Ann Clin Biochem*, 2007; **44**: 417–31.
72. Almond CSD, Shin AY, Fortescue EB, Mannix RC, Wypij D, Binstadt BA, *et al.* Hyponatraemia among runners in the Boston marathon. *N Engl J Med*, 2005; **353**: 1550–6.
73. Siegel AJ, Verbalis JG, Clement S, Mendelson JH, Mello NK, Adner M, *et al.* Hyponatremia in marathon runners due to inappropriate arginine vasopressin secretion. *JAMA*, 2007; **120**: 461e11–17.
74. Feldman BJ, Rosenthal SM, Vargas GA, Fenwick RG, Huang EA, Matsuda-Abedini M, *et al.* Nephrogenic syndrome of inappropriate antidiuresis. *N Engl J Med*, 2005; **352**: 1884–90.
75. Decaux G, Vandergheynst F, Bouko Y, Parma J, Vassart G, Vilain C, *et al.* Nephrogenic syndrome of inappropriate antidiuresis in adults: high phenotypic variability in men and women from a large pedigree. *J Am Soc Nephrol*, 2007; **18**: 606–12.
76. Palmer BF. Hyponatraemia in patients with central nervous system disease: SIADH versus CSW. *Trends Endocrinol Metab*, 2003; **14**: 182–7.
77. Verbalis JG, Goldsmith SR, Greenberg A, Schrier RW, Sterns RH, *et al.* Hyponatraemia treatment guidelines 2007: expert panel recommendations. *Am J Med*, 2007; **120**: S1–S21.
78. Schrier RW, Gross P, Gheorghiade M, Berl T, Verbalis JG, Czerwiec FS, *et al.* Tolvaptan, a selective oral vasopressin V2-receptor antagonist, for hyponatraemia. *N Engl J Med*, 2006; **355**: 2099–112.
79. Decaux G, Soupart A, Vassart G. Non-peptide arginine-vasopressin antagonists: the vaptans. *Lancet*, 2008; **371**: 1624–32.
80. Ball SG, Vaidja B, Baylis PH. Hypothalamic adipsic syndrome: diagnosis and management. *Clin Endocrinol*, 1997; **47**: 405–9.

2.3

Aetiology, pathogenesis, and management of disease of the pituitary

Contents

2.3.1 Development of the pituitary and genetic forms of hypopituitarism

Kyriaki S. Alatzoglou, Mehul T. Dattani

Introduction

Pituitary development occurs in distinct and sequential developmental steps, leading to the formation of a complex organ containing five different cell types secreting six different hormones. During this process the sequential temporal and spatial expression of a cascade of signalling molecules and transcription factors play a crucial role in organ commitment, cell proliferation, patterning, and terminal differentiation. Complex regulatory networks govern the process during which distinct cell types emerge from a common primordium. The mechanisms are not fully elucidated but it seems that opposing signalling gradients induce expression of interacting transcriptional regulators (activators or repressors) in overlapping patterns that act synergistically. Spontaneous or artificially induced mutations in the mouse and identification of mutations associated with human pituitary disease have contributed to defining the genetic cascades responsible for pituitary development.

Development of the pituitary gland

The pituitary gland has a dual embryonic origin: the anterior and intermediate lobes are derived from the oral ectoderm whereas the posterior pituitary is derived from the neural ectoderm. The development of the pituitary gland has been studied extensively in the mouse

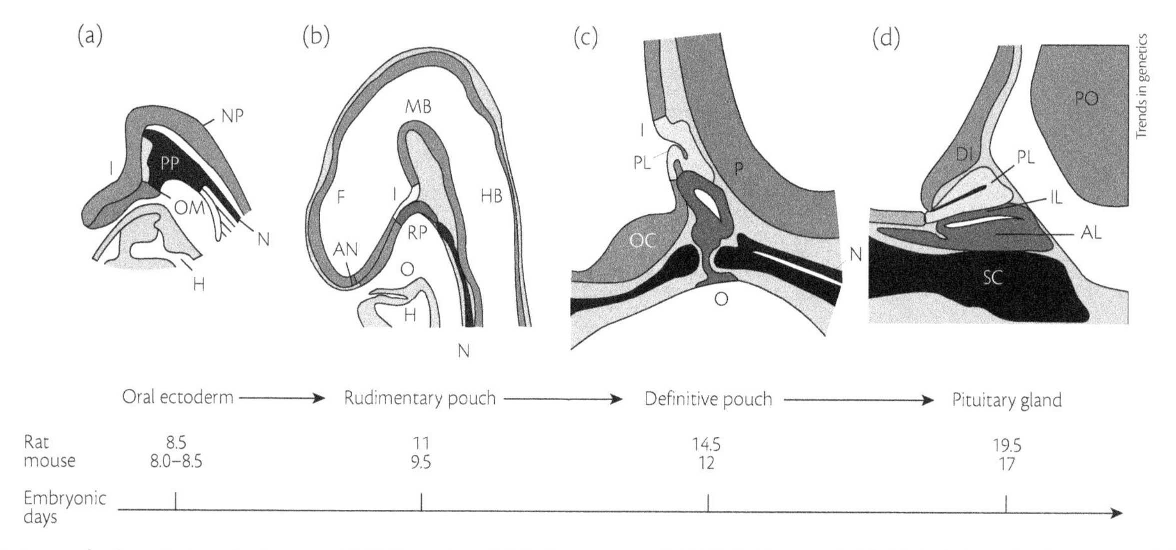

Fig. 2.3.1.1 Stages of rodent pituitary development. (a) Oral ectoderm. (b) Rudimentary pouch. (c) Definitive pouch. (d) Adult pituitary gland. AL, anterior lobe; AN, anterior neural pore; DI, diencephalon; F, forebrain; H, heart; HB, hindbrain; I, infundibulum; IL, intermediate lobe; MB, midbrain; N, notochord; NP, neural plate; O, oral cavity; OC, optic chiasm; OM, oral membrane; P, pontine flexure; PL, posterior lobe; PO, pons; PP, pituitary placode; RP, Rathke's pouch; SC, sphenoid cartilage. (Adapted from Sheng HZ, Westphal H. Early steps in pituitary organogenesis. *Trends Genet*, 1999; **15**: 236–40, with permission.)

and although relatively little is known about human pituitary development, it seems that it mirrors that in rodents (1) (Fig. 2.3.1.1).

The anterior pituitary develops from the hypophyseal or pituitary placode, one of the six cranial placodes that appear transiently as localized ectodermal thickenings in the prospective head of the developing embryo. The pituitary placode appears at embryonic day (E) 7.5 and is located ventrally in the midline of the anterior neural ridge and in continuity with the future hypothalamo-infundibular region, which is located posteriorly, in the rostral part of the neural plate. By E8.5 the neural tube has bent at the cephalic end and the placode appears as a thickening of the roof of the primitive oral cavity. At E9.0 the placode invaginates dorsally to form a rudimentary Rathke's pouch, from which the anterior and intermediate lobes of the pituitary are derived. The definitive pouch is formed by E10.5, whereas the evagination of the neural ectoderm at the base of the developing diencephalon will give rise to the posterior pituitary. Between E10.5 and E12 the pouch epithelium continues to proliferate and separates from the underlying oral ectoderm at E12.5. The progenitors of the hormone-secreting cell types proliferate ventrally from the pouch between E12.5 and E15.5 and populate what will form the anterior lobe. The remnants of the dorsal portion of the pouch will form the intermediate lobe, whereas the lumen of the pouch remains as the pituitary cleft, separating the intermediate from the anterior lobe (2).

Early developmental genes and transcription factors

The development of the anterior pituitary gland is dependent upon a carefully orchestrated genetic cascade that then encodes extrinsic and intrinsic transcription factors and signalling molecules that are expressed in a temporally and spatially restricted manner (Fig. 2.3.1.2 and Fig. 2.3.1.3).

Extrinsic molecules from the ventral diencephalon (Bmp4, Fgf8, Fgf4, Nkx2.1, Wnt5α) as well as ventral signals from the oral ectoderm (Sonic hedgehog (Shh)), surrounding mesenchyme (Bmp2, Indian hedgehog IHH, chordin) and the pouch itself (Bmp2, Wnt4) create a network of signalling gradients, which is important for morphogenesis during early pituitary development (3, 4).

Induction of Rathke's pouch and morphogenetic signals

At least two sequential inductive signals from the diencephalon are required for the induction and formation of Rathke's pouch (5). Bone morphogenetic protein 4 (Bmp4) is the earliest secreted signalling molecule detected at E8.5, followed by a second signal, fibroblast growth factor 8 (Fgf8). Fgf8 activates two key regulatory genes, LIM homoeobox 3 (*Lhx3*) and LIM homoeobox 4 (*Lhx4*), both of which are essential for subsequent development of the

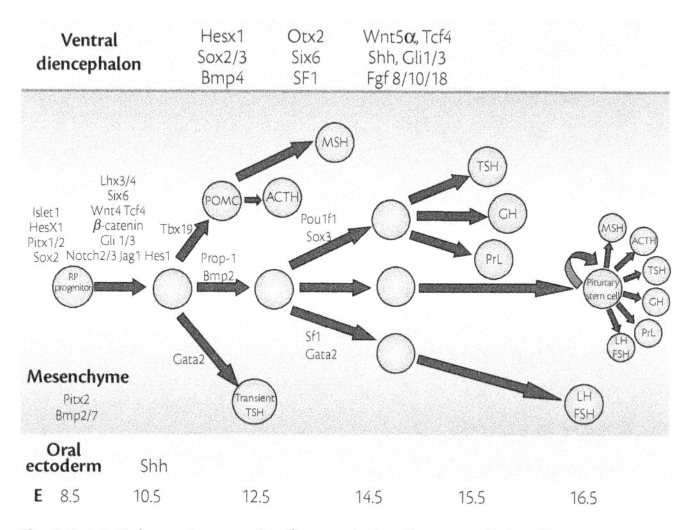

Fig. 2.3.1.2 Schematic cascade of transcription factors and signalling molecules highlighting some of the known genes and their expression domains. ACTH, adrenocorticotropic hormone; E, embryonic day; FSH, follicle-stimulating hormone; GH, growth hormone; LH, luteinizing hormone; MSH, melanocyte stimulating hormone; POMC, proopiomelanocortin; PrL, prolactin; RP, ; TSH, thyroid stimulating hormone. Adapted from Kelberman D et al. Genetic regulation of pituitary gland development in human and mouse. End Reviews 2009; **30**(7): 790–829, with permission.

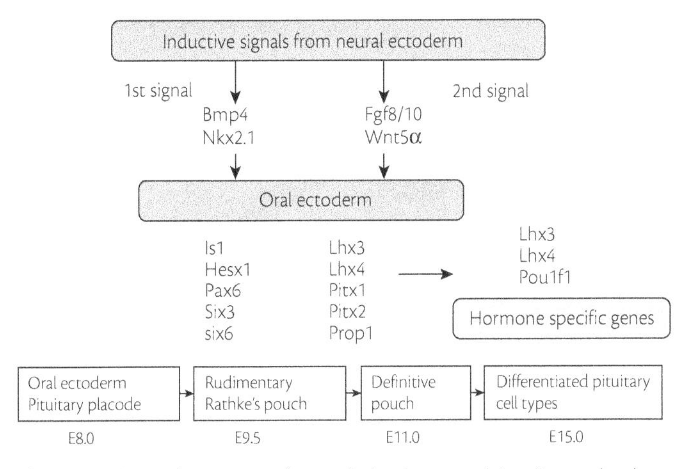

Fig. 2.3.1.3 Expression pattern of transcription factors and signalling molecules during early pituitary development.

rudimentary pouch into a definitive pouch. Signalling from the ventral diencephalon is critical for normal anterior pituitary, e.g. murine mutations within the thyroid-specific enhancer binding protein (*Ttf1* or *Nkx2.1*), only expressed in the presumptive ventral diencephalon, can cause severe defects in the development of not only the diencephalon but also the anterior pituitary gland.

At the early steps of pituitary development, Shh and its signalling pathway are also important for the patterning and morphogenesis of the gland as well as specification and expansion of ventral cell types. *Shh* null mice exhibit cyclopia and loss of midline structures of the brain. Shh binds to the transmembrane receptor Patched (PTC). This binding results in the release of the coreceptor Smoothened (SMO) and the activation of the downstream Gli transcription factors, which in turn act as activators (*Gli1*, *Gli2*) or repressors (*Gli3*). Shh is expressed in the ventral diencephalon and the oral ectoderm but its expression is excluded within Rathke's pouch as soon as the pouch appears. Its expression is maintained throughout the ventral diencephalon until E14.9, when it disappears. However, its receptor (PTC) is expressed in Rathke's pouch and Gli1-3 is expressed in the ventral diencephalon and the pouch (6). This pattern indicates that the developing gland can receive and respond to Shh signalling.

The Notch signalling pathway is an evolutionarily conserved mechanism implicated in many developmental processes. Molecules involved in Notch signalling (*Jag1*, *Notch2*, *Notch3*) and their downstream targets (*Hes1*) play critical roles in early steps of pituitary development. Notch signalling is required for maintaining expression of *Prop1* which in turn is required for generation of the *Pou1f1* (*Pit-1*) lineage. In the later phases of pituitary development, down-regulation of Notch signalling is necessary to permit terminal differentiation of the *Pou1f1* cell lineage and maturation and proliferation of the GH-producing somatotrophs (7).

Lhx3 and Lhx4

Lhx3 and *Lhx4* are members of the LIM transcription factor family of homoeobox genes characterized by the presence of a unique cysteine/histidine-rich zinc-binding LIM domain (8). *Lhx3* is one of the earliest transcription factors expressed in Rathke's pouch (E9.5) and its expression is maintained forming a gradient of expression with higher levels being observed in the dorsal region. By E16.5, *Lhx3* is expressed in the developing anterior and intermediate pituitary, but not in the posterior gland. Its expression persists throughout development and into adulthood. This highlights its importance for the establishment of hormone producing cell-types and may also play a role in the maintenance of some cell types in the mature pituitary. In addition, *Lhx3* expression has also been detected in restricted regions of the central nervous system (CNS) and inner ear (9).

Lhx4 is closely related to *Lhx3* and is also expressed in Rathke's pouch at E9.5. However, expression of *Lhx4* is restricted to the future anterior lobe, and is down-regulated at E15.5, therefore not persisting in the mature gland. *Lhx4* is also expressed in specific fields in the developing hindbrain, cerebral cortex, and motor neurons of the spinal cord (10). *Lhx3* null mice show early lethality and the anterior and intermediate lobes of the pituitary are lacking. Although Rathke's pouch is initially formed, pituitary development is then arrested as there is failure to maintain *Hesx1* expression and induce *Pou1f1*. There are some residual corticotrophs, but proopiomelanocortin (POMC)-expressing cells fail to proliferate, probably due to reduced expression of *Tbx19* (*T-Pit*) (11). In *Lhx4* null mice, Rathke's pouch is formed and there is specification of all the anterior pituitary cell lines. However, their numbers are markedly reduced leading to anterior pituitary hypoplasia. *Lhx3*$^{-/-}$, *Lhx4*$^{-/-}$ double mutant mice show a more severe phenotype than either single mutant, with an early arrest of pituitary development (1). This suggests that there is redundancy in their actions during pituitary development.

Hesx1

Hesx1 is a member of the paired-like class of homoeobox genes and one of the earliest markers of the pituitary primordium. During murine development *Hesx1* is expressed early during gastrulation in a region that will become the forebrain and from E9.0 to 9.5 it is restricted to the ventral diencephalon and the developing Rathke's pouch. From E12.5 its expression gradually disappears in a spatio-temporal sequence that corresponds to progressive pituitary cell differentiation and becomes undetectable by E15.5. *Hesx1* is a transcriptional repressor and this activity is mediated by a conserved region in the N-terminal domain (the engrailed homology domain; eh-1) and the homoeodomain. The N-terminal domain binds TLE, a mammalian homologue of the *Drosophila* corepressor protein Groucho, whereas the homoeodomain interacts with the nuclear corepressor complex NCoR1/Sin3/HDAC, thus increasing *Hesx1* repressor activity (12).

Lhx3 is important for maintaining *Hesx1* expression, whereas Prop1/β-catenin is required for its repression (13). Down-regulation of *Hesx1* is important for activation of other downstream genes such as *Prop1* and the temporal regulation of their expression is critical for normal pituitary development. Prolonged expression of *Hesx1* can block *Prop1*-dependent activation, whereas premature expression of *Prop1* can block pituitary organogenesis.

The role of *Hesx1* in pituitary development was elucidated by its targeted disruption in mice. Homozygous null animals had a reduction in the prospective forebrain tissue, absence of developing optic vesicles, optic cups, and olfactory placodes, markedly decreased head size, reduced telencephalic vesicles, severe microphthalmia, hypothalamic abnormalities, and abnormal morphogenesis of Rathke's pouch. Although a small percentage (5%) of the most severely affected null mutants had complete lack of the pituitary, the majority had multiple oral ectodermal invaginations resulting in the apparent formation of multiple pituitary glands.

The phenotype was variable and reminiscent of patients with septo-optic dysplasia (14).

In humans, homozygous and heterozygous mutations in *HESX1* are associated with varying phenotypes characterized by isolated growth hormone deficiency, combined pituitary hormone deficiency, and septo-optic dysplasia.

SOX2 and SOX3

The SOX family of transcription factors is characterized by the presence of a 79 amino acid high mobility group (HMG) DNA-binding domain which is similar to the HMG domain of the mammalian sex determining gene *SRY*. More than 20 SOX proteins and their genes have been identified and classified into eight groups, A–H. *SOX3* was among the first of the SOX genes to be identified, and along with *SOX1* and *SOX2*, belongs to the SOXB1 group, which exhibits the highest degree of similarity to *SRY* (15, 16).

During pituitary development *SOX3* is expressed in the ventral diencephalon and infundibulum, but not in Rathke's pouch. Targeted disruption of *Sox3* in mice results in mutants with a variable phenotype, including craniofacial abnormalities, midline defects, and reduction in size and fertility. Mutant mice have variable endocrine deficits, including reduced growth hormone, luteinizing hormone, follicle-stimulating hormone (FSH), and thyroid-stimulating hormone, which correlates to body weight. The pituitary gland has an abnormal morphology with a hypoplastic anterior lobe and presence of additional abnormal clefts. In *Sox3* mutants, Rathke's pouch is bifurcated and the evagination of the infundibulum is less pronounced (17).

In the mouse, *Sox2* expression is first detected before gastrulation at E2.5 at the morula stage. Following gastrulation, it is restricted to the presumptive neuroectoderm and by E9.5 it is expressed throughout the brain, CNS, sensory placodes, branchial arches, gut endoderm, the oesophagus, and the trachea. Homozygous loss of *Sox2* results in peri-implantation lethality, whereas *Sox2* heterozygous mice appear relatively normal but show a reduction in size and male fertility. Further studies that have resulted in the reduction of *Sox2* expression levels below 40%, compared with normal levels, result in anophthalmia in the affected mutants (18). This highlights the fact that *Sox2* function is dose dependent. Given the observation of growth retardation and reduced fertility, the role of *Sox2* in murine pituitary development has been studied in detail. *Sox2* expression is detected in the infundibulum and Rathke's pouch at E11.5 but, as cell differentiation occurs, expression is confined to proliferative zones. In heterozygous mutant mice the morphogenesis of the gland was abnormal with bifurcation of Rathke's pouch in a third of mutants at E12.5 and subsequent extra clefts in some of the adult pituitaries. Embryonic pituitaries at E18.5 were smaller and had significantly reduced numbers of somatotrophs and gonadotrophs, with reduced growth hormone content. Evaluation of hormonal content in 3-month-old heterozygotes showed that there was moderate reduction in growth hormone and luteinizing hormone, which was significant for males, whereas there was evidence that corticotrophs, lactotrophs, and thyrotrophs were also affected (19). In humans, mutations in *SOX2* and *SOX3* lead to variable hypopituitarism, as is described in the next section.

Terminal cell differentiation

Terminal differentiation of cells in the anterior pituitary is the result of complex interactions between extrinsic signalling molecules and transcription factors (Lhx3, Lhx4, Gata2, Isl1, Prop1, Pou1f1). Differentiated hormone-producing pituitary cells emerge sequentially, at distinct positions in the anterior pituitary. Corticotrophs expressing POMC are the first to appear (E12.5), followed by thyrotrophs (E14.5), somatotrophs (E15.5), lactotrophs (E16.5), and finally gonadotrophs at around E16.5 (20, 21) (Fig. 2.3.1.4). Among the number of transcription factors involved, Prop1 and Pou1f1 are best characterized in terms of function in both humans and mice.

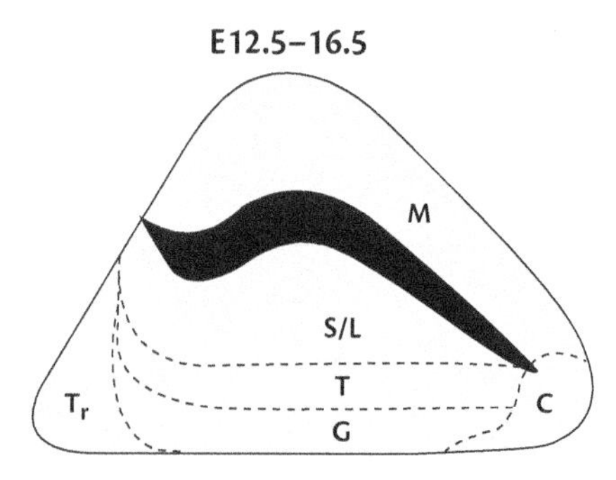

Fig. 2.3.1.4 Cell types arise in a spatial and temporal specific manner. C, corticotrophs; G, gonadotrophs; L, lactotrophs; M, melanotrophs; S, somatotrophs; T, thyrotrophs; Tr, thyrotrophs at rostral tip. (Adapted from Scully KM, Rosenfeld MG. Pituitary development: regulatory codes in mammalian organogenesis. *Science* 2002; **295**: 2231–5, with permission.)

Prop1

Prop1 (Prophet of *Pit1*) is a pituitary-specific paired-like homoeodomain transcription factor initially detected in the dorsal portion of Rathke's pouch at E10–10.5. Its expression peaks at E12 and becomes undetectable by E15.5. *Prop1* is both a transcriptional activator and repressor. Depending on associated cofactors, the β-catenin/Prop1 complex is important for activation of *Pou1f1(Pit1)* and repression of *Hesx1*. Temporal regulation of *Prop1* expression is important for normal pituitary development. Premature expression of *Prop1* in Rathke's pouch leads to agenesis of the anterior pituitary, probably by repressing Hesx1 (13).

The Ames dwarf (*df*) mouse has a naturally occurring mutation in *Prop1* that results in an eightfold reduction in DNA-binding activity compared with wild-type protein. Analysis of these animals showed that *Prop1* is important for the determination of the three *Pou1f1*-dependent cell types and is also required for the generation of gonadotrophs. Homozygous Ames *df* mice exhibit severe proportional dwarfism, hypothyroidism, and infertility, and the emerging anterior pituitary gland is reduced in size by about 50% displaying an abnormal looping appearance. The adult Ames *df* mouse exhibits growth hormone, TSH, and prolactin deficiency resulting from a severe reduction of somatotroph, lactotroph, and caudomedial thyrotroph lineages. In addition, they exhibit reduced gonadotrophin expression correlating with low plasma luteinizing hormone and FSH concentrations (22).

Differentiation of *Pou1f1 (Pit-1)* lineage

Pou1f1 (Pit-1) is a pituitary specific transcription factor which belongs to the POU-homoeodomain family (23). It is expressed late during pituitary development (E13.5) and its expression persists throughout adulthood. Autoregulation of *Pou1f1* is required to sustain its expression, once it has reached a critical threshold. The role of *Pou1f1* in pituitary development has been elucidated by the study of two naturally occurring murine models, the Snell and

Jackson *df* mice. In the Snell *df* mouse a recessive point mutation results in absence of somatotrophs, lactotrophs, and thyrotrophs. A similar phenotype results in the Jackson *df* mouse that harbours a recessive null mutation due to rearrangement of *Pou1f1*.

Pou1f1 is important for: terminal differentiation and expansion of somatotrophs, lactotrophs, and thyrotrophs in the intermediate caudomedial field; repression of gonadotroph cell fate; and transcriptional regulation of genes encoding the hormones produced by the above cell types (*GH1*, *PRL*, *TSHβ*, *GHRHR*) (24).

Differentiation of gonadotrophs

The emergence of the gonadotroph cell lineage does not depend on *Pou1f1*. Gonadotrophs arise in the most ventral part of the anterior pituitary and are the last cells to differentiate. A number of transcription factors have been shown to determine the gonadotroph cell fate, including GATA2, SF1, Egr1, Pitx1, Pitx2, Prop1, and Otx1. The result is terminal cell differentiation and expression of the markers LHβ, FSFβ, and GnRHR.

In the most ventral aspect of the anterior pituitary high levels of GATA2 restrict *Pou1f1* expression. In the absence of *Pou1f1*, GATA2 induces transcription factors that will determine gonadotroph differentiation, including *SF1*, *P-Frk*, and *Isl-1*. Conversely, in the dorsal aspect the absence of GATA2 is critical for the differentiation of the Pou1f1-positive cells (somatotrophs and lactotrophs); this induced gradient of GATA2 expression determines gonadotroph and thyrotroph cell lineages (25).

Steroidogenic factor 1 (SF1) is expressed in the gonadotrophs as well as in the developing gonads, adrenal glands and the ventromedial hypothalamus. It is a zinc-finger nuclear receptor that regulates a number of genes involved in sex determination, steroidogenesis, and reproduction, including αGSU, LHβ, FSHβ, and GnRHR. In the developing pituitary, GATA2 is capable of inducing *SF1* expression in gonadotrophs (E13.5). *SF1*-knockout mice exhibit adrenal and gonadal agenesis, male-to-female sex reversal, ablation of the ventromedial hypothalamic nucleus and selective loss of gonadotrophin, αGSU and *Gnrhr* expression.

Pituitary specific inactivation of *SF1* results in mice with hypoplastic gonads, a dramatic decrease in pituitary gonadotropin expression, and failure to develop normal secondary sexual characteristics, while the adrenal glands and hypothalamus are unaffected. In these models, expression of LHβ and FSHβ can be restored by high-dose gonadotropin-releasing hormone (GnRH), demonstrating that SF1 is necessary for maturation of gonadotrophs but not cell fate specification (26).

The function of gonadotrophs in the anterior pituitary is under the control of hypothalamic GnRH; it is synthesized by neurons in the preoptic region, which project axons to the median eminence, where they secrete GnRH. Neuroendocrine GnRH cells arise from the olfactory placode. It has been shown that *Pax6* is required for the generation of GnRH neurons, as a mouse strain with mutation in *Pax6* shows failure to develop both optical and olfactory placodes. Following their generation, GnRH cells migrate along the olfactory nerve pathway across the cribriform plate, towards the olfactory bulb and their final position in the hypothalamus (27). In humans, it is estimated that migration of the GnRH cells begins during the sixth week of gestation. An increasing number of genes are implicated in the migration and maturation of GnRH neurons (i.e. *KAL1*, *FGFR1*, *FGF8*, *PROK2*, *PROKR2*, *Kiss-1*, *GPR54*, *leptin*, *CHD7*, *TAC3*, *TACR3*). Their role is highlighted by mutations found in cases of isolated hypogonadotropic hypogonadism, as is mentioned later as well as in the relevant chapter.

Differentiation of corticotrophs

Corticotrophs producing adrenocorticotropic hormone (ACTH) are the first cell type to reach terminal differentiation. However, relatively little is known about the factors that determine the specification of corticotrophs and melanotrophs and the control of POMC expression (28). Tbx19 (T-Pit) is a member of the T-box transcription factors. During mouse pituitary development, Tbx19 is expressed at E11.5, in the most ventral region of Rathke's pouch, in corticotrophs and melanotrophs; along with Pitx1, Tbx19 activates the POMC promoter (29).

Genetic forms of hypopituitarism

Congenital hypopituitarism encompasses a group of different disorders and may manifest as an isolated hormone deficiency, or alternatively several pituitary hormone axes may be defective resulting in combined pituitary hormone deficiency (CPHD). Isolated hormone deficiencies include isolated growth hormone deficiency (IGHD), ACTH deficiency, gonadotropin deficiency (hypogonadotropic hypogonadism), TSH deficiency or central diabetes insipidus. Combined pituitary hormone deficiencies may occur in isolation or be associated with extra-pituitary defects such as optic nerve hypoplasia or midline forebrain abnormalities.

An increasing number of genes are implicated in the aetiology of congenital hypopituitarism (Table 2.3.1.1). Although mouse models have enhanced our understanding of the genetic basis of hypopituitarism in humans, the correlation with disease phenotypes is variable. In general, mutations in genes involved in early development and patterning of the forebrain and pituitary tend to result in syndromic forms of hypopituitarism in association with extrapituitary defects and midline abnormalities. On the other hand, mutations in genes encoding specific hormone subunits or required for specification of particular cell types give rise to isolated pituitary hormone deficiencies (24, 30, 31).

Combined pituitary hormone deficiencies

The majority of cases of combined pituitary hormone deficiencies have no identified genetic aetiology. Among the genetic causes, a number of genes have been implicated, which result in (1) nonsyndromic combined pituitary hormone deficiencies (*PROP1*, *POU1F1*) or (2) syndromic combined pituitary hormone deficiencies in association with ocular defects, midline abnormalities or other features. The timing and combination of pituitary hormone deficiencies, neuroimaging, and associated features may guide the diagnosis. In many cases, however, the phenotype is variable and overlapping. Table 2.3.1.2 compares the phenotype in patients with hypopituitarism as a result of mutations in some of these genes.

Mutations in PROP1

PROP1 lies on chromosome 5q and consists of three exons encoding a protein of 226 amino acids. Recessive mutations in *PROP1* are the commonest cause of CPHD, identified in approximately 50% of familial cases. In sporadic cases, however, the incidence is much lower (32). More than 20 mutations have been reported in *PROP1*. The most frequent (50–72%) is a 2 bp deletion (GA or AG) among three tandem GA repeats (296-GAGAGAG-302)

Table 2.3.1.1 Summary of genetic disorders of hypothalamo-pituitary development in humans.

Gene	Phenotype	Inheritance
Isolated hormone deficiencies		
GH1	GHD	AR, AD
GHRHR	GHD	AR
TSHβ	TSH deficiency	AR
TRHR	TSH deficiency	AR
T-PIT	ACTH deficiency	AR
PC1	ACTH deficiency, hypoglycaemia, hypogonadotropic hypogonadism, obesity	AR
POMC	ACTH deficiency, obesity, red hair	AR
GnRHR	Normosmic HH	AR
GPR54	Normosmic HH	AR
Kisspeptin	Normosmic HH	AR
Leptin	Normosmic HH, obesity	AR
Leptin-R	Normosmic HH, obesity	AR
KAL1	Kallmann's syndrome, unilateral renal agenesis, synkinesia	XL
FGFR1	Kallmann's syndrome, normosmic HH, variable gonadotrophin deficiency, cleft lip and palate, abnormalities of corpus callosum	AD
FGF8	Kallmann's syndrome, normosmic HH, variable gonadotrophin deficiency, cleft lip/palate, camptodactyly	AD
PROK2	Kallmann's syndrome, obesity	AD, AR
PROKR2	Kallmann's syndrome	AD, AR
TAC3	HH	AR
TAC3R	HH	AR
CHD7	HH, Kallmann's syndrome, CHARGE variants	AD
FSHβ	Primary amenorrhoea, defective spermatogenesis, low FSH	AR
LHβ	Delayed puberty, low or elevated LH	AR
DAX1	HH and adrenal hypoplasia congenita	XL
AVP-NPII	Diabetes insipidus	AR, AD
CRH	CRH deficiency	AR
Combined pituitary hormone deficiencies		
POU1F1	GH, TSH and prolactin deficiencies	AR, AD
PROP1	GH, TSH, LH, FSH, PRL, and evolving ACTH deficiencies	AR
Specific syndromes		
LHX3	GH, TSH, LH, FSH, PRL, and ACTH deficiencies, limited neck rotation	AR
LHX4	GH, TSH, ACTH deficiencies, cerebellar abnormalities	AD
GLI2	Holoprosencephaly and multiple midline defects	AD
GLI3	Pallister-Hall syndrome	AD
PITX2	Rieger's syndrome	AD

(continued)

Table 2.3.1.1 *(Cont'd)* Summary of genetic disorders of hypothalamo-pituitary development in humans.

Gene	Phenotype	Inheritance
HESX1	Septo-optic dysplasia, IGHD, CPHD	AR, AD
SOX3	IGHD, CPHD, learning difficulties	XL
SOX2	HH, anophthalmia, learning difficulties, oesophageal atresia, sensorineural hearing loss	AD
OTX2	Anophthalmia/severe microphthalmia, CPHD, partial GHD	AD

ACTH, adrenocorticotropic hormone; AD, autosomal dominant; AR, autosomal recessive; CPHD, combined pituitary hormone deficiencies; FSH, follicle-stimulating hormone; GH, growth hormone; GHD, growth hormone deficiency; HH, hypogonadotropic hypogonadism; IGHD, isolated growth hormone deficiency; LH, luteinizing hormone; PRL, prolactin; TSH, thyroid stimulating hormone; XL, X-linked.

within exon 2. This results in a frame shift at codon 109 and generates a truncated protein (S109X) which disrupts DNA-binding and transcriptional activation. The mutation has been detected in multiple unrelated families and represents a mutational hot spot; along with the 150delA mutation it accounts for approximately 97% of all mutations in *PROP1*.

The first reported mutations in *PROP1* were in members of four unrelated pedigrees with growth hormone, TSH, prolactin, luteinizing hormone, and FSH deficiencies (33). In patients with mutations in *PROP1*, the timing and severity of hormonal deficiencies is variable. In general, deficiency in growth hormone, TSH, and prolactin is milder in patients with mutations in *PROP1* rather than in *POU1F1*. Most patients present with early-onset growth hormone deficiency, however, normal growth in early childhood and normal final height has been reported in an untreated patient with a *PROP1* mutation. The TSH deficiency varies and may not be present from birth. Although PROP1 is essential for the differentiation of gonadotrophs in fetal life, the spectrum of gonadotrophin deficiency is highly variable. It ranges from presentation with microphallus and undescended testes, hypogonadism with lack of puberty, to spontaneous pubertal development with subsequent arrest, and infertility. This variation in timing and severity of gonadotrophin deficiency suggests that *PROP1* is required for maintenance or differentiation of gonadotrophs, rather than the cell fate determination. Individuals with mutations in *PROP1* exhibit normal ACTH and cortisol concentrations in early life but often demonstrate an evolving cortisol deficiency associated with increasing age, although it has also been described in a 7-year-old patient. The underlying mechanism for cortisol deficiency is unknown, especially as *PROP1* is not expressed in corticotrophs, but appears to be required for maintenance of the corticotroph population (34–36).

Most patients with mutations in *PROP1* have a small or normal anterior pituitary, with normal pituitary stalk and posterior lobe. However, in some cases, an enlarged anterior pituitary has also been reported. Longitudinal analyses of anterior pituitary size have revealed that a significant number of patients demonstrate pituitary enlargement in early childhood, which can wax and wane in size, with subsequent involution in older patients. This pituitary enlargement consists of a mass lesion between the anterior and posterior lobes, possibly originating from the intermediate lobe (37).

Table 2.3.1.2 Clinical features of hypopituitarism due to mutations in *PROP1*, *POU1F1*, *LHX3*, and *LHX4*

	PROP1	*POU1F1*	*LHX3*	*LHX4*
Growth hormone	Deficient	Deficient	Deficient	Deficient
Thyroid-stimulating hormone	Deficient	Deficient	Deficient	Deficient
Prolactin	Deficient	Deficient	Deficient	Normal
Luteinizing hormone/follicle-stimulating hormone	Deficient	Normal	Deficient	Normal
Adrenocorticotropic hormone	May evolve	Normal	Normal/Deficient	Deficient
Pituitary	APH, N, E	APH, N	APH, N, E	APH, EPP
Other	–	–	Short cervical spine, sensorineural deafness	Cerebellar abnormalities

APH, anterior pituitary hypoplasia; E, enlarged; EPP, ectopic posterior pituitary; N, normal.

Mutations in POU1F1

POUIFI is on chromosome 3p11 and consists of six exons encoding a 291 amino acid protein. The first mutation within *POUIFI* was identified in a child with growth hormone, prolactin, and profound TSH deficiency. To date, the majority of identified mutations are recessive, although a number of heterozygous mutations have also been reported. Among them, the dominant R271W seems to be a mutational 'hot spot'. Functional analysis suggests that some mutations disrupt DNA binding whereas others disrupt transcriptional activation or other properties such as autoregulation (38). Patients with *POUIF1* mutations present with growth hormone, TSH, and prolactin deficiency, however, the spectrum of hormone deficiencies varies. Growth hormone and prolactin deficiencies present early in life, whereas TSH deficiency can present later in childhood, or TSH secretion may even be preserved. The anterior pituitary may be small or normal with no other extrapituitary or midline abnormalities (39).

Syndromic CPHD

Mutations in LHX3/LHX4

Mutations in *LHX3* and *LHX4* are rare causes of hypopituitarism. *LHX3* is located on chromosome 9q34. Homozygous mutations in *LHX3* have been described in patients with growth hormone, prolactin, TSH, and luteinizing hormone/FSH deficiencies (40). Although ACTH secretion has been reported to be usually spared, there has been a recent report of ACTH deficiency in patients with *LHX3* mutations. In addition to combined pituitary hormone deficiencies, patients present with a short rigid cervical spine with limited head rotation and trunk movement (41). Recently, sensorineural deafness of varying severity has been reported in association with homozygous loss of *LHX3* (42). Pituitary morphology is also variable, ranging from a small to a markedly enlarged anterior pituitary, whereas a hypointense lesion with a 'microadenoma' has also been described.

LHX4 extends over 45 kb on chromosome 1q25. Heterozygous mutations within *LHX4* have been described in patients with growth hormone deficiency and variable additional endocrine deficits and extrapituitary abnormalities. The first reported patient presented with growth hormone, TSH, and ACTH deficiency (43). The anterior pituitary was hypoplastic with an ectopic posterior pituitary and absent stalk. However, other affected patients from the same family presented with isolated growth hormone deficiency and normal posterior pituitary. Additional manifestations included a poorly formed sella and pointed cerebellar tonsils. Since then, patients with variable hypopituitarism, with or without an ectopic posterior pituitary and Chiari malformation have been reported (44, 45)

Septo-optic dysplasia

Septo-optic dysplasia is defined by any combination of optic nerve hypoplasia, midline forebrain defects (i.e. agenesis of the corpus callosum, absent septum pellucidum), and pituitary hypoplasia with variable hypopituitarism. It is a highly heterogeneous condition with a reported incidence of 1:10 000, and although it is generally sporadic, familial cases have been described. Approximately 30% of patients with septo-optic dysplasia manifest the complete clinical triad, 62% have some degree of hypopituitarism, and 60% have an absent septum pellucidum. Optic nerve hypoplasia may be unilateral (12%) or bilateral (88%) and may be the first presenting feature, with the later onset of endocrine dysfunction. In rare cases the eye abnormalities may be more severe (microphthalmia, anophthalmia). Neurological manifestations are common in patients with septo-optic dysplasia (75–80%) and range from focal deficits to global developmental delay.

Endocrine abnormalities vary from isolated growth hormone deficiency to panhypopituitarism. It is worth noting, however, that the endocrinopathy may be evolving with a progressive loss of endocrine function over time. The commonest endocrine defect is growth hormone deficiency followed by TSH and ACTH deficiency, whereas gonadotropin secretion may be retained. Either sexual precocity or failure to develop in puberty may occur and it has been noted that in children with septo-optic dysplasia, commencement of growth hormone treatment may be associated with accelerated pubertal maturation. In addition, abnormal hypothalamic neuroanatomy or function and diabetes insipidus may occur (46).

Genetic and environmental factors have been implicated in the aetiology of septo-optic dysplasia, including viral infections, vascular or degenerative disorders, and antenatal exposure to alcohol and drugs. The condition presents more commonly in children born to younger mothers and clusters in geographical areas with a high frequency of teenage pregnancies. As forebrain and pituitary development are closely linked and occur as early as 3–6 weeks' gestation in the human embryo, any insult at this critical stage of development could account for the features of septo-optic dysplasia.

Genetic causes of septo-optic dysplasia

HESX1, *SOX2*, and *SOX3* have all been implicated in the aetiology of SOD and its variants (46). *HESX1* is located on chromosome

3p21.1-3p21.2; its coding region consists of four exons and spans 1.7 kb. Autosomal dominant and recessive mutations have been described in a number of patients, resulting in variable phenotype, without clear genotype–phenotype correlation (Table 2.3.1.3). The overall frequency of *HESX1* mutations in septo-optic dysplasia is low (approximately 1%) suggesting that mutations in other genes may contribute to this complex disorder (14, 47).

Mutations in SOX2

Heterozygous *de novo* mutations in *SOX2* have been reported in patients with bilateral anophthalmia or severe microphthalmia and additional abnormalities (developmental delay, learning difficulties, oesophageal atresia, and genital abnormalities) (48). Kelberman *et al.* first described in detail the pituitary phenotype in six patients with heterozygous loss of function mutations in *SOX2*, which comprised bilateral eye abnormalities, anterior pituitary hypoplasia and hypogonadotropic hypogonadism (HH) (49). Patients with *SOX2* mutations may present with forebrain abnormalities and associated developmental disorders (Table 2.3.1.4). They are at high risk of developing HH, even if it is not manifest at diagnosis, and long-term follow-up is recommended (49).

Table 2.3.1.3 Reported mutations in *HESX1*

Mutation	Inheritance	Endocrine deficiencies	Neuroradiology
Q6H	AD	GH, TSH, LH, FSH	AP hypoplasia, EPP
Q117P	AD	GH, TSH, ACTH, LH, FSH	AP hypoplasia, EPP
E149K	AD	GH	AP hypoplasia, EPP, infundibular hypoplasia
S170L	AD	GH	Normal AP, EPP, ONH, partial ACC
K176T	AD	GH, evolving ACTH and TSH deficiency	EPP
T181A	AD	GH	AP hypoplasia, absent PP bright spot, normal ON
g.1684delG	AD	GH	AP hypoplasia, absent PP bright spot, ONH, ACC
c.306_307insAG	AD	GH, LH, FSH; hypothyroidism	AP hypoplasia, ONH
R160C	AR	GH, TSH, ACTH, LH, FSH	AP hypoplasia, EPP, ONH, ACC
I26T	AR	GH, LH, FSH; evolving ACTH and TSH deficiency	AP hypoplasia, EPP, normal ON
c.357+2T>C	AR	GH, TSH, ACTH, PRL	AP aplasia, normal PP and ON
Alu insertion (exon 3)	AR	Panhypopituitarism	AP aplasia, normal PP and infundibulum
c.449_450delCA	AR	GH, TSH, ACTH	AP aplasia, normal PP and ON, thin CC, hydrocephalus

ACC, agenesis of corpus callosum; ACTH, adrenocorticotropic hormone; AD, autosomal dominant; AP, anterior pituitary; AR, autosomal recessive; CC, corpus callosum; EPP, ectopic posterior pituitary; FSH, follicle-stimulating hormone; GH, growth hormone; LH, luteinizing hormone; ON, optic nerve; ONH, optic nerve hypoplasia; PP, posterior pituitary; PRL, prolactin; TSH, thyroid stimulating hormone.

X-linked hypopituitarism and SOX3

A number of pedigrees have been described with X-linked hypopituitarism involving duplications of Xq26-q27, encompassing the *SOX3* gene (50). The phenotype comprises variable learning difficulties and hypopituitarism associated with anterior pituitary hypoplasia, infundibular hypoplasia, and an ectopic posterior pituitary, with variable abnormalities of the corpus callosum. Further implication of *SOX3* in hypopituitarism comes from the identification of affected patients with expansion of a polyalanine (PA) tract within the gene. In this case, as well, the phenotype is variable. PA expansion by 11 residues has been reported to be associated with isolated growth hormone deficiency, short stature, learning difficulties, and facial abnormalities in some, but not all, patients (51). However, expansion of the tract by seven alanine residues has been associated with panhypopituitarism, anterior pituitary hypoplasia, a hypoplastic infundibulum, and an ectopic/undescended posterior pituitary, but no evidence of learning difficulties or facial abnormalities. It has been demonstrated that +7PA results in partial loss of function of the mutant protein, possibly due to impaired nuclear localization (52).

Other syndromic forms of hypopituitarism

Holoprosencephaly

Holoprosencephaly (HPE) is characterized by abnormal separation of the midline structures of the brain. The phenotype is highly variable and associated with a number of midline defects, including nasal and ocular defects, abnormalities of the olfactory nerves and bulbs, hypothalamus, and pituitary gland. Other associated features may be partial agenesis of the corpus callosum, single central incisor, and postaxial polydactyly. The most common pituitary abnormality is diabetes insipidus, although anterior pituitary hormone deficiencies have also been described. Both environmental and genetic factors have been implicated in its aetiology. Mutations in components of the SHH pathway have been described in association with HPE. They include mutations in *SHH* (7q36), *GLI2* (2q14), and *PTC* (9q22.3). Mutations in *SHH* and *PTC* result in variable phenotypes that range from alobar HPE to normal individuals (53). Recently, heterozygous mutations in *GLI2* have reported in patients with variable craniofacial abnormalities, abnormal pituitary morphology (absent pituitary, hypoplasia) and function (isolated growth hormone deficiency or panhypopituitarism) (54).

Mutations in *OTX2* and variable hypopituitarism

Heterozygous mutations in *OTX2* have been implicated in the aetiology of a small percentage (2–3%) of anophthalmia/microphthalmia in humans. Recent reports have implicated *OTX2* in the aetiology of hypopituitarism (55); three mutations have been reported in four patients with variable hypopituitarism and MRI findings (Table 2.3.1.5). During normal pituitary development *OTX2* is required for anterior neural plate induction and appears to regulate the expression of *HESX1*. The mutant proteins reported

Table 2.3.1.4 Pituitary phenotype in patients with *SOX2* mutations

Mutation	Sex	Eye phenotype	Pituitary phenotype	Other
c.70del20	F	Left anophthalmia, right microphthalmia	HH, APH, Hippocampal abnormalities	DD
c.70del29	F	Bilateral anophthalmia	HH	
c.60_61insG	F	Bilateral anophthalmia	HH, APH, hypothalamic hamartoma	DD, oesophageal atresia, spastic diplegia
p.Q61X	F	Bilateral anophthalmia	HH	DD
p.L75Q	F	Right anophthalmia	HH	
c.387delC	M	Left microphthalmia, right coloboma	HH, APH, hypothalamic hamartoma, cryptorchidism, micropenis	DD, mild spastic diplegia
c.479delA	M	Bilateral anophthalmia	HH, APH, micropenis	DD, sensorineural deafness
p.Y160X	M	Bilateral anophthalmia	HH, APH, cryptorchidism, micropenis	Severe DD, spastic and dystonic quadriparesis
p.Q177X	M	Bilateral anophthalmia	HH, cryptorchidism, micropenis	Severe DD, mild facial dysmorphism
SOX2 deletion	F	Right anophthalmia, left microphthalmia	APH, thin corpus callosum	DD, mild pulmonary stenosis

APH, anterior pituitary hypoplasia; DD, developmental delay; F, female; HH, hypogonadotropic hypogonadism; M, male.

so far exhibit absent or reduced transcriptional activation of their putative target promoters.

Rieger's syndrome

Mutations in *PITX2* in humans are associated with Rieger's syndrome, an autosomal dominant heterogeneous condition (56). Abnormalities include malformations of the anterior chamber of the eye, dental hypoplasia, a protuberant umbilicus, and learning difficulties. In some patients reduced growth hormone concentrations and a small sella turcica have been noted, but the significance of these observations remains unclear.

Isolated hormone deficiencies

Isolated growth hormone deficiency

Congenital isolated growth hormone deficiency has a reported prevalence of 1:4000- 1:10 000 livebirths. Although most cases are sporadic, a genetic aetiology is suggested in 3–30% of cases. Congenital isolated growth hormone deficiency may result from mutations in the genes encoding growth hormone (*GH1*) or growth hormone-releasing hormone receptor (*GHRHR*). In addition, isolated growth hormone deficiency may result from mutations within the genes encoding the transcription factors *SOX3* and *HESX1*, or it may be the presenting symptom in some cases of combined pituitary hormone deficiencies. So far, no mutations in *GHRH* have as yet been described.

GH1 is located on chromosome 17q23, within a cluster of five related genes that include human chorionic somatomammotropic hormone pseudogene 1 (*CSHP1*), human chorionic somatomammotropic hormone 1 (*CSH1*), *GH2*, and human chorionic somatomammotropic hormone 2 (*CSH2*). *GH1* consists of five exons, encoding a mature molecule of 22 kDa that represents 85–90% of circulating growth hormone. Alternative splicing of mRNA generates a 20 kDa form of growth hormone that accounts for 10–15% of circulating growth hormone. Its expression is regulated by a proximal promoter and by a locus control region (LCR) located 15–32 kb upstream of the gene, which confers pituitary-specific, high-level expression of human growth hormone. Both the proximal promoter and LCR contain binding sites for the pituitary-specific transcription factor Pou1f1. *GHRHR* consists of 13 exons spanning approximately 15 kb, mapped to chromosome 7p15. GHRHR is a 423 amino acid G-protein-coupled receptor that contains seven transmembrane domains. Expression of *GHRHR* is up-regulated by *POU1F1* and is required for proliferation of somatotrophs.

There are four distinct types of congenital isolated growth hormone deficiency (57) (Table 2.3.1.6). Patients with isolated growth hormone deficiency type IA present with early and profound growth failure and undetectable or extremely low growth hormone concentrations on provocation. They develop antibodies to growth hormone treatment, resulting in a markedly decreased

Table 2.3.1.5 Pituitary phenotype in patients with *OTX2* mutations

Mutation	Eye phenotype	Sex	Endocrine deficits	Neuroradiology
c.576_577insCT	Bilateral anophthalmia	M	GH, TSH, ACTH, LH, FSH	APH, EPP, absent stalk, Chiari malformation
c.402insC	Bilateral anophthalmia	F	Partial GHD	Normal pituitary
p.N233S	Normal	M	GH, TSH, ACTH, LH, FSH	APH, EPP, hypoplastic stalk
p.N233S	Normal	F	GH, TSH, ACTH, LH, FSH	APH

ACTH, adrenocorticotropic hormone; APH, anterior pituitary hypoplasia; EPP, ectopic posterior pituitary; F, female; FSH, follicle-stimulating hormone; GH, growth hormone; GHD, growth hormone deficiency; LH, luteinizing hormone; M, male; TSH, thyroid stimulating hormone.

Table 2.3.1.6 Genetic forms of isolated growth hormone (GH) deficiency

Type	Inheritance	Phenotype	Gene	Mutations
IA	AR	Undetectable GH, anti-GH antibodies on treatment	*GH1*	Deletions (6.7kb-7.0kb-7.6kb-45 kb) Frameshift and nonsense mutations
IB	AR	Low detectable GH, no antibodies	*GH1, GHRHR*	Splice site, missense mutations
II	AD	Less severe short stature, variable phenotype	*GH1*	Splice site, splice site enhancers, missense mutations
III	X-linked	Agammaglobulinaemia/ hypogammaglobulinaemia	Not known; (?*SOX3*)	

AD, autosomal dominant; AR, autosomal recessive.

final height as an adult. The majority of these patients have large homozygous deletions within *GH1*, ranging from 6.7 to 45 kb. However, microdeletions leading to an altered reading frame, premature termination of translation, and a truncated protein have also been described.

Congenital isolated growth hormone deficiency type IB is also associated with a prenatal onset of growth hormone deficiency, but is milder than type IA, with detectable concentrations of growth hormone after provocation testing. It is also autosomal recessive and results from homozygous mutations in *GH1* or *GHRHR*. The first reported cases of *GHRHR* mutations were described in patients from the Indian subcontinent. Since then, a number of mutations have been reported, including missense, nonsense, and splice site mutations. Patients with mutations in *GHRHR* present with severe growth failure and proportionate dwarfism, but only minimal facial hypoplasia and no hypoglycaemia or microphallus. Pubertal delay has also been reported. They have low growth hormone, insulin-like growth factor 1 (IGF-1) and anterior pituitary hypoplasia on MRI.

Isolated growth hormone deficiency type II is inherited in an autosomal dominant manner. The patients present with short stature and respond well to exogenous human growth hormone (hGH) treatment with no formation of antibodies. Isolated growth hormone deficiency type II is most commonly the result of splice site mutations in intron 3 (IVS3) within the *GH1* gene, although missense mutations and mutations in the exon splice enhancer within exon 3 of the *GH1* have also been implicated in its aetiology. The phenotype associated with these mutations is highly variable and evolution of endocrinopathy over time has been described (58). In most cases, mutations result in aberrant splicing, skipping of exon 3, and generation of a 17.5 kDa molecule which lacks amino acids 32–71. This molecule has a dominant negative effect preventing secretion of normal wild-type 22 kDa GH with a consequent deleterious effect on pituitary somatotrophs. Analysis of different mutations identified in IGHD type II showed different mechanisms of secretory pathophysiology at a cellular level (59). This might be caused by differences in folding or aggregation, processes that are necessary for sorting, packaging, or secretion through the regulated secretory pathway. In addition, invasion by activated macrophages lead to significant bystander cell damage, which in time may compromise the other cell lineages. Treatment with recombinant hGH may suppress the growth hormone-releasing hormone drive and hence production of the mutant 17.5 kDa protein, although it is unclear whether the evolution of the phenotype can be prevented.

Isolated growth hormone deficiency type III is inherited as an X-linked disorder and in addition to growth hormone deficiency patients may also present with agammaglobulinaemia. In these cases no abnormalities have been documented within the *GH1* gene and the mechanism for the phenotype is unknown. Expansion of the PA tract within *SOX3* has been described in association with X-linked learning difficulties and growth hormone deficiency, as described earlier in this chapter.

Central hypothyroidism

Central hypothyroidism has a reported prevalence of 1:50 000 livebirths. It is a rare disorder characterized by insufficient TSH secretion resulting in low concentrations of thyroid hormones (60). Familial cases have been reported, although the condition may also be sporadic. The first homozygous nonsense mutation in exon 2 of the TSH-subunit gene has been reported in three children with congenital TSH-deficient hypothyroidism within two related Greek families. Inactivating mutations in the TRH receptor gene have also been described as a cause for isolated central hypothyroidism. Patients present with absence of TSH and prolactin responses to Thyrotropin-releasing hormone (TRH). Central hypothyroidism is generally milder than primary hypothyroidism and neonates may present with nonspecific symptoms such as lethargy, poor feeding, failure to thrive, prolonged hyperbilirubinaemia, and cold intolerance.

Isolated ACTH deficiency

Congenital isolated ACTH deficiency is rare and is more commonly associated with other pituitary hormone deficiencies. The clinical features are poorly defined and patients usually present in the neonatal period with nonspecific symptoms (poor feeding, failure to thrive, hypoglycaemia) or more acute signs of adrenal insufficiency (vascular collapse, shock). Abnormalities in salt excretion are unusual, as aldosterone secretion is largely controlled by the renin–angiotensin system.

Only a few cases of isolated ACTH deficiency have been reported to date; these can be due to mutations in *POMC* and *TBX19* (*T-PIT*). Patients with homozygous or compound heterozygous mutations in *POMC* present with early-onset isolated ACTH deficiency, obesity, and red hair due to the lack of MSH production (61). *TBX19* is located on chromosome 1q23-24, and encodes the transcription factor TPIT. Mutations in this gene are the principal molecular cause of congenital neonatal isolated ACTH deficiency. Recessive mutations result in severe ACTH deficiency, profound hypoglycemia associated with seizures and prolonged cholestatic jaundice (62). Neonatal deaths have been reported in up to 25% of families with *TBX19* mutations, suggesting that isolated ACTH deficiency may be an underestimated cause of neonatal death. Patients with *TBX19* mutations present with very low basal plasma

ACTH and cortisol levels, with no significant ACTH response to corticotropin-releasing hormone (63).

Mutations in *PC1* are rare and lead to ACTH deficiency in association with hypogonadotropic hypogonadism and a complex phenotype. A compound heterozygous mutation in *PC1* has been described in a female patient with extreme early-onset obesity and ACTH deficiency. In addition she presented with hypogonadotropic hypogonadism, defective processing of other prohormones and type 1 diabetes mellitus. *PC1* mutations were also reported in a child with isolated ACTH deficiency, red hair, and severe enteropathy.

Isolated gonadotrophin deficiency: hypogonadotropic hypogonadism

Isolated hypogonadotropic hypogonadism may be sporadic or inherited in an autosomal dominant, autosomal recessive, or X-linked manner. As the maturation and migration of GnRH and olfactory neurons are closely linked during development, it is not surprising that isolated hypogonadotropic hypogonadism may be associated with abnormal smell (anosmia/hyposmia).

Kallmann's syndrome

Kallmann's syndrome consists of the association between isolated hypogonadotropic hypogonadism and anosmia, with approximately 75% of patients demonstrating agenesis of the olfactory bulbs on neuroimaging. It is a clinically heterogeneous condition, with a reported prevalence of 1:10 000 in males and 1: 50 000 in females. Mutations in five genes (*KAL1*, *FGFR1*, *FGF8*, *PROKR2*, and *PROK2*) account for about 30% of cases of Kallmann's syndrome, indicating that other genes are also implicated in its aetiology (64). Mutations in *KAL1*are responsible for the X-linked form of Kallmann's syndrome. The gene is located on chromosome Xp22.3 and encodes the extracellular matrix glycoprotein anosmin-1, which has a role in the control of the migratory process of the GnRH neurons, although the molecular mechanisms of this action are not fully elucidated. In addition to isolated hypogonadotropic hypogonadism, patients with *KAL1* mutations may present with unilateral renal agenesis (30%), bimanual synkinesia (75%), sensorineural hearing loss, midline defects, and high arched palate (65).

Mutations in the receptor for fibroblast growth factor 1 (*FGFR1*) and in fibroblast growth factor 8 (*FGF8*) account for the autosomal dominant form of Kallmann's syndrome. To date, more than 40 mutations have been reported in *FGFR1* (10% of patients with Kallmann's syndrome) and six in *FGF8* (two of which are in association with *FGFR1* mutations). The phenotype of the autosomal dominant form of KS is characterized by variable penetrance. Mutations in *FGFR1* have been reported in association with complete absence of puberty, normal reproductive function, isolated anosmia or even normosmic isolated hypogonadotropic hypogonadism. Cleft lip and palate, agenesis of the corpus callosum, dental agenesis, skeletal abnormalities, and absent nasal cartilage may be associated features, whereas only two patients with bimanual synkinesia have been reported so far. Similarly, loss of function mutations in *FGF8* have been recently reported both in association with Kallmann's syndrome, normosmic hypogonadotropic hypogonadism, and variable degrees of GnRH deficiency. Their manifestation ranged from absent puberty to reproductive failure after completion of sexual maturation; cleft lip and palate, skeletal defects, and hearing loss have also been described in association with *FGF8* mutations (66). There is evidence from animal models that FGF signalling is important for the GnRH cell specification, migration, and survival; this requirement at multiple levels may account for the wide spectrum of clinical phenotypes.

In addition, homozygous, heterozygous, or compound heterozygous mutations in prokineticin2 (*PROK2*) and prokineticin-2 receptor (*PROKR2*) have recently been identified in patients with Kallmann's syndrome (MIM 612370) (9%). In animal models, *Prok2*$^{-/-}$ mice exhibit dysgenesis of the olfactory bulb, decreased numbers of GnRH neurons, and infertility. In addition, *in vitro* experiments have demonstrated that missense mutations have deleterious effect on prokineticin signalling. However, many mutations have also been found in apparently unaffected individuals, thus raising questions about their significance (67). The heterogeneity of Kallmann's syndrome does not allow for correlation between genotype and phenotype. However, it seems that patients with *KAL1* mutations have severe and permanent hypogonadotropic hypogonadism, whereas those with mutations in *FGFR1*, *FGF8*, *PROKR2*, and *PROK2* have greater variability.

Patients with Kallmann's syndrome (MIM 214800) may have features which are also part of CHARGE syndrome (deafness, dysmorphic ears, hypoplasia or aplasia of the semicircular canals). Conversely anosmia or hyposmia have been noted in cases of CHARGE. These observations prompted the screening of *CDH7* (chromodomain helicase DNA-binding protein-7), mutations of which have been identified in almost 70% of patients with CHARGE syndrome. So far heterozygous mutations in *CDH7* have been reported in a small number of patients with Kallmann's syndrome (three patients) or sporadic normosmic HH (four patients) (68). Animal studies have demonstrated high levels of *CDH7* expression in the olfactory placode and in a pattern consistent with its involvement in the migratory pathway of GnRH neurons. However, its role remains to be established.

Normosmic hypogonadotropic hypogonadism

Hypogonadotropic hypogonadism in association with normal olfaction has been reported in association with mutations in the GnRH receptor (*GnRHR*), GPR54/Kisspeptin, *LHβ*, and *FSHβ*. As mentioned before, mutations in *FGFR1* and *FGF8* have also been reported in association with normosmic hypogonadotropic hypogonadism. Mutations in *DAX-1* and leptin result in hypogonadotropic hypogonadism with a complex phenotype, whereas recently identified genes (*TAC3*, *TAC3R*) expand the spectrum of genetic changes in hypogonadotropic hypogonadism.

Approximately 20 homozygous or compound heterozygous mutations in *GnRHR* have been described. The gene, located on 4q13.2-2, encodes a 328 amino acid G-protein-coupled receptor. Mutations result in variable phenotypes that range from complete hypogonadism with undescended testes and presentation at birth to mild pubertal delay (65).

Hypogonadotropic hypogonadism may also result from mutations in the G-protein-coupled receptor *GPR54* and its endogenous ligands, kisspeptins. Kisspeptins are products of the *KiSS1* gene, derived after post-translational modification of kisspeptin-1.The longest of these peptides, kisspeptin-54, is also known as metastatin. GnRH neurons express Gpr54 and, in turn, KiSS1 expression has been detected in the arcuate and periventricular nuclei of the hypothalamus. Mice lacking GPR54 exhibit hypogonadism, but GnRH neurons migrate normally and have normal GnRH content. The role of Kiss1/GPR54 in the reproductive axis and pubertal timing is complex. Kisspeptins have a direct effect on GnRH neurons and their central administration results in GnRH release and LH secretion *in vivo*. In 2003, two independent groups reported deletions and inactivating mutations in *GPR54* in patients with HH. Since then, loss-of function mutations described in *GPR54* account for almost 5% of cases with normosmic HH. In these cases patients present with variable phenotypes that ranges from partial to severe hypogonadism (69). Recently, homozygous loss of function mutations in neurokinin-B (*TAC3*) and its receptor (*TACR3*) have been reported in eight patients from consanguineous families. They were in the second decade of life, or older, and demonstrated failure of pubertal progression. Neurokinin-B is expressed in hypothalamic neurons that also express kisspeptin; therefore, it is postulated that its function may affect the hypothalamic release of GnRH (70).

DAX1 (dosage-sensitive sex reversal, adrenal hypoplasia congenita critical region on the X chromosome) mutations in humans cause hypogonadotropic hypogonadism and adrenal hypoplasia congenita, which can result in severe neonatal adrenal crises. The condition is inherited as an X-linked disorder. *DAX1* is a transcription factor that is expressed in several tissues, including the hypothalamus and pituitary, and interacts with SF1. Duplications of *DAX1* result in persistent müllerian structures and XY sex reversal suggesting that the gene acts in a dosage-sensitive manner (71).

Leptin is secreted from adipocytes and, apart from its role in regulating nutrition, it appears to play an important role in several neuroendocrine functions by acting at a hypothalamic level. Congenital leptin deficiency, secondary to mutations in leptin or its receptor, are associated with obesity, marked hyperphagia, metabolic abnormalities, and hypogonadotropic hypogonadism (72). There is evidence that treatment with leptin results in significant weight loss and normalization of nocturnal luteinizing hormone secretion.

Central diabetes insipidus

Central diabetes insipidus is commonly due to acquired disorders. Congenital central diabetes insipidus is rare and it may be a feature of midline disorders (septo-optic dysplasia, HSE) or due to mutations in genes involved in the secretion of arginine vasopressin (AVP). A number of mutations have been described in the gene that encodes the AVP preprohormone, *prepro-AVP-NPII* (arginine vasopressin-neurophysin II), resulting in autosomal dominant diabetes insipidus (73). The gene is located on chromosome 20 and consists of three exons. Exon 1 encodes the signal peptide of the preprohormone and AVP, exon 3 encodes the glycoprotein copeptin, whereas the carrier protein NPII is encoded by all three exons. In this rare familial disorder of AVP secretion, patients present usually in the first 10 years of life, whilst neonatal manifestations are uncommon. This suggests that the pathophysiology of familial central diabetes insipidus involves progressive postnatal degeneration of AVP-producing magnocellular neurons. More than 50 different mutations have been identified so far, mainly affecting amino acid residues important for the proper folding and/or dimerization of the NP moiety of the AVP pro-hormone. The proposed mechanism is that the mutant allele exerts a dominant negative effect; the misfolded mutant hormone precursor is accumulated in the endoplasmic reticulum resulting in progressive toxic damage of the vasopressin neurons and the clinical manifestation of diabetes insipidus.

Central diabetes insipidus is also a feature of Wolfram's syndrome, a rare recessive disorder characterised by diabetes mellitus, diabetes insipidus, optic atrophy, sensorineural hearing loss, and progressive neurodegeneration. The gene, *WFS1*, is located on 4p16.1 and encodes wolframin. The protein is localized in the endoplasmic reticulum and is a component of the 'misfolded protein/stress response' machinery. In the brain, WFS1 expression has been detected in selected neurons in the hippocampus, amygdala, and olfactory tubercle.

Conclusion

Pituitary development depends on complex regulatory networks and the sequential expression of transcription factors and signalling molecules in a space- and time-specific manner. An ever-increasing number of genes are implicated in this process. Spontaneous or artificially induced mutations in the mouse and identification of mutations associated with human pituitary disease contribute to defining the genetic cascades responsible for pituitary development.

References

1. Sheng HZ, Westphal H. Early steps in pituitary organogenesis. *Trends Genet*, 1999; **15**: 236–40.
2. Rizzoti K, Lovell-Badge R. Early development of the pituitary gland: induction and shaping of Rathke's pouch. *Rev Endocr Metab Disord*, 2005; **6**: 161–72.
3. Zhu X, Gleiberman AS, Rosenfeld MG. Molecular physiology of pituitary development: signaling and transcriptional networks. *Physiol Rev*, 2007; **87**: 933–63.
4. Dasen JS, Rosenfeld MG. Signaling and transcriptional mechanisms in pituitary development. *Annu Rev Neurosci*, 2001; **24**:327–55.
5. Takuma N, Sheng HZ, Furuta Y, Ward JM, Sharma K, Hogan BL, *et al.* Formation of Rathke's pouch requires dual induction from the diencephalon. *Development*, 1998; **125**: 4835–40.
6. Treier M, O'Connell S, Gleiberman A, Price J, Szeto DP, Burgess R, *et al.* Hedgehog signaling is required for pituitary gland development. *Development*, 2001; **128**: 377–86.
7. Zhu X, Zhang J, Tollkuhn J, Ohsawa R, Bresnick EH, Guillemot F, *et al.* Sustained Notch signaling in progenitors is required for sequential emergence of distinct cell lineages during organogenesis. *Genes Dev*, 2006; **20**: 2739–53.
8. Mullen RD, Colvin SC, Hunter CS, Savage JJ, Walvoord EC, Bhangoo AP, *et al.* Roles of the LHX3 and LHX4 LIM-homeodomain factors in pituitary development. *Mol Cell Endocrinol*, 2007; **265–266**:190–5.
9. Hume CR, Bratt DL, Oesterle EC. Expression of LHX3 and SOX2 during mouse inner ear development. *Gene Expr Patterns*, 2007; **7**: 798–807.
10. Raetzman LT, Ward R, Camper SA. Lhx4 and Prop1 are required for cell survival and expansion of the pituitary primordia. *Development*, 2002; **129**: 4229–39.
11. Ellsworth BS, Butts DL, Camper SA. Mechanisms underlying pituitary hypoplasia and failed cell specification in Lhx3-deficient mice. *Dev Biol*, 2008; **313**: 118–29.
12. Dasen JS, Barbera JP, Herman TS, Connell SO, Olson L, Ju B, *et al.* Temporal regulation of a paired-like homeodomain repressor/TLE corepressor complex and a related activator is required for pituitary organogenesis. *Genes Dev*, 2001; **15**: 3193–207.
13. Olson LE, Tollkuhn J, Scafoglio C, Krones A, Zhang J, Ohgi KA, *et al.* Homeodomain-mediated beta-catenin-dependent switching events dictate cell-lineage determination. *Cell*, 2006; **125**: 593–605.
14. Dattani MT, Martinez-Barbera JP, Thomas PQ, Brickman JM, Gupta R, Martensson IL, *et al.* Mutations in the homeobox gene HESX1/Hesx1

associated with septo-optic dysplasia in human and mouse. *Nat Genet*, 1998; **19**: 125–33.
15. Pevny LH, Placzek M. SOX genes and neural progenitor identity. *Curr Opin Neurobiol*, 2005; **15**: 7–13.
16. Lefebvre V, Dumitriu B, Penzo-Mendez A, Han Y, Pallavi B. Control of cell fate and differentiation by Sry-related high-mobility-group box (Sox) transcription factors. *Int J Biochem Cell Biol*, 2007; **39**: 2195–214.
17. Rizzoti K, Brunelli S, Carmignac D, Thomas PQ, Robinson IC, Lovell-Badge R. SOX3 is required during the formation of the hypothalamo-pituitary axis. *Nat Genet*, 2004; **36**: 247–55.
18. Taranova OV, Magness ST, Fagan BM, Wu Y, Surzenko N, Hutton SR, *et al.* SOX2 is a dose-dependent regulator of retinal neural progenitor competence. *Genes Dev*, 2006; **20**: 1187–202.
19. Kelberman D, de Castro SC, Huang S, Crolla JA, Palmer R, Gregory JW, *et al.* SOX2 plays a critical role in the pituitary, forebrain, and eye during human embryonic development. *J Clin Endocrinol Metab*, 2008; **93**: 1865–73.
20. Scully KM, Rosenfeld MG. Pituitary development: regulatory codes in mammalian organogenesis. *Science*, 2002; **295**: 2231–5.
21. Zhu X, Wang J, Ju BG, Rosenfeld MG. Signaling and epigenetic regulation of pituitary development. *Curr Opin Cell Biol*, 2007; **19**: 605–11.
22. Ward RD, Raetzman LT, Suh H, Stone BM, Nasonkin IO, Camper SA. Role of PROP1 in pituitary gland growth. *Mol Endocrinol*, 2005; **19**: 698–710.
23. Andersen B, Rosenfeld MG. POU domain factors in the neuroendocrine system: lessons from developmental biology provide insights into human disease. *Endocr Rev*, 2001; **22**: 2–35.
24. Kelberman D, Dattani MT. The role of transcription factors implicated in anterior pituitary development in the aetiology of congenital hypopituitarism. *Ann Med*, 2006; **38**: 560–77.
25. Charles MA, Saunders TL, Wood WM, Owens K, Parlow AF, Camper SA, *et al.* Pituitary-specific Gata2 knockout: effects on gonadotrope and thyrotrope function. *Mol Endocrinol*, 2006; **20**: 1366–77.
26. Zhao L, Bakke M, Parker KL. Pituitary-specific knockout of steroidogenic factor 1. *Mol Cell Endocrinol*, 2001; **185**: 27–32.
27. Tobet SA, Schwarting GA. Minireview: recent progress in gonadotropin-releasing hormone neuronal migration. *Endocrinology*, 2006; **147**: 1159–65.
28. Liu J, Lin C, Gleiberman A, Ohgi KA, Herman T, Huang HP, *et al.* Tbx19, a tissue-selective regulator of POMC gene expression. *Proc Natl Acad Sci U S A*, 2001; **98**: 8674–9.
29. Pulichino AM, Vallette-Kasic S, Couture C, Gauthier Y, Brue T, David M, *et al.* Human and mouse TPIT gene mutations cause early onset pituitary ACTH deficiency. *Genes Dev*, 2003; **17**: 711–16.
30. Kelberman D, Dattani MT. Hypopituitarism oddities: congenital causes. *Horm Res*, 2007; **68** (Suppl 5): 138–44.
31. Dattani MT. Novel insights into the aetiology and pathogenesis of hypopituitarism. *Horm Res*, 2004; **62** (Suppl 3): 1–13.
32. Turton JP, Mehta A, Raza J, Woods KS, Tiulpakov A, Cassar J, *et al.* Mutations within the transcription factor PROP1 are rare in a cohort of patients with sporadic combined pituitary hormone deficiency (CPHD). *Clin Endocrinol (Oxf)*, 2005; **63**: 10–18.
33. Wu W, Cogan JD, Pfaffle RW, Dasen JS, Frisch H, O'Connell SM, *et al.* Mutations in PROP1 cause familial combined pituitary hormone deficiency. *Nat Genet*, 1998; **18**: 147–9.
34. Vallette-Kasic S, Barlier A, Teinturier C, Diaz A, Manavela M, Berthezene F, *et al.* PROP1 gene screening in patients with multiple pituitary hormone deficiency reveals two sites of hypermutability and a high incidence of corticotroph deficiency. *J Clin Endocrinol Metab*, 2001; **86**: 4529–35.
35. Bottner A, Keller E, Kratzsch J, Stobbe H, Weigel JF, Keller A, *et al.* PROP1 Mutations Cause Progressive Deterioration of Anterior Pituitary Function including Adrenal Insufficiency: A Longitudinal Analysis. *J Clin Endocrinol Metab*, 2004; **89**: 5256–65.
36. Reynaud R, Gueydan M, Saveanu A, Vallette-Kasic S, Enjalbert A, Brue T, *et al.* Genetic screening of combined pituitary hormone deficiency: experience in 195 patients. *J Clin Endocrinol Metab*, 2006; **91**: 3329–36.
37. Voutetakis A, Argyropoulou M, Sertedaki A, Livadas S, Xekouki P, Maniati-Christidi M, *et al.* Pituitary magnetic resonance imaging in 15 patients with Prop1 gene mutations: pituitary enlargement may originate from the intermediate lobe. *J Clin Endocrinol Metab*, 2004; **89**: 2200–6.
38. Turton JPG, Reynaud R, Mehta A, Torpiano J, Saveanu A, Woods KS, *et al.* Novel mutations within the POU1F1 gene associated with variable combined pituitary hormone deficiency. *J Clin Endocrinol Metab*, 2005; **90**: 4762–70.
39. Cohen LE, Radovick S. Molecular basis of combined pituitary hormone deficiencies. *Endocr Rev*, 2002; **23**: 431–42.
40. Netchine I, Sobrier ML, Krude H, Schnabel D, Maghnie M, Marcos E, *et al.* Mutations in LHX3 result in a new syndrome revealed by combined pituitary hormone deficiency. *Nat Genet*, 2000; **25**: 182–6.
41. Pfaeffle RW, Savage JJ, Hunter CS, Palme C, Ahlmann M, Kumar P, *et al.* Four novel mutations of the LHX3 gene cause combined pituitary hormone deficiencies with or without limited neck rotation. *J Clin Endocrinol Metab*, 2007; **92**: 1909–19.
42. Rajab A, Kelberman D, de Castro SC, Biebermann H, Shaikh H, Pearce K, *et al.* Novel mutations in LHX3 are associated with hypopituitarism and sensorineural hearing loss. *Hum Mol Genet*, 2008; **17**: 2150–9.
43. Machinis K, Pantel J, Netchine I, Leger J, Camand OJ, Sobrier ML, *et al.* Syndromic short stature in patients with a germline mutation in the LIM homeobox LHX4. *Am J Hum Genet*, 2001; **69**: 961–8.
44. Pfaeffle RW, Hunter CS, Savage JJ, Duran-Prado M, Mullen RD, Neeb ZP, *et al.* Three novel missense mutations within the LHX4 gene are associated with variable pituitary hormone deficiencies. *J Clin Endocrinol Metab*, 2008; **93**: 1062–71.
45. Tajima T, Hattori T, Nakajima T, Okuhara K, Tsubaki J, Fujieda K. A novel missense mutation (P366T) of the LHX4 gene causes severe combined pituitary hormone deficiency with pituitary hypoplasia, ectopic posterior lobe and a poorly developed sella turcica. *Endocr J*, 2007; **54**: 637–41.
46. Kelberman D, Dattani MT. Septo-Optic Dysplasia - Novel Insights into the Aetiology. *Horm Res*, 2008; **69**: 257–65.
47. McNay DE, Turton JP, Kelberman D, Woods KS, Brauner R, Papadimitriou A, *et al.* HESX1 mutations are an uncommon cause of septooptic dysplasia and hypopituitarism. *J Clin Endocrinol Metab*, 2007; **92**: 691–7.
48. Williamson KA, Hver AM, Rainger J, Rogers RC, Magee A, Fiedler Z, *et al.* Mutations in SOX2 cause anophthalmia-esophageal-genital (AEG) syndrome. *Hum Mol Genet*, 2006; **15**: 1413–22.
49. Kelberman D, Rizzoti K, Avilio A, bitner-Glindzicz M, Cianfarani S, Collins J, *et al.* Mutations within Sox2/SOX2 are associated with abnormalities in the hypothalamo-pituitary-gonadal axis in mice and humans. *J Clin Invest*, 2006; **116**: 2442–5.
50. Solomon NM, Ross SA, Morgan T, Belsky JL, Hol FA, Karnes PS, *et al.* Array comparative genomic hybridisation analysis of boys with X linked hypopituitarism identifies a 3.9 Mb duplicated critical region at Xq27 containing SOX3. *J Med Genet*, 2004; **41**: 669–78.
51. Laumonnier F, Ronce N, Hamel BC, Thomas P, Lespinasse J, Raynaud M, *et al.* Transcription factor SOX3 is involved in X-linked mental retardation with growth hormone deficiency. *Am J Hum Genet*, 2002; **71**: 1450–5.
52. Woods KS, Cundall M, Turton J, Rizzoti K, Mehta A, Palmer R, *et al.* Over- and underdosage of SOX3 is associated with infundibular hypoplasia and hypopituitarism. *Am J Hum Genet*, 2005; **76**: 833–49.
53. Fernandes M, Hebert JM. The ups and downs of holoprosencephaly: dorsal versus ventral patterning forces. *Clin Genet*, 2008; **73**: 413–23.
54. Roessler E, Du YZ, Mullor JL, Casas E, Allen WP, Gillessen-Kaesbach G, *et al.* Loss-of-function mutations in the human GLI2 gene are

associated with pituitary anomalies and holoprosencephaly-like features. *Proc Natl Acad Sci U S A*, 2003; **100**: 13424–9.
55. Tajima T, Ohtake A, Hoshino M, Amemiya S, Sasaki N, Ishizu K, *et al.* OTX2 Loss of Function Mutation Causes Anophthalmia and Combined Pituitary Hormone Deficiency with a Small Anterior and Ectopic Posterior Pituitary. *J Clin Endocrinol Metab*, 2009; **94**: 314–19.
56. Lin CR, Kioussi C, O'Connell S, Briata P, Szeto D, Liu F, *et al.* Pitx2 regulates lung asymmetry, cardiac positioning and pituitary and tooth morphogenesis. *Nature*, 1999; **401**: 279–82.
57. Mullis PE. Genetic control of growth. *Eur J Endocrinol*, 2005; **152**: 11–31.
58. Mullis PE, Robinson IC, Salemi S, Eble A, Besson A, Vuissoz JM, *et al.* Isolated autosomal dominant growth hormone deficiency: an evolving pituitary deficit? A multicenter follow-up study. *J Clin Endocrinol Metab*, 2005; **90**: 2089–96.
59. McGuinness L, Magoulas C, Sesay AK, Mathers K, Carmignac D, Manneville JB, *et al.* Autosomal dominant growth hormone deficiency disrupts secretory vesicles in vitro and in vivo in transgenic mice. *Endocrinology*, 2003; **144**: 720–31.
60. Yamada M, Mori M. Mechanisms related to the pathophysiology and management of central hypothyroidism. *Nat Clin Pract Endocrinol Metab*, 2008; **4**: 683–94.
61. Krude H, Biebermann H, Luck W, Horn R, Brabant G, Gruters A. Severe early-onset obesity, adrenal insufficiency and red hair pigmentation caused by POMC mutations in humans. *Nat Genet*, 1998; **19**: 155–7.
62. Metherell LA, Savage MO, Dattani M, Walker J, Clayton PE, Farooqi IS, *et al.* TPIT mutations are associated with early-onset, but not late-onset isolated ACTH deficiency. *Eur J Endocrinol*, 2004; **151**: 463–5.
63. Asteria C. T-box and isolated ACTH deficiency. *Eur J Endocrinol*, 2002; **146**: 463–5.
64. Hardelin JP, Dode C. The complex genetics of Kallmann syndrome: KAL1, FGFR1, FGF8, PROKR2, PROK2, *et al. Sex Dev*, 2008; **2**: 181–93.
65. Trarbach EB, Silveira LG, Latronico AC. Genetic insights into human isolated gonadotropin deficiency. *Pituitary*, 2007; **10**: 381–91.
66. Falardeau J, Chung WC, Beenken A, Raivio T, Plummer L, Sidis Y, *et al.* Decreased FGF8 signaling causes deficiency of gonadotropin-releasing hormone in humans and mice. *J Clin Invest*, 2008; **118**: 2822–31.
67. Cole LW, Sidis Y, Zhang C, Quinton R, Plummer L, Pignatelli D, *et al.* Mutations in prokineticin 2 and prokineticin receptor 2 genes in human gonadotrophin-releasing hormone deficiency: molecular genetics and clinical spectrum. *J Clin Endocrinol Metab*, 2008; **93**: 3551–9.
68. Kim HG, Kurth I, Lan F, Meliciani I, Wenzel W, Eom SH, *et al.* Mutations in CHD7, encoding a chromatin-remodeling protein, cause idiopathic hypogonadotropic hypogonadism and Kallmann syndrome. *Am J Hum Genet*, 2008; **83**: 511–19.
69. Seminara SB, Messager S, Chatzidaki EE, Thresher RR, Acierno JS, Jr., Shagoury JK, *et al.* The GPR54 gene as a regulator of puberty. *N Engl J Med*, 2003; **349**: 1614–27.
70. Topaloglu AK, Reimann F, Guclu M, Yalin AS, Kotan LD, Porter KM, *et al.* TAC3 and TACR3 mutations in familial hypogonadotropic hypogonadism reveal a key role for Neurokinin B in the central control of reproduction. *Nat Genet*, 2008; **41**: 354–8.
71. Achermann JC, Gu WX, Kotlar TJ, Meeks JJ, Sabacan LP, Seminara SB, *et al.* Mutational analysis of DAX1 in patients with hypogonadotropic hypogonadism or pubertal delay. *J Clin Endocrinol Metab*, 1999; **84**: 4497–500.
72. Farooqi IS, O'Rahilly S. Mutations in ligands and receptors of the leptin-melanocortin pathway that lead to obesity. *Nat Clin Pract Endocrinol Metab*, 2008; **4**: 569–77.
73. Davies JH, Penney M, Abbes AP, Engel H, Gregory JW. Clinical features, diagnosis and molecular studies of familial central diabetes insipidus. *Horm Res* 2005; **64**:231–7.

2.3.2 Molecular pathogenesis of pituitary tumours

Ines Donangelo, Shlomo Melmed

Introduction

Pituitary adenomas are discovered in up to 25% of unselected autopsies, however, clinically apparent tumours are considerably less common. The pituitary gland is composed of differentiated cell types: somatotrophs, lactotrophs, corticotrophs, thyrotrophs, and gonadotrophs. Tumours may arise from any of these cell types and their secretory products depend on the cell of origin. The functional classification of pituitary tumorus is based on identification of cell gene products by immunostaining or mRNA detection, as well as measurement of circulating tumour and target organ hormone levels. Oversecretion of adrenocorticotropic hormone (ACTH) results in cortisol excess with Cushing's disease. Growth hormone overproduction leads to acromegaly with typical acral overgrowth and metabolic abnormalities. Prolactin hypersecretion results in hypogonadism and galactorrhoea. Rarely, thyroid-stimulating hormone (TSH) hypersecretion leads to goitre and thyrotoxicosis, and gonadotropin excess results in gonadal dysfunction (1). Mixed tumours cosecreting growth hormone with prolactin, TSH, or ACTH may also arise from single cells. Clinically nonfunctional tumours are those that do not efficiently secrete their gene products, and most commonly they are derived from gonadotroph cells. Pituitary tumours are further defined radiographically as microadenomas (<1 cm in diameter) or macroadenomas (>1 cm in diameter). However, this classification does not reflect whether the pituitary tumour is amenable to total resection and limits assessment of invasive progression during serial imaging. Therefore, it is useful to apply the classification proposed by Hardy in 1973 and modified by Wilson in 1990 (Table 2.3.2.1), whereby pituitary tumours are classified into one of five grades and one of six stages, providing important preoperative information.

Table 2.3.2.1 Anatomic (radiographic and operative) classification of pituitary adenomas

Extension (stage)	Site of adenoma (grade)
Suprasellar extension	*Floor of sella intact*
0: None	I: Sella normal or focally expanded; tumour <10 mm
A: Occupies cistern	II: Sella enlarged; tumour ≥10 mm
B: Recesses of third ventricle obliterated	*Sphenoid*
C: Third ventricle grossly displaced	III: Localized perforation of sellar floor
Parasellar extension	IV: Diffuse destruction of sellar floor
D: Intracranial (intradural)	Distant spread
E: Into and beneath cavernous sinus (extradural)	V: Spread via cerebrospinal fluid or bloodborne

Adapted from Wilson CB Role of surgery in the management of pituitary tumors. *Neurosurg Clin North Am*,1990; **1**: 139–59 (2)

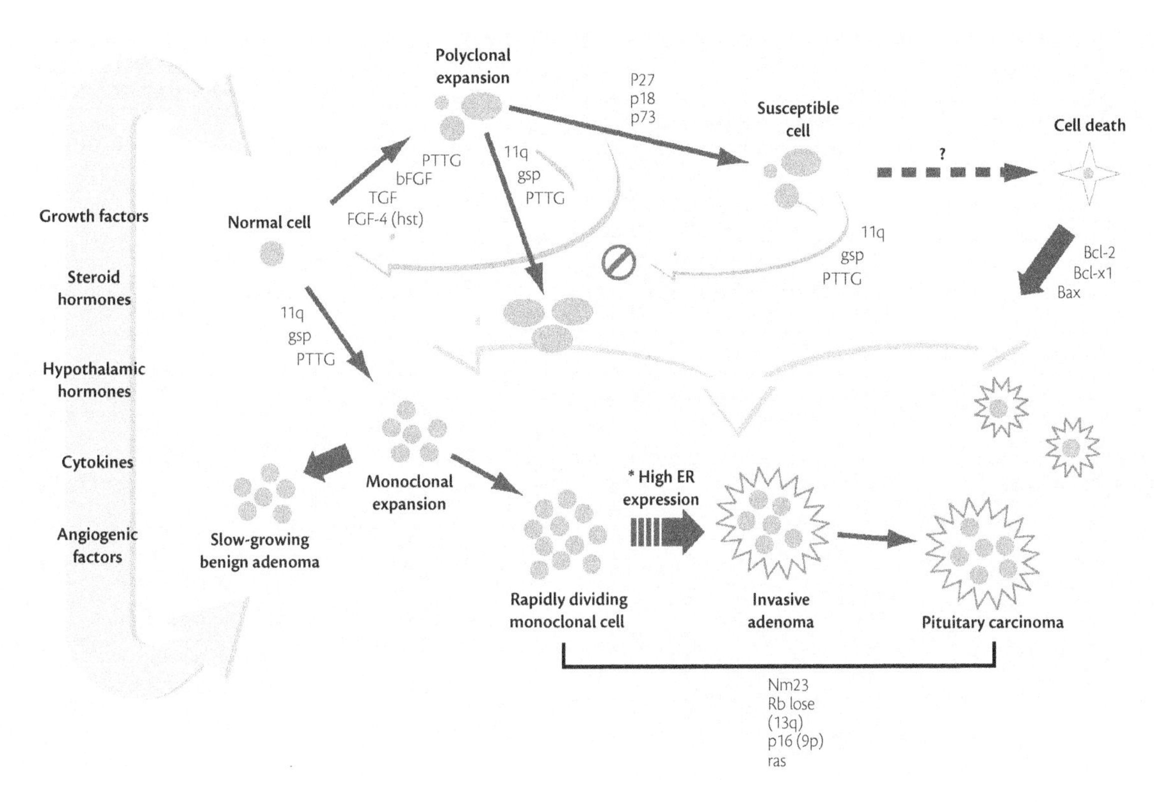

Fig. 2.3.2.1 Model of pituitary tumorigenesis. Cells responding to endocrine or paracrine stimuli (green) may expand in a polyclonal manner (top sequence). As a consequence of increased proliferation, their susceptibility to acquire activating mutations (red) or loss of inactivating mutations (blue) is increased prompting the emergence of a rapidly expanding monoclonal cell population (downward-shaded arrows). At some point in the polyclonal cell expansion, cells susceptible to acquiring the 'hit' develop, which will foster emergence of the monoclonal population (susceptible cell). Alternatively, a normal cell may acquire sufficient activating mutations or loss of inactivating events to prompt a rapidly expanding monoclonal cell population from onset (lower sequence). Following additional genetic events, this monoclonal expansion may evolve into an invasive pituitary tumour, with further events promoting the progression to metastatic pituitary carcinoma. The progress of both these pathways will be driven by a variety of hormonal stimuli, growth, and angiogenic factors, and altered receptor expression (blue shading).

Pituitary tumours cause morbidity by both abnormal hormone secretion as well as compression of regional structures. As a considerable proportion of patients do not achieve optimal therapeutic control of mass effects and/or hormone hypersecretion despite advances in therapeutic approaches, understanding pathogenesis and pituitary tumour growth patterns in individual patients will enable identification of subcellular treatment targets, ultimately decreasing tumour-related morbidity and mortality.

Determinants of initiation and progression of pituitary adenomas are not fully understood. This chapter describes a spectrum of mechanisms implicated in pituitary tumorigenesis, including the role of pituitary plasticity, imbalances in cell cycle regulation, transcription factors, signalling pathways, and angiogenesis (Fig. 2.3.2.1). Molecular events related to tumorigenesis in human pituitary adenoma subtypes are summarized in Table 2.3.2.2. The causal role for selected genetic imbalances leading to development of pituitary tumours has been confirmed in several transgenic mouse models (Table 2.3.2.3).

Pituitary plasticity

Although commitment of pituitary cell function is under cell-specific transcriptional control, resulting in differentiated mature cell types (Fig. 2.3.2.2), the pituitary gland responds to central and peripheral signals that regulate plastic pituitary cell hormone production and proliferation. Under physiological conditions, hypothalamic and peripheral hormones act in concert to regulate pituitary trophic activity. Age (puberty) and pregnancy/lactation results in increased pituitary volume, and prolonged target gland failure (e.g. hypothyroidism) and oestrogen excess are recognized causes of pituitary hyperplasia. However, there is no direct evidence in humans that pituitary hyperplasia is a necessary prerequisite for pituitary tumour development. Hyperplastic proliferation of prolactin-secreting cells during pregnancy and lactation does not increase the frequency of prolactinomas, and untreated primary hypothyroidism and exogenous oestrogen administration are infrequently associated with adenoma development. Pituitary hyperplasia caused by ectopic tumour production of growth hormone-releasing hormone (GHRH) (2) is very rarely associated with discrete adenoma formation. In general, adenohypophyseal tissue surrounding pituitary tumours is normal, supporting the notion that multiple independent cellular events such as generalized hyperplasia do not necessarily precede adenoma formation. Excess pituitary hormone secretion is usually associated with invariably benign monoclonal adenomas arising from a specific cell type supporting intrinsic pituitary defect in the process of tumour development (Box 2.3.2.1).

Hypothalamic hormones, local growth factors, and circulating sex steroid hormones are likely implicated in enabling a permissive environment which potentiates cell mutation and subsequent tumour growth. Although pituitary trophic stimuli do not frequently originate tumours in humans, they may influence the

Table 2.3.2.2 Selected molecular events related to tumorigenesis in human pituitary adenoma subtypes.

	Tumour type	Mechanism of activation/ inactivation
Activating		
Gsp	GH adenomas	Activating mutation
CREB	GH adenomas	Increased Ser-phosphorylated CREB promoted by gsp overexpression
Cyclin B2 (*CCNB2*)	All tumour types examined	Overexpression
Cyclin D1 (*CCND1*)	Nonfunctioning	Overexpression
EGF/EGFR	Nonfunctioning	Overexpression
PTTG	All tumour types examined	Overexpression
Gal-3	Prolactinomas ACTH adenomas	Overexpression
HMGA2	Nonfunctioning ACTH adenomas Prolactinomas	Overexpression
FGF-4	Prolactinomas	Overexpression
Inactivating		
RB1	Negative pRB in ~25% GH adenomas	Promoter methylation
13q14	Aggressive tumours	13q14 loss of heterozygosity
AIP	15% of FIPA 2% sporadic GH adenomas	Inactivating mutation
MEN1	Prolactinomas in familial MEN 1	Inactivating mutation
P16INK4a (*CDKN2A*)	All tumour types examined	Promoter methylation
P27KIP1 (*CDKN1B*)	All tumour types examined	Reduced expression
MEG3a	Nonfunctioning GH adenomas	Promoter methylation
Gadd45-γ	Nonfunctioning GH adenomas Prolactinomas	Promoter methylation

ACTH, adrenocorticotropic hormone; FIPA, familial isolated pituitary adenomas; GH, growth hormone; MEN, multiple endocrine neoplasia.

intra-pituitary milieu to either enhance or attenuate expansion of a monoclonal tumour cell population (3).

Because *PTTG* abundance correlates with pituitary gland trophic status, regulation of this gene may subserve a mechanism for affecting tumour formation (Fig. 2.3.2.3). *PTTG*, identified as the index mammalian securin, regulates sister chromatid separation during mitosis (4). PTTG function is discussed below. Mice with pituitary directed transgenic human *PTTG1* expression driven by the α-subunit glycoprotein (αGSU) promoter develop plurihormonal pituitary hyperplasia with small microadenomas. In contrast, global *Pttg* inactivation results in hypotrophic effects, i.e. pituitary, pancreatic β cell, splenic, and testicular hypoplasia. *Pttg* inactivation in $Rb^{+/-}$ also protects mice from pituitary tumour development, and combined $Rb^{+/-}$ and targeted pituitary *PTTG*

Table 2.3.2.3 Transgenic mouse models for pituitary tumours

	Hyperplasia/Adenoma[b]
Gene overexpression[a]	
CMV.*HMGA1*	GH, PRL
CMV.*HMGA2*	GH, PRL
Ubiquitin C.*hCG*	PRL
αGSU.*bLH*	Pit1 Lineage
GH.*galanin*	GH, PRL
PRL.*galanin*	PRL[c]
PRL.*TGFα*	PRL
αGSU.*PTTG1*	LH, GH, TSH
αGSU.*Prop1*	Nonfunctioning
PRL.*pdt-FGFR4*	PRL
Gene inactivation	
p27/Ki p1$^{-/-}$	ACTH, αMSH
p18/INK4c$^{-/-}$	ACTH, αMSH
Rb$^{+/-}$	ACTH, αMSH αGSU, GH, βTSH
D2R-deficient	PRL
Men1$^{+/-}$	PRL
PRL$^{-/-}$	Nonfunctioning

[a] Genes are listed in italics, and are preceded by the promoter that determines transcriptional control.
[b] Hormone immunoreactivity/secreting profile.
[c] Pituitary hyperplasia, with no tumour formation.
CMV, cytomegalovirus; HMGA, high mobility group A; Men1: multiple endocrine neoplasia type 1; pdt-FGFR4, pituitary tumour-derived fibroblast growth factor receptor 4; PRL, prolactin; PTTG, pituitary transforming gene; TGF, transforming growth factor.
From Donangelo I, Melmed S Molecular pathogenesis of pituitary tumors. In: Hay I, Turner H, Wass J, eds. *Clinical Endocrine Oncology*. 2nd edn. Blackwell Publishing: Massachusetts, 2008: 187–93 (3), with permission.

overexpression further enhances pituitary hyperplasia and tumour prevalence (5). Mechanisms underlying pituitary plasticity therefore provide insight for disrupting development and progression of pituitary tumours.

Cell cycle regulation

Retinoblastoma susceptibility gene (*Rb1, OMIN 180200*)

The protein encoded by this gene (pRB) is a negative regulator of the cell cycle and behaves as tumour suppressor. In its active, hypophosphorylated form pRB binds the E2F transcription factors, restraining cell cycle progression from the G1 to S phase. Mice with homozygous loss of *Rb1* are nonviable, however, those with heterozygous *Rb1* inactivation develop pituitary tumours with high penetrance, and less frequently thyroid medullary carcinoma, and phaeochromocytoma. Interestingly, mice with deregulated intermediate lobe E2F activity develop tissue hyperplasia that does not progress to tumour formation, likely because sustained E2F activity ultimately triggers premature senescence in a pRB, p16, and p19-dependent manner (6).

Individuals who inherit a defective copy of *RB1* gene are at high risk for developing retinoblastoma at an early age, however, interestingly these patients do not exhibit a predisposition to

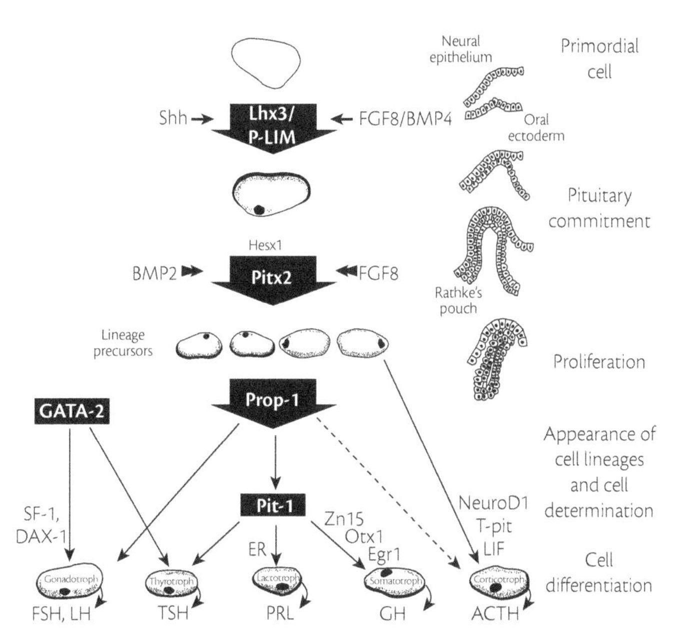

Fig. 2.3.2.2 Model for development of human anterior pituitary cell lineage determination by a temporally controlled cascade of transcription factors. Trophic cells are depicted with transcription factors known to determine cell-specific human or murine gene expression. (From Melmed S Mechanisms for pituitary tumorigenesis: the plastic pituitary. *J Clin Invest*, 2003; **112**: 1603–18 (1), with permission.)

development of pituitary adenomas. Aggressive human pituitary tumours and rarely encountered metastasis exhibit loss of heterozygosity of region 13q14 (*RB1* locus), however pRB usually remains expressed suggesting that a tumour suppressor gene other than *RB1* present in the same chromosomal region may be related to pituitary tumour progression. Studies based on immunodetection in tumour sections found normal expression of pRB in most nonfunctioning pituitary adenomas, however approximately 25% of Growth hormone-secreting adenomas exhibit loss of pRB expression, and this finding did not correlate with tumour behaviour. In some cases decreased *RB1* expression correlated with its promoter hypermethylation (7). Therefore, *RB1* inactivation may be involved in human pituitary tumour development in a small subset of adenomas.

INK4 family

Cell cycle is regulated by two families of CDK inhibitors (CKIs), the INKA4 family and the Cip/Kip family. The INK4 family (p16INK4a

Box 2.3.2.1 Evidence for an intrinsic pituitary defect in the pathogenesis of pituitary tumours

- Pituitary adenomas are monoclonal
- Absence of pituitary hyperplasia in tissue surrounding pituitary adenomas
- Surgical resection of well-circumscribed pituitary adenomas controls >75% of patients
- Adenoma formation is rarely associated with generalized pituitary hyperplasia
- Unrestrained pituitary hormonal hypersecretion occurs independently of physiological hypothalamic feedback regulation
- Normalization of hormonal pulsatility pattern often occurs after adenoma resection

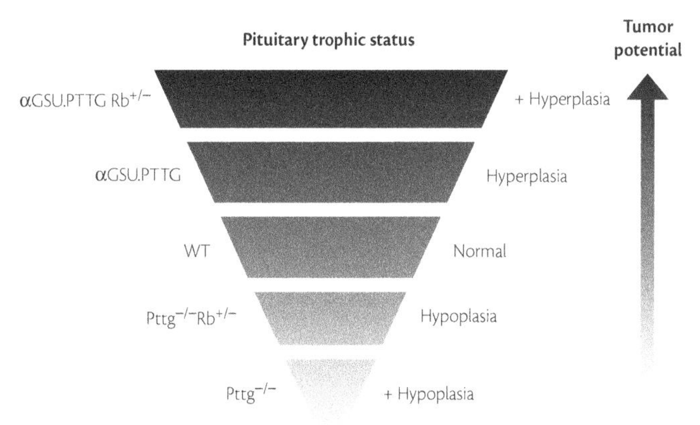

Fig. 2.3.2.3 Pituitary *PTTG* content correlates with gland plasticity and with tumour formation potential. On the left side of the inverted triangle are listed mouse models with descending pituitary *PTTG* content, with or without the combination with tumorigenic $Rb^{+/-}$. Horizontal bars composing the inverted triangle represent the observed effects of the different genotypes on pituitary trophic status, which correlates with pituitary tumorigenic potential (arrow). (From Donangelo I, Gutman S, Horvath E, Kovacs K, Wawrowsky K, Mount M, *et al*. Pituitary tumor transforming gene overexpression facilitates pituitary tumor development. *Endocrinology*, 2006; **147**: 4781–91 (6), with permission.)

OMIN 600160, p15INK4b OMIN 600431, and p18INK4c OMIN 603369) inhibit G1/S progression by binding CDK4 and CDK6.

The protein p16INK4a, encoded by the *CDKN2A* gene on chromosome 9p21, maintains pRB unphosphorylated (active) by blocking CDK4. p16INK4a is not synthesized due to promoter hypermethylation in most nonfunctioning pituitary tumours and in a smaller subset of other pituitary tumour subtypes. Loss of p16INK4a and pRB in tumours tend to be mutually exclusive, probably because functional pRB is required for cell cycle inhibition by p16INK4a and loss of both regulators of the cell cycle would not provide an additive growth advantage. Promoter hypermethylation of the *CDKN2B* gene that encodes p15INK4b has also been noted in a subset of pituitary tumours (8). p18INK4c-deficient mice develop gigantism and widespread organomegaly, and POMC intermediate lobe pituitary hyperplasia and tumours. P18INK4c is significantly underexpressed in human ACTH-secreting adenomas (9).

Cip/Kip family

Members of the Cip/Kip family (p21Cip1 OMIN 116899, p27Kip1 OMIN 600778, and p57kip2 OMIN 600856) restrain cell cycle progression by associating with CDK1 and CDK2 complexes. Mice with disrupted *CDKN1B* gene, which encodes p27Kip1, develop overall increased body weight, multiorgan hyperplasia, female infertility, POMC intermediate lobe pituitary tumours, and hyperplasia of haematopoietic organs (10). Intermediate lobe tumours derived from p27Kip1 null mice differ from those derived from $Rb+^{/-}$ mice in that they are more vascular, exhibit lower proliferation rates, and are oligoclonal or polyclonal (vs monoclonal in $Rb+^{/-}$ mice). Down-regulation of p27Kip1 protein expression is common in corticotroph tumours and pituitary carcinomas, and p27kip1 levels are lower in recurrent pituitary adenomas compared with nonrecurrent adenomas. p27kip1 mRNA expression is generally not decreased in pituitary tumours, suggesting that decreased p27kip1 expression is probably due to post-translational factors. P21-deficient mice develop increased risk for multiple neoplasias in late adult life, however pituitary tumours are uncommon, and p21Cip deletion or mutation is not commonly encountered in human tumours. The role of p21Cip in oncogene-induced pituitary senescence is discussed below.

p53

p53 inhibits cell cycle progression or induces apoptosis, however, p53 appears not to play a major role in the pathogenesis of pituitary adenomas.

Cyclins

Cyclins D and E regulate the G1 to S phase of cell cycle progression. Cyclin D1, D2, and D3 are the first wave of cyclins to be upregulated when quiescent cells (G0) enter the proliferative cell cycle. Cyclin-CDK complexes induce phosphorylation (inactivation) of pRB, releasing E2F to prompt cell cycle transition to S phase. *CCND1* (OMIN 168461) encoding cyclin D1 has been studied in pituitary tumours. Allelic imbalance at the *CCND1* locus was found to be more frequent among invasive, while cyclin D is more expressed in aggressive and nonfunctioning pituitary adenomas, than in growth hormone-secreting adenomas (11). However, *CCND1* allelic imbalance and cyclin D1 expression may not coexist in the same tumour, suggesting that it may not be a primary event in pituitary tumorigenesis. Similarly, cyclin A, B, and E are also more abundant in larger, highly proliferative pituitary adenomas.

Pituitary tumour transforming gene (*PTTG*)

Pttg was isolated from rat growth hormone-secreting pituitary tumour cells line by mRNA differential PCR display, and *Pttg* overexpression induces cellular transformation *in vitro* and tumour formation in nude mice. PTTG is a mammalian securin, a key regulator of metaphase to anaphase transition during mitosis, and overexpression or suppression of *PTTG* (OMIN 604147) directly causes aneuploidy by inhibiting sister chromatid separation. PTTG also plays a role in pathways responsible for DNA break repair (12–14).

PTTG is abundantly expressed in most pituitary tumours. Examination of *PTTG1* mRNA expression in 54 pituitary tumours by real time-polymerase chain reaction (PCR) revealed overexpression in most pituitary tumours (23/30 of nonfunctioning, 13/13 growth hormone-secreting, 9/10 prolactinoma, and 1/1 ACTH-secreting), and *PTTG* expression correlated well with clinical tumour invasiveness. Sequence analysis has not shown mutations of the *PTTG1*-coding or promoter regions as a major cause of *PTTG1* overexpression in pituitary tumours.

Transgenic mice with human *PTTG* targeted to the pituitary under the α-subunit of glycoprotein hormone (αGSU) promoter exhibited gonadotroph, thyrotroph and, somatotroph focal hyperplasia and small adenomas, with elevated serum luteinizing hormone, testosterone, growth hormone, and/or insulin-like growth factor 1 (IGF-1) levels, and prostate and seminal vesicles hypertrophy. Confocal microscopy of αGSU.*PTTG1* and particularly bitransgenic αGSU.*PTTG1*; $Rb^{+/-}$ mice (αGSU.*PTTG1* mice crossbred with $Rb^{+/-}$ mice) pituitaries revealed nuclear enlargement and marked redistribution of chromatin (Fig. 2.3.2.4a,b), and enlarged gonadotrophs with prominent Golgi complexes and numerous secretory granules were noted under electron microscopy. These cell morphology changes are indicative of functionally active cells, consistent with pituitary growth noted imaging studies. Pituitary MRI showed that pituitaries derived from compound double transgenic αGSU.*PTTG1*;$Rb^{+/-}$ are enlarged as early as 2 months of age, and the incidence of anterior lobe tumours increased 3.5-fold (Figure 2.3.2.4c), suggesting that *PTTG* overexpression in anterior lobe αGSU cells facilitates tumour formation (5).

Transcription factors

The process of adenohypophyseal differentiation is a highly specific and temporally regulated series of events. Expression of transcription factors, such as PROP1, Pit1 (POU1F1), and DAX-1, in pituitary adenomas reflects the origin of tumour cells, and possibly their level of differentiation. However, whether or not dysregulation of these transcription factors plays a causal role on the development of human pituitary tumours remains unclear.

Signalling pathways

Guanine nucleotide-activating α-subunit (*GNAS*)

The McCune–Albright syndrome comprises defects in bony skeleton and skin, precocious puberty, thyrotoxicosis, acromegaly, gigantism, or Cushing's syndrome. The molecular defect is a mutation in the *GNAS* gene that encodes Gs-α protein, termed oncogene *gsp*, which induces constitutive adenylate cyclase activation. In growth hormone-secreting cells, *gsp* activates GHRH postreceptor pathways, i.e. cell proliferation and hormone secretion without necessarily requiring ligand binding to the GHRH receptor.

Although *gsp* mutations are reported in 30–40% of growth hormone-secreting adenomas, major clinical differences between *gsp*+ and *gsp*– pituitary tumours have not been identified. *GNAS* is imprinted in normal pituitary tissue and only the maternal allele is expressed. In growth hormone-secreting adenomas, *gsp* activating mutations mostly occur in the maternal allele. The *gsp* oncogene has been detected in <10% of nonfunctioning or ACTH-secreting tumours.

Activated cAMP-response element binding proteins (CREB)

The direct mechanism by which cAMP stimulates somatotroph growth hormone transcription may be mediated by the cAMP-responsive nuclear transcription factor (CREB), which binds as a dimer to cAMP-response elements (CRE). Transgenic mice overexpressing a phosphorylation-deficient and transcriptionally inactive mutant of CREB in the anterior pituitary exhibit dwarfism and somatotroph hypoplasia, indicating that phosphorylated CREB plays a role as a biochemical intermediate in the somatotroph proliferative response. Significantly higher amounts of Ser^{133}-phosphorylated, and hence, activated CREB was detected in a series of growth hormone-secreting pituitary tumours compared to a group of nonfunctioning tumours, suggesting that constitutively activated CREB, possibly promoted by Gs-α overexpression, may be another factor facilitating somatotroph transformation (15).

Dopamine receptors

The dopamine 2 receptor (D2R) mediates inhibitory effects of dopamine on pituitary prolactin synthesis and secretion.

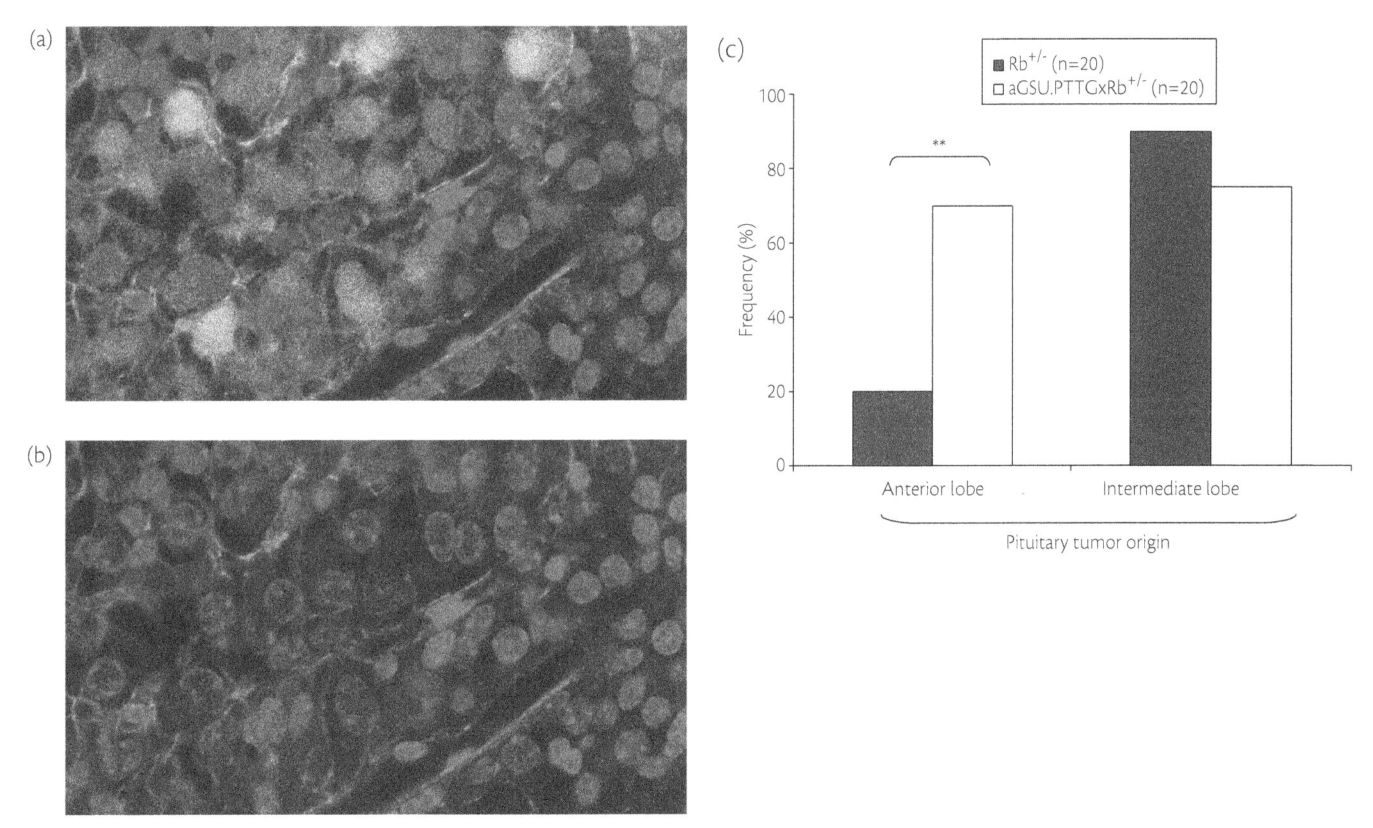

Fig. 2.3.2.4 Targeted *PTTG* overexpression to anterior lobe pituitary cells results in cell hyperplasia and increased tumour formation. Fig. 2.3.2.4(a) and (b) are duplicates of the same image, overview of pituitary cells expressing *aGSU.PTTG1.IRESeGFP* transgene. (a) is the untouched image, and in (b) the green layer (eGFP) has been hidden for better visualization of nuclear morphology. Contrast between eGFP positive (overexpressing PTTG) and eGFP negative (normal PTTG content) can be appreciated, notably presence of macronuclei and reorganization of chromatin suggestive of hyperplastic cells. (See also Plate 1) Fig. 2.3.2.4(c) depicts that bitransgenic *aGSU.PTTG;Rb*$^{+/-}$ mice exhibit higher prevalence of anterior lobe and similar prevalence of intermediate lobe pituitary tumours when compared with *Rb*$^{+/-}$ mice. Pathological analysis of pituitary tumours reveals that frequency of tumours arising from anterior lobe is higher in *aGSU.PTTG;Rb*$^{+/-}$ (white bars) than in *Rb*$^{+/-}$ (black bars) pituitary tumours (**, p = 0.0036), but frequency of tumours arising from the intermediate lobe (where there was no *PTTG* overexpression) is similar. n, total number of pituitary tumours analyzed. (From Donangelo I, Gutman S, Horvath E, Kovacs K, Wawrowsky K, Mount M, *et al.* Pituitary tumor transforming gene overexpression facilitates pituitary tumor development. *Endocrinology*, 2006; **147**: 4781–91 (6), with permission.)

D2R-deficient mice exhibit hyperprolactinaemia and lactotroph hyperplasia with late progression to pituitary tumours, suggesting that loss of dopamine inhibition induces murine neoplastic transformation. This finding probably cannot be extrapolated to pituitary tumour development in humans as D2R mutations have not been identified. Decreased D2R expression has been linked to dopamine agonist resistance in prolactinomas.

Somatostatin receptors

Somatostatin receptors (SSTR) 1–5 are expressed in all pituitary tumour types. Prolactinomas exhibit high SSTR1 expression compared with other tumour types. SSTR3 is frequently detected in nonfunctioning adenomas, while SSTR4 expression is relatively infrequent in pituitary tumours. In growth hormone-secreting adenomas, SSTR2 and SSTR5 expression does not correlate with tumour behaviour; however lower SSTR2 content is observed in adenomas less responsive to somatostatin analogue therapy. A germline mutation in the coding sequence of SSTR5 was reported in a single patient with acromegaly resistant to somatostatin analogue therapy, and no mutations have been identified in other SSTR subtypes. Polymorphisms in the coding (c1044t) and promoter (t-461c) regions of SSTR5 influence basal growth hormone and IGF-1 levels in patients with acromegaly, but SSTR2 and SSTR5 variants do not correlate with responsiveness to somatostatin analogue therapy. Therefore, SSTRs expression may correlate with responsiveness to medical treatment, but their role in the pathogenesis of pituitary adenomas, if any, remains unproven.

GHRH receptor

Mice bearing a GHRH transgene develop mammosomatotroph hyperplasia that may convert to adenomas in older mice. Extra-hypothalamic tumours secreting ectopic GHRH induce somatotroph hyperplasia and acromegaly, which rarely progress to somatotroph adenomas (16). The GHRH receptor (GHRHR) may be overexpressed in growth hormone-secreting adenomas compared with normal pituitary tissue (17), but the significance of increased expression of GHRHR in the pathogenesis of growth hormone-secreting adenomas is not clear.

Angiogenesis and growth factors

Vascularization is decreased in pituitary tumours compared with normal tissue, in marked contrast to the pattern observed in other tumour types where cancer development is linked to increased angiogenesis. This observation may be related to the slow growth of pituitary adenomas, i.e. enlargement of this benign tumour with low metabolic demands is likely not limited by the vascularization index. Moreover, in contrast to the normal pituitary, which is predominantly supplied by the hypothalamic-pituitary portal vein, pituitary adenomas receive a direct systemic blood supply, and the relatively low vascular density in these tumours may occur in parallel to an ingrowth of systemic capillaries, which may in fact dilute intrapituitary concentrations of hypothalamic factors.

Although microvascular density is decreased in pituitary adenoma tissue, vascularization and tumour are related, particularly in prolactinomas, which are more vascularized than growth hormone- or FSH-positive adenomas. Macroprolactinomas, invasive prolactinomas, or pituitary carcinomas have higher microvascular density compared, respectively, to microprolactinomas, noninvasive prolactinomas, or pituitary adenoma. Conversely, angiogenesis does not increase with tumour size in growth hormone-secreting adenomas. This is consistent with the notion that microprolactinomas may represent a pathological and clinical entity distinct from macroprolactinomas, whereas different-sized growth hormone-secreting adenomas are components of the same disease spectrum (18).

Vascular endothelial growth factor (VEGF)

VEGF increases proliferation and migration of endothelial cells, as well as endothelial permeability and fenestrations, and functions as an antiapoptotic factor promoting vessel endothelial cells survival. VEGF is detected in both the normal pituitary gland and in pituitary adenomas, and levels correlate with tumour behaviour, as VEGF is higher in carcinomas and macroprolactinomas. Dopamine, signalling through the endothelial cell DR2, inhibits VEGF-action, probably by endocytosis of VEGF receptor. In addition, pituitary glands derived from DR2-knockout female mice have increased VEGF expression compared with wild-type mice.

Fibroblast growth factors (FGFs)

FGFs participate in cell development, growth and angiogenesis, and basic FGF (bFGF or FGF2) is abundantly expressed in the pituitary and brain. During the hyperplastic phase of prolactinoma development, pituitary expression of both PTTG and bFGF is increased in a time- and dose-dependent manner in oestrogen-treated rats, and bFGF synthesis is induced in NIH-3T3 cells overexpressing PTTG. Its localization within the pituitary varies between species. In the rodent pituitary bFGF has been localized primarily to the folliculostellate cells and regulates growth hormone, prolactin, and TSH secretion. In murine folliculostelate cells, FGF2 induced positive autofeedback with protein kinase C-mediated FGF2 autoinduction, and stimulates cell proliferation and increased PTTG expression. bFGF immunoreactivity has been demonstrated in pituitary adenomas.

FGF4 is encoded by heparin-binding secretory transforming (*hst*) gene and is expressed in about 30% of PRL-secreting pituitary adenomas. FGF4 expression in prolactinomas correlates with tumour invasiveness, and GH4 cells transfected with *hst* form more aggressive tumours *in vivo* (19). No *hst* gene rearrangement has been detected in human prolactinomas, and the mechanism by which *hst*/FGF4 complex initiates or promotes lactotroph proliferation and prolactin secretion is unclear.

ErbB receptors

ErbB receptors comprise four subtypes: epidermal growth factor receptor (EGFR), p185her2/neu (or ErbB2), ErbB3, and ErbB4. Correlation between increased ErbB receptor expression and aggressive pituitary tumour behaviour has been suggested. EGF has potent mitogenic activity in pituitary cells, and both EGF and EGFR may be overexpressed in pituitary tumours, particularly in nonfunctioning adenomas. An examination of ErbB2 and ErbB3 expression in prolactinomas revealed positive results for both ErbB2 (seven of eight tumours) and ErbB3 (four of eight tumours) especially in aggressive, recurrent tumours (20). Whether ErbB receptors participate in pituitary tumour cell transformation is unknown.

EGF activates EGFR and ErbB signalling in lacto-somatotroph rat GH3 cells, with resulting increased prolactin and growth hormone expression. EGFR antagonist gefitinib decreases GH3 cell proliferation and prolactin secretion *in vitro*, and attenuates growth and hormone production of GH3-derived tumours in nude mice through blockage of EGFR/ERK signalling pathway (21). These results suggest that targeted ErbB receptor inhibition could be a potential therapeutic alternative for controlling growth and hormone secretion in aggressive prolactinomas resistant to dopamine agonists.

Familial syndromes

Multiple endocrine neoplasia type 1 (MEN 1)

Pituitary adenomas occur in a familial setting in about 5% of all cases, and over half of the cases are due to MEN 1. MEN 1 is an autosomal dominant genetic disease characterized by parathyroid adenoma, pancreatic endocrine tumours, and pituitary adenomas. Pituitary adenomas occur in approximately 25% of patients and these tumours may be larger and more aggressive that sporadic counterparts. Most secrete prolactin, with or without secretion of excess growth hormone, followed by those secreting growth hormone alone, nonfunctional tumours, and those secreting excessive ACTH. MEN 1 is caused by inactivating mutations of the tumour suppressor gene, *MEN1* (22). *MEN1* encodes Menin, a nuclear protein expressed in all organs and tissues of the body that interacts with both nuclear and cytoplasmic partners to regulate gene transcription, DNA repair, and cytoskeletal organization. Hundreds of inactivating *MEN1* mutations have been indentified, and it is unclear why *MEN1* mutations cause selected endocrine tumours while Menin is ubiquitously expressed. Homozygous murine *Men1* deletions result in embryonic lethality while heterozygous *Men1* deletion results in pituitary tumour formation.

Approximately 20% of patients harbouring clinical diagnosis of MEN 1 do not exhibit identifiable *MEN1* mutations. Generally, *MEN1* germline mutations are identified with an average prevalence of 70% in the familial forms, whereas the sporadic cases, associated with *de novo* mutation of the *MEN1* gene, represent about 10% of cases. Thus, mutations of other genes may also confer MEN 1. Rarely the gene for p27Kip1/*CDKN1B* functions as a tumour suppressor gene in patients with clinical MEN 1 but without *MEN1* mutations (23). Rare mutations in other CKI genes, p15INK4b/CDKN2B, p18INK4c/CDKN2C, p21CIP1/CDKN1A, have been identified in families with MEN 1 phenotypes with no identifiable germline *MEN1* mutations (24).

Carney complex

Carney complex is rare autosomal dominant genetic disease with myxomas of the heart, skin hyperpigmentation, and endocrine overactivity. Growth hormone-secreting adenomas are the most common pituitary tumours encountered in these patients. Up to 75% of patients have elevated levels of growth hormone, IGF-1, or prolactin, and 10% of patients exhibit clinical acromegaly. Somatotroph hyperplasia is followed by growth hormone-secreting tumour formation associated with inactivating mutations of *PRKAR1A*, the regulatory subunit isoform 1A of protein kinase A (PKA). Inactivating *PRKAR1A* mutations result in constitutive activation of PKA catalytic subunit. Mice with a specific homozygous deletion of *PRKAR1A* develop somatotroph hyperplasia, elevated growth hormone levels, and growth hormone-secreting adenomas. In some patients, and in animal models, the wild-type *PRKAR1A* allele is retained in tumour tissue and it appears that decreased expression, i.e. haploinsufficiency, rather than absence of the PKA regulatory subunit is sufficient to cause tumorigenesis.

Aryl hydrocarbon receptor interacting protein (AIP)

Familial isolated pituitary adenomas is a syndrome defined as two or more members in a family harbouring anterior pituitary tumours without evidence of MEN 1 or Carney complex. Whole-genome single-nucleotide polymorphism genotyping was performed on three Finish families with very-low-penetrance susceptibility to pituitary adenomas. Linkage analysis provided evidence for linkage in chromosome 11q12-11q13, a region previously implicated in isolated familial somatotropinomas (IFS) (25). No mutations or altered expression in *MEN1* were detected in representative blood samples from this cohort. Mapping of the linked chromosomal region identified *AIP*, or aryl hydrocarbon receptor interacting protein gene, with loss of heterozygosity detected in pituitary adenomas with *AIP* germline mutations, suggesting that AIP may behave as a tumour suppressor gene. A heterozygous nonsense germline mutation Q14X mutation was found in affected members of these Finnish families, but mutations were not found in unaffected family members or in the general population. Of 73 families with the syndrome of familial isolated pituitary adenomas, 11 (15.1%) harbour at least 10 different germline mutations in the *AIP* gene however penetrance of AIP mutations could not be established (26). Sixteen per cent of patients (7/45) with sporadic acromegaly exhibited either Q14X or IVS3-1G→A *AIP* mutations indentified in the original Finland study. However only ~2% of patients with sporadic pituitary tumours have *AIP* mutations in germline DNA, suggesting that the majority of sporadic pituitary tumours are not related to *AIP* mutations.

Other molecular events

Galectin-3

Galectin-3 (Gal-3), a β-galactoside-binding protein involved in cancer progression and metastasis, is expressed in ACTH-, prolactin-secreting and folliculostellate cells in the normal pituitary gland, and ACTH- and prolactin-producing pituitary adenomas and carcinomas are positive for Gal-3. Gal-3 expression is higher in pituitary carcinomas than in adenomas, indicating a role in pituitary tumour progression.

Growth arrest and DNA damage-inducible gene 45γ (*Gadd45-γ*)

GADD45-γ as identified as a candidate tumour suppressor gene for pituitary adenomas by cDNA-representational difference analysis (cDNA-RDA), and is expressed in the normal pituitary gland, but absent in most nonfunctioning, growth hormone-, and prolactin-secreting adenomas, as well as in immortalized pituitary cell lines. *GADD45-γ* is a p53-responsive gene induced by DNA damage and involved in growth suppression and apoptosis. Pituitary tumours positive and negative for GADD45-γ do not differ in clinical parameters. Introducing *GADD45-γ* into a rat pituitary tumour cell line decreases cell proliferation and anchorage-independent colony formation. Silencing of *GADD45-γ* in pituitary tumours probably occurs by epigenic changes, i.e. methylation of CpG islands in the *GADD45-γ* promoter (27).

Maternally expressed 3 gene (*MEG3*)

An isoform of *MEG3* contains an extra exon (*MEG3a*), and has been identified by cDNA-RDA, and is expressed in normal human pituitary, brain, and other tissues, but is diminished or absent in pituitary tumours and human cancer cell line (28). MEG3a is undetectable in both nonfunctioning and growth hormone-secreting pituitary adenomas, while introduction of *MEG3a* in cancer cells inhibits proliferation and decreases colony formation. Hence, loss of *MEG3a* in pituitary adenomas probably confers a tumour growth advantage. *MEG3* silencing in nonfunctioning pituitary adenomas is likely due to hypermethylation of the promoter region.

High mobility group A (*HMGA*)

The HMGA family includes the related HMGA1 and HMGA2 proteins. These are nonhistone chromosomal proteins that regulate transcription by altering chromatin structure. The *HMGA* genes are abundantly expressed during embryogenesis, but not in normal adult tissues, including the pituitary gland. Transgenic *HMGA1* and *HMGA2* overexpression in mice causes growth hormone-secreting adenomas and prolactinomas. Trisomy of chromosome 12, which harbours *HMGA2*, represents the most frequent cytogenetic alteration in human prolactin-secreting pituitary adenomas, and *HMGA2* overexpression was detected in a number of prolactinomas harbouring rearrangement of regions 12q14-15. Qian *et al.* noted that *HMGA2* expression was present in 38 of 98 (39%) pituitary adenomas, and was more frequent in FSH/luteinizing hormone cell adenomas (15/22, 68%), prolactinomas (5/15, 31%), and ACTH-secreting adenomas (12/18, 18%); however, it was rarely detected in growth hormone or mixed growth hormone/prolactin-secreting adenomas (29). High *HMGA2* levels correlate with tumour size, invasiveness, and cell proliferation marker. *HMGA2* tumorigenic effects may be mediated by stimulation of cyclin B2 expression by HMGA2 binding to the *CCNB2* promoter (30), and by activation of the E2F pathway. There is also evidence that *HMGA2* is suppressed by microRNA *Let7*, a putative tumour suppressor, and *HMGA2* and *Let7* expression correlate inversely in human pituitary adenoma samples (29).

Senescence

Cellular senescence is characterized by cell growth arrest induced by diverse mechanisms including age-linked telomere shortening, DNA damage, oxidative stress, chemotherapy and oncogene activation, and has emerged as a potential new component of cancer-protective response to oncogenic events. In response to oncogene activation, protective cellular mechanisms subject the cell to apoptosis and senescence. Apoptosis of cells with oncogene removes them from the tissue population thereby completely preventing tumorigenesis. Oncogene-induced senescence is a largely irreversible process in which proliferative arrest is mediated thorough upregulation of cell

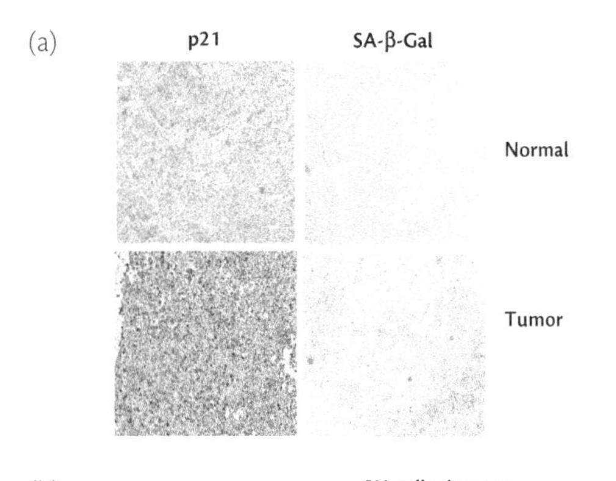

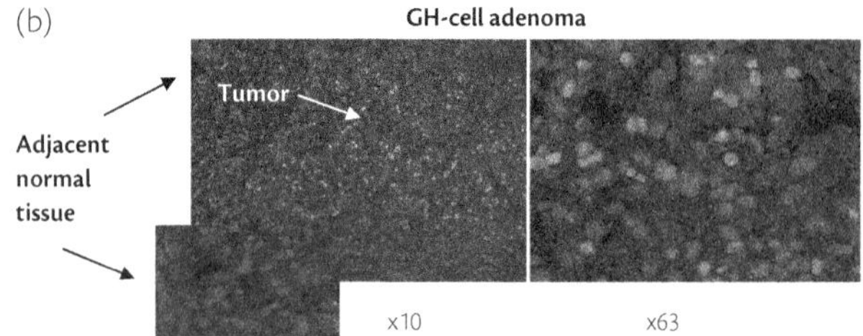

Fig. 2.3.2.5 Senescence markers in human growth hormone (GH)-producing pituitary adenomas. (a) Immunohistochemistry of the same GH-secreting human adenoma sections stained for p21 (brown) and SA-β-gal activity (blue). (b) Confocal image of double fluorescence immunohistochemistry of p21 (green) and β-galactosidase (red) proteins coexpression in human pituitary adenoma but not in normal adjacent tissue (left panel). High resolution (×63) image of the same slide (right panel). (From Chesnokova V, Zonis S, Kovacs K, Ben-Shlomo A, Wawrowsky K, Bannykh S, et al p21(Cip1) restrains pituitary tumor growth. *Proc Natl Acad Sci U S A*, 2008; **105**: 17498–503 (34), with permission.) (See also Plate 2)

cycle inhibitors, including p16INK4A, p15INK4B, p21CIP1, p53 and pRB. Oncogene-induced senescence also involves participation of cytokine and chemokine pathways that may be protective for malignant transformation (31).

Cellular senescent markers are noted to be elevated in benign tumours but not in malignant carcinomas. Indeed, p21Cip1 and senescence activity have been found to be elevated in human growth hormone-secreting adenomas and in rat GH3 pituitary cells (32). In 38 growth hormone-secreting adenomas, 29 exhibited strong and 9 weak p21 staining. In contrast, p21 was not detected in growth hormone-producing pituitary carcinomas, nonsecreting pituitary oncocytomas, null cell adenomas, or in aggressive breast carcinoma. Senescence-associated β-galactosidase activity (SA-β-gal), a marker of senescence, is strongly positive in growth hormone-secreting adenomas (Fig. 2.3.2.5). P21 and PTTG levels strongly correlated in these pituitary tumours.

Activation of the p21/p53 senescence pathway is noted to occur with both pituitary PTTG overexpression and deficiency. *Pttg*-null mice exhibit pituitary activation of senescence-like features, including increased SA-β-gal activity, upregulation of p21, pRB, and p19, and apoptosis blockage, which result in the pituitary hypoplasia phenotype. Telomere shortening was not noted in *Pttg*-null pituitaries, indicating that activation of senescence pathway is not due to early cell ageing. Upregulation of p21 is associated with relative protection from pituitary formation in $Rb^{+/-}$ mice with *Pttg* deletion ($Rb^{+/-}Pttg^{-/-}$ mice). In both *PTTG* deletion and overexpression, activation of p21/p53 senescence pathway occurs in a background on aneuploidy and DNA damage. Taken together, these findings suggest that p21 may exert a tissue-specific tumour-suppressing function, unmasked under conditions where other pituitary genetic alterations or stresses are present. Activation of the pituitary senescence pathway may constrain pituitary tumour growth, and provides an explanation for the invariably benign nature of these tumours.

References

1. Melmed S. Mechanisms for pituitary tumorigenesis: the plastic pituitary. J Clin Invest, 2003; 112: 1603–18.
2. Wilson CB Role of surgery in the management of pituitary tumors. Neurosurg Clin North Am,1990; 1: 139–59.
3. Donangelo I, Melmed S Molecular pathogenesis of pituitary tumors. In: Hay I, Turner H, Wass J, eds. Clinical Endocrine Oncology. 2nd edn. Blackwell Publishing: Massachusetts, 2008:187–93.
4. Thorner MO, Perryman RL, Cronin MJ, Rogol AD, Draznin M, Johanson A, *et al.* Somatotroph hyperplasia. Successful treatment of acromegaly by removal of a pancreatic islet tumor secreting a growth hormone-releasing factor. *J Clin Invest*, 1982; **70**: 965–77.
5. Alexander JM, Biller BM, Bikkal H, Zervas NT, Arnold A, Klibanski A. Clinically nonfunctioning pituitary tumors are monoclonal in origin. *J Clin Invest*, 1990; **86**: 336–40.
6. Donangelo I, Gutman S, Horvath E, Kovacs K, Wawrowsky K, Mount M, *et al* Pituitary tumor transforming gene overexpression facilitates pituitary tumor development. *Endocrinology*, 2006; **147**: 4781–91.
7. Zou H, McGarry TJ, Bernal T, Kirschner MW. Identification of a vertebrate sister-chromatid separation inhibitor involved in transformation and tumorigenesis. *Science*, 1999; **285**: 418–22.
8. Ogino A, Yoshino A, Katayama Y, Watanabe T, Ota T, Komine C, *et al.* The p15(INK4b)/p16(INK4a)/RB1 pathway is frequently deregulated in human pituitary adenomas. *J Neuropathol Exp Neurol*, 2005; **64**:398–403.
9. Morris DG, Musat M, Czirják S, Hanzély Z, Lillington DM, Korbonits M, *et al.* Differential gene expression in pituitary adenomas by oligonucleotide array analysis. *Eur J Endocrinol*, 2005; **153**:143–51.
10. Lazzerini Denchi E, Attwooll C, Pasini D, Helin K Deregulated E2F activity induces hyperplasia and senescence-like features in the mouse pituitary gland. *Mol Cell Biol*, 2005; **25**: 2660–72.
11. Simpson DJ, Hibberts NA, McNicol AM, Clayton RN, Farrell WE Loss of pRb expression in pituitary adenomas is associated with methylation of the RB1 CpG island. *Cancer Res*, 2000; **60**: 1211–6.
12. Kiyokawa H, Kineman RD, Manova-Todorova KO, Soares VC, Hoffman ES, Ono M, *et al* Enhanced growth of mice lacking the cyclin-dependent kinase inhibitor function of p27(Kip1). *Cell*, 1996; **85**: 721–32.
13. Hibberts NA, Simpson DJ, Bicknell JE, Broome JC, Hoban PR, Clayton RN, *et al* Analysis of cyclin D1 (CCND1) allelic imbalance and overexpression in sporadic human pituitary tumors. *Clin Cancer Res*, 1999; **5**: 2133–9.
14. Romero F, Multon MC, Ramos-Morales F, Dominguez A, Bernal JA, Pintor-Toro JA, *et al* Human securin, hPTTG, is associated with Ku heterodimer, the regulatory subunit of the DNA-dependent protein kinase. *Nucleic Acids Res*, 2001; **29**: 1300–7.
15. Bertherat J, Chanson P, Montminy M. The cyclic adenosine 3',5'-monophosphate-responsive factor CREB is constitutively activated in human somatotroph adenomas. *Mol Endocrinol*, 1995; **9**:777–83.
16. Kim DS, Franklyn JA, Smith VE, Stratford AL, Pemberton HN, Warfield A, *et al* Securin induces genetic instability in colorectal cancer by inhibiting double-stranded DNA repair activity. *Carcinogenesis*, 2007; **28**: 749–59.
17. Vlotides G, Eigler T, Melmed S Pituitary tumor-transforming gene: physiology and implications for tumorigenesis. *Endocr Rev*, 2007; **28**: 165–86.
18. Nasr C, Mason A, Mayberg M, Staugaitis SM, Asa SL Acromegaly and somatotroph hyperplasia with adenomatous transformation due to pituitary metastasis of a growth hormone-releasing hormone-secreting pulmonary endocrine carcinoma. *J Clin Endocrinol Metab*, 2006; **91**: 4776–80.
19. Lopes MB, Gaylinn BD, Thorner MO, Stoler MH Growth hormone-releasing hormone receptor mRNA in acromegalic pituitary tumors. *Am J Pathol*, 1997; **150**: 1885–91.

20. Turner HE, Harris AL, Melmed S, Wass JA Angiogenesis in endocrine tumors. *Endocr Rev*, 2003; **24**: 600–32.
21. Shimon I, Hüttner A, Said J, Spirina OM, Melmed S Heparin-binding secretory transforming gene (hst) facilitates rat lactotrope cell tumorigenesis and induces prolactin gene transcription. *J Clin Invest*, 1996; **97**: 187–95.
22. Vlotides G, Cooper O, Chen YH, Ren SG, Greenman Y, Melmed S Heregulin regulates prolactinoma gene expression. *Cancer Res*, 2009; **69**: 4209–16.
23. Vlotides G, Siegel E, Donangelo I, Gutman S, Ren SG, Melmed S Rat prolactinoma cell growth regulation by epidermal growth factor receptor ligands. *Cancer Res*, 2008; **68**: 6377–86.
24. Agarwal SK, Mateo CM, Marx SJ. Rare germline mutations in cyclin-dependent kinase inhibitor genes in multiple endocrine neoplasia type 1 and related states. *J Clin Endocrinol Metab*, 2009; **94**:1826–34.
25. Agarwal SK, Kennedy PA, Scacheri PC, Novotny EA, Hickman AB, Cerrato A, *et al* Menin molecular interactions: insights into normal functions and tumorigenesis. *Horm Metab Res*, 2005; **37**: 369–74.
26. Pellegata NS, Quintanilla-Martinez L, Siggelkow H, Samson E, Bink K, Hofler H, *et al* Germ-line mutations in p27Kip1 cause a multiple endocrine neoplasia syndrome in rats and humans. *Proc Natl Acad Sci U S A*, 2006; **103**: 15558–63.
27. Vierimaa O, Georgitsi M, Lehtonen R, Vahteristo P, Kokko A, Raitila A, *et al* Pituitary adenoma predisposition caused by germline mutations in the AIP gene. *Science*, 2006; **312**: 1228–30.
28. Daly AF, Vanbellinghen JF, Khoo SK, Jaffrain-Rea ML, Naves LA, Guitelman MA, *et al* Aryl hydrocarbon receptor-interacting protein gene mutations in familial isolated pituitary adenomas: analysis in 73 families. *J Clin Endocrinol Metab*, 2007; **92**: 1891–6.
29. Zhang X, Sun H, Danila DC, Johnson SR, Zhou Y, Swearingen B, *et al* Loss of expression of GADD45 gamma, a growth inhibitory gene, in human pituitary adenomas: implications for tumorigenesis. *J Clin Endocrinol Metab*, 2002; **87**: 1262–7.
30. Zhang X, Zhou Y, Mehta KR, Danila DC, Scolavino S, Johnson SR, *et al* A pituitary-derived MEG3 isoform functions as a growth suppressor in tumor cells. *J Clin Endocrinol Metab*, 2003; **88**: 5119–26.
31. Qian ZR, Asa SL, Siomi H, Siomi MC, Yoshimoto K, Yamada S, *et al* Overexpression of HMGA2 relates to reduction of the let-7 and its relationship to clinicopathological features in pituitary adenomas. *Mod Pathol*, 2009; **22**: 431–41.
32. De Martino I, Visone R, Wierinckx A, Palmieri D, Ferraro A, Cappabianca P, *et al* HMGA proteins up-regulate CCNB2 gene in mouse and human pituitary adenomas. *Cancer Res*, 2009; **69**: 1844–50.
33. Kuilman T, Michaloglou C, Vredeveld LC, Douma S, van Doorn R, Desmet CJ, *et al* Oncogene-induced senescence relayed by an interleukin-dependent inflammatory network. *Cell*, 2008; **133**: 1019–31.
34. Chesnokova V, Zonis S, Kovacs K, Ben-Shlomo A, Wawrowsky K, Bannykh S, *et al* p21(Cip1) restrains pituitary tumor growth. *Proc Natl Acad Sci U S A*, 2008; **105**: 17498–503.

2.3.3 Histopathology of pituitary tumours

Eva Horvath, Kalman Kovacs

Introduction

The human pituitary gland consists of two major components: the adenohypophysis comprising the hormone producing cells of the pars anterior, pars intermedia, and pars tuberalis, and the neurohypophysis, also called pars nervosa or posterior lobe (1). In contrast to most mammalian species, the human gland has no anatomically distinct pars intermedia (2). The exclusively proopiomelanocortin (POMC)-producing cells of the pars intermedia are sandwiched between the anterior and posterior lobes in the majority of mammals, whereas in the human they are incorporated within the pars anterior, thereby constituting the pars distalis (3). The pars tuberalis is a minor upward extension of the adenohypophysis attached to the exterior of the lower pituitary stalk. In this chapter we deal only with adenohypophyseal tumours.

Histologically, the adenohypophysis consists of a central median (or mucoid) wedge flanked by the two lateral wings. The hormone-producing cell types are distributed in an uneven, but characteristic manner. The cells are arranged within evenly sized acini surrounded by a delicate but well-defined reticulin fibre network giving the pituitary its distinct architecture (4). In the center of the acini is the long-neglected pituitary follicle composed of the agranular nonendocrine folliculo-stellate cells (5).

Cell types

Growth hormone cells or somatotrophs take up about 50% of the gland occupying chiefly the lateral wings. They show strong acidophilia by histology and growth hormone immunoreactivity by immunocytochemistry. Contingents of somatotrophs also express prolactin or the α-subunit of the glycoprotein hormones. Prolactin cells or lactotrophs account for 10–30% of cell population. The chromophobic or slightly acidophilic and prolactin-immunoreactive lactotrophs are evenly scattered with focal accumulation in the posterolateral rim of lateral wings. The majority of corticotrophs or adrenocorticotropic (ACTH) cells reside within the median wedge. They are basophilic, positive with the periodic acid–Schiff (PAS)-method and immunoreactive for 1-39 ACTH as well as for other POMC -peptides (β-endorphin, β-lipotrophic hormone (LPH), corticotropin-like intermediate peptide (CLIP), etc). Approximately 12% of adenohypophyseal cells are immunopositive for POMC-peptides, which include a small but undetermined percentage of pars intermedia-derived POMC cells as well. Thyroid-stimulating hormone (TSH) cells or thyrotrophs, occupying mainly the anterior one-third of the median wedge, represent only about 5% of adenohypophyseal cells. The slightly basophilic, angular thyrotrophs are strongly immunoreactive for β-TSH and α-subunit. Gonadotrophs producing follicle-stimulating hormone (FSH) and/or luteinizing hormone account for an estimated 15–20% of cells distributed quite evenly throughout the pars distalis. The basophilic, PAS-positive gonadotrophs are immunoreactive for β-FSH, β-luteinizing hormone and their α-subunit. The hormonal function of the adenohypophyseal cell types displays considerable flexibility depending on the functional demand placed on them. Even a reversible transdifferentiation is proven to occur between members of the Pit1 group: growth hormone cells to prolactin-cells (pregnancy) and growth hormone cells to TSH cells (hypothyroidism) (6, 7).

Pituitary cell types differ not only in their function, structure, and hormone content, but also in their morphological responses to functional stimulation or suppression. Thus, no extrapolation of findings from one cell type to another is appropriate (4). The folliculostellate cells have no hormonal function but both *in vitro* biochemical and morphological studies have documented that the small simple cells are not only unexpectedly versatile but frankly indispensable (5, 8).

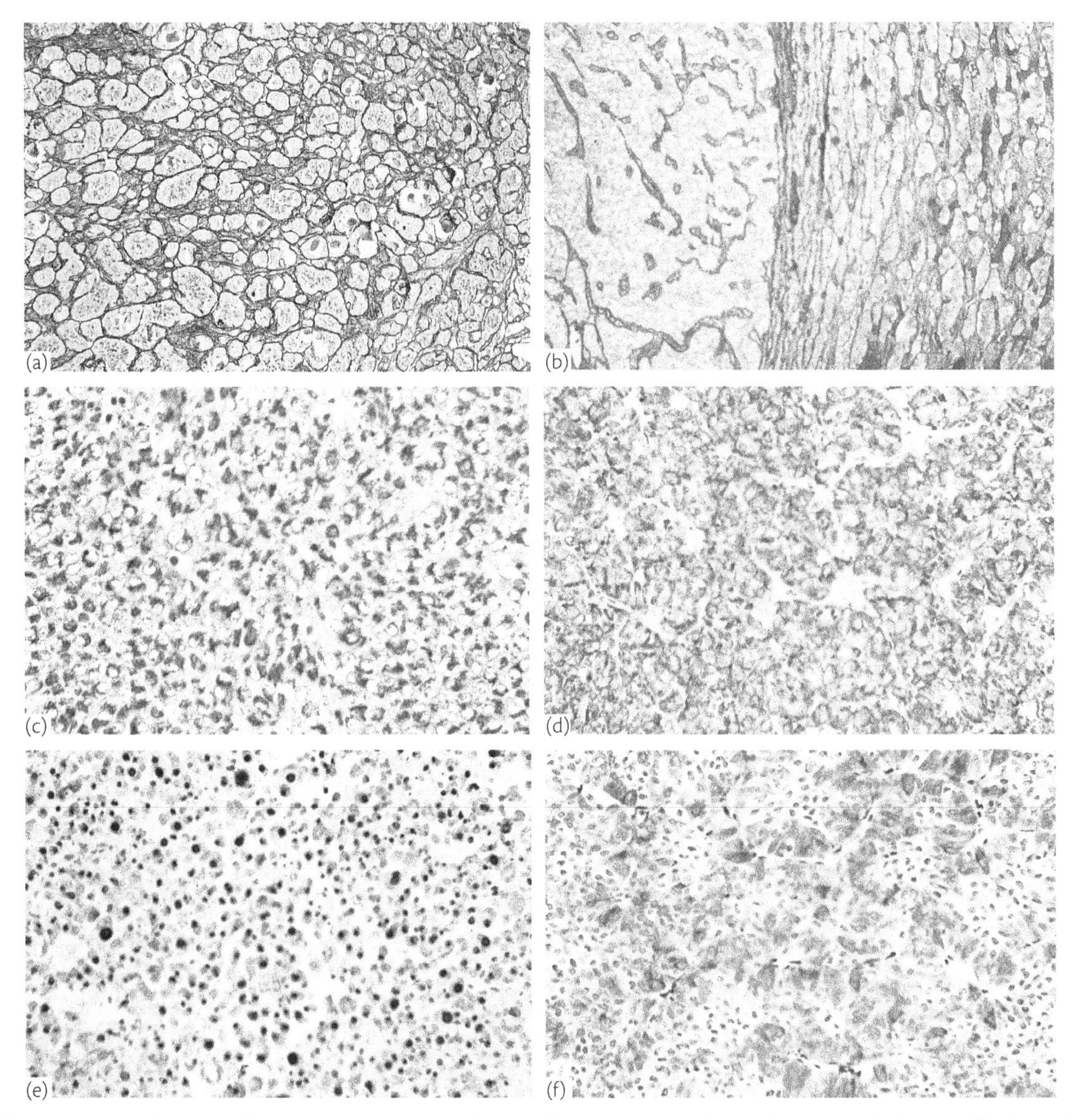

Fig. 2.3.3.1 (a) Normal acinar architecture of human adenohypophysis as shown by the Gordon–Sweet silver technique for reticulin (magnification ×10). (b) Within adenomas, the normal reticulin fibre network is broken down (left), whereas the reticulin fiber network of the surrounding nontumorous gland (right) is stretched and condensed into a so-called pseudocapsule (Gordon–Sweet reticulin technique, magnification ×10). (c) The characteristic pattern of prolactin immunoreactivity, outlining the Golgi apparatus, is shown in a prolactin cell adenoma (magnification × 40). (d) Densely granulated growth hormone cell adenoma displaying generalized immunoreactivity for growth hormone (magnification ×25). (e) Immunostaining for cytokeratin demonstrates strong immunopositivity in the intracytoplasmic spherical fibrous bodies in a sparsely granulated growth hormone cell adenoma (magnification ×25). (f) Immunostaining for follicle-stimulating hormone demonstrates immunoreactivity as well as the characteristic pseudorosette arrangement of the polar adenoma cells of a gonadotroph cell adenoma (magnification ×25).

Pituitary adenomas

General aspects

Adenomas—benign neoplasms arising in all types of hormone-producing cell of the adenohypophysis—are common, accounting for approximately 15% of intracranial tumours. Adenomas occur as small incidental findings in 5–20% of pituitaries at autopsy (1). Regardless of their size, a total dissolution of the normal acinar architecture (Fig. 2.3.3.1a) is evident in every adenoma. Pituitary adenomas are not encapsulated, but, if large enough, the tumours compress the reticulin framework of the surrounding normal gland into a pseudocapsule (Fig. 2.3.3.1b). By histology, adenomas are acidophilic, basophilic, or chromophobic. The tinctorial properties of tumours are largely unrelated to their hormonal function. Demonstration of hormone content (immunohistochemistry), assessment of ultrastructure (electron microscopy), and the increasingly popular molecular/genetic techniques are utilized for the functional classification of pituitary adenomas (9–11).

Pituitary tumours may be referred to as microadenomas (less than 10 mm in diameter), or macroadenomas (more than 10 mm in diameter). The growth pattern of these tumours may be expansive resulting in a slowly growing mass exerting increasing pressure on the surrounding normal gland and the bony sella. In contrast, invasive adenomas spread into the surrounding normal gland, dura or other parasellar structures (sphenoid sinus, cavernous sinus) regardless of their size. Adenomas extending into the suprasellar space may compress or infiltrate the optic chiasm causing visual disturbances, a frequent clinical manifestation of macroadenomas. Exceptionally large adenomas may grow into the anterior or posterior cranial fossa or downwards into the nasopharynx (12, 13).

Adenomas associated with hypersecretory syndromes

Prolactin cell adenoma

The sparsely granulated form is the most common adenoma type accounting for 27–30% of pituitary tumours (1, 9–11). It is associated with hyperprolactinaemia, primary or secondary amenorrhoea, galactorrhoea, and infertility in women. The less specific symptoms in men—decreasing libido and impotence—usually mean delay in diagnosis and development of macroadenomas whereas the majority of tumours in women are small and classified as microadenoma. Prolactin cell adenoma is most frequent in the third and fourth decade of life in both sexes (14). However, the incidence of the tumour type is significantly higher in women in their main childbearing years. Prolactin cell adenomas are associated with wide-ranging biological behaviours from indolent to highly aggressive, usually not reflected in their morphology. The prolactin blood levels are roughly proportional to the tumour mass. The frequency of the tumour type in autopsy material is around 40% in both sexes.

Histologically, the large majority of prolactin cell adenomas are chromophobic with a diffuse pattern. The other two patterns (papillary and the type with abundant hyalinous connective tissue stroma) occur mostly as incidental autopsy findings suggesting slow growth rate and/or later onset. Immunostaining demonstrates strong immunopositivity tracing the sacculi of the prominent Golgi apparatus, characteristic of prolactin cells (Fig. 2.3.3.1c). Ultrastructurally the three salient features are: masses of rough surfaced endoplasmic reticulum, prominent Golgi apparatus, and extrusion of the small, sparse secretory granules. The latter is the specific marker of prolactin differentiation (Fig. 2.3.3.2a) (1, 9–11).

Additional features Although calcification is extremely rare in other adenoma types, an estimated 10–15% of prolactin-producing adenomas display varying degrees of calcification. The alteration may be extreme ('pituitary stone'). Deposition of endocrine amyloid occurs infrequently.

Morphological effects of dopamine agonist treatment Adequate therapeutic response is associated with striking morphological changes in adenoma cells: the nucleus becomes heterochromatic, the cytoplasm shows marked shrinkage due to loss and involution of the hormone-producing apparatus (rough endoplasmic reticulum, Golgi complex) of the cells. Prolactin immunoreactivity is reduced or lost and, with the exception of granule extrusions, the cells have no ultrastructural markers of prolactin differentiation. Effects of treatment with long-acting form of bromocriptine can be exceptionally severe. Theoretically the morphological changes are reversible. However, portions of neoplasms may permanently lose their responsiveness and retain their suppressed features even when

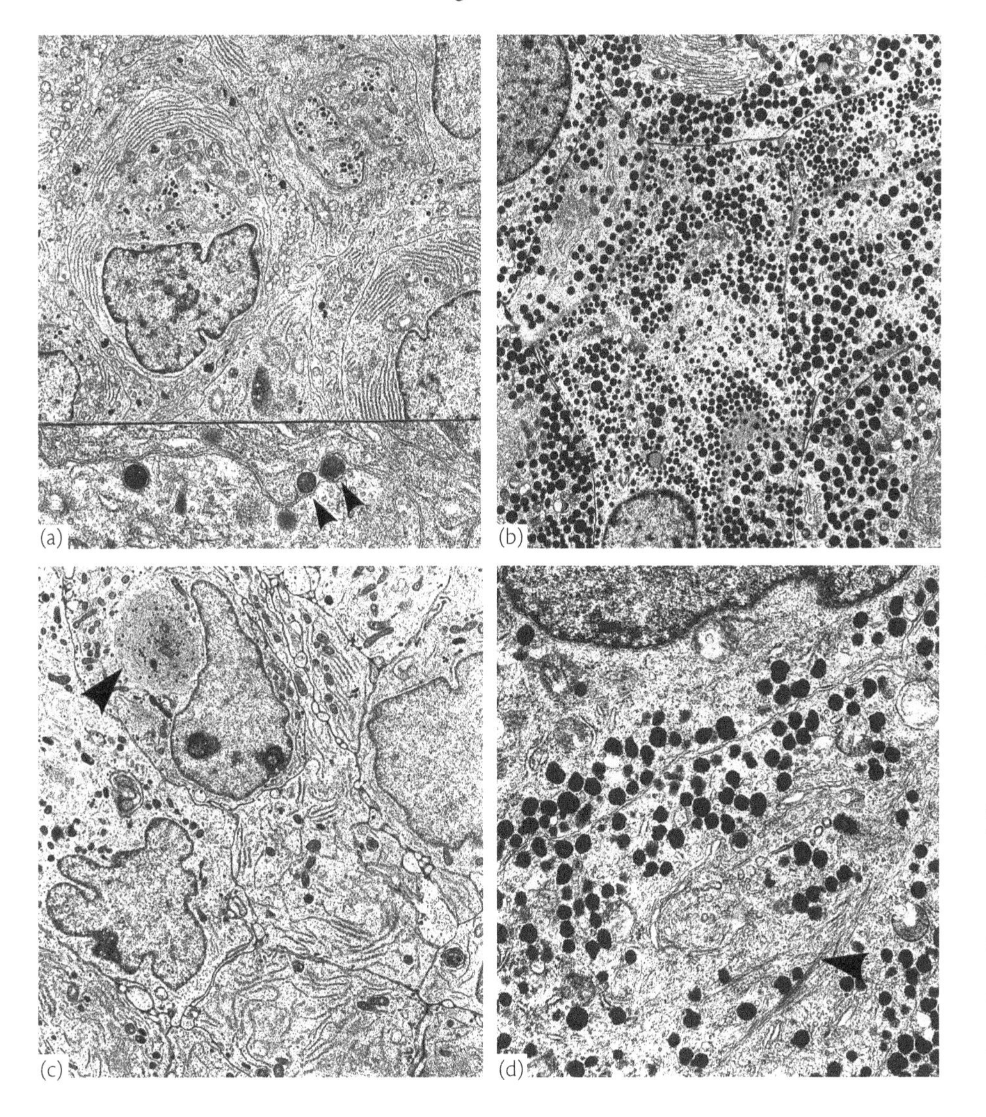

Fig. 2.3.3.2 (a) Ultrastructure of sparsely granulated prolactin cell adenoma displaying abundant rough endoplasmic reticulum, prominent Golgi complex and secretory granule extrusions (inset; arrowheads) (magnification ×4300, insert ×17 000). (b) Densely granulated growth hormone cell adenoma possessing numerous predominantly spherical large secretory granules (magnification ×4650). (c) Electron microscope view of a sparsely granulated growth hormone cell adenoma. Note fibrous body (arrowhead) and scanty, small secretory granules (magnification ×4320). (d) The distinguishing ultrastructural features of corticotroph cell adenoma are the unique morphology of secretory granules and bundles of cytokeratin filaments (arrowhead) (magnification ×10 200).

treatment is discontinued. Long-term administration of dopamine agonists may also cause varying degrees of fibrosis and calcification (15, 16) apparent as psammoma bodies.

Variants The densely granulated form of prolactin cell adenoma is very rare and clinically behaves similarly to the sparsely granulated variant (9, 10).

Growth hormone cell adenoma

Approximately 15% of surgically removed pituitary adenomas represent two forms of growth hormone cell adenoma (1, 9, 10). Most of these tumours are associated with physical stigmata and clinical signs of acromegaly, whereas tumours in children and adolescents causing gigantism are rare. Although the clinical manifestations and incidence of the two tumour types are similar, there are major differences in their morphology.

The densely granulated growth hormone cell adenoma occurs with the same frequency in both sexes peaking at the same time (in the sixth decade). The tumours display slow, expansive growth resulting in the typical 'ballooning of the sella' and may remain intrasellar for several years. Histologically, the densely granulated form is strongly acidophilic displaying diffuse or, less frequently, trabecular pattern. An extensive immunoreactivity for growth hormone (Fig. 2.3.3.1d) is usually accompanied by similarly strong positivity for α-subunit (1, 9, 10, 17). Scattered immunopositivity for prolactin and β-TSH is usually not associated with oversecretion of these hormones. The ultrastructure of adenomatous densely granulated growth hormone cells is similar to that of the normal phenotype, featuring well-developed rough endoplasmic reticulum, prominent Golgi complex and numerous large secretory granules mostly in the 350–500 nm range (see Fig. 2.3.3.2b).

The sparsely granulated growth hormone cell adenoma is more common in women, and is also diagnosed earlier peaking in the fourth decade (14). The tumours tend to be macroadenomas at the time of diagnosis and are often invasive. Histology detects chromophobic adenomas invariably displaying a diffuse pattern. Nuclear pleomorphism may be evident and adenoma cells frequently harbour a homogeneous, spherical juxtanuclear, practically unstained structure (18). This 'fibrous body' is strongly immunopositive for cytokeratin (Fig. 2.3.3.1e). The striking polkadot-pattern thereby generated is the best histological marker of the tumour type, since growth hormone immunoreactivity is often scanty. As opposed to the densely granulated type, multiple immunoreactivities for pituitary hormones are rarely noted. The ultrastructural phenotype of the sparsely granulated growth hormone cell adenoma—the spherical filamentous aggregate of the fibrous body nesting in the concavity of the eccentric crescent-shaped nucleus and scanty, small (less than 250 nm) secretory granules—is not seen in the normal gland (Fig. 2.3.3.2c).

Morphologic effects of treatment with a long-acting somatostatin analogue are neither severe nor consistent (16, 18). Remarkable shrinkage of cells and marked fibrosis are infrequent. Most common findings are the increase in size and number of secretory granules and/or increased lysosomal activity whereas significant fibrosis is less frequent. The close correlation observed between clinical response and tumour morphology in cases of prolactinomas treated with dopamine agonists does not exist in examples of octreotide treatment.

Additional features Both types of growth hormone cell adenoma may engage in usually focal, rarely massive production of endocrine amyloid. Approximately 2–3% of morphologically typical sparsely granulated adenomas are clinically silent, the reason for which is unknown (9, 10). Rare examples of the sparsely granulated tumours contain variable amounts of nervous tissue (neuron-like cells and neuropil) as a likely result of neuronal differentiation within the adenoma (9, 10).

Adenomas producing growth hormone and prolactin

The mixed (growth hormone cell/prolactin cell) adenoma, a tumour comprising two distinct cell types, is the most important in this group (1, 9, 10), accounting for an approximate 5% of surgically removed adenomas. The tumours are associated with acromegaly and varying degrees of hyperprolactinaemia. They tend to be aggressive and are difficult to treat. Mixed adenomas usually consist of densely granulated growth hormone cells and sparsely granulated prolactin cells. Other combinations may occur but they are rare. Accordingly, they are composed of acidophilic and chromophobic cells by histology displaying immunoreactivity for growth hormone and prolactin, α-subunit positivity is common, as well. By electron microscopy, the cell types constituting mixed adenomas have the features of densely granulated growth hormone cells and sparsely granulated prolactin cells as described earlier in this chapter. The infrequent (2%) mammosomatotroph cell adenoma is monomorphous, that is, it consists of one cell type displaying markers of both growth hormone and prolactin differentiation (1, 9, 10). Clinically they are associated with acromegaly and variable, usually mild hyperprolactinaemia. The acidophilic tumours are immunoreactive for growth hormone and α-subunit and, to a much lesser extent, for prolactin. At the ultrastructural level the densely granulated cells possess unusually large (up to 1000 nm and over) secretory granules and display granule extrusions, a prolactin cell marker. The slow-growing mammosomatotroph adenomas show biological behaviour similar to that of densely granulated growth hormone adenomas. They should be considered a morphological variant of densely granulated growth hormone cell adenoma with no difference in the clinical presentation.

The acidophil stem cell adenoma is a rare (2%) monomorphous type with morphological signs of prolactin and growth hormone differentiation (1, 9, 10). The tumour is associated chiefly with hyperprolactinaemia, but the serum prolactin levels may be disproportionately low for the size of the tumour. Physical stigmata of acromegaly and significant elevation of growth hormone levels are infrequent. These tumours grow aggressively in young subjects with tendency to invade infrasellar areas. Histology demonstrates chromophobic adenomas with moderate to strong immunoreactivity for prolactin. Immunopositivity for growth hormone is weak or negative, but immunostain for cytokeratin reveals the dot-like positivity of fibrous bodies. The striking ultrastructure is characterized by oncocytic change with formation of giant mitochondria, sparse, small secretory granules with extrusion (prolactin marker) and fibrous bodies (growth hormone marker).

Adenomas producing ACTH

Corticotroph or ACTH-cell adenomas responsible for pituitary dependent Cushing's disease account for 10–12% of surgically removed adenomas. The tumours show marked (4–5:1) female preponderance. The age-related occurrence of corticotroph adenoma is similar in the two sexes peaking in the fourth decade (14).

Most corticotroph lesions are small microadenomas causing florid Cushing's disease (1, 9, 10, 19). The tumours, often measuring only a few millimetres in diameter, may be too small to conclusively detect by imaging or to clearly identify by the neurosurgeon (20). Therefore serial sectioning of the biopsied tissue fragments is often needed and it may not result in the demonstration of the tumour in every case.

Histologically, corticotroph adenomas are basophilic and PAS positive with a sinusoidal or diffuse pattern (1, 9, 10, 19). Immunoreactivity can be demonstrated not only for 1-39 ACTH, but for other POMC-derived peptides, (β-endorphin, β-LPH, CLIP, etc.) as well. Electron microscopy documents cells densely granulated with secretory granules ranging up to 450–500 nm similar to those of normal ACTH cells. The best markers are: (1) the morphology of the secretory granules being spherical as well as notched, drop-shaped, and heart-shaped often displaying variable electron density; (2) perinuclear bundles of cytokeratin filaments, characteristic for the human corticotroph (Fig. 2.3.3.2d).

In a minority of cases pituitary dependent Cushing's disease is brought about by larger tumours. These neoplasms are often associated with a milder form of hypercorticism, but the tumours grow aggressively, and they often invade and are frequently macroadenomas at the time of diagnosis (21). Histologically they exhibit variable, often weak PAS positivity and immunoreactivity for ACTH. A few examples of aggressive macroadenomas display immunoreactivity for luteinizing hormone and/or α-subunit. Morphological features of corticotroph adenomas in cases of Nelson's syndrome are similar to those of densely granulated corticotroph adenomas in Cushing's disease with few or no cytokeratin filaments.

Variants Crooke's hyalinization, i.e. excessive accumulation of cytokeratin filaments, is the ubiquitous response of the normal human ACTH cell to longlasting elevation of circulating glucocorticoid levels (4). Accordingly, Crooke's hyalinization is noted in (1) nontumorous corticotrophs adjacent to corticotroph adenomas, (2) in ectopic ACTH/corticotrophin releasing hormone (CRH) syndrome, (3) in patients with glucocorticoid secreting adrenocortical tumours, (4) and in subjects having been treated with pharmacological doses of glucocorticoids. Crooke's hyalinization is not expected to develop in corticotroph tumours. Yet, a minority of such adenomas contains variable percentage of adenoma cells displaying the alteration (9, 10). Crooke's cell adenomas do not represent an entity and have no clinical correlates. Such tumors may be associated with mild, moderate, or severe hypercorticism and with variable biological behaviour (22).

Adenomas producing thyrotropin

A mere 1% of surgically removed adenomas derive in TSH cells (5, 9, 23, 24). These tumours are associated either with hyperthyroidism and inappropriately elevated levels of TSH or they develop in hypothyroid subjects, probably preceded by thyrotroph hyperplasia. Inexplicably, some adenomas bearing immunohistochemical characteristics of thyrotroph adenomas occur in euthyroid subjects. At the time of diagnosis, these tumours are often macroadenomas with a tendency to invade. The morphology of the small group of thyrotroph adenomas exhibit surprising diversity. Histologically, the adenomas are chromophobic and negative or mildly positive with PAS. They may be highly differentiated comprising elongate polar cells forming pseudorosettes around vessels. Alternatively, the pattern may be diffuse in some cases with considerable nuclear pleomorphism. Yet another variant is markedly fibrotic. Minute calcifications may be evident as well. Immunoreactivity for TSH is variable; it is often patchy or scattered, rarely extensive. Scattered cells may exhibit immunoreactivity for α-subunit, growth hormone, and prolactin. No specific ultrastructural markers exist for the tumours. They are sparsely granulated (granule size: up to 250); the secretory granules are often confined to the cell periphery outlining cell contours.

Treatment Thyrotroph adenomas possess somatostatin receptors and may show clinical improvement to octreotide therapy (25).

Adenomas unassociated with overt signs of hormone overproduction

Adenomas producing FSH and luteinizing hormone

The incidence of gonadotroph adenomas in surgical material is about 10%; they occur with similar frequency in the two sexes (5, 9). The majority of FSH/luteinizing hormone tumours appear as slow-growing, expansive macroadenomas causing local symptoms (12). Discrepancy between clinical parameters and morphological signs of gonadotroph differentiation is common; tumours displaying FSH/luteinizing hormone immunoreactivity and signs of high degree of functional differentiation by electron microscopy, may be unassociated with elevated serum FSH/luteinizing hormone levels.

The morphology of gonadotroph adenomas is variable (1, 5, 9). Histology may reveal polar cells forming pseudorosettes around vessels (Fig. 2.3.3.1f) or a diffuse pattern. Oncocytic change, i.e. undue increase of number and volume density of mitochondria is frequent. Immunoreactivity for FSH and/or luteinizing hormone is variable, often patchy; α-subunit, which is a useful clinical indicator, is not a reliable morphological marker. Electron microscopy documents unique sex-linked dimorphism. Many tumours in both sexes consists of polar cells having small (100–200 nm) secretory granules accumulating in cell processes. The Golgi complex has regular features in tumours of males, whereas it shows vacuolar transformation (honeycomb Golgi) in females. Adenomas comprising nonpolar cells have regular Golgi complex in both sexes.

Null cell adenoma and oncocytoma

These two adenoma types are the morphological variants of the same tumour (5, 9). The hormonally inactive adenomas account for approximately 25% of surgically removed tumours. They are twice as common in males peaking in the sixth decade in both sexes (14). Most of the tumours are slowly growing expansive macroadenomas causing local symptoms and varying degrees of hypopituitarism (12). Low-grade hyperprolactinaemia may occur ('stalk section effect').

Null cell adenoma is the nononcocytic form. Histologically it is chromophobic with predominantly diffuse pattern. Pseudorosette formation, characteristic of glycoprotein hormone producing tumours, may also occur. Immunostainings may detect scattered positivity for various pituitary hormones, particulary β-FSH, β-luteinizing hormone and α-subunit, or they may be immunonegative. Electron microscopy documents small cells having poorly developed cytoplasmic organelles and small (100–200 nm) scanty randomly distributed secretory granules, but no markers of cellular derivation (26).

Oncocytomas always show diffuse pattern by histology. The adenoma cells are larger than null cells and may display acidophilia due to non-specific binding of acidic stains by mitochondria. The pattern of immunoreactivities is the same as seen in null cells. By electron microscopy the sole ultrastructural marker is the extensive accumulation of mitochondria, whereas the other organelles are poorly developed. The secretory granules are sparse, small (100–200 nm) and are often displaced to the cell periphery by the crowding mitochondria.

Uncommon adenoma types

The term silent adenoma refers to three types of well-differentiated, morphologically well-characterized adenomas which are unassociated with any known hormonal hypersecretory syndromes and are not derived from any of the known anterior pituitary cell types (1, 5, 9). Silent adenomas and null cell adenomas are not synonymous, although clinically they cannot be distinguished.

Silent 'corticotroph' adenoma subtype 1 (3) (frequency less than 2%) is unassociated with clinical signs and symptoms of Cushing's disease. It shows a lesser degree of female preponderance and different age-related occurrence than corticotroph adenomas associated with Cushing's disease. The tumours display high propensity for haemorrhage and may present with pituitary apoplexy. Morphologically the adenomas have the same basophilia, PAS positivity, ACTH and β-endorphin immunoreactivity, and ultrastructural features as corticotroph tumours associated with Cushing's disease.

Silent 'corticotroph' adenoma subtype 2 (3) has a frequency of 1.5–2.0% and shows marked male preponderance. The tumours appear as nonfunctioning masses and are usually diagnosed at the macroadenoma stage. Histology reveals chromophobic tumours comprising small cells, which exhibit only modest PAS positivity and scattered immunoreactivity for ACTH and β-endorphins. Ultrastructurally the small cells possess small to midsize secretory granules (200–400 nm) showing similarity to POMC granules. However, no cytokeratin filaments are present.

The two adenoma types described above probably derive in cells of the pars intermedia, which in the human pituitary are incorporated within the pars distalis (2, 3). The physiological function of those cells is unknown.

The silent adenoma subtype 3 has a frequency of approximately 2% and is clinically more important owing to its fairly aggressive behaviour occurring mainly in young women (27). The tumour is equally frequent in the two sexes but it has strikingly different age-related distribution. In men, the tumour may occur at any age from the second to the seventh decade. The overwhelming majority of adenomas in women present between 20 and 40 years, peaking in the late twenties, but they rarely occur after 40 years of age. Silent adenoma subtype 3 consistently mimics prolactin cell adenoma in women, being associated with low-grade hyperprolactinaemia (usually less than 100 ng/ml) at the microadenoma stage. The serum prolactin levels do not increase proportionally with tumour size. Dopamine agonist treatment is not indicated; it returns to normal levels of prolactin (probably released from the non-neoplastic pituitary), but it does not cause tumour shrinkage and does not inhibit tumour progression.

Histologically, subtype 3 silent tumours are often acidophilic and may show mild PAS positivity. The large adenoma cells form diffuse, or lobular pattern. Immunocytochemistry may demonstrate scattered, minor positivity for various adenohypophyseal hormones owing to plurihormonal differentiation, but the majority of tumour cells are immunonegative for all known pituitary hormones. The ultrastructure of adenomas displays features of glycoprotein hormone differentiation and often marked accumulation of smooth endoplasmic reticulum. Owing to unspecific and variable immunoreactivities, electron microscopy is indispensable for diagnosis. The cell derivation of this adenoma type is unknown.

Unclassified plurihormonal adenomas are rare tumours, often with unique ultrastructure (5, 9). They may consist of one morphological cell type (monomorphous), or more than one phenotype (plurimorphous). The most common combinations are: growth hormone-TSH-prolactin or prolactin-TSH.

Spindle cell oncocytoma

In 2002, Roncaroli *et al.* (28) described a previously unknown type of primary oncocytic adenohypophyseal tumour in five elderly patients. The neoplastic cells were immunoreactive for vimentin, S100 protein, epithelial membrane antigen, and galectin-3, immunohistochemical markers of the folliculostellate cells of the pituitary. Immunostains for endocrine markers and pituitary hormones were negative. At the ultrastructural level, the tumour cells were markedly oncocytic but having no membrane specializations (junctional complexes) consistent with follicle formation. Roncaroli *et al.* (28) suggested derivation of the tumour from folliculostellate cells.

We have also observed a primary pituitary tumour having histological and immunohistochemical characteristics of spindle cell oncocytoma (unpublished observation). However, at the ultrastructural level widespread follicle formation and multifocal endocrine differentiation was evident as well. These findings further support the neoplastic potential of folliculostellate cells.

Pituitary carcinoma

Pituitary carcinoma can be diagnosed only when a pituitary neoplasm gives rise to distant, craniospinal, or, less frequently, extracranial metastasis (13, 29). Such tumours are extremely rare associated with dire prognosis. The majority of pituitary carcinomas produce either prolactin or ACTH. Other types, including those unassociated with signs of hormonal overproduction, are exceptionally rare. Pituitary carcinomas are not accompanied by specific histological features: enhanced mitotic activity, nuclear and cellular pleomorphism do not necessarily herald malignancy and vice versa, neoplasms with bland features might give rise to metastasis. Application of the proliferation marker, Ki-67 using the MIB-1 antibody is more useful; carcinomas display nuclear labelling consistently higher than adenomas (30). Immunoreactivities of pituitary carcinomas follow the pattern of the nonmalignant phenotype, although the degree of immunopositivity may be variably reduced. Relatively few cases have been investigated by electron microscopy revealing marked variability. In some carcinomas enough ultrastructural characteristics are retained to recognize the cell type, whereas other tumours have appearance of endocrine carcinoma of undetermined origin.

References

1. Kovacs K, Horvath E. *Tumors of the Pituitary Gland*. Washington DC: Armed Forces Institute of Pathology, 1986.
2. Horvath E, Kovacs K, Lloyd RV. Pars intermedia of the human pituitary revisited: morphologic aspects and frequency of hyperplasia of POMC-peptide immunoreactive cells. *Endocr Pathol*, 1999; **10**: 55–64.
3. Horvath E, Kovacs K. Lost and found: the pars intermedia of the human pituitary and its role in the histogenesis of silent 'corticotroph' adenomas. In: Gaillard RC, ed. *The ACTH Axis. Pathogenesis, Diagnosis and Treatment*. Norwell, Mass: Kluwer Academic Publishers, chapter 13, 2003: 259–75.
4. Horvath E, Kovacs K. Fine structural cytology of the adenohypophysis in rat and man. *J Electron Microsc Tech*, 1988; **8**: 401–32.
5. Horvath E, Kovacs K. Folliculo-stellate cells of the human pituitary: a type of adult stem cell? *Ultrastruct Pathol*, 2002; **26**: 219–28.
6. Vidal S, Horvath E, Kovacs K, Lloyd RV, Smyth HS. Reversible transdifferentiation: interconversion of somatotrophs and lactotrophs in pituitary hyperplasia. *Mod Pathol*, 2001; **14**: 20–8.
7. Vidal S, Horvath E, Kovacs K, Cohen SM, Lloyd RV, Scheithauer BW. Transdifferentiation of somatotrophs to thyrotrophs in the pituitary of patients with protracted primary hypothyroidism. *Virchows Arch*, 2000; **436**: 43–51.
8. Allaerts Wm, Vankelecom H. History and perspectives of pituitary folliculo-stellate cell research. *Eur J Endocrinol*, 2005; **153**: 1–12.
9. Horvath E, Scheithauer BW, Kovcs K, Lloyd RV. Hypothalamus and pituitary. In: Graham DI, Lantos PL, eds. *Greenfield's Neuropathology*. vol 1. 7th edn. New York, NY: Arnold Publishers, chapter 17, 2002:983–1051.
10. Horvath E, Kovacs K. The adenohypophysis. In: Kovacs K, Asa SL, eds. *Functional Endocrine Pathology*. 2nd edn. Boston: Blackwell Science, 1998:247–81.
11. Horvath E. Ultrastructural markers in the pathologic diagnosis of pituitary adenomas. *Ultrastruct Pathol*, 1994; **18**: 171–9.
12. Scheithauer BW, Kovacs KT, Laws ER Jr, Randall RV. Pathology of invasive pituitary tumors with special reference to functional classification. *J Neurosurg*, 1986; **65**: 733–44.
13. Pernicone PJ, Scheithauer BW. Invasive pituitary adenomas and pituitary carcinomas. In: Lloyd RV, ed. *Surgical Pathology of the Pituitary Gland. Philadelphia PA*, WB Saunders, 1993: 121–36.
14. Horvath E, Kovacs K. Age-related occurrence of various types of pituitary adenoma in surgical material. In: Hiroshige T, Fujimoto S, Honma K, eds. *Endocrine Chronobiology*. Sapporo: Hokkaido University Press, 1992: 185–93.
15. Kovacs K, Stefaneanu L, Horvath E, Lloyd RV, Lancranjan I, Buchfelder M, *et al*. Effect of dopamine agonist medication on prolactin producing pituitary adenomas. A morphological study including immunocytochemistry, electron microscopy and in situ hybridization. *Virchows Archiv Patholog Anat Histopathol*, 1991; **418**: 439–46.
16. Kovacs K, Horvath E. Effects of medical therapy on pituitary tumors. *Ultrastruct Pathol*, 2005; **29**: 163–7.
17. Scheithauer BW, Horvath E, Kovacs K, Laws ER Jr, Randall RV, Ryan N. Plurihormonal pituitary adenomas. *Semin Diagnos Pathol*, 1986; **3**: 69–82.
18. Ezzat S, Horvath E, Harris AG, Kovacs K. Morphological effects of octreotide on growth hormone-producing pituitary adenomas. *J Clin Endocrinol Metab*, 1994; **79**: 113–18.
19. Saeger W. Surgical pathology of the pituitary in Cushing's disease. *Pathol Res Pract*, 1991; **187**: 613–16.
20. Laws ER Jr, Thapar K. Surgical management of pituitary adenomas. *Bailliere's Clin Endocrinol Metab*, 1995; **9**: 391–405.
21. Thapar K, Kovacs K, Muller PJ. Clinical-pathological correlations of pituitary tumors. *Bailliere Clin Endocrinol Metab*, 1995; **9**: 243–70.
22. George DH, Scheithauer BW, Kovacs K, Horvath E, Young WF Jr, Lloyd RV, *et al*. Crooke's cell adenoma of the pituitary: an aggressive variant of corticotroph adenoma. *Am J Surg Pathol*, 2003; **27**: 1330–6.
23. Greenman Y, Melmed S. Thyrotropin secreting pituitary tumors: In: Melmed S, ed. *The Pituitary*. Cambridge, Mass: Blackwell Science, 1995: 546–58.
24. Beck-Peccoz P, Brucker-Davis F, Persani L, Smallridge RC, Weintraub BD. Thyrotropin-secreting pituitary tumors. *Endocr Rev*, 1996; **17**: 610–38.
25. Chanson P, Weintraub B, Harris A. Octreotide therapy for thyroid-stimulating hormone-secreting pituitary adenomas. *Ann Intern Med*, 1993; **119**: 236–40.
26. Kovacs K *et al*. Null cell adenomas of the pituitary: attempts to resolve their cytogenesis. *Endocr Pathol Update*, 1990; **1**: 17–31.
27. Horvath E, Kovacs K, Smyth HS, Cusimano M, Singer W. Silent adenoma subtype 3 of the pituitary-immunohistochemical and ultrastructural classification: a review of 29 cases. *Ultrastruct Pathol*, 2005; **29**: 1–14.
28. Roncaroli F, Scheithauer BW, Cenacchi G, Horvath E, Kovacs K, Lloyd RV, *et al*. 'Spindle cell oncocytoma' of the adenohypophysis. A tumor of folliculostellate cells? *Am J Surg Pathol*, 2002; **26**: 1048–55.
29. Pernicone PJ, Scheithauer BW, Sebo TJ, Kovacs KT, Horvath E, Young WF Jr, *et al*. Pituitary carcinoma. A clinico-pathologic study of 15 cases. *Cancer*, 1997; **79**: 804–12.
30. Thapar K, Kovacs K, Scheithauer BW, Stefaneanu L, Horvath E, Pernicone PJ, *et al*. Proliferative activity and invasiveness among pituitary adenomas and carcinomas. An analysis using the MIB-1 antibody. *Neurosurgery*, 1996; **38**: 99–107.

2.3.4 Pituitary assessment strategy

W.M. Drake, P.J. Trainer

Introduction

The optimum methods of testing anterior and posterior pituitary function and the interpretation of the results are subjects of continuing debate. The syndromes associated with and consequences of hypo- and hyperpituitarism, and the diagnosis and treatment of diabetes insipidus are all discussed elsewhere in this book. The intention of this chapter is to describe the physiological basis and evidence in favour of the various available tests of anterior pituitary function, discuss the limitations of using artificial assessments on which to base patient management decisions and, ultimately, endeavour to produce a rational approach to the investigation of suspected hypopituitarism.

The need for pituitary function tests is not disputed as, untreated, the morbidity and mortality of hypopituitarism is high, mainly as a consequence of secondary adrenal insufficiency. There are two broad groups of patients for whom pituitary function tests are required. The first group comprises all new patients with suspected hypopituitarism. This, in turn, includes patients with target organ failure (such as hypoadrenalism, hypothyroidism, and hypogonadism) in whom low levels of cortisol, thyroxine and sex steroid, respectively, are not associated with an appropriate elevation of the relevant pituitary trophic hormone: patients with cranial diabetes insipidus; patients presenting with the mechanical consequences of pituitary tumours, such as headache and visual failure; and patients in whom a pituitary mass is found incidentally during the course of radiological investigation for an unrelated symptom.

The second group of patients includes those with known pituitary disease in whom an evolving endocrine deficit is anticipated. This mainly comprises patients who have received radiotherapy as treatment for a pituitary tumour, and also includes patients with conditions in which progressive hypothalamo-pituitary destruction may occur, such as sarcoidosis or Langerhans' cell histiocytosis. Hypopituitarism usually evolves in a predictable way with, typically, growth hormone deficiency preceding gonadotropin deficiency with subsequent failure of adrenocorticotropic hormone (ACTH) and thyroid-stimulating hormone (TSH) secretion. This order is less predictable in patient with hypopituitarism consequent upon traumatic brain injury and lymphocytic hypophysitis; the latter, in particular may be characterized by isolated ACTH deficiency. In all patients, pituitary function testing may help identify those patients whose hypopituitarism is sufficiently severe to threaten their safety, irrespective of symptoms; or exclude hormonal deficiencies as a cause of symptoms such as lethargy and fatigue. For example, an asymptomatic patient with a basal serum cortisol of 120 nmol/l rising to 175 nmol/l during insulin-induced hypoglycaemia requires hydrocortisone replacement therapy and should have the reasons for such treatment carefully explained. In contrast, a patient with a pituitary mass and symptoms of lethargy who has normal thyroid hormone levels, a basal serum cortisol above 450 nmol/l and normal gonadal function does not require endocrine replacement therapy. A sound knowledge of the principles of pituitary function testing is mandatory for the accurate diagnosis and optimal treatment of pituitary failure.

The anterior pituitary gland secretes six known hormones: growth hormone, ACTH, luteinizing hormone, follicle-stimulating hormone (FSH), TSH, and prolactin, all of which are under regulatory feedback control. Regulation of secretion of each hormone is complex with, in most cases, at least two hypothalamic peptides directly acting on the appropriate pituitary cell type to influence secretion, which in turn may be pulsatile, with underlying circadian or ultradian rhythm. In the case of ACTH, for example, this phenomenon is striking with plasma levels of its target hormone, cortisol, varying in health between undetectable and 700 nmol/l over 24 h. For other pituitary hormones, such as TSH, the circadian variation is modest and there is no diurnal change in serum thyroxine concentrations. This means that a single, random blood sample is unlikely to provide sufficient diagnostic information about the function of the pituitary–adrenal axis; whereas it is rare for investigations other than basal samples to be required in the assessment of the pituitary–thyroid axis. In general, the more dynamic the physiological system in health, the more likely will be the need for a dynamic test to investigate its possible malfunction in disease. In all cases, the fundamental question being posed is: is the functioning of this 'endocrine unit' adequate for this patient's health and, if not, does it require replacement/support? This chapter will describe the physiological basis of the various tests of anterior pituitary function, discuss the evidence in favour of their interpretation and, ultimately, produce a rational, reliable and safe strategy for pituitary function testing.

General principles of pituitary assessment

The diagnostic evaluation of pituitary function has several complementary limbs involving laboratory and radiological investigations. First, it is necessary to demonstrate target organ hormonal insufficiency, such as low levels of thyroid hormone or gonadal steroid. Paired testing of both hormones in the pituitary–target organ feedback loop, sometimes in combination with provocative testing, will prove that target organ failure is consequent on lack of stimulation by the relevant pituitary trophic hormone. Additional tests may occasionally be performed in order to determine whether the pituitary itself is at fault, or whether pituitary failure is secondary to understimulation by the hypothalamus. However, this distinction is seldom useful clinically and is irrelevant to the need for hormone replacement therapy. Sophisticated radiological imaging is required to look for possible causes of hypothalamo-pituitary destruction and, together with careful neuro-ophthalmological assessment, will help determine the mechanical effects of any hypothalamo-pituitary mass lesion. Lastly, in cases of pituitary failure where the cause is believed to be a systemic illness (such as sarcoidosis or tuberculous hypophysitis) more specific investigations may be needed. These are discussed in the relevant sections elsewhere (Chapter 2.4.5).

Types of laboratory test

Basal pituitary function tests

Basal blood tests refer to samples taken with the patient resting, unstressed and with no physiological or pharmacological manipulation of the mechanisms that control the pituitary cell–target cell interaction. Hence basal samples are taken between 07.00 and 09.00 h, when serum cortisol and testosterone levels are highest. Given that the decision to proceed to dynamic testing is based on the results of basal samples, it is logical to maximize the chances of basal investigations yielding sufficient information to avoid the need for more complex tests. Paired measurement of both limbs of a pituitary hormone–target hormone loop are required for interpretation of the target hormone level. Low levels of target hormone in association with low or normal levels of the relevant pituitary trophic hormone indicate that target gland failure is consequent on understimulation by the pituitary.

Provocative tests

Provocative (stimulation) tests are employed when hypofunction of a pituitary cell type is suspected and basal investigations have not yielded sufficient information. Such tests assess the ability of a given cell type to respond acutely to a stimulus, but do not necessarily provide information about the adequacy of day-to-day hormone production by that cell type under basal conditions. Two types of provocative tests are used: those that stimulate hormone release indirectly (such as the insulin tolerance and glucagon tests) and direct stimulation tests in which pharmacological doses of synthetically manufactured peptide are injected and the target cell hormone response measured. Examples of these include hypothalamic-releasing hormone tests and the short Synacthen test (see below). The virtue of indirect provocation tests is that the integrity of an entire hypothalamo–pituitary–target cell loop is tested. Hypothalamic-releasing hormone tests with thyrotropin-releasing hormone (TRH), gonadotropin-releasing hormone, and growth hormone-releasing hormone (GHRH) are discussed briefly in the relevant sections. When introduced to clinical practice, it was thought that they would facilitate the diagnosis of hypopituitarism and forewarn of insidious pituitary failure. However, experience has shown that they have no value in diagnosing hypopituitarism and they cannot be used to predict future pituitary failure. They may occasionally be of value in differentiating hypothalamic from pituitary disease, as a normal response to the injection of hypothalamic-releasing hormone implies that the defect lies at a hypothalamic level. The major use of releasing hormone testing has been as a tool for the study of the neuroregulation of pituitary hormone secretion.

Assessing ACTH reserve (the hypothalamic–pituitary–adrenal axis)

Of all the aspects of pituitary function testing, this is the most controversial, mainly because assessment of the adequacy of the hypothalamic–pituitary–adrenal axis and the provision of replacement therapy (if required) has the most far-reaching consequences of all the anterior pituitary hormones. The laboratory assessment of the hypothalamic–pituitary–adrenal axis is performed in two distinct clinical settings, although the aim of establishing whether cortisol production is adequate is common to both. The first clinical scenario is that of a patient with symptoms suggestive of adrenal insufficiency (such as tiredness, listlessness and malaise), where the question being posed is: 'Are the symptoms due to cortisol deficiency?' The second clinical setting is one in which the patient is known to be at risk of developing secondary adrenal insufficiency. This, in turn, may occur in patients previously treated with supraphysiological doses of corticosteroids, or in patients with known hypothalamo-pituitary disease who may, in addition, have received appropriate treatment with surgery and/or radiotherapy. In the second of these clinical settings ('at-risk patients'), it is necessary to assess the adequacy of the patient's response to physiological stress, even in the absence of any symptoms of adrenal insufficiency. If the test used predicts that the patient will not be able to mount an adequate stress response, then the patient requires education about the implications of ACTH deficiency and adequate steroid cover must be provided in the event of emergency. The dynamic tests described below assess the ability to respond to physiological stress, but do not assess the appropriateness of basal, unstressed cortisol levels, and their relationship to symptoms such as lethargy and malaise. An inadequate 'stress response' necessitates steroid cover for surgery, sepsis and accidental trauma, but should not automatically be taken to indicate a need for lifelong glucocorticoid replacement therapy. A satisfactory method for assessing the adequacy of the day-to-day cortisol production rate has not yet been identified. Isotope dilution methods are accurate but complex and not widely available, while measurements of urinary free cortisol lack sensitivity for the detection of insufficiency. Interpretation of the basal and dynamic tests used to assess the two separate aspects of glucocorticoid replacement therapy is usually straightforward. However, the limitations of the assessment of the basal cortisol production rate must be borne in mind and consideration given to patients' symptoms and wellbeing when instigating lifelong glucocorticoid replacement therapy.

Physiological background

Although there is considerable debate about many aspects of assessing ACTH reserve, the aim of establishing whether cortisol production is adequate for the patient's health is not disputed. Measurement of the target hormone (cortisol) is common to all tests of the hypothalamic–pituitary–adrenal axis. Cortisol has a multitude of actions, including regulation of protein and carbohydrate metabolism, maintenance of vascular tone and modulation of the immune system. Its synthesis and secretion is controlled by ACTH, whose release from the pituitary is, in turn, regulated by hypothalamic corticotropin-releasing hormone and vasopressin. Hypothalamic function is influenced by a complex array of factors including neural stimuli (particularly from the limbic system) and humoral inputs (such as inflammatory cytokines). A change in cortisol production rate is the 'final common pathway' for all of these complex modulatory factors: hence the use of cortisol levels for the assessment of ACTH reserve. It has the added practical advantage of ease of collection, as ACTH samples require cold centrifugation and flash-freezing whereas cortisol is measured in serum.

General aspects of cortisol measurements

In virtually all laboratories, cortisol is measured by radioimmunoassay. Administered hydrocortisone, prednisolone/prednisone, and methylprednisolone will all interfere with the measurement of endogenous cortisol, such that samples for cortisol assay should not be taken within 24 h of the patient taking any of the above. There is increasing interest in the use of tandem mass spectroscopy to measure serum cortisol, as a means of eliminating cross-reactivity with other glucocorticoids and reducing between assay bias.

Only 5–10% of cortisol is free, the remainder being bound to cortisol-binding globulin. Hence plasma cortisol-binding globulin levels significantly alter measurements of serum cortisol. Cortisol-binding globulin is synthesized in the liver and, like sex hormone-binding globulin (SHBG), production is increased by oral oestrogens that pass through the liver. However, while SHBG is routinely measured along with testosterone in the assessment of the pituitary–gonadal axis, cortisol-binding globulin is not routinely measured along with cortisol. Total serum cortisol levels are therefore significantly raised in pregnancy and in patients taking oral oestrogens. Hence oral oestrogens should be discontinued prior to assessment of the hypothalamic–pituitary–adrenal axis and most authorities accept that six weeks are required for their effect on cortisol-binding globulin levels to disappear completely (1). Accurate assessment of the hypothalamic–pituitary–adrenal axis in pregnancy is extremely difficult. Other circumstances in which cortisol-binding globulin levels may complicate assessment of the hypothalamic–pituitary–adrenal axis include conditions of protein loss, such as nephrotic syndrome and protein losing enteropathy; and failure of protein synthesis, such as hepatic cirrhosis. Growth hormone decreases circulating cortisol-binding globulin, such that levels are low in acromegaly and fall with initiation of growth hormone therapy in adults with growth hormone deficiency.

The laboratory assessment of the integrity of the hypothalamic–pituitary–adrenal axis relies on several aspects of its normal physiology. First, cortisol is part of a short (pituitary) and a long (hypothalamic) feedback loop, such that falling cortisol levels stimulate a rise in ACTH and corticotropin-releasing hormone secretion from the pituitary and hypothalamus, respectively, and vice versa. Second, the zona fasciculata of the adrenal gland is dependent on ACTH stimulation for cortisol production and in the absence of a trophic signal undergoes reversible atrophy, with secondary failure of cortisol production. Last, the normal, diurnal pattern of ACTH and cortisol secretion may be greatly modified by a variety of pathophysiological stimuli such as trauma and sepsis.

Failure of ACTH secretion leads to adrenal insufficiency, the clinical spectrum of which may vary between cardiovascular collapse and a more subtle dysfunction that is apparent only during the physiological stress of sepsis, major surgery, or accidental trauma. The first question to consider is what is a 'satisfactory' serum cortisol level under such circumstances? A study of the cortisol response to major abdominal surgery in normal and corticosteroid treated individuals showed that the peak serum cortisol was at least 580 nmol/l (1). This study used the fluorimetric method of Mattingley (2) for measurement of serum cortisol, a technique that, unlike modern radioimmunoassays, also detects cortisone. In the same study (3), serum cortisol responses to hypoglycaemia were shown to correlate well with the peak perisurgical serum cortisol measurement. Since then, controlled iatrogenic hypoglycaemia has widely been accepted as the 'gold standard' by which to judge whether a given individual will be capable of mounting an adequate cortisol response to physiological stress. The 'cut-off' serum cortisol level thought to be adequate for physiological stress should be lowered from 580 to 500 nmol/l on account of the change in methodology used for cortisol measurement. This is on the basis of comparative data, suggesting that serum cortisol measured by radioimmunoassay is 0.87 of that measured by fluorimetry (580×0.87=505) (4) and is supported by the lower mean serum cortisol peak found in normal volunteers by Hurel and colleagues (5), although no comparison with cortisol levels during stress was not undertaken in that study.

Having established a minimum serum cortisol level that is adequate for acute physiological stress, the question arises as to what is the most appropriate stimulation test for the prediction that the patient will be able to achieve such a cortisol response when required. Several tests exist, each with its own merits and shortfalls, including measurements of basal serum cortisol, the insulin tolerance test, glucagon stimulation test, short Synacthen test (standard and low dose), and the metyrapone test.

There is considerable variability in the results of serum cortisol measurements according to the assay methodology employed. Clark *et al.* (6) documented a 26% difference between basal serum cortisol results using different assays, with highly significant differences also noted in serum cortisol levels 30 and 60 min after injection of Synacthen. Such findings make comparisons of cortisol responses between different centres extremely difficult and emphasize the need for every centre to establish robust local reference ranges, as opposed to selecting rigid 'cut-off' values on the basis of population studies, which may have used different methodologies.

Measurements of basal serum cortisol

Having established a minimum cortisol level that is adequate for acute illness or trauma, is it possible to infer from measurements of basal serum cortisol whether the hypothalamic–pituitary–adrenal axis is capable of responding normally to stress in a given individual? Conversely, below which level does a basal cortisol measurement make dynamic testing unnecessary to confirm ACTH deficiency? Endogenous hypothalamic–pituitary–adrenal activity is maximal in the early morning and samples should be drawn between 08.00 and 09.00 h. In cases of suspected pituitary insufficiency, a basal morning serum cortisol of less than 100 nmol/l strongly indicates ACTH deficiency, dynamic testing is not necessary and glucocorticoid replacement should commence immediately. In most patients, the requirement for steroid replacement is likely to be permanent. However, in the case of ACTH deficiency prior to surgery for a pituitary tumour, recovery of ACTH reserve following surgical decompression may occur and so it is necessary to reassess the situation postoperatively.

The next question to answer is 'what value of basal serum cortisol indicates an individual's ability to achieve a satisfactory cortisol level during physiological stress'? Several studies have confirmed that a close correlation exists between measurements of basal, unstressed serum cortisol to peak serum cortisol levels during insulin induced hypoglycaemia. From these reports, it is clear that many patients can avoid a dynamic test on the basis of basal cortisol measurements, although the precise 'cut-off' point calculated from these studies varied between 400 and 500 nmol/l (5, 7, 8).

To summarize, measurements of basal serum cortisol may identify patients for whom a dynamic test of ACTH reserve is unnecessary. Published evidence suggests that dynamic testing of ACTH reserve is required if the basal serum cortisol, measured by modern radioimmunoassay, lies between 100 and 400 nmol/l and that values outside this range indicate adrenal insufficiency and a normally functioning hypothalamic–pituitary–adrenal axis, respectively.

Emergency assessment of the hypothalamic–pituitary–adrenal axis

In the acutely sick patient with, for example, sepsis or trauma, and suspected hypoadrenalism, the clinical situation dictates that a morning cortisol and/or a dynamic test of ACTH reserve are impractical and glucocorticoid support may need to be started immediately. In such a context, circadian variation of ACTH release will be absent and activity of the hypothalamic–pituitary–adrenal axis should be maximal. If adrenal insufficiency is suspected, then random serum cortisol and plasma ACTH measure ments will suffice for an assessment of hypothalamic–pituitary–adrenal axis integrity. If, subsequently, the random cortisol level is shown to have been appropriate to the clinical situation (above 500 nmol/l) glucocorticoids may be withdrawn. If not, steroid support should continue and dynamic testing must wait until the acute clinical situation has resolved. The plasma ACTH will indicate whether the adrenal insufficiency is primary or secondary. A serum cortisol below 200 nmol/l with a plasma ACTH above 200 pmol/l is diagnostic of primary adrenal failure.

The insulin tolerance test

This test, first described in 1966 (9), seeks to simulate physiological 'stress' in a controlled, supervised environment by inducing hypoglycaemia with intravenous insulin. Hypoglycaemia is a powerful stress stimulus, which, in the intact pituitary and hypothalamus, induces ACTH and growth hormone release and a rise in serum cortisol levels. It therefore assesses the integrity of the entire hypothalamic–pituitary–adrenal axis and has traditionally been regarded as the 'gold standard' for this purpose. Its reproducibility amongst healthy volunteers is well documented (10), but not known among patients with pituitary disease. As discussed above, the assumption that the ability to respond to insulin-induced hypoglycaemia will translate into an appropriate cortisol rise in the event of acute illness or major surgery is supported by studies in which the peak cortisol levels of patients undergoing major surgery were comparable with those achieved during a preoperative insulin tolerance test (ITT) (2). Although the safety of ITT has been questioned, particularly in children, the morbidity of this investigation in experienced hands within the setting of a designated metabolic investigation unit is reassuringly low, provided that the standard criteria are adhered to (ischaemic heart disease, epilepsy/unexplained blackouts, severe longstanding hypoadrenalinism, glycogen storage disease) (8). The dose of insulin used varies between centres. Most authorities recommend a dose of 0.1–0.15 IU/kg, with higher doses (typically 0.3 IU/kg) being required for patients with acromegaly or other conditions in which insulin resistance is a feature. Patients should have normal thyroid function and no significant abnormalities on an ECG. Its major disadvantages are that it is contraindicated in patients with ischaemic heart disease or epilepsy. Many physicians are uncomfortable with its use in elderly patients and it requires careful supervision and monitoring of adrenergic and neuroglycopenic symptoms.

The immediate counterregulatory response to hypoglycaemia is characterized by catecholamine release, which, in turn, stimulates hepatic glycogenolysis and correction of hypoglycaemia. Glucocorticoids are not part of this phenomenon, although the laying down of hepatic glycogen stores does require pre-exposure to glucocorticoids. Thus, in patients with longstanding ACTH deficiency and consequent inadequate glycogen stores, recovery from hypoglycaemia may be delayed. It is therefore usual practice to administer oral glucose in the form of a sugary drink, together with a meal, at the conclusion of the test to guard against this eventuality.

A common reason to perform an ITT is to test the ability of the hypothalamic–pituitary–adrenal axis to respond to stress following the withdrawal of supraphysiological doses of corticosteroids for inflamatory conditions e.g. asthma and inflammatory bowel disease. Such doses may lead to ACTH suppression, with secondary adrenal involution and loss of responsiveness. It is therefore essential, in this situation, to perform a short Synacthen test in order to establish that the adrenals are capable of responding to ACTH. If the adrenals do not respond to ACTH, an ITT will yield no useful information.

Short Synacthen test

This investigation was originally introduced in the 1960s (11) as a test for primary adrenal failure. It involves the injection of a pharmacological dose (250 μg) of synthetic ACTH, with measurement of the serum cortisol response, and it has been advocated as an alternative to the ITT as a means of assessing ACTH reserve. The basis of its use in the context of hypopituitarism is that chronic underexposure of the adrenal glands to ACTH (either as a consequence of prolonged corticosteroid therapy or due to suspected or proven hypothalamic pituitary disease) will result in a blunted cortisol response to exogenously administered ACTH. The test does not distinguish primary from secondary adrenal insufficiency, although clinical assessment (pigmentation) and measurement of basal plasma ACTH are usually sufficient in this regard. The major argument in favour of the short Synacthen test is its simplicity, as it requires no specialist staff and takes only an hour to complete. The only reported side effect is allergy in patients with a history of atopy, although this is very rare. The test does not assess growth hormone reserve. It is universally accepted that this test cannot be used for the assessment of ACTH reserve when acute hypopituitarism develops, such as following pituitary infarction (apoplexy) or the immediate postoperative assessment of the ACTH axis. It takes at least 2 weeks for the adrenal zona fasciculata to involute following withdrawal of ACTH stimulation, during which time the adrenal cortex will remain responsive to supraphysiological doses of ACTH. In addition, it should be remembered, in the assessment of new patients with suspected hypothalamic–pituitary disease, that the duration of ACTH deficiency may be unknown and that, as following pituitary surgery or apoplexy, a falsely reassuring short Synacthen test may result.

Two main aspects of the short Synacthen test in assessing ACTH reserve have been debated: the peak serum cortisol versus increment and the level of serum cortisol that constitutes an adequate response (often referred to in the literature as the 'pass-fail cut-off'). The increase in serum cortisol following Synacthen is a poor index of adrenal responsiveness, as there is considerable overlap between normal volunteers and patients with secondary adrenal insufficiency (12). Further, the cortisol increment is inversely correlated with the basal value and hence a smaller increment is seen in the early morning when plasma ACTH and serum cortisol levels are at their highest (13). The peak serum cortisol response following Synacthen shows no diurnal variation and is now the accepted index of adrenal responsiveness and, indirectly, endogenous ACTH exposure.

Excellent correlations exist between cortisol levels 30 min after injection of Synacthen and the peak cortisol achieved during insulin-induced hypoglycaemia in patients undergoing investigation for suspected pituitary disease (16). Proponents of the use of the SST therefore suggest that an ITT can be avoided in patients who surpass a given threshold 30 min post-Synacthen cortisol level (usually between 550 and 600 nmol/l), unless simultaneous assessment of growth hormone reserve is required. This has led to its increasing use as a substitute for the ITT, such that in 1995, 50% of UK endocrinologists declared it their investigation of choice in the investigation of the hypothalamic–pituitary–adrenal axis (15) compared with 24% in 1988 (16).

However, despite its widespread use as a method of assessing ACTH reserve, there is no study showing that a normal short Synacthen test indicates that the hypothalamic–pituitary–adrenal axis is capable of responding normally to major illness or stress. Critics of the use of the short Synacthen test point to reports of patients with pituitary disease with symptoms and signs of adrenal failure, corrected by glucocorticoid replacement, having recently had a falsely reassuring 'normal' short Synacthen test. This problem cannot be corrected by application of a more 'stringent' threshold of serum cortisol as in two such reported patients the peak serum cortisol value was more than 950 nmol/l 30 min after Synacthen. However, reports also exist of patients who have developed acute adrenal crisis following a reassuringly normal ITT.

Low-dose short Synacthen test

In recent years, much interest has arisen in the use of a lower dose of ACTH (typically 1 μg) in the assessment of secondary adrenal failure. In health, the entire stored pool of pituitary ACTH is of the order of 600 μg, such that an injected bolus of 250 μg produces plasma concentrations that are unphysiological and beyond the top of the ACTH/cortisol dose–response curve. Proponents of the low-dose short Synacthen test argue that chronically understimulated adrenal glands may mount a satisfactory cortisol response to the unphysiological concentration of ACTH provided by 250 μg of Synacthen, but that only normal glands will respond to the small doses used in this test. Further, plasma ACTH levels following injection of 1 μg are comparable with those reached during an ITT in healthy volunteers (18). The test is quick (a single sample only is required 30 min after injection of ACTH) and the test may be performed at any time of day.

Abdu *et al.* (19) studied the cortisol responses to the standard and low-dose ACTH tests and to the ITT in patients with suspected or proven pituitary disease. Using a serum cortisol 500 nmol/l as a 'pass' on the ITT, the low-dose short Synacthen test has a maximum diagnostic accuracy with a sensitivity of 100% and specificity of 80% when an adequate response was defined as a serum cortisol above 600 nmol/l. In other words, there were no patients in whom a serum cortisol level above 600 nmol/l 30 min after injection of 1 μg synacthen provided false reassurance about their ability to 'pass' the ITT. Failure to achieve a serum cortisol of 600 nmol/l following 1 μg ACTH indicated the need for an ITT. The authors concluded that such a test could be used as a screening procedure for the investigation of secondary ACTH deficiency, with the ITT reserved for patients with a borderline response. Similar studies by Tjordman *et al.* (20) compared the serum cortisol response following various doses (1, 5, and 250 μg) of ACTH to the ITT or metyrapone test in healthy volunteers, patients with documented hypothalamic–pituitary–adrenal axis dysfunction due to pituitary disease and patients with pituitary disease but normal ACTH reserve. False reassurance was provided in 70% of patients with known secondary adrenal failure when the 30 min serum cortisol value following injection of 5 or 250 μg ACTH was used. In contrast, the low-dose ACTH test identified all patients with documented ACTH deficiency.

In common with the 250 μg ACTH test, variability of response is an important issue. 'Normal' 30 min values following the injection of 1 μg ACTH have, variously, been documented as lying between 480 and 600 nmol/l (21) which may, at least in part, be accounted for by the use of different protocols for the dilution of ACTH for injection. Concern about the extent to which ACTH may be adsorbed onto the plastic of syringes or saline bags dictates that further efforts at standardization and reproducibility of the low-dose ACTH test are required prior to its widespread recommendation for the assessment of ACTH deficiency. Pharmaceutical companies are being encouraged to market synthetic ACTH in 1 μg vials to allow more rigorous reference ranges for cortisol response to be established.

Glucagon stimulation test

The subcutaneous injection of glucagon causes a transient rise in plasma glucose. During the subsequent fall in glucose levels, ACTH and growth hormone are both released and this has led to its widespread use as a means of assessing the reserve of these two hormones, although mechanisms by which cortisol and growth hormone secretion are stimulated are ill-understood. Glucagon is a less powerful stimulus to ACTH release than hypoglycaemia and false negative results are a well-recognized problem. Its injection routinely makes patients feel unwell with nausea and may cause abdominal pain and vomiting. The glucagon test has not been the subject of intense study and although it is a less reliable and potent stimulus the interpretation, the interpretation of the serum cortisol response relies on criteria established for insulin-induced hypoglycaemia. However, it remains a useful method of assessing the hypothalamic–pituitary–adrenal and growth hormone axes, particularly when the ITT is contraindicated (22).

Metyrapone test

This test of adrenal reserve was first described in the 1950s (23) and its role in the assessment of ACTH reserve has therefore changed with the availability of plasma ACTH and serum cortisol assays. Metyrapone inhibits 11β-hydroxylase, the final enzyme involved in cortisol synthesis. The subsequent fall in cortisol levels following administration of metyrapone stimulates ACTH release from the intact pituitary. Corticosteroidogenesis increases and serum levels of cortisol precursors such as 11-desoxycortisol rise. 11-desoxycortisol has no glucocorticoid activity and so a rise in its level has no effect on ACTH secretion. In patients with secondary adrenal insufficiency, a fall in cortisol does not stimulate an increase in ACTH secretion and hence no rise in 11-desoxycortisol level occurs. A typical protocol entails oral administration of 30 mg/kg metyrapone in hospital at midnight. Simultaneous cortisol and 11-desoxycortisol levels are taken between 08.00 and 09.00 h and then oral glucocorticoids are administered if the index of suspicion of ACTH deficiency is high. An 11-desoxycortisol level above 200 nmol/l (7 μg/dl) indicates normal adrenal function, irrespective of the simultaneous cortisol value. Levels less than 200 nmol/l, in the presence of a low serum cortisol level, strongly suggest secondary adrenal insufficiency (24). A low serum cortisol level is required for the interpretation of the test as an indicator of the level of pituitary stimulation. Anticonvulsant therapy such as phenytoin accelerates the metabolism of metyrapone and an alternative test of the hypothalamic–pituitary–adrenal axis should be used in such patients.

A major criticism of this investigation is that it is a test of the ACTH–cortisol feedback mechanism rather than of ACTH reserve. In addition, assays for cortisol precursors are not widely available and the test is now seldom used in the UK, although it is investigation of choice in some centres for assessment of ACTH reserve.

Conclusion

It is inevitable that the debate about the optimum method for the assessment of the hypothalamic–pituitary–adrenal axis will continue. Practical issues such as cost and staff availability will, to a large extent, affect local policy but the fundamental clinical issue of patient safety remains the same. Dynamic tests of the integrity of the hypothalamic–pituitary–adrenal axis support, rather than substitute for, clinical decisions and it is important to recognize that the use of sophisticated statistical methods for the comparison of serum cortisol levels in groups of people with or without endocrine disease can never substitute for clinical awareness in the individual patient. Even the ITT, thought for so long to be the 'gold standard' for assessing ACTH reserve cannot provide complete reassurance that an individual patient will not develop secondary adrenal insufficiency during physiological stress. Changes in methodology and variation in the assays used for cortisol measurements hinder comparisons between published experiences of hypothalamic–pituitary–adrenal testing and make it difficult to recommend a single protocol for this purpose. Endocrine physicians should always educate their patients about the possible implications of pituitary disease in terms of the stress response, particularly when it is anticipated that the functioning of the hypothalamic–pituitary–adrenal axis may change over a period of time, such as following pituitary irradiation. The ITT is the single most reliable test of the hypothalamic–pituitary–adrenal axis but should only be performed under close supervision in specialist centres. If there is any doubt about the adequacy of ACTH reserve, it is sensible to err on the side of caution with respect to the provision of emergency steroid cover; and to consider a trial of oral glucocorticoid replacement therapy in patients with symptoms suggestive of chronic adrenal insufficiency and an equivocal response to dynamic testing.

Pituitary–thyroid axis

Secondary hypothyroidism can be difficult to diagnose as TSH rarely becomes undetectable in hypopituitarism and the symptoms of hypothyroidism, such as lethargy, lack diagnostic specificity. As discussed below, the TRH is of no value in diagnosing secondary hypothyroidism. The diagnosis relies on measurement of free thyroxine (fT4) and TSH, which need to be interpreted in the context of other pituitary function tests. Secondary hypothyroidism is strongly suggested by low levels of circulating fT4 in the presence of a low or low normal TSH. However in many patients the fT4 value will, by that stage have, fallen by 50% and patients may be symptomatically hypothyroid. A novel approach to diagnosing TSH deficiency has been the mathematical modelling concept of the TSH Index or 'fT4-corrected' (new reference Jostel Clinical Endocrinology 2009 71 529). Illness ('sick euthyroid' syndrome), thyroxine-binding globulin deficiency, supraphysiological doses of glucocorticoids and drugs such as phenytoin may also produce a similar picture. The interpretation of the results is dependent on the overall clinical context and is assisted by measurement of free T_4 and tissue markers of thyroid hormone action such as SHBG.

TRH testing

TRH testing is of no value in diagnosing secondary hypothyroidism or predicting imminent TSH deficiency. In normal individuals, intravenous injection of TRH produces a rise in TSH, with levels at 20 min being greater than those at 60 min. Patients with hypothalamic disease classically show a delayed response to TRH, with the 60 min value greater than that at 20 min. Patients with pituitary disease typically have an absent TSH response to TRH, although it is recognized that some patients will respond. This is thought to be because some pituitary tumours result in functional disconnection of the hypothalamus from the pituitary, thereby simulating a hypothalamic lesion. Renal failure, depression, malnutrition, and extreme illness may all be associated with delayed or absent TRH responses. Together with the widespread availability of sensitive TSH assays and the risk of syncope or precipitating pituitary apoplexy in patients with pituitary tumours, this means that the TRH test is now very seldom used in the assessment of pituitary function.

Growth hormone

The optimum method of testing for growth hormone deficiency in adults was largely academic prior to the recognition of the syndrome of adult growth hormone deficiency. Since the late 1980s, however, and particularly since 1996 when growth hormone became licensed for use in adult hypopituitarism in most European countries, accurate tests of growth hormone reserve have assumed a greater importance. Here, tests of growth hormone reserve will be described, although a more detailed discussion of their specificity and sensitivity, together with descriptions of the symptoms and signs and diagnosis of childhood and adult growth hormone deficiency can be found in Chapter 2.3.7.

Normal growth hormone secretion is pulsatile, with four to six pulses per 24 h, mostly at night in association with stage III–IV rapid eye movement sleep, punctuating long periods when growth hormone levels in blood are undetectable. As with the assessment of the hypothalamic–pituitary–adrenal axis, this means that a single basal blood sample is unlikely to yield significant diagnostic information, unless the taking of the sample coincides with a growth hormone surge. An attractive approach, therefore, might seem to measure 24 h spontaneous profiles, as has been employed in the diagnosis of growth hormone deficiency in childhood. However, this approach has proved disappointing, as there is considerable overlap in the integrated growth hormone concentration of normal subjects and those of hypopituitary patients and have little diagnostic value (25). Other physiological methods of assessing growth hormone secretion include sampling during sleep and exercise, both of which are associated with growth hormone release. However, all three of these methods are prohibitively time consuming for routine clinical use.

Most, if not all, actions of growth hormone are mediated through the peptide hormone insulin-like growth factor 1 (IGF-1). However, measurement of serum IGF-1 is of limited value in the diagnosis of adult-onset growth hormone deficiency, as 30% of patients with unequivocal growth hormone deficiency may have a serum in the lower half of the age-related reference range (26). The most recent Growth Hormone Research Society Guidelines (27) state that in the clinical context of multiple pituitary hormone deficits a very low serum IGF-1 (<2 SD below the mean) is sufficient evidence for the diagnosis of severe growth hormone deficiency that such patients may avoid a dynamic test of growth hormone reserve.

Most authorities accept that pharmacological stimulation of growth hormone release is the most practical and reproducible method of assessing growth hormone reserve. Hypoglycaemia is a powerful stimulus to growth hormone secretion and, over the years, the ITT has been the most frequently employed test in this regard. It has the advantage that ACTH reserve can be assessed simultaneously and, in experience hands, is a safe investigation provided the exclusion criteria outlined earlier are adhered to. The criterion for profound growth hormone deficiency is met if the peak growth hormone response to insulin-induced hypoglycaemia is 3 mcg/l or less (27). The marked variability in growth hormone assays makes comparison between centres difficult and must be borne in mind when applying consensus guidelines. Similarly, the endocrine physician should be alert to the confounding effect of obesity on growth hormone release which may lead to a false positive diagnosis of growth hormone deficiency (27).

Where the ITT is contraindicated, alternative provocative tests of growth hormone reserve include the glucagon, arginine+ GHRH, and arginine+ growth hormone-releasing peptide tests. It is important to appreciate that the combined tests (arginine+GHRH and arginine+GHRP) stimulate both the hypothalamus and pituitary, such that GHD due solely to hypothalamic disease may be missed, as direct stimulation of the pituitary will produce a reassuring result. This is particularly important in patients who have received cranial irradiation; in these patients the ITT shows greatest sensitivity and specificity in the first five years after treatment. If the peak GH during a combined stimulation test is normal during this period and GHD is clinically suspected then an ITT should be performed. Testing with clonidine, l-DOPA and arginine alone are of no value in diagnosing GHD in adults. Arginine alone may occasionally be used in non-obese adolescent patients.

Growth hormone secretagogue testing

In many patients with pituitary disease, growth hormone deficiency is secondary to lack of hypothalamic GHRH. Like other hypothalamic-releasing hormone tests, injection of GHRH tests the 'readily releasable' pool of pituitary hormone. Many patients with growth hormone deficiency due to pituitary tumours, hypothalamic disease, or radiotherapy have been shown to respond to GHRH administration, although fewer patients respond and the size of the response is less too than patients with isolated 'idiopathic' growth hormone deficiency. As new growth hormone secretagogue drugs are developed, it seems likely that GHRH testing will assume a more significant role in the assessment of the hypopituitary patient, particularly in units in which there is less experience and confidence in performing the ITT. They are discussed in more detail in Chapter 2.3.7 and reviewed in detail elsewhere (27).

Assessment of the pituitary–gonadal axis

Assessment of the pituitary–gonadal axis differs from other aspects of pituitary function testing. First, regular menstruation in a woman implies normal gonadotroph function and measurement of gonadotropins and oestradiol therefore add little to the clinical assessment. Associated ovulation is not necessarily implied by regular menstruation: measurement of luteal phase progesterone levels is required for the assessment of subfertility in a patient with pituitary disease and a regular cycle. Second, social and age-related factors may influence the need to correct any underlying gonadal deficiency in men and women. The avoidance of cardiovascular complications and loss of bone mineral density consequent on prolonged hypogonadism is obviously desirable, but must be set against the temporal relationship of normal physiology. For example, an 80-year-old patient with secondary hypogonadism is likely to feel differently about sex steroid replacement therapy than a patient of 30 years.

It is rare for tests other than basal measurements of gonadotropin hormones and sex steroid levels to be required for assessment of the pituitary–gonadal axis. Both oestradiol and testosterone bind to SHBG, such that simultaneous measurement of SHBG and gonadal steroid levels are required to assess 'free' (biologically active) levels of these hormones. Testosterone should be measured at 09.00 h, as levels show considerable diurnal variation. Oestradiol is best measured in the follicular phase of the menstrual cycle (if female patients are menstruating). Ovulation is assessed by measurement of progesterone in the luteal phase (days 18–25) of the cycle.

Dynamic tests are required only for the differential diagnosis of secondary gonadal failure but do not significantly alter clinical management. Previously, a combination of clomifene and luteinizing hormone-releasing hormone (LHRH) tests provided useful evidence in distinguishing hypothalamic from pituitary causes of secondary gonadal failure. However, such information has little clinical value in terms of therapy and newer, more sophisticated imaging techniques are able to distinguish these two groups of causes in the majority of cases. Central hypogonadism can be isolated, occur in the context of a hypothalamo-pituitary tumour or its treatment, or be the earliest sign of incipient panhypopituitarism. Isolated gonadotropin deficiency will either be congenital, as in Kallmann's syndrome and associated with delayed/absent pubertal development, or be acquired and secondary to systemic illness (AIDS), excessive exercise (long-distance runners) or psychological disturbance (anorexia nervosa). In all cases it is imperative to investigate pituitary function in detail.

Clomifene testing

This investigation has been used in the investigation of suspected gonadotropin deficiency. Clomifene citrate is a selective oestrogen receptor modulator (SERM) acting as a weak oestrogen-receptor antagonist at the hypothalamus and pituitary, and as an oestrogen agonist at the liver. In healthy subjects its antagonistic action at the hypothalamus stimulates gonadotropin-releasing hormone levels to rise, with consequent release of luteinizing hormone and FSH. The hepatic effect is to induce SHBG synthesis and a rise in measured total testosterone and oestradiol levels. Hence, such a rise may be misleading and does not necessarily indicate increased gonadotropin release. Clomifene should not be given to patients with liver disease because of its oestrogen-agonist effects. The test is also contraindicated in depression, because of the risk of mood disturbance, and patients should be warned of the risk of alteration of peripheral vision. In normal women, gonadotropin levels double by 10 days and menstruation usually accompanies a positive clomifene test in women. However, the test is of limited clinical value as the ability of medroxyprogesterone acetate to induce a menstrual bleed is highly predictive of the response to clomifene. A normal response to clomifene in a patient with amenorrhoea offers reassurance that the axis is intact and that the problem lies in the hypothalamus, but offers little indication of the aetiology. Patients with weight, exercise, and stress-induced amenorrhoea can have either a normal or absent response to clomifene, presumably indicative of the severity of the suppression of gonadotropin secretion.

Gonadotropin-releasing hormone testing

Gonadotropin-releasing hormone (LHRH) stimulates luteinizing hormone and FSH release from the pituitary in a dose-dependent manner between 25 and 100 μg. Following basal measurements of gonadotropins and injection of LHRH, samples for FSH and luteinizing hormone are taken according to a standard protocol and the results compared to a reference range. An absent response is indicated by a failure to rise above three times the within-assay coefficient of variation of the basal values. An impaired response is defined as a failure to rise to normal levels and an exaggerated response is seen when either the 20 or 60 min sample exceeds the normal range.

In a patient with secondary hypogonadism, a normal response to gonadotropin-releasing hormone implies that the pituitary gonadotrophs are capable of functioning normally and that hypogonadism is the result of understimulation by the hypothalamus. This in turn may be due to a hypothalamic lesion or disconnection of the pituitary from the hypothalamus by a functional pituitary stalk lesion. Although designed to stimulate pituitary gonadotrophs directly, the gonadotropin-releasing hormone test may also provide an index of hypothalamic function. Gonadotropin-releasing hormone is required for luteinizing hormone synthesis as well as its release, such that flat or subnormal responses may both be seen in hypothalamic disease if gonadotropin-releasing hormone deficiency is severe. Where gonadotropin-releasing hormone deficiency is relatively mild, the 'readily releasable pool' of gonadotropins may be normal or even increased, such that gonadotropin-releasing hormone injection produces an exaggerated response. These factors and the variability in the response to gonadotropin-releasing hormone among normal individuals means that the test is relatively seldom used in clinical practice.

Prolactin

A clinical syndrome associated with prolactin deficiency is not recognized and the clinical consequences of hyperprolactinaemia are discussed elsewhere. The principal value in serum prolactin measurement is as a guide to the aetiology of hypopituitarism. Prolactin physiology differs from that of other anterior pituitary hormones in that its secretion is principally under tonic inhibition by release of dopamine from the hypothalamus. Levels do not show significant diurnal variation and so tests other than basal measurements are very rarely required. Physiological stress and various medications that interfere with dopamine action, such as metoclopramide, prochlorperazine, and several antipsychotics, raise serum prolactin. TRH stimulates prolactin release, but provides no extra information compared to random serum prolactin measurements, on three separate occasions to minimize the risk of falsely elevated stress-induced hyperprolactinaemia.

Conclusion

Accurate assessment of anterior pituitary function requires a sound knowledge of its normal physiology together with careful integration of clinical and biochemical information. As discussed above, certain aspects of the optimum method of pituitary function testing, notably the assessment of ACTH reserve, are still disputed, with local circumstances and personal preference often dictating the final choice. Physicians are advised to acquaint themselves with their local laboratory reference ranges and never to allow a single hormonal measurement in a single patient on a single day to substitute for clinical awareness, particularly where an evolving endocrinopathy is anticipated, such as following pituitary irradiation. A reliable and safe strategy for the assessment of suspected hypopituitarism is shown in Box 2.3.4.1.

Box 2.3.4.1 Protocol for assessment of suspected hypopituitarism

New patients

- Basal investigations, at 7–9 a.m.: cortisol
- Serum
  - T_4, TSH
  - Prolactin
  - Luteinizing hormone, FSH, testosterone/oestradiol, SHBG
  - Insulin-like growth factor-1
  - Urine/plasma osmolality

If basal serum cortisol is >100 but <450 nmol/l and/or growth hormone deficiency is suspected, proceed to ITT. If there is an abnormality in any of the above tests, one should proceed to pituitary imaging.

At risk patients

In such patients (e.g. those who have received pituitary radiotherapy), pituitary function tests should be performed regularly in order to detect asymptomatic hypopituitarism, although there is a paucity of data on the optimum frequency with which this should be done. Our practice is to check thereafter basal pituitary function (07.00–09.00 h) every 2 years, with a dynamic test of ACTH reserve if the basal serum cortisol is less than 450 nmol/l. If patients exhibit the syndrome of growth hormone deficiency, then the dynamic test of choice will be the ITT. Growth hormone deficiency occurs early after radiotherapy and, once it has been proven, many physicians use sequential short Synacthen tests to document the subsequent evolution of ACTH deficiency. Note: data in this regard are scarce such that accurate, robust local reference ranges are essential.

References

1. Plumpton FS, Besser GM. The adrenocortical response to surgery and insulin-induced hypoglycaemia in corticosteroid-treated and normal subjects. *Br J Surg*, 1969; **56**: 216–19.
2. Mattingley D. A simple fluorimetric method for the estimation of free 11-hydroxycorticoids in human plasma. *J Clin Pathol*, 1962; **15**: 374–9.
3. Brien TG. Human corticosteroid binding globulin. *Clin Endocrinol*, 1981; **14**: 193–212.
4. Gashell SJ, Collins CJ, Thorne GC, Groom GV. External quality assessment of assays for cortisol in plasma: use of target data obtained by GC/mass spectrometry. *Clin Chem*, 1983; **29**: 862–7.
5. Hurel SJ, Thompson CJ, Watson MJ, Baylis PH, Kendall-Taylor P. The short synacthen and insulin stress tests in the assessment of the hypothalamic–pituitary–adrenal axis. *Clin Endocrinol* 1996; **44**: 141–6.
6. Clark PM, Neylon I, Raggatt PR, Sheppard MC, Stewart PM. Defining the normal cortisol response to the short synacthen test: implications for the investigation of hypothalamic–pituitary disorders. *Clin Endocrinol*, 1998; **49**: 287–92.
7. Pavord SR, Girach A, Price DE, Absalom SR, FalconerSmith J, Howlett TA. A retrospective audit of the combined pituitary function test, using the insulin stress test, TRH and GnRH in a district laboratory. *Clin Endocrinol*, 1992; **26**: 135–9.
8. Jones SL, Trainer PJ, Perry L, Wass JA, Besser GM, Grossman A. An audit of the insulin tolerance test in adult subjects in an acute investigation unit over one year. *Clin Endocrinol*, 1995; **42**: 101–2.
9. Greenwood FC, Landon J, Stamp TCB. The plasma sugar, free fatty acid, cortisol and growth hormone response to insulin. *J Clin Invest*, 1966; **4**: 429–36.
10. Vestergara P, Hoeck HC, Jakobsen PE, Laurber P. Reproducibility of growth hormone and cortisol response to the insulin tolerance test and the short ACTH test in normal adults. *Horm Metab Res*, 1997; **29**: 106–10.
11. Wood JB, Frankland AW, James VHT, Landon J. A rapid test of adrenocortical function. *Lancet*, 1965; i: 243–5.
12. Speckart PF, Nicolff JT, Bethune JE. Screening for adrenocortical insufficiency with cosyntropin (synthetic ACTH). *Arch Intern Med*, 1971; **128**: 761–3.
13. May ME, Carey RM. Rapid adrenocorticotropic hormone test in practice. *Am J Med*, 1985; **79**: 679–84.
14. Lindholm J, Kehlet H. Re-evaluation of the clinical value of the 30 min ACTH test in assessing hypothalamo–pituitary–adrenal function. *Clin Endocrinol*, 1987; **26**: 53–9.
15. Clayton RN. Short synacthen test versus insulin stress test for assessment of the hypothalamo–pituitary–adrenal axis: controversy revisited. *Clin Endocrinol*, 1996; **44**: 147–9.
16. Stewart PM, Corrie J, Seckl JR, Edwards CR, Padfield PL. A rational approach for assessing the hypothalamo–pituitary–adrenal axis. *Lancet*, 1988; **1**: 1208–10.
17. Streeton DHP, Anderson GH, Bonaventura MM. The potential for serious consequences from misinterpreting normal responses to the rapid adrenocorticotropin test. *J Clin Endocrinol Metab*, 1996; **81**: 285–90.
18. Darmon P, Dadoun F, Frachebios C, Velut JG, Boullu S, Dutour A, *et al.* On the meaning of the low-dose ACTH (1–24) tests to assess the functionality of the hypothalmic–pituitary–adrenal axis. *Eur J Endocrinol*, 1999; **140**: 51–5.
19. Abdu TAM, Elhadd TA, Neary R, Clayton RN. Comparison of low dose short synacthen test (1μg), conventional dose short synacthen test (250 mg) and insulin tolerance test for the assessment of the

hypothalamo–pituitary–adrenal axis in patients with pituitary disease. *J Clin Endocrinol Metab*, 1999; **84**: 838–43.
20. Tordjman K, Jaffe A, Grazas N, Apter C, Stern N. The role of low dose (1 μg) adrenocorticotrophin test in the evaluation of patients with pituitary diseases. *J Clin Endocrinol Metab*, 1995; **80**: 1301–5.
21. Streeten DHP. Shortcomings in the low-dose (1 μg) ATH test for the diagnosis of ACTH deficiency states. *J Clin Endocrinol Metab*, 1999; **84**: 835–7.
22. Littley MD, Gibson S, White A, Shalet SM. Comparison of the ACTH and cortisol responses to provocative testing with glucagon and insulin hypoglycaemia in normal subjects. *Clin Endocrinol*, 1989; **31**: 527–33.
23. Liddle GW, Estep HL, Hendall JW, Wiliams WC, Townes AW. Clinical application of a new test of pituitary reserve. *J Clin Endocrinol Metab*, 1959; **19**: 875–94.
24. Spiger M, Jubiz W, Meidle W, West CD, Tylor FJ. Single-dose metyrapone test. *Arch Intern Med*, 1975; **135**: 698–700.
25. Shalet SM, Toogood A, Rahim A, Brennan BMD. The Diagnosis of GH deficiency in children and adults. *Endocr Rev*, 1998; **19**: 203–23.
26. Hoffman DM, O'Sullivan AJ, Baxter RC, Ho KY. Diagnosis of growth hormone deficiency in adults. *Lancet*, 1994; **343**: 1064–8.
27. Ho KYY. Consensus guidelines for the diagnosis and treatment of adults with growth hormone deficiency II. *Eur J Endocrinol*, 2007; **157**: 695–700.
28. Trainer PJ, Besser GM. *The Bart's Endocrine Protocols*. Edinburgh: Churchill Livingstone: 1995.
29. Consensus Statement of a Working Party. *Pituitary Tumours*: Recommendations for service provision, guidelines for management of patients. London: Royal College of Physicians, 1997.

2.3.5 Imaging of the pituitary

J.V. Byrne

Imaging methods

MRI is the optimum method of imaging the pituitary of patients with suspected pituitary disease though CT is an acceptable alternative. The advantages of MRI are: direct multiplanar scanning, lack of ionizing radiation, and good anatomical tissue discrimination. Imaging the pituitary gland and hypothalamus is best performed in the sagittal and coronal planes because they show the relationships between gland and adjacent structures. Scanning in the axial plane alone is a poor technique for demonstrating vertical relationships between structures lying between the floor of the third ventricle and sella turcica. Computer-generated three-dimensional (3D) reconstructions of axially acquired data (by MR or CT) and can be viewed in any plane can compensate but usually direct scanning gives better resolution images.

The disadvantage of MRI in this situation is its relative insensitivity to pathological calcification, and lack of signal from corticated bone. CT or even plain film radiography may be required to demonstrate or exclude pathological calcification. In this respect CT is far more sensitive than plain film radiography and the only remaining role for the latter in pituitary imaging, is to exclude metallic implants that might be contraindications to MRI. For surgical planning and intraoperative guidance some surgeons prefer the level of bony detail that 3D CT images provide (1). Conventional catheter angiography is rarely indicated because both MR and CT angiography (MRA, CTA) are capable of identifying the positions of the intracavernous and supraclinoid carotid arteries and differentiate pituitary mass lesions from aneurysms. Very rarely the diagnoses of a substantially thrombosed aneurysm requires intra-arterial digital subtraction angiography. Angiography continues to have a role during catheter navigation for venous sampling in patients being investigated for causes of Cushing's syndrome.

MRI techniques

Various technical refinements to pituitary MRI have been advocated but given the enormous number of potentially useful MRI sequence protocols', basic scanning methods are remarkably similar in different centres. It is generally agreed that the structures of the sella region are best imaged using T_1-weighted sequences which are constructed to produce images with dark cerebrospinal fluid (CSF), grey brain and white fat. Corticated bone returns low signal and appears dark but bone marrow fat returns high signal and therefore appears white. The pituitary gland returns signal similar to cerebral white matter and flowing blood little or no signal and therefore is black. The latter is the basis for MRA (see Fig. 2.3.5.1).

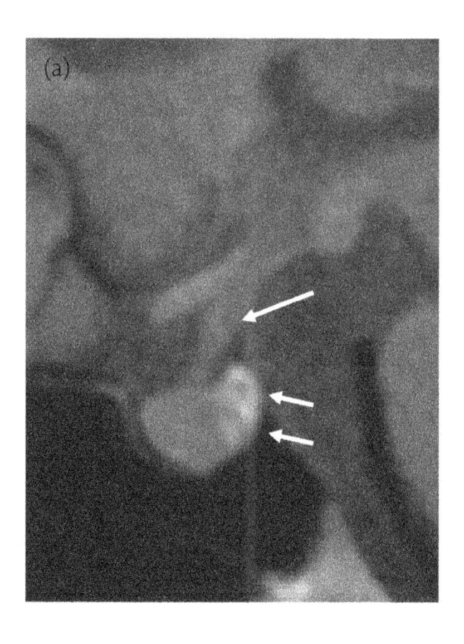

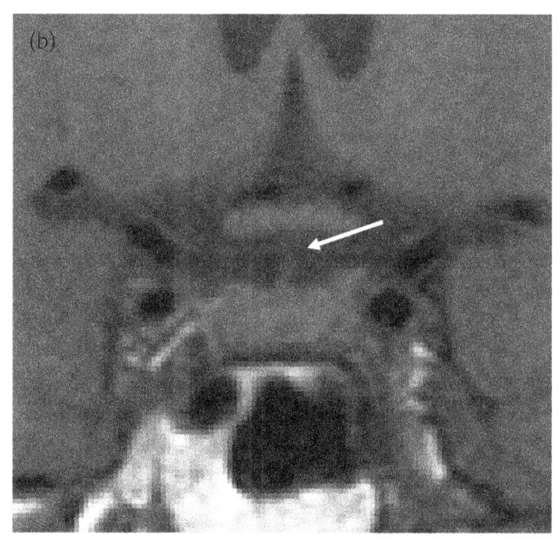

Fig. 2.3.5.1 (a) Sagittal and (b) coronal T_1-weighted MR images showing the normal pituitary gland and stalk (arrow). In the sagittal view the posterior lobe returns hyperintense signal at the site of antidiuretic hormone storage (short arrows).

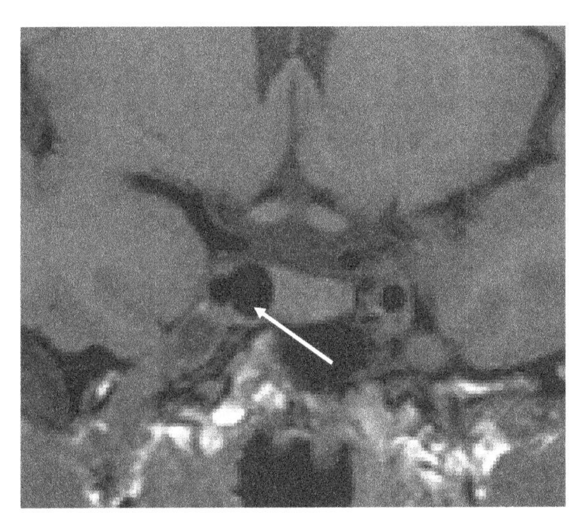

Fig. 2.3.5.2 Sagittal MR sequence showing a small aneurysm of the right internal carotid artery which points medially and extends into the sella (arrow). Flowing blood does not return signal and so appears black on MRI. Note the how the parent and contralateral carotid arteries also appear black on this sequence.

The anatomical relationships of the infundibulum of the hypophysis and hypothalamus are easily identified. Using T_1-weighted sequences the nuclei of the hypothalamus cannot usually be distinguished. Areas of bright signal in the stalk and posterior lobe are evident in up to 50% of T_1-weighted scans performed in patients without endocrine diseases. The observed frequency declines with increasing age (2) and without this chemical difference in magnetic property the anterior and posterior lobes of the gland cannot be readily distinguished. The effect identifies the site of antidiuretic hormone storage (Fig. 2.3.5.2), and has been variously ascribed to vasopressin, neurophysin, or phospholipid vesicles in the neurohypophysis (3).

The power of MRI to resolve different structures depends on the signal-to-noise ratio (SNR) of the acquired signal. A high SNR is required to detect small abnormalities and small anatomical structures. Simply increasing the matrix size, i.e. the number of pixel (or voxel) elements will not improve the SNR though decreasing the pixel size will improve the spatial resolution of the image. To improve the SNR and spatial resolution it is necessary to increase the magnet gradient strengths and to acquire more data by lengthening the scan time (3). Pituitary MRI is therefore best performance in high field strength imagers using longer echo time (TE) sequences (4). In practice T_1-weighted spin echo sequences are performed with repetition times (TR) of 500–600 ms, echo times (TE) of 15 ms and two or more excitations. Scanning is performed in coronal and sagittal planes using a minimum matrix size 256 × 256, to give 3 mm thick contiguous slices. Typically scanning takes 5–8 min at 1.5 T for each sequence. An alternative approach is to use a T_1-weighted gradient echo technique with a 3D Fourier synthesis so that subsequent computer manipulation allows the imaged sample to be viewed in any plane and the reader can review and clarify any suspicious areas. Some centres perform complementary T_2-weighted sequences in order to use the high signal returned from the CSF to outline structures in the chiasmatic and other basal cisterns and to assess signal return from tumours (Fig. 2.3.5.3).

The IV administration of paramagnetic agents such as gadolinium, which are taken up by the gland and surrounding tissues is useful but its routine use is controversial. These agents, like radiographic contrast media used in CT scanning, do not cross the blood–brain barrier. The pituitary gland and stalk therefore enhance and appear whiter on T_1-weighted images. The hypothalamus and optic chiasm do not enhance if the blood–brain barrier is intact. Blood vessels, meninges and mucosa of the paranasal sinuses will enhance. The role of gadolinium-enhanced MRI in the investigation of different pathologies will be considered below. Dynamic MRI has been used to study the timing of intravenously administered gadolinium uptake by the pituitary gland. Obtaining rapid single slice images, Sakamoto *et al.* (5) demonstrated that the stalk and posterior lobe enhanced 20 s after an intravenous injection and that this extended into the anterior portion of the gland within 80 s. Using this technique can increase the detection rate of microadenomas and is used in patients with suspected Cushing's disease and apparently normal glands on conventional scanning (6).

CT scanning techniques

Apart from its complementary role in detecting pathological calcification, CT scanning remains the primary imaging modality for the small proportion of patients who are unable to undergo MRI. Patients who are extremely claustrophobic, have cardiac pacemakers or other implants such as intracranial aneurysms clips and traumatic metallic fragments, which are sensitive to the effects of the magnetic field, cannot be scanned. CT is then used and multislice imagers with helical scanning are able to acquire axial images

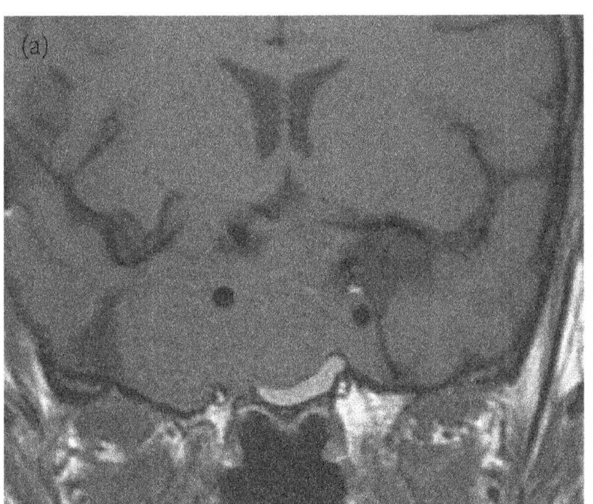

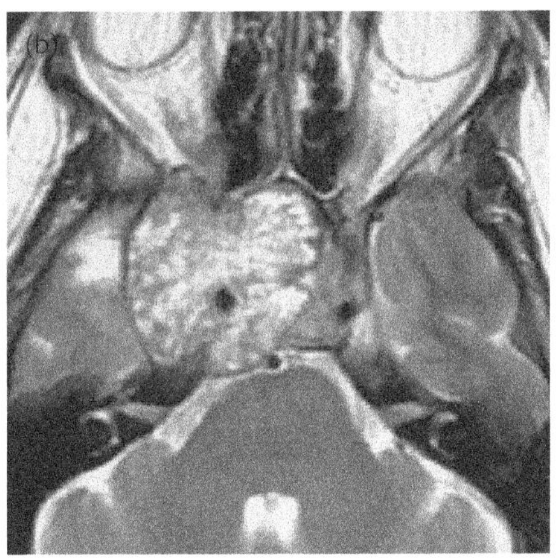

Fig. 2.3.5.3 (a) Coronal T_1-weighted and (b) axial T_2-weighted MR images showing a macroadenoma invading the right cavernous sinus. The tumour is also extending into the chiasmatic cistern but not the left cavernous sinus. Note how the tumour surrounds the right carotid artery and returns a mixed signal on the T_2-weighted sequence.

in less than a minute. These are displayed in 2D or 3D views by computer post processing. Currently available scanners generally produce images of sufficient quality to demonstrate sella anatomy on unenhanced images but intravenous injection of iodinated contrast media is generally used to improve tissue contrast. It is taken up by the hypophysis in the same way as the MRI contrast agent, gadolinium. Thus microadenomas, craniopharyngiomas, and tumours of the hypothalamus enhance and are better delineated but demonstration of microadenomas within a morphologically normal pituitary depends on differential uptake rates.

CT, unlike MRI, cannot demonstrate blood vessels without the injection of contrast agents. CTA is performed during 'first-pass' after an intravenous bolus injection of radiographic contrast media. It requires accurate timing to differentiate arteries and veins, particularly within the cavernous sinus and occasionally CTA may not give an accurate assessment of the position of the carotid arteries. Preoperative digital subtraction angiography may then be necessary and angiography should always be performed when CT raises the possibility of an aneurysm and MRA is contraindicated.

Nuclear isotope imaging techniques

Nuclear medicine techniques, such as positron emission tomography (PET) or single-photon emission tomography (SPECT), have been used to obtain *in vivo* characterization of tissue. The presence of octreotide-binding somatostatin receptors in nonfunctioning adenomas cause them to take up ^{111}In-DTPA-octreotide but meningiomas may also express somatostatin receptors and take up somatostatin receptor-specific isotopes (7). However tracers that bind to the enzyme monoamino-oxidase β have been used to differentiate meningioma from pituitary adenoma using PET and more recently a D_2 dopamine receptor specific isotope [^{18}F]fluoroethyl-spiperone has been reported to differentiate nonfunctioning adenomas from craniopharyngioma and meningioma (8). PET using tracers such as [^{18}F]fluorodeoxyglucose and [^{11}C]methionine can be used to study rates of glucose metabolism and protein synthesis. It can be used to assess tumours after treatment by differentiating viable tumour from scar tissue and monitoring pharmacological treatments. In the UK, the current availability of scanners limits the use of PET to selected patients and research.

Pituitary macroadenoma

Adenomas larger than 1 cm in maximum diameter are conventionally classified as macroadenomas irrespective of their endocrine characteristics. Imaging for diagnosis is performed to demonstrate the cause of an endocrine disturbance or for symptoms and signs of pituitary region pathology, e.g. visual loss. It is therefore directed at identifying the tumour and its extent. In cases of nonfunctioning adenoma the differential diagnosis includes other causes of pituitary region masses (see below). Once a macroadenoma is diagnosed the role of imaging is to localize the tumour for surgical or radiotherapy planning and to monitor the effects of therapy.

The imaging features of macroadenomas are generally similar for functioning and nonfunctioning pituitary tumours. They may extend well beyond the pituitary fossa but will cause expansion of the fossa as evidence of their origin (Fig. 2.3.5.4). On CT, solid tumours are isodense or hypodense relative to brain tissue and show variable patterns of enhancement after radiographic contrast media administration, on MRI signal return is typically

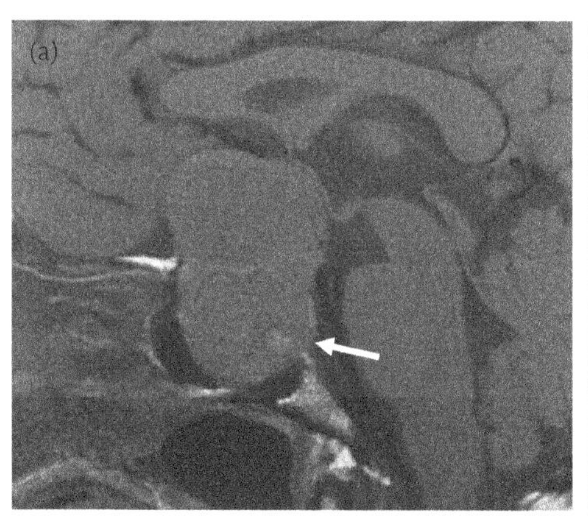

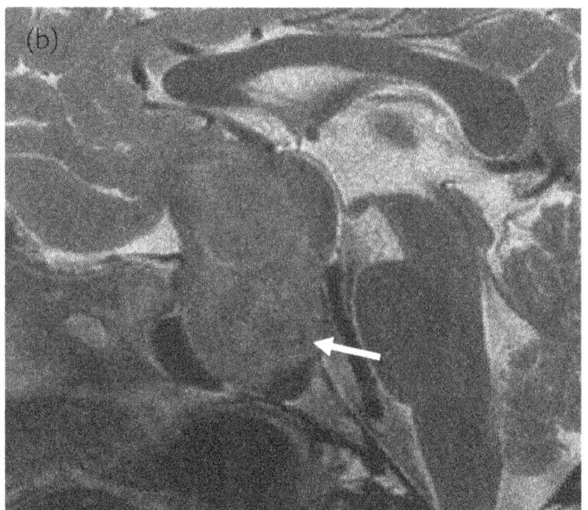

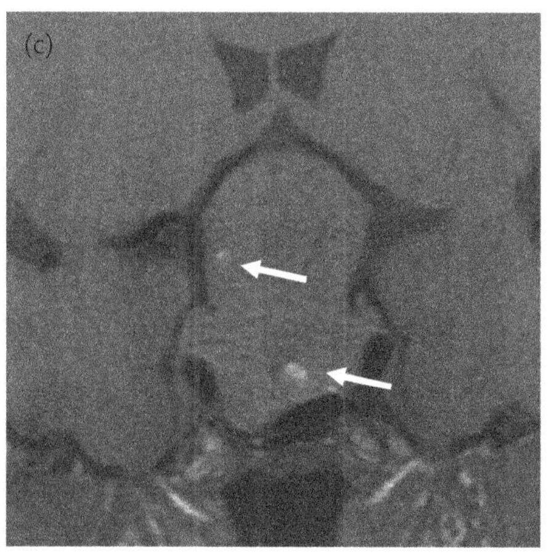

Fig. 2.3.5.4 (a) Sagittal and (c) coronal T_1-weighted and sagittal T_1-weighted MR images showing a macroadenoma. The tumour had resulted in expansion of the sella and is extending into the chiasmatic cistern. The optic chiasm is so compressed that it cannot be seem. Within the solid tumour are small foci of bright signal on the T_1-weighted sequences (a,c), which appear darker that the rest of the tumour on the T_2-weighted sequence (b). These represent areas of necrosis and haemorrhage (arrows).

similar to that of brain on both T_1- and T_2-weighted sequences (9). Gadolinium administration causes signal change due to shortening of the recovery time and brightening of tumour and gland. This is best demonstrated on T_1-weighted sequences and usually normal gland enhances more avidly than tumour aiding its localization. Cysts or areas of necrosis cause foci of moderate hypointensity on T_1-weighted and hyperintensity on T_1-weighted sequences with heterogeneous enhancement after gadolinium administration.

Signal due to haemorrhage may produce a more specific pattern but these are complex because the magnetic effects of iron in haemoglobin, changes as the molecule degrades after red blood cell lysis. In general, these are best appreciated on T_1-weighted MRI since within days of haemorrhage increased concentrations of methaemoglobin within areas of haemorrhage causes T_1 recovery time shortening and bright signal on this sequence. The appearance is therefore similar to that seen after gadolinium administration and may only be recognized if unenhanced imaging is performed. In the acute period after haemorrhage (<3 days) MR changes are nonspecific but acute haemorrhage is hyperdense on CT. Thereafter methaemoglobin forms which has a characteristic signal and can persist for weeks so that subacute and chronic haemorrhage is more easily identified on T_1-weighted MRI. It is due to shortening of the T_1 signal recovery time and termed a paramagnetic effect. It is similar to the signal returned by fat and some tumour products secreted by lesions such as craniopharyngiomas. Physiological bright or hyperintense signal on T_1-weighted sequences can be seen in the posterior lobe and stalk, as described above. This property of phospholipids is also described as paramagnetic and is due to similar shortening of T_1 recovery time. Less intense and smaller areas of bright signal are not uncommon in tumours of patients without a history suggestive of apoplexy. These asymptomatic haemorrhages have been confirmed surgically in a proportion of patients. The scan appearances of tumours in patients presenting acutely with pituitary apoplexy will reflect the relative extent of haemorrhage or necrosis, with gadolinium enhancement evident at the margins of necrotic areas (10) (see Fig. 2.3.5.4).

There have been attempts to correlate tumour appearances on imaging with hormonal activity. Imaging features such as tumour size, evidence of local invasion, CT density, and MR signal have been correlated with hormone production (9). Correlations have thus been based on general imaging features such as extreme size in gonadotroph adenomas and the presence of hypointense foci (probably due to haemorrhage or necrosis) on T_2-weighted scans in growth hormone-secreting tumours. But MR, although capable of measuring fundamental chemical characteristics does not give a hormone-specific image (11). Its contribution to patient management is currently to accurately delineate tumour extent and effect on adjacent structures. The preoperative MRI appearances are helpful in directing the surgeon to likely areas of local invasion. Administration of gadolinium aids the identification of normal pituitary gland from tumour. Tumour invasion of the cavernous sinus, sphenoid bone, and extension into the chiasmatic cistern are evident on MRI. Such behaviour has been identified surgically and histologically in all tumour types. Scotti *et al.* studied the MRI features useful in the preoperative diagnosis of cavernous sinus invasion. Encasement of the carotid artery was the most specific sign of cavernous sinus invasion. Asymmetry of the cavernous sinuses, displacement of the lateral wall and of the carotid artery were inconsistent features of invasion. An indistinct medial sinus wall was an unreliable feature, being common in controls. Intraoperative MRI is being developed for determining the completeness of transsphenoidal resections but because magnets of low field strengths have to be used, image quality remains a concern (12).

After surgery, the timing of follow-up scans is important since early postsurgical changes due to local swelling (in the first 1–2 weeks) and surgical packing materials, used in the transsphenoidal exposure, may be confused with remnant tumour (13). Gelfoam packing material returns hypointense or hyperintense signal and enhances on early postoperative MRI after gadolinium. Its reabsorption takes 4–15 months. Biological packing material returns mixed signal with fat being hyperintense and muscle isointense on T_1-weighted MRI. Re-alignment of the normal pituitary gland and reabsorption of packing material is usually evident on follow-up scans at 3 months. Early scanning is therefore only useful to investigate possible surgical complications and scanning to identify residual tumour is best delayed for at least 3 months.

Demonstration of tumour regression or recurrence relies on comparisons between follow-up scans. The protocols for postoperative follow-up imaging involves a baseline study obtained 3 months after hypophysectomy followed by interval MRI according to tumour type (usually annually for 5 years). More frequent scans are obtained if the patient's visual fields change or histological examination of the resected tumour suggests local invasion. Patients treated medically for functional macroadenomas are also monitored by serial imaging, in combination with biochemical and clinical follow-up assessments. A reduction in the size of prolactin-secreting macroadenomas after treatment with dopamine agonists may be accompanied by haemorrhage and therefore changes in signal returned by the tumour on MRI (14). Growth hormone-secreting tumours may also shrink in response to treatment with somatostatin analogues but this is less consistent and changes of necrosis or haemorrhage are infrequent. Reductions in tumour size can be demonstrated within weeks but continued shrinkage has been documented up to 3 years after starting treatment. Early follow-up imaging is therefore useful to document tumour response. A baseline study is obtained when the patient starts treatment and is then repeated 3 and 12 months later. Subsequent imaging is performed in regard to the response to therapy and dictated by the clinical and biochemical examinations.

Microadenomas

The demonstration of pituitary microadenoma remains a major diagnostic challenge for pituitary imaging. To identify adenomas less than 10 mm in size demands the highest standards of technique and interpretation. In most patients the presence of a microadenoma is assumed from biochemical testing and imaging is undertaken to confirm an intrasellar source and to guide its transsphenoidal excision. MRI is superior to CT for both diagnosis and localization (15) of microadenomas, since they show little inherent contrast to normal pituitary tissue on CT and scanning require injection of intravenous radiographic contrast agents to demonstrate nonenhancement of the microadenoma against a background of normal gland enhancement (Fig. 2.3.5.5). On MRI, microadenomas are typically spherical or oval in shape and return signal hypointense relative to normal anterior lobe on T_1-weighted and hyperintense on T_2-weighted sequences. Prolactinomas usually appear bright on T_2-weighted sequences, whereas growth

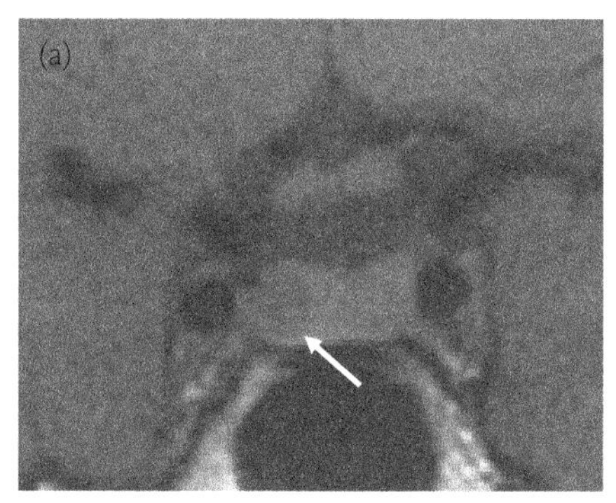

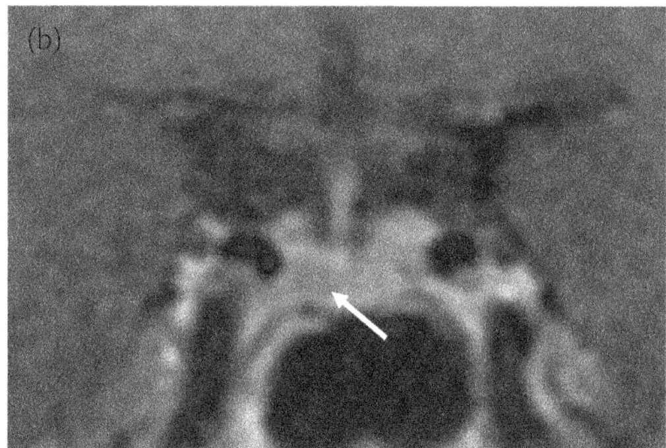

Fig. 2.3.5.5 Coronal (a) T_1-weighted and (b) T_1-weighted gadolinium-enhanced MR images showing marked enhancement of the normal sized gland after gadolinium administration. There is a microadenoma (arrows) in the right side of the gland. This enhances less avidly than the gland and so appears less bright.

hormone-secreting tumours are more likely to be isointense or hypointense on T_2-weighted sequences (16).

The need for high precision scanning has stimulated research to develop better MRI techniques. Most centres perform scans in the coronal and sagittal planes, initially without gadolinium enhancement. The coronal plane is best and typical parameters for a T_1-weighted spin echo sequence are TR 500 ms, TE 25 ms, 3 mm contiguous slice thickness with four excitations, which requires 8–9 min scan time. A 3D volume scan has the theoretical advantage of allowing postprocessing of images in different planes, higher resolutions and better SNRs but adds to the overall scan time. Techniques such as 3D-SPGR and 3D-FLASH have demonstrated the utility of this approach. The value of T_1-weighted sequences with IV gadolinium enhancement is limited by the relatively poor uptake of gadolinium by adenomas. So after gadolinium administration, microadenomas are usually evident as hypointense lesions within an enhancing gland. If the tumour is very small the gland enhancement may mask its relative hypointensity and use of half-dose (0.05 mmol/kg) gadolinium and delayed scanning techniques are performed to improve detection rates (16). Simply increasing the magnetic field strength and the SNR of the scan does not appear to solve the problem (17).

An alternative approach to improve microadenoma detection rates is dynamic MRI. This technique employs rapid sequential imaging to show temporal differences in gadolinium uptake between adenoma and normal gland. In this way, microadenomas which enhance later than the surrounding normal gland can be identified. Early studies showed that normal pituitary enhanced before adenomas, and using faster acquisition times (5–10 s per image) Yuh *et al.* found that macroadenoma enhanced at the same time as the posterior lobe and before the anterior lobe suggesting that they have a direct blood supply (18). Dynamic scanning with various fast imaging techniques have been used to identify microadenomas not detected on scanning with conventional enhancement protocols but there is an increased rate of false positives (19). The sensitivity of nonenhanced high-resolution MRI for pituitary microadenoma is in the order of 60–80%. Conventional scanning with contrast enhancement detects 5–10% more lesions and dynamic scanning a further 5–10% of lesions (20). Detection rate can thus be improved but at the expense of a higher rate of false-positive results. The problems associated with imaging at this level are both technical and biological. Technically dynamic MRI demands the maximum of humans and machines and both can be frustrated by the occurrence of small coincidental pituitary lesions, the so-called incidentalomas. Their frequency is difficult to gauge from the literature but Chong *et al.* found focal hypointensities in the pituitary glands of 38% of normal volunteers (21). That such 'lesions' exist, whatever their incidence, means that we are unlikely to ever achieve 100% specificity rates on imaging alone.

Patients with Cushing's syndrome and negative imaging may be further investigated by the venous effluent of the pituitary to differentiate Cushing's disease from ectopic sources of adrenocorticotropic hormone (22). Simultaneous bilateral sampling after stimulation with corticotropin-releasing hormone is highly accurate but the test is invasive and carries a small risk of neurological complications. The technique is reserved for patients with normal pituitary imaging but the reader should appreciate that the extent to which imaging is pursued in order to exclude a microadenoma varies from centre to centre (19).

Other tumours of the suprasellar and parasellar regions

The preoperative differentiation of pituitary adenomas from other causes of sellar and parasellar tumours relies on imaging. The most common problem in practice, is to distinguish nonfunctioning pituitary macroadenomas from craniopharyngiomas, meningioma, and rarer causes of tumour in this region. Clinical symptoms and signs are usually unhelpful, with the exceptions of diabetes insipidus, which suggests craniopharyngioma and precocious puberty which suggests a primary hypothalamic lesion. There is a wide gamut of pathologies that may simulate nonfunctioning pituitary tumour and the position of mass lesions, relative to the optic chiasm, is a useful way of refining the differential diagnosis.

Lesions arising above optic chiasm

Lesions that arise above the chiasm include ependymoma, craniopharyngioma, haemangioblastoma, glioma (usually astrocytoma), hamartoma of the hypothalamus and lipoma. Ependymoma and haemangioblastoma and rarely craniopharyngioma may arise within the anterior part of the third ventricle (Fig. 2.3.5.6). Involvement of the hypothalamus by hamartomas, glioma, teratoma, or lipoma causes precocious puberty. Local pressure effects from optic chiasm tumour or an arachnoid cyst may also cause precocious puberty. In children with precocious puberty, hypothalamic hamartoma will be the cause in a third of cases though paradoxically larger hamartomas are less likely to cause this endocrine disturbance. Unlike other tumours in the region of the hypothalamus, hamartomas are isodense on CT and isointense on MRI relative to grey matter (see Fig. 2.3.5.6). They also, neither calcify nor enhance after administration of IV contrast media and thereby can usually be distinguished from craniopharyngioma and glioma.

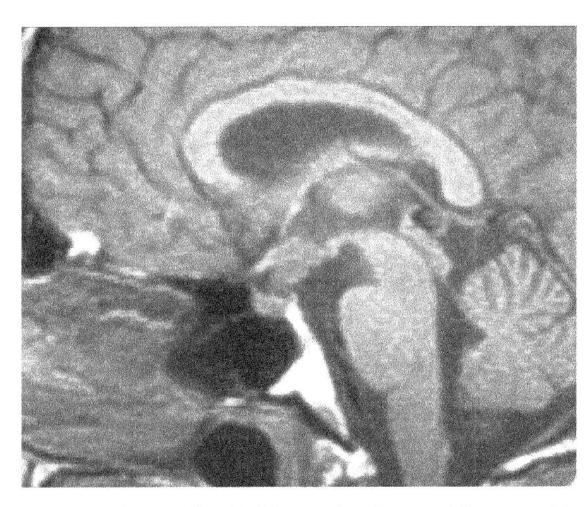

Fig. 2.3.5.6 Sagittal T_1-weighted MR image showing a nodular mass arising from the floor of the third ventricle. The lesion has the typical appearance of a hamartoma being isointense with brain.

Lesions arising below optic chiasm

The optic chiasm will be depressed by lesions arising in the floors of the third ventricle but elevated by suprasellar extension of intrasellar or parasellar tumours. The latter include meningioma, aneurysm, schwannoma (particularly of the trigeminal nerve), lymphoma, metastases, and tumours arising in bone. These lesions should be considered in the differential diagnosis of pituitary macroadenomas as well as the rare tumours of the neurohypophysis: pilocystic astrocytoma and granular cell tumour or choristoma. Imaging must distinguish intracranial aneurysm and the possibility of this diagnosis was, prior to MRI, an indication for preoperative intra-arterial angiography (IA-DSA). Blood flow in an aneurysm sac should be evident on MRI, which can be supplemented by MR or CT angiography. However if doubt remains, and rarely is this the case, intra-arterial angiography should be performed. Meningioma in this region may be parasellar and invade the cavernous sinus or arises from the tuberculum sellae. CT may show calcification and hyperostosis of bone but MRI is best at defining tumour extent. Meningiomas typically enhance homogeneously after gadolinium administration. Tumour arising in the sphenoid bone and clivus, such as chordoma, giant cell tumour and chondrosarcoma, or carcinomas arising in the nasopharynx, are associated with bone destruction, calcification, and a variable degree of enhancement. They may simulate bone invasion by pituitary macroadenoma. Imaging by both CT and MRI is helpful, since the former will demonstrate bone erosion and the latter the effects of the tumour on adjacent tissues (Fig. 2.3.5.7). Intrasellar or suprasellar metastases should always be considered in the differential diagnosis since their CT and MRI appearance is variable and they can be indistinguishable on imaging from other tumour types.

Lesions arising in the chiasmatic cistern

Finally, tumours may arise in the chiasmatic cistern and simulate suprasellar extension of a macroadenoma. The differential diagnosis includes: optic nerve glioma, meningioma, craniopharyngioma (Fig. 2.3.5.8), aneurysm, and metastasis. Again MRI has made a substantial contribution to refining the preoperative diagnosis in this region. Its key attribute lies in its ability to identify the anterior optic pathway and thereby distinguish optic nerve glioma from extra-axial tumour. This largely depends on using T_1-weighted coronal images to follow the pathway from the optic nerves to the tracts. Sumida *et al.* found that the optic nerves, chiasm, and tracts could be visualized in over 84% of patients with pituitary adenoma, craniopharyngioma, or Rathke's cleft cyst (23) (Fig. 2.3.5.9). The chiasm and tracts could be identified in 85% of 14 patients with meningioma but in only 50% were the optic nerves visible,

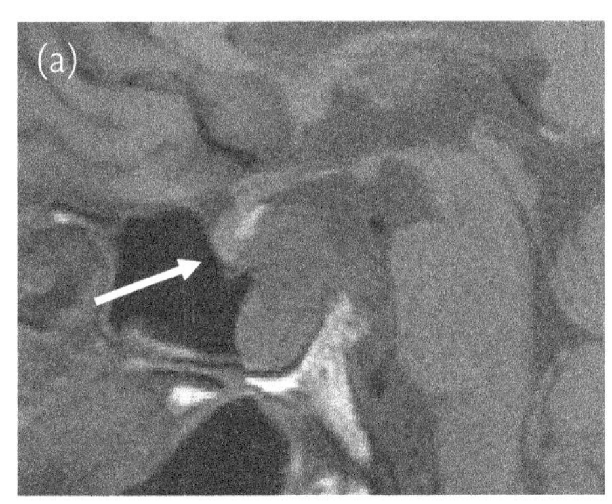

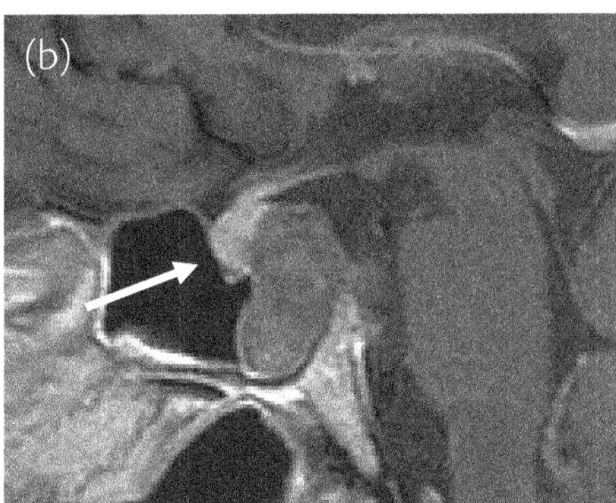

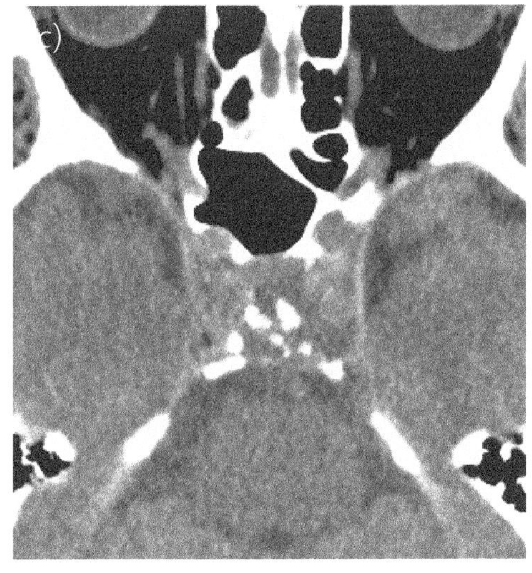

Fig. 2.3.5.7 Chordoma arising in the sphenoid bone. Sagittal (a) T_1-weighted and (b) T_1-weighted gadolinium-enhanced, and (c) axial CT showing a well-defined calcified tumour elevating and displacing the pituitary gland (arrows) anteriorly. Note how the gland enhances but there is no enhancement of the tumour.

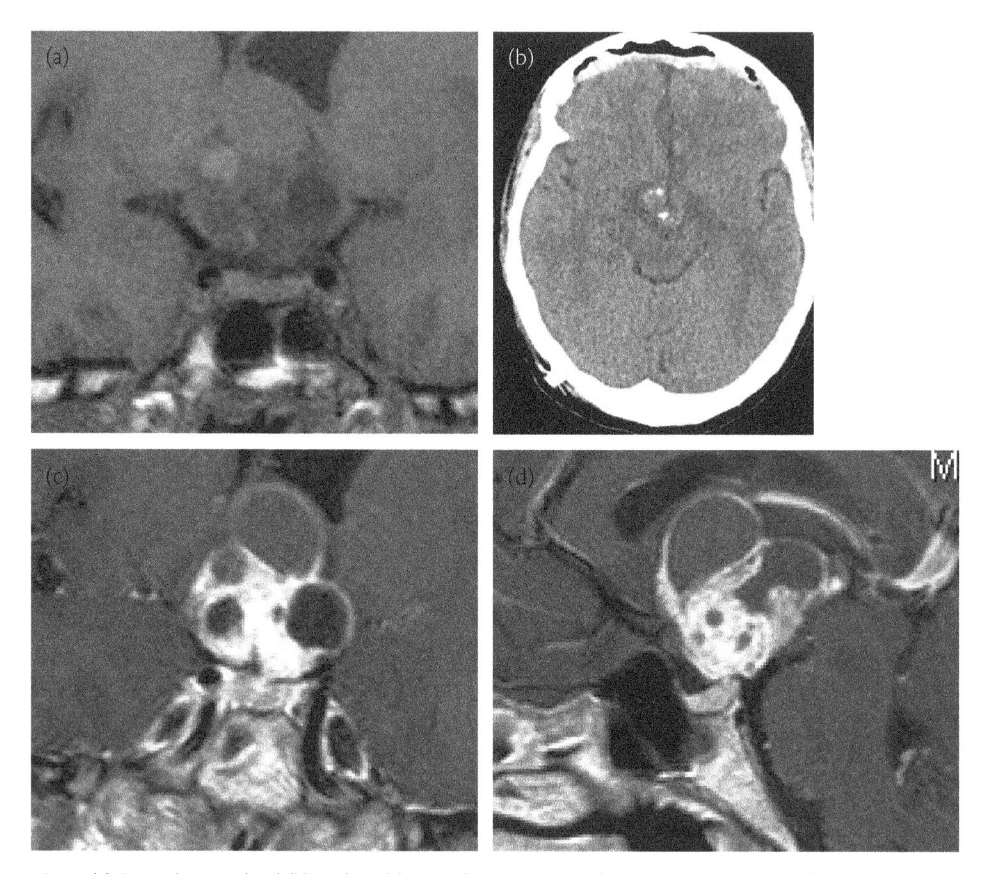

Fig. 2.3.5.8 Craniopharyngioma: (a) Coronal T_1-weighted, (b) axial CT, (c) coronal T_1-weighted gadolinium-enhanced, and (d) sagittal MR image. The imaging appearances of craniopharyngioma depend on how much of the tumour is cystic and how much solid. Typically tumours have a relatively circumscribed outline; cystic areas do not enhance but they may be septated with thick enhancing walls whereas solid elements do enhance. Calcification patterns vary from solid lumps to popcorn-like foci or less commonly an eggshell pattern lining the wall of a cyst. In addition to calcification these tumours may contain paramagnetic substances which, like gadolinium enhancement, appear bright on T_1-weighted MR images. Craniopharyngioma cysts contain variously, cholesterol, triglycerides, methaemoglobin, and desquamated epithelium. High concentrations of protein or methaemoglobin affect the MR signal and produce this characteristic T_1-weighted hyperintensity of a paramagnetic substance, as evident in one of the cystic components in (a). Imaging protocols therefore need to include both CT and MR scanning, since the former is the more sensitive means of detecting calcification. Craniopharyngiomas on CT are typically of mixed alternative with or without calcification. Contrast enhancement with gadolinium improves tumour definition from normal structures. The signal of solid tumour is isointense or hypointense relative to brain on precontrast T_1-weighted sequences and enhances after gadolinium administration. On T_1-weighted sequences it is usually of mixed hypo or hyperintensity. Larger areas of calcification are usually hypointense on both T_1- and T_2-weighted sequences. Cysts are hyperintense on T_2-weighted and hypointense on T_1-weighted sequences but if they contain paramagnetic substances, particularly breakdown products of haemoglobin, this pattern will be reversed or they may appear hyperintense on both T_2-weighted and T_1-weighted sequences.

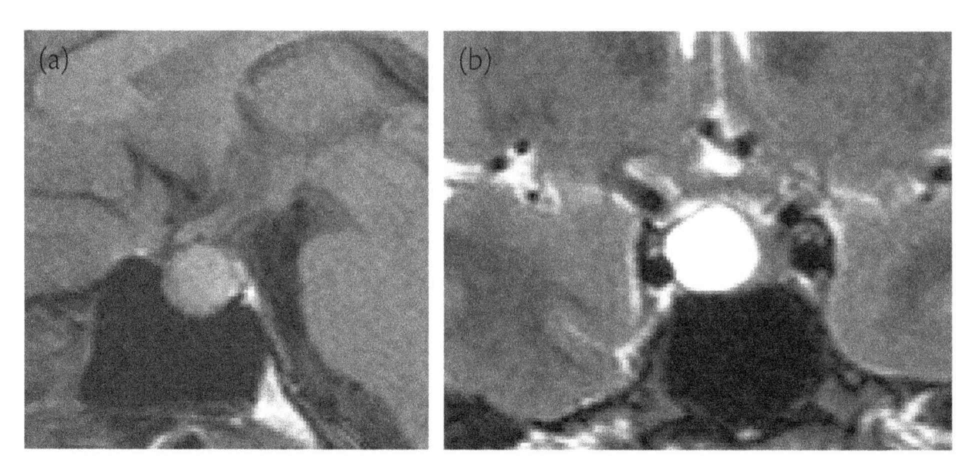

Fig. 2.3.5.9 Rathke's cleft cyst: (a) sagittal T_1-weighted and (b) coronal T_2-weighted MR images showing a cyst in the right side of the sella. Symptomatic Rathke's cleft cysts are pathological enlargements of remnant of Rathke's pouch and typically arise between the two lobes of the pituitary. They are lined by cuboidal or columnar epithelium and contain a variety of fluid types with differing magnetic properties. On MRI, the signal returned is variable; it may follow that of cerebrospinal fluid (i.e. hypointense on T_1-weighted and hyperintense on T_2-weighted sequences) or have signal characteristic of a protein-rich fluid (i.e. hyperintense on both T_1- and T_2-weighted sequences) or that of altered haemorrhage (i.e. hyperintense on T_1-weighted and hypointense on T_2-weighted sequences). Although the cyst wall does not usually enhance, intravenous administration of gadolinium is useful in order to exclude craniopharyngioma and to show the position of the normal pituitary (24). The CT appearance is typically of a noncalcified intrasellar cystic mass but showing that a lesion is not calcified is helpful in distinguishing from a craniopharyngioma. Cysts in atypical locations may make differentiation from an arachnoid cyst of the chiasmatic cistern (which also do not enhance) difficult. Rarely, they are found in the nasopharynx associated with persistent remnants of the craniopharyngeal duct. Another atypical feature of these cysts is the occasional finding of a central hypointense or isointense focus within the cyst. This is presumed to be due to desquamatized epithelium forming a 'waxy nodule' (25).

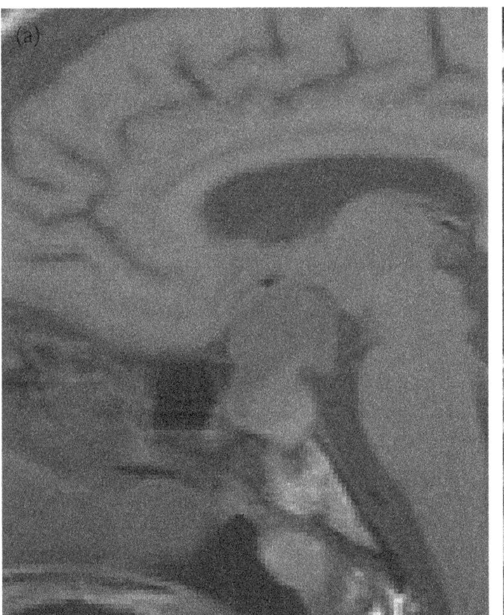

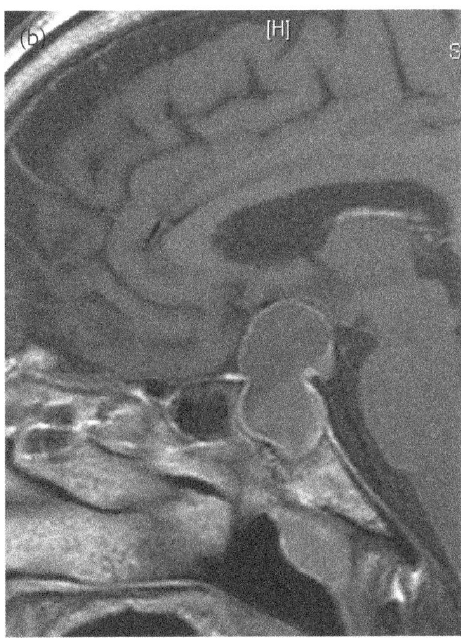

Fig. 2.3.5.10 Craniopharyngioma of adamantinous type. Craniopharyngioma arises from remnants of Rathke's pouch. The peak age at diagnosis is 5–15 years with a second peak in late middle age (55–75 years). This bimodal age distribution of incidence has been linked to histological tumour variants: an adamantinous type being commoner in children and young adults and a squamous-papillary type in older patients (26). Approximately 50% of patients present under the age of 20 years and calcification is commoner in younger patients; being demonstrable in 70% of tumours. Tumour usually are found above the sella, with 5% purely intrasellar, 20% purely suprasellar, and 75% both intrasellar and extrasellar. There have been attempts to correlate the heterogeneous MR images with the two histological variants (27). The adamantinous types were either mixed solid-cystic or mainly cystic tumours with hyperintense cysts on T_1-weighted MR images. The squamous-papillary types were solid or mixed solid-cystic tumours with hypointense cysts on T_1-weighted MR images. Imaging features found to be discriminating were: encasement of vessels, a lobulated shape, and hyperintense cyst signal for the former and a round shape, hypointense cysts and a predominantly solid appearance for the latter. Calcification is commoner in the adamantinous tumour but not discriminatory.

reflecting the frequent anterior location of this tumour. Gadolinium-enhanced scanning is useful for the identification of meningioma and metastases. Optic nerve glioma involving the chiasm rarely enhances and the imaging diagnosis depends on identifying enlargement of the optic pathway as spread is transneural. Other features of neurofibromatosis type 1 are evident in a quarter of patients with optic nerve gliomas, so imaging should include the whole cranium. Optic nerve and chiasm gliomas are isointense to grey matter on T_1-weighted and isointense or hyperintense on T_2-weighted sequences. Involvement of the optic tracts and brain parenchyma is identified as hyperintense signal on T_1-weighted sequences. Unless tumours are very large it is usually possible to see CSF between the inferior tumour margin from the diaphragma sellae and so to exclude suprasellar extension of an intrasellar mass.

Inflammatory diseases of the pituitary chiasmatic cistern

Involvement of the pituitary region by sarcoidosis, Langerhans' cell histiocytosis, tuberculous meningitis or abscesses may cause endocrine symptoms such as diabetes insipidus and abnormalities on imaging. In Langerhans' cell histiocytosis (also called eosinophilic granulomatosis) patients present with diabetes insipidus and bone lesions. The former frequently leads to imaging of the hypothalamic pituitary axis and on MRI the normal posterior pituitary high signal is typically absent (7). The diagnosis may be made by recognition of bone lesions which often occur in the skull—one of the rare situations when plain skull radiographs may be helpful in diagnosis of pituitary region disease.

Granulomatous leptomeningitis is more frequently evident in the basal cisterns than elsewhere in the cranium and involvement

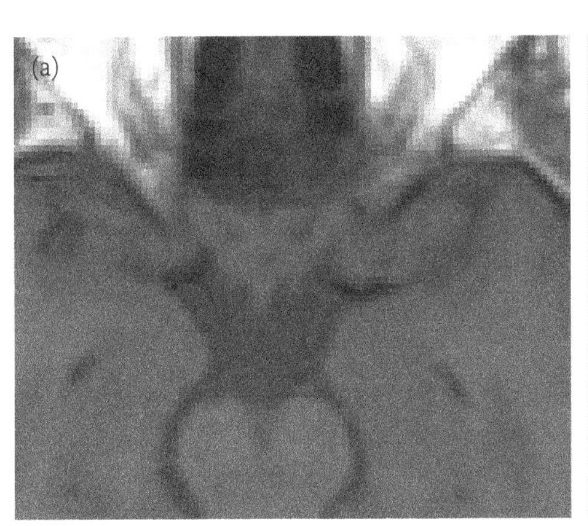

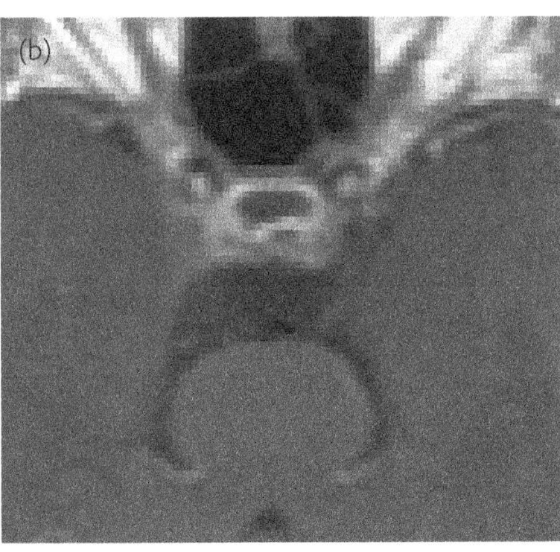

Fig. 2.3.5.11 Axial (a) T_1-weighted and (b) T_1-weighted gadolinium-enhanced MR images showing an intrasellar abscess. The appearances are of a mass replacing the gland with prominent enhancement of the margins of the abscess and the stella meininges.

of the chiasmatic cistern is more likely to be recognized because patients present with visual or endocrine symptoms. Sarcoid granulomas may be identified as meningeal masses isodense on CT and isointense on MRI, relative to grey matter (8). They are best demonstrated on T_1-weighted MRI with gadolinium enhancement. Other foci of meningeal enhancement should be sought since it may be necessary to resort to biopsy to confirm the diagnosis and a more superficial focus would be more accessible. The differential for pathological meningeal enhancement in the suprasellar region includes metastatic tumour and it is important to keep this possibility in mind. In a report of two patients (28), initial imaging performed for idiopathic diabetes insipidus was negative, but 1–2 years later, metastatic germinoma was demonstrated in the hypothalamus. Interval imaging and a high degree of suspicion is therefore warranted.

Diffuse enhancement of the pituitary occurs in lymphocytic hypophysitis and other rare forms of hypophysitis on MRI (Fig. 2.3.5.11). The gland and in particular the anterior lobe are usually moderately enlarged so hypophysitis is difficult to distinguish from adenoma on imaging alone. This rare form of autoimmune endocrine disease has probably been under diagnosed in the past because it was mistaken for adenoma or unrecognized prior to MRI being more available (29).

References

1. Fox WC, Wawrzyniak S, Chandler WF. Intraoperative acquisition of three-dimensional imaging for frameless stereotactic guidance during transsphenoidal pituitary surgery using the Arcadis Orbic System. *J Neurosurg*, 2008; **108**: 746–50.
2. Brooks BS, el Gammal T, Allison JD, Hoffman WH. Frequency and variation of the posterior pituitary bright signal on MR images. *AJNR Am J Neuroradiol*, 1989; **10**: 943–8.
3. Kucharczyk W, Lenkinski RE, Kucharczyk J, Henkelman RM. The effect of phospholipid vesicles on the NMR relaxation of water: an explanation for the MR appearance of the neurohypophysis?. *AJNR Am J Neuroradiol*, 1990; **11**: 693–700.
4. Scott WA. Magnetic Resonance Imaging of the Brain and Spine. Philadelphia, New York: Lippincott-Raven, 1996:59–63.
5. Sakamoto Y, Takahashi M, Korogi Y, Bussaka H, Ushio **Y**. Normal and abnormal pituitary glands: gadopentetate dimeglumine-enhanced MR imaging. *Radiology*, 1991; **178**: 441–5.
6. Friedman TC, Zuckerbraun E, Lee ML, Kabil MS, Shahinian H. Dynamic pituitary MRI has high sensitivity and specificity for the diagnosis of mild Cushing's syndrome and should be part of the initial workup. *Horm Metab Res*, 2007; **39**: 451–6.
7. Tien RD, Naston TH, McDermott MW, Dillon WP, Kucharczyk J. Thickened pituitary stalk on MR images in patients with diabetes insipidus and Langerhaus cell histiocytosis. *AJNR Am J Neuroradiol*, 1990; **11**: 703–8.
8. Engelken JD, Yuh WTC, Carter KD, Nerad JA. Optic nerve sarcoidosis. MR findings. *AJNR Am J Neuroradiol*, 1992; **13**: 228–30.
9. Davis PC, Hoffman JC Jr., Tindall, GT, Braun IF. CT-surgical correlation in pituitary adenomas: evaluation in 113 patients. *AJNR Am J Neuroradiol*, 1985; **6**: 711–16.
10. Semple PL, Jane JA, Lopes MB, Laws ER. Pituitary apoplexy: correlation between magnetic resonance imaging and histopathological results. *J Neurosurg*, 2008; **108**: 909–15.
11. Lundin P, Nyman R, Burman P, Lundberg PO, Muhr C. MRI of pituitary macroadenomas with reference to hormonal activity. *Neuroradiology*, 1992; **34**: 43–51.
12. Ahn JY, Jung JY, Kim J, Lee KS, Kim SH. How to overcome the limitations to determine the resection margin of pituitary tumours with low-field intra-operative MRI during trans-sphenoidal surgery: usefulness of Gadolinium-soaked cotton pledgets. *Acta Neurochir (Wien)*, 2008; **150**: 763–71.
13. Dina TS, Feater SH, Laws ER, Davis DO. MR of the pituitary gland postsurgery: serial MR studies following transspheniodal resection. *AJNR Am J Neuroradiol*, 1993; **14**: 763–9.
14. Lundin P, Bergström K, Nyman R, Lundberg PO, Muhr C. Macroprolactinomas: serial MR imaging in long-term bromocriptine therapy. *AJNR Am J Neuroradiol*, 1992; **13**: 1279–91.
15. Johnson MR, Hoare RD, Cox T, Dawson JM, Maccabe JJ, Llewelyn DE, *et al.* The evaluation of patients with a suspected pituitary microadenoma: computer tomography compared to magnetic resonance imaging. *Clin Endocrinol*, 1992; **36**: 335–8.
16. Bonneville JF, Bonneville F, Cattin F. Magnetic resonance imaging of pituitary adenomas. *Eur Radiol*, 2005; **15**: 543–8.
17. Stadnik T, Stevenaert A, Beckers A, Luypaert R, Buisseret T, Osteaux M. Pituitary microadenomas: diagnosis with two- and three-dimensional MR imaging at 1.5T before and after injection of gadolinium. *Radiology*, 1990; **176**: 419–28.
18. Yuh WTC, Fisher DJ, Nguyen HD, Tali ET, Gao F, Simonson TM, *et al.* Sequential MR enhancement pattern in normal pituitary gland and pituitary adenoma. *AJNR Am J Neuroradiol*, 1994; **15**: 101–8.
19. Tabarin A, Laurent F, Catargi B, Olivier-Puel F, Lescene R, Berge J, *et al.* Comparative evaluation of conventional and dynamic magnetic resonance imaging of the pituitary gland for the diagnosis of Cushing's disease. *Clin Endocrinol*, 1998; **49**: 293–300.
20. Elster AD. High-resolution, dynamic pituitary MR imaging: standard of care or academic pastime?. *AJR Am J Roentgenol*, 1994; **163**: 680–2.
21. Chong BW, Kucharczyk W, Singer W, George S. Pituitary gland MR: a comparative study of healthy volunteers and patients with microadenomas. *AJNR Am J Neuroradiol*, 1994; **15**: 675–9.
22. Oldfield EH, Doppman JL, Nieman LK, Chrousos GP, Miller DL, Katz DA, *et al.* Petrosal sinus sampling with and without corticotrophin-releasing hormone for differential diagnosis of Cushing's syndrome. *N Eng J Med*, 1991; **325**: 897–905.
23. Sumida M, Arita K, Migita K, Iida K, Kurisu K, Uozumi T. Demonstration of the optic pathway in sellar/juxtasellar tumours with visual disturbance on MR imaging. *Acta Neurochir(Wien)*, 1998; **140**: 541–8.
24. Krenning EP, Kwekkeboom DJ, Bakker WH, Breeman WA, Kooij PP, Oei HY, *et al.* Somatostatin receptor scintigraphy with ^{111}In-DTPA-D-Pne and ^{123}I-Tyr3-octeotride: the Rotterdam experience in more than 1000 patients. *Eur J Nucl Med*, 1993; **20**: 716–31.
25. Lucignani G, Losa M, Moresco RM, Del Sole A, Matarrese M, Bettinardi V, *et al.* Differentiation of clinically non-functioning pituitary adenomas from meningiomas and craniopharyngiomas by positron emission tomography with [^{18}F]fluoro-ethyl-spiperone. *Eur J Nucl Med*, 1997; **24**: 1149–55.
26. Sumida M, Uozumi T, Mukada K, Arita. K, Kurisu K, Eguchi K, *et al.* Rathke cleft cysts: correlation of enhanced MR and surgical findings. *AJNR Am J Neuroradiol*, 1994; **15**: 525–32.
27. Kucharczyk W, Peck WW, Kelly WM, Norman D, Newton TH, *et al.* Rathke cleft cysts: CT, MR imaging and pathological features. *Radiology*, 1987; **165**: 491–5.
28. Appignani B, Landy H, Barnes P. MR in central idiopathic diabetes insipidus in children. *AJNR Am J Neuroradiol*, 1993; **14**: 1407–10.
29. Rivera JA. Lymphocytic hypophysitis: disease spectrum and approach to diagnosis and therapy. *Pituitary* 2006; **9**: 35–45.

30. Buchfelder M, Nistor R, Fahlbusch R, Huk WJ. The accuracy of CT and MR evaluation of the sella turcica for detection of adrenocorticotropic hormone-secreting adenomas in Cushing disease. *AJNR Am J Neuroradiol*, 1992; **14**: 1183–90.
31. Adamson TE, Wiestler OD, Kleihues P, Yasargil MG. Correlation of clinical and pathological features in surgically treated craniopharyngiomas. *J Neurosurg*, 1990; **73**: 12–17.
32. Sartoretti-Schefer S, Wichmann W, Aguzzi A, Valavanis A. MR differentiation of adamantinous and squamous-papillary craniopharyngiomas. *AJNR Am J Neuroradiol*, 1997; **18**: 77–87.

2.3.6 Hypopituitarism: replacement of adrenal, thyroid, and gonadal axes

Trevor A. Howlett

Introduction

Hormone replacement of anterior pituitary hormone deficiency is one of the most frequent clinical interventions in pituitary disease, yet is an area which has rarely been the subject of rigorous scientific evaluation. Even in an era of 'evidence-based' medicine, recommendations for patient management are frequently based predominantly on clinical experience, consensus guidelines and occasional retrospective reviews rather than on controlled, prospective clinical trials. Within these limitations, this chapter will attempt to give a balanced view on current best management of adrenocorticotropic hormone (ACTH), thyroid-stimulating hormone (TSH) and gonadotropin deficiency.

Adrenal replacement in ACTH deficiency

Choice and timing of glucocorticoid replacement

Hydrocortisone, the generic pharmaceutical name for cortisol, is the standard form of glucocorticoid replacement for ACTH deficiency, and directly replaces the missing active hormone. Cortisone acetate was previously widely used, but is metabolized to cortisol to achieve its glucocorticoid activity, so that its onset of action is slower than hydrocortisone (a slight disadvantage) and biological half-life slightly longer (potentially a slight advantage).

The normal pattern of diurnal cortisol secretion is difficult to mimic precisely with oral therapy and there is no universal agreement regarding the appropriate dose, timing, and monitoring of hydrocortisone replacement, although the need for close attention has been highlighted (1). Normal individuals demonstrate undetectable cortisol and ACTH when asleep at midnight, with a sharp rise during the last hours of sleep to reach a peak at 08.00–09.00 h, followed by a steady decline throughout the rest of the waking day, with superimposition of variable peaks of cortisol secretion due other factors such as stress, meals, and exercise. Some approximation to this pattern can be achieved with thrice-daily regimens (hydrocortisone on rising, mid-day, and early evening) which appear to achieve more 'physiological' plasma cortisol levels (see below) compared with a traditional twice-daily regimen, which usually results in very low cortisol levels in late afternoon before the evening dose.

Two groups have reported progress in the development of a slow-release or tailored-release form of hydrocortisone, which might be capable of mimicking normal physiological cortisol profiles more accurately (2–4), but as yet neither form is available for routine clinical practice. Use of prednisolone or dexamethasone has been advocated on the basis of the longer half-life of these more potent synthetic glucocorticoids. However, these drugs cannot be monitored precisely and, in the case of dexamethasone, the potential for fine dose adjustment is limited by the pharmaceutical preparations available so that Cushingoid side effects are more frequent. Although these drugs may be preferred when suppression of an abnormal adrenal is required (e.g. in congenital adrenal hyperplasia), they have no advantage for routine replacement of hypopituitarism.

Assessment of hydrocortisone replacement

Criteria for deciding optimum hydrocortisone regimens are inevitably a compromise between theory, practicality, and patient convenience. Glucocorticoid replacement with hydrocortisone may be monitored using plasma cortisol measurements at multiple times throughout the day—a hydrocortisone day curve (HCDC). Studies using frequent sampling for plasma cortisol have identified wide interindividual variations in plasma cortisol levels obtained after the same dose of hydrocortisone and highlighted the need for individual adjustment of hydrocortisone dose, but such frequent sampling is rarely possible or necessary in routine practice. Simpler HCDC regimens are advocated by many centres to adjust and compare hydrocortisone replacement regimens (1, 5) although others have questioned their value and argued that clinical assessment may be equally effective (6).

My practice is to monitor hydrocortisone replacement with a simple HCDC involving collection of a 24-h urine for free cortisol (UFC) on the day prior to the test, and three plasma cortisols during a daycase attendance; patients take their morning hydrocortisone dose at the normal time, at home, on wakening and cortisol is measured at 09.00 h, 12.30 h (prior to any lunchtime dose),and 17.30 h (prior to the evening dose). For optimal replacement, I aim for a hydrocortisone dose which achieves a UFC and 09.00 h cortisol within the reference range for the normal population (28–220 nmol/24 h and 100–700 nmol/l, respectively, in our laboratory)—to avoid over-replacement—combined with 12.30 h and 17.30 h cortisol above 50 nmol/l, and ideally above 100 nmol/l—to avoid under-replacement. Using these criteria in a retrospective review of 130 patients (5) we demonstrated that thrice-daily regimens compared with twice-daily regimes are more likely to achieve 09.00 h plasma cortisol and UFC in the reference range for the normal population, more likely to avoid significant biochemical cortisol deficiency prior to the evening dose, and achieve the highest overall score for attainment of all four criteria. Overall, optimal replacement was most often achieved on hydrocortisone 10 mg on rising, 5 mg at lunchtime, and 5 mg in early evening, and this is therefore my usual starting dose for a new patient requiring replacement. This dose is lower than traditional recommendations but has also been derived by others using different empirical criteria for assessment and correlates with the oral hydrocortisone dosage equivalent of current estimates of the cortisol production rate in normal individuals (7).

After commencing hydrocortisone, individual dose adjustment is essential and a HCDC should be performed, doses adjusted, and HCDC repeated until the optimal hydrocortisone dose for an individual patient is identified. Thereafter I do not perform repeated measurement of cortisol unless clinical conditions change or symptoms indicate the need; others have advocated repeating measurements on a regular basis but there is no objective evidence comparing these two approaches.

Even thrice-daily regimens fail to accurately mimic the normal physiological circadian rhythm of cortisol and attention has been focused on the differences in circulating cortisol levels overnight in patients on hydrocortisone replacement (where levels are low or undetectable throughout the night) compared with normal individuals (where levels rise substantially during the last hours of sleep). These differences would be hard to avoid using standard preparations of hydrocortisone, since few patients would be prepared to wake to take a tablet during the night, but certainly represent an unphysiological feature of current replacement regimens, may contribute to an overnight deficiency of a variety of metabolic fuels (8), and are potentially an area where slow-release preparations could have advantages in future (although clinical trial evidence is still awaited). In practical terms, patients should certainly be advised to take hydrocortisone as soon as possible after wakening to avoid prolonged activity with low circulating cortisol levels, and those who habitually wake in the early hours some time before rising might benefit from taking their hydrocortisone dose at that time.

Mineralocorticoid replacement

Patients with ACTH deficiency should not require mineralocorticoid replacement, since the renin–angiotensin–aldosterone axis is not disrupted by pituitary disease. Studies have confirmed normal aldosterone levels in hypopituitary patients on replacement—although there may be subtle differences in dynamic responses to physiological stimuli.

Replacement during intercurrent illness

Glucocorticoid replacement is essential during intercurrent illness, and doses need to be increased for all but the most minor illness in order to mimic the normal increase in ACTH and cortisol secretion that occurs during stress and illness. Appropriate patient education on this aspect of replacement is a vital part of management of hypoadrenalism. Patients must be advised to double their normal oral dose of hydrocortisone during common pyrexial illnesses, and understand the need for parenteral glucocorticoid replacement if illness, operation, vomiting, or diarrhoea prevents the effective administration or absorption of oral glucocorticoid. Patients should seek medical advice if symptoms worsen in spite of increased oral hydrocortisone, should keep an 'emergency' ampoule of hydrocortisone at home, and if possible they or their family should be taught to give the injection if medical help is unavailable. Some patients also find a symptomatic need for increased glucocorticoid replacement during psychological stress, but this is much more difficult to define or regulate. During severe intercurrent illness or major surgery, hydrocortisone 100 mg, intramuscularly every 6 h will provide consistent, high levels of circulating cortisol comparable with those found in normal individuals during such stress; intravenous boluses of hydrocortisone produce wide swings in cortisol levels and are therefore less desirable, but stable, high plasma cortisol levels can be achieved by an IV infusion of hydrocortisone 5 mg/h (preceded by a 25 mg IV bolus) (9), although this is only appropriate in circumstances where an IV infusion can be reliably maintained and monitored.

Patient support groups have developed clearly formatted guidance on replacement for intercurrent illness and during surgery and other procedures which are readily available on the internet and invaluable when providing advice to patients and surgical colleagues (10).

Adverse effects

Adverse effects of supraphysiological doses of glucocorticoid are serious and well known, as are those of severe deficiency. In theory perfect physiological replacement should lead to no adverse effects, since circulating cortisol levels would be no different from normal subjects, but close attention to replacement doses is essential in order to achieve this.

Gross Cushingoid side effects and symptoms of severe hypoadrenalism are certainly clinically obvious and any competent clinical endocrinologist can avoid such extremes of inappropriate replacement, but minor degrees of over- or under-replacement could easily be clinically undetectable, yet give rise to important morbidity or even mortality. Several studies support this view: glucose tolerance and insulin secretion alter with hydrocortisone replacement (11), and blood pressure rises with replacement therapy (12) and may show qualitative differences between regimens although some workers have found no obvious changes related to hydrocortisone dose (13). Therefore, if minor over-replacement caused a slight worsening cardiovascular risk factors such as glucose intolerance, central obesity or blood pressure, then this might be undetectable in an individual yet have a significant influence on overall cardiovascular morbidity.

Bone mineral density may be subnormal in some patients on glucocorticoid replacement (14) although this is not confirmed by other more recent studies (6); excessive steroid replacement is a possible aetiological factor, and markers of bone metabolism normalize after reduction of hydrocortisone replacement dose to more 'appropriate' levels, although subsequent changes in bone mineral density are variable (7, 15). These factors indicate the need to avoid even subclinical glucocorticoid over-replacement and aim for the lowest total dose of hydrocortisone replacement compatible with good health. Conversely, avoidance of very low cortisol levels before the next dose seems advisable to minimize the risk of hypoadrenalism if intercurrent illness or stress occurs at that time.

Interactions with other therapy

Drugs that induce CYP3A4 liver enzyme drug metabolism (e.g. many anticonvulsants, rifampicin) increase hydrocortisone metabolism and patients taking these drugs may require higher doses of hydrocortisone to achieve adequate circulating levels. Concomitant growth hormone replacement therapy has been shown to reduce cortisol levels on a constant dose of hydrocortisone. This effect appears to be mediated by a reduction in levels of cortisol-binding globulin and so may not be of clinical importance, but may indicate the need for revised criteria for assessment in these patients.

DHEA replacement

Dehydroepiandrosterone (DHEA) is normally the most abundant circulating adrenal steroid and levels are low in ACTH deficiency.

Several clinical trials (16–18) have suggested improvements in general wellbeing, mood, subjective health status, and bone density with DHEA replacement (25–50 mg daily), particularly in women. However, some other studies have shown no benefit and the detail of effects on mood and wellbeing appears to vary between studies. Although DHEA is now regularly advocated as an important part of full adrenal replacement (19), the area remains controversial. Furthermore DHEA is not available as a licensed pharmaceutical preparation but only as a 'nutritional supplement' (which can therefore be readily purchased directly by the general public). No long-term follow-up data are available and routine replacement cannot currently be advocated—but the possibility of an individual therapeutic trial of replacement may be reasonably discussed with patients who have unresolved symptoms despite full and satisfactory conventional pituitary replacement therapy.

Thyroid replacement in TSH deficiency

Choice of replacement therapy

Levothyroxine is the routine replacement used for treatment of TSH deficiency. Its long plasma half-life ensures stable levels of thyroid hormones on once-daily administration, and conversion to T_3 *in vivo* results in appropriate blood levels of both T_4 and T_3. Liothyronine (T_3; triiodothyronine) can be used, but has no advantage in most circumstances. Combined T_4 and T_3 replacement and use of 'natural' thyroid extracts has been advocated in print and on the internet by a variety of 'alternative' clinicians and groups, but clinical trial evidence is limited and where available suggests no benefit (20).

Commencing levothyroxine replacement

Starting dose and regimen of levothyroxine replacement depends on the clinical circumstances. Prior to commencing levothyroxine it is essential to know the status of the ACTH–adrenal axis, because starting levothyroxine without glucocorticoid replacement in a patient with severe ACTH deficiency may precipitate a hypoadrenal crisis. If ACTH deficiency is present, hydrocortisone must be started before levothyroxine. Thereafter, many patients with TSH deficiency have serum free T_4 levels only slightly below the reference range, and in patients with such mild deficiency and no evidence of cardiovascular disease, replacement can be simply commenced with a near-full replacement dose of levothyroxine 100 µg once daily. In patients with more profound reductions of serum free T_4, a lower starting dose of 50 µg daily, increased after a few weeks to 100 µg may be better tolerated. In elderly patients, or any patient with known cardiovascular disease—particularly ischaemic heart disease, greater care is required: in most cases a starting dose of 25 µg will be well tolerated, increased slowly in 25 µg increments over several weeks until the target dose is achieved.

Monitoring levothyroxine replacement

Defining the optimal replacement dose of levothyroxine in TSH deficiency is problematical, and little scientific evidence is available to guide the clinician. Unlike primary hypothyroidism, where serum TSH is a sensitive marker of under- or over-replacement, there is no biochemical marker to indicate precise physiological levels of replacement for an individual patient—indeed serum TSH may be low, normal, or even slightly elevated in untreated TSH deficiency. Therefore, adjustment is based on the clinical response and on measurement of circulating thyroid hormone levels, which are limited by the very wide reference ranges in the normal population. Serum free T_4 appears the most appropriate marker with which to adjust the levothyroxine dose and a conventional recommendation is to maintain free T_4 in the middle or upper part of the reference range for normal individuals, although this is certainly not 'evidence based' and begs the question of the criteria used to define TSH deficiency since it implies that patients with pituitary disease (and indeed 50% of the normal population!) with a free T_4 in the lower half of the normal range might benefit from levothyroxine replacement therapy. Some workers have advocated using a levothyroxine dose based on body weight (1.6 µg/kg) (21) but in doing so increased free T_4 levels close to the upper limit of the reference range.

We have recently audited free T_4 levels in over 340 patients with pituitary disease at risk of TSH deficiency in our clinic (defined as evidence of macroadenoma and/or pituitary surgery, and/or pituitary radiotherapy) and compared them with those in 1800 patients with primary thyroid disease being monitored via our 'thyroid shared-care' register. Over 95% of pituitary patients had a free T_4 within the reference range at latest follow-up and 38% of patients were taking levothyroxine treatment. In contrast, using samples in patients with primary thyroid disease with a serum TSH in the laboratory normal range (and therefore assumed euthyroid) as controls, serum free T_4 was below the 10th centile of controls on no treatment in 17% of pituitary patients who were not on levothyroxine and below the 10th centile of controls on levothyroxine in 39% of pituitary patients on thyroid replacement (note that controls on levothyroxine treatment with a normal TSH had considerably higher free T_4 than controls who were not) (22) (Fig. 2.3.6.1). This audit suggests that TSH deficiency may be substantially underdiagnosed and undertreated in routine clinical practice. The 20–80th centile range for controls on levothyroxine was a free T_4 level of 14–19 pmol/l in our laboratory and we propose to use this as target range for replacement levels in TSH deficiency in the future.

Ultimately, such controversies regarding appropriate levothyroxine replacement dosage and monitoring can only be answered by a controlled trial. In the meantime, I accept a serum free T_4 anywhere in the middle centiles of the normal range when the patient is asymptomatic, but I will push the free T_4 into the upper part of the reference range if the patient continues to have symptoms suggestive of hypothyroidism.

Adverse effects of thyroid replacement

There are no specific data on adverse effects of excessive thyroid replacement in hypopituitarism, but data in patients with primary hypothyroidism are reassuring. Although thyrotoxicosis is a well-documented risk factor for osteoporosis, bone density remains normal even in patients on deliberate supraphysiological replacement with levothyroxine (23). However, thyrotoxicosis is also a risk factor for cardiovascular disease and, although there is no direct evidence of such adverse effects of levothyroxine replacement, the association of suppressed TSH levels and risk of atrial fibrillation in older patients in population-based studies (24) indicates the need for caution to avoid unnecessary over-replacement.

Interaction with other therapy

Other than changes induced by the restoration of the euthyroid state and normal metabolic rate, levothyroxine has few interactions with other therapy. A variety of other drugs raise (e.g. oral oestrogen

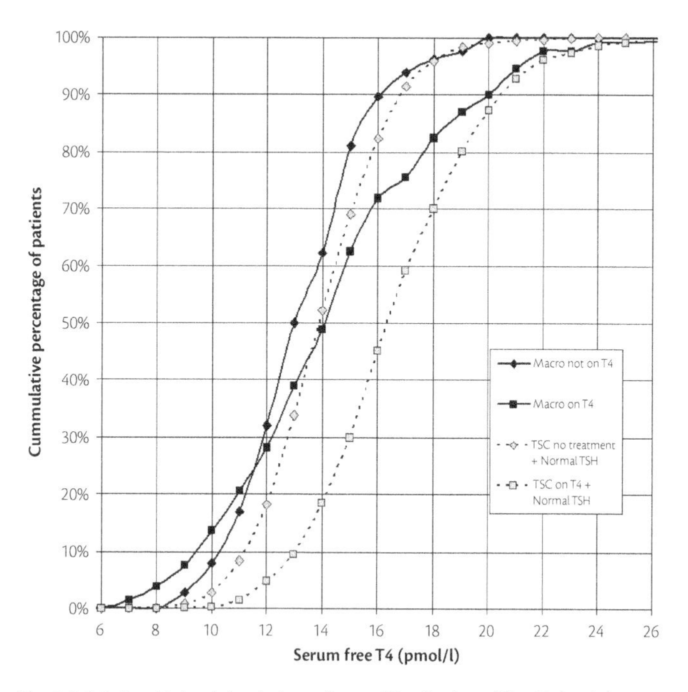

Fig. 2.3.6.1 Free T_4 levels in pituitary disease. Distribution of free T_4 levels in 344 patients with pituitary macroadenoma and/or surgery and/or radiotherapy (solid lines) compared to euthyroid samples (in which thyroid stimulating-hormone (TSH) level was normal) from 1800 patients with primary thyroid disease being monitored in a thyroid shared-care (TSC) register in the same period (dotted lines). ♦, patients not taking levothyroxine (nor antithyroid drugs); ■, patients receiving levothyroxine. Although most pituitary patients have free T_4 within the reference range (9–25 pmol/l), the levels are substantially lower than patients with an intact pituitary axis (22).

therapy) or lower (e.g. anticonvulsant therapy) the levels of total T_4 in serum by altering binding to Thyroid-Binding Globulin (TBG) which could lead to inappropriate dose adjustment, but free T_4 is rarely affected in reliable assays. Concomitant growth hormone replacement causes a fall in total and free T_4 (usually with a rise in T_3 levels due to increased extrathyroidal conversion); levels usually remain within the normal range but dose adjustment may be required.

Simultaneous use of proton pump inhibitors or antacids, calcium carbonate, and ferrous sulfate may reduce absorption of levothyroxine and result in altered dose requirements.

Gonadal steroid and gonadotropin replacement in gonadotropin deficiency

Unlike adrenal and thyroid replacement, replacement of gonadotropin deficiency offers an extensive choice of gonadal steroid replacement therapy for both sexes, and the choice of gonadotropin or gonadotropin-releasing hormone (GnRH) therapy if and when fertility is desired. Direct, oral replacement of the missing gonadal steroids is not possible due to rapid first-pass liver metabolism and short half-life. Again, in most cases the choice between different treatment modalities is largely a matter of patient and physician preference rather than 'evidence based'.

Therapy in females

Choice of replacement regimen

All female patients of premenopausal age with gonadotropin deficiency require oestrogen replacement to avoid the long-term consequences of oestrogen deficiency; cyclical progestagen is also essential in patients with an intact uterus to avoid endometrial hyperplasia and neoplasia.

Oral therapy

Choice of oral replacement is extensive, including all forms of oral oestrogen marketed for postmenopausal oestrogen deficiency and all combined oestrogen–progesterone contraceptive pills. Almost any such preparation represents acceptable replacement, and there is little or no objective evidence to choose between regimens. In younger women the low dose (20–35 μg ethinylestradiol) oestrogen-progesterone pill is often preferred since there are extensive data on its safety in long-term use in women of this age, due to its lower cost, and since in some cases taking the 'pill' may feel more 'normal' psychologically than taking 'HRT'. Monitoring of blood levels is impossible or unreliable with most preparations, but all give adequate levels of oestrogen to avoid effects of deficiency, and in an individual patient a regular menstrual withdrawal bleed is considered an adequate bioassay of oestrogen effect. When future pregnancy is planned it may be appropriate to monitor uterine size and endometrial thickness by ultrasonography to ensure that the uterus is indeed adequately oestrogenized.

Transdermal therapy

A variety of transdermal oestradiol delivery systems are available—some of which also deliver transdermal progestagen. Gel preparations are available but have not been widely used. Such regimens have the advantage of achieving lower physiological levels of natural oestradiol, but the disadvantage of skin reactions and unsatisfactory skin adherence in some patients, and of increased cost in all. This form of oestrogen replacement has advantages as first line in patients with complex pituitary disease since it avoids the effects of oral oestrogen on other hormone-binding proteins and shows less interaction with growth hormone replacement levels (see below). Transdermal oestrogen may also be particularly appropriate in patients where direct hepatic effects need to be avoided (e.g. in rare patients who develop hepatic adenomas on oral oestrogen, or in young patients with known thrombophilia or previous thromboembolic disease).

Implant regimens

Oestradiol implants achieve high circulating levels of oestrogen over long periods, but the problems with tachyphylaxis, which are well established in routine postmenopausal oestrogen replacement, make this form of replacement suboptimal.

Risk–benefit analysis

In recent years large studies of hormone replacement in postmenopausal women have suggested that, although HRT certainly reduces the risk of osteoporosis and probably bowel cancer, the increased risk of thromboembolism and cardiovascular disease at postmenopausal age means that the overall effect on health may be negative. These conclusions do not, however apply to younger women with oestrogen deficiency, including those with gonadotropin deficiency, since the risk of osteoporosis is greater and the risk of cardiovascular events lower due to younger age; indeed it is still hoped that oestrogen replacement should reduce the risk of premature vascular disease. Resolution of local and systemic symptoms of oestrogen deficiency provides additional drivers for routine oestrogen replacement in all gonadotropin-deficient women of premenopausal age. Balanced against these positive effects is a slight increase in risk of venous thromboembolism compared with the deficient state (which nevertheless remains a very low absolute risk), and mixed evidence on a possible slight increase in risk of breast cancer. In addition, some women will suffer from unwelcome cyclical changes similar to those which may be experienced the normal cycle. In the younger women the balance of risks seems overwhelmingly in favour of routine oestrogen replacement. In women of postmenopausal age the choice of whether or not to take oestrogen replacement is ultimately no different from that in women without pituitary disease.

Interactions with other therapy

Oral oestrogen raises plasma total T_4 and cortisol levels by inducing increases in thyroid- and cortisol-binding globulin, respectively. This does not influence active levels of these hormones or change the necessary dose of replacement, but does make biochemical monitoring of thyroid and adrenal reserve and/or replacement doses of these hormones more difficult. It is therefore usually best to fully assess thyroid and adrenal axes and/or optimize replacement levels before oral oestrogen is started (or during a 2–3-month break in therapy), or to use transdermal oestradiol as an alternative. Oral oestrogen also causes a slight reduction in insulin-like growth factor 1 (IGF-1) and rise in growth hormone levels, which may require dose adjustment to concomitant growth hormone replacement therapy to maintain IGF-1 in the target range.

Therapy in males

Men with gonadotropin deficiency usually require androgen replacement not only for relief of the symptoms of hypogonadism but also to prevent the long-term consequences of gonadotropin deficiency—particularly osteoporosis. More recent evidence that low testosterone levels may be associated with increased risk of cardiovascular disease and which may be reduced by replacement (25), provides an additional reason to advocate replacement even if the patient is apparently asymptomatic.

Choice of replacement regimen

In recent years a wide range of forms of testosterone replacement have become available (26).

Intramuscular depot testosterone

Depot testosterone ester preparations were the traditional form of androgen replacement, typically given as testosterone enantate, 250 mg IM every 3 weeks (range 2–4 weeks) or mixed testosterone esters (Sustanon) IM every 3 weeks. These regimens are certainly the cheapest preparations but do not mimic normal physiology, resulting in high or high normal levels of plasma testosterone in the days immediately following injection falling to low normal or subnormal levels before the next dose. Most patients will notice some changes in mood, libido, muscle strength, or general 'drive' consistent with these hormonal fluctuations, and some find this troublesome. The need for IM injections also usually necessitates regular visits to the surgery which may be inconvenient, although occasionally patients may self-administer.

These disadvantages mean that newer forms of testosterone replacement, which have become available in recent years have become the preferred methods of replacement in many countries. A depot preparation of testosterone undecanoate 1000 mg administered every 3 months (Nebido) is now a popular alternative that gives much more stable and physiological testosterone levels, achieved more rapidly if the second injection is given after 6 weeks (27). Timing of doses can be adjusted by measuring trough levels of testosterone prior to injection. Long-term experience of this formulation is still awaited.

Oral therapy

Testosterone undecanoate is a 17α-hydroxyl ester which is active orally since its highly polar side chain and oily vehicle allows direct absorption into the lymphatic system bypassing hepatic metabolism. The half-life remains relatively short, and multiple daily doses are necessary—typically 40 mg, 2–3 times daily—but oral therapy is preferred by some patients. This preparation is not currently approved for use in the USA but is available widely elsewhere. Other oral formulations of testosterone are either ineffective or have an unacceptable incidence of hepatic side effects and are no longer used.

Implant therapy

Testosterone pellets can be implanted subcutaneously by trocar and provide stable testosterone levels, typically using testosterone 600 mg every 6 months. The need for repeated surgical procedures means that this form of replacement is now largely superseded by long-acting depots.

Transdermal therapy

Transdermal gel preparations (typically 50 mg in 5 ml of 1% gel) have become increasingly popular in recent years. They are available in a variety of formulations including sachet, tube, and pump dispenser—all of which have their advantages and disadvantages in terms of convenience and ability to adjust doses. In each case the gel is applied by the patient to the shoulders, arms, or abdomen after bathing or showering, typically first thing in the morning. Contact of gel, or gel-treated areas, with females or children needs to be avoided. This form of treatment is very convenient for many patients but can be problematic for individuals who need to wash or shower frequently. Transdermal patch preparations are still available, but their niche has been largely overtaken by gel preparations. The patch may cause troublesome skin reactions in 5–10% of patients. All forms of transdermal therapy achieve physiological peak levels of testosterone and can even mimic the normal testosterone circadian rhythm.

Monitoring replacement

Testosterone levels can be measured in blood on all forms of replacement. With conventional intramuscular depot, I advocate measuring levels 1 week after injection (which should be in the upper part of the reference range for normal individuals) and just prior to injection (which will usually be low normal); frankly subnormal levels prior to injection may indicate the need for more frequent injection, while very high peak levels may necessitate a reduction in dose. On the 3-monthly depot a preinjection level is most informative. Testosterone levels in the morning on transdermal preparations should be in the mid-reference range. Random testosterone measurements are often low or low normal on oral testosterone undecanoate, but the short half-life makes these measurements less reliable, and dihydrotestosterone levels may be preferentially raised.

Sexual function

Severe androgen deficiency causes a reduction in libido and potency, which are usually restored by appropriate replacement therapy. In patients who have been hypogonadal for many years, counselling of the patient and their partner will be necessary before starting therapy. However, a proportion of men presenting with sexual dysfunction will also be found to have testosterone levels in the borderline low range, without elevation of gonadotropins, but with no other evidence of pituitary disease; improvement in libido and particularly potency is far less certain with replacement in these patients.

Adverse effects

Excess androgen replacement will cause polycythaemia, and this can also occur in elderly men, in chronic obstructive airways disease and in sleep apnoea with high-normal replacement doses, so that haemoglobin levels need to be monitored in such patients. Sleep apnoea may also be worsened by testosterone replacement. The possibility of long-term adverse effects on the prostate remains controversial. Hypogonadal men have lower prostate volume and prostate-specific antigen levels than the normal population, and induction of hypogonadism in patients with established prostate cancer induces temporary disease remission and reduction in prostate volume—thus raising the possibility that testosterone replacement might increase the incidence of prostate cancer and prostatic hypertrophy. While it seems likely that replacement will raise the incidence of these conditions to those of the normal population there is currently no evidence to suggest an absolute increased risk of either condition with appropriate replacement. In spite of this, and the current lack of evidence that screening for prostate cancer is beneficial in the normal population, some form of prostate monitoring is usually recommended in older men on testosterone replacement; I favour monitoring serum prostate-specific antigen (PSA), with further investigation only if PSA levels rise above normal, but others recommend repeated rectal examination and/or prostate imaging.

Previous concerns about the possibility of increased cardiovascular risk arose from the increased risk of cardiovascular disease in men compared with women—but evidence now suggests that low testosterone itself may be associated with the metabolic syndrome and increased cardiovascular risk and that testosterone replacement may therefore be beneficial to cardiovascular health (25). Long-term clinical trial evidence is still awaited.

Puberty induction

Where gonadotropin deficiency develops before puberty, special care is required to induce pubertal developmental at an appropriate speed in both sexes. Simply commencing full adult replacement doses will result in inappropriately rapid pubertal development with insufficient time for usual psychological adaptation, in less satisfactory secondary sexual development and in possible attenuation of the pubertal growth spurt and final height.

Gonadal steroid replacement is commenced in low doses in both sexes. In females, low doses of oral oestrogen (e.g. ethinyloestradiol 10 μg daily, or even lower doses where available) or transdermal oestradiol (e.g. 25 μg or less, twice weekly) is commenced, and usually continued at very low dose for 6–12 months before increasing steadily to full replacement dosage with eventual addition of cyclical progestagen. Males may commence with testosterone enantate 100 mg IM every 3–4 weeks, again continued at this low dose for many months before increasing towards adult replacement dosage; similar low-dose regimens can be devised using transdermal testosterone or oral testosterone undecanoate. Other factors sometimes require attention: girls with prepubertal panhypopituitarism may fail to develop pubic hair, and use of topical testosterone creams has been described if normal hair growth is desired; boys may need reassurance that pubertal gynaecomastia is common, and that normal adult facial and body hair develop slowly over many years once testosterone levels have reached the normal adult range.

Growth

Normal individuals show a pubertal growth spurt associated with gonadal steroids, particularly in males, yet gonadal steroids are also responsible for epiphyseal fusion and the cessation of linear growth. Appropriate adjustment of replacement doses of gonadal steroid and growth hormone are therefore essential in patients with hypopituitarism during induction of puberty. Overall, studies indicate that although early puberty (spontaneous or induced) reduces final height, deliberately delaying puberty induction to allow increased time for growth probably does not increase final height significantly, and may be associated with obvious adverse psychological consequences.

Fertility induction

Gonadal steroid replacement does not induce fertility, but ovulation and spermatogenesis can be stimulated by therapy with gonadotropin injections (initially human menopausal, now increasingly recombinant) or by pulsatile GnRH administered subcutaneously by infusion pump.

Therapy in females

Use of gonadotropin therapy and pulsatile GnRH are both highly successful, resulting in fertility rates approximating normal levels with repeated cycles of treatment in expert hands (28). GnRH therapy is mostly used where the gonadotropin deficiency is considered primarily 'hypothalamic', but may also be successful in patients considered to have primary pituitary disease. As always, such therapy should only be undertaken with close biochemical and ultrasound monitoring of the ovarian response, and in centres with extensive experience of ovarian stimulation techniques; precise description of treatment regimens is beyond the scope of this book.

Therapy in males

Gonadotropin and GnRH therapy can both induce spermatogenesis, but induction of adequate spermatogenesis takes a minimum of 3 months and may require 1–2 years. Luteinizing hormone therapy is usually used first in the form of human chorionic gonadotropin (hCG) (typically 1000–2000 IU, 2–3 times/week); this should result in adequate testosterone levels and may sometimes be sufficient to allow spermatogenesis, but follicle-stimulating hormone activity is usually required for adequate fertility. A wide variety of regimens have been recommended with successful fertility in a majority of patients which may occur at surprisingly low total sperm counts. Coexistent primary testicular defects (e.g. related to cryptorchidism) may cause failure. The need to wear an infusion pump or attend for regular intramuscular injections over many months is clearly a disadvantage, but self-administration of low doses of gonadotropins subcutaneously may also be successful in both induction of fertility and increase in testicular size (29). When pregnancy is achieved, spermatogenesis may occasionally be maintained by testosterone replacement alone although usually continued or repeated gonadotropin therapy is required. Sperm may also be frozen after successful treatment for use in future attempts at fertility.

Pituitary coma

Pituitary coma is a rare, but life-threatening, presentation of severe, longstanding, untreated hypopituitarism, usually precipitated by stress including infection, trauma, surgery, or infarction, or by an acute pituitary insult such as apoplexy. Treatment is firstly full replacement with parenteral hydrocortisone (as above), followed by correction of other factors which may precipitate or worsen coma, including hypothermia, salt and water depletion due to hypoadrenalism, and/or diabetes insipidus, hyponatraemia due to excessive desmopressin or hypothalamic dysfunction, and (slow) replacement of hypothyroidism.

Patient education and participation

Pituitary disease and the investigation and replacement of pituitary deficiencies are complex and optimal management is only possible when the patient is fully aware of the nature and consequences of the disorder and can participate actively in the adjustment of replacement therapy. Patient education is therefore an essential part of management, and patients should also be encouraged to obtain further information and support from groups such as the Pituitary Foundation (UK) (www.pituitary.org.uk) or Pituitary Network Association (USA) (www.pituitary.org).

Self-medication and dose adjustment

Replacement therapy may be very complex in patients with panhypopituitarism and patients must be aware of the nature, indications, and administration schedule for all replacement therapies that they require. For those on glucocorticoid replacement it is essential that they understand the need to increase doses during intercurrent illness (see above), and carry a steroid card and MedicAlert/SOS bracelet or pendant. When injection or infusion pump therapy is indicated patients must be fully conversant with the techniques. Gonadal steroid replacement is often neglected by both physicians and patients, and patients should be fully aware of the benefits and risks of replacement. Patients in the U.K should also be made aware than hypopituitarism is currently an indication for exemption from National Health Service (NHS) prescription charges.

Management of equivocal or borderline deficiency

The biochemical assessment of pituitary deficiency remains regrettably imprecise and many patients will have evidence of equivocal or borderline deficiency. Other patients will have normal tests but have a pituitary disorder in which progressive hypopituitarism is possible or likely (e.g. following pituitary radiotherapy). All such patients must be fully aware of the symptoms and consequences of hypopituitarism (particularly hypoadrenalism which might be life-threatening), should participate actively in the decision to commence or withhold replacement therapy, and report promptly the development of new symptoms that might indicate worsening deficiency. Asymptomatic patients with borderline or equivocal ACTH deficiency who are not on regular glucocorticoid replacement should have a supply of hydrocortisone for intercurrent illness with clear information about when and how it should be used.

References

1. Monson JP. The assessment of glucocorticoid replacement therapy. *Clin Endocrinol (Oxf)*, 1997; **46**: 269–70.
2. Debono M, Ghobadi C, Rostami-Hodjegan A, Huatan H, Campbell MJ, Newell-Price J, *et al.* Modified-release hydrocortisone to provide circadian cortisol profiles. *J Clin Endocrinol Metab*, 2009; **94**: 1548–54.
3. Newell-Price J, Whiteman M, Rostami-Hodjegan A, Darzy K, Shalet S, Tucker GT, *et al.* Modified-release hydrocortisone for circadian therapy: a proof-of-principle study in dexamethasone-suppressed normal volunteers. *Clin Endocrinol (Oxf)*, 2008; **68**: 130–5.
4. Johannsson G, Bergthorsdottir R, Nilsson AG, Lennernas H, Hedner T, Skrtic S. Improving glucocorticoid replacement therapy using a novel modified-release hydrocortisone tablet: a pharmacokinetic study. *Eur J Endocrinol*, 2009; **161**: 119–30.
5. Howlett TA. An assessment of optimal hydrocortisone replacement therapy. *Clin Endocrinol (Oxf)*, 1997; **46**: 263–8.
6. Arlt W, Rosenthal C, Hahner S, Allolio B. Quality of glucocorticoid replacement in adrenal insufficiency: clinical assessment vs. timed serum cortisol measurements. *Clin Endocrinol (Oxf)*, 2006; **64**: 384–9.
7. Peacey SR, Guo CY, Robinson AM, Price A, Giles MA, Eastell R, *et al.* Glucocorticoid replacement therapy: are patients over treated and does it matter?. *Clin Endocrinol (Oxf)*, 1997; **46**: 255–61.
8. Al-Shoumer KA, Ali K, Anyaoku V, Niththyananthan R, Johnston DG. Overnight metabolic fuel deficiency in patients treated conventionally for hypopituitarism. *Clin Endocrinol (Oxf)*, 1996; **45**: 171–8.
9. Symreng T, Karlberg BE, Kagedal B, Schildt B. Physiological cortisol substitution of long-term steroid-treated patients undergoing major surgery. *Br J Anaesth*, 1981; **53**: 949–54.
10. Addison's Disease Self Help Group. Information Index 2009. Available at: http://www.addisons.org.uk/info/i_index1.html (accessed 16 August 2009).
11. Al-Shoumer KA, Beshyah SA, Niththyananthan R, Johnston DG. Effect of glucocorticoid replacement therapy on glucose tolerance and intermediary metabolites in hypopituitary adults. *Clin Endocrinol (Oxf)*, 1995; **42**: 85–90.
12. Matsumura K, Abe I, Fukuhara M, Fujii K, Ohya Y, Okamura K, *et al.* Modulation of circadian rhythm of blood pressure by cortisol in patients with hypopituitarism. *Clin Exp Hypertens*, 1994; **16**: 55–66.
13. Dunne FP, Elliot P, Gammage MD, Stallard T, Ryan T, Sheppard MC, *et al.* Cardiovascular function and glucocorticoid replacement in patients with hypopituitarism. *Clin Endocrinol (Oxf)*, 1995; **43**: 623–9.
14. Zelissen PM, Croughs RJ, van Rijk PP, Raymakers JA. Effect of glucocorticoid replacement therapy on bone mineral density in patients with Addison disease. *Ann Intern Med*, 1994; **120**: 207–10.
15. Peacey SR, Yuan GC, Eastell R, Weetman AP. Optimization of glucocorticoid replacement therapy: the long-term effect on bone mineral density. *Clin Endocrinol (Oxf)*, 1999; **50**: 815–17.
16. Arlt W, Callies F, van Vlijmen JC, Koehler I, Reincke M, Bidlingmaier M, *et al.* Dehydroepiandrosterone replacement in women with adrenal insufficiency. *N Engl J Med*, 1999; **341**: 1013–20.
17. Gurnell EM, Hunt PJ, Curran SE, Conway CL, Pullenayegum EM, Huppert FA, *et al.* Long-term DHEA replacement in primary adrenal insufficiency: a randomized, controlled trial. *J Clin Endocrinol Metab*, 2008; **93**: 400–9.
18. Hunt PJ, Gurnell EM, Huppert FA, Richards C, Prevost AT, Wass JA, *et al.* Improvement in mood and fatigue after dehydroepiandrosterone replacement in Addison's disease in a randomized, double blind trial. *J Clin Endocrinol Metab*, 2000; **85**: 4650–6.
19. Arlt W. The approach to the adult with newly diagnosed adrenal insufficiency. *J Clin Endocrinol Metab*, 2009; **94**: 1059–67.
20. Grozinsky-Glasberg S, Fraser A, Nahshoni E, Weizman A, Leibovici L. Thyroxine-triiodothyronine combination therapy versus thyroxine monotherapy for clinical hypothyroidism: meta-analysis of randomized controlled trials. *J Clin Endocrinol Metab*, 2006; **91**: 2592–9.

21. Slawik M, Klawitter B, Meiser E, Schories M, Zwermann O, Borm K, *et al.* Thyroid hormone replacement for central hypothyroidism: a randomized controlled trial comparing two doses of thyroxine (T4) with a combination of T4 and triiodothyronine. *J Clin Endocrinol Metab*, 2007; **92**: 4115–22.
22. Koulouri O, Auldin MA, Agarwal R, Kieffer V, Robertson C, Falconer-Smith J, *et al.* Patients with pituitary disease are at risk of under-replacement with levothyroxine. *Endocr Abstr*, 2010; **21**: 287.
23. Franklyn JA, Betteridge J, Daykin J, Holder R, Oates GD, Parle JV, *et al.* Long-term thyroxine treatment and bone mineral density. *Lancet*, 1992; **340**: 9–13.
24. Sawin CT, Geller A, Wolf PA, Belanger AJ, Baker E, Bacharach P, *et al.* Low serum thyrotropin concentrations as a risk factor for atrial fibrillation in older persons. *N Engl J Med*, 1994; **331**: 1249–52.
25. Mathur A, Malkin C, Saeed B, Muthusamy R, Jones T, Channer K. Long term benefits of testosterone replacement therapy on angina thresholdand atheroma in men. *Eur J Endocrinol*, 2009; **161**: 443–9.
26. Nieschlag E. Testosterone treatment comes of age: new options for hypogonadal men. *Clin Endocrinol (Oxf)*, 2006; **65**: 275–81.
27. Moisey R, Swinburne J, Orme S. Serum testosterone and bioavailable testosterone correlate with age and body size in hypogonadal men treated with testosterone undecanoate (1000 mg IM—Nebido). *Clin Endocrinol (Oxf)*, 2008; **69**: 642–7.
28. Martin KA, Hall JE, Adams JM, Crowley WF, Jr. Comparison of exogenous gonadotropins and pulsatile gonadotropin-releasing hormone for induction of ovulation in hypogonadotropic amenorrhea. *J Clin Endocrinol Metab*, 1993; **77**: 125–9.
29. Jones TH, Darne JF. Self-administered subcutaneous human menopausal gonadotrophin for the stimulation of testicular growth and the initiation of spermatogenesis in hypogonadotrophic hypogonadism. *Clin Endocrinol (Oxf)*, 1993; **38**: 203–8.

2.3.7 Adult growth hormone deficiency

Aurora Aragon-Alonso, Mark Sherlock, Andrew A. Toogood

Introduction

It has been known for many years that growth hormone is essential for normal linear growth, but over the past few years, with the advent of recombinant human growth hormone therapy, the importance of growth hormone during adult life has been described in detail. The growth hormone peptide was first isolated from bovine pituitaries in the 1940s (1), but was found to be species specific and inactive in humans. In 1956, growth hormone was extracted from human cadaveric pituitary tissue (2) and a year later was administered to a 13-year-old boy with hypopituitarism, resulting in an increased growth velocity (3). The first report suggesting growth hormone could have beneficial actions in adulthood was published in 1962 in which a 35-year-old woman with hypopituitarism reported increased vigour, ambition, and wellbeing after 2 months treatment with cadaveric growth hormone (4). However, the limited supply of pituitary-derived growth hormone confined its use to the treatment of children with severe growth failure caused by proven growth hormone deficiency (GHD). In 1985, the association of cadaveric growth hormone treatment with Creutzfeldt–Jakob disease led to its withdrawal from use worldwide (5). Since then, all growth hormone in clinical use has been produced using recombinant DNA technology.

The first placebo-controlled trials of growth hormone replacement therapy in adults with GHD were published in 1989 (6, 7). These and subsequent studies have led to the recognition of adult GHD as a specific clinical syndrome and the impact of GHD and replacement therapy in adults with GHD has been studied in detail.

Pathophysiology

Growth hormone is a 191 amino acid single chain polypeptide hormone synthesized and secreted by somatotrophs in the anterior pituitary in a pulsatile fashion, with peaks separated by nadirs during which growth hormone levels fall below the sensitivity of routine assays and are only detectable with sensitive chemiluminescent assays (8). Two hypothalamic hormones are the predominant regulators of growth hormone secretion: growth hormone-releasing hormone (GHRH), which stimulates both growth hormone synthesis and growth hormone release, and somatostatin, which inhibits growth hormone release (but not its biosynthesis) (9). A third factor is thought to be ghrelin, the natural ligand of the endogenous growth hormone secretagogue receptor, distinct from that for GHRH (10). The stomach is the principal source of circulating ghrelin, and as well as its growth hormone-releasing role, ghrelin has orexigenic activity among other functions (11). It has been shown that ghrelin stimulates growth hormone secretion synergistically with GHRH, which is required for ghrelin to exert its effect as a growth hormone secretagogue (12, 13), however, the physiological role of endogenous ghrelin in growth hormone regulation remains to be determined. Multiple neurotransmitter pathways as well as a variety of metabolic and hormonal factors are also involved in the regulation of growth hormone secretion, either by acting directly on the somatotrophs and/or modulating GHRH or somatostatin release. It is through these pathways that stress, sleep, exercise, hypoglycaemia, and high levels of circulating amino acids (such as arginine) stimulate growth hormone secretion, while high levels of glucose and free fatty acids inhibit its secretion. Other hormones influence growth hormone secretion: oestradiol increases growth hormone secretion when administered orally and glucocorticosteroids and thyroid hormone excess impair growth hormone release (9). Growth hormone secretion is known to be higher in premenopausal women than in age-matched men (14) and is inversely associated with increasing age and adiposity (15, 16), in particular abdominal obesity (17).

Growth hormone circulates bound to a growth hormone-binding protein, which is homologous to the extracellular domain of the growth hormone receptor (GHR) (18). Growth hormone exerts its effects directly by binding to the extracellular domain of the GHR, at the cell surface which causes dimerization of two GHR molecules and initiates the intracellular signalling pathway which includes Janus kinase and the signal transducers and activators of transcription (STAT) pathway (19). The metabolic effects of growth hormone are mediated through the subsequent production of insulin-like growth factor 1 (IGF-1). The liver is the dominant source of circulating IGF-1 although it can also be generated in many other tissues, where it appears to act in an autocrine/paracrine fashion (20). A small proportion of IGF-1 circulates in a free state, but the majority is associated with a tertiary complex consisting of IGFBP3 and the acid-labile subunit (ALS), significantly prolonging its half-life, maintaining stable circulating levels, and regulating its availability to target tissues (21). These three peptides, IGF-1, IGFBP-3, and ALS, are all growth hormone dependent. Many factors affect both hepatic and local tissue IGF-1 production in response to a given growth hormone stimulus, including sex steroids, thyroxine, glucocorticoids, insulin, and liver disease. Androgens enhance the IGF-1 response to growth hormone, and oestrogens attenuate growth hormone action by reducing IGF-1 in a dose-dependent fashion following oral administration (22).

Somatostatin, GHRH, growth hormone, and IGF-1 are maintained homoeostatically in the hypothalamus, pituitary, and circulation by a complex interplay of feedback signals. Growth hormone inhibits its own secretion indirectly by regulation of GHRH and somatostatin release from the hypothalamus, as well as directly acting on the somatotrophs. IGF-1 inhibits growth hormone secretion through a negative feedback action on the pituitary and less clearly on the hypothalamus (9).

Aetiology of adult GHD

Adults with GHD are primarily divided into those who develop the condition during childhood and those diagnosed during adulthood. Patients who previously had childhood GHD account for 15–27% of the patients with adult GHD (23, 24), idiopathic being the most common cause in this group (25). Isolated, idiopathic GHD of childhood appears to be reversible in a large proportion of cases when retested at the completion of linear growth. Up to 80% of cases demonstrate a normal growth hormone response when retested in young adult life. Individuals with structural disease of the hypothalamic pituitary axis are less likely to recover their growth hormone axis and in many cases the severity of GHD may increase (25). It has been shown that between 40% and 60% of young adults who have completed growth hormone replacement therapy in childhood continue to have a degree of GHD. Therefore, reassessment of growth hormone status once linear growth is completed is mandatory (26).

The causes of GHD that occur in adulthood are summarized in Table 2.3.7.1, using data derived from 1034 patients enrolled in the KIMS database, a multinational, pharmacoepidemiological survey of patients receiving growth hormone replacement (23). Although GHD may occur in isolation, it is often observed in the context of multiple pituitary hormone deficiencies, where growth hormone is typically the first hormone to become clearly deficient. In this way, in patients with organic hypothalamic-pituitary disease, the likelihood of GHD increases with the increasing number of pituitary hormone deficits from approximately 45% if no other deficits are present to 95% if three or four pituitary hormone deficiencies are present (27, 28) (Fig. 2.3.7.1). Adult-onset GHD usually results from damage to the pituitary gland or the hypothalamus, the most common cause being a pituitary adenoma or its treatment with surgery or radiotherapy (25). Pituitary microadenomas are rarely associated with hypopituitarism, and patients with this condition may not need assessment of GHD unless other pituitary hormone deficits are present or unless there is a strong clinical suspicion of GHD (27). Radiotherapy induces damage to the neuroendocrine axes and growth hormone axis is the most susceptible, being the earliest and most frequent pituitary hormone affected following radiotherapy. The severity and speed of onset of radiation-induced GHD is dose and time (elapsed postirradiation) dependent (29). Children appear to be more radiosensitive than adults and GHD is found less frequently following irradiation in adulthood (30).

Table 2.3.7.1 Aetiology of GHD in 1034 hypopituitary adult patients according to KIMS

Cause	Per cent
Pituitary adenoma	53.9
Craniopharyngioma	12.3
Idiopathic	10.2
Central nervous system (CNS) tumour	4.4
Empty sella syndrome	4.2
Sheehan's syndrome	3.1
Head trauma	2.4
Hypophysitis	1.6
Surgery other than for pituitary treatment	1.5
Granulomatous diseases	1.3
Irradiation other than for pituitary treatment	1.1
CNS malformation	1
Perinatal trauma or infection	0.5
Other	2.5

(Reproduced with permission, from Abs R, Bengtsson BA, Hernberg-Stahl E, Monson JP, Tauber JP, Wilton P, *et al.* GH replacement in 1034 growth hormone deficient hypopituitary adults: demographic and clinical characteristics, dosing and safety. *Clin Endocrinol (Oxf)* 1999; **50**: 703–13).

Traumatic brain injury (TBI) and subarachnoid haemorrhage (SAH) have been reported to produce some degree of hypopituitarism which can be permanent in 27.5 and 47% of patients respectively (31). In several of these studies, GHD has been identified as the most frequent pituitary deficiency, with GHD reported in 12.4% and 25.4% of the patients after TBI and SAH, respectively (31). Severe GHD has also been reported in 8% to 21% of TBI patients (32). Isolated GHD is rarer in adults than in children, accounting for approximately 10% of cases of GHD in adulthood (23, 33). In this group of patients, nonfunctioning and secreting pituitary adenomas are the most common primary diagnosis (33). Idiopathic isolated GHD occurring *de novo* in adults is not a recognized entity (34).

Clinical features of adult GHD

Adult GHD is recognized as a clinically relevant syndrome associated with a variety of symptoms and signs, which are summarized in Box 2.3.7.1. It causes abnormalities that affect multiple systems, but three areas are most relevant clinically: quality of life (QoL), cardiovascular risk (including disturbance of body composition), and skeletal health.

GHD and quality of life

Adults with GHD report reduced psychological wellbeing and quality of life compared with matched healthy controls, particularly low energy levels, social isolation, greater emotional liability, impaired socioeconomic performance, and greater difficulties forming relationships (35). The aspect of quality of life most

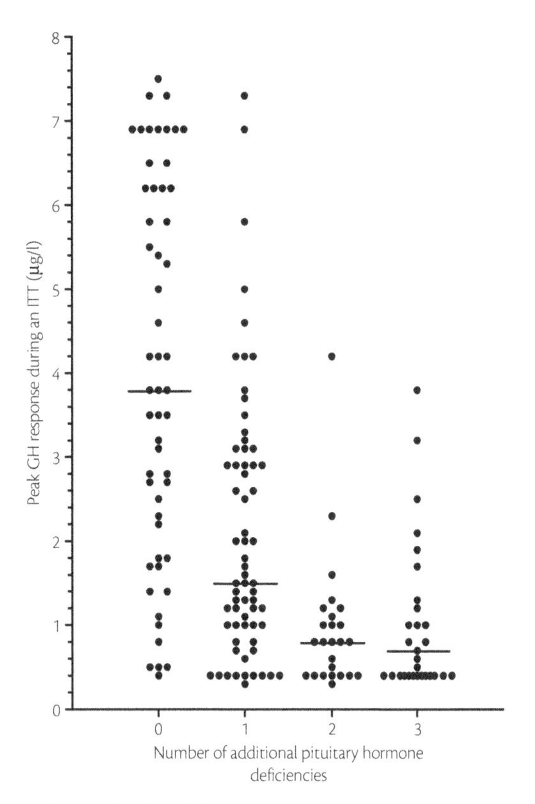

Fig. 2.3.7.1 The distribution of the peak serum growth hormone in response to an insulin tolerance test (ITT) in 190 patients divided into groups according to the degree of hypopituitarism present (i.e. number of anterior pituitary hormone deficiencies) in each patient. Of patients with two or three additional pituitary hormone deficits, 95% have a peak growth hormone <3 μg/l. Horizontal bars represent medians. (Adapted with permission from Toogood AA, Beardwell CG, Shalet SM. The severity of growth hormone deficiency in adults with pituitary disease is related to the degree of hypopituitarism. *Clin Endocrinol* 2004; **41**: 511–16).

frequently affected by GHD is energy and vitality (25). Initial studies evaluating quality of life in GHD used a variety of generic questionnaires designed for subjects with long-term illness, but condition-generated questionnaires focusing on quality of life issues that are relevant to patients with GHD have been developed (35). One of these questionnaires which is now widely used for the baseline and follow-up of patients, is the Quality of Life Assessment in Growth Hormone Deficient Adults (QoL-AGHDA), a disease-generated questionnaire developed from interviews with patients with GHD (36). It consists of 25 questions, with a yes/no response, the score being determined by the number of positive answers. A score of 25/25 indicates poor quality of life, scores of 4/25 or less have been reported in a normal control population (37). However, quality of life evaluations of GHD have shown a high degree of variability, and while some GHD patients report severe impairment of quality of life, others demonstrate a normal quality of life (25). This disparity may be because of many other possible influences on the quality of life, such as the age of onset of GHD. Impairment of quality of life is less frequently found in patients with childhood-onset GHD (38) and in older patients (39).

GHD and cardiovascular risk

Growth hormone has important effects on lipid, protein, and carbohydrate metabolism (40, 41). Consequently, GHD is associated

Box 2.3.7.1 The clinical features of GHD in adults

Impaired quality of life
- Low energy levels
- Social isolation
- Emotional liability
- Impaired socioeconomic performance
- Difficulties forming relationships

Abnormal body composition
- Increased fat mass, particularly central fat deposition
- Decreased lean mass
- Decreased total body water

Abnormal lipid profile
- Increased total and low-density lipoprotein-cholesterol
- Increased triglycerides
- Increased apolipoprotein B-100
- Decreased high-density lipoprotein-cholesterol in some studies

Reduced insulin sensitivity

Hypertension in some studies

Decreased fibrinolysis
- Increased fibrinogen
- Increased plasminogen activator inhibitor 1
- Increased tissue plasminogen activatort

Endothelial dysfunction (decreased NO formation)

Increased levels of inflammatory markers (C-reactive protein and IL-6)

Increased carotid intima media thickness and abnormal wall dynamics

Microvascular abnormalities
- Reduced capillary density
- Microvascular perfusion
- Capillary leakage

Changes in cardiac size and function
- Reduced left ventricular mass
- Left ventricular systolic dysfunction

Reduced bone mineral density
- Increased risk of nonvertebral fractures and vertebral deformities

Dry, thin, and cool skin

Decreased resting energy expenditure in some studies

Defective sweating

Reduced isometric muscle strength

Reduced/lower normal range isokinetic muscle strength

Reduced exercise capacity

Reduced red blood cell volume

Decreased glomerular filtration rate

with substantial changes in body composition; body fat mass is increased (by approximately 7%) (42), with a propensity towards visceral fat deposition (43). This central obesity is known to increase cardiovascular risk via several mechanisms including atherothrombotic and proinflammatory abnormalities, insulin resistance, hypertension, and dyslipidaemia (43). The cause of central obesity in adult GHD is not clear, although it has been suggested that increased local tissue exposure to cortisol could play a role. IGF-1 inhibits the enzyme 11B-hydroxysteroid dehydrogenase type 1 (11β-HSD1), responsible for conversion of inactive cortisone into active cortisol in liver and adipose tissue (44). Patients with GHD in the context of hypopituitarism have an increased cortisol/cortisone metabolite ratio and reduction in circulating cortisol concentrations in patients receiving hydrocortisone replacement (44). In GHD, central obesity (as well as insulin resistance and other cardiovascular abnormalities) could be a consequence of exposure to raised cortisol levels at key target tissues, and therefore the reported benefits of growth hormone replacement on cardiovascular risk factors may be an indirect effect of alterations in cortisol metabolism (44).

Lean body mass has been shown to be reduced by 7% in GHD (42), which may explain the reductions in muscle strength and exercise capacity observed in these patients. Some of the decrease in lean mass could be due to the reduction in total body water seen in adults with GHD, as growth hormone has antinatriuretic properties (45). Growth hormone also affects lipoprotein metabolism, and adult GHD is associated with an atherogenic lipid profile. Increased levels of total and low-density lipoprotein (LDL) cholesterol, triglycerides, and apolipoprotein B-100, with normal or decreased high-density lipoprotein (HDL) cholesterol have been reported in GHD adults (25, 46).

Although low, normal and high basal levels of insulin have been found in GHD adults, probably reflecting different degrees of obesity, it has also been demonstrated using the hyperinsulinaemic euglycaemic clamp method that there is a twofold to threefold reduction in insulin sensitivity in GHD patients compared with controls, despite normal fasting glucose and insulin levels (43). Blood pressure has not consistently been shown to be increased in patients with GHD, and the possible mechanism of hypertension is not clear (35).

GHD is associated with decreased fibrinolysis, with augmented levels of fibrinogen, plasminogen activator inhibitor 1 (PAI-1), and tissue plasminogen activator antigen (tPA) (46). These changes in thrombogenic proteins may contribute to the development of atherosclerosis and cardiovascular events. Patients with GHD have endothelial dysfunction, which is an early step in the atherogenic process and is associated with decreased nitric oxide production (47). Indeed, IGF-1 has a direct stimulatory effect on nitric oxide synthesis, and nitric oxide formation is decreased in GHD patients (46, 47). Furthermore, GHD is associated with elevated levels of inflammatory markers also associated with cardiovascular risk, such as C-reactive protein (CRP) and interleukin 6 (IL-6) (35). GHD patients also have abnormal parameters of vascular integrity, such as increased arterial intima-medial thickness (independent risk marker for myocardial infarction and cerebrovascular accident (48)), reduced endothelium-derived flow-mediated dilation, reduced muscle blood flow and increased vascular resistance associated with increased sympathetic nerve activity (49). Adults with GHD in addition to the above effects on large- and medium-sized vessels show reduced capillary density, microvascular perfusion, and capillary leakage (49).

Finally, GHD is associated with changes in cardiac size and function, and although there are conflicting results in patients with adulthood-onset GHD, reductions in left ventricular mass (50, 51) and left ventricular systolic dysfunction (51, 52) have been described in some studies. GHD exerts adverse effects upon several cardiovascular risk factors, and it has been shown that both cerebrovascular and cardiovascular morbidity are increased in GHD patients (53). Several studies have reported a twofold increase in the overall mortality rate (mainly due to increased cardiovascular mortality) in hypopituitary adults without growth hormone replacement (53–56). Although GHD may contribute to the increase in morbidity and mortality observed in these patients, multiple factors are likely to be involved, such as the underlying disease, untreated hypogonadism, excessive glucocorticoid or thyroxine replacement, and previous treatment with surgery or radiotherapy.

GHD and bone

Growth hormone has an important effect on bone metabolism. Initially stimulating bone resorption followed by bone deposition the overall effect of growth hormone-dependent bone remodelling is anabolic. Growth hormone is involved in the promotion of linear growth in childhood, achievement of peak bone mass after cessation of linear growth, and maintenance of bone density through life (57). Adult patients with GHD have a marked reduction in bone turnover, demonstrated by bone biopsies which show reduced osteoid and mineralization surfaces and decreased bone formation rate and by the finding of diminished levels of both markers of osteoclastic and osteoblastic activity (57).

Bone mineral density (BMD) in adults with GHD is approximately 1 SD score below those of age- and sex-matched controls, even when the possible effect of hypogonadism or glucocorticoid over-replacement are corrected for (25). The severity of the observed bone loss is related to the age of the patient the severity of GHD and the age of onset of GHD (25, 57). Patients with childhood-onset GHD have a more severe reduction in bone mass than those developing GHD in adulthood. Achievement of optimal peak bone mass requires growth hormone. In young adults, GHD prevents the acquisition of optimal bone mass resulting in a relatively severe osteopenia (57). As age increases the severity of osteopenia associated with GHD declines until it is no longer apparent after the age of 55 or 60 years (58, 59).

There have been reports of an increased risk of nonvertebral fractures (frequently localized in the radius) as well as radiological vertebral deformities (suggesting vertebral fractures) in GHD patients (57). The prevalence of bone fractures is related to the degree of GHD and seems not to be affected by concomitant hypopituitarism or by replacement of other pituitary hormones (57).

Other clinical features

There are conflicting data suggesting resting energy expenditure (REE) is affected by GHD, as decreased REE and REE expressed in terms of lean body mass have been described in some, but not all studies (60). In contrast, GHD patients show reduced exercise capacity, evidenced by cycle ergometry, with a 20–30% reduction in maximum oxygen uptake compared to those predicted for age, gender, and height. This could be attributed to the reduction in lean body mass that leads to decreased muscle strength, the diminished cardiac capacity, the decreased oxygen transport capacity (as IGF-1 stimulates erythropoiesis), as well as an impaired ability to dissipate heat by sweating after heat or exercise (60). Adults with GHD have reduced isometric muscle strength (static contraction of a muscle without any visible movement in the angle of the joint) and reduced or low normal isokinetic muscle strength (muscle contracts and shortens at constant speed) when compared with normal controls (35). Moreover, local muscle endurance has also been found to be either reduced or in the lower normal range in adults with GHD (35).

In addition to the effects of GHD described above, GHD patients have been reported to have a dry, thin, and cool skin, probably related to the loss of direct anabolic actions of growth hormone on skin, decreased cardiac output, and decreased sweating (61). Finally decreased glomerular filtration rate has also been described in GHD patients (62).

Diagnosis of GHD in adults

The manifestations of GHD in adults, in contrast to the reduced growth velocity observed in children, are subtle and none is pathognomonic. In the absence of a good clinical indicator that will reliably discriminate a GHD patient from the normal population the diagnosis of adult GHD is based on the results of biochemical testing in an appropriate clinical context (27). Current consensus guidelines identify two groups of patients who should be tested for GHD in adult life; those at risk of hypothalamic-pituitary dysfunction, in whom there is an intention to treat with growth hormone replacement, and those with childhood-onset of GHD who have reached final height (34) (Fig.2.3.7.2). The first group includes patients with evidence of hypothalamic-pituitary disease (endocrine, structural, and/or genetic causes), those who have received cranial radiotherapy, which impacts on the hypothalamic-pituitary axis, and those with TBI or subarachnoid haemorrhage. For those patients with childhood-onset GHD, the need for continuation of growth hormone replacement should be assessed once final height has been achieved, although repeat growth hormone testing is not required for those with a transcription factor mutation, those with more than three pituitary hormone deficits, and those with isolated GHD associated with an identified mutation (34). All other patients should undergo growth hormone testing after at least 1 month off growth hormone therapy (34). Idiopathic isolated GHD in adulthood is not a recognized clinical entity, so adults who do not fulfil the criteria outlined above should not undergo assessment of their growth hormone status.

Growth hormone is secreted in a pulsatile fashion and has a short half-life, which renders assessment of random serum growth hormone concentrations worthless for the diagnosis of GHD, although a single growth hormone measurement taken fortuitously at the time of a secretory peak may exclude GHD (63). Because of this pulsatile secretion, multiple sampling of growth hormone levels would be ideal (24-h profile with a minimum of 20-min sampling), but is impractical in routine clinical practice (25), so endocrinologists rely on dynamic function tests to determine growth hormone status.

A number of agents have been used to stimulate the release of a growth hormone pulse. The insulin tolerance test (ITT) is regarded as the 'gold standard', as it distinguishes GHD from the reduced growth hormone secretion that accompanies normal ageing and obesity, provided adequate hypoglycaemia is achieved (27). The ITT should be carried out in dedicated units, under supervision by experienced staff (27). The ITT is contraindicated in patients with electrocardiographic evidence or a clinical history of ischaemic heart disease or seizures and in elderly people (34). The ITT should be performed with caution in brain-injured patients (64). There are other accepted and validated alternative tests when the ITT is contraindicated, including the glucagon stimulation test, GHRH with arginine, and GHRH with growth hormone-releasing peptide 6 (GHRP-6). The glucagon stimulation test is as reliable as the ITT, and has the same validated cut-off for GHD in adults: a peak growth hormone response of <3 μg/l (34, 65) (Table 2.3.7.2). The other tests consist of the combined administration of GHRH with either arginine (that seems to reduce hypothalamic somatostatin secretion) or a synthetic growth hormone secretagogue such as GHRP-6 (34, 65), although the latter is not available for use in normal clinical practice. Both tests provide a potent stimulus to growth hormone secretion and constitute appropriate alternatives to the ITT, with a very good safety profile and relatively fewer contraindications (65). It must be noted though, that these combined tests may miss GHD due to hypothalamic disease (e.g. those having received irradiation of the hypothalamic-pituitary region), as they stimulate both the hypothalamus and the pituitary. Therefore, they are not recommended for the diagnosis of severe GHD in patients

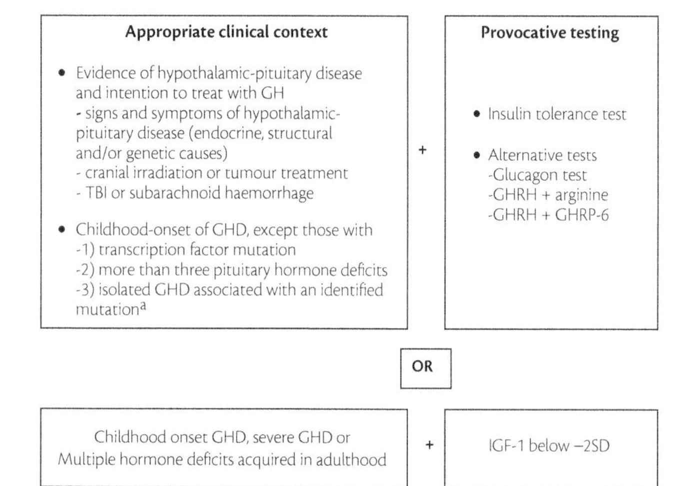

Fig. 2.3.7.2 The diagnosis of adult growth hormone deficiency (GHD).

Table 2.3.7.2 Diagnostic thresholds for severe growth hormone deficiency (GHC) during the insulin tolerance test, glucagon stimulation test and combined GHRH + arginine test

Provocative test	Severe GHD cut-off levels: peak growth hormone response
Insulin tolerance test	<3 μg/l
Glucagon	<3 μg/l
GHRH + arginine:	
BMI <25 kg/m^2	<11 μg/l
BMI 25–30 kg/m^2	<8 μg/l
BMI >30 kg/m^2	<4 μg/l

with cranial irradiation, the ITT being the preferred test to be used in this situation, as this test shows the greatest sensitivity and specificity within the first 5 years of irradiation (25, 34, 65) following which all tests seem to be reliable and generally concordant (65).

As growth hormone secretion is affected by age, gender, and body mass index (BMI), the majority of tests are limited by the lack of validated normative data based on these parameters. Obesity is particularly important, as both spontaneous and stimulated growth hormone secretion is negatively associated with BMI, and sometimes the growth hormone response to provocative stimuli is as impaired to the same degree as in hypopituitary patients with severe GHD. This constitutes a clinical problem in the interpretation of the growth hormone response to provocative tests in obese patients in whom GHD is suspected, particularly as GHD is often associated with obesity. It is recommended that diagnostic thresholds appropriate to lean, overweight, and obese subjects are used, in order to achieve an appropriate diagnosis in obese adults and lean GHD adults (65). For the ITT, the diagnostic threshold is <3 μg/l and can be applied to all as it has been shown to distinguish normal subjects (including those who are obese) from patients with severe GHD (65). Cut-off levels of growth hormone response validated by BMI are not available for the glucagon test, but are clearly defined in the GHRH + arginine test (34, 65) (see Table 2.3.7.2).

Serum levels of the growth hormone-responsive molecules IGF-1 and IGFBP3 are stable through the day, show minimal diurnal variation and need not be drawn fasting (61). IGF-1 and IGFBP3 effectively provide integrated markers of growth hormone secretion that can be utilized as indicators of growth hormone status. Of the two, IGF-1 is the most sensitive marker of growth hormone action, but its diagnostic value in adults is limited by the significant overlap in IGF-1 values between GHD and normal controls; this overlap is more prevalent in GHD patients with adult-onset than those with childhood-onset GHD (65, 66). Therefore, a normal age-adjusted IGF-1 value does not exclude the diagnosis of GHD in adults (25, 27, 65) (Fig. 2.3.7.3). Nonetheless, in the absence of conditions that may decrease IGF-1 generation, including malnutrition, hepatic disease, hypothyroidism, or poorly controlled diabetes mellitus, an IGF-1 below the reference range in the presence of multiple pituitary hormone deficits confirms the diagnosis of GHD (27). Thus, although it is widely accepted that the diagnosis of adult GHD is established by provocative testing of growth hormone secretion, it is accepted that, in patients at risk of GHD (childhood-onset GHD, severe GHD, or multiple hormone deficits acquired in adulthood), a serum IGF-1 below the age-specific normal range is diagnostic (65) (see Fig. 2.3.7.2).

Finally, it is important to note that the actual value reported for the growth hormone concentration in a specific's serum sample is determined to a great extent by the assay method used, limiting the applicability of international consensus guidelines to local clinical practice. Some of the reasons for the difficulty in growth hormone assays standardization are the heterogeneity of the analyte itself, the availability of different reference preparations for calibration and the interference from matrix components such as GHBP (67). In a recent study more than twofold variation in growth hormone and IGF-1 values measured in different laboratories was found, probably due to variability in assay performance, coupled with use of inappropriate conversion factors and reference ranges (68). The Growth Hormone Research Society (GRS) recommends the adoption of universal growth hormone and IGF-1 calibrators (recombinant 22 kDa growth hormone calibrator, International Reference Preparation 98/574 and a recombinant human IGF-1 of the highest purity) by all growth hormone and IGF-1 assays manufacturers, in order to reduce this substantial heterogeneity among existing assays (34).

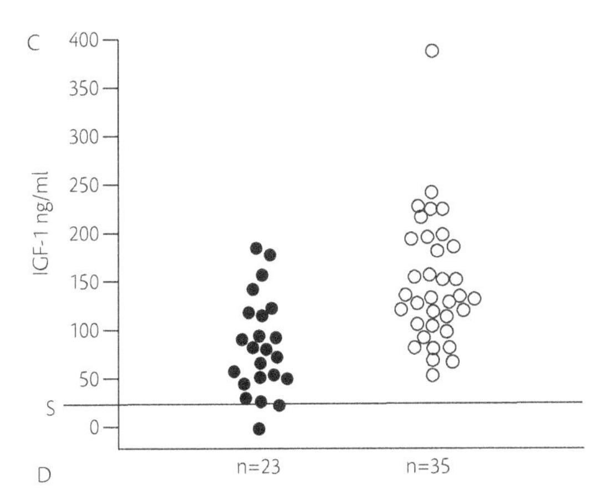

Fig. 2.3.7.3 Distribution of serum insulin-like growth factor 1 (IGF-1) concentrations in 35 normal (○) and 23 hypopituitary (•) subjects. There is an overlap of serum IGF-1 concentration between the two groups with 70% (16 of 23) of hypopituitary individuals having concentrations within the range of normal subjects. (Adapted with permission, from Hoffman DM, O'Sullivan AJ, Baxter RC, Ho KKY. Diagnosis of growth-hormone deficiency in adults. *Lancet* 1994; **343**: 1065–8).

Treatment of GHD in adults

Rationale for treating GHD in adults

The rationale for treating adults with GHD is primarily based on the improvement of the features discussed above. To date, there is no evidence that treatment of adult GHD results in normalization of the increased mortality observed in this patient population (37, 63). In contrast to other endocrine replacement used in hypopituitarism, for which there is general agreement regarding its use and efficacy, there remains considerable variation in the use of growth hormone between centres and between countries. Some endocrinologists advocate the blanket approach, adopted by the GRS consensus guidelines, which suggest all patients with documented severe GHD are eligible for growth hormone treatment and should be treated (27, 34). The approach adopted by the UK and other European countries is to select patients for growth hormone replacement based on impaired quality of life or to optimize bone mass. (37) (Box 2.3.7.2). In the UK, current guidance for growth hormone replacement in adults was issued by the National Institute of Clinical Excellence (NICE) in 2003 (Box 2.3.7.3), (69). These guidelines restrict access to growth hormone replacement therapy to patients with an impaired quality of life, defined as a baseline QoL-AGHDA score of 11 or more.

Effects of growth hormone replacement therapy

Growth hormone replacement therapy and quality of life

The benefits of growth hormone replacement therapy on psychological wellbeing and perceived health have been described in some double-blind, placebo-controlled trials, and in a meta-analysis of open studies of growth hormone replacement (35). The findings of double-blind, placebo-controlled studies are not consistent; some

Box 2.3.7.2 Treatment of patients with adult GHD

Indication

- All patients with documented severe GHD (GRS approach)
- Only those GHD patients with impaired quality of life and/or BMD (many European countries approach)

Dose

- Starting dose: 0.2 mg/day in young men, 0.3 mg/day in women, 0.1 mg/day in older patients
- Dose escalation gradual, individualized, guided by clinical and biochemical response

Monitoring of treatment

- Biochemical marker: IGF-1
  - Initially to be measured every 1–2 months; at least yearly once stable dose is reached
  - IGF-1 assessment no sooner than 6 weeks after a GH growth hormone dose change
  - IGF-1 levels to be maintained below the age-and gender-related upper limit of normal
- Body composition changes
  - Anthropometric measures (BMI, waist, and hip circumferences)
  - Bioelectrical impedance
  - DEXA
- Plasma lipids
- Insulin sensitivity

Quality of life:

- Clinical history with attention to quality of life parameters
- Specific quality of life questionnaire
- Consider clinical evaluation of glucocorticoid status and measurement of free T3 and T4 within the first months/long-term

Contraindications:

- Active malignancy
- Benign intracranial hypertension
- Proliferative or preproliferative diabetic retinopathy

Side effects

- Most common: fluid retention (paraesthesias, join stiffness, peripheral oedema, arthralgia, myalgia, carpal tunnel syndrome)
- Rare: atrial fibrillation, gynaecomastia, congestive heart failure, benign cranial hypertension, retinopathy
- Possible increase of insulin resistance and worsening of glucose tolerance: careful monitoring of GHD patients with high risk of type 2 diabetes mellitus or already having diabetes

have shown a definite benefit in quality of life, others have reported a more limited improvement or no change in quality of life after growth hormone therapy (25). On the other hand, some long-term postmarketing surveillance studies that have compared the quality

Box 2.3.7.3 Guidelines for the use of recombinant human growth hormone in England and Wales (adapted from NICE guidelines)

Patients being considered for GH growth hormone replacement therapy should fulfil the following criteria:

- Severe GHD a peak GH growth hormone response of less than 9 9 mU/litre (3 μg/l) during an ITT or equivalent using alternative test.
- Impaired quality of life, as demonstrated by a reported score of ≥11 QoL-AGHDA
- They are already receiving treatment for any other pituitary hormone deficiencies as required.

Quality of life should be reassessed 9 months after the initiation of therapy. Growth hormone treatment should be discontinued for those people who demonstrate a quality of life improvement of less than 7 points in QoL-AGHDA score.

Patients who develop GHD in early adulthood, after linear growth is completed but before the age of 25 years, should be given growth hormone treatment until adult peak bone mass has been achieved, provided they satisfy the biochemical criteria for severe GHD. After adult peak bone mass has been achieved, the decision to continue growth hormone treatment should be based on all the criteria in point 1.

At completion of linear growth (that is, growth rate < 2 cm/year), Growth hormone treatment should be stopped for 2–3 months, and then growth hormone status should be reassessed. Growth hormone treatment at adult doses should be restarted only in those satisfying the biochemical criteria for severe GHD and continued until adult peak bone mass has been achieved (normally around 25 years of age). After adult peak bone mass has been achieved, the decision to continue growth hormone treatment should be based on all the criteria set out above.

Initiation of growth hormone treatment, dose titration, and assessment of response during trial periods should be undertaken by a consultant endocrinologist with a special interest in the management of growth hormone disorders. Thereafter, if maintenance treatment is to be prescribed in primary care, it is recommended that this should be under an agreed shared care protocol.

of life in GHD adults treated with long-term growth hormone replacement with general population data from several European countries have shown a sustained improvement in quality of life towards the normative country-specific values (35). Finally, a sustained improvement in overall psychological wellbeing in GHD patients after 10 years of growth hormone therapy has also been demonstrated (70)

In general, the degree of improvement in quality of life is proportional to the degree of impairment at the outset, but shows no correlation with the degree of improvement in IGF-1 levels; this means that if the quality of life at baseline is normal, no improvement will be seen with growth hormone replacement (25). It is worth noting, that concomitant obstructive sleep apnoea syndrome (which is a common finding in hypopituitary adults) may confound quality of life evaluation; therefore in severe GHD patients not responding adequately to growth hormone treatment this syndrome should be ruled out (35).

In addition to the beneficial effects upon quality of life, improvements on cognitive performance in GHD patients during growth hormone replacement have also been described, particularly in attention and memory (35). In practice, there are patients who perceive a benefit from growth hormone replacement therapy and report an improvement in their quality of life which can be measured, while others perceive no benefit and will chose to discontinue therapy.

Growth hormone therapy and cardiovascular risk

Body composition

The beneficial effects of growth hormone replacement on body composition have been consistently observed. Total body fat (especially visceral fat) is reduced, and lean mass is increased (Table 2.3.7.3) (35, 71). Some of the increase of lean body mass is accounted for by growth hormone-mediated fluid retention (61); however, there is also a genuine increase in skeletal muscle mass (61). Long-term studies of growth hormone replacement (over 5–10 years) have confirmed a sustained improvement in lean body mass, although in some of these studies the increase in total body nitrogen, which reflects total body protein, seemed to be transient. After 10 years of growth hormone therapy, body weight has been found to increase, and total body fat returns towards baseline values. These changes may reflect the changes in body composition associated with normal ageing rather than a waning of the effects of growth hormone replacement (35).

Lipid metabolism

Short-term studies of growth hormone replacement therapy in GHD adults have shown a reduction or no change in serum total cholesterol concentrations, a reduction of serum LDL cholesterol and apoprotein B concentrations (35). Serum HDL cholesterol concentrations are generally unchanged although some have demonstrated an increase. Serum triglyceride levels have mostly been unchanged (35) (Table 2.3.7.3) (71). The magnitude of the reduction of both total and LDL cholesterol is greater in those patients with higher baseline serum cholesterol levels, and it occurs even in those patients receiving concurrent lipid-lowering agents (HMG CoA-reductase inhibitors) (72). Long-term growth hormone replacement studies also show that the beneficial changes in serum lipoprotein profile are maintained following 10 years of growth hormone therapy, and that the improvement of serum lipid levels may even be progressive over that period (35). Serum lipoprotein(a), a proposed independent risk factor for cardiovascular disease, is increased after initiation of growth hormone replacement, although this observation has not been uniform (73). Although this contradictory data could be due to lipoprotein (a) assay differences (73), its overall significance regarding cardiovascular risk remains to be determined.

Carbohydrate metabolism

During short-term (<6 months) growth hormone replacement therapy, there is an initial period during which insulin resistance is adversely affected, due to increased lipolysis with elevated circulating free fatty acid concentrations (35, 47). Insulin sensitivity returns towards baseline values after 3 months of growth hormone treatment as the beneficial effect upon body composition become apparent (35). The long-term (≥1 year) effect of growth hormone replacement therapy on insulin sensitivity is not clear. Some studies have demonstrated unchanged insulin sensitivity compared to baseline and others reported that insulin sensitivity is still compared to baseline assessments (35). As individual patients have differential sensitivity in these parameters, it is not surprising that with growth hormone administration, some show a worsening of insulin sensitivity, while others show little change (25). A meta-analysis of blinded, randomized, placebo-controlled trials of growth hormone treatment in adults with GHD showed that growth hormone therapy significantly increases both fasting insulin levels and plasma glucose, although mean glucose levels remained in the normal range (71) (Table 2.3.7.3). However, this

Table 2.3.7.3 Results of a meta-analysis of blinded, randomized, placebo-controlled trials of growth hormone treatment on cardiovascular risk factors in GHD adults

Factors	No of trials	Treatments		Q test	Weighted mean change (GH placebo)	Globla effect size (95% CL)
		GH	Placebo			
Lean mass	19	473	474	ns	2.82 kg (2.68)	
Fat Mass	13	352	345	ns	−3.05kg (3.29)	
Body mass index	8	134	134	ns	−0.12 kg/m^2 (1.40)	
Triglycerides	11	202	203	ns	0.07mmol/l (0.36)	
HDL cholesterol	13	267	261	ns	0.06 mmol/l (0.09)	
LDL cholesterol	13	255	248	ns	−0.53 mmol/l (0.29)	
Total cholesterol	15	310	306	ns	−0.34 mmol/l (0.31)	
Diastolic Blood Pressure	10	200	201	ns	−1.80 mmHg (3.77)	
Systolic Blood Pressure	9	190	191	ns	2.06 mmHg (5.34)	
Insulin	11	192	194	ns	8.66 pmol/l (6.98)	
Glucose	13	254	257	ns	0.22 mmol/l (0.14)	

HDL, high-density lipoprotein; LDL, low-density lipoprotein.

Adapted with permission, from Maison P, Griffin S, Nicoue-Beglah M, Haddad N, Balkau B, Chanson P. Impact of growth hormone (GH) treatment on cardiovascular risk factors in GH-deficient adults: a metaanalysis of blinded, randomized, placebo-controlled trials. *J Clin Endocrinol Metab* 2004; **89**: 2192–2199.

meta-analysis included very few studies with a prolonged follow-up (≥12 months), and insulin sensitivity was assessed in only one long-term trial (74) showing that the initial increase of both insulin levels and insulin-to-glucose ratios reported after growth hormone therapy, was not maintained at 18 months, and the HbA_{1c} did not change significantly.

Finally, there are contradictory results of glucose metabolism in several long-term trials of growth hormone replacement; while two of them reported no changes in glucose homoeostasis (assessed by glucose tolerance and insulin concentrations on the first one (75), and by fasting glucose, insulin and C peptide on the second (70)) after 7 and 10 years, respectively, of growth hormone therapy, others showed an increase (76) and reduction (77) of HbA_{1c}, respectively, after 10 years' of growth hormone replacement.

Cardiac morphology and function

There are discordant data about the medium and long-term effects of growth hormone replacement on cardiovascular abnormalities (78). However, in a meta-analysis reviewing 16 trials (nine blinded, placebo-controlled trials and seven open studies) of growth hormone treatment in GHD adults, growth hormone treatment was found to have a positive effect on many cardiac parameters assessed by echocardiography, such as a significant increase in left ventricular mass, interventricular septum thickness, left ventricular posterior wall, left ventricular end-diastolic diameter, and stroke volume (79).

Peripheral vascular effects, blood pressure, inflammation, and other cardiovascular risk markers

GHD is associated with endothelial dysfunction with impairment of nitric oxide production. Although growth hormone therapy is not associated with a very impressive effect on circulating markers of endothelial dysfunction (35), it does normalize urinary nitrate excretion (47), endothelium-derived flow mediated dilation, and brachial artery blood flow (49). There are conflicting results of growth hormone replacement effect on blood pressure, as some studies have reported reduction of blood pressure, while others have shown no change or even an increase of blood pressure after growth hormone therapy (35) (Table 2.3.7.3) (71). On the other hand, administration of growth hormone can, at least partly, reverse the pathological fibrinolysis and restore the augmented sympathetic nerve activity found in untreated GHD adults (35). In addition, growth hormone replacement therapy has also been shown to reduce circulating CRP and IL-6 levels (35), as well as normalizing the microvascular abnormalities described in patients with GHD (49). Growth hormone replacement has been shown to reverse early atherosclerotic changes in the carotid arteries in GHD adults such as the increase of carotid intima media thickness(35). Moreover, it has been reported that this beneficial effect is sustained even after 10 years of treatment (70) (Fig. 2.3.7.4).

Cardiovascular and cerebrovascular morbidity and mortality

Although growth hormone replacement therapy improves most of the adversely affected cardiovascular risk factors observed in GHD patients, there are still limited data regarding the effect of growth hormone therapy on cardiovascular morbidity and mortality. In fact, Svensson *et al.* have reported an increased rate of cerebrovascular events in GHD patients receiving growth hormone therapy (53), although the rate of myocardial infarctions as well as the overall mortality were lower and similar respectively to those of the normal background population. This increased risk ratio for cerebrovascular events could be related to radiation angiopathy, which, again, demonstrates that factors other than growth hormone may have an important effect on outcome in patients with hypopituitarism (53).

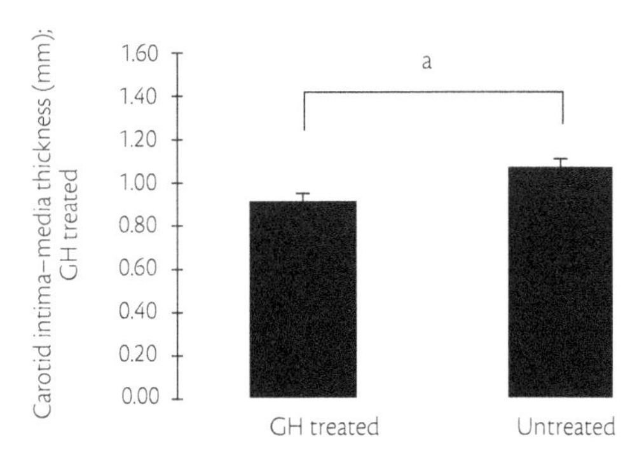

Fig. 2.3.7.4 Mean carotid intima media thickness assessed at the 10-year point only in the growth hormone-treated and untreated groups. a, $p<0.05$ between groups. (Modified with permission, from Gibney J, Wallace JD, Spinks T, Schnorr L, Ranicar A, Cuneo RC, *et al.* The effects of 10 years of recombinant human growth hormone (GH) in adult GH-deficient patients. *J Clin Endocrinol Metab* 1999; **84**: 2596–602).

In conclusion, current data suggest that the standardized mortality rate is not increased in adults receiving growth hormone replacement, although the duration of therapy is relatively short. However it remains unclear whether growth hormone replacement will normalize the mortality rate observed in hypopituitary patients over the longer term.

Growth hormone therapy and bone

Growth hormone replacement in GHD patients produces a biphasic increase in bone turnover, causing a maximal effect on bone resorption after 3 months, and on bone formation after 6 months, which leads to a net gain of bone mass after 6–12 months in children, and after 18–24 months in adults (as the initial bone loss must first be replaced) (35, 57). Furthermore, studies of up to 10 years of growth hormone replacement show a sustained increase of BMD. It has been demonstrated that BMD continues to increase 18 months after discontinuation of growth hormone therapy (57).

Patients with lower BMD prior to growth hormone therapy respond with a higher increase in BMD, and the increase in BMD is slower in women than in men (35). The impact of growth hormone replacement on bone is greater on cortical than on trabecular bone (35). Unfortunately, measurement of BMD in GHD may not be a reliable predictor of fracture risk, and there is a lack of prospective studies documenting a reduction in fracture rates (57). A few cross-sectional studies have shown that growth hormone therapy reduces the risk of morphometric vertebral and nonvertebral fractures in GHD patients, even in those with untreated hypogonadism (57). This beneficial effect of bone fracture reduction seems to only occur in patients receiving growth hormone treatment shortly after being diagnosed with GHD (57). Finally, the addition of conventional osteoporosis therapy to GHD patients with confirmed osteoporosis, who already receive growth hormone replacement therapy, is also beneficial (35).

The GRS recommends assessment of BMD before initiating growth hormone therapy, and subsequently every 2 years (34) although this may be excessive. In order to monitor the skeletal response to growth hormone therapy, some authors also recommend an independent baseline assessment of fractures, as BMD may not be a good predictor of fractures in GHD (57). Additionally, the measurement of serum calcium, phosphate, alkaline phosphatase activity, and osteocalcin levels after the initiation of growth hormone treatment could be useful to evaluate the achievement of a therapeutic response (57).

Growth hormone therapy and other clinical features

In addition to the effects of growth hormone replacement discussed above, growth hormone has effects on many other areas of the body. Skin thickness and sweat secretion increase (60). Growth hormone affects deiodinase activity, increasing circulating triiodothyronine (T_3) levels (60) (35). This together with increase protein synthesis and fat oxidation (60) may explain the rapid 12–18% increase in REE which cannot be accounted for by increased lean body mass alone (61). Some, but not all studies, have shown increases in isometric and isokinetic strength (25); these changes become apparent after approximately 1 year and persist after 5 years of growth hormone therapy (35). This increase in muscle strength seems to be caused by an increment in muscle volume, and not by changes in muscle morphology or metabolism (35). Moreover, the degree of augmentation of muscle strength seems to be greater in childhood-onset GHD patients (35). In addition, local muscle endurance returns to baseline values after long-term growth hormone replacement (over 5 years), despite an initial decrease observed during the first 2 years of growth hormone treatment (35).

Finally, some but not all short- and long-term growth hormone replacement studies have shown an improvement in exercise capacity and physical performance, with marked increments in maximum oxygen uptake as well as maximum work capacity (25). Growth hormone therapy seems to increase exercise capacity through several mechanisms, including an increment in muscle mass, increased cardiac capacity, decreased fat mass, augmented red cell volume by IGF-1 stimulated erythropoiesis, and possibly by improved sweating (61).

Dosing strategies and long-term monitoring

The goal for growth hormone replacement in adults is to correct the abnormalities associated with adult GHD, maximizing benefits and minimizing side effects (34). As growth hormone secretion is greater in younger individuals than older ones, and in women than men, it is recommended that the starting dose of growth hormone in young men and women be 0.2 and 0.3 mg/day, respectively, and in older patients 0.1 mg/day (34) (see Box 2.3.7.2). Dose determination based on body weight is not recommended due to large interindividual variation in absorption and sensitivity to growth hormone, as well as the lack of evidence that a larger replacement dose is required for heavier individuals in adulthood (34). Dose escalation should be gradual, individualized, and guided by clinical and biochemical response (34). Measurement of serum IGF-1 provides the most useful marker for growth hormone dose titration in adults and it should be measured at least yearly. During the initial stages of dose titration, frequent measures are required; following a change in dose, IGF-1 assessment should be undertaken after 6 weeks (27, 34). The aim of dose titration is to achieve a serum IGF-1 level within the upper half of the age related normal range (34).

Despite IGF-1 being considered the most sensitive serum marker of growth hormone action, it may not reflect appropriately the growth hormone status of the patient, because as already described, normal serum IGF-1 concentrations are found in a considerable proportion of severe GHD patients. Moreover, the relationship between serum IGF-1 response during growth hormone therapy and other treatment effects such as metabolic endpoints and body composition is poor (35). Thus, it can be observed that the same dose of growth hormone can be suboptimal in one patient but cause side effects of over-dosage in another, and that normalization of serum IGF-1 can induce side effects attributable to growth hormone excess in some individuals (35). Hence, it is recommended to monitor other aspects of growth hormone therapy to assess both the efficacy and side effects of growth hormone treatment, and therefore to perform an individual dose titration (growth hormone dose titration against both clinical features of GHD and evidence of over-treatment determined by serum IGF-1 and the appearance of side effects) (35).

Since changes in body composition have been consistently found in growth hormone replacement trials in adults with GHD, the assessment of body composition, in particular extracellular water, could be used to monitor growth hormone replacement (35, 80). The GRS recommends performing a careful clinical examination and recording of anthropometric measures (weight, height, and BMI) before the start of the growth hormone replacement therapy, and the assessment of body composition to monitor growth hormone treatment response (34). The GRS considers that quantification of body composition changes (including bone mineral density) should preferably be made by dual X-ray absorptiometry (DEXA) where available, at baseline, and every 2 years after (34). However, body composition can also be assessed using anthropometric measures (including measurement of waist and hip circumferences), as well as with bioelectrical impedance evaluation (35). In addition, the GRS considers that cardiovascular risk markers should be measured yearly (34). Thus, some authors recommend measuring plasma lipids before growth hormone therapy starts, and subsequently on a regular basis, particularly in patients with baseline abnormalities, or those with other cardiovascular risk factors (35). Insulin sensitivity monitoring should be undertaken, which can be done by calculation of the homoeostasis model assessment (HOMA), by measurement of fasting levels of glucose, insulin, and HbA_{1c} (35). In contrast to the NICE guidelines, GRS usually reserves the use of disease-specific quality of life questionnaires for research purposes, although it recommends undertaking a detailed history with attention to quality of life parameters to monitor the efficacy of growth hormone replacement therapy (34). However, other authors recommend the use of a specific questionnaire before starting growth hormone treatment, which could be repeated every year in the follow up of GHD patients to evaluate the sustained response of quality of life to growth hormone therapy (63). In reality, the monitoring of patients receiving growth hormone replacement undertaken in clinical practice is determined by the rationale for treatment and safety.

Both GRS and NICE guidelines agree that adult patients receiving growth hormone replacement should be followed by an endocrinologist with special experience in pituitary disease/special interest in the management of growth hormone disorders, although it can be managed in partnership or 'shared-care' agreement with an internist or general practitioner. Growth hormone replacement is considered to most likely be for life; GRS recommends that a trial of withdrawal should be considered if any patient perceives no benefit (34), while NICE advises that growth hormone treatment should be discontinued in those patients who demonstrate inadequate improvement in quality of life score (<7 points on the QoL-AGHDA scale) after the first 9 months of therapy (69). There are concerns over the sole use of quality of life as a determinant of who receives growth hormone therapy and for the evaluation of its efficacy in GHD patients, as this practice fails to consider the other benefits of growth hormone replacement such as the improvement in markers of cardiovascular risk or bone health. Strategies for growth hormone replacement based solely on quality of life may deny patients these benefits which may have a consequence for their long term health.

The growth hormone dose may need to be reduced during long-term treatment, mimicking the decline in growth hormone secretion associated with ageing, reflected by the fall in the upper limit of the age specific normal range for IGF-1 (35). Growth hormone requirements may also change because of initiation or discontinuation of oral oestrogen (35). Other endocrine replacement may need to be adjusted. Initiation of growth hormone replacement may modify the dose of thyroxine or unmask the presence of central hypothyroidism (by increasing conversion of T_4 to T_3). More importantly the action of growth hormone and IGF-1 on 11-βHSD type 1 can lead to cortisol deficiency, particularly in patients on fixed-dose glucocorticoid replacement, which should be increased if indicated clinically (35).

Side effects and safety of growth hormone

Growth hormone replacement therapy in adults appears to be safe, when standards of care are followed (34). Recombinant human growth hormone is identical to the endogenous hormone and therefore it does not produce hypersensitivity reactions (61) although some patients may be sensitive to components of the diluent used. Absolute contraindications for growth hormone treatment include active malignancy, benign intracranial hypertension, and proliferative or preproliferative diabetic retinopathy (27). Although early pregnancy is not a contraindication, growth hormone should be discontinued in the second trimester as growth hormone is produced by the placenta (27).

Common side effects

Most adverse effects are dose related and are rarely seen in clinical practice if the dose of growth hormone is titrated carefully (25). Fluid retention, caused by the antinatriuretic effect of growth hormone, is the most frequent side effect, occurring in 5–18% of patients and includes paraesthesias, joint stiffness, peripheral oedema, arthralgia, and myalgia (25). In addition, 2% of treated GHD adults develop carpal tunnel syndrome (25). These fluid retention complications are more frequently seen in older, heavier, and female GHD adult patients, and most of them will resolve with dose reduction (25).

Diabetes mellitus

Growth hormone replacement therapy is not associated with an increased incidence of either type 1 or type 2 diabetes mellitus in adults (34), although data suggests it may be in children (35). However, growth hormone increases insulin resistance, so GHD patients with high risk of developing type 2 diabetes (positive family history, obese or older) require careful monitoring (34). These patients should be given a very low dose of growth hormone at initiation of therapy, which should be followed by a gradual increase in dose based on the clinical response (35). If type 2 diabetes is diagnosed, it should be managed similarly to any other patient with this disease, and growth hormone replacement therapy can be continued (34). Patients who have pre-existing diabetes mellitus require careful monitoring as their requirements for hypoglycaemic agents may increase during initiation of growth hormone therapy (25).

Rare side effects

Other reported side effects of growth hormone replacement include atrial fibrillation, gynaecomastia, congestive heart failure and benign intracranial hypertension, all of which are more likely to occur in the elderly (61) (with the exception of intracranial hypertension, which occurs primarily in children and adolescents) (25). Again, all these mentioned side effects are dose related (61). Retinopathy is an extremely unusual complication, but can also improve after growth hormone therapy withdrawal (25).

Tumour recurrence

There is no evidence that hypothalamic or pituitary tumour recurrence is influenced by growth hormone replacement therapy (34). Thus, although data of tumour recurrence and regrowth during growth hormone replacement is still limited (small studies and limited follow-up periods), the findings are reassuring (35). Consensus guidelines for the diagnosis and treatment of adults with GHD (34) recommend undertaking pituitary imaging before starting growth hormone therapy with appropriate follow-up imaging determined by the nature of the underlying condition. The use of growth hormone replacement does not require additional monitoring of residual disease (34).

Malignancy risk

There are conflicting results regarding the incidence of malignancies in hypopituitary patients not receiving growth hormone, as decreased and increased rates of malignancies have been reported in these patients (53). Some second tumours, such as meningioma, may be attributable to treatment with radiotherapy rather than hypopituitarism *per se* (53).

There is also an important concern regarding the possibility of increased risk of *de novo* cancer with growth hormone treatment, due to the mitogenic and growth-promoting actions of growth hormone and IGF-1. However, to date there is no evidence that growth hormone replacement in adults increases the risk of *de novo* malignancy, although growth hormone treatment during childhood slightly increases the relative risk of secondary neoplasia among cancer survivors (34). However, as reported by authors of the study that suggested an increased incidence of second neoplasms in survivors of acute leukaemia (81), the data need to be interpreted with caution given the small number of events (3 osteogenic sarcomas in 122 leukemia/lymphoma survivors treated with growth hormone vs 2 cases in 4545 leukemia/lymphoma survivors not treated with growth hormone). In the same study, growth hormone replacement did not appear to increase the risk of disease recurrence or death in survivors of childhood cancer. In a long-term follow-up study of 1848 patients treated in childhood and early adulthood with growth hormone (82), two patients died from colorectal cancer and two from Hodgkin's disease.

Extensive long-term, postmarketing surveillance of thousands of children and adults treated with growth hormone has not shown any increase in cancer rates (83). If growth hormone replacement treatment does result in a small increase in cancer risk compared with untreated patients with GHD, it is unlikely that, with careful dosing and monitoring, it will exceed that observed in the general population (83). Patients treated with growth hormone do not require screening for malignant disease beyond that recommended for the normal population.

Conclusion and the future

Over the past 20 years understanding of the impact of GHD in adults has increased and it is now a recognised clinical entity that affects a wide range of pathophysiological parameters. Although growth hormone replacement has become routine in modern endocrine practice there are still many questions that need to be answered. Long-term observational studies will determine whether the observed increased mortality in hypopituitarism will be reduced to levels seen in the normal population. Other work is required to determine whether the 'treatment for all' approach should be adopted universally or whether a more focused, symptom related approach is more appropriate. As new causes of pituitary dysfunction are identified, e.g. TBI, the role of growth hormone in rehabilitation needs to be explored. Finally, the features of GHD and the response to treatment described above are derived from patients with severe GHD. Future studies are required to determine whether patients with partial GHD would benefit from growth hormone replacement.

References

1. Li CH, Evans HM, Simpson ME. Isolation and properties of anterior hypophyseal growth hormone. *J Biol Chem*, 1945; **159**: 353–66.
2. Li CH, Papkoff, H. Preparation and properties of growth hormone from human and monkey pituitary glands. *Science*, 1956; **124**: 1293–4.
3. Raben MS. Treatment of a pituitary dwarf with human growth hormone. *J Clin Endocrinol Metab*, 1958; **18**: 901–3.
4. Raben MS. Growth hormone (concluded). 2 Clinical use of human growth hormone. *N Engl J Med*, 1962; **266**: 82–6.
5. Raiti S. Human growth hormone and Creutzfeldt-Jakob disease [editorial]. *Ann Intern Med*, 1985; **103**: 288–9.
6. Salomon F, Cuneo RC, Hesp R, Sönksen PH. The effects of treatment with recombinant human growth hormone on body composition and metabolism in adults with growth hormone deficiency. *N Engl J Med*, 1989; **321**:1797–803.
7. Jorgensen JOL, Pedersen SA, Thuesen L, Jorgensen J, Ingemann-Hansen T, Skakkebaek NE, *et al.* Beneficial effects of growth hormone treatment in GH-deficient adults. *Lancet*, 1989; **1**: 1221–5.
8. Iranmanesh A, Grisso B, Veldhuis JD. Low basal and persistent pulsatile growth hormone secretion are revealed in normal and hyposomatotropic men studied with a new ultrasensitive chemiluminescence assay. *J Clin Endocrinol Metab*, 1994; **78**: 526–35.
9. Giustina A, Veldhuis JD. Pathophysiology of the neuroregulation of growth hormone secretion in experimental animals and the human. *Endocr Rev*, 1998; **19**: 717–97.
10. Kojima M, Hosoda H, Date Y, Nakazato M, Matsuo H, Kangawa K. Ghrelin is a growth-hormone-releasing acylated peptide from stomach. *Nature*, 1999; **402**: 656–60.
11. Wren AM, Small CJ, Abbott CR, Dhillo WS, Seal LJ, Cohen MA, *et al.* Ghrelin causes hyperphagia and obesity in rats. *Diabetes*, 2001; **50**: 2540–7.
12. Arvat E, Maccario M, Di Vito L, Broglio F, Benso A, Gottero C, *et al.* Endocrine activities of ghrelin, a natural growth hormone secretagogue (GHS), in humans: comparison and interactions with hexarelin, a nonnatural peptidyl GHS, GH-releasing hormone. *J Clin Endocrinol Metab*, 2001; **86**: 1169–74.
13. Tannenbaum GS, Epelbaum J, Bowers CY. Interrelationship between the novel peptide ghrelin and somatostatin/growth hormone-releasing hormone in regulation of pulsatile growth hormone secretion. *Endocrinology*, 2003; **144**: 967–74.
14. van den Berg G, Veldhuis JD, Frölich M, Roelfsema F. An amplitude-specific divergence in the pulsatile mode of growth hormone (GH) secretion underlies the gender difference in mean GH concentrations in men and premenopausal women. *J Clin Endocrinol Metab*, 1996; **81**: 2460–7.
15. Iranmanesh A, Lizarralde G, Veldhuis JD. Age and relative adiposity are specific negative determinants of the frequency and amplitude of growth hormone (GH) secretory bursts and the half-life of endogenous GH in healthy men. *J Clin Endocrinol Metab*, 1991; **73**: 1081–8.
16. Rudman D, Kutner MH, Rogers CM, Lubin M, Fleming GA, Bain RP. Impaired growth hormone secretion in the adult population: relation to age and adiposity. *J Clin Invest*, 1981; **67**: 1361–9.
17. Clasey JL, Weltman A, Patrie J, Weltman JY, Pezzoli S, Bouchard C, *et al.* Abdominal visceral fat and fasting insulin are important predictors of 24-hour GH release independent of age, gender, and other physiological factors. *J Clin Endocrinol Metab*, 2001; **86**: 3845–52.
18. Leung DW, Spencer SA, Cachianes G, Hammonds RG, Collins C, Henzel WJ, *et al.* Growth hormone receptor and serum binding protein: purification, cloning and expression. *Nature*, 1987; **330**: 537–43.
19. Smit LS, Meyer DJ, Billestrup N, Norstedt G, Schwartz J, Carter-Su C. The role of the growth hormone (GH) receptor and JAK1 and JAK2 kinases in the activation of Stats 1, 3, and 5 by GH. *Mol Endocrinol*, 1996; **10**: 519–33.
20. D'Ercole AJ, Stiles AD, Underwood, LE. Tissue concentrations of somatomedin C: further evidence for multiple sites of synthesis and paracrine or autocrine mechanisms of action. *Proc Natl Acad Sci U S A*, 1984; **81**: 935–9.
21. Boisclair YR, Rhoads RP, Ueki I, Wang J, Ooi GT. The acid-labile subunit (ALS) of the 150 kDa IGF-binding protein complex: an important but forgotten component of the circulating IGF system. *J Endocrinol*, 2001; **170**: 63–70.
22. Meinhardt UJ, Ho KK. Modulation of growth hormone action by sex steroids. *Clin Endocrinol (Oxf)*, 2006; **65**: 413–22.
23. Abs R, Bengtsson B-Å, Hernberg-Ståhl E, Monson JP, Tauber JP, Wilton P, Wüster C. GH replacement in 1034 growth hormone deficient hypopituitary adults: demographic and clinical characteristics, dosing and safety. *Clin Endocrinol (Oxf)*, 1999; **50**: 703–13.
24. Webb SM, Strasburger CJ, Mo D, Hartman ML, Melmed S, Jung H, *et al.* Changing Patterns of the Adult Growth Hormone Deficiency Diagnosis Documented in a Decade-Long Global Surveillance Database. *J Clin Endocrinol Metab*, 2008; **94**: 392–9.
25. Molitch ME, Clemmons DR, Malozowski S, Merriam GR, Shalet SM, Vance ML. Evaluation and treatment of adult growth hormone deficiency: an Endocrine Society Clinical Practice Guideline. *J Clin Endocrinol Metab*, 2006; **91**: 1621–34.
26. Nicolson A, Toogood AA, Rahim A, Shalet SM. The prevalence of severe growth hormone deficiency in adults who received growth hormone replacement in childhood [see comment]. *Clin Endocrinol (Oxf)*, 1996; **44**: 311–16.
27. Consensus guidelines for the diagnosis and treatment of adults with growth hormone deficiency: summary statement of the Growth Hormone Research Society Workshop on Adult Growth Hormone Deficiency. *J Clin Endocrinol Metab*, 1998; **83**: 379–81.
28. Toogood AA, Beardwell, CG, Shalet, SM. The severity of growth hormone deficiency in adults with pituitary disease is related to the degree of hypopituitarism. *Clin Endocrinol (Oxf)*, 1994; **41**: 511–16.
29. Toogood AA. Endocrine consequences of brain irradiation. *Growth Horm IGF Res*, 2004; **14** Suppl A: S118–24.

30. Agha A, Sherlock M, Brennan S, O'Connor SA, O'Sullivan E, Rogers B, *et al.* Hypothalamic-pituitary dysfunction after irradiation of nonpituitary brain tumors in adults. *J Clin Endocrinol Metab*, 2005; **90**: 6355–60.
31. Schneider HJ, Kreitschmann-Andermahr I, Ghigo E, Stalla GK, Agha A. Hypothalamopituitary dysfunction following traumatic brain injury and aneurysmal subarachnoid hemorrhage: a systematic review. *JAMA*, 2007; **298**: 1429–38.
32. Agha A, Thompson, CJ. Anterior pituitary dysfunction following traumatic brain injury (TBI). *Clin Endocrinol (Oxf)*, 2006; **64**: 481–8.
33. Abs R, Mattsson AF, Bengtsson BA, Feldt-Rasmussen U, Góth MI, Koltowska-Häggström M, *et al.* Isolated growth hormone (GH) deficiency in adult patients: baseline clinical characteristics and responses to GH replacement in comparison with hypopituitary patients. A sub-analysis of the KIMS database. *Growth Horm IGF Res*, 2005; **15**: 349–59.
34. Ho KK. Consensus guidelines for the diagnosis and treatment of adults with GH deficiency II: a statement of the GH Research Society in association with the European Society for Pediatric Endocrinology, Lawson Wilkins Society, European Society of Endocrinology, Japan Endocrine Society, and Endocrine Society of Australia. *Eur J Endocrinol*, 2007; **157**: 695–700.
35. Nilsson AG, Svensson J, Johannsson G. Management of growth hormone deficiency in adults. *Growth Horm IGF Res*, 2007; **17**: 441–62.
36. McKenna SP, Doward LC, Alonso J, Kohlmann T, Niero M, Prieto L, *et al.* The QoL-AGHDA: an instrument for the assessment of quality of life in adults with growth hormone deficiency. *Qual Life Res*, 1999; **8**: 373–83.
37. Drake WM, Howell SJ, Monson JP, Shalet SM. Optimizing gh therapy in adults and children. *Endocr Rev*, 2001; **22**: 425–50.
38. Attanasio AF, Lamberts SW, Matranga AM, Birkett MA, Bates PC, Valk NK, *et al.* Adult growth hormone (GH)-deficient patients demonstrate heterogeneity between childhood onset and adult onset before and during human GH treatment. Adult Growth Hormone Deficiency Study Group. *J Clin Endocrinol Metab*, 1997; **82**: 82–8.
39. Toogood AA, Shalet SM. Growth hormone replacement therapy in the elderly with hypothalamic-pituitary disease: a dose-finding study. *J Clin Endocrinol Metab*, 1999; **84**: 131–6.
40. Davidson MB. Effect of growth hormone on carbohydrate and lipid metabolism. *Endocr Rev*, 1987; **8**: 115–31.
41. Russell-Jones DL, Weissberger AJ, Bowes SB, Kelly JM, Thomason M, Umpleby AM, *et al.* The effects of growth hormone on protein metabolism in adult growth hormone deficient patients. *Clin Endocrinol (Oxf)*, 1993; **38**: 427–31.
42. Salomon F, Wiles CM, Hesp R, Sonksen PH. The effects of treatment with recombinant human growth hormone on body composition and metabolism in adults with growth hormone deficiency. *N Engl J Med*, 1989; **321**: 1797–803.
43. McCallum RW, Petrie JR, Dominiczak AF, Connell JM. Growth hormone deficiency and vascular risk. *Clin Endocrinol (Oxf)*, 2002; **57**: 11–24.
44. Stewart PM, Toogood AA, Tomlinson JW. Growth hormone, insulin-like growth factor-I and the cortisol-cortisone shuttle. *Horm Res*, 2001; **56** Suppl 1: 1–6.
45. Rosen T, Bosaeus I, Tolli J, Lindstedt G, Bengtsson BA. Increased body fat mass and decreased extracellular fluid volume in adults with growth hormone deficiency. *Clin Endocrinol (Oxf)*, 1993; **38**: 63–71.
46. Colao A, Di Somma C, Savanelli MC, De Leo M, Lombardi G. Beginning to end: cardiovascular implications of growth hormone (GH) deficiency and GH therapy. *Growth Horm IGF Res*, 2006; **16** Suppl A: S41–8.
47. Gola M, Bonadonna S, Doga M, Giustina A. Clinical review: Growth hormone and cardiovascular risk factors. *J Clin Endocrinol Metab*, 2005; **90**: 1864–70.
48. Toogood A. Safety and efficacy of growth hormone replacement therapy in adults. *Expert Opin Drug Saf*, 2005; **4**: 1069–82.
49. Murray RD. Adult growth hormone replacement: current understanding. *Curr Opin Pharmacol*, 2003; **3**: 642–9.
50. Beshyah SA, Shahi M, Foale R, Johnston DG. Cardiovascular effects of prolonged growth hormone replacement in adults. *J Intern Med*, 1995; **237**: 35–42.
51. Amato G, Carella C, Fazio S, Montagna GL, Gittadini A, Sabatini D, *et al.* Body composition, bone metabolism, and heart structure and function in growth hormone (GH)-deficient adults before and after GH replacement therapy at low doses. *J Clin Endocrinol Metab*, 1993; **77**: 1671–6.
52. Colao A, Vitale G, Pivonello R, Ciccarelli A, Di Somma C, Lombardi G. The heart: an end-organ of GH action. *Eur J Endocrinol*, 2004; **151**(Suppl 1): S93–101.
53. Svensson J, Bengtsson BA, Rosen T, Oden A, Johannsson G. Malignant disease and cardiovascular morbidity in hypopituitary adults with or without growth hormone replacement therapy. *J Clin Endocrinol Metab*, 2004; **89**: 3306–12.
54. Bulow B, Hagmar L, Mikoczy Z, Nordstrom CH, Erfurth EM. Increased cerebrovascular mortality in patients with hypopituitarism. *Clin Endocrinol (Oxf)*, 1997; **46**: 75–81.
55. Rosen T, Bengtsson, BA. Premature mortality due to cardiovascular disease in hypopituitarism. *Lancet*, 1990; **336**: 285–8.
56. Tomlinson JW, Holden N, Hills RK, Wheatley K, Clayton RN, Bates AS, *et al.* Association between premature mortality and hypopituitarism. West Midlands Prospective Hypopituitary Study Group. *Lancet*, 2001; **357**: 425–31.
57. Giustina A, Mazziotti G, Canalis E. Growth hormone, insulin-like growth factors, and the skeleton. *Endocr Rev*, 2008; **29**: 535–59.
58. Rosen T, Hansson T, Granhed H, Szucs J, Bengtsson BA. Reduced bone mineral content in adult patients with growth hormone deficiency. *Acta Endocrinol (Copenh)*, 1993; **129**: 201–6.
59. Murray RD, Columb B, Adams JE, Shalet SM. Low bone mass is an infrequent feature of the adult growth hormone deficiency syndrome in middle-age adults and the elderly. *J Clin Endocrinol Metab*, 2004; **89**: 1124–30.
60. Carroll PV, Christ ER, Bengtsson BA, Carlsson L, Christiansen JS, Clemmons D, *et al.* Growth hormone deficiency in adulthood and the effects of growth hormone replacement: a review. Growth Hormone Research Society Scientific Committee. *J Clin Endocrinol Metab*, 1998; **83**: 382–95.
61. Cummings DE, Merriam GR. Growth hormone therapy in adults. *Annu Rev Med*, 2003; **54**: 513–33.
62. Jorgensen JO, Muller J, Moller J, Wolthers T, Vahl N, Juul A, *et al.* Adult growth hormone deficiency. *Horm Res*, 1994; **42**: 235–41.
63. Doga M, Bonadonna S, Gola M, Mazziotti G, Giustina A. Growth hormone deficiency in the adult. *Pituitary*, 2006; **9**: 305–11.
64. Ghigo E, Masel B, Aimaretti G, Léon-Carrión J, Casanueva FF, Dominguez-Morales MR, *et al.* Consensus guidelines on screening for hypopituitarism following traumatic brain injury. *Brain Inj*, 2005; **19**: 711–24.
65. Ghigo E, Aimaretti G, Corneli G. Diagnosis of adult GH deficiency. *Growth Horm IGF Res*, 2008; **18**: 1–16.
66. Roberts B, Katznelson L. Approach to the evaluation of the GH/IGF-axis in patients with pituitary disease: which test to order. *Pituitary*, 2007; **10**: 205–11.
67. Bidlingmaier M, Strasburger CJ. Growth hormone assays: current methodologies and their limitations. *Pituitary*, 2007; **10**: 115–19.
68. Pokrajac A, Wark G, Ellis AR, Wear J, Wieringa GE, Trainer PJ. Variation in GH and IGF-I assays limits the applicability of international consensus criteria to local practice. *Clin Endocrinol (Oxf)*, 2007; **67**: 65–70.

69. National Institute for Health and Clinical Excellence. Human growth hormone (somatropin) in adults with growth hormone deficiency. London: National Institute for Health and Clinical Excellence, 2003.
70. Gibney J, Wallace JD, Spinks T, Schnorr L, Ranicar A, Cuneo RC,*et al.* The effects of 10 years of recombinant human growth hormone (GH) in adult GH-deficient patients. *J Clin Endocrinol Metab*, 1999; **84**: 2596–602.
71. Maison P, Griffin S, Nicoue-Beglah M, Haddad N, Balkau B, Chanson P, *et al.* Impact of growth hormone (GH) treatment on cardiovascular risk factors in GH-deficient adults: a Metaanalysis of Blinded, Randomized, Placebo-Controlled Trials. *J Clin Endocrinol Metab*, 2004; **89**: 2192–9.
72. Florakis D, Hung V, Kaltsas G, Coyte D, Jenkins PJ, Chew SL, *et al.* Sustained reduction in circulating cholesterol in adult hypopituitary patients given low dose titrated growth hormone replacement therapy: a two year study. *Clin Endocrinol (Oxf)*, 2000; **53**: 453–9.
73. Abrams P, Abs R. The lipid profile in adult hypopituitary patients with growth hormone deficiency. *Growth Hormone Deficiency in Adults.10 years of KIMS*, ed. F.-R.U. Abs R. Oxford: Oxford PharmaGenesis TM Ltd. 2004; **349**: 127–138.
74. Sesmilo G, Biller BM, Llevadot J, Hayden D, Hanson G, Rifai N, *et al.* Effects of growth hormone administration on inflammatory and other cardiovascular risk markers in men with growth hormone deficiency. A randomized, controlled clinical trial. *Ann Intern Med*, 2000; **133**: 111–22.
75. Chrisoulidou A, Beshyah SA, Rutherford O, Spinks TJ, Mayet J, Kyd P, *et al.* Effects of 7 years of growth hormone replacement therapy in hypopituitary adults. *J Clin Endocrinol Metab*, 2000; **85**: 3762–9.
76. Arwert LI, Roos JC, Lips P, Twisk JW, Manoliu RA, Drent ML. Effects of 10 years of growth hormone (GH) replacement therapy in adult GH-deficient men. *Clin Endocrinol (Oxf)*, 2005; **63**: 310–16.
77. Gotherstrom G, Bengtsson BA, Bosaeus I, Johannsson G, Svensson J. A 10-year, prospective study of the metabolic effects of growth hormone replacement in adults. *J Clin Endocrinol Metab*, 2007; **92**: 1442–5.
78. Fideleff HL, Boquete HR. Growth hormone deficiency and GH replacement therapy: effects on cardiovascular function. in Growth Hormone Deficiency in Adults:10 Years of KIMS, ed Feldt-Rasmussen U, Abs R. Oxford: Oxford Pharmagenesis. 2004; 149–159.
79. Maison P, Chanson P. Cardiac effects of growth hormone in adults with growth hormone deficiency: a meta-analysis. *Circulation*, 2003; **108**: 2648–52.
80. Bengtsson BA, Johannsson G, Shalet SM, Simpson H, Sonken PH. Treatment of growth hormone deficiency in adults. *J Clin Endocrinol Metab*, 2000; **85**: 933–42.
81. Sklar CA, Mertens AC, Mitby P, Occhiogrosso G, Qin J, Heller G, *et al.* Risk of disease recurrence and second neoplasms in survivors of childhood cancer treated with growth hormone: a report from the Childhood Cancer Survivor Study. *J Clin Endocrinol Metab*, 2002; **87**: 3136–41.
82. Swerdlow AJ, Higgins CD, Adlard P, Preece MA. Risk of cancer in patients treated with human pituitary growth hormone in the UK, 1959–85: a cohort study. *Lancet*, 2002; **360**: 273–7.
83. Jenkins PJ, Mukherjee A, Shalet SM. Does growth hormone cause cancer? *Clin Endocrinol (Oxf)*, 2006; **64**: 115–21.

2.3.8 Surgery of pituitary tumours

Ian F. Dunn, Edward R. Laws Jr.

Introduction

Pituitary tumours have both endocrine and neuro-oncologic sequelae. Secretory tumours may liberate physiological hormones to pathological excess, generating a full spectrum of metabolic aberrations and hallmark clinical syndromes. Other pituitary tumours are endocrinologically inactive and generate instead a variety of compressive phenomena such as pituitary hypofunction and neurological compromise. Although advances continue to be made in the pharmacological and radiotherapeutic management of pituitary tumours, surgery remains the treatment of choice for most of these lesions. Of the available surgical options, the trans-sphenoidal route is the dominant surgical approach to these tumours. Shaped by the brilliant insight of individual surgeons and technological innovation, transsphenoidal surgery for the sellar and parasellar regions is a fascinating chronicle in surgical history whose evolution continues unabated. We herein review surgical approaches to pituitary tumours, emphasizing the transsphenoidal approach.

History

Transcranial surgical approaches to the sella preceded widespread adoption of the transphenoidal approach. The first reported surgical intervention for pituitary tumour was in 1892, when an English general surgeon performed a temporal decompression for headache in an acromegalic patient (1). Fedor Krause of Berlin described the details of a frontal transcranial approach to the sella in 1905; varying modifications of frontal and subtemporal approaches by such pioneering surgeons as Sir Victor Horsley, Walter Dandy, and Harvey Cushing followed (2).

The morbidity of these transcranial approaches, however, catalysed the development of extracranial approaches to the sella. Schloffer reported the first transsphenoidal approach to the sella in 1907 (3); he was followed by von Eiselsberg (4) and Hochenegg, who also used external rhinotomy incisions for access. Kocher soon after provided the first description of a submucosal dissection of the nasal septum. Endonasal and sublabial approaches performed without a disfiguring rhinotomy incision were pivotal advances introduced by Hirsch (5) and Halstead (6), respectively, *en route* to Cushing's introduction of his sublabial submucosal transseptal approach (7); these approaches are the direct progenitors of today's techniques. Cushing would famously abandon transsphenoidal surgery in favour of transcranial techniques in 1927, but his transsphenoidal approaches were sustained and refined by Norman Dott, his trainee Gerard Guiot—who would introduce fluoroscopy—and Jules Hardy, whose titanic contributions included the introduction of the operating microscope, the concept of the microadenoma, and the notion of selective tumour removal, while preserving normal pituitary tissue and function (5). The pioneering work of Guiot and Hardy formally established the technical and conceptual aspects of transsphenoidal surgery that form the basis of modern-day pituitary surgery.

Transsphenoidal surgery for pituitary tumours continues to develop. While the addition of image guidance in the form of frameless stereotaxy and ultrasonography have added to the safety and precision of the approach, the most significant refinement of the transsphenoidal approach in recent times has been the introduction of the purely endoscopic transsphenoidal approach (8–11). Although used intermittently as an adjunct to microscopic transsphenoidal surgery (12), the concept of a pure endoscopic transsphenoidal technique was introduced in the 1990s and has expanded the breadth of pathological entities approachable through the transsphenoidal corridor (9–11, 13, 14).

Whether performed microscopically or endoscopically, the transsphenoidal approach represents the preferred approach for more that 95% of pituitary tumours and for an expanding proportion of parasellar pathologies as well. In this chapter, we review the essential details of surgery for pituitary tumours, drawing on the personal experience of the senior author (ERL) that includes over 5000 transsphenoidal operations.

Epidemiology

Pituitary tumours are the third most common primary central nervous system tumour, accounting for 10–15% of all primary brain tumours; unselected autopsy studies have shown that 20–25% of the general population harbours small pituitary microadenomas (15). Data from academic medical centres suggest that pituitary tumours represent as many as 20% of surgically resected primary brain tumours (16). As a general rule, functioning pituitary tumours tend to be more common among younger adults, whereas nonfunctioning adenomas become more prominent with increasing age. Pituitary tumours are more common among women and are rare in the paediatric population.

Classification

The simplest approach to clinically classifying pituitary adenomas is the functional classification that broadly distinguishes tumours as functional or nonfunctional, based on their secretory activity. Functional adenomas are those that secrete prolactin, growth hormone, thyroid-stimulating hormone (TSH), or adrenocorticotropic hormone (ACTH), producing their respective clinical phenotypes of amenorrhoea-galactorrhoea syndrome, acromegaly or gigantism, secondary hyperthyroidism, and Cushing's disease or Nelson's syndrome. Tumours unassociated with a clinical hypersecretory state (i.e. gonadotroph adenomas, null cell adenomas, oncocytomas, and various silent adenomas) are collectively designated as clinically nonfunctional. More recently, a seven-tiered classification system comprising these features in addition to neuroimaging and intraoperative data, histological features, immunohistochemical profile, ultrastructural type, and molecular biology genetics has been developed by the WHO as a more universally applicable nomenclature (17).

From a surgical standpoint, classification systems that stress pituitary tumour size and growth characteristics are highly relevant. The most general system divides tumours purely based on size into microadenomas (<1 cm in diameter) or macroadenomas (>1 cm). The most enduring classification is that devised by Jules Hardy in 1969 and modified by Charles Wilson (18). This radiological classification first differentiates tumours as microadenomas or macroadenomas, with distinction made among microadenomas with abnormal sellar appearance. Macroadenomas causing diffuse enlargement, focal destruction, and extensive destruction of sella are referred to as grade II, grade III, and grade IV tumours, respectively. In this system macroadenomas are further staged according to the degree and direction of extrasellar extension.

Clinical presentation

The clinical manifestation of pituitary adenomas usually centres on one or more of three clinical scenarios: hypersecretion, hypopituitarism, or mass effect. The first involves pituitary hyperfunction in the form of several characteristic hypersecretory states. Hypersecretion of prolactin, growth hormone, ACTH, and TSH produces their corresponding clinical syndromes: amenorrhoea galactorrhoea syndrome, acromegaly or gigantism, Cushing's disease, and secondary hyperthyroidism. Because as many as 70% of pituitary adenomas are endocrinologically active, the presence of a hypersecretory endocrine state is the most common mode of presentation. As a rule, prolactin levels in excess of 200 ng/ml are generally the result of prolactin-producing tumour. Below this level, the lesion may still be a small prolactinoma, but any of a variety of other sellar pathologies may also give rise to elevated prolactin levels owing to the 'stalk effect'.

The second type of manifestation involves pituitary insufficiency and is typically associated with larger tumours that compress the nontumorous pituitary gland or its stalk or, as in the case of giant pituitary adenomas, compress areas of the hypothalamus. Only the anterior pituitary is compromised; regardless of how large the tumour is or how extreme the glandular or stalk compression, posterior pituitary failure (i.e. diabetes insipidus) is exceedingly rare.

A third pattern of manifestation is mass effect, with or without coexisting endocrinopathy. Headache is commonly an early symptom and has been attributed to stretching of the overlying diaphragma sellae. Suprasellar growth may compress the optic nerves and confer a bitemporal hemianopsia with diminished acuity. Continued suprasellar growth may compromise hypothalamic function and cause obstructive hydrocephalus. Lateral expansion into the cavernous sinus may lead to facial pain, diplopia, ptosis, or ocular symptoms due to cranial nerve involvement. Massive tumours can extend toward the temporal lobes and cause complex partial seizures.

Increasing numbers of adenomas are diagnosed incidentally by MRI and CT for evaluation of sinus disorders, trauma, and headache. Careful clinical and endocrinological correlations are required for such *incidentalomas* as these incidentally discovered adenomas may be symptomatic; up to 15% of incidentally discovered tumours are associated with endocrinopathy (19). These patients should be followed, as over 25% of incidentally discovered macroadenomas show considerable growth over time (19–21).

Diagnosis

An anatomical and endocrine diagnosis must be established in patients with pituitary tumours. MRI is used to establish an anatomical diagnosis and elucidate pertinent surgical details including the relationship of the tumour to the cavernous sinus, path of the carotid arteries, suprasellar extension and optic nerve compression, and sphenoid anatomy. Endocrine testing ordinarily includes serum hormone levels and provocative tests of the hypothalamic–pituitary–target organ axes. As an initial endocrine screen, basal measurements of prolactin, growth hormone, ACTH, luteinizing hormone, follicle-stimulating hormone (FSH), TSH, α-subunit, thyroxine, cortisol, insulin-like growth factor type 1 (IGF-1), testosterone, and oestradiol should be obtained to assess for pituitary dysfunction or hypersecretion. Thereafter, additional provocative, dynamic, and special hormonal assays are performed to define precisely a specific endocrinopathy.

Diagnosing Cushing's disease may be more complicated. Endocrinological findings suggestive of Cushing's disease include an elevated 24-h urine free cortisol level, loss of the diurnal variation in blood cortisol levels, and lack of suppression of serum cortisol levels after low-dose dexamethasone administration. Inferior petrosal sinus sampling after corticotropin-releasing factor stimulation may be required to help localize a pituitary source, though this may be accurate in only 60–70% of cases (22). In Cushing's disease patients without identifiable tumours, work-up for an ectopic hormone-secreting tumour in the chest, abdomen, or retroperitoneum is required.

Surgery

In general, therapy for pituitary tumours should be directed at the following goals:

- reversing endocrinopathy and restoring normal pituitary function
- eliminating a mass effect and restoring normal neurological function
- eliminating or minimizing the possibility of tumour recurrence
- obtaining a definitive histologic diagnosis

Therapeutic options for pituitary tumours include surgical resection, pharmacotherapy, and radiation therapy (i.e. conventional and stereotactic). Pharmacotherapy and radiotherapy are reviewed elsewhere in this volume.

Surgical indications

Surgery is considered first-line treatment in all symptomatic pituitary tumours except prolactinomas; in patients with these tumours, surgery may be required in the event of intolerance to, or failure of, medical therapy. Surgery should be performed urgently in pituitary apoplexy with compressive symptoms, regardless of the tumour type. In apoplexy, the presentation includes sudden headache, precipitous visual loss, ophthalmoplegia, altered level of consciousness, and collapse from acute adrenal insufficiency. In such situations, urgent glucocorticoid replacement and surgical decompression constitute the most reliable and effective forms of therapy. Another clear surgical indication is progressive mass effect from a large macroadenoma. These patients should always have a serum prolactin determination because prompt and dramatic shrinkage of prolactinomas can occur with appropriate pharmacological management. More often, the prolactin level is only modestly elevated, and the patient has a clinically nonfunctioning pituitary tumour or other sellar mass; such patients require decompression. An additional indication for surgery is the need to establish a tissue diagnosis.

Choice of surgical approach

Surgical approaches to the sellar region can be broadly categorized into three basic groups: transphenoidal approaches, conventional craniotomy, and alternative skull base approaches (Box 2.3.8.1).

Box 2.3.8.1 Surgical options for sellar and parasellar lesions

- Standard transsphenoidal approaches
- Endonasal submucosal transseptal transsphenoidal approach
- Endonasal submucosal septal "'pushover"' approach
- Sublabial transseptal transsphenoidal approach
  - Endoscopic transsphenoidal approach
- Standard transcranial approaches
- Pterional craniotomy
- Subfrontal craniotomy
  - Subtemporal craniotomy
- Alternative skull base approaches
- Fronto-orbital-zygomatic osteotomy approach
- Transbasal approach of Derome
- Extended transsphenoidal approach
- Lateral rhinotomy or paranasal approaches
- Sublabial transseptal approach with nasomaxillary osteotomy
- Transethmoidal and extended transethmoidal approaches
  - Sublabial transantral approach

The overwhelming majority of all pituitary adenomas can be approached through a transphenoidal approach. The remainder usually require a pterional or subfrontal craniotomy.

The choice of surgical approach depends on several factors. The most important of these includes the size of the sella, the size and pneumatization of the sphenoid sinus, the position and tortuosity of the carotid arteries, the presence and direction of any intracranial tumour extensions, whether any uncertainty exists about the pathology of the lesion, and whether prior therapy has been administered (i.e. surgery, pharmacological, or radiotherapeutic). Craniotomy may be preferred if the tumour has significant anterior or middle fossa extension or if a tumour with suprasellar extension is suspected to be of sufficiently fibrous consistency so as to prevent descent of the lesion inferiorly through the diaphragm. Occasionally, the configuration of the tumour is such that a single approach, transphenoidal or transcranial, is insufficient to effect complete tumour removal; in these cases, a combined transcranial-transphenoidal approach may prove effective.

Below, we review the surgical approaches for pituitary tumours, with specific emphasis on transphenoidal approaches.

Transsphenoidal approaches

For most pituitary tumours, a transsphenoidal approach is the most appropriate route. Major considerations in the approach to the sella through the sphenoid sinus include entry through the nostril directly (endonasal) or through the nostril via a midline incision under the lip (sublabial) and whether the microscope and/or endoscope is used. In our practice, the endonasal endoscopic approach has become our standard approach.

Advantages of the microscope include its familiarity to the neurosurgeon and three-dimensional view. The microscope itself is out of the surgical field and does not impair the manoeuvrability of instruments. Instruments can be brought in and out of the field easily without injuring the mucosa or nares, which are protected by a nasal speculum. The disadvantages include the limitations created by line of sight. Removal of tumour out of view is performed by feel, which is a factor requiring not only surgical skill but also experience.

Advantages of the endoscope include the panoramic and angled views that allow the surgeon to remove a greater portion of the tumour by direct visualization. The endoscopic approach is also well tolerated, rarely requires nasal packing, and avoids most anterior sinonasal complications. A disadvantage is that current endoscopic technology permits only two-dimensional viewing. Moreover, the surgeon must create enough room not only for the standard operating instruments as used in the microscopic approaches, but also for the endoscope itself. Because more instruments are in place than the microscopic approach, the exposure must necessarily be larger to accommodate the addition of the endoscope. Below, we review the sequential steps of the transsphenoidal approach.

Positioning

The patient's head is supported by a Mayfield headrest with a horseshoe (Fig. 2.3.8.1). Because the head is not fixed, gentle lateral movements of the head can be used to optimize intraoperative visualization, especially of the cavernous sinus area. This is not as significant a factor in endoscopic cases, in which the endoscope provides a panoramic view. Fixation of the head may be necessary when certain forms of image guidance are used.

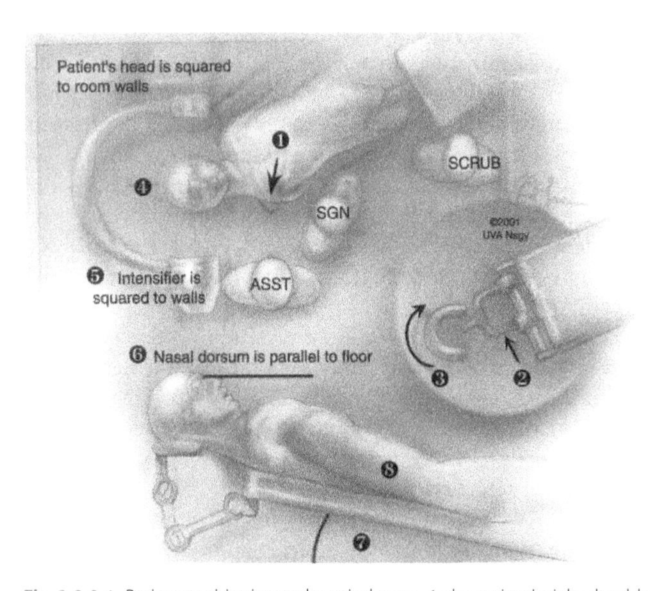

Fig. 2.3.8.1 Patient positioning and surgical team. 1, the patient's right shoulder is positioned in the top right-hand corner of the operative table; 2, the headrest frame is positioned to the far left; 3, the horseshoe headrest is rotated so that the patient's head is oriented toward the surgeon; 4 and 5, the patient's head is oriented at a right angle to the walls of the room to facilitate lateral intraoperative videofluoroscopy on the draped patient; 6, the head is positioned so that the trajectory is toward the sella. This is most easily accomplished by positioning the neck such that the dorsum of the nose is parallel with the floor; 7, the beach-chair position is used with the table angled approximately 20°; 8, the patient's right hand is carefully positioned in an unobtrusive manner under the buttocks. We have recently altered our team's positioning slightly in that the scrub now stands across the table from the surgeon to facilitate instrument handling. SGN, surgeon; ASST, assistant.

A semirecumbent position is used with the back at a 20° angle from the horizontal with the head above the heart (see Fig. 2.3.8.1). This facilitates venous drainage and decreases venous pressure within the cavernous sinus. The right shoulder is placed at the upper right hand corner of the bed and the patient's left ear is pointed toward the left shoulder and the bed turned so that the patient's head remains parallel to the wall of the room. The head may is gently tilted to the right.

Preoperative phase

Special consideration must be given to the intubation of acromegalic patients, who may require awake intubation to safely secure an airway. Perioperative prophylactic antibiotics are routinely employed. We administer steroids only in patients who show adrenal insufficiency on preoperative testing. In all others we no longer administer perioperative exogenous steroids. Instead, patients are monitored for clinical symptoms of adrenal insufficiency and morning serum cortisol levels are drawn on each postoperative day to determine the hypothalamic–pituitary–adrenal (HPA) axis reserve. Levels less than 8 µg/dl are considered low and replaced accordingly.

Prior to and immediately after induction, patients are given oxymetazoline intranasally for nasal decongestion. During positioning, cocaine-soaked patties are placed in both nostrils. The pledgets are allowed to remain in contact with the nasal mucosa for 5–10 minutes, during which draping of the patient is completed. The patties are removed after prepping and draping.

Sphenoid sinus access and exposure

Microscopic approaches

The next major consideration in the transsphenoidal procedure is the precise route of entry into the sphenoid sinus. For microscopic approaches, the two basic options are the endonasal approach and the sublabial approach. Selection of one over the other depends on the size of the nostril, the size of the lesion, and the preference of the surgeon. We tend to favour endonasal approaches in most instances, reserving the sublabial incision for paediatric patients or adults with small nostrils in whom the broader corridor afforded by the piriform aperture improves the visualization of the surgical field and the manoeuvrability of the surgical instruments. The endonasal microscopic approaches include the transeptal submucosal, the septal pushover, and the direct sphenoidotomy. These essentially differ based on the location of the initial incision. With the transeptal submucosal technique (Fig. 2.3.8.2a,b) the incision is made just within the nostril posterior to the columella; with the septal pushover (Fig. 2.3.8.2c) it is fashioned at the junction of the bony and cartilaginous septum; and with the direct sphenoidotomy, the incision is made at the junction of the septum and the rostrum of the sphenoid (23). As the incision is carried farther back, the amount of septal dissection, and therefore nasal complications, necessarily decreases. This decrease in septal dissection does come at the cost of a progressively more narrow and potential off-midline trajectory to the sella.

Endonasal microscopic approaches

The endonasal submucosal transseptal approach begins with a right-sided hemitransfixion incision in the nostril with the columella retracted to the patient's left and the ala retracted toward the right (see Fig. 2.3.8.2a,b). The inferior border of the cartilaginous septum is exposed with sharp dissection, and one side of the septum

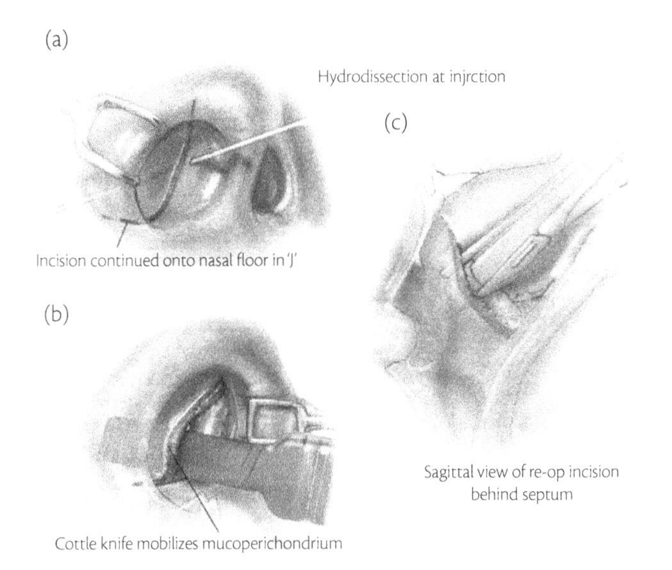

Fig. 2.3.8.2 Endonasal endoscopic approach: (a, b) submucosal endonasal approach; (c) septal displacement approach). Re-op, reoperation.

is exposed submucosally with a combination of sharp and blunt dissection, thereby creating a unilateral anterior tunnel. The dissection continues posteriorly, elevating the nasal mucosa away from the cartilaginous septum back to its junction with the bony septum. A vertical incision is then made at this junction, and bilateral posterior submucosal tunnels are created on either side of the perpendicular plate of the ethmoid. The articulation of the cartilaginous septum with the maxilla is then dissected free, and an attempt is made to raise the inferior mucosal tunnel on the opposite side so that the cartilaginous septum can be displaced laterally without creating inferior mucosal tears. A self-retaining nasal speculum can then be introduced to straddle the perpendicular plate of the ethmoid, exposing the face of the sphenoid sinus.

In some patients, particularly those who have had previous nasal, septal, or transsphenoidal surgery, we have used an alternative endonasal approach called the endonasal septal pushover technique (24) (Fig. 2.3.8.2c). Instead of a submucosal incision for creation of an anterior nasal tunnel, the nostril is entered, and an incision is made though the lateral mucous membrane of the nasal septum at the base of the septal insertion onto the maxillary ridge. The incision is carried back to the junction of the cartilaginous and bony septi or back to the face of the sphenoid if this bone has previously been removed. The nasal septum is carefully disarticulated, an opposite-side inferior tunnel is developed, and the septum together with the two layers of attached mucous membrane is reflected laterally to expose the perpendicular plate of the ethmoid and the sphenoid face. This is a rapid method of reaching the sphenoid, which we employ commonly. The most rapid of all endonasal approaches is the direct sphenoidotomy (23). In this approach a speculum is inserted directly anterior to the sphenoid rostrum. A sharp incision is be made at the attachment of the septum to the sphenoid rostrum and the septum is then reflected laterally exposing the rostrum of the sphenoid. As there is no submucosal septal dissection, there is rarely a need for nasal packing with its resultant postoperative discomfort. The primary advantages of the septal pushover and direct sphenoidotomy are the rapidity of the approaches and the avoidance of anterior septal dissection and its potential complications. However, these more direct approaches provide a more narrow exposure and an off-midline trajectory.

Sublabial microscopic approach

We reserve the sublabial approach for patients with small nasal apertures, including paediatric patients, and for patients with large tumours with significant extension into the cavernous sinuses and clivus which may be inadequately visualized through an endonasal approach. After the upper lip is retracted, an incision is made in the buccogingival junction from one canine tooth to the other (Fig. 2.3.8.3). Subperiosteal dissection is used to carefully elevate the mucosa from the maxillary ridge and the anterior nasal spine until the inferior border of the piriform aperture is exposed. Two inferior nasal tunnels are created by dissecting the mucosa away from the superior surface of the hard palate. With sharp dissection, a right anterior tunnel is created, and connected with the right inferior tunnels, and the entire right side of the nasal septum is exposed back to the perpendicular plate of the ethmoid. Using firm, blunt dissection along the right side of the base of the nasal septum, the cartilaginous portion of the nasal septum is dislocated and reflected to the left, and a left posterior mucosal tunnel is developed along the left side of the bony septum. At this point, it should be possible to insert the transsphenoidal retractor. After the retractor is in place, the vomer, with its distinctive keel shape, should be visualized.

Endoscopic approaches

Whereas the transsphenoidal approach has always been considered minimally invasive, particularly when compared with conventional transcranial approaches, the concept has been redefined in the context of endoscopic approaches to the sella (8). These approaches use straight and angled endoscopes as the sole visualization tools (i.e. pure endoscopic approach) or as a supplement to the operating microscope (i.e. endoscopic-assisted microscopic approach).

Several endoscopic approaches to the sella are used (8, 14, 25, 26). The iterations include mono- or bi-narial techniques, two-handed approaches with or without the endoscope holder, or three-handed or four-handed approaches without the holder. Some surgeons advocate a unilateral partial middle turbinectomy to improve the maneuverability of instruments. Our bias is to perform a three-handed binarial technique with a partial posterior septectomy without routine middle turbinectomy.

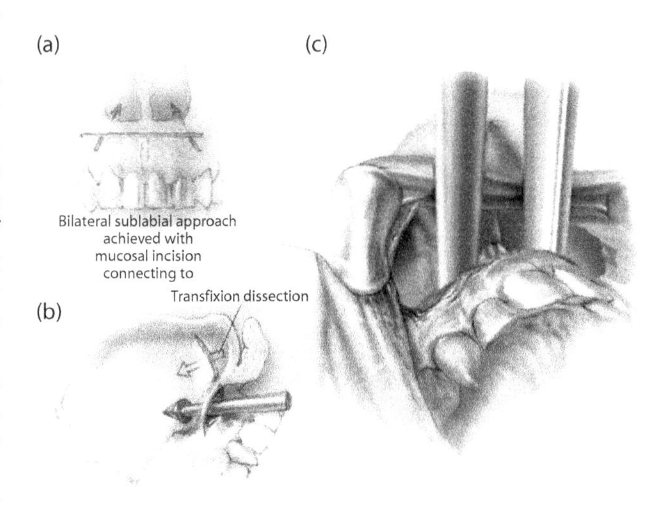

Fig. 2.3.8.3 Sublabial approach: (a, b) anterior and lateral conceptualization of trajectory to sella turcica; C, nasal speculum inserted.

The 0° endoscope is used for the majority of the exposure and tumour resection. The endoscope is brought within the nostril and the sinonasal anatomy is identified including the nasal floor and both the inferior and middle turbinates. The middle turbinate is lateralized and the choana and the spheno-ethmoid recess are identified. The sphenoid ostium is then identified posterior to the inferior third of the superior turbinate (Fig. 2.3.8.4a). Once identified, the posterior septum can be incised and reflected contralaterally to identify the contralateral sphenoid ostium (Fig. 2.3.8.4b). The bone between the two ostia is then removed providing the initial sphenoidotomy. A posterior septectomy is then completed, with care to not remove septum more anterior than the anterior limit of the middle turbinate.

Sphenoidotomy

Microscopic approach

Once the anterior face of the sphenoid sinus is reached, videofluoroscopy or neuronavigational image guidance is used to make any necessary adjustments to the final position and trajectory of the retractor blades. Midline orientation is crucial at this stage, and CT images of the sphenoidal region are extremely helpful in delineating the bony anatomy and planning sphenoidal entry. Portions of the bony nasal septum present in the operative field should be resected with a Lillie–Koeffler tool or a Ferris–Smith punch. Any cartilage and bone that has been resected should be preserved so it can be used during closure. For experienced surgeons, the nasal spine anteriorly does not represent a major obstacle, and from a cosmetic standpoint, it is preferable to preserve this structure rather than chisel it away. With the sphenoid retractors in position, the keel of the vomer and the face of the sphenoid are seen. On either side of the central ridge, the ostia of the sphenoid sinuses can be identified.

After the operating microscope is introduced, the anterior wall of the sphenoid is opened. Fracturing into the sphenoid sinus is usually possible by grasping the vomer with a Lillie–Koffler forceps, Ferris–Smith punch, or chisel, if necessary. Once within the sphenoid sinus, the exposure is widened with a right-angled punch. The mucosa within the sinus is resected with a cup forceps. Resection of the mucosa aids in reducing bleeding and decreases the risk of postoperative mucocele formation. With all internal bony landmarks clearly visible, the surgeon reorients himself or herself with respect to the position of the carotid arteries, sellar floor, anterior fossa floor, and clivus, correlating the operative anatomy with the imaging studies and navigational adjuncts, ensuring that the appropriate midline trajectory is maintained.

Endoscopic approach

The endoscopic anterior sphenoidotomy is generally larger than is required for microscopic approaches. Once the initial sphenoidotomy has been performed the intersphenoid sinus septae should be removed so that the sella can be identified. The extent of the sphenoidotomy can then be tailored to the location of the sella. The inferior extent of the sphenoidotomy should allow a suction to be placed on the clivus below the level of the tumour. The proximal vomer should be protected as a reference point for the anatomical midline. Care must also be taken to not injure the posterior nasal branches of the sphenopalatine artery at the inferolateral margins of the sphenoidotomy. The superior extent of the sphenoidotomy provides room for the endoscope during the tumour resection. The sphenoidotomy should continue superiorly until the tuberculum sellae, lateral opticocarotid recesses, and planum sphenoidale are readily observed (Fig. 2.3.8.4c).

Sellar entry

The sellar floor should be clearly visible in the microscopic and endoscopic approach (Fig. 2.3.8.4c). With some tumours, the sellar floor is eroded or is extraordinarily thin, and it can be fractured with a blunt hook. Occasionally, a midline septum within the sphenoid sinus can be used to gain entry into the sella by grasping its base and gently twisting as the bone is removed. If the floor of the sella is thick, a small chisel can be used to remove a square of bone. In cases of an even thicker sellar floor and when the sphenoid sinus is poorly pneumatized, a high-speed drill can be used to provide exposure. In the setting of recurrence, the appearance of the sellar floor can vary considerably. In more difficult instances, it may consist entirely of scar tissue, seemingly in continuity with the scarring encountered in the sphenoid sinus. In other cases, the sellar floor may have been fully reconstituted, appearing as if no prior procedure had been performed. In microscopic cases, the surgeon should use careful videofluoroscopic control or image guidance to continually monitor sellar entry, exposure, and trajectory. The panoramic endoscopic views generally provide adequate information regarding the anatomical midline and trajectory except in repeat surgery or tumours with significant sphenoid sinus invasion.

After the sellar floor has been penetrated, the opening is widened with a Kerrison-type punch. An adequate bony exposure is

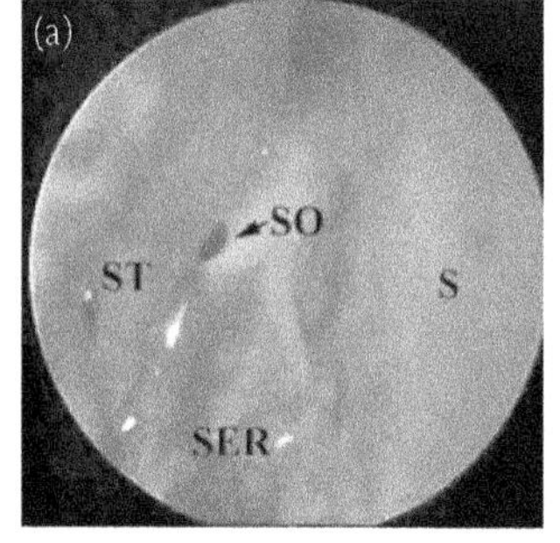

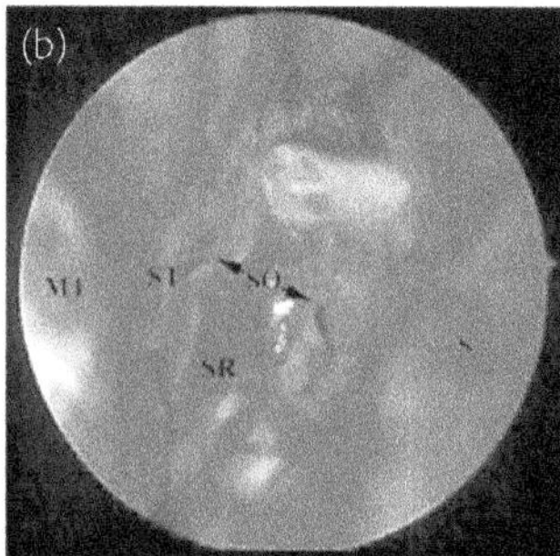

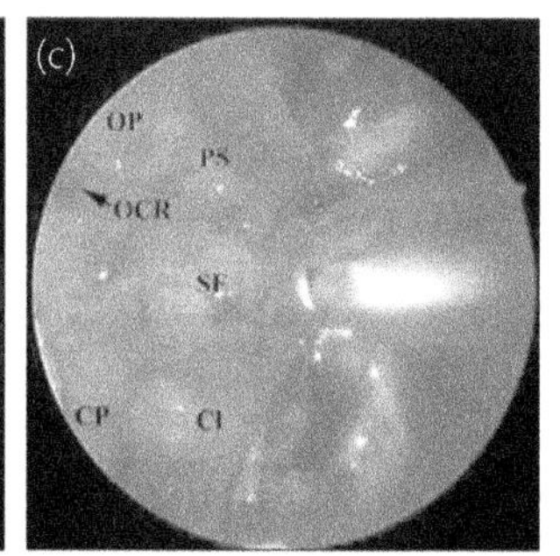

Fig. 2.3.8.4 (a) Endoscopic view of the right sphenoid ostium (SO). The sphenoid ostium (arrow) can be found at the inferior third portion of the superior turbinate (ST) and provides an important landmark for the level of the sphenoid sinus. (b) Endoscopic view following the posterior septectomy but prior to the anterior sphenoidotomy. Both sphenoid ostia (arrows) are visible with the endoscope in the right nasal cavity. An instrument placed through the left nostril can be seen above both ostia. (c) After the anterior sphenoidotomy, the panoramic view of the sphenoid anatomy with the optic and carotid protuberances (OP, CP respectively), opticocarotid recess (OCR, arrow), clivus (CI), planum sphenoidale (PS), and sellar impression. SER, sphenoethmoid recess; SF, sellar floor; SR, sphenoid rostrum.

crucial to the success of the transsphenoidal approach, particularly when dealing with large tumours. For recurrent tumours in particular, a wide bony opening can allow virgin dura to be uncovered. Identification of the latter is a real comfort and greatly assists in establishing a plane between dura and scar tissue. In general, we favour a wide removal of the sellar floor in virtually every case extending from one cavernous sinus to the other. A small, bony margin of the sellar floor should be left, because this facilitates sellar reconstruction at the end of the procedure.

An invasive tumour may erode through the anterior dura of the sella, but in most cases, the dura is intact. It is exposed as widely as is feasible, and careful attention is paid to its appearance. Transverse, blue intracavernous sinuses traversing the sella at the top and bottom of the anterior dura are common, particularly in cases of microadenomas. The anterior dura may appear blue and very thin, indicating the possible presence of a cyst or an empty sella. After the dura is exposed completely, it should be opened with great care. A partial empty sella is sometimes present, and a cerebrospinal fluid (CSF) leak early in the operation can be a major deterrent to success. Before the dural incision is made, it is prudent to use Doppler ultrasound and to review the imaging studies to assess the position of the carotid arteries so that they are not injured on durotomy. In dealing with some cystic pituitary adenomas, a helpful manoeuvre is to use a long needle to evacuate and evaluate cyst contents before dural opening.

The site of dural opening is then selected and incised in a cruciate or X-shaped fashion or with the excision of a dural window. Next, an attempt is made to establish a definite subdural cleavage plane between the pituitary gland or tumour and the underlying dura. A plane of dissection between the two leaves of the dura should be carefully avoided, because this practice allows entrance into the cavernous sinus, and heavy venous bleeding will result. The dural perimeter is widened by shrinking the dural margins with cautery, providing an unobstructed view into the sella.

Tumour removal

For the typical macroadenoma, the tumour is entered with a ring curet; tissue is loosened and then removed with a relatively blunt curet and forceps. Regardless of whether a microscopic or endoscopic surgery is performed, the surgeon should attempt tumour removal in an orderly fashion (see Fig. 2.3.8.6c below). Our practice has been to first remove tumour in the inferior aspect and then to proceed laterally, from inferior to superior aspects on both sides, removing tumour along the medial side of the cavernous sinus. The main distinction during endoscopic removal is the ability to directly visualize tumour removal from the cavernous sinus walls and suprasellar space (Fig. 2.3.8.5). The surgeon must resist coring out the central and most accessible portion of the tumour first, because this may cause premature descent of the diaphragma and entrapment of more laterally situated tumour. It is also important to delay the superior dissection until the lesion is relatively free elsewhere, because this minimizes trauma to the pituitary stalk and secondarily transmitted trauma to the hypothalamus. The surgeon occasionally may be required to follow tumour into a cavernous sinus or to deal with tumour directly involving the diaphragma. Decompression of the intrasellar portion of the tumour frequently permits a suprasellar extension to prolapse into view within the sella. After this has been resected, the diaphragma subsequently prolapses and generally signifies that the resection is complete. When spontaneous prolapse of the tumour capsule or diaphragma

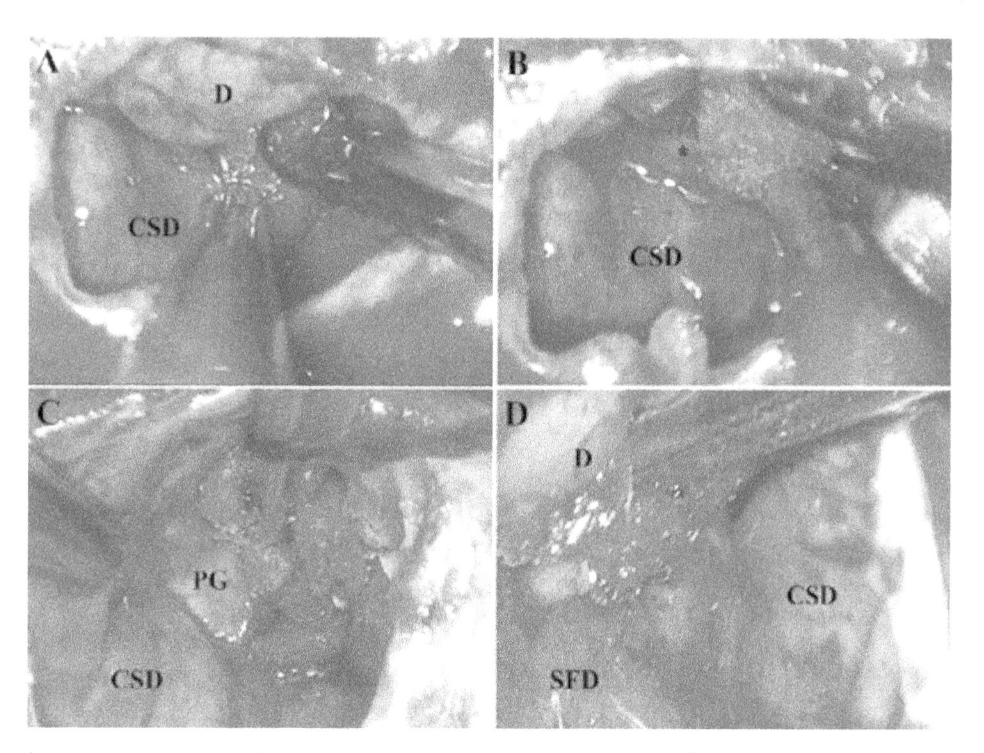

Fig. 2.3.8.5 Intrasellar endoscopic views. Using the endoscope, the resection cavity can be fully inspected. (a) View using the 30° endoscope looking toward the right cavernous sinus wall. The redundant diaphragma sellae (D) obstructs the full view. (b) Still using the 30° endoscope with the same vantage point, the diaphragma is elevated, which exposes residual tumour (asterisk). (c) View after the tumour residual has been removed. Note the compressed pituitary gland against the diaphragm. (d) Endoscopic view of the left cavernous sinus wall and a portion of the sellar floor using the 30° endoscope after tumour resection. The cavernous sinus wall appears to be intact and free of tumour residue. CSD, cavernous sinus dura; SFD, sellar floor dura.

does not occur, instillation of 15–20 ml of air or lactated Ringer's solution into a lumbar subarachnoid catheter may facilitate descent. Alternatively, bilateral jugular vein compression or application of positive end expiratory pressure can also help in delivering suprasellar tumour. If the tumour still fails to descend, a ring curet can be used cautiously in the intracranial space. These manoeuvres are well suited for the endoscopic technique which allows both cavernous sinus and suprasellar portions of tumours to be removed under direct visualization. Bleeding from the tumour bed can usually be controlled by precise tamponade with cotton patties or Gelfoam. In all cases, a concerted effort is made to preserve normal pituitary tissue. In a large, diffuse adenoma, normal glandular tissue usually appears as a thin membrane, situated superolaterally against the sellar wall. The orange-yellow gland, together with its firm consistency, distinguishes it from the greyish colour and finely granular texture typical of the tumour (Fig. 2.3.8.5).

Microadenomas necessitate a different operative strategy because many are not immediately visualized on opening the dura. A systematic search through a seemingly normal-appearing gland is often required. We begin with a transverse glandular incision, followed by subdural dissection and mobilization of the lateral wings. If the incision in the gland is deep enough, lateral pressure with a Hardy dissector usually causes the microadenoma to herniate into the operative field. Its location can therefore be delineated, its cavity entered, and its removal completed by use of a small ring curet and cup forceps. All suspicious tissue is removed, and a biopsy specimen is occasionally obtained from the residual and presumably normal pituitary gland.

Reconstruction and closure

This phase begins with a careful inspection for the presence of CSF leaks—these can occur during all types of intrasellar explorations. If a CSF leak is present or suspected, a fat graft is obtained from a subumbilical incision, prepared as described below. The fat is cut into appropriate-sized pieces soaked in 10% chloramphenicol solution, patted on a cotton ball in order to incorporate a few wisps of cotton fibres (which provoke a fibrotic reaction), and rolled in Avitene haemostatic collagen powder. The fat is packed into the sellar cavity, avoiding excessive packing but placing enough to occlude the sella, to prevent spinal fluid leak, and to achieve haemostasis. The sellar floor is then reconstructed (Fig. 2.3.8.6). One can use bone from the initial operative phase or artificial constructs such as a MedPor-tailored plate (27, 28). The MedPor plate is a thin polyethylene plate with a perpendicularly oriented tab to facilitate implant placement and manoeuvring; its micropores allow for tissue ingrowth and it features a very low signal intensity on MRI (28). This is placed epidurally if a CSF leak was present and otherwise is placed intradurally; other groups also stress the importance of the extradural layer in preventing CSF leak (29).

One carefully suctions blood and surgical debris from the sphenoid cavity and the nasopharynx prior to closure, and if no packing is necessary, the turbinates are then medialized. We place Merocel nasal packs in patients who have undergone submucosal dissection or in whom haemostasis was challenging. The abdominal incision is closed with subcuticular technique. The oropharynx is carefully suctioned prior to extubation of the patient.

Adjuncts

If significant suprasellar extension is present, a catheter may be placed into the lumbar subarachnoid space, into which an infusion of air may be used to facilitate descent of the tumour's superior extent into the sella. Similar results may be accomplished with Valsalva's manoeuvre or with jugular vein compressions.

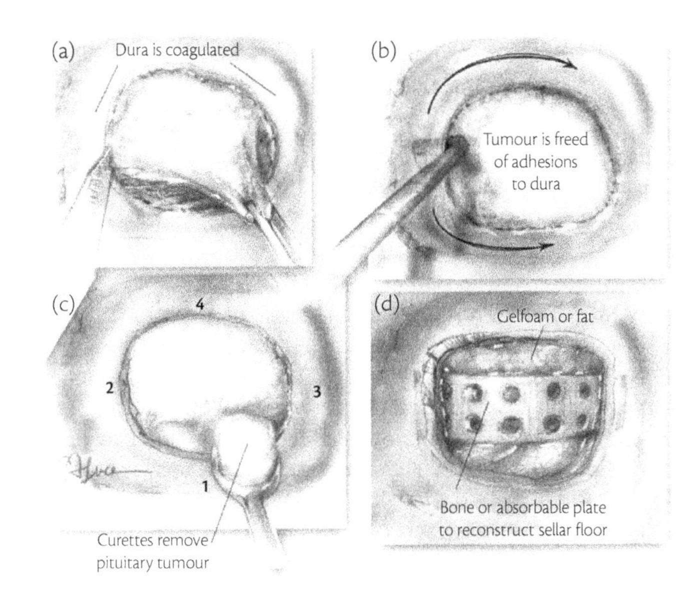

Fig. 2.3.8.6 Schematic showing the steps of tumour resection. (a) Dural incision. (b) Subdural plane developed. (c) Sequential removal of tumour inferiorly, laterally, then superiorly. (d) Reconstruction of sella with fat or Gelfoam pieces buttressed by a bioabsorbable plate.

Image guidance

The most widely used intraoperative imaging device is the C-arm videofluoroscope. Most often, a lateral image confirms the appropriate trajectory to the sella turcica and is also used to confirm its superior and inferior confines. Knowing the superior and inferior limits of the sella turcica allows the surgeon to confirm adequate exposure and prevents unnecessary opening of the planum sphenoidale and CSF leak. One disadvantage of the C-arm is the inability to image adjacent neurovascular structures and tumour. The increasing sophistication of image-guidance platforms allowing highly accurate and precise instrument tracking on a co-registered preoperative MRI scan has influenced our and others' practice, and we now perform virtually every transsphenoidal operation with the aid of frameless stereotaxy. Its main utility is in the initial stages of the transsphenoidal approach to the sella, as such systems provide very accurate information regarding operative trajectory and adherence to the midline, proximity to the sphenoid, sella, and carotids. The sagittal view is especially helpful in tracking the trajectory to the sphenoid and sellar face, while the coronal and axial views are useful in verifying proximity to the midline and helping to prevent errant entry into the cavernous sinus or carotid arteries (30–32).

Another useful adjunct in an attempt to avoid cavernous carotid injury is a bayoneted micro-Doppler probe (33, 34). This has proven to be a helpful tool in identifying the carotid arteries prior to incising the sellar dura and during removal of lateral portions of sellar lesions.

Postoperative care

For all patients, vigilant postoperative monitoring of water and electrolyte balance is mandatory. Diuresis of various degrees regularly occurs in the postoperative period, but it does not necessarily imply a diagnosis of diabetes insipidus nor a need for vasopressin. This state must be distinguished from true diabetes insipidus, which is accompanied by a brisk diuresis, defined by characteristic alterations in the serum sodium and serum or urine osmolalities and for which prompt fluid replacement and vasopressin are crucial. When it does occur, diabetes insipidus is usually temporary. Patients without preoperative evidence of hypothalamic–pituitary–adrenal axis deficits are not given exogenous steroids. Instead, they are monitored for signs of cortisol deficiency and morning serum cortisol levels are drawn on each postoperative day. Levels less than 8 ug/dl are considered low and patients are then given physiological steroid replacement.

Prophylactic antibiotics are continued until the nasal packing is removed, usually on the first or second postoperative day. In uncomplicated cases, the patient can be discharged from hospital by the second day. The first follow-up visit occurs about 8 weeks after surgery, at which time endocrine testing is performed and endocrine replacement therapy administered for any deficiencies identified. Follow-up gadolinium-enhanced MRI of the sella is usually performed at this time and then on an annual basis as necessary. Formal visual field examinations are also performed at the 2-month visit for patients who had preoperative visual deficits.

Outcomes

Nonfunctioning pituitary adenomas most often present as macroadenomas and cause visual field deficits and hypopituitarism. Of patients presenting with visual deficits, surgery improves visual loss in approximately 87% (Table 2.3.8.1). Postoperative worsening of vision occurs in 4% of patients, and in the remainder vision is unchanged. Twenty-seven per cent of patients presenting with hypopituitarism experience postoperative normalization of hormone secretion. Operative mortality for these larger, and often more invasive, tumours is higher than for the hyperfunctioning adenomas and reaches just over 1%. For similar reasons, tumour recurrence is also an issue. Ten-year recurrence/persistence rates are approximately 16%, although only 6% require reoperation. Long-term follow-up finds 83% of patients alive and well without evidence of disease (35).

Criteria for reporting remission from acromegaly require normalization of age-adjusted IGF-1 levels; random growth hormone less than 2.5 ng/ml; and nadir growth hormone during an oral glucose tolerance test of less than 1 ng/ml. Using these strict criteria, transsphenoidal surgery obtains remission in 88% of patients with microadenomas and 65% of patients with macroadenomas. Acromegalic symptoms are improved in 95%. Recurrence at 10 years is less than 2%. Ninety-seven per cent of patients have preserved normal pituitary function. Seventy-two per cent of patients with greater than 10-year follow-up, including those with adjunctive therapy, are alive and well without evidence of active disease.

Patients with prolactinomas who present for surgery are most often those who have failed medical management. Prolactin levels are normalized in 87% of patients with microadenomas and 56% of those with macroadenomas. The recurrence rate among those patients who are normalized after a transsphenoidal operation is 13% at 10 years. Preserved pituitary function occurs in all but 3%.

Surgical management of Cushing's disease achieves a 91% remission rate for patients with microadenomas, but falls to 65% for those with macroadenomas. Although up to 12% of adults might experience recurrence after 10 years, a higher percentage of children develop recurrence of Cushing's disease. Adjunctive radiosurgery has achieved remission in approximately 68% of patients whose disease either did not remit after surgery or recurred (35).

Table 2.3.8.1 Postoperative remission and recurrence after transsphenoidal surgery for pituitary adenomas: results of transsphenoidal surgery, 1972–2000 (n = 3093)

Clinical entity	Remission (%)	Recurrence at 10 years (%)	No disease at 10 years (%)
Nonfunctioning adenoma	NA	16	83
Growth hormone adenoma		1.3	72
Microadenoma	88		
Macroadenoma	65		
Prolactin adenoma		13	65
Microadenoma	87		42% (children)
Macroadenoma	56		
ACTH adenoma		12 (adults), 42 (paediatric)	75
Microadenoma	91		
Macroadenoma	65		

ACTH, adrenocorticotropic hormone (corticotropin).

Complications

The transsphenoidal approach is a safe operation with a well-established complication profile (Table 2.3.8.2). In a carefully analysed series of over 2500 transsphenoidal cases, the mortality rate was 1% and the rate of major complications 3.4%, comprising vascular injury and its sequelae, visual loss, cranial nerve injury, CSF leak, and meningitis. Transient diabetes insipidus occurs in 18% of cases, with 2% requiring long-term treatment (36). Anterior septal perforations are becoming less common as surgeons adopt progressively more direct approaches to the sphenoid sinus.

Intraoperative CSF leak is common during transsphenoidal surgery, and an adequate repair during surgery is essential to avoid a postoperative leak. Upon confirmation or suspicion of an intraoperative CSF leak, we harvest a fat graft as described above. Patients with postoperative CSF leaks are usually taken back promptly to the operating room for exploration, repacking, and reconstruction of the sellar floor.

Iatrogenic injury to the internal carotid artery is arguably the most feared complication of transsphenoidal surgery; exuberant cavernous sinus bleeding and sphenopalatine artery injury are among other vascular complications encountered. Carotid injury occurs in 1–2% of cases, with patients who have had prior craniotomy, transsphenoidal surgery, or radiation therapy at greater risk (37, 38). Careful study of preoperative imaging to appreciate the course of the carotids and operating from a true midline position are critical; intraoperative image guidance can help confirm midline positioning during surgery, particularly in reoperations or in other cases where normal anatomy appears distorted. A micro-Doppler can help confirm carotid location. Should the carotid be injured during surgery, options include direct repair and non-obliterative packing, with the latter more commonly employed. Immediate angiography should be performed to delineate possible cavernous-carotid fistula or pseudoaneurysm and a balloon occlusion test performed should the carotid require sacrifice. If the angiogram is normal, it should be repeated in 1 week.

Table 2.3.8.2 Complications of transsphenoidal surgery[a]

Complications	Patients
Operative mortality (30 day)	
Hypothalamic injury or haemorrhage	5
Meningitis	2
Vascular injury or occlusion	4
CSF leak or pneumocephalus, SAH or spasm, myocardial infarction	1
Postoperative myocardial infarction, postoperative seizure	2
Total	14 (1.0%)
Major morbidity	
Vascular occlusion, stroke, SAH, or spasm	5
Visual loss (new)	11
Vascular injury (repaired)	8
Meningitis (nonfatal)	8
Sellar abscess	1
Sellar pneumatocele	1
Sixth cranial nerve palsy	2
Third cranial nerve palsy	1
CSF rhinorrhea	49
Total	86 (3.4%)
Lesser morbidity	
Hemorrhage (intraoperative or postoperative)	9
Postoperative psychosis	5
Nasal septal perforation	16
Sinusitis, wound infection	5
Transient cranial nerve palsy (III or IV)	5
Diabetes insipidus (usually transient)	35
Cribriform plate fracture	2
Maxillary fracture	2
Hepatitis	1
Symptomatic SIADH	37
Total	117 (4.6%)

[a] From the authors' series of 2562 pituitary adenomas.
CSF, cerebrospinal fluid; SAH, subarachnoid haemorrhage; SIADH, syndrome of inappropriate antidiuretic hormone.

Transcranial approaches

There are three basic transcranial approaches to pituitary tumours: pterional, subfrontal, and subtemporal. Selection of one approach over the others depends on the precise geometry and growth trajectory of the tumour, as well as the preference and experience of the surgeon. Probably the most versatile approach, and the one that we prefer most is the pterional approach. Occasionally other skull base craniotomy approaches are useful (see Box 2.3.8.1); however, their review is beyond the scope is this chapter.

Pterional approach

For most tumours, except those with significant left-sided extensions, we use a right-sided pterional approach. The placement of a lumbar drain is optional, but it can be of help with brain relaxation during the intradural portion of the procedure. The head is placed in a three-point pinion headrest and turned 20° to the left side such that the lateral aspect of the malar eminence is brought to an uppermost position. The position of the neck relative to the body is such that venous drainage of the head is uncompromised. This position, too, usually places the ipsilateral optic nerve perpendicular to the floor.

The scalp incision is placed behind the hairline, using a coronal or curved Dandy incision. We turn a standard pterional bone flap which spans the Sylvian fissure but often include a generous frontal extension, with the craniotomy extending to just above the supraorbital rim. The sphenoid ridge is generously drilled from lateral to medial aspects. The dura is opened in a C-shaped fashion and reflected anteriorly.

Attention is then turned to achieving adequate brain relaxation. This requires osmotic diuresis or withdrawal of CSF, or both, through a lumbar drain or directly from the basal cisterns or from the lateral ventricle if hydrocephalus coexists. Ordinarily, we begin by gently elevating the frontal lobe, identifying the optic nerve and carotid artery and sharply incising their respective arachnoid cisterns. This step is performed with patience, gradually withdrawing sufficient CSF to optimize brain relaxation and minimize retraction pressures. Microdissection and opening of the sylvian fissure is almost always worthwhile, because it releases the frontal lobe and allows it to more freely fall backward with gravity. Self-retaining retractors are placed as necessary.

In most instances, obvious tumour is encountered behind the tuberculum and between the optic nerves. The pituitary stalk, with its portal vessels producing a characteristic vertically striated appearance, can usually be identified behind the tumour in the triangle between the lateral border of the right optic nerve and the carotid triangle. Every effort is made not to disturb this structure. The tumour capsule is then carefully dissected away from surrounding structures. Great care should be exercised in dealing with portions of the tumour attached to the optic apparatus, the dissection of which may damage these structures or their microvasculature. The tumour can be entered through several operative corridors. Usually, the capsule is incised between the optic nerves. The tumour is entered and its contents removed by curettes, suction, or for unusually fibrous tumours, with sharp dissection. Manipulation of the capsule and additional internal decompression can be performed though the opticocarotid triangle as well. A translaminar terminalis approach can also be performed if a third ventricular component fails to descend.

After the tumour has been removed and haemostasis ensured, particularly from within the sella, the dura is closed in a watertight fashion. If the frontal sinus has been transgressed, it should be exenterated and isolated with a pericranial flap. The bone flap is replaced, the temporalis muscle reapproximated, and the scalp closed in the usual two-layered fashion.

The postoperative care of these patients, like those undergoing transsphenoidal surgery, centres on careful monitoring of fluid and electrolytes, recognition and management of diabetes insipidus if it develops, and replacement therapy for pituitary insufficiency. These patients, like all patients undergoing craniotomy for any reason, must also be monitored for brain swelling, postoperative haemorrhage, seizures, CSF leak, and infection. Mortality and major morbidity rates with transcranial procedures are generally less than 3%, and the overall complication rate is usually less than 10%.

Summary

Contemporary surgery for pituitary tumours is the product of over a century of innovation and technical refinement. The transsphenoidal approach is used in over 95% of cases of pituitary tumour, with craniotomies only rarely performed for these tumours; substantial surgical series have shown the transsphenoidal variations to be remarkably safe and effective. The increasing prevalence of the endoscope in transsphenoidal surgery will only enhance the safety and flexibility of this skull base approach.

References

1. Caton R, Paul F. Notes on a case of acromegaly treated by operation. *Br Med J*, 1893; **2**: 1421–3.
2. Kanter AS, Dumont AS, Asthagiri AR, Oskouian RJ, Jane JA Jr, Laws ER, Jr. The transsphenoidal approach. A historical perspective. *Neurosurg Focus*, 2005; **18**: e6.
3. Schloffer H. Erfolgreiche Operationen eines Hypophysentumors auf Nasalem Wege. *Wien Klin Wochenschr*, 1907; **20**: 621–4.
4. von Eiselsberg A. The operative cure of acromegaly by removal of a hypophysial tumor. *Laryngoscope*, 1908; **102**: 951–3.
5. Lanzino G, Laws ER Jr. Key personalities in the development and popularization of the transsphenoidal approach to pituitary tumors: an historical overview. *Neurosurg Clin N Am*, 2003; **14**: 1–10.
6. Halstead AE. Remarks on the operative treatment of tumors of the hypophysis. With the report of two cases operated on by an oronasal method. *Trans Am Surg Assoc*, 1910; **28**: 73–93.
7. Cushing H. The Weir Mitchell Lecture. Surgical experiences with pituitary adenoma. *JAMA*, 1914; **63**: 1515–25.
8. Jho HD, Carrau RL. Endoscopic endonasal transsphenoidal surgery: experience with 50 patients. *J Neurosurg*, 1997; **87**: 44–51.
9. Kassam A, Snyderman CH, Mintz A, Gardner P, Carrau RL. Expanded endonasal approach: the rostrocaudal axis. Part II. Posterior clinoids to the foramen magnum. *Neurosurg Focus*, 2005; **19**: E4.
10. Kassam A, Snyderman CH, Mintz A, Gardner P, Carrau RL. Expanded endonasal approach: the rostrocaudal axis. Part I. Crista galli to the sella turcica. *Neurosurg Focus*, 2005; **19**: E3.
11. Cappabianca P, Alfieri A, de Divitiis E. Endoscopic endonasal transsphenoidal approach to the sella: towards functional endoscopic pituitary surgery (FEPS). *Minim Invasive Neurosurg*, 1998; **41**: 66–73.
12. Apuzzo ML, Heifetz MD, Weiss MH, Kurze T. Neurosurgical endoscopy using the side-viewing telescope. *J Neurosurg*, 1977; **46**: 398–400.
13. Jane JA Jr, Han J, Prevedello DM, Jagannathan J, Dumont AS, Laws ER Jr. Perspectives on endoscopic transsphenoidal surgery. *Neurosurg Focus*, 2005; **19**: E2.
14. Jho HD. Endoscopic pituitary surgery. *Pituitary*, 1999; **2**: 139–54.
15. McComb DJ, Ryan N, Horvath E, Kovacs K. Subclinical adenomas of the human pituitary. New light on old problems. *Arch Pathol Lab Med*, 1983; **107**: 488–91.
16. Jane JA Jr, Sulton LD, Laws ER Jr. Surgery for primary brain tumors at United States academic training centers: results from the Residency Review Committee for neurological surgery. *J Neurosurg*, 2005; **103**: 789–93.
17. Louis DN, Ohgaki H, Wiestler OD, Cavenee WK, Burger PC, Jouvet A, *et al.* The (2007) WHO classification of tumours of the central nervous system. *Acta Neuropathol*, 2007; **114**: 97–109.
18. Hardy J. Transphenoidal microsurgery of the normal and pathological pituitary. *Clin Neurosurg*, 1969; **16**: 185–217.
19. Feldkamp J, Santen R, Harms E, Aulich A, Modder U, Scherbaum WA. Incidentally discovered pituitary lesions: high frequency of macroadenomas and hormone-secreting adenomas-results of a prospective study. *Clin Endocrinol (Oxf)*, 1999; **51**: 109–13.
20. Donovan LE, Corenblum B. The natural history of the pituitary incidentaloma. *Arch Intern Med*, 1995; **155**: 181–3.
21. Molitch ME, Russell EJ. The pituitary 'incidentaloma'. *Ann Intern Med*, 1990; **112**: 925–31.
22. Oldfield EH, Doppman JL, Nieman LK, Chrousos GP, Miller DL, Katz DA, *et al.* Petrosal sinus sampling with and without corticotropin-releasing hormone for the differential diagnosis of Cushing's syndrome. *N Engl J Med*, 1991; **325**: 897–905.
23. Zada G, Kelly DF, Cohan P, Wang C, Swerdloff R. Endonasal transsphenoidal approach for pituitary adenomas and other sellar lesions: an assessment of efficacy, safety, and patient impressions. *J Neurosurg*, 2003; **98**: 350–8.
24. Wilson WR, Laws ER Jr. Transnasal septal displacement approach for secondary transsphenoidal pituitary surgery. *Laryngoscope*, 1992; **102**: 951–3.
25. Heilman CB, Shucart WA, Rebeiz EE. Endoscopic sphenoidotomy approach to the sella. *Neurosurgery*, 1997; **41**: 602–7.
26. Sethi DS, Pillay PK. Endoscopic management of lesions of the sella turcica. *J Laryngol Otol*, 1995; **109**: 956–62.
27. Jane JA Jr, Thapar K, Kaptain GJ, Maartens N, Laws ER, Jr. Pituitary surgery: transsphenoidal approach. *Neurosurgery*, 2002; **51**: 435–42.
28. Park J, Guthikonda M. The Medpor sheet as a sellar buttress after endonasal transsphenoidal surgery: technical note. *Surg Neurol*, 2004; **61**: 488–92; discussion 493.
29. Cavallo LM, Messina A, Esposito F, de Divitiis O, Dal Fabbro M, de Divitiis E, *et al.* Skull base reconstruction in the extended endoscopic transsphenoidal approach for suprasellar lesions. *J Neurosurg*, 2007; **107**: 713–20.
30. Elias WJ, Chadduck JB, Alden TD, Laws ER, Jr. Frameless stereotaxy for transsphenoidal surgery. *Neurosurgery*, 1999; **45**: 271–5.
31. Jagannathan J, Prevedello DM, Ayer VS, Dumont AS, Jane JA Jr, Laws ER. Computer-assisted frameless stereotaxy in transsphenoidal surgery at a single institution: review of 176 cases. *Neurosurg Focus*, 2006; **20**: E9.
32. Jane JA Jr, Thapar K, Alden TD, Laws ER, Jr. Fluoroscopic frameless stereotaxy for transsphenoidal surgery. *Neurosurgery*, 2001; **48**: 1302–7; discussion 1307-8.
33. Dusick JR, Esposito F, Malkasian D, Kelly DF. Avoidance of carotid artery injuries in transsphenoidal surgery with the Doppler probe and micro-hook blades. *Neurosurgery*, 2007; **60**(4 Suppl 2): 322–8; discussion 328-9.
34. Yamasaki T, Moritake K, Hatta J, Nagai H. Intraoperative monitoring with pulse Doppler ultrasonography in transsphenoidal surgery: technique application. *Neurosurgery*, 1996; **38**: 95–7; discussion 97–8.
35. Jane JA Jr, Laws ER Jr. The surgical management of pituitary adenomas in a series of 3,093 patients. *J Am Coll Surg*, 2001; **193**: 651–9.
36. Nemergut EC, Zuo Z, Jane JA Jr, Laws ER Jr. Predictors of diabetes insipidus after transsphenoidal surgery: a review of 881 patients. *J Neurosurg*, 2005; **103**: 448–54.
37. Laws ER Jr. Vascular complications of transsphenoidal surgery. *Pituitary*, 1999; **2**: 163–70.
38. Ciric I, Ragin A, Baumgartner C, Pierce D. Complications of transsphenoidal surgery: results of a national survey, review of the literature, and personal experience. *Neurosurgery*, 1997; **40**: 225–36; discussion 236–7.

2.3.9 Pituitary radiotherapy

Thankamma Ajithkumar, Michael Brada

Introduction

External beam radiotherapy remains an important component of management of patients with pituitary adenoma and a considerable proportion of patients receive it during the course of their illness. Traditional policy had been to use radiotherapy for all patients with residual nonfunctioning pituitary adenoma after surgery as the majority were considered to progress (1). With improvement in surgical techniques and access to MRI, postoperative radiotherapy is no longer routinely employed even in the presence of residual tumour. The use of radiotherapy is based on relative risk assessment, generally withholding further treatment until progression unless there is a perceived threat to function, particularly vision, if the tumour was to progress. Currently radiotherapy is used in patients with progressive nonfunctioning adenoma demonstrated on interval imaging and achieves tumour control in over 90% of patients at 10 years and 85–92% in 20 years (1–9). Radiotherapy remains an integral component of treatment of patients with secreting adenoma who fail to achieve biochemical cure following surgery and medical treatment and in patients with progressive/recurrent tumour mass regardless of the status of hypersecretion. The slow rate of decline in hormone levels means that normalization takes months to years and the delay is primarily related to pretreatment hormone levels. Nevertheless radiotherapy leads to normalization of excess hormone secretion in the majority of patients.

The past two decades have seen developments in radiotherapy, which can largely be considered as refinement of existing technology. The principal aim of modern high-precision, localized radiotherapy is to treat less normal tissue to significant radiation doses therefore minimizing the risk of late normal tissue injury. The higher precision relies on increased accuracy of tumour delineation using modern imaging. The overall success of modern high-precision treatment is more likely to be related to the treatment centre infrastructure and expertise and the accuracy in identifying the tumour than the exact equipment used.

Modern radiotherapy techniques

The current standard of care is the use of three-dimensional (3D) conformal radiotherapy (CRT) using CT and MRI, computerized 3D planning, and the use of multiple shaped beams. The practical steps prior to treatment delivery include noninvasive methods of patient immobilization, coregistered 3D imaging with CT and MRI, and 3D computerized treatment planning followed by quality assurance procedures to ensure the accuracy of the whole process both before and during treatment.

Immobilization is critical to the accuracy of treatment and the device should be well tolerated and minimize movement during the preparation steps and during treatment. Patients are usually immobilized in a custom-made, closely fitting plastic mask made of lightweight thermoplastic material applied directly to the face in a single procedure. The repositioning accuracy is in the region of 3–5 mm (10) and can be reduced to 2–3 mm with a more closely fitting but less comfortable mask (11).

Imaging for the purpose of treatment planning is performed in the immobilization device and includes an unenhanced thin-slice MR image (Fig. 2.3.9.1) and a coregistered CT scan. The extent of the pituitary adenoma identified as visible tumour on MRI is outlined in all orthogonal planes. It should take into account all previous imaging, particularly preoperative scans, to ensure that all areas of uncertainty, which may contain residual tumour, are included. It is not standard practice to include the whole extent of tumour prior to a debulking procedure especially when normal anatomical structures have returned to their normal position. The outline of the visible and presumed tumour is defined as the gross tumour volume (GTV). A margin of 5–10 mm is added in the treatment planning process to account for the technical uncertainty of immobilization, treatment planning, and delivery, and this is defined as the planning target volume (PTV). The exact margin applied should be based on the measurement of uncertainty specific to each centre and the system used. Surrounding normal structures, such as the optic chiasm and optic nerves, the brain stem, and the hypothalamus may also be outlined.

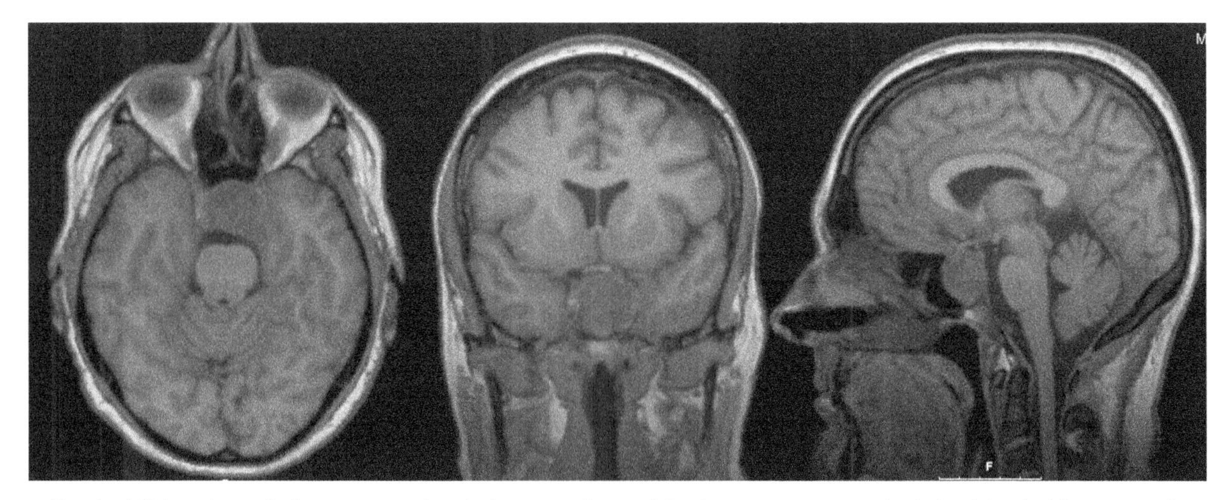

Fig. 2.3.9.1 Planning MRI (unenhanced) of a recurrent nonfunctioning macroadenoma following surgery 3 years previously, involving the left cavernous sinus and not compressing the chiasm.

The computerized treatment planning process defines the number, shaping, and orientation of radiation beams to achieve uniform dose within the PTV and as low a dose as possible to the surrounding normal tissue. With conventionally fractionated radiotherapy the dose to the adenoma is below the radiation tolerance of the surrounding neural structures with the exception of hypothalamus and in fractionated CRT no specific measures are generally taken to avoid the optic apparatus, hypothalamus, and brain stem, particularly as in many patients requiring radiotherapy, some or all of the structures are within or in close proximity to the adenoma. Nevertheless the preferred beam paths tend to avoid the eyes.

The usual CRT arrangement is three fixed radiation beams shaped to conform to the PTV with a multileaf collimator (MLC). The MLC leaves are automatically preset to the shape of the PTV as defined in the planning process. Radiation dose intensity can also be altered across the beam by MLC leaves placed in the beam path and this is described as intensity-modulated radiotherapy (IMRT). IMRT is a form of conformal radiotherapy which can spare critical structures within a concave PTV. This is rarely required for pituitary adenomas and IMRT offers neither technical nor clinical advantage compared with conformal radiotherapy for most sellar and suprasellar tumours (12).

Stereotactic conformal radiotherapy and radiosurgery

Stereotactic techniques are a refinement of conformal radiotherapy with improved immobilization, more accurate image coregistration, and high-precision treatment delivery. The term 'stereotactic' derived from neurosurgery, denotes the method of determining the position of a lesion within a space defined by coordinates based on the immobilization system, usually a stereotactic frame.

Stereotactic irradiation can be given in multiple doses as fractionated stereotactic radiotherapy (fSRT), as fractionated stereotactic conformal radiotherapy (fSCRT) or in a single dose when it is described as stereotactic radiosurgery, although this remains a radiation and not a surgical procedure. fSRT/SCRT are generally delivered using a linear accelerator. Stereotactic radiosurgery can be delivered using either a multiheaded cobalt unit (gamma knife) or a linear accelerator. The precision of modern linear accelerators does not require modification for stereotactic irradiation. Smaller linear accelerators have been mounted on a robotic arm (Cyberknife) which allow for nonisocentric movement. However, the access to the lesion is restricted by the robotic arm geometry and the small size of the accelerator produces smaller beams at a lower dose rate. In comparative studies the robotic arm mounted linear accelerator does not offer better target and normal tissue dose distribution (13) and no advantage in the accuracy of treatment delivery compared with other high-precision techniques.

Fractionated treatment

For fractionated stereotactic radiotherapy, patients are immobilized in a noninvasive relocatable frame with a relocation accuracy of 1–2 mm (14, 15) or a precisely fitting mask system with accuracy of 2–3 mm (11). As in conventional radiotherapy, GTV is outlined on MRI coregistered with a CT scan. The PTV margin is smaller than for conventional radiotherapy, usually in the region of 3 mm and this is based on the overall accuracy of the system of which the principal determinant is the repositioning accuracy of the patient in the immobilization device (16). Precise definition of the tumour is of paramount importance to avoid treatment failure due to exclusion of a part of the tumour from the high-dose volume.

SRT employs larger number of beams than conventional radiotherapy (usually four to six) (Fig. 2.3.9.2), each conforming to the shape of the tumour using a narrow-leaf MLC (5 mm width described as mini MLC or 3 mm width as micro MLC). fSRT/SCRT combine the precision of the stereotactic positioning and treatment delivery, treating less normal neural tissue, with fractionation, which preferentially spares damage to normal tissue. In addition, complete avoidance of critical structures such as the

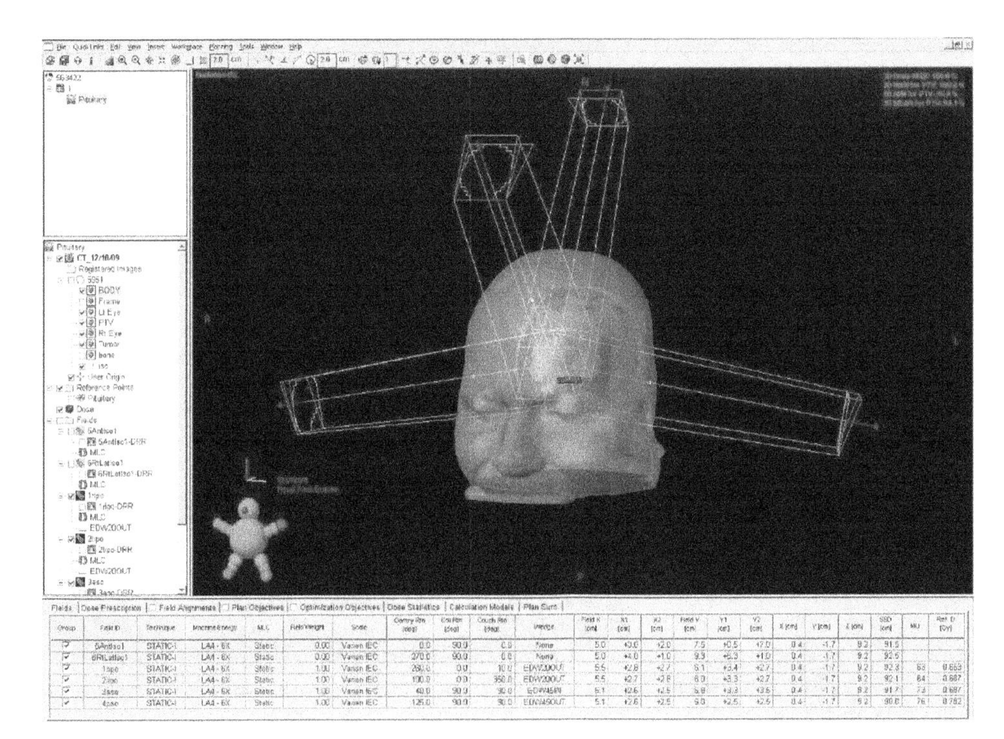

Fig. 2.3.9.2 Screenshot of 3D reconstruction of four-field stereotactic conformal radiotherapy of a large recurrent nonfunctioning adenoma on a planning computer. Individual fields are shaped with a multileaf collimator.

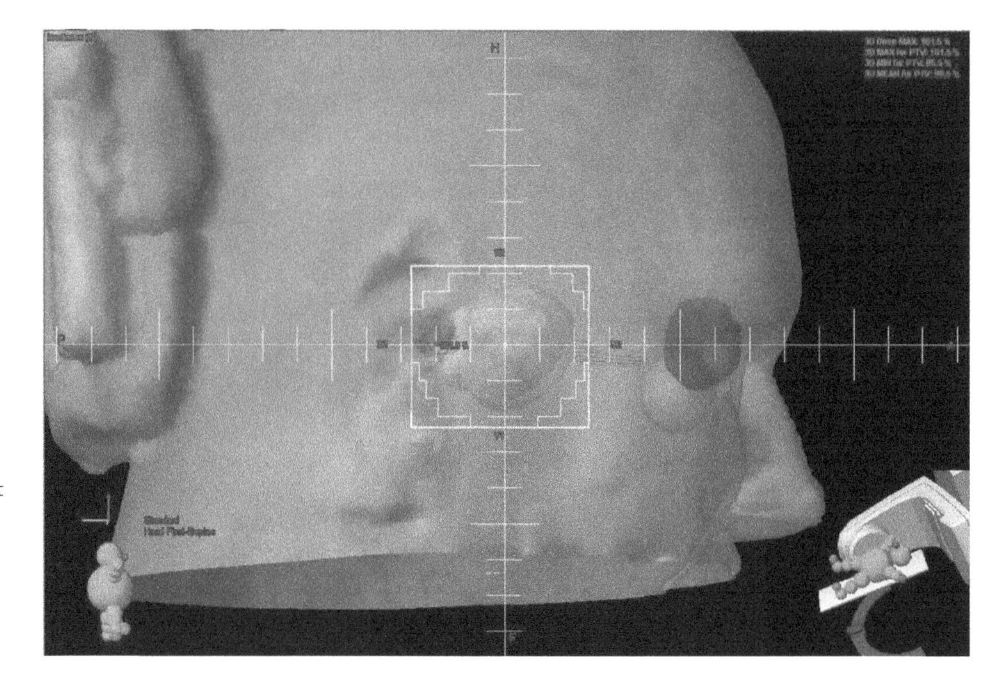

Fig. 2.3.9.3 Beam's eye view of a right inferior oblique field with position of multileaf collimator leaves. Eyes, optic nerves, and chiasm are also outlined. The optic chiasm is treated to below tolerance doses and does not need to be avoided.

optic apparatus is not necessary especially as the dose fractionation schemes as used for conventional radiotherapy are below radiation tolerance of the normal central nervous system (Fig. 2.3.9.3 (Fig. 2.3.9.4 and Fig. 2.3.9.5)). Fractionated stereotactic radiotherapy technique is therefore suitable for pituitary adenomas of all sizes regardless of the relationship to critical structures.

Single fraction treatment

For single fraction SRS, patients are immobilized in an invasive neurosurgical frame fixed to the skull. It requires all the preparation procedures and treatment delivery to be carried out in 1 day. The gamma knife delivers a spherical dose distribution of 6–18 mm diameter. Larger nonspherical tumours, which represent the majority of pituitary adenomas, are treated by combining several radiation spheres using a multiple isocentres technique. The appropriate number and distribution of isocentres is defined using a 3D computer planning system, which also allows for selective plugging of some of the source positions to enable shaping of the high-dose volume envelope. The use of multiple isocentres results in dose inhomogeneity within the target with small areas of high radiation dose (hot spots) in the region of overlap of the radiation dose spheres. This may lead to radiation damage if critical normal structures such as cranial nerves are within the hot spots of the target.

Linear accelerator-based radiosurgery can be carried out either in a relocatable or a fixed stereotactic frame. Computerised treatment planning defines the arrangement of beams as in SRT/SCRT. This can be either as multiple arcs of rotation, simulating gamma knife treatment producing small spherical dose distributions, or as multiple fixed conformal fields. Multiple arc SRS with a linear accelerator, employing multiple isocentres, is cumbersome and rarely employed. The use of multiple fixed fields is generally confined to fractionated treatment although it can also be used for single fraction SRS.

Because of the potential damaging effect of large single radiation doses to normal neural structures, SRS is only suitable for small pituitary adenomas, 3–5 mm away from the optic chiasm.

Proton therapy

The biological effect of protons is equivalent to the ionization damage caused by photons. The principal benefit is more localized deposition of energy of a mono-energetic proton beam described as the Bragg peak with little ionizing radiation beyond the peak (17). The preparation steps are as would be used for other CRT techniques.

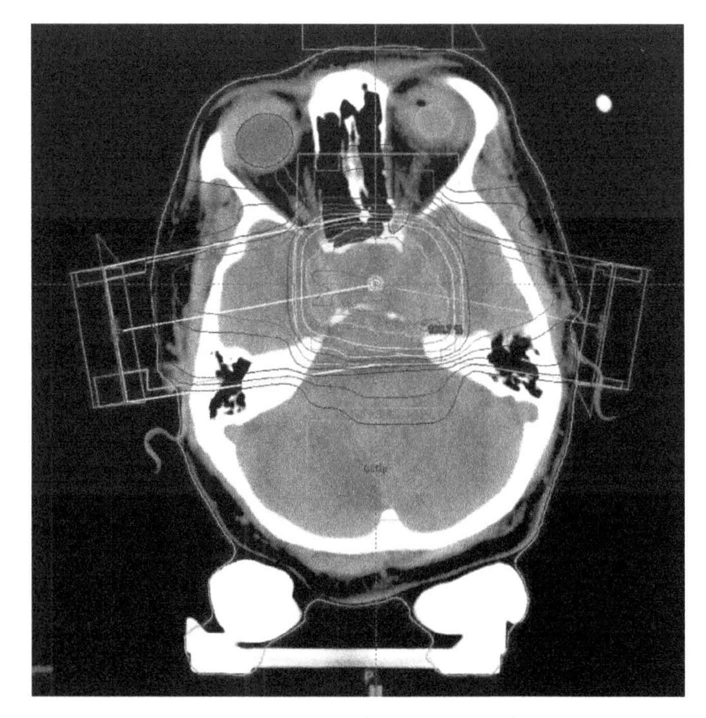

Fig. 2.3.9.4 Transverse isodose plan of a four-noncoplanar field conformal technique.

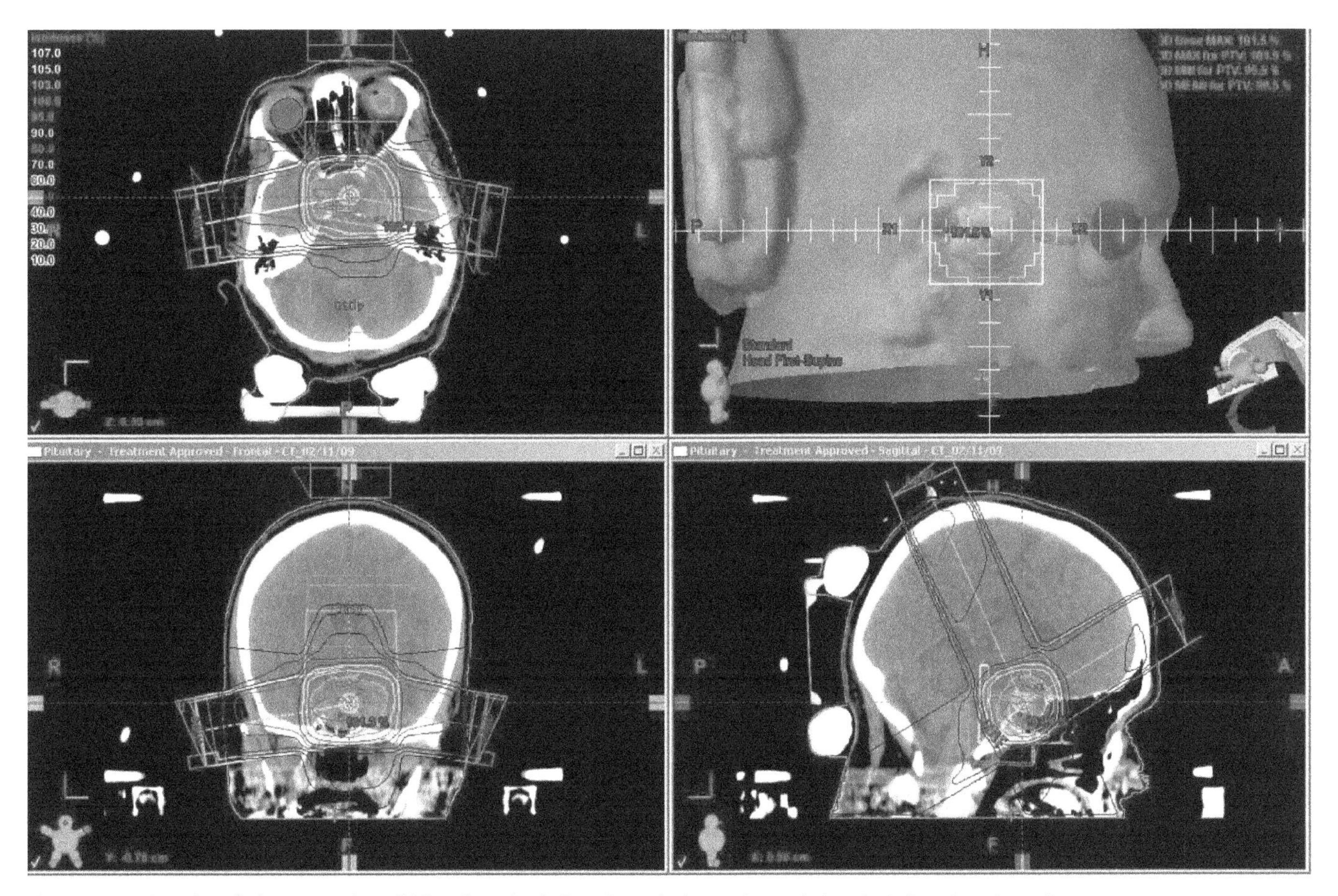

Fig. 2.3.9.5 Isodose plan of a four-noncoplanar field conformal technique shown in three orthogonal planes including a beam's eye view.

Dose fractionation of radiotherapy

The therapeutic benefit of radiotherapy in malignant tumours is considered to be due to cell attrition either as apoptosis or reproductive cell death as a consequence of radiation-induced DNA damage. The time taken to manifest radiation effects is related to the rate of cell proliferation in the tissue irradiated. In rapidly proliferating cells, radiation effects are expressed either during or immediately after the course of radiotherapy, while in slowly proliferating cell population they take months or years to manifest. It is assumed that the beneficial effects of radiation in pituitary adenomas conform to the same mechanism with depletion of tumour cells where adenomas are considered as slowly proliferating tissue. The surrounding normal brain parenchyma is also considered to consist largely of slow proliferating cell population although critical cell populations with faster turnover such as blood vessels are also present and affected by radiation.

Conventional radiotherapy and fractionated SCRT are given to total dose of 45–50 Gy at 1.8 Gy per fractionation, once a day 5 days per week. The dose is below the tolerance of the central nervous system and the risk of structural damage is <1%.

While single large doses of radiation may result in higher cell kill than the same dose given in a small number of fractions, this is also true for normal tissue cell population leading to toxicity which may not be acceptable if affecting eloquent regions such as optic chiasm. As the majority of pituitary adenomas requiring radiation lie in close proximity to the optic apparatus and the nerves in the cavernous sinus, radiosurgery is suitable only for small lesions located away from the critical structures and the optic apparatus should not exceed doses beyond 8–10 Gy.

Clinical outcome of pituitary radiotherapy

The clinical efficacy of radiotherapy for pituitary adenoma should be assessed in terms of survival, actuarial tumour control (progression-free survival (PFS)), and quality of life. The commonly reported endpoints for nonfunctioning pituitary adenoma are local tumour control measured as PFS and long-term morbidity. In patients with secreting pituitary adenoma the principal endpoint, in addition to PFS and morbidity, is the normalization of elevated hormone levels. The rate of hormonal decline after radiotherapy varies with the type of secreting tumour and the time to reach normal levels is dependent on the initial hormone level. The appropriate comparative measure for each hormone is the time to reach 50% of pretreatment hormone level and this should be corrected for the confounding effect of medical treatment. Surrogate endpoints such as 'control rate', without indication of time and duration of follow-up and the proportion of patients achieving normal hormone levels without a clear relationship to pre-radiotherapy values do not provide appropriate information on the efficacy of different radiotherapy approaches and are potentially misleading (18).

The reporting of efficacy of various techniques of radiotherapy is also subject to selection bias. While fractionated radiotherapy is suitable for all pituitary tumours, irrespective of size, shape or

Table 2.3.9.1 Summary of results of published series on conventional radiotherapy for pituitary adenomas[a]

Authors	Type of adenoma	Number of patients	Follow-up, median (years)	Actuarial PFS, %	Late toxicity, %	
					Visual	Hypopituitarism
Grigsby *et al.*, 1989	NFA, SA	121	11.7	89.9 at 10 years	1.7	NA
McCollough *et al.*, 1991	NFA, SA	105	7.8	95 at 10 years	NA	NA
Brada *et al.*, 1993	NFA, SA	411	10.8	94 at 10 years	1.5	30 at 10 years
				88 at 20 years		
Tsang *et al.*, 1994	NFA, SA	160	8.7	87 at 10 years	0	23[c]
Zierhut *et al.*, 1995	NFA, SA	138	6.5	95 at 5 years	1.5	27[c]
Estrada *et al.*, 1997	SA (ACTH)	30	3.5	73 at 2 years[b]	0	48[c]
Rush *et al.*, 1997	NFA, SA	70	8	NA	NA	42[c]
Breen *et al.*, 1998	NFA	120	9	87.5 at 10 years	1	NA
Gittoes *et al.*, 1998	NFA	126	7.5	93 at 10 and 15 years	NA	NA
Barrande *et al.*, 2000	SA (GH)	128	11	53 at 10 years[b]	0	50 at 10 years
Biermasz *et al.*, 2000	SA (GH)	36	10	60 at 10 years[b]	0	54 at 10 years
Sasaki *et al.*, 2000	NFA, SA	91	8.2	93 at 10 years	1	NA
Epaminonda *et al.*, 2001	SA (GH)	67	10	65 at 15 years[b]	0	NA
Minniti *et al.*, 2005	SA (GH)	45	12	52 at 10 years[b]	0	45 at 10 years
Langsenlehner *et al.*, 2007	NFA, SA	87	15	93 at 15 years	0	88 at 10 years
Minniti *et al.*, 2007	SA (ACTH)	40	9	78 and 84 at 5 and 10 years[b]	0	62 at 10 years

[a] For details of individual papers, see Brada M, Ajithkumar TV, Minniti G. Radiosurgery for pituitary adenomas. *Clin Endocrinol (Oxf)*, 2004; **61**: 531–43 (19) and Minniti G, Gilbert DC, Brada M. Modern techniques for pituitary radiotherapy. *Rev Endocr Metab Disord*, 2009; **10**: 135–44 (20).
[b] Hormone concentration normalization
[c] No time specified.
ACTH, Cushing's; GH, acromegaly; NA, not assessed; NFA, nonfunctioning adenoma; SA, secreting adenoma;

proximity to critical structures, radiosurgery is only suitable for small tumours away from the optic chiasm. Studies reporting efficacy of stereotactic radiosurgery mostly deal with small tumours often associated with lower hormone levels, if secretory, and the results do not apply to the generality of adenomas.

Efficacy and toxicity of conventional radiotherapy

Tumour control

The long-term results following conventional fractionated radiotherapy are listed in Table 2.3.9.1 (19, 20). The actuarial PFS is in the region of 80–90% at 10 years and 75–90% at 20 years (19, 20). The largest series of patients with pituitary adenoma treated at the Royal Marsden Hospital reported a 10-year PFS of 92% and a 20-year PFS of 88% (4).

Endocrine control

Fractionated irradiation leads to normalization of excess hormone secretion in the majority of patients albeit with delay. In acromegaly normalization of growth hormone/insulin-like growth factor 1 (IGF-1) levels is achieved in 30–50% of patients at 5–10 years and 75% of patients at 15 years after treatment (see Table 2.3.9.1) (19, 20), and the time to normalization of growth hormone is related to pretreatment growth hormone. The time to achieve a 50% reduction is in the region of 2 years with IGF-1 reaching half of pretreatment level later (21, 22). Following conventional fractionated radiotherapy in Cushing's disease, urinary free cortisol (UFC) reduces to 50% of its pretreatment value in 6–12 months and plasma cortisol in 12 months (23). The median time to reaching normal cortisol level is in the region of 24 months (23). The reported tumour and hormone control at a median follow-up of 8 years are 97% and 74%, respectively (see Table 2.3.9.1).

Radiotherapy is rarely employed in patients with prolactinoma. Occasional patients who fail surgery and medical therapy have been treated with fractionated radiotherapy and the 10-year tumour and biochemical control is 90% and 50%, respectively (24–26).

Toxicity of conventional radiotherapy

The toxicity of conventional radiotherapy with doses of 45–50 Gy at <2 Gy per fraction is low. The reported incidence of presumed radiation optic neuropathy resulting in visual deficit is 1–3% (5, 27) and risk of necrosis of normal brain structures is almost unknown although reported in 0.2% of patients (28). Hypopituitarism represents the most commonly reported late complication of radiotherapy, occurring in 30–60% of patients 10 years after radiotherapy (4, 5, 20). Growth hormone secretion appears to be most frequently affected, followed by gonadotropins, adrenocorticotropic hormone (ACTH), and thyroid-stimulating hormone (TSH). Long-term routine testing for pituitary deficiency of all pituitary axes is therefore an essential component of management of patients receiving all types of pituitary radiotherapy.

Table 2.3.9.2 Summary of results of published series on stereotactic radiosurgery for nonfuntioning pituitary adenomas[a]

Authors	Number of patients	Follow-up median (months)	Tumour growth control rate, %	Late toxicity, %	
				Visual	Hypopituitarism
Martinez *et al.*, 1998	14	26–45	100	0	0
Pan L *et al.*, 1998	17	29	95	0	0
Ikeda *et al.*, 1998	13	45	100	0	0
Mokry *et al.*, 1999	31	20	98	NA	NA
Sheehan *et al.*, 2002	42	31[a]	97	2.3	0
Wowra and Stummer, 2002	45	55	93 at 3 years	0	14
Petrovich *et al.*, 2003	56	36	94 at 3 years	4	NA
Pollock and Carpenter, 2003	33	43	97 at 5 years	0	28 and 41 at 2 and 5 years
Losa *et al.*, 2004	56	41[b]	88 at 5 years	0	24
Iwai *et al.*, 2005	34	60	93 at 5 years	0	6
Mingione *et al.*, 2006	100	45[b]	92	0	25
Liscak *et al.*, 2007	140	60	100	0	2
Pollock *et al.*, 2008	62	64	95 at 3 and 7 years	0	32 at 5 years
Kobayashi 2009 (37)	60	>3 years	97	4.3	8.2 worsening

[a] For details of individual papers, see Brada M, Ajithkumar TV, Minniti G. Radiosurgery for pituitary adenomas. *Clin Endocrinol (Oxf)*, 2004; **61**: 531–43 (19) and Minniti G, Gilbert DC, Brada M. Modern techniques for pituitary radiotherapy. *Rev Endocr Metab Disord*, 2009; **10**: 135–44 (20).

[b] Mean follow-up.

NA, not available.

An increased incidence of cerebrovascular accidents, and excess cerebrovascular mortality, have been reported in patients with pituitary adenoma treated with conventional radiotherapy. The cause is multifactorial, including the metabolic and cardiovascular consequences of hypopituitarism, the effects of individual endocrine syndromes, the consequences of surgical intervention, and vascular effects of radiotherapy. The relative contribution of radiation to its frequency remains to be determined (29–32).

Radiation is associated with the development of a second, radiation-induced brain tumour. The reported cumulative incidence of development of gliomas and meningiomas following treatment of pituitary adenoma is in the region of 2% at 20 years (32–34). Radiotherapy to large volumes of normal brain, particularly in children, is associated with neurocognitive impairment. The effect of small-volume irradiation on neurocognitive function in adults is not clear, particularly as the effect of radiotherapy cannot be clearly differentiated from the effect of other interventions and the tumour itself (35, 36).

Efficacy and toxicity of radiosurgery

Tumour control

The published results of stereotactic radiosurgery in patients with nonfunctioning and secreting pituitary adenomas have been summarized in systematic reviews (19, 20) and are shown in Table 2.3.9.2 (19, 20, 37). The majority of published reports provide information on 'control rate' without specifying a time and provide little useful information on the efficacy of SRS. The summary figure of the actuarial 5-year control rate (PFS) following SRS for nonfunctioning adenomas is in the region of 94% (there are few reliable 10-year results). This rate of tumour control, when only small tumours suitable for SRS are treated, is below those reported following fractionated radiotherapy for adenomas of all sizes.

Endocrine control

The outcome of gamma knife stereotactic radiosurgery in acromegaly is shown in Table 2.3.9.3 (19, 20, 37, 38). In the summary of published literature 37% of patients achieved normalization of serum growth hormone, at a median follow-up of 39 months. The time to reach 50% of baseline serum growth hormone, reported in only three studies, is in the region of 1.5–2 years with a slower reduction in IGF-1 levels (39–41), which is similar to the rate reported following conventional fractionated radiotherapy suggesting the rate of decline in growth hormone level following stereotactic radiosurgery is no faster than following conventional radiotherapy.

Fifty-one per cent of patients with Cushing's disease achieved biochemical remission (as defined by plasma cortisol and 24-h UFC levels) at a corrected median follow-up of 42 months after stereotactic radiosurgery (Table 2.3.9.4) (19, 20, 37, 38). The reported time to hormonal response ranged from 3 months to 3 years with no clear difference in the rate of decline of hormone level compared with conventional radiotherapy. Stereotactic radiosurgery for Cushing's disease recorded a remission rate of 54% with 20% of patients who achieved remission subsequently relapsing, suggesting a higher failure rate than following fractionated treatment (42).

In patients with prolactinoma undergoing stereotactic radiosurgery the reported time to hormonal response ranges from 5 months to 40 months (Table 2.3.9.5) (19, 20, 37, 43, 44). At a corrected median follow-up of 29 months (median range 6–55 months), 33% of patients had normalization of serum prolactin concentrations following stereotactic radiosurgery (20). One study of 35 patients reported a hormonal normalization of 80% at a median of 96 months and tumour control of 97% (44). There is insufficient information to assess the rate of decline of prolactin in comparison with fractionated radiotherapy.

Table 2.3.9.3 Summary of results of published series on stereotactic radiosurgery for growth hormone-secreting pituitary adenomas

Authors	Number of patients	Follow-up median (months)	Hormone normalization,[b] %	Late toxicity, %	
				Visual	Hypopituitarism
Thoren M *et al.*, 1991	21	64	10	0	15
Martinez *et al.*, 1998	7	26–45	NA	0	0
Pan L *et al.*, 1998	15	29	NA	0	0
Morange Ramos *et al.*, 1998	15	20	20	6	16
Lim *et al.*, 1998	20	26	30	5	5
Kim *et al.*, 1999	11	27	35	NA	NA
Landolt *et al.*, 1998	16	17	50	0	16
Mokry *et al.*, 1999	16	46	31	0	NA
Hayashi *et al.*, 1999	22	>6	41	0	0
Inoue *et al.*, 1999	12	> 24	58	0	0
Zhang *et al.*, 2000	68	> 12	40	NA	NA
Izawa *et al.*, 2000	29	>6	41	0	0
Pollock *et al.*, 2002	26	36	47	4	16
Attanasio *et al.*, 2003	30	46	23	0	6
Choi *et al.*, 2003	12	43	30	0	0
Jane *et al.*, 2003	64	> 18	36	0	28
Petrovich *et al.*, 2003	6	36	100	0	NA
Castinetti *et al.*, 2005	82	49.5[b]	17	0	18
Gutt *et al.*, 2005	44	22	48	NA	NA
Kobayashi *et al.*, 2005	67	63	17	0	NA
Jezkova *et al.*, 2006	96	54	50	0	26
Pollock *et al.*, 2007	46	63	11 and 60 at 2 and 5 years	0	33 at 5 years
Jagannathan *et al.*, 2009 (38)	95	57 (mean)	53	5[c]	34 (new)
Kobayashi 2009 (37)	49	63	17 (normal or nearly normal)	11	15

[a] For details of individual papers, see Brada M, Ajithkumar TV, Minniti G. Radiosurgery for pituitary adenomas. *Clin Endocrinol (Oxf)*, 2004; **61**: 531–43 (19) and Minniti G, Gilbert DC, Brada M. Modern techniques for pituitary radiotherapy. *Rev Endocr Metab Disord*, 2009; **10**: 135–44 (20).

[b] Mean follow-up.

[c] Three had previous radiotherapy.

NA, not assessed.

Early studies of linear accelerator stereotactic radiosurgery report a small number of patients and the results are broadly equivalent to those reported for gamma knife stereotactic radiosurgery (12). The largest study of 175 patients with pituitary adenoma treated with linear accelerator stereotactic radiosurgery with a single dose of 20 Gy reported local tumour control rate of 97% at a minimum of 12 months' follow-up (45). Actuarial 5-year PFS is not reported. Hormonal normalization rates were 47% for growth hormone-secreting adenomas, 65% with Cushing's disease, and 39% with prolactinomas with a mean time for hormone normalization of 36 ± 24 months. Within the limited follow-up, 12% developed additional pituitary dysfunction, 3% developed radiation-induced tissue damage, and 1% developed radiation-induced neuropathy. These results are difficult to evaluate but are broadly similar to those achieved with gamma knife stereotactic radiosurgery.

Toxicity of gamma knife stereotactic radiosurgery

The most commonly observed complication following stereotactic radiosurgery is hypopituitarism, with a crude incidence ranging from 0% to 66% (19, 20); the actuarial incidence is not fully defined. The frequency of visual complications should be low if stereotactic radiosurgery is only offered to patients with adenoma a safe distance from the optic chiasm and nerves (~5 mm). Nevertheless, studies in patients with Cushing's disease reported 10% incidence of new cranial nerve deficit with 6% incidence of optic neuropathy, and in patients with prolactinoma, 10% incidence of cranial nerve deficit is not seen following fractionated treatment (42, 46). Long-term risks of cerebrovascular events and the incidence of second tumours are not yet defined.

Efficacy and toxicity of SCRT

SCRT data for 490 patients with either nonfunctioning or secreting pituitary adenomas have been reported in eight studies (Table 2.3.9.6) (12, 19, 20). At a corrected median follow-up of 39 months (median range 10–60 months) tumour control was achieved in 98% of patients. The 5-year actuarial PFS of 92 patients (67 nonfunctioning, 25 secreting) treated at the Royal Marsden Hospital was 97% (47). The results are similar to patient cohorts treated with conventional radiotherapy (see Table 2.3.9.1).

Table 2.3.9.4 Summary of results of published series on stereotactic radiosurgery for ACTH-secreting pituitary adenomas[a]

Authors	Number of patients	Follow-up, median (months)	Tumour growth control rate, %	Hormone normalization,[b] %	Late toxicity, %	
					Visual	Hypopituitarism
Degerblad *et al.*, 1986	29	3–9 years	76	48	NA	55
Ganz *et al.*, 1993	4	18	NA	NA	0	NA
Seo *et al.*, 1995	2	24	100	NA	0	NA
Martinez *et al.*, 1998	3	26–45	100	100	0	0
Pan L *et al.*, 1998	4	29	95	NA	0	0
Morange Ramos *et al.*, 1998	6	20	100	66	0	16
Lim *et al.*, 1998	4	26	NA	25	2	2
Mokry *et al.*, 1999	5	26	93	20	0	2
Kim *et al.* 1999	8	26	100	60	NA	NA
Hayashi *et al.*, 1999	10	>6	100	10	0	5%
Inoue *et al.*, 1999	3	>24	100	100	0	0
Izawa *et al.*, 2000	12	>6	100	17	NA	0
Sheehan *et al.*, 2000	43	44	100	63	2	16
Hoybye *et al.*, 2001	18	17 yr	100	83	0	66
Kobayashi *et al.*, 2002	20	60	100	35	NA	NA
Pollock *et al.*, 2002	11	36	85	35	35	8
Choi *et al.*, 2003	9	43	100	55	0	0
Jane *et al.*, 2003	45	>18	100	63	1	31
Petrovich *et al.*, 2003	4	36	NA	50	0	NA
Devin *et al.*, 2004	35	35	91	49	0	40
Castinetti *et al.*, 2007	40	54	100	42	0	NA
Jagannathan *et al.*, 2009 (38)	90	45	96	54	5	22
Kobayashi 2009 (37)	25	64 (mean)	100	35	NA	NA

[a] For details of individual papers, see Brada M, Ajithkumar TV, Minniti G. Radiosurgery for pituitary adenomas. *Clin Endocrinol (Oxf)*, 2004; **61**: 531–43 (19) and Minniti G, Gilbert DC, Brada M. Modern techniques for pituitary radiotherapy. *Rev Endocr Metab Disord*, 2009; **10**: 135–44 (20).
[b] Time not specified.
NA, not assessed.

In the Royal Marsden series six of 18 acromegalic patients (35%) had normalization of growth hormone/IGF-1 at a median follow-up of 39 months (47). Similarly, in a study of 20 patients treated with SCRT, normalisation of growth hormone levels was reported in 70% and local control 100% at a median follow up of 26 months (48). Data on the rate of decline is not available, although it is expected to be similar to that seen following conventional radiotherapy as the same dose-fractionation is used. There are limited data on SCRT in patients with Cushing's disease. In a small series of 12 patients, control of elevated cortisol was reported in nine out of 12 patients (75%) at a median time of 29 months (49). Hypopituitarism was reported in 20% of patients at an overall corrected median follow-up of 60 months. Other late complications were rarely recorded. While the incidence appears low, longer follow-up is necessary to detect toxicity appearing many years after treatment.

In summary, SCRT achieves tumour control and normalization of hormone hypersecretion at rates similar to the best reported rates following conventional fractionated radiotherapy. Longer follow-up is required to demonstrate the presumed lower incidence of long-term morbidity compared with conventional CRT.

Proton beam radiotherapy

An early study of 30 patients with acromegaly reported 80% decrease in growth hormone at 4.5 years while pituitary deficiency as well as oculomotor nerve palsies were more common with protons (50). The use of proton stereotactic radiosurgery in 22 patients with acromegaly reported 59% normalization of growth hormone at a median of 42 months. New pituitary deficiency was reported in 38% of patients (51). A study of 47 patients treated with fractionated proton radiotherapy reported tumour stabilization in only 41 (87%) patients at a minimum 6-month follow-up: 1 patient developed temporal lobe necrosis, 3 new significant visual deficits and 11 hypopituitarism. The available peer review reports of protons for pituitary adenoma demonstrate disappointing efficacy and toxicity.

Reirradiation for recurrent pituitary adenoma

Reirradiation for progression of pituitary adenoma after radiotherapy is considered risky because of the presumed cumulative radiation damage to optic apparatus, cranial nerves, and normal

Table 2.3.9.5 Summary of results of published series on stereotactic radiosurgery for prolactin-secreting pituitary adenomas[a]

Authors	Number of patients	Follow-up, median (months)	Hormone normalization, %	Late toxicity, %	
				Visual	Hypopituitarism
Ganz *et al.*, 1993	3	18	0	0	NA
Martinez *et al.*, 1998	5	26–45	0	0	0
Pan L *et al.*, 1998	27	29	30	0	0
Morange Ramos *et al.*, 1998	4	20	0	0	16
Lim *et al.*, 1998	19	26	50	NA	NA
Mokry *et al.*, 1999	21	31	57	0	19
Kim *et al.*, 1999	18	27	16	NA	NA
Hayashi *et al.*, 1999	13	>6	15	NA	5
Inoue *et al.*, 1999	2	>24	50	0	0
Landolt 2000	20	29	25	0	NA
Pan L *et al.*, 2000	128	33	41	0	NA
Izawa *et al.*, 2000	15	>6	16	0	NA
Polllock *et al.*, 2002	7	26	29	14	16
Choi *et al.*, 2003	21	43	23	0	0
Jane *et al.*, 2003	19	>18	11	0	21
Petrovich *et al.*, 2003	12	36	83	0	NA
Pouratian *et al.*, 2006	23	55	26	7	28
Jezkova *et al.*, 2009 (44)	35	96	80	NA	NA
Kobayashi 2009 (37)	27	37 (mean)	17	0	0

[a]For details of individual papers, see Brada M, Ajithkumar TV, Minniti G. Radiosurgery for pituitary adenomas. *Clin Endocrinol (Oxf)*, 2004; **61**: 531–43 (19) and Minniti G, Gilbert DC, Brada M. Modern techniques for pituitary radiotherapy. *Rev Endocr Metab Disord*, 2009; **10**: 135–44 (20).
NA, not assessed.

brain. Fractionated reirradiation using conventional or stereotactic techniques is feasible with acceptable toxicity (18), provided there is 3–4-year gap from primary radiotherapy to doses of 45 Gy at <1.8 Gy fraction. Stereotactic radiosurgery has also been used for small recurrent lesions (52). While the impression is that late toxicity of reirradiation is uncommon there are insufficient long-term data to demonstrate it.

Radiotherapy in pituitary adenoma—conclusion

Fractionated radiotherapy is an effective treatment achieving excellent disease control and normalization of hormone levels. While overall safe, it is not devoid of side effects and it should only be employed when the risks from the disease itself are considered

Table 2.3.9.6 Summary of results on published studies on stereotactic conformal radiotherapy for pituitary adenomas[a]

Authors	Number of patients	Follow-up, median (months)	Tumour growth control rate, %	Late toxicity, %	
				Visual	Hypopituitarism
Coke *et al.*, 1997	19[b]	9	100	0	0
Mitsumori *et al.*, 1998	30[b]	33	86 at 3 years	0	20
Milker-Zabel *et al.*, 2001	68[b]	38	93 at 5 years	7	5
Paek *et al.*, 2005	68	30	98 at 5 years	3	6
Colin *et al.*, 2005	110[b]	48	99 at 5 years	2	29 at 4 years
Minniti *et al.*, 2006	92[b]	32	98 at 5 years	1	22
Selch *et al.*, 2006	39[b]	60	100	0	15
Kong *et al.*, 2007	64[b]	37	97 at 4 years	0	11
Snead *et al.*, 2008	100[b]	6.7 years	98 at 10 year for NFA and 73 SA	1	35

[a] For details of individual papers, see Brada M, Ajithkumar TV, Minniti G. Radiosurgery for pituitary adenomas. *Clin Endocrinol (Oxf)*, 2004; **61**: 531–43 (19) and Minniti G, Gilbert DC, Brada M. Modern techniques for pituitary radiotherapy. *Rev Endocr Metab Disord*, 2009; **10**: 135–44 (20).
[b] Series include secreting pituitary adenomas.
NFA, nonfunctioning adenoma; SA, secreting adenoma.

to outweigh the risks from the treatment. The balance of risks should not only consider early consequences of the disease and treatment, measured in terms of disease control and immediate morbidity, but also late effects particularly in terms of the influence on survival and quality of life, both of which are not so well defined.

Residual tumours, most of which have indolent natural history, pose little threat to function, unless close to the optic apparatus or when destructively invading surrounding structures, which is an uncommon event. The risks are therefore minimal and in the absence of progression or hormone hypersecretion, there is currently little justification to offer adjuvant treatment whether in the form of fractionated or single fraction treatment. However the policy of surveillance requires close monitoring usually in the form of annual MRI, proceeding with timely irradiation, prior to the need for further surgery. The aim is to arrest tumour growth without the additional risks of reoperation.

In secreting tumours irradiation is generally offered to patients with persistent hormone elevation not decreasing at the expected rate following previous intervention. That generally means persistent elevation in patients with acromegaly, Cushing's disease and other secreting adenomas, regardless of the actual level as the aim in most instances is to reach normalization. In patients with acromegaly treated with somatostatin analogues, the expense and inconvenience of protracted systemic treatment would also argue for early radiotherapy to allow for gradual withdrawal of medical treatment. The alternative is to continue medical management indefinitely without radiotherapy. It is not clear which policy is associated with better long-term survival and quality of life and this should ideally be tested in a prospective randomized trial.

The current practice is therefore to offer treatment to patients with progressive nonfunctioning (or secretory) adenomas considered to be of threat to function and to patients with secretory adenomas with persistent hypersecretion. On the evidence available, single fraction radiosurgery, while apparently more convenient, is less effective in achieving long-term disease control of adenoma tumour masses and without faster decline in hormone levels in secreting tumours. In addition, single fraction treatment of larger adenomas close to critical structures carries a considerable risk of radiation-induced damage. Fractionated irradiation either as CRT or SCRT therefore remains the standard of care with stereotactic radiosurgery considered as an experimental and in some instances less effective treatment.

The availability of radiosurgery has in some centres led to the policy of adjuvant single fraction radiosurgery in patients with small residual tumours. It is not clear that such practice is appropriate as the risks from small nonfunctioning adenomas are unlikely to be greater than the risks of stereotactic radiosurgery. Similarly, some patients with slow decline in hormone levels, particularly in acromegaly, have been offered additional stereotactic radiosurgery. There is no clear evidence that further irradiation markedly speeds up the hormone decline while carrying additional morbidity of reirradiation.

Modern conformal techniques of fractionated irradiation have become standard practice with many centres offering the additional accuracy of high precision treatment with 'stereotactic' guidance. Such practice relies on the expertise of accurate target definition using modern imaging, on the precision of the system based on exhaustive quality assurance programme and infrastructure particularly in the form of expertise of staff in complex techniques of treatment planning and delivery. In the final analysis it is likely that the expertise at all levels of staff is more important to the success of pituitary radiotherapy than the equipment and the precise technique of treatment.

References

1. Gittoes NJ, Bates AS, Tse W, Bullivant B, Sheppard MC, Clayton RN, *et al.* Radiotherapy for non-function pituitary tumours. *Clin Endocrinol (Oxf)*, 1998; **48**: 331–7.
2. Grigsby PW, Simpson JR, Emami BN, Fineberg BB, Schwartz HG. Prognostic factors and results of surgery and postoperative irradiation in the management of pituitary adenomas. *Int J Radiat Oncol Biol Phys*, 1989; **16**: 1411–17.
3. McCollough WM, Marcus RB Jr, Rhoton AL Jr, Ballinger WE, Million RR. Long-term follow-up of radiotherapy for pituitary adenoma: the absence of late recurrence after greater than or equal to 4500 cGy. *Int J Radiat Oncol Biol Phys*, 1991; **21**: 607–14.
4. Brada M, Rajan B, Traish D, Ashley S, Holmes-Sellors PJ, Nussey S, *et al.* The long-term efficacy of conservative surgery and radiotherapy in the control of pituitary adenomas. *Clin Endocrinol (Oxf)*, 1993; **38**: 571–8.
5. Tsang RW, Brierley JD, Panzarella T, Gospodarowicz MK, Sutcliffe SB, Simpson WJ. Radiation therapy for pituitary adenoma: treatment outcome and prognostic factors. *Int J Radiat Oncol Biol Phys*, 1994; **30**: 557–65.
6. Zierhut D, Flentje M, Adolph J, Erdmann J, Raue F, Wannenmacher M. External radiotherapy of pituitary adenomas. *Int J Radiat Oncol Biol Phys*, 1995; **33**: 307–14.
7. Rush S, Cooper PR. Symptom resolution, tumor control, and side effects following postoperative radiotherapy for pituitary macroadenomas. *Int J Radiat Oncol Biol Phys*, 1997; **37**: 1031–4.
8. Breen P, Flickinger JC, Kondziolka D, Martinez AJ. Radiotherapy for nonfunctional pituitary adenoma: analysis of long-term tumor control. *J Neurosurg*, 1998; **89**: 933–8.
9. Sasaki R, Murakami M, Okamoto Y, Kono K, Yoden E, Nakajima T, *et al.* The efficacy of conventional radiation therapy in the management of pituitary adenoma. *Int J Radiat Oncol Biol Phys*, 2000; **47**: 1337–45.
10. Khoo VS, Oldham M, Adams EJ, Bedford JL, Webb S, Brada M. Comparison of intensity-modulated tomotherapy with stereotactically guided conformal radiotherapy for brain tumors. *Int J Radiat Oncol Biol Phys*, 1999; **45**: 415–25.
11. Karger CP, Jakel O, Debus J, Kuhn S, Hartmann GH. Three-dimensional accuracy and interfractional reproducibility of patient fixation and positioning using a stereotactic head mask system. *Int J Radiat Oncol Biol Phys*, 2001; **49**: 1493–504.
12. Ajithkumar T, Brada M. Stereotactic linear accelerator radiotherapy for pituitary tumors. *Treat Endocrinol*, 2004; **3**: 211–16.
13. Cozzi L, Clivio A, Bauman G, Cora S, Nicolini G, Pellegrini R, *et al.* Comparison of advanced irradiation techniques with photons for benign intracranial tumours. *Radiother Oncol*, 2006; **80**: 268–73.
14. Gill SS, Thomas DG, Warrington AP, Brada M. Relocatable frame for stereotactic external beam radiotherapy. *Int J Radiat Oncol Biol Phys*, 1991; **20**: 599–603.
15. Graham JD, Warrington AP, Gill SS, Brada M. A non-invasive, relocatable stereotactic frame for fractionated radiotherapy and multiple imaging. *Radiother Oncol*, 1991; **21**: 60–2.
16. Kumar S, Burke K, Nalder C, Jarrett P, Mubata C, A'Hern R, *et al.* Treatment accuracy of fractionated stereotactic radiotherapy. *Radiother Oncol*, 2005; **74**: 53–9.
17. Greco C, Wolden S. Current status of radiotherapy with proton and light ion beams. *Cancer*, 2007; **109**: 1227–38.
18. Brada M, Jankowska P. Radiotherapy for pituitary adenomas. *Endocrinol Metab Clin North Am*, 2008; **37**: 263–75, xi.
19. Brada M, Ajithkumar TV, Minniti G. Radiosurgery for pituitary adenomas. *Clin Endocrinol (Oxf)*, 2004; **61**: 531–43.

20. Minniti G, Gilbert DC, Brada M. Modern techniques for pituitary radiotherapy. *Rev Endocr Metab Disord*, 2009; **10**: 135–44.
21. Biermasz NR, Dulken HV, Roelfsema F. Postoperative radiotherapy in acromegaly is effective in reducing GH concentration to safe levels. *Clin Endocrinol (Oxf)*, 2000; **53**: 321–7.
22. Minniti G, Jaffrain-Rea ML, Osti M, Esposito V, Santoro A, Solda F, *et al.* The long-term efficacy of conventional radiotherapy in patients with GH-secreting pituitary adenomas. *Clin Endocrinol (Oxf)*, 2005; **62**: 210–16.
23. Minniti G, Osti M, Jaffrain-Rea ML, Esposito V, Cantore G, Maurizi Enrici R. Long-term follow-up results of postoperative radiation therapy for Cushing's disease. *J Neurooncol*, 2007; **84**: 79–84.
24. Tsagarakis S, Grossman A, Plowman PN, Jones AE, Touzel R, Rees LH, *et al.* Megavoltage pituitary irradiation in the management of prolactinomas: long-term follow-up. *Clin Endocrinol (Oxf)*, 1991; **34**: 399–406.
25. Johnston DG, Hall K, Kendall Taylor P, Ross WM, Crombie AL, Cook DB, *et al.* The long-term effects of megavoltage radiotherapy as sole or combined therapy for large prolactinomas: studies with high definition computerized tomography. *Clin Endocrinol (Oxf)*, 1986; **24**: 675–85.
26. Mehta AE, Reyes FI, Faiman C. Primary radiotherapy of prolactinomas. *Eight- to 15-year follow-up. Am J Med*, 1987; **83**: 49–58.
27. Brada M, Rajan B, Traish D, Ashley S, Holmes Sellors PJ, Nussey S, *et al.* The long term efficacy of conservative surgery and radiotherapy in the control of pituitary adenomas. *Clin Endocrinol (Oxf)*, 1993; **38**: 571–8.
28. Becker G, Kocher M, Kortmann RD, Paulsen F, Jeremic B, Muller RP, *et al.* Radiation therapy in the multimodal treatment approach of pituitary adenoma. *Strahlenther Onkol*, 2002; **178**: 173–86.
29. Brada M, Ashley S, Ford D, Traish D, Burchell L, Rajan B. Cerebrovascular mortality in patients with pituitary adenoma. *Clin Endocrinol (Oxf)*, 2002; **57**: 713–17.
30. Brada M, Burchell L, Ashley S, Traish D. The incidence of cerebrovascular accidents in patients with pituitary adenoma. *Int J Radiat Oncol Biol Phys*, 1999; **45**: 693–8.
31. Tomlinson JW, Holden N, Hills RK, Wheatley K, Clayton RN, Bates AS, *et al.* Association between premature mortality and hypopituitarism. West Midlands Prospective Hypopituitary Study Group. *Lancet*, 2001; **357**: 425–31.
32. Erfurth EM, Bulow B, Svahn-Tapper G, Norrving B, Odh K, Mikoczy Z, *et al.* Risk factors for cerebrovascular deaths in patients operated and irradiated for pituitary tumors. *J Clin Endocrinol Metab*, 2002; Nov; **87**: 4892–9.
33. Tsang R, Laperriere N, Simpson W, Brierley J, Panzarella T, Smyth H. Glioma arising after radiation therapy for pituitary adenoma: a report of four patients and estimation of risk. *Cancer*, 1993; **72**: 2227–33.
34. Brada M, Ford D, Ashley S, Bliss JM, Crowley S, Mason M, *et al.* Risk of second brain tumour after conservative surgery and radiotherapy for pituitary adenoma. *BMJ*, 1992; **304**: 1343–6.
35. Peace KA, Orme SM, Padayatty SJ, Godfrey HP, Belchetz PE. Cognitive dysfunction in patients with pituitary tumour who have been treated with transfrontal or transsphenoidal surgery or medication. *Clin Endocrinol (Oxf)*, 1998; **49**: 391–6.
36. Guinan EM, Lowy C, Stanhope N, Lewis PD, Kopelman MD. Cognitive effects of pituitary tumours and their treatments: two case studies and an investigation of 90 patients. *J Neurol Neurosurg Psychiatry*, 1998; **65**: 870–6.
37. Kobayashi T. Long-term results of stereotactic gamma knife radiosurgery for pituitary adenomas. Specific strategies for different types of adenoma. *Prog Neurol Surg*, 2009; **22**: 77–95.
38. Jagannathan J, Yen CP, Pouratian N, Laws ER, Sheehan JP. Stereotactic radiosurgery for pituitary adenomas: a comprehensive review of indications, techniques and long-term results using the Gamma Knife. *J Neurooncol*, 2009; **92**: 345–56.
39. Attanasio R, Epaminonda P, Motti E, Giugni E, Ventrella L, Cozzi R, *et al.* Gamma-knife radiosurgery in acromegaly: a 4-year follow-up study. *J Clin Endocrinol Metab*, 2003; **88**: 3105–12.
40. Castinetti F, Taieb D, Kuhn JM, Chanson P, Tamura M, Jaquet P, *et al.* Outcome of gamma knife radiosurgery in 82 patients with acromegaly: correlation with initial hypersecretion. *J Clin Endocrinol Metab*, 2005; **90**: 4483–8.
41. Jagannathan J, Sheehan JP, Pouratian N, Laws ER Jr, Steiner L, Vance ML. Gamma knife radiosurgery for acromegaly: outcomes after failed transsphenoidal surgery. *Neurosurgery*, 2008; **62**: 1262–9; discussion 9–70.
42. Jagannathan J, Sheehan JP, Pouratian N, Laws ER, Steiner L, Vance ML. Gamma Knife surgery for Cushing's disease. *J Neurosurg*, 2007; **106**: 980–7.
43. Pollock BE, Brown PD, Nippoldt TB, Young WF Jr. Pituitary tumor type affects the chance of biochemical remission after radiosurgery of hormone-secreting pituitary adenomas. *Neurosurgery*, 2008; **62**: 1271–6; discussion 6–8.
44. Jezkova J, Hana V, Krsek M, Weiss V, Vladyka V, Liscak R, *et al.* Use of the Leksell gamma knife in the treatment of prolactinoma patients. *Clin Endocrinol (Oxf)*, 2009; **70**: 732–41.
45. Voges J, Kocher M, Runge M, Poggenborg J, Lehrke R, Lenartz D, *et al.* Linear accelerator radiosurgery for pituitary macroadenomas: a 7-year follow-up study. *Cancer*, 2006; **107**: 1355–64.
46. Pouratian N, Sheehan J, Jagannathan J, Laws ER, Jr., Steiner L, Vance ML. Gamma knife radiosurgery for medically and surgically refractory prolactinomas. *Neurosurgery*, 2006; **59**: 255–66; discussion -66.
47. Minniti G, Traish D, Ashley S, Gonsalves A, Brada M. Fractionated stereotactic conformal radiotherapy for secreting and nonsecreting pituitary adenomas. *Clin Endocrinol (Oxf)*, 2006; **64**: 542–8.
48. Milker-Zabel S, Debus J, Thilmann C, Schlegel W, Wannenmacher M. Fractionated stereotactically guided radiotherapy and radiosurgery in the treatment of functional and nonfunctional adenomas of the pituitary gland. *Int J Radiat Oncol Biol Phys*, 2001; **50**: 1279–86.
49. Colin P, Jovenin N, Delemer B, Caron J, Grulet H, Hecart AC, *et al.* Treatment of pituitary adenomas by fractionated stereotactic radiotherapy: a prospective study of 110 patients. *Int J Radiat Oncol Biol Phys*, 2005; **62**: 333–41.
50. Ludecke DK, Lutz BS, Niedworok G. The choice of treatment after incomplete adenomectomy in acromegaly: proton—versus high voltage radiation. *Acta Neurochir (Wien)*, 1989; **96**: 32–8.
51. Petit JH, Biller BM, Coen JJ, Swearingen B, Ancukiewicz M, Bussiere M, *et al.* Proton stereotactic radiosurgery in management of persistent acromegaly. *Endocr Pract*, 2007; **13**: 726–34.
52. Edwards AA, Swords FM, Plowman PN. Focal radiation therapy for patients with persistent/recurrent pituitary adenoma, despite previous radiotherapy. *Pituitary*, 2009; **12**: 30–4.

2.3.10 Prolactinomas and hyperprolactinaemia (including macroprolactinaemia)

John S. Bevan

Introduction

Prolactin promotes milk production in mammals. It was characterized as a hormone distinct from growth hormone, which also has lactogenic activity, as recently as 1971. In humans, the predominant prolactin species is a 23 kDa, 199 amino acid polypeptide synthesized and secreted by lactotroph cells in the anterior pituitary gland. Prolactin is produced also by other tissues including decidua, breast, T lymphocytes, and several regions of the brain, where its functions are largely unknown and its gene regulation different from that of the pituitary gene. Pituitary prolactin production is under tonic inhibitory control by hypothalamic dopamine, such that pituitary stalk interruption produces hyperprolactinaemia. The neuropeptides thyrotrophin-releasing hormone (TRH) and vasoactive intestinal peptide (VIP) exert less important stimulatory effects on pituitary prolactin release (1).

Following the discovery of prolactin as a separate hormone it became apparent that many apparently functionless 'chromophobe' pituitary adenomas were prolactinomas. Indeed, prolactinoma is the commonest type of functioning pituitary tumour diagnosed in humans. There is a marked female preponderance and prolactinoma is relatively rare in men. Several studies have revealed small prolactinomas in approximately 5% of autopsy pituitaries, most of which are undiagnosed during life. From a clinical standpoint, prolactinomas are divided arbitrarily into microprolactinomas (≤10 mm in diameter) and macroprolactinomas (>10 mm). This is a useful distinction which predicts tumour behaviour and indicates appropriate management strategies. Generally, microprolactinomas run a benign course. Some regress spontaneously, most stay unchanged over many years, and very few expand to cause local pressure effects. In contrast, macroprolactinomas may present with pressure symptoms, often increase in size if untreated and rarely disappear. Some clinicians find an intermediate category of *meso*-prolactinoma useful (10–20 mm in diameter), since this tumour group may have a more favourable treatment outcome than for larger macroprolactinomas.

Prolactinomas are usually sporadic tumours. Molecular genetics has shown nearly all to be monoclonal, suggesting that an intrinsic pituitary defect is likely to be responsible for pituitary tumorigenesis (see Chapter 2.3.2). Occasionally, prolactinoma may be part of a multiple endocrine neoplasia syndrome type I, but this occurs too infrequently to justify screening in every patient with a prolactinoma. Mixed growth hormone and prolactin-secreting tumours are well recognized and give rise to acromegaly in association with hyperprolactinaemia. Most contain separate growth hormone and prolactin-secreting cells whereas a minority secrete growth hormone and prolactin from a single population of cells, the mammosomatotroph adenomas. Prolactin-secreting adenomas may produce other hormones such as thyroid-stimulating hormone (TSH) or adrenocorticotropic hormone (ACTH), but such tumours are uncommon. Malignant prolactinomas are also very rare. A few cases have been described which have proved resistant to aggressive treatment with surgery, radiotherapy, and dopamine agonists. In a small proportion, extracranial metastases in liver, lungs, bone, and lymph nodes have been documented. The alkylating agent temozolomide is effective against some aggressive prolactinomas (2).

Clinical features of prolactinoma

The clinical features of prolactinoma are attributable to three main factors: hyperprolactinaemia, space occupation by the tumour, and varying degrees of hypopituitarism (Box 2.3.10.1). The individual clinical picture will be determined by the sex and age of the patient, and the tumour size. In brief, hyperprolactinaemia stimulates milk production, particularly from the oestrogen-primed breast, and inhibits hypothalamic gonadotropin-releasing hormone release, which leads to hypogonadotropic hypogonadism.

Premenopausal women, most of whom will have microprolactinomas, usually present with oligomenorrhoea or amenorrhoea (90%) and/or galactorrhoea (up to 80%). Anovulatory infertility is common. Excluding pregnancy, hyperprolactinaemia accounts for 10–20% cases of secondary amenorrhoea. It should be noted that most women with galactorrhoea do not have menstrual disturbance, hyperprolactinaemia, or a pituitary tumour. Postmenopausal women are, by definition, already hypogonadal and markedly hypo-oestrogenaemic. Hyperprolactinaemia in this age group does not present with classic symptoms and a prolactinoma

Box 2.3.10.1 Clinical features of prolactinoma

Caused by prolactin excess

Women

- Oligomenorrhoea/amenorrhoea
- Galactorrhoea
- Infertility
- Hirsutism/acne[a]

Men

- Reduced libido
- Impotence
- Infertility
- Galactorrhoea[a]

Caused by tumour size (usually in men)

- Headache
- Visual failure, classically bitemporal hemianopia
- Cranial nerve palsies

Caused by other pituitary hormone deficiency

- Microprolactinoma—other pituitary function usually normal
- Macroprolactinoma—varying degrees of hypopituitarism may be present

[a] Less common features.

may be recognized only when it grows large enough to produce headache and/or visual disturbance.

The presentation of hyperprolactinaemia in men is with reduced libido, impotence (75%), and infertility associated with a reduced sperm count. Such symptoms are quite often concealed or ignored, particularly by older men, so men tend to present later with larger tumours causing pressure symptoms. Galactorrhoea is very uncommon in men but does occur occasionally. Weight gain is noted frequently by hyperprolactinaemic men.

Long-term hyperprolactinaemic hypogonadism may reduce bone mineral density (BMD) in either sex and is an important cause of secondary osteoporosis. Prolactinoma is an unusual cause of delayed puberty in both sexes and some advocate the routine measurement of serum prolactin in this situation.

Diagnostic investigations

Causes of hyperprolactinaemia

The causes of hyperprolactinaemia can be divided simply into physiological, pharmacological, and pathological (Box 2.3.10.2). The normal prolactin range for nonpregnant women is below 500 mU/l (20 μg/l) and below 300 mU/l (12 μg/l) for men. The finding of mild hyperprolactinaemia should always be rechecked in a second blood sample to exclude possible venepuncture stress elevation, although the importance of this effect has probably been overemphasized. Pregnancy is the commonest cause of hyperprolactinaemic amenorrhoea and serum prolactin concentrations may rise as high as 8000 mU/l (320 μg/l) during the third trimester. Normal lactation is also associated with quite marked elevation of serum prolactin. As predicted from the physiological dopaminergic inhibition of prolactin secretion, treatment with dopamine receptor antagonist drugs commonly induces hyperprolactinaemia. Serum prolactin levels may rise as high as 5000 mU/l (200 μg/l). This is a particular problem with the major tranquillizers (for example, chlorpromazine) and antiemetics (such as metoclopramide) (3). It is a lesser problem with newer atypical antipsychotics such as quetiapine and olanzapine (4). There is potential for confusion if a patient does not reveal that he or she is taking an 'over-the-counter' preparation, such as a combined medication for the treatment of migraine which contains both an analgesic and an antiemetic. Similarly, some nonprescribed herbal or alternative remedies contain ingredients that cause prolactin elevation. Thus, a comprehensive drug history is essential. With regard to pathological causes of hyperprolactinaemia, it is important to exclude primary hypothyroidism. Modest hyperprolactinaemia is present in 40% of patients, although only 10% have levels above 600 mU/l (24 μg/l). Nevertheless, some hypothyroid young women may present with menstrual disturbance and galactorrhoea, together with very few 'typical' hypothyroid symptoms. Once venepuncture stress, pregnancy, interfering drugs, and primary hypothyroidism have been excluded, significant hyperprolactinaemia is usually associated with a pituitary adenoma (Box 2.3.10.2).

Box 2.3.10.2 Causes of hyperprolactinaemia

Physiological
- Stress (venepuncture?)
- Pregnancy
- Lactation

Pharmacological
- Anti-emetics (for example, metoclopramide, domperidone, prochlorperazine)
- Phenothiazines (for example, chlorpromazine, risperidone)
- Many others (see Ref. 3)

Pathological
- Primary hypothyroidism
- Pituitary tumours
  - Prolactinoma
  - Growth hormone-secreting (30% of acromegalics)
  - Non-functioning ('stalk pressure' or 'disconnection' hyperprolactinaemia)
- Polycystic ovarian syndrome (10% of PCOS)
- Hypothalamic lesions (rare)
  - Sarcoidosis
  - Langerhan's cell histiocytosis
  - Hypothalamic tumours
- Chest wall stimulation
  - Repeated breast self-examination
  - Post-herpes zoster
- Liver or renal failure

Interpretation of prolactin immunoassay results

Macroprolactin

Prolactin in human serum exists in multiple molecular forms, with three dominant species identified by gel filtration chromatography: monomeric prolactin (23 kDa), big prolactin (50–60 kDa), and big-big prolactin (macro-prolactin, 150–170 kDa). Macroprolactin is a complex of prolactin with an IgG antibody which is detected to a greater or lesser extent by all prolactin immunoassays (5). This prolactin species is present in significant amounts in ~25% of hyperprolactinaemic sera (Fig. 2.3.10.1) (5,6) and ~1% of the normal population. *In vivo*, macroprolactin has little prolactin bioactivity and many patients with macroprolactinaemia do not have typical hyperprolactinaemic symptoms (7). Macroprolactinaemia is not associated with macroprolactinoma.

Failure to recognize that hyperprolactinaemia may be due to macroprolactinaemia may lead to unnecessary investigation, incorrect diagnosis, and inappropriate management in patients presenting with common symptoms suggesting possible prolactin excess, such as amenorrhoea or impotence. The presence of macroprolactin can be confirmed by polyethylene glycol (PEG) precipitation and most UK biochemistry laboratories screen hyperprolactinaemic sera using this simple method (8). PEG precipitates high-molecular-weight compounds, including immunoglobulins, and repeat assay of the treated serum gives the residual monomeric prolactin concentration. At the present state of knowledge, there is no justification for detailed pituitary investigation or long-term follow-up of an individual shown to have macroprolactinaemia.

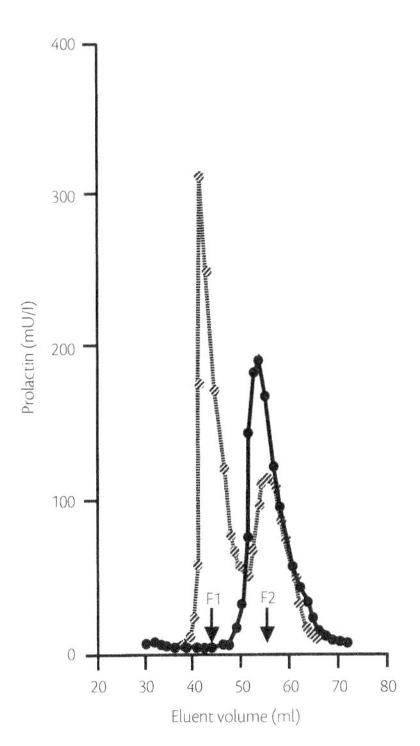

Fig. 2.3.10.1 Gel filtration of two serum samples containing monomeric prolactin (dark line), and a combination of macroprolactin and monomeric prolactin (grey line). Macroprolactin is contained in the F1 fractions. (Modified with permission from Fahie-Wilson MN, Soule SG. Macroprolactinaemia: contribution to hyperprolactinaemia in a district general hospital and evaluation of a screening test based on precipitation with polyethylene glycol. *Ann Clin Biochem*, 1997; **34**: 252–8.)

Prolactin 'hook effect'

If serum prolactin concentrations are extremely high (as in some men with giant prolactinomas), the amount of prolactin antigen may cause antibody saturation in prolactin immunoradiometric assays (IRMAs), leading to artefactually low prolactin results. This is known as the high-dose 'hook effect' and has been recognized some time in other immunoassays (e.g. B-human chorionic gonadotrophin, hCG). This artefact may lead to misdiagnosis and inappropriate surgery for some patients with macroprolactinoma. Serum prolactin should always be assayed in dilution in any patient with a large pituitary lesion which might be a prolactinoma (9).

Dynamic prolactin function tests

A number of dynamic tests have been proposed for the evaluation of hyperprolactinaemia but few UK clinical endocrinologists routinely use dynamic prolactin function tests. In my experience, the intravenous administration of a dopamine antagonist (such as 10 mg domperidone or metoclopramide) is a simple, well-tolerated procedure which provides clinically useful information, particularly for patients with modest elevations of serum prolactin. As illustrated in Fig. 2.3.10.2, dopamine antagonist administration to normal individuals results in a marked rise in serum prolactin concentration (to at least three times basal) together with little or no change in serum TSH (less than 2 mU/l rise). In contrast, patients with pituitary micro- and macro-lesions have blunted prolactin responses. Patients with microprolactinomas may, in addition, show exaggerated TSH responses due to enhanced dopaminergic

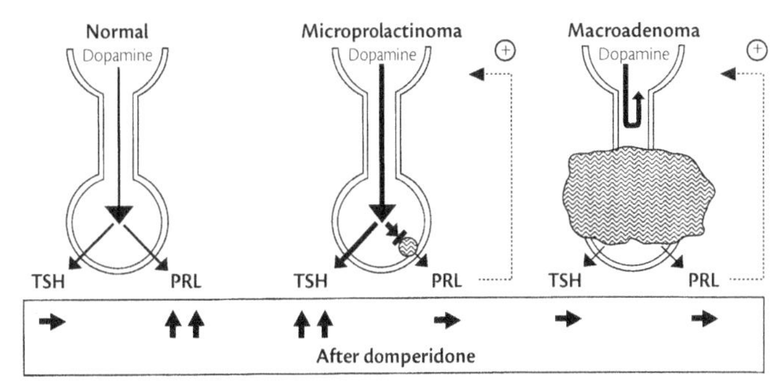

Fig. 2.3.10.2 Serum prolactin (PRL) and thyroid-stimulating hormone (TSH) responses to the intravenous administration of domperidone or metoclopramide in normal subjects (left), patients with microprolactinomas (centre) and patients with macrolesions (either prolactin- or nonsecreting) (right). In normal subjects, hypothalamic dopamine exerts dominant inhibition on lactotroph prolactin secretion and has relatively little effect on thyrotroph secretion—typical dopamine antagonist responses are therefore characterized by a marked rise in prolactin and a relatively small TSH increment. In patients with microprolactinomas, hypothalamic dopamine output is increased in response to the significant hyperprolactinaemia. This has little effect on the prolactinoma which has a separate arterial blood supply, but exerts increased inhibitory tone on the normal thyrotrophs. Dopamine antagonist administration therefore has little effect on serum prolactin but causes release of thyrotroph inhibition, with an exaggerated rise in serum TSH. In patients with macrolesions, the increased hypothalamic dopamine output is prevented from reaching the normal lactotrophs and thyrotrophs; consequently, prolactin/TSH levels do not rise after dopamine antagonism.

tone on the anterior pituitary thyrotrophs (via short-loop hypothalamic feedback).

Sawers and co-workers reviewed 84 hyperprolactinaemic patients whose investigation had included a domperidone test and high-resolution MRI (10). Eighteen of 20 patients with normal prolactin responses to domperidone had normal MR scans and the other two had only microadenomas, possibly incidentalomas. In contrast, 18 of the remaining 64 patients with abnormal prolactin responses had lesions greater than 10 mm diameter. Of the remainder, 63% had microadenomas. Dopamine antagonist testing can therefore identify a subset of hyperprolactinaemic patients for whom detailed pituitary imaging is mandatory. Conversely, a normal prolactin response to domperidone identifies those who do not require pituitary imaging.

Dopamine antagonist testing can also be informative before and after surgery for microprolactinoma. Webster and colleagues described a series of 82 hyperprolactinaemic patients who underwent surgery for suspected prolactinoma (11). No tumour was found in three cases, including the only two patients with normal prolactin and TSH responses to domperidone. Overall, 79% of patients had early postoperative normalization of serum prolactin but there were three relapses during long-term follow-up. Two of these had persistently abnormal prolactin and TSH responses to domperidone, even when basal prolactin levels remained normal.

Thus, although few patients with microprolactinoma are now treated surgically, these data are important because they indicate that dopamine antagonist testing can confirm (or refute) the presence of a microprolactinoma with reasonable certainty. Clinicians may regard this confirmatory biochemical evidence to be helpful in the medical management of such patients when histological proof of the diagnosis is not forthcoming and MRI may be negative. TRH testing is less discriminatory and generally unhelpful in the

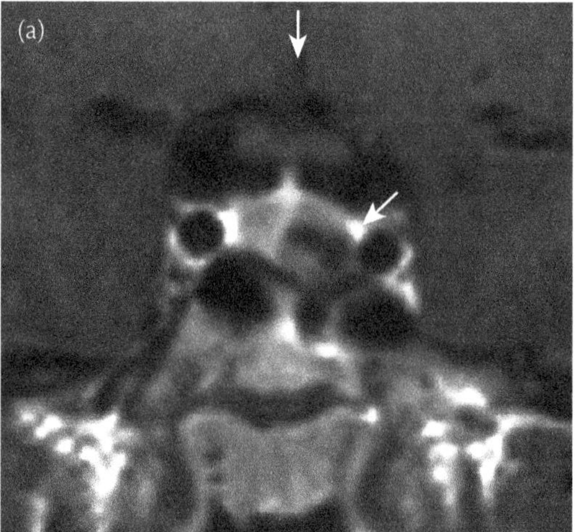

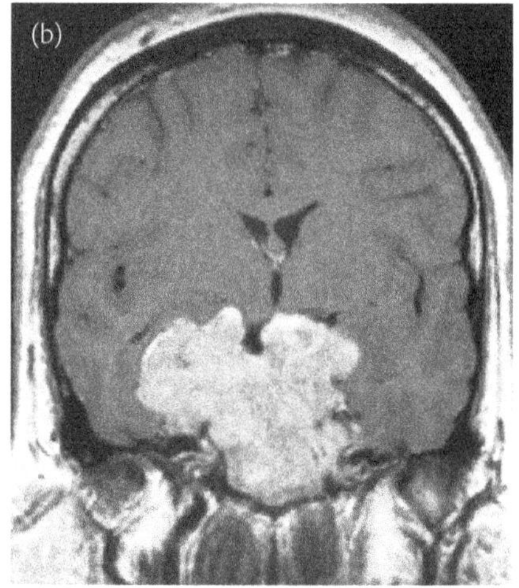

Fig. 2.3.10.3 High-resolution MRI of prolactinoma. (a) Microprolactinoma (9 mm) in a 14-year-old girl with secondary amenorrhoea (serum prolactin 4700 mU/l). The adenoma is indicated by the solid arrow and has a necrotic area within it. The optic chiasm is marked by the open arrow (the pituitary stalk is positioned centrally, and is visible below the chiasm). (b) Giant macroprolactinoma in a 28-year-old man with headaches and seizures (serum prolactin 850 000 mU/l). The tumour is several centimetres in diameter and extends into the suprasellar region and right temporal lobe.

investigation of hyperprolactinaemia. However, the test may have limited use in the evaluation of patients with growth hormone or gonadotropin-secreting tumours, a proportion of whom will show paradoxical stimulation of hormone release.

Pituitary imaging

Pituitary imaging is best performed using MRI with gadolinium enhancement. Compared with high-resolution CT, this technique provides superior detail of the optic chiasm, suprasellar masses, and cavernous sinus invasion. It does not involve the use of ionizing radiation and has a limit of resolution of approximately 2 mm. With MRI, the majority of microadenomas appear as focal hypodense lesions within the pituitary on T_1-weighted images (Fig. 2.3.10.3a). It should be noted that microadenomas are present in a significant proportion of the normal population and small 'incidentalomas' may be revealed by high-resolution MRI in up to 20% of healthy subjects. Conversely, a normal MRI examination does not exclude a microadenoma. Macroadenomas have a variety of appearances but are usually obvious on MRI (Fig. 2.3.10.3b). Imaging provides no information on tumour function or pathology, and macroprolactinoma, nonfunctioning macroadenoma, and craniopharyngioma may have identical appearances on MRI.

Diagnostic value of the basal serum prolactin concentration

Most patients with microprolactinomas have basal serum prolactin concentrations less than 5000 mU/l (200 µg/l). In patients with pituitary macrolesions, the basal serum prolactin is of considerable diagnostic value. A value greater than 5000 mU/l is virtually diagnostic of a macroprolactinoma and with a level greater than 10 000 mU/l there is no other possible diagnosis. A serum prolactin concentration lower than 2000 mU/l in a patient with a pituitary macrolesion usually indicates 'disconnection' hyperprolactinaemia rather than tumoural secretion of the hormone. This is due most commonly to a nonfunctioning pituitary macroadenoma, although intrasellar craniopharyngiomas and numerous other neoplastic and inflammatory pathologies may masquerade as 'pseudo-pituitary adenomas' (12).

An intermediate serum prolactin level (2000–5000 mU/l) in a patient with a large pituitary lesion produces an area of some diagnostic uncertainty which dynamic prolactin function tests cannot resolve. Most of these patients will have true prolactinomas and the remainder 'disconnection' hyperprolactinaemia (13). This has implications for management strategies as discussed below in the section on macroprolactinoma. Figure 2.3.10.4 shows the range of serum prolactin levels in a group of patients with pituitary

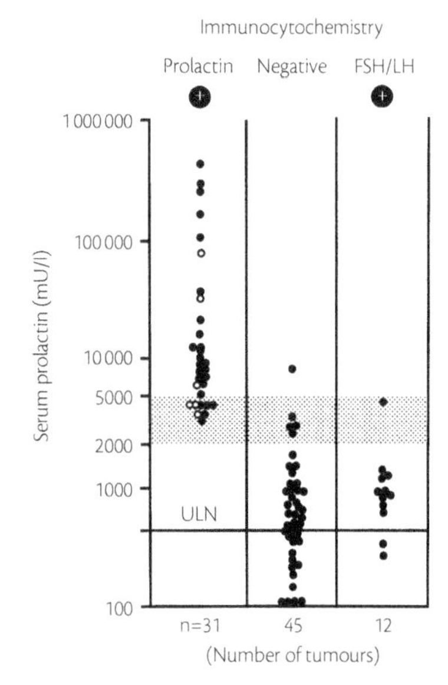

Fig. 2.3.10.4 Preoperative serum prolactin concentrations and pituitary tumour immunocytochemistry in 88 patients. Open symbols indicate undiluted prolactin values. The highest prolactin levels were found in patients with true prolactinomas (left-hand column). More than half of the patients with clinically functionless tumours had elevated serum prolactin values (middle and right-hand columns). The shading highlights the area of preoperative diagnostic uncertainty (serum prolactin 2000–5000 mU/l) with subsequent pathology revealing eight prolactin-secreting and five nonprolactin-secreting adenomas. In this series two patients with non-adenomas also had prolactin levels in this range. (Adapted with permission from Bevan JS, Burke CW, Esiri MM, Adams CBT. Misinterpretation of prolactin levels leading to management errors in patients with sellar enlargement. *Am J Med*, 1987; **82**: 29–32).

macroadenomas who underwent surgery and thus provided corroborative immunohistochemistry (12).

Ophthalmological assessment

There is usually about 10 mm between the top of the normal pituitary and the optic chiasm. All patients with pituitary macrolesions and suprasellar extension should therefore undergo specialist ophthalmological assessment, including Goldman perimetry. Since there is great variation in the pattern of suprasellar tumour growth (and the position of the chiasm may also vary) the pattern of visual impairment may range from the classic bitemporal hemianopia to partial quadrantic defects or scotomas. No pattern of visual loss is specific to prolactinoma, compared with other tumour types.

General pituitary function

Larger pituitary masses may cause hypopituitarism either by direct pituitary compression or by disruption of hypothalamic control mechanisms. Patients with microprolactinomas usually have normal growth hormone, ACTH, and TSH function. However, with macroprolactinomas the degree of hypopituitarism is likely to be proportional to the size of the tumour. With the largest tumours, ACTH and TSH deficits may be present at diagnosis in approximately 20% of patients and growth hormone deficiency is almost invariable. All patients with macroprolactinomas should have full pituitary function testing.

Management of prolactinoma

Treatment indications

Most patients with prolactinoma require treatment. Infertility, menstrual disturbance with longstanding hypogonadism (risk of secondary osteoporosis), troublesome galactorrhoea, an enlarging pituitary tumour, and tumour pressure effects (particularly visual failure) are all indications for treatment. Dopamine agonist drugs are now indicated as primary medical therapy for patients with prolactinomas of all sizes. However, an important exception is the patient with a pituitary macrolesion and minor elevation of prolactin, who is most likely to have a nonfunctioning pituitary adenoma requiring surgery for decompression and histological diagnosis. It may be reasonable to simply observe some patients with microprolactinomas, particularly if circulating sex steroid concentrations are judged to be adequate.

Dopamine agonists

The introduction of medical therapy with dopamine agonists revolutionized the treatment of patients with prolactinoma. The first dopamine agonist was bromocriptine, a semisynthetic ergopeptine derivative, introduced in 1971. On a global basis, this probably remains the most commonly used dopamine agonist, but other longer-acting and better tolerated drugs, such as cabergoline and quinagolide, are now widely available. Most endocrinologists use cabergoline as first-choice dopamine agonist; a large comparative study with bromocriptine convincingly demonstrated its superiority in terms of tolerability, patient convenience and efficacy (14). Similar data favour the use of quinagolide over bromocriptine (15). Pregnancy is a special situation, since there are many more safety data for bromocriptine than for the newer agents. Many endocrinologists select bromocriptine as first-line treatment for hyperprolactinaemic infertility.

Bromocriptine is used in a dose of 2.5 mg twice or thrice daily. The doses of 20–40 mg per day used in early studies are no more efficacious and produce more side-effects. Cabergoline is usually effective in a dose of 0.5–1.0 mg once or twice weekly and quinagolide in a once-daily dose of 75–150 μg. In order to minimize side-effects, patients can be advised to take these two drugs, together with a supper snack, just before retiring to bed.

Adverse effects of dopamine agonists

All dopamine agonists may produce unwanted side effects including, in decreasing order of importance, upper gastrointestinal disturbance (especially nausea), postural hypotension, constipation, nasal stuffiness and Raynaud's phenomenon (Box 2.3.10.3). These can be minimized by using an incremental dosage schedule and taking tablets with food. In a double-blind comparison of bromocriptine and cabergoline, 12% of patients stopped bromocriptine because of intolerance whereas only 3% stopped cabergoline (14).

Acute psychotic reactions have been described with quinagolide, albeit rarely. It is unclear whether this important side effect is drug-specific since acute psychosis was encountered occasionally in earlier patients treated with large bromocriptine doses. Sleep and mild mood disturbances can occur with all the dopamine agonists (Box 2.3.10.3).

Recent studies of parkinsonian patients treated with dopamine agonists revealed restrictive valvular heart disease in about one third of patients taking pergolide. The valvulopathy was mostly

Box 2.3.10.3 Potential dopamine agonist adverse effects during prolactinoma treatment

Common side effects

- Gastrointestinal—nausea, constipation
- Postural hypotension
- Nasal congestion
- Raynaud's phenomenon

Central nervous system/psychiatric side effects

- Sleepiness
- Fatigue
- Pathological gambling
- Hypomania
- Psychosis

Adverse events due to dopamine agonist-induced changes within a macroprolactinoma

- Cerebrospinal fluid rhinorrhoea
- Traction ophthalmopathy
- Pituitary apoplexy

Long-term side effects (controversial at prolactinoma doses—see section 'Adverse effects of dopamine agonists')

- Pulmonary fibrosis
- Retroperitoneal fibrosis
- Fibrotic valvulopathy

mild, but correlated with the cumulative dose, and a similar effect was demonstrated with cabergoline. However, much higher doses of dopamine agonist are used in Parkinson's disease (typically 20–30 times the dose used to treat prolactinoma), patients tend to be older (perhaps with altered cardiac susceptibility) and a large cumulative dose is attained more quickly than in prolactinoma patients. Nevertheless, European medicines regulatory agencies issued a drug alert in late 2008 related to potential valvulopathy in endocrine patients on ergot-derived dopamine agonists (16–18). Of seven published studies of endocrine patients treated with cabergoline, with appropriate age and sex matched controls, only one showed a significantly increased risk of valve disease. This study also showed rates of moderate tricuspid regurgitation *in controls* that were sixfold greater those in the other studies, suggesting the investigators may have used more stringent echocardiographic criteria. The results from the controlled studies show valvular abnormalities in 50 of 450 (11%) of endocrine patients taking cabergoline compared with 33 of 416 (8%) for controls ($p = 0.13$). If uncontrolled data are added for the patients on cabergoline, the percentage with valvular abnormalities falls to 8% (61/645). Overall, the cardiac risks associated with low-dose cabergoline seem to be low but further studies are required for reassurance. The need for echocardiographic surveillance in endocrine patients remains unproven. At the present state of knowledge, it would seem reasonable to focus on patients taking more than 2 mg cabergoline per week but there are no data to inform the best screening protocol.

Microprolactinomas

Dopamine agonists

Medical therapy is remarkably effective in the treatment of microprolactinoma (19–21). In early studies of patients treated with bromocriptine, normoprolactinaemia or ovulatory cycles were restored in 80–90% of patients. Fertility returned within two months in 70% of women. Galactorrhoea disappeared or was greatly reduced in the majority, usually within a few days or weeks. In comparative studies of cabergoline and bromocriptine, resumption of ovulatory cycles or occurrence of pregnancy was documented in 72% of cabergoline patients (up to 1.0 mg twice weekly) compared with 52% in the bromocriptine group (up to 5.0 mg twice daily) (14). The number of women with stable normoprolactinaemia was also higher in the cabergoline group (83% vs 58%). Bone mineral density (BMD) has been shown to increase during long-term dopamine agonist therapy, presumably in response to restoration of normal ovarian oestrogen secretion, although there are no prospective data on fracture reduction (19).

Tumour shrinkage occurs during long-term treatment, although this is less critical than for patients with macroprolactinomas. Importantly, a minority of patients may be 'cured' after a period of dopamine agonist treatment. The mechanism is unknown. The probability of 'cure' remains unclear but at least one-third of microprolactinomas seem to remit with time (22–23). A dopamine-agonist induced pregnancy may increase the chances of remission (24). For these reasons, most endocrinologists interrupt dopamine agonist treatment every 3 years, for further clinical assessment and prolactin testing. In doing so, one should remember that women may continue to have ovulatory cycles for 3–6 months after withdrawal of the long-acting drug cabergoline.

Transsphenoidal surgery

In some centres, transsphenoidal surgery may be offered as an alternative to medical therapy. Indeed, surgery may be essential if the patient is intolerant of or resistant to dopamine receptor agonists. Surgical success is critically dependent on surgical experience and the size of the tumour. In most large centres, normoprolactinaemia is achieved post operatively in 60–90% of patients, with results for larger microprolactinomas (4–9 mm diameter) being significantly better than for smaller ones. Previous dopamine agonist therapy may hamper surgery but this is less troublesome for micro- than it is for macroprolactinomas. Recurrence of hyperprolactinaemia, usually without radiologically evident tumour, is well recognized. Using normoprolactinaemia as the main criterion of cure, it is probably reasonable to speak of a long-term surgical cure rate of between 50% and 70% when counselling patients with respect to choice of therapy. It is important to mention the small but measurable morbidity of transsphenoidal surgery (discussed elsewhere in this volume), together with the small risk of loss of normal pituitary function. The latter would be particularly important if the patient wished fertility.

Due to the excellent therapeutic responses to either dopamine agonists or transsphenoidal surgery, radiotherapy is no longer considered acceptable primary therapy for microprolactinoma.

Observation (including oral contraception)

Longitudinal studies suggest only 5% of microprolactinomas progress to larger lesions. Hence, in a woman with a microprolactinoma who has normal menses and libido, non-troublesome galactorrhoea, and who does not wish to become pregnant, there may be no clear indication for antiprolactinoma therapy. Before recommending simple observation of a microprolactinoma, most endocrinologists would wish to confirm 'adequate' circulating sex steroid concentrations (mean oestradiol above 200 pmol/l in a woman and testosterone above 7 nmol/l in a man), together with BMD within 1 SD of age-related mean values. In this situation it would be reasonable to monitor the patient with 6–12 monthly serum prolactin and oestradiol/testosterone estimations, supplemented with bone densitometry every 3–5 years, thus enabling individualized timing of any intervention. The question of oral contraceptive safety often arises. There are good data confirming safety of the oral contraceptive in combination with a dopamine agonist in women with microprolactinomas but no satisfactory prospective studies of treatment with an oral contraceptive alone. If the latter course of action is taken, serum prolactin should be checked every 3–6 months, with the addition of dopamine agonist therapy should the serum prolactin level rise above an arbitrary target level (e.g. twice the basal level).

Macroprolactinomas

Dopamine agonists

These drugs directly activate pituitary D2 dopamine receptors, mimicking the action of endogenous hypothalamic dopamine. In addition to reducing prolactin secretion, D2 receptor stimulation results in rapid involution of the cellular protein synthetic machinery and thus marked reduction in lactotroph cell size. This effect, together with an antimitotic action, accounts for the rapid and sustained tumour shrinkage which enables these drugs to be used as primary therapy for patients with larger prolactinomas, even those with pressure effects. Dopamine agonist treatment is followed typically by a rapid fall in serum prolactin (within hours) and tumour shrinkage (within days or weeks). Tumour regression is often followed by an improvement in visual function over a (short) time-course which rivals that seen after surgical decompression of the chiasm. Thus, patients with macroprolactinomas presenting with visual failure are no longer the neurosurgical emergencies they were previously regarded to be. Nevertheless, it is vitally important that all patients with a pituitary macrolesion producing chiasmal compression should have serum prolactin measured urgently (and checked in dilution–see section on prolactin immunoassay). Four illustrative patients are shown in Fig. 2.3.10.5, Fig. 2.3.10.6, Fig. 2.3.10.7, and Fig. 2.3.10.8.

Shrinkage rates

A meta-analysis of 271 well-characterized macroprolactinomas treated with dopamine agonists showed that 79% of tumours shrank by more than a quarter, and 89% shrank to some degree. The pretreatment prolactin level is not a reliable predictor of tumour shrinkage, since 83% of tumours showed significant tumour shrinkage in both the 'above 100 000 mU/l' and '5000–10 000 mU/l' groups. Of the macroprolactinomas large enough to produce chiasmal compression, 85% showed significant tumour shrinkage (25).

Time course of shrinkage

Tumour shrinkage can be demonstrated within a week or two of starting dopamine agonist therapy and most shrinkage takes place during the first three months of treatment (Fig. 2.3.10.9) (25–26). However, in many patients, shrinkage continues at a slower rate over many months (see tumours in Fig. 2.3.10.6 and Fig. 2.3.10.7). It is recommended to repeat MRI 3 months after commencing dopamine agonist therapy and, if there has been an acceptable response, again at 1 and 2 years.

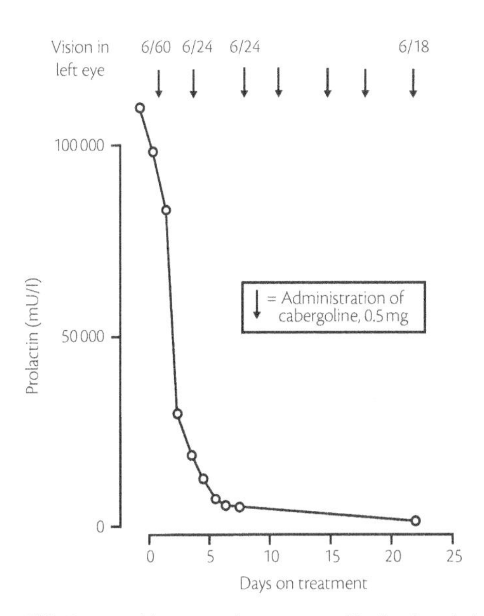

Fig. 2.3.10.5 This 68-year-old man was impotent and had reduced visual acuity in his left eye; serum prolactin was greatly elevated at 109 000 mU/l, and a 3 cm macroadenoma was shown on MRI. He was commenced on treatment with cabergoline, 0.5 mg twice weekly. His left visual acuity started to improve after just one tablet, and his serum prolactin was close to normal after two tablets. Follow up MRIs over a four year period showed approximately 80% tumour shrinkage.

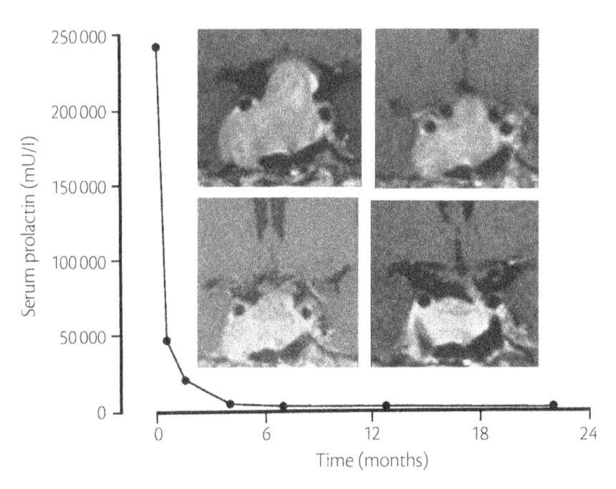

Fig. 2.3.10.6 This 61-year-old woman had headaches and a right temporal visual field defect: serum prolactin was greatly elevated at 240 000 mU/l, and a macroadenoma with suprasellar extension was shown on MRI. She was treated with cabergoline in an initial dose of 0.5 mg twice weekly, increased to 1.0 mg twice weekly after 2 months. Her vision was virtually normal after 1 month. The rapid fall in serum prolactin is shown in the main figure, although levels have remained slightly elevated. Marked tumour shrinkage is shown in the figure insert. MRI scans at baseline (top left), 3 months (top right), 1 year (bottom left) and 2 years (bottom right) are shown. The optic chiasm is stretched over the suprasellar extension at baseline and clearly decompressed after 2 years. Rest of pituitary function improved during this time course without the need for hormone replacement: free thyroxine (T_4) rose from 8 to 15 pmol/l and peak serum cortisol 30 min after tetracosactrin from 450 to 770 nmol/l.

Amount of shrinkage and visual recovery

Approximately 40% of macroprolactinomas treated with dopamine agonists for 1–3 months show tumour size reduction by at least one half. Of those treated for 1 year or longer, almost 90% show such shrinkage (25). Visual field defects improve in approximately 90% of patients in whom they were abnormal before treatment.

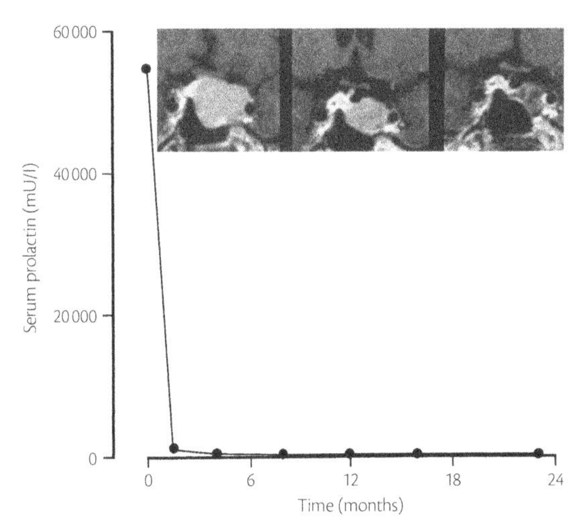

Fig. 2.3.10.7 This 47-year-old man had left-sided trigeminal neuralgia, lassitude, weight gain of 12.7 kg (28 lb) and reduced libido: serum prolactin was raised at 55 000 mU/l, and MRI showed a macroadenoma invading the left cavernous sinus. He was treated with cabergoline 0.5 mg twice weekly and was pain-free within 1 day of taking the first tablet. As shown in the figure, serum prolactin has normalized and this has been accompanied by a rise in serum testosterone from 9 to 14 nmol/l. The figure insert shows MRI scans at baseline (left), 3 months (centre), and 9 months (right). The latest scan shows a markedly shrunken tumour remnant. He had a trial withdrawal of cabergoline after 8 years treatment but serum prolactin rose to 700 mU/l and his neuralgia returned after 6 months; he continues to take cabergoline 0.5 mg per week.

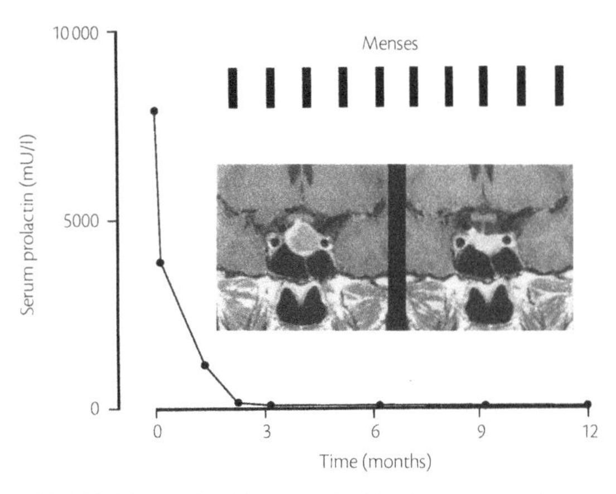

Fig. 2.3.10.8 This 16-year-old girl presented with primary amenorrhoea and galactorrhoea: serum prolactin was raised at 8000 mU/l, and MRI showed a macroadenoma with a low-density centre abutting the optic chiasm. Under a clinical trial protocol, cabergoline was incremented to 1.0 mg twice weekly over a 1-month period. Prolactin normalization and onset of menses occurred after 2 months of treatment. The figure insert shows MRI scans at baseline (left) and after 3 months (right): there has been marked tumour shrinkage, and the optic chiasm and central pituitary stalk are clearly seen.

Although early visual improvement occurs frequently, it may be several months before maximum benefit accrues. Thus, persistence of a visual field defect is not an absolute indication to proceed to surgery.

Serum prolactin responses

Suppression of serum prolactin usually accompanies successful tumour shrinkage. Indeed, all of the responsive patients in the meta-analysis showed a fall in serum prolactin of at least 50%, and in 58% of patients serum prolactin became entirely normal (25).

Effects on pituitary function

Several investigators have demonstrated recovery of impaired anterior pituitary function in association with tumour shrinkage. Importantly, these data have been extended to include recovery of growth hormone reserve, which may obviate the need for expensive growth hormone replacement in a proportion of these patients (27). In contrast, it is worth noting that at least two-thirds of men with successfully treated prolactinomas have persistently subnormal testosterone levels and require androgen supplementation (25). In premenopausal women with medically treated macroprolactinomas cyclical menses return in over 90%.

Dopamine agonist resistance

Overall, the acquisition of dopamine agonist resistance during therapy appears to be very rare, even with treatment periods of 10 or more years (28). A handful of cases have, however, been described (25). Primary resistance to cabergoline occurs in fewer than 10% of patients (19) but most patients will normalize prolactin if the drug is tolerated and the dose can be increased (29–31).

Dopamine agonist withdrawal

Although prolactinomas usually remain sensitive to dopamine agonists, the drugs do not provide a definitive cure for most patients with macroprolactinoma and many have to remain on long-term therapy. Immediate tumour re-expansion may occur after drug withdrawal following medium-term therapy (up to 1 year) but re-expansion is less common after long-term treatment (several years) (23, 32). Recent withdrawal studies have suggested that up to 40% of macroprolactinomas may remain in remission after withdrawal of long-term cabergoline therapy, particularly in those patients who achieved prolactin normalization and near tumour disappearance during treatment (Fig. 2.3.10.10) (23). In patients who need to remain on treatment, the dose of dopamine agonist can often be reduced considerably once initial tumour regression has been achieved, with ongoing satisfactory control of tumour size.

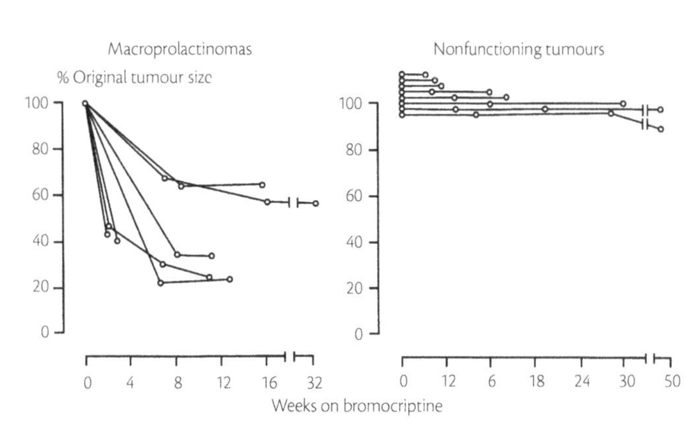

Fig. 2.3.10.9 Tumour volume changes (expressed as a percentage of the pretreatment volume) during bromocriptine therapy in seven patients with macroprolactinomas (left-hand panel) and eight patients with non-functioning tumours, several of whom had 'disconnection' hyperprolactinaemia (right-hand panel). Note that all of the prolactinomas shrank, by an average of approximately 50%, and that most shrinkage took place during the first 3 months of treatment. None of the nonfunctioning tumours shrank. (With permission from Bevan JS, Adams CB, Burke CW, Morton KE, Molyneux AJ, Moore RA, *et al.* Factors in the outcome of transsphenoidal surgery for prolactinoma and non-functioning pituitary tumour, including pre-operative bromocriptine therapy. *Clin Endocrinol*, 1987; **26**: 541–56).

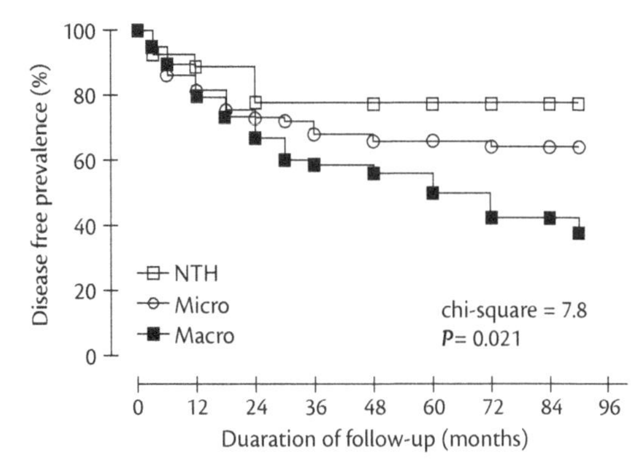

Fig. 2.3.10.10 Kaplan-Meier stimulation of recurrence of hyperprolactinaemia after 8 years cabergoline withdrawal in 221 patients. Patients were eligible for withdrawal if they maintained a normal serum prolactin level and showed tumour disappearance or at least 50% tumour volume reduction on MRI scan, after their maintenance cabergoline dose had been reduced to 0.5 mg/week. The initial diagnosis was non-tumoural hyperprolactinaemia (NTH, n = 27), microprolactinoma (n = 115) or macroprolactinoma (n = 79). Persistent remission of hyperprolactinaemia without evidence of tumour regrowth occurred in the majority of patients with small tumours and in about 40% of those with macroprolactinomas. (Modified with permission from: Colao A, Di Sarno A, Guerra E, Pivonello R, Cappabianca P, Caranci F, *et al.* Predictors of remission of hyperprolactinaemia after long-term withdrawal of cabergoline therapy. *Clin Endocrinol* 2007; **67**: 426–33).

Nonshrinking prolactinomas

Approximately 10% of genuine macroprolactinomas fail to regress during dopamine agonist therapy. The mechanism is obscure since most patients with nonshrinking tumours have marked suppression of serum prolactin levels. However, patients with little or no fall in serum prolactin often show minimal reductions in tumour size and a few continue to grow. Some nonshrinking tumours have large cystic components, some have atypical histology and some appear to have a deficiency of membrane-bound D2 dopamine receptors (25).

Choice of dopamine agonist

Macroprolactinoma shrinkage has been demonstrated with all of the clinically available dopamine agonists including bromocriptine, quinagolide, and cabergoline. Studies of cabergoline show that over 80% of previously untreated macroprolactinomas undergo significant tumour regression. Significant success rates were recorded also in patients previously resistant to or intolerant of other dopamine agonists, including bromocriptine (19). Some examples of cabergoline-induced shrinkage are shown in Fig. 2.3.10.6, Fig. 2.3.10.7, and Fig. 2.3.10.8. It is worth trying an alternative dopamine agonist in the event of drug resistance or intolerance (15).

Management strategies

Macroprolactinoma is virtually certain if serum prolactin is greater than 5000 mU/l in a patient with a pituitary macrolesion and primary treatment with a dopamine agonist has an excellent chance of tumour volume reduction. As noted earlier, a serum prolactin level between 2000 and 5000 mU/l presents some diagnostic uncertainty. Closely supervised dopamine agonist therapy is appropriate, provided surgery is performed in the event of any visual deterioration. Dopamine agonists reduce prolactin secretion from both normal and tumorous lactotrophs; therefore, serum prolactin is likely to fall irrespective of the cause of the hyperprolactinaemia. Pituitary macrolesions associated with prolactin levels less than 2000 mU/l are rarely prolactinomas and surgery should be undertaken to decompress the lesion and provide a histological diagnosis. Some of these important practice points are illustrated by the case shown in Fig. 2.3.10.11.

Medical treatment alone is an acceptable option for most patients with macroprolactinoma, particularly those with fertility needs in whom adjunctive therapy might compromise gonadotropin function. Physicians should be aware of the infrequent complication of cerebrospinal fluid (CSF) rhinorrhoea, which may occur after shrinkage of inferiorly invasive tumours and may be very difficult to correct surgically (33). Traction ophthalmopathy may occur rarely if the optic chiasm is adherent to the upper part of a shrinking tumour (34). Pituitary apoplexy may occur in a cystic tumour as it shrinks (35) (Box 2.3.10.3).

The present role of radiotherapy and surgery

A minority of endocrinologists consider that dopamine agonist therapy alone is unsuitable for long-term management of macroprolactinoma and recommend external beam radiotherapy. Although prolactin levels fall over a period of several years after radiotherapy, enabling dopamine agonist withdrawal in a proportion of patients, this treatment is likely to be followed by varying degrees of hypopituitarism (see Chapter 2.3.6).

A meta-analysis of 2226 macroprolactinomas treated with primary surgery showed prolactin normalization in only 34% of patients (19). Certainly, one would not anticipate a curative surgical procedure in patients with giant, invasive macroprolactinomas, such as that illustrated in Fig. 2.3.10.3b. Consequently, in view of the effectiveness of medical treatment, only a minority of patients with large tumours should now require surgical intervention. There are a few selected situations in which some clinicians might consider surgery and a cautionary note on the effect of dopamine agonists on macroprolactinoma fibrosis is necessary. There is a direct relationship between tumour fibrosis and duration of medical treatment such that surgery is made much more difficult—and may even be hazardous—if dopamine agonists have been given for longer than 3 months (26, 36). Overall, it is prudent to limit preoperative dopamine agonist therapy to a maximum of 3 months if surgery is to be undertaken.

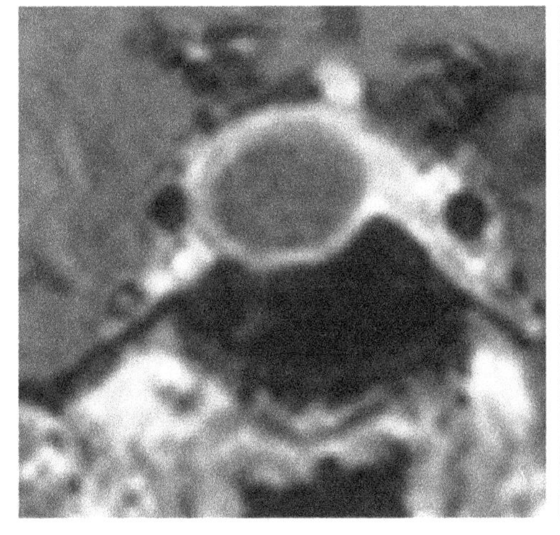
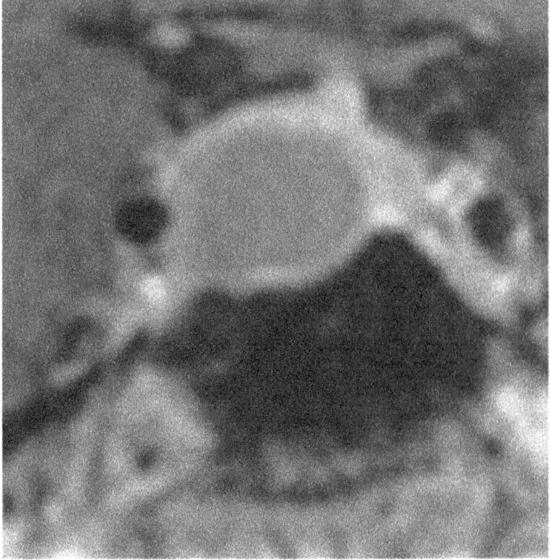

Fig. 2.3.10.11 This 37-year-old woman presented with secondary amenorrhoea; serum prolactin was elevated at 1380 mU/l with an impaired response to domperidone. MRI revealed a 14 mm macrolesion with a possibly necrotic centre (left-hand panel). She had a trial of cabergoline during which prolactin suppressed to below 40 mU/l and her periods recommenced. However, repeat MRI 3 months later showed no change in the size of the lesion (right-hand panel). Transsphenoidal surgery revealed a functionless macroadenoma with negative prolactin immunostaining and evidence of haemorrhagic infarction.

Pregnancy and prolactinomas

Management recommendations

Oestrogens have a stimulatory effect on prolactin synthesis and secretion, and the hormonal changes of normal pregnancy cause marked lactotroph hyperplasia. MRI studies have confirmed a gradual doubling in pituitary volume during the course of gestation. In view of these effects of pregnancy on normal lactotrophs it is not surprising that prolactinomas may also increase in size.

The potential risk to the patient depends on the prepregnancy size of the prolactinoma. For women with microprolactinomas the risk of clinically relevant tumour expansion is very small indeed—less than 2%. Dopamine agonists can be safely stopped in such patients as soon as pregnancy has been confirmed. Nevertheless, patients should be advised to report for urgent assessment in the event of severe headache or any visual disturbance. Routine endocrine review may be arranged on two or three occasions during the pregnancy, but formal charting of visual fields is unnecessary and measurement of serum prolactin provides no useful information, given the considerable prolactin rise during normal gestation. Women can safely breastfeed their infants.

There has been some controversy concerning the risk of pregnancy for women with larger prolactinomas. In early reviews, macroprolactinoma expansion was reported to occur in nearly 40%, but many of these women received ovulation induction with gonadotropins and not dopamine agonists. More recent reviews suggest that symptomatic macroprolactinoma expansion occurs in fewer than 20% of women. The figure is probably 10% or lower in women given a several-month course of dopamine agonist prior to conception

Some clinicians continue to recommend conservative debulking surgery or even radiotherapy before pregnancy in women with macroprolactinomas to reduce the likelihood of major tumour expansion. However, dopamine agonists may be safely employed as sole therapy, using the following strategy. Medical treatment should be used for a minimum of 6 months, and preferably 12 months, together with follow-up MRI to assess residual suprasellar extension, before conception is attempted. If the tumour has shrunk to within the fossa, the dopamine agonist can be withdrawn once pregnancy is confirmed, with a less than 10% chance of re-expansion problems. If neurological problems do occur, bromocriptine should be started during the pregnancy and this will restore tumour control in nearly all cases. If there is significant suprasellar tumour before conception, the choice is between debulking surgery or continuing bromocriptine throughout the pregnancy. The latter seems to be effective but present experience is still relatively limited.

Dopamine agonist safety in pregnancy

There is no evidence of teratogenicity in the offspring of women treated with simple bromocriptine-induced ovulation or those treated throughout pregnancy with the drug. Nevertheless, it is prudent not to use the drug during pregnancy unless absolutely necessary. Safety data for cabergoline and quinagolide are limited to a few hundred pregnancies, compared with several thousand for bromocriptine. Outcomes of 380 pregnancies following cabergoline treatment during a 12-year observational study have been reported recently (37). The spontaneous abortion rate in 329 pregnancies with known outcome was 9.1%, well within the expected range. The fetal malformation rate also fell within reported ranges for the general population with no pattern of type or severity. Since clinical experience is limited in relation to pregnancy and since the drug has a long half-life, the manufacturer still recommends that cabergoline be stopped 1 month prior to intended conception. However, this is clinically inconvenient and requires repeated monitoring of prolactin and ovarian status. There seems to be little risk in women who become pregnant while taking cabergoline. Pregnancy safety data on quinagolide are limited and perhaps less reassuring than those for cabergoline. In a recent review of 176 pregnancies in women treated with the drug, 14% ended in spontaneous abortion. Nine fetal malformations were diagnosed, including two infants with Down's syndrome (38). Quinagolide has an intermediate duration of action and, in acknowledgement of the limited pregnancy experience, the manufacturer recommends that the drug be withdrawn as soon as pregnancy is confirmed.

References

1. Molitch ME. Prolactin. In: Melmed M, ed. *The Pituitary*. 2nd edn. Malden, Massachusetts: Blackwell Science, 2002:119–71 ***Review of prolactin basic physiology with 902 references.***
2. Neff LM, Weil M, Cole A, Hedges TR, Shucart W, Lawrence D, *et al.* Temozolomide in the treatment of an invasive prolactinoma resistant to dopamine agonists. *Pituitary*, 2007; **10**: 81–6.
3. Molitch ME. Medication-induced hyperprolactinaemia. *Mayo Clin Proc*, 2005; **80**: 1050–7.
4. Wieck A, Haddad P. Hyperprolactinaemia caused by antipsychotic drugs. *BMJ*, 2002; **324**: 250–2.
5. Fahie-Wilson MN, John R, Ellis AR. Macroprolactin; high molecular mass forms of circulating prolactin. *Ann Clin Biochem*, 2005; **42**: 175–92. ***Review of laboratory and clinical aspects of macroprolactin with 105 references.***
6. Fahie-Wilson MN, Soule SG. Macroprolactinaemia: contribution to hyperprolactinaemia in a district general hospital and evaluation of a screening test based on precipitation with polyethylene glycol. *Ann Clin Biochem*, 1997; **34**: 252–8.
7. Pinto LP, Hanna FWF, Evans LM, Davies JS, John R, Scanlon MF. The TSH response to domperidone reflects the biological activity of prolactin in macroprolactinaemia and hyperprolactinaemia. *Clin Endocrinol*, 2003; **59**: 580–4.
8. McKenna TJ. Should macroprolactin be measured in all hyperprolactinaemic sera? *Clin Endocrinol*, 2009; **71**: 466–9.
9. St-Jean E, Blain F, Comtois R. High prolactin levels may be missed by immunoradiometric assay in patients with macroprolactinomas. *Clin Endocrinol*, 1996; **44**: 305–9.
10. Sawers HA, Robb OJ, Walmsley D, Strachan FM, Shaw J, Bevan JS. An audit of the diagnostic usefulness of PRL and TSH responses to domperidone and high resolution magnetic resonance imaging of the pituitary in the evaluation of hyperprolactinaemia. *Clin Endocrinol*, 1997; **46**: 321–6.
11. Webster J, Page MD, Bevan JS, Richards SH, Douglas-John AG, Scanlon MF. Low recurrence rate after partial hypophysectomy for prolactinoma; the predictive value of dynamic prolactin function tests. *Clin Endocrinol*, 1992; **36**: 35–44.
12. Bevan JS, Burke CW, Esiri MM, Adams CBT. Misinterpretation of prolactin levels leading to management errors in patients with sellar enlargement. *Am J Med*, 1987; **82**: 29–32.
13. Karavitaki N, Thanabalasingham G, Shore HC, Trifanescu R, Ansorge O, Meston N, *et al.* Do the limits of serum prolactin in disconnection hyperprolactinaemia need re-definition? A study of 226 patients with histologically verified non-functioning pituitary macroadenoma. *Clin Endocrinol*, 2006; **65**: 524–9.

14. Webster J, Piscitelli G, Polli A, Ferrari CI, Ismail I, Scanlon MF. A comparison of cabergoline and bromocriptine in the treatment of hyperprolactinemic amenorrhea. *N Engl J Med*, 1994; **331**: 904–9.
15. Abraham P and Bevan JS. Prolactinoma. In: Powell MP, Lightman SL, Laws ER. eds. *Management of Pituitary Tumors: The Clinician's Practical Guide*. Totowa, New Jersey, Humana Press, 2003:21–41.
16. Sherlock M, Steeds R, Toogood AA. Dopamine agonist therapy and cardiac valve dysfunction. *Clin Endocrinol*, 2007; **67**: 643–4.
17. Herring N, Szmigielski C, Becher H, Karavitaki N, Wass JA. Valvular heart disease and the use of cabergoline for the treatment of prolactinoma. *Clin Endocrinol*, 2009; **70**: 104–8.
18. British National Formulary. *Bromocriptine and Other Dopaminergic Drugs*, 2009:421–3. Available at www.bnf.org (accessed).
19. Gillam MP, Molitch ME, Lombardi G, Colao A. Advances in the treatment of prolactinomas. *Endocr Rev*, 2006; **27**: 485–534. ***Comprehensive and up-to-date prolactinoma review with 626 references.***
20. Casanueva FF, Molitch ME, Schlechte JA, Abs R, Bonert V, Bronstein MD, *et al.* Guidelines of the Pituitary Society in the diagnosis and management of prolactinomas. *Clin Endocrinol*, 2006; **65**: 265–73.
21. Snyder PJ. *Treatment of hyperprolactinaemia due to lactotroph adenoma and other causes.* Available at: www.uptodate.com (accessed) (most recent update—May 2010).
22. Biswas M, Smith J, Jadon D, McEwan P, Rees DA, Evans LM, *et al.* Long-term remission following withdrawal of dopamine agonist therapy in subjects with microprolactinomas. *Clin Endocrinol*, 2005; **63**: 26–31.
23. Colao A, Di Sarno A, Guerra E, Pivonello R, Cappabianca P, Caranci F, *et al.* Predictors of remission of hyperprolactinaemia after long-term withdrawal of cabergoline therapy. *Clin Endocrinol*, 2007; **67**: 426–33.
24. Jeffcoate WJ, Pound N, Sturrock NDC, Lambourne J. Long-term follow-up of patients with hyperprolactinaemia. *Clin Endocrinol*, 1997; **45**: 299–303.
25. Bevan JS, Webster J, Burke CW, Scanlon MF. Dopamine agonists and pituitary tumor shrinkage. *Endocr Rev*, 1992; **13**: 220–40. ***Comprehensive meta-analysis of the responses of 271 well-characterized macroprolactinomas to dopamine agonist therapy with 219 references.***
26. Bevan JS, Adams CB, Burke CW, Morton KE, Molyneux AJ, Moore RA, *et al.* Factors in the outcome of transsphenoidal surgery for prolactinoma and non-functioning pituitary tumour, including pre-operative bromocriptine therapy. *Clin Endocrinol*, 1987; **26**: 541–56.
27. Popovic V, Simic M, Ilic L, Micic D, Damjanovic S, Djurovic M, *et al.* Growth hormone secretion elicited by GHRH, GHRP-6 or GHRH plus GHRP-6 in patients with microprolactinoma and macroprolactinoma before and after bromocriptine therapy. *Clin Endocrinol*, 1998; **48**: 103–8.
28. Molitch ME. Pharmacologic resistance in prolactinoma patients. *Pituitary*, 2005; **8**: 43–52.
29. Ono M, Miki N, Kawamata T, Makino R, Amano K, Seki T, *et al.* Prospective study of high-dose cabergoline treatment of prolactinomas in 150 patients. *JCEM*, 2008; **93**: 4721–7.
30. Molitch ME. The cabergoline-resistant prolactinoma patient: new challenges. *JCEM*, 2008; **93**: 4643–5.
31. Delgrange E, Daems T, Verhelst J, Abs R, Maiter D. Characterization of resistance to the prolactin-lowering effects of cabergoline in macroprolactinomas: a study in 122 patients. *Eur J Endocrinol*, 2009; **160**: 747–52.
32. Johnston DG, Hall K, Kendall-Taylor P, Patrick D, Watson M, Cook DB. Effect of dopamine agonist withdrawal after long-term therapy in prolactinomas. *Lancet*, 1984; **2**: 187–92.
33. Suliman SG, Gurlek A, Byrne JV, Sullivan N, Thanabalasingham G, Cudlip S, *et al.* Non-surgical cerebrospinal fluid rhinorrhoea in invasive macroprolactinoma: incidence, radiological and clinicopathological features. *J Clin Endocrinol Metab*, 2007; **92**: 3829–35.
34. Jones SE, James RA, Hall K, Kendall-Taylor P. Optic chiasmal herniation, an under-recognised complication of dopamine agonist therapy for macroprolactinoma. *Clin Endocrinol*, 2000; **53**: 529–34.
35. Balarini Lima GA, Machado Ede O, Dos Santos Silva CM, Filho PN, Gadelha MR. Pituitary apoplexy during treatment of cystic prolactinomas with cabergoline. *Pituitary*, 2008; **11**: 287–92.
36. Esiri MM, Bevan JS, Burke CW, Adams CBT. Effect of bromocriptine treatment on the fibrous tissue content of prolactin-secreting and non-functioning macroadenomas of the pituitary gland. *J Clin Endocrinol Metab*, 1986; **63**: 383–8.
37. Colao A, Abs R, Bárcena DG, Chanson P, Paulus W, Kleinberg DL. Pregnancy outcomes following cabergoline treatment: extended results from a 12-year observational study. *Clin Endocrinol*, 2008; **68**: 66–71.
38. Webster J. A comparative review of the tolerability profiles of dopamine agonists in the treatment of hyperprolactinaemia and inhibition of lactation. *Drug Safety*, 1996; **14**: 228–38.

2.3.11 Acromegaly

John A.H. Wass, Peter J. Trainer, Márta Korbonits

Definition

Acromegaly is the condition most often associated with an anterior pituitary tumour, which results from growth hormone and insulin-like growth factor 1 (IGF-1) excess. It causes most characteristically enlargement of the hands and feet (Greek: *akron*, extremities; *megas*, great). Gigantism, which is the juvenile counterpart of acromegaly, is also caused by a pituitary tumour secreting growth hormone, but it causes excessive growth before epiphyseal fusion. It occurs less frequently than acromegaly because pituitary tumours in children are much less common than in adults.

History

Goliath was the first giant to be recorded (290 cm/9 ft 6½ inches). The pharaoh Akhenaten—the iconoclast who moved the capital of Egypt and originated monotheism in favour of the sun—is often suggested to have acromegaloid features, but probably did not have acromegaly. It is more likely that his acromegalic appearances were a family trait and anyway he was fertile. The Irish giant James Byrne, whose skeleton is exhibited in the Royal College of Surgeons of England, was 234 cm. Cushing correctly suggested that he would have an enlarged pituitary fossa. The tallest man recorded was Robert Wadlow, an American who died in 1940 at the age of 22 years (272 cm). Comprehensive historical and illustrated descriptions of acromegaly and gigantism are available (1–3).

Acromegaly was first described in 1886 by Marie (Fig. 2.3.11.1) a pupil of Charcot. Although there had been previous cases described, it was Marie who gave the name to the condition. He did not at the time realize that the pituitary was the cause of the problem and the first recognition of an enlarged pituitary is attributed to Minkowski (1887). The first attempt at surgical treatment was by Caton and Paul in Liverpool (1893). They attempted to

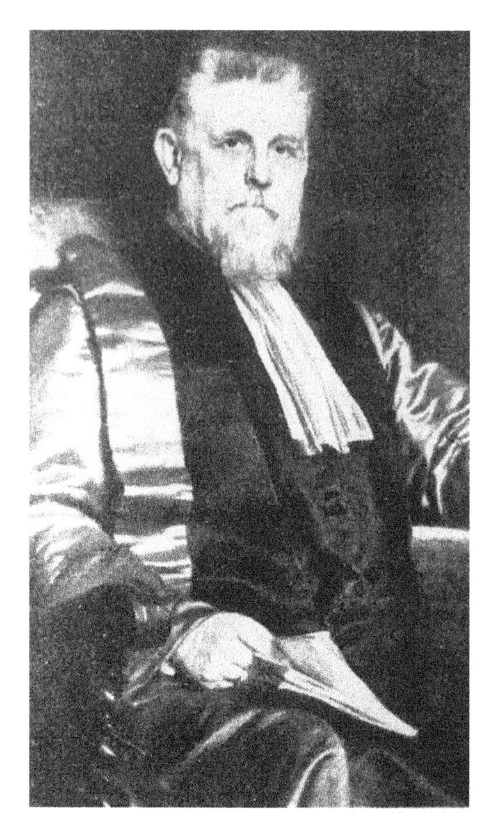

Fig. 2.3.11.1 Pierre Marie, the describer of acromegaly.

relieve the headache simply by surgical removal of part of the skull vault. Harvey Cushing was convinced that acromegaly was a form of hyperpituitarism and he operated for the first time, via the trans-sphenoidal route, to improve the condition. Radiation therapy was reported first in 1909 by Béclère. The development of radioimmunoassays for growth hormone in the 1960s provided the tools for the more accurate assessment of the disease. Medical therapy with dopamine agonists was introduced by Liuzzi and colleagues in Milan in 1972. In 1986, the first somatostatin analogues were described as providing more effective lowering of growth hormone levels in acromegaly. In 2000 a growth hormone receptor antagonist was shown to be very effective (4).

Epidemiology

Several epidemiological studies have been published (5). The mean incidence per million is 3.3 per year with a mean prevalence ranging from 38 to 69 cases per million. More recently, a higher prevalence of about 130 per million has been suggested by a study with more active surveillance for pituitary adenomas (6). Acromegaly occurs in all races with an approximately equal sex incidence. Peak age at diagnosis is 44 but patients with acromegaly can present at all ages. The mean time to diagnosis is 8 years with a range of 6–10 years. Larger, more aggressively behaving tumours secreting growth hormone tend to be present in younger patients. Patients with family history with pituitary adenomas present at an earlier age (7, 8).

Aetiology

Acromegaly is most frequently caused by a pure growth hormone-secreting adenoma. A third of patients with pituitary tumours have mixed growth hormone- and prolactin-secreting adenomas. Very rarely growth hormone and thyroid-stimulating hormone (TSH) are secreted together, causing acromegaly with thyrotoxicosis and a detectable TSH (Box 2.3.11.1).

Less than 1 % of patients with acromegaly have a growth hormone-releasing hormone (GHRH) secreting tumour. This is usually a carcinoid tumour either in the pancreas or in the lung. These are associated with pituitary somatotroph hyperplasia which histologically often gives the clue to the presence of the GHRH-secreting lesion, which may also present on its own accord. In such cases, the pituitary is globally enlarged, with no focal tumour detected. Very rarely hypothalamic GHRH-producing tumours have been described, such as, gangliocytoma. Carcinoma of pituitary secreting growth hormone has been described but is very rare (see below).

Acromegaly can occur as part of a genetic condition due to (1) Carney complex, (2) familial isolated pituitary adenoma (FIPA) (3) multiple endocrine neoplasia type 1 (MEN 1) or (3) McCune–Albright syndrome (see below). Acromegaloidism (insulin-mediated pseudo-acromegaly) refers to the development of acromegaly-like features (e.g. jaw, hand, and feet enlargement) together with acanthosis nigricans caused by very severe insulin resistance. Growth hormone and IGF-1 values are normal (9). Rarely pachydermoperiostosis (OMIM 1671002) or a familial condition with variable acromegaloid features and abnormalities of chromosome 11 (10) can present as differential diagnostic problems.

Pathology

Somatotroph cells are usually located in the posterolateral region of the pituitary often explaining the cavernous sinus invasion of these adenomas. In normal somatotroph cells the growth hormone-containing vesicles are 400 nm in mean diameter. Somatotroph adenomas can either be sparsely or densely granulated. The sparsely granulated somatotroph adenomas occur more often in young patients, tend to be more aggressive with cells showing less differentiation and have a greater tendency to tumour invasiveness.

Box 2.3.11.1 Lesions associated with excessive secretion of growth hormone and insulin-like growth factor 1

Pituitary
- Adenoma
  - Growth hormone-secreting adenoma
  - Growth hormone and prolactin mixed adenoma
  - Growth hormone and TSH secreting adenoma
- Carcinoma
  - Growth hormone-secreting carcinoma

Ectopic
- GHRH producing carcinoid such as in pancreas and lung

Hypothalamic
- GHRH producing tumours such as in gangliocytoma

GHRH: growth hormone-releasing hormone.

Approximately one-third of patients with acromegaly present with hyperprolactinaemia due to increased prolactin secretion from a tumour or alternatively loss of dopamine inhibition from stalk compression because of a macroadenoma. Prolactin secretion from the tumour can be due to mixed somatotroph and lactotroph adenomas, with discrete populations of growth hormone or prolactin-secreting cells or due to mammosomatotroph tumours, which are composed of cells that produce both growth hormone and prolactin. Mixed somatotroph and thyrotroph adenomas are associated rarely with acromegaly and thyrotoxicosis.

Pituitary carcinoma

There have been at least 10 reported instances of metastasizing pituitary carcinomas secreting growth hormone. Most often the metastases are found in the cerebrospinal axis but they have been described outside the central nervous system. The incidence probably lies between 0.1 and 0.5% of clinically diagnosed anterior pituitary adenomas (11).

Molecular endocrinology of growth hormone-secreting pituitary adenomas

The molecular pathogenesis of sporadic growth hormone secreting pituitary tumours is best considered by discussing changes which activate factors leading to increased tumour formation, e.g. oncogenes, or alterations which inactivate cell proliferation controlling genes, e.g. tumour suppressor genes. Amongst the described activating genetic alterations are stimulatory guanine nucleotide-binding protein (G-protein) α-subunit gene (*GNAS*), cyclin D (*CCDN1*), fibroblast growth factor receptor 4 (*FGFR4*), and pituitary tumour transforming gene (*PTTG*).

The G-protein is involved in the activation of adenylate cyclase which mediates the regulatory actions of GHRH to stimulate growth hormone synthesis and secretion. Missense mutations of *GNAS* at codons 201 and 227 (termed 'gsp' mutations) most commonly result in inhibition of the intrinsic GTPase activity of the α-subunit of the G protein adenyl cyclase which is persistently activated resulting in high intracellular levels of cyclic AMP and its downstream pathway including increased protein kinase A and cyclic AMP-response element binding protein (CREB) activity (12). This results in autonomous growth hormone secretion (Fig. 2.3.11.2). This somatic mutation has been demonstrated in 40% of human growth hormone secreting pituitary adenomas and is the most commonly described the genetic defect. If the *GSP* mutation occurs in embryonic stage and is found in a mosaic form in various organs contributing to activation of various G_s-coupled receptors, the patient develops McCune–Albright syndrome (see below). Increased PTTG mRNA expression has been demonstrated in somatotroph adenomas and correlates with tumour size. FGFR4 and cyclin D overexpression have been described in pituitary tumours; however, this is not specific for somatotroph adenomas.

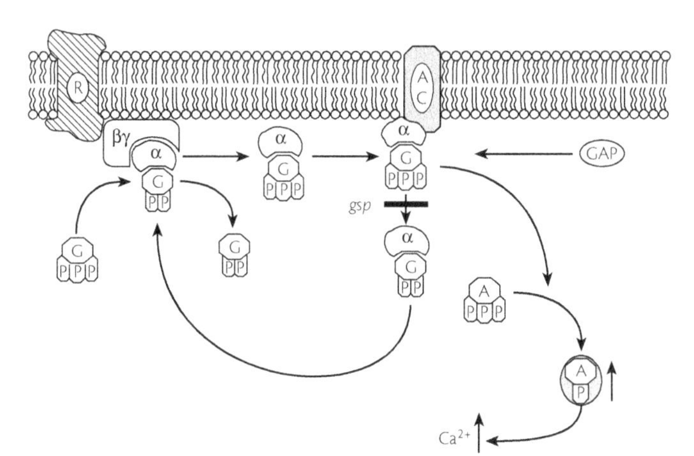

Fig. 2.3.11.2 The G-protein abnormality seen in the pituitary of 40% of Caucasian patients with acromegaly.

Tumour suppressor genes that may be involved in pituitary tumour pathogenesis include the retinoblastoma (*Rb*) gene, cyclin-dependant kinase inhibitors such as p27 (*CDKN1B*) and p16 (*CDKN2A*) as well as growth arrest and DNA damage-inducible protein (*GADD45γ*) and maternal imprinting gene 3 (*MEG3*). Some of these proteins are lost in pituitary tumours due to epigenetic mechanism such as hypermethylation. p27 expression is reduced in all types of pituitary adenomas including somatotrophs. GADD45γ is a proapoptotic factor which is lost in growth hormone-secreting adenomas. MEG3 is an imprinted gene encoding a noncoding RNA that suppresses tumour cell growth; it is lost in nonfunctioning pituitary adenomas but not in somatotroph tumours. Aryl hydrocarbon receptor-interacting protein (AIP) germline mutations have been described in families with isolated pituitary adenomas and *in vitro* studies confirm that loss of function of this protein is in the pathogenesis of these adenomas. Occasionally seemingly sporadic cases are also positive for AIP mutation but the change is detectable in germline DNA and in one of the parents as well (8, 13).

Theoretically it is possible that there is a role of hypothalamic factors and GHRH in the autocrine or paracrine role in growth hormone-secreting tumour pathogenesis, and this has been shown in a mouse model of GHRH overexpression. However, this has not been shown in humans.

Genetic alterations associated with acromegaly

McCune–Albright syndrome

This is characterized by polyostotic fibrous dysplasia, hyperpigmented cutaneous patches, and endocrinological abnormalities including precocious puberty, thyrotoxicosis, gigantism, and Cushing's syndrome. The genetic defect is a somatic mosaicism for the *gsp* mutation which results in autonomous activation of adenylate cyclase generally causing growth hormone hypersecretion and somatotroph hyperplasia. Growth hormone excess is observed up to 20% of the patients and somatotorph and lactotroph hyperplasia have been described but detectable pituitary adenomas are identified in only few patients (14).

Carney complex

This is an autosomal dominant condition caused by a mutation in the protein kinase A regulatory subunit gene (*PRKAR1a* on 17q22-24) in 60% of the cases with the other 40% mapped to 2p16. It is characterized by spotty cutaneous pigmentation, cardiac and other myxomas, and endocrine overactivity, particularly Cushing's syndrome due to nodular adrenal cortical hyperplasia. Similar to McCune–Albright syndrome, abnormal growth hormone dynamics can be detected in a high proportion of cases and somatotroph hyperplasia has been documented but patients only rarely develop true adenomas (14).

Familial isolated pituitary adenomas

This is an autosomal dominant disorder with incomplete penetrance characterised by familial occurrence of pituitary adenomas but no other endocrine abnormality, therefore clearly distinguished from MEN 1 and Carney complex. Most often family members have acromegaly but mixed acromegaly-prolactinoma families and more rarely nonfunctioning adenoma families have also been found. In 30–50% of the cases a mutation can be identified in the AIP gene (15), while in the rest of the families mutations in probably other gene(s) cause the disease. Patients with AIP mutations usually have early-onset disease, the penetrance is 30%, and the responsiveness to somatostatin analogues is poor. In families without AIP mutations the age of onset is higher and the penetrance is lower, with a more mixed picture of the type of adenomas presenting in the family members (6).

Multiple endocrine neoplasia type 1

This is an autosomal dominant disorder which is described elsewhere (see Part 4). Acromegaly is not the commonest of the pituitary hypersecretory syndromes to occur in MEN 1.

Symptoms of acromegaly

Gross acromegaly is easily recognized. The diagnosis in younger patients is more of a test of clinical acumen. Growth hormone and IGF-1 enlarge everything except the nervous system. The most noticeable feature is usually a change in facial appearance. Vague symptoms such as fatigue may predominate. Increased sweating and sebaceous activity can be noticed in the face. There is enlargement of the supraorbital ridges, prognathism, and macroglossia (see Fig. 2.3.11.4); interdental separation occurs. This together with the obvious changes in the hands and feet often makes the diagnosis easy (see Box 2.3.11.2). Often headache is a typical symptom, more commonly than other types of pituitary adenoma. Patients are commonly recognized by rheumatologists, orthopaedic surgeons (joint pain and abnormalities), dentists (separation of the teeth), neurologists (carpal tunnel syndrome), or by physicians treating the patient's sleep apnoea, hypertension, or diabetes. Often the symptoms are present and progress insidiously over several years. It can be useful to review serial old photographs to show the presence and progress of subtle facial appearances.

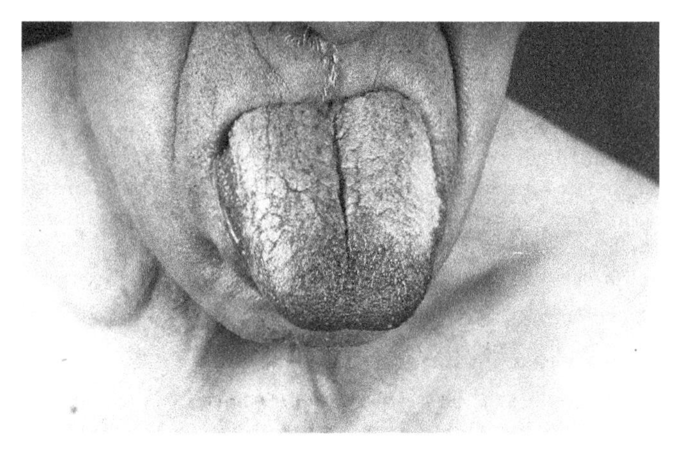

Fig. 2.3.11.4 Macroglossia in a patient with acromegaly. The patient had to have surgical tongue reduction.

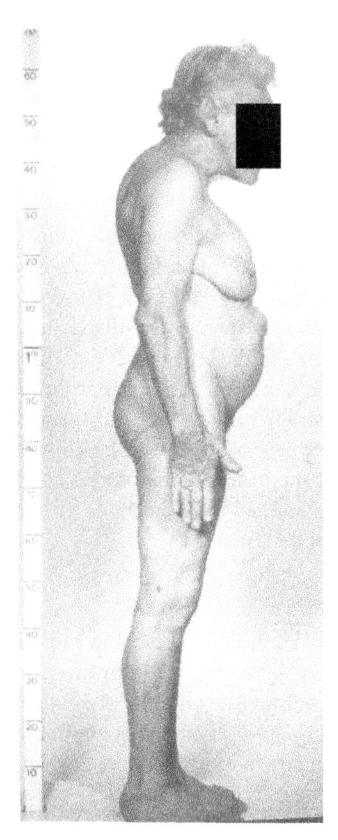

Fig. 2.3.11.3 Kyphosis in a patient with acromegaly.

Symptoms of an enlarged pituitary fossa are the same as with nonfunctioning tumours and are discussed on page 209. They include visual filed defects, headache, and pituitary apoplexy (more often in younger patients) can be a rare presenting feature of acromegaly.

Effects of growth hormone excess

The skin on the back of the hand is thickened and this may be a very useful bedside test. Increased sweating occurs in 80% and patients look older than their years.

In the cardiovascular system, hypertension is present in 50% due to a direct effect of growth hormone on sodium absorption, and there is also increased left ventricular muscle mass. Ischaemic heart disease is also present, possibly exacerbated by insulin resistance and is a major cause of morbidity and mortality. Myocardial hypertrophy with fibrosis leading to ventricular dilatation and biventricular failure are features of an acromegalic cardiomyopathy.

Respiratory symptoms are also common and account for part of the increased mortality of the condition. Sleep apnoea may result from significant airway obstruction caused by prognathism, macroglossia, and hypertrophied nasal structures. Difficulty in tracheal intubation is often encountered in acromegalic patients undergoing anaesthesia. There may also be a central element to sleep apnoea and narcolepsy may be a presenting symptom in patients with acromegaly.

In the alimentary tract macroglossia and visceromegaly are common. A high prevalence of colonic polyps in acromegaly is reported

Box 2.3.11.2 Clinical features of acromegaly

Acral enlargement
- Increased hand-, shoe- and ring size
- Prominent nasolabial fold
- Frontal bossing
- Prominent supra orbital ridge

Skin
- Increased sweating
- Oiliness and increased sebaceous activity
- Thickened skin
- Skin tags

Cardiovascular
- Hypertension
- Congestive heart failure
- Ventricular hypertrophy
- Cardiomyopathy

Respiratory
- Sleep apnoea

Musculoskeletal
- Arthropathy, knee, hip, lumbar spine
- Kyphosis (Fig. 2.3.11.3)
- Prognathism
- Dental malocclusion
- Muscle weakness

Alimentary
- Macroglossia (Fig. 2.3.11.4)
- Visceromegaly
- Colonic polyps

Neurological
- Headache
- Carpal tunnel syndrome (Fig. 2.3.11.5)

Reproductive
- Amenorrhoea
- Impotence
- Prostatic hypertrophy

Metabolic alterations
- Increased insulin resistance, diabetes mellitus
- Hypercalciuria
- Hypercalcaemia (due to MEN 1)

Endocrine system
- Cosecretion of prolactin or thyroid-stimulating hormone
- Galactorrhoea

Box 2.3.11.2 *(Continued)* Clinical features of acromegaly

- Hypopituitarism
- Multinodular goitre

Psychological effects
- Anxiety due to distorted body image

Local tumour effects
- Headache
- Visual field defects (bitemporal hemianopsia)
- Cranial nerve palsy

and these may progress to colonic neoplasia. Hence vigilance is important and full-length colonoscopy recommended on presentation or at aged 50. With careful preparation and appropriate equipment the technical difficulties due to the enlarged bowel can be overcome. Growth hormone and/or IGF-1 may possess direct mitogenic effects on colonic epithelial cells. The latter is expressed in colonic carcinomas where IGF-1 receptors are present.

The musculoskeletal changes predominantly involve the weight-bearing joints. Proliferation of chondrocytes occurs in response to increased growth hormone and IGF-1 levels. The osteoarthritis that subsequently develops can be extremely debilitating and this is one complication of acromegaly that is difficult to reverse.

Metabolic consequences of elevated growth hormone levels

Increased insulin resistance occurs because of direct anti-insulin effects of growth hormone. Acromegalic patients may develop type II diabetes mellitus and carbohydrate tolerance is considerably improved with successful therapy after lowering of growth hormone. Frank diabetes mellitus occurs in about a third of patients. Hypercalciuria occurs in 80% of patients because of growth hormone being facultative in the synthesis of 1,25-dihydroxyvitamin D. Hyperphosphataemia may occur due to the direct effect of GH/IGF-1 on renal phosphate reabsorption. If hypercalcaemia is detected hyperparathyroidism and MEN 1 (3%) need to be investigated. Multinodular goitre occurs with increased frequency in acromegaly.

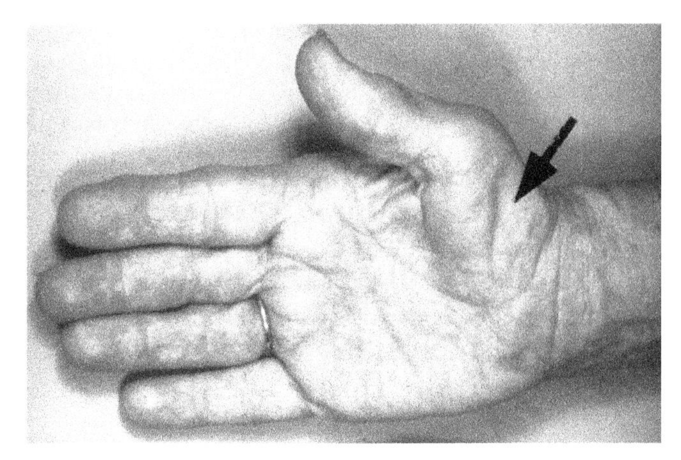

Fig. 2.3.11.5 Carpal tunnel syndrome in acromegaly. Thenar wasting is clearly seen (arrow).

IGF-1 is a major determinant of thyroid cell growth. Thyroid dysfunction (hyperthyroidism) occurs in acromegaly and is most commonly due to a multinodular goitre but TSH secretion from a mixed pituitary tumour should be considered if the TSH is inappropriately normal/elevated in association with thyrotoxicosis.

Acromegaly is associated with a decreased life expectancy. This was first shown in the 1950s and later it was confirmed that that these patients have an increased cardiovascular and respiratory mortality (16). More recently the possibility of increased mortality due to malignant disease has been raised. Overall mortality of untreated disease is approximately double normal. As the tumours tend to be larger and have a greater frequency for being extrasellar in younger patients, particularly those with extrasellar tumours are more difficult to treat successfully. This applies to all modalities of treatment, including surgery, medical treatments, and radiotherapy.

Cardiovascular and respiratory risk

This increased risk relates to hypertension and diabetes. There is no characteristic lipid disturbance in acromegaly. Before 1966, 50% of acromegalic patients died before the age of 50, cardiovascular disease being the commonest cause of death. Cardiovascular disorders accounted for about 25% of deaths, followed by respiratory (20%) and cerebrovascular disease (15%). More recent data suggest a twofold risk of cardiovascular disease and no increased respiratory mortality (17).

Mortality from malignancy

Most previous series show an increased risk of malignant disease (Table 2.3.11.1), but it is interesting that the largest cohort did not show this, although it did show an increased risk of colonic cancer (relative risk 1.68) (18).

Diagnosis of acromegaly

The diagnosis of acromegaly is made with observing an elevated IGF-1 level as matched for age and gender, and failure to suppress growth hormone in response to an oral glucose tolerance test (OGTT) usually to a level of less than 1 μg/l (19). But for early detection of the disease when using sensitive growth hormone assays the threshold should be lowered to 0.4 μg/l (20). In patients with acromegaly there may even be a paradoxical rise in growth hormone in response to OGTT. False positives do occur (Box 2.3.11.3) but few conditions apart from adolescence are likely to cause diagnostic confusion. However, in tall adolescents, possibly associated with large growth hormone pulses, growth hormone levels may not become undetectable during an OGTT, thus raising the possibility of acromegaly. In these patients IGF-1 is not elevated.

Box 2.3.11.3 Conditions associated with a failure of suppression after a glucose load

- Adolescence
- Diabetes mellitus
- Liver failure
- Renal failure
- Malnutrition
- Laron dwarfism
- Anorexia nervosa

Table 2.3.11.1 Acromegaly and malignancy

Author	Date	No. of patients	Incidence of malignancy (Observed versus expected)
Alexander *et al.*	1980	164	6 versus 1.3 ($p<0.01$)
Nabarro *et al.*	1987	256	11 versus 11.5
Bengtsson *et al.*	1988	166	15 versus 5.5 ($p<0.05$)
Brazilay *et al.*	1991	87	17 versus 7.8 ($p<0.05$)
Orme *et al.*	1998	1362	79 versus 104.12

Growth hormone levels even if elevated, are not individually adequate to diagnose acromegaly. Multiple samples during the day, however, always show detectable levels of growth hormone, whereas in normals 75% of the samples during the day are undetectable. The IGF-1 level is invariably high in acromegaly. Occasionally patients who are very ill with acromegaly and in whom IGF-1 is measured, may not demonstrate an elevation, but this becomes apparent later when they recover from the intercurrent illness.

Insulin-like growth factor binding protein 3 is not so growth hormone dependent as IGF-1 and does not give the same clear differences between acromegaly and normality (Fig. 2.3.11.6). In 80% of the patients with acromegaly there is a paradoxical release of growth hormone (by 50% over basal, or an increment of at least 3 μg/l) after thyrotrophin-releasing hormone (TRH) and less frequently after gonadotropin-releasing hormone (GnRH). This and the paradoxical fall in growth hormone seen in acromegaly in response to dopamine and dopamine agonists are rarely required to confirm the diagnosis of acromegaly.

The suspicion of acromegaly can be based on typical acromegalic features (35%) but often on associated abnormalities such as amenorrhoea, visual field defect, carpal tunnel syndrome, joint problems, or headache. About 50% of patients are diagnosed when seeking medical advice for an unrelated complain.

Investigations

Growth hormone levels tend to be higher in younger patients presenting with larger tumours (Box 2.3.11.4). In those who present after the age of 50, the tumour is often smaller and intrasellar. There is a

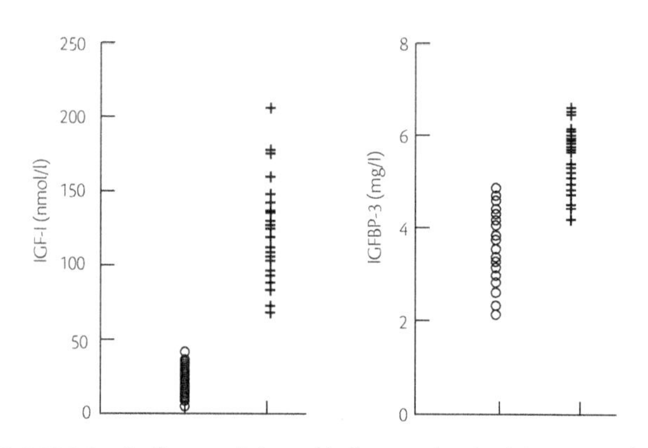

Fig. 2.3.11.6 Insulin-like growth factor binding protein 3 levels in acromegaly do not differentiate patients with acromegaly from normal.

Box 2.3.11.4 Investigation of acromegaly

Establish diagnosis
- 75 g OGTT
- IGF-1

Establish growth hormone levels
- Mean of several growth hormones (day curve)

Metabolic consequences of high growth hormone
- OGTT (for glucose)
- HbA1c
- 24-h urine calcium

Pituitary function
- LH/FSH, testosterone/oestradiol
- fT4, TSH
- Cortisol
- ITT for cortisol (not growth hormone)

Pituitary anatomy
- MRI
- Visual fields

Other (coexistent) diagnoses
- Serum calcium (multiple endocrine neoplasia)
- Urine catecholamines (phaeochromocytoma)
- Sleep apnoea

fT4, free thyroxine; ITT, insulin-tolerance test; LH/FSH, luteinizing hormone/follicle-stimulating hormone; OGTT, oral glucose tolerance test; TSH, thyroid-stimulating hormone.

relationship between serum IGF levels and the log of the serum growth hormone. Saturation of IGF-1 occurs above a growth hormone level of 20 μg/l whereafter, little further rise in IGF-1 occurs. Plasma GHRH should be measured if an ectopic source of acromegaly is suspected, or if occasionally, pituitary histology reveals hyperplasia.

Tumour size

About 40% of patients present with microadenomas, the rest are macroadenomas that may extend outside the fossa.

Other associations

Essential hypertension is common in acromegaly, often associated with an increase in intravascular volume and low renin and increased aldosterone secretion. Phaeochromocytoma is not associated with acromegaly; however, it is important to exclude a phaeochromocytoma in a hypertensive patient with acromegaly, particularly prior to surgery.

Treatment of acromegaly

Ideal treatment

The ideal treatment will render growth hormone secretion normal, completely ablate the pituitary tumour mass, whilst preserving normal pituitary function resulting in complete reversal of acral and other systematic complications of growth hormone excess. There should be no biochemical or tumour recurrence. No currently available treatment effectively fulfils all these criteria.

Modes of treatment

Primary treatment is usually surgical. Most often this is accomplished through the transsphenoidal route. If this fails, medical treatments to reduce growth hormone and IGF levels to normal should be initiated (50–60% overall) (Box 2.3.11.5). Usually this is first attempted using an analogue of somatostatin (octreotide or lanreotide). If unsuccessful, cabergoline the best tolerated dopamine agonist is added up to a weekly dose of 3 mg, although one should be aware of possible cardiac valve effects of long-term high-dose cabergoline treatment. Then pegvisomant should be added if possible. At this stage radiotherapy is considered.

Treatment goals

Abundant epidemiological evidence suggests that a growth hormone level of 1 μg/l or less is associated with a normal life expectancy (21). The most important determinant of outcome is the most recent growth hormone or IGF-1 level. Normalization of IGF-1 is associated with no difference in survival from a control sample. Other factors which have been associated with increased mortality include duration of symptoms prior to diagnosis, duration of disease, older age at diagnosis, and the presence of cardiovascular disease, diabetes, and hypertension at diagnosis.

After surgery, growth hormone pulses are often not normal. Growth hormone deficiency may occur and in most patients growth hormone secretion is not normal. After radiotherapy too, growth hormone pulses become absent and there is often a constant low-grade level of elevated growth hormone secretion resulting in higher IGF-1 than one would expect from the ambient growth hormone. These facts have led to the concept of a safe growth hormone level (mean of less than 1.7 μg/l) rather than talking specifically about a cure which in terms of normalization of growth hormone secretory dynamics virtually never occurs.

Transsphenoidal surgery

Growth hormone results

Table 2.3.11.2 shows the effects on growth hormone levels of surgery in various surgical centres throughout the world. It is evident

Box 2.3.11.5 Modes of treatment of acromegaly

Surgery
- Transsphenoidal
- Transfrontal

Drugs
- Somatostatin analogues
- Dopamine agonists
- Growth hormone receptor antagonists

Radiotherapy
- Three-field, multi-fractional
- Stereotactic, e.g. gamma knife and SMART

Table 2.3.11.2 Effect of surgery on growth hormone levels

Study	Microadenoma cure rate (%)	Macroadenoma cure rate (%)	Criteria
Manchester UK1974–98	38.8	11.8	OGTT GH<1.7 μg/l
Newcastle UK 1980–91	64	48	OGTT GH<0.7 μg/l
Oxford UK 1974–95	91	45	OGTT GH<0.7 μg/l or mean GH<1.7 μg/l
Massachusetts USA 1978–96	91	48	OGTT GH<1.7 μg/l or random GH <1.7 μg/l or normal IGF-1
Charlottesville USA 1972–93	65	55	OGTT GH<2 μg/l
Erlangen-Nurnberg, Germany 1972–93	72	50	OGTT GH<1.4 μg/l
Tindall *et al.* 1993	N/A	N/A	GH<5 μg/l and/or normal IGF-1 level
Davis *et al.* 1993	N/A	N/A	GH£2 μg/l (basal or OGTT)
Sheaves *et al.* 1996	61	23	GH≤ 2.5 μg/l
Abosch *et al.* 1998	75	71	GH<5 μg/l
Freda *et al.* 1998	88	53	GH<2 μg/l (OGTT) or normal IGF-1 level
Laws *et al.* 2000	87	50.5	GH≤2.5 μg/l, GH≤1 μg/l (OGTT), normal IGF-1 level
Kreutzer *et al.* 2001	N\A	N\A	GH≤2.5 μg/l, GH≤1 μg/l (OGTT), normal IGF-1 level
De *et al.* 2003	72	50	GH≤2.5 μg/l, GH≤1 μg/l (OGTT), normal IGF-1 level
Mortini *et al.* 2005	83	53	GH<1 μg/l (OGTT), normal IGF-1 level
Nomikos *et al.* 2005	78	50	Basal GH £2.5 μg/l, GH≤1 μg/l (OGTT), normal IGF-1 level

from these figures that the outcome for microadenomas is better than that for macroadenomas. In addition, the criteria used to judge success differ widely. A mean of several growth hormone levels of 1.7 μg/l or less are equivalent to a nadir achieved during oral glucose tolerance of levels less than 0.5 μg/l (22). Given these figures, it is clear that there is quite a wide disparity in outcomes, but the best available figures in the best surgical hands show that between 70% and 90% with microadenomas and between 45% and 50% of macroadenomas should have levels of growth hormone rendered into the safe range with surgery (23).

Complications

The most common complication is hypopituitarism. This can involve anterior or posterior pituitary function and complication rates appear to be higher with bigger tumours. New hypopituitarism develops in between 12% and 18% of patients undergoing transsphenoidal surgery for acromegaly. These patients may require lifelong pituitary hormone replacement therapy. Occasionally pituitary function may recover (22). Other complications include transient or permanent diabetes insipidus, cerebrospinal fluid leaks, haemorrhage, and meningitis. Recurrence of acromegaly occasionally occurs (5.5% at 3 years).

Factors affecting outcome

Pretreatment growth hormone levels in a large number of series have been shown to affect outcome such that high levels are associated with a less successful surgical outcome. In a series by Sheaves *et al.* (24) postoperative growth hormone levels fell below 1.7 μg/l in 65% of patients in whom pretreatment growth hormone levels were less than 6 μg/l, and in only 18% of those in whom pretreatment levels were greater than 33 μg/l. Table 2.3.11.2 also shows the effect of tumour size (micro vs macroadenoma) on surgical outcome.

Surgical experience has been shown to have a significant impact on the outcome of surgery. With large numbers of surgeons doing a small number of operations annually, the outcome is less good and in several centres the outcome has been improved considerably following the policy of adopting one or two surgeons to do all pituitary surgery. Complications are also less common with experienced surgeons(23, 25).

Transcranial surgery

Transcranial surgery is occasionally necessary when there is a very large suprasellar extension or a tumour extending out laterally which is unreachable transsphenoidally, although the use of endoscopic surgery increases the reachable areas in the lateral direction. In cases where transcranial surgery is indicated the reduction of growth hormone to safe levels is virtually never obtained.

Drugs

Somatostatin analogues

Octreotide and lanreotide are synthetic octapeptide analogues of somatostatin which share some amino acid homology with it. They exhibit pharmacological effects similar to somatostatin, although with a much longer duration of action than the parent compound (Fig. 2.3.11.7). Unlike the parent compound there is no rebound hypersecretion of growth hormone and other hormone secretions following cessation of their action. There are five somatostatin receptor (SSTRs) subtypes. The main SSTR subtypes on the anterior pituitary are SSTR2 and SSTR5, and octreotide and lanreotide bind specifically with high affinity to these receptors. A newer somatostatin analogue, pasireotide (SOM230), has a wider activity on all SSTRs except SSTR3. Whether newer analogues of somatostatin, like SOM230, which stimulate other somatostatin receptors, are more effective has yet to be established.

Initially somatostatin analogues were given thrice daily, as subcutaneous injections. Longer acting somatostatin analogues have been developed which need to be administered once a month.

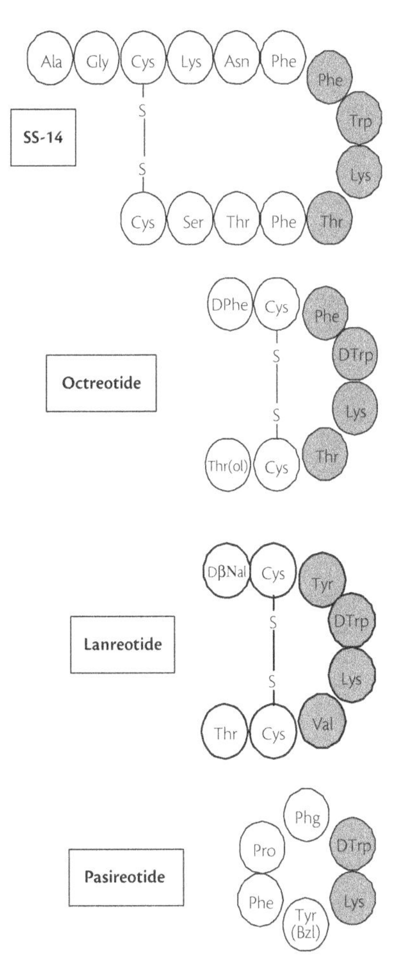

Fig. 2.3.11.7 The structures of native somatostatin (SS-14) and the somatostatin analogues

Octreotide LAR and Lanreotide Autogel are two such analogues. Lanreotide exhibits a two phase pattern with an instant release of the analogue localized at the surface of the copolymer, followed by a second period with a slower and more prolonged liberation by enzymatic breakdown of microcapsules.

Effect on growth hormone

The effect of somatostatin analogues on growth hormone production in acromegaly can be predicted by a single subcutaneous dose of octreotide which in responsive patients shows a fall to less than 1.7 μg/l.

Octreotide LAR is started with a dose of 20 mg per month. After 3 months, growth hormone levels are re-assessed and if greater than 1.7 μg/l the dose should be increased to 30 mg, and if less than 1.7 μg/l reduced to 10 mg. Between 50 and 80% of patients on this drug, attain safe growth hormone levels of 1.7 μg/l or less. Around 50% achieve a normal age-related IGF-1. In general, patients starting with high growth hormone levels are less likely to achieve safe values on octreotide or lanreotide than those starting with lower values. Comparison of octreotide LAR and Lanreotide Autogel show similar numbers of patients who attain growth hormone levels of less than 1.7 μg/l (27)Patients with sparsely granulated tumours and patients from families with familial isolated pituitary adenomas are less responsive to somatostatin analogues (8, 28, 29).

Patients on somatostatin analogue therapy can be followed by IGF-1 and by mean growth hormone levels but the response to OGTT is variable (19). For patients who were treated with radiotherapy and are currently on medical therapy 12–24-monthly temporary cessation of medical treatment is suggested for the assessment of growth hormone/IGF-1 status unless it is still high despute on going somatostatin analogues treatment.

Effect on carbohydrate tolerance and prolactin

Despite suppression of insulin, the effect on growth hormone predominates and in the majority of patients, somatostatin analogues improve carbohydrate tolerance. In contrast to the effect of dopamine agonists, somatostatin analogues usually do not have an effect on prolactin levels. Somatomammotropic tumours treated with long-acting somatostatin analogues may show a fall in prolactin levels as well as growth hormone.

Side effects

Diarrhoea and abdominal pain occur in 30% of patients to a mild or moderate degree initially but in the vast majority these usually settles (Box 2.3.11.6). The most important chronic side effect is gallstones, which complicates long-term therapy with octreotide and the somatostatin analogues. The rate varies widely between 14% and 60% and probably depends on the length of treatment. They develop because octreotide decreases gallbladder contractility by suppressing cholecystokinin (CCK) release. Bile also becomes abnormal, possibly in relation to prolonged intestinal transit and altered bacterial flora. The abrupt withdrawal of octreotide may be associated with the development of acute pancreatitis or gallstone colic. Otherwise, gall stones developing on somatostatin analogues very rarely cause symptoms (30). Antibody formation occurs but rarely and is very infrequently significant in terms of altering growth hormone levels. Dependency has been described but very rarely. The compound acts at opiate receptors. For this reason, in occasional patients with severe headache it is very effective at relieving this and often at minimum doses. In these patients headache is improved by frequent subcutaneous doses of 100 μg. However,

Box 2.3.11.6 Side effects of somatostatin analogues in the treatment of acromegaly

Local
- Stinging at the injection site (warm prior to injection)

Gastrointestinal
- Short term
  - Diarrhoea
  - Abdominal pain
- Long term
  - Gall stones
  - Gastritis

Biochemical
- Antibody formation

Endocrinological
  - Worsening carbohydrate tolerance
  - Hypoglycaemia
  - Dependency

formal studies comparing subcutaneous and long-acting analogues have not been carried out in this context.

Place of treatment

Octreotide and lanreotide are currently the best available medical treatments for acromegaly. Most frequently they are used postoperatively if operations have been unsuccessful at rendering growth hormone levels safe. There is increasing interest in the preoperative use of somatostatin analogues either as an alternative to surgery or for a limited time preoperatively with the desire to reduce morbidity and possibly, by shrinking the tumour, improve the surgical cure rate. Prospective studies of octreotide-LAR in treatment-naïve patients with micro- or macroadenomas have demonstrated normalization of growth hormone or IGF-1 levels in 40% to 70% of patients in the first year with rates improving with longer duration of therapy. A reduction in tumour size of at least 20% is seen in 75% of the patients with a significant improvement in signs and symptoms of disease. However, the overall response rates, particularly in patients with small tumours and low growth hormone levels are lower than surgery and their use would need to be prolonged and therefore expensive. They may also be used following radiotherapy, until radiotherapy has effectively reduced growth hormone and IGF-1 levels to normal.

Dopamine agonists

Pharmacology

Bromocriptine, cabergoline, and quinagolide are selective agonist at the D_2 dopamine receptors. Their administration results in the paradoxical fall of growth hormone levels in acromegalic patients, while in normals they stimulate growth hormone levels. Bromocriptine is the only dopamine agonist licensed for the treatment of acromegaly but cabergoline is the most potent and best tolerated.

Effects on growth hormone

It is not possible to predict the response to bromocriptine or cabergoline. Overall between 10% and 20% of patients have growth hormone levels that are safe on treatment with bromocriptine (usually 20–40 mg daily) or cabergoline (1–3 mg weekly).

Carbohydrate tolerance improves because of the lowering of growth hormone levels and prolactin levels are suppressed to below normal.

Side effects

Dopamine agonists may cause acute postural hypotension, nausea, and vomiting. Usually these settle with time. Very rarely, particularly on high doses, psychosis and digital vasospasm may also develop. Cardiac fibrosis has been described with the high doses of cabergoline used for Parkinson's disease and it is recommended that all patients treated with ergot-derived dopamine agonists (eg. cabergoline) have an annual echocardiogram. No effects on the heart have been found in patients with acromegaly and prolactinoma who are routinely given much lower doses.

Place of treatment

Dopamine agonists are less expansive than somatostatin analogues and are available orally. When medical treatment is indicated it should theoretically be the case that dopamine agonists are tried first. In practice, because the response rate is low this does not happen. However, it should be noted that occasionally patients who are not responsive to a somatostatin analogue respond to a dopamine agonist.

Growth hormone receptor antagonist (pegvisomant)

A novel growth hormone receptor antagonist has been developed and has undergone evaluation for the treatment of acromegaly (4). Reversible binding to the growth hormone receptor leads to inhibition of signal transduction and therefore lowering of IGF-1. This drug is a recombinant protein with structural similarity to wild-type human growth hormone, but substitutions have been made at the sites of interaction with the preformed growth hormone receptor dimer to leave the receptor inactivated and unresponsive to endogenous growth hormone. An arginine to glycine substitution at position 120 is crucial to inhibition of activation of the growth hormone–receptor complex, while pegylation of the protein increasing its half-life from 11 min to greater than 70 h reduces immunogenicity. The drug is administered subcutaneously and since it does not lower circulating growth hormone, serum IGF-1 is the principal biochemical means of monitoring effectiveness of treatment. With daily dosing and adequate dose titration a satisfactory IGF-1 level can be achieved in over 90% of patients (including those who do not respond to somatostatin analogue therapy). The drug is generally well tolerated with no overall significant change in MRI appearances of the pituitary or the development of antibodies to the drug or to growth hormone. Although there has been some concern that pituitary tumour growth can be observed, the majority of patients included in the studies have had pituitary surgery and/or radiotherapy to the exact frequency cannot be assessed but it appears rare. Liver function tests can also become abnormal, so these as well as pituitary size need monitoring on treatment. Lipohypertrophy at the site of injection has been reported. Control of acromegaly is possible in the majority of patients requiring medical treatment with pegvisomant.

Place of treatment

Pegvisomant is indicated for patients unresponsive to somatostatin analogues, and the choice is whether to add it to ongoing somatostatin analogue or substitute pegvisomant in place of the somatostatin analogue. The decision depends on individual patient circumstances, e.g. good tumour shrinkage with a somatostatin analogue would be a reason for combination treatment whilst deteriorating glucose tolerance argues for monotherapy (31).

Radiotherapy

Indications

There are two indications for radiotherapy in patients with acromegaly: to control postoperative tumour growth and to control growth hormone secretion and thereby, with time, allow withdrawal of expensive medical treatment. This is particularly the case if drug therapy cannot attain safe levels of growth hormone and IGF-1 (Box 2.3.11.7). In the absence of radiotherapy, medical treatment is possible but by implication, very expensive option.

Conventional multifractional external beam irradiation

Growth hormone results

There is little doubt that external beam radiation (Fig. 2.3.11.8) is effective in lowering growth hormone (32). Recently there has been some controversy, however, when the current criteria for safe growth hormone levels (1.7 μg/l) are applied to the results that are published. Overall growth hormone levels decline exponentially (Fig. 2.3.11.9) from the beginning of treatment. This is a slow process and at 10 years around 50% of patients have a growth

Box 2.3.11.7 Treatment paradigms in acromegaly

Surgery

- 70–90% growth hormone levels less than 1.7 μg/l (microadenoma)
- 45–50% growth hormone levels less than 1.7 μg/l (macroadenoma)

Medical – if growth hormone levels greater than 1.7 μg/l

- Somatostatin analogues – ↓ growth hormone less than 1.7 μg/l in 50–60%
- Dopamine agonist therapy – growth hormone less than 1.7 μg/l in 10–20%
- Pegvisomant – ↓ IGF-1 in >90%

Consider external beam radiotherapy

- Failed medical therapy (growth hormone greater than 1.7 μg/l)
- Residual tumour
- Large extrasellar tumour

hormone level of less than 1.7 μg/l and a normal IGF-1. IGF-1 levels may be slower to normalize than growth hormone, which reflects continuous low-grade growth hormone secretion without pulses.

Various parameters have been suggested which help predict the kind of patients who will respond to irradiation. Although pretreatment concentrations of prolactin do not reliably predict response, the major determinant is the preirradiation growth hormone level. If, in pretreatment, the growth hormone level is 3–10 μg/l it will take a mean of 4.5 years to achieve a growth hormone of 1.7 μg/l, but if the starting growth hormone is greater than 20 μg/l this level will not be achieved for 7 years or more, if ever. IGF-1 levels postradiotherapy are currently not so well studied. Recent data of the UK acromegaly database do suggest that 56% are normal at 10 years.

Radiotherapy, although it does not always control growth hormone and IGF-1 levels, does prevent further tumour growth and it is very rare to observe tumour growth after external beam irradiation in acromegaly.

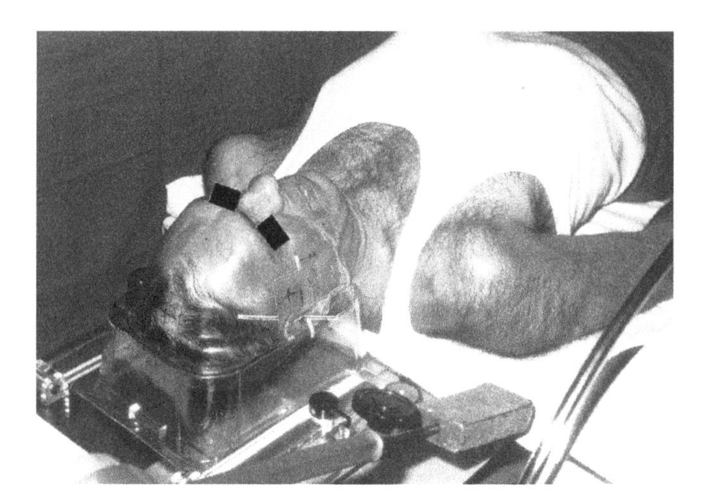

Fig. 2.3.11.8 A patient in a shell, specially made, undergoing radiotherapy for acromegaly.

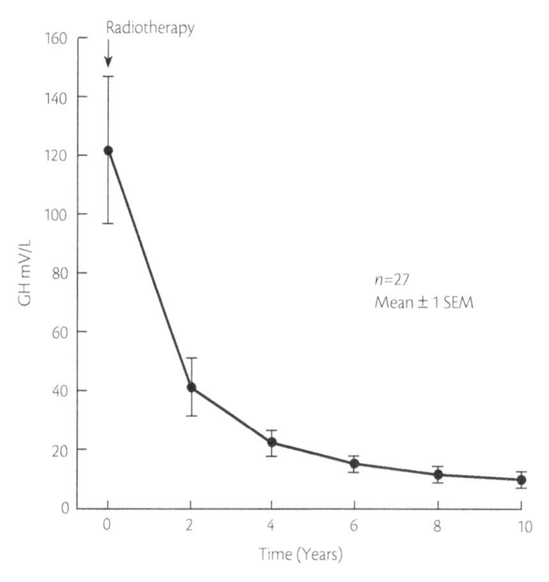

Fig. 2.3.11.9 The exponential fall in growth hormone (GH) levels after radiotherapy in patients with acromegaly studied over 10 years.

Side effects

In general external beam radiotherapy is well tolerated. Hypopituitarism is common and after exclusion of patients with preirradiation hormone deficiency; postradiotherapy, gonadal, adrenal, and thyroid deficiency occur in 50, 35, and 35%, respectively, at 10 years. Pituitary function deterioration develops gradually so that it is necessary for regular (usually annual) assessment. Visual loss and late malignancy are discussed elsewhere and there is no specific increased risk associated with acromegaly. The effect of external pituitary radiotherapy on memory and mental function requires further study.

Stereotactic radiotherapy

Gamma knife therapy and SMART (stereotactic multiple arc radiotherapy) radiotherapy are given in a single session to ablate tumours invading the cavernous sinus and are effective methods of delivering radiation therapy to growth hormone secreting tumours (33). There is a theoretical possibility that because of the steep fall-off of irradiation to surrounding tissues, radiosurgery will be less likely to cause second brain tumours and neurocognitive complications. Further studies in this area are needed. The available data suggest that pituitary hypersecretion may resolve faster with gamma knife therapy, but more longer-term data are required both on this and the effect on pituitary function, but significant numbers develop pituitary complications (34).

Treatment paradigms (35)

For macroadenoma, surgery is 'curative' in around 55%. Thus surgery renders growth hormone levels safe in this group. Surgery is usually performed for macroadenoma even if surgical cure is unlikely, because debulking surgery improves the outcome of treatment with somatostatin analogues (36). There are a significant number of patients who require further therapy in these circumstances because elevated IGF-1 and growth hormone levels are associated with an increase in mortality and morbidity. In these circumstances somatostatin analogue therapy or dopamine agonist therapy should be considered. Somatostatin analogue therapy is more likely to render growth hormone levels safe, but occasionally in non-somatostatin analogue responsive patients, dopamine agonists may be effective. The usual first lines are octreotide LAR or Lanreotide Autogel or cabergoline, respectively. It is important to consider external beam radiotherapy in patients whose medical therapy does not render growth hormone levels safe. It should also be considered in patients whose growth hormone levels postsurgery are higher than 1.7 µg/l, and in patients with large extrasellar tumours post surgery (see Box 2.3.11.7). In patients with persisting active disease, pegvisomant, either as monotherapy or in combination with a somatostatin analogue, should be considered. Microadenomas are treated similarly but many more are cured surgically.

Follow-up

Patients with acromegaly should be kept under review, either annually or once every 2 years, probably for life. If at surgery, hyperplasia of the pituitary is found and there is no tumour, a GHRH-secreting tumour, most commonly in the pancreas or in the lung needs to be sought or the possibility of McCune–Albright syndrome or Carney complex considered. This is a very uncommon surgical finding, but it is important that the necessary action is taken.

In patients whose growth hormone and IGF-1 levels are rendered safe and normal, annual review is sufficient when growth hormone and IGF-1 are measured. Recurrence is uncommon but may necessitate further surgery, medical or radiotherapy treatment. Once the level of the rest of the pituitary function is established post-surgery, this does not need to be repeatedly tested because it will not change, unless radiotherapy is given.

If surgery is not curative, further medical treatment and radiotherapy need to be considered as above. Monitoring of both growth hormone and IGF-1 levels should take place after radiotherapy, and caution should be taken as after radiotherapy IGF-1 and growth hormone assessments are often discordant (37). After radiotherapy annual assessment of pituitary function should be carried out (see Chapter 2.3.4). Colonoscopy needs to be undertaken on acromegalic patients at presentation or at age 50 but only needs to be repeated if polyps are found or symptoms develop.

The future

There is a general acceptance that the utility of IGF-1 measurement in the diagnosis and monitoring of acromegaly has been compromised by a lack of standardization, in part due to a lack of a recombinant reference material, and inadequate age-related reference ranges. The recent release of a recombinant IGF-1 reference material (WHO 02/254) and the recognition of the need for more robustly established reference ranges offers the prospect of a new generation of IGF-1 assays in which clinicians can have confidence.

In the near term there are likely to be additional pharmaceutical agents. Pasireotide is a novel somatostatin analogue that is at an advanced stage of clinical development while clinical trials have begun on a chimeric molecule directed at the dopamine and somatostatin receptors.

Increasing numbers of patients are recognized with familial acromegaly. Careful biochemical and genetic screening can identify patients at risk and at very subclinical, early stages of the disease where appropriate intervention can prevent morbidity in these usually aggressive adenoma cases.

Surgical techniques have been refined considerably. In the field of radiotherapy, we need a more detailed assessment of the effects of stereotactic radiotherapy, and from the epidemiological point of view, we need to know more about the effects of hypopituitarism on mortality in acromegaly as well as a number of other disease variables, e.g., hypertension, diabetes, and their effect on mortality. The prospect of being able to control virtually every acromegalic patient, in terms of normalization of IGF-1 levels with the new growth hormone receptor antagonists is exciting.

References

1. Sheaves R. A history of acromegaly. *Pituitary*, 1999; **2**: 7–28.
2. de Herder WW. Acromegaly and gigantism in the medical literature. Case descriptions in the era before and the early years after the initial publication of Pierre Marie (1886). *Pituitary*, 2009; **12**: 236–44.
3. de Herder WW. Endocrinology and Art. 4 movie actors with acromegaly/gigantism. *Endocrinol Invest*, 2009; **32**(9):791–2.
4. Trainer PJ, Drake WM, Katznelson L, Freda PU, Herman-Bonert V, van der Lely AJ, *et al.* Treatment of acromegaly with the growth hormone-receptor antagonist pegvisomant. *N Eng J Med*, 2000; **342**: 1171–7.
5. Holdaway IM, Rajasoorya C. Epidemiology of acromegaly. *Pituitary*, 1999; **2**: 29–41.
6. Daly AF, Rixhon M, Adam C, Dempegioti A, Tichomirowa MA, Beckers A. High prevalence of pituitary adenomas: a cross-sectional study in the province of Liege, Belgium. *J Clin Endocrinol Metab*, 2006; **91**: 4769–75.
7. Daly AF, Vanbellinghen JF, Khoo SK, Jaffrain-Rea ML, Naves LA, Guitelman MA, *et al.* Aryl hydrocarbon receptor-interacting protein gene mutations in familial isolated pituitary adenomas: analysis in 73 families. *J Clin Endocrinol Metab*, 2007; **92**: 1891–6.
8. Leontiou CA, Gueorguiev M, van der SJ, Quinton R, Lolli F, Hassan S, *et al.* The role of the aryl hydrocarbon receptor-interacting protein gene in familial and sporadic pituitary adenomas. *J Clin Endocrinol Metab*, 2008; **93**: 2390–401.
9. Yaqub A, Yaqub N. Insulin-mediated pseudoacromegaly: a case report and review of the literature. *W V Med J*, 2008; **104**: 12–15.
10. Stratakis CA, Turner ML, Lafferty A, Toro JR, Hill S, Meck JM, *et al.* A syndrome of overgrowth and acromegaloidism with normal growth hormone secretion is associated with chromosome 11 pericentric inversion. *J Med Genet*, 2001; **38**: 338–43.
11. Kaltsas GA, Nomikos P, Kontogeorgos G, Buchfelder M, Grossman AB. Clinical review: Diagnosis and management of pituitary carcinomas. *J Clin Endocrinol Metab*, 2005; **90**: 3089–99.
12. Bertherat J, Chanson P, Montminy M. The cyclic adenosine 3',5'-monophosphate-responsive factor CREB is constitutively activated in human somatotroph adenomas. *Mol Endocrinol*, 1995; **9**: 777–83.
13. Cazabat L, Libe R, Perlemoine K, Rene-Corail F, Burnichon N, Gimenez-Roqueplo AP, *et al.* Germline inactivating mutations of the aryl hydrocarbon receptor-interacting protein gene in a large cohort of sporadic acromegaly: mutations are found in a subset of young patients with macroadenomas. *Eur J Endocrinol*, 2007; **157**: 1–8.
14. Horvath A, Stratakis CA. Clinical and molecular genetics of acromegaly: MEN1, Carney complex, McCune-Albright syndrome, familial acromegaly and genetic defects in sporadic tumors. *Rev Endocr Metab Disord*, 2008; **9**: 1–11.
15. Vierimaa O, Georgitsi M, Lehtonen R, Vahteristo P, Kokko A, Raitila A, *et al.* Pituitary adenoma predisposition caused by germline mutations in the AIP gene. *Science*, 2006; **312**: 1228–30.
16. Wright AD, Hill DM, Lowy C, Fraser TR. Mortality in acromegaly. *Q J Med*, 1970; **39**: 1–16.

17. Holdaway IM, Rajasoorya RC, Gamble GD. Factors influencing mortality in acromegaly. *J Clin Endocrinol Metab*, 2004; **89**: 667–74.
18. Renehan AG, Brennan BM. Acromegaly, growth hormone and cancer risk. *Best Pract Res Clin Endocrinol Metab*, 2008; **22**: 639–57.
19. Carmichael JD, Bonert VS, Mirocha JM, Melmed S. The utility of oral glucose tolerance testing for diagnosis and assessment of treatment outcomes in 166 patients with acromegaly. *J Clin Endocrinol Metab*, 2009; **94**: 523–27.
20. Freda PU, Reyes CM, Nuruzzaman AT, Sundeen RE, Bruce JN. Basal and glucose-suppressed GH levels less than 1 microg/L in newly diagnosed acromegaly. *Pituitary*, 2003; **6**: 175–80.
21. Holdaway IM, Bolland MJ, Gamble GD. A meta-analysis of the effect of lowering serum levels of GH and IGF-I on mortality in acromegaly. *Eur J Endocrinol*, 2008; **159**: 89–95.
22. Ahmed S, Elsheikh M, Stratton IM, Page RC, Adams CB, Wass JA. Outcome of transphenoidal surgery for acromegaly and its relationship to surgical experience. *Clin Endocrinol (Oxf)*, 1999; **50**: 561–7.
23. Wass JA, Turner HE, Adams CB. The importance of locating a good pituitary surgeon. *Pituitary*, 1999; **2**: 51–4.
24. Sheaves R, Jenkins P, Blackburn P, Huneidi AH, Afshar F, Medbak S, *et al.* Outcome of transsphenoidal surgery for acromegaly using strict criteria for surgical cure. *Clin Endocrinol (Oxf)*, 1996; **45**: 407–13.
25. Ciric I, Ragin A, Baumgartner C, Pierce D. Complications of transsphenoidal surgery: results of a national survey, review of the literature, and personal experience. *Neurosurgery*, 1997; **40**: 225–36.
26. Buchfedlder M, Schlaffer S. Surgical management of acromegaly. In: Wass JAH, ed. *Acromegaly*. Bristol: Bioscientifica; 2009:139–51.
27. Murray RD, Melmed S. A critical analysis of clinically available somatostatin analog formulations for therapy of acromegaly. *J Clin Endocrinol Metab*, 2008; **93**: 2957–68.
28. Bhayana S, Booth GL, Asa SL, Kovacs K, Ezzat S. The implication of somatotroph adenoma phenotype to somatostatin analog responsiveness in acromegaly. *J Clin Endocrinol Metab*, 2005; **90**: 6290–5.
29. Stefaneanu L, Kovacs K, Thapar K, Horvath E, Melmed S, Greenman Y. Octreotide effect on growth hormone and somatostatin subtype 2 receptor mRNAs of the human pituitary somatotroph adenomas. *Endocr Pathol*, 2000; **11**: 41–8.
30. Veysey MJ, Thomas LA, Mallet AI, Jenkins PJ, Besser GM, Wass JA, *et al.* Prolonged large bowel transit increases serum deoxycholic acid: a risk factor for octreotide induced gallstones. *Gut*, 1999; **44**: 675–81.
31. Melmed S, Colao A, Barkan A, Molitch M, Grossman AB, Kleinberg D, *et al.* Guidelines for acromegaly management: an update. *J Clin Endocrinol Metab*, 2009; **94**: 1509–17.
32. Jenkins PJ, Bates P, Carson MN, Stewart PM, Wass JA. Conventional pituitary irradiation is effective in lowering serum growth hormone and insulin-like growth factor-I in patients with acromegaly. *J Clin Endocrinol Metab*, 2006; **91**: 1239–45.
33. Jagannathan J, Sheehan JP, Pouratian N, Laws ER Jr, Steiner L, Vance ML. Gamma knife radiosurgery for acromegaly: outcomes after failed transsphenoidal surgery. *Neurosurgery*, 2008; **62**: 1262–9.
34. Pollock BE, Brown PD, Nippoldt TB, Young WF, Jr. Pituitary tumor type affects the chance of biochemical remission after radiosurgery of hormone-secreting pituitary adenomas. *Neurosurgery*, 2008; **62**: 1271–6.
35. *Acromegaly*. Bristol: Bioscientifica; 2009.
36. Karavitaki N, Turner HE, Adams CB, Cudlip S, Byrne JV, Fazal-Sanderson V, *et al.* Surgical debulking of pituitary macroadenomas causing acromegaly improves control by lanreotide. *Clin Endocrinol (Oxf)*, 2008; **68**: 970–5.
37. Sherlock M, Aragon AA, Reulen RC, Ayuk J, Clayton RN, Holder G, *et al.* Monitoring disease activity using GH and IGF-I in the follow-up of 501 patients with acromegaly. *Clin Endocrinol (Oxf)*, 2009; **71**: 74–81.

2.3.12 Clinically nonfunctioning pituitary tumours and gonadotropinomas

W.W. de Herder, R.A. Feelders, A.J. van der Lely

The significant progress that has been made in the past years in the medical treatment of all pituitary adenomas is in stark contrast with the lack of progress in the medical treatment of clinically nonfunctioning pituitary tumours, or adenomas. In fact, only secreting, or functioning, tumours can be treated by medical therapy with at least modest to very impressive effect. Clinically nonfunctioning pituitary adenomas do not produce clinical signs of hormonal hypersecretion. Therefore, signs and symptoms will depend on the mass effect of these adenomas over the central nervous system (1–3).

Due to the lack of hypersecretion of hormones, nonfunctioning pituitary adenomas present themselves because of their mass effect and compression or destruction of surrounding tissues. This could also lead to hypopituitarism, which can be the presenting symptom as well (1–3). Despite their histologically benign nature, giant and 'invasive' nonfunctioning pituitary adenomas are one of the most complex neurosurgical challenges. Large nonfunctioning pituitary tumours are usually confined inferiorly by the sellar dura, superiorly by the elevated sellar diaphragm, and laterally by an intact medial wall of the cavernous sinus. If the anatomical extensions of the tumour are understood and a radical tumour resection is achieved, the visual and long-term outcome can be very rewarding. The goals of surgery are twofold: first to make a pathological diagnosis, and second, because these tumours are endocrinologically silent, to decompress the neural tissue (4). The vast majority of nonfunctioning pituitary adenomas are gonadotroph cell adenomas, as demonstrated by immunocytochemistry. However, they are rarely associated with increased levels of dimeric luteinizing hormone or follicle-stimulating hormone. Increased levels of subunits (free α-subunit mainly, LH-B subunit more rarely), however, are more frequently encountered, but are generally modest (5).

In this chapter the term 'clinically nonfunctioning pituitary adenomas' is used to describe pituitary tumours, which in most instances produce low quantities of hormones causing no clinically recognizable symptomatology. In the few instances, in which such tumours produce intact gonadotropins that activate testicular or ovarian activity, the term 'gonadotropinomas' is used.

Pathology

In the late 1970s and early 1980s, much work has been done on defining the pathological properties of pituitary tumours (6–9). The work of Asa and Kovacs is specially known for the accurate description of the microscopic findings of nonfunctioning pituitary adenomas (10). These tumours are morphologically classified into two groups, those which have hormone immunoreactivity and ultrastructural features of known adenohypophyseal cell types but are clinically silent, and those composed of cells that do not resemble nontumorous adenohypophyseal cell types. Among the former are the silent somatotroph adenomas, silent corticotroph adenomas, and silent gonadotroph adenomas; the latter include the silent type III adenomas, null cell adenomas, and oncocytomas (10). It is now known that nonfunctioning adenomas represent a heterogeneous group. By immunocytochemistry, the large majority of these tumours are glycoprotein producing and less commonly they are nonfunctioning somatotroph, lactotroph, or corticotoph adenomas (10–19). Their aetiopathogenesis is complex and their development is probably influenced by several factors, such as hypothalamic hormones (growth hormone-releasing hormone), growth factors (fibroblast growth factor), proliferation factors (proliferative cell nuclear antigen and Ki-67), protein p53, and the proto-oncogene *c*-erb-B2 (20).

Gsp and MEN1 genes play a role in the initiation and promotion of pituitary adenomas, while p53, ras, Rb, and nm23 genes play some role in the progression of the tumour. *Gsp* gene may play an important role in activation of 10% of nonfunctioning tumours (21). Gsp produces cAMP, which later produce cdk2 and cdk4 respectively, and stimulates cell progression from G1 to S phase. cAMP also induces *ras* gene, which inhibits binding of pRb with E2F, which is necessary to prevent action of E2F in th eaccelerating cell cycle (21).

A substantial proportion of tumours with particularly aggressive behaviour are the so-called 'silent subtype 3 adenoma'. Its diagnosis requires ultrastructural confirmation. Although once included among silent corticotroph adenomas, this aggressive, morphologically distinctive tumour is now recognized as a major form of plurihormonal adenoma and, in fact, some patients might present with clinical hormonal excess. In a recent report from the Mayo Clinics on 27 confirmed examples of silent subtype three adenomas, most of these tumours were plurihormonal, featuring immunoreactivity for PRL prolactin (n=17), growth hormone (n=15), thyroid-stimulating hormone (TSH) (n=16), or adrenocorticotropic hormone (ACTH) (n=3), while only 1 lesion was immunonegative (22).

Symptomatology

Nonfunctioning pituitary tumours are relatively common. A large number of these tumours are incidentally found pituitary microadenomas (<1 cm) and are usually of no clinical importance. Those tumours that require treatment are generally macroadenomas and come to medical attention because of mass effect and/or hypopituitarism. Visual field defects are present in roughly 70% of patients with nonfunctioning macroadenoma at the time of diagnosis and the majority of these patients have at least growth deficiency and hypogonadism (3).

Hyperstimulation by excessive FSH secretion of gonadotropinomas has been described in only a few patients. An example of this is the observation of high serum FSH concentrations, but normal luteinizing hormone and testosterone and large testes in four men with pituitary macroadenomas (23). After pituitary surgery there were decreases in serum gonadotropin and testosterone levels, which were accompanied by decreases in testicular volume (23). In females, a similar example was the description of a woman whose gonadotroph adenoma caused supranormal serum concentrations of FSH, which resulted in the development of multiple ovarian cysts, persistent elevation of her serum oestradiol concentration, and endometrial hyperplasia (24).

Diagnostic evaluations

Except for gonadotropins and their free subunits that may be increased in the case of gonadotropinomas, markers of endocrine secretory activity are lacking. In subjects with nonfunctioning pituitary adenomas, only 11% have elevated basal chromogranin A (CgA) levels, so serum CgA levels do not provide a helpful marker for the clinical management of these tumours (25). As stated in the introduction, the vast majority of nonfunctioning pituitary adenomas are gonadotroph cell adenomas, as demonstrated by immunocytochemistry. Increased levels of uncombined subunits are more frequently encountered, but are generally modest (5).

Sellar masses are associated most commonly with pituitary adenomas. Many other neoplastic, inflammatory, infectious, and vascular lesions, however, may affect the sellar region and mimic pituitary tumours. These lesions must be considered in a differential diagnosis of especially nonfunctioning pituitary adenomas (26). The diagnosis of such lesions involves a multidisciplinary approach, and detailed endocrinological, ophthalmological, neuroimaging, neurological, and finally histological studies are required (27). Examples of immune diseases that can present as nonfunctioning pituitary adenomas are sarcoidosis (28, 29), lymphocytic hypophysitis (30), plasma cell granulomas (31), and idiopathic granulomatous hypophysitis (32).

Relatively frequent encountered inflammatory lesions of the sellar region are isolated tuberculomas (33), while the wide spectrum of benign nonpituitary sellar tumours ranges in diagnosis from myofibroblastic tumours (34), ependymomas (35), osteochondromas (36), and pituitary blastomas (37) to paragangliomas (38) and angiolipomas (39). Malignant lesions are almost always metastases of which mammary cancer and prostate cancer are the most frequently observed ones (40). Probably the most frequent and important sellar lesion that is often confused with a nonfunctioning pituitary adenoma is the lymphocytic hypophysitis. Pituitary autoimmunity encompasses a spectrum of conditions ranging from histologically proven forms of lymphocytic hypophysitis to the presence of pituitary antibodies in apparently healthy subjects. Hypophysitis is a rare but increasingly recognized disorder that typically presents as a mass in the sella turcica. It mimics clinically and radiologically other nonfunctioning sellar masses, such as the more common pituitary adenoma (41). Hypophysitis shows a striking temporal association with pregnancy (42), and it has been recently described during immunotherapies that block CTLA-4. Several candidate pituitary autoantigens have been described in recent years, although none has proven useful as a diagnostic tool (41).

Hypophysitis has been histologically classified into five types: lymphocytic hypophysitis, granulomatous hypophysitis, xanthogranulomatous hypophysitis, xanthomatous hypophysitis, and necrotizing hypophysitis (43).

Therapy

Therapeutic modalities for nonfunctioning pituitary adenoma include surgery, radiotherapy, and medical therapy. In patients with relatively small adenomas, i.e. intrasellar adenomas or adenomas with limited extrasellar extension, a wait and see policy can be applied with careful radiological follow-up (44). Microadenomas (<10 mm) rarely grow and convert to a macroadenoma (45, 46). Macroadenomas, in contrast, tend to grow and the tumour volume of macroadenomas increases gradually in approximately 50% of patients (14, 47). In patients with a growing adenoma or with complications due to mass effects of the tumour, surgery is indicated eventually followed by radiotherapy and/or medical therapy.

Surgery

Suprasellar and parasellar extension of nonfunctioning pituitary adenoma can lead to compression of the optic chiasm and the ophthalmic motor nerves (cranial nerves III, IV, and VI), respectively, which can result in a decreased visual acuity, temporal visual field defects and ophthalmoparesis. The aims of pituitary surgery for nonfunctioning pituitary adenoma are recovery of visual function, to obtain tumour tissue for pathological diagnosis, and to achieve long-term tumour control. Urgent decompression is indicated in patients with a pituitary apoplexia, a syndrome caused by acute bleeding and/or infarction of the adenoma resulting in a sudden tumour expansion with acute visual loss and cranial nerve palsy. Pituitary surgery is primarily performed by the transsphenoidal approach (Fig. 2.3.12.1) (48). Also tumours with a large suprasellar component can successfully be resected via the transsphenoidal route. A transcranial approach via the pterional or subfrontal route may be indicated in case of a dominant extrasellar tumour compartment and a small sella turcica, a large eccentric tumour extension into the middle, anterior or posterior cranial fossa, or a coexisting aneurysm of the carotid artery (49). Transcranial surgery is, however, accompanied by a higher morbidity and mortality rate compared with the transsphenoidal approach (49).

After transsphenoidal resection, improvement of visual function is achieved in 85–90% of patients with normalization of vision in approximately 40% of patients (50, 51). The rapidity of visual recovery depends in part on the duration of optic nerve compression. Recovery of visual function can already be observed in the first days postoperatively and can continue up to a year after surgery (52–54). In patients with pre-existing (partial) hypopituitarism, pituitary function is not likely to restore after resection of the adenoma although in some patients improvement can be demonstrated (44, 55). In experienced hands, transsphenoidal surgery is a safe procedure with a perioperative mortality of 0.5–1% (56). Postoperative complications are cerebrospinal fluid leakage, meningitis, (transient) diabetes insipidus, and new anterior pituitary deficiency (48). Recent developments in pituitary surgery include the endoscopic approach and the use of neuro-navigation and intraoperative MRI (48, 57). Advantages of endoscopic surgery are a wider and closer view of the surgical area, also of the supra- and parasellar regions, and less nasal traumatism with no need for postoperative nasal packing (57). Future studies will reveal whether these new techniques will improve surgical outcome.

Radiotherapy

Complete removal of a macroadenoma is achieved in only a minority of patients. The optimal treatment strategy of patients with a residual tumour after transsphenoidal surgery (example shown in Fig. 2.3.12.1b) is still a matter of debate. Observational studies on the natural course of macroadenoma remnants show variable results with tumour regrowth rates between 6% and 46% (50, 58–62). Factors predictive of regrowth are parasellar invasion before surgery and (the degree of) suprasellar extension of the postoperative remnant adenoma (62). Unfortunately, no morphological tumour features or molecular markers of cell proliferation are

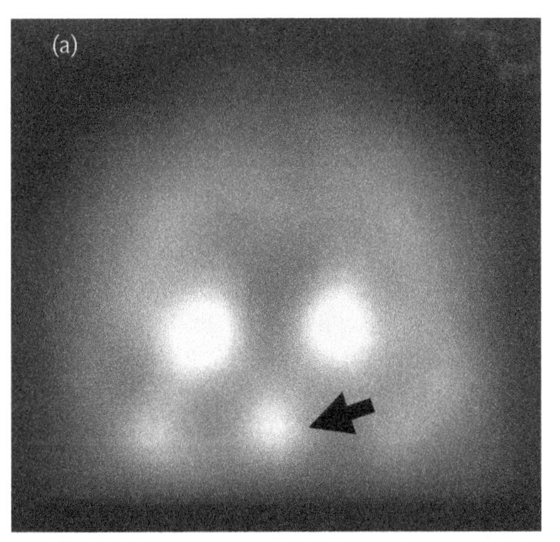

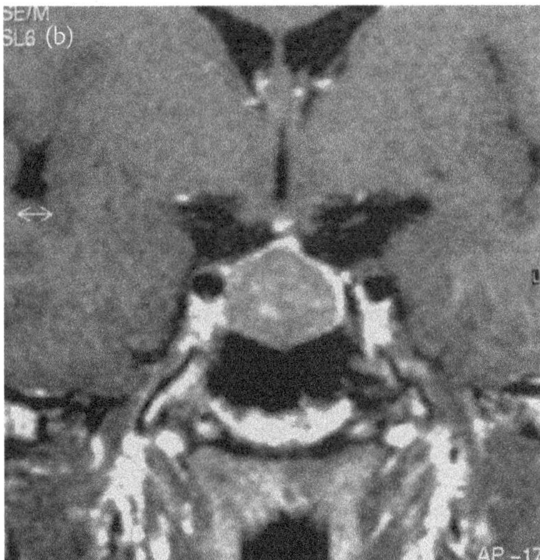

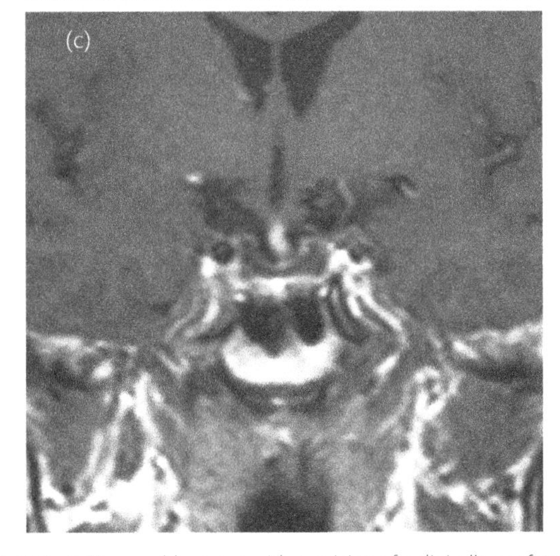

Fig. 2.3.12.1 A 48-year-old woman with suspicion of a clinically nonfunctioning pituitary macroadenoma with compression of the optic chiasm leading to impaired visual acuity and bitemporal visual field defects. Postoperatively, visual function recovered while anterior pituitary function remained intact. (a) Baseline MR image. (b) Following transsphenoidal subtotal resection. Note the tumour remnant encasing the right carotid artery (arrow). However, significant tumour reduction has been achieved with complete decompression of the optic chiasm.

available that predict tumour growth (63, 64). Postoperative external radiotherapy is applied in nonfunctioning pituitary adenoma to achieve long-term tumour control by induction of tumour shrinkage or stabilization. In patients who receive conventional radiotherapy, progression free survival at 10 years is more than 90%, significantly higher compared to patients who where only observed (65–68). On the other hand, radiotherapy can not control tumour growth in each patient. Studies vary with respect to follow-up duration, amount of invasive tumours, etc., but regrowth of residual adenomas in patients treated with radiotherapy has been observed in 2–36% of patients (50, 61, 62). Overall, although no randomized trials have been performed that compare radiotherapy with a wait and see policy. Adjuvant radiotherapy has beneficial effects on tumour regrowth but this should be balanced against the complications of radiotherapy, i.e. radiation damage to the optic nerves with visual impairment, development of (partial) hypopituitarism in up to 50% of patients, increased risk of cerebrovascular events and an increased risk on secondary brain tumours (65, 69–73). Therefore, the treatment strategy in patients with a residual adenoma after transsphenoidal surgery should be individualized and factors such as age, comorbidity, remnant tumour size, tumour distance to the optic chiasm, and status of pituitary function should be involved in the decision on adjuvant radiotherapy. Patients not treated with radiotherapy should carefully be observed with MRI and ophthalmological evaluation. If regrowth occurs, radiotherapy is still effective, but repeat surgery can also be considered (74).

Stereotactic radiotherapy is a more recently developed radiation technique with radiosurgery and fractionated stereotactic radiotherapy as treatment modalities (75). The advantage of stereotactic radiotherapy is that more accurate tumour localization is achieved with consequently less exposure of surrounding brain tissue to radiation. With radiosurgery a high-dose focused radiation is given in a single treatment session. Radiosurgery is suitable for small adenomas with sufficient distance to the optic nerves and optic chiasm which are radiosensitive tissues. Fractionated stereotactic radiotherapy can be applied in larger tumours and tumours with a smaller proximity to the optic chiasm (75). With both forms of stereotactic radiotherapy tumour control can be achieved in more than 90% (76–79). No data are available yet that compare recurrence rates and long-term safety and complications of conventional radiotherapy and stereotactic radiotherapy.

Medical treatment

In analogy with medical treatment of prolactinomas and somatotroph pituitary adenomas, the possibility of medical treatment in patients with clinically nonfunctioning pituitary adenomas has been investigated. Several different drugs (combinations) have been investigated.

Dopamine agonists

Clinically nonfunctioning pituitary adenomas express dopamine receptors on their cell membranes (1, 80). The D_2 receptor is the predominantly expressed subtype, and mainly as its long version (D_2 long, D_2Lh). The D_2 short isoform (D_2Sh), or combinations of both D_2Lh and D_2Sh isoforms are expressed in a minority of cases. The D_4 receptor can also be expressed by these tumours (81–83).

Based on these findings, the effects of various dopamine agonists have been investigated in these tumours, both *in vitro* and *in vivo*. Addition of high pharmacological concentrations of bromocriptine, quinagolide, or cabergoline to cultures of tumour cells of gonadotroph origin suppressed the release and synthesis of gonadotropins and their α-subunits (82, 84). These results closely correlated with D_2 expression on the tumour cells (82).

In patients with nonfunctioning pituitary adenoma, dopamine agonist therapy causes tumour shrinkage in approximately 28% of patients. There is, however, a huge variation in this response between the different studies, depending on patient's selection, size of the study population (generally very small), choice of the dopamine agonist and its dose and the treatment period (82, 85–101). The results of the different studies are shown in Table 2.3.12.1. In line with this observation of tumour shrinkage occurring in selected cases, improvements in visual field defects have also been observed in a similar percentage (20%). Tumour growth was observed in 9% of cases (Table 2.3.12.1).

D_2 receptor scintigraphy of pituitary adenomas is feasible by single photon emission computed tomography (SPECT) using ^{123}I-S-(−)-N-[(1-ethyl-2-pyrrolidinyl)-methyl]-2-hydroxy-3-iodo-6-methoxybenzamide (^{123}I-IBZM) and ^{123}I-(S)-N-[(1-ethyl-2-pyrrolidinyl) methyl]-5-iodo-2, 3-dimethoxybenzamide (^{123}I-epidepride) (Fig. 2.3.12.2). ^{123}I-epidepride is superior to ^{123}I-IBZM for the visualization of D_2 receptors on pituitary macroadenomas (102–104). Although it was initially suggested that D_2 receptor scintigraphy might be a useful tool for predicting inhibition of hormonal hypersecretion and tumour shrinkage by dopamine D_2 agonists in patients with clinically nonfunctioning adenomas, more recent studies could not confirm these results. However, there seems to be a correlation between the intensity of the tumour uptake of the radioligand and tumour shrinkage with dopamine agonist treatment (97, 98, 105). These findings are in line with studies showing a positive correlation between dopamine D_2 expression in surgically removed tumour tissue and postoperative tumour remnant shrinkage with cabergoline (82). The post-surgery use of dopamine agonists to prevent tumour regrowth of nonfunctioning pituitary adenoma is, therefore, also advocated by other experts in the field (101, 106).

Somatostatin analogues

Somatostatin receptors are expressed in nonfunctioning pituitary adenoma, with a predominance of the somatostatin receptor subtype 3 (sst_3), followed by sst_2 and sst_5 and infrequent expression of sst_1, sst_4 and sst_5 (107–109). The expression of sst_2 is required for achieving a tumour response to the currently available octapeptide somatostatin analogues, octreotide and lanreotide. These drugs show a high affinity for sst_2 and sst_5 and a low affinity for sst_3 and no affinity for sst_1 and sst_4 (110, 111). Both somatostatin analogues have demonstrated promising results *in vitro* with regard to their effects on growth of cells derived from nonfunctioning pituitary adenoma and suppression of their secretory products (112–114).

The effects of immediate release octreotide on the size and secretion of clinically nonfunctioning pituitary adenomas have been tested in several clinical trials (115–123). The study results are summarized in Table 2.3.12.2. Like in the trials studying the effects of dopamine agonists, a huge variation in tumour and/or biochemical response between the different studies, depending on patient's selection, size of the study population (generally very small), and dose and treatment period existed. Medication was either given as

Table 2.3.12.1 Dopamine agonist trials in patients with clinically non-functioning pituitary adenomas

Visual fields			Tumour volume			Drug	Reference
Improved	**Stable**	**Worsened**	**Growth**	**Stable**	**Shrinkage**		
			0/11	2/11	9/11	Bromocriptine	85
			0/12	6/12	6/12	Bromocriptine	86
			0/15	15/15	0/15	Bromocriptine/mesulergine/pergolide	87
1/5	4/5	0/5	0/5	1/5	4/5	Bromocriptine	88
1/20	15/20	4/20	0/20	19/20	1/20	Bromocriptine	89
			0/7	7/7	0/7	Bromocriptine	90
3/3	0/3	0/3				Bromocriptine	91
			0/8	8/8	0/8	Bromocriptine	92
			0/4	2/4	2/4	Bromocriptine	93
1/25	23/25	1/25	1/25	20/25	4/25	Bromocriptine	95
2/5	3/5	0/5	0/5	4/5	1/5	Quinagolide	96
			0/6	4/6	2/6	Quinagolide	97
0/10	6/10	4/10	6/10	4/10	0/10	Quinagolide	99
3/10	7/10	0/10	0/10	8/10	2/10	Quinagolide/cabergoline	98
2/13	11/13	0/13	0/13	6/13	7/13	Cabergoline	100
4/9	5/9	0/9	3/9	1/9	5/9	Cabergoline	82
			7/33	15/33	11/33	Bromocriptine	101
17/100	74/100	9/100	17/193	122/193	54/193		Overall
17%	74%	9%	9%	63%	28%		

Modified from Colao A, Di Somma C, Pivonello R, Faggiano A, Lombardi G, Savastano S. Medical therapy for clinically non-functioning pituitary adenomas. *Endocr Relat Cancer*, 2008; **15**: 905–15. (1).

primary therapy or as adjuvant therapy. Tumour reduction was reported in 3% of cases. The great majority of patients (86%) had stable (remnant) tumours (Table 2.3.12.2). In 11% of the patients tumour (re-)growth was observed despite treatment.

^{111}In-pentetreotide scintigraphy (OctreoScan) has been used for demonstrating the presence of the sst_2 subtype on pituitary adenomas. In contrast with dopamine receptor scintigraphy, the normal, nonpathological, pituitary can also be visualized as

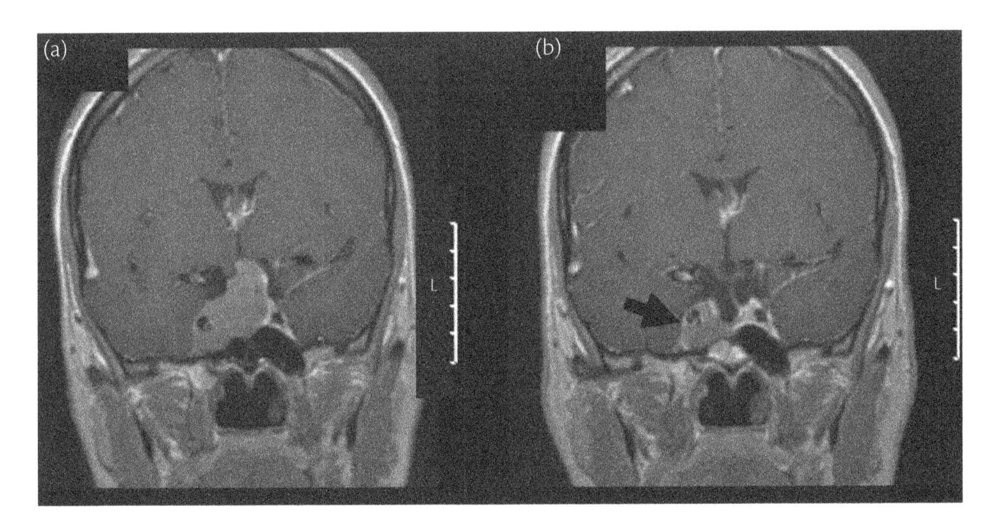

Fig. 2.3.12.2 A 50-year-old man with clinical suspicion of a clinically nonfunctioning pituitary macroadenoma, with follicle-stimulating hormone and α-subunit hypersecretion, hypopituitarism, and nonelevated circulating prolactin levels. There were neither visual field defects nor impairment of the visual acuity. (a) ^{123}I-epidepride scintigraphy showing intense uptake in the pituitary area (arrow). (b) Baseline coronal T_1-weighted MR image after the administration of gadolinium-DTPA showing a pituitary macroadenoma with dimensions 1.8 × 1.8 × 2.0 cm, without compression of the optic chiasm. (c) Coronal T_1-weighted MR image after the administration of gadolinium-DTPA obtained after 10 years' treatment with 300 µg quinagolide/day showing impressive regression of the pituitary adenoma.

Table 2.3.12.2 Trials using immediate release octreotide in patients with clinically nonfunctioning pituitary adenomas

Visual fields			Tumour volume			Reference
Improved	**Stable**	**Worsened**	**Growth**	**Stable**	**Shrinkage**	
3/5	2/5	0/5	0/2	2/2	0/2	115
3/4	1/4	0/4	0/4	4/4	0/4	116
1/3	2/3	0/3				117
1/5	3/5	1/5	2/8	6/8	0/8	118
1/9	8/9	0/9	0/19	18/19	1/19	119
			2/14	12/14	0/14	120
9/22	9/22	4/22	3/7	3/7	1/7	123
8/16	6/16	2/16	0/16	16/16	0/16	121
			2/9	7/9	0/9	122
26/64	31/64	7/64	9/79	68/79	2/79	Overall
41%	48%	11%	11%	86%	3%	

Modified from Colao A, Di Somma C, Pivonello R, Faggiano A, Lombardi G, Savastano S. Medical therapy for clinically non-functioning pituitary adenomas. *Endocr Relat Cancer*, 2008; **15**: 905–15. (1).

a receptor-positive area using this technique. This might partly explain the contradictory findings obtained by using this imaging technique in different studies in patients with nonfunctioning pituitary adenoma for predicting the effects of somatostatin analogues on these adenomas (120, 122–125). ^{111}In-pentetreotide scintigraphy is generally not recommended and also not required for the clinical work-up of a clinically nonfunctioning pituitary macroadenomas. Interestingly, improvement in headaches and visual disturbances generally occurring shortly after introduction of octreotide treatment and despite the absence of a clear tumour response has been reported in two studies. This effect is more likely caused by a direct effect of this drug on the retina and the optic nerve (115, 116, 126).

Recently a new, so-called universal, somatostatin analogue has been introduced for clinical use. Pasireotide (SOM230) is a somatostatin analogue with high binding affinity to sst_1, sst_2, sst_3 and sst_5. *In vitro*, this drug was able to inhibit the viability of nonfunctioning pituitary adenoma cells by inhibiting vascular endothelial growth factor (VEGF) secretion (127). Of now, *in vivo* data with this promising compound are lacking.

Combined treatment with somatostatin analogues and dopamine agonists, or with chimeric compounds

In line with monotherapy with somatostatin analogues or dopamine agonists, combinations of both drugs in patients with nonfunctioning pituitary adenoma can also produce tumour shrinkage and improvement of visual field defects (128, 129). A new chimeric D_2 agonist/sst_2 and sst_5 analogue, BIM-23A760, was effective in inhibiting cell proliferation in two-thirds of clinically nonfunctioning pituitary adenomas *in vitro* (80, 130, 131). Until now, no clinical trials in patients with nonfunctioning pituitary adenoma have been performed with this promising new drug.

Gonadotropin-releasing hormone agonists and antagonists

The release of gonadotrophins by normal anterior pituitary cells is regulated by pulsatile secretion of gonadotropin-releasing hormone by the hypothalamus. The chronic administration of gonadotropinreleasing hormone to normal individuals produces an initial rise in gonadotropin levels, followed by gonadotroph desensitization, leading to efficient suppression of gonadotrophin release. Several case reports describe the occurrence of pituitary apoplexy after the administration of gonadotropinreleasing hormone as a test agent or as an agonist for the treatment of prostate cancer (132–137). Long-term treatment with gonadotropinreleasing hormone analogues had no effect on tumour size or visual fields in patients with nonfunctioning pituitary adenoma (138, 139). This treatment modality is currently not anymore under clinical investigation.

Temozolomide

Temozolomide has been proposed as a treatment option for pituitary carcinomas and aggressive pituitary adenomas. In addition, it has been suggested that the responsiveness of pituitary tumours to temozolomide depends on the expression of O(6)-methylguanine DNA methyltransferase (MGMT). A recent study has shown that in patients with progressive, regrowing nonfunctioning pituitary adenoma, about half of these tumour cells exhibited low MGMT expression and, therefore, are potential candidates for treatment with temozolomide (140).

References

1. Colao A, Di Somma C, Pivonello R, Faggiano A, Lombardi G, Savastano S. Medical therapy for clinically non-functioning pituitary adenomas. *Endocr Relat Cancer*, 2008; **15**: 905–15.
2. Turner HE, Adams CB, Wass JA. Pituitary tumours in the elderly: a 20 year experience. *Eur J Endocrinol*, 1999; **140**: 383–9.
3. Jaffe CA. Clinically non-functioning pituitary adenoma. *Pituitary*, 2006; **9**: 317–21.
4. Agrawal A, Cincu R, Goel A. Current concepts and controversies in the management of non-functioning giant pituitary macroadenomas. *Clin Neurol Neurosurg*, 2007; **109**: 645–50.
5. Chanson P, Brochier S. Non-functioning pituitary adenomas. *J Endocrinol Invest*, 2005; **28**: 93–9.
6. Gray AB, Doniach I, Leigh PN. Correlation of diameters of secretory granules in clinically non-functioning chromophobe adenomas of the pituitary with those of normal thyrotrophs. *Acta Endocrinol (Copenh)*, 1975; **79**: 417–20.

7. Lipson LG, Beitins IZ, Kornblith PL, McArthur JW, Friesen HG, Kliman B, *et al.* Tissue culture studies on human pituitary tumours: long term release of anterior pituitary hormones into the culture medium. *Acta Endocrinol (Copenh)*, 1979; **90**: 421–33.
8. Dufy B, Israel JM, Zyzek E, Dufy-Barbe L, Guerin J, Fleury H, *et al.* An electrophysiological study of cultured human pituitary cells. *Mol Cell Endocrinol*, 1982; **27**: 179–90.
9. Iwaki T, Kondo A, Takeshita I, Nakagaki H, Kitamura K, Tateishi J. Proliferating potential of folliculo-stellate cells in human pituitary adenomas. Immunohistochemical and electron microscopic analysis. *Acta Neuropathol*, 1986; **71**: 233–42.
10. Asa SL, Kovacs K. Clinically non-functioning human pituitary adenomas. *Can J Neurol Sci*, 1992; **19**: 228–35.
11. Saeger W, Ludecke B, Ludecke DK. Clinical tumor growth and comparison with proliferation markers in non-functioning (inactive) pituitary adenomas. *Exp Clin Endocrinol Diabetes*, 2008; **116**: 80–5.
12. Ribeiro-Oliveira A Jr, Franchi G, Kola B, Dalino P, Pinheiro SV, Salahuddin N, *et al.* Protein western array analysis in human pituitary tumours: insights and limitations. *Endocr Relat Cancer*, 2008; **15**: 1099–114.
13. Honegger J, Zimmermann S, Psaras T, Petrick M, Mittelbronn M, Ernemann U, *et al.* Growth modelling of non-functioning pituitary adenomas in patients referred for surgery. *Eur J Endocrinol*, 2008; **158**: 287–94.
14. Dekkers OM, Hammer S, de Keizer RJ, Roelfsema F, Schutte PJ, Smit JW, *et al.* The natural course of non-functioning pituitary macroadenomas. *Eur J Endocrinol*, 2007; **156**: 217–24.
15. Suzuki M, Minematsu T, Oyama K, Tahara S, Miyai S, Sanno N, *et al.* Expression of proliferation markers in human pituitary incidentalomas. *Endocr Pathol*, 2006; **17**: 263–75.
16. Hanson PL, Aylwin SJ, Monson JP, Burrin JM. FSH secretion predominates in vivo and in vitro in patients with non-functioning pituitary adenomas. *Eur J Endocrinol*, 2005; **152**: 363–70.
17. Baldeweg SE, Pollock JR, Powell M, Ahlquist J. A spectrum of behaviour in silent corticotroph pituitary adenomas. *Br J Neurosurg*, 2005; **19**: 38–42.
18. Wolfsberger S, Wunderer J, Zachenhofer I, Czech T, Bocher-Schwarz HG, Hainfellner J, *et al.* Expression of cell proliferation markers in pituitary adenomas—correlation and clinical relevance of MIB-1 and anti-topoisomerase-IIalpha. *Acta Neurochir (Wien)*, 2004; **146**: 831–9.
19. Pawlikowski M, Pisarek H, Kunert-Radek J, Radek A. Immunohistochemical detection of somatostatin receptor subtypes in 'clinically nonfunctioning' pituitary adenomas. *Endocr Pathol*, 2003; **14**: 231–8.
20. Ferreira JE, de Mello PA, de Magalhaes AV, Botelho CH, Naves LA, Nose V, *et al.* [Non-functioning pituitary adenomas: clinical features and immunohistochemistry]. *Arq Neuropsiquiatr*, 2005; **63**: 1070–8.
21. Suhardja AS, Kovacs KT, Rutka JT. Molecular pathogenesis of pituitary adenomas: a review. *Acta Neurochir (Wien)*, 1999; **141**: 729–36.
22. Erickson D, Scheithauer B, Atkinson J, Horvath E, Kovacs K, Lloyd RV, *et al.* Silent subtype 3 pituitary adenoma: a clinicopathologic analysis of the Mayo Clinic experience. *Clin Endocrinol (Oxf)*, 2009; **71**: 92–9.
23. Heseltine D, White MC, Kendall-Taylor P, De Kretser DM, Kelly W. Testicular enlargement and elevated serum inhibin concentrations occur in patients with pituitary macroadenomas secreting follicle stimulating hormone. *Clin Endocrinol (Oxf)*, 1989; **31**: 411–23.
24. Djerassi A, Coutifaris C, West VA, Asa SL, Kapoor SC, Pavlou SN, *et al.* Gonadotroph adenoma in a premenopausal woman secreting follicle-stimulating hormone and causing ovarian hyperstimulation. *J Clin Endocrinol Metab*, 1995; **80**: 591–4.
25. Gussi IL, Young J, Baudin E, Bidart JM, Chanson P. Chromogranin A as serum marker of pituitary adenomas. *Clin Endocrinol (Oxf)*, 2003; **59**: 644–8.
26. Glezer A, Paraiba DB, Bronstein MD. Rare sellar lesions. *Endocrinol Metab Clin North Am*, 2008; **37**: 195–211.
27. Kaltsas GA, Evanson J, Chrisoulidou A, Grossman AB. The diagnosis and management of parasellar tumours of the pituitary. *Endocr Relat Cancer*, 2008; **15**: 885–903.
28. Cannavo S, Romano C, Buffa R, Faglia G. Granulomatous sarcoidotic lesion of hypothalamic-pituitary region associated with Rathke's cleft cyst. *J Endocrinol Invest*, 1997; **20**: 77–81.
29. Bullmann C, Faust M, Hoffmann A, Heppner C, Jockenhovel F, Muller-Wieland D, *et al.* Five cases with central diabetes insipidus and hypogonadism as first presentation of neurosarcoidosis. *Eur J Endocrinol*, 2000; **142**: 365–72.
30. Moskowitz SI, Hamrahian A, Prayson RA, Pineyro M, Lorenz RR, Weil RJ. Concurrent lymphocytic hypophysitis and pituitary adenoma. *Case report and review of the literature. J Neurosurg*, 2006; **105**: 309–14.
31. Murakami K, Muraishi K, Ikeda H, Yoshimoto T. Plasma cell granuloma of the pituitary gland. *Case report. Surg Neurol*, 2001; **56**: 247–51.
32. Gazioglu N, Tuzgen S, Oz B, Kocer N, Kafadar A, Akar Z, *et al.* Idiopathic granulomatous hypophysitis: are there reliable, constant radiological and clinical diagnostic criterias?. *Neuroradiology*, 2000; **42**: 890–4.
33. Yilmazlar S, Bekar A, Taskapilioglu O, Tolunay S. Isolated intrasellar tuberculoma mimicking pituitary adenoma. *J Clin Neurosci*, 2007; **14**: 477–81.
34. Yamagami K, Yoshioka K, Isaka Y, Inoue T, Hosoi M, Shakudo M, *et al.* A case of hypopituitarism due to inflammatory myofibroblastic tumor of the sella turnica. *Endocr J*, 2008; **55**: 339–44.
35. Scheithauer BW, Swearingen B, Whyte ET, Auluck PK, Stemmer-Rachamimov AO. Ependymoma of the sella turcica: a variant of pituicytoma. *Hum Pathol*, 2009; **40**: 435–40.
36. Inoue T, Takahashi N, Murakami K, Nishimura S, Kaimori M, Nishijima M. Osteochondroma of the sella turcica presenting with intratumoral hemorrhage. *Neurol Med Chir (Tokyo)*, 2009; **49**: 37–41.
37. Scheithauer BW, Kovacs K, Horvath E, Kim DS, Osamura RY, Ketterling RP, *et al.* Pituitary blastoma. *Acta Neuropathol*, 2008; **116**: 657–66.
38. Ozum U, Egilmez R, Yildirim A. Paraganglioma in pituitary fossa. *Neuropathology*, 2008; **28**: 547–50.
39. Kolenc D, Zarkovic K, Jednacak H, Ozretic D, Habek M. Sellar angiolipomas: two case reports and a review of the literature. *J Neurooncol*, 2008; **89**: 109–12.
40. Komninos J, Vlassopoulou V, Protopapa D, Korfias S, Kontogeorgos G, Sakas DE, *et al.* Tumors metastatic to the pituitary gland: case report and literature review. *J Clin Endocrinol Metab*, 2004; **89**: 574–80.
41. Caturegli P, Lupi I, Landek-Salgado M, Kimura H, Rose NR. Pituitary autoimmunity: 30 years later. *Autoimmun Rev*, 2008; **7**: 631–7.
42. Kidd D, Wilson P, Unwin B, Dorward N. Lymphocytic hypophysitis presenting early in pregnancy. *J Neurol*, 2003; **250**: 1385–7.
43. Tashiro T, Sano T, Xu B, Wakatsuki S, Kagawa N, Nishioka H, *et al.* Spectrum of different types of hypophysitis: a clinicopathologic study of hypophysitis in 31 cases. *Endocr Pathol*, 2002; **13**: 183–95.
44. Dekkers OM, Pereira AM, Romijn JA. Treatment and follow-up of clinically nonfunctioning pituitary macroadenomas. *J Clin Endocrinol Metab*, 2008; **93**: 3717–26.
45. Burrow GN, Wortzman G, Rewcastle NB, Holgate RC, Kovacs K. Microadenomas of the pituitary and abnormal sellar tomograms in an unselected autopsy series. *N Engl J Med*, 1981; **304**: 156–8.
46. Sanno N, Oyama K, Tahara S, Teramoto A, Kato Y. A survey of pituitary incidentaloma in Japan. *Eur J Endocrinol*, 2003; **149**: 123–7.
47. Karavitaki N, Collison K, Halliday J, Byrne JV, Price P, Cudlip S, *et al.* What is the natural history of nonoperated nonfunctioning pituitary adenomas? *Clin Endocrinol*, 2007; **67**: 938–43.
48. Joshi SM, Cudlip S. Transsphenoidal surgery. *Pituitary*, 2008; **11**: 353–60.
49. Buchfelder M, Kreutzer J. Transcranial surgery for pituitary adenomas. *Pituitary*, 2008; **11**: 375–84.

50. Dekkers OM, Pereira AM, Roelfsema F, Voormolen JH, Neelis KJ, Schroijen MA, *et al.* Observation alone after transsphenoidal surgery for nonfunctioning pituitary macroadenoma. *J Clin Endocrinol Metab*, 2006; **91**: 1796–801.
51. Mortini P, Losa M, Barzaghi R, Boari N, Giovanelli M. Results of transsphenoidal surgery in a large series of patients with pituitary adenoma. *Neurosurgery*, 2005; **56**: 1222–33. discussion 1233.
52. Jakobsson KE, Petruson B, Lindblom B. Dynamics of visual improvement following chiasmal decompression. *Quantitative pre- and postoperative observations. Acta Ophthalmol Scand*, 2002; **80**: 512–16.
53. Kerrison JB, Lynn MJ, Baer CA, Newman SA, Biousse V, Newman NJ. Stages of improvement in visual fields after pituitary tumor resection. *Am J Ophthalmol*, 2000; **130**: 813–20.
54. Gnanalingham KK, Bhattacharjee S, Pennington R, Ng J, Mendoza N. The time course of visual field recovery following transphenoidal surgery for pituitary adenomas: predictive factors for a good outcome. *J Neurol, Neurosurg Psychiatry*, 2005; **76**: 415–19.
55. Webb SM, Rigla M, Wagner A, Oliver B, Bartumeus F. Recovery of hypopituitarism after neurosurgical treatment of pituitary adenomas. *J Clin Endocrinol Metab*, 1999; **84**: 3696–700.
56. Barker FG, 2nd, Klibanski A, Swearingen B. Transsphenoidal surgery for pituitary tumors in the United States, 1996–2000: mortality, morbidity, and the effects of hospital and surgeon volume. *J Clin Endocrinol Metab*, 2003; **88**: 4709–19.
57. Cappabianca P, Cavallo LM, de Divitiis O, Solari D, Esposito F, Colao A. Endoscopic pituitary surgery. *Pituitary*, 2008; **11**: 385–90.
58. Lillehei KO, Kirschman DL, Kleinschmidt-DeMasters BK, Ridgway EC. Reassessment of the role of radiation therapy in the treatment of endocrine-inactive pituitary macroadenomas. *Neurosurgery*, 1998; **43**: 432–8.
59. Turner HE, Stratton IM, Byrne JV, Adams CB, Wass JA. Audit of selected patients with nonfunctioning pituitary adenomas treated without irradiation - a follow-up study. *Clin Endocrinol*, 1999; **51**: 281–4.
60. Ebersold MJ, Quast LM, Laws ER Jr, Scheithauer B, Randall RV. Long-term results in transsphenoidal removal of nonfunctioning pituitary adenomas. *J Neurosurg*, 1986; **64**: 713–19.
61. Woollons AC, Hunn MK, Rajapakse YR, Toomath R, Hamilton DA, Conaglen JV, *et al.* Non-functioning pituitary adenomas: indications for postoperative radiotherapy. *Clin Endocrinol*, 2000; **53**: 713–17.
62. Greenman Y, Ouaknine G, Veshchev I, Reider G II, Segev Y, Stern N. Postoperative surveillance of clinically nonfunctioning pituitary macroadenomas: markers of tumour quiescence and regrowth. *Clin Endocrinol*, 2003; **58**: 763–9.
63. Buch HN, Raskauskiene D, Bahar A, Bicknell EJ, Farrell WE, Clayton RN. Prediction of recurrence of nonfunctioning pituitary tumours by loss of heterozygosity analysis. *Clin Endocrinol*, 2004; **61**: 19–25.
64. Dubois S, Guyetant S, Menei P, Rodien P, Illouz F, Vielle B, *et al.* Relevance of Ki-67 and prognostic factors for recurrence/progression of gonadotropic adenomas after first surgery. *Eur J Endocrinol*, 2007; **157**: 141–7.
65. Brada M, Rajan B, Traish D, Ashley S, Holmes-Sellors PJ, Nussey S, *et al.* The long-term efficacy of conservative surgery and radiotherapy in the control of pituitary adenomas. *Clin Endocrinol*, 1993; **38**: 571–8.
66. Gittoes NJ, Bates AS, Tse W, Bullivant B, Sheppard MC, Clayton RN, *et al.* Radiotherapy for non-function pituitary tumours. *Clin Endocrinol*, 1998; **48**: 331–7.
67. Tsang RW, Brierley JD, Panzarella T, Gospodarowicz MK, Sutcliffe SB, Simpson WJ. Radiation therapy for pituitary adenoma: treatment outcome and prognostic factors. *Int J Radiat Oncol Biol Phys*, 1994; **30**: 557–65.
68. van den Bergh AC, van den Berg G, Schoorl MA, Sluiter WJ, van der Vliet AM, Hoving EW, *et al.* Immediate postoperative radiotherapy in residual nonfunctioning pituitary adenoma: beneficial effect on local control without additional negative impact on pituitary function and life expectancy. *Int J Radiat Oncol Biol Phys*, 2007; **67**: 863–9.
69. al-Mefty O, Kersh JE, Routh A, Smith RR. The long-term side effects of radiation therapy for benign brain tumors in adults. *J Neurosurg*, 1990; **73**: 502–12.
70. Littley MD, Shalet SM, Beardwell CG, Ahmed SR, Applegate G, Sutton ML. Hypopituitarism following external radiotherapy for pituitary tumours in adults. *Q J Med*, 1989; **70**: 145–60.
71. Nelson PB, Goodman ML, Flickenger JC, Richardson DW, Robinson AG. Endocrine function in patients with large pituitary tumors treated with operative decompression and radiation therapy. *Neurosurgery*, 1989; **24**: 398–400.
72. Erfurth EM, Bulow B, Svahn-Tapper G, Norrving B, Odh K, Mikoczy Z, *et al.* Risk factors for cerebrovascular deaths in patients operated and irradiated for pituitary tumors. *J Clin Endocrinol Metab*, 2002; **87**: 4892–9.
73. Minniti G, Traish D, Ashley S, Gonsalves A, Brada M. Risk of second brain tumor after conservative surgery and radiotherapy for pituitary adenoma: update after an additional 10 years. *J Clin Endocrinol Metab*, 2005; **90**: 800–4.
74. Park P, Chandler WF, Barkan AL, Orrego JJ, Cowan JA, Griffith KA, *et al.* The role of radiation therapy after surgical resection of nonfunctional pituitary macroadenomas. *Neurosurgery*, 2004; **55**: 100–6. discussion 106–7.
75. Kanner AA, Corn BW, Greenman Y. Radiotherapy of nonfunctioning and gonadotroph adenomas. *Pituitary*, 2009; **12**: 15–22.
76. Pollock BE, Carpenter PC. Stereotactic radiosurgery as an alternative to fractionated radiotherapy for patients with recurrent or residual nonfunctioning pituitary adenomas. *Neurosurgery*, 2003; **53**: 1086–91. discussion 1091–4.
77. Sheehan JP, Kondziolka D, Flickinger J, Lunsford LD. Radiosurgery for residual or recurrent nonfunctioning pituitary adenoma. *J Neurosurg*, 2002; **97**: 408–14.
78. Colin P, Jovenin N, Delemer B, Caron J, Grulet H, Hecart AC, *et al.* Treatment of pituitary adenomas by fractionated stereotactic radiotherapy: a prospective study of 110 patients. *Int J Radiat Oncol Biol Phys*, 2005; **62**: 333–41.
79. Minniti G, Traish D, Ashley S, Gonsalves A, Brada M. Fractionated stereotactic conformal radiotherapy for secreting and nonsecreting pituitary adenomas. *Clin Endocrinol*, 2006; **64**: 542–8.
80. Ferone D, Pivonello R, Resmini E, Boschetti M, Rebora A, Albertelli M, *et al.* Preclinical and clinical experiences with the role of dopamine receptors in the treatment of pituitary adenomas. *Eur J Endocrinol*, 2007; **156** Suppl 1: S37–43.
81. Renner U, Arzberger T, Pagotto U, Leimgruber S, Uhl E, Muller A, *et al.* Heterogeneous dopamine D2 receptor subtype messenger ribonucleic acid expression in clinically nonfunctioning pituitary adenomas. *J Clin Endocrinol Metab*, 1998; **83**: 1368–75.
82. Pivonello R, Matrone C, Filippella M, Cavallo LM, Di Somma C, Cappabianca P, *et al.* Dopamine receptor expression and function in clinically nonfunctioning pituitary tumors: comparison with the effectiveness of cabergoline treatment. *J Clin Endocrinol Metab*, 2004; **89**: 1674–83.
83. Pivonello R, Ferone D, Lombardi G, Colao A, Lamberts SW, Hofland LJ. Novel insights in dopamine receptor physiology. *Eur J Endocrinol*, 2007; **156** Suppl 1: S13–21.
84. Kwekkeboom DJ, Hofland LJ, van Koetsveld PM, Singh R, van den Berge JH, Lamberts SW. Bromocriptine increasingly suppresses the in vitro gonadotropin and alpha-subunit release from pituitary adenomas during long term culture. *J Clin Endocrinol Metab*, 1990; **71**: 718–24.

85. Wollesen F, Andersen T, Karle A. Size reduction of extrasellar pituitary tumors during bromocriptine treatment. *Ann Intern Med*, 1982; **96**: 281–6.
86. Barrow DL, Tindall GT, Kovacs K, Thorner MO, Horvath E, Hoffman JC Jr. Clinical and pathological effects of bromocriptine on prolactin-secreting and other pituitary tumors. *J Neurosurg*, 1984; **60**: 1–7.
87. Grossman A, Ross R, Charlesworth M, Adams CB, Wass JA, Doniach I, *et al.* The effect of dopamine agonist therapy on large functionless pituitary tumours. *Clin Endocrinol (Oxf)*, 1985; **22**: 679–86.
88. Pullan PT, Carroll WM, Chakera TM, Khangure MS, Vaughan RJ. Management of extra-sellar pituitary tumours with bromocriptine: comparison of prolactin secreting and non-functioning tumours using half-field visual evoked potentials and computerised tomography. *Aust N Z J Med*, 1985; **15**: 203–8.
89. Verde G, Oppizzi G, Chiodini PG, Dallabonzana D, Luccarelli G, Liuzzi A. Effect of chronic bromocriptine administration on tumor size in patients with 'nonsecreting' pituitary adenomas. *J Endocrinol Invest*, 1985; **8**: 113–15.
90. Zarate A, Moran C, Kleriga E, Loyo M, Gonzalez-Angulo A, Aquilar-Parada E. Bromocriptine therapy as pre-operative adjunct of non-functional pituitary macroadenomas. *Acta Endocrinol (Copenh)*, 1985; **108**: 445–50.
91. D'Emden MC, Harrison LC. Rapid improvement in visual field defects following bromocriptine treatment of patients with non-functioning pituitary adenomas. *Clin Endocrinol (Oxf)*, 1986; **25**: 697–702.
92. Bevan JS, Adams CB, Burke CW, Morton KE, Molyneux AJ, Moore RA, *et al.* Factors in the outcome of transsphenoidal surgery for prolactinoma and non-functioning pituitary tumour, including pre-operative bromocriptine therapy. *Clin Endocrinol (Oxf)*, 1987; **26**: 541–56.
93. Klibanski A, Shupnik MA, Bikkal HA, Black PM, Kliman B, Zervas NT. Dopaminergic regulation of alpha-subunit secretion and messenger ribonucleic acid levels in alpha-secreting pituitary tumors. *J Clin Endocrinol Metab*, 1988; **66**: 96–102.
94. Garcia-Luna PP, Leal-Cerro A, Pereira JL, Montero C, Acosta D, Trujillo F, *et al.* Rapid improvement of visual defects with parenteral depot-bromocriptine in a patient with a non-functioning pituitary adenoma. *Horm Res*, 1989; **32**: 183–7.
95. van Schaardenburg D, Roelfsema F, van Seters AP, Vielvoye GJ. Bromocriptine therapy for non-functioning pituitary adenoma. *Clin Endocrinol (Oxf)*, 1989; **30**: 475–84.
96. Kwekkeboom DJ, Lamberts SW. Long-term treatment with the dopamine agonist CV 205–502 of patients with a clinically non-functioning, gonadotroph, or alpha- subunit secreting pituitary adenoma. *Clin Endocrinol (Oxf)*, 1992; **36**: 171–6.
97. Ferone D, Lastoria S, Colao A, Varrella P, Cerbone G, Acampa W, *et al.* Correlation of scintigraphic results using 123I-methoxybenzamide with hormone levels and tumor size response to quinagolide in patients with pituitary adenomas. *J Clin Endocrinol Metab*, 1998; **83**: 248–52.
98. Colao A, Ferone D, Lastoria S, Cerbone G, Di Sarno A, Di Somma C, *et al.* Hormone levels and tumour size response to quinagolide and cabergoline in patients with prolactin-secreting and clinically non-functioning pituitary adenomas: predictive value of pituitary scintigraphy with 123I-methoxybenzamide. *Clin Endocrinol (Oxf)*, 2000; **52**: 437–45.
99. Nobels FR, de Herder WW, van den Brink WM, Kwekkeboom DJ, Hofland LJ, Zuyderwijk J, *et al.* Long-term treatment with the dopamine agonist quinagolide of patients with clinically non-functioning pituitary adenoma. *Eur J Endocrinol*, 2000; **143**: 615–21.
100. Lohmann T, Trantakis C, Biesold M, Prothmann S, Guenzel S, Schober R, *et al.* Minor tumour shrinkage in nonfunctioning pituitary adenomas by long-term treatment with the dopamine agonist cabergoline. *Pituitary*, 2001; **4**: 173–8.
101. Greenman Y, Tordjman K, Osher E, Veshchev I, Shenkerman G, Reider G II, *et al.* Postoperative treatment of clinically nonfunctioning pituitary adenomas with dopamine agonists decreases tumour remnant growth. *Clin Endocrinol (Oxf)*, 2005; **63**: 39–44.
102. de Herder WW, Reijs AE, de Swart J, Kaandorp Y, Lamberts SW, Krenning EP, *et al.* Comparison of iodine-123 epidepride and iodine-123 IBZM for dopamine D2 receptor imaging in clinically non-functioning pituitary macroadenomas and macroprolactinomas. *Eur J Nucl Med*, 1999; **26**: 46–50.
103. de Herder WW, Reijs AE, Kwekkeboom DJ, Hofland LJ, Nobels FR, Oei HY, *et al.* In vivo imaging of pituitary tumours using a radiolabelled dopamine D2 receptor radioligand. *ClinEndocrinol (Oxf)*, 1996; **45**: 755–67.
104. de Herder WW, Lamberts SW. Imaging of pituitary tumours. [Review]. *Baillieres Clin Endocrinol Metab*, 1995; **9**: 367–89.
105. de Herder WW, Reijs AE, Feelders RA, van Aken MO, Krenning EP, Tanghe HL, *et al.* Dopamine agonist therapy of clinically non-functioning pituitary macroadenomas. Is there a role for 123I-epidepride dopamine D2 receptor imaging? *Eur J Endocrinol*, 2006; **155**: 717–23.
106. Greenman Y. Dopaminergic treatment of nonfunctioning pituitary adenomas. *Nat Clin Pract Endocrinol Metab*, 2007; **3**: 554–5.
107. Greenman Y, Melmed S. Heterogeneous expression of two somatostatin receptor subtypes in pituitary tumors. *J Clin Endocrinol Metab*, 1994; **78**: 398–403.
108. Greenman Y, Melmed S. Expression of three somatostatin receptor subtypes in pituitary adenomas: evidence for preferential SSTR5 expression in the mammosomatotroph lineage. *J Clin Endocrinol Metab*, 1994; **79**: 724–29.
109. Hofland LJ, Lamberts SW. Somatostatin receptor subtype expression in human tumors. *Ann Oncol*, 2001; **12** Suppl 2: S31–6.
110. van der Hoek J, Lamberts SW, Hofland LJ. Preclinical and clinical experiences with the role of somatostatin receptors in the treatment of pituitary adenomas. *Eur J Endocrinol*, 2007; **156** Suppl 1: S45–51.
111. Taboada GF, Luque RM, Bastos W, Guimaraes RF, Marcondes JB, Chimelli LM, *et al.* Quantitative analysis of somatostatin receptor subtype (SSTR1–5) gene expression levels in somatotropinomas and non-functioning pituitary adenomas. *Eur J Endocrinol*, 2007; **156**: 65–74.
112. Florio T, Thellung S, Arena S, Corsaro A, Spaziante R, Gussoni G, *et al.* Somatostatin and its analog lanreotide inhibit the proliferation of dispersed human non-functioning pituitary adenoma cells in vitro. *Eur J Endocrinol*, 1999; **141**: 396–408.
113. Padova H, Rubinfeld H, Hadani M, Cohen ZR, Nass D, Taylor JE, *et al.* Effects of selective somatostatin analogs and cortistatin on cell viability in cultured human non-functioning pituitary adenomas. *Mol Cell Endocrinol*, 2008; **286**: 214–18.
114. Pawlikowski M, Lawnicka H, Pisarek H, Kunert-Radek J, Radek M, Culler MD. Effects of somatostatin-14 and the receptor-specific somatostatin analogs on chromogranin A and alpha-subunit (alpha-SU) release from 'clinically nonfunctioning' pituitary adenoma cells incubated in vitro. *J Physiol Pharmacol*, 2007; **58**: 179–88.
115. Warnet A, Timsit J, Chanson P, Guillausseau PJ, Zamfirescu F, Harris AG, *et al.* The effect of somatostatin analogue on chiasmal dysfunction from pituitary macroadenomas. *J Neurosurg*, 1989; **71**: 687–90.
116. de Bruin TW, Kwekkeboom DJ, Van't Verlaat JW, Reubi JC, Krenning EP, Lamberts SW, *et al.* Clinically nonfunctioning pituitary adenoma and octreotide response to long term high dose treatment, and studies in vitro. *J Clin Endocrinol Metab*, 1992; **75**: 1310–17.

117. Katznelson L, Oppenheim DS, Coughlin JF, Kliman B, Schoenfeld DA, Klibanski A. Chronic somatostatin analog administration in patients with alpha-subunit-secreting pituitary tumors. *J Clin Endocrinol Metab*, 1992; **75**: 1318–25.
118. Gasperi M, Petrini L, Pilosu R, Nardi M, Marcello A, Mastio F, *et al.* Octreotide treatment does not affect the size of most non- functioning pituitary adenomas. *J Endocrinol Invest*, 1993; **16**: 541–3.
119. Merola B, Colao A, Ferone D, Selleri A, Di Sarno A, Marzullo P, *et al.* Effects of a chronic treatment with octreotide in patients with functionless pituitary adenomas. *Horm Res*, 1993; **40**: 149–55.
120. Plockinger U, Reichel M, Fett U, Saeger W, Quabbe HJ. Preoperative octreotide treatment of growth hormone-secreting and clinically nonfunctioning pituitary macroadenomas: effect on tumor volume and lack of correlation with immunohistochemistry and somatostatin receptor scintigraphy. *J Clin Endocrinol Metab*, 1994; **79**: 1416–23.
121. Broson-Chazot F, Houzard C, Ajzenberg C, Nocaudie M, Duet M, Mundler O, *et al.* Somatostatin receptor imaging in somatotroph and non-functioning pituitary adenomas: correlation with hormonal and visual responses to octreotide. *Clin Endocrinol (Oxf)*, 1997; **47**: 589–98.
122. Colao A, Lastoria S, Ferone D, Varrella P, Marzullo P, Pivonello R, *et al.* The pituitary uptake of (111)In-DTPA-D-Phe1-octreotide in the normal pituitary and in pituitary adenomas. *J Endocrinol Invest*, 1999; **22**: 176–83.
123. Warnet A, Harris AG, Renard E, Martin D, James-Deidier A, Chaumet-Riffaud P. A prospective multicenter trial of octreotide in 24 patients with visual defects caused by nonfunctioning and gonadotropin-secreting pituitary adenomas. French Multicenter Octreotide Study Group. *Neurosurgery*, 1997; **41**: 786–95.
124. Faglia G, Bazzoni N, Spada A, Arosio M, Ambrosi B, Spinelli F, *et al.* In vivo detection of somatostatin receptors in patients with functionless pituitary adenomas by means of a radioiodinated analog of somatostatin ([123I]SDZ 204–090). *J Clin Endocrinol Metab*, 1991; **73**: 850–6.
125. Duet M, Mundler O, Ajzenberg C, Berolatti B, Chedin P, Duranteau L, *et al.* Somatostatin receptor imaging in non-functioning pituitary adenomas: value of an uptake index. *Eur J Nucl Med*, 1994; **21**: 647–50.
126. Lamberts SW, de Herder WW, van Koetsveld PM, Koper JW, van der Lely AJ, Visser-Wisselaar HA, *et al.* Somatostatin receptors: clinical implications for endocrinology and oncology. *Ciba Found Symp*, 1995; **190**: 222–36.
127. Zatelli MC, Piccin D, Vignali C, Tagliati F, Ambrosio MR, Bondanelli M, *et al.* Pasireotide, a multiple somatostatin receptor subtypes ligand, reduces cell viability in non-functioning pituitary adenomas by inhibiting vascular endothelial growth factor secretion. *Endocr Relat Cancer*, 2007; **14**: 91–102.
128. Andersen M, Bjerre P, Schroder HD, Edal A, Hoilund-Carlsen PF, Pedersen PH, *et al.* In vivo secretory potential and the effect of combination therapy with octreotide and cabergoline in patients with clinically non-functioning pituitary adenomas. *Clin Endocrinol (Oxf)*, 2001; **54**: 23–30.
129. Colao A, Hofland LJ. The role of somatostatin and dopamine receptors as molecular targets for the treatment of patients with pituitary adenomas. *Eur J Endocrinol*, 2007; **156** Suppl 1: S1.
130. Zatelli MC, Ambrosio MR, Bondanelli M, Uberti EC. Control of pituitary adenoma cell proliferation by somatostatin analogs, dopamine agonists and novel chimeric compounds. *Eur J Endocrinol*, 2007; **156** Suppl 1: S29–35.
131. Florio T, Barbieri F, Spaziante R, Zona G, Hofland LJ, van Koetsveld PM, *et al.* Efficacy of a dopamine-somatostatin chimeric molecule, BIM-23A760, in the control of cell growth from primary cultures of human non-functioning pituitary adenomas: a multi-center study. *Endocr Relat Cancer*, 2008; **15**: 583–96.
132. Hands KE, Alvarez A, Bruder JM. Gonadotropin-releasing hormone agonist-induced pituitary apoplexy in treatment of prostate cancer: case report and review of literature. *Endocr Pract*, 2007; **13**: 642–6.
133. Reznik Y, Chapon F, Lahlou N, Deboucher N, Mahoudeau J. Pituitary apoplexy of a gonadotroph adenoma following gonadotrophin releasing hormone agonist therapy for prostatic cancer. *J Endocrinol Invest*, 1997; **20**: 566–8.
134. Chanson P, Schaison G. Pituitary apoplexy caused by GnRH-agonist treatment revealing gonadotroph adenoma. *J Clin Endocrinol Metab*, 1995; **80**: 2267–8.
135. Masson EA, Atkin SL, Diver M, White MC. Pituitary apoplexy and sudden blindness following the administration of gonadotrophin releasing hormone. *Clin Endocrinol (Oxf)*, 1993; **38**: 109–10.
136. Arafah BM, Taylor HC, Salazar R, Saadi H, Selman WR. Apoplexy of a pituitary adenoma after dynamic testing with gonadotropin-releasing hormone. *Am J Med*, 1989; **87**: 103–5.
137. Drury PL, Belchetz PE, McDonald WI, Thomas DG, Besser GM. Transient amaurosis and headache after thyrotropin releasing hormone. *Lancet*, 1982; **1**: 218–19.
138. Colombo P, Ambrosi B, Saccomanno K, Bassetti M, Cortelazzi D, Faglia G. Effects of long-term treatment with the gonadotropin-releasing hormone analog nafarelin in patients with non-functioning pituitary adenomas. *Eur J Endocrinol*, 1994; **130**: 339–45.
139. Roman SH, Goldstein M, Kourides IA, Comite F, Bardin CW, Krieger DT. The luteinizing hormone-releasing hormone (LHRH) agonist [D-Trp6-Pro9-NEt]LHRH increased rather than lowered LH and alpha-subunit levels in a patient with an LH-secreting pituitary tumor. *J Clin Endocrinol Metab*, 1984; **58**: 313–19.
140. Widhalm G, Wolfsberger S, Preusser M, Woehrer A, Kotter MR, Czech T, *et al.* O(6)-methylguanine DNA methyltransferase immunoexpression in nonfunctioning pituitary adenomas: are progressive tumors potential candidates for temozolomide treatment? *Cancer*, 2009; **115**: 1070–80.

2.3.13 Thyrotropinomas

Paolo Beck-Peccoz, Luca Persani

Introduction

Thyrotropinomas are rare tumours, accounting for no more than 1% of all secreting or nonsecreting pituitary adenomas (1, 2). Since the prevalence of pituitary tumours in the general population is about 0.03%, 1–3 thyrotropinomas are expected to be seen per million people. The number of reported thyrotropinomas increased exponentially in the past years, as a consequence of the introduction of ultrasensitive immunometric assays for thyroid-stimulating hormone (TSH) as first-line test for evaluating thyroid function (1). Based on the finding of measurable serum TSH levels in the presence of elevated thyroid hormone concentrations, many patients previously thought to be affected with Graves' disease or toxic nodular goitre could be correctly diagnosed as patients with central hyperthyroidism. In our opinion, this latter term is preferable to 'inappropriate secretion of TSH', as it more precisely reflects the pathophysiological events underlying such an unusual disorder, where the thyroid hormone negative feedback mechanism is clearly disrupted and TSH itself is responsible for the hyperstimulation of the thyroid gland and the consequent hypersecretion of thyroid hormones (Fig. 2.3.13.1).

Central hyperthyroidism is mainly due to autonomous TSH hypersecretion from a thyrotropinoma. However, signs and symptoms of hyperthyroidism along with biochemical findings similar to those found in thyrotropinoma, may be recorded in the minority of patients with resistance to thyroid hormones (RTH) (3, 4). This form of RTH is called pituitary RTH (PRTH), as the resistance to thyroid hormone action appears more severe at the pituitary than at the peripheral tissue level (see Fig. 2.3.13.1). The clinical importance of these rare entities is based on the diagnostic and therapeutic challenges they present. Failure to recognize these different disorders may result in undesirable consequences, such as improper thyroid ablation in patients with central hyperthyroidism or unnecessary pituitary surgery in patients with RTH. Conversely, early diagnosis and correct treatment of thyrotropinomas may prevent the occurrence of complications (visual defects by compression of the optic chiasm, hypopituitarism, etc.) and should improve the rate of cure.

Pathology and aetiopathogenesis

The great majority of thyrotropinomas (79.3%) are macroadenomas with a diameter of more than 10 mm at the time of diagnosis. Extrasellar extension in the supra- and/or parasellar direction is present in more than two-thirds of cases. Most of the tumours show localized or diffuse invasion of the surrounding structures, especially into the dura mater and bone. The occurrence of invasive macroadenomas is particularly high in patients with previous thyroid ablation by surgery or radioiodine, a fact illustrating the deleterious effects of incorrect diagnosis and treatment of these

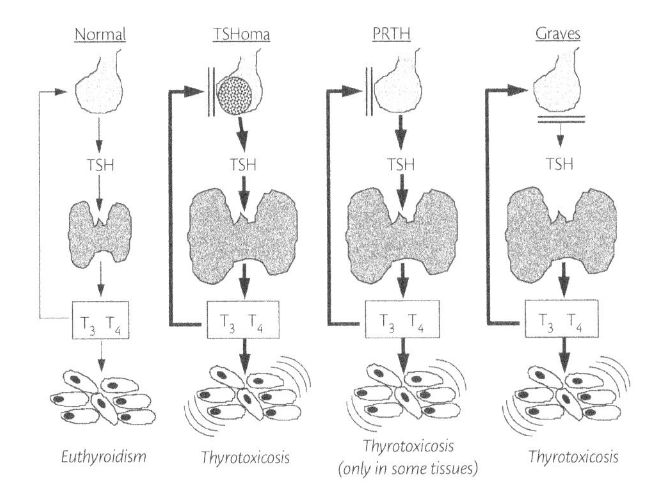

Fig. 2.3.13.1 Schematic representation of pathophysiological mechanisms operating in normal subjects (Normal), patients with thyrotropinoma (TSHoma), pituitary resistance to thyroid hormones (PRTH), and Graves' disease (Graves). In patients with thyrotropinoma or PRTH, the feedback mechanism is clearly disrupted and thyroid-stimulating hormone (TSH) itself is responsible for the hyperstimulation of the thyroid gland (goitre) and the consequent hypersecretion of the thyroid hormones. On the contrary, the feedback mechanism is normal in patients with Graves'disease, so that TSH secretion is completely blocked. In all the three pathological conditions, signs and symptoms of thyrotoxicosis are recorded. However, in PRTH patients, some tissues, such as liver and bone, appear resistant to thyroid hormone action, whereas others, in particular the heart, are normally responsive to the high circulating levels of the thyroid hormones.

rare adenomas. In fact, microadenomas (diameter <10 mm) and intrasellar macroadenomas have been found in 34% of untreated patients versus 19% in those with thyroid ablation, while the opposite proportions were seen in patients with invasive macroadenomas. Therefore, previous thyroid ablation may induce an aggressive transformation of the tumour, which resembles that occurring in Nelson's syndrome after adrenalectomy for Cushing's disease. Almost all thyrotropinomas originate from pituitary thyrotrophs. Indeed, two cases of ectopic nasopharyngeal thyrotropinoma causing hyperthyroidism have so far been reported (5, 6).

Thyrotropinomas are benign tumours and until now transformation of a thyrotropinoma into a carcinoma with multiple metastases and loss of pituitary glycoprotein hormone α-subunit (α-GSU) has been reported in one patient (7), while in another case TSH-secreting carcinoma developed from a previously nonfunctioning pituitary adenoma (8). Thyrotropinomas may present with very fibrous consistency and may be densely calcified. On light microscopy, chromofobic adenoma cells appear large and arranged in cords, with frequent nuclear atypies and mitoses, thus being often mistakenly recognized as pituitary malignancy or metastasis from distant carcinomas (9).

About 70% of thyrotropinomas secrete TSH alone, frequently accompanied by an unbalanced hypersecretion of α-GSU. Cosecretion of other anterior pituitary hormones occurs in about 30% of thyrotropinomas. Hypersecretion of growth hormone and prolactin, resulting in acromegaly and amenorrhea/galactorrhea syndrome, are seen in 21% and 9% of patients, respectively. This may be because growth hormone and prolactin are known to share with TSH common transcription factors, such as PROP1, Pit1, and HESX1 (10). Double immunostaining studies have shown that TSH frequently colocalizes with other pituitary hormones in the same tumoural cell or even in the same secretory granule (11).

Similar to most pituitary tumours, the aetiopathogenesis of thyrotropinoma remains largely unknown. Inactivation analysis of the X chromosome has demonstrated that most pituitary adenomas, including the small number of thyrotropinomas investigated (12), derive from the clonal expansion of a single initially transformed cell. Screening studies for genetic abnormalities resulting in transcription activation have yielded negative results. In particular, no activating mutations of putative proto-oncogenes, such as *ras*, G-protein, TRH, and *PIT1* gene, or loss of genes with tumour suppressor activity, such as *p53*, have been reported in thyrotropinomas (1). Recently, mutations of the aryl hydrocarbon receptor-interacting protein (*AIP*) gene, which are known to cause a low-penetrance pituitary adenoma predisposition, were reported in a single sporadic thyrotropinoma (A. Beckers, personal communication, 2010). Another candidate gene is menin, whose mutations are responsible for multiple endocrine neoplasia type 1 (MEN 1). In fact, about a fourth of sporadic pituitary adenomas show loss of heterozygosity (LOH) on 11q13, where menin is located, and LOH on this chromosome seems to be associated with the transition from the noninvasive to the invasive phenotype. Interestingly, hyperthyroidism due to thyrotropinomas has been reported in five cases within a familial setting of MEN 1.

The extreme refractoriness of tumoral thyrotropes to the inhibitory action of thyroid hormones led to search for alterations in the thyroid hormone receptor function. Absence of TRa1, TRα2, and TRβ1 expression was reported in one thyrotropinoma, but aberrant alternative splicing of TRβ2 mRNA encoding TRβ variant lacking T_3-binding activity was recently shown as a mechanism for impaired T_3-dependent negative regulation of both TSHβ and α-GSU in tumoral tissue (13). Moreover, recent data suggest that somatic mutations of TRβ may be responsible for the defect in negative regulation of TSH secretion in some thyrotropinomas (14).

Finally, somatostatin receptor subtypes have been studies in few adenomas. The presence of subtypes 1, 2A, 3, and 5 were documented, a figure that may explain the high efficacy on hormone hypersecretion and tumour shrinkage during somatostatin analogue treatment in the majority of patients with thyrotropinoma (15). Moreover, it has been shown that LOH and particular polymorphisms at the somatostatin receptor type 5 gene locus are associated with an aggressive phenotype and resistance to somatostatin analogue treatment, possibly due to lack of somatostatin-induced inhibition of TSH secretion (16). Overexpression of basic fibroblast growth factor by some thyrotropinomas suggests the possibility that it may play a role in the development of fibrosis and tumour cell proliferation of this unusual type of pituitary neoplasm (17).

Clinical manifestations

The clinical presentation of thyrotropinomas depends on the pituitary hormone secretory profile, the biological potency of secreted TSH, and the size of the tumour. Almost all patients with thyrotropinoma present with signs and symptoms of hyperthyroidism, frequently associated with those related to the pressure effects of the adenoma on the surrounding structures.

Most patients have a long history of thyroid dysfunction, often misdiagnosed as Graves' disease, and about a third have had inappropriate thyroidectomy or radioiodine thyroid ablation (Table 2.3.13.1) (1, 18, 19). In some acromegalic patients, signs and symptoms of hyperthyroidism may be overshadowed by those of acromegaly. Cardiac failure and atrial fibrillation, as well as episodes of periodic paralysis, are rare events.

The presence of goitre is the rule, even in patients with previous thyroidectomy, since thyroid residue may regrow as a consequence of TSH hyperstimulation. Occurrence of uni- or multinodular goitre is frequent (about a third of reported cases), whereas differentiated thyroid carcinomas have been documented in two cases (1). Bilateral exophthalmos occurred in a few patients who subsequently developed autoimmune thyroiditis, while unilateral exophthalmos due to orbital invasion by thyrotropinoma was reported in three patients. Thyrotropinoma as part of MEN 1 has been rarely seen, but clinical and biochemical features of parathyroid and endocrine pancreas hyperfunction should be accurately investigated in each patient bearing a pituitary tumour.

Patients with a TSH-secreting macroadenoma may seek medical attention with signs or symptoms of an expanding intracranial tumour (see Table 2.3.13.1). Indeed, as a consequence of tumour suprasellar extension or invasiveness, signs and symptoms of tumour mass prevail over those of thyroid hyperfunction in many patients. Visual field defects are present in about 30% and headache in 25% of patients. Partial or total hypopituitarism is seen in about 35% of cases.

Table 2.3.13.1 Clinical characteristics of patients with thyrotropinoma never treated by thyroid or pituitary surgery, or radioiodine[a]

	n/total (%)[b]
Age range (years)	8–84
Female/male ratio	1.15
Severe thyrotoxicosis	28/104 (26.9)
Goitre	90/98 (91.8)
Thyroid nodule(s)	40/63 (63.5)
Macroadenomas	111/140 (79.3)
Acromegaly	38/184 (20.6)
Galactorrhoea	6/68 (8.8)
Hypopituitarism (partial or combined)	32/95 (33.7)
Visual field defects	24/78 (30.8)
Headache	20/81 (27.7)
Normal TSH levels	74/168 (38.0)
High α-GSU levels	58/88 (65.9)
High α-GSU/TSH molar ratio	66/84 (78.6)
High SHBG levels	24/27 (88.8)
Blunted TSH response to TRH test	97/112 (86.6)
Abnormal TSH response to T_3 suppression tets[c]	30/30 (100)

[a] Data from reports published until December 2008 and personal unpublished observations.
[b] n/total refers to the number of patients in whom the information was available.
[c] Lack of complete TSH inhibition after 8–10 days of L-T_3 administration (80–100 μg/day).
α-GSU, glycoprotein hormone α-subunit; SHBG, sex hormone-binding globulin; TRH, thyrotrophin-releasing hormone; TSH, thyroid-stimulating hormone.

Diagnosis

Serum thyroid hormone and TSH levels

Serum TSH levels in untreated patients with thyrotropinoma may be elevated or in the normal range, whereas total and free thyroid hormone levels are definitely high (see Table 2.3.13.1). Variations of the biological activity of secreted TSH molecules most likely account for the findings of normal TSH in the presence of high free T_4 and T_3 levels, and goitre (20). Patients whose thyroid was previously ablated by thyroidectomy or radioiodine have TSH levels much higher than in untreated patients, even though thyroid hormone levels still remained into the hyperthyroid range. Therefore, tumoral thyrotrophs which are totally resistant to the inhibitory action of elevated thyroid hormone levels still show a preserved or even increased sensitivity to the reduction of circulating thyroid hormone levels (19).

Certain clinical situations and possible interference in TSH and TH thyroid hormone measurement methods may cause biochemical profiles evocative of central hyperthyroidism (1, 4). Since these conditions are more common than thyrotropinomas, they must be excluded before embarking on the cumbersome and expensive clinical investigations required for patients with suspected thyrotropinoma. Indeed, alterations of thyroxine-binding globulin, albumin, or transthyretin leading to increases in TH thyroid hormone levels are in either congenital or drug-induced conditions. These conditions are easily recognized by measuring with direct methods the circulating free moiety of thyroid hormone, instead of their total concentration (1, 4). Circulating anti-T_4 and/or anti-T_3 autoantibodies can interfere in some immunometric assays, leading to an overestimation of the actual levels of both total and free TH thyroid hormones. Only the measurement of free T_4 and

T_3 concentrations by equilibrium dialysis or by direct 'two-step' methods prevents autoantibody interference (1, 4). Lastly, the more common factors interfering in TSH measurement are heterophilic antibodies directed against or cross-reacting with mouse IgG, and the anti-TSH autoantibodies, which may be discovered by appropriate laboratory techniques.

Glycoprotein hormone α-subunit

The measurement of α-GSU and the calculation of α-GSU/TSH molar ratio are helpful tools for the diagnosis of thyrotropinoma (see Table 2.3.13.1). Although previous studies have suggested that an α-GSU/TSH molar ratio above 1 is indicative of the presence of a thyrotropinoma, similar values may be recorded in normal subjects, particularly in euthyroid postmenopausal women, indicating the need for appropriate control groups matched for TSH and gonadotropin levels (1, 4). Interestingly, microadenomas, that frequently have α-GSU levels within the normal range (2), may show a high α-GSU/TSH molar ratio, further strengthening the importance of this index (18, 19).

Parameters of peripheral thyroid hormone action

Patients with central hyperthyroidism may present with mild signs and symptoms of thyrotoxicosis. Therefore, the measurement of several parameters of peripheral thyroid hormone action both *in vivo* (basal metabolic rate, cardiac systolic time intervals, Achilles' reflex time) and *in vitro* (sex hormone-binding globulin (SHBG), cholesterol, angiotensin-converting enzyme, soluble interleukin-2 receptor, osteocalcin, C-terminal cross-linked telopeptide of type I collagen (ICTP), etc.), have been proposed to quantify the degree of peripheral hyperthyroidism (2–4, 21, 22). Some of these parameters, and in particular SHBG and ICTP, have been widely used to differentiate hyperthyroid patients with thyrotropinoma from those with PRTH. In fact, as it occurs in the common forms of hyperthyroidism, patients with thyrotropinomas have high SHBG and ICTP levels, while they are into the normal range in patients with hyperthyroidism due to PRTH (see Table 2.3.13.1) (21, 22).

Testing

None of several stimulatory and inhibitory tests is of clear-cut diagnostic value, but the combination of some of them may increase the testing specificity and sensitivity. Classically, a lack of inhibition of TSH secretion in response to T_3 suppression test (80–100 μg L-T_3 daily for 8–10 days) is a common finding in patients with thyrotropinoma (see Table 2.3.13.1). In patients with previous thyroid ablation, T_3 suppression is the most sensitive and specific test in assessing the presence of a thyrotropinoma (18, 19). Obviously, this test is strictly contraindicated in elderly patients or those with coronary heart disease. TRH test has been widely used to investigate the presence of a thyrotropinoma. In 87% of patients, TSH levels do not increase after TRH injection. The lack of TSH response to TRH may also be useful in unusual situation where thyrotropinoma coexists with primary hypothyroidism (23, 24).

As most thyrotropinomas maintain the sensitivity to native somatostatin and its analogues (25, 26), we have recently treated a series of patients with thyrotropinomas or PRTH with multiple injections of long-acting somatostatin analogues and documented a marked decrease of free T_3 and T_4 levels in all patients but one with pituitary adenoma, while all patients with PRTH did not respond. Thus, administration of these long-acting analogues for at least 2 months can be useful in the differential diagnosis of problematic cases of central hyperthyroidism (27). Nevertheless, since none of these tests is of clear-cut diagnostic value, it is recommend to use both the T_3 suppression and TRH tests whenever possible, because the combined results increase the specificity and sensitivity of the diagnostic work-up (1, 2, 18).

Imaging studies

Full imaging studies are mandatory in the diagnostic work-up of thyrotropinomas, particularly nuclear MRI or high-resolution CT. Various degrees of suprasellar extension or sphenoid sinus invasion are present in two-thirds of cases. Microadenomas are now reported with increasing frequency, accounting for about 20% of all recorded cases in both clinical and surgical series. Recently, pituitary scintigraphy with radiolabelled octreotide has been shown to successfully image thyrotropinomas (18, 28). However, the specificity of these scintigrams is very low, since pituitary tumours of different types, either secreting or nonsecreting, and even nonspecific pituitary lesions, may show positive scans due to the presence of somatostatin receptors.

Differential diagnosis

In a patient with signs and symptoms of hyperthyroidism, the presence of elevated thyroid hormone and detectable TSH levels rules out primary hyperthyroidism. In patients on L-T_4 replacement therapy, the finding of measurable TSH in the presence of high thyroid hormone levels may be due to poor compliance or to an incorrect high L-T_4 dosage assumed before blood sampling. The measurement of free thyroid hormone concentration by direct 'two-step' methods is mandatory in the case of euthyroid hyperthyroxinaemia and whenever methodological interferences are suspected (1).

When the existence of central hyperthyroidism has been confirmed, several diagnostic steps have to be carried out to differentiate a thyrotropinoma from PRTH (Table 2.3.13.2). Indeed, the possible presence of neurological signs and symptoms (visual defects, headache) or clinical features of concomitant hypersecretion of

Table 2.3.13.2 Tests useful in the differential diagnosis of thyrotropinomas (TSHomas) and pituitary resistance to thyroid hormones (PRTH)

Parameter	TSHomas	RTH
Clinical thyrotoxicosis	Present	Present
Family history	Absent	Present
α-GSU levels	Elevated	Normal
α-GSU/TSH molar ratio	Elevated	Normal
TSH response to TRH	Blunted	Normal
(n = 23)		(n = 42)
TSH response to T_3 suppression test	No change	Decrease
Parameters of peripheral thyroid hormone action	Elevated	Normal
Pituitary imaging	Tumour	Normal

α-GSU: glycoprotein hormone α-subunit; TRH: thyrotrophin-releasing hormone; TSH, thyroid-stimulating hormone.

other pituitary hormones (acromegaly, galactorrhoea/amenorrhoea) points to the presence of a thyrotropinoma. The presence of pituitary alteration at MRI or CT scan strongly supports the diagnosis of thyrotropinoma, though the differential diagnosis may be difficult when the adenoma is undetectable by CT scan or MRI, or in the case of confusing lesions such as empty sella or incidentalomas. The finding of the same biochemical alteration in some relatives of the patient suggests PRTH, as familial cases of thyrotropinoma have never been reported. Moreover, TSH unresponsiveness to dynamic testing favours the presence of a thyrotropinoma. The parameters of peripheral thyroid hormone action are in the hyperthyroid range in patients with thyrotropinoma whereas they are into the normal range in PRTH.

Finally, an apparent association between thyrotropinoma and RTH has been recently reported, though genetic investigations of possible mutations in TRβ1 were not carried out (29). Nonetheless, the occurrence of thyrotropinoma in RTH patients is theoretically possible and, therefore, should be carefully considered.

Treatment, criteria for cure, and follow-up

Surgical resection is the recommended therapy for TSH-secreting pituitary tumours, with the aim of removing neoplastic tissues and restoring normal pituitary and thyroid function. However, a radical removal of the large tumours, which still represent the majority of thyrotropinomas, is particularly difficult because of the marked fibrosis of these tumours and their local invasiveness. Patient should be prepared for surgery with prescription of antithyroid drugs or somatostatin analogues, aiming the restoration of the euthyroidism. If surgery is contraindicated or the patient declines, as well as in the case of surgical failure, pituitary radiotherapy is mandatory. The recommended dose is no less than 45 Gy fractionated at 2 Gy per day or 10–25 Gy in a single dose if a stereotactic gamma unit is available.

With the above therapeutic approaches, normalization of thyroid hormone circulating levels and apparent complete removal of tumour mass has been observed in a third of patients who may therefore be considered apparently cured. An additional third of patients were judged improved, as normalization of thyroid hormone circulating levels was achieved in all, though there was no complete removal of the adenoma. Evaluation of pituitary function, particularly adrenocorticotropic hormone (ACTH) secretion, should be carefully investigated soon after surgery and checked again every year, especially in patients treated with radiotherapy. In addition, in the case of surgical cure, postoperative TSH is undetectable and may remain low for weeks or months, causing central hypothyroidism. A permanent central hypothyroidism, as well as partial or complete hypopituitarism, may also occur due to the compression exerted by the tumour on the surrounding pituitary cells or the pituitary stalk, or to surgical damage of the normal pituitary cells. Thus, transient or permanent hormone replacement therapy may be necessary. Finally, in few patients total thyroidectomy has been performed after pituitary surgery failure, as the patients were at risk of thyroid storm.

Although earlier diagnosis has significantly improved the surgical/radiation cure rate of thyrotropinomas, about a third of patients require medical therapy to control a persistent hyperthyroidism. Dopaminergic drugs have been employed in few patients with variable results, positive effects being mainly observed in patients with mixed prolactin/TSH adenoma. Today, the medical treatment of thyrotropinomas rests on long-acting preparations of somatostatin analogues, such as octreotide-LAR, lanreotide-SR and lanreotide-Autogel (1, 2, 15, 25–28, 30). Treatment with these analogues leads to a restoration of the euthyroid state in the majority of patients and tumour shrinkage occurs in about a half of them with vision improvement in 75% (25, 28, 30). Resistance to somatostatin analogue treatment has been documented in only 4% of cases. Patients on somatostatin analogues have to be carefully monitored, as untoward side effects, such as cholelithiasis and carbohydrate intolerance, may become manifest. The dose administered should be tailored for each patient, depending on therapeutic response and tolerance (including gastrointestinal side effects). Whether somatostatin analogue treatment may be an alternative to surgery and irradiation in patients with thyrotropinoma remains to be established.

Due to the rarity of the disease and the great heterogeneity of parameters used, the criteria for cure and follow-up of patients operated and/or irradiated for thyrotropinomas have not been clearly established. Clinical remission of hyperthyroidism, disappearance of neurological symptoms, resolution of neuroradiological alterations, and normalization of thyroid hormones, TSH, or α-GSU/TSH molar ratio are reliable parameters. It is obvious that previous thyroid ablation makes some of these criteria inapplicable. However, the restoration of clinical and biochemical euthyroidism in untreated hyperthyroid patients is not *per se* synonymous with complete removal of tumoral cells, since transient clinical remission accompanied by normalization of thyroid function tests has been observed (19). In our experience, T_3 suppression appears to be the most sensitive and specific test to document the complete removal of the adenoma. In fact, only those patients appear to be truly cured in whom T_3 administration completely inhibits basal and TRH-stimulated TSH secretion (19).

Recurrence of the adenoma does not appear to be frequent, at least in the first years after successful surgery (18, 19). In general, the patient should be evaluated clinically and biochemically two or three times the first year postoperatively, and then every year. Pituitary imaging should be performed every two or three years, but should be promptly done whenever an increase in TSH and thyroid hormone levels, or clinical symptoms occur. In the case of persistent macroadenoma, a close visual fields follow-up is required, as the visual function is threatened.

Acknowledgements

This work was supported by Ricerca Corrente Funds of Fondazione Policlinico IRCCS (Milan, Italy) and Istituto Auxologico Italiano IRCCS (Milan, Italy).

References

1. Beck-Peccoz P, Brucker-Davis F, Persani L, Smallridge RC, Weintraub BD. Thyrotropin-secreting pituitary tumours. *Endocr Rev*, 1996; **17**: 610–38.
2. Socin HV, Chanson P, Delemer B, Tabarin A, Rohmer V, Mockel J, *et al.* The changing spectrum of TSH-secreting pituitary adenomas: diagnosis and management in 43 patients. *Eur J Endocrinol*, 2003; **148**: 433–42.
3. Refetoff S, Weiss RE, Usala SJ. The syndromes of resistance to thyroid hormone. *Endocr Rev*, 1993; **14**: 348–99.
4. Gurnell M, Beck-Peccoz P, Chatterjee VK. Resistance to thyroid hormone. In: DeGroot LJ, Jameson JL, eds. *Endocrinology*. 5th edn. Philadelphia: Elsevier Saundres, 2006:2227–37
5. Cooper DS, Wenig BM. Hyperthyroidism caused by an ectopic TSH-secreting pituitary tumor. *Thyroid*, 1996; **6**: 337–43.

6. Pasquini E, Faustini-Fustini M, Sciarretta V, Saggese D, Ron- caroli F, Serra D, *et al.* Ectopic TSH-secreting pituitary adenoma of the vomerosphenoidal junction. *Eur J Endocrinol*, 2003; **148**: 253–7.
7. Mixson AJ, Friedman TC, David AK, Feuerstein IM, Taubenberger JK, Colandrea JM, *et al.* Thyrotropin-secreting pituitary carcinoma. *J Clin Endocrinol Metab*, 1993; **76**: 529–33.
8. Brown RL, Muzzafar T, Wollman R, Weiss RE. A pituitary carcinoma secreting TSH and prolactin: a non-secreting adenoma gone awry. *Eur J Endocrinol*, 2006; **154**: 639–43.
9. Bertholon-Grégoire M, Trouillas J, Guigard MP, Loras B, Tourniaire J. Mono- and plurihormonal thyrotropic pituitary adenomas: pathological, hormonal and clinical studies in 12 patients. *Eur J Endocrinol*, 1999; **140**: 519–27.
10. Cohen LE, Radovick S. Molecular bases of pituitary hormone deficiencies. *Endocr Rev*, 2002; **23**: 431–42.
11. Terzolo M, Orlandi F, Bassetti M, Medri G, Paccotti D, Cortelazzi D, *et al.* Hyperthyroidism due to a pituitary adenoma composed of two different cell types, one secreting alpha-subunit alone and another cosecreting alpha-subunit and thyrotropin. *J Clin Endocrinol Metab*, 1991; **72**: 415–21.
12. Ma W, Ikeda H, Watabe N, Kanno M, Yoshimoto T. A plurihormonal TSH-producing pituitary tumor of monoclonal origin in a patient with hypothyroidism. *Horm Res*, 2003; **59**: 257–61.
13. Ando S, Sarlis NJ, Krishnan J, Feng X, Refetoff S, Zhang MQ, *et al.* Aberrant alternative splicing of thyroid hormone receptor in a TSH-secreting pituitary tumor is a mechanism for hormone resistance. *Mol Endocrinol*, 2001; **15**: 1529–38.
14. Ando S, Sarlis NJ, Oldfield EH, Yen PM. Somatic mutation of TRbeta can cause a defect in negative regulation of TSH in a TSH-secreting pituitary tumor. *J Clin Endocrinol Metab*, 2001; **86**: 5572–6.
15. Horiguchi K, Yamada M, Umezawa R, Satoh T, Hashimoto K, Tosaka M, *et al.* Somatostatin receptor subtypes mRNA in TSH-secreting pituitary adenomas: a case showing a dramatic reduction in tumor size during short octreotide treatment. *Endocr J*, 2007; **54**: 371–8.
16. Filopanti M, Ballaré E, Lania AG, Bondioni S, Verga U, Locatelli M, *et al.* Loss of heterozygosity at the SS receptor type 5 locus in human GH- and TSH-secreting pituitary adenomas. *J Endocrinol Invest*, 2004; **27**: 937–42.
17. Ezzat S, Horvath E, Kovacs K, Smyth HS, Singer W, Asa SL. Basic fibroblast growth factor expression by two prolactin and thyrotropin-producing pituitary adenomas. *Endocr Pathol*, 1995; **6**: 125–34.
18. Brucker-Davis F, Oldfield EH, Skarulis MC, Doppman JL, Weintraub BD. Thyrotropin-secreting pituitary tumors: diagnostic criteria, thyroid hormone sensitivity, and treatment outcome in 25 patients followed at the National Institutes of Health. *J Clin Endocrinol Metab*, 1999; **84**: 476–86.
19. Losa M, Giovanelli M, Persani L, Mortini P, Faglia G, Beck-Peccoz P. Criteria of cure and follow-up of central hyperthyroidism due to thyrotropin-secreting pituitary adenomas. *J Clin Endocrinol Metab*, 1996; **81**: 3084–90.
20. Beck-Peccoz P, Persani L. Variable biological activity of thyroid-stimulating hormone. *Eur J Endocrinol*, 1994; **131**: 331–40.
21. Beck-Peccoz P, Roncoroni R, Mariotti S, Medri G, Marcocci C, Brabant G, *et al.* Sex hormone-binding globulin measurement in patients with inappropriate secretion of thyrotropin (IST): evidence against selective pituitary thyroid hormone resistance in nonneoplastic IST. *J Clin Endocrinol Metab*, 1990; **71**: 19–25.
22. Persani L, Preziati D, Matthews CH, Sartorio A, Chatterjee VKK, Beck-Peccoz P. Serum levels of carboxyterminal cross-linked telopeptide of type I collagen (ICTP) in the differential diagnosis of the syndromes of inappropriate secretion of TSH. *Clin Endocrinol*, 1997; **47**: 207–14.
23. Langlois M-F, Lamarche JB, Bellabarba D. Long-standing goiter and hypothyroidism: an unusual presentation of a TSH-secreting adenoma. *Thyroid*, 1996; **6**: 329–35.
24. Losa M, Mortini P, Minelli R, Giovanelli M. Coexistence of TSH-secreting pituitary adenoma and autoimmune hypothyroidism. *J Endocrinol Invest*, 2006; **29**: 555–9.
25. Bertherat J, Brue T, Enjalbert A, Gunz G, Rasolonjanahary R, Warnet A, *et al.* Somatostatin receptors on thyrotropin-secreting pituitary adenomas: comparison with the inhibitory effects of octreotide upon in vivo and in vitro hormonal secretions. *J Clin Endocrinol Metab*, 1992; **75**: 540–6.
26. Gancel A, Vuillermet P, Legrand A, Catus F, Thomas F, Kuhn JM. Effets of a slow-release formulation of the new somatostatin analogue lanreotide in TSH-secreting pituitary adenomas. *Clin Endocrinol*, 1994; **40**: 421–8.
27. Mannavola D, Persani L, Vannucchi G, Zanardelli M, Fugazzola L, Verga U, *et al.* Different response to chronic somatostatin analogues in patients with central hyperthyroidism. *Clin Endocrinol*, 2005; **62**: 176–81.
28. Losa M, Magnani P, Mortini P, Persani L, Acerno S, Giugni E, *et al.* Indium-111 pentetreotide single-photon emission tomography in patients with TSH-secreting pituitary adenomas: correlation with the effect of a single administration of octreotide on serum TSH levels. *Eur J Nucl Med*, 1997; **24**: 728–31.
29. Watanabe K, Kameya T, Yamauchi A, Yamamoto N, Kuwayama A, Takei I, *et al.* Thyrotropin-producing adenoma associated with pituitary resistance to thyroid hormone. *J Clin Endocrinol Metab*, 1993; **76**: 1025–30.
30. Kuhn JM, Arlot S, Lefebvre H, Caron P, Cortet-Rudelli C, Archambaud F, *et al.* Evaluation of the treatment of thyrotropin-secreting pituitary adenomas with a slow release formulation of the somatostatin analog lanreotide. *J Clin Endocrinol Metab*, 2000; **85**: 1487–91.

2.3.14 Pituitary carcinoma

John Ayuk, Christopher J. McCabe, Neil J.L. Gittoes

Introduction

Most pituitary adenomas are slow-growing, benign tumours. Some do, however, demonstrate aggressive growth characteristics that include infiltration of the dura, bone, and surrounding tissues. Despite such apparent aggressive features, these invasive adenomas are not considered to be truly malignant. To make a diagnosis of pituitary carcinoma requires the presence of a pituitary tumour associated with central nervous system or systemic metastases. Little is known of the pathogenesis of these tumours and the prognostication of future tumour behaviour through clinical, histopathological, or molecular analyses remains challenging (1).

Incidence

Pituitary carcinomas are very rare, representing only 0.10–0.25% of all pituitary tumours (2–4). Only around 150 cases having been reported in the English literature (4, 5). Although these tumours generally occur in the context of previously diagnosed invasive macroadenomas, the diagnosis of pituitary carcinoma requires the demonstration of cerebrospinal metastases (Fig. 2.3.14.1) and/or systemic metastases, and not simply evidence of local invasion, which is a common finding with pituitary adenomas (7).

Pathogenesis

The pathogenesis of pituitary carcinoma is unclear and there are no established markers that reliably predict later malignant transformation. Most cases of pituitary carcinoma arise from macroadenomas (8), and given the long latency to the development of metastases, current opinion suggests that they arise from benign adenomas rather than appear *de novo* as malignant tumours (2, 8). The adenoma-to-carcinoma hypothesis is supported by the observation that in most cases, similar histological findings and molecular markers are found in primary pituitary tumours and their metastases (Fig. 2.3.14.2), although some studies have reported metastatic deposits of pituitary carcinoma of distinct clonal origin from the primary tumour (9, 10).

Histopathological characteristics

The distinction between pituitary adenoma and carcinoma cannot be made on the basis of histological or ultrastructural features alone, as significant similarities exist in the ultrastructural appearance of pituitary carcinomas and their benign counterparts (11). However, increased mitotic activity and higher labelling indices for proliferation (MIB1, PCNA) have been observed in pituitary carcinomas (2), and although no particular threshold exists, brisk mitotic activity is associated with aggressive growth and malignant potential (12). Estimation of the cell cycle-specific antigen Ki-67, using the MIB1 antibody, has been shown to correlate best with invasiveness and probably prognosis (12, 13). Thapar *et al.* demonstrated that malignant and invasive tumours exhibit much higher Ki-67 labelling indices (LI) than benign adenomas (11.9% vs 4.7% vs 1.4%, respectively), with a Ki-67 index of less than 3% exhibiting a 97% specificity in distinguishing invasive from noninvasive pituitary tumours (13). Pituitary carcinomas did have significantly higher mean Ki-67 LI, but there was wide variability and overlap with the other groups, with measurements ranging from 0 to 21.9% (Fig. 2.3.14.3). This suggests that although assessment of proliferation may be helpful in arousing suspicion of subsequent tumour invasiveness and/or malignant potential, it cannot be reliably used to predict future malignant behaviour (13, 14).

Microvascular density, a marker of angiogenesis, has been examined as a potential prognostic marker of metastatic potential. A study by Vidal *et al.* showed a trend toward increased vascularity with more invasive tumours, but the trend did not reach statistical significance (15). No correlation was found between the MIB1 LI and microvascular density.

Molecular characteristics

The prediction of future tumour behaviour through molecular analysis remains challenging (1). Paradoxically, genes implicated in hereditary syndromes of pituitary tumorigenesis are rarely mutated in sporadic tumours (16), and genes involved in the initiation of pituitary tumorigenesis are not necessarily predictive of future aggressiveness or metastasis (17). Thus, molecular markers in pituitary tumours might inform us of the underlying processes driving growth and expansion of pituitary cells; however, they will not always

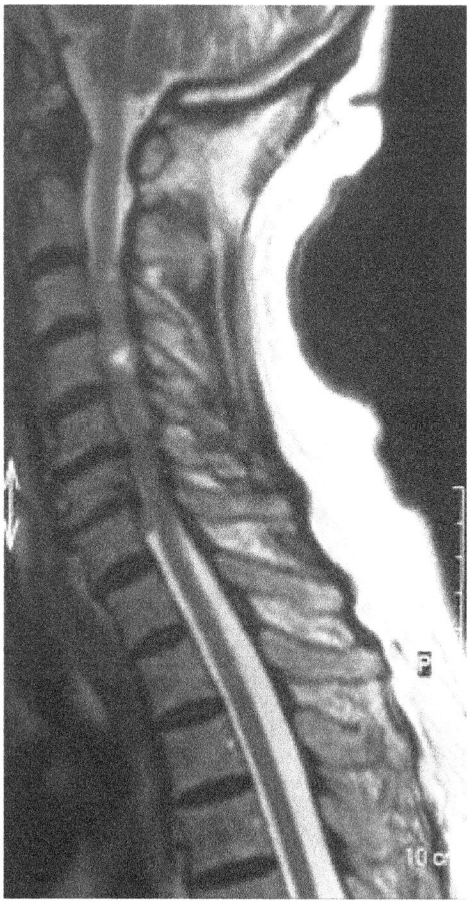

Fig. 2.3.14.1 MRI of cervical spine showing intradural, extramedullary metastatic disease between C2 and C4 from pituitary carcinoma (6).

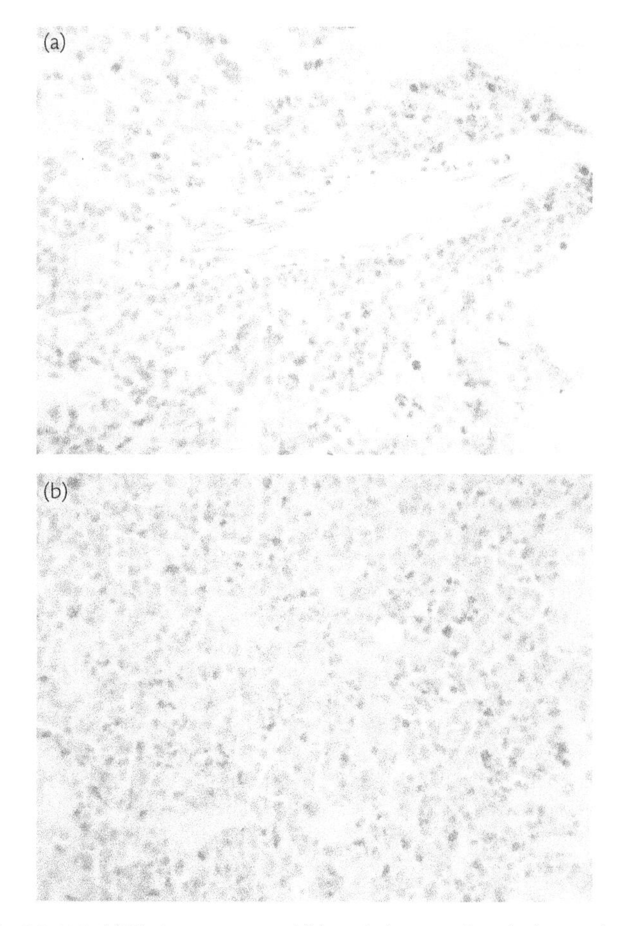

Fig. 2.3.14.2 (a) Pituitary tumour and (b) cervical metastasis excised 4 years later, both showing positive (brown) immunostaining for prolactin (6). (See also Plate 3)

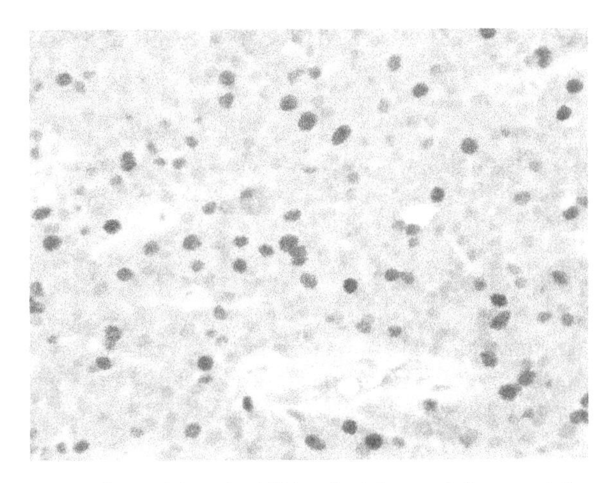

Fig. 2.3.14.3 Ki-67 staining using MIB1 antibody in a cervical metastasis from a pituitary carcinoma; the MIB1 proliferation index is around 10% (6). (See also Plate 4)

be useful in identifying the subset of tumours that will subsequently become metastatic carcinomas because, as with many tumour types, discrete processes may govern the early initiation of pituitary cell growth and the late drive towards invasion and metastasis.

Because pituitary tumours often acquire different functional characteristics as they evolve, it is likely that a number of sequential molecular events lead to ultimate carcinogenesis. As in most other tumour types, 'late stage' genes may be involved in the progression to carcinoma from an existing adenoma. Because of the relative rarity of pituitary carcinoma, large scale examination of late stage molecular events have been confined to disparate studies examining small numbers of carcinomas. However, several genes classically associated with pituitary tumorigenesis have been studied simultaneously in the context of expression and mutation in adenomas and carcinomas, enabling insight into earlier and later molecular events. Due to a dearth of data pertaining to human pituitary carcinoma, mouse models of pituitary tumorigenesis will be considered where appropriate in the following sections.

Pituitary cell proliferation and the cell cycle

Mitotic activity is generally low in pituitary tumours, even in those that are relatively aggressive, in contrast to tumours arising from more rapidly replicating tissues. The cell cycle—the process by which cells divide into daughter cells—is divided into four phases: S phase (synthesis of DNA), during which the genome is duplicated, M phase (mitosis), in which the duplicated genetic material segregates into two daughter cells, and two intervening gap (G) phases, G1 and G2. In human cells, a number of well-characterized protein kinases regulate the transition through G1, S, G2, and M. Recently, several mouse models of cell cycle regulation have revealed that pituitary tumours may show profound cell cycle dysregulation (18). Numerous other studies have dissected the contribution of other related cell cycle genes such as p27, p16, p18, and PTTG, which have provided an intricate insight into the importance of correct cell cycle regulation in pituitary cell function (18).

Rb

The original link between cell cycle regulation and the pituitary came from analysis of the retinoblastoma (Rb) mouse. The retinoblastoma protein inhibits entry into the cell cycle and progression from the G1 phase into S. Mice heterozygous for Rb demonstrate highly prevalent pituitary tumours (19), and the frequent occurrence of pituitary carcinomas, suggesting the possibility that Rb is involved in the development of these tumours. Although Rb dysregulation is not as prevalent as might have been predicted from murine data, studies have nonetheless reported loss of heterozygosity of Rb (20), and hypomethylation of the Rb promoter (21) in human pituitary tumours. One interesting case reported a woman who presented with two adjacent but histologically discrete sella tumours, one a benign adrenocorticotropic hormone (ACTH) adenoma and the other a poorly differentiated ACTH-positive carcinoma that eventually metastasized (22, 23). Interestingly, the adenoma was shown to express the Rb protein, while the carcinoma did not, suggesting that loss of Rb expression may be important in the development of some pituitary carcinomas. However, there are currently no compelling data to suggest that Rb is a frequent inducer of progression from adenoma to pituitary carcinoma.

p27

p27, in particular, has been associated with malignant change in the pituitary. The cyclin-dependent kinase inhibitor $p27^{Kip1}$ (p27) is an essential participant in the regulation of cell cycle progression. Reduced synthesis of p27 protein has been frequently observed in a variety of human malignancies, and a significant correlation between low p27 protein synthesis and high tumour grade has been described (24). p27-null mice develop pituitary adenomas (25), and reduced protein synthesis has been reported by several groups, with a particular relevance to malignant pituitary tumours (26–28), indicating that *p27* may be a strong candidate gene in pituitary tumour progression to carcinoma.

p53

p53 has previously been implicated in pituitary carcinogenesis. In a clinicopathological study of 15 cases of pituitary carcinoma, Pernicone *et al.* (2) demonstrated an increase in the percentage of nuclear staining for p53 in pituitary metastases (mean 7.3%) as compared with solitary pituitary adenomas (mean 1%). Supporting these data, Thapar *et al.* (12) described a significant association between p53 expression and tumour invasiveness, which demonstrated p53 immunohistochemical labelling in 0% of noninvasive adenomas, 15.2% of invasive tumours, and 100% of metastases. These data suggest that p53 expression analysis may be a promising avenue for assessing aggressive tumour behaviour, although one recent report failed to detect p53 expression in a malignant prolactin-secreting macroadenoma (29).

MAPK (Ras/ERK) and PI3K/Akt

The Ras/Raf/MEK/ERK and Ras/PI3K/PTEN/Akt pathways interact with each other to regulate growth, and in some cases directly promote mechanisms of tumorigenesis. The roles of MAPK and PI3K/Akt pathways in pituitary tumorigenesis are far from being fully deciphered. Although there is some evidence that there may be increased activity in both pathways, a lack of consistency across many studies suggests the existence of a complex network of several regulatory mechanisms and feedback loops that are not yet fully understood. That said, mutation of the H-ras oncogene has been observed in a subset of aggressive pituitary adenomas. In one case of a pituitary carcinoma, a mutated H-ras oncogene was detected (30), and in a separate study three distant metastatic pituitary tumour secondary deposits were shown to harbour H-ras mutations (31), together suggesting a potential role of H-ras in the progression of pituitary adenomas into their aggressive and metastatic variants. However, subsequent studies have not identified H-ras mutations as common molecular events in pituitary carcinomas.

Pik3ca

The phosphoinositide 3-kinase (PI3K)/AKT signalling pathway regulates fundamental cellular process linked to tumorigenesis, including cell proliferation, adhesion, survival, and motility (32). Mutations in the *PIK3CA* gene of the phosphoinositide 3-kinase (PI3K)/AKT pathway have been found in many human tumours. *PIK3CA* mutations occurred exclusively in invasive pituitary tumours but not in noninvasive pituitary tumours, suggesting that the PI3K/AKT pathway, when aberrantly activated by *PIK3CA* mutations, may play a role in the invasiveness of pituitary tumours (33). This finding, although important, needs to be addressed in a wide series of pituitary carcinomas.

nm23

The *nm23* gene, which is located on the long arm of chromosome 17 (17q24-25), was one of the first metastasis suppressor genes identified. In colorectal tumours, for example, reduced *nm23* expression has been demonstrated in tumour cells invading the stroma at the tumour margin compared with the centre, indicating that decreased expression of *nm23* may participate in local invasion as well (34). Reduced expression of *nm23* has also been detected in two studies of aggressive and invasive pituitary tumours (23, 35), suggesting a potential role in the progression of adenoma to metastatic carcinoma.

Non-genomic changes

Epigenetic changes in gene expression result from altered methylation and histone regulation, rather than genetic changes such as mutation. Numerous gene expression changes in pituitary tumours may in fact arise not from mutation or other genetic mechanisms, but rather from the inappropriate silencing of genes with critical functions in cell cycle and metabolism. For example, the mitotic inhibitor *p16* has been shown to be underexpressed in pituitary adenomas through hypermethylation of its promoter (36), and the tumour suppressor *MEG3* is similarly repressed through epigenetic mechanisms in nonfunctioning tumours (37). Numerous other genes, including *Rb*, have been shown to be epigenetically silenced in pituitary tumours (for a comprehensive review see Ezzat (38)). The exact impact of epigenetic changes on pituitary carcinoma may be critical, but as yet remains to be defined.

Given that genes such as *p53*, *PIK3CA*, *nm23*, and *H-ras* have been implicated in the aetiology of pituitary carcinoma, it is likely that carcinomas follow a progressive change from adenoma to carcinoma, a sequence in keeping with that found in numerous other tumour types. For example, *p53* is relatively unimportant in well-differentiated papillary and follicular thyroid tumours, but appears critical in the progression to anaplastic thyroid cancer (39); *PIK3CA* also appears particularly important in anaplastic thyroid progression (40); *nm23* has been particularly associated with malignant progression in cervical cancer (41) and *H-ras* has been shown to be predictive of oral carcinoma progression (42). The nature of the progressive change from pituitary adenoma to carcinoma has been examined through histological, molecular and loss-of heterozygosity studies, providing compelling evidence that carcinoma follows adenoma (2, 25, 27, 43). Against this, an elegant case report previously described the distinct clonal composition of a primary and metastatic ACTH-producing pituitary carcinoma (8). However, until more evidence for a potential multiclonal origin of pituitary carcinoma is generated, the consensus remains that pituitary carcinomas represent rare progressive changes in existing adenomas, whose precise molecular changes remain to be defined given their relative scarcity.

Extrinsic factors

Radiation therapy and surgery have been linked to possible malignant transformation and tumour metastatic potential, however, a significant number of reported cases of pituitary carcinoma have not been subjected to either form of treatment (7, 44). In addition, if radiation therapy and surgery were important aetiological factors, one would expect a higher incidence of cases of pituitary carcinoma, given the number of patients with pituitary adenomas treated with one or both of these treatment modalities.

Clinical features

An extensive review of the English-language literature up to 2004 identified 140 well-documented cases of pituitary carcinoma (4). Since then a further 13 cases have been reported (5, 6, 45–55) (Table 2.3.14.1). Mean age at diagnosis was 44.5 years (range 1.5–75), although reports suggest patients with GH-secreting carcinomas tend to present at a younger age (8). Both sexes were equally affected. The majority of carcinomas were endocrinologically active (88%), with 63 (41%) ACTH-secreting, 51 (33%) prolactin-secreting, 10 (7%) growth hormone-secreting, 9 (6%) luteinizing hormone/follicle-stimulating hormone (FSH)-secreting, and 2 (1%) thyroid-stimulating hormone (TSH)-secreting lesions. One tumour was reported to be cosecreting prolactin and TSH (45). Only 18 cases (12%) were reported as null-cell carcinoma, and the true proportion of endocrinologically inactive lesions is likely to be even lower, as it is possible that a significant number of those classified as clinically nonfunctioning in earlier reports may actually have represented prolactin-secreting tumours (2).

Pituitary carcinomas generally present in a similar manner to other pituitary adenomas, with symptoms due to mass effect on surrounding tissues and/or effects of hormone hypersecretion. Commonly occurring features include visual field defects, reduction in visual acuity, cranial nerve palsies, and headache. The most common features associated with hormonal hypersecretion include symptoms/signs of Cushing's syndrome, menstrual irregularities, hypopituitarism, and features of acromegaly (8).

Table 2.3.14.1 Classification of reported cases of pituitary carcinoma based on hormone secreted/cell type(4–6, 45–55)

Tumour type	n	Proportion (%)
ACTH-secreting	63	41
PRL-secreting	51	33
GH-secreting	10	7
LH/FSH-secreting	9	6
TSH-secreting	2	1
Null cell	18	12

ACTH, adrenocorticotropic hormone; GH, growth hormone; LH/FSH, luteinizing hormone/follicle-stimulating hormone; PRL, prolactin; TSH, thyroid-stimulating hormone.

Natural history

Almost all cases of pituitary carcinoma initially present as macroadenomas confined to the sella. The time interval between initial presentation with a pituitary adenoma and the diagnosis of metastatic pituitary carcinoma varies widely, ranging between 4 months and 9 years, with a median of 7 years (mean of 5 years) (2, 8). In a series of 15 pituitary carcinomas, latency interval was longest in ACTH-secreting lesions (mean 9.5 years), while the mean latency period for prolactin-secreting lesions was 4.7 years (2).

Pituitary carcinomas display a greater tendency toward systemic metastasis than craniospinal metastasis, although 13% show both patterns of spread (2). A notable exception is null-cell pituitary carcinomas, which are more predisposed to craniospinal than to systemic metastases (56). Metastasis has been reported to the cerebral cortex, cerebellum, spinal cord, leptomeninges, cervical lymph nodes, liver, lungs, ovaries, and bone.

The endocrine behaviour of pituitary carcinomas is variable and generally does not permit differentiation from adenomas. However, in secretory tumours, the finding of very high levels of prolactin, ACTH, or growth hormone in spite of surgical clearance or necrosis of the primary tumour may indicate the presence of metastases (57). Worsening of the secretory state has been observed in patients with partial or complete resistance to dopamine agonists in malignant prolactinomas and to somatostatin analogues in patients with growth hormone-secreting carcinomas (13). Sudden or progressive reduction of tumour hormonogenesis, presumably due to tumour dedifferentiation, has also been described (13).

Survival

The diagnosis of pituitary carcinoma carries a poor prognosis. Fewer than 40% of patients survive beyond 1 year following identification of metastases (2). Mean survival ranges between 2 and 4 years (2, 13), although outcomes are worse for patients with ACTH-secreting tumours (mean survival 17 months) (58) and those with systemic metastatic disease (2). Occasionally, however, long-term survival has been reported (58).

Management of pituitary carcinoma

The rarity of pituitary carcinoma means that most published data exist in the form of case reports, rendering it a difficult subject for audit; hence there are no evidence-based standards of optimum care for these patients. Current imaging modalities, notably CT and MRI allow detection of pituitary pathology with high sensitivity. More recently, ^{111}In-labelled octreotide scintigraphy and positron emission tomography scanning using ^{18}F-labelled deoxyglucose as radiolabelled tracer have been used to identify metastases from pituitary carcinomas (13). Regular use of these and other imaging modalities may lead to the identification of clinically unapparent metastases; however, the clinical significance of this is yet to be established.

Surgery is rarely curative, although repeated resections of recurrent metastases have been reported to prolong survival in some cases (2), and even achieve complete tumour removal (8). In most cases, radiation therapy only has a palliative effect, although radiotherapy to central nervous system metastases may arrest growth or even induce partial regression (59, 60). Experience with stereotactic radiotherapy (8, 61) and gamma-knife radiosurgery (62, 63) to date has been limited, with variable but generally poor results.

Dopamine agonists have a role in the early management of PRL prolactin-producing pituitary carcinomas, but the tumours typically develop drug resistance (2, 8). A significant number of neuroendocrine tumours express somatostatin receptors, and labelled somatostatin analogues have been used to detect metastatic lesions from pituitary carcinomas (64, 65). However, expression of somatostatin receptors and uptake of labelled octreotide does not necessarily translate into somatostatin analogue-induced tumour growth suppression, and to date the use of octreotide has had little therapeutic effect in the management of pituitary carcinomas (8).

Various regimens of cytotoxic chemotherapy have been used, particularly in patients with systemic metastases, Temozolomide is an oral alkylating agent which has been used successfully in the management of several central nervous system malignancies. It readily crosses the blood–brain barrier and is not cell-cycle specific, which confers an advantage when treating relatively slow-growing pituitary tumours (52). Several recent case studies have reported on successful use of temozolomide in the management of aggressive pituitary tumours (80,81) and pituitary carcinomas (52,55,65). In four cases of pituitary carcinoma, treatment with temozolomide resulted in reduction in tumour mass and metastases, as well as a return to near-normal prolactin levels in the three subjects with prolactin-secreting pituitary carcinomas (52,55,65). These effects persisted for up to 24 months following treatment. An interesting finding in a number of these cases was that tumours expressing low levels of O(6)-methylguanine-DNA methyltransferase (MGMT), a DNA repair protein that counteracts the effect of temozolomide, were more likely to respond to treatment (65,82). Given the small number of cases reported, further studies are required to validate the use of temozolomide for the treatment of pituitary carcinomas and to determine the full utility of MGMT immunohistochemistry in predicting response to temozolomide therapy in these patients.

Conclusions

Pituitary carcinoma is rare but an awareness of the diagnosis is important in patients with previously diagnosed pituitary adenoma who present with neurological dysfunction or other signs of disseminated malignancy. Although several genes classically associated with pituitary tumorigenesis have been studied in the context of expression and mutation in adenomas and carcinomas, none have so far been found to reliably identify the subset of tumours that will subsequently become metastatic carcinomas. Increased mitotic activity and higher labelling indices for proliferation have been observed in pituitary carcinomas, but although assessment of proliferation may be helpful in arousing suspicion of subsequent tumour invasiveness and/or malignant potential, it cannot be reliably used to predict future malignant behaviour. Current therapeutic modalities are rarely curative, and once metastases develop, the prognosis is relatively poor. Surgery and radiotherapy are generally palliative, although repeated resections of recurrent metastases have been reported to prolong survival in some cases. Somatostatin analogues generally fail to control tumour growth in hormone-secreting pituitary carcinomas, and overall response to currently used chemotherapeutic agents is relatively poor, although initial reports on the use of temozolomide are promising. Further research is required, directed principally at identifying reliable prognostic markers for pituitary carcinoma and developing effective treatment strategies.

References

1. Grossman AB. The 2004 World Health Organization classification of pituitary tumors: is it clinically helpful? *Acta Neuropathol*, 2006; **111**: 76–7.

2. Pernicone PJ, Scheithauer BW, Sebo TJ, Kovacs KT, Horvath E, Young WF Jr, *et al.* Pituitary carcinoma: a clinicopathologic study of 15 cases. *Cancer*, 1997; **79**: 804–12.
3. Kaltsas GA, Grossman AB. Malignant pituitary tumours. *Pituitary*, 1998; **1**: 69–81.
4. Ragel BT, Couldwell WT. Pituitary carcinoma: a review of the literature. *Neurosurg Focus*, 2004; **16**: E7.
5. Pinchot SN, Sippel R, Chen H. ACTH-producing carcinoma of the pituitary with refractory Cushing's Disease and hepatic metastases: a case report and review of the literature. *World J Surg Oncol*, 2009; **7**: 39.
6. Ayuk J, Natarajan G, Geh JI, Mitchell RD, Gittoes NJ. Pituitary carcinoma with a single metastasis causing cervical spinal cord compression. Case report. *J Neurosurg Spine*, 2005; **2**: 349–53.
7. Scheithauer BW, Kovacs KT, Laws ER Jr, Randall RV. Pathology of invasive pituitary tumors with special reference to functional classification. *J Neurosurg*, 1986; **65**: 733–44.
8. Kaltsas GA, Grossman AB. Malignant pituitary tumours. *Pituitary*, 1998; **1**: 69–81.
9. Zahedi A, Booth GL, Smyth HS, Farrell WE, Clayton RN, Asa SL, *et al.* Distinct clonal composition of primary and metastatic adrencorticotrophic hormone-producing pituitary carcinoma. *Clin Endocrinol (Oxf)*, 2001; **55**: 549–56.
10. Buch H, El Hadd T, Bicknell J, Simpson DJ, Farrell WE, Clayton RN. Pituitary tumours are multiclonal from the outset: evidence from a case with dural metastases. *Clin Endocrinol (Oxf)*, 2002; **56**: 817–22.
11. Scheithauer BW, Fereidooni F, Horvath E, Kovacs K, Robbins P, Tews D, *et al.* Pituitary carcinoma: an ultrastructural study of eleven cases. *Ultrastruct Pathol*, 2001; **25**: 227–42.
12. Thapar K, Scheithauer BW, Kovacs K, Pernicone PJ, Laws ER Jr. p53 expression in pituitary adenomas and carcinomas: correlation with invasiveness and tumor growth fractions. *Neurosurgery*, 1996; **38**: 763–70.
13. Kaltsas GA, Nomikos P, Kontogeorgos G, Buchfelder M, Grossman AB. Clinical review: Diagnosis and management of pituitary carcinomas. *J Clin Endocrinol Metab*, 2005; **90**: 3089–99.
14. Turner HE, Wass JA. Are markers of proliferation valuable in the histological assessment of pituitary tumours?. *Pituitary*, 1999; **1**: 147–51.
15. Vidal S, Kovacs K, Horvath E, Scheithauer BW, Kuroki T, Lloyd RV. Microvessel density in pituitary adenomas and carcinomas. *Virchows Arch*, 2001; **438**: 595–602.
16. Grossman AB. The molecular biology of pituitary tumors: a personal perspective. *Pituitary*, 2008; **14**: 757–63.
17. Al-Shraim MA, sa SL. The 2004 World Health Organization classification of pituitary tumors: what is new? *Acta Neuropathol*, 2006; **111**: 1–7.
18. Quereda V Malumbres M. Cell cycle control of pituitary development and disease. *J Mol Endocrinol*, 2009; **42**: 75–86.
19. Jacks T, Fazeli A, Schmitt EM, Bronson RT, Goodell MA, Weinberg RA. Effects of an Rb mutation in the mouse. *Nature*, 1992; **359**: 295–300.
20. Pei L, Melmed S, Scheithauer B, Kovacs K, Benedict WF, Prager D. Frequent loss of heterozygosity at the retinoblastoma susceptibility gene (RB) locus in aggressive pituitary tumors: evidence for a chromosome 13 tumor suppressor gene other than RB. *Cancer Res*, 1995; **55**: 1613–16.
21. Simpson DJ, Hibberts NA, McNicol AM, Clayton RN, Farrell WE. Loss of pRb expression in pituitary adenomas is associated with methylation of the RB1 CpG island. *Cancer Res*, 2000; **60**: 1211–16.
22. Hinton DR, Hahn JA, Weiss MH, Couldwell WT. Loss of Rb expression in an ACTH-secreting pituitary carcinoma. *Cancer Lett*, 1998; **126**: 209–14.
23. Takino H, Herman V, Weiss M, Melmed S. Purine-binding factor (nm23) gene expression in pituitary tumors: marker of adenoma invasiveness. *J Clin Endocrinol Metab*, 1995; **80**: 1733–8.
24. Sgambato A, Cittadini A, Faraglia B, Weinstein IB. Multiple functions of p27(Kip1) and its alterations in tumor cells: a review. *J Cell Physiol*, 2000; **183**: 18–27.
25. Nakayama K, Ishida N, Shirane M, Inomata A, Inoue T, Shishido N, *et al.* Mice lacking p27(Kip1) display increased body size, multiple organ hyperplasia, retinal dysplasia, and pituitary tumors. *Cell*, 1996; **85**: 707–20.
26. Korbonits M, Chahal HS, Kaltsas G, Jordan S, Urmanova Y, Khalimova Z, *et al.* Expression of phosphorylated p27(Kip1) protein and Jun activation domain-binding protein 1 in human pituitary tumors. *J Clin Endocrinol Metab*, 2002; **87**: 2635–43.
27. Lidhar K, Korbonits M, Jordan S, Khalimova Z, Kaltsas G, Lu X, *et al.* Low expression of the cell cycle inhibitor p27Kip1 in normal corticotroph cells, corticotroph tumors, and malignant pituitary tumors. *J Clin Endocrinol Metab*, 1999; **84**: 3823–30.
28. Scheithauer BW, Gaffey TA, Lloyd RV, Sebo TJ, Kovacs KT, Horvath E, *et al.* Pathobiology of pituitary adenomas and carcinomas. *Neurosurgery*, 2006; **59**: 341–53.
29. Crusius PS, Forcelini CM, Mallmann AB, Silveira DA, Lersch E, Seibert CA, *et al.* Metastatic prolactinoma: case report with immunohistochemical assessment for p53 and Ki-67 antigens. *Arq Neuropsiquiatr*, 2005; **63**: 864–9.
30. Karga HJ, Alexander JM, Hedley-Whyte ET, Klibanski A, Jameson JL. Ras mutations in human pituitary tumors. *J Clin Endocrinol Metab*, 1992; **74**: 914–19.
31. Pei L, Melmed S, Scheithauer B, Kovacs K, Prager D. H-ras mutations in human pituitary carcinoma metastases. *J Clin Endocrinol Metab*, 1994; **78**: 842–6.
32. Samuels Y Ericson K. Oncogenic PI3K and its role in cancer. *Curr Opin Oncol*, 2006; **18**: 77–82.
33. Lin Y, Jiang X, Shen Y, Li M, Ma H, Xing M, *et al.* Frequent mutations and amplifications of the PIK3CA gene in pituitary tumors. *Endocr Relat Cancer*, 2009; **16**: 301–10.
34. Campo E, Miquel R, Jares P, Bosch F, Juan M, Leone A, *et al.* Prognostic significance of the loss of heterozygosity of Nm23-H1 and p53 genes in human colorectal carcinomas. *Cancer*, 1994; **73**: 2913–21.
35. Pan LX, Chen ZP, Liu YS, Zhao JH. Magnetic resonance imaging and biological markers in pituitary adenomas with invasion of the cavernous sinus space. *J Neurooncol*, 2005; **74**: 71–6.
36. Farrell WE, Clayton RN. Epigenetic change in pituitary tumorigenesis. *Endocr Relat Cancer*, 2003; **10**: 323–30.
37. Gejman R, Batista DL, Zhong Y, Zhou Y, Zhang X, Swearingen B, *et al.* Selective loss of MEG3 expression and intergenic differentially methylated region hypermethylation in the MEG3/DLK1 locus in human clinically nonfunctioning pituitary adenomas. *J Clin Endocrinol Metab*, 2008; **93**: 4119–25.
38. Ezzat S. Epigenetic control in pituitary tumors. *Endocr J*, 2008; **55**: 951–7.
39. Taccaliti A, Boscaro M. Genetic mutations in thyroid carcinoma. *Minerva Endocrinol*, 2009; **34**: 11–28.
40. Santarpia L, El-Naggar AK, Cote GJ, Myers JN, Sherman SI. Phosphatidylinositol 3-kinase/akt and ras/raf-mitogen-activated protein kinase pathway mutations in anaplastic thyroid cancer. *J Clin Endocrinol Metab*, 2008; **93**: 278–84.
41. Branca M, Giorgi C, Ciotti M, Santini D, Di BL, Costa S, *et al.* Down-regulated nucleoside diphosphate kinase nm23-H1 expression is unrelated to high-risk human papillomavirus but associated with progression of cervical intraepithelial neoplasia and unfavourable prognosis in cervical cancer. *J Clin Pathol*, 2006; **59**: 1044–51.
42. Shah NG, Trivedi TI, Tankshali RA, Goswami JA, Shah JS, Jetly DH, *et al.* Molecular alterations in oral carcinogenesis: significant risk predictors in malignant transformation and tumor progression. *Int J Biol Markers*, 2007; **22**: 132–43.
43. Gaffey TA, Scheithauer BW, Lloyd RV, Burger PC, Robbins P, Fereidooni F, *et al.* Corticotroph carcinoma of the pituitary: a clinicopathological study. Report of four cases. *J Neurosurg*, 2002; **96**: 352–60.
44. Taylor WA, Uttley D, Wilkins PR. Multiple dural metastases from a pituitary adenoma. *Case report. J Neurosurg*, 1994; **81**: 624–6.

45. Brown RL, Muzzafar T, Wollman R, Weiss RE. A pituitary carcinoma secreting TSH and prolactin: a non-secreting adenoma gone awry. *Eur J Endocrinol*, 2006; **154**: 639–43.
46. Tena-Suck ML, Salinas-Lara C, Sanchez-Garcia A, Rembao-Bojorquez D, Ortiz-Plata A. Late development of intraventricular papillary pituitary carcinoma after irradiation of prolactinoma. *Surg Neurol*, 2006; **66**: 527–33.
47. Fadul CE, Kominsky AL, Meyer LP, Kingman LS, Kinlaw WB, Rhodes CH, *et al*. Long-term response of pituitary carcinoma to temozolomide. Report of two cases. *J Neurosurg*, 2006; **105**: 621–6.
48. Siddiqui A, ABashir SH. Giant pituitary macroadenoma at the age of 4 months: case report and review of the literature. *Childs Nerv Syst*, 2006; **22**: 290–4.
49. Kumar K, Wilson JR, Li Q, Phillipson R. Pituitary carcinoma with subependymal spread. *Can J Neurol Sci*, 2006; **33**: 329–32.
50. Sivan M, Nandi D, Cudlip S. Intramedullary spinal metastasis (ISCM) from pituitary carcinoma. *J Neurooncol*, 2006; **80**: 19–20.
51. Koyama J, Ikeda K, Shose Y, Kimura M, Obora Y, Kohmura E. Long-term survival with non-functioning pituitary carcinoma - case report -. *Neurol Med Chir (Tokyo)*, 2007; **47**: 475–8.
52. Guastamacchia E, Triggiani V, Tafaro E, De Tommasi A, De Tommasi C, Luzzi S, *et al*. Evolution of a prolactin-secreting pituitary microadenoma into a fatal carcinoma: a case report. *Minerva Endocrinol*, 2007; **32**: 231–6.
53. Brown RL, Wollman R, Weiss RE. Transformation of a pituitary macroadenoma into to a corticotropin-secreting carcinoma over 16 years. *Endocr Pract*, 2007; **13**: 463–71.
54. Manahan MA, Dackiw AP, Ball DW, Zeiger MA. Unusual case of metastatic neuroendocrine tumor. *Endocr Pract*, 2007; **13**: 72–6.
55. Mamelak AN, Carmichael JD, Park P, Bannykh S, Fan X, Bonert HV. Atypical pituitary adenoma with malignant features. *Pituitary*, 24 October 2008; [Epub ahead of print]
56. Sivan M. Metastases from nonfunctioning pituitary carcinomas. *Neurosurg Focus*, 2005; **19**: E11.
57. Doniach I. Pituitary carcinoma, In: Sheaves R, Jenkins P, Wass JA, eds. *Clinical Endocrine Oncology*. Oxford: Blackwell Science, 1997: 225–7
58. Landman RE, Horwith M, Peterson RE, Khandji AG, Wardlaw SL. Long-term survival with ACTH-secreting carcinoma of the pituitary: a case report and review of the literature. *J Clin Endocrinol Metab*, 2002; **87**: 3084–9.
59. Martin NA, Hales M, Wilson CB. Cerebellar metastasis from a prolactinoma during treatment with bromocriptine. *J Neurosurg*, 1981; **55**: 615–19.
60. Wilson DF. Pituitary carcinoma occurring as middle ear tumor. *Otolaryngol Head Neck Surg*, 1982; **90**: 665–6.
61. Hurel SJ, Harris PE, McNicol AM, Foster S, Kelly WF, Baylis PH. Metastatic prolactinoma: effect of octreotide, cabergoline, carboplatin and etoposide; immunocytochemical analysis of proto-oncogene expression. *J Clin Endocrinol Metab*, 1997; **82**: 2962–5.
62. Cartwright DM, Miller TR, Nasr AJ. Fine-needle aspiration biopsy of pituitary carcinoma with cervical lymph node metastases: a report of two cases and review of the literature. *Diagn Cytopathol*, 1994; **11**: 68–73.
63. Harada K, Arita K, Kurisu K, Tahara H. Telomerase activity and the expression of telomerase components in pituitary adenoma with malignant transformation. *Surg Neurol*, 2000; **53**: 267–74.
64. Greenman Y, Woolf P, Coniglio J, O'Mara R, Pei L, Said JW, *et al*. Remission of acromegaly caused by pituitary carcinoma after surgical excision of growth hormone-secreting metastasis detected by 111-indium pentetreotide scan. *J Clin Endocrinol Metab*, 1996; **81**: 1628–33.
65. Garrao AF, Sobrinho LG, Pedro O, Bugalho MJ, Boavida JM, Raposo JF, *et al*. ACTH-producing carcinoma of the pituitary with haematogenic metastases. *Eur J Endocrinol*, 1997; **137**: 176–80.

2.3.15 Pituitary incidentalomas

Niki Karavitaki

Definition

A pituitary incidentaloma is defined strictly as a 'totally asymptomatic nonfunctional tumour, clinically and biochemically silent, which was discovered incidentally on a patient who is asymptomatic' or, less strictly, a pituitary mass discovered in the course of evaluation for an unrelated problem (1, 2). Based on the second definition, the term incidentaloma may not be appropriate to many of these lesions, as an incidentally detected macroadenoma may still be clinically relevant.

Frequency of detection—pathology

Pituitary masses in autopsy series have been described in 1.5–26.7% of cases (3). The detection of incidental pituitary lesions on imaging depends on the modality used, the administration of contrast agents, and the slice thickness used (4). Pituitary incidentalomas have been reported with increasing frequency paralleling the advances in imaging techniques and the wider use of brain scans. The prevalence of pituitary incidentalomas found by CT ranges from 3.7% to 20% and of those found by MRI is 10% (5). In a recent community-based, cross-sectional study including 81 149 inhabitants, two out of 63 pituitary adenomas (3.2%) were incidentally

Box 2.3.15.1 Differential diagnoses of pituitary incidentalomas

- Pituitary adenomas (functioning (growth hormone, prolactin, follicle-stimulating hormone/luteinizing hormone, adrenocorticotropic hormone, thyroid-stimulating hormone), nonfunctioning)
- Germ cell tumours (germinoma, dermoid, teratoma)
- Gliomas
- Craniopharyngioma
- Rathke's cleft cyst
- Meningioma
- Chordoma
- Primary lymphoma
- Pituitary carcinoma
- Metastasis
- Arachnoid cyst
- Haemorrhage
- Inflammatory lesions (e.g. sarcoidosis, hypophysitis, histiocytosis X)
- Infectious lesions (e.g. abscess, tuberculosis)
- Aneurysm
- Hypertrophy

found giving a prevalence of 2.5 cases/100 000 inhabitants (6). They are more common with increasing age (7). The majority of lesions reported in autopsy studies are microadenomas. Interestingly, among a total of 12 411 pituitaries from autopsy studies, the average frequency of finding an adenoma was 11.3% and all but three tumours had a diameter less than 10 mm (3). Furthermore, radiological studies on individuals undergoing imaging for reasons not related to the pituitary have found a frequency of macroadenomas between 0.16% and 0.20% (2). Apart from adenomas, the differential diagnosis is extensive and is shown in Box 2.3.15.1. Autopsy specimens have shown that in case of adenomas, the immunohistochemical staining is negative in 41–50% (4) and prolactin positive in 25–41% (8).

Diagnostic evaluation

A cost-effective approach is required to exclude potentially harmful conditions, as well as to decrease patient anxiety. Imaging techniques are helpful in the diagnostic evaluation of an incidentally found pituitary mass. MRI has been proven to be more sensitive than CT for the detection of pituitary adenomas (9). CT is superior in detecting calcifications and is therefore, helpful for the diagnosis of craniopharyngiomas and meningiomas (10). There are no studies providing correlation between MRI and pathological features of pituitary masses. Nevertheless, specific MRI features of a number of sellar masses (including meningiomas, metastatic disease, craniopharyngiomas, Rathke's cleft cysts, arachnoid cysts, hypophysitis, abscess) may be useful in the differentiation from an adenoma (11).

Given that the most common lesion in the sella area is a pituitary adenoma, assessment for hormonal hypersecretion is recommended. This includes clinical evaluation for relevant manifestations combined with biochemical screening for hormonal excess:

- prolactin (two to three measurements) for prolactinomas
- insulin-like growth factor 1, which in cases of suspected acromegaly could be combined with an oral glucose tolerance test
- 24-h urine free cortisol and overnight dexamethasone suppression test for Cushing's disease
- thyroid-stimulating hormone (TSH), free T_4 and free T_3 for TSH-secreting tumour
- follicle-stimulating hormone, luteinizing hormone, α-subunit, oestradiol, or testosterone for functioning gonadotroph adenomas

Notably, epidemiological data (although limited) suggest that functioning adenomas are uncommon among the incidentalomas (12). Microadenomas do not generally compromise the pituitary function and therefore, evaluation for hypopituitarism in warranted in patients with larger lesions. In such cases, assessment of the visual fields should also be performed.

Table 2.3.15.1 Natural history of pituitary incidentalomas.

Series	Number of subjects	Size of lesion	Follow-up duration	Outcome
Reincke *et al.*, 1990 (13)	14	≥1 cm, n = 7 <1 cm, n = 7	Median 22 months	Increase (all with intact visual acuity): • 14% of those with mass <1 cm, • 29% of those with mass >1 cm. Regression: • 14% of those with mass <1 cm, • 0% of those with mass >1 cm
Donovan and Corenblum, 1995 (14)	31	>1 cm, n = 16 <1 cm, n = 15	>1 cm mean 6.7 years >1 cm mean 6.1 years	Increase: • 25% of those with mass >1 cm (one developed visual deterioration and was treated surgically), • 0% of those with mass <1 cm
Nishizawa *et al.*, 1998 (15)	28	>1 cm, n = 28 (n = 24 grade A and n = 4 grade B, Hardy's classification)	Mean 5.6 years	Increase: • 7% (both grade B) (developed apoplexy, treated surgically)
Feldkamp *et al.*, 1999 (16)	50	>1 cm, n = 19 <1 cm, n = 31	Mean 2.7 years	Increase: • 3% of those with mass <1 cm, • 26% of those with mass >1 cm Decrease: • 3% of those with mass <1 cm, • 5% of those with mass >1 cm
Sanno *et al.*, 2003 (17)	242	–	Mean 26.9 months	Increase: • 12% (among them, 67% had initial size >1 cm and none had shown visual disturbance) Decrease: • 12%
Arita *et al.*, (2006) (18)	42	<1 cm, n = 5 >1 cm, n = 37	61.9 months	Lesion's height surpassing 110% of its initial measured height (48% had visual deterioration, diplopia or hypopituitarism): • 40% of those with mass <1 cm, • 51% of those with mass >1 cm • Apoplexy developed in 9.5% of total group

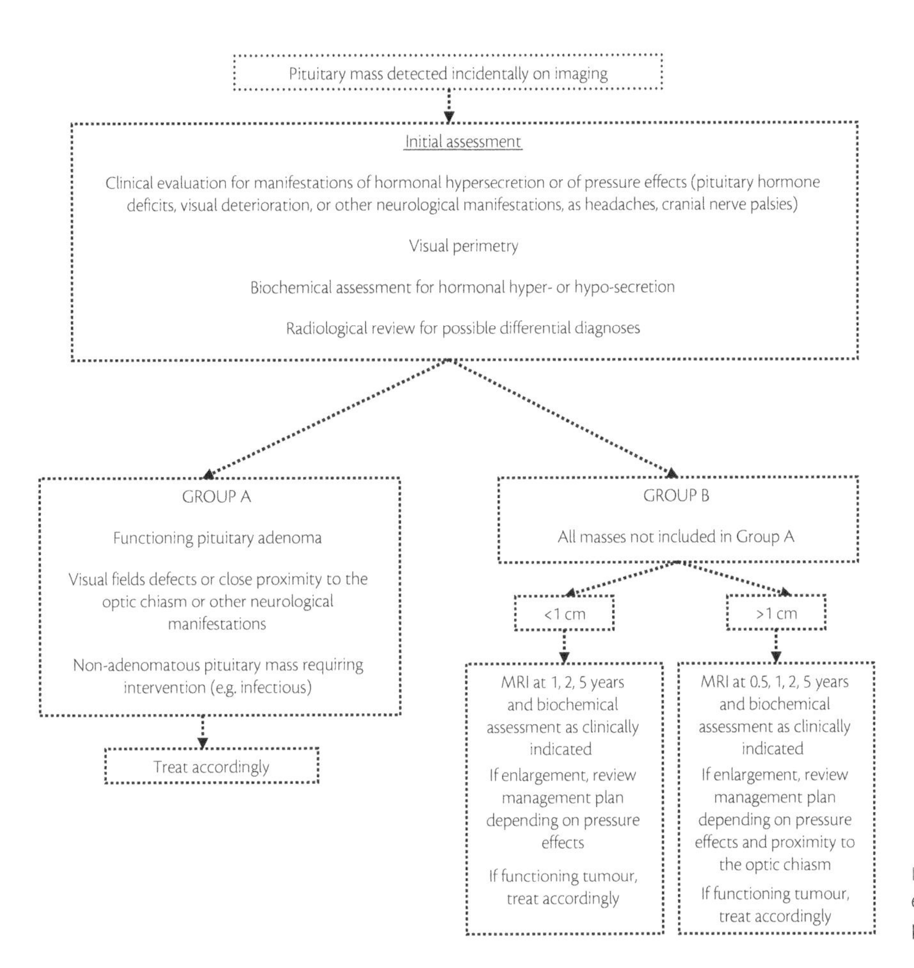

Fig. 2.3.15.1 Algorithm for the evaluation and management of pituitary incidentalomas.

Natural history

Studies on the natural history of pituitary incidentalomas are limited. Their results, including masses of various pathologies, are summarized in Table 2.3.15.1. With the exception of the Arita *et al.* series (18), in which the number of lesions less than 1 cm in size was small, published data suggest that microincidentalomas follow a benign course. In contrast, masses greater than 1 cm in size are associated with higher risk of enlargement often leading to pressure effects and requiring neurosurgical intervention. These data are in accord with the reported outcome of nonoperated nonfunctioning pituitary adenomas (during a mean follow-up period of 42 months, 12.5% of the microadenomas and 50% of the macroadenomas increased in size) (19). Furthermore, the risk of apoplexy should also be taken into consideration, particularly in patients exposed to predisposing factors (e.g. anticoagulation).

The potential of incidentally found adenomas to become hormonally active at a later stage has not been fully elucidated and reliable data on the chance of developing relevant endocrinopathy is lacking.

Management

The long-term natural history of incidentally detected pituitary masses is still unclear and hence, a clear consensus on their best approach has not been established as yet. Based on the significant literature available, the proposed protocol for the initial evaluation and management of these lesions is shown in Fig. 2.3.15.1. As the optimum duration of follow-up is unknown, the decisions on monitoring any mass remaining stable 5 years after its initial detection should be individualized. Finally, the cost-effectiveness of the suggested or other approaches remains to be elucidated.

References

1. Mirilas P, Skandalakis JE. Benign anatomical mistakes: incidentaloma. *Am Surg*, 2002; **68**: 725–40.
2. Krikorian A, Aron D. Evaluation and management of pituitary incidentalomas–revisiting an acquaintance. *Nat Clin Pract Endocrinol Metab*, 2006; **2**: 138–45.
3. Molitch ME. Pituitary Incidentalomas. *Endocrinol Metab Clin North Am*, 1997; **26**: 725–40.
4. Turner HE, Moore NR, Byrne JV, Wass JAH. Pituitary, adrenal and thyroid incidentalomas. *Endocr Relat Cancer*, 1998; **5**: 131–50.
5. Aron DC, Howlett TA. Pituitary Incidentalomas. *Endocrinol Metab Clin North Am*, 2000; **29**: 205–21.
6. Fernandez A, Karavitaki N, Wass JAH. Prevalence of pituitary adenomas: a community-based, cross-sectional study in Banbury (Oxfordshire, UK). *Clin Endocrinol (Oxf)*, 2010; **72**: 377–82.
7. Parent AD, Rebin J, Smith RR. Incidental pituitary adenomas. *J Neurosurg*, 1981; **54**: 228–31.
8. Ezzat S, Asa SL, Couldwell WT, Barr CE, Dodge WE, Vance ML, *et al.* The prevalence of pituitary adenomas. *Cancer*, 2004; **101**: 613–19.
9. Johnson MR, Hoare RD, Cox T, Dawson JM, Maccabe JJ, Llewelyn DE, *et al.* The evaluation of patients with suspected pituitary microadenoma: computed tomography compared to magnetic resonance imaging. *Endocrinol (Oxf)*, 1992; **36**: 335–8.
10. Karavitaki N, Cudlip S, Adams CBT, Wass JAH. (2006). Craniopharyngiomas. *Endocr Rev*, **27**: 371–97.

11. Connor SE, Penney CC. MRI in the differential diagnosis of a sellar mass. *Clin Radiol*, 2003; **58**: 20–31.
12. Chidiac RM, Aron DC. Incidentalomas: A disease of modern technology. *Endocrinol Metab Clin North Am*, 1997; **26**: 233–53.
13. Reincke M, Allolio B, Saeger W, Menzel J, Winkelmann W. The 'incidentaloma' of the pituitary gland. Is neurosurgery required? *JAMA*, 1990; **263**: 2772–6.
14. Donovan LE, Corenblum B. The natural history of the pituitary incidentaloma. *Arch Intern Med*, 1995; **155**: 181–83.
15. Nishizawa S, Ohta S, Yokoyama T, Uemura K. Therapeutic strategy for incidentally found pituitary tumours ('pituitary incidentalomas'). *Neurosurgery*, 1998; **43**: 1344–50.
16. Feldkamp J, Santen R, Harms E, Aulich A, Modder U, Scherbaum WA. Incidentally discovered pituitary lesions: high frequency of macroadenomas and hormone-secreting adenomas-results of a prospective study. *Endocrinol (Oxf)*, 1999; **51**: 109–113.
17. Sanno N, Oyama K, Tahara S, Teramoto A,Kato Y. A survey of pituitary incidentaloma in Japan. *Eur J Endocrinol*, 2003; **149**: 123–7.
18. Arita K, Tominaga A, Sugiyama K, Eguchi K, Iida K, Sumida M› *et al*. Natural course of incidentally found non-functioning pituitary adenoma, with special reference to pituitary apoplexy during follow-up examination. *J Neurosurg*, 2006; **104**: 884–91.
19. Karavitaki N, Collison K, Halliday J, Byrne JV, Price P, Cudlip S, *et al*. What is the natural history of nonoperated nonfunctioning pituitary adenomas?. *Endocrinol (Oxf)*, 2007; **67**: 938–43.

2.4

Aetiology, pathogenesis, and management of diseases of the hypothalamus

Contents

2.4.1 Hypothalamic dysfunction (hypothalamic syndromes)

M. Guftar Shaikh

Introduction

The hypothalamus is a complex area of the brain and is important in co-coordinating signals between the nervous system and the endocrine system, primarily via the pituitary gland. Various processes throughout life, such as birth, puberty, and pregnancy, as well as neurological and psychiatric disorders are regulated by the hypothalamus (1). It influences many hormonal and behavioural circadian rhythms, as well as being involved in the control of body temperature, hunger, and thirst. Damage to the hypothalamus whether it is congenital or acquired will lead to significant clinical morbidity (Box 2.4.1.1). Recent advances in molecular techniques and improved neuroimaging, particularly MRI and positron emission tomography (PET) have given us a better understanding of hypothalamic syndromes and their clinical manifestations.

It may be very difficult to differentiate between hypothalamic and pituitary disease as the endocrine abnormalities are often similar. As the hypothalamus regulates both endocrine and autonomic function, there is usually a combination of endocrine and neurological disturbance in hypothalamic damage. This includes abnormal behaviour, eating disorders, and thermoregulation.

The hypothalamus consists of a number of different nuclei which have very specific functions and also secretion of hypothalamic hormones and neuropeptides (1). The clinical syndrome will depend on the location and extent of the underlying lesion. The lesion may be very small and only affect specific hypothalamic nuclei which will result in discrete symptoms; however larger lesions, which are more likely, will present with a variety of problems (Fig. 2.4.1.1). The endocrine abnormalities seen in hypothalamic syndromes usually result in pituitary hyposecretion; however due to loss of inhibitory factors hypersecretion can also occur.

Children and adolescents usually present with growth failure and disorders of puberty, which can be both delayed and precious. Adults with hypothalamic dysfunction can present with dementia, disturbances in appetite and sleep, as well as hormonal deficiencies. Causes of hypothalamic damage, particularly the anterior hypothalamus, include tumours such as craniopharyngiomas, optic nerve gliomas, and inflammatory conditions such as histiocytosis and sarcoidosis.

Clinical features

These include both endocrine and nonendocrine neurological features (Box 2.4.1.2). It can be difficult to distinguish between them, as endocrine dysfunction can also lead to hypothermia, lethargy, and abnormalities in sodium and water balance, which may be due to inadequate replacement of pituitary hormones.

Due to the variability of presentation of hypothalamic dysfunction, the clinician needs to maintain a high index of suspicion, particularly when there is a combination of endocrine and neurological abnormalities. A history of cranial surgery, especially pituitary, cranial radiotherapy and trauma to the head are risk factors

Box 2.4.1.1 Aetiology of hypothalamic syndromes

Congenital*[a]

- Septo-optic dysplasia
- Prader–Willi syndrome
- Hypothalamic trophic factor deficiency
- Disorders of regulation of growth
  - Isolated GHRH deficiency
  - GH-RH receptor mutations

Acquired

- Panhypopituitarism
- Meningitis
- Granulomatous disorders
- Lesions of pituitary stalk
- Craniopharyngioma
- Hypothalamic tumours
- Disorders of luteinizing hormone-releasing hormone regulation
- Precocious puberty
  - Delayed puberty
- Male
  - Kallman's syndrome
  - GnRH receptor mutations
  - Idiopathic hypogonadotrophic hypogonadism
- Female
  - Anorexia nervosa
  - Functional amenorrhoea
  - Disorders of regulation of prolactin-regulating factors
- Tumour
- Sarcoidosis
- Drug therapy
- Hypothyroidism
- Chronic irritation of chest wall, e.g. herpes zoster
- Nipple manipulation
- Disorders of regulation of corticotrophin-releasing hormone
- Loss of circadian rhythm
- Depression
- Antidiuretic hormone deficiency
  - Idiopathic/acquired

[a] Some congenital causes may not manifest themselves until later in life.

for hypothalamic damage. Symptoms and signs of hypopituitarism may be due to an abnormality in the hypothalamus rather than the pituitary gland. Visual field defects may indicate a mass lesion causing hypothalamic disturbance.

Biochemical assessment

If there is a suggestion of an endocrinopathy, either at the pituitary or hypothalamic level, basal assessment is essential, although dynamic tests may be more appropriate. In cases of cranial tumours where surgery is imminent, it should be assumed that the patient has adrenocorticotropic hormone (ACTH) deficiency and is treated with glucocorticoids during surgery and the postoperative period. The patient should remain on replacement glucocorticoid therapy until they are well enough for formal dynamic testing, which may be a few months later.

Unfortunately, dynamic assessment will not necessarily differentiate between a pituitary and hypothalamic aetiology of the hormonal deficiencies. A thyrotropin-releasing hormone (TRH) test may provide useful information. An exaggerated and delayed rise in thyroid-stimulating hormone (TSH) following administration of TRH suggests hypothalamic disruption. The need for the TRH test has been debated and its usefulness questioned as diagnosis of central hypothyroidism can be made on serial measurements of serum thyroxine alone (2, 3).

Neuroimaging

CT or MR scans are mandatory in the investigation of hypothalamic disorders to exclude mass lesions. Unfortunately no imaging techniques are easily able to diagnose hypothalamic dysfunction, although PET scans using radiolabels have demonstrated the hypothalamus to be involved in the early stages of some neurological disorders, such as Huntingdon's disease (4). PET scans together with appropriate radiolabels may be more helpful in the future. Advances in MRI such as the use of pulse sequences and perfusion weighted images may allow better evaluation of neuroendocrine disorders (5). In a study by Manuchehri and colleagues, where prolactinomas were treated with dopamine antagonists, reductions in vascularity preceded tumour shrinkage (6). This form of imaging may provide earlier information about response to treatment and the need to intensify therapy.

Endocrine abnormalities

Hypothalamic hormone deficiencies consist of TRH, corticotropin-releasing hormone (CRH), gonadotropin-releasing hormone (GnRH), and growth hormone-releasing hormone (GHRH). These can occur in isolation or in combination and without obvious hypothalamic damage, particularly if the abnormality is due to a genetic defect, such as GHRH receptor gene. The management of these hypothalamic hormone deficiencies is no different from pituitary hormone deficiencies. Hormone replacement therapy in the form of thyroxine, glucocorticoids, sex steroids, and growth hormone is recommended if indicated. In addition, desmopressin may also be needed if there is evidence of central diabetes insipidus.

Disruption of hypothalamic hormone secretion may occur due to psychosocial disorders. Children subjected to severe emotional distress can demonstrate low growth hormone levels on testing, however, when the child is placed in a better environment their growth hormone levels return to normal (7). Another situation where reversible hypothalamic disruption occurs is in anorexia and severe weight loss. This results in secondary amenorrhoea, and menstruation returns after appropriate weight gain. A similar situation is also seen in female athletes. The majority of hormonal

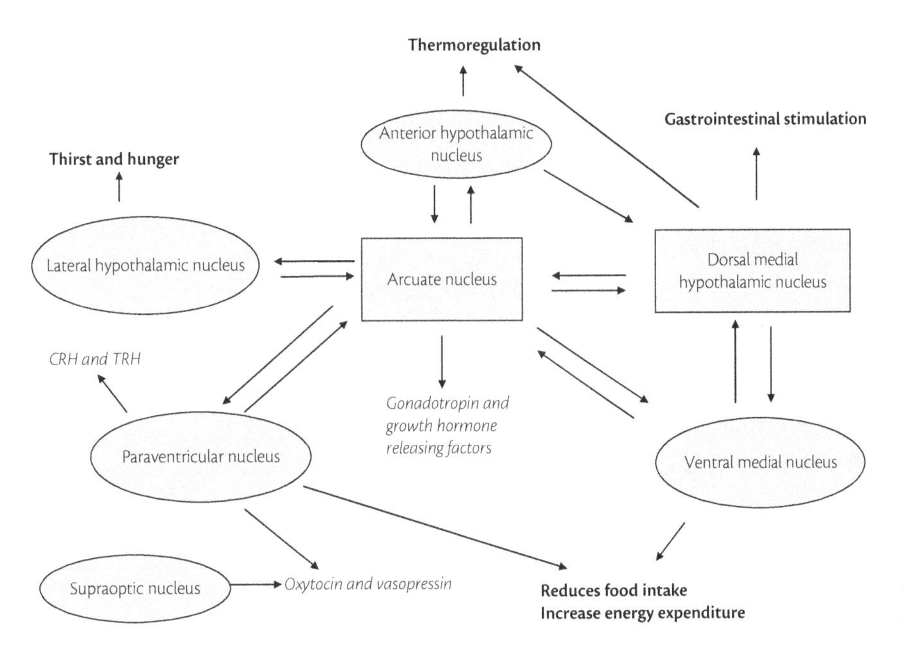

Fig. 2.4.1.1 The hypothalamic nuclei network and functions.

problems result due to loss of function, however, hypersecretion of pituitary hormones may also occur in hypothalamic disease.

Excessive GHRH secretion, due to a tumour, has been reported to cause acromegaly and gigantism. Increased secretion of GnRH will result in precocious puberty in children and may be due to a hypothalamic hamartoma. An underlying cause must always be sought in boys with precocious puberty, although a cause may not always be found in girls.

Box 2.4.1.2 Nonendocrine manifestations of hypothalamic dysfunction

Eating disorders
- Obesity
- Hyperphagia
- Anorexia

Water/sodium balance
- Adipsia/hypodipsia
- Essential hypernatraemia

Temperature regulation
- Hypothermia/hyperthermia

Behavioural problems
- Rage
- Memory loss

Sleep disorders
- Insomnia
- Somnolence

Autonomic dysfunction
- Excessive sweating
- Blood pressure control
- Cardiac arrhythmias

Hyperprolactinaemia can occur due in hypothalamic dysfunction, possibly as a result of reduced dopamine secretion. Raised prolactin levels may present with delayed puberty in children, together with galactorrhoea in girls and gynaecomastia in boys. Headaches and visual disturbance may also be a presenting feature. The prolactinomas may be part of an inherited syndrome such as multiple endocrine neoplasia type 1 (MEN 1). Prolactin level needs to be measured in any patient with a pituitary mass, as treatment for a prolactinoma is primarily medical and not surgical.

Eating disorders

Several hypothalamic sites, including the arcuate nucleus (ARC), ventromedial nucleus (VMH), paraventricular nucleus (PVN), and the lateral hypothalamic nucleus (LHN) are important in regulating feeding behaviour (8). The obesity may be due to genetic causes resulting in abnormal hypothalamic signalling or more commonly due to damage to the hypothalamus from tumours, either directly or as a result of subsequent surgery and/or radiotherapy. Damage to the LHN results in aphagia and even death by starvation, whereas damage to the other sites, particularly the VMH, leads to hyperphagia and obesity. A variety of orexigenic and anorectic peptides are produced within these hypothalamic nuclei and it is these signals that influence the neural circuitry within the hypothalamus, resulting in energy homoeostasis (8).

Leptin, secreted by adipose tissue, together with insulin, leads to the suppression of appetite via the hypothalamus, by inhibiting neuropeptide Y (NPY) and Agouti-related protein (AgRP) expression (9). NPY is a potent stimulator of food intake and this is confirmed in animals (9). Melanocortin-concentrating hormone (MCH) and AgRP also stimulate food intake (8, 9). AgRP blocks the binding of α-melanocyte stimulating hormone (α-MSH) to melanocortin receptors and reduces the anorectic activity of the melanocortin pathway (10). The increased adiposity signals, leptin and insulin, lead to neuronal synthesis of peptides such as α-MSH and cocaine and amphetamine related transcript (CART), which promote negative energy balance through the α-melanocortin pathway, by either reducing food intake or increasing energy expenditure (8, 9).

Anorexia/failure to thrive

Although anorexia nervosa is a psychiatric illness which can be related to hypothalamic dysfunction, it is important to remember hypothalamic disease may present with symptoms of anorexia. Neuroimaging may be needed to exclude hypothalamic tumours. The endocrine abnormalities associated with anorexia nervosa are not always reversible despite adequate weight gain (11).In childhood, diencephalic syndrome may present with severe failure to thrive. This is despite a normal or even excessive calorie intake. Features include emaciation, hyperactivity, and inappropriate euphoric effect. The syndrome is a result of a hypothalamic tumour near the optic chiasm, usually a glioma, and can be associated with neurofibromatosis 1. The prognosis for these children is very poor and even if they survive initially, hyperphagia and obesity usually occur.

Obesity

Hypothalamic obesity is severe and difficult to manage. Craniopharyngioma patients and patients who have received surgery and/or radiotherapy for treatment of their tumours are most at risk of developing hypothalamic damage and subsequent obesity (12–14). These individuals are also at increased risk of developing the metabolic syndrome due to the obesity and growth hormone deficiency (15). The degree of hypothalamic damage on neuroimaging is also a significant risk factor for the development of obesity (16). It is clear that damage to the VMH in rats leads to hyperinsulinaemia, hyperphagia, and insulin resistance, although the exact pathogenesis remains unclear (17). The autonomic hypothesis proposed by Bray *et al.* (18) suggests a reduction in sympathetic activity and an increase in parasympathetic activity occurs after VMH lesioning. A similar hypothesis proposed by Lustig is that damage to the VMH results in disinhibition of vagal tone at the pancreatic level (19, 20), leading to insulin hypersecretion by the pancreas and resultant obesity.

Lustig and colleagues have used octreotide, a somatostatin receptor agonist, to inhibit β cell insulin release by the pancreas. This demonstrated a reduction in weight gain and body mass index (BMI), together with improvements in insulin responses (21). These initial results were promising, however, more recent studies using a long acting form of octreotide have been variable and disappointing (22). It important to remember octreotide is expensive and not without complications.

It is still not clear whether the hyperinsulinaemia seen in these individuals is the primary driving force behind the obesity or whether the increased adiposity causes the hyperinsulinaemia. Some studies have shown no differences in insulin levels between hypothalamic obese individuals and those with simple obesity suggesting hyperinsulinaemia is a secondary phenomenon (23).

Another hormone which influences appetite is ghrelin. This is the hormone of hunger, with elevated levels during fasting. Elevated ghrelin levels have been reported in Prader–Willi syndrome, however, Kanumakala and colleagues demonstrated ghrelin levels were not raised in obesity following hypothalamic damage (24), suggesting it is not ghrelin that causes the hyperphagia.

Receptors within the hypothalamus may be affected as a result of the surgery and/or the radiation. Hypothalamic insulin receptors are important in the regulation of food intake. Knockout mice without central nervous system insulin receptors (25) and mice where hypothalamic insulin receptors are reduced (26) also develop hyperphagia and obesity.

Leptin levels have been shown to be elevated following hypothalamic obesity. This appears to be more than a reflection of the underlying obesity as the leptin levels are much higher compared to simple obese controls (23). Dysfunctional insulin and leptin receptors within the hypothalamus may have a role in hypothalamic obesity. As well as the leptin pathway, another pathway that is important in weight regulation is the melanocortin pathway.

The melanocortin pathway accounts for the gene causing the majority of genetic obesity. The mutated gene, which was discovered more than 100 years ago, is called Agouti or Agouti-signalling protein (ASIP) (27). It was not until more recently that its effect on obesity was discovered. ASIP blocks the binding of α-MSH to melanocortin receptor 1 (MC1R). ASIP was found to also block the binding of a-MSH to MC3R and MC4R, which are found within the hypothalamus and regulate food intake. MC4R mutations have been mainly identified through studies in severely obese children and account for the commonest form of genetic obesity (28).

α-MSH is produced by proteolysis of pro-opiomelanocortin C (POMC). As α-MSH binds to MC3R and MC4R to reduce food intake, mutations in *POMC* also result in obesity. Children with certain *POMC* mutations also have adrenal insufficiency, as α-MSH is composed of the first 13 amino acids of ACTH, and have red hair, as binding of α-MSH in skin (MC1R) is responsible for the hair colour (29, 30). POMC needs to be converted into different hormones including α-MSH by a protease prohormone convertase-1 (PCSK1). Mutations in PCSK1 have been reported causing hypogonadism, adrenal insufficiency, as well as obesity (31).

The genetic mutations in MC3R and MC4R, which are found within the hypothalamus, regulate food intake (27). These are expressed within the brain and result in abnormal signalling within the hypothalamus. More recently, the endocannabinoid system has been shown to be involved in appetite and energy metabolism. The cannabinoid receptors within the hypothalamus have been shown to stimulate food. Receptor antagonists have been shown to reduce appetite, together with improvements in diabetic control which cannot be due to reductions in weight alone, suggesting the cannabinoid system has an effect on a variety of organs and metabolic processes. Unfortunately, one of these drugs, rimonabant, was recently withdrawn due to an increased suicide risk.

Energy expenditure

The hypothalamus is not only involved in appetite control, but also energy expenditure (32, 33). The resting metabolic rate (which is highly variable between individuals but is consistent within individuals (34)) typically accounts for 50–65% of total daily expenditure in sedentary individuals and can be influenced by the hypothalamus, primarily through the sympathetic nervous system. Leptin deficiency, either primarily or receptor abnormalities may lead to impaired sympathetic activity and decreased thermogenesis, and although this has been demonstrated in rodents, it is unclear whether or not this occurs in humans (35). Adipocytokines, in particular adiponectin, also seem to increase energy expenditure in animals (36). Damage to the hypothalamus has been shown to result in a reduced basal metabolic rate and physical activity which will further exacerbate the obesity (37). Supra-physiological doses of thyroxine have used in the treatment of hypothalamic obesity (38).

Autonomic dysfunction

The hypothalamus and in particular the paraventricular nucleus has been shown to be an important regulator of the autonomic nervous system and can also influence gastrointestinal and cardiac function. The anterior nuclei, such as the medial preoptic nucleus, reduce heart rate and blood pressure through parasympathetic activity, whereas the posterior nucleus increases blood pressure by increasing sympathetic activity. This autonomic stimulation is mediated via a complex integrated circuitry, with influences also from nonendocrine neurons (39).Recently, a number of cytokines and hormones have been shown to stimulate neurons within the hypothalamus. This includes angiotensin II and adiponectin, which have an effect on blood pressure and glucose metabolism, respectively. Drugs which modify angiotensin II action, such as angiotensin-converting enzyme inhibitors may have a role within the hypothalamus and not just a direct cardiac action (39).

The autonomic nervous system through the hypothalamus may influence the cortisol-cortisone shuttle. Tiosano and colleagues demonstrated enhanced activity of 11β-hydroxysteroid dehydrogenase-1 (HSD) in patients with hypothalamic obesity, suggesting the hypothalamus regulates the peripheral activity of 11β-HSD (40). The increased conversion of cortisone to the active metabolite cortisol, possibly through CRF and ACTH deficiency, together with increased sympathetic tone (41), may lead to increased side effects of glucocorticoids, one of which is obesity.

Fluid balance and thirst

Osmoreceptors within the hypothalamus are involved in the regulation of sodium and water balance through the secretion of antidiuretic hormone (ADH). Deficiency of ADH leads to diabetes insipidus, causing polyuria and polyuria, which further result in hypernatraemia. The patient may maintain normal serum sodium levels and serum osmolality by drinking excessively through thirst. If the patient loses the perception of thirst, a fixed daily fluid requirement is needed in addition to desmopressin therapy. It is important to remember ADH deficiency may not manifest itself if there is also underlying ACTH deficiency. Diabetes insipidus will become evident once glucocorticoid therapy is initiated.

Disturbances in hypothalamic function may also lead to the syndrome of inappropriate ADH (SIADH), resulting in hyponatraemia, but this is usually transient.

Regulation of sleep

Sleep can be altered due to hypothalamic damage. There are both sleep promoting and arousal systems within the hypothalamus. The posterior hypothalamus is involved in the arousal network, whereas neurons in the preoptic hypothalamus have been shown to secrete the inhibitory neurotransmitter γ-aminobutyric acid (GABA) resulting in modulation of the arousal system, leading to sleep promotion and maintenance (42). Damage to the anterior hypothalamus will result in insomnia, and damage to the posterior hypothalamus will result in a hypersomnolent state.

Abnormal sleeping patterns will have an effect not only on the individual patient but also on the rest of the family, particularly parents and other siblings. If there is significant problems sleeping, a trial of melatonin is recommended, however, it is not effective in all patients, which may be related to the degree of hypothalamic disruption. If excessive sleepiness, particularly during the day is a problem, central nervous system stimulants such as modafinil can be used, although it should be used with caution as long-term use may result in dependence.

Recently discovered neuropeptides known as orexins and hypocretins may be involved not only in sleep, as they promote wakefulness, but they may also be involved in breathing. Mice lacking the orexin gene have been found to be less responsive to carbon dioxide induced increases in breathing, together with more sleep apnoeas (43). Orexins may have a role in the treatment of respiratory disorders. Disruption of sleep will also have an impact on circadian rhythms.

Temperature regulation

The anterior/preoptic and dorsomedial areas of the hypothalamus have been shown to be involved in thermoregulation. The anterior area, which contains the warm sensitive neurons, seems to the primary thermosensitive region (44). Activity within these neurons results in a fall in temperature, whereas activity in the dorsomedial nucleus leads to a rises in core temperature. The exact mechanisms by which the hypothalamus maintains core temperature remains unclear. Hypothermia can be a feature of hypothalamic disease and may reflect damage to the posterior hypothalamus (45). Paroxysmal hypothermia may also occur in association with hyperhidrosis, and is characterized by episodes of hypothermia with excessive sweating. This may be due to a resetting of the temperature set point or possibly due to increased firing of the warm sensitive neurons resulting in excessive sweating and hypothermia. There has been some beneficial effect of using muscarinic cholinergic receptor blockers to reduce sweating, such as oxybutynin or glycopyrrolate. Other drugs which have been used include clonidine, chlorpromazine, and cyproheptadine, although these centrally acting drugs have been reported to have varying success (45). It is important to ensure optimum pituitary hormone deficiencies before considering any of the above drugs.

Genetic/syndromic causes of hypothalamic dysfunction

A number of signalling molecules and transcription factors have been reported to be involved in the development of the hypothalamus and pituitary gland (46). These are discussed in more detail in Chapters 2.1 and 2.2. Although most of these affect the pituitary gland, some also lead to hypothalamic dysfunction.

Kallmann's syndrome

Classic Kallmann's syndrome is characterized by hypogonadotropic hypogonadism and is associated with anosmia/hyposmia and occasionally optic features. It can be inherited as an X-linked recessive disorder due to an abnormality in the in the *KAL1* gene, which maps to chromosome Xp22.3. This gene encodes anosmin-1, which is required to promote migration of GnRH neurons into the hypothalamus. This results in hypothalamic GnRH deficiency. Other genes which have been implicated in Kallmann's syndrome include fibroblast growth factor receptor 1 (*FGFR1*) gene and mutations in the pro-kineticin receptor-2 gene (*PROKR2*) and its ligand prokineticin 2 (PROK2) (47).

Prader–Willi syndrome

This syndrome is due to a paternal deletion of chromosome 15 or unimaternal disomy. It is associated with dysmorphic features, together with short stature, hypotonia, and hypogonadism. These children develop hyperphagia, despite having difficulty in feeding during early infancy. Growth hormone is licensed for these children primarily to improve body composition, however, provocative testing may demonstrate growth hormone deficiency possibly due to hypothalamic dysfunction (48).

Septo-optic dysplasia

This is a triad of absent septum pellucidum, optic nerve hypoplasia, and hypopituitarism, although for diagnosis only two of the triad are required. The spectrum of the disorder is variable with varying degrees of visual impairment and pituitary deficiencies. Vascular insults during embryonic development have been implicated, together with maternal drug abuse. Mutations in *HESX1* have been found in children with septo-optic dysplasia, however this accounts for a very small proportion (49). These patients can have significant hypothalamic dysfunction in the form of hyperphagia, sleep disturbance and temperature regulation as well as hormonal deficiencies. The degree of hypothalamic dysfunction is not necessarily related to the anatomical abnormality seen on neuroimaging (50).

Acquired causes of hypothalamic dysfunction

These are primarily tumours such as craniopharyngiomas, germinomas, and hamartomas and are discussed in more detail in other chapters. Other causes include inflammatory conditions such as histiocytosis and sarcoidosis. Histiocytosis is a granulomatous disorder with different clinical types and can affect skin, muscle and bone, as well as other organs. Diabetes insipidus can be a presenting feature. Pituitary hormones deficiencies although less common can occur and are usually permanent. Treatment consists of glucocorticoids and or chemotherapy depending on the response to initial therapy and histological findings at diagnosis.

Sarcoidosis, which is a systemic disease, can be associated with hyperprolactinaemia. The exact reasons for elevated prolactin levels remain unclear, but it may be due to production by T lymphocytes causing disruption of the hypothalamic dopaminergic feedback mechanism. Thyroid disease both hypothyroidism and hyperthyroidism is also common in women with sarcoidosis.

Radiotherapy for treatment of nasopharyngeal and intracranial tumours is an important cause of hypothalamic damage (51). The effects of radiotherapy on hypothalamic function may not become evident until several years after treatment. The damage to the hypothalamus is dose dependent and also the field of therapy. Somatotrophs are the most sensitive cells to radiotherapy and children present with growth failure, followed by damage to gonadotrophs, which usually presents with delayed puberty. However children who have cranial tumours may also develop precocious puberty.

Traumatic brain injury is now increasingly recognized as a cause of growth hormone deficiency and other pituitary hormones (52). This may be due to damage at the hypothalamic or pituitary level, or a combination of both.

Management

Management of hypothalamic dysfunction is primarily aimed at replacing hormonal deficiencies. Standard replacement therapy in terms of thyroxine, glucocorticoids, and, where appropriate, growth hormone and sex steroids should be initiated. Desmopressin may also be required. It is important to remember that the endocrinopathies may evolve with time in certain hypothalamic syndromes, particularly in those individuals who have had cranial tumours and subsequent radiotherapy. If glucocorticoid deficiency is suspected, replacement therapy should be started without delay, particularly if surgical intervention is urgently needed. Surgery for hypothalamic dysfunction may be appropriate, especially where tumours are responsible for the hypothalamic syndrome. The non-endocrine manifestations are more difficult to manage and usually involve a trial of therapy (Table 2.4.1.1).

Table 2.4.1.1 Medications used in the management of hypothalamic dysfunction (21, 38, 45, 53, 54)

Obesity	Octreotide Triiodothyronine Dextroamphetamine Rimonabant[a] Fenfluramine[a]
Temperature	Oxybutynin
Regulation	Glycopyrrolate Clonidine Chlorpromazine Cyproheptadine
Sleep disorders	Melatonin Modafinil

[a] These drugs are no longer available.

Octreotide and sibutramine has been used in the treatment of hypothalamic obesity with some success (21, 53). Triiodothyronine has been shown to be of benefit in a few individuals (38). Future strategies to increase energy expenditure, in particular resting metabolic rate, together with the manipulation of neuropeptides involved in appetite and weight regulation may lead to improvements in the management of hypothalamic obesity.

The autonomic dysfunction of hypothalamic syndromes is particularly difficult to manage and usually involves a trial of medication, some of which have already been mentioned. Unfortunately a lot of these therapies are not very successful. Better understanding of the neuropeptides involved in hypothalamic dysfunction, such as orexins, may result in pharmacotherapies in the future.

References

1. Swaab DF. Neuropeptides in hypothalamic neuronal disorders. *Int Rev Cytol*, 2004; **240**: 305–75.
2. Mehta A, Hindmarsh PC, Stanhope RG, Brain CE, Preece MA, Dattani MT. Is the thyrotropin-releasing hormone test necessary in the diagnosis of central hypothyroidism in children. *J Clin Endocrinol Metab*, 2003; **88**: 5696–703.
3. van Tijn DA, de Vijlder JJ, Vulsma T. Role of the thyrotropin-releasing hormone stimulation test in diagnosis of congenital central hypothyroidism in infants. *J Clin Endocrinol Metab*, 2008; **93**: 410–19.
4. Politis M, Pavese N, Tai YF, Tabrizi SJ, Barker RA, Piccini P. Hypothalamic involvement in Huntington's disease: an in vivo PET study. *Brain*, 2008; **131**: 2860–9.
5. Keogh BP. Recent advances in neuroendocrine imaging. *Curr Opin Endocrinol Diabetes Obes*, 2008; **15**: 371–5.
6. Manuchehri AM, Sathyapalan T, Lowry M, Turnbull LW, Rowland-Hill C, Atkin SL. Effect of dopamine agonists on prolactinomas

and normal pituitary assessed by dynamic contrast enhanced magnetic resonance imaging (DCE-MRI). *Pituitary*, 2007; **10**: 261–6.

7. Mouridsen SE, Nielsen S. Reversible somatotropin deficiency (psychosocial dwarfism) presenting as conduct disorder and growth hormone deficiency. *Dev Med Child Neurol*, 1990; **32**: 1093–8.
8. Sahu A. Minireview: A hypothalamic role in energy balance with special emphasis on leptin. *Endocrinology*, 2004; **145**: 2613–20.
9. Sahu A. Leptin signaling in the hypothalamus: emphasis on energy homeostasis and leptin resistance. *Front Neuroendocrinol*, 2003; **24**: 225–53.
10. Wynne K, Stanley S, McGowan B, Bloom S. Appetite control. *J Endocrinol*, 2005; **184**: 291–318.
11. Lawson EA, Klibanski A. Endocrine abnormalities in anorexia nervosa. *Nat Clin Pract Endocrinol Metab*, 2008; **4**: 407–14.
12. Tiulpakov AN, Mazerkina NA, Brook CG, Hindmarsh PC, Peterkova VA, Gorelyshev SK. Growth in children with craniopharyngioma following surgery. *Clin Endocrinol (Oxf)*, 1998; **49**: 733–8.
13. Sorva R. Children with craniopharyngioma. Early growth failure and rapid postoperative weight gain. *Acta Paediatr Scand*, 1988; **77**: 587–92.
14. Karavitaki N, Brufani C, Warner JT, Adams CB, Richards P, Ansorge O, *et al.* Craniopharyngiomas in children and adults: systematic analysis of 121 cases with long-term follow-up. *Clin Endocrinol (Oxf)*, 2005; **62**: 397–409.
15. Srinivasan S, Ogle GD, Garnett SP, Briody JN, Lee JW, Cowell CT. Features of the Metabolic Syndrome after Childhood Craniopharyngioma. *J Clin Endocrinol Metab*, 2004; **89**: 81–6.
16. de Vile CJ, Grant DB, Hayward RD, Kendall BE, Neville BG, Stanhope R. Obesity in childhood craniopharyngioma: relation to post-operative hypothalamic damage shown by magnetic resonance imaging. *J Clin Endocrinol Metab*, 1996; **81**: 2734–7.
17. Inoue S, Bray GA. An autonomic hypothesis for hypothalamic obesity. *Life Sci*, 1979; **25**: 561–6.
18. Bray GA, Inoue S, Nishizawa Y. Hypothalamic obesity. The autonomic hypothesis and the lateral hypothalamus. *Diabetologia*, 1981; **20**(Suppl): 366–77.
19. Lustig RHM. Hypothalamic Obesity: The Sixth Cranial Endocrinopathy. [Review]. *Endocrinologist*, 2002; **12**: 210–17.
20. Lustig RH. Pediatric endocrine disorders of energy balance. *Rev Endocr Metab Disord*, 2005; **6**: 245–60.
21. Lustig RH, Hinds PS, Ringwald-Smith K, Christensen RK, Kaste SC, Schreiber RE, *et al.* Octreotide therapy of pediatric hypothalamic obesity: a double-blind, placebo-controlled trial. *J Clin Endocrinol Metab*, 2003; **88**: 2586–92.
22. Lustig RH, Greenway F, Velasquez-Mieyer P, Heimburger D, Schumacher D, Smith D, *et al.* A multicenter, randomized, double-blind, placebo-controlled, dose-finding trial of a long-acting formulation of octreotide in promoting weight loss in obese adults with insulin hypersecretion. *Int J Obes (Lond)*, 2006; **30**: 331–41.
23. Shaikh MG, Grundy RG, Kirk JM. Hyperleptinaemia rather than fasting hyperinsulinaemia is associated with obesity following hypothalamic damage in children. *Eur J Endocrinol*, 2008; **159**: 791–7.
24. Kanumakala S, Greaves R, Pedreira CC, Donath S, Warne GL, Zacharin MR, *et al.* Fasting Ghrelin Levels Are Not Elevated in Children with Hypothalamic Obesity. *J Clin Endocrinol Metab*, 2005; **90**: 2691–5.
25. Bruning JC, Gautam D, Burks DJ, Gillette J, Schubert M, Orban PC, *et al.* Role of brain insulin receptor in control of body weight and reproduction. *Science*, 2000; **289**: 2122–5.
26. Obici S, Feng Z, Karkanias G, Baskin DG, Rossetti L. Decreasing hypothalamic insulin receptors causes hyperphagia and insulin resistance in rats. *Nat Neurosci*, 2002; **5**: 566–72.
27. Warden NA, Warden CH. Biological influences on obesity. *Pediatr Clin North Am*, 2001; **48**: 879–91.
28. Farooqi IS, O'Rahilly S. Recent advances in the genetics of severe childhood obesity. *Arch Dis Child*, 2000; **83**: 31–4.
29. Barsh GS, Farooqi IS, O'Rahilly S. Genetics of body-weight regulation. *Nature*, 2000; **404**: 644–51.
30. Krude H, Biebermann H, Luck W, Horn R, Brabant G, Gruters A. Severe early-onset obesity, adrenal insufficiency and red hair pigmentation caused by POMC mutations in humans. *Nat Genet*, 1998; **19**: 155–7.
31. O'Rahilly S, Gray H, Humphreys PJ, Krook A, Polonsky KS, White A, *et al.* Impaired Processing of Prohormones Associated with Abnormalities of Glucose Homeostasis and Adrenal Function. *N Engl J Med*, 1995; **333**: 1386–91.
32. Richard D. Energy expenditure: a critical determinant of energy balance with key hypothalamic controls. *Minerva Endocrinol*, 2007; **32**: 173–83.
33. Park AJ, Bloom SR. Neuroendocrine control of food intake. *Curr Opin Gastroenterol*, 2005; **21**: 228–33.
34. Goran MI, Treuth MS. Energy expenditure, physical activity, and obesity in children. *Pediatr Clin North Am*, 2001; **48**: 931–53.
35. Eikelis N, Esler M. The neurobiology of human obesity. *Exp Physiol*, 2005; **90**: 673–82.
36. Qi Y, Takahashi N, Hileman SM, Patel HR, Berg AH, Pajvani UB, *et al.* Adiponectin acts in the brain to decrease body weight. *Nat Med*, 2004; **10**: 524–9.
37. Shaikh MG, Grundy RG, Kirk JM. Reductions in basal metabolic rate and physical activity contribute to hypothalamic obesity. *J Clin Endocrinol Metab*, 2008; **93**: 2588–93.
38. Fernandes JK, Klein MJ, Ater JL, Kuttesch JF, Vassilopoulou-Sellin R. Triiodothyronine supplementation for hypothalamic obesity. *Metabolism*, 2002; **51**: 1381–3.
39. Ferguson AV, Latchford KJ, Samson WK. The paraventricular nucleus of the hypothalamus - a potential target for integrative treatment of autonomic dysfunction. *Expert Opin Ther Targets*, 2008; **12**: 717–27.
40. Tiosano D, Eisentein I, Militianu D, Chrousos GP, Hochberg Z. 11 beta-Hydroxysteroid dehydrogenase activity in hypothalamic obesity. *J Clin Endocrinol Metab*, 2003; **88**: 379–84.
41. Friedberg M, Zoumakis E, Hiroi N, Bader T, Chrousos GP, Hochberg Z. Modulation of 11{beta}-Hydroxysteroid Dehydrogenase Type 1 in Mature Human Subcutaneous Adipocytes by Hypothalamic Messengers. *J Clin Endocrinol Metab*, 2003; **88**: 385–93.
42. Szymusiak R, McGinty D. Hypothalamic regulation of sleep and arousal. *Ann N Y Acad Sci*, 2008; **1129**: 275–86.
43. Williams RH, Burdakov D. Hypothalamic orexins/hypocretins as regulators of breathing. *Expert Rev Mol Med*, 2008; **10**: e28.
44. Morrison SF, Nakamura K, Madden CJ. Central control of thermogenesis in mammals. *Exp Physiol*, 2008; **93**: 773–97.
45. Benarroch EE. Thermoregulation: recent concepts and remaining questions. *Neurology*, 2007; **69**: 1293–7.
46. Kelberman D, Dattani MT. Hypothalamic and pituitary development: novel insights into the aetiology. *Eur J Endocrinol*, 2007; **157**(Suppl 1): S3–14.
47. Mehta A, Dattani MT. Developmental disorders of the hypothalamus and pituitary gland associated with congenital hypopituitarism. *Best Pract Res Clin Endocrinol Metab*, 2008; **22**: 191–206.
48. Swaab DF. Prader-Willi syndrome and the hypothalamus. *Acta Paediatr Suppl*, 1997; **423**: 50–4.
49. McNay DE, Turton JP, Kelberman D, Woods KS, Brauner R, Papadimitriou A, *et al.* HESX1 mutations are an uncommon cause of septooptic dysplasia and hypopituitarism. *J Clin Endocrinol Metab*, 2007; **92**: 691–7.
50. Borchert M, Garcia-Filion P. The syndrome of optic nerve hypoplasia. *Curr Neurol Neurosci Rep*, 2008; **8**: 395–403.
51. Gleeson HK, Shalet SM. The impact of cancer therapy on the endocrine system in survivors of childhood brain tumours. *Endocr Relat Cancer*, 2004; **11**: 589–602.
52. Behan LA, Phillips J, Thompson CJ, Agha A. Neuroendocrine disorders after traumatic brain injury. *J Neurol Neurosurg Psychiatry*, 2008; **79**: 753–9.
53. Danielsson P, Janson A, Norgren S, Marcus C. Impact sibutramine therapy in children with hypothalamic obesity or obesity with aggravating syndromes. *J Clin Endocrinol Metab*, 2007; **92**: 4101–6.
54. Ismail D, O'Connell MA, Zacharin MR. Dexamphetamine use for management of obesity and hypersomnolence following hypothalamic injury. *J Pediatr Endocrinol Metab*, 2006; **19**: 129–34.

2.4.2 Craniopharyngiomas

Niki Karavitaki

Epidemiology

Craniopharyngiomas are rare tumours with a reported incidence of 0.13 cases per 100 000 person-years. They account for 2–5% of all the primary intracranial neoplasms, 5.6–15% of the intracranial tumours in childhood populations, in which they are the commonest lesion involving the hypothalamo-pituitary region. They may be detected at any age, even in the pre- and neonatal periods and almost half of the total cases have been described in adults. They show a bimodal age distribution with peak incidence rates in children aged 5–14 and adults aged 50–74 years (1).

Pathogenesis

Craniopharyngiomas are epithelial tumours arising along the path of the craniopharyngeal duct (the canal connecting the stomodeal ectoderm with the evaginated Rathke's pouch). Neoplastic transformation of embryonic squamous cell rests of the involuted craniopharyngeal duct or metaplasia of adenohypophyseal cells in the pituitary stalk or gland are the proposed theories (1). B-catenin gene mutations have been identified in the adamantinomatous subtype affecting exon 3, which encodes the degradation targeting box of B-catenin; this is compatible with an accumulation of nuclear B-catenin protein (a transcriptional activator of the Wnt signalling pathway). Strong B-catenin expression has been shown in the adamantinomatous subtype indicating re-activation of the Wnt signalling pathway, which is implicated in the development of several neoplasms (2).

Pathology

Craniopharyngiomas are grade I tumours according to the WHO classification. Rare cases of malignant transformation (possibly triggered by previous irradiation) have been described. Two main pathological subtypes have been reported: the adamantinomatous and the papillary, but transitional or mixed forms have also been described (1, 3).

The adamantinomatous type is the most common subtype and may occur at any age. Macroscopically these tumours have cystic and/or solid components, necrotic debris, fibrous tissue and calcification. The cysts may be multiloculated and contain liquid ranging from 'machinery oil' to shimmering cholesterol-laden fluid consisting of desquamated squamous epithelial cells, rich in membrane lipids and cytoskeleton keratin. They tend to have sharp and irregular margins, often merging into a peripheral zone of dense reactive gliosis, with abundant Rosenthal fiber formation (consisting of irregular masses of granular deposits within astrocytic processes) in the surrounding brain tissue and the vascular structures. The epithelium of the adamantinomatous type is composed of three layers of cells: a distinct palisade basal layer of small cells with darkly staining nuclei and little cytoplasm (somewhat resembling the basal cells of the epidermis of the skin), an intermediate layer of variable thickness composed of loose aggregates of stellate cells (termed stellate reticulum), whose processes traverse empty intercellular spaces, and a top layer facing into the cyst lumen with abruptly enlarged, flattened, and keratinized to flat plate-like squamous cells (Fig. 2.4.2.1). The flat squames are desquamated singly or in distinctive stacked clusters and form nodules of 'wet' keratin, which are often heavily calcified and appear grossly as white flecks. The keratinous debris may elicit an inflammatory and foreign body giant cell reaction. The presence of the typical adamantinomatous epithelium or of the 'wet' keratin alone are diagnostic, whereas features only suggestive of the diagnosis in small or non-representative specimens include fibrohistiocytic reaction, necrotic debris, calcification, and cholesterol clefts (1).

The papillary variety has been almost exclusively described in adult populations (accounts for 14–50% of the adult cases and for up to 2% of the paediatric ones). Calcification is rare and the cyst content is usually viscous and yellow. It is generally well circumscribed and infiltration of adjacent brain tissue by neoplastic epithelium is less frequent than in the adamantinomatous type. It consists of mature squamous epithelium forming pseudopapillae and an anastomosing fibrovascular stroma without the presence of peripheral palisading of cells or stellate reticulin (Fig. 2.4.2.2). The differential diagnosis between a papillary craniopharyngioma and a Rathke's cleft cyst may be difficult, particularly in small biopsy specimens, as the epithelial lining of the Rathke's cysts may undergo squamous differentiation; however, the lack of a solid component and the presence of extensive ciliation and/or mucin production are suggestive of Rathke's (1, 3).

Location/imaging

Most of the craniopharyngiomas are located in the sellar/parasellar region. The majority (94–95%) has a suprasellar component (purely suprasellar 20–41%/both supra- and intrasellar 53–75%), whereas the purely intrasellar ones represent the least common variety (5–6%). Other rare locations include the nasopharynx, the paranasal area, the sphenoid bone, the ethmoid sinus, the intrachiasmatic area, the temporal lobe, the pineal gland, the posterior cranial fossa,

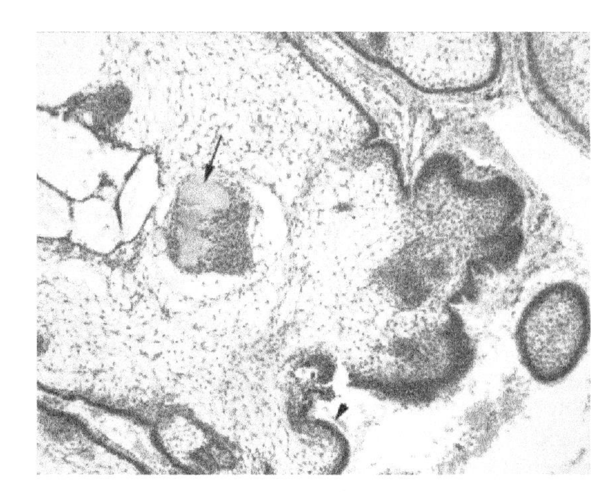

Fig. 2.4.2.1 Adamantinomatous craniopharyngioma. The epithelium consists of a palisaded basal layer of cells (arrowhead), an intermediate stellate reticulum, and a layer of flattened, keratinized squamous cells. Nodules of 'wet' keratin (arrow) are also shown. (Reprinted from Karavitaki N, Cudlip S, Adams CBT, Wass JAH. Craniopharyngiomas. *Endocr Rev*, 2006; **27**: 371–97 (1) with permission. Copyright 2006, The Endocrine Society.) (See also Plate 5)

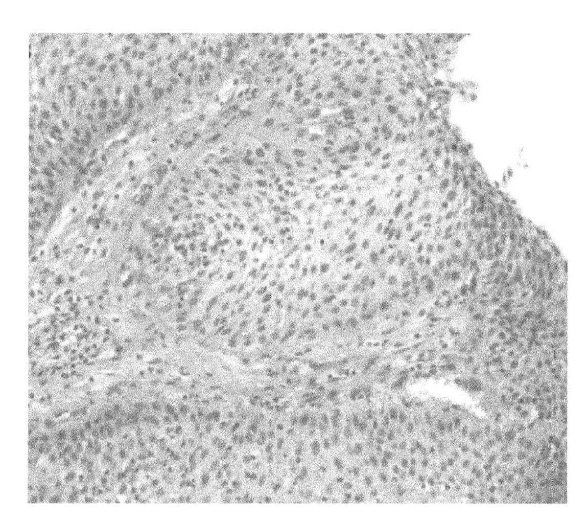

Fig. 2.4.2.2 Papillary craniopharyngioma. The epithelium is mature squamous forming pseudopapillae downward into the underlying tissues. (Reprinted from Karavitaki N, Cudlip S, Adams CBT, Wass JAH. Craniopharyngiomas. *Endocr Rev*, 2006; **27**: 371–97 (1) with permission. Copyright 2006, The Endocrine Society.) (See also Plate 6)

the cerebellopontine angle, the midportion of the midbrain, or completely within the third ventricle (1, 4).

Imaging tools for the diagnosis of craniopharyngiomas include plain skull X-rays, CT, MRI, and occasionally, cerebral angiography. Plain skull X-rays, although seldom used nowadays, may show calcification and abnormal sella (1). CT is helpful for the evaluation of the bony anatomy, the identification of calcifications and the discrimination of the solid and the cystic components; they are usually of mixed attenuation, the cyst fluid has low density and the contrast medium enhances any solid portion, as well as the cyst capsule (1) (Fig. 2.4.2.3). The MRI is particularly useful for the topographic and structural analysis of the tumour. The appearance of the craniopharyngioma depends on the proportion of the solid and cystic components, the content of the cyst(s) (cholesterol, keratin, haemorrhage) and the amount of calcification present. A solid lesion appears as iso- or hypointense relative to the brain on precontrast T_1-weighted images, shows enhancement following gadolinium administration and is usually of mixed hypo- or hyperintensity on T_2-weighted sequences. Large amounts of calcification may be visualized as areas of low signal on both T_1- and T_2-weighted images. A cystic element is usually hypointense on T_1- and hyperintense on T_2-weighted sequences. On T_1-weighted images a thin peripheral contrast-enhancing rim of the cyst is demonstrated. Protein, cholesterol, and methaemoglobin may cause high signal on T_1-weighted images, while very concentrated protein and various blood products may be associated with low T_2-weighted signal (1) (Fig. 2.4.2.4).

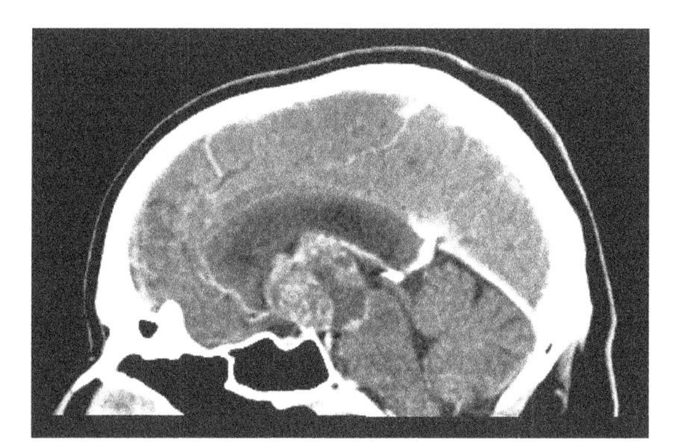

Fig. 2.4.2.3 CT head: craniopharyngioma in the suprasellar area associated with mass effect on the third ventricle and hypothalamus. The lesion shows a multicystic appearance with calcifications and a marked inhomogeneous enhancement.

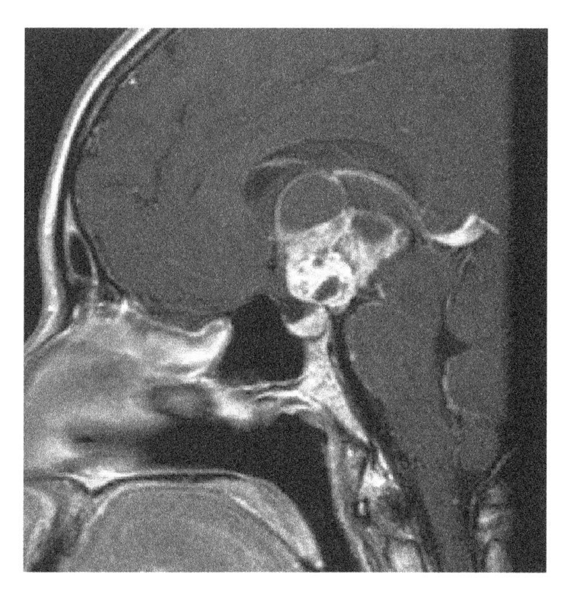

Fig. 2.4.2.4 MRI of pituitary: large suprasellar craniopharyngioma with complex internal signal. There is cyst formation and enhancement after contrast.

The size of craniopharyngiomas has been reported to be more than 4 cm in 14–20% of the cases, 2–4 cm in 58–76%, and less than 2 cm in 4–28%. Their consistency is purely or predominantly cystic in 46–64%, purely or predominantly solid in 18–39% and mixed in 8–36%. Calcification has been demonstrated in 45–57% and is probably more common in children (78–100%). The calcification patterns vary from solid lumps to popcorn-like foci or less commonly, to an eggshell pattern lining the cyst wall. Hydrocephalus has been reported in 20–38% and is probably more frequent in childhood-diagnosed disease (41–54%). There is no agreement on the radiological features discriminating the two histological subtypes. The differential diagnosis includes a number of sellar or parasellar lesions, including Rathke's cleft cyst, dermoid cyst, epidermoid cyst, pituitary adenoma, germinoma, hamartoma, suprasellar aneurysm, arachnoid cyst, suprasellar abscess, glioma, meningioma, sacroidosis, tuberculosis, and Langerhans cell histiocytosis. Differention from a Rathke's cleft cyst (typically small, round, purely cystic lesion lacking calcification), or from a pituitary adenoma (in the rare case of a homogeneously enhancing solid craniopharyngioma) may be particularly difficult (1, 4–7).

Presenting manifestations

Patients with craniopharyngioma may present with a variety of clinical manifestations attributed to pressure effects on vital structures of the brain (visual pathways, brain parenchyma, ventricular system, major blood vessels and hypothalamo-pituitary system). Their severity depends on the location, the size, and the growth potential of the tumour. The duration of the symptoms until diagnosis ranges between 1 week to 372 months (1). The presenting clinical manifestations (neurological, visual, hypothalamo-pituitary) and the pituitary function in a large series of cases are shown in Tables 2.4.2.1

Table 2.4.2.1 Presenting clinical features in children and adults with craniopharyngioma

	Children (%)	Adults (%)	Total (%)
Headaches	78	56	64
Menstrual disorders		57	
Visual field defects	46	60	55
Decreased visual acuity	39	40	39
Nausea/vomiting	54	26	35
Growth failure	32		
Poor energy	22	32	29
Impaired sexual function		28	
Impaired secondary sexual characteristics			24
Lethargy	17	26	23
Other cranial nerves palsies	27	9	15
Polyuria/polydipsia	15	15	15
Papilloedema	29	6	14
Cognitive impairment (memory, concentration, orientation)	10	17	14
Anorexia/weight loss	20	8	12
Optic atrophy	5	14	10
Hyperphagia/excessive weight gain	5	13	10
Psychiatric symptoms/change in behaviour	10	8	8
Somnolence	5	10	8
Galactorrhoea		8	
Decreased consciousness/ coma	10	4	6
Cold intolerance	0	8	5
Unsteadiness/ataxia	7	3	4
Hemiparesis	7	1	3
Blindness	3	3	3
Meningitis	0	3	2

Adapted with permission from Karavitaki N, Brufani C, Warner JT, Adams CBT, Richards P, Ansorge O, *et al.* Craniopharyngiomas in children and adults: systematic analysis of 121 cases with long-term follow-up. *Clin Endonol*, 2005; **62**: 97–409 (4).

and 2.4.2.2. Headaches, nausea/vomiting, visual disturbances, growth failure (in children) and hypogonadism (in adults) are the most frequently reported.

Treatment

Surgical removal combined with or not combined with external beam irradiation

Surgery combined with or not combined with adjuvant external beam irradiation is currently one of the most widely used first therapeutic modalities for craniopharyngiomas. These remain challenging tumours, even in the era of modern neurosurgery. This is mainly attributed to their sharp, irregular margins and to their tendency to adhere to vital neurovascular structures making surgical manipulations potentially hazardous to vital brain areas. The attempted extent of excision has been a subject of significant debate and depends on the size (achieved in 0% of lesions >4 cm) and location (particularly difficult for retrochiasmatic or within the third ventricle) of the tumour, the presence of hydrocephalus, of greater than 10% calcification and of brain invasion, as well as on the experience, the individual judgement during the operation and the general treatment policy (aggressive or not) adopted by each neurosurgeon (1, 6, 7). Reasons for incomplete removal, as reported in 56 patients who underwent primary surgery, include firm adherence to hypothalamus (26.8%), obstructed view (21.4%), major calcifications (14.3%), adherence to perforating vessels (10.7%), adherence to major vessels (7.1%), severe bradycardia during dissection (5.4%), advanced age of the patient (3.6%), high blood loss because of coexistent aneurysm (1.8%), very thin capsule (1.8%), and impression of complete removal (7.1%) (6). The perioperative morbidity ranges between 1.7% and 5.4% for primary operations (1, 4, 5, 8). The irradiation of cystic craniopharyngiomas carries the risk of enlargement, which may later regress or necessitate further intervention (4, 9).

Table 2.4.2.2 Pituitary function at presentation in children and adults with craniopharyngioma

	Children (%)	Adults (%)	Total (%)
Growth hormone deficiency	100	86	95
Follicle-stimulating hormone/ Luteinizing hormone deficiency		74	
Adrenocorticotropic hormone deficiency	68	58	62
Thyroid-stimulating hormone deficiency	25	42	36
Hyperprolactinaemia		55	
Diabetes insipidus	22	17	18

Adapted with permission from Karavitaki N, Brufani C, Warner JT, Adams CBT, Richards P, Ansorge O, *et al.* Craniopharyngiomas in children and adults: systematic analysis of 121 cases with long-term follow-up. *Clin Endonol*, 2005; **62**: 97–409 (4).

Recurrent tumors may arise even from small islets of craniopharyngioma cells in the gliotic brain adjacent to the tumour, which can remain even after gross total resection. The mean interval for their diagnosis after various primary treatment approaches ranges between 1 and 4.3 years and relapses as late as 36 years after initial therapy have been reported. Remote recurrences after apparent successful removal have been described with possible mechanisms including transplantation during the surgical procedures and dissemination by meningeal seeding or cerebrospinal fluid spreading (1, 4).

Series with radiological confirmation of the extent of resection show that the recurrence rates following gross total removal range between 0 and 62% at 10 years follow-up. These are significantly lower than those reported after partial or subtotal resection (25–100% at 10 years follow-up). In cases of limited surgery, adjuvant radiotherapy improves significantly the local control rates (recurrence rates 10–63% at 10 years follow-up). Series with statistical comparisons of the recurrences achieved by gross total removal or combination of surgery and radiotherapy have not provided consistent results. Finally, radiotherapy alone, which, however, can be offered to selected tumours, provides 10-year recurrence rates ranging between 0 and 23% (1, 4–14) (Table 2.4.2.3). In cases of predominantly cystic tumours, fluid aspiration provides relief of the obstructive manifestations and facilitates the removal of the solid tumour portion; the latter should not be delayed for more than a few weeks, as there is significant risk of cyst refilling (reported in up to 81% of the cases at a median period of 10 months) (4, 6). The interpretation of the data on the effectiveness of each therapeutic modality has to be done with caution, since the published studies are retrospective, nonrandomized and often specialty-biased. Although not widely accepted, it has been suggested that the tumor control correlates with the irradiation dose and doses of and below 5400 cGy are associated with poorer outcome. The growth rate of craniopharyngiomas varies considerably and reliable clinical, radiological, and pathological criteria predicting their behaviour are lacking. Thus, apart from significant impact of the treatment modality, attempts to identify other prognostic factors (age group at diagnosis, sex, imaging features, pathological subtypes, immunoreactivity of the tumor proliferation marker MIB1) have not provided consistent data (1).

The management of recurrent tumours remains difficult, as scarring/adhesions from previous surgeries or irradiation decrease the chance of successful excision. In such cases, total removal is achieved in a significantly lower rate when compared with primary surgery (0–25%) and is associated with increased perioperative morbidity and mortality (10.5–24%), suggesting that for many recurrent lesions palliative surgery is the most realistic target. The beneficial effect of radiotherapy (preceded or not by second surgery) in recurrent lesions has been clearly shown (1, 4, 13, 14).

Other treatment options

Intracavitary irradiation (brachytherapy) is a minimally invasive approach involving stereotactically guided instillation of β-emitting isotopes into cystic craniopharyngiomas and delivering higher radiation dose to the cyst lining than the one offered by external beam radiotherapy. It causes destruction of the secretory epithelial lining leading to elimination of the fluid production and cyst shrinkage. A number of β- and γ-emitting isotopes (mainly phosphate-32, yttrium-90, rhenium-186, gold-198) have been used; as none of them has the ideal physical and biological profile (i.e. pure β emitter with short half-life and with tissue penetrance limited to cover only the cyst wall), there is no consensus on which is the most suitable therapeutic agent. Based on studies with the largest series of patients and with relatively long follow-up periods, brachytherapy seems to offer a good prospect for the reduction/stabilization of cystic craniopharyngiomas. This combined with its reported low surgical morbidity and mortality render intracavitary irradiation an attractive option for predominantly cystic tumors, and particularly the monocystic ones. Its impact on the quality of survival and long-term morbidity (particularly vision, neuroendocrine, and cognitive function) remain to be assessed (1, 15, 16).

The intracystic installation of the antineoplasmatic agent bleomycin has been proposed for the management of cystic tumours. However, in published reports the tumour control rates range between 0 and 100%. Direct leakage of the drug to surrounding tissues during the installation procedure, diffusion though the cyst wall or high drug dose have been associated with various toxic (hypothalamic damage, blindness, hearing loss, ischaemic attacks, peritumoral oedema) or even fatal effects. The value of this treatment option in the tumour control or even in the delaying of potentially harmful surgery and/or radiotherapy, as well as the optimal protocol and the clear-cut criteria predicting the long-term outcome remain to be established in large series with appropriate follow-up (1, 17, 18).

Stereotactic radiosurgery delivers a single fraction of high-dose ionizing radiation on precisely mapped targets keeping the exposure of adjacent structures to a minimum. Tumour volume and close attachment to critical structures are limiting factors for its application with 10 and 15 Gy being the maximum tolerated doses to the optic apparatus and the other cranial nerves, respectively. Published studies suggest that it achieves tumour control in a substantial number of patients with small volume lesions (complete/partial resolution: 67–90%). Stereotactic radiosurgery may be particularly useful for well-defined residual disease following surgery or for the treatment of small solid recurrent tumuors, particularly after failure of the conventional radiotherapy. In cases of large cystic portions multimodality approaches with instillation of radioisotopes or bleomycin may offer further benefits. Studies with long-term follow-up evaluating the optimal marginal dose, its role in the prevention of tumour growth and its effects on the neurocognitive and neuroendocrine functions are required (1, 19–21).

Systemic chemotherapy has been offered in a limited number of patients mainly with aggressive tumours with relative success (1). Its application remains rather experimental and its place, particularly in the treatment of aggressive tumours, remains to be assessed.

Table 2.4.2.3 Recurrence rates at 10 years' follow-up after treatment of craniopharyngioma by surgery and/or radiotherapy

Primary treatment	Range of 10-year recurrence rate (%)
Gross total removal	0–62
Partial/subtotal removal	25–100
Partial/subtotal removal + radiotherapy	10–63
radiotherapy	0–23

Long-term outcome after surgery with or without conventional external beam irradiation

Morbidity

Patients with craniopharyngioma suffer from significant long-term morbidity (mainly endocrine, visual, hypothalamic, neurobehavioural, and cognitive) attributed to the damage of critical neuronal structures by the primary or recurrent tumour and/or to the adverse effects of the therapeutic interventions (Table 2.4.2.4). Notably, the severity of the radiation-induced late toxicity (endocrine, visual, hypothalamic, neurocognitive) is associated with the total and per fraction doses, the volume of the exposed normal tissue and the young age in childhood populations (1).

In series including subjects with various treatment modalities and follow-up periods, the frequency of pituitary hormone deficits ranges between 88% and 100% for growth hormone, 80–95%

Table 2.4.2.4 Probability of various morbidities and compromised functional outcome at 10 years' follow-up in patients with craniopharyngioma

Outcome	Rate at 10 years follow-up (%)
Major visual filed defects (i.e. at least quadrantanopia)	48
Hyperphagia-excessive weight gain	39
Hemiparesis or monoparesis	11
Epilepsy	12
Complete dependency for basal daily activities	9
Unable to work in previous occupation	23
School status behind the expected level	28
Depression or mood disorders necessitating treatment for various periods	15
Growth hormone deficiency	88
Follicle-stimulating hormone/Luteinizing hormone deficiency	90
Adrenocorticotropic hormone deficiency	86
Thyroid-stimulating hormone deficiency	80
Diabetes insipidus	65

Adapted from Karavitaki N, Brufani C, Warner JT, Adams CBT, Richards P, Ansorge O, *et al.* Craniopharyngiomas in children and adults: systematic analysis of 121 cases with long-term follow-up. *Clin Endonol*, 2005; **62**, 97–409 (4) (with permission).

for follicle-stimulating hormone/luteinizing hormone, 55–88% for adrenocorticotropic hormone, 39–95% for thyroid-stimulating hormone and 25–86% for antidiuretic hormone (ADH). Apart from symptomatic diabetes insipidus, which is probably more common in surgically treated patients, the long-term endocrine morbidity is not affected by the type of tumour therapy. Interestingly, restoration of pre-existing hormone deficits after surgical removal is absent or uncommon. The phenomenon of growth without growth hormone has been reported in some children with craniopharyngioma, who show normal or even accelerated linear growth, despite their untreated growth hormone deficiency. The pathophysiological mechanism has not been clarified; the obesity-associated hyperinsulinaemia or the presence of hyperprolactinaemia have been proposed as factors stimulating growth by affecting serum concentrations of insulin-like growth factor 1 (IGF-1) or by binding directly to the IGF-1 receptor. Finally, a number of studies support the view that growth hormone replacement in children and adults does not increase the risk of tumour recurrence (1, 4, 22, 23). Compromised vision has been reported in up to 62.5% of the patients treated by surgery combined with or not combined with radiotherapy during an observation period of 10 years. The visual outcome is adversely affected by the presence of visual symptoms at diagnosis and by daily irradiation doses above 2 Gy (1).

Hypothalamic damage may result in hyperphagia and uncontrollable obesity, disorders of thirst and water/electrolyte balance, behavioural and cognitive impairment, loss of temperature control and disorders in the sleep pattern. Obesity is the most frequent manifestation affecting 26–61% of the patients treated by surgery combined or not with radiotherapy. It is a consequence of the disruption of the mechanisms controlling satiety, hunger, and energy balance, and it often results in devastating metabolic and psychosocial complications. This necessitates provision of dietary and behavioural modifications, encouragement of regular physical activity, psychological counselling, and antiobesity drugs. Diabetes insipidus with an absent or impaired sense of thirst confers a significant risk of serious electrolyte imbalance and is one of the most difficult complications to manage. In this group of patients, the maintenance of the osmotic balance has been shown to be precarious with recurrent episodes of hyper- or hyponatraemia contributing to morbidity and mortality. Careful fluid balance in and out and regular weighting are important. Factors associated with significant hypothalamic morbidity have been proposed to be young age at presentation in children, manifestations of hypothalamic disturbance at diagnosis, hypothalamic invasion, tumour height greater than 3.5 cm from the midline, attempts to remove adherent tumour from the region of hypothalamus, multiple operations for recurrence and hypothalamic radiation doses greater than 51 Gy (1, 4, 5, 7).

The compromised neuropsychological, and cognitive function in patients with craniopharyngioma contributes significantly to poor academic and work performance, disrupted family and social relationships, and impaired quality of life. In a series of 121 patients treated by surgery with or without adjuvant radiotherapy and followed up for a mean period of 10 years, 40% had poor outcome (the assessment was based on motor and visual deficits, dependence for activities of daily living, Karnofsky Performance Scale, school and work status, debilitating psychological or emotional problems) (5). It has also been shown that the mean morbidity scores (based on endocrine deficiencies, vision, motor disorders and epilepsy, learning difficulties, behavioral problems, IQ, hypothalamic dysfunction) of children with additional surgery for recurrence were higher than the ones after their initial surgery and higher than those of children without recurrence (7). There is no consensus on the therapeutic option with the least adverse impact on the neurobehavioural outcome necessitating prospective studies with formal neuropsychological testing and specific behavioural assessment prior and after any intervention (1). These data are particularly important for young children, in whom the uncertainties of whether delaying irradiation is a reasonable policy, and whether the neurotoxicity of the recurrent disease and the subsequent surgery is higher than the one associated with irradiation offered to prevent relapse, need to be answered.

Mortality

The overall mortality rates of patients with craniopharyngioma have been reported to be three to six times higher than that of the general population with survival rates ranging between 83% and 92.7% at 10 years. Apart from the deaths directly attributed to the tumour (pressure effects to critical structures) and to the surgical interventions, the risk of cardio-/cerebrovascular and respiratory mortality is increased. It has also been suggested that in childhood populations the hypoadrenalism and the associated hypoglycaemia, as well as the metabolic consequences of ADH deficiency and absent thirst may contribute to the excessive mortality. The impact of tumour recurrence on the long-term mortality is widely accepted and the 10-year survival rates in such cases range between 29% and 70% (depending on the subsequent treatment modalities) (1, 4, 24).

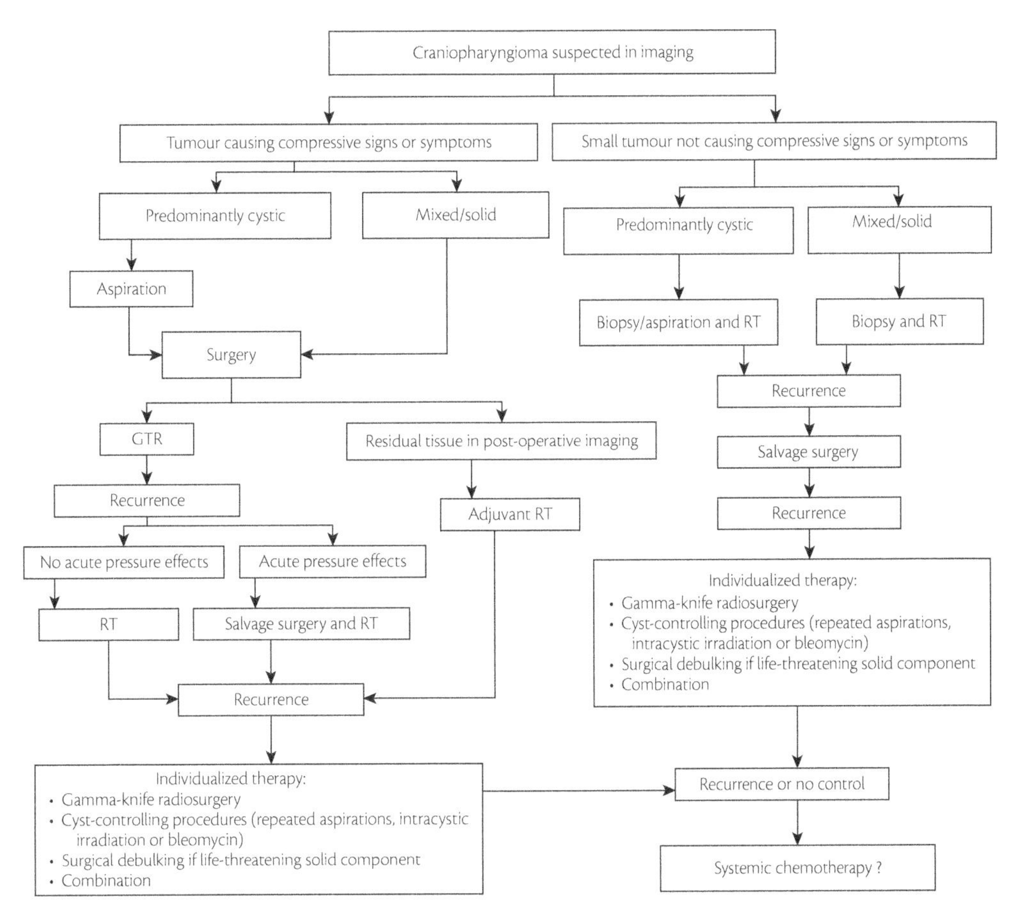

Fig. 2.4.2.5 Treatment algorithm for craniopharyngiomas. (Modified from Karavitaki N, Cudlip S, Adams CBT, Wass JAH. Craniopharyngiomas. *Endocr Rev*, 2006; **27**: 371–97 (1) with permission. Copyright 2006, The Endocrine Society.)

Treatment algorithm

The proposed treatment algorithm, which is based on the significant available literature, is shown in Fig. 2.4.2.5 (1). Surgical removal is suggested for all craniopharyngiomas causing compressive signs or symptoms (if a predominantly cystic lesion, the resection may be facilitated by previous aspiration of the cyst fluid). Gross total removal is a reasonable aim provided it is performed by experienced neurosurgical hands and hazardous manipulations to vital brain structures are avoided. If residual tumour remains following surgery, adjuvant irradiation is recommended; this is because of the high risk of recurrence and its adverse impact on morbidity and mortality. Although this strategy may be debated for the young children, the radiation toxicity to the developing brain needs to be balanced with the consequences of relapse and subsequent possible multiple surgical procedures. In small tumours not causing pressure effects (visual, neurological, hypothalamic), radiotherapy (preceded by biopsy for confirmation of the diagnosis) is an attractive approach avoiding the risks of surgery. In predominantly cystic tumours, previous fluid aspiration may reduce the adverse sequelae of possible cyst enlargement during irradiation.

The treatment of recurrent disease depends on the previous interventions and the severity of the clinical manifestations. In recurrent lesions not previously irradiated, radiotherapy provides satisfactory local control rates. In view of the high morbidity and mortality of a second surgery, such an intervention is advocated only in cases of acute pressure effects. The treatment of further recurrence(s) should be individualized and could include gamma-knife radiosurgery, cyst-controlling procedures, surgical debulking (for significant solid life-threatening component), and systemic chemotherapy (1).

References

1. Karavitaki N, Cudlip S, Adams CBT, Wass JAH. Craniopharyngiomas. *Endocr Rev*, 2006; **27**, 371–97.
2. Buslei R, Nolde M, Hofman B, Meissner S, Eyupoglu IY, Sie-bzehnrubl F, *et al.* Common mutations of beta-catenin in adamantinomatous but not in other tumours originating from the sellar region. *Acta Neuropathol (Berl)*, 2005; **109**: 589–97.
3. Crotty TB, Scheithauer BW, Young WF, Davis DH, Shaw EG, Miller GM, *et al.* Papillary craniopharyngioma: a clinico-pathological study of 48 cases. *J Neurosurg*, 1995; **83:** 206–14.
4. Karavitaki N, Brufani C, Warner JT, Adams CBT, Richards P, Ansorge O, *et al.* Craniopharyngiomas in children and adults: systematic analysis of 121 cases with long-term follow-up. *Clin Endonol*, 2005; **62**: 97–409.
5. Duff JM, Meyer FB, Ilstrup DM, Laws ER Jr, Scleck CD, Scheithauer BW. (2000). Long-term outcomes for surgically resected craniopharyngiomas. *Neurosurg*, 2000; **46**: 291–305.
6. Fahlbush R, Honegger J, Paulus W, Huk W, Buchfelder M. Surgical treatment of craniopharyngiomas: experience with 168 patients. *J Neurosurg*, 1999; **90**: 37–250.
7. De Vile CJ, Grant DB, Kendall BE, Ne-ville BGR, Stanhope R, Watkins KE, *et al.* Management of childhood craniopharyngioma: can the morbidity of radical surgery be predicted? *J Neurosurg*, 1996; **85**: 73–81.

8. Van Effenterre R, Boch AL. Craniopharyngioma in adults and children. *J Neurosurg*, 2002; **97**: 3–11.
9. Minniti G, Saran F, Traish D, Soomal R, Sardell S, Gonsalves A, *et al.* Fractionated stereotactic conformal radiotherapy following conservative surgery in the control of craniopharyngiomas. *Radiother Oncol*, 2007; **82:** 90–5.
10. Tomita T, Bowman RM. Craniopharyngiomas in children: surgical experience at Children's Memorial Hospital. *Childs Nerv Syst*, 2005; **21**: 729–46.
11. Rajan B, Ashley S, Gorman C, Jose CC, Horwich A, Bloom HJG, *et al.* Craniopharyngioma - long-term results following limited surgery and radiotherapy. *Radiother Oncol*, 1993; **26:** 1–10.
12. Kim SK, Wang KC, Shin SH, Choe G, Chi JG, Cho BK. Radical excision of pediatric craniopharyngioma: recurrence pattern and prognostic factor. *Childs Nerv Syst*, 2001; **17:** 531–6.
13. Kalapurakal JA, Goldman S, Hsieh YC, Tomita T, Marymont MH. Clinical outcome in children with craniopharyngioma treated with primary surgery and radiotherapy deferred until relapse. *Med Pediatr Oncol*, 2003; **40:** 214–18.
14. Stripp DC, Maity A, Janss AJ, Belasco JB, Tochner ZA, Goldwein JW, *et al.* Surgery with or without radiation therapy in the management of craniopharyngiomas in children and young adults. *Int J Radiat Oncol Biol Phys*, 2004; **28:** 714–20.
15. Julow J, Backlund EO, Lanyi F, Hajda M, Bálint K, Nyáry I, *et al.* Long-term results and late complications after intracavitary yttrium-90 colloid irradiation of recurrent cystic craniopharyngiomas. *Neurosurgery*, 2007; **61:** 288–95.
16. Hasegawa T, Kondzilka D, Hadjipanayis CG, Lunsford LD. Management of cystic craniopharyngiomas with phosphous-32 intracavitary irradiation. *Neurosurgery*, 2004; **54:** 813–22.
17. Takahashi H, Yamaguchi F, Teramoto A. Long-term outcome and reconsideration of intracystic chemotherapy with bleomycin for craniopharyngioma in children. *Childs Nerv Syst*, 2005; **21**: 701–4.
18. Hukin J, Steinbok P, Lafay-Cousin L, Hendson G, Strother D, Mercier C, *et al.* Intracystic bleomycin therapy for craniopharyngioma in children: the Canadian experience. *Cancer*, 2007; **109**: 2124–31.
19. Chung WY, Pan DHC, Shiau CY, Guo WY, Wang LW. Gamma knife radiosurgery for craniopharyngiomas. *J Neurosurg*, 2000; **93**: 47–56.
20. Kobayashi T, Kida Y, Mori Y, Hasegawa T. Long-term results of gamma knife surgery for the treatment of craniopharyngioma in 98 consecutive cases. *J Neurosurg*, 2005; **103;** 482–488.
21. Gopalan R, Dassoulas K, Rainey J, Sherman JH, Sheehan JP. Evaluation of the role of Gamma Knife surgery in the treatment of craniopharyngiomas. *Neurosurg Focus*, 2008; **24**: E5.
22. Honegger J, Buchfelder M, Fahlbusch R. Surgical treatment of craniopharyngiomas: endocrinological results. *J Neurosurg*, 1999; **90**:251–7.
23. Karavitaki N, Warner JT, Shine B, Ryan F, Turner HE, Wass JAH. GH replacement does not increase the risk of recurrence in patients with craniopharyngiomas. *Clin Endocrinol*, 2006; **64**: 556–60.
24. Tomlinson JW, Holden N, Hills RK, Wheatley K, Clayton RN, Bates AS, *et al.* Association between premature mortality and hypopituitarism. *Lancet*, 2001; **357**: 425–31.

2.4.3 Perisellar tumours including cysts, hamartomas, and vascular tumours

Jürgen Honegger, Rudi Beschorner, Ulrike Ernemann

Introduction

Approximately 80% of symptomatic tumours in the pituitary region are pituitary adenomas and further 10% are craniopharyngiomas. Among the remaining 10%, a considerable number of rare tumour entities have to be considered (Box 2.4.3.1) which makes the differential diagnosis sometimes difficult. Endocrinological, neuroradiological, and ophthalmological evaluation is the indispensable diagnostic triad to identify typical features in nonadenomatous perisellar tumours, and to provide diagnostic accuracy. This chapter presents typical clinical aspects of various nonadenomatous sellar tumours and the differential diagnostic value of specific symptoms. The current therapeutic strategies are also described.

Rathke's cleft cysts

It is assumed that Rathke's cleft cysts are related to embryonal pituitary development and consist of remnants of Rathke's pouch. Microscopic Rathke's cysts are found during autopsies in 30% of normal pituitary glands. However, it is relatively uncommon for Rathke's cysts to enlarge considerably in size and become clinically symptomatic. Rathke's cysts can become symptomatic in childhood or in adulthood.

Symptoms and endocrinological findings

Essentially, Rathke's cysts cause three symptoms. In order of frequency these are: hormonal impairments (Fig. 2.4.3.1 and Fig. 2.4.3.2), headache, and impaired vision (1). In the largest published series on 28 symptomatic Rathke's cleft cysts, endocrine symptoms at presentation were amenorrhea (37.5%), hypopituitarism (14.3%), retarded growth (7.1%), decreased libido and impotence (8.3%) and diabetes insipidus (3.6%) (1). Perception of amenorrhea may explain the more common finding of Rathke's cysts in women.

Neuroradiological diagnostics

MRI is the best technique for evaluation of perisellar cysts. Usually, Rathke's cleft cysts are rounded lesions. The hyperintense appearance of the protein-rich cyst contents on T_1-weighted images is characteristic but not obligatory. There are two typical locations:

- Intrasellar, possibly with suprasellar extension.
- Purely suprasellar, around the hypophyseal stalk.

Figure 2.4.3.3 shows a typical suprasellar Rathke's cleft cyst above the pituitary body and rostral to the hypophyseal stalk. After contrast administration, the thin wall of the cyst may show a moderate enhancement.

Box 2.4.3.1 Perisellar tumours

Pituitary and hypothalamic tumours
- Craniopharyngioma
- Gangliocytoma
- Hamartoma, hypothalamic
- Granular cell tumour
- Optico-hypothalamic glioma
- Pituicytoma
- Pituitary adenoma
- Rathke's cleft cyst
- Sellar colloid cyst

Extradural tumours
- Bone umours (e.g. Paget's disease, fibrous dysplasia)
- Chondrosarcoma
- Chordoma
- Esthesioneuroblastoma
- Mucocele
- Myeloma
- Naso-pharyngeal carcinoma
- Sarcoma

Vascular lesions
- Aneurysm
- Cavernous haemangioma

Other perisellar tumours
- Angiolipoma
- Arachnoid cyst
- Dermoid cyst
- Epidermoid cyst
- Germ cell tumour (non-germinomatous)
- Germinoma, suprasellar
- Haemangiopericytoma
- Lipoma, hypothalamic
- Lymphoma
- Meningioma
- Metastasis

Therapy

Surgery is indicated for these benign cysts only when there is evidence of hormonal or opthalmological deficits or a large space-occupying cyst is present. The vast majority of Rathke's cysts can be removed by transsphenoidal surgery. Purely suprasellar cysts around the pituitary stalk can be excised using the transsphenoidal, transtuberculum sellae approach. The objective of surgery is drainage of the cyst and biopsy or partial excision of the cyst wall. Radical resection

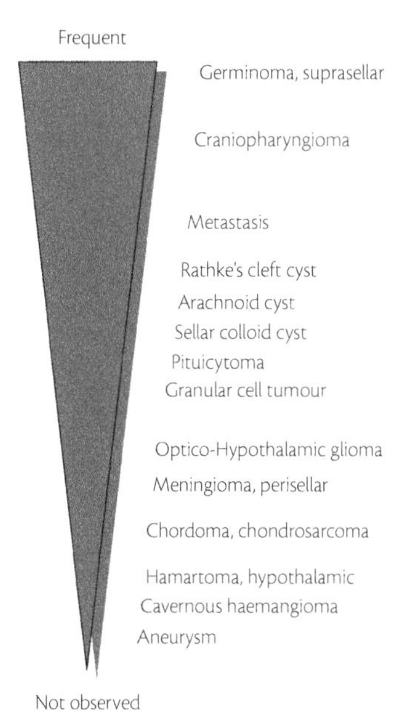

Fig. 2.4.3.1 Frequency of hypopituitarism in perisellar tumours.

of the often adherent and thin capsule is usually not performed due to the increased morbidity, e.g. nasal cerebrospinal fluid (CSF) fistula, pituitary deficiency. Histologically, the wall of the cyst is mainly lined by columnar ciliated and globlet cells and occasionally with pituitary hormone-producing cells (2). Cases with secondary inflammatory reaction, possibly as a result of a ruptured capsule, have been described.

Outcome

Hypopituitarism and visual impairment often improve postoperatively. As in the case of pituitary adenomas, however, it is observed that the chances of recovery are limited in cases with serious preoperative deficits (1). The recurrence rate is also relatively low, even in incomplete resection of the cyst wall.

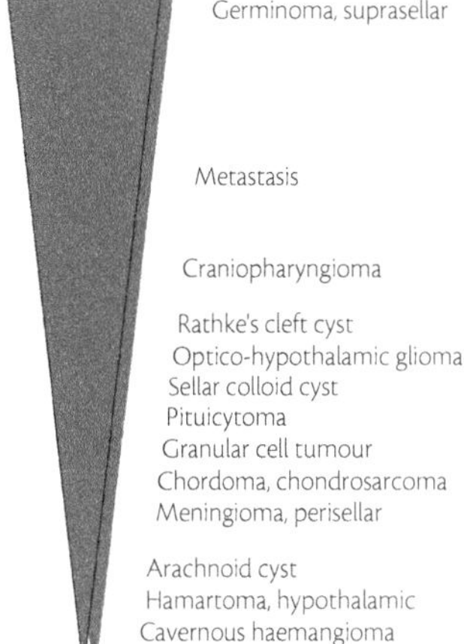

Fig. 2.4.3.2 Frequency of diabetes insipidus in perisellar tumours.

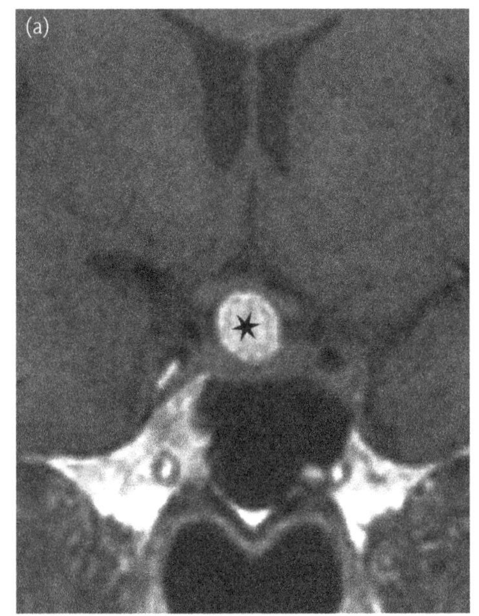

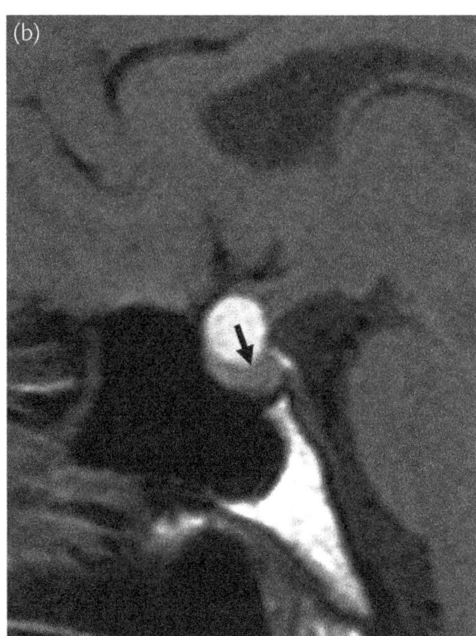

Fig. 2.4.3.3 Suprasellar Rathke's cleft cyst. (a) Coronal and (b) sagittal T_1-weighted MR image shows the hyperintense signal of the cyst (*) and the pituitary gland below (arrow).

Sellar colloid cysts

Sellar colloid cysts are often misinterpreted as pituitary adenomas.

Symptoms and endocrinological findings

Usually, sellar colloid cysts are a chance finding and there are no endocrinological impairments. Surgical treatment is only indicated in cases of symptomatic colloid cysts. In neurosurgical series, the patients are mostly women with menstrual period disruption, galactorrhoea, and headache as the main presenting symptoms. Endocrine deficits are usually mild. In one study, formal endocrinological examination revealed hyperprolactinaemia and hypogonadism in 72% of the symptomatic cases (3). Panhypopituitarism is an exceptional finding.

Neuroradiological diagnostics

The oval configuration (like a rugby ball) and localization between the anterior lobe and the posterior lobe of the pituitary are characteristic and reliable features to consider in the differential diagnosis (Fig. 2.4.3.4). Larger cysts may extend into the suprasellar region. In T_1-weighted images, colloid cysts appear hypointense and there is no contrast accumulation at the cyst boundaries.

Therapy

Surgical draining of symptomatic colloid cysts is performed by transsphenoidal approach. Colloid material is removed. Sellar colloid cysts do not exhibit an epithelial lining but normal pituitary tissue is usually found in specimens of the adjacent tissue (3).

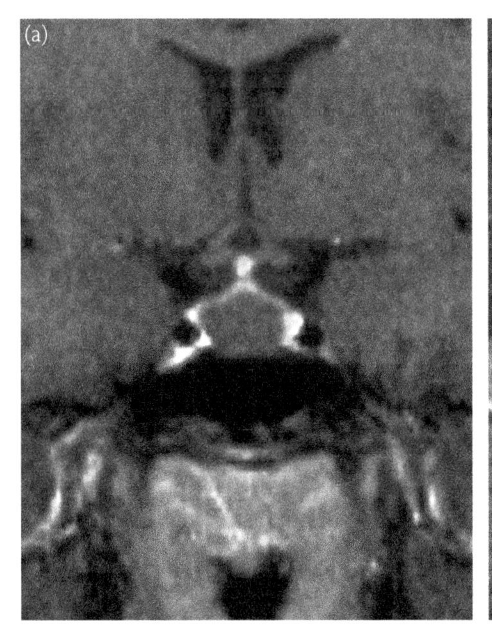

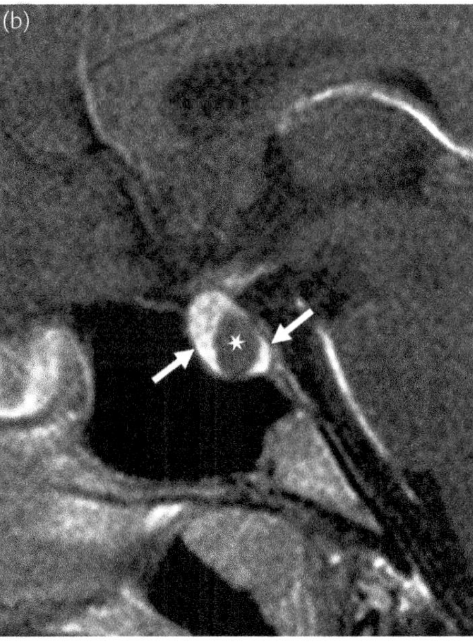

Fig. 2.4.3.4 Characteristic configuration of a sellar colloid cyst (*). T_1-weighted MR image with contrast: (a) coronal and (b) sagittal view. The sagittal view clearly depicts the localization of the cyst between the anterior lobe and posterior lobe of the pituitary (arrows).

Therefore, sellar colloid cysts must be regarded as 'pseudocysts'. This is probably the reason why they do not appear in current histopathological classifications of sellar tumours and cysts. However, they are relatively frequent sellar lesions and represent a clearly distinct clinical entity. The pathogenesis has not yet been completely elucidated. It has been suggested that sellar colloid cysts are a result of cellular degeneration (3). They must not be confused with colloid cysts of the third ventricle, which are a totally different entity.

Outcome

Headaches often subside postoperatively. The endocrinological deficits mostly regress and normal prolactin levels are restored. No recurrence is usually expected.

Arachnoid cysts

Arachnoid cysts constitute a nonproliferative anomaly of the arachnoidea. An expansile, 'tumour-like' cyst can arise due to a loculated collection of cerebrospinal fluid (CSF) within the duplication of the arachnoidal membrane. The pathophysiological mechanism behind the development of intrasellar arachnoid cysts is not fully understood and they are relatively uncommon. In 2007, Dubuisson *et al.* (4) reported on 14 published series and case reports which included a total of 42 operated intrasellar arachnoid cysts since 1980.

Symptoms and endocrinological findings

Visual impairment and headache are the main presenting symptoms in sellar arachnoid cysts (4). Visual compromise is explained by suprasellar bulging of the cyst. In a recent publication on intrasellar arachnoid cysts (4), hypogonadism and growth hormone deficiency were described in four of eight (50%) previously untreated cases (see Fig. 2.4.3.1). Hyperprolactinaemia is another frequent finding. However, panhypopituitarism is rarely observed. Diabetes insipidus is not mentioned in the relevant literature as a symptom of sellar arachnoid cysts (see Fig. 2.4.3.2).

Neuroradiological diagnostics

MRI shows the typical findings of a cystic space-occupying lesion. Arachnoid cysts may be localized in the suprasellar region or intrasellar with secondary suprasellar arching. The signal of the cyst contents corresponds to the CSF signal (Fig. 2.4.3.5). Due to the thin arachnoidal capsule, no peripheral contrast enhancement is found. The space-occupying character manifests as displacement and compression of the neighbouring anatomical structures, such as the optic chiasm and the pituitary stalk. This also enables diagnostic differentiation from a communicating CSF-filled defect, such as the empty sella.

Therapy

Surgical treatment of sellar arachnoid cysts is challenging. Most neurosurgeons prefer transsphenoidal surgery despite the high risk of postoperative rhinorrhoea. Wide fenestration of the cyst wall toward the suprasellar CSF spaces has been recommended for communicating arachnoid cysts that refill with CSF after cyst evacuation (4). In noncommunicating arachnoid cysts, only cyst evacuation is performed, leaving the suprasellar capsule in place. For closure, meticulous sellar floor reconstruction is paramount and additional sellar packing (e.g. with a fat graft) is often carried out (4, 5).

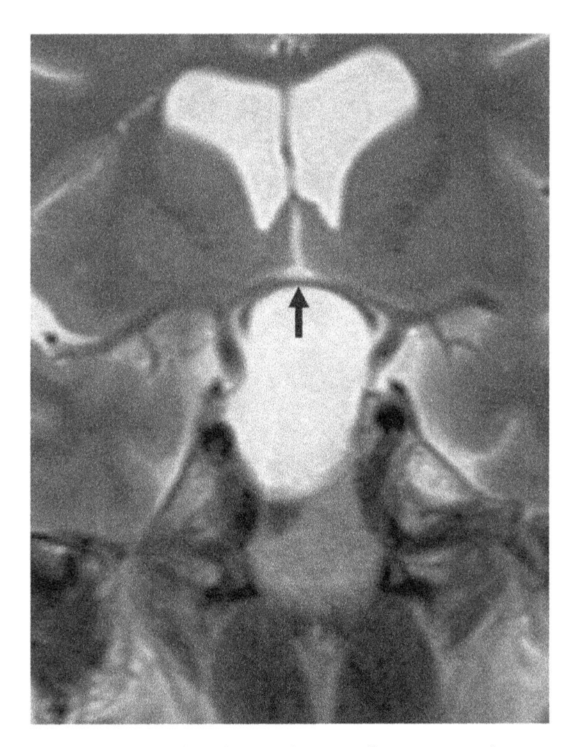

Fig. 2.4.3.5 Intrasellar arachnoid cyst with suprasellar extension. The optic chiasm is elevated (arrow). The coronal T_2-weighted MR image shows the cerebrospinal fluid signal of the cyst contents.

Dermoid and epidermoid cysts

Dermoid and epidermoid cysts arise from scattered remnants of embryonal epithelial cells. In both, the cyst wall is lined by benign keratinizing squamous epithelium. Cutaneous adnexa (e.g. hair follicles, sudoriferous or sebaceous glands) are present in dermoid cysts and their presence excludes the diagnosis of an epidermoid cyst. Intracranial dermoid and epidermoid cysts are typically found in the area of the cerebellopontine angle. Very rarely, however, sellar dermoid and epidermoid cysts are observed. Only a few cases of sellar dermoid and epidermoid cysts are described in the literature. Therefore definitive statements cannot be made about the probability of endocrinological impairments. Chemical meningitis may be elicited by rupture of the cyst capsule. Analysis of the signal behaviour on MRI enables neuroradiological differentiation from other sellar masses. Dermoid cysts usually contain fat, which is hyperintense on both T_1- and T_2-weighted images. Epidermoid cysts typically reveal a hyperintense signal on diffusion-weighted MRI due to restricted diffusion within the cyst. Surgical therapy in intrasellar cysts is via the transsphenoidal approach. Care must be taken during the operation that the cyst contents are not spilled into the subarachnoid space. If capsule remnants are not removed, there is danger of recurrence.

Meningiomas

Perisellar meningiomas

Meningiomas are by far the most frequent nonpituitary tumours with secondary spread into the pituitary fossa and encroachment on the pituitary gland or stalk. Consequently, endocrine dysfunction may follow. Meningiomas arise from arachnoid cover cells of the meninges. In the WHO classification of tumours of the central nervous system, the more frequently occurring benign grade I tumours are differentiated from atypical meningiomas (grade II) and anaplastic meningiomas (grade III). The higher-grade meningiomas (grades II and III) are more aggressive and have a greater tendency to recur.

Suprasellar meningiomas

In addition to the histological classification, meningiomas are also subdivided according to their location. The most important and common meningiomas which may cause hypopituitarism are the so-called suprasellar meningiomas. Dependent on the precise tumour origin, these can be further subdivided into:

- planum sphenoidale meningiomas (frequent)
- tuberculum sellae meningiomas (frequent)
- diaphragma sellae meningiomas (infrequent)

The ratio of occurrence in females and males is 5:1.

Symptoms

The main symptom of suprasellar meningiomas is visual impairment, which can be unilateral because of a prechiasmatic lesion or bilateral due to a chiasmal syndrome.

Endocrinological findings

Pituitary failure is rare in planum sphenoidale and tuberculum sellae meningiomas despite their often considerable size. In some cases, hypogonadism is observed or hyperprolactinaemia, due to displacement of the pituitary stalk (6). Serious hypopituitarism or diabetes insipidus are only very rarely present at the time of diagnosis. Hypopituitarism and diabetes insipidus are more likely in diaphragma sellae meningiomas that originate immediately anterior or posterior to the pituitary stalk (7). However, diaphragma sellae meningiomas represent an infrequent subtype of suprasellar meningiomas.

Neuroradiological diagnostics

A frequent error in differential diagnostics is misdiagnosing a suprasellar meningioma as a pituitary adenoma. The patients then attend the neurosurgical appointment with the false hope that the tumour can be removed through the nose. Therefore, precise inspection of sagittal MR images is paramount, which will show the meningioma resting with a broad base above the sella turcica, but not growing into the pituitary fossa. The pituitary is located underneath and can be delineated from the tumour (Fig. 2.4.3.6). Meningiomas often show dural enhancement (so-called *dural tail* or *dural sign*). The dural tail is explained by tumour spread and also by the increased vascularization of the neighbouring meninges. If the presence of a meningioma is suspected, CT, in addition to MRI, is appropriate to identify tumour calcifications and the hyperostosis that is typically found around the tumour attachment area.

Therapy

The treatment of first choice is microsurgical resection of suprasellar meningiomas via a pterional or subfrontal craniotomy. In the majority of cases, suprasellar meningiomas can be completely resected. The mortality rate is low in modern microsurgical series.

Outcome

The chance of postoperative improvement in vision is up to 80% (6). Hyperprolactinaemia and hypogonadism may regress postoperatively. The risk of recurrence is less than 5%.

Sinus cavernosus meningiomas

Meningiomas are also frequently found in the cavernous sinus.

Symptoms

The main symptom of such cavernous sinus meningiomas are ocular motor nerve palsies. Facial numbness due to involvement of branches of the trigeminal nerve is a typical finding. Retro-orbital pain is often reported due to dural involvement and distension of the cavernous sinus.

Endocrinological findings

Hormone deficits occur when the direction of growth is medial. The most frequent endocrine abnormality is hyperprolactinaemia (8).

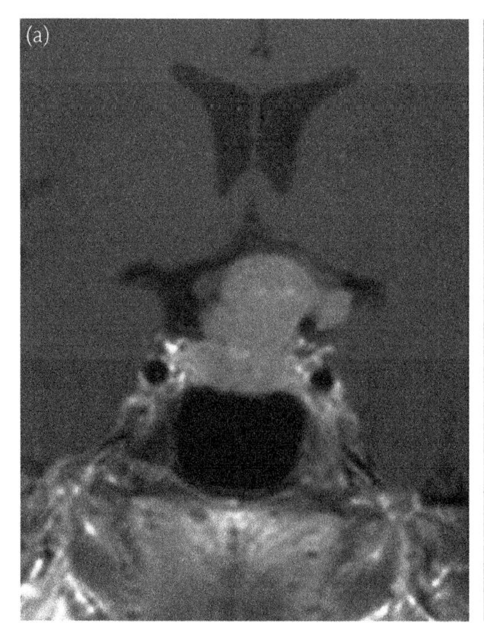

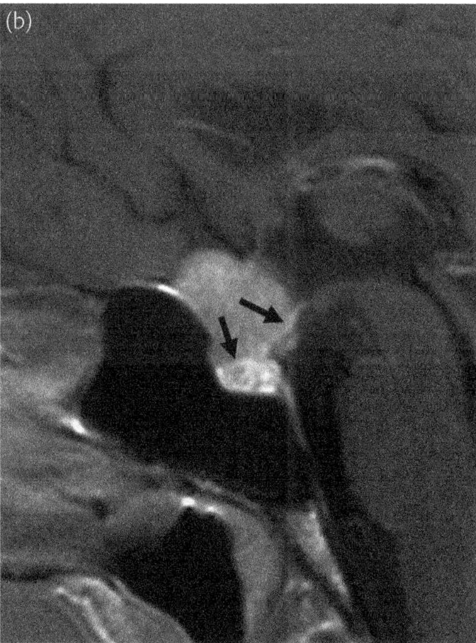

Fig. 2.4.3.6 Suprasellar meningioma of dural origin located at the tuberculum sellae. T_1-weighted MR image with contrast: (a) coronal and (b) sagittal view. The pituitary can be identified below the tumour (arrow), and the pituitary stalk is also displaced (arrow).

Neuroradiological diagnostics

Neuroradiologically, the expansile tumour within the cavernous sinus shows strong contrast enhancement. The marked dural tail, which extends to the tentorium, is characteristic of cavernous sinus meningiomas.

Therapy

Whereas suprasellar meningiomas can be removed surgically with low morbidity, radical resection of meningiomas of the cavernous sinus is problematical. The radical cavernous sinus surgery performed in the 1980s has been abandoned due to the high morbidity and tendency to recurrence. Surgical debulking is done in cases of exophytic tumour expansion and in compression of the optic pathways or growth into the optic canal. Thanks to modern MRI techniques, there is usually adequate diagnostic certainty so that histological confirmation of diagnosis is not necessary in typical cavernous sinus meningiomas (9). Symptomatic tumours or growing meningiomas of the cavernosus sinus are currently treated primarily with radiosurgery with a gamma knife or linear accelerator, or with fractionated stereotactic radiation (9, 10).

Outcome

Tumour control rates of more than 90% can be achieved with the above-mentioned radiation modalities.

In light of the close proximity to the hypothalamo-pituitary system, radiation of perisellar meningiomas requires close attention to radiation-related endocrinological deficits, which may manifest several years after treatment. Endocrinological postprocedural follow-up is required.

Intrasellar meningiomas

Purely intrasellar meningiomas are rare. It is assumed that this entity arises from the lower side of the diaphragma sellae. Thus, it is a special variant of diaphragma sellae meningiomas.

Symptoms

Kinjo *et al.* (7) reported on a total of 14 published cases. The most frequent symptoms were visual impairment, hormone impairment, and headache. Diagnostic differentiation from pituitary adenomas is difficult.

Endocrinological findings

Hypopituitarism and hyperprolactinaemia are present in more than 40% of patients with intrasellar meningiomas (8). Thus, hormonal deficits are much more frequent than in meningiomas of suprasellar or parasellar origin.

Neuroradiological diagnostics

The stronger contrast enhancement compared with pituitary adenomas may help in the differential diagnosis of an intrasellar meningioma.

Therapy

Most intrasellar meningiomas have been treated by the transsphenoidal approach (8), but resection of these often highly vascular tumours is more difficult than resection of pituitary adenomas. Additional transcranial operation may possibly be necessary. If the correct diagnosis has been made preoperatively, a primary transcranial operation can also be taken into consideration (7).

Other perisellar meningiomas

Meningiomas of the anterior clinoid process (so-called *clinoidal meningiomas*) or medial sphenoid wing meningiomas can also spread to hypothalamo-pituitary structures. In such cases, examination of the pituitary hormone status is required.

Metastases

Metastases are reported in published autopsy series of patients with malignant disease with a frequency of 1% to 11.8%. By contrast, metastases in the pituitary and hypothalamus are relatively rare in surgical series. It is assumed that metastasis to the bone, in particular into the clivus, usually occurs with secondary spread to the pituitary. Other sites of predilection for metastasis are also the pituitary itself and the pituitary stalk. Breast and lung cancer are predominant among the cancers that metastasize to the pituitary region (11).

Clinical signs and symptoms

It is important to differentiate these tumours from pituitary adenomas because the diagnosis often impacts on the treatment offered: metastases require early therapy, while slow-growing pituitary adenomas can often simply be kept under observation. Preoperatively, there are usually certain factors that point to metastasis and against the presence of pituitary adenoma. Among these are:

- *History of malignant tumour*: About half of the patients have a history of malignant tumour (12).
- *Occurrence of ocular motor palsy*: Eye muscle pareses ranging to ophthalmoplegia are characteristic of malignant tumours in the sellar region.
- *Osteodestructive growth*: Osteodestructive growth is an important criterion in the differential diagnosis, and its presence indicates a malignant tumour. It can be confirmed by CT (Fig. 2.4.3.7).
- *Expansion along the hypophyseal stalk*: MRI often shows tumour expansion along the hypophyseal stalk.

Other frequent complaints are retro-orbital pain and visual impairment. MRI usually shows strong, homogeneous contrast enhancement. Fig. 2.4.3.7 shows a malignant tumour of the clivus encroaching on the pituitary gland.

Endocrinological findings

Diabetes insipidus is clinically found in 40–60% of patients presenting with pituitary metastases (11, 12). This might be explained by the destructive nature of malignant tumours, or by direct haematogenic metastasis to the posterior pituitary lobe. Anterior pituitary insufficiency is encountered with almost equal frequency and panhypopituitarism is fairly common (11, 12). Mild hyperprolactinaemia is often found (11).

Therapy

Indication for surgery depends on the clinical context. The main arguments for surgery are relief of visual deficits and pain, confirmation of diagnosis, and removal of the tumour mass if considered beneficial for the overall outcome. The transsphenoidal approach is most often used (12). Usually, the indication is given for adjuvant radiation therapy after surgical treatment and confirmation of diagnosis (11, 12). Administration of chemotherapy depends on the underlying malignant disease.

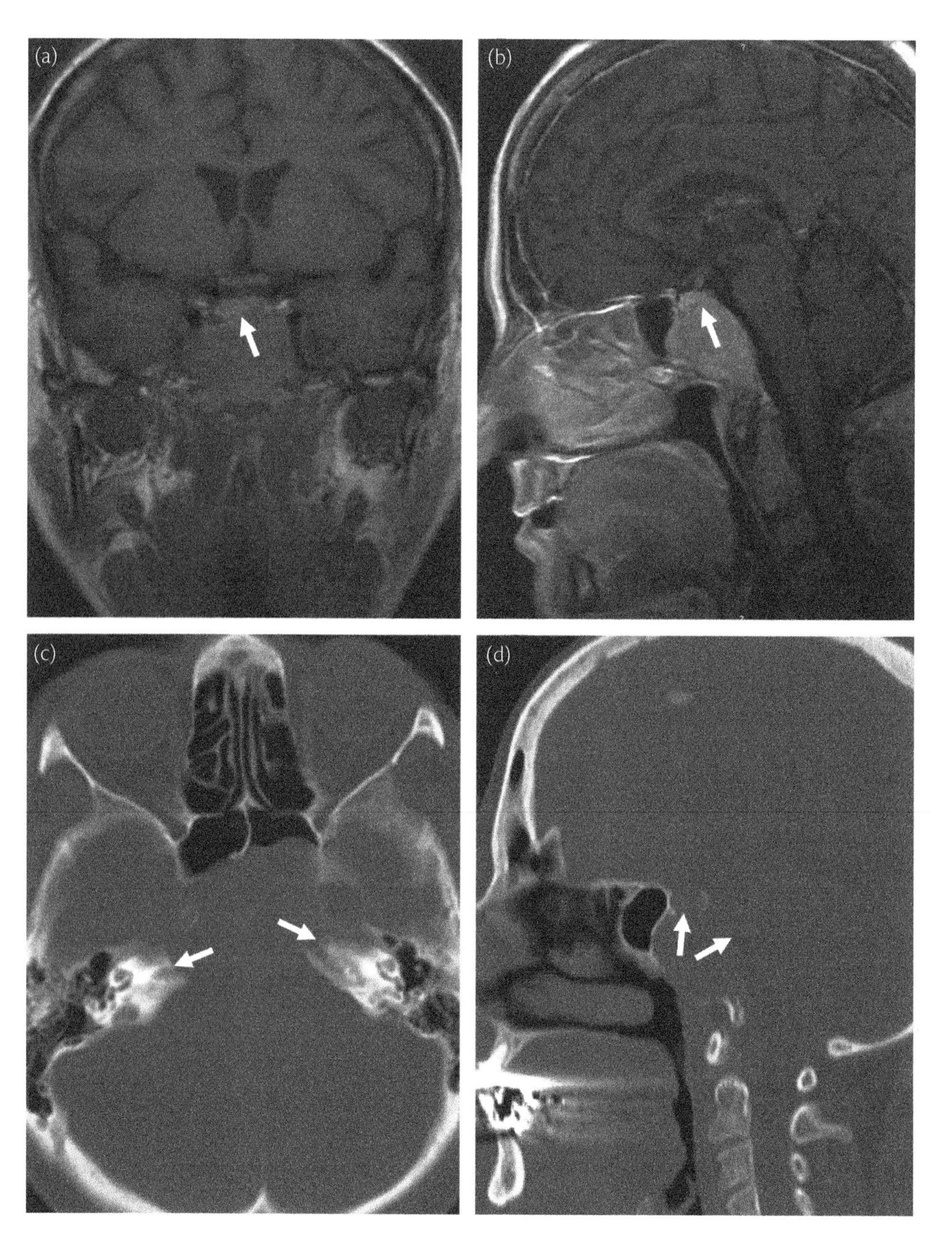

Fig. 2.4.3.7 Malignant tumour of the clivus with secondary spread to the pituitary. T_1-weighted MRI with contrast: (a) coronal and (b) sagittal view. The tumour is encroaching upon the pituitary gland (arrows). (c) Axial and (d) sagittal CT with bone window shows the destruction of the sellar floor, of the apex of the petrous bone, and of the clivus (arrows).

Outcome

While ophthalmological symptoms are likely to improve after surgical decompression, endocrinological deficits are usually not reversible. In two large series, the mean survival time has been reported to be 6 and 17 months, respectively (11, 12). The prognosis strongly depends on the origin and type of malignant tumour.

Chordomas and chondrosarcomas

Chondrosarcomas and chordomas are often reported together in the literature since they show similar clinical and imaging characteristics and the same therapeutic modalities are used.

Chordomas

Chordomas arise from persisting remnants of the notochord and consist of typical so-called physaliphorous tumour cells (Fig.c 2.4.3.8). They can occur everywhere along the neuraxis although the sites of predilection are the sacrum and the clivus. Chordomas of the clivus may expand toward the pituitary fossa as well as in a suprasellar direction toward the pituitary stalk and hypothalamus, and thus cause hormonal impairments.

Symptoms and endocrinological findings

The main symptom of chordoma in the upper clivus area is a one- or two-sided abducens nerve palsy, since the abducens nerve enters the clivus via the Dorello canal. Visual impairments occur with suprasellar expansion. Depending on the direction of growth, other cranial nerves may also be affected (13). Hypothalamo-hypophyseal endocrinological deficits are relatively rare (see Fig. 2.4.3.1). Hyperprolactinaemia can occur.

Neuroradiological diagnostics

MRI shows a tumour which is typically hyperintense on T_2-weighted images and enhances nonhomogeneously after contrast

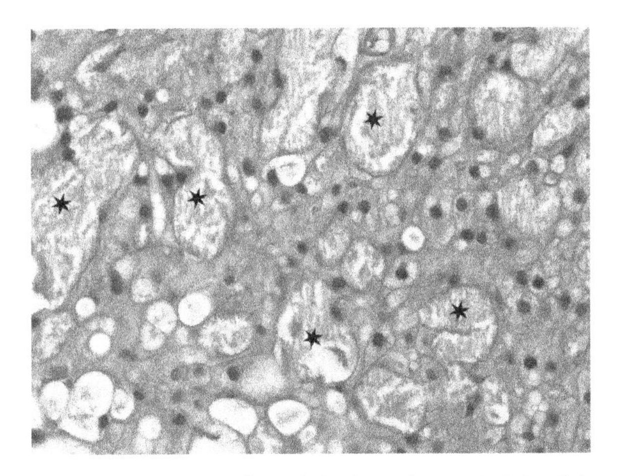

Fig. 2.4.3.8 Histologic section of a clival chordoma shows typical physaliphorous tumour cells with cytoplasmic vacuoles and distinct cell margins lying on a mucinous matrix (*). Haematoxylin and eosin, original magnification ×400.

administration. In chordomas, too, in addition to MRI, CT is appropriate as it will reveal the typical osteodestructive growth. Expansive growth with convex arching of the clivus dura toward the brain stem and pons cerebri is typical. Suprasellar expansion may occur starting from involvement of the dorsum sellae. The pituitary gland which is displaced in large tumours, can usually still be identified.

Therapy

Chordomas are characterized by their local, relatively slow but aggressive and destructive growth, and by a high tendency to recurrence. Metastasis is rarely observed. The primary treatment is surgical. In chordomas near the midline in the upper and middle third of the clivus, resection is initially transsphenoidal. Gross total or near-total tumour removal is accomplished using the transsphenoidal approach in 67–89% of patients with clival chordoma (13).

In such procedures, which go well beyond the operative corridor of classical pituitary surgery, we refer to extended transsphenoidal surgery. The entire area of the clivus and also the parasellar area can be reached via such extended approaches. Depending on experience and preference of the individual surgeon, microsurgical or endoscopic techniques, or both techniques in a complementary fashion, are used.

Depending on the expansion, other skull base approaches or combined procedures may be necessary. Complete cure by means of surgery is usually not possible. Usually the patients undergo radiotherapy after surgical treatment, preferably with heavy particles, such as proton radiation. Radiosurgery may also be considered in the case of small tumours or discrete recurrences (14).

Due to the tendency to recur, repeated surgical procedures and radiotherapy are often necessary.

Chondrosarcomas

Chondrosarcomas arise from primitive mesenchymal cells of the chondral matrix. At the skull base, chondrosarcomas usually arise in the clivus or in close vicinity. The tumour control rate after surgery and radiation is more favourable for chondrosarcomas than for chordomas. In a large series of skull base chondrosarcomas treated by surgery and consecutive fractionated radiation therapy, the 5- and 10-year local control rates were 99% and 98%, respectively (15).

Optico-hypothalamic gliomas

Optic pathway gliomas account for approximately 5% of all brain tumours in children and are frequently associated with neurofibromatosis 1. The majority of optico-hypothalamic gliomas occur during the first decade of life (16), but they are, however, also observed in later childhood and in adults (17).

Symptoms

Clinically, visual impairments are in the foreground. Deficits in field of vision are often unsystematic due to growth within the optic nerve, optic chiasma, or optic tract. Headache and nausea are the second most-common, caused in cases of large tumours by an occlusive hydrocephalus secondary to foramen of Monro occlusion (Fig. 2.4.3.9).

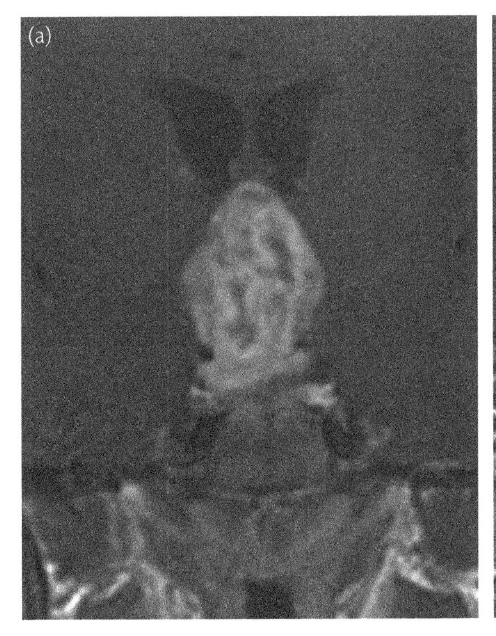

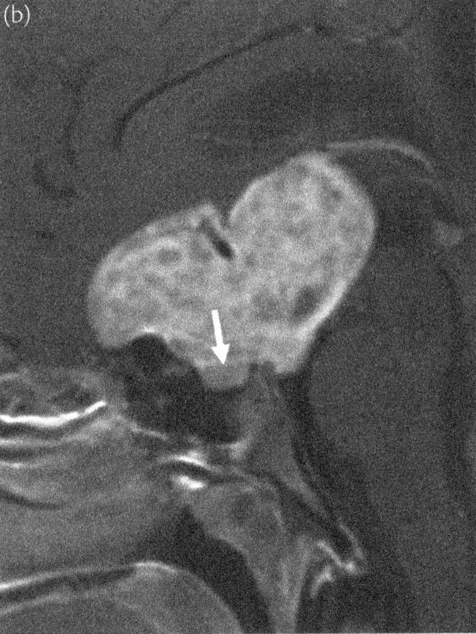

Fig. 2.4.3.9 Pilocytic optico-hypothalamic astrocytoma with marked, heterogeneous contrast uptake. (a) The coronal view shows hydrocephalus due to occlusion of the foramen of Monro. (b) The sagittal view depicts the pituitary gland and fossa below the tumour (arrow).

Endocrinological findings

Preoperative differentiation from craniopharyngiomas may be difficult. Contrary to craniopharyngiomas, hypopituitarism is relatively rarely seen preoperatively (see Fig. 2.4.3.1). In a series of 38 cases, only seven patients (18.4%) showed endocrine deficiency (17). More than one hormonal axis is rarely affected. Diabetes insipidus is relatively rare (see Fig. 2.4.3.2). Hyperprolactinaemia is the most frequent endocrinological abnormality. However, in cases of optico-hypothalamic gliomas, attention must be paid to hypothalamic syndrome, which occurs in about 20% of the patients (17). Among hypothalamic disorders, cachexia prevails. However, hypothalamic obesity or precocious puberty may also occur (17).

Neuroradiological diagnostics

Typical distension of the optic pathways by optico-hypothalamic gliomas should be watched for on MRI while compression and displacement are found in craniopharyngiomas. Sometimes the tumour has already attained a gigantic size at the time of diagnosis. The numerically dominant pilocytic astrocytomas show both cystic and solid portions with areas of high contrast uptake (see Fig. 2.4.3.9).

Therapy and outcome

Pilocytic astrocytomas (WHO grade I) of the optic pathways and hypothalamus region present a very heterogeneous growth tendency. Spontaneous remissions have been described. The unpredictable growth pattern has led to divergence of opinion about management (16). The approach can be conservative and therapy withheld if tumour size and vision are stable. This policy has particularly been recommended for patients with optico-hypothalamic gliomas associated with neurofibromatosis 1, who have a much better prognosis (16).

Surgery is generally indicated in patients with progressive tumours and with visual deterioration or severe visual compromise. Initial surgical treatment ranges from biopsy to large-scale resection (17). Due to the intrinsic growth in the area of the visual pathways and the hypothalamus, radical operation is often not possible. If the tumour is very large, tumour debulking should be attempted. Radiotherapy and chemotherapy are effective and established treatment modalities and can often result in tumour control (16). In very young patients, radiotherapy is avoided where possible due to the adverse long-term sequelae on the developing brain, and chemotherapy is performed instead. An overall 5-year survival rate of 40–88% in patients with optico-hypothalamic gliomas has been reported (16).

In addition to low-grade pilocytic astrocytomas, higher-grade optico-hypothalamic astrocytomas are also seen. As in other locations, radiotherapy or radiochemotherapy is required in addition to surgical therapy in anaplastic astrocytomas (WHO grade III) or glioblastomas (WHO grade IV).

Suprasellar germinomas

Suprasellar germinomas (also called *ectopic pinealomas*) are extragonadal germ cell tumours, which are primarily observed in children. They are corresponding tumours to seminomas in the testis and to dysgerminomas in the ovary. The incidence is especially high in Japan.

Symptoms and endocrinological findings

The triad of anterior pituitary insufficiency, diabetes insipidus, and visual compromise is found in practically all those affected. Often, panhypopituitarism is present. Diabetes insipidus with no imaging evidence of a lesion may be a nascent germinoma and requires close monitoring.

Neuroradiological diagnostics

MRI reveals a tumour with marked contrast uptake in the area of the pituitary stalk. In some cases, a second lesion is found in the area of the pineal gland and raises strong suspicion of a germinoma (Fig. 2.4.3.10). If a germinoma is suspected, MRI of the entire cranio-spinal axis is indicated.

The differential diagnosis from other lesions with contrast uptake in the area of the pituitary stalk, such as infundibulo-hypophysitis, Langerhans' cell histiocytosis (formerly known as *histiocytosis X*), or metastases is often difficult. A detailed CSF analysis with examination for tumour cells, inflammatory cells, and tumour markers is mandatory in such cases. If an intracranial germ cell tumour is suspected, analysis of the tumour markers α-fetoprotein and β-human chorionic gonadotropin (hCG) in CSF and serum is required. Raised levels of α-fetoprotein and β-hCG indicate the presence of a nongerminomatous germ cell tumour which is, however, extremely rare in the suprasellar location.

Therapy and outcome

If a germinoma is suspected, stereotactic or endoscopic biopsy confirmation of the histopathological diagnosis is obligatory. In small lesions, open biopsy via craniotomy under direct vision is to

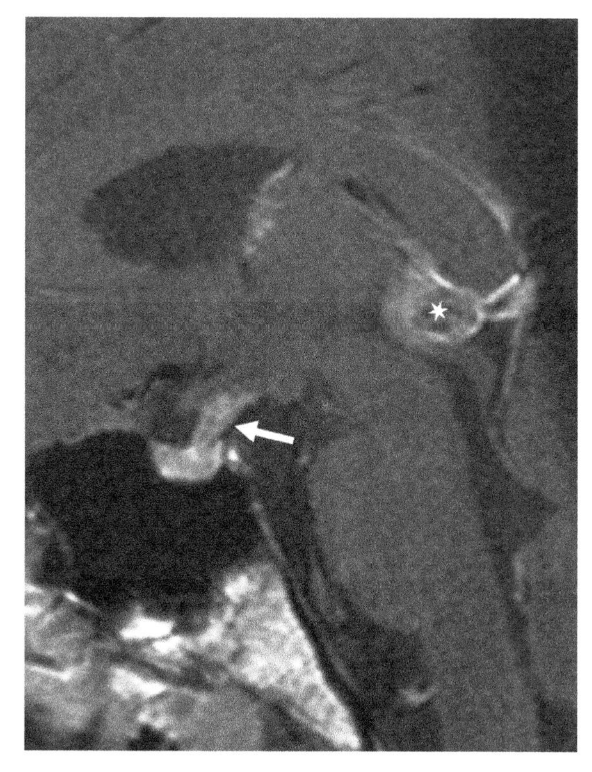

Fig. 2.4.3.10 Suprasellar germinoma at the hypophyseal stalk (arrow). T_1-weighted MRI: (a) coronal and (b) sagittal view A second lesion in the pineal area (*) raises strong suspicion of a germinoma.

be preferred due to the vicinity of critical vascular and neural structures. Radical operation is not justified in the light of the radiosensitivity of suprasellar germinomas. Pathological examination of germinomas shows large undifferentiated tumour cells with vesicular nuclei resembling primordial germinal elements and often abundant lymphocytic infiltration (18).

Fractionated radiation is the treatment of choice in suprasellar germinomas (19). In intracranial germinomas, 5-year survival rates of 80–100% are attained (20). Whether local, whole-brain, or cranio-spinal radiotherapy is required for isolated suprasellar germinomas is a matter of controversy. The occurrence of distant recurrences after local radiation of suprasellar germinomas does not appear to be common (19). Some centres first administer chemotherapy and select the dose of subsequent radiotherapy based on the response. This concept is especially appropriate in very young patients to reduce the detrimental sequelae of radiotherapy (20).

Hypothalamic hamartomas

Hypothalamic hamartoma is a non-neoplastic, malformed mass, which consists of atypically differentiated glial and neural tissue. The diagnosis can usually be made based on the characteristic clinical symptoms and typical neuroradiological signs.

Clinical signs and symptoms

Clinically, precocious puberty and gelastic ('laughing') seizures predominate. Those affected by hypothalamic hamartomas usually become clinically symptomatic in early childhood. Gonadotropin-releasing hormone (GnRH)-positive neurons have been found in some hypothalamic hamartomas, so that a heterotopic GnRH pulse generator is assumed to be the cause of precocious puberty. As an alternative hypothesis, substances such as GnRH or transforming growth factor α (TGFα), which are excreted by hypothalamic hamartomas, may elicit premature activation of the adjoining endogenous GnRH pulse generator (21).

The laughing seizures constitute a specific epileptic disorder (so-called *gelastic epilepsy*), which is pathognomonic for the presence of a hypothalamic hamartoma. Gelastic epilepsy is pharmacoresistant and leads to secondary epileptogenesis with additional types of seizures. In addition, cognitive impairment and behavioural disturbances occur varying in severity up to serious psychiatric symptoms. Hypothalamic hamartomas may also elicit further hypothalamic syndromes, such as polyphagia and obesity.

Neuroradiological diagnostics

MRI reveals a tumour without contrast uptake in the area of the tuber cinereum or the mamillary bodies, which appears isointense to grey matter on T_1-weighted images. Neuroradiological follow-up does not show progression. Pediculated and small hamartomas lead more often to precocious puberty, while broad-based and large hamartomas with intrahypothalamic expansion and involvement of the third ventricle more often elicit gelastic epilepsy (21).

Treatment of precocious puberty

Precocious puberty is usually treated nowadays with GnRH analogues. A few authors prefer operative resection via a transcranial approach in the case of pedunculated hamartomas, and report a good rate of success in regression of precocious puberty.

Treatment of epilepsy

Due to the serious pharmaco-refractory course of the gelastic epilepsy, operative or radiotherapeutic treatment is required.

Operative treatment

In open surgery, the hamartoma is resected or the attachment disconnected. Hamartomas extending into the third ventricle can be treated via a transcallosal approach, while hamartomas at the floor of the hypothalamus with exophytic expansion into the CSF cisterns are operated via a pterional approach. The surgical results reported in the literature vary widely. The cited rate of freedom from seizure ranges from 15 to 67%. The complication rate is between 0 and 54% and includes endocrinological and neurological deficits. The complication rate of treatment by experienced surgeons appears, however, to be quite low.

Endoscopic disconnection is used especially for hamartomas with expansion into the third ventricle. Using a navigation system, the endoscope is inserted into the third ventricle via the foramen of Monro. The low rate of complications has been reported for the endoscopic technique.

In a leading centre, freedom from seizures was achieved in 48.5% of the patients using combined open surgical and endoscopic procedures (22).

Single-session radiosurgery

This technique is especially suited for the treatment of small and medium-sized hamartomas. Régis *et al.* (23) conducted a prospective study with 60 patients and achieved total freedom from seizures in 37%.

Interstitial radiosurgery (brachytherapy)

A radioactive source is placed stereotactically in the hamartoma. The success rate appears to be lower than that of the other procedures described above.

Gangliocytomas

Gangliocytomas consist of neural cells. In addition to gangliocytomas in the brain, gangliocytomas are also observed in the hypophysis. Of the sellar gangliocytomas, 65% are associated with adjacent pituitary adenomas which are mostly hormone secreting (Fig. 2.4.3.11). Associated growth hormone-secreting pituitary adenomas, leading to acromegaly, prevail (24). As the hypothalamic-releasing hormone corresponding to the hormonal oversecretion syndrome has been demonstrated in gangliocytomas, the formation of the adenoma as a result of stimulation by the gangliocytoma is assumed (24). The exact histogenesis of sellar gangliocytomas has not, however, been completely elucidated. A common progenitor cell with transformation into two cell types is also discussed. Some investigators propose that adenohypophyseal cells transform into neuronal cells (25, 26). The diagnosis of two distinct tumours (i.e. gangliocytoma and adenoma) is difficult to establish on the basis of preoperative imaging studies. The mainstay of therapy is transsphenoidal surgery, and the double lesion can be removed. A review of the literature found a 63% chance to normalize the associated hypersecretory endocrinopathy by surgery (24).

Granular cell tumours

Granular cell tumours consist of lysosome-rich granular cells and may arise at various sites of the body, most frequently on the tongue.

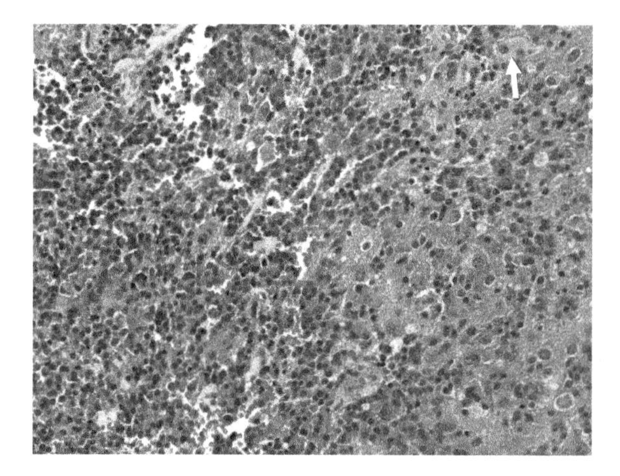

Fig. 2.4.3.11 Pituitary gangliocytoma and adenoma. Histological section showing the border zone between the distinct parts of two different tumours. On the right, the tumour consists of mature ganglion cells including single binucleated ganglion cell (arrow). On the left, small epithelial cells are seen as part of a pituitary adenoma. Haematoxylin and eosin, original magnification ×200.

Granular cell tumours are the most common primary lesions of the neurohypophysis and pituitary stalk. They are classified as WHO grade I tumours. The histogenesis of granular cell tumours at different sites of the body is still unclear. It is assumed that granular cell tumours of the sellar region develop from pituicytes, specialized glial cells in the infundibulum, and the neurohypophysis.

While small granular cell tumours are often observed in autopsy series, large and symptomatic granular cell tumours of the pituitary occur only rarely (27, 28). No reliable clinical features exist to distinguish granular cell tumours from other sellar tumours. Visual compromise prevails among presenting symptoms. Partial pituitary insufficiency and hyperprolactinaemia is present in 33% and 7% of symptomatic cases, respectively (28). Diabetes insipidus is surprisingly rare despite the infundibular or posterior lobe origin (28). Symptomatic granular cell tumours are treated by transsphenoidal surgery. Radiotherapy is beneficial in cases with less than total removal (28).

Pituicytomas

Pituicytomas are extremely rare neoplasms that arise from pituicytes. The pituicytoma is now accepted as a distinct entity and is included in the new WHO classification of tumours of the nervous system. The pituicytoma is classified as grade I tumour. Histological features are different from granular cell tumours, but pituicytomas and granular cell tumours may be related neoplasms. Wolfe *et al.* (29) reported on only 28 cases in the literature that met the histological criteria. Pituicytoma have a male to female ratio of approximately 1.6:1 and occur most often during the middle decades of life. Pituicytomas are slow-growing tumours and 39% of the reported patients presented with impaired visual acuity and visual field defects, and 53% with signs of pituitary insufficiency (29). On MRI, these intrasellar or suprasellar tumours are circumscribed with strong and homogeneous contrast enhancement.

As pituicytomas are firm and highly vascular, surgical removal is difficult. Gross total removal can be curative (29). Mostly a transsphenoidal approach has been used, but transcranial and extended procedures have also been reported. Given the low number of reported cases, the role of adjuvant radiotherapy following less than total resection is not well established.

Aneurysms

After traversing the skull base, the carotid artery travels in close proximity to the pituitary over a longer distance. Initially it runs extradural in the cavernous sinus and is called the carotid siphon at that point due to its convoluted course. After entering the intradural space, the carotid artery runs into the suprasellar cisterns on both sides and then divides at its bifurcation into the anterior cerebral artery and the middle cerebral artery.

Extradural aneurysms of the carotid artery

Symptoms

Extradural aneurysms of the carotid artery in a medial direction result in a sellar 'tumour' with compression of the pituitary gland and stalk. They can thus also induce hyperprolactinaemia or hypopituitarism. More frequent symptoms, however, are ocular motor nerve palsies. Deficits are not elicited primarily by compression of the structures, but rather by continuous arterial pulsations.

Neuroradiological diagnostics

On MRI, aneurysms can be recognized by their position in relation to the vessels and by their flow signal (Fig. 2.4.3.12). It is extremely important to recognize the neuroradiological signs, since aneurysms may imitate pituitary tumours. The transnasal operation of a wrongly-interpreted aneurysm could have fatal consequences. If an aneurysm is suspected, digital subtraction angiography (DSA) is the gold standard to confirm the diagnosis (Figure 2.4.3.12). CT angiography and MR angiography are increasingly used alternative non-invasive methods to investigate vascular lesions.

Therapy

Surgical access to extradural carotid aneurysms is difficult. Symptomatic or growing aneurysms are usually treated by endovascular means. Since extradural aneurysms often present with a wide neck, endovascular coil embolization of the aneurysm is usually assisted by stenting to reconstruct the vessel wall. Recently, stents with very tight meshes (so-called *flow diverters*) have been successfully employed to induce thrombosis and shrinkage of the aneurysm by altering the haemodynamics in the parent artery. If cross-flow via the contralateral carotid artery is adequate, endovascular occlusion of the carotid artery can also be considered.

Intradural aneurysms of the carotid artery

Symptoms and endocrinological findings

Intradural aneurysms of the carotid artery can lead to visual impairment due to compression of the optic nerves and optic chiasm. Endocrinological deficits are only rarely reported in the case of intradural aneurysms of the carotid artery without subarachnoid haemorrhage (SAH), but they have not yet been subjected to systematic investigation. Intradural aneurysms of the carotid artery can also imitate a pituitary tumour, as can aneurysms of the anterior communicating artery and basilar artery if they project towards the pituitary area.

Therapy

Intradural aneurysms are classically treated by microsurgical clipping. Endovascular coil embolization has become an alternative.

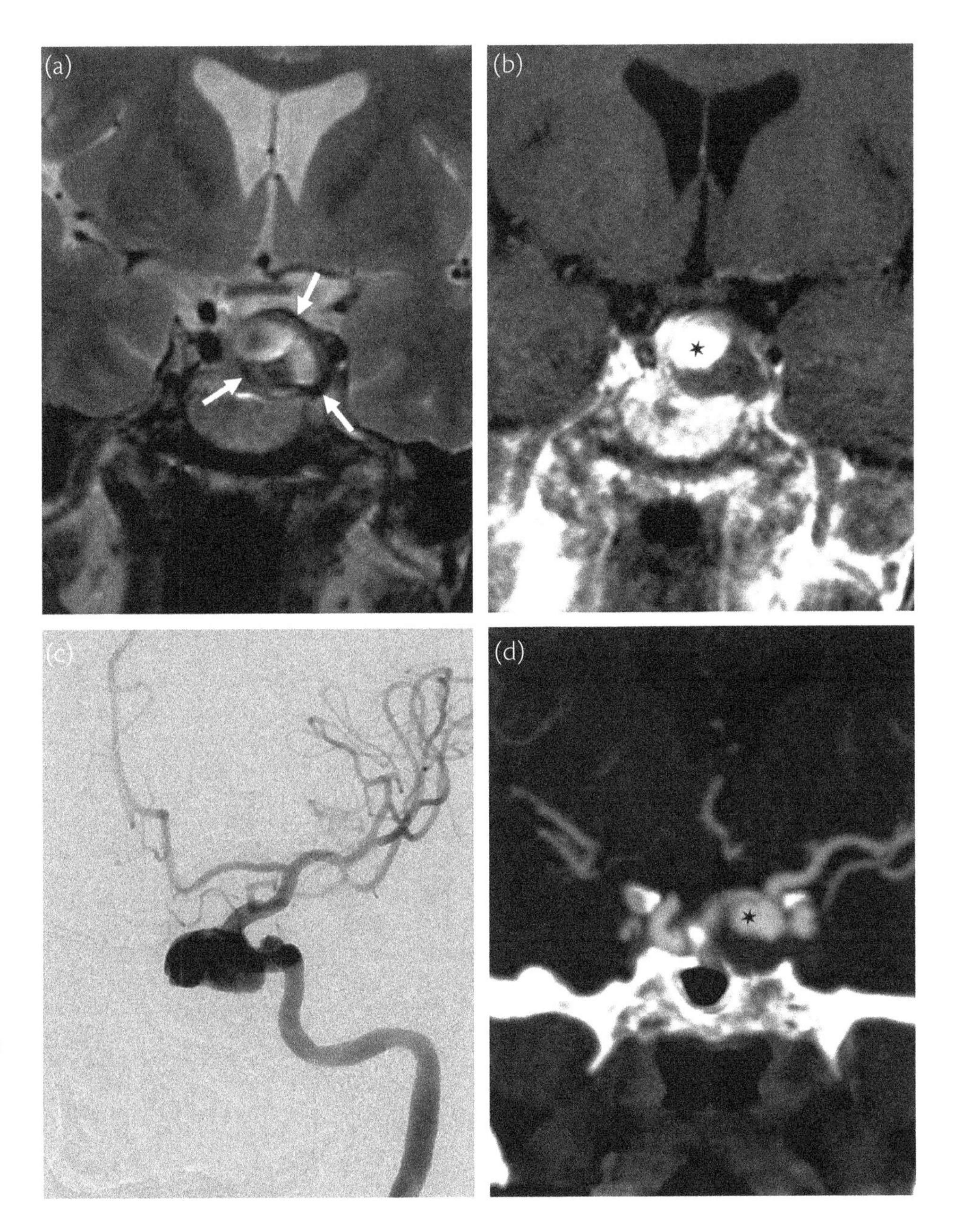

Fig. 2.4.3.12 Aneurysm of the left carotid artery directed medially with compression of the pituitary and the pituitary stalk. (a) The T_2-weighted image shows a mixed flow signal due to the turbulent flow in the aneurysm (arrows). (b) The bright signal on the T_1-weighted image represents the contrast agent within the aneurysm lumen (*). (c) Digital subtraction angiography (DSA) and (d) CT angiography depict the aneurysm (*).

Increasing attention is being paid to endocrinological deficits after SAH in ruptured intracranial aneurysms. Speculation about the cause is about not only direct damage due to SAH but also secondary vascular events elicited by vasospasms. The exact incidence of endocrinological deficits after SAH, including in dependence on the site of the aneurysm, is currently the subject of intensive research.

Cavernous haemangiomas

Cavernous hemangiomas are vascular malformations composed of closely apposed dilated vascular channels, which appear as discrete tumours. In the perisellar region, there are two rare but well-defined entities of cavernous haemangiomas, namely *haemangiomas of the cavernous sinus* and *haemangiomas of the optic chiasm*.

Cavernous haemangiomas of the cavernous sinus

Cavernous haemangiomas of the cavernous sinus are rare lesions that account for 2% of cavernous sinus tumours. They mostly affect females.

Symptoms

Clinically, cranial neuropathies, visual compromise, and headaches are in the foreground (30). Pituitary insufficiency may occur with medial expansion toward the pituitary.

Neuroradiological diagnostics

Unlike cavernous haemangiomas of the brain, these lesions rarely manifest by bleeding. MRI is the first choice examination method in these cases, too. Cavenous haemangiomas appear strongly hyperintense on T_2-weighted images (Fig. 2.4.3.13), and show

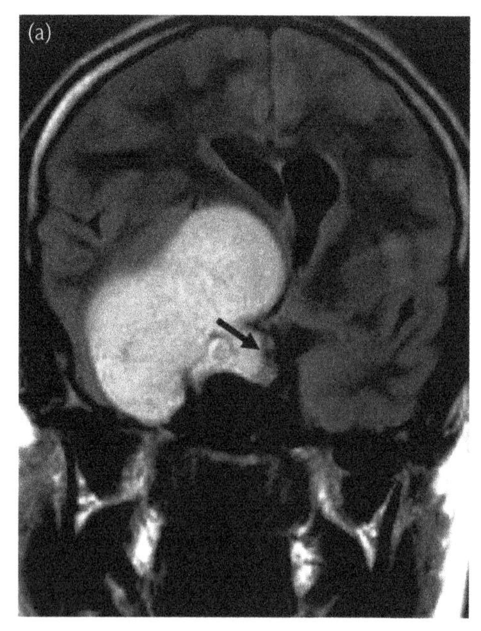

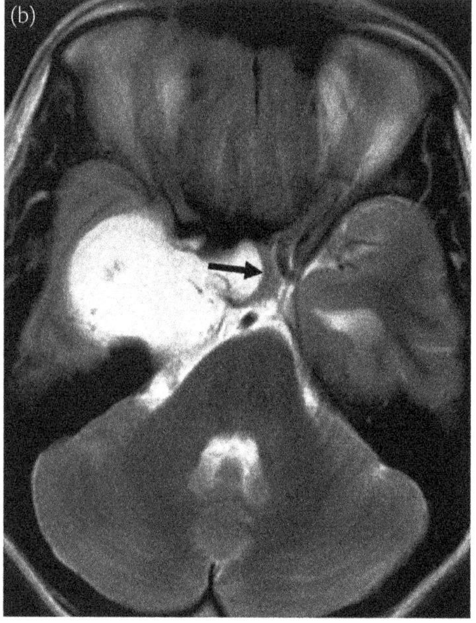

Fig. 2.4.3.13 Haemangioma of the cavernous sinus with lateral expansion towards the temporal lobe and medial expansion with compression of the pituitary (arrow). (a) The coronal fluid attenuated inversion recovery (FLAIR) T_2-weighted image shows the hyperintense signal of the tumour. (b) Similarly, the lesion appears strongly hyperintense on the axial T_2-weighted image.

marked contrast uptake. In the differential diagnosis, cavernous haemangiomas must be differentiated from meningiomas of the cavernous sinus and, in cases with medial expansion, from pituitary adenomas as well.

Therapy and outcome

Cavernous sinus haemangiomas are approached by a fronto-temporal or pterional craniotomy. Extensive blood loss must be anticipated in these highly vascular lesions. Total removal has been reported in 44% of the cases (30). Radiotherapy should be considered after subtotal removal. Postoperative improvement and deterioration of cranial neuropathies has been reported with equal frequency (30). Due to the low number of reported cases, there are no valid data on endocrinological outcome.

Cavernous haemangiomas of the optic chiasm

Cavernous haemangiomas of the optic chiasm are a relatively rare differential diagnosis in suprasellar tumours. Clinically, acute or subacute visual impairment due to acute bleeding occurred in most of the cases described in the literature. MRI may reveal bleeding into the optic chiasm, with a berry-shaped 'tumour' arising in the optic chiasm. Therapeutically, evacuation of a haematoma and resection of the lesion is performed via a transcranial approach.

Summary

With today's experience, the differential diagnosis of sellar tumours can often be made with a high degree of certainty even before histological confirmation. In particular, use of modern endocrinological diagnostics and increasing experience with MRI is of paramount importance in differentiating between the various tumours that can be encountered in the perisellar area. In parallel, the histopathological classification has further developed and now allows a more precise distinction and definition of tumour entities.

The differing frequency of endocrinological deficits can be used in the differential diagnosis. The differential diagnosis and classification of pituitary and hypothalamic tumours is important for planning the therapeutic procedures and prognostic evaluation.

References

1. El-Mahdy W, Powell M. Transsphenoidal management of 28 symptomatic Rathke's cleft cysts, with special reference to visual and hormonal recovery. *Neurosurgery*, 1998; **42**: 7–17.
2. Burger PC, Scheithauer BW. *Tumors of the Central Nervous System*. Washington, DC: ARP Press, 2007.
3. Nomikos P, Buchfelder M, Fahlbusch R. Intra- and suprasellar colloid cysts. *Pituitary*, 1999; **2**: 123–6.
4. Dubuisson AS, Stevenaert A, Martin DH, Flandroy PP. Intrasellar arachnoid cysts. *Neurosurgery*, 2007; **61**: 505–13.
5. Cavallo LM, Prevedello D, Esposito F, Laws ER Jr, Dusick JR, Messina A, *et al*. The role of the endoscope in the transsphenoidal management of cystic lesions of the sellar region. *Neurosurg Rev*, 2008; **31**: 55–64.
6. Fahlbusch R, Schott W. Pterional surgery of meningiomas of the tuberculum sellae and planum sphenoidale: surgical results with special consideration of ophthalmological and endocrinological outcomes. *J Neurosurg*, 2002; **96**: 235–43.
7. Kinjo T, Al-Mefty O, Ciric I. Diaphragma sellae meningiomas. *Neurosurgery*, 1995; **36**: 1082–92.
8. Honegger J, Fahlbusch R, Buchfelder M, Huk WJ, Thierauf P. The role of transsphenoidal microsurgery in the management of sellar and parasellar meningioma. *Surg Neurol*, 1993; **39**: 18–24.
9. Pollock BE, Stafford SL. Results of stereotactic radiosurgery for patients with imaging defined cavernous sinus meningiomas. *Int J Radiat Oncol Biol Phys*, 2005; **62**: 1427–31.
10. Selch MT, Ahn E, Laskari A, Lee SP, Agazaryan N, Solberg TD, *et al*. Stereotactic radiotherapy for treatment of cavernous sinus meningiomas. *Int J Radiat Oncol Biol Phys*, 2004; **59**: 101–11.
11. Heshmati HM, Scheithauer BW, Young WF. Metastases to the pituitary gland. *Endocrinologist*, 2002; **12**: 45–9.
12. Morita A, Meyer FB, Laws ER. Symptomatic pituitary metastases. *J Neurosurg*, 1998; **89**: 69–73.
13. Fatemi N, Dusick JR, Gorgulho AA, Mattozo CA, Moftakhar P, De Salles AA, *et al*. Endonasal microscopic removal of clival chordomas. *Surg Neurol*, 2008; **69**: 331–8.
14. Martin JJ, Niranjan A, Kondziolka D, Flickinger JC, Lozanne KA, Lunsford D. Radiosurgery for chordomas and chondrosarcomas of the skull base. *J Neurosurg*, 2007; **107**: 758–64.

15. Rosenberg, AE, Nielsen GP, Keel SB, Renard LG, Fitzek MM, Munzenrider JE, *et al.* Chondrosarcoma of the base of the skull: a clinicopathologic study of 200 cases with emphasis on its distinction from chordoma. *Am J Surg Pathol*, 1999; **23**: 1370–8.
16. Alshail E, Rutka JT, Becker LE, Hoffman HJ. Optic chiasmatic-hypothalamic glioma. *Brain Pathol*, 1997; **7**: 799–806.
17. Martinez R, Honegger J, Fahlbusch R, Buchfelder M. Endocrine findings in patients with optico-hypothalamic gliomas. *Exp Clin Endocrinol Diabetes*, 2003; **111**: 162–7.
18. Wei YQ, Hang ZB, Liu KF. In situ observation of inflammatory cell-tumor cell interaction in human seminomas (germinomas): light, electron microscopic, and immunohistochemical study. *Hum Pathol*, 1992; **23**: 421–8.
19. Fuller BG, Kapp DS, Cox R. Radiation therapy of pineal region tumors: 25 new cases and a review of 208 previously reported cases. *Int J Radiat Oncol Biol Phys*, 1994; **28**: 229–45.
20. Fouladi M, Grant R, Baruchel S, Chan H, Malkin D, Weitzman S, *et al.* Comparison of survival outcomes in patients with intracranial germinomas treated with radiation alone versus reduced-dose radiation and chemotherapy. *Childs Nerv Syst*, 1998; **14**: 596–601.
21. Jung H, Probst EN, Hauffa BP, Partsch CJ, Dammann O. Association of morphological characteristics with precocious puberty and/or gelastic seizures in hypothalamic hamartoma. *J Clin Endocrinol Metab*, 2003; **88**: 4590–5.
22. Procaccini E, Dorfmüller G, Fohlen M, Bulteau C, Delalande O. Surgical management of hypothalamic hamartomas with epilepsy: the stereoendoscopic approach. *Neurosurgery*, 2006; **59** [ONS Suppl 4]: ONS336–ONS346.
23. Régis J, Scavarda D, Tamura M, Nagayi M, Villeneuve N, Bartolomei F, *et al.* Epilepsy related to hypothalamic hamartomas: surgical management with special reference to gamma knife surgery. *Childs Nerv Syst*, 2006; **22**: 881–95.
24. Puchner MJA, Lüdecke DK, Saeger W, Riedel M, Asa SL. Gangliocytomas of the sellar region–a review. *Exp Clin Endocrinol Diabetes*, 1995; **103**: 129–49.
25. Asa SL, Kovacs K, Kontogeorgos G, Lloyd RV, Sano T, Trouillas J. Gangliocytoma. In: DeLellis RA, Lloyd RV, Heitz PU, Eng C, eds. *World Health Organization Classification of Tumours: Pathology and Genetics. Tumours of Endocrine Organs.* Lyon: IARC Press, 2004: 40.
26. Kontogeorgos G, Mourouti G, Kyrodimou E, Liapi-Avgeri G, Parasi E. Ganglion cell containing pituitary adenomas: signs of neuronal differentiation in adenoma cells. *Acta Neuropathol*, 2006; **112**: 21–8.
27. Lopes MBS, Scheithauer BW, Saeger W. Granular cell tumour. In: DeLellis RA, Lloyd RV, Heitz PU, Eng C, eds. *World Health Organization Classification of Tumours: Pathology and Genetics. Tumours of endocrine organs.* Lyon: IARC Press, 2004: 44–5.
28. Schaller B, Kirsch E, Tolnay M, Mindermann T. Symptomatic granular cell tumor of the pituitary gland: case report and review of the literature. *Neurosurgery*, 1998; **42**: 166–71.
29. Wolfe SQ, Bruce J, Morcos JJ. Pituicytoma: case report. *Neurosurgery*, 2008; **63**: E173–4.
30. Linskey ME, Sekhar LN. Cavernous sinus hemangiomas: a series, a review, and an hypothesis. *Neurosurgery*, 1992; **30**: 101–7.

2.4.4 Lymphocytic hypophysitis and other inflammatory conditions of the pituitary

Jelena Kravarusic, Mark E. Molitch

Introduction

Inflammatory lesions of the pituitary are far less common than pituitary adenomas. Although the most common of these, lymphocytic hypophysitis, is limited to the pituitary and pituitary stalk, many of the other lesions are usually part of a systemic process. Nonetheless, even these lesions, such as Langerhans' cell histiocytosis (LCH) and sarcoidosis, sometimes present as part of disease limited to the central nervous system (CNS) and, rarely, present as isolated lesions of the hypothalamic/pituitary area. When lesions are located in the base of the hypothalamus or in the stalk, they commonly present with a combination of diabetes insipidus and hypopituitarism. In some cases, hypothalamic infiltration may be more widespread, affecting a variety of additional hypothalamic functions, such as satiety, sleep, and temperature regulation. These inflammatory lesions tend to be progressively destructive, resulting ultimately in fibrosis but the rate of progression is highly variable. When hypopituitarism or diabetes insipidus occur, they rarely recover even if the underlying process is directly treated. Thus, these lesions present more with endocrine hypofunction than with mass effects, although in early stages lymphocytic hypophysitis may well present with mass effects to the point where it can be confused with a pituitary adenoma.

Lymphocytic hypophysitis

Lymphocytic hypophysitis is a rare but increasingly recognized disease associated with hypopituitarism and a sellar mass. It is most commonly seen in the peri- or postpartum period but it has also been reported after menopause (1). About 15% of reported cases occur in males. The diagnosis may be challenging, as the clinical and radiographic distinction from pituitary adenomas and other sellar masses is often not obvious. The disease is presumably autoimmune in aetiology, although there has never been a specific target antigen identified (1).

Pituitary lymphoplasmacytic infiltration and panhypopituitarism was first described by Rapp and Pashkis in 1953 (2), but the concept of endocrine autoimmunity had not yet been considered and was only introduced several years later for Hashimoto's thyroiditis. In 1962, Goudie and Pinkerton reported a case of a young woman with hypothyroidism and amenorrhoea, who died at of adrenal insufficiency 14 months postpartum at the time of appendectomy; her autopsy showed lymphocytic thyroiditis, severely atrophic adrenals, and a small atrophic pituitary with extensive lymphocytic infiltration. As it is most commonly seen in young women after childbirth it can be confused with Sheehan's syndrome and its true incidence is unknown. However, the number of reported cases has increased in the recent years, likely due to improved imaging criteria and techniques (3).

Epidemiology

About 500 patients with primary lymphocytic hypophysitis have been described in the literature (4). It affects women more frequently than men, with a reported ratio of about 5:1; however, the female:male ratio has been decreasing in recent years as more male cases are reported. When lymphocytic hypophysitis affects women of the reproductive age, it shows a striking temporal association with pregnancy. The mean age at diagnosis is approximately 35 years for women and 45 years for men (4). Of the 57% of patients developing the disorder in association with pregnancy, most occur during the last month of pregnancy or during the first 2 months postpartum (1, 5).

Classification and pathology

Hypophysitis can be classified based on anatomical distribution and whether it is a primary disorder of the pituitary gland or a secondary manifestation of a systemic disease.

Anatomically, the most common form is lymphocytic adenohypophysitis, where anterior pituitary cells and hormones are affected but posterior pituitary involvement is absent or minimal. With the much less common lymphocytic infundibulo-neurohypophysitis, the posterior pituitary is primarily involved, causing diabetes insipidus, and anterior pituitary function is usually preserved (1, 6–8). Lymphocytic infundibulo-panhypophysitis is even more rare, with lymphocytic infiltration and destruction present in both the anterior and posterior pituitary. These patients present with a combination of diabetes insipidus and anterior pituitary deficiency (1, 6–8).

Pathologically, primary hypophysitis has been described in three forms: lymphocytic, granulomatous, and xanthomatous. Lymphocytic hypophysitis is characterized by a dense lymphocytic infiltration of the anterior pituitary with destruction of the normal pituitary architecture and replacement with fibrosis (1, 6–9) as illustrated in the Fig. 2.4.4.1. The lymphocytes are predominantly cytotoxic T lymphocytes (CD8+), suggesting that T cell-mediated cytotoxicity is critical in the pathogenesis of the disorder (10).

Granulomas and multinucleated giant cells are not found in lymphocytic hypophysitis and, if observed, suggest an alternative diagnosis of granulomatous hypophysitis. This rare disorder has an incidence of 1/1 000 000. Granulomatous hypophysitis occurs in men and women with equal frequency and is not particularly associated with pregnancy. It may also present as a mass lesion with hypopituitarism and pathologically is characterized by giant cell granulomas (1, 6–10).

Xanthomatous hypophysitis, is exceedingly rare, with fewer than a dozen cases having been reported. The pathology of xanthomatous hypophysitis is characterized by a predominance of foamy macrophages, lymphocytes and single plasma cells (1, 10). Other more rare types of hypophysitis appear to be part of a more generalized inflammatory process and include Rosai–Dorfman disease and fibrosing inflammatory pseudotumor (also called Tolosa–Hunt syndrome and parasellar chronic inflammatory disease) (11).

Although hypophysitis is usually thought of as a primary process, it may occur secondarily in relation to infection (viral, bacterial, fungal, tuberculosis, syphilis) or other processes such as LCH, sarcoidosis, Wegener's granulomatosis, Crohn–Takayasu disease and ruptured cysts (1, 6–8). It has also been documented to follow treatment with ipilimumab, a monoclonal antibody used in treatment of melanoma and renal cancer (12).

Pathogenesis

The aetiology of lymphocytic hypophysitis is unknown but it has been speculated to have an autoimmune basis (1, 6–8, 6–10). Nearly 30% of patients have a history of coexisting autoimmune diseases such as Hashimoto's thyroiditis, Addison's disease, type 1 diabetes, and pernicious anaemia (1, 6–9), and the condition is now considered a component of the type 1 polyglandular autoimmune syndrome (1, 6–8). Cytotoxic T lymphocyte-associated antigen 4 (CTLA4) blockade using the human anti-CTLA4 monoclonal antibody, ipilimumab, has antitumour activity in melanoma and renal

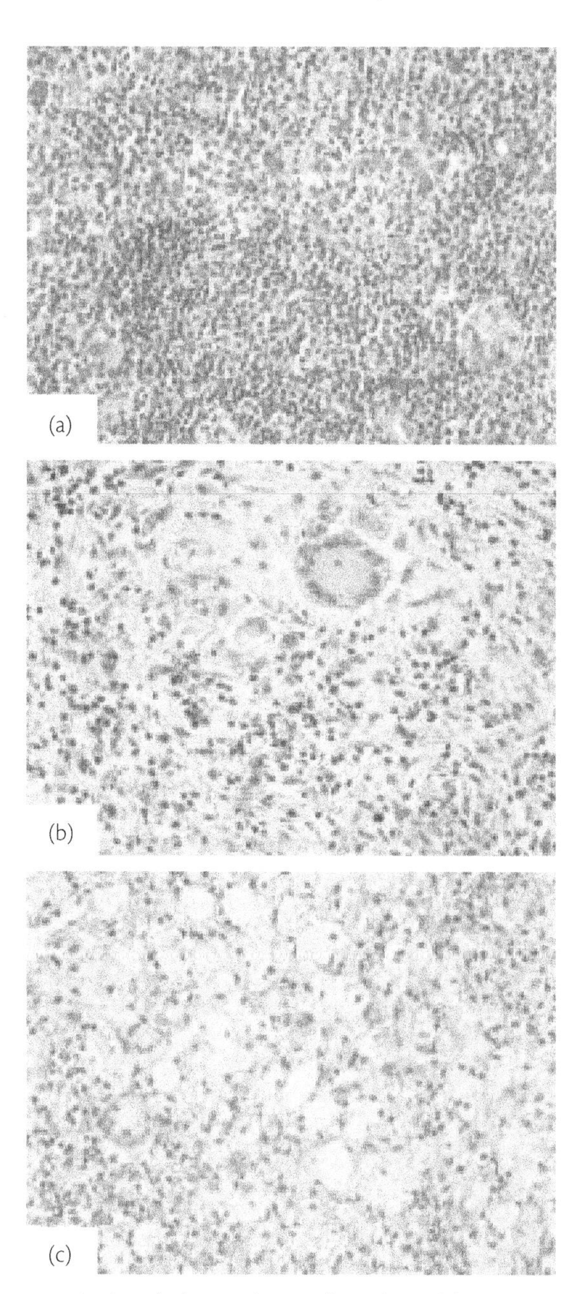

Fig. 2.4.4.1 Histological subtypes of primary hypophysitis. (a) Lymphocytic hypophysitis. Note massive lymphocytic infiltration of pituitary with scattered islands of preserved pituitary cells. (b) Idiopathic granulomatous hypophysitis. Characteristic multinucleated giant cells and granuloma surrounded by fibrosis; there is sparse infiltration of plasma cells. (c) Xanthomatous hypophysitis. Predominance of foamy macrophages, a few lymphocytes, and single plasma cells. Haematoxylin and eosin, original magnification ×40. (10). (See also Plate 7)

cancer and has been found to be associated with lymphocytic hypophysitis (12), supporting an immune aetiology for the disorder.

Although antipituitary antibodies have been demonstrated in some patients with lymphocytic hypophysitis, their specificity for hypophysitis is poor, as they are also present in patients with non-autoimmune pituitary disease, other nonpituitary autoimmune disease (13, 14), and in normal postpartum women who do not develop hypophysitis. The pathogenic pituitary autoantigen(s) remain to be elucidated, although several candidates have been proposed (4).

Presentation

When associated with pregnancy, lymphocytic hypophysitis typically presents in the third trimester of pregnancy or within 1 year postpartum, with symptoms usually related to a pituitary mass (headaches or visual symptoms) or hypopituitarism. The disorder often comes to attention due to failure of either lactation or menses following delivery (1, 3, 6–8). Neurohypophyseal involvement, manifesting as diabetes insipidus, occurs in 15% of cases (1, 3, 6–9). Other rare presentations of lymphocytic hypophysitis include meningeal irritation, diplopia due to cavernous sinus involvement, and occlusion of the internal carotid arteries.

Symptoms resulting from partial or panhypopituitarism occur in approximately 80% of cases, and multiple deficiencies are found in approximately 75% of cases (1, 3, 6–9) as illustrated in the Table 2.4.4.1.

There is an inexplicable unique predilection for the corticotrophs and thyrotrophs to be affected while the gonadotrophs may be spared. Prolactin levels range from unmeasurable to elevated; low levels are attributable to destruction of the lactotrophs, while hyperprolactinaemia is expected during pregnancy and the early postpartum period. However, elevated prolactin levels have been reported in cases of lymphocytic hypophysitis in men and non-pregnant women (9, 15), which is likely secondary to compression of the pituitary stalk.

Table 2.4.4.1 Lymphocytic hypophysitis: clinical presentation

Symptoms	Frequency (%)
Mass effects	
Headache	60
Visual disturbance	40
Bitemporal hemianopsia	32
Impaired visual acuity	16
Diplopia	<5
Endocrine dysfunction	80
Adrenal insufficiency	65
Hypothyroidism	60
Growth hormone deficiency	54
Hypogonadism	40
Hyperprolactinaemia	30
Diabetes insipidus	15

Data abstracted from Beressi *et al.* (3), based on analysis of 145 cases of clinically suspected and biopsy-proven lymphocytic hypophysitis.

Radiology

MRI in hypophysitis commonly shows an enlarged pituitary gland, often with suprasellar extension and stalk thickening (1, 6–9) as shown in the Fig. 2.4.4.2. With hypophysitis, the gland is generally symmetrically enlarged, and administration of gadolinium homogeneously enhances the gland. In contrast, in adenomas gadolinium enhances the gland more focally as described in Table 2.4.4.2. In lymphocytic hypophysitis, the pituitary displays a relative low signal on T_1- and a relatively high signal on T_2-weighted images. By comparison, in macroadenomas a low signal on T_1-weighted images is uncommon, but a high signal on T2 -weighted images is occasionally seen. Often, the dura mater adjacent to the mass in lymphocytic hypophysitis shows a unique, marked contrast enhancement referred to as a 'dural tail'. In late stages, these MRI findings may be absent due to shrinkage of the mass with resolution of the inflammatory process, and fibrotic changes and an empty sella may be seen (15).

Diagnosis

Lymphocytic hypophysitis should be considered in the differential diagnosis of pituitary masses and/or hypopituitarism in females who are pregnant or in the early postpartum period. This is especially true in cases associated with other autoimmune diseases or unusual patterns of hormone deficiencies. In the past many individuals with postpartum hypopituitarism who lacked a history of hypovolaemic shock were inadvertently labelled as having Sheehan's syndrome when, in fact, they had hypophysitis.

A definitive diagnosis of lymphocytic hypophysitis requires tissue biopsy. However, it may be possible to make a presumptive clinical diagnosis in patients who meet the following criteria: (1) a history of gestational or postpartum hypopituitarism, especially after a delivery uncomplicated by hemorrhage or hypotension; (2) a contrast enhancing sellar mass with imaging features characteristic of lymphocytic hypophysitis; (3) a pattern of pituitary hormone deficiency with early loss of adrenocorticotropic hormone (ACTH)

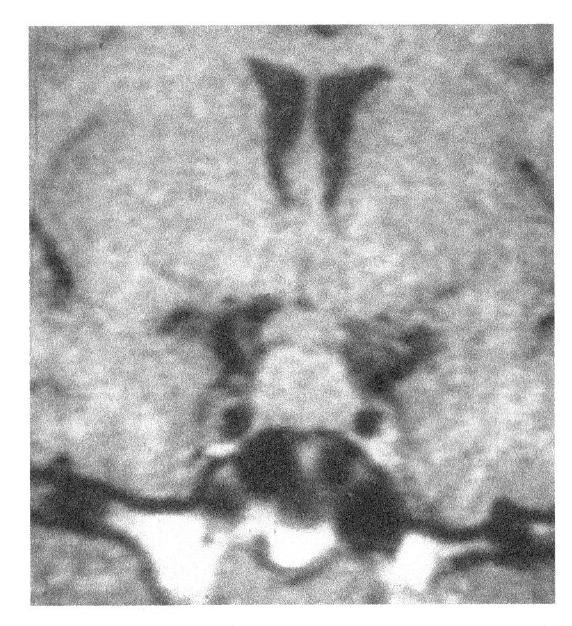

Fig. 2.4.4.2 Lymphocytic hypophysitis on coronal section in T_1 phase. The pituitary gland is diffusely and symmetrically enlarged, extending into the suprasellar region. The floor of the sella is intact (7).

Table 2.4.4.2 MRI characteristics of lesions of the hypothalamus/pituitary

Type of lesion	Signal intensity on T_1	Signal intensity on T_2	Contrast enhancement	Pattern of enhancement	Shape	Dural enhancement
Hypophysitis	Relatively low	High	Marked	Homogeneous	Symmetric	Common
Histiocytosis	Isointense	Hyperintense	Moderate	Nonspecific	Stalk thickening	Common
Sarcoidosis	Isointense	Hyperintense	Moderate	Nonspecific	Stalk thickening	Leptomeningae
Wegener's granulomatosis	Isointense	Hyperintense	Intense	Homogeneous	Superior infundibulum thickening	Common, linear
Tuberculosis	Isointense to hypointense	Hyperintense	Marked	Nonspecific	Nodular stalk thickening	Common
Pituitary Adenoma	Isointense	Usually isointense	Moderate	Focal	Variable	Rare

Data abstracted from Lury (7), Saiwai *et al.* (16), Shimono *et al.* (17), Kaltsas *et al.* (18), Bullmann *et al.* (19), Hoffman *et al.* (20), Murphy *et al.* (21), Lam *et al.* (22), Yilmazlar *et al.* (23).

and thyroid-stimulating hormone (TSH)—unlike that typically found with macroadenomas (i.e. sequential loss of growth hormone, luteinizing hormone (LH)/follicle-stimulating hormone (FSH), ACTH, and TSH); (4) relatively rapid development of hypopituitarism in contrast to the expected slow development of hypopituitarism that would be expected with an adenoma; and (5) a degree of pituitary failure disproportionate to the size of the mass. Nevertheless, biopsy may be required in situations in which a distinction cannot be made between lymphocytic hypophysitis and a nonfunctioning macroadenoma or prolactinoma and when neurological signs develop.

Lymphocytic infundibulo-neurohypophysitis

Lymphocytic hypophysitis and infundibulo-neurohypophysitis likely represent distinctly separate pathological entities, as the latter tends to occur in older patients and is less likely to be associated with pregnancy (1, 6–9). Lymphocytic infundibulo-neurohypophysitis causes central diabetes insipidus and spares the anterior pituitary as a result of an inflammatory process confined to the stalk and posterior pituitary (17). The radiological features are generally more clearly delineated: thickening of the pituitary stalk or neurohypophysis and homogeneous enhancement of the pituitary stalk or neurohypophysis after the administration of contrast material (24).

Management

The natural history of lymphocytic hypophysitis is variable and unpredictable. Typically, the pituitary initially becomes inflamed, oedematous, and enlarged, and the patient develops symptoms secondary to mass effects. Progressive fibrosis causing destruction of the parenchyma leads to hypopituitarism. In some cases, the course is aggressive and neurological deficits progress rapidly (1, 6–9). However, cases of spontaneous partial or full recovery of pituitary function, as well as resolution of pituitary masses in the absence of any intervention, have been well documented (25–27). Because the natural history of lymphocytic hypophysitis is so variable, appropriate management remains controversial.

Controlled therapeutic trials are not feasible due to the rarity of hypophysitis, an inability to make definitive diagnoses without histological proof, and the considerable variability in the natural history of the disorder. Until recently, preoperative suspicion of the diagnosis was rare due to under-recognition, and the traditional diagnostic and therapeutic approach involved transsphenoidal biopsy, exploration, and/or pituitary resection. Consequently, cases illustrating only transient compressive effects and endocrine dysfunction support a case for conservative management. With a greater knowledge of the course of lymphocytic hypophysitis and the ability to make a presumptive diagnosis in highly suggestive cases, it is possible to avoid routine neurosurgical exploration in many cases.

Corticosteroid therapy has been advocated as a means of attenuating inflammation and, in some patients, has been associated with return of pituitary function and reduction of the mass (28, 29). Conversely, cases have also been reported in which lymphocytic hypophysitis failed to improve with glucocorticoid therapy (9, 30). There are also a few documented cases of improvement in symptoms with administration of corticosteroids followed by a relapse when therapy was discontinued (31). It is unclear, however, whether improvement in the clinical course is directly attributable to corticosteroid treatment or simply reflects the natural course of the disease (25–27). Given the uncertainty regarding the efficacy of corticosteroid treatment and its known adverse effects, such therapy does not seem justified for most patients.

Patients with a presumed diagnosis of lymphocytic hypophysitis should be observed closely and undergo serial visual field examinations or an MRI if they are managed medically. Surgical decompression of the pituitary mass may be required if the patient fails conservative therapy as demonstrated by progressive radiological or neurological deterioration or by signs of optic nerve compression. However, in this situation some would argue for a short course of steroids (1, 6–9). The optimal surgical strategy involves only partial resection of the mass to decompress the surrounding structures via a transsphenoidal approach rather than an attempt at complete resection, because surgery rarely improves endocrine dysfunction. All patients with lymphocytic hypophysitis require appropriate replacement therapy for deficient hormones. Long-term follow-up is mandatory to monitor for the development of other hormonal deficits. Because hypopituitarism is temporary in a subset of patients, a careful attempt should be made to withdraw hormone replacement after resolution of the inflammatory stage if progression to fibrosis does not result in irreversible hypopituitarism.

Langerhans' cell histiocytosis

LCH is a rare disorder characterized by clonal proliferation of abnormal dendritic antigen-presenting histiocytes, known as

Langerhans' cells, with an accompanying infiltrate of lymphocytes, eosinophils, and neutrophils resulting in the destruction of a variety of tissues. LCH is also regarded as an inflammatory disease because an altered expression of cytokines and cellular adhesion molecules important for the migration and homing of Langerhans' cells has been demonstrated (32, 33).

Epidemiology

LCH is usually considered to be a disease of childhood, with a peak incidence at the ages of 1 to 3 years (34). Overall, the incidence is 3–5 cases per million per year, with a male to female ratio of 2:1 (34). In adults, the mean age at diagnosis is 33 years and it is seen even more rarely, the estimated prevalence being 1–2 cases per million (35).

Classification and pathology

LCH encompasses a group of diseases that have been referred to as Hand–Schüller–Christian disease, Letterer–Siwe disease, eosinophilic granuloma, histiocytosis X, Hashimoto–Pritzker syndrome, self-healing histiocytosis, pure cutaneous histiocytosis, Langerhans' cell granulomatosis, type II histiocytosis, and nonlipid reticuloendotheliosis (36). Letterer–Siwe disease usually presents in the first 2 years of life and is an acute disseminated form of LCH with extensive cutaneous lesions classically resembling seborrhoeic dermatitis, and is associated with fever, anaemia, lymphadenopathy, osteolytic lesions, and hepatosplenomegaly. Hand–Schuller–Christian disease is a chronic, multisystem disease seen in older children, and the classic, although rare, triad consists of bone disease, diabetes insipidus, and exophthalmos. Eosinophilic granuloma presents in older children and adults, and the granulomatous lesions most often affect bone. Hashimoto–Pritzker disease, also known as congenital, self-healing reticulocytosis, is limited to the skin and resolves rapidly over a period of weeks. Two different phenotypes are usually seen in adults and children with LCH; involvement of bone, lung, skin and diabetes insipidus usually predominates in adults, whereas involvement of liver, spleen, lymph nodes and bone marrow is more common in children (37).

Presentation

In adults, LCH has a predilection for the hypothalamus and pituitary. When only patients with multisystem disease are included, the prevalence of diabetes insipidus can be as high as 40% and diabetes insipidus is considered to be the most common disease-related permanent consequence (38). Diabetes insipidus can also be the presenting feature, pre-dating the diagnosis of LCH. Established diabetes insipidus is generally permanent and does not respond to any disease-modifying treatment; hence the only treatment is desmopressin (39). Diabetes insipidus associated with structural abnormalities of the hypothalamus and pituitary often heralds the development of anterior pituitary hormone deficiencies and CNS involvement (18). Anterior pituitary dysfunction is found in up to 20% of patients with LCH, and is almost always associated with diabetes insipidus (39, 40). Once established, anterior pituitary deficiencies seem to be permanent and are not affected by any form of LCH disease-modifying treatment (18).

The most frequent anterior pituitary hormone deficiency is that of growth hormone, which is found in up to 42% of patients and generally diagnosed with a latency of 1 year from the diagnosis of diabetes insipidus. Deficiencies of luteinizing hormone/FSH are next most common, with a latency of 7 years from the diagnosis of diabetes insipidus (40). Therefore if a partial pituitary hormone deficiency is identified in a patient with LCH, regular monitoring for the remaining hormones is advised. In addition to pituitary involvement, up to 40% of patients with diabetes insipidus have hypothalamic infiltration which results in nonendocrine hypothalamic manifestations, including abnormal eating patterns, morbid obesity, and disturbances in social behaviour, temperature, sleep pattern, and thirst. Diabetes insipidus may be particularly difficult to manage in patients with impaired memory.

Radiology

Patients with LCH and diabetes insipidus commonly demonstrate a loss of the hyperintense signal of the posterior pituitary on T_1-weighted images ('bright spot') on MRI (39). Infundibular enlargement is present in up to 71% of patients at the time of diagnosis of diabetes insipidus (41) as illustrated in the Fig. 2.4.4.3. Hypothalamic mass lesions have been described in 8–18% of patients exhibiting one or more pituitary hormone deficiencies (41). The LCH lesions typically are isointense on T_1 images, hyperintense on T_2 images and enhance with gadolinium (41).

Diagnosis

In order to make the diagnosis of LCH, one must search for extracranial manifestations of LCH with a radiographic skeletal survey, skull series, chest X-ray, and bone scan so that these lesions can be biopsied. Osteolytic lesions due to LCH may be present in the jaw or mastoid, so radiographs of the jaw are a worthwhile part of the diagnostic evaluation. When biopsies of other tissues show LCH and the MRI and clinical picture are compatible, biopsy of the hypothalamic/stalk lesion is rarely necessary.

To establish a diagnosis according to the published criteria of the Histiocytosis Society, a tissue biopsy must either show presence of pathognomonic Birbeck granules on electron microscopy or stain positive for CD1a (43). Birbeck granules are pentalaminar cell inclusions that sometimes have a 'tennis racquet' dilated terminal appearance (44). Their exact function is unknown, but some studies implicate them in antigen processing.

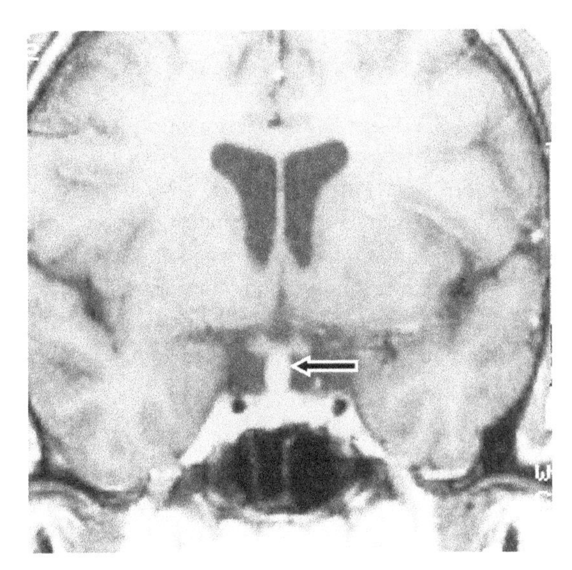

Fig. 2.4.4.3 Thickening of pituitary stalk (arrow) due to biopsy-proven Langerhans' cell histiocytosis. (42).

Management

The course of LCH is often unpredictable, varying from spontaneous regression and resolution to rapid progression and death or repeated recurrence with a considerable risk of permanent sequelae. Patients with disease that is localized to one organ system—single system disease—usually in the bone, skin, or lymph nodes, have a good prognosis and seem to need minimal or even no treatment. In contrast, multiple organ involvement—multisystem disease—carries a risk of a poor outcome, including 10–20% mortality and a 50% risk of life-impairing morbidity. Therefore an early diagnosis and close follow-up is critical. The mainstays of treatment of LCH have been surgery and radiation over the years. However, vinblastine in combination with steroids is now the most frequently used initial therapy for multisystem disease (40). Reports have shown that the purine analogue cladribine (2-chlorodeoxyadenosine) can be effective for adults with recurrent and/or disseminated disease (45).

Anterior and posterior pituitary hormonal deficits are replaced as necessary. With disease limited to the stalk, panhypopituitarism and diabetes insipidus may be present early and need immediate treatment. As with other infiltrative diseases of the hypothalamus, the anterior pituitary hormone deficits may gradually appear. Therefore, periodic testing for many years and then treatment of new deficits may be necessary.

Sarcoidosis

The prevalence of CNS involvement in sarcoidosis is 5–15% and most of these patients are found to have non-caseating granulomas in the hypothalamo-pituitary region in addition to the leptomeninges and cranial nerves (46). The most commonly found hormonal abnormality is diabetes insipidus (17–90% of patients), followed by hyperprolactinemia (3–32%) (19). Hypothalamic involvement may also cause obesity, somnolence with disruption of sleep cycle, alteration in the thirst centre, and loss of short-term memory (47).

MRI usually shows pituitary stalk thickening and enhancement as well as pituitary enlargement. Periventricular lesions and leptomeningeal enhancement can be seen in sarcoidosis and this can help distinguish it from lymphocytic hypophysitis. Significant laboratory findings that may aid in diagnosis are elevated levels of serum and cerebrospinal fluid angiotensin-converting enzyme (ACE). As with LCH, a search for other systemic tissue involvement is important, so that a biopsy can be obtained.

Management of sarcoidosis frequently involves the use of steroids, but recovery of anterior and posterior pituitary function usually does not occur (19). Recently, cladribine was also found to reverse diabetes insipidus caused by sarcoidosis (48). The hypothalamic/pituitary involvement may be gradual and progressive, so that periodic testing is necessary and hormonal deficits treated as they develop.

Wegener's granulomatosis

Wegener's granulomatosis is a systemic vasculitis affecting small- and medium-sized vessels, most commonly in the respiratory tract and kidneys; the pituitary is involved in less than 1% of cases (20). Involvement of the pituitary can occur via direct extension from nasal, paranasal, or orbital disease, from remote granulomatous involvement, or from vasculitis of the hypothalamus. Patients most frequently present with diabetes insipidus, but hyperprolactinaemia and panhypopituitarism have also been reported (7).

The finding of high titres of antineutrophil cytoplasmic antibody (c-ANCA) can be diagnostic but in some cases biopsy of affected tissue is required. When there is hypothalamic/pituitary involvement, MRI reveals an enlarged pituitary with homogeneous enhancement, thickening,and enhancement of the pituitary stalk, and enhancement of the optic chiasm (7, 21).

Wegener's granulomatosis is usually treated with glucocorticoids and/or cyclophosphamide. However, such treatment does not usually lead to reversal of the hypopituitarism. Similar to other infiltrative disease, the destruction may be gradual, necessitating repeated testing and treatment of hormonal deficits as they develop.

Tuberculosis

Since the introduction of antibiotics sellar tuberculomas have become rare, now constituting only 0.15–4.0% of all intracranial mass lesions (49). However, CNS tuberculosis is still relatively common in developing countries. Interestingly, pituitary tuberculomas are found more commonly in women.

Patients may have both anterior and posterior pituitary hormone deficiencies as well as manifestations of other hypothalamic dysfunction. In some cases, these disorders may manifest very gradually over many years, as depicted in Fig. 2.4.4.4. In one series of patients followed up after having had tuberculous meningitis, 20% were found to have anterior pituitary hormone deficiencies (22).

Imaging can reveal involvement of the paranasal sinuses or pituitary fossa, enhancing lesions in the hypothalamus, thickening of the pituitary stalk, pituitary atrophy, and adjacent meningeal enhancement. Pituitary abscesses may also have peripheral contrast enhancement. Tuberculomas are isointense to hypointense on T_1-weighted images and hyperintense on T_2-weighted images. However, these signal characteristics are not unique to tuberculomas and can be seen in pituitary adenomas as well.

Therapy with antituberculous drugs along with surgery when indicated has been used; improvement in pituitary function has been reported in rare cases (23). Pituitary hormonal deficits should be treated when they develop.

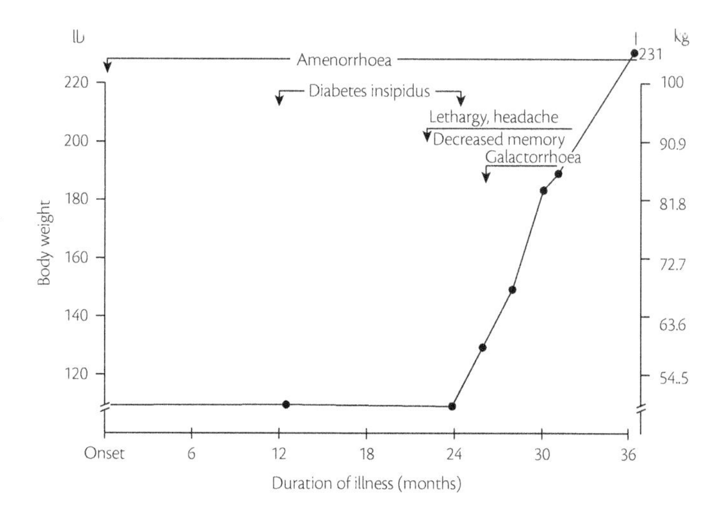

Fig. 2.4.4.4 Progressive dysfunction from hypothalamic tuberculosis in an 18 year old woman(50).

References

1. Caturegli P, Newschaffer C, Olivi A, Pomper MG, Burger PC, Rose NR. Autoimmune hypophysitis. *Endocr Rev*, 2005; **26**: 599–614.
2. Rapp JJ, Pashkis KE. Panhypopituitarism with idiopathic hypoparathyroidism. *Ann Intern Med*, 1953; **39**: 1103–7.
3. Beressi N, Beressi JP, Cohen R, Modigliani E. Lymphocytic hypophysitis: a review of 145 cases. *Ann Med Interne*, 1999; **150**: 327–41.
4. Caturegli P, Lupi I, Landek-Salgado M, Kimura H, Rose NR. Pituitary autoimmunity: 30 years later. *Autoimmun Rev*, 2008; **7**: 631–7.
5. Cheung CC, Ezzat S, Smyth HS, Asa SL. The spectrum and significance of primary hypophysitis. *J Clin Endocrinol Metab*, 2001; **86**: 1048–53.
6. Bellastella A, Bizzarro A, Coronella C, Bellastella G, Sinisi AA, De Bellis A. Lymphocytic hypophysitis: a rare or underestimated disease?. *Eur J Endocrinol*, 2003; **149**: 363–76.
7. Lury KM. Inflammatory and infectious processes involving the pituitary gland. *Top Magn Reson Imaging*, 2005; **16**: 301–6.
8. Rivera J-A. Lymphocytic hypophysitis: disease spectrum and approach to diagnosis and therapy. *Pituitary*, 2006; **9**: 35–45.
9. Thodou E, Asa SL, Kontogeorgos G, Kovacs K, Horvath E, Ezzat S. Clinical case seminar: lymphocytic hypophysitis: clinicopathological findings. *J Clin Endocrinol Metab*, 1995; **80**: 2302–11.
10. Gutenberg A, Buslei R, Fahlbusch R, Buchfelder M, Brück W. Immunopathology of primary hypophysitis. Implications for pathogenesis. *Am J Surg Pathol*, 2005; **29**: 329–38.
11. Hansen I, Petrossians P, Thiry A, Flandroy RC, Gaillard K, Kovacs F, *et al*. Extensive inflammatory pseudotumor of the pituitary. *J Clin Endocrinol Metab*, 2001; **86**: 4603–10.
12. Shaw SA, Camacho LH, McCutcheon IE, Waguespack SG. Transient hypophysitis after cytotoxic T lymphocyte-associated antigen 4 (CTLA4) blockade. *J Clin Endocrinol Metab*, 2007; **92**: 1201–2.
13. Crock PA. Cytosolic autoantigens in lymphocytic hypophysitis. *J Clin Endocrinol Metab*, 1998; **83**: 609–18.
14. Komatsu M, Kondo T, Yamauchi K, Yokokawa N, Ichikawa K, Ishihara M, *et al*. Antipituitary antibodies in patients with the primary empty sella syndrome. *J Clin Endocrinol Metab*, 1988; **67**: 633–8.
15. Cebelin MS, Velasco ME, de las Mulas JM, Druet RL. Galactorrhea associated with lymphocytic adenohypophysitis. Case report. *Br J Obstet Gynaecol*, 1981; **88**: 675–80.
16. Saiwai S, Inoue Y, Ishihara T, Matsumoto S, Nemoto Y, Tashiro T, *et al*. Lymphocytic adenohypophysitis: skull radiographs and MRI. *Neuroradiology*, 1998; **40**: 114–20.
17. Shimono T, Yamaoka T, Nishimura K, Koshiyama H, Sakamoto M, Koh T, *et al*. Lymphocytic hypophysitis presenting with diabetes insipidus: MR findings. *Eur Radiol*, 1999; **9**: 1397–400.
18. Kaltsas GA, Powles TB, Evanson J, Plowman PN, Drinkwater JE, Jenkins PJ, *et al*. Hypothalamo–pituitary abnormalities in adult patients with Langerhans cell histiocytosis: clinical, endocrinological, and radiological features and response to treatment. *J Clin Endocrinol Metab*, 2000; **85**: 1370–6.
19. Bullmann C, Faust M, Hoffmann A, Heppner C, Jockenhovel F, Muller-Wieland D, *et al*. Five cases with central diabetes insipidus and hypogonadism as first presentation of neurosarcoidosis. *Eur J Endocrinol*, 2000; **142**: 365–72.
20. Hoffman GS, Kerr GS, Leavitt RY, Hallahan CW, Lebovics RS, Travis WD, *et al*. Wegener granulomatosis: an analysis of 158 patients. *Ann Intern Med*, 1992; **116**: 488–98.
21. Murphy JM, Gomez-Anson B, Gillard JH, Antoun NM, Cross J, Elliott JD, *et al*. Wegener granulomatosis: MR imaging findings in brain and meninges. *Radiology*, 1999; **213**: 794–9.
22. Lam KS, Sham MM, Tam SC, Ng MM, Ma HT. Hypopituitarism after tuberculous meningitis in childhood. *Ann Intern Med*, 1993; **118**: 701–6.
23. Yilmazlar S, Bekar A, Taskapilioglu O, Tolunay S. Isolated intrasellar tuberculoma mimicking pituitary adenoma. *J Clin Neurosci*, 2007; **14**: 477–81.
24. Abe T. Lymphocytic infundibulo-neurohypophysitis and infundibulo-panhypophysitis regarded as lymphocytic hypophysitis variant. *Brain Tumor Pathol*, 2008; **25**: 59–66.
25. Ishihara T, Hino M, Kurahachi H, Kobayashi H, Kajikawa M, Moridera K, *et al*. Long-term clinical course of two cases of lymphocytic adenohypophysitis. *Endocr J*, 1996; **43**: 433–40.
26. Castle D, de Villiers JC, Melvill R. Lymphocytic adenohypophysitis. Report of a case with demonstration of spontaneous tumour regression and a review of the literature. *Br J Neurosurg*, 1988; **2**: 401–5.
27. Leiba S, Schindel B, Weinstein R, Lidor I, Friedman S, Matz S. Spontaneous postpartum regression of pituitary mass with return of function. *JAMA*, 1986; **255**: 230–2.
28. Feigenbaum SL, Martin MC, Wilson CB, Jaffe RB. Lymphocytic adenohypophysitis: a pituitary mass lesion occurring in pregnancy. Proposal for medical treatment. *Am J Obstet Gynecol*, 1991; **164**: 1549–55.
29. Kristof RA, Van Roost D, Klingmüller D, Springer W, Schramm J. Lymphocytic hypophysitis: non-invasive diagnosis and treatment by high dose methylprednisolone pulse therapy? *J Neurol Neurosurg Psychiatry*, 1999; **67**: 398–402.
30. Reusch JE, Kleinschmidt-DeMasters BK, Lillehei KO, Rappe D, Gutierrez-Hartmann A. Preoperative diagnosis of lymphocytic hypophysitis (adenohypophysitis) unresponsive to short course dexamethasone: case report. *Neurosurgery*, 1992; **30**: 268–72.
31. Parent AD. The course of lymphocytic hypophysitis [letter; comment]. *Surg Neurol*, 1992; **37**: 71.
32. Arceci RJ. The histiocytoses: the fall of the Tower of Babel. *Eur J Cancer*, 1999; **35**: 747–67.
33. Aricò M, Egeler RM. Clinical aspects of Langerhans cell histiocytosis. *Hematol Oncol Clin North Am*, 1998; **12**: 247–58.
34. Broadbent V, Egeler RM, Nesbit ME Jr. Langerhans cell histiocytosis–clinical and epidemiological aspects. *Br J Cancer*, 1994; **Suppl 23**: S11–S16.
35. Malpas JS. Langerhans cell histiocytosis in adults. *Hematol Oncol Clin N Amer*, 1998; **12**: 259–68.
36. Howarth DM, Gilchrist GS, Mullan BP, Wiseman GA, Edmonson JH, Schomberg PJ. Langerhans cell histiocytosis: diagnosis, natural history, management and outcome. *Cancer*, 1999; **85**: 2278–90.
37. Newman B, Hu W, Nigro K, Gilliam AC. Aggressive histiocytic disorders that can involve the skin. *J Am Acad Dermatol*, 2007; **56**: 302–16.
38. Haupt R, Nanduri V, Calevo MG, Bernstrand C, Braier JL, Broadbent V, *et al*. Permanent consequences in Langerhans cell histiocytosis patients: a pilot study from the Histiocyte Society–Late Effects Study Group. *Pediatr Blood Cancer*, 2004; **42**: 438–44.
39. Aricò M, Girschikofsky M, Généreau T, Klersy C, McClain K, Grois N, *et al*. Langerhans cell histiocytosis in adults. Report from the International Registry of the Histiocyte Society. *Eur J Cancer*, 2003; **39**: 2341–8.
40. Makras P, Alexandraki KI, Chrousos GP, Grossman AB, Kaltsas GA. Endocrine manifestations in Langerhans cell histiocytosis. *Trends Endocrinol Metab*, 2007; **18**: 252–7.
41. Ouyang DL, Roberts BK, Gibbs IC, Katznelson L. Isolated Langerhans cell histiocytosis in an adult with central diabetes insipidus: case report and review of literature. *Endocr Pract*, 2006; **12**: 660–3.
42. Purdy LP, Molitch ME. Sudden onset of diabetes insipidus in an adolescent. *Endocr Trends*, 1998; **5**: 1–7.
43. Favara B, Feller A, Paulli M, Jaffe ES, Weiss LM, Arico M, *et al*, for the WHO Committee on Histiocytic/Reticulum cell proliferations, the Reclassification Working Group of the Histiocyte Society. Contemporary classification of histiocytic disorders. *Med Pediatr Oncol*, 1997; **29**: 157–66.
44. Davis SE, Rice DH. Langerhans' cell histiocytosis: current trends and the role of the head and neck surgeon. *Ear Nose Throat J*, 2004; **83**: 340–2.

45. Pardanani A, Phyliky RL, Li CY, Tefferi A. 2-Chlorodeoxyadenosine therapy for disseminated Langerhans cell histiocytosis. *Mayo Clin Proc*, 2003; **78**: 301–6.
46. Agbogu B, Stern BJ, Sewell C, Yang G. Therapeutic considerations in patients with refractory neurosarcoidosis. *Arch Neurol*, 1995; **52**: 875–9.
47. Stuart CA, Neelon FA, Lebovitz HE. Disordered control of thirst in hypothalamic-pituitary sarcoidosis. *N Engl J Med*, 1980; **303**: 1078–82.
48. Tikoo RK, Kupersmith MJ, Finlay JL. Treatment of refractory neurosarcoidosis with cladribine. *N Engl J Med*, 2004; **350**: 1798–9.
49. DeAngelis LM. Intracranial tuberculoma: case report and review of the literature. *Neurology*, 1981; **31**: 133–6.
50. Bray GA, Gallagher TF Jr. Manifestations of hypothalamic obesity in man: a comprehensive investigation of eight patients and a review of the literature. *Med (Balt)*, 1975; **54**: 301–30.

2.5

Pineal physiology and pathophysiology, including pineal tumours

Anna Aulinas, Cristina Colom, Susan M. Webb

Pineal physiology

The pineal gland is innervated mainly by sympathetic nerve fibres that inform the gland of the prevailing light-dark cycle and acts as a neuroendocrine transducer. The gland is located behind the third ventricle in the centre of the brain and is a highly vascular organ formed by neuroglial cells and parenchymal cells or pinealocytes. The latter synthesize melatonin as well as other indoleamines and peptides.

The main pineal hormone melatonin (*N*-acetyl-5-methoxytryptamine) exhibits an endogenous circadian rhythm, reflecting signals originating in the suprachiasmatic nucleus; environmental lighting entrains the rhythm, by altering its timing. Independently of sleep, pineal melatonin is inhibited by light and stimulated during darkness, thanks to the neural input by a multisynaptic pathway that connects the retina, through the suprachiasmatic nucleus of the hypothalamus, preganglionic neurons in the upper thoracic spinal cord and postganglionic sympathetic fibres from the superior cervical ganglia, with the pineal gland.

Melatonin deficiency may produce sleeping disorders, behavioural problems, or be associated with precocious or delayed puberty in children, while chronically elevated melatonin has been observed in some cases of hypogonadotropic hypogonadism (1, 2).

Pineal tumours

The main clinical problem related to the pineal gland is that of pineal tumours. They are rare, and 10 times more common in children than in adults and mainly derive from the three types of cell (3, 4) (Box 2.5.1).

Astrocytic tumours may affect children and adults of any age. Pylocytic astrocytomas usually present before the age of 20 years, with no sex predilection, while other types are more frequent in adults.

While parenchymal tumours secrete melatonin, they differ in their degree of malignancy, pineoblastomas (WHO grade IV, Table 2.5.1) being highly malignant, aggressive and of rapid growth (similar to other primitive neuroectodermal tumours such as neuroblastomas or medulloblastomas), while pinealocytomas are mostly benign (WHO grade I, Table 2.5.1). Histologically, pineocytomas characteristically present pineocytomatous rosettes, while pineoblastomas are populated by small, highly undifferentiated cells, often present with haemorrhagic or necrotic components, but rarely calcifications. However, most parenchymal tumours are either mixed or show intermediate differentiation (WHO grades II and III, Table 2.5.1).

Germ cell tumours, histologically and biologically homologous to gonadal germ cell neoplasms, will characteristically present positive markers for α-fetoprotein (AFP) and β-human chorionic gonadotrophin (β-hCG), with more (teratomas) or less differentiation (germinomas), as well as intermediate degrees (yolk sac tumours).

Very rarely, pineal region tumours may derive from meningothelial, mesenchymal, ependymal, choroid plexus elements and peripheral nerves, giving rise to gangliogliomas, melanocytic neoplasms, atypical teratoid/rhabdoid tumours, meningiomas, cavernous angiomas, haemangiopericytomas or neurinomas/neurofibromas, apart from lymphomas or metastases.

Clinical presentation

Clinical presentation of pineal tumours depends on age at onset and histology (7). Over 90% present with raised intracranial pressure, often with obstructive hydrocephalus; initial symptoms are frequently headache, nausea, vomiting, and decreased vision; 50–70% of patients refer visual signs such as diplopia, cranial nerve palsies, papilloedema, and ptosis or Parinaud's syndrome (failure of upward gaze, pupillary dilatation and diminution of pupillary light reflex) due to pressure on the pretectal region. Compression on the brain, cerebellum, hypothalamus, and pituitary may cause paralysis of other cranial nerves, ataxia, diabetes insipidus, and hypopituitarism. Pineal tumours may interfere with puberty, due to either pressure of the tumour on the hypothalamic centres which govern gonadotrophin secretion, excessive melatonin secretion by pinealocyte tumours causing delayed puberty in adolescents, or reduction of the potential antigonadotropic effect of melatonin, which, together with β-hCG secretion by destructive germ cell tumours could explain precocious puberty in prepubertal children.

Parenchymal tumours (8–11). The recent WHO classification of these tumours grade them from I to IV (Table 2.5.1) (3, 4).

Box 2.5.1 Classification of pineal tumours

Neuroglial cells (20%)
- Low-grade astrocytomas (juvenile pilocytic)
- Intermediate diffuse and anaplastic astrocytomas
- High-grade malignant glioblastomas

Parenchymal tumours (15–30%) (see Table 2.5.1)
Germ cell tumours (80% in Japan, 30–50% in western Europe and USA)
- Germinomas
- Nongerminomatous germ cell tumours
  - Embryonal carcinoma
  - Yolk sac tumour
  - Choriocarcinoma
  - Teratomas
- Benign teratomas
- Immature
- Mature
- Teratoma with malignant transformation
- Mixed germ cell tumours

Pineocytomas (grade I) present more often in adults over the age of 25 years, without sex predilection, evolve slowly (interval between onset of symptoms and surgery may be of several years), do not invade contiguous tissue, or seed the cerebrospinal fluid (CSF). Nonspecific presenting manifestations reflect compression of neighbouring structures (tectal plate, aqueduct of Sylvius, cerebellum, brainstem, hypothalamus, pituitary) such as increased intracranial pressure, changes in mental status, neuro-ophthalmological, brain stem, and/or cerebellum dysfunction, hypopituitarism, and hyperprolactinaemia. Rarely intratumoral haemorrhage (pineal apoplexy) with subarachnoid extravasation may occur. Concurrent uveoretinitis in occasional patients with pineocytomas probably reflects the common photoreceptor activity of pineal and retinal cells. No metastases and a 5-year survival >90% have been reported.

Pineoblastomas (grade IV) typically appear before the age of 20 years, most often in young children, but there are reports in adults, with a slight male preponderance. Presenting symptoms of this least differentiated and most aggressive pineal parenchymal tumour are more rapidly progressive and of shorter duration (interval between initial symptoms and surgery may be less than a month). Median postsurgical survival varies from 24 to 30 months. They are locally invasive and prone to disseminate through the CSF, often fatal, but may be controlled in some cases by a multimodality combination of aggressive surgery, radiotherapy, and chemotherapy. The association of a pineoblastoma in a child with familial bilateral retinoblastoma (due to a germline retinoblastoma gene mutation) is known as a trilateral retinoblastoma, with a median survival of only 6 months. Intermediate grades II and III represent different degrees of differentiation and prognosis (Table 2.5.1).

Table 2.5.1 Parenchymal pineal tumour classification (3–6); the current WHO classification does not provide strict criteria to distinguish grade II and III tumours

WHO grade	Histological type	Indicators of differentiation (from more to less)	Prognosis
I	Pineocytoma	No mitoses/very positive NF protein staining	Good
II III	Intermediate differentiation (20%)	Moderate nuclear atypia/low to moderate mitotic activity/ <2 mitoses per HPFs/ positive NF protein staining/MIB1 proliferation indices 3–10% >6 mitoses per HPF/necrosis/ negative NF protein staining	↓
IV	Pineoblastoma	Variable plus positive or negative NF	Bad

Germ cell tumours These arise around the third ventricle, most commonly in the pineal region, but may also be seen in the suprasellar compartment; 5–10% of patients harbour both lesions. Ninety per cent appear under the age of 20 years and are more frequent in males than females (2.5:1), except suprasellar lesions, which are more common in females. An increased risk of intracranial germ cell tumours has been associated with Klinefelter's syndrome, Down's syndrome, and neurofibromatosis type 1 (12, 13).

Other tumours Pineal meningiomas, gangliogliomas, ependymomas, lipomas and pineal metastases, most frequently of breast or lung origin, may occur, often with other brain metastases; symptoms and signs reflect the extent of the disease (14, 15).

Diagnosis

An appropriate tissue specimen for accurate histological diagnosis and determining tumour type is critical to optimize subsequent management. Serum AFP (synthesized mainly by yolk sac tumours, and teratomas) and β-hCG (in choriocarcinomas or germinomas) concentrations are of diagnostic utility if markedly elevated in serum and/or cerebrospinal fluid (CSF). Measurement of these markers in CSF for initial staging, and if positive, for follow-up are useful. CSF cytological examination should be delayed at least 2 weeks after surgery to increase the chance of reflecting true dissemination of viable tumour rather than postoperative tumour spillage. If these markers are clearly raised, histological verification may not be required.

Biopsies may be obtained by classic surgical routes (posterior interhemispheric transcallosal, suboccipital transtentorial, and infratentorial-supracerebellar routes) or by microsurgical techniques, with significantly reduced perioperative mortality rates (<2%). A neuroendoscopic or stereotactic biopsy is reasonably safe and well tolerated (7, 16) in experimented hands, but the diagnosis of mixed or intermediate tumours may be difficult without extensive tissue sampling. In any case, operative risk should be balanced with the risk of not obtaining an accurate histological diagnosis, with prognostic implications. In cases of nondiagnostic or equivocal biopsies or indicative of a benign tumour (mature teratoma, meningioma), surgery is recommended.

Imaging

An MRI will disclose the size and extension of the tumour and possible metastases, but cannot accurately identify the histological nature, which relies on biopsy or serum/CSF tumour markers. In the more malignant tumours (pineoblastomas, germinomas, teratomas)

the spine as well as the brain should be imaged, since spread into the subarachnoid space and the spine is frequent.

Neuroimaging of astrocytic tumours can vary; MRI usually shows hypodensity on T_1-weighted images and hyperintensity on T_2-weighted images; gadolinium enhancement is uncommon, except if active tumour progression occurs. Among parenchymal tumours, pineocytomas appear as noninvasive, solid masses in the posterior third ventricular region, and tend to be smaller (<3 cm in general), rounder, hypodense, homogeneous masses with dispersed calcifications, particularly peripheral, which enhance heterogeneously or diffusely on CT and MRI, and present a lesser degree of hydrocephalus. Macrocystic presentation is rare but small cysts may be present. T_1-weighted images are hypointense while T_2 are hyperintense. Haemorrhage and necrosis are exceptional.

Pineoblastomas are larger, lobulated, homogeneous tumours, rarely calcified and present with a greater degree of hydrocephalus and local invasion of contiguous brain or leptomeninges; they may exhibit distant subarachnoid and extracranial metastases, more frequently in young females; they are hyperdense and enhance homogeneously on CT (Fig. 2.5.1), while on MRI they appear as hypointense to isointense on T_1-weighted images and enhance diffusely or heterogeneously with contrast (Fig. 2.5.2, Fig. 2.5.3, and Fig. 2.5.4). Haemorrhage and necrosis are common (Fig. 2.5.5).

Germ cell tumours (except teratomas) appear as solid masses on MRI, iso- or hyperdense, and enhance after contrast (Fig. 2.5.6 and Fig. 2.5.7); small nodular calcifications may be seen on CT-scans. Teratomas tend to contain intratumoral cysts next to calcifications and low attenuation signals, typical of fat. Haemorrhages are common in choriocarcinomas and mixed neoplasms.

Treatment

Surgery, chemotherapy and radiation are used in the treatment of pineal region tumours. Surgery, either open, stereotactic or endoscopic, is used to obtain a biopsy, mandatory in the majority of cases to obtain a definite histological diagnosis (7). Morbidity and cure rates have improved over the past years thanks to a greater understanding of the nature of the different tumours, more accurate neurosurgical experience, selective use of chemotherapy, and the introduction of modern irradiation techniques. However, because of the rarity of pineal tumours, it is difficult to conduct large, prospective, multicentre international studies to define their optimal management.

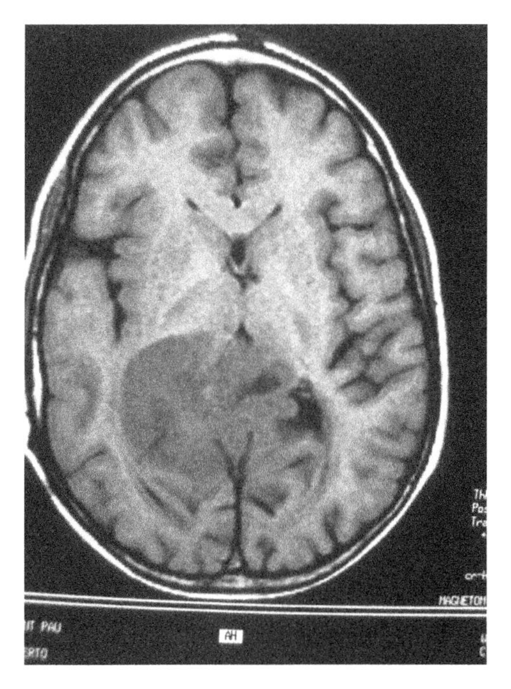

Fig. 2.5.2 Noncontrast T_1-weighted MR image of a recurrent pineoblastoma in a 16-year-old boy.

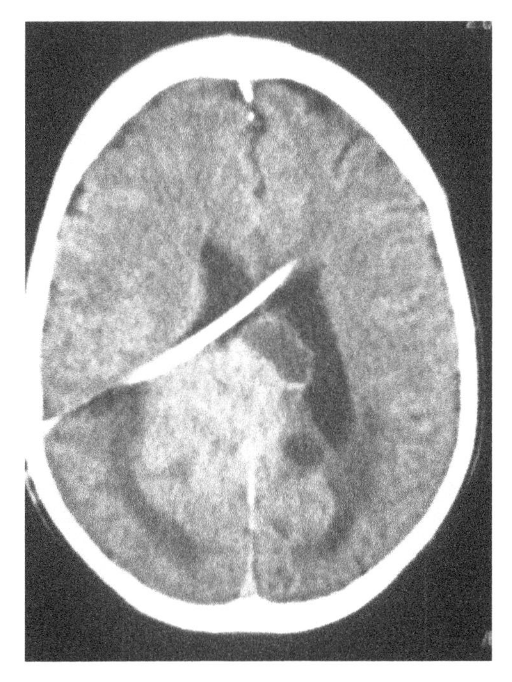

Fig. 2.5.1 Contrast-enhanced CT scan of a recurrent pineoblastoma in a 16-year-old boy with ventricular shunt. (Courtesy of Dr E. Guardia.)

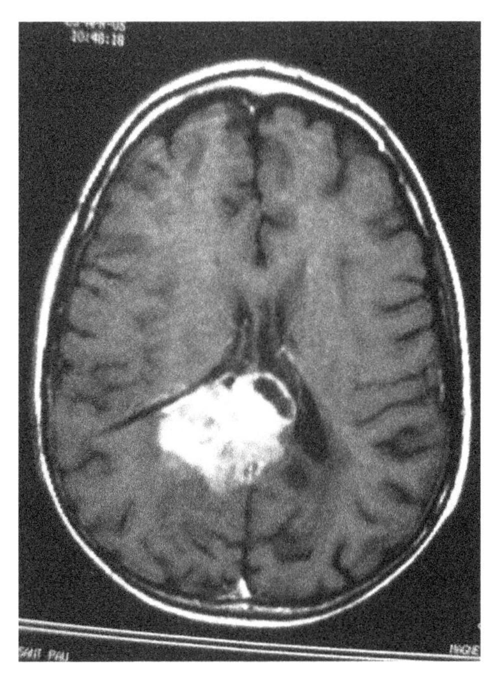

Fig. 2.5.3 T_1-weighted gadolinium-enhanced MR image of a recurrent pineoblastoma showing the ventricular shunt.

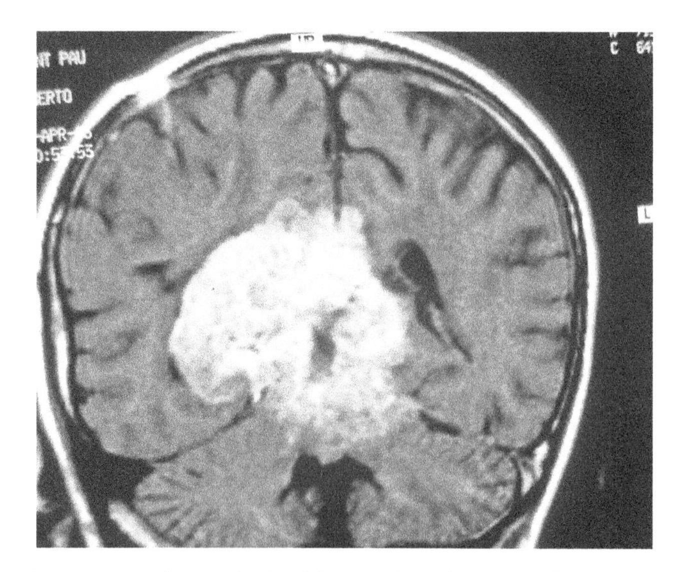

Fig. 2.5.4 Coronal T_1-weighted gadolinium-enhanced MR image of a recurrent pineoblastoma.

Treatment depends on histology obtained after surgery, which apart from the biopsy can resolve intracranial hypertension with a ventricular shunt (atrial or peritoneal) and perform partial debulking of the tumour if possible; total resection is rarely possible (Table 2.5.2).

Astrocytomas

Treatment for astroglial-derived malignant gliomas is local radiotherapy to the tumor (54 Gy), either conventional or stereotaxic, while surgery may be curative for the more benign pylocytic astrocytomas.

Pineal parenchymal tumors

Pineocytomas only require local radiotherapy to the tumor (54 Gy). In pinealoblastomas, a high probability of spinal seedlings should lead to craniospinal radiotherapy, since they are radiosensitive (25–30 Gy on the neuroaxis with a pineal boost of 40 Gy aimed at more effective local disease control). However, routine craniospinal irradiation has been questioned and may not be necessary in patients with negative staging. Stereotaxic radiosurgery may control local progression and minimize damage to the surrounding brain, which is especially important in prepubertal patients, in whom total brain irradiation is associated with neurocognitive dysfunction, endocrinopathy, second malignancies, vascular complications, and spinal growth impairment. However, it may be associated with a high risk of marginal recurrence and distant metastases, and is not considered the treatment of choice for

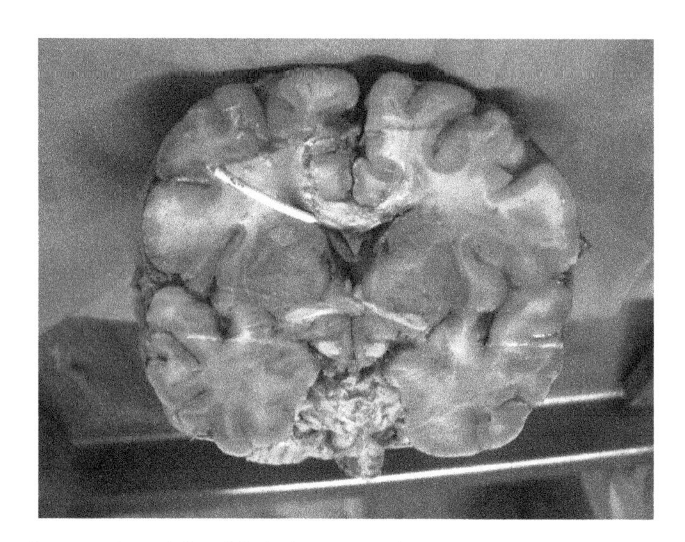

Fig. 2.5.5 Coronal slice of the brain corresponding to Fig. 2.5.1, showing the pineoblastoma and the ventricular shunt. (Courtesy of Dr E. Guardia.)

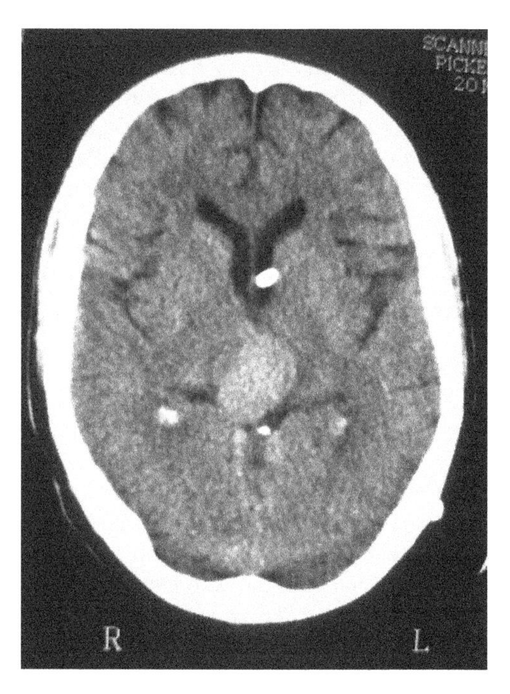

Fig. 2.5.6 CT scan of a recurrent pineal germinoma in a 57-year-old man, with a ventriculoperitoneal shunt. (Courtesy of Dr E. Guardia.)

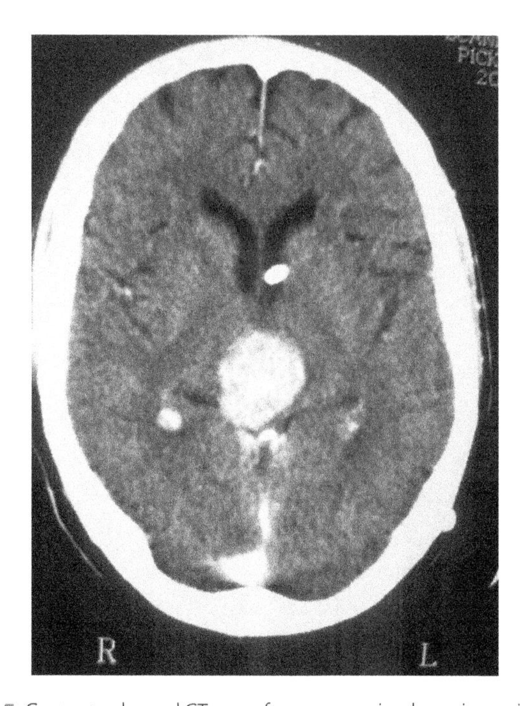

Fig. 2.5.7 Contrast-enhanced CT scan of a recurrent pineal germinoma in a 57-year old man.

Table 2.5.2 Treatment guidelines for pineal tumours. Surgery for histologic biopsy and subtyping and if necessary cerebrospinal fluid (CSF) diversion (ventriculoperitoneal shunt or ventriculostomy) should always be performed, with the possible exception of germ cell tumours with diagnostically elevated tumour markers.

Tumour type	Radiotherapy	Chemotherapy[a]	Surgery
Glial origin			
Juvenile pilocytic astrocytoma	No	No	Complete resection
Intermediate/diffuse/anaplastic/ Astrocytomas/glioma	Local	No	Debulking
Malignant glioblastoma	Local	No	Debulking
Parenchymal tumours			
Pineocytoma	Local	No	Biopsy
Intermediate or mixed tumour	Local ± craniospinal	Yes in more undifferentiated tumours	Biopsy
Pineoblastoma	Local Routine craniospinal not always indicated. Age <5 years: Lower dose, after initial chemotherapy	Yes (role on final outcome unclear)	Biopsy
Germ cell tumours			
Germinoma	Local + craniospinal (unless convinced of negative staging)	Yes (alone not curative)	Biopsy
Nongerminatous tumours	Local + craniospinal	Yes (pre- or post-surgery)	Resection as much as possible, without ↑ morbidity

[a] Chemotherapy includes cisplatin, etoposide and cyclophosphamide or isofosfamide.

infiltrative but curable tumours. Furthermore, complications such as ataxic gait and gaze palsy have been reported after radiosurgery, In young children chemotherapy with cisplatin, etoposide, cyclophosphamide and vincristine, which alone is not curative, may allow a lower dose of radiotherapy to have similar effects. In older children with pineoblastoma, craniospinal irradiation is followed by chemotherapy (even though its role on final outcome is not fully defined). Autologous haematopoietic stem cell-supported high-dose chemotherapy is currently being investigated with some initial promising results, although experience is limited (17).

In mixed or intermediate pineal parenchymal cells (grade II or III, Table 2.5.1), apart from local radiotherapy, craniospinal irradiation and chemotherapy should be considered with increasing number of mitoses and less differentiation (7–11).

Germ cell tumours

Surgery is not considered curative in germinomas, which are radiosensitive and should therefore receive local radiotherapy (7, 12, 13). Unless firmly confident of negative staging (by negative tumour markers AFP and β-hCG in blood and CSF, and negative MRI), craniospinal radiotherapy should be offered given the high probability of spinal seedlings. Germinomas are also highly chemosensitive, and excellent responses to postoperative cisplatin and cyclophosphamide have been reported. Survival is high (>90% at 5 years) in patients with localized pure germinomas, using either chemotherapy or focal radiotherapy or craniospinal irradiation, while focal irradiation alone has a worse outcome. In metastatic germinomas, craniospinal irradiation is the treatment of choice (25–35 Gy to the spine and a local pineal boost of 40 Gy). Lower irradiation doses are currently being considered, especially if adjuvant chemotherapy is offered (12). Bifocal lesions in the pineal and hypothalamus should be considered localized germinomas rather than metastatic disease, and receive irradiation to both locations.

Other germ cell tumours are less radiosensitive than germinomas, with a poor survival after radiotherapy alone (median survival of under 2 years) and require multimodality treatment (12, 13). Surgical resection after tumour reduction with initial chemotherapy with cisplatin, etoposide, and isofosfamide is a modern alternative. Tumour markers are useful for follow-up. Combining chemotherapy with radiotherapy (local up to 54 Gy or craniospinal up to 36 Gy) may increase long-term survival to 80%.

Surgery is the treatment of choice of pineal meningiomas and other localized pineal tumours if possible; alternatively localized stereotactic radiosurgery may be offered with good long-term prognosis (7).

Pineal cysts

Masses in the pineal region are most commonly non-neoplastic cysts, incidentally discovered at autopsy or on a radiographic work-up for symptoms not reasonably attributed to the cyst. Very rarely they act as a mass lesion and produce signs of increased intracranial pressure, by compressing the aqueduct (obstructive hydrocephalus) or tectal plate (Parinaud's syndrome). On MRI they appear as a 1–3 cm mass, equally or slightly more dense than CSF in T1-weighted image studies and which brightly enhance in T2-weighted images, reflecting their fluid nature; evidence of haemorrhage and peripheral calcification may be found. If asymptomatic, pineal cysts do not generally require treatment; if large enough to increase intracranial pressure, resection may be necessary, with an excellent long-term outcome (7).

References

1. Webb SM, Puig-Domingo M. Melatonin in health and disease. *Clin Endocrinol*, 1995; **42**: 221–34.
2. Macchi MM, Bruce JN. Human pineal physiology and functional significance of melatonin. *Front Neuroendocrinol*, 2004; **25**: 177–95.

3. Louis DN, Ohgaki H, Wiestler OD, Cavenee WK, Burger PC, Jouvet A, *et al.* The 2007 WHO classification of tumours of the central nervous system. *Acta Neuropatho*, 2007; **114**: 97–109.
4. Brat DJ, Parisi JE, Kleinschmidt-DeMasters BK, Yachnis AT,. Montine TJ, Boyer PJ, *et al.* Neuropathology Committee, College of American Pathologists Surgical neuropathology update: a review of changes introduced by the WHO classification of tumours of the central nervous system, 4th edition. *Arch Pathol Lab Med*, 2008; **132**: 993–1007.
5. Fauchon F, Jouvet A, Paquis P, Saint-Pierre G, Mottolese C, Ben Hassel M, *et al.* Parenchymal pineal tumors: A clinicopathological study of 76 cases. *Internat J Rad Oncol Biol Phys*, 2000; **46**: 959–68.
6. Jouvet A, Saint-Pierre G, Fouchon F, Privat K, Bouffet E, Ruchoux MM, *et al.* Pineal parenchymal tumors: A correlation of histological features with prognosis in 66 cases. *Brain Pathol*, 2000; **10**: 49–60.
7. Balmaceda C, Loeffler JS, Wen PY. Pineal Gland Masses. UpToDate Version 16.3, 2008. Available at: www.uptodate.com (accessed January 2009).
8. Chang SM, Lillis-Hearne PK, Larson DA, Wara WM, Bollen AW, Prados MD. Pineoblastoma in adults. *Neurosurgery*, 1995; **37**: 383–90.
9. Schild SE, Scheithauer BW, Schomberg PJ, Hook CC, Kelly PJ, Frick L, *et al.* Pineal parenchymal tumors. Clinical, pathologic and therapeutic aspects. *Cancer*, 1993; **72**: 870–80.
10. Cohen BH, Zeltzer PM, Boyett JM, Geyer JR, Allen JC, Finlay JL, *et al.* Prognostic factors and treatment results for supratentorial primitive neuroectodermal tumors in children using radiation and chemotherapy: A children's cancer group randomized trial. *J Clin Oncol*, 1995; **13**: 1687–96.
11. Jackacki RI, Zeltzer PM, Boyett JM, Albright AL, Allen JC, Geyer JR, *et al.* Survival and prognostic factors following radiation and/or chemotherapy for primitive neuroectodermal tumors of the pineal region in infants and children: A report of the Children's Cancer Group. *J Clin Oncol*, 1995; **13**: 1377–83.
12. Echevarría ME, Fangusaro J, Goldman S. Pediatric central nervous system germ cell tumors: a review. *Oncologist*, 2008; **13**: 690–9.
13. Matsutani M, Sano K, Takakura K, Fujimaki T, Nakamura O, Funata N, *et al.* Primary intracranial germ cell tumors: A clinical analysis of 153 histologically verified cases. *J Neurosurg*, 1997; **86**: 446–55.
14. Bailey S, Skinner R, Lucraft HH, Perry RH, Todd N, Pearson AD. Pineal tumours in the North of England 1968–93. *Arch Dis Child*, 1996; **75**: 181–5.
15. Mena H, Nakazato Y, Scheithauer BW. Pineal parenchymal tumors. In Kleihues P, Cavenee WK, eds. *Pathology and Genetics. Tumors of the nervous system.* Lyon, France: International Agency for Research on Cancer, 1997: 115–21.
16. Oi S, Shibata M, Tominaga J, Honda Y, Shinoda M, Takei F, *et al.* Efficacy of neuroendoscopic procedures in minimally invasive preferential management of pineal region tumors: a prospective study. *J Neurosurgery*, 2000; **93**: 245–53.
17. Gururangan S, McLaughlin C, Quinn J, Rich J, Reardon D, Halperin EC, *et al.* High-dose chemotherapy with autologous stem-cell rescue in children and adults with newly diagnosed pineoblastomas. *J Clin Oncol*, 2003; **21**: 2187–91.

2.6

Neuropsychiatric endocrinological disorders

Contents

2.6.1 Endocrinology, sleep and circadian rhythms

G. Brabant

Introduction

Endogenous circadian rhythms enable organisms to prepare for environmental changes and to temporally modify behavioural and physiological functions. A variation in energy demands appears to be the most important common denominator of these circadian changes, which renders the intimate reciprocal relation of circadian behaviour and endocrine rhythms no surprise. One of the most obvious examples of circadian behaviour is the sleep–wake cycle, closely linked to diurnal variations of locomotor activity, temperature regulation, and water/food intake. Already subtle changes in these circadian cycles may lead to detrimental effects in human biology. Such causative relationship between these changes and adverse biological effects have been obtained not only from mutations characterized in genes responsible for the generation and the integration of circadian rhythms but also from observational studies where circadian rhythmicity was experimentally changed. Life in modern societies tends to increasingly ignore the natural time cues and these environmental insults are increasingly recognized as the underlying mechanism for many pathophysiological changes and a higher susceptibility to disease. Focusing on endocrine-related effects, this chapter will highlight our current understanding of the genetic background of circadian rhythms, their integration with the light–dark cycle and their links to sleep-related changes (1).

Mechanisms underlying circadian behaviour and definitions

Definitions

Rhythmic circadian behaviour is not restricted to humans but can be detected in the entire animal kingdom, starting with bacteria. These rhythms synchronize biological processes to the day–night (or light–dark) cycle of the natural environment. In humans, it was originally believed that only specialized neurons of the suprachiasmatic nucleus (SCN) are able to induce circadian behaviour but recent detection of rhythmicity in most peripheral organs or cells have challenged this view. The detection of clock and clock-output-genes in these peripheral cells and of rhythmic behaviour when time cues from the SCN are missing suggest a general endogenous pattern. Approximately 5–10% of all peripherally expressed genes show such cyclical behaviour. However, in contrast to the SCN, which integrates time cues from the light circle, peripheral cells are not sensitive to light and are predominantly regulated by hormonal time cues. The time interval between two peaks of an individual rhythm defined as the *period* is regulated to a 24-h cycle by external time cues, so-called *Zeitgeber*. When these are missing, individual circadian rhythms may dissociate. These *free running rhythms* have been detected in experiments with volunteers kept for long time in isolation of all Zeitgebers, especially the two most powerful Zeitgebers, light and food. One of the most striking acute conditions where synchronization of circadian rhythms is temporarily lost is jetlag due to a transmeridian flight. There are multiple other examples for a weakening of the coordination of rhythms. With the recent characterization of the molecular mechanism underlying circadian rhythmicity mutational changes have been described affecting the circadian mechanism in all cells. This may result either in a shorter or a longer than expected underlying rhythm, and external time cues may no longer be able to optimally synchronize circadian rhythmicity. The so-called 'phase', which is defined as interval between a fixed event like the beginning of the night and the peak of a given rhythm, is shifted. This can be either shifted to an earlier time, i.e. *phase advanced*, or may be prolonged or *phase delayed* (2).

Molecular mechanism

Seminal work in plants, flies, mice, and humans on periodicity genes governing circadian behaviour led to the independent discovery of the first genes involved in circadian behaviour in mammals. Subsequently, the molecular components of the circadian clock were unravelled in much greater detail even though there are still many inconsistencies remaining. A gene named *c*ircadian *l*ocomoter *o*utput *c*ycles *k*aput or *CLOCK* and its paralogue *n*euronal *PAS* domain protein *2*, *NPAS2* have been characterized as integral parts of the circadian machinery, which further needs *BMAL1* (also known as aryl hydrocarbon receptor nuclear translocator-like; Arntl), period homologue 1 (*Per1*), *Per2*, and cryptochrome 1 and 2 (*Cry1, Cry2*) (Table 2.6.1.1). Under conditions of light, *CLOCK* (or *NPAS2*) activates transcription of Per and Cyr proteins by interaction with bmAL1. Per and Cry proteins heterodimerize at high protein levels, and on translocation to the nucleus inhibit their own transcription following interaction with the Clock–Bmal1 complex. Subsequently during the dark period the repressor complex of Per–Cry is degraded, and a new cycle of transcription is activated by Per/Cry. The period of the entire process approximates 24 h. This primary feedback loop is stabilized by a second negative feedback through nuclear hormone receptor Rev-erba. Rev-erba, a direct target of Clock-Bmal1, is a strong inhibitor of Bmal1 transcription. This basic regulation is modulated by a large number of additional factors that change the kinetics of the feedback by altering the stoichiometry of the complexes. During the late afternoon and night Per1 and Per2 proteins are progressively phosphorylated through key kinases such as casein kinase 1δ and ε (CSNK1δ; CSNK1ε). These phosphorylation steps are crucial for the degradation of clock proteins via the proteosomal pathway. Mutants in any members of these regulators may alter the kinetic of the circadian process and result in either short or long periods. Fig. 2.6.1.1 schematically illustrate the process. In addition, more recently the critical importance of circadian changes in histone H3 acetylation and chromatin remodelling for circadian transcription of Clock–Bmal1 target genes has been recognized. It supports an intimate link between the autoregulatory feedback loop and chromatin remodelling (for reviews see Schibler(1), Takahashi et al. (2), Brown et al. (3), and Hussain and Pan (4)).

Intriguing work in a human fibroblast model indicated that these clock genes continue to work as a self-sustained oscillator even outside of the body. It appears that every individual has a given period length which governs its chronotrope. Morning ('lark') or evening ('owl') types have been characterized in humans who differ by up to 4 h in their optimal cognitive function due to the set-up of the molecular clock (5, 6).

Table 2.6.1.1 Genetic links between genes involved in circadian behaviour, sleep, and metabolism

Gene	Seq.variant	Phenotype
Metabolic disorders		
BMAL1	SNPs rs7950226 rs6486121	Type 2 diabetes Hypertension
CLOCK	SNPs rs486454 rs1801260	Metabolic syndrome and obesity Mood/behavioural disorders
ARNTL/BMAL1	SNPs rs3789327 rs2278749	Associated with bipolar disorder
NPAS2	L471S[1]	Diurnal preference/SAD
PER3	SNPs rs228729 rs228642 rs228666 rs2859388 rs228697	Associated with bipolar disorder
ASMT (HIOMT)	SNPs rs4446909 rs5989681	Autism spectrum disorder

SAD, See the supplement to Takahashi JS, Hong HK, Ko CH, McDearmon EL. The genetics of mammalian circadian order and disorder: implications for physiology and disease. *Nat Rev Genet* 2008; **9**(+ Supplement): 764–75 (2).

Role of light and the suprachiasmatic nucleus

Despite the characterization of clock genes in many mammalian cells the key importance of the hypothalamus for the integration of circadian rhythms is undisputed. Targeted deletion of hypothalamic nuclei including SCN, the ventrolateral preoptic, and dorsomedial nucleus clearly indicates that a normal patterning of sleep–wake cycle, locomotor behaviour, feeding, and the secretion of circadian hormones is no longer observed. Using the same molecular instrumentarium observed in many cells, the SCN appears to be the master regulator of circadian behaviour. This may be based on its ability to respond to light which has been shown for the SCN expression of the clock genes, *Per1* and *Per2*. This sensitivity is detectable only during the night period when

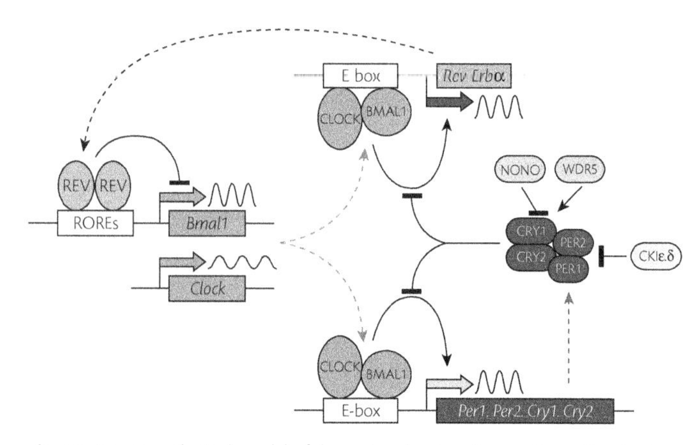

Fig. 2.6.1.1 Hypothetical model of the molecular circadian oscillator. The rhythm generating circuitry is thought to be based on molecular feedback loops within a positive limb (*CLOCK, BMAL1*) and a negative oscillator limb (Per and Cry proteins) that are interconnected via the nuclear orphan receptor Rev-erba (1). NONO, RNA-binding proteins; REV, nuclear receptor subfamily 1 group D; RORE, retinoic acid related orphan receptor; WDR5, histone methyltransferase-binding protein. (2).

levels are low whereas the high levels during the day are not changed by additional light exposure (7).

Role of food and the dorsomedial hypothalamus

Studies in nocturnal animals show that a shift in the availability of food has a dominant effect on locomotor activity and the circadian patterns of liver, lung, and heart. This supports the notion that a food-entrainable oscillator exists distinct from the well-characterized light-dependent entrainment of circadian rhythms. Ablation studies indicate that the dorsal medial hypothalamus and not the SCN is critical for food-dependent effects on circadian rhythmicity. A gut–brain communication either via humoral or neural pathways is postulated. Clock genes expressed in the intestinum appear to be independent of the light–dark cycle and processing of food. The circadian rhythmicity observed in triglyceride levels even in the fasting state exemplifies such endogenous diurnal behaviour (4).

Sleep and circadian rhythms

The daily pattern of activity versus sleep is the most obvious circadian rhythm in humans. Sleep is controlled by two interacting processes: during the wake phases sleep propensity rises and this dissipates during sleep. This flip-flop mechanism is driven during wakefulness by the monoaminergic systems which inhibit sleep promoting neurons in the ventricular-lateral preoptic regions (VLPO). The firing rate of these sleep promoting, mainly γ-aminobutyric acid (GABA)ergic neurons is high during sleep under the stimulation of adenosine whereas orexinergic and monoaminergic neurons are inhibited. The distribution of neurons that produce orexins (also referred to as hypocretins) is restricted to the perifornical area, the lateral and posterior hypothalamus. Experimental evidence supports a dominant influence of orexin on wake-inducing monoaminergic neurons. Fitting to this pattern, it has been shown in animal models that orexin neurons fire during wake state. They are virtually completely inactive during rapid eye movement (REM) and non-REM sleep (NREMS), a condition associated with atonia. Monoaminergic neurons in turn inhibit sleep-promoting neurons in the VLPO but have also an inhibitory role on orexin neurons, forming a delicate double inhibitory circuit (8). This complex interaction is highlighted by mutations of orexin or orexin 2 receptors in animal models and humans. In both conditions, daytime sleepiness, narcolepsy, and obstructive sleep apnoea may be induced. Narcolepsy with a prevalence of roughly 1 in 2000 is characterized by excessive daytime sleepiness but also a sudden onset of weakness/atonia, cataplexy, fitting to orexin effects on muscle tone. Orexin stimulates locomotor behaviour and energy homoeostasis. Orexin partly stimulates food intake via neuropeptide Y (NPY) but exerts as well an inhibitory action on proopiomelanocortin (POMC) neurons, which will dominantly decrease energy expenditure (8).

In addition to narcolepsy the genetic basis of some other human sleep disorders have been elucidated and linked to circadian alterations in the timing of sleep. The molecular defect in familial advanced sleep phase syndrome (FASPS) has been established as a mutation in the *PER2* gene. Patients with this autosomal dominant disease have persistent 3–4-h advanced sleep onset which, however, only leads to clinically apparent problems under a forced sleep–wake schedule. Another clearly genetically based disease, the delayed sleep phase syndrome (DSPS), has been linked to mutations in the *CLOCK* gene even though the pathophysiology is still not completely unravelled (2, 8, 9).

Again, a close relation to changes in activity/inactivity and food/fasting rhythms, energy homoeostasis, and metabolism is apparent with these mutations. Orexin/ataxin 3 neuron-ablated mice show significantly lower expression of the clock genes *Per2*, *Bmal*, and *nPas2*, along with hypophagia, reduced locomotor activity, and altered energy expenditure. The stimulatory effects of orexin on food anticipation, hunger, locomotor activity, and food intake fit to the close links of the orexin system to multiple metabolic key regulators. Neuronal inputs from the arcuate nucleus through NPY, Agouti, α-melanocyte-stimulating hormone (α-MSH) and also inhibitory inputs from the preoptic GABAergic neurons from leptin and glucose are part of this integrated system. The role of orexin highlights this intimate interplay between sleep–wakefulness, locomotion, and central as well as peripheral metabolic control into a sensitively regulated circadian system. It implies that any disturbance of the sleep–wake cycle, of energy homoeostasis, and of the interfering endocrine regulation may lead to substantial changes in other components of this highly integrated system (8, 9; Fig. 2.6.1.2).

Circadian endocrine rhythms and their relation to sleep and energy homoeostasis

Multiple hormonal systems show pronounced circadian rhythmicity (see Fig. 2.6.1.3 for examples and the link to other circadian rhythms). The physiological relevance of these rhythms is only in part elucidated so far. Multidirectional interactions between sleep, energy homoeostasis, and the endocrine system are currently best characterized, and the following section will thus focus on these interactions. As the capacity of endocrine signals to affect energy homoeostasis are reviewed in more detail in other parts of this book, the following will only review the relevance of energy shifts in relation to circadian behaviour and sleep.

Ghrelin and leptin

Ghrelin and leptin are among the most important regulators of energy homoeostasis. Both hormones show a significant diurnal variation in lean subjects. Leptin secretion follows a circadian pattern. Both, in lean and obese subjects, a nightly increase of leptin has been shown with peak levels reached at around 02.00 h in the morning hours. Leptin levels decrease thereafter to reach a nadir in the hours between waking and noon. These changes have been viewed as important for the well-known regulatory effects of leptin on energy homoeostasis but also on leptin's action on other hypothalamic/pituitary hormones (10, 11).

Leptin secretion is linked to another important hormone in appetite control, ghrelin. Ghrelin is released with a marked nocturnal increase with peak fhrelin levels reached after waking in the morning. This diurnal pattern of ghrelin secretion is restricted to lean persons only. An analysis of synchrony between ghrelin and leptin levels neither revealed any copulsatility nor a clear phase shift between the diurnal rhythm found for ghrelin and leptin. It is interesting that the diurnal ghrelin pattern is lost in obese subjects (10).

Ghrelin is known to activate orexin neurons and thus plays an important role in the regulation of food searching behaviour and locomotive activity. Ghrelin also has direct effects on the machinery of circadian behaviour by inducing a phase advance and shifting

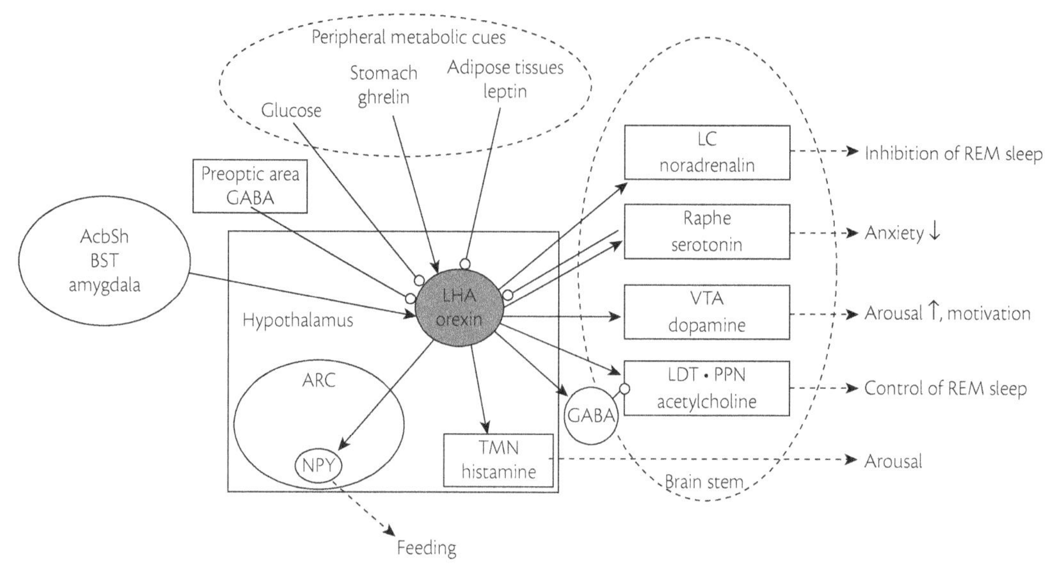

Fig. 2.6.1.2 Orexin-centred view of sleep–wake regulation, energy homoeostasis, arousal, and locomotion (9). ARC, arcuatus nucleus; BST, bed nucleus of the stria terminalis; LC, locus coeruleus; LDT, laterodorsal tegmental nucleus; LHA, lateral hypothalamic area; PPT, pedunculopontine tegmental nucleus; TMN, tuberomammillary nucleus; VTA, ventral tegmental area.

per2 expression. On the contrary, leptin exerts an inhibitory influence on the firing of orexin neurons and counteracts feeding behaviour by activating POMC. Leptin as well acts directly via periodicity genes as shown in the example of mice deficient in per or Cry in their osteoblasts. At least in this example clear phenotypic changes are found under leptin treatment indicating that leptin acts on osteoblast proliferation via sympathetic nervous pathways and periodicity gene activation (8, 12–14).

Growth hormone

With growth hormone-releasing hormone (GHRH) and somatostatin, ghrelin is an important regulator of growth hormone. Growth hormone secretion shows a marked diurnal variation.

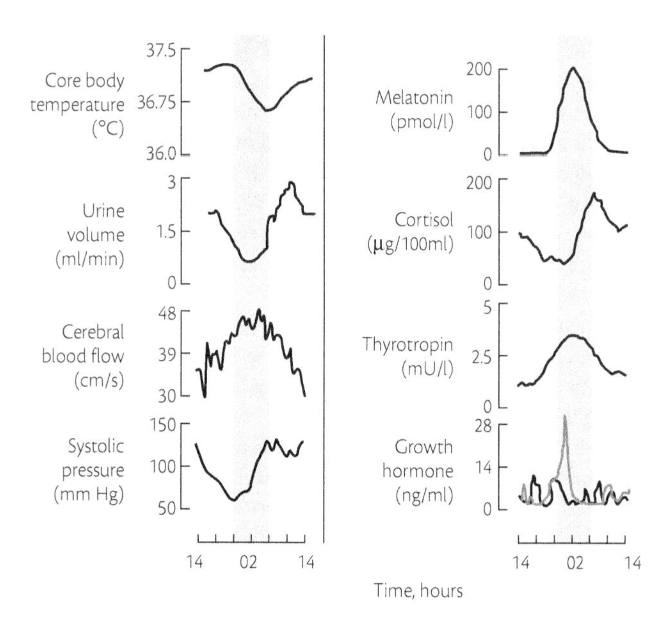

Fig. 2.6.1.3 Examples of prominent endocrine and nonendocrine circadian rhythms (7).

Using high frequency sampling techniques in several hundreds of volunteers and patients it has been shown that growth hormone is released in secretory pulses, and that these pulses form the basis of a circadian pattern. Modulation of frequency and amplitude of these secretory pulses and their fusion form the circadian rhythm; a common pattern observed in many hormonal systems (13).

Growth hormone in humans is closely linked to sleep. Quantifying the amount of NREMS revealed that GH is robustly associated with the duration and deepness of NREMS but this relation depends on age and gender. It typically develops at about 3 months of age, reaches a peak in adolescence, and progressively decreases after 30 years of age. Despite the fact that there is a marked sex-related difference with a markedly closer relation in males than in females, the decline in slow wave sleep parallels the almost complete decline in nightly growth hormone secretion above the age of 50 in both sexes (14).

These observational studies on a close link between growth hormone and sleep were recently supported by investigations in mutant and transgenic animals. Growth hormone secretion in spontaneous dwarf rats (SDR) is almost completely lost due to a mutation of the *GH* gene. At variance to expectations NREMS is not reduced in these animals, but rather increased during the rest period. This suggests that growth hormone/insulin-like growth factor 1 (IGF-1) is only indirectly responsible for the reduction in spontaneous NREMS. The suspicion that a major part of this activity is mediated by GHRH- dependent pathways is supported by several mouse models with deletions of the GHRH receptor, such as the lit/lit mice or the dw/dw rats. Growth hormone and IGF-1 productions in both animals are greatly decreased along with significantly reduced spontaneous NREMS. As no GHRH action is expected in these animals chronic growth hormone replacement in these animals allows to dissect GHRH action from growth hormone/IGF-1 responses. Despite successful correction of growth hormone deficiency, growth hormone replacement is unable to stimulate NREMS to normal indicating an important role of GHRH in the regulation of NREMS. This assumption fits to the detection of a circadian and sleep-related variation of GHRH in the hypothalamus. In contrast, REM sleep seems to be directly stimulated by GH secretion (15).

Adrenal axis

Endogenous cortisol secretion rises sharply between 02.00 and 04.00 h at night with a peak serum concentration approximately 1 h after wakening. Cortisol is secreted in a diurnal pattern which generally reflects the pattern of adrenocorticotropic activity (ACTH). Its high variation between nadir and peak secretions and its high reproducibility allow to use the circadian pattern as a window to evaluate changes in circadian rhythmicity in order to capture pathophysiology. This is exemplified in the diagnosis of Cushing's syndrome where the circadian variation is markedly dampened or even abolished. Whereas a morning cortisol may still be within the normal range, typically the midnight cortisol level is increased (16). Similarly, circadian secretion is altered in normal ageing with an increased nightly secretion. This is a mild alteration whereas in depressive illnesses, as well as in chronic alcohol abuse, more pronounced shifts in circadian pattern reminiscent of Cushing's syndrome are observed. In cortisol deficiency stimulation of the entire corticotropin-releasing hormone (CRH)–ACTH–cortisol axis may be achieved by administration of the 11β-hydroxylase antagonist metyrapone, which blocks the conversion of 11-deoxycortisol to cortisol. The reduced negative feedback inhibition of cortisol on CRH and ACTH secretion can be used diagnostically in partial pituitary insufficiency. It is, however, highly dependent on the circadian timing. Deoxycortisol has been shown to be maximally induced when the drug is applied at 20.00 h. This stimulation was significantly higher than after administration during the morning hours. Similarly, suppression of ACTH secretion by cortisol or synthetic analogues depends on the timing of their administration. Maximal inhibitory effects on ACTH secretion are observed just prior to the endogenous nightly rise in ACTH secretion. These effects have implications for the timing of corticosteroid treatment.

For physiological replacement therapy a slow-release preparation has recently been developed which is able to mimic the nightly cortisol increase (17). Application of the preparation when going to sleep will release peak cortisol levels at the physiological peak secretion time in the early morning hours. It is hoped, but still remains to be proven that these promising preparations will improve the impaired quality of life of patients with Addison's disease. In pharmacotherapy with glucocorticoids it is evident that the effectiveness depends on the timing. Nightly application improves the effect/dose but side effects are higher as well. Bearing in mind interindividual variations on the sensitivity to glucocorticoids it is currently not worked out which minimal dose is effective at which time of the day (18). In addition, this may vary due to disease specific factors.

Thyroid hormone axis

Thyrotropin (thyroid-stimulating hormone (TSH)) exhibits a marked circadian rhythm that governs a similar 24-h rhythm of free triiodothyronine (19). Data on the circadian thyroxine rhythm are less clear. There are early observations suggesting a light–dark cycle in total thyroxine but more recent data on free thyroxine could not confirm such dark–night cycle. There are no data on the influence of light on TSH secretion but the important impact of sleep on TSH has been well investigated. Sleep withdrawal induces an acute increase and prolonged release of nocturnal TSH

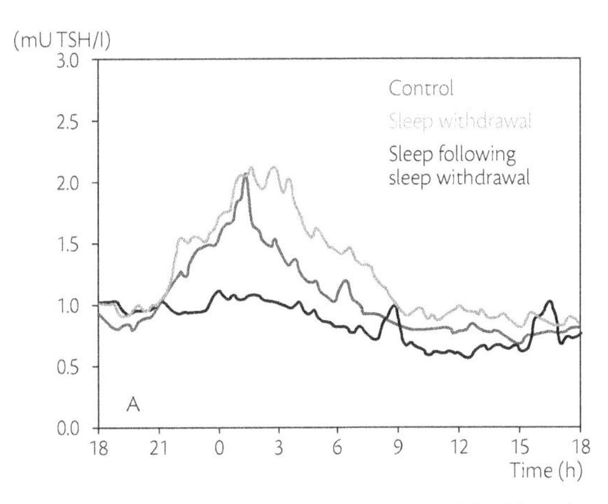

Fig. 2.6.1.4 Effects of sleep modulation on TSH secretion in healthy volunteers. Comparing normal sleep to acute sleep withdrawal and to sleep in the night following sleep withdrawal. (Adapted from Brabant G, Prank K, Ranft U. Physiological regulation of circadian and pulsatile thyrotropin secretion in normal man and woman. *J Clin Endocrinol Metab*, 1990; **70**: 403–9 (20)).

secretion (20; Fig. 2.6.1.4). This is independent of total thyroid hormone levels. In contrast, TSH is almost completely suppressed if the volunteers slept significantly more and deeper in the night following a night of sleep withdrawal. This recovery of hormonal changes in acute total sleep deprivation is observed for other hormonal systems as well and raises the possibility that chronic sleep loss may result in long-term adverse effects via alterations in the circadian rhythmicity. A direct link to energy homoeostasis is currently elusive. Short-term activation of the axis as in acute sleep withdrawal may, however, be linked to an activation of energy stores via the thyroid hormone system, an assumption fitting to data on fasting. Decreased energy availability following a 3-day fast almost completely suppresses circadian TSH release. Effects on the sympathetic nervous system are clearly important in this context but detailed studies are missing to date (21).

Melatonin

Melatonin, which is, exclusively derived from the pineal gland is secreted with a circadian rhythm. Ganglionic photoreceptor cells in the retina integrate information on the light-dark cycle and signal via the retinohypothalamic pathway to the SCN where duration, phase, and amplitude of melatonin hormone production are modulated. Light suppresses melatonin secretion with blue light in the range 460–470 nm having the most pronounced effect. Circulating melatonin dominantly bound to albumin levels shows high interindividual variability which presumably is genetically determined. A circadian rhythm with an increase in the evening hours between 19.00 and 21.00 h, a peak between 02.00and 04.00 h and lowest values during daytime hours seems to be preserved until old age with large interindividual variations (22).

Melatonin exerts its physiological actions through G-protein-coupled specific cell membrane receptors, MT1 and MT2 melatonin receptor. The functions of the subtypes differ and is not restricted to sleep and circadian behaviour where MT1 receptor decreases neuronal firing rates, whereas the MT2 receptor regulates phase shifts. In addition, melatonin is a major regulator of the circadian rhythm of core body temperature in humans. This pattern is linked to sleep. In normal adults, the deepest level of sleep and the lowest core body temperature are reached simultaneously.

Melatonin represents the classical example of a light–dark-driven hormone. It is thought to synchronize circadian rhythms. Investigations in totally blind patients with no recognition of light demonstrate that the coordination of endogenous rhythms is lost. Synchronized endogenous circadian rhythms are important for a normal quality of life. Totally blind persons lose this synchrony and exhibit cyclical sleeplessness associated with daytime sleepiness (23).

Exogenous melatonin affects sleep regulation largely through a phase-resetting mechanism. By its capability to readjust disturbed circadian rhythms to their correct phase position melatonin decreases daytime sleepiness and normalizes sleep quality. Furthermore, other biological rhythms are entrained by melatonin treatment, indicating a general normalizing effect and suggesting a role of melatonin in the coordination of light-dependent effects on the endocrine system. Circadian rhythm sleep disorders, either advance or delayed sleep phase syndrome, have been successfully treated with melatonin (24). A common denominator of these conditions is the loss of coordination between endogenous rhythms. Jet lag induced by a transmeridian flight across several time zones is a well known but transient condition of such loss of entrainment as a mismatch occurs between the endogenous circadian rhythms and the new environmental light–dark cycle (25). Endogenous rhythms shift in the direction of the flight with a phase advance on eastbound flights but a phase delay when flying westwards. Symptoms typically include a disturbed night-time sleep, impaired daytime alertness and performance, irritability, distress and appetite changes, along with other physical symptoms such as disorientation, fatigue, gastrointestinal disturbances and light-headedness. Modification of melatonin secretion has been used to synchronize endogenous rhythms in jetlag and in shift workers. The convincing positive data in the totally blind on a coordinating role of melatonin have recently been paralleled in healthy volunteers treated with a melatonin agonist. The dose-dependent effect on sleep propensity supports an important coordinating function of melatonin on the sleep–wake cycle and on other circadian rhythms. To understand melatonin action in normal physiology, further mechanisms such as the activation of the sympathetic nerve system which suppress melatonin secretion from the pineal gland, may play a crucial role. Light, even dim light at night leads to a suppression of melatonin and feedback on other rhythms. Recent data on melatonin secretion in postmenopausal women highlights this complex relation. Absolute 24-h melatonin secretion is enhanced in depressed postmenopausal women. In addition, timing of melatonin secretion is altered, showing a delayed morning offset of melatonin. This longer melatonin secretion time fits to results in seasonal affective disorders where a dissociation of endogenous rhythms is observed via a shift in the timing of the circadian rhythmicity. These patients also have an increased melatonin secretion during the winter months. In both groups mood disturbance and sleep are improved by bright light therapy (26).

Altered sleep, circadian rhythmicity, and metabolism

Increased melatonin secretion may further impact on the risk of insulin resistance and diabetes mellitus. Recent data from three independent groups reveal that a polymorphism of the melatonin receptor 1B, which leads to chronic overactivity of the intracellular melatonin dependent signalling pathways, is an independent and strong risk factor for glucose intolerance and type 2 diabetes mellitus. The mechanism behind this is not entirely clarified but inhibition of insulin secretion from pancreatic β cells and a negative impact on incretins seem to cooperate.

Glucose tolerance, which critically depends on the ability of the pancreatic β cell to respond to a given glucose challenge, varies over the day in healthy individuals. It is much lower in the evening than in the morning. There is a further increase in plasma glucose when tested in the middle of the night, suggesting minimal glucose tolerance during sleep. Whereas reduced glucose tolerance in the evening hours is attributed to both, a reduction in insulin sensitivity and a reduced insulin secretory response to glucose, the further deterioration of glucose tolerance during the night depends on sleep related processes to maintain stable glucose levels during the extended overnight fast. During NREMS glucose utilization is lowest; it increases during REM sleep and is highest in the wake period. The underlying multifactorial causes of this circadian change in glucose tolerance are only partly unravelled. Insulin sensitivity decreases in the evening predominantly due to a decreased pancreatic insulin secretory response to glucose. Melatonin-mediated effects may significantly contribute to this regulation. Glucose production and utilization fall in association with sleep during the first half of the night and increase again in the latter part. Insulin-dependent and -independent glucose disposal is reduced during sleep. In parallel, growth hormone secretion is increased with the initiation of slow-wave sleep, cortisol is inhibited, sympathetic nerve activity is decreased, and vagal tone stimulated.

Moderate alteration of night sleep with a reduction to only 4 h/night over a period of 6 nights has been shown experimentally to profoundly affect energy metabolism. It acutely reduces insulin release predominantly via an increased sympathetic outflow and decreases peripheral insulin sensitivity on several levels. Importantly, counteractive hormone release is activated with an augmented nightly growth hormone, TSH, and cortisol secretion, and also with a higher level of cytokines and inflammatory markers (14). It is not surprising that testing for insulin resistance in such a state of sleeplessness revealed a metabolic state well comparable with metabolic syndrome and prediabetes. Similar data have subsequently been obtained in subjects where selective suppression of slow-wave sleep decreased the quality but not the duration of sleep.

The sleep reduction best investigated in obstructive sleep apnoea is further associated with a dysregulation of the neuroendocrine control of appetite. A combined alteration of ghrelin, orexin, and leptin secretion is part of the pathomechanism leading to excessive food intake, decreased energy expenditure and, as recent data indicate, to hypertension (see Fig. 2.6.1.5 for schematic integration of mechanisms). There is further evidence that metabolic changes in the polycystic ovary syndrome are a result of obstructive sleep apnoea. The experimental studies on partial sleep loss and their impact on energy conservation parallel epidemiological findings on the greatly increased risk of obesity and diabetes mellitus in societies. It is tempting to speculate but remains to be proven that sleep curtailment by modern lifestyle changes is a primary force behind the adverse metabolic effects via their impact on diurnal endocrine regulation (27, 28).

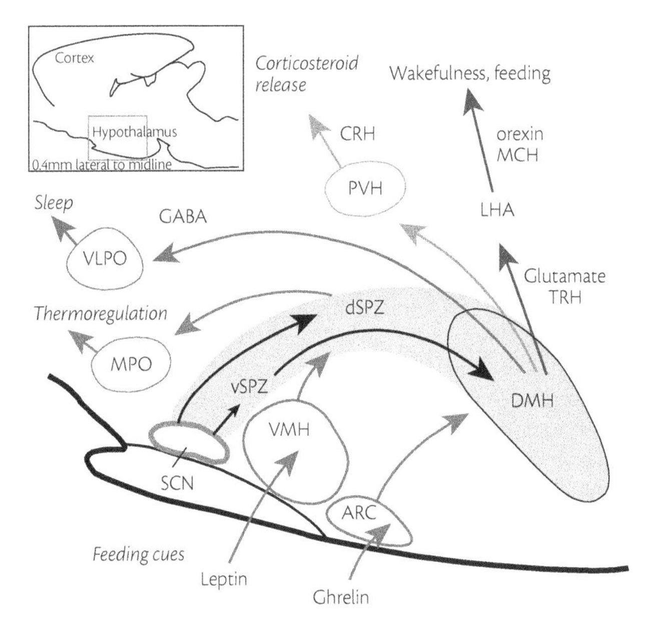

Fig. 2.6.1.5 Integration of endocrine signals with sleep and food regulating hypothalamic circuits (from Saper (27)). ARC, arcuate nucleus; DMH, dorsomedial hypothalamus; dSPZ, dorsal subparaventricular zone; GABA, γ-aminobutyric acid; LHA, lateral hypothalamic area; MCH, melanin-concentrating hormone; MPO, medial preoptic area; PVH, periventricular hypothalamus; SCN, suprachiasmatic nucleus; TRH, thyrotropin-releasing hormone; VLPO, ventrolateral preoptic area; VMH, ventromedial hypothalamus; vSPZ, ventral subparaventricular zone.

In summary, these latter examples clearly demonstrate a powerful circadian regulation of the endocrine/metabolic system interlinked with sleep. Evidence is accumulating that the common curtailment of normal sleep in modern society has important consequences for metabolic and endocrine functions. Data on shift workers who most frequently experience gastrointestinal disturbances support the importance of food-entrained rhythms in addition to the light–dark cycle for the timing of many endocrine rhythms and sleep-associated cycles. Constant violation of these patterns may lead to detrimental effects. The example of treatment with melatonin and melatonin agonists suggests that a better understanding of the pathophysiology of the circadian patterns may help to develop new means to endocrinologically modulate these cycles for the benefit of patients.

References

1. Schibler U. Circadian time keeping: the daily ups and downs of genes, cells and organisms. *Prog Brain Res*, 2006; **153**: 271–82.
2. Takahashi JS, Hong HK, Ko CH, McDearmon EL. The genetics of mammalian circadian order and disorder: implications for physiology and disease. *Nat Rev Genet*, 2008; **9**(+ Supplement): 764–75.
3. Brown SA, Kunz D, Dumas A, Westermark PO, Vanselow K, Wahnschaffe A, *et al.* Molecular insights into human daily behavior. *Proc Natl Acad Sci U S A* 2008; **105**:1602–7.
4. Hussain MM, Pan X. Clock genes, intestinal transport and plasma lipid homeostasis. *Trends Endocrinol Metab*, 2009; **20**: 147–202.
5. Schmidt C, Collette F, Leclercq Y, Sterpenich V, Vandewalle G, Berthomier P, *et al.* Homeostatic Sleep Pressure and Responses to Sustained Attention in the Suprachiasmatic Area *Science*, 2009; **324**: 516–19.
6. Phillips ML. Circadian rhythms: Of larks, owls and alarm clocks. *Nature*, 2009; **458**: 142–4.
7. Maywood ES, O'Neill JS, Chesham JE, Hastings MH. Minireview: The circadian clockwork of the suprachiasmatic nuclei—analysis of a cellular oscillator that drives endocrine rhythms. *Endocrinology*, 2007; **148**: 5624–34.
8. Adamantidis A, de Lecea L. The hypocretins as sensors for metabolism and arousal. *J Physiol*, 2009; **587**: 33–40.
9. Ohno K, Sakurai T. Orexin neuronal circuitry: role in the regulation of sleep and wakefulness. *Front Neuroendocrinol*, 2008; **29**: 70–87.
10. Yildiz BO,Suchard MA, Wong ML, McCann SM, Licinio J. Alterations in the dynamics of circulating ghrelin, adiponectin, and leptin in human obesity. *Proc Natl Acad Sci U S A*, 2004; **101**:10434–9.
11. Spiegel K, Tasali E, Penev P, van Cauter E. Brief Communication: Sleep Curtailment in Healthy Young Men Is Associated with Decreased Leptin Levels, Elevated Ghrelin Levels, and Increased Hunger and Appetite. *Ann Intern Med*, 2004; **141**: 846–50.
12. Fu L, Patel MS, Bradley A, Wagner EF, Karsenty G. The molecular clock mediates leptin-regulated bone formation. *Cell*, 2005; **122**: 803–15.
13. Schofl C, Prank K, Wiersinga W, Brabant G. Pulsatile hormone secretion: Analysis and biological significance. *Trends Endocrinol Metab*, 1995; **6**: 113–14.
14. Knutson KL, Spiegel K, Penev P, Van Cauter E. The metabolic consequences of sleep deprivation. *Sleep Med Rev*, 2007; **11**: 163–78.
15. Obal F, Krueger JM. Physiology of sleep: GHRH and sleep Sleep. *Med Rev*, 2004; **8**: 367–77.
16. Carroll T, Raff H, Findling JW. Late-night salivary cortisol measurement in the diagnosis of Cushing's syndrome. *Nat Clin Pract Endocrinol Metab*, 2008; **4**: 344–50.
17. Debono M, Ghobadi C, Rostami-Hodjegan A, Huatan H, Campbell MJ, Newell-Price J, *et al.* Modified-release hydrocortisone to provide circadian cortisol profiles. *J Clin Endocrinol Metab*, 2009; **94**: 1548–54.
18. Haus E. Chronobiology in the endocrine system. *Ad Drug Deliv Rev*, 2007; **59**: 985–1014.
19. Russell W, Harrison RF, Smith N, Darzy K, Shalet S, Weetman AP, *et al.* Free triiodothyronine has a distinct circadian rhythm that is delayed but parallels thyrotropin levels. *J Clin Endocrinol Metab*, 2008; **93**: 2300–6.
20. Brabant G, Prank K, Ranft U. Physiological regulation of circadian and pulsatile thyrotropin secretion in normal man and woman. *J Clin Endocrinol Metab*, 1990; **70**: 403–9.
21. Behrends J, Prank K, Dogu E, Brabant G. Central Nervous System Control of Thyrotropin Secretion during Sleep and Wakefulness. *Horm Res*, 1998; **49**: 173–7.
22. Pandi-Perumal SR, Trakht I, Spence DW, Srinivasan V, Dagan Y, Cardinali DP. The roles of melatonin and light in the pathophysiology and treatment of circadian rhythm sleep disorders. *Nat Clin Pract Neurol*, 2008; **4**: 436–47.
23. Sack RL, Brandes RW, Kendall AR, Lewy AJ. Entrainment of free-running circadian rhythms by melatonin in blind people. *N Engl J Med*, 2000; **343**: 1070–7.
24. Rajaratnam SM, Polymeropoulos MH, Fisher DM, Roth T, Scott C, Birznieks G, *et al.* Melatonin agonist tasimelteon (VEC-162) for transient insomnia after sleep-time shift: two randomised controlled multicentre trials. *Lancet*, 2009; **373**: 482–91.
25. Copinschi G, Spiegel K, Leproult R, van Cauter E. Pathophysiology of human circadian rhythms. *Novartis Found Symp*, 2000; **227**: 143–57.
26. Parry BL, Meliska CJ, Sorenson DL, Lopez AM, Martinez LF, Nowakowski S, *et al.* Increased melatonin and delayed offset in menopausal depression: role of years past menopause, follicle-stimulating hormone, sleep end time, and body mass index. *J Clin Endocrinol Metab*, 2008; **93**: 54–60.
27. Saper CB. Staying awake for dinner: hypothalamic integration of sleep, feeding, and circadian rhythms. *Prog Brain Res*, 2006; **153**: 243–52.
28. Ramsey KM, Bass J. Obeying the clock yields benefits for metabolism. *Proc Natl Acad Sci U S A*, 2009; **106**: 4069–70.

2.6.2 Endocrinology of eating disorders

Gerasimos E. Krassas, Luigi Bartalena

Introduction

Eating disorders affect about five million Americans every year. There are three different eating disorders: anorexia nervosa, bulimia nervosa, and binge eating disorder. Eating disorders are complex conditions deriving from a complex interplay of long-standing behavioural, emotional, psychological, interpersonal, and social factors. The neuronal circuits that control the ingestion of food are mainly related to catecholaminergic, serotoninergic, and peptidergic systems. In this respect, while serotonin, dopamine and prostaglandin promote the ingestion of food, by contrast, neuropeptide Y, noradrenaline, γ-aminobutyric acid (GABA), and opioid peptides inhibit food ingestion, thus causing the development of eating disorders (1).

Eating disorders typically occur in adolescent girls or young women, although 5–15% of cases of anorexia nervosa and bulimia nervosa and 40% of cases of binge eating disorder occur in boys and men. Approximately 3% of young women are affected with these disorders, and probably twice that number has clinically important variants. Although early disorders mostly develop in adolescence or young adulthood, they can occur after the age of 40 years and are increasingly seen in young children (2). Eating disorders are more prevalent in industrialized societies than in nonindustrialized societies, and occur in all socioeconomic classes and major ethnic groups in the USA. About half of those who have anorexia nervosa or bulimia nervosa fully recover, approximately 30% have a partial recovery, and 20% have no substantial improvement in symptoms (2).

The aim of this chapter is to give an overview of the endocrinology of eating disorders leading to excessive weight gain or excessive weight loss in humans. It is of note that despite the strong association between obesity and eating disorders, the increase in obesity is not followed by an increase in eating disorders (3).

Anorexia nervosa

Anorexia nervosa, i.e. 'nervous loss of appetite', was described for the first time by Richard Morton in 1689, although the name anorexia nervosa is attributed to Sir William Gull and Charles Lassegue during the late 19th century (4). It is a psychiatric disorder characterized by disordered food intake, purging behaviour, and distorted body image. The person with this condition presents with a classic triad: amenorrhoea, weight loss, and behavioural changes. This group of symptoms usually presents together, although any one of these basic symptoms may precede another. It is the only psychiatric disorder that requires an endocrine disturbance, amenorrhoea, as a diagnostic criterion (5). It is generally seen in young white women under 25 and is particularly common in adolescence. It is the third most frequent cause of chronic disease in adolescent girls (6). Although the true prevalence of the disease is not well established internationally, most researchers agree that anorexia nervosa has increased at least fivefold during the past 30 years in Western industrialized countries (4).

In general, the overall incidence of anorexia nervosa is 0.24–1.64 per 100 000 persons, but the incidence differs greatly in different population groups. This syndrome occurs in 1 of every 100 middle-class adolescent girls, and professional ballet dancers have an incidence ranging from 1 in 20 to 1 in 5 depending on the competitive level of the company from which the survey originated. Recent work also indicates that some ethnic groups have a much lower incidence of anorexia nervosa; for instance, it is rare among black people, including black ballet dancers, who are exposed to the same rigid standards of competition and weight restriction. The low incidence of this problem among black people may relate to different sociocultural influences, or, conceivably, this group may possess more efficient metabolic mechanisms for dealing with the high activity level and lowered caloric intake (4).

It is of interest in this regard that studies on monozygous twins have suggested a genetic factor in the pathogenesis of the syndrome. The risk for female siblings is 6%, suggesting that inborn metabolic factors may contribute to the syndrome. There is also an increased incidence in association with Turner's syndrome, diabetes mellitus, and Cushing's disease suggesting that factors associated with these conditions may predispose to the development of the illness. Although rare in men (male: female ratio is 9:1), the syndrome has been reported in men who are training for competitive activities while restricting their weight (4).

The mortality of the disease also varies. An 11-year, outpatient follow-up study of eating disorders in Boston showed a mortality of 5.1% for anorexia nervosa (7). A 6-year course and outcome study of anorexia nervosa conducted in 103 German patients found that 34.7% had a good outcome, 38.6% an intermediate outcome, 20.8% a poor outcome, and 6 of 101 patients (5.9%) died (8). Body mass index (BMI) in average was still low (17.9 ± 2.8 kg/m^2) at the 6-year follow-up, and amenorrhoea was still present in 23.9% (8). Moreover, a follow-up study of patients with severe anorexia nervosa in London, 5.7 years after compulsory hospitalization reported a mortality rate of 13% (9).

Usually the diagnosis of anorexia nervosa is not difficult. In 1972, Feighner *et al.* (10) outlined diagnostic criteria that were used for many years and were fairly restrictive. The main criteria, suggested in 1994 by the American Psychiatric Association, are presented in Box 2.6.2.1.

Box 2.6.2.1 Diagnostic criteria for anorexia nervosa

- Body weight <85% of expected weight
- Body mass index ≤18
- Intense fear of gaining weight/of becoming fat
- Refuse to maintain body weight at or above a minimally normal weight for age and height
- Disturbance in the way in which one's body weight or shape is experienced
- Amenorrhoea in post-menarche females

Adapted from Becker AE, Grinspoon SK, Klibanski A, Herzog DB. Eating disorders. *N Engl J Med*, 1999; **340**: 1092–8 (2).

Endocrinology of anorexia nervosa

The endocrine changes associated with anorexia nervosa have been studied in depth and provide strong evidence of hypothalamic dysfunction. It now seems clear that the endocrine disturbances are all secondary, i.e. there is no evidence of primary dysfunction in the pituitary, thyroid, adrenal, or gonads. Overall endocrine changes in anorexia nervosa are presented in Box 2.6.2.2.

Hypothalamic–pituitary–gonadal axis

Secondary amenorrhoea is a cardinal manifestation of anorexia nervosa and is most often the result of disturbances in the hypothalamic–pituitary–gonadal axis (HPG) axis. Puberty, including the onset of menarche, may be delayed in adolescents with anorexia nervosa, leading to arrest of linear growth. In men, low weight is also associated with clinical hypogonadism and decreased levels of serum testosterone (2). In general, even early abnormal eating behaviours, particularly with restrictive fat intake, can disrupt gonadotropin secretion and cause amenorrhoea (11).

Regarding gonadotropin secretion, low plasma levels of luteinizing hormone and follicle-stimulating hormone (FSH), accompanied by a marked oestrogen deficiency have been reported. In addition, there is a lack of the normal episodic variation of luteinizing hormone secretion and, in some cases, a reversion to a prepubertal low pattern of secretion over a 24-h period. Nocturnal spurt of luteinizing hormone is also seen in adults, a pattern usually observed only in early puberty (12). A reversion to the normal adult-like pattern occurs with refeeding. Artificially, the pattern of gonadotropin secretion can be reverted to a normal adult-like secretion by the pulsatile administration of gonadotropin-releasing hormone (GnRH). If this drug is given intravenously or subcutaneously every 2 h, a normal adult-like pattern of gonadotropin secretion results, and menstrual bleeding and ovulation can be induced (13). Recent findings suggest that the amenorrhoea seen in anorexia nervosa is probably due to faulty signals reaching the medial central hypothalamus from the arcuate nucleus, the centre most likely responsible for the important episodic stimulation of GnRH.

Also of interest is the fact that the response of the pituitary to GnRH is reduced by a factor that is directly correlated with the weight loss. In addition, the pattern of response to GnRH is immature, resembling that seen in prepubertal children; the FSH response is much greater than the luteinizing hormone response. With refeeding, the normal ratios develop, with the luteinizing hormone response being much greater than that of FSH. This adult-like response can also be induced artificially with the episodic administration of GnRH (13). Recent evidence indicates that the pituitary gonadotrophs have become sluggish owing to the lack of endogenous stimulation with GnRH and that the episodic stimulation may be important in determining the relative amounts of luteinizing hormone and FSH secreted. Moreover, patients who have partially recovered from anorexia nervosa tend to have an exaggerated response to GnRH. These changes have been seen in children in early puberty, suggesting that the hypothalamic signals of the central nervous system (CNS) revert to a prepubertal or pubertal stage.

Prolactin basal levels are normal. Thyrotropin-releasing hormone (TRH)-stimulated prolactin levels are also normal, although the time of the peak prolactin response is delayed. However, the response of prolactin to luteinizing hormone-releasing hormone (LHRH) stimulation test was positive (peak prolactin levels greater than 1.125 nmol/L and delta increase in prolactin greater than 0.045 nmol/L) in 16.9% of 65 patients with anorexia nervosa and negative in all controls. With weight gain the described endocrine abnormalities revert to normal (14).

Despite the return of normal gonadotropin secretory patterns, amenorrhoea may persist in almost 30% of patients with anorexia nervosa. This suggests that other mechanisms, yet unknown, are involved (4). Establishing regular menstrual cycles is an important milestone for women in recovery from anorexia nervosa (11).

Amenorrhoea in active anorexia nervosa is a protective physiological adaptation to prevent pregnancy at a time of compromised nutrition. Luteal deficiency has been observed historically in times of famine and food rationing such as during the first and second world wars (11). Infertility results from both anovulation and self-imposed restrictions on sexual activity in anorexia nervosa. The initial serum

Box 2.6.2.2 Overall endocrine changes in anorexia nervosa

Growth hormone ↑ or →

IGF-1 ↓

IGF-2 ↓ or →

GH BP ↓

IGFBP-1 ↑

IGFBP-2 ↑

IGFBP-3 ↓

LH ↓ (response to GnRH ↓)

FSH ↓

Oestradiol ↓

Oestrone ↓

Progesterone ↓

Testosterone ↓

PRL → (delayed response to TRH)

T_4 ↓

T_3 ↓

TSH → (↓ delayed response to TRH)

rT_3 ↑

Cortisol → or ↑

Urinary free cortisol → or ↑

ACTH → (↓ response to CRH)

Leptin ↓

Ghrelin ↑

↓, decreased; ↑, increased; →, normal

ACTH, adrenocorticotropic hormone; CRH, corticotropin-releasing hormone; FSH, follicle-stimulating hormone; GHBP, growth hormone binding protein; GnRH, gonadotropin-releasing hormone; IGF, insulin-like growth factor; IGFBP, IGF binding protein; LH, luteinizing hormone; PRL, prolactin; TRH, thyrotropin-releasing hormone; TSH, thyroid-stimulating hormone.

concentrations of FSH, inhibin-B and anti-müllerian hormone may also correlate with the degree of ovarian suppression and may predict the resumption of ovulation with weight gain (11). Of note, silent eating disorder (ED) is not uncommon in women seeking therapy for infertility. In one study, 58% of women with either amenorrhoea or oligomenorrhoea had evidence of an eating disorder (15).

GH–IGFs and IGFBPs axis

In the majority of patients with anorexia nervosa, basal growth hormone levels are increased. Støving *et al.* (16) using multiple parameter deconvolution analysis tried to evaluate neuroregulation of pulsatile growth hormone secretion in anorexia nervosa. They found that the pituitary growth hormone secretory burst frequency, growth hormone burst mass, and growth hormone burst duration were increased in women with anorexia nervosa compared with those in normal weight healthy women. A fourfold increase in 24-h pulsatile growth hormone secretion was accompanied by a remarkable 20-fold increase in the basal growth hormone secretion rate (nonpulsatile secretion). These dynamics of augmented growth hormone release were specific, because the half-life of growth hormone did not change in anorexia nervosa. They postulated that the observed elevation in nonpulsatile growth hormone secretion probably indicates a reduced hypothalamic somatostatin releasing inhibiting hormone (SRIH) tone, whereas the increase in growth hormone pulse frequency could indicate an increased frequency of hypothalamic growth hormone-releasing hormone (GHRH) discharges. They further hypothesized that the pathogenesis of augmented pulsatile growth hormone secretion in anorexia nervosa is caused by two distinct mechanisms: one related to the weight loss preferably increasing burst mass, and one related to hypo-oestrogenism preferably increasing pulse frequency. Støving *et al.* also found no significant differences in mean half-life of growth hormone disappearance resolved by deconvolution analysis in patients with anorexia nervosa compared with controls. It is well known that in normal subjects, half-life of growth hormone is not altered by fasting (16). Confirming earlier studies they also found low circulating total insulin growth factor 1 (IGF-1) levels, presumably resulting in diminished feedback inhibition of growth hormone secretion. They did not find a significant inverse correlation between IGF-1 and growth hormone levels. They finally suggested that enhanced growth hormone secretion in anorexia nervosa is due to markedly altered neuroendocrine regulation of growth hormone axis dynamics, resulting in jointly increased hypothalamic GHRH discharges and reduced hypothalamic somatostatinergic tone (16).There are conflicting reports on the level of free IGF-1 in anorexia nervosa, and it is not know to what extent free IGF-1 serum concentrations reflect IGF-1 tissue levels.

De Marinis *et al.* (17) studied the plasma growth hormone responses to direct stimulation with GHRH before and after a standard meal in anorexic women. They found that such women had elevated basal plasma growth hormone levels and a normal response after GHRH stimulation that was inversely correlated to body weight ($r = -0.59$; $p < 0.05$). They also found that feeding exerts differential effects on the growth hormone responses to GHRH in anorexia nervosa; the plasma growth hormone response was blunted when the meal was given at 08.15 h, and it was augmented when the meal was given at 13.15 h (15). The latter has also found in obese subjects. An absent growth hormone response to L-dopa, apomorphine, and insulin-induced hypoglycaemia has also been reported, while prompt release of growth hormone was reported after TRH stimulation.

In a very interesting study Counts *et al.* (18) studied the relationship of serum IGF-1, IGF-2, the IGF-binding proteins (IGFBP-1, -2, -3), and GHBP in patients with anorexia nervosa before and after a refeeding programme. Serum GHBP, IGF-1 and BP-3 were all significantly decreased in patients with anorexia nervosa and returned to nearly normal levels with refeeding. Fasting serum G2H and serum IGFBP-1 and -2 were significantly increased in patients with anorexia nervosa and also nearly normalized with refeeding. Serum IGF-2 was 27% lower in patients with anorexia nervosa than in controls but this difference was not statistically significant. Both serum IGF-1 and 2 were positively correlated with serum IGFBP-3 and negatively correlated with serum IGFBP-1 and -2. They concluded that nutritional deprivation alters the GH–IGF axis by down-regulating the GH receptor or its postreceptor mechanisms, and that this effect is reversible with refeeding (18).

Argente *et al.* (19) investigated growth hormone, IGF-1, free IGF-1, IGF-2, IGFBP-1, -2, and -3 and GHBP levels in 50 patients with anorexia nervosa at the time of clinical diagnosis and two points after nutritional therapy, i.e. after regaining between 6% and 8% (n=42) and 10% or less of the initial weight (n=20). They demonstrated that patients with anorexia nervosa are not homogeneous in their pattern of growth hormone secretion. Two distinct groups were seen, those who significantly hypersecreted growth hormone and those whose growth hormone secretion was reduced significantly. Argente *et al.* postulated that this abnormality is an epiphenomenon of the disease, as nutritional recovery restores it to normal, although patients are still affected with the psychiatric problems associated with anorexia nervosa. The peripheral GH–IGF axis, however, is altered similarly in all patients, indicating that this is not totally dependent on growth hormone secretion (19). Although serum insulin and total IGF-1 levels were profoundly diminished, free IGF-1 and -2 levels were in the normal range. In addition, all the IGFBPs studied as well as GHBP were modified. Although after nutritional therapy these patients are no long undernourished, some of the parameters reported here remain abnormal. Hence, it is clear that recovery does not immediately restore these functions (19).

Støving *et al.* (20) investigated the IGFBP-3 proteolytic activity in 24 patients with anorexia nervosa, and found it to be normal. They concluded that the mechanisms responsible for the adaptation of the GH–IGF–IGFBP axis in anorexia nervosa may be different from other catabolic conditions, because the low levels of free and total IGF-1 in anorexia nervosa are not associated with increased IGFBP-3 proteolysis.

Gianotti *et al.* (21) studied the effects of (rh)IGF-1 on spontaneous and GHRH-stimulated GH secretion in nine women with anorexia nervosa. They demonstrated that a low (rh) IGF-1 dose inhibits, but does not normalize, spontaneous and GHRH-stimulated growth hormone secretion, pointing also to the existence of a defective hypothalamic control of growth hormone release. Moreover, they suggested that the increased IGFBP-1 levels might curtail the negative IGF-1 feedback in anorexia nervosa.

Grinspoon *et al.* (22) investigated the effects of (rh) IGF-I and oestrogen on IGF binding protein -2 and -3 in 65 osteopenic women with anorexia nervosa: IGFBP-2 increased while IGFBP-3 decreased during therapy. The change in IGFBP-2 was inversely associated with the change in total hip bone density (22). The clinical sequelae of the above-mentioned disturbances are controversial and difficult to define.

Finally, Fazeli *et al.* (23) conducted a randomized, placebo, controlled study the aim of which was to investigate whether supraphysiological rhGH increases IGF-I levels in AN. They investigated 21 women with AN, 10 treated with rhGH and 11 treated with placebo. The mean maximum daily dose of rhGH was 1.4±0.12 mg/d). Their data demonstrated that doses of rhGH greater than 5 times the dose used to treat GH-deficient patients do not increase levels of IGF-I and therefore are not able to overcome the GH resistance state in AN. Although weight was similar in both groups at the end of the study, the loss in fat mass observed in the rhGH group suggests that rhGH is unlikely to provide therapeutic benefit to women with AN, while acts as a mediator on lipolysis independent of IGF-I.

Hypothalamic–pituitary–thyroid axis

Despite the low basal metabolic rate and slow pulse that characterize anorexia nervosa there is no evidence of hypothyroidism. Usual findings (see Box 2.6.2.2) include low-normal thyroxine (T_4), low triiodothyronine (T_3), and increased reverse T_3 levels, abnormalities which resemble to sick euthyroid syndrome (4). This is due to the fact that in anorexia nervosa the peripheral deiodinative convertion of T_4 is directed from formation of the active T_3 to the production of the metabolically inactive reverse T_3. Evidence also indicates that fasting decreases hepatic uptake of T_4, with a proportionate decrease in T_3 production. The low T_4 value is somewhat more difficult to be explained. Low T_4 euthyroidism has been seen in seriously ill patients. Some studies indicate that in ill patients there is a unique dysfunctional state with abnormal T_4 binding, with a normal free T_4 availability to peripheral tissue sites, while tissue hypothyroidism cannot be excluded. Presumably, similar mechanisms may be operative in anorexia nervosa. Interestingly, the so-called 'low-T3 syndrome" may mask hyperthyroidism, although this condition is rare. Secretion of thyroid-stimulating hormone (TSH), however, appears to be normal, but the peak TSH response to TRH stimulation is delayed from 20–30 to 60–120 min and is also augmented. This may reflect an altered set point for endogenous TRH regulation and is also characteristic of hypothalamic hypothyroidism. All the above abnormalities generally normalize following weight regain (4).

Hypothalamic–pituitary–adrenal axis

Biochemical findings suggest hypercortisolism (see Box 2.6.2.2), but no clinical features of cortisol excess are present. Plasma cortisol levels are high-normal or elevated. Urinary free cortisol is also elevated. The half-life of plasma cortisol is prolonged, and urinary metabolites are decreased. Cortisol production rates are normal or slightly elevated, particularly, if body mass is considered. Many explanations for elevated cortisol levels have been provided, including peripheral resistance to the hormone (24).

Cortisol binding in plasma is normal. The consensus is that the primary defect is localized in the hypothalamus, but the mechanism is unknown. Dexamethasone suppression is abnormal in anorexia nervosa and the corticotropin response to corticotropin-releasing hormone (CRH) is blunted. CRH levels in the cerebrospinal fluid are elevated, whereas corticotropin (ACTH) levels are low. The proposed mechanism is that the initial lesion is hypersecretion of CRH, hypersecretion of ACTH, overproduction of cortisol, and hyperplasia of the adrenals, with subsequent feedback of cortisol on the pituitary so that ACTH levels fall into the normal range (24). It is postulated that feedback on the hypothalamus is impaired, which could account for the elevated CRH levels. Although the ACTH response to synthetic CRH is blunted, the cortisol response expected from a given rise in ACTH is increased (24). The observation of a retained circadian rhythm at higher cortisol levels suggests that a new set point has been determined by the hypothalamus–pituitary–adrenal (HPA) axis.

In conclusion, in anorexia nervosa HPA axis arousal, an increased secretion of cortisol under basal conditions or after stress stimuli, and reduced or absent suppression at dexamethasone suppression test have been observed. These findings seem to be directly associated with weight loss. Alterations seem to be more relevant as the disease becomes more severe, weight recovery does not normalize HPA functions, and the concurrent comorbid pathology does not influence HPA axis function in anorexia nervosa.

Miscellaneous hormones: melatonin, glucagon, leptin, and ghrelin

Melatonin levels have generally been found to be increased with higher than normal day/night ratios (25) although night concentrations were not increased in one study. The response of glucagon to hypoglycaemia is impaired, whereas release after administration of arginine is normal.

In anorexia nervosa leptin levels are lower because of reduced body weight and fat mass (11) and diurnal variation in leptin is decreased. Soluble leptin receptor levels are increased, resulting in a lower free leptin index. Nutritional rehabilitation increases serum leptin levels, which correlates with increasing gonadotropin levels. Resumption of menses is associated with a significant increase in the free leptin index suggesting that free leptin may be an important determinant of menstrual recovery (4).

Notably, Wabitsch *et al.* (26) described three men with anorexia nervosa whose serum concentrations of leptin, gonadotropins, and testosterone and the free androgen index (FAI) were analysed longitudinally during extreme underweight and therapeutically induced weight gain. They found that leptin levels at low BMI values were below the 5th percentile. During weight gain, leptin levels reached or surpassed the 95th percentile. Leptin increments were paralleled by increments of gonadotropins, testosterone, and FAI. They suggested that leptin might also play an important role in the regulation of the hypothalamo-pituitary-gonadal axis and fertility in underweight men as previously shown in underweight women (25).

Fasting ghrelin levels are elevated in patients with anorexia nervosa and normalize after partial weight recovery (11). High ghrelin levels appear compensatory to increase food intake and to induce a state of positive energy balance. Patients with anorexia nervosa are less sensitive to ghrelin administration than healthy women with respect to growth hormone response and appetite. A meta-analysis on ghrelin that included a total of 28 studies revealed that persons with anorexia nervosa and bulimia nervosa have higher baseline levels of ghrelin (large effect). However, there was large heterogeneity among the studies and the results were highly variable and subject to multiple confounding factors (27). In a recent paper Tolle *et al.* (28) investigated ghrelin plasma levels in patients with anorexia nervosa before and after renutrition. The relationships between plasma ghrelin levels and other neuroendocrine and nutritional parameters, such as growth hormone, leptin, T_3 and cortisol, were also assessed. In anorexia nervosa, morning fasting plasma ghrelin levels were doubled compared with controls and after renutrition. Twenty-four-hour plasma ghrelin, growth hormone, and cortisol levels determined every 4 h were significantly increased, whereas 24-h plasma leptin levels were decreased in anorexia nervosa patients compared with controls. Both ghrelin and leptin levels returned to control values in anorexia nervosa patients after renutrition. Ghrelin was negatively correlated with BMI, leptin, and T_3 in anorexia nervosa patients and controls, whereas no correlation was found between growth hormone and ghrelin or between cortisol and ghrelin. Ghrelin and BMI or T_3 were still correlated after refeeding, suggesting that ghrelin is also a good nutritional indicator.

Finally, Karczewska-Kupczewska *et al.* (29) investigated serum ghrelin concentration in the fasting state and after hyperinsulinemia in women with AN. They investigated 19 women with AN, 26 lean healthy women, and 25 women who were overweight or obese. Serum ghrelin concentration was measured in the fasting state and after euglycemic hyperinsulinemic clamp. They concluded that women with AN have an increased suppression of serum ghrelin by hyperinsulinemia. This phenomenon may lead to an increased and more rapid feeling of satiety in AN.

Bone metabolism

Women with anorexia nervosa have evidence of reduced bone of more than 90% density and 38% meet the diagnostic criteria for osteoporosis. Abnormal bone metabolism is multifaceted and appears to result from osteoblastic abnormalities. Severe nutritional deficiency, excessive exercise, hormonal aberrancies and elevated catecholamines and glucocorticoid levels contribute to decreased bone density levels (11).

Recently it was reported that serum levels of osteoprotegerin (OPG) in anorexia nervosa patients were significantly higher than those in controls and negatively correlated with BMI, E_2, IGF-1, or leptin. Serum levels of free RANKL could not be detected except for only one healthy control in both groups. The results suggest that serum OPG levels may be increased by a compensatory mechanism for malnutrition and oestrogen deficiency, which induces an increase in bone resorption (30).

Finally, Estour *et al.* (31) evaluated the hormonal profiles in a large cohort of AN and their relationship with critical states. They investigated 210 young female subjects with restrictive-type AN and 42 female controls of comparable age. They measured thyroid hormones, GH, IGF-I, cortisol, oestradiol, FSH, LH, SHBG, DHEA-S, plasma metanephrines and bone markers. They concluded that the hormonal response to undernutrition is heterogeneous in a large population with restrictive AN. In clinical practice, metanephrines, GH, and/or cortisol data could be used as important predictors for severe short-term outcome.

Bulimia nervosa

Bulimia nervosa shares many clinical and biological features with anorexia nervosa. A major difference between those two diagnostic categories is that patients with bulimia nervosa maintain normal body weight. Clinically manifest bulimia nervosa is usually preceded by prolonged attempts to restrain eating that are eventually interrupted by episodes of binge eating and compensation mechanisms to avoid weight gain (purging), such as self-induced vomiting, misuse of laxatives, diuretics, enemas, and excessive exercising, and fasting the day following a binge. Diagnostic criteria for bulimia nervosa are presented in Box 2.6.2.3. It is of note that what makes a person bulimic—as opposed to anorexic—is not the purging, but the cycle of bingeing and purging.

Box 2.6.2.3 Diagnostic criteria for bulimia nervosa

Recurrent episodes of binge eating

- Recurrent inappropriate compensatory behaviour in order to prevent weight gain (purging), such as self-induced vomiting; misuse of laxatives, diuretics, enemas, or other medications; fasting; or excessive exercise

The binge eating and purging both occur, on average, at least twice a week for 3 months

Self-evaluation is unduly influenced by body shape and weight

Two types

- Purging type
- Nonpurging type

Most bulimia nervosa patients are young women; only occasionally does the disorder develop in men. Prevalence rates are greater than those of anorexia nervosa, ranging from 1% to 2%. Almost 30% of bulimic patients have a previous history of anorexia nervosa. Regarding outcome, 50% of bulimia nervosa patients are asymptomatic 2–10 years after cognitive-behavioural therapy; there is a group of 20% of patients who remain persistently symptomatic. The mortality rate in bulimia nervosa is much lower than that of anorexia nervosa (5). Patients with bulimia nervosa generally have fewer serious medical complications than those with anorexia nervosa.

Endocrinology of bulimia nervosa

The endocrine abnormalities found in bulimia nervosa are less consistent than those found in anorexia nervosa, and there are some discrepancies among various studies. The possible reason may be the fact that bulimia nervosa is characterized not only by bingeing and purging, but also by intermittent dieting and starvation; accordingly, endocrine changes associated with malnutrition might not be present in the same patients all the time. It would therefore be logical to expect different studies would yield different results if they examined patients in various stages of dieting and at various levels of weight loss or gain.

Reproductive system

Amenorrhoea occurs in only about 50% of patients. Almost half of the patients have anovulatory cycles. A reduced luteinizing hormone pulse frequency during the early follicular phase has been reported, which suggests a deficient hypothalamic drive. Prolactin is normal. However, bulimia nervosa patients have a significant reduction in nocturnal prolactin levels. Additionally, patients who are bingeing and vomiting have increased prolactin levels, compared with controls who eat normally (5).

Hypothalamic–pituitary–thyroid axis

In bulimia nervosa, thyroid function varies according to the binge-eating-fasting cycle of the disorder (32). During the bingeing phase of the illness patients have lower total T_3 values than controls. After 7 weeks of normalized behaviour, patients have lower total

T_3, free T_3, free T_4, reverse T_3, and thyroxine-binding globulin (TBG) values compared with controls and significant reductions in total T_3, total T_4, free T_4, and TBG compared to themselves in the active phase of the illness. Binge-purge behaviour may transiently increase thyroid indices in patients with bulimia nervosa because there is a positive correlation between caloric intake and TSH values during the bingeing phase of the illness (32). On the other hand, decreases in thyroid function following abstinence may be related to diminished caloric consumption or may reflect a trait hypothalamic-pituitary dysregulation in these patients.

Gendall *et al.* (33) examined the T_4 and free T_4 status of 135 bulimic women and its value as a predictor of outcome. They concluded that low T_4 levels at pretreatment may be a predictor of poor outcome in bulimia nervosa.

Hypothalamic–pituitary–adrenal axis

Women with bulimia nervosa have transverse 24-h plasma cortisol concentrations that have been reported to be normal or increased. Similarly, the ACTH response to CRH has been reported to be normal or blunted. In the bulimic women, cortisol levels remained unchanged, whereas growth hormone concentrations have been found to rise significantly after a glucose load (5).

In general, unlike anorexic patients, bulimia nervosa patients do not display a clear association between the eating disorder symptoms and HPA axis dysfunction. In fact, different studies suggested that bingeing and vomiting do not substantially influence hormonal secretion, as the peak rise in cortisol during bingeing is proportionally comparable to that of healthy control women consuming a large meal. Moreover, purging behaviour does not alter cortisol or ACTH levels, so hyperactivation of the HPA axis in bulimia nervosa seems to be related to psychological stress and the chronic and repeated ingestion of large amounts of food (34).

GH-IGF-1 axis

Patients with bulimia nervosa have increased growth hormone plasma concentrations, and enhanced growth hormone response to TRH. Despite this growth hormone elevation, their mean IGF-1 concentration is within the normal range. This suggest that IGF-1 generation is resistant to the elevated circulating growth hormone and IGF-1 is not inhibiting growth hormone secretion in the pituitary-hypothalamic axis (5).

Miscellaneous hormones: melatonin, leptin, ghrelin

Melatonin levels are increased with higher than normal day/night rations. Patients with bulimia nervosa also show a strong positive correlation between plasma levels of leptin and BMI although there may be a decreased contribution of leptin in signalling acute changes in energy balance in bulimia nervosa (5). Interestingly, the pattern of food intake, including binges and disruption of mealtimes, alters the diurnal pattern of plasma leptin levels.

In anorexia nervosa and bulimia nervosa there are decreased plasma glucose and insulin levels throughout the 24-h period. Bone mineral density is normal in bulimia nervosa even though menstrual dysfunction is frequently found among those patients (5).

Binge eating disorder

Binge eating disorder is a newly designated condition that probably affects million of Americans. People with binge eating disorder frequently eat large amounts of food, while feeling a loss of control over their eating. This disorder is different from bulimia nervosa because people with binge eating disorder usually do not purge afterward by vomiting or using laxatives. The diagnostic criteria are presented in Box 2.6.2.4.

Although it has only recently been recognized as a distinct entity, binge eating disorder is probably the most common eating disorder. Most patients with binge eating disorder are obese (more than 20% above a healthy body weight), but normal weight people also can be affected. Binge eating disorder probably affects 2% of all adults (about one to two million Americans). Among mildly obese people in self-help or commercial weight loss programmes, 10–15% have binge eating disorder. The disorder is even more common in those with severe obesity. Binge eating disorder is slightly more common in women, with 3 women affected for every 2 men. The disorder affects black people as often as white people. Obese people with binge eating disorder often become overweight at a younger age than those without the disorder. They also may have more frequent episodes of losing and regaining weight (yo-yo dieting) (35).

Endocrinology of binge eating disorder

Type 2 diabetes and its complications are a real health problem for patients with binge eating disorder. Other endocrine disturbances which have been reported in patients with binge eating disorder

Box 2.6.2.4 Diagnostic criteria for binge eating disorder

Recurrent episodes of binge eating. An episode of binge eating is characterized by both of the following:

- Eating, in a discrete period of time (e.g. within any 2-h period), an amount of food that is definitely larger than most people would eat during a similar period of time under similar circumstances
- A sense of lack of control during the episodes (e.g. a feeling that one cannot stop eating or control what or how much one is eating).

The binge eating episodes are associated with at least three of the following behavioural indications of loss of control:

- Eating much more rapidly than usual
- Eating until feeling uncomfortably full
- Eating large amounts of food when not feeling physically hungry
- Eating alone because of being embarrassed by how much one is eating
- Feeling disgusted with oneself, depressed or feeling very guilty after overeating

Marked distress regarding binge eating

The binge eating occurs, on average, at least 2 days a week for a 6-month period

The binge eating is not associated with the regular use of inappropriate compensatory behaviours (e.g. purging, fasting, excessive exercise) and does not occur exclusively during the course of anorexia nervosa or bulimia nervosa await confirmation because they may reflect the nutritional status rather than specific patterns of disordered eating behaviour.

Hypothalamic–pituitary–thyroid axis

No significant differences have been observed between obese bingers and nonbingers in resting metabolic rate or thyroid hormones (36).

Hypothalamic–pituitary–adrenal axis

Different HPA axis abnormalities have been observed in binge eating disorder and obese subjects, and in general these alterations are considered to be mainly due to excess weight (34). Specifically, binge eating disorder was not associated with increased levels of salivary cortisol. In women with binge eating disorder salivary cortisol correlated significantly with Binge Eating Scale. Although obesity is associated with decreased levels of cortisol, the relationship may be lost in patients with binge eating disorder, in whom binge eating severity may be a more relevant regulator of cortisol secretion than obesity itself. Gluck *et al.* (37) assessed cortisol, hunger, and the desire to binge eat after a cortisol pressor test among women with binge eating disorder. They found that the binge eating disorder group had a higher basal cortisol concentration than the nonbinge eating disorder group, but cortisol did not differ after dexamethasone suppression test. Also, they had greater area under the curve (AUC) for hunger and desire to binge eat after the cortisol pressure test. These observations suggest that in binge eating disorder there is a hyperactivity of the HPA axis which may contribute to increase hunger and binge eating.

Miscellaneous hormones: oestradiol, prolactin, leptin

Monteleone *et al.* (38) investigated 67 women, 21 with anorexia nervosa, 32 with bulimia nervosa, 14 with binge eating disorder, and 25 healthy controls: circulating levels of leptin were significantly enhanced in women with binge eating disorder, whereas oestradiol and prolactin concentrations were reduced. A strong positive correlation revealed between plasma leptin and BMI or body weight, suggesting that factors other than body weight may play a role in the determination of leptin changes in eating disorders. All these findings await confirmation.

Conclusions

Eating disorders affect million of Americans and Europeans every year, when the three different disorders, anorexia nervosa, bulimia nervosa, and binge eating disorder, are considered. Behavioural, emotional, psychological, interpersonal, and social factors are involved in the aetiopathogenesis of eating disorders. The associated endocrine abnormalities may involve the HPG axis, the GH-IGFs axis, the HPT axis, the HPA axis, and different peptides and hormones such as melatonin, glucagon, leptin and ghrelin. Bone metabolism may be abnormal in anorexia nervosa, but not in bulimia nervosa or binge eating disorder. It is worth noting that the results of endocrine investigations may vary according to the different stages of dieting and the different degrees of weight loss or gain in the subjects.

References

1. Capasso A, Putrella C, Milano W. Recent clinical aspects of eating disorders. *Rev Recent Clin Trials*, 2009; **4**: 63–9.
2. Becker AE, Grinspoon SK, Klibanski A, Herzog DB. Eating disorders. *N Engl J Med*, 1999; **340**: 1092–8.
3. Zachrisson HD, Vedul-Kjelsås E, Götestam KG, Mykletun A. Time trends in obesity and eating disorders. *Int J Eat Disord*, 2008; **41**: 673–80.
4. Krassas GE. Endocrine abnormalities in Anorexia Nervosa. *Pediatr Endocrinol Rev*, 2003; **1**: 46–54.
5. Negrão AB, Licinio J. Anorexia nervosa and bulimia nervosa. In: Arnold A, Etgen A, Rubin R, eds. *Hormones, Brain and Behavior, Section: Endocrinologically Important Behavioral Syndromes*. San Diego: Academic Press, 2002:515–30.
6. Lucas AR, Beard CM, O'Fallon WM, Kurland LT. 50-year trends in the incidence of anorexia nervosa in Rochester, Minn.: a population-based study. *Am J Psychiatry*, 1991; **148**: 917–22.
7. Herzog DB, Greenwood DN, Dorer DJ, Flores AT, Ekeblad ER, Richards A, *et al.* Mortality in eating disorders: a descriptive study. *Int J Eat Disord*, 2000; **28**: 20–6.
8. Fichter MM, Quadflieg N. Six-year course and outcome of anorexia nervosa. *Int J Eat Disord*, 1999; **26**: 359–85.
9. Ramsay R, Ward A, Treasure J, Russell GF. Compulsory treatment in anorexia nervosa. Short-term benefits and long-term mortality. *Br J Psychiatry*, 1999; **175**: 147–53.
10. Feighner JP, Robins E, Guze SB, Woodruff RA Jr, Winokur G, Munoz R. Diagnostic criteria for use in psychiatric research. *Arch Gen Psychiatry*, 1972; **26**: 57–63.
11. Usdan LS, Khaodhiar L, Apovian CM. The endocrinopathies of anorexia nervosa. *Endocr Pract*, 2008; **14**: 1055–63.
12. Boyar RM, Katz J, Finkelstein JW, Kapen S, Weiner H, Weitzman ED, *et al.* Anorexia nervosa. Immaturity of the 24-hour luteinizing hormone secretory pattern. *N Engl J Med*, 1974; **291**: 861–5.
13. Marshall JC, Kelch RP. Low dose pulsatile gonadotropin-releasing hormone in anorexia nervosa: a model of human pubertal development. *J Clin Endocrinol Metab*, 1979; **49**: 712–18.
14. Tamai H, Karibe C, Kiyohara K, Mori K, Takeno K, Kobayashi N, *et al.* Abnormal serum prolactin responses to luteinizing hormone-releasing hormone (LHRH) in patients with anorexia nervosa and bulimia. *Psychoneuroendocrinology*, 1987; **12**: 281–7.
15. Stewart DE, Robinson E, Goldbloom DS, Wright C. Infertility and eating disorders. *Am J Obstet Gynecol*, 1990; **163**: 1196–9.
16. Støving RK, Veldhuis JD, Flyvbjerg A, Vinten J, Hangaard J, Koldkjaer OG, *et al.* Jointly amplified basal and pulsatile growth hormone (GH) secretion and increased process irregularity in women with anorexia nervosa: indirect evidence for disruption of feedback regulation within the GH-insulin-like growth factor I axis. *J Clin Endocrinol Metab*, 1999; **84**: 2056–63.
17. De Marinis L, Folli G, D'Amico C. Differential effects of feeding on the ultradian variation of the growth hormone (GH) response to GH-releasing hormone in normal subjects and patients with obesity and anorexia nervosa. *J Clin Endocrinol Metab*, 1988; **66**: 598–604.
18. Counts DR, Gwirtsman H, Carlsson LM, Lesem M, Cutler GB Jr. The effect of anorexia nervosa and refeeding on growth hormone-binding protein, the insulin-like growth factors (IGFs), and the IGF-binding proteins. *J Clin Endocrinol Metab*, 1992; **75**: 762–7.
19. Argente J, Caballo N, Barrios V. Multiple endocrine abnormalities of the growth hormone and insulin-like growth factor axis in patients with anorexia nervosa: effect of short- and long-term weight recuperation. *J Clin Endocrinol Metab*, 1997; **82**: 2084–92.
20. Støving RK, Flyvbjerg A, Frystyk J. Low serum levels of free and total insulin-like growth factor I (IGF-I) in patients with anorexia nervosa are not associated with increased IGF-binding protein-3 proteolysis. *J Clin Endocrinol Metab*, 1999; **84**: 1346–50.
21. Gianotti L, Pincelli AI, Scacchi M, Rolla M, Bellitti D, Arvat E, *et al.* Effects of recombinant human insulin-like growth factor I

administration on spontaneous and growth hormone (GH)-releasing hormone-stimulated GH secretion in anorexia nervosa. *J Clin Endocrinol Metab*, 2000; **85**: 2805–9.
22. Grinspoon S, Miller K, Herzog D, Clemmons D, Klibanski A. Effects of recombinant human insulin-like growth factor (IGF)-I and estrogen administration on IGF-I, IGF binding protein (IGFBP)-2, and IGFBP-3 in anorexia nervosa: a randomized-controlled study. *J Clin Endocrinol Metab*, 2003; **88**: 1142–9.
23. Farezi KP, Lawson EA, Prabhakaran R, Miller KK, Donoho DA, Clemmon DR, *et al.* Effects of recombinant human growth hormone in anorexia nervosa: a randomized, placebo-controlled study. *J Clin Endocrinol Metab*, 2010 Jul 28. [Epub ahead of print]
24. Gold PW, Gwirtsman H, Avgerinos PC. Abnormal hypothalamic-pituitary-adrenal function in anorexia nervosa. Pathophysiologic mechanisms in underweight and weight-corrected patients. *N Engl J Med*, 1986; **314**: 1335–42.
25. Tortosa F, Puig-Domingo M, Peinado MA, Oriola J, Webb SM, de Leiva A. Enhanced circadian rhythm of melatonin in anorexia nervosa. *Acta Endocrinol (Copenh)*, 1989; **120**: 574–8.
26. Wabitsch M, Ballauff A, Holl R. Serum leptin, gonadotropin, and testosterone concentrations in male patients with anorexia nervosa during weight gain. *J Clin Endocrinol Metab*, 2001; **86**: 2982–8.
27. Prince AC, Brooks SJ, Stahl D, Treasure J. Systematic review and meta-analysis of the baseline concentrations and physiologic responses of gut hormones to food in eating disorders. *Am J Clin Nutr*, 2009; **89**: 755–65.
28. Tolle V, Kadem M, Bluet-Pajot MT. Balance in ghrelin and leptin plasma levels in anorexia nervosa patients and constitutionally thin women. *J Clin Endocrinol Metab*, 2003; **88**: 109–16.
29. Karczewska-Kupczewska M, Straczkowski M, Adamska A, Nikolajuk A, Otziomek E, Gorska M, *et al.* Increased suppression of serum ghrelin concentration by hyperinsulinemia in women with anorexia nervosa. *Eur J Endocrinol*, 2010; **162**: 235–9.
30. Ohwada R, Hotta M, Sato K, Shibasaki T, Takano K. The relationship between serum levels of estradiol and osteoprotegerin in patients with anorexia nervosa. *Endocr J*, 2007; **54**: 953–9.
31. Estour B, Germain N, Diconne E, Frere D, Cottet-Emard JM, Carrot G, *et al.* Hormonal profile heterogeneity and short-term physical risk in restrictive anorexia nervosa. *J Clin Endocrinol Metab*, 2010; **95**: 2203–10.
32. Altemus M, Hetherington M, Kennedy B, Licinio J, Gold PW. Thyroid function in bulimia nervosa. *Psychoneuroendocrinology*, 1996; **21**: 249–61.
33. Gendall KA, Joyce PR, Carter FA, McIntosh VV, Bulik CM. Thyroid indices and treatment outcome in bulimia nervosa. *Acta Psychiatr Scand*, 2003; **108**: 190–5.
34. Lo Sauro C, Ravaldi C, Cabras PL, Faravelli C, Ricca V. Stress, hypothalamic-pituitary-adrenal axis and eating disorders. *Neuropsychobiology*, 2008; **57**: 95–115.
35. Mental Health Consumer. Mental Health Disorders and Conditions. *Binge Eating Disorder*. Available at: www.athealth.com/consumer/disorders/bingeeating.html (accessed 26 February 2009).
36. Wadden TA, Foster GD, Letizia KA, Wilk JE. Metabolic, anthropometric, and psychological characteristics of obese binge eaters. *Int J Eat Disord*, 1993; **14**: 17–25.
37. Gluck ME, Geliebter A, Hung J, Yahav E. Cortisol, hunger, and desire to binge eat following a cold stress test in obese women with binge eating disorder. *Psychosom Med*, 2004; **66**: 876–81.
38. Monteleone P, Di Lieto A, Tortorella A, Longobardi N, Maj M. Circulating leptin in patients with anorexia nervosa, bulimia nervosa or binge-eating disorder: relationship to body weight, eating patterns, psychopathology and endocrine changes. *Psychiatry Res*, 2000; **94**: 121–9.

2.6.3 The endocrine response to stress

David E. Henley, Joey M. Kaye, Stafford L. Lightman

Introduction

In the face of any threat or challenge, either real or perceived, an organism must mount a series of coordinated and specific hormonal, autonomic, immune, and behavioural responses that allow it to either escape or adapt (1–3). To be successful, the characteristics and intensity of the response must match that posed by the threat itself and should last no longer than is necessary. A response that is either inadequate or excessive in terms of its specificity, intensity or duration may result in one or more of a multitude of psychological or physical pathologies (2–5). This concept of threat and the organism's response to it is frequently recognized and understood as 'stress' but is so diverse that it lacks a universally accepted definition (2) and thus is difficult to investigate or study (6).

In the early 1900s, Walter Cannon introduced the concept of homoeostasis (4)—an ideal steady state for all physiological processes. Stress has been defined as the state where this ideal is threatened. More easily appreciated, however, are those factors, both intrinsic and extrinsic, which represent a challenge to homoeostasis (termed stressors) and the complex physiological, hormonal, and behavioural responses that occur to restore the balance, the stress response (1). The importance of endocrine systems in this stress response was emphasized by Hans Selye (7), who described the need for multiple, integrated systems to respond in a coordinated fashion following exposure to a particular stressor. Nonspecific activation of the hypothalamic–pituitary–adrenal (HPA) and sympatho-adrenomedullary (SAM) axes occurred following initial exposure to a noxious stimulus. Continued exposure to the same agent has been shown to have lasting and damaging effects on various endocrine, immune, and other systems, although recovery from this state was possible provided the stress was terminated (7). In addition to various noxious agents, numerous potential stressors exist including exertion, physical extremes, trauma, injury, and psychological stress. Indeed, psychological stressors are some of the most potent stimuli of the endocrine stress response particularly when they involve elements of novelty, uncertainty, and unpredictability. This has been highlighted by the observation that anticipating an event can be as potent an activator of the stress response as the event itself (7).

Anatomy and physiology of the endocrine response to stress

The HPA and SAM axes are the principal endocrine effector arms of the stress response (Fig. 2.6.3.1). However, a number of other hormone axes and neurotransmitter systems are either directly stress responsive themselves, or modulate these other hormone systems.

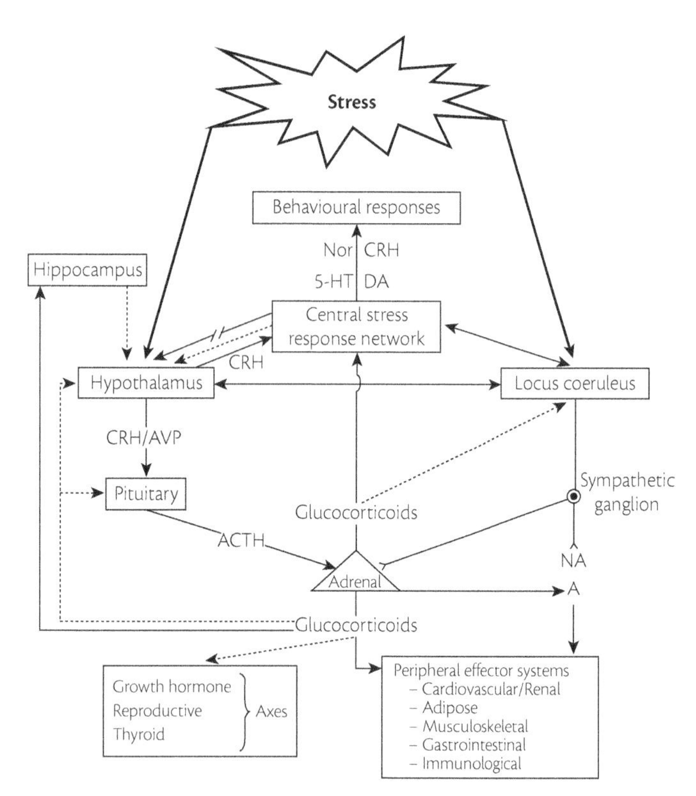

Fig. 2.6.3.1 Chronic stress response. Simplified overview of the chronic stress response and its two main effector arms, the hypothalamic–pituitary–adrenal axis and the sympatho-neural/sympatho-adrenomedullary system. Note the glucocorticoid feedforward and feedback regulatory loops, reciprocal interaction of corticotropin-releasing hormone (CRH) and the locus coeruleus, together with the putative central stress response network in effecting peripheral and central adaptive responses. Components of the central brain stress response network include: parvocellular neurons in the paraventricular nuclei, central nucleus of the amygdala, bed nuclei of the stria terminalis, Barrington's nucleus, ventral tegmental area, dorsal raphe, locus coeruleus and the A1/A2 medullary noradrenergic cell groups. Solid lines indicate stimulation; dashed lines indicate inhibition; broken line indicates indirect projections. A, adrenaline; ACTH, adrenocorticotropic hormone; AVP, arginine vasopressin; DA, dopamine; NA, noradrenaline; 5-HT, 5-hydroxytryptamine (serotonin).

The hypothalamic–pituitary–adrenal axis

Corticotropin-releasing hormone (CRH), identified by Vale and others (8) in 1981, is a 41 amino acid peptide responsible for promoting the synthesis and release of anterior pituitary adrenocorticotropin (ACTH). Hypophyseotropic CRH neurons project to the median eminence from the paraventricular hypothalamic nucleus (PVN). CRH is also widely distributed throughout the CNS, being found within the cortex where it has important effects on behaviour and cognitive processing. Within the brainstem interactions with sympathetic and parasympathetic centres influence autonomic functioning while within limbic and paralimbic regions such as the amygdala, CRH influences the expression of mood and anxiety-type behaviours (9). Arginine vasopressin (AVP), synthesized in parvocellular cells of the PVN, acts synergistically with CRH to stimulate the release of ACTH (9).

ACTH release from the anterior pituitary acts directly on the adrenal cortex to promote the release of adrenal glucocorticoids into the circulation (1, 3, 9). Glucocorticoids, in general, have two fundamental roles in the stress response. First, during stress-free periods, basal levels have a role in preparing the organism for future stress exposure. The circadian rise in glucocorticoids actually occurs prior to activity and thus in humans starts at about 03.00 h and peaks around 09.00 h (see below). This anticipatory activity results in energy storage and conservation by promoting glucose and fat uptake and opposing energy utilization, and prepares the organism for the activities of the next waking day. The glucocorticoids also prime the immune system for future activation and promote memory formation of previous stressors so that future exposure to the same or similar stressor may facilitate a more rapid and efficient response (10).

The second role of the HPA response is to modulate events at the time of stress exposure itself. Initially glucocorticoids enhance the cardiovascular effects of catecholamines and AVP, promote energy provision and utilization, influence and enhance appropriate stress-related behaviours, and stimulate certain aspects of the immune response (10). It is perhaps even more important that once the stress response has been initiated, some of the principal actions of glucocorticoids are to suppress and restrain the activity of these systems, in particular the SAM and immune systems. In doing so, glucocorticoids provide an essential regulatory balance to ensure the stress response is appropriate in terms of both its intensity and duration and that all these responses are 'switched off' when the stress has been successfully dealt with (2, 10).

Glucocorticoid secretion is precisely controlled by a complex feedback system that involves a direct action on the hypothalamus and anterior pituitary reducing the amount of releasing hormone (CRH and ACTH, respectively) produced, and consequently limiting the amount of further glucocorticoid released into the circulation. In addition, a further level of feedback activity occurs at the level of the hippocampus, a site that is also important in memory formation. A subset of hippocampal neurons that release the neurotransmitter γ-aminobutyric acid (GABA), project to the hypothalamus where GABA inhibits CRH release, thus contributing to the negative feedback effect on cortisol (1).

There are two known glucocorticoid receptors in the brain, the glucocorticoid receptor (GR) and the mineralocorticoid receptor (MR) which are involved in the feedback system. GRs are found throughout the brain but are most abundant in the hypothalamic CRH neurons and pituitary corticotrophs while MR expression is highest in the hippocampus. The low affinity GR is occupied during periods of intermediate to high glucocorticoid secretion (e.g. during the circadian peak and following stress) while the high affinity MR will be extensively bound even during periods of basal secretion (11). Therefore MR is thought to regulate tonic HPA activity while GR (in coordination with MR) mediates the response to stress.

Three time domains of corticosteroid feedback have been described (12). Fast, rate sensitive feedback occurs within seconds to minutes, during the period of increasing plasma corticosteroid concentrations, and probably controls the rate and magnitude of ACTH and corticosteroid response to stimuli. This may be mediated by membrane-associated MRs via rapid, nongenomic mechanisms (13). Disruption of fast feedback has been demonstrated in ageing humans and in depressed patients, and thus may have a role in the maintenance of homoeostasis (13). Intermediate feedback occurs over 2–10 h and may limit the response of the system to repeated stimulation within a relatively short period of time (hours) while slow feedback (over hours to days) may have the same role during prolonged stress (12).

Circadian and ultradian rhythms of HPA activity

As with virtually all endocrine systems, ACTH and cortisol show fluctuation in their secretory activity. The classic circadian (24-h) rhythm describes the pattern of HPA activity with hormone concentrations reaching a nadir around midnight, commencing to rise about 03.00 h to reach a peak around 09.00 h before gradually falling throughout the day toward the nadir levels. However, this circadian rhythm is subserved by an underlying ultradian (less than 24-h) rhythm of secretory pulses which can only be detected by frequent blood sampling.

The episodic, pulsatile secretion of ACTH and cortisol has been known for some time (14). More recently specific mathematical models such as deconvolution analysis (15) provide quantitative estimates of *in vivo* hormone secretion such as the number, amplitude, and duration of underlying secretory bursts. Modulation of the amplitude of both ACTH and cortisol secretory pulses gives rise to their respective nyctohemeral rhythms (16). Under physiological conditions ACTH secretion is characterized by episodic pulses of activity separated by intervals of low basal (nonpulsatile) secretion.

Cortisol is synthesized and secreted from zona fasciculata cells of the adrenal cortex in response to ACTH secreted by the corticotroph cells of the anterior pituitary. There is a high temporal concordance between ACTH and cortisol secretion peaks, with the latter lagging those of ACTH by 10 min (14, 16, 17) (Fig. 2.6.3.2). Secretory bursts of both hormones are episodic in that they are independent events produced randomly over time (16, 18). Sexual diergism in ACTH pulsatility has been demonstrated with males showing greater pulse frequency (18 vs 10 per 24 h), mean peak amplitude and area under the 24-h profile (19). Cortisol secretory bursts occur more frequently in the early hours of the morning (shortly before arising from sleep) and least frequently during late afternoon (18).

Until recently the relevance of episodic ultradian signalling has been unclear. It had been postulated that the quiescent interpulse interval period may allow intracellular synthesis, processing, transport, and storage of ACTH by the metabolically replete and unstressed corticotroph, providing readily releasable hormone in the event of an acute stressful stimulus (20). It is now emerging that corticosteroid pulsatility is important in steroid signalling in that it provides scope for a digital, in addition to analogue, signal for tissue glucocorticoid receptors (21). Hippocampal GR and MR receptors have been shown to translocate rapidly from the cytoplasm to the nucleus and bind DNA in response to a corticosteroid pulse (22). Since GR dissociated rapidly from DNA and disappears from the nucleus within a 1-h interpulse interval, in contrast to MR which remains bound to DNA, changes in pulse frequency will have differential effects on MR and GR binding to DNA. Given the presence of different transcription factors and molecular chaperones in cells of different tissues there is scope for multiple cell specific responses to different digital signals (23).

The sympatho-neural and sympatho-adrenomedullary axis

The hallmark sympathetic 'fight or flight' response is characterized by global activation of the SAM system and features typical physiological and behavioural activation including accelerated heart rate, increased blood pressure, and rapid breathing. Fear, vigilance, sensory arousal, and motor activation often with trembling, goose bumps, and piloerection also occur. Catecholamines, the effector hormones of this system, act through specific cell surface receptors that are widely distributed and account for the rapid effects these hormones have on multiple physiological processes (1, 3). Release of glucose stores, immune activation, and increased blood flow to essential organs such as the brain while inhibiting nonessential activity such as digestion together produce a 'state of emergency', which can rapidly attend to a sudden change in physiological balance (3). This response is characterized by its speed of onset, its ability to begin in anticipation of an event being stressful, and by its interaction with other stress-responsive systems (3). This interaction can occur either through neural connections or through increased blood flow that transports other messengers (such as hormones and cytokines) more rapidly to their respective sites of action (3).

The sympathetic nervous system originates from nuclei in the lower brainstem that use noradrenaline as their principal neurotransmitter (see Fig. 2.6.3.1). These noradrenergic nuclei, centred on the locus coeruleus (LC), project downward to the intermediolateral columns of the spinal cord. Cell bodies from here send

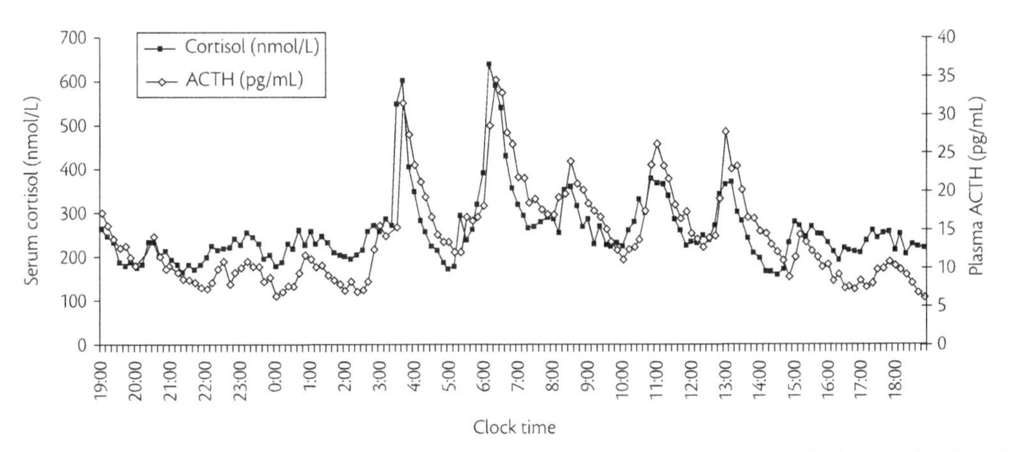

Fig. 2.6.3.2 Plasma ACTH and serum cortisol concentration curves. Superimposed ACTH and cortisol concentration profiles from two healthy male volunteers demonstrate the close concordance between these two interlinked hormones. Note the circadian rhythm subserved by an underlying ultradian rhythm. (Adapted from Henley DE, Leendertz JA, Russell GM, Wood SA, Taheri S, Woltersdorf WW, *et al*. Development of an automated blood sampling system for use in humans. *J Med Eng Technol*, 2009; **33**: 199–208 (17)).

preganglionic fibres to the paraspinal ganglia chain from where postganglionic fibres give rise to sympathetic nerves that supply the heart, blood vessels, lungs, gut, kidneys, and other organ systems. These nerves principally release noradrenaline from their terminals close to their site of action. Other preganglionic fibres also innervate the adrenal medulla and regulate the release of adrenaline into the general circulation.

Acute stress

The stress response system has evolved as both an early warning system capable of recognizing potential or existing threats, and as a response system that can initiate and drive the necessary processes required to escape or confront the threat. By its very nature, the response must be dynamic, beginning rapidly with brain and behavioural activation followed quickly by physiological activation. These processes are characterized by positive feedback and feedforward loops that enhance and reinforce themselves as well as recruiting other arms of the stress response. Slower acting hormone systems are recruited into the cascade providing checks and balances to the already active, but energy expensive systems, putting a brake on the whole response to ensure it is kept appropriate to the type of stress faced, to its intensity and duration, and to ensure the response is switched off when the threat has been adequately dealt with (10, 24).

Changes in the internal or external environment that represent either real or potential threats are recognized with the parts of the brain responsible for receiving, integrating, interpreting, and then relaying this information on to those areas responsible for coordinating the necessary response. This brain activation can be detected within milliseconds and proceeds over seconds to minutes as the response continues to unfold. Stereotypical orienting behaviour, initiated within seconds, gradually gives way to more goal-directed behaviour that is specific to the stressor being faced and the environment in which it is occurring (24).

Activation of the autonomic nervous system occurs within seconds, mediated by the release of catecholamines from sympathetic nerves and the adrenal medulla and enhanced by a withdrawal of parasympathetic activity. These systems promote the immediate physiological, motor, and behavioural responses needed in the face of acute physical or psychological stress. Within minutes of the onset of this cascade of events occurring, hypothalamic-releasing hormones stimulate the release of pituitary hormones with the appearance of ACTH signalling the recruitment of the HPA axis into the process (1, 9). Cortisol levels begin to rise within 2–5 min (25), with peak levels not seen for 15–20 min after the onset of the stress (26) (Fig. 2.6.3.3). Early actions of the HPA system provide additional energy resources for the stress response, while slower gene-related effects over the next few minutes to hours serve to restrain ongoing actions of the stress response which, if left unchecked, may prove to be unsustainable for the individual (1, 3).

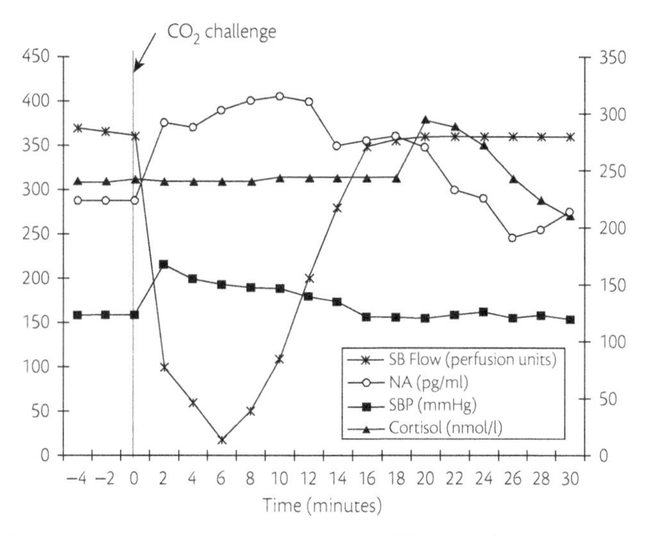

Fig. 2.6.3.3 Acute stress response. Time course of the sympatho-adrenomedullary and HPA axis response to an acute stressor (single breath of 35% CO_2) in a single healthy individual. Noradrenaline release peaks at 2 min with corresponding vasoconstriction (fall in peripheral skin blood flow) and an acute pressor (rise in systolic blood pressure) response. Cortisol rise peaks later at 20 minutes. NA, noradrenaline; SB flow, skin blood flow; SBP, systolic blood pressure.

Chronic stress

Terminology

Stress is an ambiguous term with many connotations and does not distinguish between the experiences of daily life and major life events such as abuse or trauma (27). The term 'allostasis' was therefore introduced to define the active process by which the body responds to daily events and maintains homoeostasis; literally, achieving stability through change. Since a chronic increase or dysregulation of allostasis may lead to disease, the term 'allostatic load or overload' was coined to describe the 'wear and tear' that results from either too much stress or the inefficient management of allostasis (27). Four situations are associated with allostatic load (2): (1) frequent stress; (2) lack of adaptation to a homotypic (same) stressor; (3) inability to shut off allostatic responses after a stress is terminated; and (4) inadequate response by one allostatic system triggering a compensatory increase in another. The advantage of this terminology arises from the fact that behavioural changes (such as poor sleep, eating/drinking too much, smoking, lack of physical activity) that are part of the allostatic load/overload concept are not obvious in the use of the word 'stress' (27). With the superimposition of unpredictable events in the environment, disease, human disturbance, and social interactions then allostatic load can significantly increase, becoming allostatic overload and predisposing the individual to disease (28).

Chronic stress and the brain

There is a marked change in the hypothalamic response to chronic stress with a greater role for AVP (23). In the hypothalamus there is an increase in AVP synthesis, in the proportion of CRH neurons coexpressing AVP, and in the ratio of AVP to CRH immunoreactivity in neurosecretory vesicles as well as colocalization of AVP and CRH in neurosecretory axon terminals (29). Furthermore, AVP stimulation of ACTH secretion is less sensitive to glucocorticoid feedback than is CRH (30). Pituitary changes with chronic stress paradigms include a reduction in CRH receptor numbers and sustained elevations in V1b (AVP) receptor mRNA (29). It appears in some chronic stress paradigms that CRH has a permissive role whereas AVP is the dynamic mediator of ACTH secretion.

It is important for survival that the HPA axis responds adequately during chronic stress. Rodent stress models reveal three basic patterns of response, depending on the type of stress (31): (1)

desensitization of ACTH responses to the sustained stimulus, but hyperresponsiveness to a novel stress despite elevated plasma glucocorticoid levels; (2) corticotroph hyperresponsiveness to a novel stimulus, with no desensitization to the primary repeated stress; and (3) small and transient increases in basal ACTH, followed by marked hyporesponsiveness to novel stimuli. The level of response is determined by the differential regulation of CRH and AVP. The increase in AVP during chronic stress (where glucocorticoid negative feedback down-regulates CRH and ACTH responses) appears to be an important mediator of ACTH release upon new demand. Decreased sensitivity of glucocorticoid feedback is critical for the maintenance of ACTH responses in the presence of increased plasma glucocorticoid levels during chronic stress. It appears that the increase in number of pituitary V1b receptors is the main determining factor for the responsiveness of the corticotroph during adaptation to chronic stress (31).

Involvement of the limbic system in HPA axis regulation is complex (see Fig. 2.6.3.1). The role of limbic structures is both region- and stimulus-specific, they all express both GR and MR and they all exert their effects via subcortical intermediaries (32). Typically, the hippocampus and anterior cingulate/prelimbic cortex inhibit stress-induced HPA axis activation, whereas the amygdala and possibly the infralimbic cortex may enhance glucocorticoid secretion (32). Furthermore, the HPA axis is also subject to glucocorticoid-independent inhibition from neuronal sources. For example, the PVN is richly innervated by GABAergic neurons from the bed nucleus of the stria terminalis, medial pre-optic area, dorsomedial hypothalamus and lateral hypothalamic area. However, the degree to which these GABAergic inhibitory circuits respond to neural vs. glucocorticoid inhibition has not been fully elucidated (32).

The concept of a *central stress response network* recruited by glucocorticoids and chronic stress has recently been described (25). There is a critical role for extrahypothalamic CRH neuronal cell groups, in particular the amygdala. Elevated glucocorticoids acting in a feedforward manner at the amygdala increase CRH expression and secretion, and this increased amygdalar CRH expression is tightly coupled to hypersensitivity of the HPA axis to stressors. The CRH acts on receptors in structures throughout the brain, in particular monoaminergic cell groups that widely innervate the forebrain, resulting in behavioural changes (e.g. more cautious, more ready to be diverted from tasks at hand, adopt alternative strategies, enjoy rewards and remember fearful situations) that make the organism chronically exposed to stress more capable of adapting to the stressful conditions (see Fig. 2.6.3.1).

Reciprocal neural connections exist between CRH and the locus coerulus/noradrenergic neurons of the central stress system, with each one stimulating the other (4) (see Fig. 2.6.3.1). Chronic stress increases CRH content in the locus coerulus. Thus, CRH may induce mechanisms that result in HPA axis facilitation via increased catecholaminergic input to CRH cells, preparing the organism for the capacity to maintain CRH responses to acute stress during periods of chronic stress when the corticosteroid feedback signal is high (30).

Clinical manifestations of chronic stress

Throughout the history of medicine, reference has been made to the influence of stress, particularly in the form of negative emotions and psychological distress, on physical health (6). Relevant examples include psychiatric conditions such as depression and post-traumatic stress disorder (1), vascular disease such as coronary heart disease, immune-mediated conditions including asthma, and other conditions such as osteoporosis, diabetes, dementia, and premature death (1, 6). Why some individuals manifest stress as psychiatric illness, whilst others are more prone to physical disease and yet others seem resistant to the effects of stress exposure is not well understood.

The implication from these associations is that all stress is ultimately damaging with negative consequences for the individual in whom it is occurring. It is clear, however, that there is a protective role for the stress response in the short term (2), and the associated learning and adaptation (a process that requires plasticity of brain responses) that follows stress exposure is critical to the longer term health and survival of the individual. It is only when these responses occur in excess of the body's requirements, or continue for longer than is necessary that damaging effects occur (2).

Psychosocial stress

The importance of the concept of allostatic load can be seen in the fact that there is an association between socioeconomic status and health at every level of the socioeconomic status hierarchy (33). This was classically demonstrated in the Whitehall study of coronary heart disease (CHD) mortality (34) which classified 17 530 UK civil servants according to employment grade and recorded their CHD mortality over 7.5 years. Employment grade was a stronger predictor of subsequent risk of CHD death than any other major coronary risk factor. Depression and depressive symptoms are both inversely related to socioeconomic status and depression is linked to health outcomes, particularly CHD (33). As explained by Adler *et al.* (33) there are two mechanisms by which higher placement in the socioeconomic status hierarchy can reduce stress and its somatic consequences: (1) by diminishing the likelihood that individuals will experience negative events; and (2) through greater social and psychological resources to cope with stressful life events, therefore being less susceptible to the subjective experience of stress.

Mood disorders

Melancholic depression has been described as the prototypic example of chronic activation of the stress system (both HPA axis and SAM) (4). Cortisol secretion is increased, the plasma ACTH response to exogenous CRH is decreased and autopsy studies have shown a marked increase in the number of PVN CRH and AVP neurons (1). Depression is also associated with increased pituitary vasopressinergic responsivity and the locus coerulus of depressed patients contains elevated CRH concentrations (35) Repeated stress that causes frequent surges in blood pressure and catecholamine release is associated with accelerated atherosclerosis and an increased risk of myocardial infarction. Patients with melancholic depression develop varying degrees of atherosclerosis and cardiovascular disease (1) and there is evidence that patients with depression that is associated with chronic hyperactivity of the HPA axis have a reduced life expectancy predominantly as a result of an excess of cardiovascular deaths (1, 6, 36). Furthermore, patients with melancholic depression may develop metabolic syndrome, osteoporosis and Th1 immunosuppression (1) consistent with chronic hyperactivation of the stress system. In addition to depression, hypercortisolism is associated with other mood and affective disorders including anorexia nervosa, chronic anxiety, obsessive-compulsive disorder, chronic alcoholism, and other situations such as childhood sexual abuse (1). Hyperactivity of the locus coerulus and other central noradrenergic centres have been shown to influence anxiety and behavioural arousal, with dysregulation of this system postulated as contributing to the pathogenesis of mood disorders particularly depression and with noradrenaline levels being an important predictor of outcome in major depression (1).

Animal experiments of chronic stress provided evidence that glucocorticoid overexposure affects the hippocampus with respect to neuronal viability and function—decreased neurogenesis, degenerative loss in pyramidal neurons, reduced dendritic branching, and atrophy (27, 35). This led to the so-called 'glucocorticoid cascade hypothesis' (35) where stress-induced HPA activation and elevated glucocorticoid levels were purported to act in a feedforward manner causing hippocampal damage, resulting in disinhibition of glucocorticoid negative feedback, further rise in glucocorticoid levels and accumulating damage to the hippocampus. This was supported in principle by the fact that patients with Cushing's disease (resulting in excess adrenal glucocorticoid production) exhibit both hippocampal atrophy and depression, both of which are reversed with treatment. In addition, depressed patients experience cognitive dysfunction consistent with hippocampal damage and most antidepressant treatments enhance neurogenesis (37). However, although reduced hippocampal volumes have been seen on MRI scans of depressed patients, significant histological damage has not been found on postmortem studies (35). Thus, despite compelling animal data linking stress induced hypercortisolism with modulation of neurogenesis in the pathogenesis of depression, evidence for translation to human depression is inconclusive, but is currently an active area of ongoing research. It is also increasingly apparent that HPA dysregulation appears well before clinical symptomatology and is a predictor of treatment resistance in depression. Similarly, failure to normalize HPA axis responses with treatment is a strong predictor of relapse (38).

Obesity and the metabolic syndrome

Chronic stress has been linked to obesity and the metabolic syndrome which is characterized by the combination of central obesity, insulin resistance, dyslipidaemia, and hypertension (39). Glucocorticoids regulate adipocyte differentiation and stress-induced excess cortisol is associated with increased abdominal fat accumulation (39). In humans, chronic stress-induced increases in cortisol, catecholamines, and interleukin (IL)-6 in combination with associated suppression of the growth hormone-, gonadal- and thyroid-axes produces a hormonal milieu conducive to the development of visceral obesity, hypertension, atherosclerosis, osteoporosis, and immune dysfunction (39). Corticosteroids stimulate behaviours that are mediated by dopaminergic mesolimbic 'reward' pathways and the central stress response network (25). In fact, glucocorticoids stimulate caloric intake and 'comfort foods' may result in a metabolic feedback signal that damp brain stress responses (25). In the current era of chronic social stress and allostatic load, together with the availability of high-calorie palatable foods (acquired with ever-decreasing physical effort), this adaptive mechanism proposed to enable many species to survive may be occurring at a significant (maladaptive) metabolic cost to contemporary humans.

Sleep disorders

According to McEwen (27) the experience of feeling 'stressed out' is associated with elevations in cortisol, sympathetic activity and proinflammatory cytokines that result in an allostatic overload, classically exemplified by sleep deprivation. In animal models with varying degrees of sleep deprivation there has been a consistent pattern of cognitive impairment, namely in learning and retention (40). This has been associated with increased brain levels of proinflammatory cytokines (IL-1β mRNA), and hippocampal oxidative stress and structural changes. Clinical studies have confirmed elevated evening cortisol and day time growth hormone levels with increased sympathetic nervous activity for both total and partial sleep deprivation (41). The resultant increased insulin resistance and reduced glucose tolerance promotes the risk of developing diabetes. This is further compounded by the dysregulation of the neuroendocrine control of appetite promoting obesity.

Evidence is emerging that obstructive sleep apnoea (OSA) represents a chronically stressed state. OSA is characterized by intermittent upper airway obstruction and subsequent hypoxia during sleep. A cyclical sequence of events consisting of upper airway obstruction, progressive hypoxaemia, autonomic, and EEG arousal occurs. This is sufficient to prompt the individual to open and clear the airway to reverse the asphyxia, followed by successive relaxation of the airway and subsequent constriction (42). This results in fragmented sleep which in turn results in daytime sleepiness and fatigue. Other associated symptoms include morning headache, poor concentration, irritability, depression, forgetfulness, overweight, and sexual dysfunction. Morbidity and mortality from OSA is primarily due to cardiovascular disease. It has also been associated with significant metabolic dysfunction including insulin resistance and the metabolic syndrome.

We have found evidence of HPA axis dysfunction in OSA that is altered with continuous positive airways pressure (CPAP) therapy. Obese male subjects with moderately severe or severe OSA had ultradian ACTH and cortisol measured every 10 min over 24 h pre- and 3 months post-CPAP under basal conditions using an automated blood sampling system (17). Hormone secretory characteristics were estimated using multi-parameter deconvolution analysis. There was no change in the number of predicted secretory episodes, secretion pulse height or frequency, however, there was a significant reduction in pulsatile and total ACTH and cortisol production post-CPAP (Henley *et al.*, unpublished data). There was an increased mean pulse mass pre-treatment and this was due to a longer duration of the individual secretory episodes. This is consistent with impaired fast feedback affecting pulse duration (13). This may be due to metabolic/hypoxic insults on the hippocampus, alterations in hippocampal MR expression due to SAM hyperactivity or result from an AVP effect on ACTH pulse duration. Further evidence of HPA axis hyperresponsiveness in untreated OSA is provided by the single breath 35% CO_2 stress test, a validated method for evaluating the stress response in humans (26). There was a markedly exaggerated response to CO_2 pre-CPAP which was reduced to normal levels after treatment (Henley *et al.*, unpublished data) (43). It is therefore likely that the activation of the stress system in OSA contributes to the metabolic complications of this condition.

Other effects

CRH hypersecretion and HPA axis activation has also been shown to influence the activity of other systems and may have a role in producing some of the other clinical manifestations of stress. CRH hyperactivity is associated with gastrointestinal symptoms such as pain, increased gut motility and diarrhoea—typical features of the irritable bowel syndrome that is commonly associated with stress (1). Similarly, glucocorticoids inhibit the growth axis and it has been postulated that the severe growth retardation associated with psychosocial abuse or deprivation during childhood is, in part, related to chronic HPA axis activation (1).

Chronic hypoactivation of the HPA axis in contrast is also associated with specific disease states. Post-traumatic stress disorder, chronic fatigue syndrome and atypical depression (1, 36) are associated with CRH hypoactivity and reduced cortisol production. Similarly, immune dysregulation is an important consequence of altered HPA axis activity. Differential levels of hypothalamic CRH in the high CRH Fischer and lower CRH Lewis rats are associated with enhanced immune response and resistance to infections and tumours in the Lewis rats, but also an increased susceptibility to some autoimmune conditions (6). In human studies, rheumatoid arthritis appears to be associated with HPA axis hypoactivation (44) with blunted cortisol diurnal rhythms and reduced ACTH and cortisol levels.

Summary

Stress may be considered as a real or perceived threat to homoeostasis. The two primary arms of the stress response are the HPA axis and the SAM systems. These two systems are interlinked and regulated by complex feedback and feedforward processes. The acute stress response is protective and promotes survival in the short term. However, prolonged activation of the stress response is implicated in the pathogenesis of illness, in particular mood and affective disorders, and also obesity, the metabolic syndrome, and more recently obstructive sleep apnoea.

References

1. Chrousos GP. Stressors, stress, and neuroendocrine integration of the adaptive response. The 1997 Hans Selye Memorial Lecture. *Ann N Y Acad Sci*, 1998; **851**: 311–35.
2. McEwen BS. Protective and damaging effects of stress mediators. *N Engl J Med*, 1998; **338**: 171–9.
3. Habib KE, Weld KP, Rice KC, Pushkas J, Champoux M, Listwak S, *et al.* Oral administration of a corticotropin-releasing hormone receptor antagonist significantly attenuates behavioral, neuroendocrine, and autonomic responses to stress in primates. *Proc Natl Acad Sci U S A*, 2000; **9711**: 6079–84.
4. Chrousos GP, Gold PW. The concepts of stress and stress system disorders. Overview of physical and behavioral homeostasis. *JAMA*, 1992; **267**: 1244–52.
5. Vanitallie TB. Stress: a risk factor for serious illness. *Metabolism*, 2002; **51**(6 Suppl 1): 40–5.
6. Sternberg EM. Emotions and disease: from balance of humors to balance of molecules. *Nat Med*, 1997; **3**: 264–7.
7. Levine S. Influence of psychological variables on the activity of the hypothalamic-pituitary-adrenal axis. *Eur J Pharmacol*, 2000; **405**: 149–60.
8. Vale W, Spiess J, Rivier C, Rivier J. Characterization of a 41-residue ovine hypothalamic peptide that stimulates secretion of corticotropin and beta-endorphin. *Science*, 1981; **213**: 1394–7.
9. Harbuz MS, Lightman SL. Stress and the hypothalamo-pituitary-adrenal axis: acute, chronic and immunological activation. *J Endocrinol*, 1992; **134**: 327–39.
10. Sapolsky RM, Romero LM, Munck AU. How do glucocorticoids influence stress responses? Integrating permissive, suppressive, stimulatory, and preparative actions. *Endocr Rev*, 2000; **21**: 55–89.
11. Reul JM, de Kloet ER. Two receptor systems for corticosterone in rat brain: microdistribution and differential occupation. *Endocrinology*, 1985; **117**: 2505–11.
12. Keller-Wood ME, Dallman MF. Corticosteroid inhibition of ACTH secretion. *Endocr Rev*, 1984; **5**: 1–24.
13. Atkinson HC, Wood SA, Castrique ES, Kershaw YM, Wiles CC, Lightman S. Corticosteroids mediate fast feedback of the rat hypothalamic-pituitary-adrenal axis via the mineralocorticoid receptor. *Am J Physiol Endocrinol Metab*, 2008; **294**: E1011–E22.
14. Gallagher TF, Yoshida K, Roffwarg HD, Fukushima DK, Weitzman ED, Hellman L. ACTH and cortisol secretory patterns in man. *J Clin Endocrinol Metab*, 1973; **36**: 1058–68.
15. Johnson ML, Virostko A, Veldhuis JD, Evans WS. Deconvolution analysis as a hormone pulse-detection algorithm. *Methods Enzymol*, 2004; **384**: 40–54.
16. Veldhuis JD, Iranmanesh A, Johnson ML, Lizarralde G. Amplitude, but not frequency, modulation of adrenocorticotropin secretory bursts gives rise to the nyctohemeral rhythm of the corticotropic axis in man. *J Clin Endocrinol Metab*, 1990; **71**: 452–63.
17. Henley DE, Leendertz JA, Russell GM, Wood SA, Taheri S, Woltersdorf WW, *et al.* Development of an automated blood sampling system for use in humans. *J Med Eng Technol*, 2009; **33**: 199–208.
18. Veldhuis JD, Iranmanesh A, Lizarralde G, Johnson ML. Amplitude modulation of a burstlike mode of cortisol secretion subserves the circadian glucocorticoid rhythm. *Am J Physiol*, 1989; **257**: E6–14.
19. Horrocks PM, Jones AF, Ratcliffe WA, Holder G, White A, Holder R, *et al.* Patterns of ACTH and cortisol pulsatility over twenty-four hours in normal males and females. *Clin Endocrinol (Oxf)*, 1990; **32**: 127–34.
20. Veldhuis JD. The neuroendocrine control of ultradian rhythms. In: Conn PM, Freeman ME, eds. *Neuroendocrinology in Physiology and Medicine*. 1st ed. Totowa: Humana Press, 2000: 453–72.
21. Lightman SL, Wiles CC, Atkinson HC, Henley DE, Russell GM, Leendertz JA, *et al.* The significance of glucocorticoid pulsatility. *Eur J Pharmacol*, 2008; **583**: 255–62.
22. Conway-Campbell BL, McKenna MA, Wiles CC, Atkinson HC, de Kloet ER, Lightman SL. Proteasome-dependent down-regulation of activated nuclear hippocampal glucocorticoid receptors determines dynamic responses to corticosterone. *Endocrinology*, 2007; **148**: 5470–7.
23. Lightman SL. The neuroendocrinology of stress: a never ending story. J Neuroendocrinol, 2008; **20**: 880–4.
24. Eriksen HR, Olff M, Murison R, Ursin H. The time dimension in stress responses: relevance for survival and health. *Psychiatry Res*, 1999; **85**: 39–50.
25. Dallman MF, Pecoraro NC, la Fleur SE, Warne JP, Ginsberg AB, Akana SF, *et al.* Glucocorticoids, chronic stress, and obesity. *Prog Brain Res*, 2006; **153**: 75–105.
26. Kaye J, Buchanan F, Kendrick A, Johnson P, Lowry C, Bailey J, *et al.* Acute carbon dioxide exposure in healthy adults: evaluation of a novel means of investigating the stress response. *J Neuroendocrinol*, 2004; **16**: 256–64.
27. McEwen BS. Central effects of stress hormones in health and disease: Understanding the protective and damaging effects of stress and stress mediators. *Eur J Pharmacol*, 2008; **583**: 174–85.
28. McEwen BS. Protection and damage from acute and chronic stress: allostasis and allostatic overload and relevance to the pathophysiology of psychiatric disorders. *Ann N Y Acad Sci*, 2004; **1032**: 1–7.
29. Scott LV, Dinan TG. Vasopressin and the regulation of hypothalamic-pituitary-adrenal axis function: implications for the pathophysiology of depression. *Life Sci*, 1998; **62**: 1985–98.
30. Dallman MF. Adaptation of the hypothalamic-pituitary-adrenal axis to chronic stress. *Trends Endocrinol Metab*, 1993; **4**: 62–9.
31. Aguilera G. Regulation of pituitary ACTH secretion during chronic stress. *Front Neuroendocrinol*, 1994; **15**: 321–50.
32. Herman JP, Ostrander MM, Mueller NK, Figueiredo H. Limbic system mechanisms of stress regulation: hypothalamo-pituitary-adrenocortical axis. *Prog Neuropsychopharmacol Biol Psychiatry*, 2005; **29**: 1201–13.

33. Adler NE, Boyce T, Chesney MA, Cohen S, Folkman S, Kahn RL, *et al.* Socioeconomic status and health. The challenge of the gradient. *Am Psychol*, 1994; **49**: 15–24.
34. Marmot MG, Rose G, Shipley M, Hamilton PJ. Employment grade and coronary heart disease in British civil servants. *J Epidemiol Community Health*, 1978; **32**: 244–9.
35. Swaab DF, Bao AM, Lucassen PJ. The stress system in the human brain in depression and neurodegeneration. *Ageing Res Rev*, 2005; **4**: 141–94.
36. Miller DB, O'Callaghan JP. Neuroendocrine aspects of the response to stress. *Metabolism*, 2002; **51**(6 Suppl 1): 5–10.
37. Thomas RM, Peterson DA. Even neural stem cells get the blues: evidence for a molecular link between modulation of adult neurogenesis and depression. *Gene Expr*, 2008; **14**: 183–93.
38. Holsboer F. The corticosteroid receptor hypothesis of depression. *Neuropsychopharmacology*, 2000; **23**: 477–501.
39. Kyrou I, Chrousos GP, Tsigos C. Stress, visceral obesity, and metabolic complications. *Ann N Y Acad Sci*, 2006; **1083**: 77–110.
40. McEwen BS. Sleep deprivation as a neurobiologic and physiologic stressor: Allostasis and allostatic load. *Metabolism*, 2006; **55**(10 Suppl 2): S20–23.
41. Knutson KL, Van CE. Associations between sleep loss and increased risk of obesity and diabetes. *Ann N Y Acad Sci*, 2008; **1129**: 287–304.
42. Buckley TM, Schatzberg AF. On the interactions of the hypothalamic-pituitary-adrenal (HPA) axis and sleep: normal HPA axis activity and circadian rhythm, exemplary sleep disorders. *J Clin Endocrinol Metab*, 2005; **90**: 3106–14.
43. Henley DE, Russell GM, Douthwaite JA, Wood SA, Buchanan F, Gibson R, *et al.* Hypothalamic-pituitary-adrenal axis activation in obstructive sleep apnea: The effect of continuous positive airway pressure therapy. *J Clin Endocrinol Metab*, 2009; **94**: 4234–42.
44. Eijsbouts AM, van den Hoogen FH, Laan RF, Hermus AR, Sweep CG, van de Putte LB. Hypothalamic-pituitary-adrenal axis activity in patients with rheumatoid arthritis. *Clin Exp Rheumatol*, 2005; **23**: 658–64.

2.6.4 Endocrinology and alcohol

Margit G. Proescholdt, Marc Walter

Introduction

Alcohol has widespread effects on multiple organs, including the endocrine organs, potentially impairing endocrine function and affecting the entire endocrine milieu. Endocrine impairment may be observed with acute alcohol ingestion, excessive chronic alcohol consumption, and during alcohol withdrawal. Whereas many effects of alcohol on the endocrine organs are reversible following cessation of alcohol consumption, some changes may extend into abstinence. Importantly, endocrine dysfunction observed in alcoholism, is no longer considered to simply result from hepatic failure or chronic malnutrition, but, at least partially, from direct, toxic actions of alcohol on the endocrine organs themselves. In addition, there is increasing evidence that the endocrine system itself may play a crucial role in the pathogenesis of addictive behaviour.

Ethanol and its metabolite acetaldehyde directly affect cell membranes and influences intracellular metabolism. Indirect effects include stress, nausea, and vomiting during acute intoxication and withdrawal. Whereas the list of alcohol-induced endocrine dysfunction is long, scientific and epidemiological evidence is frequently controversial. Controversies may result from the highly heterogenic group of alcohol-dependent individuals regarding dose and duration of alcohol consumption, periods of abstinence, age, gender, nutritional status, cigarette smoking, use of other drugs, presence of other diseases, particularly liver disease, and the complexity of endocrine regulation in general.

Hypothalamic–pituitary–adrenal (HPA) axis and alcohol

Alterations in the hypothalamic-pituitary-adrenal (HPA) axis have long been reported in alcohol-dependent patients. In healthy volunteers alcohol effects on the HPA axis are dose-dependent. Alcohol amounts corresponding to social drinking attenuate HPA axis activity, whereas alcohol-induced HPA stimulation can only be seen if nausea occurs which markedly triggers vasopressin (AVP) secretion, thereby stimulating adrenocorticotropic hormone (ACTH). By contrast, chronic alcohol consumption may result in increased serum cortisol levels (Table 2.6.4.1). Plasma concentrations of ACTH may be normal or increased, and urinary excretion of free cortisol is frequently increased. Furthermore, alcohol-dependent patients show a persisting cortisol hyporeactivity to a wide range of stressors (1).

Rarely, alcohol-dependent patients develop pseudo-Cushing's syndrome, which is indistinguishable from true Cushing's syndrome, but may present with fewer biochemical alterations and fewer clinical symptoms. Hormonal testing shows an increased secretion of cortisol which is not suppressed by the overnight dexamethasone test. Importantly, both the physical and the hormonal abnormalities improve after discontinuation of alcohol use, which is why abstention from alcohol not only is curative but also an important diagnostic tool.

Acute alcohol withdrawal results in immediate increases of circulating plasma levels of cortisol and ACTH, disruption of the normal diurnal cortisol secretion pattern, and a blunted response of ACTH to various stressors including intravenous (i.v.) corticotropin-releasing factor (CRF). Accordingly, it has been suggested that enhanced ACTH and cortisol, as well as extrahypothalamic CRF levels (animal studies), contribute to the stressful and anxiogenic state observed during alcohol withdrawal (2). As the withdrawal syndrome wanes, cortisol and ACTH levels, as well as the diurnal secretion pattern normalize. However, HPA regulation may not be completely normal even after the diurnal pattern has recovered, as shown by deficient cortisol responses to HPA stimulation by CRF

Table 2.6.4.1 Hypothalamic–pituitary–adrenal axis and alcoholism

Clinical findings	Pseudo-Cushing syndrome: *rare*
Laboratory findings	Serum cortisol: normal or increased
	Adrenocorticotropic hormone: normal or increased
	Urinary free cortisol: increased
	Cortisol hyporeactivity to various stressors
CRF system	Suggested key role in facilitating and maintaining substance use disorders

in abstinent alcohol-dependent patients. Furthermore, low baseline serum cortisol levels, and a blunted cortisol stress response were shown to correlate with increased craving for alcohol, and an increased risk for relapse, respectively (2). In abstinent alcohol-dependent patients (day 40), cortisol levels in the cerebrospinal fluid were shown to decrease compared with normal controls, and relapsers showed higher levels than abstainers (3).

In addition, there is increasing evidence that the HPA axis—with particular emphasis on the CRF system—plays a key role in facilitating and maintaining substance use disorders, and may therefore qualify as a major target for its treatment. To date the mechanisms by which alcohol interferes with the HPA axis are not fully understood, and include direct effects of alcohol on all levels of the HPA axis, as well as genetic, and environmental factors (2, 4).

Male gonadal function and alcohol

It is well known that chronic and excessive alcohol consumption eventually results in gonadal failure (hypogonadism). Although overt alcohol-induced hypogonadism is more frequent in alcohol-dependent men with advanced liver disease, gonadal dysfunction is also observed in the absence of liver cirrhosis. Hypogonadism is manifested by testicular atrophy, infertility, loss of libido, and impotence. In particular, seminiferous tubular atrophy, and marked abnormal seminal determinations are frequent findings in alcohol-dependent men independent of liver disease (5). Likewise, sexual disorders are frequently reported, with prevalence estimates ranging from 8% to 58%. In the absence of significant hepatic or gonadal failure, abstention may result in the recovery of normal sexual function even after a history of prolonged and severe alcohol abuse (6), although persistent sexual dysfunction has been reported as well.

Feminization, by contrast, is distinct from hypogonadism, and is manifested by gynaecomastia, female body habitus changes, spider angiomata, palmar erythema, and changes in body hair patterns. Feminization occurs later in the course of chronic alcohol disease, and is seen only occasionally in the absence of liver disease. Clinical reports on sex hormone profiles are somewhat inconclusive. The most common findings are shown in Table 2.6.4.2 (7, 8).

In general, acute administration of alcohol to healthy male volunteers results in decreased testosterone levels. Decreased testosterone levels are also common in alcoholic liver disease. By contrast, in the absence of liver impairment, total testosterone levels are mostly within the normal range. Yet, concentrations of the sex hormone-binding globulin (SHBG) are usually increased in actively drinking men. Accordingly, some studies report a reduced free androgen index (FAI: total testosterone/SHBG), indicating a reduced free-to-total plasma testosterone ratio, and thus a condition of relative hypoandrogenism. Concentrations of the gonadotropins (luteinizing hormone and follicle-stimulating hormone (FSH)) are reported normal or increased when compared to healthy individuals. In addition, studies have found inadequately normal or raised luteinizing hormone concentrations in the presence of reduced or increased testosterone levels, respectively, indicating a disturbance of the testosterone-mediated adenohypophyseal feedback mechanism (9). During withdrawal, testosterone levels were shown to increase (8, 10) while concentrations of SHBG and oestradiol decrease. However, sustained increases in serum testosterone in the presence of inadequately raised luteinizing hormone concentrations were still observed up to 4 months after cessation of drinking (10).

Table 2.6.4.2 Hypothalamic–pituitary–gonadotropic axis in men and alcoholism

Clinical findings	Hypogonadism
	Feminization[a]
Laboratory findings	Testosterone: normal, decreased[a]
	Free testosterone: normal, decreased
	SHBG: increased
	FAI: normal, decreased
	FSH: normal, increased
	LH: normal, increased
	Androstendione: normal, increased
	Oestradiol: normal, increased

[a] Particularly in patients with advanced liver disease. FAI, free androgen index; FSH, follicle-stimulating hormone; LH, luteinizing hormone; SHBG, sex hormone-binding globulin.

Although the underlying mechanisms have not been completely identified, alcohol-induced hypogonadism is attributed to a direct (toxic) alcohol-induced primary gonadal injury and to an alcohol-associated hypothalamic pituitary dysfunction. Feminization, by contrast, may result from the combined effects of altered enterohepatic circulation of biliary excreted steroids as a result of portal hypertension and liver disease, and conversion of weak adrenal androgens to oestrogens.

Female gonadal function and alcohol

Premenopausal women

Chronic heavy consumption of alcohol can contribute to a multitude of reproductive disorders. These include amenorrhoea, anovulation, menstrual cycle irregularities, loss of libido, early menopause, and increased risk of spontaneous abortions. These dysfunctions can be caused by alcohol's interfering directly with the hormonal regulation of the reproductive system or indirectly through other disorders associated with alcohol consumption, such as liver disease, pancreatic disease, malnutrition, or fetal abnormalities. Prospective and well-designed studies on the effects of alcohol on female hormone levels in premenopausal alcohol-dependent women are sparse, and data available so far are still inconclusive. In detail, oestradiol levels are reported increased, normal, or reduced. Progesterone levels are more consistently reported reduced, especially during the luteal phase. Testosterone levels are reported increased or decreased. Gonadotropins (luteinizing hormone and FSH) are reported unchanged or decreased (11).

Acute alcohol ingestion is shown to substantially increase plasma testosterone levels, whereas reports on oestradiol (increased or normal) and progesterone (decreased or normal) levels are less conclusive (12, 13).

In 'modest' alcohol consumption, studies indicate an alcohol-induced rise in oestrogen levels, however, the positive (for example, protection against osteoporosis and cardiovascular disease) and/or negative (for example, breast cancer) implications of these findings on female health need further evaluation. Further studies are also needed to clarify the effects of modest alcohol consumption on the onset of menopause (suggested to be delayed) and fecundity (suggested to be unaltered or reduced). In the specific case of reproductive health, binge drinking may be most detrimental at certain times, namely puberty, the cyclical selection of follicles for maturation, ovulation, and the implantation and subsequent survival of the blastocyst (12). Furthermore, studies indicate that alcohol consumption during early adolescence may delay puberty and adversely affect the maturation of the female reproductive system. The latter findings clearly emphasize the risks of underage drinking and the importance of its prevention.

Postmenopausal women

In postmenopausal women with alcohol-induced cirrhosis, oestradiol and prolactin levels are significantly increased, and levels of testosterone, luteinizing hormone, and FSH are decreased compared to abstaining postmenopausal women or postmenopausal women with moderate alcohol consumption. Whereas the decreased levels of luteinizing hormone and FSH may result from the increased oestradiol levels, the decreases in luteinizing hormone and FSH may also reflect a more subtle alcohol-induced central defect at the level of the hypothalamus and pituitary (14). In postmenopausal women with 'moderate' alcohol consumption (0.1 to 28 drinks/week), oestradiol levels are increased, and testosterone levels are decreased, compared to abstaining postmenopausal women. Luteinizing hormone, FSH, and prolactin levels do not differ between these two groups. Furthermore, moderate alcohol consumption (no more than one drink per day) is being suggested to increase oestradiol levels in postmenopausal women with respective positive (for example, protection from osteoporosis and cardiovascular disease) and negative (increased risk for breast cancer) implications. However, so far, a firm relationship between moderate alcohol consumption and oestrogen levels in postmenopausal women has not been established (15). By contrast, effects of alcohol on oestrogen levels in postmenopausal women exposed to oestrogen replacement therapy (ERT) are more consistent, but variable. In oral ERT, alcohol administration was shown to result in robust increases in blood oestradiol levels. Increased circulating oestradiol levels, however, may increase the risk of breast cancer in postmenopausal women (15).

Alcohol and breast cancer

Several studies have noted an association between alcohol and breast cancer, and risk estimates are shown in Table 2.6.4.3. Despite the well-established fact that breast cancer is multifactorial in nature, and despite a relatively moderate excess risk, the high incidence of breast cancer results in more women with breast cancer attributable to alcohol than for any other type of cancer (16).

The exact mechanisms by which alcohol causes breast cancer are still unknown. Several hypotheses exist, and include perturbation of oestrogen metabolism and response, induction of mutagenesis by acetaldehyde derived from oxidation of ethanol by alcohol dehydrogenase, stimulation of oxidative damage through ethanol metabolism, and/or affection of folate and one-carbon metabolism pathways. By contrast, alcohol does not seem to increase the risk of endometrial cancer. A possible protective effect of alcohol on the risk of ovarian cancer needs further investigation (16).

Table 2.6.4.3 Relative risk for major chronic disease categories, by gender and average drinking category

	Drinking category[a]		
Disease	**I**	**II**	**III**
Hypertensive disease			
Females	1.40	2.0	2.0
Males	1.40	2.0	4.10
Breast cancer	1.14	1.41	1.59
Under 45 years of age	1.15	1.41	1.46
45 years and over	1.14	1.38	1.62
Diabetes mellitus			
Females	0.92	0.87	1.13
Males	1.0	0.57	0.73

[a] Drinking category: females: I, 0–19,99; II, 20–39.99; III, 40 or more g pure alcohol per day; males: I, 0–39.99; II, 40–59.99; III, 60 or more g pure alcohol per day.

Modified from Rehm J, Gmel G, Sempos CT, Trevisan M. Alcohol-related morbidity and mortality. *Alcohol Res Health*, 2003; **27**: 39–51 (17).

Hypothalamic–pituitary–thyroid (HPT) axis and alcohol

In alcohol-dependent patients, thyroid dysfunction is a frequent finding. However, consensus on clinical relevance and mechanisms has not been achieved. Thyroid dysfunction is particularly evident during chronic alcohol consumption and early abstinence (less than 3 weeks), and usually normalizes during abstinence. In individuals, where thyroid dysfunction persists into abstinence, other nonalcohol-related thyroid diseases should be excluded (e.g. autoimmune thyroid disease). In patients with pre-existing hyperthyroidism, acute alcohol intoxication may promote the manifestation of a thyrotoxic crisis, warranting immediate analysis of thyroid hormones and adequate medical treatment. Furthermore, alcohol-associated HPT axis dysfunction has been associated with relapse prediction, the severity of withdrawal symptoms, and considered a trait marker for the risk to develop alcohol dependence, the latter being controversial.

Regarding thyroid hormones (Table 2.6.4.4), the most consistent findings include a reduction in total thyroxin (T_4), total (T_3) and free triiodothyronine (fT_3) concentrations during early abstinence, normal thyroid-stimulating hormone (TSH) levels, and a blunted TSH response following administration of

Table 2.6.4.4 Thyroid gland and alcoholism

Clinical findings	**Usually absence of overt clinical signs of hypothyroidism**
	Thyroid volume reduced
Laboratory findings	Basal thyroid-stimulating hormone: usually normal
	Free or total T_3: may be reduced
	Free or total T_4: usually normal
	Thyrotropin-releasing hormone test: frequently blunted

thyrotropin-releasing hormone (TRH, TRH test). Reductions in peripheral thyroid hormones and TRH blunting are particularly evident during withdrawal. During abstinence, peripheral hormones usually normalize, whereas TRH blunting may still be observed after several weeks thereafter (18). Independent of liver disease, thyroid volumes are significantly decreased in alcohol-dependent patients, indicating a direct toxic and dose-dependent effect of alcohol on the thyroid gland (19).

The exact mechanisms by which alcohol causes dysfunction of the HPT axis are still unknown. However, evidence suggests direct toxic effects of alcohol on the thyroid gland and its metabolism, as well as central effects at the level of the hypothalamus and/or pituitary (18).

Water and electrolyte balance and alcohol

The main regulator of blood and urine osmolality, the antidiuretic hormone arginine vasopressin (AVP), is profoundly altered by alcohol. In alcohol-naïve individuals, mild to moderate alcohol ingestion leads to a dose-dependent suppression of AVP resulting in water diuresis. After cessation of alcohol intake, AVP suppression and diuresis resolve resulting in a normalization of water balance and plasma osmolality (Table 2.6.4.5). By contrast, single large doses of alcohol increase plasma AVP levels. When alcohol concentrations are kept steady in normal volunteers, additional doses of alcohol produce progressively smaller and eventually negligible diuretic responses.

Chronic alcohol ingestion does no longer suppress baseline AVP levels, but rather results in the development of tolerance to the effects of alcohol. Clinical studies measuring AVP levels in alcohol-dependent patients, however, show conflicting results with elevated, normal, and decreased AVP levels. Furthermore, chronic alcohol consumption may be associated with isosmotic overhydration although dehydration has been suggested as well (21).

Table 2.6.4.5 Effects of alcohol on water and sodium homoeostasis

Ascending plasma alcohol concentrations	**Plasma AVP: decrease**
	Water diuresis: increase
	Plasma osmolality: increase
Descending plasma alcohol concentrations	AVP: increase
	Voluntary fluid intake: increase
	Water diuresis: decrease
	Plasma osmolality: normalization
Chronic alcohol intake	Possible overhydration
Acute alcohol withdrawal	Plasma AVP: increase
	Possible overhydration
After alcohol withdrawal	Plasma AVP: decrease
	Water, sodium, chloride excretion: increase
	Body volumes: normalization

AVP, argenine vasopressin.

Modified from Vamvakas S, Teschner M, Bahner U, Heidland A. Alcohol abuse: potential role in electrolyte disturbances and kidney diseases. *Clin Nephrol*, 1998; **49**: 205–13 (20).

In particular, persons who consume large quantities of beer with low total solute intake (sodium content of beer: less than 2 mmol/l) are at risk to develop life-threatening water intoxication with serum sodium levels as low as 100 mmol/l.

During withdrawal, AVP levels increase to high levels within a few hours, reaching highest levels in delirium tremens, and return to normal levels within 4–10 days. The high AVP levels are not associated with appreciable changes in plasma osmolality (22), and elevated plasma AVP levels during withdrawal were associated with overhydration. Therefore, administration of parenteral fluid to withdrawing patients should be undertaken with caution. In addition, because alcohol withdrawal may cause substantial disturbances in electrolyte homoeostasis, blood electrolytes should be monitored closely. After alcohol withdrawal, AVP levels decrease, and excretion of water, sodium and chloride increase resulting in normalization of the expanded extracellular fluid volume within several days.

Remarkably, AVP levels are persistently decreased in long-term abstinent alcoholics, and it has been suggested that the suppressed AVP levels may reflect a dysregulation in the brain that influences the function of the HPA axis, mood, memory, addiction behaviour, and craving during alcohol abstinence (23).

The mechanisms by which alcohol interferes with AVP secretion are not entirely understood. Possible mechanisms include genetically determined or alcohol-induced reduced AVP expression in hypothalamic neurons, insufficient secretion of AVP by the posterior pituitary, alcohol-induced resetting of osmoreceptors, and renal hypersensitivity to AVP. In addition, regulation of fluid balance and electrolyte homeostasis is highly complex and particularly in chronic alcoholism influenced by many factors. Additional factors include atrial natriuretic peptide, possible chronic hypervolaemia, alterations in the renin–angiotensin–aldosterone system, increased plasma cortisol levels, liver and/or renal failure, cardiomyopathy, malnutrition, vomiting, diarrhoea, and others.

Hypertension and alcohol

The recent literature has consistently shown a firm association between hypertensive disease and chronic alcohol consumption. The relative risk estimates for alcohol-induced hypertension in females and males are shown in Table 2.6.4.3 (17). Whereas acute alcohol intake causes peripheral vasodilatation with a consequent fall of blood pressure, chronic alcohol consumption increases the blood pressure in a dose-dependent manner. Several studies have established chronic consumption of three standard drinks (8–10 g of alcohol per drink) as the threshold for raising blood pressure. Below this threshold, results have been less consistent. Alcohol increases systolic and—to a somewhat smaller degree—diastolic blood pressure. Most studies show a linear relationship between blood pressure and alcohol intake, although J- and U-shaped curves have also been reported.

The exact mechanisms by which alcohol raises blood pressure are not entirely understood, and it is likely that different mechanisms are effective in different people. Possible mechanisms of alcohol-induced hypertension include impairment of baroreceptor control, increase of sympathetic activity, activation of the renin–angiotensin–aldosterone system, increase in cortisol levels, increased shift of calcium to the intracellular space, increased release of endothelin (potent vasoconstrictors, from endothelium), inhibition of endothelium-dependent nitric oxide production (vasodilator), and chronic subclinical withdrawal (20).

Reduction in alcohol intake is effective in lowering blood pressure in both hypertensives and normotensives and may help to prevent the development of hypertension. Therefore, cessation or at least marked reduction of alcohol consumption is the first step in the treatment of alcohol-induced hypertension. Pharmacological treatment should be considered if blood pressure continues to be elevated 2–4 weeks after cessation of alcohol intake. By contrast, hypotension may develop in alcoholics with alcohol-induced autonomic neuropathy and/or late-stage cardiomyopathy.

Growth hormone and alcohol

Alcohol clearly impairs the spontaneous secretion of growth hormone, although the underlying aetiology remains unresolved. Ethanol administration to healthy human volunteers results in a significant and dose-dependent decrease of the nocturnal growth hormone surge. Studies in alcohol-dependent patients have shown a significantly blunted growth hormone response to challenge (e.g. apomorphine). The blunted growth hormone response appears related to alcohol dependence rather than the severity of alcohol withdrawal symptoms, and is associated with early relapse. The association between early relapse and a lower growth hormone response to challenge was suggested to reflect an altered balance of somatostatin to somatotropin releasing hormone (GHRH) that also affects slow wave sleep (SWS) in alcohol-dependent patients. During SWS δ wave activity, the hypothalamus releases GHRH, which causes the pituitary to release growth hormone. Alcohol-dependent patients have lower levels of SWS power and growth hormone release than normal patients (24).

Insulin-like growth factor 1 (IGF-1) is an important anabolic agent, and an essential component of the endocrine system responsible for maintaining lean body mass. Physiological and pathophysiological fluctuations in IGF-1 can markedly influence whole body and muscle protein balance. In addition, IGF-1 is now recognized as an important immunomodulator. The synthesis and secretion of IGF-1 by the liver can be stimulated by elevations in growth hormone or decreased by an elevation in glucocorticoids. Studies in humans with alcoholic hepatitis and alcoholic cirrhosis have shown marked reductions in IGF-1 concentrations. While nutritional status and liver dysfunction are important contributors to this decrease, a reduction in IGF-1 has also been demonstrated in long-term alcohol users without evidence of significant liver disease or malnutrition (25). Disruption of IGF-1 signalling is implicated in the aetiology of alcoholic myopathy. However, further research is needed to establish the role of the IGF system in human alcohol disease.

Parathyroid hormone and alcohol

Reports on parathyroid hormone show inconsistent results in chronic alcoholism. Transient hypothyroidism has been observed with acute alcohol intoxication, followed by a rebound hyperparathyroidism. Disturbances in electrolyte homoeostasis (calcium, magnesium, phosphorus, and potassium) are frequent findings in alcoholism, and mainly due to poor intake, vomiting, diarrhoea, and increased urinary loss. Severe magnesium depletion can result in reduced secretion of parathyroid hormone and end-organ (in bone and kidney) resistance to parathyroid hormone, and thus cause hypocalcaemia. In this case, magnesium administration alone leads to clinical improvement and normalization of calcium abnormalities (26). Calcium and vitamin D supplementation are not appropriate for the treatment of hypocalcaemia secondary to magnesium deficiency. Furthermore, as magnesium is a predominantly intracellular cation, serum magnesium does not always correlate with total body depletion. Therefore, intraerythrocytic magnesium determination is sometimes needed (26).

Bone disease and alcohol

Chronic and heavy alcohol consumption eventually results in an osteopenic skeleton, and increased risk for osteoporosis. Frequent findings include a low bone mass (osteopenia), decreased bone formation, increased frequency of fractures from falls, and delayed and/or complicated fracture healing. The onset of bone loss precedes the increased risk of fractures by one or two decades, and is asymptomatic during this interval. However, when it is exacerbated by various factors, especially liver disease, symptoms of osteoporosis and osteomalacia often manifest. Additional confounding factors include malnutrition, malabsorption, liver disease, hypogonadism, cigarette smoking, age, gender, and others, although their contributory role is still controversial (27). Rare manifestations of skeletal pathology in alcoholism include aseptic necrosis of the femur head, and bone disease resulting from hypercortisolism in pseudo-Cushing's syndrome, or secondary hyperparathyroidism in alcohol-induced renal failure.

Alcohol-induced osteopenia is distinct from disuse osteoporosis and postmenopausal osteoporosis, where the rate of bone remodelling is increased. Plasma osteocalcin, a marker of bone formation, is reduced and restored during abstinence, whereas calcium-regulating hormones (parathyroid hormone, calcitonin, and vitamin D metabolites) show inconsistent results (27). By contrast, moderate alcohol consumption may result in increased bone mass, particularly in postmenopausal women. In addition, persons who consume 0.5–1.0 drink per day have a lower risk of hip fracture compared with abstainers and heavier drinkers. However, the available literature is insufficient to determine the precise range of alcohol consumption that would maximize bone density and minimize hip fracture (28).

The mechanisms by which alcohol induces bone disease are not fully understood. Clinical and experimental studies indicate that alcohol directly suppresses osteoblast activity and disturbs cell signalling, thus leading to decreased bone formation, and decreased synthesis of an ossifiable matrix, resulting in deficient healing, while probably only small changes occur in bone resorption. The toxic effects of alcohol on osteoblast activity are dose dependent and some studies show that bone loss is greater with longer duration of alcohol consumption. Despite remaining unsolved issues, therapeutic recommendations clearly must highlight the importance of abstinence from alcohol consumption in affected alcohol-dependent individuals (27).

Diabetes mellitus and alcohol

Intake of light to modest amounts of alcohol (10–30 g/day) is associated with enhanced insulin sensitivity, and may thus contribute to some beneficial effects of alcohol in type 2 diabetes. Therefore, light to modest consumption of alcohol in people with type 1 and type 2 diabetes must not be restricted. Larger doses of alcohol, however, were shown to impair glucose uptake by peripheral tissues (29), but there is little evidence from epidemiological studies (24) that chronic alcohol consumption *per se* increases the risk to develop diabetes mellitus, in general (Table 2.6.4.3). By contrast, diabetes mellitus is frequently found in patients with alcoholic liver cirrhosis. In animals, chronic alcohol administration also increases secretion of glucagon and other hormones that raise blood glucose levels. In addition, alcohol can induce diabetes mellitus through pancreatic destruction (29). Moreover, in a Japanese study alcoholics with diabetes had a significantly lower survival rate than other alcoholics. Treatment of alcohol-associated diabetes mellitus must emphasize abstinence from alcohol, which—in the absence of severe pancreatic or liver disease—may be curative. When pharmacological treatment includes metformin, patients must be instructed to avoid consuming excessive amounts of alcohol because of the increased risk to develop a potentially life-threatening lactic acidosis.

References

1. Lovallo WR. Cortisol secretion patterns in addiction and addiction risk. *Int J Psychophysiol*, 2006; **59**: 195–202.
2. Kiefer F, Wiedemann K. Neuroendocrine pathways of addictive behaviour. *Addict Biol*, 2004; **9**: 205–12.
3. Walter M, Gerhard U, Gerlach M, Weijers HG, Boening J, Wiesbeck GA. Cortisol concentrations, stress-coping styles after withdrawal and long-term abstinence in alcohol dependence. *Addict Biol*, 2006; **11**: 157–62.
4. Heilig M, Koob GF. A key role for corticotropin-releasing factor in alcohol dependence. *Trends Neurosci*, 2007; **30**: 399–406.
5. Villalta J, Ballesca JL, Nicolas JM, Martinez de Osaba MJ, Antunez E, Pimentel C. Testicular function in asymptomatic chronic alcoholics: relation to ethanol intake. *Alcohol Clin Exp Res*, 1997; **21**: 128–33.
6. Schiavi RC, Stimmel BB, Mandeli J, White D. Chronic alcoholism and male sexual function. *Am J Psychiatry*, 1995; **152**: 1045–51.
7. Heinz A, Rommelspacher H, Graf KJ, Kurten I, Otto M, Baumgartner A. Hypothalamic-pituitary-gonadal axis, prolactin, and cortisol in alcoholics during withdrawal and after three weeks of abstinence: comparison with healthy control subjects. *Psychiatry Res*, 1995; **56**: 81–95.
8. Walter M, Gerhard U, Gerlach M, Weijers HG, Boening J, Wiesbeck GA. Controlled study on the combined effect of alcohol and tobacco smoking on testosterone in alcohol-dependent men. *Alcohol Alcohol*, 2007; **42**: 19–23.
9. Bannister P, Handley T, Chapman C, Losowsky MS. Hypogonadism in chronic liver disease: impaired release of luteinising hormone. *Br Med J (Clin Res Ed)*, 1986; **293**: 1191–3.
10. Hasselblatt M, Krieg-Hartig C, Hufner M, Halaris A, Ehrenreich H. Persistent disturbance of the hypothalamic-pituitary-gonadal axis in abstinent alcoholic men. *Alcohol Alcohol*, 2003; **38**: 239–42.
11. Augustynska B, Ziolkowski M, Odrowaz-Sypniewska G, Kielpinski A, Gruszka M, Kosmowski W. Menstrual cycle in women addicted to alcohol during the first week following drinking cessation—changes of sex hormones levels in relation to selected clinical features. *Alcohol Alcohol*, 2007; **42**: 80–3.
12. Gill J. The effects of moderate alcohol consumption on female hormone levels and reproductive function. *Alcohol Alcohol*, 2000; **35**: 417–23.
13. Sarkola T, Makisalo H, Fukunaga T, Eriksson CJ. Acute effect of alcohol on estradiol, estrone, progesterone, prolactin, cortisol, and luteinizing hormone in premenopausal women. *Alcohol Clin Exp Res*, 1999; **23**: 976–82.
14. Gavaler JS, Van Thiel DH. Hormonal status of postmenopausal women with alcohol-induced cirrhosis: further findings and a review of the literature. *Hepatology*, 1992; **16**: 312–19.
15. Purohit V. Moderate alcohol consumption and estrogen levels in postmenopausal women: a review. *Alcohol Clin Exp Res*, 1998; **22**: 994–7.
16. Boffetta P, Hashibe M. Alcohol and cancer. *Lancet Oncol*, 2006; **7**: 149–56.
17. Rehm J, Gmel G, Sempos CT, Trevisan M. Alcohol-related morbidity and mortality. *Alcohol Res Health*, 2003; **27**: 39–51.
18. Hermann D, Heinz A, Mann K. Dysregulation of the hypothalamic-pituitary-thyroid axis in alcoholism. *Addiction*, 2002; **97**: 1369–81.
19. Hegedus L, Rasmussen N, Ravn V, Kastrup J, Krogsgaard K, Aldershvile J. Independent effects of liver disease and chronic alcoholism on thyroid function and size: the possibility of a toxic effect of alcohol on the thyroid gland. *Metabolism*, 1988; **37**: 229–33.
20. Vamvakas S, Teschner M, Bahner U, Heidland A. Alcohol abuse: potential role in electrolyte disturbances and kidney diseases. *Clin Nephrol*, 1998; **49**: 205–13.
21. Ragland G. Electrolyte abnormalities in the alcoholic patient. *Emerg Med Clin North Am*, 1990; **8**: 761–73.
22. Trabert W, Caspari D, Bernhard P, Biro G. Inappropriate vasopressin secretion in severe alcohol withdrawal. *Acta Psychiatr Scand*, 1992; **85**: 376–9.
23. Doring WK, Herzenstiel MN, Krampe H, Jahn H, Pralle L, Sieg S, *et al.* Persistent alterations of vasopressin and N-terminal proatrial natriuretic peptide plasma levels in long-term abstinent alcoholics. *Alcohol Clin Exp Res*, 2003; **27**: 849–61.
24. Lands WE. Alcohol, slow wave sleep, and the somatotropic axis. *Alcohol*, 1999; **18**: 109–22.
25. Lang CH, Fan J, Lipton BP, Potter BJ, McDonough KH. Modulation of the insulin-like growth factor system by chronic alcohol feeding. *Alcohol Clin Exp Res*, 1998; **22**: 823–9.
26. Hermans C, Lefebvre C, Devogelaer JP, Lambert M. Hypocalcaemia and chronic alcohol intoxication: transient hypoparathyroidism secondary to magnesium deficiency. *Clin Rheumatol*, 1996; **15**: 193–6.
27. Chakkalakal DA. Alcohol-induced bone loss and deficient bone repair. *Alcohol Clin Exp Res*, 2005; **29**: 2077–90.
28. Berg KM, Kunins HV, Jackson JL, Nahvi S, Chaudhry A, Harris KA Jr, *et al.* Association between alcohol consumption and both osteoporotic fracture and bone density. *Am J Med*, 2008; **121**: 406–18.
29. Greenhouse L, Lardinois CK. Alcohol-associated diabetes mellitus. A review of the impact of alcohol consumption on carbohydrate metabolism. *Arch Fam Med* 1996; **5**: 229–33.

PART 3

The thyroid

3.1

Evaluation of the thyroid patient

Contents

3.1.1 The history and iconography relating to the thyroid gland

Robert Volpé and Clark Sawin

Introduction

This chapter is a brief summary of the history and art related to the thyroid gland. The reader is referred to other sources for an exhaustive exposition of these matters (1–3).

Early years

Knowledge of goitre (which was not known to be a thyroid enlargement until about the 16th century) goes back into antiquity. In 1600 BC, burnt sponge and seaweed was used for the treatment of goitre in China (2). In the fourth century BC, the Ayur Veda, a Hindu system of medicine in India, contained a discussion of goitre (1,2). In Greece, in the days of Hippocrates, goitre was regarded purely as a deformity, and was attributed to the drinking of snow water (2). In ancient Greece, swellings in the region of the thyroid gland (and presumably swellings elsewhere in the neck) were referred to as 'bronchocoele' or 'struma'. Galen (AD 130–200), considered the greatest medical practitioner in antiquity after Hippocrates, regarded the thyroid as a lubricant for the larynx (2). Later, Julius Caesar (2) noted that Gauls had large necks as one of their characteristics. Celsus (25 BC to AD 50) in Rome defined bronchocele (a tumour in the neck, most likely goitre) and he also described cystic goitre, as well as surgery for these lesions (2). At the same time, in Egypt, Egyptian coins showed the presence of goitres, (4) and an Egyptian relief of Cleopatra likewise depicted her with what appears to be a goitre.

Even in these early years several writers (1,2) referred to epidemics of goitre in the Alps, which was a forerunner to a wide literature from this region regarding goitres and their relationship to Alpine culture. The Chinese also were well aware of goitre in those early years, and recommended seaweed for the treatment of goitre as early as AD 340. Much later, the treatment of goitre with desiccated thyroid was advocated as early as AD 1475 by Wang Hei in China (2).

In Switzerland in the 16th century, Paracelsus (5) (1493–1541) recognized the connection between cretinism, endemic goitre, and congenital idiocy. He attributed goitre to mineral impurities in the drinking water. Later in that century and the next century, also in Switzerland, many writers described cretins in Swiss cantons and related them to the presence of goitre (3). In 1656 (6) at St Thomas's Hospital, London, Thomas Wharton named the lobes of the thyroid, 'glandulae thyroidiaeae' because of their anatomical proximity to the thyroid cartilage, and not because of their shape. He felt that the fact that women generally had larger thyroid glands than men was for the purpose of making their necks 'more even and beautiful'.

During the mid and late medieval period in Europe, goitre and cretinism played a significant part in the social history of middle Europe, particularly in Alpine areas where these conditions were quite prevalent. Indeed, there was a connotation that those people with goitres were somehow inherently evil, and this was reflected in the folk art of the period. Indeed, depictions of goitre and cretinism in art and sculpture at that time were commonplace, and form the subject of an entire volume (3).

The discovery of iodine at the beginning of the 19th century was a landmark event in relation to the thyroid gland. In 1811, Bernard Courtois (1777–1838), a self-taught chemist and dealer in chemicals and manufacturer of saltpetre in Paris, was using vitriol to clean the vats used for making potash from seaweed, when he noted violet fumes. This violet gas condensed into crystals on cooling; he called the crystals substance X. The substance was soon identified as a new halogen element by Sir Humphrey Davy (1778–1829), (7) who happened to be in Paris at the time (despite the ongoing Napoleonic War). As mentioned above, seaweed or burnt sponge had been employed in the treatment of goitre for centuries (2). However, the credit for using iodine itself in the treatment of goitre appears to go to Coindet (1774–1834) (8) of Geneva in 1820, after he had determined that the substance in burnt sponge that acted against 'bronchocoele' was actually iodine. In his 'tincture of iodine', he used 48 grains of iodine to one ounce of spirit of wine. For adults, he prescribed 10 drops of the tincture in half a tumbler of 'syrup of capillaire' and water three times a day, the dose being increased after a few weeks to 15 or even 20 drops. He noted that bronchocoele would usually subside and be destroyed within the space of 6–10 weeks. A few years later, Lugol (1786–1851) in 1829 (2) also recommended and used (what we now call) Lugol's solution for the treatment of goitre, with considerable success.

With the spread of iodine usage, toxic effects soon appeared, as described by Coindet in 1821, and later by Frederic Rilliet (1814–1861) (9). These ill effects of iodine led to a great deal of anxiety about its use for goitre under any circumstance; for some, it was completely proscribed.

Surgical treatment of goitre had been mentioned by Celsus (25 BC to AD 50) (2). It was also mentioned in the Turkish manuscript of Charaf Eddin in 1465. Johann A. W. Hedenus (1760–1836) (2) reported in 1822 on six cases of successful excision of a goitre for impending suffocation. Joseph Henry Green (1791–1863) reported the removal of the right lobe of the thyroid gland in St Thomas's Hospital, London, in 1829, but the patient died of sepsis 2 weeks later.

Structure and function

In a paper by T. W. King (1809–47) (10) of Guy's Hospital, London, there is a description of what was thought to be the secretion of the thyroid as passing into its lymphatics and so into the great veins. King noted that this had been indirectly surmised by Morgagni. He also remarked prophetically that we should be able one day to show that a particular material is slowly formed and partially kept in reserve and that this principle is also supplementary, when poured into the descending inferior vena cava, to important functions in the course of the circulation. Thus he had a conception of the internal secretion by the thyroid. In notes appended to King's paper, Astley Cooper (1768–1841), a surgeon at the same hospital, agreed with King about this idea.

John Simon (1818–97) (1) in 1844, while assistant surgeon at King's College Hospital and demonstrator of anatomy at King's College, London, published a paper on the comparative anatomy of the thyroid. He stated that in addition to its copious vascular supply, it had the structure of a secreting gland. Several decades later, based on thyroidectomies performed on monkeys and other mammals, Victor Horsley (1857–1916) (11) in 1885 supported the generalization of Felix Semon (1849–1921) in 1883 that myxoedema, cretinism, and operative cachexia strumipriva were all due to thyroid deficiency, and not due to chronic asphyxia (as Theodor Kocher, a surgeon in Bern, Switzerland, originally believed) or due to injury of the sympathetic or other nervous structures. Horsley thought that the thyroid controlled the metabolism of mucus, and that the effects of thyroid insufficiency were due to an accumulation of mucus. Others thought that the function of the thyroid was to neutralize or remove poisons, and so thyroid insufficiency was presumed to produce toxaemia. Horsley, in his report to the Clinical Society's Committee on Myxoedema (1888) divided the effects of complete thyroidectomy on monkeys into (1) the acute effects, which consisted of nervousness, tremor, clonic spasm, contracture, paresis, paralysis, and which came on between the second and the twelfth day (now in retrospect clearly the result of damage to the parathyroid glands) and (2) chronic experimental myxoedema. After Gley's (12) rediscovery in 1891 of the parathyroid glands, it became evident that the effect of complete removal of the thyroid resulted in myxoedema, and that removal of the parathyroids was responsible for what had previously been called tetania thyreopriva.

The dramatic results of replacement treatment of myxoedema by thyroid preparations by George Murray (1865–1939) (13) (Fig. 3.1.1.1) in the UK in 1891, and Magnus-Levy's(14) demonstration

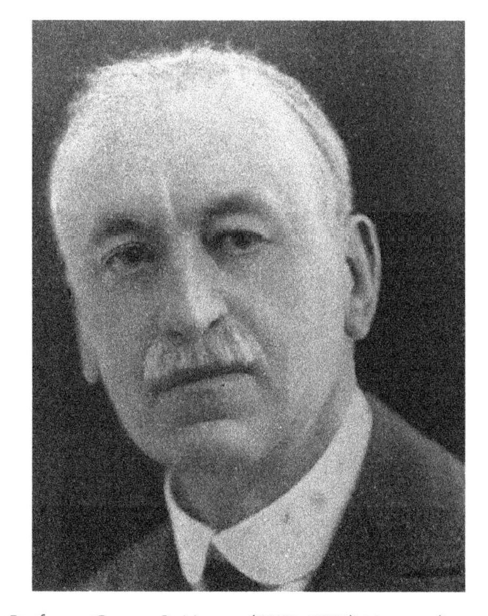

Fig. 3.1.1.1 Professor George R. Murray (1865–1939), Newcastle-upon-Tyne, England, who first used extracts of sheep thyroid for the treatment of myxoedema in 1891. (Reproduced with permission from Rolleston HD. *The Endocrine Organs in Health and Disease, with a Historical Review*. London: Oxford University Press, 1936. (3))

in France in 1895 that thyroid medication accelerated metabolism, led to the conclusion that the thyroid and its internal secretion had definite powers other than detoxification.

Theodor Kocher (1841–1917)(2) suggested in 1895 that the thyroid might contain iodine. In the same year, Tschirch (2) was unable to establish this point. However, Eugen Baumann (1846–96), (15) apparently quite independently of Kocher's suggestion, investigated the chemistry of the thyroid, and was much surprised to find iodine. He published his findings in 1896, (15) called the extracted compound that contained iodine 'thyreo-iodin', and considered it to be the active principle of the thyroid. This led to the isolation by Kendall (16) in 1914 of an active principle which was initially called thyroxyindole and later thyroxin. In 1926, Harington (1897–1972) (17) proved that it was derived from tyrosine and not, as Kendall thought, from tryptophane, and was found to be a basic substance, now called thyroxine. Thyroxine was subsequently shown by Harington (2) and Salter (2) to be less powerful than desiccated thyroid. It was of interest that Harington was not able to accept the possibility that a principle other than thyroxine might exist to explain the metabolic effects of desiccated thyroid. It was not until 1952 that Gross and Pitt-Rivers (18) discovered triiodothyronine, which proved to be that elusive second principle.

Cretinism

The term cretin is thought by some to derive from Christianus, in that the cretinous patients were 'incapable of sin' (2). They were considered as simple, innocent creatures, '*gens du bon Dieu*' (2). Cretinism was one of the diseases first recognized in early life before it was realized that adults were also affected. The observation that cretinoid conditions occurred in adult life in women occurred much later, and was particularly recognized by Sir William Gull (1816–90) (19) in 1873. He was instrumental in leading the commission (which he initially chaired) to the conclusion that myxoedema was actually due to thyroid deficiency. William Ord (1834–1902) (20) gave the name 'myxoedema' to the adult form in 1877 and was the chairman of the commission at the time of the report (1888).

Significant differences were noticed between the adult and the childhood form. In the latter, there was arrest of development in growth both in body and brain. Because cretinism was found more commonly in the deep mountain valleys, there were many theories as to the relationship of air, water, and food, as noted by Hoefer (1614–81), DeSaussure (1740–99), and Malacarne (1744–1816) (1). A Royal Commission in Sardinia (1) in 1848 found that the incidence of cretinism was 28% of the population in the District of Aosta but much lower elsewhere.

Causes of hypothyroidism

The causes of the hypothyroidism were not fully understood throughout the 19th century. W. M. Ord (20,21) described the appearance of the thyroid gland in this condition in 1878, and 13 cases were examined after death in the Report of the Clinical Society of London in 1888. The thyroid showed fibroid atrophy and great diminution in size and weight. There was evidence of chronic inflammation, lymphocytic infiltration, fibrosis, and disappearance of the acini and colloid. However, in 1912, it was Hakaru Hashimoto (1888–1934) (22,23) a surgeon from Fukuoka, Japan, who described four cases of goitre associated with hypothyroidism in which lymphocytic infiltration of the thyroid gland was an important feature. The most common cause of spontaneous hypothyroidism in areas of the world where there is no iodine deficiency is that of (what is now termed) Hashimoto's thyroiditis or autoimmune thyroiditis. Only much later, in 1956, was autoimmune thyroiditis produced experimentally by Rose and Witebsky in Buffalo, New York, (24) and in that same year, thyroid antibodies were found in the circulation of patients with Hashimoto's thyroiditis by Roitt and Doniach (25) in the UK. These findings helped to usher in the era of autoimmunity.

Toxic goitre

Few diseases can have more synonyms and none more eponyms. C. P. Howard (26) collected more than 20 such terms.

Looking back into antiquity, the Persian writer, Sayyid Ismail Al-Jurjani in 1136 (1,2) may have been the first to connect exophthalmos with goitre. Flajani's (1741–1808) (27) description in 1802 in Ascoli, Italy, failed to associate the goitre, exophthalmos, and palpitations as one disease, and his account failed to attract much attention. Indeed, Antonia Testa's (1756–1814) (28) reference in 1800 to the coincidence of prominent eyes and a cardiac disorder likewise did not attract much attention. Testa was the professor of medicine and surgery at Bologna and was said to be a learned theorist, but a mediocre clinician. Caleb Hillier Parry (29,30) (1755–1822) of Bath, England observed a case in August 1786, but his description of eight cases of 'enlargement of the thyroid gland in connection with enlargement or palpitation of the heart' was not published until 1825, 3 years after his death. His second case, seen in 1802, was of particular interest as it seemed to be precipitated by an acute stress, a factor that still exercises the interest of many observers. He considered that the thyroid was acting as a reservoir for the blood being pumped out by the hyperactive heart. This posthumous report in 1825 still preceded Graves' publication by a decade.

Robert J. Graves (31,33) (1796–1853) of Dublin, Ireland, gave a clinical lecture at the Meath Hospital in Dublin and subsequently published a short article on 'palpitation of the heart with enlargement of the thyroid gland' in 1835. He then included these accounts in textbooks that he later wrote. These texts drew considerable attention to the disorder. This attention was later amplified in 1840 by Karl Adolf von Basedow (1799–1854) (34) of Merseburg, Germany, who described four patients with exophthalmos, goitre, and palpitations; his description eave rise to the phrase 'the Merseburg triad'. William Stokes (1804–78), a colleague and friend of Graves in Dublin, actually described hyperthyroidism much more fully than Graves in his text, *Diseases of the Heart* in 1854 (35).

In France, the first description of the disease was provided in 1856 by Jean-Martin Charcot (1825–93), (36) employing the term 'cachexia exophthalmica' to describe the condition. Charcot's older colleague, Armand Trousseau (1801–67) mentioned in a lecture at the Hotel Dieu in Paris in 1860, that iodine, which had been 'inappropriately' prescribed for hyperthyroidism had actually caused marked amelioration of the disease (37). Nevertheless, he felt that the use of iodine in toxic goitre was dangerous, and warned against it.

The credit for the precedence for the description of this disease is scarcely resolved to this day. Sir William Osler (38,39) in his third edition of his famous textbook of medicine belatedly gave the credit for the first important description of this disease to Parry. However, Trousseau (37) had been impressed with the books written by Graves (who was highly regarded as an academic physician) and felt that Graves should be given the credit. In mid-Europe, many observers have given that honour to Basedow. Thus although the term Graves' disease is in common usage in English-speaking countries, Basedow's disease is generally used in Europe. In Italy, the term, Flajani's disease is sometimes heard. At international meetings, the term Graves' disease is most commonly heard.

The cause of Graves' disease remained unknown, and led to many interesting hypotheses, most notably the importance of psychological factors. Rolleston (1) has summarized the various influences which were thought to be at work in causing this condition. In 1907, Charles Mayo (2) of Rochester, Minnesota, first used the term 'hyperthyroidism', to conform to the idea we hold today, namely that the disorder represents an excess of thyroid hormone. In 1910, Kocher (1,2) coined the term 'Jod-Basedow' to describe hyperthyroidism precipitated or aggravated by excess iodine. David Marine (2) also suggested that iodine might actually be a treatment for Graves' disease. A few years later, in 1913, Henry Plummer (1874–1937) (40) was able to separate Graves' disease from hyperthyroidism related to toxic nodular goitre (Plummer's disease). In 1924, Plummer and Boothby (41) showed that the preoperative use of iodine greatly simplified the operative management of Graves' disease.

Treatment of Graves' disease remained mainly surgical until 1942, when Hertz and Roberts (42,43) introduced radioactive iodine for the diagnosis and treatment of Graves' disease. The following year, Astwood (44) used thiourea and thiouracil in the medical treatment of Graves' disease, thus initiating the era of antithyroid drug therapy. In 1956, the year that thyroid autoantibodies were first identified, Adams and Purves (45) in New Zealand described the presence of an abnormal stimulator of the thyroid in Graves' disease which later proved to be an antibody directed against the thyroid-stimulating hormone receptor (thyroid-stimulating antibody). Thus Graves' disease, as well as Hashimoto's thyroiditis, proved to be an autoimmune disorder.

Other conditions

In 1896, Riedel (46,47) described invasive fibrous thyroiditis, a rare fibrosing condition of the thyroid gland and de Quervain (49) described subacute nonsuppurative thyroiditis in 1896.

Endnote

The above account is provided to give a brief overview of some of the historical and artistic highlights related to the thyroid, that lead up to the modern era. It is only recently, with a fuller understanding of biochemistry and biology, physiology, pathology, immunology and immunogenetics, that our comprehension of these matters has become reasonably rational.

References

1. Rolleston HD. *The Endocrine Organs in Health and Disease, with a Historical Review*. London: Oxford University Press, 1936.
2. Medvei VC. *A History of Endocrinology*. Lancaster, England: MTP Press, 1982.
3. Merke F. *History and Iconography of Endemic Goitre and Cretinism*. Lancaster, England: MTP Press, 1984.
4. Hart GD. Even the gods had goitre. *Can Med Assoc J*, 1967; **96**: 1432–6.
5. Paracelsus (Bombastus v. Hohenheim TPA). De Generatione Stultorum. In: *Opera*, 1603; **2**: 174–82.
6. Wharton T. *Adenographia: Sive, Glandularum Totius Corporis Descriptio*. London, 1656: 118.
7. Davy H. *Philosophical Transactions of the Royal Society of London*, 1814; 104: 74.
8. Coindet JF. Decouverte d'un nouveau remede contre le goitre. *Ann Chim Phys*, 1820; **15**: 49–59.
9. Rilliet F. Constitutional iodism. *Bulletin de l'Academie de Medicine de Paris*, 1859; **25**: 382.
10. King TW. Observations on the thyroid gland. *Guys Hosp Rep*, 1836; **1**: 429–46.
11. Horsley V. Functional nervous disorders due to loss of thyroid gland and pituitary body. *Lancet*, 1886; **2**: 5.
12. Gley E. Sur les fonctions des corps thyroide. *Comptes Rendues de la Societe Biologique*, 1891; **43**: 841–7.
13. Murray GR. Notes on the treatment of myxoedema by hypodermic injections of an extract of the thyroid gland of a sheep. *Br Med J*, 1891; **ii**: 796–7.
14. Magnus-Levy A. Ueber den respiratorischen Gaswechel unter dem Einfluss der Thyroidea sowie unter verschiedenen pathologischen Zustaenden. *Berlin Klinischen Wochenschrift*, 1895; **32**: 650–2.
15. Baumann E, Goldman E. Ist das Iodothyrin (Thyrojodin) der lebenswichtige Bestandteil der Schilddruse?. *Munch Med Wochensch*, 1896; **43**: 1153.
16. Kendall EC. Collected papers. *Mayo Clinic, Mayo Foundation*, 1917; **9**: 309–36.
17. Harington CR, Barger G. Chemistry of thyroxine. III. Constitution and synthesis of thyroxine. *Biochem J*, 1927; **21**: 169–83.
18. Gross J, Pitt-Rivers RV. Triiodothyronine. I. Isolation from thyroid gland and synthesis. *Biochem J*, 1953; **53**: 645–50.
19. Gull WW. On a cretinoid state supervening in adult life in women. *Trans Clin Soc Lond*, 1873–74; **7**: 180–5.
20. Ord WM. On myxoedema, a term proposed to be applied to an essential condition in the 'cretinoid' affection, occasionally observed in middle-aged women. *Med Chir Trans*, 1878; **61**: 57–78.
21. Ord WM. Report of a committee of the Clinical Society of London nominated December 14, 1883 to investigate the subject of myxoedema. *Trans Clin Soc Lond*, 1888; **8**: 15.
22. Hashimoto H. Zur Kenntnis der lymphomatosen Veranderung der Schilddruse (Struma lymphomatosa). *Archiv der Klinische Chirurgie*, 1912; **97**: 219.
23. Volpé R. Historical perspective: The life of Doctor Hakaru Hashimoto. *Autoimmunity*, 1989; **3**: 243–5.
24. Rose NR, Witebsky E. Studies of organ specificity. V. Changes in the thyroid glands of rabbits following active immunization with rabbit thyroid extracts. *J Immunol*, 1956; **76**: 417.
25. Roitt IM, Doniach D, Campbell RN, Hudson RV. Autoantibodies in Hashimoto's disease (lymphadenoid goitre). *Lancet*, 1956; **ii**: 820.
26. Howard CP. Hyperthyroidism. In: Barker LF, Hoskins RG, Mosenthal HO, eds. *Endocrinology and Metabolism. D.* Appleton and Co., 1922; **1**: 304.
27. Flajani G. Sopra un tumor freddo nell'anterior parte dell collo detto bronchocele. *Collezione d'osservazioni e riflessioni di chirurgia*, Roma, 1802; **3**: 270–3.

28. Testa A. *Collezione d'osservazioni e reflessioni di chirurgia*, Roma, 1800.
29. Parry CH. *Collections from the Unpublished Medical Writings of the Late Caleb Hillier Parry*. London: Underwoods, 1825; **2**: 110.
30. Volpé R. The life of Caleb Hillier Parry. *Endocrinologist*, 1994; **4**: 157–9.
31. Graves RJ. Clinical lectures. *Lond Med Surg J*, 1835; **7**: 513–20.
32. Taylor S. *Robert Graves: The Golden Years of Irish Medicine*. London: Royal Society of Medicine, 1989.
33. Coakley D. *Robert Graves: Evangelist of Clinical Medicine*. Dublin: Irish Endocrine Society, 1996.
34. Basedow CA. Exophthalmos durch hypertrophie des Zellgewebes in der augenhoehle. *Wochenschrift Ges Heilkunde*, 1840; **6**: 197–204, 220–8.
35. Stokes W. *Diseases of the Heart and Aorta*. Dublin, 1854: 278–97.
36. Charcot JM. Memoire sur une affection caractérisé par les palpitation du coeur et les arteres, la tumefavtion de la glande thyroide et une double exophthalmie. *Comptes Rendus desMemoires de la Societe Biologique*, 1857; **3**: 43.
37. Trousseau A. *Lectures on Clinical Medicine*. Paris: New Sydenham Society, 1868: 542.
38. Osler W. *Principles and Practice of Medicine*, 3rd edn. New York: D. Appleton and Co., 1898: 836.
39. Hoffenberg R. The thyroid and Osler. *J Roy Coll Phys Lond*, 1985; **19**: 80–5.
40. Plummer HS. The clinical and pathological relationship of simple and exophthalmic goiter. *Am J Med Sci*, 1913; **146**: 790.
41. Plummer HS, Boothby WM. The value of iodine in exophthalmic goitre. *Iowa Med Soc*, 1924; **14**: 66–73.
42. Hertz S, Roberts A, Evans RD. Radioactive iodine as an indicator in the study of thyroid physiology. *Proc Soc Exp Biol Med*, 1938; **38**: 510–13.
43. Hertz S, Roberts A. Application of radioactive iodine in therapy of Graves' disease. *J Clin Investig*, 1942; **21**: 624.
44. Astwood EB. Treatment of hyperthyroidism with thiourea. *J A Med A*, 1943; **122**: 78–81.
45. Adams DD, Purves HD. Abnormal responses to the assay of thyrotrophin. *Proc University of Otago Medical School*, 1956; **11**: 34.
46. Riedel BM. Die chronische zur Bildung eisenharter Tumoren fuhrende Entzundung der Schilddruse. *Verhandlungen der Deutschen Gesellschaft fur Chirurgie*, 1896; **25**: 101–5.
47. Riedel BM. Vorstellung eines Kranken mit Chronische Strumitis. *Verhandlungen der Deutschen Gesellschaft Chirurgie*, 1897; **26**: 127–9.
48. de Quervain F. Die akute nicht Eiterige Thyreoiditis und die Beteiligung der schilddruse und akuten intoxikationen und infectionen Uberhaupt. *Mitteilungen aus der Grenzgeheiten der Medizin und Chirurgie*, 1991; **2** (suppl. Bd): 1–165, 6 pt.

3.1.2 Biosynthesis, transport, metabolism, and actions of thyroid hormones

Theo J. Visser

Introduction

In healthy humans with a normal iodine intake, the thyroid follicular cells produce predominantly the prohormone thyroxine (3,3′,5,5′-tetraiodothyronine; T_4), which is converted in peripheral tissues to the bioactive hormone 3,3′,5-triiodothyronine (T_3) or to the inactive metabolite 3,3′,5′-triiodothyronine (reverse T_3). The bioavailability of thyroid hormone in target tissues depends to a large extent on the supply of plasma T_4 and T_3, the activity of transporters mediating the cellular uptake and/or efflux of these hormones, as well as the activity of deiodinases and possibly other enzymes catalyzing their activation or inactivation. Thyroid function is regulated most importantly by the hypophyseal glycoprotein thyroid-stimulating hormone (TSH), also called thyrotropin. In turn, TSH secretion from the anterior pituitary is stimulated by the hypothalamic factor thyrotropin-releasing hormone (TRH). TSH secretion is down-regulated by negative feedback action of thyroid hormone on the hypothalamus and the pituitary. The contribution of locally produced T_3 versus uptake of plasma T_3 is much greater for some tissues such as the brain and the pituitary than for most other tissues. Plasma TSH is an important parameter for the diagnosis of thyroid dysfunction but is not representative for the thyroid state of all tissues. In this chapter various aspects will be discussed of: (a) the neuroendocrine regulation of thyroid function, (b) the biosynthesis of thyroid hormone (i.e. the prohormone T_4), (c) the activation and inactivation of thyroid hormone in peripheral tissues, and (d) the mechanism by which T_3 exerts it biological activity. A schematic overview of the hypothalamus–pituitary–thyroid–periphery axis is presented in Fig. 3.1.2.1.

Regulation of thyroid function

Thyrotropin-releasing hormone

TRH is a tripeptide with the structure pyroglutamyl-histidyl-proline amide (pGlu-His-Pro-NH_2) in which the C-terminal carboxyl group is blocked by amidation and the N-terminal α-amino group is blocked by cyclization. Beside stimulating TSH secretion, TRH also stimulates prolactin secretion and, under certain pathological conditions, growth hormone secretion from the anterior pituitary. TRH is not only produced in the hypothalamus but is widely distributed through the central nervous system where it functions as a neurotransmitter or neuromodulator. Centrally mediated actions of TRH include neurobehavioural, haemodynamic, and gastrointestinal effects. TRH is also detected in the posterior pituitary and

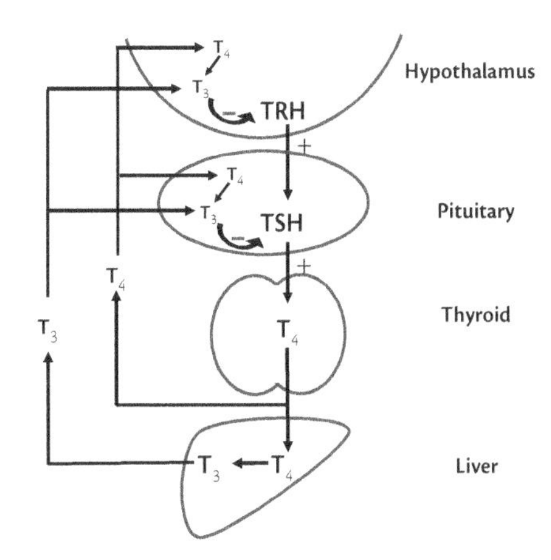

Fig. 3.1.2.1 Overview of the regulation of the production and metabolism of thyroid hormone in the hypothalamus–pituitary–thyroid–periphery axis, showing the liver as a major T_3-producing tissue.

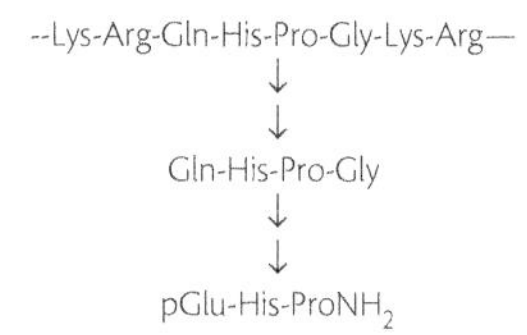

Fig. 3.1.2.2 Biosynthesis of TRH. The figure shows the several steps by which the TRH progenitor sequences in proTRH are processed to mature TRH.

in different peripheral tissues, such as the pancreas, the heart, the testis, the adrenal, and the placenta. Little is known about the function of TRH in these tissues.

Hypophysiotropic TRH is produced in neurons, the cell bodies of which are located in the paraventricular nucleus of the hypothalamus (1). The biosynthesis of TRH involves the production of a large precursor protein (proTRH) which, in humans, consists of a sequence of 242 amino acids. This proTRH contains six copies of the TRH progenitor sequence Gln-His-Pro-Gly, flanked at both sides by pairs of the basic amino acids Arg and/or Lys (Fig. 3.1.2.2). Cleavage of proTRH at the basic amino acids by prohormone convertases (e.g. PC1 and PC2) and further removal of remaining basic residues by carboxypeptidases results in the liberation of the progenitor sequences. A specific glutaminyl cyclase catalyses the formation of the pGlu ring at the N-terminus and a so-called peptidylglycine α-amidating mono-oxygenase converts Pro-Gly to ProNH$_2$ at the C-terminus (2). The processing of proTRH takes place in vesicles that transport mature TRH and intervening peptides along the axons of the TRH neurons to the median eminence, where they are released into the portal vessels of the hypophyseal stalk.

TRH is transported over a short distance through the hypophyseal stalk to the anterior lobe of the pituitary, where it stimulates the production and secretion of TSH (and prolactin). These actions of TRH are initiated by its binding to the type 1 TRH receptor (TRHR1), which is expressed on both the thyrotroph (TSH-producing cell) and the lactotroph (prolactin-producing cell) (3). This receptor belongs to the family of G-protein-coupled receptors, characteristically containing seven transmembrane domains. Human TRHR1 is a protein consisting of 398 amino acids, and binding of TRH induces a change in its interaction with the trimeric G-protein, resulting in the stimulation of phospholipase C activity. The activated phospholipase C catalyses the hydrolysis of phosphatidylinositol-4,5-diphosphate to the second messengers inositol-1,4,5-triphosphate and diacylglycerol, which initiate a cascade of reactions, including an increase in cellular Ca^{2+} levels and protein kinase C activity, that ultimately stimulates the release as well as the synthesis of TSH (and prolactin) (3). TRH stimulation of TSHβ gene expression is also dependent on the pituitary-specific transcription factor 1.

In addition to the TRHR1 expressed in the anterior pituitary, a second TRH receptor (TRHR2) has been cloned and characterized in rat and mouse brain which probably mediates most central actions of TRH (3). In humans, only one type of TRH receptor exists, namely TRHR1.

TRH is subject to rapid degradation in the blood as well as in different tissues. Although multiple enzymes are involved, a very important role is played by the TRH-degrading ectoenzyme TRHDE, which catalyses the cleavage of the pGlu-His bond (4):

$$\text{pGlu-His-ProNH}_2 \rightarrow \text{pGlu} + \text{His-ProNH}_2$$

This enzyme has been characterized as a zinc-containing metalloproteinase, which in humans consists of 1024 amino acids. It has a single transmembrane domain and is inserted in the plasma membrane such that most of the protein is exposed on the cell surface (ectopeptidase), in particular in brain, pituitary, liver, and lung. Enzymatic cleavage of the protein close to the cell membrane releases most of the protein in a soluble and enzymatically active form into the circulation, representing the origin of plasma TRHDE. Plasma TRHDE appears to be derived mostly from the liver. In the brain and the pituitary, where the enzyme is probably located in close vicinity of the TRH receptor, TRHDE supposedly plays an important role in the local regulation of TRH bioavailability. Interestingly, TRHDE activity in the pituitary and in plasma is increased in hyperthyroidism and decreased in hypothyroidism, which may contribute to the negative feedback control of TSH secretion by thyroid hormone (4).

Thyroid-stimulating hormone

TSH is a glycoprotein produced by the thyrotropic cells of the anterior pituitary. Like the other hypophyseal hormones, luteinizing hormone and follicle-stimulating hormone, it is composed of two subunits. The α-subunit is identical and the β-subunit is homologous among the three hormones (5). Although hormone specificity is conveyed by the β-subunit, dimerization with the α-subunit is required for biological activity. Human TSH consists of 205 amino acids; 92 in the α-subunit and 113 in the β-subunit. It has a molecular weight of 28 kDa, 20% of which is contributed by three complex carbohydrate groups: two on the α-subunit and one on the β-subunit. The structure of these carbohydrate groups is important for the biological activity of TSH and is dependent on the stimulation of the thyrotroph by TRH (5).

In addition to the stimulation by TRH and negative feedback by thyroid hormone, TSH production and secretion is also subject to negative regulation by hypothalamic somatostatin and dopamine, and by cortisol (6). The inhibitory effect of cortisol is exerted to an important extent at the hypothalamic level.

TSH binds to a specific TSH receptor located in the plasma membrane of the follicular cell. Like the TRH receptor, this is also a G-protein-coupled receptor which, in humans, is a protein consisting of 764 amino acids with an exceptionally long extracellular N-terminal domain (7). The TSH receptor is preferentially coupled to a $G_s\alpha$-subunit of the trimeric G-protein. Binding of TSH to its receptor induces the dissociation of the G-protein subunits, resulting in the activation of the membrane-bound adenylate cyclase and, thus, in the stimulation of cAMP formation as second messenger. The increased cAMP levels induce a series of events, including the activation of protein kinase A activity, that ultimately results in the stimulation of the biosynthesis and secretion of thyroid hormone (8). In particular, the expression of genes coding for key proteins for hormone production (e.g. the iodide transporter, thyroglobulin, and thyroid peroxidase) is increased through mechanisms that also involve different thyroid-specific transcription factors such as TTF1, TTF2, and PAX8. At high TSH concentrations, the TSH receptor also couples to the $G_q\alpha$-subunit, resulting in the activation of the phosphoinositide pathway, which is also involved in the regulation of thyroid function and growth (8).

As discussed elsewhere in this section, hyperthyroidism is often caused by an autoimmune process in which TSH receptor-stimulating antibodies play an important role. Hyperthyroidism may also be caused by a hyperfunctioning adenoma. In most patients with a toxic adenoma, somatic mutations have been identified in the TSH receptor, which result in the constitutive activation of this receptor (9). In other patients, somatic mutations have been found in the $G_s\alpha$-subunit that result in the constitutive activation of the G-protein in the absence of TSH. Together, mutations in the TSH receptor and the $G_s\alpha$-subunit account for the majority of toxic thyroid adenomas. Also, germline, gain-of-function mutations have been identified in patients with congenital, nonautoimmune hyperthyroidism. Conversely, germline, loss-of-function mutations have been described in patients with TSH resistance (9). Such a loss-of-function mutation has also been identified as the cause of the hypothyroidism in the *hyt/hyt* mouse. However, patients with TSH resistance may be clinically euthyroid because the partial defect in TSH receptor function is compensated by increased plasma TSH levels (9).

Biosynthesis of thyroid hormone

The functional unit of the thyroid gland is the follicle, composed of a single layer of epithelial cells surrounding a colloidal lumen in which thyroid hormone is stored as an integral part of its precursor protein thyroglobulin. The biosynthesis of thyroid hormone comprises the following steps, which are depicted schematically in Fig. 3.1.2.3 (8, 10):

1. Uptake of iodide through the basolateral membrane and export through the apical membrane.
2. Clustering of thyroglobulin, thyroid peroxidase (TPO), and the dual oxidase DUOX2 in a 'thyroxisome' at the luminal surface of the apical membrane (11).
3. Formation of H_2O_2 by DUOX2.
4. H_2O_2-dependent iodination of tyrosine residues in thyroglobulin by TPO.
5. H_2O_2-dependent coupling of iodotyrosine to iodothyronine residues in thyroglobulin by TPO.
6. Resorption of thyroglobulin from the lumen and hydrolysis in lysosomes.
7. De-iodination of iodotyrosines and reutilization of iodide.
8. Secretion of iodothyronines, predominantly T_4.

Iodide uptake

Iodine is an essential trace element required for the synthesis of thyroid hormone. It is not surprising, therefore, that the basolateral membrane of the follicular cell contains an active transporter that mediates uptake of I^- together with Na^+. This sodium-iodide symporter (NIS) has been characterized as a protein consisting, in humans, of 618 amino acids and 13 transmembrane domains (12). Supposedly, these domains form a channel through which I^- and Na^+ are transported in a stoichiometry of 1:2. The surplus of positive charge indicates that I^- transport is electrogenic and further driven by the Na^+ gradient. TSH stimulates the expression of the *NIS* gene to such an extent that the intracellular iodide concentration may be up to 500 times higher than its extracellular level. The NIS is not completely specific for iodide but also binds other anions, some of which are even transported (12).

An important example is perchlorate (ClO_4^-) which potently inhibits iodide uptake by the NIS, an effect utilized in the perchlorate discharge test used for the diagnosis of an organification defect, i.e. impaired incorporation of iodine in thyroglobulin. Perchlorate inhibits the uptake but not the release of iodide from the thyroid. Therefore, if perchlorate is administered after a dose of radioactive iodide, it will provoke a marked release of radioactivity from the thyroid in case of an organification defect but not from a normal thyroid gland. Pertechnetate (TcO_4^-) is another anion transported by the NIS, and this observation is utilized in the scanning of the thyroid gland using radioactive $^{99m}TcO_4^-$. Of course, the latter is not incorporated in thyroglobulin and, thus, cannot be used to test the hormone production capacity of the thyroid.

It is not sufficient that iodide is transported across the plasma membrane. Since the iodination of thyroglobulin takes place at the luminal surface of the apical membrane, iodide also has to pass this

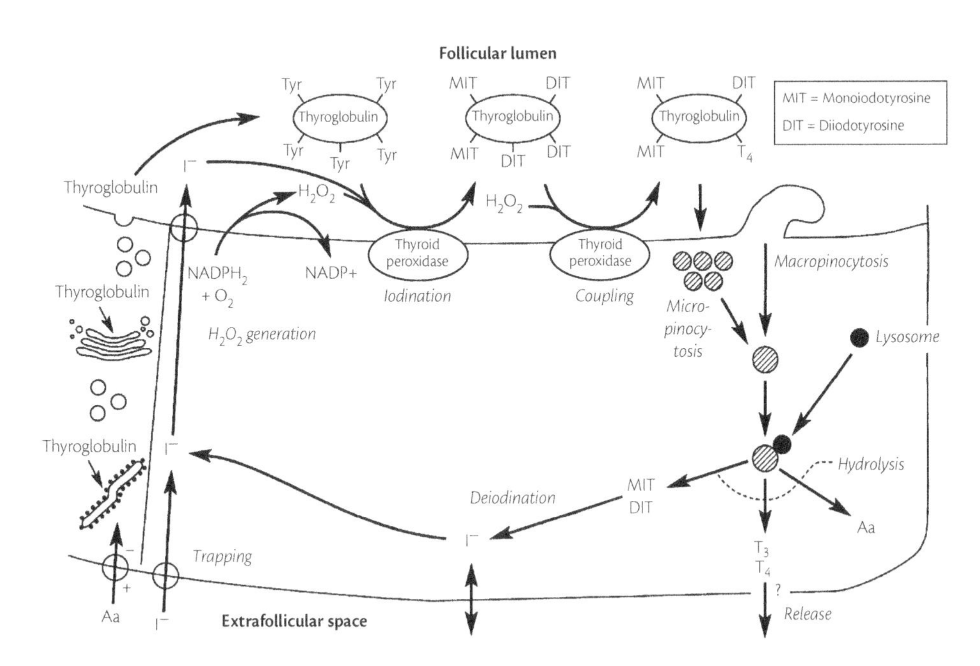

Fig. 3.1.2.3 Schematic presentation of a thyroid follicular cell and important steps in the synthesis of thyroid hormone. DIT, 3,5-diiodotyrosine; MIT, monoiodotyrosine. (Courtesy of Prof. J. Dumont, Brussels).

membrane. A transporter putatively involved in this process has been identified and termed pendrin, since the gene coding for this protein is mutated in patients with Pendred's syndrome (13). This is a congenital condition characterized by deafness due to a cochlear defect and hypothyroidism due to an organification defect as indicated by a positive perchlorate discharge test. Pendrin is capable of transporting bicarbonate, chloride, and iodide (13), and is expressed only in the thyroid and the cochlea. The exact function of pendrin in the transport of iodide across the apical membrane is subject to debate. Most likely, it is not the only protein capable of releasing iodide into the follicular lumen. Efflux of iodide from thyroid follicular cells is acutely stimulated by TSH, which may involve recruitment and/or activation of an iodide exporter such as pendrin. The function of pendrin in the cochlea probably lies in the secretion of bicarbonate into the endolymph.

Thyroglobulin, DUOX2, and TPO

Thyroglobulin is an exceptionally large glycoprotein consisting of two identical subunits. Each mature subunit in human thyroglobulin contains 2748 amino acids and has a molecular weight of approximately 330 kDa (14). The *TG* gene is located on human chromosome 8q24.2-q24.3; it covers about 300 kb of genomic DNA and consists of 48 exons.

DUOX2 is a large and complex glycoprotein embedded in the apical membrane of the thyrocyte. Mature human DUOX2 contains 1527 amino acids and has seven putative transmembrane domains, an NADPH-binding domain, an FAD-binding domain, a haem-binding domain, two calcium-binding EF hands, and a peroxidase domain (15). It catalyses the oxidation of NADPH from the cytoplasm and delivers its product H_2O_2 to the luminal surface of the membrane. The haem group appears to be the site of H_2O_2 generation and its location within transmembrane domains fits with the vectorial (enzyme/transport) function of DUOX2. Functional expression of DUOX2 requires the presence of the maturation factor DUOXA2, a protein consisting of 320 amino acids and five putative transmembrane domains (16). The *DUOX2* and *DUOXA2* genes are clustered together with the homologous *DUOX1* and *DUOXA1* genes on human chromosome 15q15.

TPO is a glycoprotein consisting of 933 amino acids and featuring a single transmembrane domain. A short C-terminal domain is located in the cytoplasm but most of the protein is exposed on the luminal surface of the apical membrane, which also contains a haem-binding domain, the active centre of the enzyme (17). Functional TPO may exist as a homodimeric structure linked through a disulfide bond. The human *TPO* gene covers about 150 kb on chromosome 2p25, distributed over 17 exons. In addition to full-length TPO1, the TPO2 splice variant is generated by the skipping of exon 10, resulting in the loss of 57 amino acids in the middle of the protein (17). TPO2 has no enzyme activity and its function is unknown.

Formation of iodothyronines

Thyroid hormone synthesis takes place at the luminal surface of the apical membrane in the scaffold of the thyroglobulin molecule and consists of two important reactions that are both catalysed by TPO, i.e. the iodination of Tyr residues and the subsequent coupling of iodotyrosine to iodothyronine residues (17). The structures of these compounds are illustrated in Fig. 3.1.2.4. The prosthetic haem group of TPO undergoes a two-electron oxidation

MIT

DIT

T_3

T_4

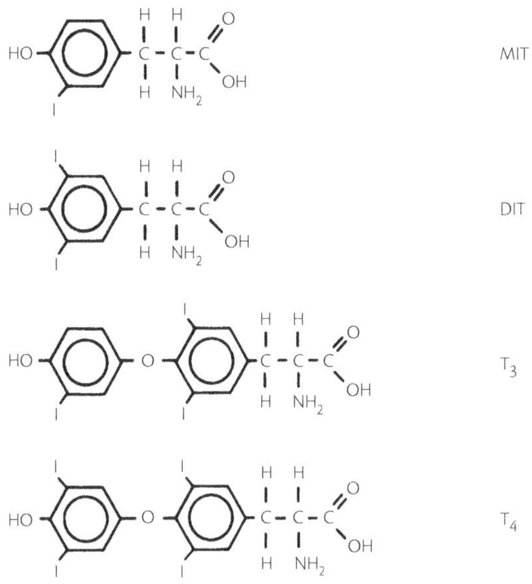

Fig. 3.1.2.4 Structures of the iodotyrosines MIT and DIT and the iodothyronines T_3 and T_4.

by H_2O_2 (supplied by DUOX2) to the intermediate compound 1 (Cpd1). Cpd1 may carry out either a one-electron oxidation reaction, by which it is converted to the intermediate Cpd2, or a two-electron oxidation by which native TPO is regenerated. TPO-catalysed iodination probably involves a two-electron oxidation of I^- to I^+ with subsequent electrophilic substitution of Tyr residues in thyroglobulin, producing 3-iodotyrosine (monoiodotyrosine, MIT). Substitution of MIT residues with a second iodine produces 3,5-diiodotyrosine (DIT).

Coupling of two suitably positioned iodotyrosine residues results in the formation of an iodothyronine residue at the site of the acceptor iodotyrosine, leaving a dehydroalanine residue at the site of the donor iodotyrosine (17). It is generally believed that coupling involves the one-electron oxidation of each donor and acceptor iodotyrosine residue, generating radicals that rapidly combine to produce an iodothyronine residue. Coupling of the diiodophenol moiety of one DIT residue to the phenolic oxygen of a second DIT residue results in the formation of T_4, while coupling of the iodophenol moiety of MIT to a DIT residue yields T_3. Coupling of DIT and MIT to generate reverse T_3 is apparently a rare event, since thyroidal secretion of reverse T_3 is negligible. This probably also holds for formation of 3,3′-T_2 by coupling of two MIT residues.

Although Tyr is the building block of thyroid hormone, the Tyr content of thyroglobulin is not greater than that of most other proteins. Of the 67 Tyr residues per thyroglobulin subunit, about 20–25 are available for iodination, but the capacity for iodothyronine formation is limited (17). Each thyroglobulin subunit has only four hormonogenic sites, Tyr residues that can ultimately be transformed into iodothyronines. At three sites (positions 5, 1290, and 2553 in the mature protein) T_4 can be formed, while at the fourth site (position 2746) T_3 is preferentially produced. However, at normal levels of iodination the average yield is 1–1.5 molecules of T_4 and approximately 0.1 molecule of T_3 per thyroglobulin subunit. At this stage the iodothyronines are still in peptide linkage with the thyroglobulin backbone and remain stored as such in the lumen until their secretion is required.

Release of thyroid hormone

In response to TSH stimulation, thyroglobulin is resorbed from the lumen largely by both macro- and micropinocytosis (8, 10). The former type of endocytosis is associated with the formation of large pseudopodia that engulf colloid and the thyroglobulin contained therein, resulting in the formation of large cytoplasmic vesicles also known as colloid droplets. The second process concerns the receptor-mediated endocytosis of thyroglobulin, involving the binding of thyroglobulin to apical membrane proteins. Megalin, a very large (*c.*600 kDa) cargo protein located in the apical membrane of different cell types, including thyrocytes, may be involved although it appears to function primarily in the transcellular transport of poorly iodinated thyroglobulin (18).

Both types of endosomes fuse with lysosomes, generating so-called phagolysosomes. In these vesicles thyroglobulin is hydrolysed by lysosomal proteases, i.e. cathepsins (19), resulting in the liberation of T_4, a small amount of T_3, as well as excess MIT and DIT molecules. MIT and DIT are probably exported from the vesicles via a specific transporter (20). Thus, they have access to the iodotyrosine dehalogenase (DEHAL1 or IYD), located in the endoplasmic reticulum, which catalyses their deiodination by NADH (21, 22). The iodide thereby released is reutilized for iodination of thyroglobulin.

Human DEHAL1 is a homodimer of a 289-amino acid protein containing an N-terminal membrane anchor and a conserved nitroreductase domain with an FMN-binding site (21, 22). The *DEHAL1* gene is located on chromosome 6q24-q25 and consists of five exons. Since DEHAL1 lacks an NADH-binding sequence, iodotyrosine deiodinase activity requires the involvement of a reductase, which has not yet been identified. DEHAL1 is also expressed in the liver and kidneys.

Surprisingly little is still known about the exact mechanism of thyroid hormone secretion. One option involves the transcellular transport of the thyroglobulin-liberated iodothyronines in vesicles, which fuse with the basolateral membrane and release their content in the extracellular compartment. Alternatively, iodothyronines may be released via transporters from the vesicles into the cytoplasm, and subsequently secreted through transporters located in the basolateral membrane. In the latter route, some T_4 may be converted before secretion to T_3 by iodothyronine deiodinases present in the thyrocyte (see below). Recent findings suggest that the transporter MCT8 (see below) plays an important role in thyroid hormone secretion.

In an average human subject, T_4 and T_3 are secreted in a ratio of about 15:1, i.e. about 100 μg (130 nmol) T_4 and 6 μg (9 nmol) T_3 per day. The latter represents approximately 20% of daily total T_3 production (23). Hence, most T_3 is produced by deiodination of T_4 in peripheral tissues.

Inhibitors of thyroid hormone production and/or secretion

Administration of a large amount of iodide usually results in an acute but transient decrease in thyroid hormone secretion (8, 10). The mechanism of this inhibition of thyroid hormone secretion by excess iodide is unknown. Excess iodide will also induce an inhibition of the synthesis of thyroid hormone; this phenomenon is known as the Wolff–Chaikoff effect (8, 10). The mechanism appears to involve, among other things, the formation of an iodinated lipid (iodolactone) that inhibits several steps in thyroid hormone synthesis. This includes the inhibition of iodide uptake by the NIS, which results in a decrease in the intracellular iodide concentration and, thus, a decrease in iodolactone formation. This relieves the inhibited hormone synthesis, known as the escape from the Wolff–Chaikoff effect, that occurs despite the continued administration of excess iodide.

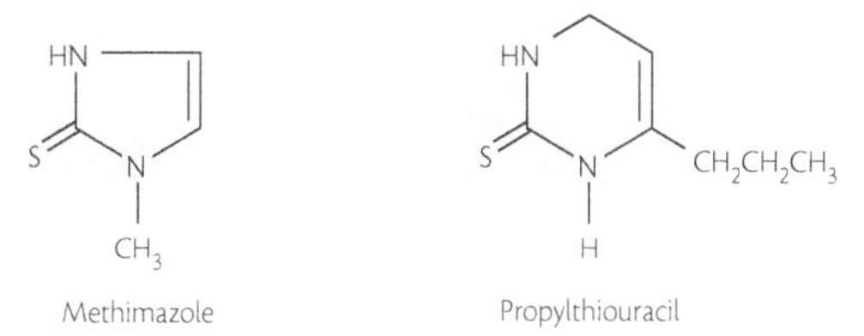

Fig. 3.1.2.5 Structures of the TPO inhibitors methimazole and propylthiouracil. The thiourea moiety of the drugs is shaded.

Thiourea derivatives have been known since the pioneering work of Astwood in the 1940s as potent inhibitors of thyroid hormone synthesis (24). Two of these, methimazole and 6-propyl-2-thiouracil are widely used in the medical treatment of patients with hyperthyroidism (Fig. 3.1.2.5). Their antithyroid activity is based on the potent inhibition of TPO, the mechanism of which depends on the available iodide concentration (17). In the presence of iodide, the thiourea inhibitors compete with the Tyr residues in thyroglobulin for the TPO–I^+ iodination complex, preventing the formation of thyroid hormone. The thiourea inhibitors are thus converted to the sulfenyl iodide derivatives which undergo further oxidation of the sulfur ultimately to sulfate.

Methimazole is a more potent inhibitor of TPO than propylthiouracil (17), and lower doses of methimazole (or the prodrug carbimazole) are required for the treatment of hyperthyroidism compared with propylthiouracil. Besides inhibiting thyroid hormone (i.e. T_4) synthesis by TPO, propylthiouracil also inhibits conversion of T_4 to T_3 by the type 1 iodothyronine deiodinase located not only in the thyroid but also in liver and kidney (see below). In contrast, methimazole does not affect D1 activity.

Transport of thyroid hormone

Plasma transport

In plasma, thyroid hormone is bound to three proteins, thyroxine-binding globulin (TBG), transthyretin (TTR, previously known as thyroxine-binding prealbumin (TBPA)), and albumin (Table 3.1.2.1) (25). Human TBG is a 54-kDa glycoprotein produced in the liver and consists of 395 amino acids and four carbohydrate residues. The *TBG* gene is located on the human chromosome Xq22.2, spans about 5.5 kb, and contains five exons (26). Among the different thyroid hormone transport proteins it shows by far the highest affinity for T_4, with an equilibrium dissociation constant (K_d) of approximately 0.1 nM, but also the lowest plasma concentration (*c.*15 mg/l) (25).

TTR is composed of four identical subunits, each consisting of 127 amino acids. The *TTR* gene is located on human chromosome 18q11.2-q12.1, covers about 7 kb, and contains four exons (27). TTR has a cigar-shaped structure with two identical binding channels, each formed by two symmetrically positioned subunits, with ligand entry sites at opposite ends of the TTR molecule. Binding of a T_4 molecule in one site hinders the binding of another T_4 molecule in the second site. Binding of the first T_4 molecule to TTR is characterized by a K_d value of approximately 10 nM, and the plasma concentration of TTR amounts to approximately 250 mg/l (25).

Table 3.1.2.1 Characteristics of T_4-binding proteins in human plasma

Protein	Concentration in plasma (mg/l)	Dissociation constant (K_d) (μmol/l)	T_4 distribution (mol/l)	Percentage
TBG	*c*.15	*c*.0.3	*c*.10^{-10}	75
TTR	*c*.250	*c*.5	10^{-8}	10
Albumin	*c*.40 000	*c*.600	10^{-6} to 10^{-5}	15

TBG, T_4-binding globulin; TTR, transthyretin (formerly known as T_4-binding prealbumin, TBPA).

Plasma TTR is produced in the liver, but the protein is also expressed in the choroid plexus where it is probably involved in T_4 transfer from plasma to the cerebrospinal fluid. Furthermore, TTR is expressed in trophoblasts where it may participate in the transplacental transfer of maternal T_4 to the fetus. TTR also binds retinol-binding protein and thus also plays an important role in vitamin A transport (27).

Albumin has multiple low-affinity binding sites for thyroid hormone, with K_d values for T_4 of 1–10 μM, but it has by far the highest plasma concentration (*c*.40 g/l) (25). Iodothyronines also bind to lipoproteins, in particular high-density lipoprotein. Although the proportion of plasma T_4 and T_3 bound to lipoproteins is low compared with the other plasma transport proteins, it may be important to target thyroid hormone specifically to lipoprotein receptor-expressing tissues (25).

The resultant of the concentrations and affinities of the different thyroid hormone-binding proteins is that in normal human subjects approximately 75% of plasma T_4 is bound to TBG, approximately 15% is bound to albumin, and approximately 10% is bound to TTR (25). The total binding capacity of these proteins is so high that only approximately 0.02% of plasma T_4 is free (non-protein-bound). The affinity of T_3 for the different proteins is roughly 10% of that of T_4. Therefore, plasma T_3 shows a similar distribution to T_4 over the different proteins, and the free T_3 fraction in normal plasma amounts to approximately 0.2%. Thus, while the mean normal plasma total T_4 (*c*.100 nmol/l) and T_3 (*c*.2 nmol/l) levels differ about 50-fold, the difference in the mean normal free T_4 (*c*.20 pmol/l) and free T_3 (*c*.5 pmol/l) is only about fourfold. Reverse T_3 binds with intermediate affinity to the plasma proteins (25).

Since it is the plasma free T_4 and free T_3 concentrations that determine the tissue availability of thyroid hormone, they are more important parameters than the plasma total T_4 and T_3 concentrations in the assessment of thyroid status. Both concentration and thyroid hormone-binding affinity of the different plasma proteins are influenced by a variety of (patho)physiological factors (25). Since it binds most thyroid hormone in plasma, variations in TBG concentration are more important than variations in TTR or albumin concentrations. Inherited TBG excess is a rare phenomenon caused by *TBG* gene duplication. Inherited TBG deficiency is often caused by a single base mutation in the *TBG* gene, resulting in a decreased T_4 affinity or a decreased protein stability. More severe *TBG* gene defects are responsible for a complete lack of serum TBG in affected hemizygous males (26). Beside genetic variation, TBG levels are also influenced by various endogenous and exogenous factors. Notably, plasma TBG levels are increased by oestrogens, whereas they are decreased by androgens. In addition, different endogenous factors, such as free fatty acids, and drugs, such as salicylates, competitively inhibit T_4 binding to TBG (25).

A large number of mutations have also been identified in the *TTR* gene, some of which are associated with a decrease in T_4 binding affinity, whereas others (e.g. Ala109Thr and Thr119Met) result in an increased affinity for T_4 (28). More importantly, however, *TTR* mutations often cause neuropathic or cardiomyopathic amyloidosis, resulting from the deposition of insoluble TTR fibrils in nerves or the heart (28). Finally, binding of thyroid hormone to albumin is subject to genetic variation. In particular, a specific increase in the binding of T_4 to albumin is frequently observed in otherwise healthy subjects, which may lead to the false diagnosis of hyperthyroidism if inadequate methods for analysis of plasma free T_4 are used (25). This phenomenon of familial dysalbuminaemic hyperthyroxinaemia has been attributed to mutations in the albumin gene, resulting in a marked increase in T_4 affinity (29).

Perturbation of plasma iodothyronine binding provokes an adaptation of the hypothalamus–pituitary–thyroid axis until normal free T_4 and free T_3 concentrations are again obtained. Therefore, measurement of plasma free T_4 rather than total T_4 levels is, together with analysis of plasma TSH, the cornerstone of the diagnosis of thyroid disorders.

Tissue transport

Because iodothyronines are lipophilic compounds, it has been generally assumed that they readily pass the plasma membrane by simple diffusion. However, the polar nature of the alanine side chain ('zwitterion') is a serious obstacle for passage through the lipid bilayer of the cell membrane. However, studies in recent years have established that tissue uptake of thyroid hormone does not take place by diffusion but is mediated by specific plasma membrane transporters (30). Most studies have been carried out in isolated rat hepatocytes, but carrier-mediated uptake of iodothyronines has been demonstrated in a variety of cells, including neuronal cells, astrocytes, erythrocytes, thymocytes, choriocarcinoma cells, fibroblasts, (cardio)myocytes, and anterior pituitary (tumour) cells (30).

The kinetics of T_4 and T_3 uptake by isolated rat hepatocytes suggest the involvement of multiple mechanisms with different affinities (30). The high-affinity components are characterized by K_m values in the nanomolar range and most likely represent cellular uptake of the iodothyronines by specific transporters. The low-affinity components are characterized by K_m values in the micromolar range and may represent uptake of the iodothyronines by nonspecific transporters or binding to the cell surface. Although T_3 is capable of inhibiting T_4 uptake, and vice versa, the large difference between the K_m and K_i values for each iodothyronine suggests the involvement of different transporters (30).

High-affinity transport of thyroid hormone into rat liver cells is an active process, dependent on the ATP content of the cells. A decrease in cellular ATP has a greater effect on T_4 and reverse T_3 uptake than on T_3 uptake, supporting the involvement of different transporters. *In vitro* studies in isolated human hepatocytes as well as *in vivo* studies in human subjects also suggest energy-dependent thyroid hormone uptake into the human liver. Uptake of iodothyronines by hepatocytes is inhibited by the Na^+,K^+-ATPase inhibitor ouabain, suggesting Na^+ dependence of the transporters involved (30). Thyroid hormone uptake in liver is inhibited by different iodinated compounds such as the antiarrhythmic drug amiodarone and the radiographic contrast agents iopanoic acid and ipodate (see below).

The mechanisms of thyroid hormone uptake appear to differ between tissues as studies in rat pituitary cells suggest a common transporter for T_4 and T_3, whereas neonatal rat cardiomyocytes show preferential uptake of T_3 over T_4 (30). In view of the iodothyronine structure, it is not surprising that thyroid hormone uptake by different cell types is mediated, at least in part, by amino acid transporters showing partial (L-type) or complete (T-type) preference for aromatic amino acids (31, 32).

Thyroid hormone transporters

Since 2000, a number of thyroid hormone transporters have been identified at the molecular level (Fig. 3.1.2.6). These include the Na-taurocholate cotransporting polypeptide (NTCP), different members of the organic anion transporting polypeptide (OATP) family, the L-type amino acid transporters (LATs), and members of the monocarboxylate transporter family (33, 34).

Of these transporters, only NTCP (SLC10A1) transports its ligands in a Na^+-dependent manner (35). It is exclusively expressed in liver and transports primarily bile acids. Human NTCP consists of 349 amino acids and has seven transmembrane domains. The *NTCP* gene is located on chromosome 14q24.1 and has five exons. There are no other thyroid hormone transporters in the SLC10 family. NTCP shows a preference for sulfated over nonsulfated iodothyronines and probably is not the major Na^+-dependent thyroid hormone transporter in liver, which therefore remains elusive.

The human OATP family contains of 11 members, most of which have been shown to transport iodothyronine derivatives (36). In general they are multispecific, transporting a variety of ligands, not only anionic but also neutral and even cationic compounds. OATPs are glycoproteins containing around 700 amino acids and 12 transmembrane domains. The human OATP1 subfamily contains four members (OATP1A2, 1B1, 1B3, 1C1) with quite interesting properties. They are encoded by a gene cluster on chromosome 12p12 containing 14–15 exons. OATP1B1 and 1B3 are expressed only in liver and show preference for sulfated over nonsulfated iodothyronines as ligands (37). The latter also holds for OATP1A2, which is expressed in different tissues. OATP1C1 is by far the most interesting transporter in this subfamily, showing a high preference for T_4 as the ligand and almost exclusive expression in the brain, especially in choroid plexus and capillaries. It thus appears very important for T_4 transport into the brain (36).

T_4 and T_3 are also transported by two members of the heterodimeric amino acid transporters LAT1 and LAT2 (38). These transporters are glycoproteins consisting of two subunits, a heavy chain and a light chain. In humans, there are two possible heavy chains (SLC3A1,2) and least 13 possible light chains (SLC7A1–11,13,14). The heavy chains contain a single transmembrane domain, and the light chains contain 12–14 transmembrane domains. LAT1 is composed of the SLC3A2 (4F2hc or CD98hc) heavy chain and the SLC7A5 light chain, and LAT2 is composed of the same heavy chain and the SLC7A8 light chain. These transporters are expressed in various tissues, and stimulated in activated immune cells and in tumours. Both LAT1 and LAT2 facilitate the bidirectional transport of a variety of aliphatic and aromatic amino acids as well as iodothyronines over the plasma membrane (38).

- **Organic anion transporters**
  NTCP (Na/taurocholate cotransporting polypeptide)
  OATPs (organic anion transporting polypeptides)
- **Amino acid/monocarboxylate transporters**
  LAT1,2 (L-type amino acid transporters)
  MCT8,10* (monocarboxylate transporters)

* MCT10=TAT1 (T-type amino acid transporter)

Fig. 3.1.2.6 Identification of human thyroid hormone transporters.

Two important thyroid hormone transporters come from an unexpected family, the monocarboxylate transporter (MCT) family, named such because MCT1–4 facilitate transport of monocarboxylates such as lactate and pyruvate (39, 40). Functional expression of MCT1–4 requires their interaction with the ancillary proteins basigin (CD147) or embigin. The MCT family contains 14 members, but the function of most of these transporters is as yet unknown. However, two members from this family, MCT8 and MCT10, have recently been identified as important thyroid hormone transporters. Of these, MCT10 also transports the aromatic amino acids Trp, Tyr, and Phe, but so far only iodothyronines have been identified as ligands for MCT8.

Human MCT8 consists of 613 or 539 amino acids, depending on which of the two possible translation start sites is used, and MCT10 has 515 amino acids. They are homologous proteins with about 50% amino acid identity between 'short' MCT8 and MCT10 (Fig. 3.1.2.7). Like the other MCTs, both MCT8 and MCT10 have 12 transmembrane domains. However, they are not glycosylated and they also do not appear to require ancillary proteins for functional expression. They have identical gene structures; the *MCT8* gene is located on human chromosome Xq13.2, and the *MCT10* gene is located on chromosome 6q21-q22. Both consist of six exons and five introns, with a large approximately 100 kb first intron. MCT8 and MCT10 show wide but different tissue distributions.

MCT8 and MCT10 are the most active and specific thyroid hormone transporters known today (34, 41, 42). MCT8 is importantly expressed in brain, where it is localized in choroid plexus, capillaries, and neurons in different brain areas. MCT8 appears to be essential for T_3 uptake in central neurons and, thus, for the crucial action of thyroid hormone during brain development. Mutations in MCT8 have recently been identified as the cause of the Allan–Herndon–Dudley syndrome that occurs in male patients and is characterized by severe psychomotor retardation in combination with highly elevated serum T_3 levels (34, 41, 42) (see Chapter **3.4.8**).

Thyroid hormone metabolism takes place intracellularly (see next section) and requires cellular uptake of iodothyronines over the plasma membrane. Thus, T_4 uptake in T_3-producing tissues is one of the factors determining peripheral T_3 production (30). A diminished liver T_4 uptake may therefore contribute to the decreased T_3 production underlying the low T_3 syndrome induced by nonthyroidal illness and fasting. This may be due in part to inhibition of T_4 transporters by plasma factors such as bilirubin and free fatty acids, which are increased in illness. Radiographic agents and other iodinated compounds such as the antiarrhythmic drug amiodarone also inhibit liver uptake of T_4 which may contribute to the decrease in serum T_3 induced by their administration. Since T_3 exerts most of its effects by binding to intracellular (nuclear)

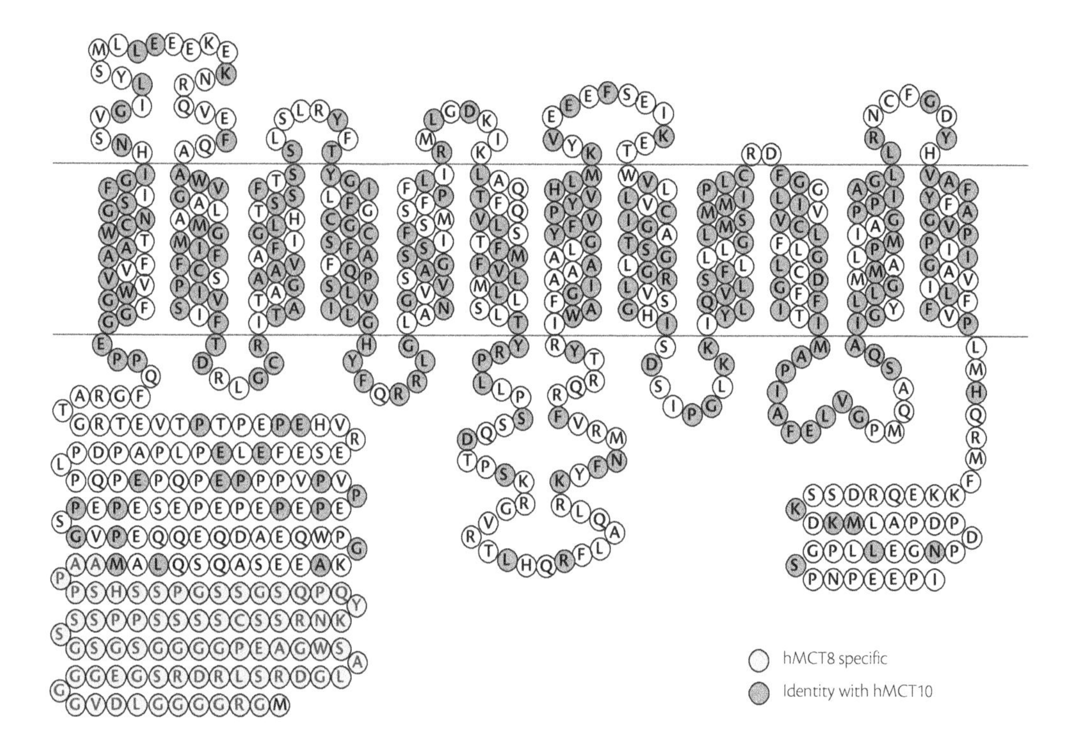

Fig. 3.1.2.7 Protein structure of human MCT8 and MCT10.

receptors, thyroid hormone bioactivity also depends on the activity of T_3 transporters in different tissues.

Metabolism of thyroid hormone

Deiodination

The thyroid gland of a healthy human adult with an adequate iodine intake produces predominantly the prohormone T_4 and only a small amount of the bioactive hormone T_3. It is generally accepted that, in humans, approximately 80% of circulating T_3 is produced by enzymatic outer ring deiodination (ORD) of T_4 in peripheral tissues (23). Alternatively, inner ring deiodination (IRD) of T_4 produces the inactive metabolite reverse T_3, thyroidal secretion of which is negligible. Deiodination is also an important pathway by which T_3 and reverse T_3 are further metabolized. T_3 largely undergoes IRD to the inactive compound T_2, which is also the main metabolite produced from reverse T_3 by ORD (Fig. 3.1.2.8). Thus, the bioactivity of thyroid hormone is determined to an important extent by the enzyme activities responsible for the ORD (activation) or IRD (inactivation) of iodothyronines.

Three iodothyronine deiodinases (D1–3) are involved in the reductive deiodination of thyroid hormone (Fig. 3.1.2.9) (43). They are homologous proteins consisting of 249–278 amino acids, with a single transmembrane domain located at the N-terminus. The deiodinases are inserted in cellular membranes such that the major part of the protein is exposed on the cytoplasmic surface. This is consistent with the reductive nature of the cytoplasmic compartment required for the deiodination process. Probably all three deiodinases are functionally expressed as homodimers (43).

The most remarkable feature of all three deiodinases is the presence of a selenocysteine (Sec) residue in the centre of the amino acid sequence. As in other selenoproteins, this Sec residue is encoded by a UGA triplet, which in mRNAs for nonselenoproteins functions as a translation stop codon. The translation of the UGA codon into Sec requires the presence of a particular stemloop structure in the 3′-untranslated region of the mRNA, termed Sec-insertion sequence (SECIS) element, Sec-tRNA, and a number of cellular proteins, including SECIS-binding protein (SBP2). A bona fide SECIS element has been identified in the mRNA of all deiodinases (43).

D1 is a membrane-bound enzyme expressed predominantly in liver, kidneys, and thyroid (43). It catalyses the ORD and/or IRD of a variety of iodothyronine derivatives, although it is most effective in the ORD of reverse T_3. In the presence of dithiothreitol (DTT) as the cofactor, D1 displays high K_m and V_{max} values. Hepatic D1 is probably a major site for the production of plasma T_3 and clearance

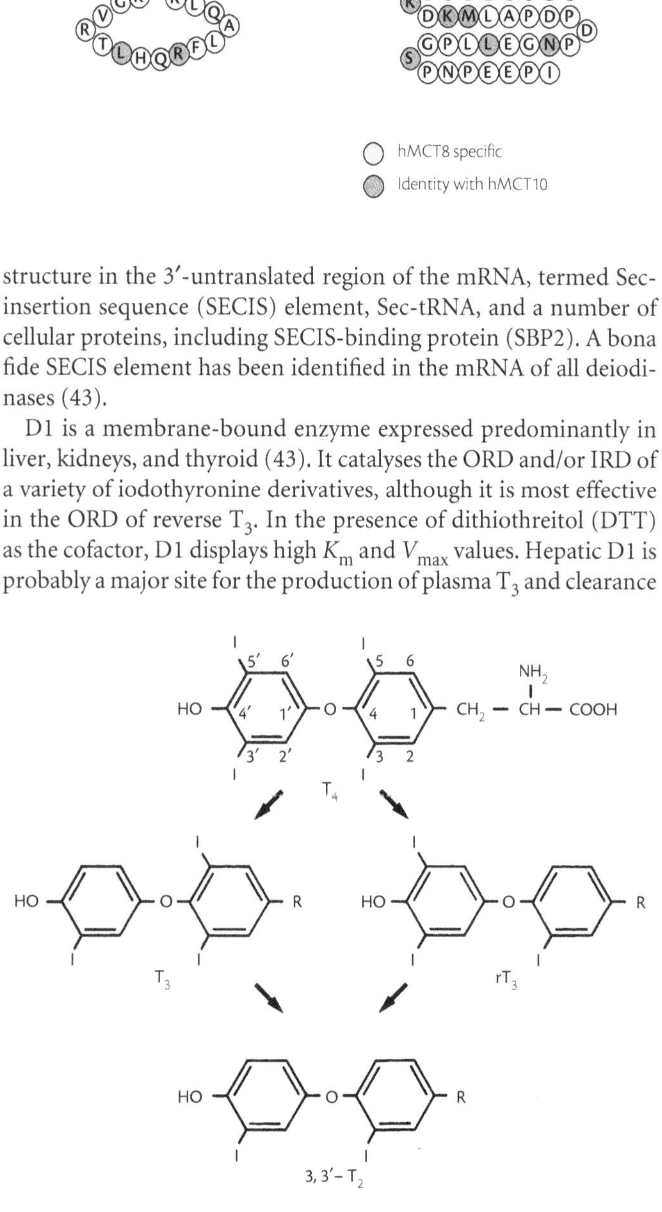

Fig. 3.1.2.8 Conversion of the prohormone T_4 by outer ring deiodination (ORD) to the bioactive hormone T_3 or by inner ring deiodination (IRD) to the metabolite reverse T_3, and further conversion of T_3 by IRD and of reverse T_3 by ORD to the common metabolite T_2.

Type	D1	D2	D3
	$T_4 \rightarrow T_3$, rT_3; T_3, $rT_3 \rightarrow T_2$	$T_4 \rightarrow T_3$; $rT_3 \rightarrow T_2$	$T_4 \rightarrow rT_3$; $T_3 \rightarrow T_2$
Tissues, e.g.	liver, kidney, thyroid	brain, pituitary, thyroid skeletal muscle, heart(?)	brain, placenta uterus, fetal tissues
Susbtrates	$rT_3 \gg T_4 \approx T_3$	$T_4 > rT_3$	$T_3 > T_4$
K_m values	≈0.1-10 μM	≈1 nM	≈10 nM
Function	plasma T_3 production	local T_3 production	T_3 degradation
Inhibitors (IC_{50}, μM)			
PTU	≈5	>1000	>1000
IAc	≈2	≈1000	≈1000
GTG	≈0.05	≈1	≈5
Hypothyroidism	decrease	increase	decrease
Hyperthyroidism	increase	decrease	increase

Fig. 3.1.2.9 Properties of the three iodothyronine deiodinases.

of plasma reverse T_3. D1 activity in liver and kidney is increased in hyperthyroidism and decreased in hypothyroidism, representing the regulation of D1 activity by T_3 at the transcriptional level.

Hepatic and renal D1 activities are strongly reduced in rats fed a selenium-deficient diet, resulting in a decrease in serum T_3 and an increase in serum T_4. The Sec residue is essential for the function of D1 since substitution with Cys reduces enzyme activity to 1%, while substitution with Leu yields a completely inactive protein. Rapid inactivation of D1 by iodoacetate is probably due to modification of the highly reactive Sec residue. Moreover, D1 activity is extremely sensitive to inhibition by very low concentrations of gold thioglucose by formation of a stable complex with the Sec residue. Thus, Sec is the catalytic centre of D1 (Fig. 3.1.2.10).

The different deiodinases require thiols as cofactor. Although reduced glutathione is the most abundant intracellular thiol, its activity is very low compared with the unnatural thiol DTT, which is often used in *in vitro* studies. Alternative endogenous cofactors include dihydrolipoamide, glutaredoxin, and thioredoxin. D1 shows ping-pong-type kinetics in catalysing the deiodination of iodothyronines by DTT. D1 activity is potently inhibited by propylthiouracil, and this inhibition is uncompetitive with substrate and competitive with cofactor. Together, these findings suggest that the catalytic mechanism of D1 involves the transfer of an iodinium ion (I^+) from the substrate to the selenolate (Se^-) group of the enzyme, generating a selenenyl iodide intermediate which is reduced back to native enzyme by thiols such as DTT or converted into a dead-end complex by propylthiouracil (Fig. 3.1.2.10).

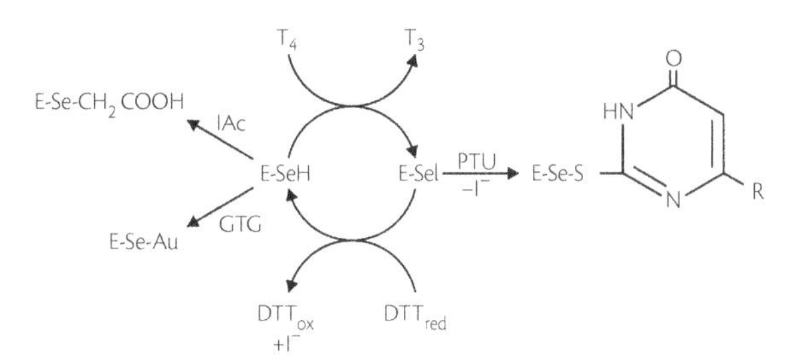

Fig. 3.1.2.10 Putative model of the catalytic mechanism of the type 1 iodothyronine deiodinase and its inhibition by propylthiouracil, iodoacetate, and gold thioglucose.

D2 is expressed primarily in brain, anterior pituitary, brown adipose tissue, thyroid, and to some extent also in skeletal muscle (43, 44). D2 mRNA is also expressed in human heart, but it is unknown to what extent this is translated into functional deiodinase. In brain, D2 mRNA has been localized in astrocytes, in particular also in tanycytes lining the third ventricle in the arcuate nucleus–median eminence region. D2 is a low-K_m, low-capacity enzyme possessing only ORD activity, with a preference for T_4 over reverse T_3 as the substrate. The amount of T_3 in brain, pituitary, and brown adipose tissue is derived to a large extent from local conversion of T_4 by D2 and to a minor extent from plasma T_3 (23, 43). The enzyme located in the anterior pituitary and the arcuate nucleus of the hypothalamus appears very important for the negative feedback regulation of TSH and TRH secretion (1).

In general, D2 activity is increased in hypothyroidism and decreased in hyperthyroidism. This is explained in part by substrate-induced inactivation of the enzyme by T_4 and reverse T_3 involving the ubiquitin-proteasome system (43). However, inhibition of D2 activity and mRNA levels by T_3 has also been demonstrated in the brain and pituitary. The substrate (T_4, reverse T_3) and product (T_3)-dependent down-regulation of D2 activity is important to maintain brain T_3 levels in the face of changing plasma thyroid hormone levels.

In mammals, D2 mRNA contains a second UGA codon just upstream of a UAA stop codon (43). It remains to be determined to what extent this second TGA codon specifies the incorporation of a second Sec residue or acts as a translation stop codon. The amino acid sequence downstream of this second Sec is not required for enzyme activity.

D3 activity has been detected in different human tissues, brain, skin, liver, and intestine, where activities are much higher in the fetal stage than in the adult stage (43). D3 is also abundantly expressed in placenta and pregnant uterus. D3 has only IRD activity, catalysing the inactivation of T_4 and T_3 with intermediate K_m and V_{max} values. D3 in tissues such as the brain is thought to play a role in the regulation of intracellular T_3 levels, while its presence in placenta, pregnant uterus, and fetal tissues may serve to protect developing organs against undue exposure to active thyroid hormone. Indeed, fetal plasma contains low T_3 (and high reverse T_3) concentrations. However, local D2-mediated T_3 production from T_4 is crucial for brain development. Also in adult subjects, D3 appears to be an important site for clearance of plasma T_3 and production of plasma reverse T_3. In brain, but not in placenta, D3 activity is increased in hyperthyroidism and decreased in hypothyroidism, which at least in brain is associated with parallel changes in D3 mRNA levels (23, 43).

In contrast to the marked decrease in hepatic and renal (but not thyroidal) D1 activities, there are only minor effects of selenium deficiency on tissue D2 and D3 activities (45). This may be explained by findings that the selenium state of different tissues varies greatly in selenium-deficient animals. In addition, the efficiency of the SECIS element to facilitate read-through of the UGA codon may differ among selenoproteins, which could result in the preferred incorporation of Sec into D2 or D3 over other selenoproteins.

The presence of Sec in a strongly conserved region of the proteins suggests the same catalytic mechanism for the different deiodinases. However, D2 and D3 are much less susceptible than D1 to the mechanism-based inhibitors propylthiouracil, iodoacetate, and gold thioglucose (43). This could be explained if the reactivity of the selenol group in D2 and D3 is much lower than that in D1. Indeed, substitution of Sec in D1 with the much less reactive Cys is associated with a dramatic decrease in its sensitivity to inhibition by gold thioglucose and propylthiouracil. Interestingly, the amino acid two positions downstream of the catalytic Sec residue (Ser in D1, Pro in D2 and D3) plays an important role in determining the reactivity of the catalytic Sec residue (43).

Alanine side chain modification

Intriguing metabolites are generated by side-chain metabolism of iodothyronines (Fig. 3.1.2.11). Presumably by action of aromatic L-amino acid decarboxylase (AADC) iodothyronines are converted into iodothyronamines. In particular two of these, 3-iodothyronamine (T_1AM) and thyronamine (T_0AM), have high affinity for the trace amine receptor TAR1, and exert acute and dramatic effects on heart rate, body temperature, and physical activity, inducing a torpor-like state (46). Thus, these thyroid hormone metabolites appear to have neurotransmitter-like properties, adding a novel dimension to the already diverse effects of the conventional thyroid hormone structures.

Presumably by further conversion of iodothyronamines by the monoamine oxidases MAO-A or MAO-B, the iodothyroacetic acid metabolites 3,3′,5,5′-tetraiodothyroacetic acid (Tetrac) and 3,3′,5-triiodothyroacetic acid (Triac) are generated from T_4 and T_3, respectively (Fig. 3.1.2.11) (47). Although, in general, oxidative deamination is an inactivating pathway for monoamines, Triac has significant thyromimetic activity and its affinity for the T_3 receptor TRα1 is equal to that of T_3 and for the TRβ receptor it is even higher that of T_3 (see next section). There may be multiple pathways leading from T_4 and T_3 to T_1AM and T_0AM with different orders for the successive decarboxylation and deiodination steps. Iodothyronamines are deiodinated by the different deiodinases (48), but it is unknown which iodothyronines are substrates for AADC or which iodothyronamines are converted by MAO-A or MAO-B. Also, the exact biological functions of the iodothyronamine and iodothyroacetic acid metabolites remain to be established.

Sulfation

In addition to deiodination, iodothyronines are metabolized by conjugation of the phenolic hydroxyl group with sulfate or glucuronic acid (Fig. 3.1.2.11). Sulfation and glucuronidation are so-called phase II detoxification reactions, which increase the water solubility of substrates and, thus, facilitate their biliary and/or urinary clearance. However, iodothyronine sulfate levels are normally very low in plasma, bile, and urine, as these conjugates are rapidly degraded by D1, suggesting that sulfate conjugation is a primary step leading to the irreversible inactivation of thyroid hormone (49, 50). Thus, the IRD of T_4 sulfate to reverse T_3 sulfate and of T_3 sulfate to T_2 sulfate is orders of magnitude faster than the IRD of nonsulfated T_4 and T_3, whereas the ORD of T_4 sulfate to T_3 sulfate is completely blocked. Plasma levels (and biliary excretion) of iodothyronine sulfates are increased if D1 activity is inhibited by drugs such as propylthiouracil, and during fetal development, nonthyroidal illness, and fasting. Under these conditions, T_3 sulfate may function as a reservoir of inactive hormone from which active T_3 may be recovered by action of tissue sulfatases and bacterial sulfatases in the intestine.

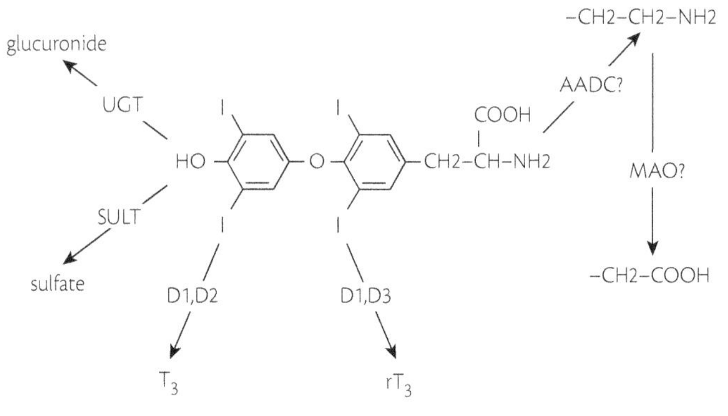

Sulfotransferases represent a family of enzymes with a monomer molecular weight of approximately 34 kDa, located in the cytoplasm of different tissues, in particular liver, kidney, intestine, and brain. They catalyse the transfer of sulfate from 3′-phosphoadenosine-5′-phosphosulfate to usually a hydroxyl group of the substrate. Different phenol sulfotransferases have been identified with significant activity towards iodothyronines. These include human SULT1A1, 1A2, 1A3, 1B1, and 1C2 (49). They have a large substrate preference for T_2, which is sulfated orders of magnitude faster than T_3 or reverse T_3, whereas sulfation of T_4 is hardly detectable.

Surprisingly, human oestrogen sulfotransferase (SULT1E1) is an important isoenzyme for sulfation of thyroid hormone. Although human SULT1E1 shows much greater affinity for oestrogens (K_m *c.*nM) than for iodothyronines (K_m *c.*μM), it sulfates T_2 and T_3 as efficiently as other SULTs, and is much more efficient in sulfating reverse T_3 and T_4 (49). Human tissues expressing SULT1E1 include liver, uterus, and mammary gland (51). In particular, the enzyme expressed in the endometrium may be a significant source of the high levels of iodothyronine sulfates in human fetal plasma. Different human SULTs have also been shown to catalyse the sulfation of iodothyronamines (52).

Glucuronidation

In contrast to the sulfates, iodothyronine glucuronides are rapidly excreted in the bile. However, this is not an irreversible pathway of hormone disposal since, after hydrolysis of the glucuronides by bacterial β-glucuronidases in the intestine, part of the liberated iodothyronines is reabsorbed, constituting an enterohepatic cycle (50, 53). Nevertheless, about 20% of daily T_4 production appears in the faeces, probably through biliary excretion of glucuronide conjugates. Glucuronidation is catalysed by UDP-glucuronyltransferases (UGTs) that utilize UDP-glucuronic acid as cofactor. UGTs are localized in the endoplasmic reticulum of predominantly liver, kidney, and intestine. Most UGTs are members of the UGT1A and UGT2B families (54).

Glucuronidation of T_4 and T_3 is catalysed by different members of the UGT1A family, 1A1, 1A3, and 1A7–10. Usually, this involves the glucuronidation of the hydroxyl group (Fig. 3.1.2.11), but human UGT1A3 also catalyses the glucuronidation of the side-chain carboxyl group, with formation of so-called acyl glucuronides (55). Interestingly, Tetrac and Triac are much more rapidly glucuronidated in human liver than T_4 and T_3, and this occurs predominantly by acyl glucuronidation (56).

Fig. 3.1.2.11 Pathways of thyroid hormone metabolism.

In rodents, metabolism of thyroid hormone is accelerated through induction of T_4-glucuronidating UGTs by different classes of compounds, including barbiturates, fibrates, and polychlorinated biphenyls (57, 58). This may result in a hypothyroid state as the thyroid gland is not capable of compensating for the increased hormone loss. In humans, thyroid function may be affected by induction of T_4 glucuronidation by antiepileptics, but overt hypothyroidism is rare (59). Administration of such drugs to T_4-replaced hypothyroid patients may necessitate an increase in the T_4 substitution dose.

Thyroid hormone actions

Role of thyroid hormone in thermogenesis

Thyroid hormone is critical for the development of different tissues, in particular the brain, but it is also essential for an optimal function of most tissues in adult life (60). It is probably the most important factor regulating thermogenesis, as reflected by the increase in the basal metabolic rate in hyperthyroid subjects and the decrease observed in hypothyroid individuals (61–63). The positive effect of thyroid hormone on the resting metabolic rate appears to be largely mediated by the stimulation of so-called futile cycles. This concerns the cycling of substrates of the intermediary metabolism as well as that of cations such as Na^+, K^+, and Ca^{2+} across cellular membranes. Such cycles result in the net hydrolysis of ATP, the energy of which is dissipated as heat. Thyroid hormone increases the synthesis as well the degradation of proteins, lipids, and carbohydrates, predominantly by stimulating the expression of key enzymes involved in these processes. Examples of these are the lipogenic enzymes, malic enzyme, fatty acid synthase, and glucose-6-phosphate dehydrogenase, and the gluconeogenic enzyme phosphoenolpyruvate carboxykinase.

Special forms of substrate cycling take place between the cytoplasm and the mitochondrion, such as the glycerol-3-phosphate/dihydroxyacetone phosphate shuttle in which cytoplasmic and mitochondrial α-glycerophosphate dehydrogenase (αGPD) isoenzymes participate (61, 62). This represents one way to enable oxidation of cytoplasmic NADH in the mitochondrion, which is impermeable to this cofactor. Thyroid hormone stimulates the expression of mitochondrial αGPD, and the increased electron flow via this enzyme is associated with an increased heat production relative to ATP synthesis.

Thyroid hormone also increases the activity of Na^+,K^+-ATPase, an enzyme located in the plasma membrane of all tissues, in particular kidney, heart, and skeletal muscle, which is responsible for the maintenance of the Na^+ and K^+ gradients across this membrane. This increased Na^+,K^+-ATPase activity is only functional if associated with—and perhaps triggered by—the activation of processes that tend to dissipate these gradients (61, 62). Tissue uptake of glucose, amino acids, fatty acids, and other nutrients predominantly occurs by cotransport with Na^+ via specific plasma membrane transporters. Stimulated cycling of these substrates by thyroid hormone, which may also involve increased expression of the transporters, is thus accompanied by a significant cellular Na^+ influx. In addition, thyroid hormone may promote the permeability of the cell membrane for Na^+ and K^+ by activation of channels for these ions. In myocytes, the increased Na^+,K^+-ATPase activity accelerates the repolarization of the sarcolemma following a depolarization stimulus that contributes to the tachycardia induced by thyroid hormone. T_3 stimulates the expression of both (α and β) subunits of Na^+,K^+-ATPase by increasing the transcription of the genes as well as by stabilization of the mRNAs (61).

Another important target for thyroid hormone action is the Ca^{2+}-ATPase located in the sarcoplasmic reticulum of muscle cells (63). Innervation of the myocyte triggers the release of large amounts of Ca^{2+} from the sarcoplasmic reticulum into the cytoplasm, where it binds to the actomyosin complex that initiates contraction. Relaxation of the muscle requires the reuptake of the Ca^{2+} into the sarcoplasmic reticulum by Ca^{2+}-ATPase at the expense of ATP. There are two Ca^{2+}-ATPase isoenzymes, SERCA1 that is characteristic for fast-type skeletal muscle and SERCA2 that is characteristic for slow-type skeletal muscle and heart. T_3 increases Ca^{2+}-ATPase activity by stimulating the transcription of both *SERCA1* and *SERCA2* genes, which explains the increased relaxation rate of the muscle induced by T_3 (63).

It is difficult to estimate how much the increased Ca^{2+}-ATPase activity accounts for the T_3-induced increase in resting energy expenditure of muscle, since the extent of futile Ca^{2+} cycling is unknown in resting muscle. This depends not only on the activity of the Ca^{2+}-ATPase but also on the rate of Ca^{2+} leak from the sarcoplasmic reticulum. However, it has been estimated that excess Ca^{2+} cycling in contracting muscle may account for up to 50% of the T_3-dependent energy expenditure during work or shivering (63). The remainder of the T_3-induced energy turnover in contracting muscle is largely accounted for by the change in the expression of two forms of the myosin heavy chain which are characterized by high (MHCα) and low (MHCβ) ATPase activities and contraction rates. T_3 stimulates the expression of the *MHCα* gene, whereas it inhibits the expression of the *MHCβ* gene (63). A similar T_3-induced shift in MHC expression is also observed in the heart (64).

In addition, T_3 increases the expression of the uncoupling protein UCP1 in brown adipose tissue (BAT) (61, 62). This is an important mechanism by which T_3 stimulates nonshivering cold-induced thermogenesis. UCP1 is an ion transporter located in the inner mitochondrial membrane which dissipates the proton gradient over this membrane generated by the respiratory chain, producing heat instead of ATP. Significant amounts of BAT were thought to be present only in small mammals and the human infant. Recently, however, significant BAT depots have also been demonstrated in the neck and shoulder region of normal adults, especially in cold-adapted subjects and more so in younger females than in older males (65). Cold exposure leads to a dramatic stimulation of D2 expression in BAT, and the resultant induction of local T_3 production plays an important role in the stimulation of BAT activity. This includes increased mobilization and burning of lipids as well as stimulated UCP1 expression, together resulting in a major increase in heat production (61, 62).

UCP1 is expressed exclusively in BAT. Other members of the UCP family are expressed in other human tissues, including UCP2 in a variety of tissues including heart and skeletal muscle, UCP3 in skeletal muscle, and UCP4 and UCP5 in brain. The expression of UCP2 and UCP3 is also under positive control of thyroid hormone, but their role in T_3-induced thermogenesis has not been established (66).

The regulation of the mitochondrial proteins UCP1 and αGPD by thyroid hormone is mediated predominantly by interaction of the nuclear T_3 receptor with the promoters of these genes (61, 66). However, there is also evidence for direct effects of thyroid hormone on the mitochondria, the mechanism of which is incompletely understood but may involve interaction of T_3 and other iodothyronines such as 3,3'-T_2 and 3,5-T_2 with cytochrome *c* oxidase (67). Many studies have reported effects of thyroid hormone on cellular processes that are not mediated by the nuclear T_3 receptor, including stimulation of transport of glucose, amino acids, and ions over the cell membrane, stimulation of actin polymerization in neurons, and stimulation of mitogen-activated protein kinase activity. The last is mediated by the binding of iodothyronines to integrin, a plasma membrane receptor. The interested reader is referred to a recent extensive review of these extranuclear actions of thyroid hormone (68).

Specific thyroid hormone-binding sites have also been detected in the cytoplasm in different tissues. A notable example is the NADPH-dependent cytoplasmic thyroid hormone-binding protein present in rat liver, which appears to be important for the trafficking of thyroid hormone to the nucleus or mitochondria (69).

Mechanism of T_3 action

Most biological actions of T_3 are initiated by its binding to nuclear T_3 receptors (70–72). These proteins are members of the superfamily of ligand-dependent transcription factors, which also includes the receptors for steroids (e.g. cortisol, oestradiol, and testosterone), 1,25-dihydroxyvitamin D_3, retinoic acid, and 9-*cis*-retinoic acid. The last, so-called retinoid X receptor (RXR) is an important member of this gene family, because it forms functional heterodimers with a number of other nuclear receptors, including T_3 receptors. Two T_3 receptor genes have been identified; the α gene is located on human chromosome 17 and the β gene on human chromosome 3. By alternative exon utilization of both genes, four major receptor isoforms, TRα1, TRα2, TRβ1, and TRβ2, are generated, which consist of 410–514 amino acids (Fig. 3.1.2.12). Although the β gene (150 kb) is much larger than the α gene (*c*.30 kb), they have similar genomic structures, comprising 10 (β) or 11 (α) exons, and their coding sequences show a high degree of homology (70–72).

As in the other members of the nuclear receptor family, functional key domains have been recognized in the T_3 receptors, in particular the DNA-binding domain (DBD), which is approximately 100 amino acids long, and the ligand-binding domain (LBD), which is approximately 250 amino acids in length (70–72). The amino acid sequences of the TRα and TRβ subtypes are most homologous in their DBD and LBD and least homologous at their N-terminus. The latter contains the ligand-independent AF1 transactivation domain, while an AF2 domain necessary for homo- and heterodimerization and ligand-dependent activation is located at the C-terminus. The short sequence between the DBD and the LBD is usually referred to as the hinge region.

The structural difference between TRα1 and TRα2 is located at the C-terminus of the proteins, where the sequences of the last 40 amino acids in TRα1 and 122 amino acids in TRα2 differ completely due to alternative splicing. The alteration in the LBD of TRα2 is associated with a complete loss of T_3 binding. Therefore, this splice variant is not a bona fide T_3 receptor, but for convenience it will still be referred to here as TRα2. TRα2 has a weak negative effect on the action of T_3 through the other T_3 receptors. The N-terminal domains of TRβ1 (106 amino acids) and TRβ2 (159 amino acids) differ almost completely due to utilization of alternative transcription start sites. Apparently, this domain provides TRβ2 with specific properties required for T_3-induced down-regulation of *TRH* and *TSH* genes (70–72).

The high homology between the LBDs of TRα1 and TRβ explains their very similar ligand specificity, with affinities decreasing in the order T_3 more than T_4 more than reverse T_3. However, the metabolite Triac also binds to the T_3 receptors with an affinity equal to (TRα1) or even greater than (TRβ1) that of T_3 (73). Nevertheless, T_3 is the major endogenous iodothyronine occupying the nuclear thyroid hormone receptors, which are thus true T_3 receptors. Recently, several TRβ-specific agonists have been developed with pharmacologically interesting and selective effects on the liver, resulting in lowering of body weight, lipid, and cholesterol without detrimental effects on the heart (72, 73). Most likely, the tissue-specific effects of these compounds is not only determined by their affinity for the T_3 receptor isoforms but also by the diverse ligand-preference of thyroid hormone transporters in different tissues. Interestingly, nonselective T_3 receptor antagonists have been developed as well (72, 73).

The different T_3 receptor isoforms show distinct tissue distributions (70–72). The TRα1 is the predominant T_3 receptor expressed in brain, heart, and bone, whereas TRβ1 is the major receptor in other tissues, including liver, skeletal muscle, kidney, and fat. TRβ2 is preferentially expressed in the anterior pituitary and the hypothalamic area of the brain. These locations suggest the particular involvement of TRβ2 in the feedback inhibition of TSH and TRH secretion by thyroid hormone. Exon utilization specifying TRβ2 expression in the anterior pituitary is under the control of pituitary-specific transcription factor 1, response elements for which are located in the TRβ gene promoter (74). Regulation of the expression of T_3-responsive genes involves the binding of the T_3 receptors to so-called T_3 response elements (TREs) in the

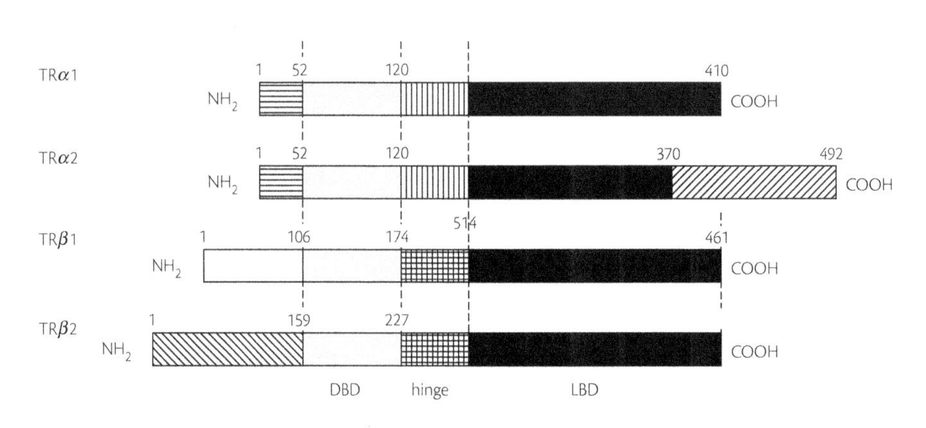

Fig. 3.1.2.12 Domain structures of the different T_3 receptor (TR) isoforms. The TRα2 variant is incapable of binding T_3. DBD, DNA-binding domain; LBD ligand-binding domain.

promoter region of these genes (70–72). TREs usually consist of two half-sites arranged as repeats or palindromes. The most prevalent TRE half-site sequence is AGGTCA, and the direct repeat of this half-site spaced by four nucleotides (DR4) is a particularly powerful TRE. However, some TREs show marked deviation from this 'consensus' half-site sequence, which, moreover, is also recognized by other receptors such as RXR and the retinoic acid receptor. This may be the basis for 'cross-talk' between different nuclear receptors and their target genes. Although T_3 receptors may bind as homodimers to the TREs, T_3 effects on gene expression are usually mediated by T_3 receptor/RXR heterodimers.

Binding of the T_3 receptor/RXR heterodimer to TRE does not require T_3 or 9-*cis*-retinoic acid, the ligand for RXR. The DBDs of these (and other) nuclear receptors contain two 'zinc fingers' (peptide loops that chelate a zinc atom) that fit in the grooves of the DNA and are, thus, very important for the specificity of the receptor-promoter interaction (70–72). In the absence of T_3 and irrespective of the presence of 9-*cis*-retinoic acid, binding of the T_3 receptor/RXR heterodimer to the TRE results in suppressed gene transcription mediated by the binding of corepressor proteins such as NCoR (nuclear corepressor) or SMRT (silencing mediator of retinoid and thyroid hormone receptors) to a specific region (CoR box) of the unliganded T_3 receptor (Fig. 3.1.2.13). These corepressors directly or indirectly inhibit the activity of the basal transcription machinery.

Binding of T_3 induces a conformational change in the T_3 receptor, which results in the release of the corepressors and the recruitment of coactivator proteins such as SRC1 (steroid receptor coactivator-1) and CBP (cAMP response element-binding protein (CREB)-binding protein) (70–72). The AF2 domain, a highly conserved 9-amino acid sequence located at the C-terminus of the different nuclear receptors, plays an important role in the binding of the coactivators. The latter directly or indirectly stimulate the activity of the basal transcription machinery. One mechanism by which transcription is stimulated involves the histone acetyltransferase activity of the coactivators or of other proteins with which they interact. Acetylation of histones loosens the chromatin structure and thus facilitates interaction of the transcription machinery with the DNA. Conversely, corepressors may recruit proteins with deacetylase activity.

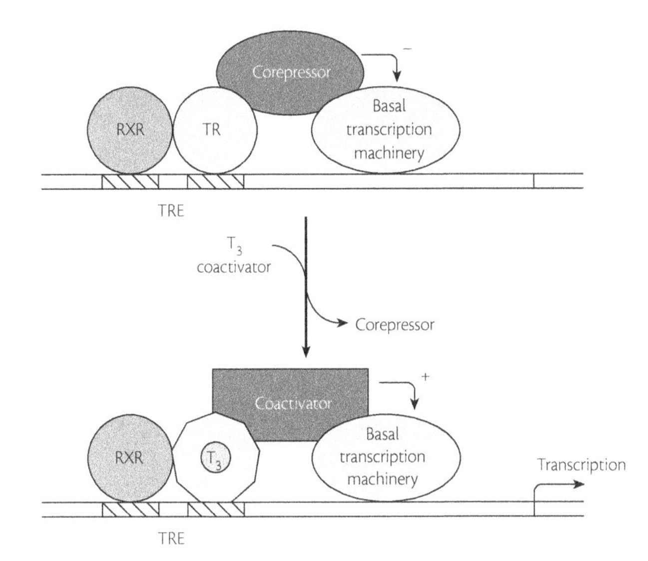

Fig. 3.1.2.13 Simplistic model of the regulation of gene transcription by T_3. RXR, retinoid X receptor; TR, T_3 receptor; TRE, T_3 response element in the promoter of a T_3-responsive gene.

T_3 *inhibition of* TSH *and* TRH *gene expression*

The above discussion of the mechanism of action of T_3 concerns the expression of genes which are under positive control of thyroid hormone. However, a roughly equal number of genes are negatively regulated by T_3, in particular those involved in the negative feedback regulation of the hypothalamus–pituitary–thyroid axis, i.e. the *TSHβ* and the *TRH* genes. In the promoter regions of these genes negative TREs have been identified that often consist of only one half-site. In the *TSHβ* gene such a negative TRE has been found in close proximity to the AP-1 site which mediates the stimulation of *TSHβ* gene transcription by TRH. As mentioned above, there appears to be a specific role for TRβ2 in the regulation of the negative TREs in the *TSHβ* and *TRH* genes (70–72). In contrast to gene regulation through positive TREs, binding of TRβ2 to negative TREs in the absence of T_3 probably results in the activation of gene transcription. In the presence of T_3, transcription is inhibited. The exact mechanism of this negative regulation of gene expression by T_3 and any T_3 receptor is still unclear.

TSHβ gene transcription is also strongly inhibited by 9-*cis*-retinoic acid, and this effect is mediated by the pituitary-specific RXRγ1 subtype, and involves both TRE-dependent and TRE-independent interactions with the *TSHβ* gene promoter. The clinical relevance of this effect is underscored by a recent study showing that treatment of patients with T-cell lymphoma with bexarotene, another RXR-selective ligand, induces central hypothyroidism (75). It is also interesting to mention that the *TRH* gene promoter contains a glucocorticoid response element. Hypothalamic TRH-producing cells also express the glucocorticoid receptor, and the interaction of this receptor with its response element appears to mediate the inhibition of TRH synthesis by glucocorticoids (76).

In addition to the regulation of TSHβ and α-subunit gene expression, T_3 also acutely inhibits TSH secretion, the exact mechanism of which is still unresolved. Although T_3 is the active hormone exerting the inhibition of TSH production and secretion, serum T_4 appears to be a major player in the negative feedback regulation of the hypothalamus–pituitary–thyroid axis by acting as a precursor for local D2-mediated generation of T_3 at these central sites (43, 77).

Recent research in two particular areas has led to important advances in our understanding of the mechanism of action of T_3. One type of study has utilized T_3 receptor knockout and mutant mice in which one or more of the different T_3 receptor isoforms is deleted or mutated (72). These studies reveal which organ functions critically depend on the type of T_3 receptors they express. Much knowledge regarding the molecular mechanisms of T_3 receptor/T_3 action has also been gained from studies in patients with thyroid hormone resistance associated with mutations in the *THRβ* gene. For a thorough discussion of this subject, the reader is referred to Chapter 3.4.8.

References

1. Fliers E, Alkemade A, Wiersinga WM, Swaab DF. Hypothalamic thyroid hormone feedback in health and disease. *Prog Brain Res*, 2006; **153**: 189–207.

2. Perello M, Nillni EA. The biosynthesis and processing of neuropeptides: lessons from prothyrotropin releasing hormone (proTRH). *Front Biosci*, 2007; **12**: 3554–65.
3. Sun Y, Lu X, Gershengorn MC. Thyrotropin-releasing hormone receptors: similarities and differences. *J Mol Endocrinol*, 2003; **30**: 87–97.
4. Heuer H, Schafer MK, Bauer K. The thyrotropin-releasing hormone-degrading ectoenzyme: the third element of the thyrotropin-releasing hormone-signaling system. *Thyroid*, 1998; **8**: 915–20.
5. Grossmann M, Weintraub BD, Szkudlinski MW. Novel insights into the molecular mechanisms of human thyrotropin action: structural, physiological, and therapeutic implications for the glycoprotein hormone family. *Endocr Rev*, 1997; **18**: 476–501.
6. Mariotti S. Normal physiology of the hypothalamic-pituitary-thyroidal system and relation to the neural system and other endocrine glands, in www.thyroidmanager.org, 20 May 2010. South Dartmouth MA: Endocrine Education Inc.
7. Kleinau G, Krause G. Thyrotropin and homologous glycoprotein hormone receptors: structural and functional aspects of extracellular signaling mechanisms. *Endocr Rev*, 2009; **30**: 133–51.
8. Dumont JE, Opitz R, Christophe D, Vassart G, Roger PP, Maenhaut C. The phylogeny, ontogeny, anatomy and regulation of the iodine metabolizing thyroid, in www.thyroidmanager.org, 20 May 2010. South Dartmouth MA: Endocrine Education Inc.
9. Davies TF, Ando T, Lin RY, Tomer Y, Latif R. Thyrotropin receptor-associated diseases: from adenomata to Graves' disease. *J Clin Invest*, 2005; **115**: 1972–83.
10. Kopp P. Thyroid hormone synthesis. In: Braverman LE, Utiger RD, eds. *Werner & Ingbar's The Thyroid*. Philadelphia: Lippincott Williams & Wilkins, 2005: 52–77.
11. Song Y, Driessens N, Costa M, De Deken X, Detours V, Corvilain B, *et al.* Roles of hydrogen peroxide in thyroid physiology and disease. *J Clin Endocrinol Metab*, 2007; **92**: 3764–73.
12. Dohan O, De la Vieja A, Paroder V, Riedel C, Artani M, Reed M, *et al.* The sodium/iodide symporter (NIS): characterization, regulation, and medical significance. *Endocr Rev*, 2003; **24**: 48–77.
13. Kopp P, Pesce L, Solis SJ. Pendred syndrome and iodide transport in the thyroid. *Trends Endocrinol Metab*, 2008; **19**: 260–8.
14. Rivolta CM, Targovnik HM. Molecular advances in thyroglobulin disorders. *Clin Chim Acta*, 2006; **374**: 8–24.
15. Moreno JC, Visser TJ. New phenotypes in thyroid dyshormonogenesis: hypothyroidism due to DUOX2 mutations. *Endocr Dev*, 2007; **10**: 99–117.
16. Grasberger H, Refetoff S. Identification of the maturation factor for dual oxidase. Evolution of an eukaryotic operon equivalent. *J Biol Chem*, 2006; **281**: 18269–72.
17. Taurog A. Hormone synthesis: thyroid iodine metabolism. In: Braverman LE, Utiger RD, eds. *Werner & Ingbar's The Thyroid*. Philadelphia: Lippincott Williams & Wilkins, 2000: 61–85.
18. Lisi S, Pinchera A, McCluskey RT, Willnow TE, Refetoff S, Marcocci C, *et al.* Preferential megalin-mediated transcytosis of low-hormonogenic thyroglobulin: a control mechanism for thyroid hormone release. *Proc Natl Acad Sci U S A*, 2003; **100**: 14858–63.
19. Friedrichs B, Tepel C, Reinheckel T, Deussing J, von Figura K, Herzog V, *et al.* Thyroid functions of mouse cathepsins B, K, and L. *J Clin Invest*, 2003; **111**: 1733–45.
20. Andersson HC, Kohn LD, Bernardini I, Blom HJ, Tietze F, Gahl WA. Characterization of lysosomal monoiodotyrosine transport in rat thyroid cells. Evidence for transport by system h. *J Biol Chem*, 1990; **265**: 10950–4.
21. Gnidehou S, Caillou B, Talbot M, Ohayon R, Kaniewski J, Noel-Hudson MS, *et al.* Iodotyrosine dehalogenase 1 (DEHAL1) is a transmembrane protein involved in the recycling of iodide close to the thyroglobulin iodination site. *FASEB J*, 2004; **18**: 1574–6.
22. Moreno JC, Klootwijk W, van Toor H, Pinto G, D'Alessandro M, Leger A, *et al.* Mutations in the iodotyrosine deiodinase gene and hypothyroidism. *N Engl J Med*, 2008; **358**: 1811–18.
23. Bianco AC, Larsen PR. Intracellular pathways of iodothyronine metabolism. In: Braverman LE, Utiger RD, eds. *Werner & Ingbar's The Thyroid*. Philadelphia: Lippincott Williams & Wilkins, 2005: 109–35.
24. Astwood EB. Landmark article 8 May (1943): treatment of hyperthyroidism with thiourea and thiouracil. *JAMA*, 1984; **251**: 1743–6.
25. Benvenga S. Thyroid hormone transport proteins and the physiology of hormone binding. In: Braverman LE, Utiger RD, eds. *Werner & Ingbar's The Thyroid*. Philadelphia: Lippincott Williams & Wilkins, 2005: 97–109.
26. Refetoff S, Murata Y, Mori Y, Janssen OE, Takeda K, Hayashi Y. Thyroxine-binding globulin: organization of the gene and variants. *Horm Res*, 1996; **45**: 128–38.
27. Richardson SJ. Cell and molecular biology of transthyretin and thyroid hormones. *Int Rev Cytol*, 2007; **258**: 137–93.
28. Saraiva MJ. Transthyretin mutations in hyperthyroxinemia and amyloid diseases. *Hum Mutat*, 2001; **17**: 493–503.
29. Petitpas I, Petersen CE, Ha CE, Bhattacharya AA, Zunszain PA, Ghuman J, *et al.* Structural basis of albumin-thyroxine interactions and familial dysalbuminemic hyperthyroxinemia. *Proc Natl Acad Sci U S A*, 2003; **100**: 6440–5.
30. Hennemann G, Docter R, Friesema EC, de Jong M, Krenning EP, Visser TJ. Plasma membrane transport of thyroid hormones and its role in thyroid hormone metabolism and bioavailability. *Endocr Rev*, 2001; **22**: 451–76.
31. Blondeau JP, Beslin A, Chantoux F, Francon J. Triiodothyronine is a high-affinity inhibitor of amino acid transport system L1 in cultured astrocytes. *J Neurochem*, 1993; **60**: 1407–13.
32. Zhou Y, Samson M, Francon J, Blondeau JP. Thyroid hormone concentrative uptake in rat erythrocytes. Involvement of the tryptophan transport system T in countertransport of tri-iodothyronine and aromatic amino acids. *Biochem J*, 1992; **281**: 81–6.
33. Friesema EC, Jansen J, Milici C, Visser TJ. Thyroid hormone transporters. *Vitam Horm*, 2005; **70**: 137–67.
34. Visser WE, Friesema EC, Jansen J, Visser TJ. Thyroid hormone transport in and out of cells. *Trends Endocrinol Metab*, 2008; **19**: 50–6.
35. Geyer J, Wilke T, Petzinger E. The solute carrier family SLC10: more than a family of bile acid transporters regarding function and phylogenetic relationships. *Naunyn Schmiedebergs Arch Pharmacol*, 2006; **372**: 413–31.
36. Hagenbuch B. Cellular entry of thyroid hormones by organic anion transporting polypeptides. *Best Pract Res*, 2007; **21**: 209–21.
37. van der Deure W, Peeters R, Visser T. Molecular aspects of thyroid hormone transporters, including MCT8, MCT10 and OATPs, and the effects of genetic variation in these transporters. *J Mol Endocrinol*, 2010; **44**: 1 11.
38. Taylor PM, Ritchie JW. Tissue uptake of thyroid hormone by amino acid transporters. *Best Pract Res*, 2007; **21**: 237–51.
39. Halestrap AP, Meredith D. The SLC16 gene family-from monocarboxylate transporters (MCTs) to aromatic amino acid transporters and beyond. *Pflugers Arch*, 2004; **447**: 619–28.
40. Meredith D, Christian HC. The SLC16 monocarboxylate transporter family. *Xenobiotica*, 2008; **38**: 1072–106.
41. Heuer H, Visser TJ. Minireview: pathophysiological importance of thyroid hormone transporters. *Endocrinology*, 2009; **150**: 1078–83.
42. Visser WE, Friesema EC, Jansen J, Visser TJ. Thyroid hormone transport by monocarboxylate transporters. *Best Pract Res*, 2007; **21**: 223–36.
43. Gereben B, Zavacki AM, Ribich S, Kim BW, Huang SA, Simonides WS, *et al.* Cellular and molecular basis of deiodinase-regulated thyroid hormone signaling. *Endocr Rev*, 2008; **29**: 898–938.
44. Larsen PR. Type 2 iodothyronine deiodinase in human skeletal muscle: new insights into its physiological role and regulation. *J Clin Endocrinol Metab*, 2009; **94**: 1893–5.

45. Kohrle J. Selenium and the control of thyroid hormone metabolism. *Thyroid*, 2005; **15**: 841–53.
46. Scanlan TS. Minireview: 3-iodothyronamine (T1AM): a new player on the thyroid endocrine team? *Endocrinology*, 2009; **150**: 1108–11.
47. Wood WJ, Geraci T, Nilsen A, DeBarber AE, Scanlan TS. Iodothyronamines are oxidatively deaminated to iodothyroacetic acids in vivo. *Chembiochem*, 2009; **10**: 361–5.
48. Piehl S, Heberer T, Balizs G, Scanlan TS, Smits R, Koksch B, *et al.* Thyronamines are isozyme-specific substrates of deiodinases. *Endocrinology*, 2008; **149**: 3037–45.
49. Kester MHA, Visser TJ. Sulfation of thyroid hormones. In: Pacifici GM, Coughtrie MWH, eds. *Human Cytosolic Sulfotransferases*. Boca Raton: CRC Press, 2005: 121–34.
50. Wu SY, Green WL, Huang WS, Hays MT, Chopra IJ. Alternate pathways of thyroid hormone metabolism. *Thyroid*, 2005; **15**: 943–58.
51. Song WC. Biochemistry and reproductive endocrinology of estrogen sulfotransferase. *Ann N Y Acad Sci*, 2001; **948**: 43–50.
52. Pietsch CA, Scanlan TS, Anderson RJ. Thyronamines are substrates for human liver sulfotransferases. *Endocrinology*, 2007; **148**: 1921–7.
53. Visser TJ. *Hormone metabolism*, in www.thyroidmanager.org, 20 May 2010. South Dartmouth MA: Endocrine Education Inc.
54. Mackenzie PI, Bock K, Burchell B, Guillemette C, Ikushiro S, Iyanagi T, *et al.* Nomenclature update for the mammalian UDP glycosyltransferase (UGT) gene superfamily. *Pharmacogenet Genomics*, 2005; **15**: 677–85.
55. Kato Y, Ikushiro S, Emi Y, Tamaki S, Suzuki H, Sakaki T, *et al.* Hepatic UDP-glucuronosyltransferases responsible for glucuronidation of thyroxine in humans. *Drug Metab Dispos*, 2008; **36**: 51–5.
56. Moreno M, Kaptein E, Goglia F, Visser TJ. Rapid glucuronidation of tri- and tetraiodothyroacetic acid to ester glucuronides in human liver and to ether glucuronides in rat liver. *Endocrinology*, 1994; **135**: 1004–9.
57. Visser TJ, Kaptein E, Gijzel AL, de Herder WW, Ebner T, Burchell B. Glucuronidation of thyroid hormone by human bilirubin and phenol UDP-glucuronyltransferase isoenzymes. *FEBS Lett*, 1993; **324**: 358–60.
58. Hood A, Allen ML, Liu Y, Liu J, Klaassen CD. Induction of T(4) UDP-GT activity, serum thyroid stimulating hormone, and thyroid follicular cell proliferation in mice treated with microsomal enzyme inducers. *Toxicol Appl Pharmacol*, 2003; **188**: 6–13.
59. Benedetti MS, Whomsley R, Baltes E, Tonner F. Alteration of thyroid hormone homeostasis by antiepileptic drugs in humans: involvement of glucuronosyltransferase induction. *Eur J Clin Pharmacol*, 2005; **61**: 863–72.
60. Hulbert AJ. Thyroid hormones and their effects: a new perspective. *Biol Rev Camb Philos Soc*, 2000; **75**: 519–631.
61. Silva JE. Thyroid hormone control of thermogenesis and energy balance. *Thyroid*, 1995; **5**: 481–92.
62. Silva JE. Thermogenic mechanisms and their hormonal regulation. *Physiol Rev*, 2006; **86**: 435–64.
63. Simonides WS, van Hardeveld C. Thyroid hormone as a determinant of metabolic and contractile phenotype of skeletal muscle. *Thyroid*, 2008; **18**: 205–16.
64. Kahaly GJ, Dillmann WH. Thyroid hormone action in the heart. *Endocr Rev*, 2005; **26**: 704–28.
65. Celi FS. Brown adipose tissue: when it pays to be inefficient. *New Engl J Med*, 2009; **360**: 1553–6.
66. Lanni A, Moreno M, Lombardi A, Goglia F. Thyroid hormone and uncoupling proteins. *FEBS Lett*, 2003; **543**: 5–10.
67. Moreno M, de Lange P, Lombardi A, Silvestri E, Lanni A, Goglia F. Metabolic effects of thyroid hormone derivatives. *Thyroid*, 2008; **18**: 239–53.
68. Davis PJ, Leonard JL, Davis FB. Mechanisms of nongenomic actions of thyroid hormone. *Front Neuroendocrinol*, 2008; **29**: 211–18.
69. Suzuki S, Mori J, Hashizume K. mu-crystallin, a NADPH-dependent T(3)-binding protein in cytosol. *Trends Endocrinol Metab*, 2007; **18**: 286–9.
70. Yen PM. Physiological and molecular basis of thyroid hormone action. *Physiol Rev*, 2001; **81**: 1097–142.
71. Bassett JH, Harvey CB, Williams GR. Mechanisms of thyroid hormone receptor-specific nuclear and extra nuclear actions. *Mol Cell Endocrinol*, 2003; **213**: 1–11.
72. Flamant F, Gauthier K, Samarut J. Thyroid hormones signaling is getting more complex: STORMs are coming. *Mol Endocrinol*, 2007; **21**: 321–33.
73. Brenta G, Danzi S, Klein I. Potential therapeutic applications of thyroid hormone analogs. *Nat Clin Pract Endocrinol Metab*, 2007; **3**: 632–40.
74. Wood WM, Dowding JM, Bright TM, McDermott MT, Haugen BR, Gordon DF, *et al.* Thyroid hormone receptor beta2 promoter activity in pituitary cells is regulated by Pit-1. *J Biol Chem*, 1996; **271**: 24213–20.
75. Sharma V, Hays WR, Wood WM, Pugazhenthi U, St Germain DL, Bianco AC, *et al.* Effects of rexinoids on thyrotrope function and the hypothalamic-pituitary-thyroid axis. *Endocrinology*, 2006; **147**: 1438–51.
76. Lee GC, Yang IM, Kim BJ, Woo JT, Kim SW, Kim JW, *et al.* Identification of glucocorticoid response element of the rat TRH gene. *Korean J Intern Med*, 1996; **11**: 138–44.
77. Bianco AC, Larsen PR. Intracellular pathways of iodothyronine metabolism. In: Braverman LE, Utiger. eds. *Werner and Ingbar's The Thyroid*. 9th edn. Philadephia: Lippincott Wlliams & Wilkins, 2005: 109–35.

3.1.3 Clinical assessment of the thyroid patient

Peter Laurberg, Inge Bülow Pedersen

Introduction

Thyroid disorders are common, especially in older people where 10–20% may have structural abnormalities of the thyroid glan and/or thyroid function tests outside the reference range (1). Evaluation of thyroid function, size, and structure is therefore an important part of any complete history and physical examination of a patient.

Deficient or excessive thyroid hormone secretion affects nearly all body systems, and examination of a patient with a proven or suspected thyroid abnormality should include a more general evaluation of the patient. For example, an episode of thyrotoxicosis in an elderly person may provoke atrial fibrillation and impair cardiac function. The abnormality may persist after treatment of the thyrotoxicosis, and supplementary therapy directed against the atrial fibrillation may be needed. In a patient with hypothyroidism, symptoms of arteriosclerotic heart disease may worsen after initiation of treatment. Both the hypothyroidism and the heart disease should be diagnosed to develop an appropriate plan of therapy.

The three key abnormalities of the thyroid gland are: (1) thyrotoxicosis with excessive thyroid hormone effects on the body, (2) hypothyroidism with thyroid hormone deficiency, (3) and goitre with a general or focal abnormal enlargement of the thyroid gland. A less common abnormality is the painful thyroid. Examination of the thyroid patient should lead to a conclusion based on symptoms and signs related to these abnormalities.

The many clinical symptoms and signs of hyper- and hypothyroidism are dealt with in detail in subsequent chapters. However, during the initial assessment symptoms and signs of a clinical condition requiring more than usual observation or even acute therapy should be identified. In a thyrotoxic patient the risk of thyrotoxic crises should be evaluated. The risk of myxoedema coma is very low in a patient with hypothyroidism; the condition certainly should not develop during the period of diagnostic investigations. Some 'warning' symptoms and signs in hyper- and hypothyroidism are shown in Box 3.1.3.1. The box also depicts some factors which increase the risk of malignancy in a patient with goitre. Their presence may indicate the need to accelerate further diagnostic evaluation.

Each of the thyroid abnormalities may be caused by a number of diseases with different prognoses, risks, and treatments. Any clinical finding giving suspicion of a thyroid abnormality should be followed by a systematic evaluation of which disease is behind the abnormality (nosological diagnosis). For example, if the patient seems to be thyrotoxic the examination should lead to a provisional conclusion on the disease leading to the thyrotoxicosis. The four most common causes of thyrotoxicosis are Graves' disease, multinodular toxic goitre, toxic adenoma, and subacute thyroiditis (2). Subsequently the diagnosis should be substantiated by further biochemical tests and often imaging procedures.

Box 3.1.3.1 Warning symptoms and signs in thyroid patients

- Untreated hyperthyroidism[a]
  - Fever
  - Diarrhoea
  - Severe tachycardia (resting pulse rate >110 beats/min)
  - Complicating severe disease
  - Resting dyspnoea
- Untreated hypothyroidism[b]
  - Somnolence
  - Hypothermia
  - Complicating severe disease
- Goitre[c]
  - Hard solitary nodule
  - Growth of nodule
  - Stridor or hoarseness
  - Fixed to surroundings
  - Enlarged lymph nodes
  - Radiation to the neck as a child

[a] In untreated hyperthyroidism imminent thyrotoxic crisis should be looked for. Another severe com plication is pulmonary embolism, in part due to dehydration.
[b] Somnolence and hypothermia may be warnings of myxoedema coma.
[c] Symptoms and signs indicating a higher risk of malignancy in a goitre.

Some of the diseases leading to thyroid abnormalities may have other manifestations which should be looked for. A common example is the orbitopathy and (less common) the pretibial myxoedema of Graves' disease. A rare example is the retroperitoneal fibrosis with ureteral obstruction encountered in some patients with Riedel's thyroiditis.

The history and clinical examination may be so typical for a specific thyroid disorder that the diagnostic sensitivity and specificity approach 100%. However, the symptoms and signs of hypo- or hyperthyroidism overlap considerably with complaints and abnormalities which are common in other diseases and also in apparently healthy people (e.g. fatigue, weight alterations, nervousness, lack of concentration, constipation). Biochemical testing of thyroid function is therefore central in the evaluation of thyroid patients.

Laboratory tests of thyroid function may be influenced by various clinical circumstances and medication. During the clinical examination, information should be obtained on such circumstances or medication to allow proper interpretation of the tests. One important example is pregnancy (3). Both total and free thyroid hormones in serum vary during normal pregnancy, and pregnancy-induced modulations of the immune system may modify autoimmune thyroid abnormalities.

Transient hypo- or hyperthyroidism as part of autoimmune postpartum thyroiditis are seen in 4–5% of women 3–9 months after delivery. Another example is severe general illness (4) which may be accompanied by various alterations in total and free thyroid hormones and thyroid-stimulating hormone (TSH) in serum even if the thyroid gland is not affected.

Many medications may alter thyroid function tests (5). Some important examples are oestrogens (high thyroxin-binding globulin with high total thyroxine (T_4) and triiodothyronine (T_3)), carbamazepine, and phenytoin (low total and free T_4 and T_3), and amiodarone (high total and free T_4, slightly depressed total and free T_3, and high normal TSH). These are the variations seen in patients without thyroid abnormalities. Amiodarone has high iodine content and is also a frequent cause of thyroid disease.

Excess iodine, whether due to iodine-containing medications, over-the-counter 'health products' with iodine, intake of seaweed, or iodine-containing radiocontrast agents, may induce hypo- or hyperthyroidism in susceptible patients. The disease is transient in most cases. In geographical areas with a high basic iodine intake hypothyroidism is the common abnormality induced, while thyrotoxicosis predominates in areas with a low basic iodine intake. This difference in type of abnormality induced by excess iodine reflects the basic difference in the epidemiology of thyroid abnormalities in low and high iodine intake areas. In low iodine intake areas nontoxic and multinodular toxic goitre are the dominating abnormalities, whereas autoimmune diseases with subclinical and clinical hypothyroidism are the most common abnormalities in high iodine intake areas. Hence the history should reveal any excess iodine intake, and additional information on the general iodine intake level in the area where the patient lives will provide clues to the probability of the various thyroid abnormalities (2).

Thyroid diseases cluster in some families and a family history is valuable for risk estimation. Information on more specific genetic defects such as those leading to thyroid hormone resistance syndromes or to alterations of hormone binding proteins in serum is important to avoid diagnostic errors. The presence in a patient of autoimmune disorders such as vitiligo, rheumatoid arthritis, type 1 diabetes, Addison's disease, and pernicious anaemia considerably enhances the risk for an autoimmune thyroid disorder.

Previous thyroid disease gives a high risk for a current thyroid abnormality. For example, both hyper- and hypothyroidism may be transient if induced by excessive iodine intake (Chapter 3.2.4). However, there may be an underlying subclinical thyroid abnormality (e.g. autonomous thyroid nodules in hyperthyroidism, autoimmune thyroiditis in hypothyroidism). Relapse is therefore common after re-exposure to excess iodine. Spontaneous development of a thyroid function abnormality may also occur.

Patients with postpartum thyroiditis typically harbour an underlying autoimmune thyroiditis. Hence a new episode of thyroiditis is common after the next pregnancy, and the risk for a permanent thyroid hypofunction is considerably increased. If a patient is in remission after previous medication for the hyperthyroidism of Graves' disease, the risk for relapse is considerable (in the order of 50%). Patients treated with radioiodine or surgery for hyperthyroidism commonly develop immediate or early hypothyroidism. If not, hypothyroidism may develop later, even after decades. Patients who have received external radiation of the neck have an increased risk of hypothyroidism, and if treated with radiation to the neck or exposed to radioactive fallout during childhood a greatly increased risk of malignant and benign thyroid nodules.

The history on tobacco smoking is pertinent because smoking may aggravate the orbitopathy of Graves' disease (6), and by interacting with iodine deficiency lead to a high frequency of goitre (7).

Physical examination of the thyroid gland

Inspection and palpation of the anterior region of the neck with the thyroid gland is performed as part of any complete physical examination. In addition, auscultation of the thyroid gland can be used to evaluate blood flow in a goitre, and percussion of the upper part of the sternum to test for the presence of a large retrosternal goitre.

The normal thyroid is situated with the upper poles of the lobes at the level of the cricoid cartilage. The lower poles are 1–2 cm above the sternoclavicular junction in young adults, but the thyroid gland tends to be located more caudally on the neck in elderly patients. The thyroid isthmus transverses the trachea 1–2 cm below the cricoid cartilage. The location varies with the general anatomy of the neck.

Inspection of the thyroid gland

The patient is examined sitting or standing with light from a window or a lamp falling obliquely on the anterior of the neck. The chin of the patient is raised moderately. The skin is inspected for scars after thyroid surgery and vascular changes suggesting impaired venous flow or previous radiation of the neck.

The thyroid region should be studied carefully for signs of thyroid enlargement, nodules, and asymmetry (Fig. 3.1.3.1a). The normal thyroid gland is not or is only barely visible in most people. In young women with a slender neck, a high and medially situated normal thyroid gland may give the clinical impression of goitre ('pseudo-goitre').

The next step is to inspect the region while the patient is swallowing. If no water for swallowing is available it may be helpful to ask the patient to imagine chewing a piece of lemon. This may induce salivation and facilitate swallowing. The thyroid gland will normally move upwards during swallowing following the trachea (compare the thyroid region before swallowing (Fig. 3.1.3.1b) with the region during swallowing (Fig. 3.1.3.1c)). Small thyroid enlargements and nodules may be identified in this way. Inspection during swallowing is an important part of characterization of a goitre. If the goitre remains fixed to the surroundings and does not move it may be a sign of malignancy (Box 3.1.3.1). If still uncertain, inspect the thyroid region while the patient swallows, with light from various angles and with the neck of the patient more or less extended.

Palpation of the thyroid gland

Palpation can be performed while the examiner and the patient are sitting or standing in front of each other or while the examiner is standing behind the sitting patient. The patient should hold the head upright but the neck should not be hyperextended. Palpation involves a superficial and a deep examination of the gland. In addition, thorough palpation for enlarged cervical lymph nodes should be performed. The superficial part of the thyroid is examined by moving the flat fingertips systematically across the thyroid region searching for swellings and nodules (Fig. 3.1.3.1d). When special care is needed the examination may be facilitated by using lubricant (e.g. gel for ultrasound examination). It may also be helpful to ask the patient to swallow while palpating softly over the gland. Nodules and enlarged lobes may be identified when they are moving.

Palpation of the thyroid lobes between the fingers is achieved by displacing the larynx (and thereby the trachea and the thyroid gland) to one side (Fig. 3.1.3.1e) and palpating the thyroid lobe behind the sternocleidomastoid muscle as illustrated in Fig. 3.1.3.1f. Nodules in the deeper parts of the thyroid lobes can be detected in this way.

If goitre or one or more nodules are observed or palpated they should be examined and described with respect to size, hardness, location, mobility, and tenderness. Proper description of location is important as it aids interpretation of the findings of the scintigram (Is this a cold nodule?). Lack of mobility during swallowing is often a sign of malignancy but several other possibilities exist. Fixation could be caused by inflammation surrounding an acute or subacute thyroiditis. Such lesions tend, however, to be painful which is rarely the case with a cancer.

Auscultation of the thyroid gland

The goitre of patients with active Graves' disease may have a very high blood flow. The flow can occasionally be heard upon auscultation as a systolic murmur over the gland. When present in the medically treated patient it indicates persistent activity of the disease despite medication and is often accompanied by a 'high serum T_3 low serum T_4' pattern. If surgery is planned, pretreatment with iodine for 7–10 days before surgery to reduce blood flow may be considered.

A similar clinical pattern may occasionally be induced if patients with Graves' disease are grossly overtreated with thyroid-blocking drugs. This is followed by a low serum T_4 and T_3, excessive TSH secretion, and induction of a 'blocking goitre' with high blood flow.

A systolic murmur over the thyroid does not always originate in the thyroid gland. Differential diagnostic possibilities are referred sound from the heart in a patient with aortic stenosis or sclerosis and a systolic murmur from an arteriosclerotic carotid artery.

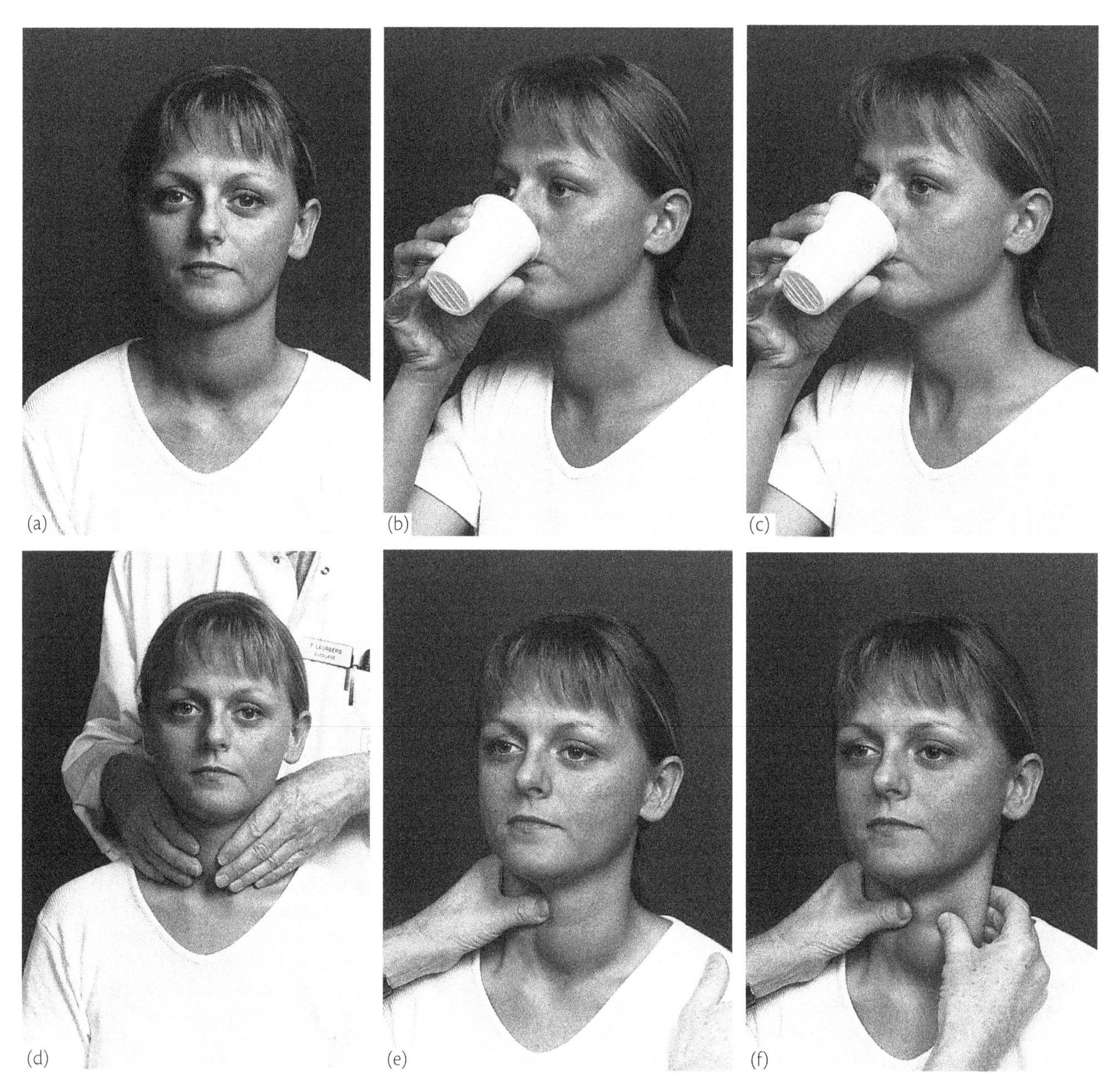

Fig. 3.1.3.1 Clinical examination of the thyroid gland in a young woman with a small goitre. (a) Inspection with oblique light, (b) inspection while the patient drinks water before swallowing, and (c) during swallowing. Note the change in position of the small goitre. (d) Palpation of the superficial part of the thyroid gland with flat fingertips. (e) Displacement of the thyroid to the left by pressure on the larynx (pressure on the trachea is more irritant). (f) Bidigital palpation of the deep parts of the left thyroid lobe behind the sternocleidomastoid muscle.

Reliability of clinical assessment in thyroid disease

In the typical Graves' disease patient—a young or middle-aged woman with family history, complaints of nervousness, heat intolerance and palpation, weight loss, high pulse rate, agility, diffuse goitre, and eye signs—the diagnosis based on clinical assessment is nearly 100% reliable. However, both hyper- and hypothyroidism may be difficult to diagnose from clinical findings, especially in elderly people where the diseases may be nearly monosymptomatic with, e.g., slow cerebration in hypothyroidism and weight loss in thyrotoxicosis. Biochemical evaluation of thyroid function is necessary and TSH measurement should be a first-line test in many clinical circumstances.

A special problem is the diagnosis of goitre. Classically goitre is a thyroid gland which is palpable or visible due to focal or general enlargement. Occasionally the goitre is not visible or palpable because the growth and extension of the gland has occurred behind the sternum as a retrosternal goitre.

A visible and/or palpable thyroid gland is not goitre if there is no general or focal enlargement. In young women this may be seen as 'pseudo-goitre'. Ultrasound examination of the thyroid gland with measurement of volume and identification or exclusion of thyroid nodules is an important supplement to the clinical evaluation of the thyroid gland, and it is most helpful in such patients. The interobserver variability of thyroid volume determinations by ultrasonography is around 10% and the reproducibility of identifying nodules is high.

The size of the thyroid gland of apparently healthy people depends considerably on the iodine intake level of the area where the investigation is performed. Upper normal values of 18 ml for

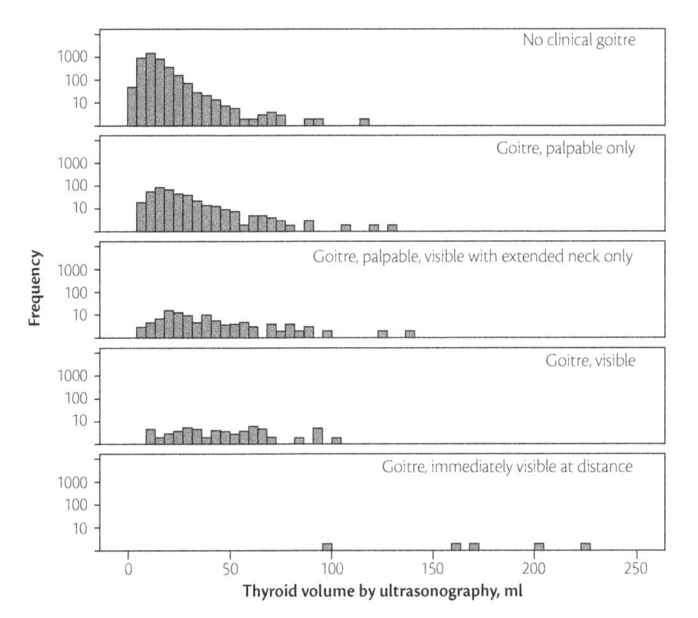

Fig. 3.1.3.2 Goitre by clinical examination and thyroid volume measured by ultrasonography in a population study of 4649 people living in an area with mild to moderate iodine deficiency. Data from the DanThyr cross-sectional study performed before the Danish iodine fortification programme (9).

women and 25 ml for men have been suggested (8). However, there is a profound discrepancy between the 'true' thyroid volume determined by ultrasound examination and the finding of no goitre or a small goitre by clinical examination. This is illustrated in Fig. 3.1.3.2, which also demonstrates that thyroid volumes several times the upper normal may be present without clinical goitre. Systematic studies of the clinical assessment of goitre have shown that estimation of thyroid size by inspection and palpation is imprecise and large intra- and interobserver variations have been found (10, 11).

Not only the estimation of size by clinical examination but also the evaluation of nodularity of the thyroid gland is difficult. Solitary thyroid nodules identified by palpation are often part of multinodular glands when examined by ultrasonography (in one investigation 50% of cases (12)). Ultrasound examination reveals more patients with thyroid nodules than clinical examination. In a follow-up study of patients who had received neck irradiation as children and therefore had a high risk of later development of thyroid cancer, only approximately 50% of nodules larger than 1.5 cm detected by ultrasonography were identified by palpation (13).

In daily clinical practice the fact that ultrasonography is such a sensitive method for detection of thyroid nodules may cause problems (14). Hence a properly performed clinical investigation for thyroid nodules remains the first-line investigation of the thyroid gland. Clinical investigation is also the primary investigation used for goitre detection. Even if the volume of the thyroid gland is not normal by ultrasound examination this is of limited clinical importance if the function of the gland is normal and if there are no signs and symptoms of goitre.

So the situation differs when considering the necessity to supplement the clinical examination for thyroid function abnormalities on the one hand and for abnormalities of thyroid structure and size on the other. Supplementary investigation of thyroid function using a measurement of serum TSH as the first-line test should be performed relatively freely in many patients with all kinds of complaints of a certain duration, even if the clinical suspicion of thyroid disease is weak. On the other hand, clinical examination of the thyroid gland remains the important first-line evaluation for goitre and thyroid nodules. Sensitive imaging procedures such as ultrasound examination should be reserved for patients with abnormal clinical and/or biochemical findings suggesting thyroid disease, as well as for patients with a special risk of developing thyroid cancer.

References

1. Laurberg P, Pedersen KM, Hreidarsson A, Sigfusson N, Iversen E, Knudsen PR. Iodine intake and the pattern of thyroid disorders: a comparative epidemiological study of thyroid abnormalities in the elderly in Iceland and in Jutland, Denmark. *J Clin Endocrinol Metab*, 1998; **83**: 765–9.
2. Laurberg P, Pedersen IB, Knudsen N, Ovesen L, Andersen S. Environmental iodine intake affects the type of nonmalignant thyroid disease. *Thyroid*, 2001; **11**: 457–69.
3. Baloch Z, Carayon P, Conte-Devolx B, Demers LM, Feldt-Rasmussen U, Henry JF, *et al.* Laboratory medicine practice guidelines. Laboratory support for the diagnosis and monitoring of thyroid disease. *Thyroid*, 2003; **13**: 3–126.
4. Chopra IJ. Clinical review 86: euthyroid sick syndrome: is it a misnomer? *J Clin Endocrinol Metab*, 1997; **82**: 329–34.
5. Wenzel KM. Disturbances of thyroid function tests by drugs. *Acta Med Austriaca*, 1996; **23**: 57–60.
6. Wiersinga WM. Management of Graves' ophthalmopathy. *Nat Clin Pract Endocrinol Metab*, 2007; **3**: 396–404.
7. Vejbjerg P, Knudsen N, Perrild H, Carlé A, Laurberg P, Pedersen IB, *et al.* The impact of smoking on thyroid volume and function in relation to a shift towards iodine sufficiency. *Eur J Epidemiol*, 2008; **23**: 423–9.
8. Gutekunst R, Becker W, Hehrmann R, Olbricht T, Pfannenstiel P. Ultraschalldiagnostik der Schilddruse. *Dtsch Med Wochenschr*, 1988; **113**: 1109–12.
9. Laurberg P, Jørgensen T, Perrild H, Ovesen L, Knudsen N, Pedersen IB, *et al.* The Danish investigation on iodine intake and thyroid disease, DanThyr: status and perspectives. *Eur J Endocrinol*, 2006; **155**: 219–28.
10. Berghout A, Wiersinga WM, Smits NJ, Touber JL. The value of thyroid volume measured by ultrasonography in the diagnosis of goitre. *Clin Endocrinol*, 1988; **28**: 409–14.
11. Jarløv EA, Hegedüs L, Gjørup T, Hansen MJ. Inadequacy of the WHO classification of the thyroid gland. *Thyroidology*, 1992; **4**: 107–10.
12. Tan GH, Gharib H, Reading CC. Solitary thyroid nodule. *Arch Intern Med*, 1995; **155**: 2418–23.
13. Schneider AB, Bekerman C, Leland J, Rosengarten J, Hyun H, Collins B, *et al.* Thyroid nodules in the follow-up of irradiated individuals: comparison of thyroid ultrasound with scanning and palpation. *J Clin Endocrinol Metab*, 1997; **82**: 4020–7.
14. Gharib H, Papini E, Paschke R. Thyroid nodules: a review of current guidelines, practices, and prospects. *Eur J Endocrinol*, 2008; **159**: 493–505.

3.1.4 Thyroid function tests and the effects of drugs

Jim Stockigt

Introduction

The assessment of thyroid function by laboratory testing began in about 1934 with the measurement of oxygen consumption or basal metabolic rate. Twenty years later measurement of protein-bound iodine became the standard technique and after a further 20 years this assay was superseded by radioimmunoassays of thyroxine (T_4) and triiodothyronine (T_3). Radioimmunoassays for thyroid-stimulating hormone (TSH) were reported from 1965, but early techniques could not distinguish normal values from the suppressed levels found in thyrotoxicosis. Until about 1990 this distinction was made by the administration of intravenous thyrotropin-releasing hormone (TRH), which fails to increase TSH to measurable levels in thyrotoxicosis, while producing a clear 5- to 15-fold increase in serum TSH in euthyroid subjects with normal pituitary function. Immunometric TSH assays now allow the suppressed serum TSH levels of thyrotoxicosis to be clearly distinguished from normal. This fundamental advance has coincided with the development of ingenious techniques to estimate the minute fraction of total serum T_4 that circulates in the unbound state, but even the best free T_4 methods offer only a marginal diagnostic advantage over the measurement of total T_4, e.g. when the concentration of thyroxine-binding globulin (TBG) is abnormal. Current enthusiasm for free T_4 and T_3 estimation needs to be tempered by an understanding of the method-dependent limitations of these techniques, particularly in situations where assessment of thyroid function is most difficult (see below).

All current methods of measuring TSH, T_4, and T_3 in serum, whether by radioimmunoassay or immunometric techniques, are comparative, i.e. they depend on the assumption that the unknown sample and the assay standards are identical in all measured characteristics other than the concentration of analyte. When this condition is not fulfilled, e.g. when the sample shows anomalous binding of tracer to serum proteins or antibodies, the assay result will be spurious and potentially misleading.

While there is little doubt that circulating TSH and T_4 should both be measured when an abnormality of thyroid function is suspected, recent recommendations suggest that it may be appropriate to apply testing more widely in a wide range of patient groups with an increased risk of thyroid dysfunction (Box 3.1.4.1). For example, neonatal screening for congenital hypothyroidism is firmly established. Routine testing of thyroid function with a single measurement of serum TSH in women over 50, the group most likely to have significant thyroid dysfunction (2), first advocated about 2000, (3) has become widely recommended (see also Chapter 3.1.7). Because current TSH assays are very sensitive in detecting either thyrotoxicosis or primary hypothyroidism, there is a trend for T_4 to be estimated in primary care only if TSH is abnormal (see below).

The recognition that an adequate level of maternal thyroxine in the first trimester of pregnancy is a crucial determinant of fetal brain development, has led to increased testing of thyroid function in preparation for pregnancy, especially in women who have impaired fertility or any risk factors for thyroid dysfunction (4) (see Chapter 3.4.5). The frequency of postpartum thyroid dysfunction places a high priority on the assessment of thyroid function for any suggestive clinical features in the first year after childbirth (5) (see Chapter 3.4.6).

The value of routine testing needs to be compared with the sensitivity and accuracy of clinical assessment. Studies of unselected patients assessed by primary care physicians show that clinical acumen alone lacks sensitivity and specificity in detecting previously undiagnosed thyroid dysfunction (6). In up to one-third of patients evaluated for suspected thyroid disease by specialists, laboratory results lead to revision of the clinical assessment (7).

Box 3.1.4.1 Groups with an increased likelihood of thyroid dysfunction (1)

- Previous thyroid disease or surgery
- Goitre
- Autoimmune disease(s)
- Other endocrine deficiencies
- Down's syndrome, Turner's syndrome
- Type 1 diabetes
- Metabolic syndrome, morbid obesity
- Irradiation of head and neck
- Impaired reproductive function in women
  - Polycystic ovarian syndrome
  - Endometriosis
  - Premature ovarian failure
  - Recurrent miscarriage
- Postpartum ill health
- Preterm infants
- Drug therapy
  - Cytotoxic therapy
  - Contrast agent or other iodine exposure
  - Amiodarone
  - Lithium
  - Highly active antiretroviral therapy
  - Sunitinib
  - Retinoids
  - Biological agents
    - Interferon α
    - Interleukin 2
    - Interferon β 1a or 1b
    - Monoclonal antibody treatment
    - Denileukin diftitox
- Pituitary abnormality
- Severe head injury

The T_4–TSH relationship

Regardless of the strategy that is used for first-line testing, serum TSH and a valid serum T_4 estimate are both necessary for definitive assessment of thyroid status. As shown in Fig. 3.1.4.1, the common types of thyroid dysfunction can be identified by diagonal deviations from the normal T_4–TSH relationship, which depends on the negative feedback interaction between target gland secretion and trophic hormone. The figure shows primary hypothyroidism due

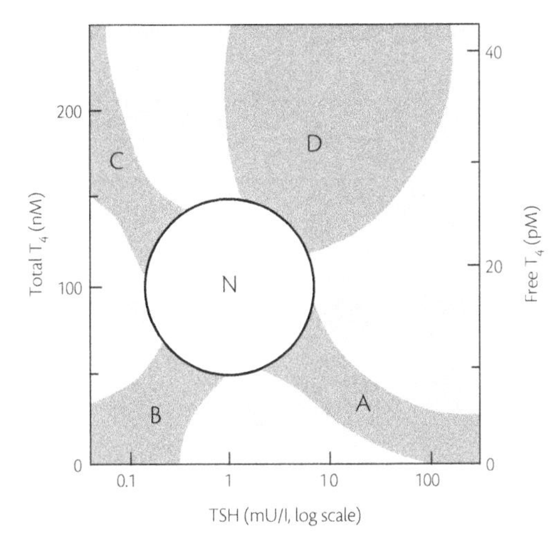

Fig. 3.1.4.1 The relationship between serum TSH and total free T_4 concentrations is shown in normal subjects (N) and in various typical abnormalities of thyroid function: primary hypothyroidism (A); central or pituitary-dependent hypothyroidism (B); thyrotoxicosis due to autonomy or abnormal thyroid stimulation (C); and TSH-dependent thyrotoxicosis or generalized thyroid hormone resistance (D). Note that linear free T_4 responses correspond to logarithmic TSH changes. Areas A and C represent primary thyroid abnormalities, while results that fall in areas B and D suggest a primary pituitary abnormality. Abnormal findings that fall in the intermediate areas suggest non-steady state sampling conditions due to the large difference in half-lives of TSH and T_4, an assay artefact, an altered T_4–TSH relationship, or the presence of another agonist, e.g. T_3.

to target gland failure (high serum TSH with low free T_4: A), failure of TSH secretion (both low: B), autonomous or abnormally stimulated target gland function (high serum free T_4 with low TSH: C), and primary excess of TSH or thyroid hormone resistance (both high: D). Abnormal results that fall outside these areas suggest that some other factor has disturbed this relationship, or that the sample has been collected under non-steady state conditions (see below). The figure shows serum free T_4 rather than T_3 because T_4 is the major circulating determinant of TSH secretion, although circulating T_3 also has an important direct inhibitory effect on TSH secretion.

The relationship shown in Fig. 3.1.4.1 allows precise diagnosis of thyroid dysfunction from a single serum sample, subject to the assumptions and limiting conditions summarized in Box 3.1.4.2. The first of these assumptions (steady-state conditions) should always be questioned when associated illness or medications perturb the pituitary–thyroid axis. The large difference between the half-lives of TSH (1 h) and T_4 (1 week) accounts for many transient nondiagnostic abnormalities in the T_4–TSH relationship. Of the six assumptions detailed in Box 3.1.4.2, only the last three can be validated in the laboratory; the first three must be verified clinically. It should be emphasized that optimal assessment of thyroid function depends on collaborative communication across the laboratory–clinical interface. Critical aspects of this approach have been summarized by Stockigt (see section 7 of Chapter 6b on this website) (1).

Assay choice and application

A general algorithm for the assessment of thyroid function based on initial measurement of TSH is shown in Fig. 3.1.4.2. The application of this strategy will vary depending on the circumstances in

Box 3.1.4.2 Assumptions that are made in using the T_4–TSH relationship to assess thyroid status. Limitations are shown in italics

- Steady-state conditions (NB difference in half-lives of TSH and T_4)
  - *Acute effects of medications*
  - *Early response to therapy*
  - *Evolution of disease*
  - *TSH pulse secretion and diurnal variation*
- Normal trophic-target hormone relationship
  - *Alternative thyroid stimulators*
    - *Immunoglobulins*
    - *Chorionic gonadotropin*
  - *Medications* (see also Table 3.1.4.3)
    - *T_3, triiodothyroacetic acid*
    - *Glucocorticoids*
    - *Dopamine*
    - *Amiodarone*
  - *Early treatment of thyrotoxicosis*
  - *Treatment of longstanding hypothyroidism* (Fig. 3.1.4.3)
  - *Variable individual set point*
  - *TSH receptor mutations*
- Tissue responses proportional to hormone concentrations
  - *Hormone resistance syndromes*
  - *Slow onset/offset of thyroid hormone action*
  - *Drug effects (amiodarone, phenytoin)*
- Accurate estimate of active hormone concentration
  - *Alternative agonist in excess (e.g. T_3)*
  - *Changes in serum binding proteins*
  - *TSH of altered biological activity*
  - *Spurious assay results*
    - *TSH: Heterophilic antibodies*
    - *Free T_4: Circulating inhibitors of binding; heparin artefact* (Fig. 3.1.4.5); *assay limitations* (8)
- Appropriate reference ranges
  - *Influence of age*
  - *Medications*
  - *Associated illness*
  - *Nutrition*
- Adequate assay sensitivity
  - *Diminished precision towards the limit of detection*

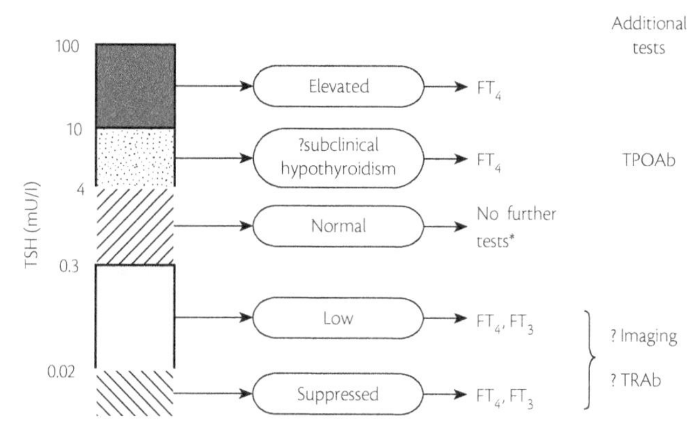

Fig. 3.1.4.2 Algorithm for the assessment of thyroid function based on initial assay of serum TSH. With highly sensitive TSH assays, the reference interval for euthyroid subjects can be clearly separated from suppressed values typical of thyrotoxicosis. For screening or case-finding studies in the absence of clinical features of thyroid dysfunction, abnormal TSH values lead to further assays as shown. Because serum TSH may give an incomplete or inaccurate assessment of thyroid status, assays of free T_4 (FT_4) are appropriate in the presence of a normal serum TSH if thyroid or pituitary dysfunction is suspected, during the early treatment of thyroid dysfunction, and with the use of drugs that influence the pituitary–thyroid axis. TPOAb, thyroid peroxidase antibody; TRAb, thyrotropin receptor antibody.

which testing is initiated. Several distinct clinical situations can be identified: (1) testing of untreated subjects in screening or case-finding studies with low prediagnostic probability, (2) when clinical features suggest thyroid dysfunction, (3) evaluation of the response to treatment, and (4) assessment when associated illness, drug therapy, or pregnancy are likely to complicate clinical and laboratory assessment.

Screening and case-finding

In the absence of associated disease, where there are no clinical features to suggest thyroid dysfunction, a normal serum TSH concentration has over 99% negative predictive value in ruling out primary hypothyroidism or thyrotoxicosis (3). Assessment of untreated subjects who have no features of thyroid dysfunction now commonly begins with measurement of TSH alone, with T_4 and/or T_3 assays added only if TSH is abnormal, or if an abnormality of TSH secretion is suspected (Fig. 3.1.4.2). According to this algorithm, free T_4 is measured to distinguish between overt and subclinical hypothyroidism when serum TSH is elevated, while a suppressed or subnormal TSH level should be followed by assay of both free T_4 and free T_3 to distinguish subclinical from overt thyrotoxicosis and to identify T_3 toxicosis.

Clinical suspicion of thyroid dysfunction

The use of serum TSH as the sole initial test of thyroid function may lead to incorrect or incomplete assessment of thyroid status in a number of situations, as summarized in Table 3.1.4.1. Initial measurement of both T_4 and TSH is appropriate whenever thyroid dysfunction is clinically suspected, because thyroid dysfunction due to pituitary disease, either hypopituitarism, or the less common situation of TSH-dependent hyperthyroidism, may be missed if TSH alone is used for initial assessment (9). The far-reaching consequences of missing these disorders are not reflected by a small percentage deficit in diagnostic sensitivity!

Table 3.1.4.1 Situations in which serum TSH alone can give a false or uncertain indication of thyroid status

Condition	TSH	Free T_4	Free T_3
Primary abnormality of TSH secretion			
Pituitary–hypothalamic disturbance	L-N	L	
Central TSH excess	N-H	H	H
Very low birth weight premature infants	L-N	L	L
Thyrotoxicosis			
Subclinical	U	N	N
Early treatment	U	H-N-L	H-N-L
Hypothyroidism			
Subclinical	H	N	
Early treatment	H	L-N	
TSH assay artefact			
Euthyroid subject	H	N	N
Thyrotoxic subject	L-N-H	H	H
Medications			
Dopamine	L	N	
Glucocorticoids	L	N	

N, normal; L, low; H, high; U, undetectable.

Evaluating and adjusting the response to treatment

In patients with newly treated thyrotoxicosis, TSH may remain suppressed for months after normalization of serum T_4 and T_3; serious overtreatment may result if TSH alone is used for adjustment of antithyroid drug dosage. Further, during drug treatment, thyrotoxicosis may persist due solely to T_3 excess. A reassessment of serum free T_4 and free T_3 levels is recommended after about 3 weeks drug treatment of thyrotoxicosis to allow appropriate dose adjustment. During long-term drug treatment of thyrotoxicosis, serum TSH may give a reliable guide to optimal drug dosage.

Serum TSH is the best single index of appropriate replacement, or suppressive therapy, during long-term treatment with thyroxine, but during the early phase of treatment of hypothyroidism, free T_4 should also be measured, because TSH may remain inappropriately elevated for several months after normalization of T_4 (Fig. 3.1.4.3). In elderly patients, especially those with cardiac ischaemia, dose adjustment is a clinical decision that need not be determined by serum TSH. During long-term replacement therapy, the best indicator of optimal dosage is a low-normal value for serum TSH, often associated with a slightly increased level of serum free T_4 that may vary depending on the time interval between dose and sampling. During suppressive therapy with T_4, periodic assessment of free T_4 and free T_3, in addition to TSH, is appropriate to identify and avoid thyroid hormone excess that may have adverse effects on the cardiovascular system or bone density.

In the treatment of hypothyroidism due to pituitary or hypothalamic disease, serum TSH is of no value in assessing T_4 dosage, which should be judged on the basis of serum free T_4 and clinical response.

Difficult diagnostic situations

Interpretation of thyroid function tests may be compromised by intercurrent illness and medications. There is a high prevalence of

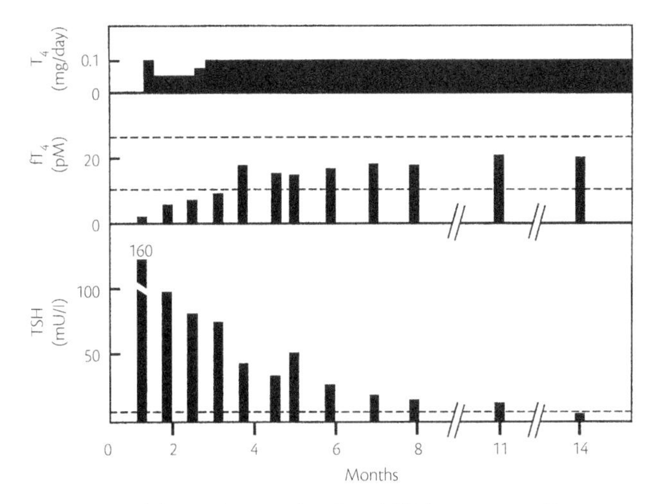

Fig. 3.1.4.3 Serial changes in serum free T_4 and TSH in response to T_4 replacement in a 68-year-old woman with longstanding severe untreated primary hypothyroidism. Normalization of serum TSH lagged 7–10 months behind normalization of serum free T_4. Imaging showed no evidence of pituitary enlargement or tumour. Dashed lines indicates limits of reference intervals.

abnormal serum free T_4 or TSH values in patients with acute medical illness (10) and in some studies of acute psychiatric illness (11). However, when TSH and free T_4 are considered together, as in Fig. 3.1.4.1, most of these abnormalities do not indicate true thyroid dysfunction. Because clinical assessment of thyroid status is difficult in the face of associated disease, some have advocated widespread testing (10), but the consensus has moved away from routine testing during critical illness without some clinical indication (12). If not due to medications (see below), the combination of low serum free T_4 and low TSH indicates a poor prognosis in critically ill patients (13), although there is no evidence that these findings can usefully influence management decisions for individuals.

During any severe illness, one or more of the assumptions outlined in Box 3.1.4.2 may not be valid, e.g. when there are wide deviations from the steady state due to acute inhibition of TSH secretion or abnormally rapid T_4 clearance. Serum TSH values are frequently subnormal in the absence of thyrotoxicosis, although highly sensitive TSH assays show higher levels than are typical of thyrotoxicosis (see below). Serum free T_4 estimates during critical illness are prone to multiple method-dependent interfering influences, e.g. due to heparin and other medications (see below). Serum total T_4 measurements are less prone to such artefacts (8).

In late pregnancy, there are clearly unresolved methodological problems in estimating serum free T_4, with strong negative bias in some methods (14, 15). A recent study has questioned the wisdom of continuing to rely on free thyroxine estimates during pregnancy (15). In contrast to various free T_4 methods (14, 15) total serum T_4 and its derivative, the free thyroxine index, showed a more robust inverse relationship with serum TSH, with consistent results in numerous reports (15). Thus, total T_4 measurement may be superior to free T_4 estimates as a guide to therapy during pregnancy, provided that the reference values are modified to take account of the normal oestrogen-induced increase in TBG. If free T_4 estimates continue to be used in pregnancy, clinicians should interpret results in relation to reference intervals that are both trimester specific and method specific. It remains to be established whether problems inherent in free thyroxine measurement during pregnancy can be resolved by using isotope dilution liquid chromatography tandem mass spectrometry after ultrafiltration (16).

Measurement of serum TSH concentrations

The secretion of TSH, a 24–30 kDa glycoprotein composed of two subunits, from the thyrotropic cells of the anterior pituitary is regulated by negative feedback from the serum free T_4 and free T_3 concentrations. In normal subjects, the serum TSH concentration shows both pulsatile and diurnal variation, with mean maximum concentrations of approximately 3 mU/l at about 02.00 with nadir values of about 1 mU/l at about 16.00; there is no significant sex difference in reference values (17). Because serum TSH fluctuates with an amplitude of 20–50% around the mean (17), it can be difficult to establish whether serial changes are relevant in follow-up studies of patients with subclinical hypothyroidism, because a change of up to 40% could reflect pulsatile secretion rather than progression of disease (18).

Between 08.00 and 21.00, reference values for serum immunoreactive TSH are generally in the range 0.3–4 mU/l (Table 3.1.4.2), with higher values in the immediate postnatal period when there is a surge of TSH secretion. The reference range should be calculated after logarithmic transformation of control values to achieve a valid estimate of the lower normal limit. Although not perfect, logarithmic transformation brings TSH reference values closer to a normal distribution that can be statistically assessed. Median values are generally at about 1 mU/l with a long tail to the right, so that the upper limit of the reference range is contentious (see below).

The introduction of immunometric assays that use two antibodies against different epitopes on the α- and β-subunits of TSH has greatly improved assay sensitivity (19). With the best current techniques, serum TSH can be precisely measured at least to 0.03 mU/l, so that the lowest concentrations in normal subjects are clearly distinguishable from those found in thyrotoxicosis. Factors that become important when clinical decisions are based on values close to the limit of detection include between-assay reproducibility or precision profile, composition of the assay matrix, possible appearance of nonspecific interference during sample storage, as well as possible carryover from one sample to the next during automated sampling (20). Analytical sensitivity can be defined from the dose response characteristics of a single assay by expressing sensitivity as 2 or 3 SD above the zero point, but this estimate is often

Table 3.1.4.2 Typical reference ranges for serum thyroid hormones and TSH in humans[a]

Hormone	Reference ranges
Thyroxine (T_4)	60–140 nmol/l
Free T_4	10–25 pmol/l
Triiodothyronine (T_3)	1.1–2.7 nmol/l[b]
Free T_3	3–8 pmol/l[b]
Reverse T_3	0.2–0.7 nmol/l
TSH	0.3–4.0 mU/l[c]
TSHα-subunit	<2 μg/l

[a] These ranges should be determined for the particular methods used in each laboratory.

[b] Higher values in childhood.

[c] Reference interval controversial (see text).

too optimistic (19). A definition of functional sensitivity as the 20% between-assay coefficient of variation has become accepted (19). Manufacturers' estimates of functional sensitivity are often not confirmed on clinical testing, and assay performance may vary between laboratories despite apparently identical technique. Laboratories should establish their own detection limit from the between-assay precision profile in the subnormal range.

Nonspecific interference in TSH assays

While immunometric TSH assays offer enhanced sensitivity, there can be important problems with nonspecific interference, e.g. in methods that use mouse monoclonal antibodies. An antimouse immunoglobulin in the test serum allows the formation of a false bridge between the solid phase and the signal antibody, thus generating a spuriously high assay value (21). Inclusion of nonspecific mouse immunoglobulin in the assay usually blocks this effect, although persistent false-positive detectable serum TSH values are still found in some samples (22).

The TSH reference range: current controversies and uncertainties

Widespread application of thyroid function testing has identified large numbers of asymptomatic subjects with abnormal TSH, with normal serum T_4, who may merit the designation 'subclinical thyroid dysfunction' (23). A sustained abnormality should be demonstrated before definite categorization (24). The merits and limitations of initiating therapy for these individuals are discussed in Chapters 3.3.4 and 3.4.4.

These considerations have become complicated because of lack of consensus on the limits of the TSH range (25, 26, 27). There is ongoing debate (26, 27) on whether the upper limit of the TSH reference range should be reduced from about 4 mU/l to 3 mU/l or even lower, based on exclusion criteria for the reference population, statistical treatment of data, inference of adverse outcome, or prospect of benefit from intervention. Similarly, for subclinical hyperthyroidism there is lack of consensus as to how subnormal TSH values should be classified. The NHANES III study (28) reserves the designation 'subclinical hyperthyroidism' for serum TSH values below 0.1 mU/l. By contrast, other guidelines for the diagnosis and management of subclinical thyroid disease classify values below the lower normal limit of 0.45 mU/l as indicating subclinical hyperthyroidism (29). Such a difference in classification may affect the health classification of up to 1% of any population. Since the gradation from normality to severe thyroid dysfunction is a continuum, studies of adverse outcomes or benefits from intervention will be critically dependent on uniform cut-off points and terminology.

Until these uncertainties are resolved, it is likely that most clinicians will recommend a period of observation rather than immediate intervention. If a trend towards overt disease is to be the cue to intervention, it is critical to establish what constitutes a significant change in serum TSH value, a hormone that is pulse-secreted and shows diurnal variation. From an analysis of serial individual variation over 1 year, the difference required for two test results to be convincingly different was 40% for TSH and 15% for free T_4 and free T_3 (18).

Serum TSH values during T_4 therapy

During standard T_4 replacement therapy a TSH value in the lower normal range usually coincides with an optimal symptomatic response. When the aim of T_4 suppressive therapy is regression of benign thyroid tissue, it may be appropriate to give sufficient T_4 to reduce serum TSH to 0.1–0.3 mU/l. In the follow-up treatment of high-risk patients with thyroid cancer, further TSH suppression is generally advocated, although the benefit of sufficient T_4 to suppress TSH to less than 0.1 mU/l remains unproven.

Serum TSH in critical illness

Critically ill patients frequently have subnormal levels of serum TSH, but with a sufficiently sensitive assay these values can be distinguished from the typical values found in thyrotoxicosis. The large majority of thyrotoxic subjects have values below 0.01 mU/l, whereas hospitalized patients with nonthyroidal illness do not show this degree of TSH suppression (30).

Indications for TRH testing

The need for TRH testing in clinical practice has almost been eliminated by the development of highly sensitive TSH assays. However, measurement of serum TSH 20–30 min after intravenous injection of 200–500 μg TRH is still useful for some purposes: (1) to assess patients whose basal serum TSH values are out of context (TSH assay artefacts, e.g. those due to heterophilic antibodies, generally fail to show a physiological response), (2) to investigate apparent thyroid hormone resistance or pituitary-dependent thyrotoxicosis (most patients with thyrotoxicosis due to TSH-secreting pituitary tumours show no increase in serum TSH after TRH (31), while those with thyroid hormone resistance usually show an increase), and (3) to identify central hypothyroidism in which a low serum free T_4 value may be associated with a normal amount of serum immunoreactive TSH that has impaired biological activity (32).

Assays for serum TSH α-subunit

Most patients with TSH-secreting pituitary tumours have increased serum α-subunit concentrations (31), but values can also be elevated in postmenopausal women and in hypogonadal men.

Assays for serum T_4 and T_3

Concentrations of total serum T_4 and T_3 reflect not only hormone production, but also the number and affinity of plasma protein binding sites. Total concentrations vary in direct relationship to protein binding, while serum free T_4 and free T_3 concentrations should not, if measured by valid methods. Serum total and free T_3 concentrations are somewhat higher in children (33). Typical reference ranges for serum total and free T_4 and T_3 are shown in Table 3.1.4.2. In late pregnancy, reference ranges for free T_4 show marked method-dependent variation; quoted ranges should be both trimester specific and method specific.

Estimation of serum free T_4 and free T_3

There have been many approaches to the assay of serum free T_4 and free T_3 concentrations, with detailed analysis of the validity of various methods (34). Two-step methods that separate a fraction of the free T_4 pool from the binding proteins as a preliminary before assay are generally least prone to analytical artefacts. Figure 3.1.4.4 outlines a two-step free T_4 method based on incubation of serum with a solid-phase T_4 antibody, followed by back titration of unoccupied antibody with labelled T_4.

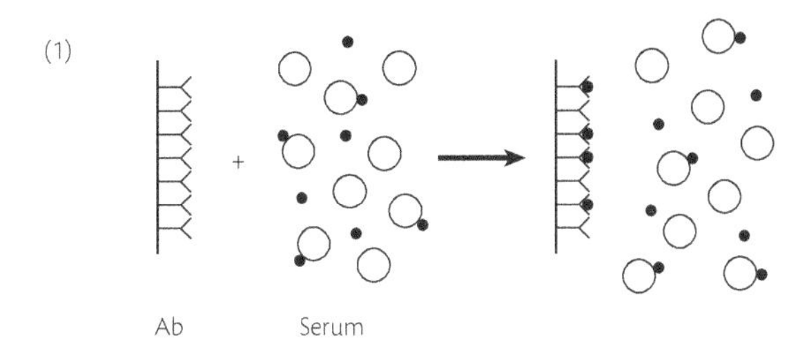

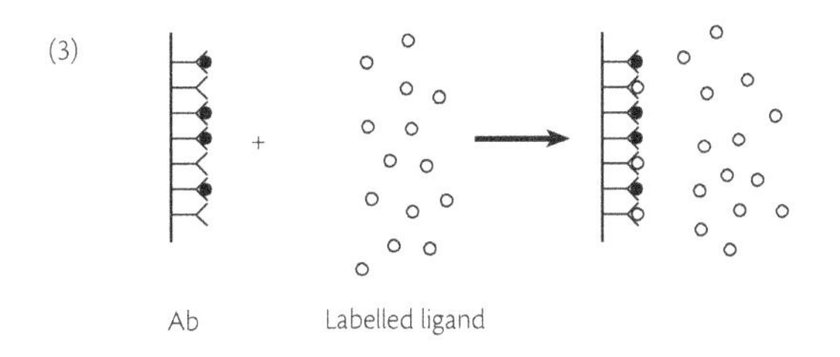

Fig. 3.1.4.4 Representation of a typical two-step serum free T_4 immunoassay. Serum is incubated with solid-phase T_4 antibody (Ab), which captures some of the free T_4. After washing to remove serum followed by back titration of the solid phase with labelled T_4, solid-phase radioactivity is inversely proportional to the serum free T_4 concentration. (Reproduced with permission from Ekins R. Measurement of free hormones in blood. *Endocr Rev*, 1990; **11**: 5–46.)

No current method conveniently measures the free T_4 concentration in undisturbed, undiluted serum in a way that reflects *in vivo* conditions. Although equilibrium dialysis is widely considered the reference method for free T_4 measurement, it is also subject to error, especially as a result of generation of fatty acids during sample storage or incubation, and the inability of diluted samples to reflect the effect of binding competitors (see below). Evaluation of novel serum free T_4 methods should include testing with various protein binding abnormalities, as well as sera that contain substances that compete for serum protein binding sites. Unexpected interference may only be noted after methods have been used for some time, as in the effect of rheumatoid factor (35), heparin (36), or drug competitors for protein binding (8).

Recent reports suggest that methods based on liquid chromatography/tandem mass spectrometry after ultrafiltration (16), or equilibrium dialysis (37) may improve the measurement of free T_4. Further evaluations, in particular details of long-term reproducibility (i.e. interassay variation) of these techniques, as well as serial dilution studies to evaluate the effect of circulating inhibitors of T_4 binding (see below) are awaited.

Measurement of serum T_3

Assays for serum total or free T_3 have no place in the diagnosis of hypothyroidism, but should be included in the diagnostic protocol in the following situations:

- in suspected thyrotoxicosis when serum T_4 is normal and serum TSH is suppressed, to distinguish T_3 toxicosis from subclinical thyrotoxicosis
- during antithyroid drug therapy to identify persistent T_3 excess, despite normal or even subnormal serum T_4 values
- for diagnosis of amiodarone-induced thyrotoxicosis, which should not be based on T_4 excess alone because of the frequent occurrence of euthyroid hyperthyroxinaemia during amiodarone treatment
- to detect early recurrence of thyrotoxicosis in the presence of suppressed TSH, after cessation of antithyroid drug therapy
- to establish the extent of hormone excess during suppressive therapy with T_4, or when an intentional T_4 overdose has been taken

The serum T_3 concentration is not useful in assessing the effectiveness of T_3 replacement. Because of its short plasma half-life, the T_3 concentration is highly dependent on the interval between dosage and sampling.

Variant binding proteins

Molecular changes in TBG, transthyretin (TTR, previously known as thyroxine-binding prealbumin), or albumin may result in altered serum concentrations of these binding proteins, or may alter their binding affinity for T_4 and/or T_3 (38). The X-linked structural TBG variants, some of which show abnormal heat lability, have either normal or reduced affinity for T_4; T_3 is usually similarly affected. Fifteen of at least 24 known X-linked variants of TBG cause complete TBG deficiency, while eight variants are associated with subnormal concentrations of immunoreactive serum TBG, often with reduced affinity for T_4 (38). In the total absence of TBG, total serum T_4 is reduced to 20–40 nmol/l (normal 50–140 nmol/l), whereas in hereditary TBG excess the concentration may increase up to 250 nmol/l (38); free T_4 remains normal. In general, the various methods of estimating serum free T_4 give a valid correction for TBG abnormalities, whether hereditary or acquired.

The albumin variant responsible for familial dysalbuminaemic hyperthyroxinaemia (FDH) (38), due to an Arg-His substitution at position 218, shows a selective increase in binding affinity for T_4 resulting in total serum T_4 in the range 180–240 nmol/l. The variant protein has increased affinity for some T_4-analogue tracers, resulting in spuriously high serum free T_4 estimates (38); equilibrium dialysis and various two-step free T_4 methods and serum TSH confirm that people with the FDH variant are euthyroid. TTR variants can increase total serum T_4 into the range 150–200 nmol/l, but are not reported to cause spurious free T_4 results.

Circulating T_3- or T_4-binding autoantibodies can cause methodological artefacts in both total and free measurements of T_4 and T_3 (8). Depending on the separation method that is used, tracer bound to the endogenous human antibody will be classified as 'bound' in absorption methods of assay separation, but falsely classified as 'free' in double antibody methods, leading, respectively, to spuriously low or high serum values (8). Assay after ethanol extraction of serum establishes the true total hormone concentration.

Euthyroid hyperthyroxinaemia and hypothyroxinaemia

These terms are used when the total or free T_4 concentrations are increased or decreased without evidence of thyroid dysfunction. The effects of medications and alterations in the T_4 binding proteins are the commonest causes (Box 3.1.4.3, Table 3.1.4.3). Hypothyroxinaemia is a normal response when TSH secretion is

Box 3.1.4.3 Euthyroid hyperthyroxinaemia

- High serum total T_4, normal free T_4
  - Increase in binding protein affinity or concentration
  - Thyroxine-binding globulin
    - Hereditary
    - Pregnancy
    - Liver diseases
    - Drugs: oestrogen, heroin, methadone, clofibrate, 5-fluorouracil, perphenazine, tamoxifen
  - Transthyretin
    - Hereditary[a]
    - Pancreatic neuroendocrine tumours
  - Albumin
    - Familial dysalbuminaemic hyperthyroxinaemia[a]
  - T_4 antibody-associated hyperthyroxinaemia
- High serum total T_4, high free T_4
  - Thyroid hormone resistance
  - Severe illness (small proportion)
  - Altered hormone synthesis, release, or clearance
    - Contrast agents
    - Amiodarone
    - Propranolol (high doses)
  - Thyroxine therapy
  - Thyroid stimulation
    - Hyperemesis gravidarum
    - Acute psychiatric illness?
- Normal serum total T_4, high free T_4
  - Drug competitors
  - Heparin (*in vitro* effect)

[a] Changes in binding affinity of the protein.

Table 3.1.4.3 Major medications and exogenous substances that influence thyroid hormone or TSH levels[a] (1)

Medication/exogenous substance	Effect
TSH secretion	
Dopamine, glucocorticoids	
Bexarotene, metformin	–
Iodine uptake	
Sunitinib gain	–
Iodine load	
Contrast agents, amiodarone, topical preparations	±
Thyroid hormone release	
Lithium, glucocorticoids	–
Deiodination	
Amiodarone, glucocorticoids, β-blockers[b]	–
Contrast agents[b]	–
Binding of T_4, T_3 to plasma proteins	
Furosemide, salicylates, nonsteroidal anti-inflammatory agents[b]	–
Phenytoin, carbamazepine, heparin[c]	–
Major medications that influence thyroid hormone or TSH levels[a]	
Altered concentration of T_4 binding globulin	
Oestrogen, raloxifene, heroin, methadone	+
Clofibrate, 5-fluorouracil, perphenazine, tamoxifen	+
Glucocorticoids, androgens	–
Altered thyroid hormone action	
Amiodarone, phenytoin	?±
Increased metabolism of iodothyronines	
Barbiturates, phenytoin, carbamazepine	+
Rifampicin, motesanib, imitanib, bexarotene	+
Sertraline?, fluoxetine?, dothiepin?	+
Impaired absorption of ingested T_4	
Aluminium hydroxide, ferrous sulfate, calcium carbonate, cholestyramine	–
Colestipol, sucralfate, soya preparations	–
Kayexalate, proton pump inhibitors, chromium picolinate, sevelamer	–

[a] Conventional antithyroid drugs excluded.
[b] Some members of the group.
[c] *In vitro* effect of *in vivo* heparin administration (see Fig. 3.1.4.5).
+, stimulatory; –, inhibitory; ±, effect depends on thyroid status.

inhibited by another thyromimetic such as T_3 or triiodothyroacetic acid. During critical illness serum T_4 may be subnormal due to inhibition of TSH secretion (39), decreased production of binding proteins, or accelerated T_4 clearance. Hypothyroxinaemia without the anticipated increase in TSH also is seen in very low birthweight premature infants, in whom the lack of TSH response appears to reflect hypothalamic–pituitary immaturity (40).

Drug effects on serum T_4 and TSH

The multiple effects of medications on the pituitary–thyroid axis (Table 3.1.4.3) have been reviewed elsewhere (1, 38, 41) Medications that present special problems include amiodarone, heparin, lithium, phenytoin, highly active antiretroviral therapy, and drugs that displace T_4 from TBG. Oestrogen, endogenous or exogenous, is the substance that most commonly affects tests of thyroid function by increasing total T_4 due to an increase in the concentration of TBG. Free T_4 remains normal. Oestrogens, including a minor effect of selective oestrogen agonists such as raloxifene (42), act to increase the glycosylation of TBG, which slows its clearance (38). Transdermal oestrogens do not show this effect (38).

Amiodarone

Amiodarone is the most complex and difficult of the drugs that can affect thyroid status (43). The clinical entities that may result from amiodarone therapy include two forms of thyrotoxicosis, one due to iodine excess and one attributed to thyroiditis (see Chapter 3.3.10). In iodine-replete regions the predominant amiodarone-induced thyroid abnormality is hypothyroidism, which is especially prevalent in those with associated autoimmune thyroiditis (see Chapter 3.2.6). The drug also causes benign euthyroid hyperthyroxinaemia in up to 25% of treated patients. There is often poor correlation between circulating thyroid hormone levels and the clinical manifestations of amiodarone-induced thyroid dysfunction, perhaps because of interaction of this drug or its metabolites with thyroid hormone receptors. In assessing the severity of amiodarone-induced thyrotoxicosis, the extent of measured thyroid hormone excess is less relevant than criteria such as muscle weakness and weight loss.

Heparin

In serum obtained from heparin-treated patients, the measured concentration of serum free T_4 may be higher than the true *in vivo* concentration, due to *in vitro* generation of nonesterified fatty acids as a result of heparin-induced lipase activity during sample storage or incubation (36) (Fig. 3.1.4.5). High serum triglyceride concentrations and sample incubation at 37°C accentuate this artefact. Low-molecular-weight heparin preparations have a similar effect (44).

Lithium

Lithium, a medication used in the management of manic-depressive illness, has multiple effects on the pituitary–thyroid axis, the most important being an effect to inhibit thyroglobulin hydrolysis and hormone release (45). It can exacerbate or may initiate autoimmune thyroid disease with development of goitre and hypothyroidism; there are also rare reports of lithium-induced thyrotoxicosis (45). Serum TSH, T_4, and T_3 assays give a true index of thyroid status during lithium treatment.

Phenytoin and carbamazepine

The antiepileptic phenytoin and carbamazepine both commonly result in subnormal serum total T_4, with an apparent lowering of free T_4, not accompanied by the anticipated increase in TSH (46).

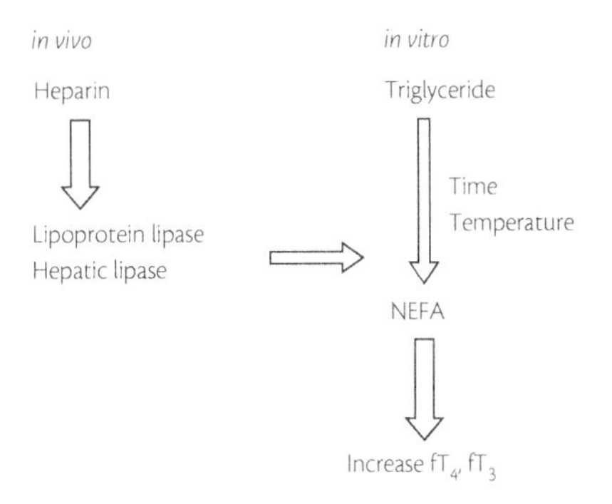

Fig. 3.1.4.5 Summary of the heparin-induced changes that can markedly increase the apparent concentration of serum free T_4. Heparin acts *in vivo* (left) to liberate lipoprotein lipase from vascular endothelium. Lipase acts *in vitro* (right) to increase the concentration of free fatty acids to levels more than 3 mmol/l, resulting in displacement of T_4 and T_3 from TBG. *In vitro* generation of free fatty acids is increased by sample storage at room temperature, or incubation at 37°C and by high concentration of serum triglyceride. The T_4-displacing effect of free fatty acids is accentuated at low albumin concentrations. NEFA, nonesterified fatty acids; fT_3, free T_3; fT_4, free T_4.

This discrepancy, which is not easily distinguishable from central hypothyroidism due to pituitary deficiency, is a methodological artefact related to underestimation of true free T_4 in diluted serum samples that contain inhibitors of T_4 protein binding (8, 46) (see below).

Antiretroviral therapy

Infection with HIV may influence tests of thyroid function by various mechanisms, occasionally as result of direct infection of the thyroid gland or alteration of immunological function, but more frequently from the effect of medications that alter metabolism of thyroxine or as a nonspecific effect of debilitating illness. Some studies (47) show a higher than expected prevalence of hypothyroidism, predominantly subclinical, during treatment with highly active antiretroviral therapy (HAART). There are reports of reduced effectiveness of thyroxine replacement during treatment for HIV infection as a result of accelerated thyroxine metabolism, as with lopinavir/ritonavir (48); there is one paradoxical report of transient over-replacement during treatment with indinavir (49). There is no consensus as to whether thyroid function should be routinely monitored in HIV-infected patients, but testing will frequently be required to assess features that could be due to thyroid dysfunction. During HAART, thyroxine replacement needs to be monitored and adjusted (47, 48).

Effects of drug competitors for thyroid hormone binding to plasma proteins

In contrast to the steroid and vitamin D binding plasma proteins, both TBG and TTR show extensive cross-reactions with a wide range of drugs (1, 38, 41). As reviewed elsewhere (8), the failure of current free T_4 and T_3 methodology to reliably reflect the effect of drug competitors that increase free T_4 and T_3 *in vivo* by displacement, remains a major limitation in the general applicability of free hormone assays. These effects are poorly reflected by standard free hormone assays because samples are generally assayed after dilution, resulting in underestimation of the free hormone concentration in the presence of competitors (8, 46). When measured by ultrafiltration of undiluted serum, therapeutic concentrations of phenytoin and carbamazepine showed an increase in free T_4 fraction by 45–65%, but these effects were obscured by 1:5 assay dilution of serum (46). This discrepancy occurs because of dissociation of bound ligand with progressive sample dilution, so that the free concentration, at first well maintained, declines steeply as the 'reservoir' of bound ligand becomes depleted (8, 46). Important drug competitors have a much smaller proportional reservoir of bound ligand than does T_4, so that their free concentration becomes negligible with progressive dilution while the free T_4 concentration remains unaltered (8). Since competition is a function of relative free ligand concentrations, the effect of a competitor to increase free T_4 is underestimated, the error being greatest in assays with the highest sample dilution (1, 8, 46).

Drug interactions

Drug effects on thyroid function may be especially potent when several agents are given together. For example, infusion of furosemide in high dosage lowers serum T_4, while concurrent dopamine infusion inhibits TSH secretion; together they can result in profound hypothyroxinaemia. Combinations of rifampicin or ritonavir or other medications that accelerate T_4 clearance, with glucocorticoid-induced inhibition of TSH secretion can have a similar effect.

Integration of tests of thyroid function with other investigations

When thyroid function is abnormal, additional diagnostic information can be gained from antibody studies, imaging techniques, and measurement of thyroglobulin. The investigation of thyroid masses *per se* is not considered here.

Antibody measurements

In subclinical hypothyroidism, the presence of thyroid peroxidase (TPO) antibodies indicates a four- to fivefold increase in the chance of developing overt hypothyroidism (2). The presence of this antibody also indicates an increased likelihood of postpartum thyroiditis or amiodarone-induced hypothyroidism. The finding of persistently positive thyrotropin receptor antibody (TRAb) is useful in indicating that apparent remission of Graves' disease is unlikely to be sustained. TRAb measurement can indicate the possibility of neonatal thyrotoxicosis in the infant of a mother with autoimmune thyroid disease and may also define the aetiology of atypical eye disease.

Thyroid imaging

The use of isotope imaging techniques in thyrotoxicosis due to Graves' disease varies widely between different centres. While some now regard routine radioisotope imaging as redundant in typical Graves' disease, negligible uptake can be a key feature in confirming thyrotoxicosis due to thyroiditis, iodine contamination, and factitious ingestion of thyroid hormone. Imaging also can confirm a 'hot' nodule as the predominant source of thyroid hormone excess. CT is valuable in identifying the extent of retrosternal extension, but contrast agents should be avoided. Colour flow Doppler has been reported to differentiate between type 1 and type 2 amiodarone-induced thyrotoxicosis (43) (see Chapter 3.3.10).

Thyroglobulin

In the follow-up of differentiated thyroid cancer, an undetectable serum thyroglobulin concentration in the presence of high serum TSH indicates effective ablation and may justify less rigorous T_4-induced suppression of TSH. Thyroglobulin is undetectable in thyrotoxicosis factitia, and generally extremely high in subacute thyroiditis and in amiodarone-induced thyrotoxicosis of the thyroiditis type.

Assay of thyroglobulin in the needle wash from suspect neck lymph nodes appears to have a higher sensitivity and specificity than cytology in establishing whether they contain metastatic thyroid tissue (50).

Indices of thyroid hormone action

While there is currently no diagnostically reliable laboratory index of peripheral thyroid hormone action, some tests (51), including sex steroid binding globulin, serum ferritin, serum angiotensin-converting enzyme, as well as measurement of oxygen consumption, systolic time interval, and ultrasonographic parameters of cardiac contractility (52), may be useful in following individual response in situations of suspected thyroid hormone resistance or during long-term suppressive therapy with T_4.

Diagnostic approach to anomalous or discordant laboratory results

When there is discordance between laboratory results and clinical findings, a distinction needs to be made between anomalous assay results due to specific or nonspecific assay interference and those that indicate previously unsuspected or subclinical disease. Consideration of the fundamental assumptions that underlie the diagnostic use of the trophic-target hormone relationship (Box 3.1.4.2) may give a clue to the discrepancy. Anomalous or unexpected assay results can be approached in the following sequence:

1. Clinical re-evaluation with particular attention to the medication history and to long-term features suggestive of thyroid disease, e.g. weight change, goitre.
2. Optimal measurement of serum TSH to identify the degree of TSH suppression.
3. Estimation of serum free T_4 and free T_3 by alternative methods with particular attention to method-dependent artefacts related to medications.
4. Follow-up sampling to establish whether the abnormality is transient or persistent.
5. Measurement of serum total T_4 to establish whether the free T_4 estimate is disproportionately high or low in relation to total T_4 (e.g. heparin artefact). (Arguably, measurement of total T_4 with correction for variations in TBG, interpreted in conjunction with TSH, could now be regarded as the gold standard where free T_4 estimates are inconclusive (8)).
6. Search for an unusual binding abnormality or hormone resistance syndrome in the propositus and family members.

References

1. Stockigt JR. Clinical strategies in the testing of thyroid function, Chapter 6b in www.thyroidmanager.org, 17 May 2010. South Dartmouth MA: Endocrine education Inc.
2. Vanderpump MPJ, Tunbridge WMG, French JM, Appleton D, Bates D, Clark F, *et al.* The incidence of thyroid disorders in the community: a twenty-year follow-up of the Whickham Survey. *Clin Endocrinol*, 1995; **43**: 55–68.
3. Helfand M, Redfern CC. Screening for thyroid disease: an update. *Ann Intern Med*, 1998; **129**: 144–58.
4. Brent GA. Diagnosing thyroid dysfunction in pregnant women: is case finding enough? *J Clin Endocrinol Metab*, 2007; **92**: 39–41.
5. Management of thyroid dysfunction during pregnancy and postpartum: an Endocrine Society Clinical Practice Guideline. *J Clin Endocrinol Metab*, 2007; **92**: S1–S47. http://www.endo-society.org/publications/guidelines/index.cfm.
6. Eggertsen R, Petersen K, Lundberg P-A, Nyström E, Lindstedt G. Screening for thyroid disease in a primary care unit with a thyroid stimulating hormone assay with a low detection limit. *Br Med J*, 1988; **297**: 1586–92.
7. Jarlov AE, Nygaard B, Hegedus L, Hartling SG, Hansen JM. Observer variation in the clinical and laboratory evaluation of patients with thyroid dysfunction and goiter. *Thyroid*, 1998; **8**: 393–8.
8. Stockigt JR, Lim CF. Medications that distort in vitro tests of thyroid function, with particular reference to estimates of serum free thyroxine. *Best Prac Res Clin Endocrinol Metab*, 2009; **23**: 753–67.

9. Beckett GJ, Toft AD. First-line thyroid function tests: TSH alone is not enough. *Clin Endocrinol*, 2003; **58**: 20–1.
10. DeGroot LJ, Mayor G. Admission screening by thyroid function tests in an acute general care teaching hospital. *Am J Med*, 1992; **93**: 558–64.
11. Ryan WG, Roddam RF, Grizzie WE. Thyroid function screening in newly admitted psychiatric patients. *Ann Clin Psychiatry*, 1994; **6**: 7–12.
12. Stockigt JR. Guidelines for diagnosis and monitoring of thyroid disease: nonthyroidal illness. *Clin Chem*, 1996; **42**: 188–92.
13. Rothwell PM, Udwadia ZF, Lawler PG. Thyrotropin concentration predicts outcome in critical illness. *Anaesthesia*, 1993; **48**: 373–6.
14. Roti E, Gardini E, Minelli R, Bianconi L, Flisi M. Thyroid function evaluation by different commercially available free thyroid hormone measurement kits in term pregnant women and their newborns. *J Endocrinol Invest*, 1991; **14**: 1–9.
15. Lee RH, Spencer CA, Mestman JH, Miller EA, Petrovic I, Braverman LE, *et al.* Free T_4 assays are flawed during pregnancy. *Am J Obstet Gynecol*, 2009; **260**: 260e1–e6.
16. Kahric-Janicic N, Soldin SJ, Soldin OP, West T, Gu J, Jonklaas J. Tandem mass spectrometry improves the accuracy of free thyroxine measurements during pregnancy. *Thyroid*, 2007; **17**: 303–11.
17. Brabant G, Prank K, Ranft U, Schuermeyer T, Wagner TO, Hauser H. Physiological regulation of circadian and pulsatile thyrotropin secretion in normal man and woman. *J Clin Endocrinol Metab*, 1990; **70**: 403–9.
18. Karmisholt J, Andersen S, Laurberg P. Variation in thyroid function tests in patients with stable untreated subclinical hypothyroidism. *Thyroid*, 2007; **18**: 303–8.
19. Spencer CA. Assay of thyroid hormones and related substances, in www.thyroidmanager.org, 17 May 2010. South Dartmouth MA: Endocrine education Inc.
20. Sadler WA, Murray LM, Turner JG. Influence of specimen carryover on sensitive thyrotropin (TSH) assays: is there a problem? *Clin Chem*, 1996; **42**: 593–7.
21. Després N, Grant AM. Antibody interference in thyroid assays: a potential for clinical misinformation. *Clin Chem*, 1998; **44**: 440–54.
22. Ross HA, Menheere PPCA, Thomas CMG, Mudde AH, Kouwenberg M, olffenbuttel BH, *et al.* Interference from heterophilic antibodies in seven current TSH assays. *Ann Clin Biochem*, 2008; **45**: 616.
23. Biondi B, Cooper DS. The clinical significance of subclinical thyroid dysfunction. *Endocr Rev*, 2008; **29**: 76–131.
24. Meyerovitch J, Rotman-Pikielny S, Sherf M, Battat E, Levy Y, Surks MI. Serum thyrotropin measurements in the community: five-year follow-up in a large network of primary care physicians. *Arch Int Med*, 2007; **167**: 1533–8.
25. Ringel MD, Mazzaferri EL. Subclinical thyroid dysfunction: can there be consensus about a consensus? *J Clin Endocrinol Metab*, 2006; **90**: 588–90.
26. Wartofsky L, Dickey RA. The evidence for a narrower thyrotropin reference range is compelling. *J Clin Endocrinol Metab*, 2005; **90**: 5489–96.
27. Surks MI, Goswami G, Daniels GH. The thyrotropin reference range should remain unchanged. *J Clin Endocrinol Metab*, 2005; **90**: 5483–8.
28. Hollowell JG, Staeling NW, Flanders WD, Hannon WH, Gunter EW, Spencer CA, *et al.* Serum TSH, T_4 and thyroid antibodies in the US population (1988–1994): national health and nutrition examination survey (NHANES III). *J Clin Endocrinol Metab*, 2002; **87**: 489–99.
29. Surks MI, Ortiz E, Daniels GH. Subclinical thyroid disease: clinical applications. *JAMA*, 2004; **291**: 239–43.
30. Spencer CA, LoPresti JS, Patel A, Guttler RB, Eigen A, Shen D, *et al.* Applications of a new chemiluminometric thyrotropin assay to subnormal measurement. *J Clin Endocrinol Metab*, 1990; **70**: 453–460.
31. Beck-Peccoz P, Brucker-Davis F, Persani L, Smallridge RC, Weintraub BD. Thyrotropin-secreting pituitary tumors. *Endocr Rev*, 1996; **17**: 610–38.
32. Beck-Peccoz P, Persani L. Variable biological activity of thyroid-stimulating hormone. *Eur J Endocrinol*, 1994; **131**: 331–40.
33. Verheecke P. Free triiodothyronine concentration in serum of 1050 euthyroid children is inversely related to their age. *Clin Chem*, 1997; **43**: 963–7.
34. Ekins R. Measurement of free hormones in blood. *Endocr Rev*, 1990; **11**: 5–46.
35. Norden AGW, Jackson RA, Norden LE, Griffin AJ, Barnes MA, Little JA, *et al.* Misleading results from immunoassays of serum free thyroxine in the presence of rheumatoid factor. *Clin Chem*, 1997; **43**: 957–62.
36. Mendel CM, Frost PH, Kunitake ST, Cavalieri RR. Mechanism of the heparin-induced increase in the concentration of free thyroxine in plasma. *J Clin Endocrinol Metab*, 1987; **65**: 1259–64.
37. Yue B, Rockwood AL, Sandrock T, La'ulu SL, Kushnir MM, Meikle AW. Free thyroid hormones in serum by direct equilibrium dialysis and online solid-phase extraction: liquid chromatography/tandem mass spectrometry. *Clin Chem*, 2008; **54**: 642–51.
38. Stockigt JR. Thyroid hormone binding and variants of transport proteins. In: DeGroot LJ, Jameson L, eds. *Endocrinology*. 6th edn. Philadelphia: Saunders, 2010: 1733–44.
39. Mebis, L, Debaveye Y, Visser TJ, Van den Berghe G. Changes within the thyroid axis during the course of critical illness. *Endocrinol Metab Clin North Am*, 2006; **35**: 807–21.
40. Williams FLR, Mires GJ, Barnett C, Ogston SA, van Toor H, Visser TJ, *et al.* Transient hypothyroxinemia in preterm infants: the role of cord sera thyroid hormone levels adjusted for prenatal and intrapartum factors. *J Clin Endocrinol Metab*, 2005; **90**: 4599–606.
41. Surks MI, Sievert R. Drugs and thyroid function. *N Engl J Med*, 1995; **333**: 1688–94.
42. Ceresini G, Morganti S, Rebecchi I, Bertone L, Ceda GP, Bacchi-Modena A, *et al.* A one-year follow-up study of the effects of raloxifene on thyroid function in postmenopausal women. *Menopause*, 2004; **11**: 176–9.
43. Han TS, Williams GR, Vanderpump MPJ. Benzofuran derivatives and the thyroid. *Clin Endocrinol*, 2009; **70**: 2–13.
44. Stevenson HP, Archbold GPR, Johnston P, Young IS, Sheridan B. Misleading serum free thyroxine results during low molecular weight heparin treatment. *Clin Chem*, 1998; **44**: 1002–1007.
45. Kirov G, Tredget J, John R, Owen MJ, Lazarus JH. A cross-sectional and a prospective study of thyroid disorders in lithium-treated patients. *J Affect Disord*, 2005; **87**: 313–17.
46. Surks MI, DeFesi CR. Normal serum free thyroid hormone concentrations in patients treated with phenytoin or carbamazepine. *JAMA*, 1996; **275**: 1495–8.
47. Madeddu G, Spanu A, Chessa F, Calia GM, Lovigu C, Solinas P, *et al.* Thyroid function in HIV patients treated with highly active antiretroviral therapy. *Clin Endocrinol*, 2006; **64**: 575–83.
48. Touzot M, Le Beller C, Touzot F, Louet AL, Piketty C. Dramatic interaction between levothyroxine and lopinavir/ritonavir in a HIV-infected patient. *AIDS*, 2006; **20**: 1210–12.
49. Lanzafame M, Trevenzoli M, Faggian F, Marcati P, Gatti F, Carolo G, *et al.* Interaction between levothyroxine and indinavir in a patient with HIV infection. *Infection*, 2002; **30**: 54–5.
50. Kim MJ, Kim E-K, Kim BM, Kwak JY, Lee EJ, Park CS, *et al.* Thyroglobulin measurements in fine-needle aspirate washouts: the criteria for neck node dissection for patients with thyroid cancer. *Clin Endocrinol*, 2009; **79**: 145–51.
51. Weiss R, Wu SY, Refetoff S. Diagnostic tests of the thyroid: tests that assess the effects of thyroid hormone on body tissues. In: DeGroot LJ, Jameson LJ, eds. *Endocrinology*. 5th edn. Philadelphia: Saunders, 2006: 1915–16
52. Fazio S, Biondi B, Carella C, Sabatini D, Cittadini A, Panza N, *et al.* Diastolic dysfunction in patients on thyroid-stimulating hormone suppressive therapy with levothyroxine: beneficial effect of β-blockade. *J Clin Endocrinol Metab*, 1995; **80**: 2222–6.

3.1.5 Nonthyroidal illness

R.P. Peeters

Introduction

A few hours after the onset of acute illness, marked changes in serum thyroid hormone levels occur. This is referred to as nonthyroidal illness (NTI). The most characteristic and persistent abnormality is a low level of serum triiodothyronine (T_3). Despite these low levels of serum T_3, patients usually have no clinical signs of thyroid disease. Other terms for this disease state have been used, e.g. the low T_3 syndrome and the euthyroid sick syndrome. In addition to nonthyroidal illness, a low T_3 in euthyroid patients is seen during caloric deprivation and after the use of certain types of medication (see Chapter 3.1.4).

Low levels of thyroid hormone in hypothyroidism are associated with a decreased metabolic rate. Both in nonthyroidal illness and in fasting there is a negative energy balance in the majority of cases. Therefore the low levels of T_3 during nonthyroidal illness and starvation have been interpreted as an attempt to save energy expenditure, and intervention is not required. However, this remains controversial and has been a debate for many years. In this chapter, the changes in thyroid hormone levels, the pathophysiology behind these changes, the diagnosis of intrinsic thyroid disease, and the currently available evidence whether these changes should or should not be corrected will be discussed (Box 3.1.5.1).

Box 3.1.5.1 Essential information

- In critical illness, marked changes in thyroid hormone levels occur.
- A decrease in T_3 and increase in reverse T_3 are the most characteristic and persistent abnormalities.
- The magnitude of these changes is related to the severity of disease and associated with a worse prognosis.
- An altered feedback setting at the hypothalamus–pituitary level and a decreased activation and an increased inactivation of thyroid hormone occur in nonthyroidal illness.
- The acute and the more chronic phase of nonthyroidal illness should be seen as two separate entities. An altered peripheral metabolism is the major player in the acute situation, whereas central dysfunction is more important in the chronic phase of severe illness.
- There is currently no evidence that nonthyroidal illness (in the acute or in the chronic phase) should be treated with thyroid hormone.
- Possible benefits of treatment with hypothalamic releasing factors should be the subject of future studies.

Serum and local thyroid parameters in nonthyroidal illness

Within 2 h of the onset of acute illness (and after 24–36 h of fasting), T_3 levels decrease and reverse T_3 levels rise (1). The magnitude of these changes is related to the severity of the disease. The characteristic pattern of changes in thyroid hormone concentrations in relation to severity of disease is shown in Fig. 3.1.5.1. T_3 levels decrease progressively with increasing severity of disease without reaching a plateau, whereas reverse T_3 increases in relation to severity of disease, but reaches a plateau. It has been reported that reverse T_3 is not invariably elevated in all causes of nonthyroidal illness. It may be normal or even low in acute and endstage renal disease, the nephrotic syndrome, AIDS, and prolonged illness (2). However, recent studies have shown significantly elevated levels of serum reverse T_3 in patients with prolonged critical illness and acute renal failure requiring renal replacement therapy (3).

In mild illness, total and free thyroxine (T_4) levels may rise initially after the onset of disease but in severely ill patients, T_4 levels drop as well. Both low T_4 and T_3 levels, as well as high reverse T_3 levels are associated with a worse prognosis (1, 4). Thyroid-stimulating hormone (TSH) levels may rise briefly for about 2 h after the onset of disease, but despite the drop in serum T_3 (and in severe illness also T_4) levels, circulating TSH usually remains within the low to normal range.

In recent years, evidence has emerged that, in addition to severity of illness, duration of illness is another important determinant of the thyrotropic profile in critical illness (5, 6). Patients requiring intensive care for several days enter a more chronic phase of severe illness, and the low levels of thyroid hormone in prolonged illness have a more neuroendocrine origin (see also next paragraph). Pulsatility and circadian variation in TSH secretion is diminished in prolonged illness, and hypothalamic thyrotropin-releasing hormone (TRH) mRNA expression in patients who died from chronic severe illness is low compared to patients who died from an acute lethal trauma (7). In prolonged illness, both low TSH secretion and TRH expression correlate with the low T_3 levels. This results in even lower levels of T_3 and a low T_4 as well. Reverse T_3 levels remain elevated or may return back to normal with the decrease in serum T_4 (see Fig. 3.1.5.2a). Obviously, severity and duration of illness are both important factors that determine the changes in nonthyroidal illness, and mixed forms of the above-mentioned changes further

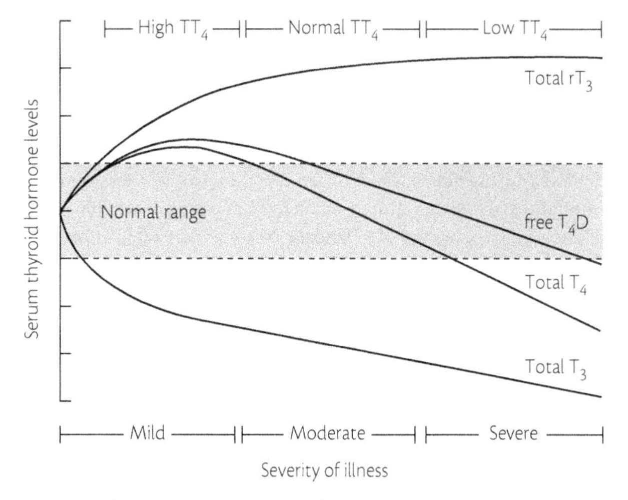

Fig. 3.1.5.1 Relationship between thyroid hormone serum levels and severity of nonthyroidal illness. TT_4, total T_4; rT_3, reverse T_3. (From Kaptein EM. Thyroid hormone metabolism in illness. In: Hennemann G, ed. *Thyroid Hormone Metabolism*. New York: Marcel Dekker, 1986: 297–333, with permission.)

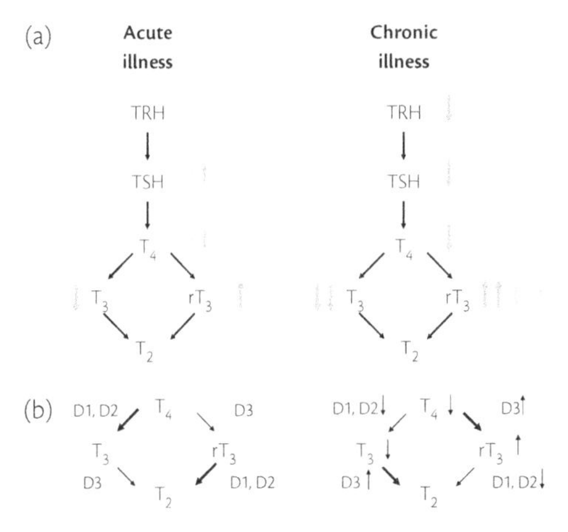

Fig. 3.1.5.2 (a) Simplified overview of the major changes occurring within the thyroid axis during the acute and chronic phase of critical illness. The normal regulation of the thyroid axis is shown in black, whereas the alterations induced by critical illness are indicated in grey. As discussed in the text, for the acute phase of critical illness, thyrotropin and T_4 levels are elevated briefly and subsequently return to normal. T_2, diiodothyronine. (Reproduced from Van den Berghe G. Novel insights into the neuroendocrinology of critical illness. *Eur J Endocrinol*, 2000; **143**: 1–13, with permission.) (b) Relationship between the different iodothyronines and the outer ring (D1, D2) and inner ring (D3) deiodination by the three deiodinases are shown on the left. Like D3, D1 has some inner ring deiodination capacity *in vitro*, but there is currently no evidence that this is of any significance *in vivo* (see also Chapter 3.1.2). This is therefore omitted from the figure. Observed changes in deiodinase activities and iodothyronine levels during critical illness, both in the acute and chronic phase of critical illness, are shown on the right. (Reproduced from Peeters RP, Debaveye Y, Fliers E, Visser TJ. Changes within the thyroid axis during critical illness. *Crit Care Clinics*, 2006; **22**: 41–55; with permission.)

complicate the interpretation of thyroid function tests in critical illness. In addition to severity and duration of illness, type of illness may also be important with regard to the changes in peripheral thyroid hormone levels (2, 3) (see below).

Both low T_4, low T_3, and high reverse T_3 levels are associated with a more severe illness and a worse prognosis. A study in 451 patients who received intensive care for at least 5 days showed that not only the absolute values but also the time course of serum thyroid parameters between survivors and nonsurvivors is completely different (4). In this study, TSH, T_4, T_3, and the T_3/reverse T_3 ratio increased in patients who survived, whereas there was no such rise in nonsurvivors (see Fig. 3.1.5.3).

Only a few studies have been reported investigating the tissue concentrations of thyroid hormone in critical illness. One study demonstrated that patients who died after critical illness had lower levels of tissue T_3 compared to patients who had died acutely, but the severity seems to vary from one organ to another (8). A different study in patients who had died in the intensive care unit showed that low levels of serum T_4 and T_3 correlated well with local concentrations in liver and skeletal muscle (9). This suggests that the decrease in serum T_3 (and in severe illness also T_4) in nonthyroidal illness also results in decreased tissue levels of thyroid hormone.

Neuroendocrine changes in nonthyroidal illness

Acute illness

In primary hypothyroidism, TSH levels rise sharply in response to low levels of circulating thyroid hormones. After the onset of acute disease, TSH levels may rise briefly for about 2 h, but despite the ongoing decrease in circulating T_3 (and in severe illness also T_4) levels, TSH usually remains within the low to normal range in nonthyroidal illness. This suggests an altered feedback setting at the level of the hypothalamus and/or pituitary. The physiological nocturnal TSH surge is absent in this acute phase of illness (5) (see Fig. 3.1.5.4). These changes in the acute phase cannot be attributed to exogenous glucocorticoids or dopamine, since serum TSH is also in the low to normal range in patients without these drugs.

Different mechanisms have been proposed for this altered feedback setting. Studies in rodents during fasting and after lipopolysaccharide injection, which is a model for acute inflammation, show no compensatory rise in TRH in contrast to hypothyroid animals (10). Local expression of thyroid hormone-activating type 2 deiodinase (D2) is increased and expression of thyroid hormone-inactivating D3 is unaltered, resulting in higher local concentrations of hypothalamic T_3 (11, 12) (see Chapter 3.1.2 for a more detailed description of the function of the different iodothyronine deiodinases). This is in agreement with a down-regulation of TRH in fasting and acute illness. MCT8, a specific thyroid hormone transporter which is important in brain development, and OATP1C1, a high-affinity T_4 transporter, are both expressed in the hypothalamus, suggesting an important role for these transporters in the hypothalamic set point (13). Animal data also show that an altered transmembrane transport of thyroid hormone at the levels of the pituitary and/or hypothalamus may be involved in the altered hypothalamus–pituitary–thyroid axis set point, as well as an enhanced occupancy of nuclear T_3 receptors in the pituitary thyrotrophs.

In the acute phase of critical illness, circulating levels of cytokines are usually high. Injection of cytokines such as interleukin (IL)-1, IL-6, and tumour necrosis factor-α (TNFα) is at least partially able to mimic the thyrotropic alterations of the acute stress response. Studies in IL-12 and IL-18 knockout mice show that these cytokines are also involved. However, cytokine antagonism fails to restore thyroid hormone levels, both in animals (IL-1, IL-6, TNFα, interferon) and in humans (IL-1) (14, 15).

High levels of endogenous cortisol may also contribute to the blunted TSH response in acute illness. In addition, endogenous thyroid hormone analogues, such as thyronamines and thyroacetic acids, may also contribute to the pathogenesis of nonthyroidal illness, by blunting the TSH response to low levels of thyroid hormone and/or by competing with thyroid hormone for binding to transport proteins, transmembrane transporters, deiodinases, and/or nuclear receptors.

Chronic illness

Patients with prolonged critical illness have a more severe central dysfunction. In addition to the absent nocturnal TSH surge, TSH pulsatility diminishes dramatically and hypothalamic TRH expression is reduced (5, 6). Both low TSH secretion and low TRH expression correlate with the low T_3 levels in prolonged critical illness (7). Patients who die after severe illness have less than one-half the concentration of hypothalamic and pituitary T_3 compared to patients who die acutely from trauma (8). This combination of a low TRH expression in the hypothalamus, a low TSH secretion from the pituitary, and low levels of T_3 in both tissues implies a major change in the hypothalamus–pituitary feedback regulation, and suggests a more central origin of the low T_3 syndrome in

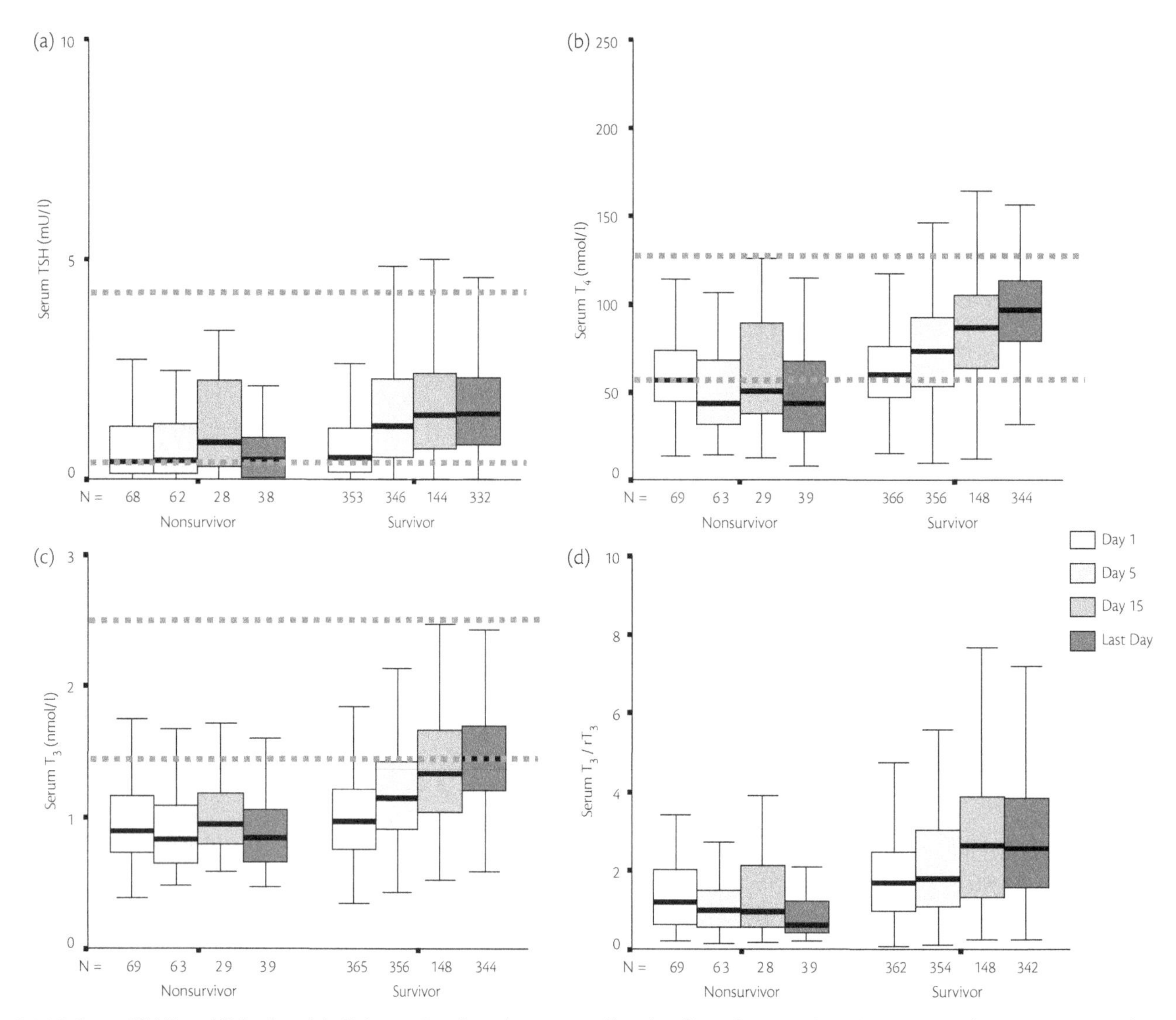

Fig. 3.1.5.3 Serum TSH, T_4, and T_3 levels and the T_3/reverse T_3 ratio at day 1, 5, 15, and last day of intensive care unit stay in survivors and nonsurvivors. From day 5 onward, serum TSH, T_4, and T_3 increased in patients who survived, whereas there was no such pattern in patients who died (a–c). The serum T_3/reverse T_3 ratio increased in survivors from day 5 to last day, whereas it did not alter or even decreased in nonsurvivors (d). On the last day of intensive care unit stay, the majority of patients had TSH and T_4 levels within the normal range, whereas T_3 was still low. The blocked line represents the normal values. (Modified from Peeters RP, Wouters PJ, van Toor H, Kaptein E, Visser TJ, Van den Berghe G. Serum 3,3′,5′-triiodothyronine (rT_3) and 3,5,3′-triiodothyronine/rT_3 are prognostic markers in critically ill patients and are associated with postmortem tissue deiodinase activities. *J Clin Endocrinol Metab*, 2005; **90**: 4559–65; with permission.)

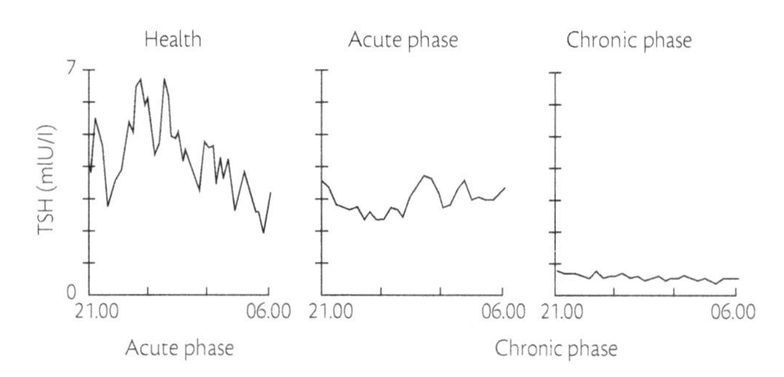

Fig. 3.1.5.4 The nocturnal serum concentration profiles of thyrotropin in critical illness are abnormal and differ markedly between the acute and chronic phase of the disease. (Modified from Van den Berghe G, de Zegher F, Bouillon R. Acute and prolonged critical illness as different neuroendocrine paradigms. *J Clin Endocrinol Metab*, 1998; **83**: 1827–34; with permission.)

prolonged illness. The positive correlation of TSH secretion and TRH expression with serum T_3 levels also points in this direction. In contrast, an increase in TSH is a marker for recovery, which suggests that recovery from the low T_3 syndrome is also initiated centrally (see Fig. 3.1.5.3 in which the recovery of TSH precedes the recovery of the T_3/reverse T_3 ratio). In addition, continuous infusion with TRH (especially when combined with a growth hormone secretagogue) is able to (partially) restore serum TSH, T_4, and T_3 in prolonged critical illness, both in humans and in animals (16).

The pathophysiology behind this suppression of the hypothalamus–pituitary–thyroid axis is not fully understood. Circulating cytokines are usually low in the chronic phase of severe illness, so other mechanisms must be involved. An up-regulation of hypothalamic D2, which is seen in animal models of acute illness, and/or a down-regulation of D3 could suppress TRH expression via relatively high concentrations of hypothalamic T_3.

However, hypothalamic and pituitary T_3 levels are low in patients who die after prolonged illness (8). This makes an important contribution of hypothalamic and pituitary deiodinases to the central suppression in prolonged critical illness less likely. Similarly, the low levels of hypothalamic T_3 in prolonged illness make an important contribution of thyroid hormone transporters to the altered set point in chronic illness less likely.

Other pathways, such as the melanocortin signalling pathway and neuropeptide Y (NPY), seem to be involved in regulating hypothalamic TRH secretion in chronic critical illness as well (6, 17, 18). However, the exact role of these neuropeptides in nonthyroidal illness is not yet elucidated. Different experimental and clinical conditions show different results. For example, patients with chronic illness showed weak immunocytochemical staining of NPY cells in the infundibular nucleus compared to patients who died acutely, and low NPY expression was associated with decreased TRH mRNA expression in the paraventricular nucleus (18). However, an inverse relationship is observed during fasting (19), again illustrating that changes in fasting and acute illness should not be extrapolated to the chronic phase of severe illness.

Exogenous glucocorticoids and dopamine are known to suppress the hypothalamus–pituitary–thyroid axis, and perhaps prolonged hypercortisolism and/or endogenous dopamine in these patients may also play a role.

Peripheral changes in nonthyroidal illness

In the acute phase of critical illness and after starvation, changes in thyroid hormone levels are mainly caused by changes in the peripheral metabolism of thyroid hormones and by alterations in the capacity of serum binding proteins (1). In the more chronic phase of critical illness, these changes persist but a decreased T_4 production by the thyroid is superimposed on the altered peripheral metabolism. The serum T_3/reverse T_3 ratio is the most accurate reflection of the peripheral metabolism, since this ratio is independent of variations in binding proteins and independent of a decreased T_4 production by the thyroid (see also Chapter 3.1.2). The decrease in serum T_3 and increase in serum reverse T_3 that occurs within a few hours of the onset of disease suggests major changes in the peripheral metabolism of thyroid hormone.

Deiodination of thyroid hormones in nonthyroidal illness

Approximately 20% of serum T_3 is produced by the thyroid, whereas the rest is derived from conversion of T_4 in peripheral tissues such as liver and skeletal muscle. The availability of T_3 for nuclear thyroid hormone receptors is largely regulated by different transmembrane transporters and by three deiodinases that catalyse deiodination of the different iodothyronines (20) (Fig. 3.1.5.2b, see also Chapter 3.1.2). D1 is present in liver, kidney, and thyroid, and plays a key role in the production of serum T_3 from T_4 and in the breakdown of the inactive metabolite reverse T_3. D2 is present in brain, anterior pituitary, thyroid, and skeletal muscle. D2 also converts T_4 to the active hormone T_3. D2 is important for local T_3 production in tissues such as the brain, but the enzyme in skeletal muscle may also contribute to plasma T_3 production. D3 is present in brain, skin, placenta, pregnant uterus, and various fetal tissues, and is the major T_3 and T_4 inactivating enzyme by converting T_4 and T_3 to reverse T_3 and T_2, respectively. D3 protects tissues from excess thyroid hormone. All three deiodinases are selenoproteins and use reductive compounds, such as reduced glutathione, as cofactors.

The fall in serum T_3 levels and increase in serum reverse T_3 levels in the acute phase of critical illness and in fasting are largely due to a decreased conversion of T_4 to T_3 and of reverse T_3 to T_2, as demonstrated by multiple kinetic studies (see reference (1) for a review of the literature). Different factors contributing to these decreased conversions have been proposed, such as a decreased tissue uptake due to a negative energy balance and increased levels of bilirubin and nonesterified fatty acids, decreased availability of selenium and/or cofactors, and drugs inhibiting deiodinase activity.

Liver and skeletal muscle biopsies obtained minutes after death of intensive care unit patients demonstrated that liver D1 activity in these patients is low compared to values observed in healthy individuals, except for patients who died acutely from severe brain damage (Fig. 3.1.5.2b) (3). Deiodinase activities were measured in tissue homogenates in the presence of excess cofactor, which suggests a down-regulation of D1 independent of the above-mentioned mechanisms. Low levels of D1 activity were clearly correlated with high levels of reverse T_3 and a low T_3/reverse T_3 ratio, independent of duration of illness (see Fig. 3.1.5.5). D1 activities also showed a clear correlation with local T_3 concentrations and T_3/reverse T_3 ratios in liver (9).

No D2 activity could be detected in skeletal muscle samples of these patients, although there is evidence that D2 activity is expressed in normal skeletal muscle. A reduced activity of D2 may therefore also contribute to the low levels of T_3 in the acute phase of nonthyroidal illness. However, other studies show some D2 expression in muscle, especially after prolonged illness (21). This suggests that an altered D2 activity may not play a role in the pathogenesis of the low T_3 syndrome in prolonged critical illness.

A clear induction of D3 activity was demonstrated in both liver and muscle samples of these patients, whereas these tissues normally do not express D3 in adult subjects (Fig. 3.1.5.2b). High liver and high muscle D3 activity was associated with high serum and local tissue reverse T_3 levels (see Fig. 3.1.5.5). D3 induction was independent of duration of illness. From these data it can be concluded that a down-regulation of thyroid hormone-activating D1 (and in the acute phase of illness also D2) and an induction of thyroid hormone-inactivating D3 are important factors contributing to the low levels of T_3 and high levels of reverse T_3 in nonthyroidal illness.

Tissue deiodinase activities and serum thyroid hormone levels are significantly associated with cause of death (3). A postmortem study in over 60 patients demonstrated that liver D1 activity and serum T_3/reverse T_3 were highest in patients who died from severe brain damage, intermediate in those who died from sepsis or excessive inflammation, and lowest in patients who died from cardiovascular collapse (see Fig. 3.1.5.6). Liver D3 showed an opposite relationship. There was no relation between deiodinase activities and a marker of inflammation (C-reactive protein), but patients who needed inotropes and/or those requiring dialysis because of acute renal failure had a lower liver D1 activity and higher liver and muscle D3 activity. This suggests that poor tissue perfusion and cellular hypoxia may be an important determinant regulating deiodinase activities *in vivo*. Recently it has been shown that D3 activity and D3 mRNA are increased by hypoxia and by hypoxia mimetics that increase hypoxia-inducible factor 1 (22). This supports the

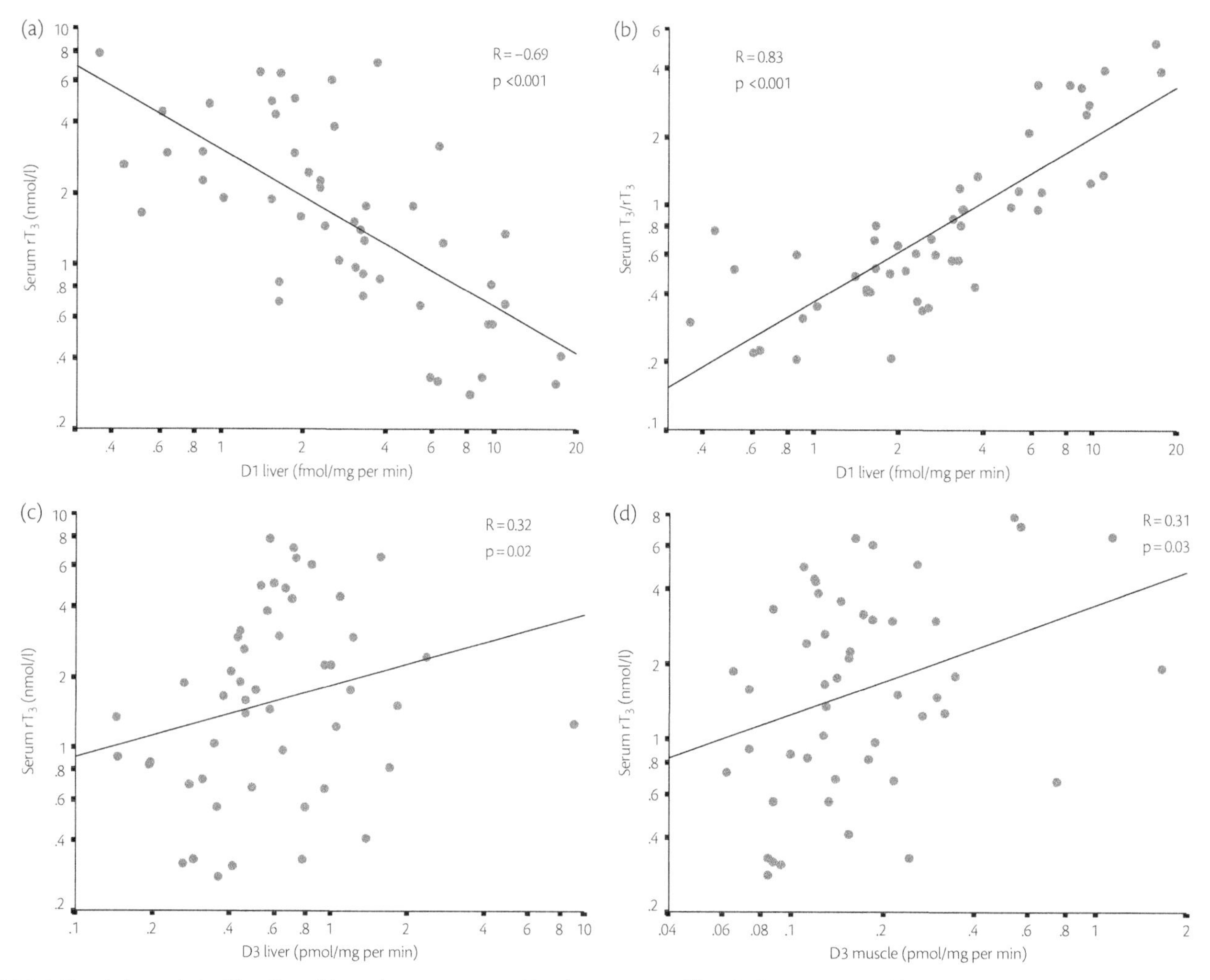

Fig. 3.1.5.5 Correlation analysis of liver D1 activity and serum reverse T_3 (a) and T_3/reverse T_3 (b), and of liver D3 activity (c), skeletal muscle D3 activity (d), and serum reverse T_3. Liver D1 showed a significant negative correlation with reverse T_3 ($p < 0.001$) and a significant positive correlation with the T_3/reverse T_3 ratio ($p < 0.001$). Both liver and skeletal muscle D3 activity were positively correlated to serum reverse T_3 levels ($p < 0.05$). R, Spearman's correlation coefficient. (Reproduced from Peeters RP, Wouters PJ, van Toor H, Kaptein E, Visser TJ, Van den Berghe G. Serum 3,3′,5′-triiodothyronine (rT_3) and 3,5,3′-triiodothyronine/rT_3 are prognostic markers in critically ill patients and are associated with postmortem tissue deiodinase activities. *J Clin Endocrinol Metab*, 2005; **90**: 4559–65; with permission.)

hypothesis that up-regulation of D3 by cellular hypoxia may be a way to alter thyroid hormone bioactivity during limited oxygen supply (see also Chapter 3.1.2).

Transmembrane transport of thyroid hormones in nonthyroidal illness

Thyroid hormone mediates its effects by binding to nuclear T_3 receptors, resulting in initiation or repression of transcription. Depending on the target tissue, nuclear T_3 is derived from plasma and/or from intracellular generation from T_4. This means that both T_3 and T_4 have to cross the plasma membrane of target cells for biological action (see Chapter 3.1.2). The process of uptake of thyroid hormones by cells is rate limiting for subsequent intracellular metabolism and nuclear T_3 binding.

Uptake of T_4 by human hepatocytes is temperature, Na^+, and energy dependent, and kinetic analyses indicate that T_4 and T_3 cross the plasma membrane by different transporters (23). Kinetic studies have shown that fasting and nonthyroidal illness result in attenuation of uptake of liver T_4 and reverse T_3, probably via decreased concentrations of intracellular ATP. Liver T_3 uptake is less sensitive to intracellular ATP concentrations. Inhibition of thyroid hormone uptake has also been shown with nonesterified fatty acids and bilirubin, both elevated in critical illness, and certain drugs such as amiodarone. It has not been studied whether these alterations in transport persist during prolonged illness, but there is no evidence to assume otherwise.

In recent years, different thyroid hormone transporters have been identified, exhibiting a different tissue distribution, substrate specificity, and selectivity. Human MCT8, with a preference for T_3 over T_4, is probably the best studied transporter. Mutations in MCT8 lead to a phenotype of severe psychomotor retardation (24). Transport activity by MCT8 is not Na^+ and/or energy dependent, but MCT8 is expressed in, among other tissues, liver and skeletal muscle. In critically ill patients, neither liver nor skeletal muscle MCT8 expression were related to the ratio of the serum over tissue concentration of T_4, T_3, or reverse T_3 (9). This suggests that MCT8 is not crucial in the transport of these iodothyronines over the plasma membrane in liver and skeletal muscle. However, this does not exclude an important regulatory function of other known (i.e. MCT10) and as yet unknown thyroid hormone

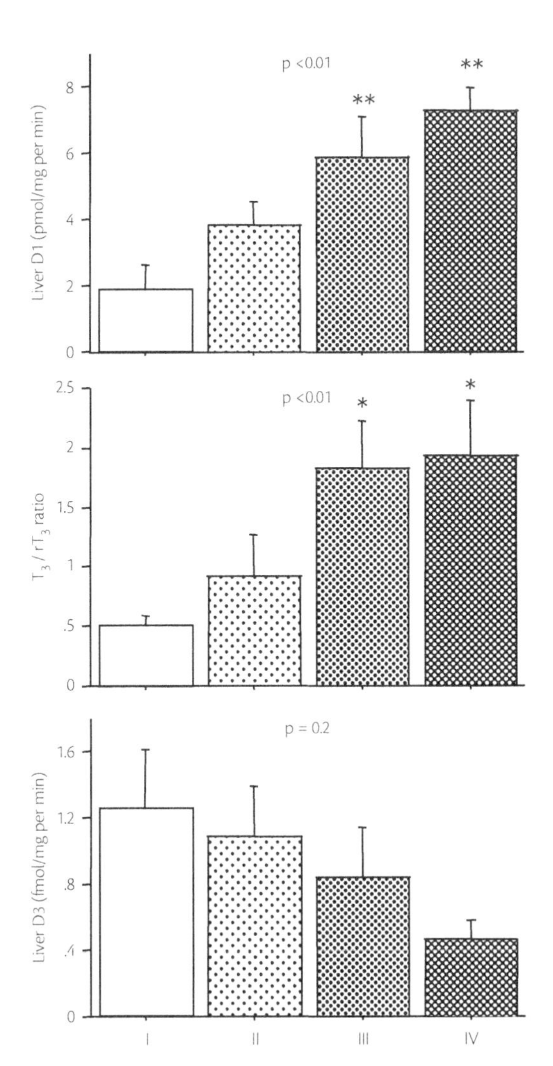

Fig. 3.1.5.6 Correlation of liver D1 (a) activity, the T_3/reverse T_3 ratio (b), and liver D3 (c) activity with cause of death. Patients are divided into four different groups based on cause of death. I, cardiovascular collapse (n = 5); II, multiple organ failure with sepsis (n = 21); III, multiple organ failure with systemic inflammatory response syndrome (n = 14); IV, severe brain damage (n = 4). Liver D1 activity and serum T_3/reverse T_3 ratio showed a significant relation with cause of death ($p < 0.01$), whereas liver D3 activity showed an opposite trend. **, $p < 0.01$ versus group I; *, $p < 0.05$ versus group I. Data represent means ± SEM and p values were obtained with ANOVA and Fisher's least significant difference for multiple comparisons. (Modified from Peeters RP, Wouters PJ, Kaptein E, van Toor H, Visser TJ, Van den Berghe G. Reduced activation and increased inactivation of thyroid hormone in tissues of critically ill patients. *J Clin Endocrinol Metab*, 2003; **88**: 3202–11; with permission.)

transporters in nonthyroidal illness, and needs to be addressed in future studies.

Thyroid hormone receptors in nonthyroidal illness

Different thyroid hormone receptor (TR) isoforms are generated from the *THRA* and *THRB* genes by alternative splicing and different promoter usage. *THRA* encodes five proteins, but only TRα1 has intact DNA- and T_3-binding domains. There is evidence that TRα2 acts as a dominant negative isoform. *THRB* encodes three proteins that can bind T_3 and DNA. The T_3-binding thyroid hormone receptors are highly homologous, except in the N-terminal α- and β-domains (25) (see Chapter 3.1.2). Both in the liganded and unliganded state, thyroid hormone receptors bind to T_3-response elements (TREs) in the promoter region of target genes. Unliganded thyroid hormone receptors repress basal transcription. Binding of T_3 releases corepressors and allows recruitment of coactivators required for gene expression above basal levels. TRα1 and TRβ1 are ubiquitously expressed; TRα1 is expressed preferentially in brain, heart, and bone, and TRβ1 preferentially in liver, kidney, and thyroid.

Little is known about the regulation of thyroid hormone receptors in nonthyroidal illness. In rats, it has been shown that starvation results in a decreased expression and occupancy of hepatic thyroid hormone receptors (26). In peripheral mononuclear cells in humans, an increased expression of both TRα and TRβ has been demonstrated in patients with chronic liver and renal disease, whereas in patients in the intensive care unit only TRβ mRNA was increased (27). In patients with liver disease, both liver TRα (20-fold) and liver TRβ (fivefold) were increased compared to healthy liver controls. A postmortem study in 58 subjects who had died in the intensive care unit showed an increased expression of the TRα1/TRα2 ratio (active isoform/dominant negative isoform), which was positively related to severity of disease and age (28). In this study, no relation between severity of disease and TRβ1 expression was observed.

The clinical relevance of these changes is not yet clear. One might argue that an increase in the expression of the active receptor isoforms is an adaptive response by the body to decreasing levels of thyroid hormone. On the other hand, a higher thyroid hormone receptor expression with low levels of T_3 will lead to an increase in the percentage of unliganded receptors, which would have an opposite effect. Interestingly, no relation was demonstrated between liver TRβ1 mRNA levels and serum thyroid hormone parameters in critically ill patients, although D1 expression is, among other things, regulated by T_3 via TRβ1 (28).

Other metabolic pathways in nonthyroidal illness

Alternate metabolic pathways of thyroid hormone metabolism include sulfation and glucuronidation. Sulfated iodothyronines do not bind to thyroid hormone receptors, and sulfation mediates the rapid and irreversible degradation of iodothyronines by D1. Inner ring deiodination (see Chapter 3.1.2) of T_4 and T_3 by D1 are markedly facilitated after sulfation, whereas outer ring deiodination of T_4 is completely blocked after sulfation. As a consequence, serum concentrations of sulfated iodothyronines are usually low. D2 and D3 are incapable of deiodinating sulfated iodothyronines.

Elevated levels of T_4 sulfate and T_3 sulfate/T_3 ratios have been reported in patients with nonthyroidal illness, and postmortem serum T_4 sulfate levels in critically ill patients were positively correlated with the length of stay in the intensive care unit (29, 30). Low hepatic D1 activity in these patients plays an important role in the increased levels of T_4 sulfate.

Glucuronidation in nonthyroidal illness may be important with regard to the use of several drugs. In particular, the anticonvulsant drugs carbamazepine and phenytoin and the antituberculous drug rifampicin have been shown to induce hepatic glucuronidation. This may lower T_4 levels, but T_3 and TSH levels are usually unaffected.

Alterations in thyroid hormone binding

More than 99% of iodothyronines are bound by serum thyroid hormone-binding proteins (see Chapter 3.1.2) leaving only a small proportion in the free form, about 0.02% of T_4 and 0.3% of T_3 and reverse T_3. As thyroxine-binding globulin (TBG) binds the bulk of circulating thyroid hormones, any change in its binding capacity will markedly affect total hormone levels. TBG, transthyretin, and albumin are decreased in nonthyroidal illness as a reflection of the catabolic state of the patient. However, increased TBG levels can be present in liver disease. Different drugs that are used in severe illness may cause alterations in serum binding of thyroid hormone, either by decreasing TBG (e.g. glucocorticoids) or by displacing thyroid hormones from binding proteins (e.g. acetylsalicylic acid, furosemide) (see also Chapter 3.1.4). However, the altered ratios of thyroid hormones that occur in critical illness must be independent of any variation in serum binding capacity.

In addition, patients in the intensive care unit are frequently treated with heparin. In these patients, the measured concentration of serum free T_4 can be higher than the true *in vivo* concentration. This is the result of heparin-induced lipase activity during sample storage and incubation, resulting in *in vitro* generation of nonesterified fatty acids which displace T_4 and T_3 from TBG (see also Chapter 3.1.4). Low-molecular-weight heparin preparations have a similar effect.

Low binding of thyroid hormone in nonthyroidal illness due to the presence of a circulating binding inhibitor has been proposed in older studies (1). However, exogenous T_4 administration can easily replenish the T_4 pool in patients with prolonged illness, making it unlikely that such a binding inhibitor is an important cause of the low levels of T_4 in prolonged nonthyroidal illness (31).

Diagnosis of thyroid disease in critical illness

Evaluation of thyroid status in nonthyroidal illness can be very difficult, especially in patients in the intensive care unit, not only regarding interpretation of laboratory results, but also on clinical grounds as signs and symptoms of the illness may imitate or mask any accompanying thyroid disease. Despite these difficulties the value of clinical examination in this respect should not be underestimated. Thus, the presence of eye signs (ophthalmic Graves' disease), goitre, and a family history of thyroid disease or autoimmune disease in general, are important points that may be supportive for the diagnosis of autoimmune thyroid disease.

Because of the changes that occur in serum thyroid parameters in critical illness and because there is currently no evidence that these changes should be treated, thyroid function should not be tested in critically ill patients unless there is strong suspicion of thyroid disease. In unselected hospitalized patients in the late 1980s, TSH was undetectable (at that time TSH assays were less sensitive, defining undetectable as <0.1 mU/l) in only 3.1% of cases, whereas TSH concentration was above 20 mU/l in only 1.6% of patients (32). When thyroid function is tested, measurement of TSH alone is often not sufficient. Most free T_4 assays are unreliable in critical illness, due to alterations in binding proteins, increased use of heparin in an intensive care unit setting, and the possible presence of circulating binding inhibitors. Therefore, the total thyroid hormone should be measured as well (Box 3.1.5.2).

Box 3.1.5.2 Diagnosis of thyroid disease in critical illness

- In critical illness, thyroid function should only be tested if there is a very strong suspicion of thyroid disease.
- A normal TSH level virtually excludes thyrotoxicosis or hypothyroidism. However, when thyroid function is tested, measurement of TSH alone is often not sufficient.
- Most free T_4 assays are unreliable in critical illness.
- Frequently administered drugs in the intensive care unit, such as dopamine and steroids, suppress TSH secretion.
- Hyperthyroidism
  - A low TSH level is compatible with both nonthyroidal illness and thyrotoxicosis.
  - Nearly all patients with a low but detectable TSH level will have normal thyroid function tests after recovery from illness.
  - Approximately 75% of patients with nonthyroidal illness and a TSH level of less than 0.01 mU/l have hyperthyroidism.
  - Serum T_4 and T_3 levels should be high (or high to normal) in hyperthyroidism, and low (or low to normal) in nonthyroidal illness.
- Hypothyroidism
  - In patients recovering from nonthyroidal illness, TSH levels may become temporarily elevated.
  - Most patients with an elevated TSH level (<20 mU/l) will have normal thyroid function tests after recovery from illness, especially when thyroid peroxidase and thyroglobulin antibodies are negative.
  - In patients with a TSH level of more than 20 mU/l, hypothyroidism is permanent in only 50% of cases.
  - T_4 and T_3 levels may help to differentiate, since patients with hypothyroidism have lower levels of T_4 and T_3 (and a relatively higher T_3/T_4 ratio) compared to patients recovering from nonthyroidal illness.
  - Serum reverse T_3 levels may also be helpful. Low reverse T_3 levels suggest hypothyroidism, whereas high reverse T_3 levels are supportive of nonthyroidal illness.
- If no definite diagnosis can be made, thyroid function tests should be repeated after recovery from illness.

Hyperthyroidism

In a patient with nonthyroidal illness suspected of having hyperthyroidism, serum TSH is the most helpful test. If serum TSH is still within the normal range, the presence of thyrotoxicosis is virtually excluded. But when serum TSH is low, this could be a consequence of nonthyroidal illness or it could be caused by hyperthyroidism. However, nonthyroidal illness almost never results in TSH levels less than 0.01 mU/l (33, 34). Nearly all patients with a low but detectable TSH level will have normal thyroid function tests after recovery from illness. On the other hand, approximately 75% of patients with the low T_3 syndrome and a TSH level of less than 0.01 mU/l have hyperthyroidism (35). Interpretation of serum TSH becomes more difficult in patients treated with TSH-suppressing agents such as dopamine and corticosteroids, which are often used in intensive care units. Additional measurement of T_4 and T_3 levels is mandatory, but should be interpreted with care. T_4 levels are low in approximately 50% of critically ill patients, and T_3 levels are low in the majority of patients, which could mask active hyperthyroidism. However, serum T_4 and T_3 levels should be high (or high to normal) in hyperthyroidism, and low (or low to normal) in nonthyroidal illness.

Hypothyroidism

The diagnosis seems straightforward for critically ill patients with suspected hypothyroidism and elevated serum TSH. However, in patients recovering from nonthyroidal illness, TSH levels may become temporarily elevated. As well as for hyperthyroidism, the magnitude of the change in TSH is important. Nevertheless, even in patients with TSH levels of more than 20 mU/l, hypothyroidism is permanent in only about 50% of cases (32). T_4 and T_3 levels may help to differentiate these patients, since patients with permanent hypothyroidism had significantly lower levels of T_4 and T_3. Most patients with an elevated TSH level (<20 mU/l) will have normal thyroid function tests after recovery from illness, especially if thyroid peroxidase and thyroglobulin antibodies are negative.

In central hypothyroidism, serum TSH is usually low and differentiation from nonthyroidal illness on the basis of these data becomes very difficult. Other pituitary deficiencies and related clinical signs are commonly present in these patients, but prolonged critical illness often leads to suppression of other neuroendocrine axes as well (5). Serum reverse T_3 may be helpful in some cases, since reverse T_3 levels are high in patients with nonthyroidal illness. However, reverse T_3 assays are not available in all centres and reverse T_3 levels may be slightly high in mild hypothyroidism as well. In general, a high T_3/T_4 ratio and a low reverse T_3 favour the presence of hypothyroidism over nonthyroidal illness and vice versa. If no definite diagnosis can be established, thyroid function tests should be repeated after recovery from illness.

Should patients with nonthyroidal illness be treated with thyroid hormone?

Both in acute and in prolonged critical illness, low levels of thyroid hormone are associated with a higher mortality rate, but it remains controversial whether nonthyroidal illness is an adaptation protecting against catabolism or a maladaptation. It is important to re-emphasize the teleological differences between the acute and chronic phase of severe illness (Fig. 3.1.5.2). Acute changes within the thyroid axis after the onset of critical illness (low T_3 and elevated reverse T_3) are similar to the changes observed in starvation. These changes have been interpreted as an attempt to save energy expenditure and protein wasting and do not need intervention. Thyroid hormone replacement in fasting subjects results in an increased nitrogen excretion and negative nitrogen balance, suggesting catabolism. Whether this also applies to the changes in the acute, and especially in the more chronic phase of critical illness, is controversial. Thyroid hormone treatment in critically ill rats shows no beneficial or even negative effects.

In humans, only a few studies have been performed, and studies were carried out in few patients. So far, no clear beneficial effect on clinical outcome has been demonstrated. Intravenous T_4 (150 μg) administration every 12 h for 48 consecutive hours in 28 patients with acute renal failure was even associated with an increased mortality compared to the control group (36). This might have been due to the suppression of TSH in the treatment group, although free T_4 and free T_3 levels were similar in both groups. Intravenous T_4 (1.5 μg/kg per day) administration to 11 patients with nonthyroidal illness for 14 days did not alter the outcome compared to 12 control patients (31). T_4 levels returned to the normal range in the treated patients, but serum T_3 concentrations remained low and did not differ between the two treatment groups. This is probably due to the decreased T_4 to T_3 conversion, which is seen in both the acute and chronic phase of critical illness, and by the accelerated breakdown of T_4 and T_3 by D3.

Because of the decreased T_4 to T_3 conversion in nonthyroidal illness, T_3 treatment may be a better choice. However, T_3 will also be degraded by D3, and T_3 treatment may be harmful as well. T_3 administration to 14 patients with burn injuries did not improve outcome compared to placebo-treated patients (37). An improved cardiac function has been observed in different studies in adult patients treated with pharmacological doses of T_3 after coronary artery bypass grafting, and in dopamine-treated children who received T_3 substitution after cardiopulmonary bypass surgery (38, 39). However, no effect on (perioperative) survival has been demonstrated.

In the chronic phase of critical illness, altered thyroid hormone levels appear to have a more central origin, although the peripheral metabolism is also altered (see Fig. 3.1.5.2). Studies performed in fasting subjects and in patients with acute critical illness should therefore not be extrapolated to the chronic phase of severe illness. Serum thyroid hormone levels in prolonged illness are negatively correlated with markers of increased protein degradation and bone resorption, suggestive of catabolism (16).

In a recent study, tissue thyroid hormone levels were measured in patients who stayed on the intensive care unit for more than 5 days (9). Some of these patients were treated with a combination of T_4 and T_3, but not in a randomized controlled study. Patients were treated if they had a serum T_4 concentration below 50 nmol/l, a normal TBG, and clinical signs of hypothyroidism. Higher serum T_3 levels in treated patients were accompanied by higher levels of tissue T_3. However, the increase in liver T_3 concentrations in patients who received thyroid hormone was disproportional compared to the increase in serum and muscle T_3 concentrations (*c.*4 times higher in liver compared to *c.*2 times higher in serum and skeletal muscle). In addition, TSH levels were suppressed in patients who were treated with thyroid hormone, suggesting overtreatment although their serum T_3 levels were still in the low or low to normal range. So, if patients are given thyroid hormone therapy, should we aim for thyroid hormone levels within or still below the normal range?

Intervention with hypothalamic releasing factors has the advantage that the negative feedback inhibition of thyroid hormone on the pituitary is maintained, thereby providing a safer therapy option. It has been shown that in patients with prolonged critical illness, and in an animal model, continuous infusion of TRH in combination with a growth hormone secretagogue is able to restore thyroid hormone levels. In these patients, this therapy resulted in a reduction of catabolic markers. Whether this also results in a beneficial effect on mortality remains to be addressed in future studies.

References

1. Docter R, Krenning EP, de Jong M, Hennemann G. The sick euthyroid syndrome: changes in thyroid hormone serum parameters and hormone metabolism. *Clin Endocrinol*, 1993; **39**: 499–518.
2. Kaptein EM. Thyroid hormone metabolism and thyroid diseases in chronic renal failure. *Endocr Rev*, 1996; **17**: 45–63.

3. Peeters RP, Wouters PJ, Kaptein E, van Toor H, Visser TJ, Van den Berghe G. Reduced activation and increased inactivation of thyroid hormone in tissues of critically ill patients. *J Clin Endocrinol Metab*, 2003; **88**: 3202–11.
4. Peeters RP, Wouters PJ, van Toor H, Kaptein E, Visser TJ, Van den Berghe G. Serum 3,3′,5′-triiodothyronine (rT_3) and 3,5,3′-triiodothyronine/rT_3 are prognostic markers in critically ill patients and are associated with postmortem tissue deiodinase activities. *J Clin Endocrinol Metab*, 2005; **90**: 4559–65.
5. Van den Berghe G, de Zegher F, Bouillon R. Clinical review 95: acute and prolonged critical illness as different neuroendocrine paradigms. *J Clin Endocrinol Metab*, 1998; **83**: 1827–34.
6. Mebis L, Debaveye Y, Visser TJ, Van den Berghe G. Changes within the thyroid axis during the course of critical illness. *Endocrinol Metab Clin North Am*, 2006; **35**: 807–21.
7. Fliers E, Guldenaar SE, Wiersinga WM, Swaab DF. Decreased hypothalamic thyrotropin-releasing hormone gene expression in patients with nonthyroidal illness. *J Clin Endocrinol Metab*, 1997; **82**: 4032–6.
8. Arem R, Wiener GJ, Kaplan SG, Kim HS, Reichlin S, Kaplan MM. Reduced tissue thyroid hormone levels in fatal illness. *Metabolism*, 1993; **42**: 1102–8.
9. Peeters RP, van der Geyten S, Wouters PJ, Darras VM, van Toor H, Kaptein E, *et al.* Tissue thyroid hormone levels in critical illness. *J Clin Endocrinol Metab*, 2005; **90**: 6498–507.
10. Boelen A, Kwakkel J, Thijssen-Timmer DC, Alkemade A, Fliers E, Wiersinga WM. Simultaneous changes in central and peripheral components of the hypothalamus-pituitary-thyroid axis in lipopolysaccharide-induced acute illness in mice. *J Endocrinol*, 2004; **182**: 315–23.
11. Diano S, Naftolin F, Goglia F, Horvath TL. Fasting-induced increase in type II iodothyronine deiodinase activity and messenger ribonucleic acid levels is not reversed by thyroxine in the rat hypothalamus. *Endocrinology*, 1998; **139**: 2879–84.
12. Fekete C, Gereben B, Doleschall M, Harney JW, Dora JM, Bianco AC, *et al.* Lipopolysaccharide induces type 2 iodothyronine deiodinase in the mediobasal hypothalamus: implications for the nonthyroidal illness syndrome. *Endocrinology*, 2004; **145**: 1649–55.
13. Alkemade A, Vuijst CL, Unmehopa UA, Bakker O, Vennstrom B, Wiersinga WM, *et al.* Thyroid hormone receptor expression in the human hypothalamus and anterior pituitary. *J Clin Endocrinol Metab*, 2005; **90**: 904–12.
14. van der Poll T, Van Zee KJ, Endert E, Coyle SM, Stiles DM, Pribble JP, *et al.* Interleukin-1 receptor blockade does not affect endotoxin-induced changes in plasma thyroid hormone and thyrotropin concentrations in man. *J Clin Endocrinol Metab*, 1995; **80**: 1341–6.
15. Boelen A, Platvoet-ter Schiphorst MC, Wiersinga WM. Immunoneutralization of interleukin-1, tumor necrosis factor, interleukin-6 or interferon does not prevent the LPS-induced sick euthyroid syndrome in mice. *J Endocrinol*, 1997; **153**: 115–22.
16. Van den Berghe G, Wouters P, Weekers F, Mohan S, Baxter RC, Veldhuis JD, *et al.* Reactivation of pituitary hormone release and metabolic improvement by infusion of growth hormone-releasing peptide and thyrotropin-releasing hormone in patients with protracted critical illness. *J Clin Endocrinol Metab*, 1999; **84**: 1311–23.
17. Lechan RM, Fekete C. Role of melanocortin signaling in the regulation of the hypothalamic-pituitary-thyroid (HPT) axis. *Peptides*, 2006; **27**: 310–25.
18. Fliers E, Unmehopa UA, Manniesing S, Vuijst CL, Wiersinga WM, Swaab DF. Decreased neuropeptide Y (NPY) expression in the infundibular nucleus of patients with nonthyroidal illness. *Peptides*, 2001; **22**: 459–65.
19. Ahima RS, Saper CB, Flier JS, Elmquist JK. Leptin regulation of neuroendocrine systems. *Front Neuroendocrinol*, 2000; **21**: 263–307.
20. Bianco AC, Salvatore D, Gereben B, Berry MJ, Larsen PR. Biochemistry, cellular and molecular biology, and physiological roles of the iodothyronine selenodeiodinases. *Endocr Rev*, 2002; **23**: 38–89.
21. Mebis L, Langouche L, Visser TJ, Van den Berghe G. The type II iodothyronine deiodinase is up-regulated in skeletal muscle during prolonged critical illness. *J Clin Endocrinol Metab*, 2007; **92**: 3330–3.
22. Simonides WS, Mulcahey MA, Redout EM, Muller A, Zuidwijk MJ, Visser TJ, *et al.* Hypoxia-inducible factor induces local thyroid hormone inactivation during hypoxic-ischemic disease in rats. *J Clin Invest*, 2008; **118**: 975–83.
23. Hennemann G, Docter R, Friesema EC, de Jong M, Krenning EP, Visser TJ. Plasma membrane transport of thyroid hormones and its role in thyroid hormone metabolism and bioavailability. *Endocr Rev*, 2001; **22**: 451–76.
24. Friesema EC, Jansen J, Heuer H, Trajkovic M, Bauer K, Visser TJ. Mechanisms of disease: psychomotor retardation and high T_3 levels caused by mutations in monocarboxylate transporter 8. *Nat Clin Pract Endocrinol Metab*, 2006; **2**: 512–23.
25. Wondisford FE. Thyroid hormone action: insight from transgenic mouse models. *J Investig Med*, 2003; **51**: 215–20.
26. Carr FE, Seelig S, Mariash CN, Schwartz HL, Oppenheimer JH. Starvation and hypothyroidism exert an overlapping influence on rat hepatic messenger RNA activity profiles. *J Clin Invest*, 1983; **72**: 154–63.
27. Williams GR, Franklyn JA, Neuberger JM, Sheppard MC. Thyroid hormone receptor expression in the "sick euthyroid" syndrome. *Lancet*, 1989; **ii**: 1477–81.
28. Thijssen-Timmer DC, Peeters RP, Wouters P, Weekers F, Visser TJ, Fliers E, *et al.* Thyroid hormone receptor isoform expression in livers of critically ill patients. *Thyroid*, 2007; **17**: 105–12.
29. Chopra IJ, Santini F, Hurd RE, Chua Teco GN. A radioimmunoassay for measurement of thyroxine sulfate. *J Clin Endocrinol Metab*, 1993; **76**: 145–50.
30. Peeters RP, Kester MHA, Wouters PJ, Kaptein E, van Toor H, Visser TJ, *et al.* Increased thyroxine sulfate levels in critically ill patients as a result of a decreased hepatic type I deiodinase activity. *J Clin Endocrinol Metab*, 2005; **90**: 6460–5.
31. Brent GA, Hershman JM. Thyroxine therapy in patients with severe nonthyroidal illnesses and low serum thyroxine concentration. *J Clin Endocrinol Metab*, 1986; **63**: 1–8.
32. Spencer C, Eigen A, Shen D, Duda M, Qualls S, Weiss S, *et al.* Specificity of sensitive assays of thyrotropin (TSH) used to screen for thyroid disease in hospitalized patients. *Clin Chem*, 1987; **33**: 1391–6.
33. Franklyn JA, Black EG, Betteridge J, Sheppard MC. Comparison of second and third generation methods for measurement of serum thyrotropin in patients with overt hyperthyroidism, patients receiving thyroxine therapy, and those with nonthyroidal illness. *J Clin Endocrinol Metab*, 1994; **78**: 1368–71.
34. Spencer CA, LoPresti JS, Patel A, Guttler RB, Eigen A, Shen D, *et al.* Applications of a new chemiluminometric thyrotropin assay to subnormal measurement. *J Clin Endocrinol Metab*, 1990; **70**: 453–60.
35. Stockigt JR. Guidelines for diagnosis and monitoring of thyroid disease: nonthyroidal illness. *Clin Chem*, 1996; **42**: 188–92.
36. Acker CG, Singh AR, Flick RP, Bernardini J, Greenberg A, Johnson JP. A trial of thyroxine in acute renal failure. *Kidney Int*, 2000; **57**: 293–8.
37. Becker RA, Vaughan GM, Ziegler MG, Seraile LG, Goldfarb IW, Mansour EH, *et al.* Hypermetabolic low triiodothyronine syndrome of burn injury. *Crit Care Med*, 1982; **10**: 870–5.
38. Bettendorf M, Schmidt KG, Grulich-Henn J, Ulmer HE, Heinrich UE. Tri-iodothyronine treatment in children after cardiac surgery: a double-blind, randomised, placebo-controlled study. *Lancet*, 2000; **356**: 529–34.
39. Mullis-Jansson SL, Argenziano M, Corwin S, Homma S, Weinberg AD, Williams M, *et al.* A randomized double-blind study of the effect of triiodothyronine on cardiac function and morbidity after coronary bypass surgery. *J Thorac Cardiovasc Surg*, 1999; **117**: 1128–34.

3.1.6 Thyroid imaging: nuclear medicine techniques

I. Ross McDougall, Andrei Iagaru

Introduction

Thyroid imaging with radio-isotopes of iodine provides functional and quantitative information. Images, scans, or scintiscans are the terms used for the pictures that are obtained. In general, a radionuclide or radiopharmaceutical is administered orally or intravenously and images of the distribution of the radioactive tracer are obtained after specific times using a gamma camera. Some clinicians employ a rectilinear scanner rather than a gamma camera to produce the images, but this should not be considered state of the art. Scintiscans do not have the resolution of ultrasonography, CT, or MRI, but they provide reasonable anatomical information as well as functional information. A numerical uptake measurement of how much of the tracer has been trapped can be obtained at the same time as the scintiscan to provide complementary quantitative information. Imaging with radio-iodine is of great value in the diagnosis and management of patients with thyrotoxicosis and differentiated thyroid cancer. It is of less value in thyroid nodules, hypothyroidism, simple goitre, and undifferentiated thyroid cancer. The chapter starts with a discussion of the radioactive tracers and the methods for scanning. Then the appearance of a normal scan followed by findings in patients with thyrotoxicosis, simple goitre, nodular goitre, and congenital defects are described. In these situations the scintiscan evaluates the region of the thyroid. Finally, the role of nuclear medicine imaging in patients with cancer of the thyroid is presented separately since the imaging is different in that it usually evaluates the whole body.

Radionuclides and radiopharmaceuticals

The thyroid is unique in its ability to trap and organify iodine. The sodium-iodide symporter (NIS) provides the mechanism for trapping (1). Scintigraphy and measurement of thyroid function relies on the NIS which cannot differentiate between radio-isotopes of iodine and the nonradioactive ^{127}I. Table 3.1.6.1 lists the clinically useful radio-isotopes and some of their properties. The thyroid can also trap technetium (^{99m}Tc) as pertechnetate ($^{99m}TcO_4$), but this radiopharmaceutical is not organified and it leaks out of the gland. As a result imaging and uptake measurements are obtained 10–20 min after intravenous injection of pertechnetate, rather than after hours or days as is the case with radio-iodines. For routine thyroid scintigraphy and uptake we prefer an oral dose of ^{123}I. Iodine-123 has a clinically useful half-life of 13 h, and a γ-photon of 159 keV that is suitable for gamma camera detection. The units of administered activity are expressed by two different terms. In the SI system the basic unit is the becquerel that is equal to one decay/s. The doses or activity administered are usually in the order of megabecquerels (MBq) for tests and gigabecquerels (GBq) for therapy. In the USA the basic unit is the curie (Ci) which is 3.7×10^{10} disintegrations/s. Diagnostic tests employ μCi to mCi doses and therapy mCi doses. An uptake and scan are usually obtained 24 h after oral administration of 100–300 μCi ^{123}I (3.7–7.4 MBq). Earlier measurements at, e.g. 3–6 h, in addition to 24 h, may give additional information such as rapid turnover of iodine (2). In some countries ^{123}I is not always available and 1–10 mCi of ^{99m}Tc (37–370 MBq) injected intravenously can be used for scintigraphy with images at 10–20 min. The percentage uptake of ^{99m}Tc can be calculated at that time and each laboratory should determine the normal range, which is usually reported to be in the range 1.5–3.5% (3). This is quite different from the measurement of radio-iodine uptake at 24 h. In our department the range is 10–30% and in regions of low dietary iodine the normative range is higher, around 30–50%. Some authorities use a tracer of 10–20 μCi (3.7–7.4 MBq) ^{131}I taken by mouth to determine the 24-h uptake as an adjunct to ^{99m}Tc imaging.

Table 3.1.6.1 Commonly used radio-isotopes for thyroid imaging

Radio-isotope	Half-life	Administered dose (activity)	Clinical uses	Comments
^{123}I	13 h	Routine scan 100–300 μCi (3.7–11.1 MBq)	Imaging thyroid gland	Oral High-quality images and functional information
		Whole body scan 2–5 mCi (74–185 MBq)	Imaging residual thyroid and functioning metastases after thyroidectomy in patients with thyroid cancer	Oral High-quality images at 24 and possibly 48 h with quantitative information Low radiation to patient
^{124}I	4.18 days	Whole-body PET/CT scan 4–5 mCi (148–185 MBq)	For PET and PET/CT scan in patients with thyroid cancer	Oral High resolution PET images that can be reconstructed in multiple planes Volumetric information
^{131}I	8.1 days	Whole-body diagnostic scan 2–4 mCi (74–148 MBq)	Imaging residual thyroid and functioning metastases in patients with thyroid cancer	Oral Low resolution images and higher radiation to patient
		Post-therapy scan 1.1 to >7.4 GBq	For imaging uptake of therapeutic ^{131}I	
$^{99m}TcO_4$	6 h	1–10 mCi (37–370 MBq)	Thyroid imaging	Intravenous Only evaluates trapping not organification
FDG	110 min	10–15 mCi (370–550 MBq)	Whole-body PET and PET/CT in patients with thyroid cancer	Intravenous Most often used for thyroglobulin-positive iodine-negative patient

Methods

Anterior images are made with the patient lying prone; a pillow can be placed under the neck and shoulders to cause extension thus pushing the thyroid forward and closer to the collimator of the camera. A gamma camera with a pinhole collimator produces images with good resolution. It is necessary to collect 10 000–50 000 counts for the image and this can be difficult in children and restless patients. The clinical findings must be correlated with the scintiscans, and palpable nodules should be marked on the scan by placing a radioactive source (cobalt or technetium) on the edges of the mass so that clinical abnormalities can be correlated unequivocally with the findings on the scintiscan. Oblique and lateral images are produced by rotating the head of the camera or by repositioning the patient. These additional projections help determine whether small nodules are functioning or nonfunctioning, since on the anterior image there can be 'shine through' of photons from normal thyroid behind the nodule. One-half of the photons are attenuated by 5 cm of tissue, the so-called half-value thickness. Therefore a small nodule with no function only attenuates a small proportion of counts from surrounding normal thyroid and on the scan it merges into the normal thyroidal activity producing a false-negative result. Scintiscans obtained with a gamma camera are superior to images obtained with a rectilinear scanner (4).

Single photon emission CT (SPECT) is useful in identifying small nodules and determining their function. This is more often the case with multinodular glands. For SPECT scans, the gamma camera rotates around the region of interest, and images are reconstructed as with CT. Tomographic images using a pinhole collimator provide better resolution, but there are significant technical considerations and for most patients planar anterior and oblique views are usually sufficient (5).

The uptake measurement can be obtained with a simple probe by measuring the number of radioactive counts emitted from the thyroid and comparing this with the quantity of radioactivity administered to the patient. It is necessary to correct the counts for radioactive decay. In addition, a correction is made for background activity in soft tissues. This is calculated by taking the radioactive counts from a region over the thigh and subtracting that number from the counts obtained over the neck. For example, the patient receives a capsule of ^{123}I that gives 500 000 counts in 1 min. The uptake is measured at 26 h (two half-lives of ^{123}I), therefore the capsule would contain 125 000 counts at that time. In a patient, the number of counts over the neck is determined to be 26 000 counts/min (cpm) and over the thigh 1000 cpm, therefore the thyroid counts would be 26 000 − 1000, i.e. 25 000. The percentage uptake is 25 000/125 000 × 100 = 20%. Alternatively, the uptake can be measured using a gamma camera image displayed on a computer console. Counts are measured from a region of interest drawn around the thyroid. This is corrected by subtracting counts from an equal area of soft tissue adjacent to the thyroid and compared to the radioactive counts from a known activity of the tracer. The percentage uptake is calculated by comparison to the known number of counts that were administered making sure that there was a correction for decay of the isotope.

Normal thyroid scan and uptake

A normal thyroid scintiscan shows homogeneous distribution of the radionuclide in both lobes (Fig. 3.1.6.1). The lobes can show a slight asymmetry of size with the right being larger more frequently than the left. The central region of each lobe can appear more intense due to the greater depth of functioning thyroid. The isthmus is often seen less well on images made with a gamma camera and sometimes there is almost no uptake in that region and the clinician has to ensure by palpation that there is no mass at that site, since reduced uptake in a thyroid mass implies a nonfunctioning or 'cold' area. The pyramidal lobe is not usually seen on a normal scintiscan but is apparent more frequently in hyperactive glands. The percentage uptake varies with the time of measurement after ingestion of the radionuclide, the function of the thyroid, and the amount of iodine in the diet. Most authorities obtain a measurement at 24 h when a radionuclide of iodine is used and between 10 and 20 min for $^{99m}TcO_4$. The greater the dietary iodine, the lower the percentage of radioiodine or $^{99m}TcO_4$ trapped. The normative range should be obtained for each geographical region. The uptake measurement is used to calculate therapeutic doses of ^{131}I in patients with hyperthyroidism, and whether ^{131}I treatment of thyroid cancer is appropriate. These are discussed below.

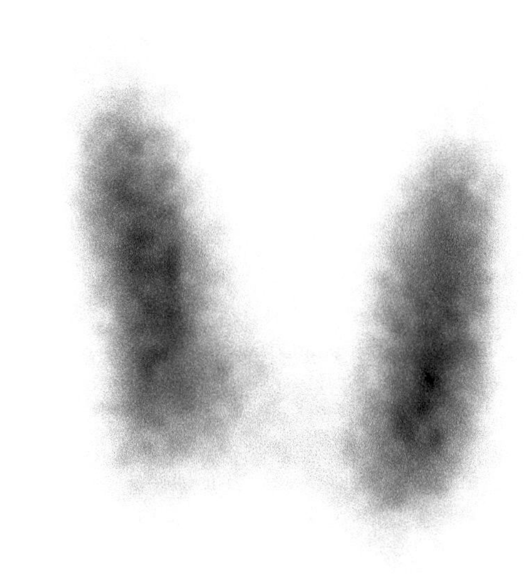

Fig. 3.1.6.1 Normal thyroid ^{123}I scintiscan showing homogeneous distribution of the radionuclide in both lobes.

Thyrotoxicosis

Graves' hyperthyroidism is the commonest cause of thyrotoxicosis. In countries where there is limited dietary iodine, the proportion of patients with single or multiple functioning nodules as the cause of thyrotoxicosis increases. Each of these conditions is associated with high uptake of iodine by measurement and by scintigraphy and each has a characteristic appearance. Figure 3.1.6.2 shows a scintiscan of Graves' disease. The gland is usually enlarged but the size can vary considerably. The lobes are broader and there is less background activity, so the contrast between the thyroid and surrounding neck is accentuated. A pyramidal lobe can be identified in many patients. The uptake measurements are increased and in our laboratory are usually between 40 and 90% at 24 h. The thyroid scan in a patient with a single functioning nodule varies depending on the thyroid status of the patient. If the nodule secretes enough hormone to suppress thyroid-stimulating hormone (TSH), the remaining normal thyroid is not imaged, i.e. it is suppressed. A spectrum from

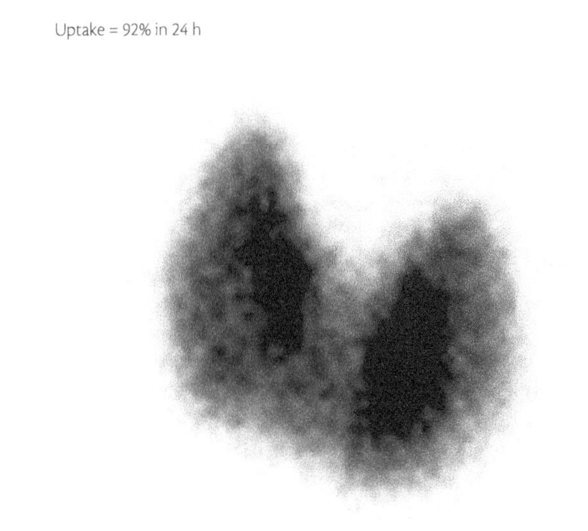

Fig. 3.1.6.2 ^{123}I scintiscan of Graves' disease.

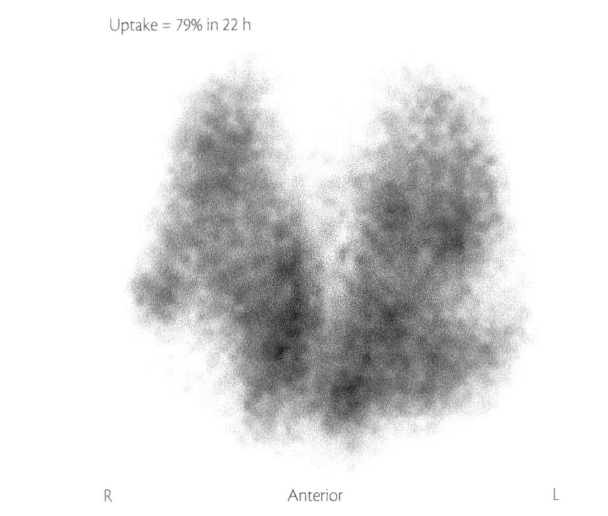

Fig. 3.1.6.3 ^{123}I scintiscan of toxic multinodular goitre.

that appearance to one where the non-nodular tissue appears normal can be seen in patients with normal TSH values. The appearance of a toxic multinodular goitre is shown in Fig. 3.1.6.3. The nodules show varying degrees of uptake of radio-iodine and when the TSH is low the normal thyroid between nodules can show no uptake. The 24-h uptake values are usually in the range 25–50%, thus overlapping with normal thyroid and with Graves' hyperthyroidism. There are conditions in which the patient is clinically and biochemically thyrotoxic, but the uptake is low and scintigraphy shows only faint or no uptake of ^{123}I (Fig. 3.1.6.4). These include subacute, silent, and postpartum thyroiditis, which are discussed below, excess exogenous thyroid hormone, and excess iodine.

Congenital abnormalities

Congenital abnormalities of the thyroid are uncommon and scintigraphy can be useful in defining both structural and functional abnormalities. Many authorities recommend thyroid scintiscan in all newborns found to be hypothyroid by biochemical screening (6). Congenital defects include agenesis, an important cause of neonatal hypothyroidism in which thyroid replacement treatment is necessary for life. In the neonate, ^{99m}Tc pertechnetate scans are simpler because the material is administered intravenously, however, swallowed radioactive saliva from ^{99m}Tc pertechnetate trapped by the salivary glands in the upper oesophagus can be misinterpreted as thyroidal tissue. This radioactivity is usually flushed into the stomach as the child drinks. In agenesis, no thyroid is imaged. Ectopic thyroid, such as lingual or suprahyoid thyroid, can be diagnosed by ^{123}I or ^{99m}Tc pertechnetate scan, which shows uptake in the maldescended organ but not in the normal cervical location. Correlation of the images and physical findings in the patient is important. Hemiagenesis is usually diagnosed by chance in a patient having a scan for some other reason, such as hyperthyroidism. The presence of a single lobe or lobe and isthmus, the so-called 'hockey stick sign or Nike sign', has to be differentiated from a functioning nodule on the same side as the lobe. This can be resolved by several approaches. First by taking a longer time to produce the scan. Alternatively the functioning tissue can be covered with a thin sheet of lead and imaging continued. In hemiagenesis there is no concentration of ^{123}I in the opposite side because there is no lobe and these additional pictures fail to show any functioning tissue. In the case of a functioning nodule the 'suppressed' lobe can be seen faintly. An ultrasound examination proves the presence or absence of thyroid tissue on the contralateral side and resolves the issue rapidly.

Inborn errors in thyroid synthesis are very rare and the diagnosis is aided by scintigraphy. There is no uptake of ^{123}I or ^{99m}Tc in thyroid

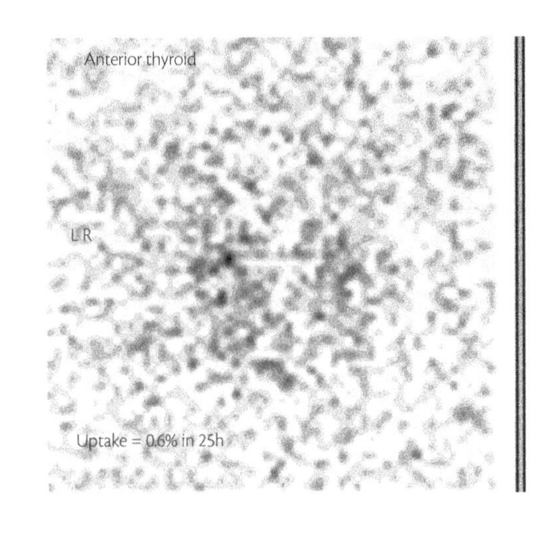

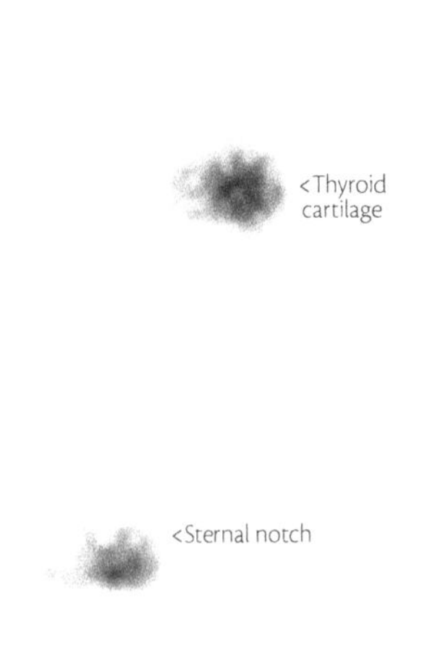

Fig. 3.1.6.4 ^{123}I scintiscan of thyroiditis.

and salivary glands in patients who have a defect in trapping. When there is a deficiency in thyroid peroxidase there is trapping of radio-iodine, but the radioactivity can be discharged from the thyroid by oral or intravenous perchlorate (7).

Hypothyroidism

Thyroid scintigraphy has a very limited role in hypothyroidism. The diagnosis is made by a high clinical suspicion and measuring serum TSH. Treatment with thyroid hormone can usually be started without imaging. Scintiscan can show a variable pattern depending on the cause of hypothyroidism and the uptake measurement is usually low but some patients have normal values. Therefore this measurement should not be used to make the diagnosis of hypothyroidism or to decide on the need for lifelong replacement treatment.

Goitre

In a patient with a diffusely enlarged thyroid and normal thyroid function, scintiscan generally does not provide useful information. In those with a multinodular thyroid, the scan demonstrates which nodules are functioning and which are nonfunctioning. The relevance is discussed in the section on thyroid nodules. In contrast, when there is evidence suggesting a substernal thyroid, frequently first recognized as a superior mediastinal mass on a chest radiograph or CT obtained for some other reason, ^{123}I scan is valuable. The scan demonstrates that substernal goitre contains functioning thyroid tissue, whereas alternative disorders such as lymphoma or thymoma do not. ^{99m}Tc pertechnetate is not advised for diagnosis of substernal goitre because the background activity in the heart and great vessels makes interpretation difficult.

Thyroiditis

There are several conditions called thyroiditis. They have different causes, clinical courses, and outcomes. The commonest cause of thyroiditis is Hashimoto's disease (chronic lymphocytic thyroiditis). The clinical and immunological features are typical and scintiscan is seldom required. The scan in Hashimoto's disease can appear normal, look like Graves' disease, have a patchy appearance, or may show solitary or multiple nodules. Hashimoto's disease has been called the great mimic on thyroid scan, and correlation with clinical, immunological, biochemical, and scintigraphic findings is important (8).

Subacute thyroiditis, silent thyroiditis, and postpartum thyroiditis have a similar course lasting 3–6 months, with a thyrotoxic phase followed by a hypothyroid phase and usually a return to normality. Clinically, the thyrotoxic phase in silent or postpartum thyroiditis can be difficult to differentiate from early or mild Graves' disease. However, uptake and scintiscan show low or no concentration of ^{123}I in thyroiditis in contrast to increased uptake in Graves' disease. Radio-isotopes should not be administered to a woman who is breastfeeding; if a woman is breastfeeding, she must be advised how long it is necessary to stop breastfeeding. Ten half-lives ensures there will be no radioactivity, but finding no radioactive counts in samples of milk might allow restoration of nursing sooner. The pattern of uptake in subacute thyroiditis is the same with low or no uptake in the involved area or the whole gland. The clinical presentation of subacute thyroiditis with pain and malaise is often diagnostic, and uptake and scintiscan should be reserved for atypical cases. There are reports of increased uptake of ^{67}Ga in subacute thyroiditis that had not been suspected clinically. However, this investigation is not necessary when the presentation is typical.

Thyroid nodules

The main clinical decision with a thyroid nodule is whether it is a cancer or not. When cancerous, the nodule and, in most patients, the thyroid are removed surgically. Benign nodules can be kept under periodic clinical evaluation provided they are not causing symptoms. Historically, scintiscan was used to help with this decision. However, it is now acknowledged that the simplistic separation of functioning nodules being benign and nonfunctioning nodules having an increased risk of being malignant is not particularly helpful. This is because in many countries the incidence of functioning nodules is small and, in addition, most nonfunctioning nodules are benign. Most authorities recommend fine-needle aspiration (FNA) and examination of a cytological sample to make the distinction of benign versus malignant. FNA under ultrasound guidance is the optimal technique. If an adult patient is clinically or biochemically thyrotoxic and has a nodule, it is reasonable to obtain a scan to prove the nodule is functioning and therefore very unlikely to be a cancer. FNA would not be required.

Thyroid cancer (differentiated thyroid cancer, papillary, follicular, and variants) and whole body scan

In patients with proven thyroid cancer, whole body scan (WBS) can be useful after thyroidectomy and also 5–10 days after ^{131}I treatment. A WBS with a dual-headed large field-of-view camera, together with spot views of neck and chest, and uptake measurements over abnormal regions provide the information necessary to decide about therapy. Multiple spot views can be obtained in place of whole body images, but they are less satisfying aesthetically and are probably less easy to interpret. Whichever technique is used, the images should be interpreted in association with knowledge of the level of TSH and thyroglobulin, the stage of cancer, and pathological findings.

A WBS is used after surgery to identify residual thyroid or functioning metastases in patients with differentiated thyroid cancers. These cancers usually retain the ability to trap iodine. This test determines whether patients have functioning thyroid that could be ablated by a therapeutic dose of radio-iodine. The diagnostic scan also defines the extent of disease and helps determine what dose of therapeutic ^{131}I to administer. We acknowledge that many authorities proceed with ^{131}I treatment without a diagnostic WBS, but we continue to recommend the procedure because some patients will have no uptake and are unlikely to benefit from radio-iodine therapy, others show metastases in distant sites and would require a larger therapy dose, and still others can show uptake in functioning breast tissues and that should not be subjected to a large dose of radiation since it is known that the breast is a radiation-sensitive organ.

It has been known for a long time that it is necessary to have an elevated thyrotropin level (TSH) to obtain a sensitive result with WBS. We like to have the TSH at 50 IU/l, but most clinicians believe 30 IU/l is acceptable. There are no evidence-based data to prove which level is superior. The high TSH was traditionally achieved by withdrawing whichever thyroid hormone the patient was taking; 4 weeks withdrawal is the most common time for thyroxine, and 2 weeks for triiodothyronine. Alternatively, recombinant human

TSH (rhTSH) can be injected and the usual regime involves two intramuscular injections, the first dose of 0.9 mg administered on a Monday and the second on Tuesday, followed by the test dose of ^{131}I on Wednesday, and the scan on Friday, i.e. 48 h later. Thus this protocol fits neatly into the working week and was promoted by the rhTSH investigators at a time when ^{131}I was the isotope used for WBS (9, 10). There has been a move to the use of ^{123}I that has superior physical characteristics with a shorter half-life, a more suitable γ-ray emission, and no particulate emissions, and is less likely to cause stunning, as discussed later. We have found that ^{123}I can be given late on the day of the second injection of rhTSH or early the following morning and scans can be completed after 24 h. The ^{123}I WBS after rhTSH has been shown to be equivalent to ^{131}I (11).

It is also advised that the patient ingest a low-iodine diet (12). The goal is to reduce the plasma inorganic iodine so that the radioactive tracers are not diluted by nonradioactive iodine. Again there are no evidence-based data to confirm this helps, but in countries where the dietary iodine intake is high we would definitely make this recommendation.

The distribution of uptake on the WBS depends on tissues that express the NIS, the route of excretion of iodine, and whether the scan is a diagnostic scan using a small dose of either ^{123}I or ^{131}I or a post-treatment scan after a large dose of ^{131}I. Sites expressing the NIS on a diagnostic scan include residual thyroid and functioning metastases in regional lymph nodes and distant sites such as the lungs and skeleton. Other nonthyroidal sites with the NIS are the salivary glands, stomach, and functioning mammary glands. These are also seen on the post-treatment scan but, because of the larger photon flux and more time for localization, uptake can also be identified in the lacrimal duct, nose, and thymus and can be misinterpreted as sites of disease. False positives are discussed below. The majority of iodine is excreted through the kidneys so the urinary tract, especially the bladder, can be identified on diagnostic and post-treatment WBS. Thyroid hormone is metabolized in the liver by deiodination and conjugation with glucuronide and sulfide, and excreted in the bile. Because it takes time for radio-iodine to be incorporated into thyroid hormone and released from the thyroid, and then be taken up by hepatocytes and metabolized, the liver is usually not seen on a diagnostic WBS but is frequently recognized on a post-treatment scan. The intensity of uptake in the liver is directly related to the quantity of thyroid left after thyroidectomy or the functioning mass of metastases. It is often overlooked that much of the radiation to the whole body derives from circulating thyroid hormone containing ^{131}I. The bowel is seen in both diagnostic and post-treatment scans. In the former it is usually radio-iodine that has not been fully absorbed, and in the latter it is radio-iodinated metabolites of thyroid hormones. There is almost no uptake in muscles, skeleton, brain, heart, or lungs unless there are functioning metastases. As a result it can sometimes be difficult to be certain where a lesion is situated. A transmission scan that is produced by placing a radioactive source such as ^{99m}Tc or ^{57}Co behind the patient to outline the body can help. A SPECT scan, especially if it is combined with a simultaneous CT scan, can define anatomy and help with interpretation.

False-positive scan

A false-positive WBS can result from uptake of radio-iodine in a nonthyroidal organ that has an NIS and that is judged to be a metastasis, as described above. Contamination by saliva, tears, milk, urine, or stool can also be misinterpreted. These have been fully tabulated in reviews (13). It is important for the person who interprets the scan to know the details of the patient's history and pathological stage of disease. For example, it would be unlikely for a 25-year-old woman with a 1.5-cm fully excised papillary cancer to have a distant metastasis. Knowledge of the thyroglobulin level when the TSH is high is also important. If that value is low or undetectable, significant abnormal uptake of ^{123}I should be fully evaluated to ensure that a false positive is excluded before making a diagnosis of metastasis. Figure 3.1.6.5 shows focal uptake in the right breast. This is not metastatic thyroid cancer but has been described in primary breast cancer (14).

False-negative scan

A false-negative whole body ^{131}I scan can be due to several factors. The cancer cells might have lost their ability to trap iodine and this likelihood increases with dedifferentiation. The volume of cancer can be too small to be imaged. There can be technical factors including failure to stop exogenous thyroid hormone or there has been an excess of iodine, in particular from radiographic contrast and mineral supplements. Patients who live in areas of high intake of dietary iodine should take a low-iodine diet for 2 weeks prior to scanning and continue until after ^{131}I treatment is prescribed. Thyroid hormone can be started 24–48 h after ^{131}I therapy because it takes several days for the serum TSH to become normal. ^{131}I is an excellent radionuclide for therapy because it has a half-life of 8 days and emits β-particles that are locally destructive. These properties are disadvantageous for diagnostic imaging because the patient receives a higher dose of radiation and the resolution of the images is poor. Iodine-123 only emits γ-rays and has a half-life of approximately 13 h; 148 MBq (4 mCi) of this isotope has the same photon flux as approximately 3.7 GBq (100 mCi) ^{131}I. We have conducted 366 ^{123}I WBS, 238 showed abnormal uptake and 128 were judged to be negative. Of the 238 patients, 228 were treated and 226 had a post-treatment scan for comparison. In our clinic it is usually possible to obtain the chosen therapy dose in capsule form within 2 h so patients are treated on the same day as the diagnostic scan. Of the paired scans, 93% were equivalent, 5% of the post-treatment scans showed some additional information, and 2% showed somewhat less. Eighteen patients with a negative diagnostic scan but high levels of thyroglobulin were treated and 15 of the post-treatment scans were also negative. These results confirm that ^{123}I diagnostic scans give a reliable analysis of the extent of disease and whether it will be amenable to therapy. The results are very similar to those published by Urhan *et al.* who had a concordance of 87% for positive scans and 75% for negative (15).

Controversies about whole body scan

The first controversy is whether a diagnostic WBS is necessary. We would argue yes, based on the premise in oncology that it is important to know what is being treated. The second controversy concerns the optimal dose of ^{131}I for diagnostic WBS. In the past, 37–74 MBq (1–2 mCi) was prescribed, but larger doses can demonstrate more extensive disease. As a result 185–370 MBq (5–10 mCi) became standard test doses for many nuclear medicine physicians. Then it was reported that larger doses could produce enough damage to thyroid tissue that therapeutic doses would not be taken up by thyroidal tissues. This has been called 'stunning',

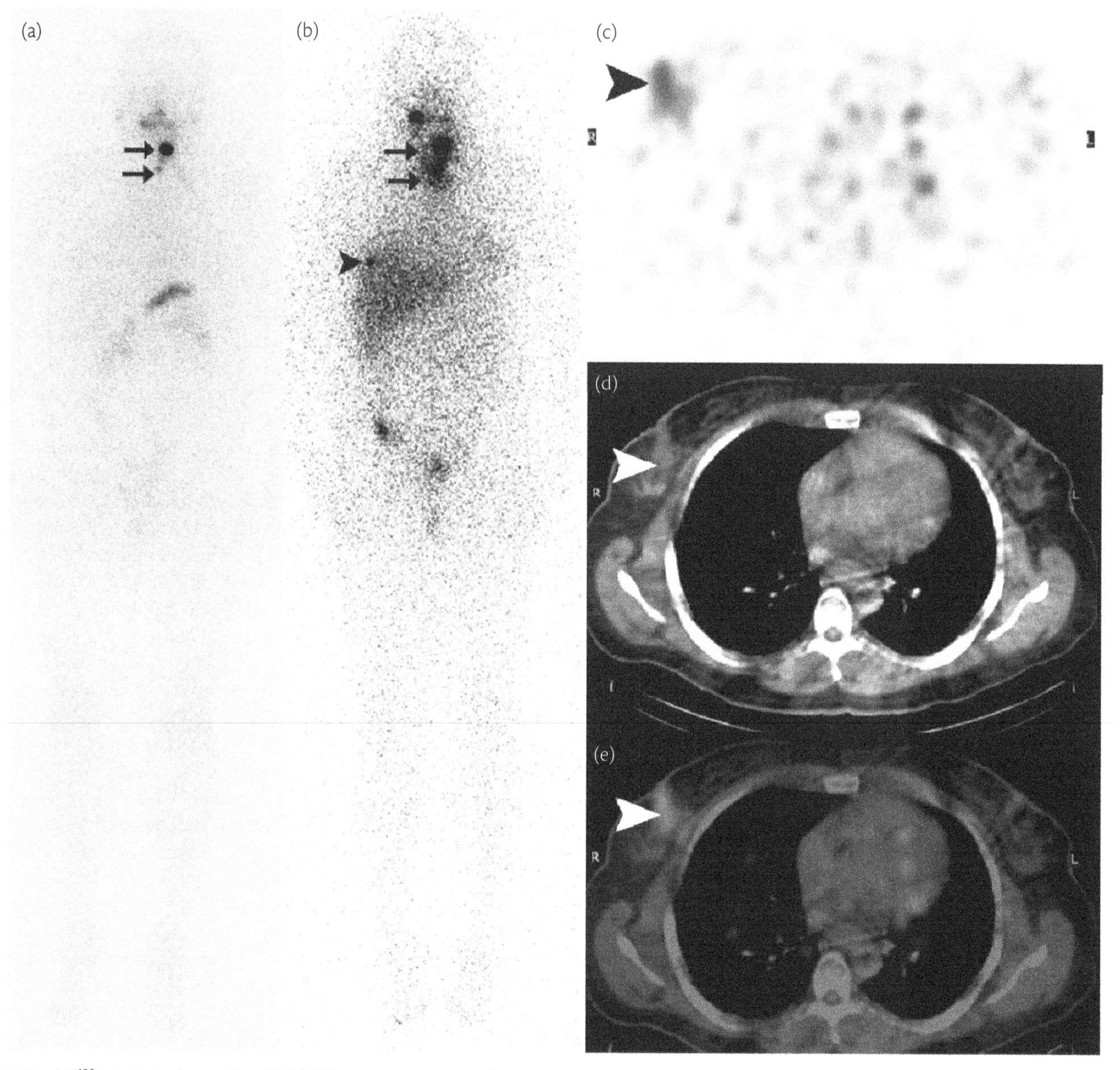

Fig. 3.1.6.5 (a) ^{123}I whole-body scan (4 mCi). (b) ^{131}I post-treatment scan showing uptake in neck and diffuse uptake in liver. There is a focus of abnormal uptake on the right side just at the superior edge of the liver. (c–e) Tomographic image at this level with a CT scan in an identical position shows this focus is in the breast. This is a false-positive for thyroid cancer but the patient will need additional testing because there might be a primary breast cancer.

and 10 mCi (370 MBq) caused this effect in 86% of 18 patients (16). We have found that 74 Mbq (2 mCi) caused stunning in only 3.5% of 300 paired diagnostic and post-treatment WBS, and this dose seldom underestimated the extent of disease. Therefore, if ^{131}I is the isotope to be used, we recommend a dose of about 74 MBq (2 mCi). The controversy of stunning has been summarized in a debate providing information for and against the concept (17). However, we now routinely use ^{123}I in a dose of 148 MBq (4 mCi) because the images are of a significantly higher quality and the patient receives considerably less radiation. Figure 3.1.6.6 shows an ^{123}I WBS before and 1 year after ^{131}I therapy.

Another controversial area is the management of the clinical problem that occurs when the whole body ^{131}I scan is negative but serum thyroglobulin elevated. The abnormal thyroglobulin might only be present when the TSH is high in preparation for WBS. Measurable thyroglobulin implies there is thyroid tissue somewhere and that this tissue has a probability of being cancerous. Most often it is in lymph nodes in the neck but it could be in lungs or skeleton. What constitutes a negative ^{131}I scan has been defined differently. There should be no uptake in the thyroid bed or in local or distant metastases. Uptake in the thyroid region of no more than 0.2% of the administered dose is a cut-off which is reasonable for ^{131}I scans made 48–72 h after administration of the isotope. Uptake values of no more than 0.5% is appropriate for ^{123}I scans at 24 h.

There are different approaches to the patient with a negative diagnostic scan but elevated thyroglobulin. Some authorities prescribe a large dose of ^{131}I based on the concept that the scan after a therapy dose sometimes shows lesions not seen on diagnostic scan (18, 19). In published reports the percentage of patients in

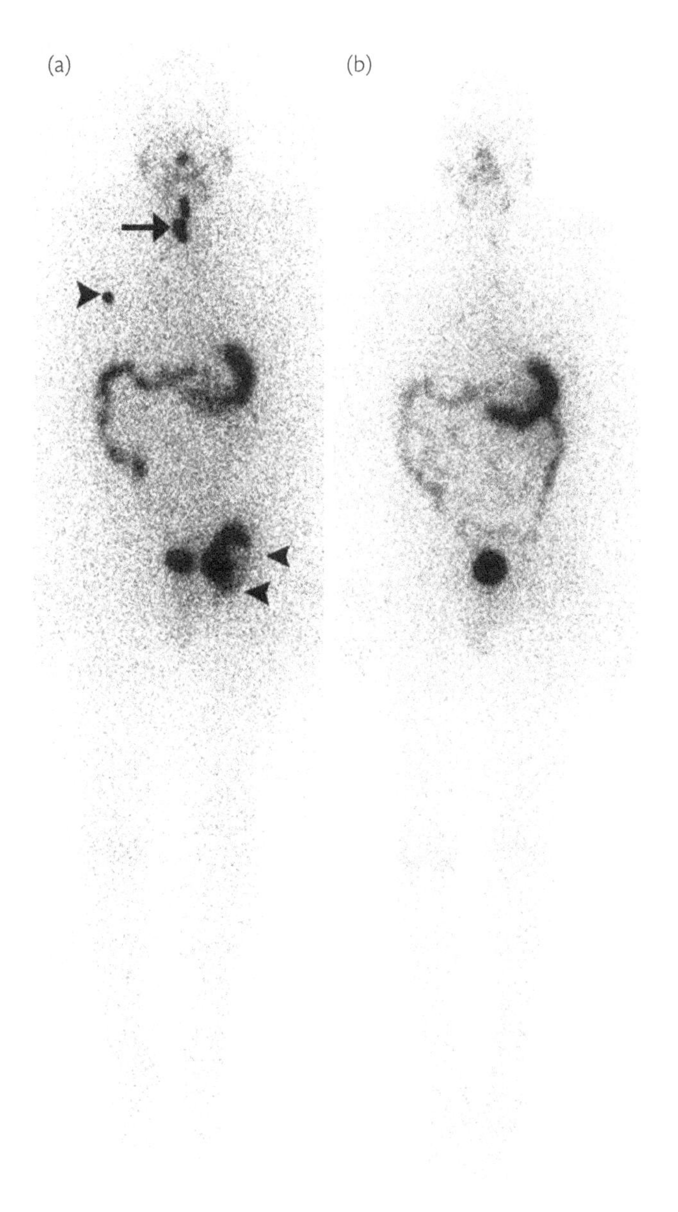

Fig. 3.1.6.6 A 67-year-old man with papillary thyroid cancer. (a) Pretreatment ^{123}I scan shows residual thyroid tissue in the neck (arrow), as well as right rib and left hip metastases (arrowheads). (b) No abnormal uptake is seen on the ^{123}I scan taken at the 1-year follow-up.

whom additional lesions are recognized varies from 10 to 25%; we found this in 17% of patients. Therefore the therapy is ineffective in about 80% of patients. As a result, alternative methods of imaging including ultrasonography and transaxial radiological methods are often used. These are not within the scope of this review. There are 'cancer-seeking' radiopharmaceuticals that are not specific for thyroid cancer. Historically, the myocardial imaging agents ^{201}Tl, ^{99m}Tc-labelled sestamibi, and tetrafosmin have been used with limited success. Positron emission tomography (PET) with deoxyglucose labelled with ^{18}F is the radiopharmaceutical of choice.

Positron emission tomography

The basis of clinical molecular imaging is to provide functional information by imaging patients after they have been injected with a radiotracer that circulates and is incorporated into various *in vivo* cellular processes. This general principle has been applied for many years in nuclear medicine using radiopharmaceuticals and gamma cameras. The advent of PET for oncology has sparked a renewed interest in molecular imaging because of its greater resolution and also because of the radiotracer [^{18}F]2-fluoro-2-deoxy-D-glucose (FDG) that has been proven to be accurate for managing a wide variety of cancers. PET imaging technology advanced further after the introduction of combined PET and CT (PET/CT) scanners in 2001 that allowed evaluation of merged complementary functional and anatomical information. The uptake of FDG into cells is proportional to the rate of glucose metabolism. Because cancers generally use more glucose, FDG is an indicator for malignancy. PET scanners are designed as rings of multiple pairs of photon detectors arranged 180° apart from each other with the patient lying in the middle of this ring. These pairs of photon detectors are electronically linked such that they accept only pairs of photons that arrive at both detectors at precisely the same time and reject the ones that arrive at incongruent times. Positron emitters emit positive electrons that almost instantaneously interact with electrons that have a negative charge. The positron and negatively charged electron annihilate each other and their mass is conserved as two photons that travel at an angle of 180°. The emitted photons produce the image and a CT scan is obtained with the patient in the identical position; this information is used for anatomical correlation and to provide data for attenuation correction of the PET images.

As discussed previously, the standard method of therapy for papillary thyroid cancer (PTC) is total thyroidectomy and in selected cases ^{131}I. Follow-up includes scintigraphy with ^{123}I and measurement of thyroglobulin, both when TSH is high or normal to low. In the setting of high or rising thyroglobulin levels and negative ^{123}I scintiscans or post-treatment ^{131}I scan, the alternative approach is to use an imaging test that does not rely on the NIS. The concept is to identify the site of thyroglobulin production and treat that by operation or external beam radiation. In recent years, the test most favoured has been FDG PET and more recently PET/CT.

There are many reports of the value of PET in PTC, with the first one as early as 1987 (20). Several published reports are focused on iodine-negative thyroglobulin-positive patients (21-30). Stokkel *et al.* have tabulated the results in 18 published series (31). The sensitivity of PET varies from about 50 to 100%, and the range is probably due to the degree of differentiation of residual cancer and the volume of tissue. In general, poorly differentiated cancers demonstrate higher uptake of FDG, whereas well-differentiated cancers that trap iodine might fail to be imaged using FDG. This has been called 'flip/flop' (32) and an illustration of this concept is presented in Fig. 3.1.6.7. The overall sensitivity of PET/CT is unlikely to be much greater than that of PET alone for identifying sites of thyroid cancer that are unable to trap iodine. However, the fused images allow potential false positives to be correctly identified. PET/CT allows regions of FDG uptake that are not due to cancer to be confidently diagnosed correctly. FDG uptake in brown fat and muscles (including muscles of speech) can be demonstrated not to be cancer by comparing anatomy with function. This produces an increased specificity compared with published results of PET alone. The summarized literature for PET in differentiated thyroid cancer (DTC) shows a specificity range of 25–80% (13). The one exception was a reported specificity of 95% (21 of 22 patients

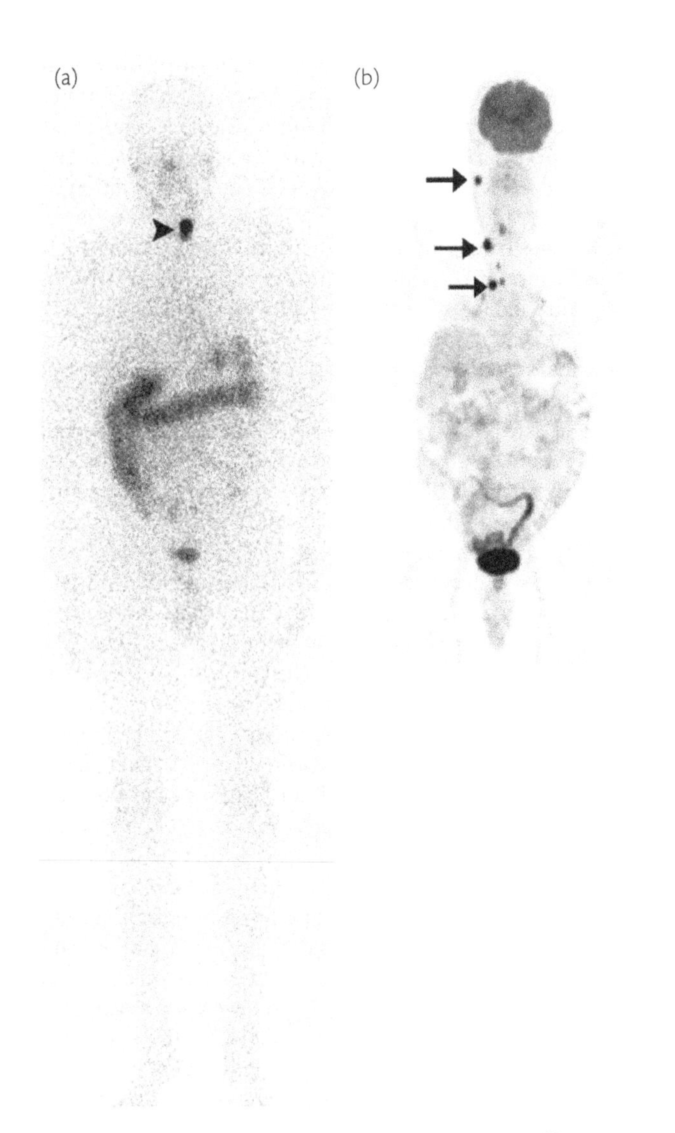

Fig. 3.1.6.7 A 74-year-old man with papillary thyroid cancer. (a) ^{123}I scan shows thyroid tissue in the left neck (arrowhead). (b) FDG PET/CT (carried out on the same day) shows extensive metastatic disease in cervical and mediastinal lymph nodes (arrows).

in remission), although six of these patients had measurable thyroglobulin (33).

Recent research explored the role of the positron emitter ^{124}I in the management of patients with PTC. Some reports suggest that ^{124}I PET/CT imaging is a promising technique to improve treatment planning in thyroid cancer and is particularly valuable in patients with advanced DTC before radio-iodine therapy, as well as in patients with suspected recurrence and potential metastatic disease (34, 35). However, there is evidence that for small disseminated iodine-avid lung metastases, additional diagnostic tests are necessary for diagnosis (36). A maximum intensity projection image from ^{124}I PET is presented in Fig. 3.1.6.8.

FDG PET and PET/CT have a role in the management of patients with medullary thyroid cancer (MTC), with high sensitivity and specificity for disease detection (37, 38). This imaging method provides additional information in a significant proportion of cases and can be used for restaging of patients with MTC and elevated levels of biomarkers (calcitonin), particularly when other imaging modalities (CT, MRI, ultrasonography) fail to demonstrate the site of recurrence.

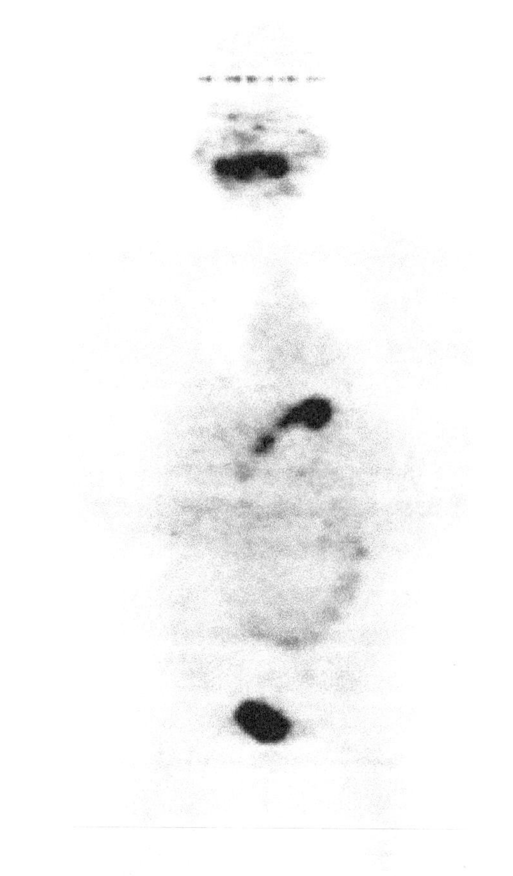

Fig. 3.1.6.8 Normal distribution of ^{124}I on PET (absent thyroid).

Anaplastic thyroid cancer (ATC) demonstrates intense FDG PET uptake. PET/CT may improve disease detection and have an impact on the management of patients with ATC relative to other imaging modalities (39). PET/CT demonstrates the extent of local disease as well as local and distant metastases when they are present. Figure 3.1.6.9 presents a patient with ATC evaluated with FDG PET/CT before and after therapy. Other rare malignancies

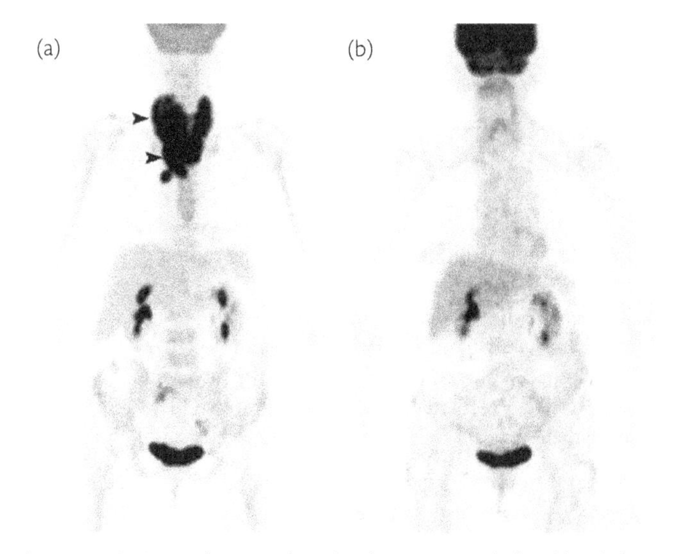

Fig. 3.1.6.9 Patient with ATC evaluated with FDG PET/CT before (a) and after (b) therapy.

involving the thyroid, such as lymphoma and melanoma, have been imaged using FDG PET and PET/CT (40, 41).

References

1. Baker CH, Morris JC. The sodium-iodide symporter. *Curr Drug Targets Immune Endocr Metabol Disord*, 2004; **4**: 167–74.
2. Morris LF, Waxman AD, Braunstein GD. Accuracy considerations when using early (four- or six-hour) radioactive iodine uptake to predict twenty-four-hour values for radioactive iodine dosage in the treatment of Graves' disease. *Thyroid*, 2000; **10**: 779–87.
3. Atkins H. Technetium-99m pertechnetate uptake and scanning in the evaluation of thyroid function. *Semin Nucl Med*, 1971; **1**: 345–55.
4. Sostre S, Ashare AB, Quinones JD, *et al.* Thyroid scintigraphy: pinhole images versus rectilinear scan. *Radiology*, 1978; **129**: 759–62.
5. Wanet PM, Sand A, Abramovici J. Physical and clinical evaluation of high-resolution thyroid pinhole tomography. *J Nucl Med*, 1996; **37**: 2017–20.
6. Verelst J, Chanoine J-P, Delange F. Radionuclide imaging in primary permanent congenital hypothyroidism. *Clin Nucl Med*, 1991; **16**: 652–5.
7. Gray HW, Hooper LA, Greig WR, McDougall IR. A twenty minute perchlorate discharge test. *J Clin Endocrinol Metab*, 1972; **34**: 594–7.
8. Ramtoola S, Maisey MN, Clarke SEM, Fogelman I. The thyroid scan in Hashimoto's thyroiditis: the great mimic. *Nucl Med Commun*, 1988; **9**: 639–45.
9. Ladenson PW, Braverman LE, Mazzaferri EL, Brucker-Davis F, Cooper DS, Garber JR, *et al.* Comparison of administration of recombinant human thyrotropin with withdrawal of thyroid hormone for radioactive iodine scanning in patients with thyroid carcinoma. *N Engl J Med*, 1997; **337**: 888–96.
10. Haugen BR, Pacini F, Reiners C, Schlumberger M, Ladenson PW, Sherman SI, *et al.* A comparison of recombinant human thyrotropin, thyroid hormone withdrawal for the detection of thyroid remnant or cancer. *J Clin Endocrinol Metab*, 1999; **84**: 3877–85.
11. Anderson GS, Fish S, Nakhoda K, Zhuang H, Alavi A, Mandel SJ. Comparison of I-123 and I-131 for whole-body imaging after stimulation by recombinant human thyrotropin: a preliminary report. *Clin Nucl Med*, 2003; **28**: 93–6.
12. Hinds SR 2nd, Stack AL, Stocker DJ. Low-iodine diet revisited: importance in nuclear medicine imaging and management. *Clin Nucl Med*, 2008; **33**: 247–50.
13. Carlisle M, Lu C, McDougall IR. The interpretation of 131I scans in the evaluation of thyroid cancer, with an emphasis on false positive findings. *Nucl Med Commun*, 2003; **24**: 715–35.
14. Wapnir IL, Goris M, Yudd A, Dohan O, Adelman D, Nowels K, *et al.* The Na^{+}/I_{-} symporter mediates iodide uptake in breast cancer metastases and can be selectively down-regulated in the thyroid. *Clin Cancer Res*, 2004; **10**: 4294–302.
15. Urhan M, Dadparvar S, Mavi A, Houseni M, Chamroonrat W, Alavi A, *et al.* Iodine-123 as a diagnostic imaging agent in differentiated thyroid carcinoma: a comparison with iodine-131 post-treatment scanning and serum thyroglobulin measurement. *Eur J Nucl Med Mol Imaging*, 2007; **34**: 1012–7.
16. Park H, Perkins OW, Edmondson JW, Schnute RB, Manatunga A. Influence of diagnostic radioiodines on the uptake of ablative dose of iodine-131. *Thyroid*, 1994; **4**: 49–54.
17. Kalinyak JE, McDougall IR. Whole-body scanning with radionuclides of iodine, and the controversy of "thyroid stunning". *Nucl Med Commun*, 2004; **25**: 883–9.
18. Pineda JD, Lee T, Ain K, Reynolds JC, Robbins J. Iodine-131 therapy for thyroid cancer patients with elevated thyroglobulin and negative diagnostic scan. *J Clin Endocrinol Metab*, 1995; **80**: 1488–92.
19. Schlumberger M, Mancusi F, Baudin E, Pacini F. 131I therapy for elevated thyroglobulin levels. *Thyroid*, 1997; **7**: 273–6.
20. Joensuu H, Ahonen A. Imaging of metastases of thyroid carcinoma with fluorine-18 fluorodeoxyglucose. *J Nucl Med*, 1987; **28**: 910–4.
21. McDougall IR, Davidson J, Segall GM. Positron emission tomography of the thyroid, with an emphasis on thyroid cancer. *Nucl Med Commun*, 2001; **22**: 485–92.
22. Jadvar H, McDougall IR, Segall GM. Evaluation of suspected recurrent papillary thyroid carcinoma with [18F]fluorodeoxyglucose positron emission tomography. *Nucl Med Commun*, 1998; **19**: 547–54.
23. Conti PS, Durski JM, Bacqai F, Grafton ST, Singer PA. Imaging of locally recurrent and metastatic thyroid cancer with positron emission tomography. *Thyroid*, 1999; **9**: 797–804.
24. Iagaru A, Quon A, Johnson D, Gambhir SS, McDougall IR. 2-Deoxy-2-[F-18]fluoro-D: -glucose Positron Emission Tomography/Computed Tomography in the Management of Melanoma. *Mol Imaging Biol*, 2007; **9**: 50–7.
25. Dietlein M, Scheidhauer K, Voth E, Theissen P, Schicha H. Fluorine-18 fluorodeoxyglucose positron emission tomography and iodine-131 whole-body scintigraphy in the follow-up of differentiated thyroid cancer. *Eur J Nucl Med*, 1997; **24**: 1342–8.
26. Alnafisi N, Driedger AA, Coates G, Moote DJ, Raphael SJ. FDG PET of recurrent or metastatic 131I-negative papillary thyroid carcinoma. *J Nucl Med*, 2000; **41**: 1010–15.
27. Grunwald F, Kalicke T, Feine U, Lietzenmayer R, Scheidhauer K, Dietlein M, *et al.* Fluorine-18 fluorodeoxyglucose positron emission tomography in thyroid cancer: results of a multicentre study. *Eur J Nucl Med*, 1999; **26**: 1547–52.
28. Wang W, Macapinlac H, Finn RD, Yeh SD, Akhurst T, Finn RD, *et al.* [18F]-2-fluoro-2-deoxy-D-glucose positron emission tomography localizes residual thyroid cancer in patients with negative diagnostic (131)I whole body scans and elevated serum thyroglobulin levels. *J Clin Endocrinol Metab*, 1999; **84**: 2291–302.
29. Schluter B, Bohuslavizki KH, Beyer W, Plotkin M, Buchert R, Clausen M. Impact of FDG PET on patients with differentiated thyroid cancer who present with elevated thyroglobulin and negative 131I scan. *J Nucl Med*, 2001; **42**: 71–6.
30. Iagaru A, Kalinyak JE, McDougall IR. F-18 FDG PET/CT in the management of thyroid cancer. *Clin Nucl Med*, 2007; **32**: 690–5.
31. Stokkel MP, Duchateau CS, Dragoiescu C. The value of FDG-PET in the follow-up of differentiated thyroid cancer: a review of the literature. *Q J Nucl Med Mol Imaging*, 2006; **50**: 78–87.
32. Fiene ULR, Hanke JP, Wohrle H, Muller-Schauenburg W. 18FDG whole-body PET in differentiated thyroid carcinoma. Flipflop in uptake patterns of 18FDG and 131I. *Nuclearmedizin*, 1995; **34**: 127–34.
33. Chung JK, So Y, Lee JS, Choi CW, Lim SM, Lee DS, *et al.* Value of FDG PET in papillary thyroid carcinoma with negative 131I whole-body scan. *J Nucl Med*, 1999; **40**: 986–92.
34. Freudenberg LS, Antoch G, Jentzen W, Pink R, Knust J, Görges R, *et al.* Value of (124)I-PET/CT in staging of patients with differentiated thyroid cancer. *Eur Radiol*, 2004; **14**: 2092–8.
35. Sgouros G, Kolbert KS, Sheikh A, Pentlow KS, Mun EF, Barth A, *et al.* Patient-specific dosimetry for 131I thyroid cancer therapy using 124I PET and 3-dimensional-internal dosimetry (3D-ID) software. *J Nucl Med*, 2004; **45**: 1366–72.
36. Freudenberg LS, Jentzen W, Muller SP, Bockisch A. Disseminated iodine-avid lung metastases in differentiated thyroid cancer: a challenge to 124I PET. *Eur J Nucl Med Mol Imaging*, 2008; **35**: 502–8.
37. Iagaru A, Masamed R, Singer PA, Conti PS. Detection of occult medullary thyroid cancer recurrence with 2-deoxy-2-[F-18]fluoro-D: -glucose-PET and PET/CT. *Mol Imaging Biol*, 2007; **9**: 72–7.
38. Bozkurt MF, Ugur O, Banti E, Grassetto G, Rubello D. Functional nuclear medicine imaging of medullary thyroid cancer. *Nucl Med Commun*, 2008; **29**: 934–42.
39. Bogsrud TV, Karantanis D, Nathan MA, Mullan BP, Wiseman GA, Kasperbauer JL, *et al.* 18F-FDG PET in the management of patients with anaplastic thyroid carcinoma. *Thyroid*, 2008; **18**: 713–19.

40. Basu S, Li G, Bural G, Alavi A. Fluorodeoxyglucose positron emission tomography (FDG-PET) and PET/computed tomography imaging characteristics of thyroid lymphoma and their potential clinical utility. *Acta Radiol*, 2009; **50**: 201–4.
41. Basu S, Alavi A. Metastatic malignant melanoma to the thyroid gland detected by FDG-PET imaging. *Clin Nucl Med*, 2007; **32**: 388–9.

3.1.6.1 *Thyroid imaging: nonisotopic techniques*

Laszlo Hegedüs, Finn N. Bennedbæk

Introduction

Clinical examination and evaluation of thyroid function remain fundamental in the evaluation of thyroid disorders, but observer variation leads to a considerable heterogeneity in the evaluation of patients with suspected thyroid disease (1). It is not surprising, therefore, that imaging of the thyroid is often performed. Although it most often cannot distinguish between benign and malignant lesions, and its clinical value is generally thought to be limited (2), a European survey demonstrated that 88% of European Thyroid Association members would use imaging in an index case of a euthyroid patient with a solitary thyroid nodule and absence of clinical suspicion of malignancy (3). In the case of a clinically benign nontoxic multinodular goitre, the figure was 91% (4).

The thyroid gland can be evaluated by several different non-isotopic imaging techniques. The most commonly used are ultrasonography, CT, and MRI. Each method has advantages and limitations, and there is no absolute clinical indication for performing any of these imaging procedures in the majority of patients. The major drawback of all techniques, in addition to expense, is that the technical advances in thyroid imaging have not been accompanied by increased specificity for tissue diagnosis. This chapter will focus on the clinical use of these methods and, as far as this is possible, compare their advantages and disadvantages (Table 3.1.6.1.1).

Box 3.1.6.1.1 Possible applications of ultrasonography in thyroid disorders

- Size determination
- Morphology (diffuse, uni- or multinodular, cyst)
- Echogenicity (hypo-, normo-, or hyperechogenic)
- Flow determination
- Aid in diagnostic biopsies
- Aid in treatment (cyst aspiration, ethanol and laser therapy)
- Evaluation of regional lymph nodes

Ultrasonography

Examination of the neck is performed with high-frequency transducers (7–15 MHz), and the patient is in the supine position with the neck hyperextended. The transducer is coupled to the skin with gel since ultrasound does not pass through air. The technique can detect thyroid lesions as small as 2 mm. It can distinguish solid from simple and complex cysts. It enables the accurate determination of thyroid size, gives a rough estimate of echogenicity, visualizes vascular flow and velocity (colour flow Doppler), and aids in the accurate placing of needles, be it for diagnostic or therapeutic purposes (Box 3.1.6.1.1). The main drawbacks are the high degree of observer dependency and the inability to visualize retroclavicular or intrathoracic extension of the thyroid (2, 5). The average investigation rarely takes more than 10 min.

Ultrasonography is based on the emission of high-frequency sound waves and subsequent reflection as they pass through the tissue. The amplitude of the reflections of the sound waves is due to differences in the acoustic impedance of the various body tissues. The depth of tissue penetration is the least for high-frequency waves. Conversely, structural resolution is best. The frequency used to visualize the thyroid (7–15 MHz) is a compromise between the need for depth of penetration and that for resolution. The use of real-time allows the differentiation of static structures (thyroid, neck muscles, lymph nodes) from that of moving or pulsating structures (blood vessels, oesophagus) (2, 5).

Table 3.1.6.1.1 Characteristics of commonly used imaging modalities in relation to disorders of the thyroid

Characteristics	Scintigraphy	Ultrasonography	CT	MRI
Physical principle	Radioactivity	Ultrasound	X-rays	Radio waves/magnetic field
Availability	Good	Good	Good	Poor
Most suited anatomical regions	Neck structures (whole body)	Neck structures	Thorax (neck structures)	Thorax (neck structures)
Ionizing irradiation	Yes	No	Yes	No
Intravenous injection	Yes	No	Possible	Possible
Dynamic picture	No	Yes	No	No
Biopsy possible	No	Yes	Yes	No
Investigation time (min)	30[a]	10[a]	20[a]	25[a]
Cost (GBP)	200[b]	100[b]	250[b]	400[b]
Operator dependency	Medium	High	Medium	Medium

[a] Varies considerably depending on type of disease and whether biopsy is performed.

[b] Varies considerably within and between countries. These rough approximations are valid for outpatients at the author's hospital.

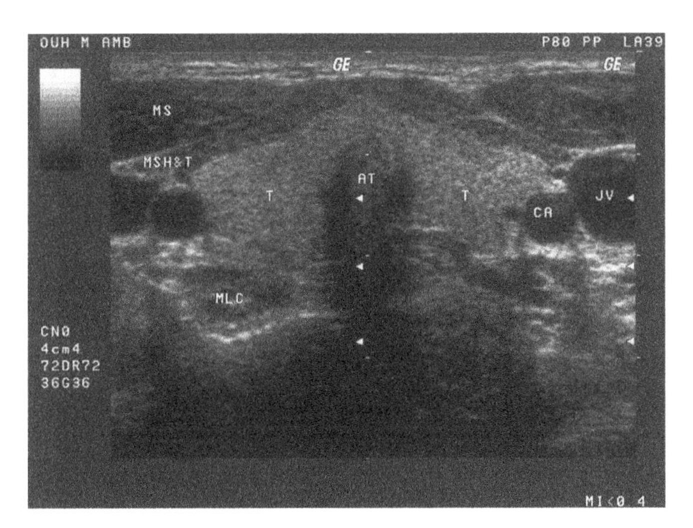

Fig. 3.1.6.1.1 Transverse sonogram of the normal thyroid gland. AT, trachea; CA, common carotid artery; JV, jugular vein; MLC, longus colli muscle, MS, sternocleid muscle; MSH&T, sternohyoid and thyrodhyoid muscle; T, thyroid.

Normal thyroid

The normal thyroid parenchyma has a characteristic homogeneous medium-level echogenicity (Fig. 3.1.6.1.1). The surrounding muscles have a lower echogenicity. Posterolaterally the thyroid is bordered by the sonolucent common carotid artery and internal jugular vein, and medially by the trachea. The oesophagus with its echogenic mucosa can be seen behind and to the left of the trachea.

A high proportion of people with a normal thyroid gland have small (1–3 mm) cystic or solid lesions, the frequency being higher in women, increasing with age, and varying between countries (5, 6). The importance of these abnormalities is unclear, but since incidental sonographic nodules ('incidentalomas') are very common, whereas thyroid cancer is not, a conservative/expectant approach is generally recommended. An incidentally disclosed nodule or cyst less than 1 cm in diameter in an asymptomatic individual with a normal neck palpation should generally not lead to biopsy or further investigations (5, 6).

Goitre, i.e. an enlarged thyroid gland, remains a clinical diagnosis. But this evaluation carries an inaccuracy of approximately 40% and cannot reliably be used for size determination (1). For this, two principally different methods are available. One employs the model of a rotation ellipsoid and can be modified to length × width × thickness × $\pi/6$ for each lobe, and carries an inaccuracy of 15–20% that increases with size and degree of irregularity (2,5). The other method is based on obtaining cross-sections of the entire thyroid gland. This method carries an inaccuracy of 5–10% and is less influenced by size and degree of irregularity (2, 5). The normal thyroid size (5–30 ml in adults) is positively related to weight and age, increases with decreasing iodine intake, and is influenced by a number of physiological as well as environmental factors (2, 5). Ultrasonography is the most sensitive technique for screening populations for goitre and is widely used for field studies (2, 5, 7).

Diffuse thyroid disease

Nonautoimmune nontoxic diffuse goitre appears diffusely enlarged with a uniform or discretely irregular echo pattern without nodules. Various degrees of hypoechogenicity may be evident, but, when marked, suggest the presence of autoimmunity. In Hashimoto's thyroiditis, hypoechogenicity is always marked but may be inhomogeneous. Ultrasonography cannot differentiate between benign autoimmune thyroiditis and lymphoma or carcinoma. Therefore, goitre growth, especially in the L-thyroxine-treated patient, should raise suspicion of lymphoma and lead to biopsy or operation. In Graves' disease, the thyroid is most often enlarged and the echo pattern homogeneous. Echogenicity can be normal to markedly decreased and the latter suggests a decreased probability of achieving remission on antithyroid drugs. Colour flow Doppler can demonstrate the rich vascularity and increased flow related to the degree of hyperthyroidism. Subacute thyroiditis leads to thyroid enlargement and areas of hypoechogenicity probably related to areas that are affected. Remission leads to normalization of size, but areas of hypoechogenicity may remain long after remission is obtained.

Multinodular goitre

Multinodular goitres are often larger than diffuse goitres and a significant number (10–20%) have a substernal or intrathoracic extension which cannot be visualized since the bony thorax prevents penetration of sound waves. The echographic structure may be heterogeneous without well-defined nodules or composed of multiple nodules interspersed throughout a normal-appearing gland. Often areas of haemorrhage, necrosis, and calcifications are seen. Most patients evaluated for a single nodule have additional small thyroid nodules when examined by ultrasonography (5, 6). The echogenicity of the nodules may vary from hyper- to iso-, to hypoechoic, even within the same patient. The presence of multiple nodules identified by ultrasound examination (or any other imaging modality) does not exclude malignancy, it is just as likely as in the solitary nodule (6, 8). Therefore, especially in view of the increasing use of nonsurgical treatment for this disorder, (6, 8) fine-needle aspiration biopsy (FNAB) should be used liberally especially in the patient with a dominant or growing nodule. Ultrasound guidance is also recommended for selection of the most suspicious nodules (6).

Thyroid cysts

Thyroid cysts are well-defined areas with greatly reduced or absent echogenicity. Varying degrees of echogenicity can often be seen due to debris or necrotic tissue. True simple cysts are extremely rare (approximately 1% of all nodules) and virtually always benign. Most, however, are complex cysts and are as likely to be a carcinoma as is a solid nodule (Fig. 3.1.6.1.2). Cystic degeneration is present in 20–30% of thyroid carcinomas and benign solid nodules. After ultrasound-guided aspiration a residual nodule should be biopsied. In case of benign cytology and recurrence of the cyst (which is seen in approximately 50% of the patients) ultrasound-guided treatment can be offered. Flushing with ethanol decreases recurrence rate (9). Malignancy cannot be excluded either by cytology of the cystic component or by the colour of the cyst fluid.

Benign thyroid nodules

There are no specific characteristics that can differentiate benign thyroid nodules from thyroid carcinomas. Neither size, echogenicity, elasticity, the finding of a sonographic halo, calcifications, nor vascularization can with acceptable specificity be used for this purpose (2, 5, 6). Therefore, the most cost-effective investigation of

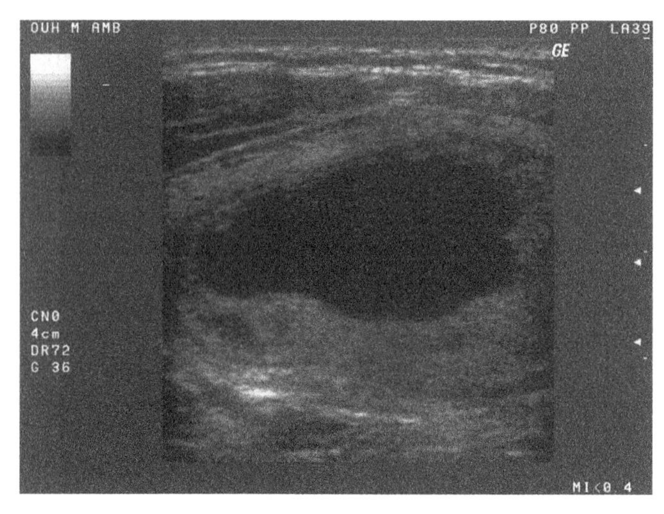

Fig. 3.1.6.1.2 Ultrasound image of a cystic–solid nodule with a central cystic part. After aspiration of the cystic part, fine-needle aspiration biopsy of the solid component is mandatory to reduce the likelihood of overlooking malignancy.

these patients is fine-needle aspiration biopsy. In Europe most thyroidologists will use ultrasound-guided fine-needle aspiration biopsy (3) and this increases the likelihood of obtaining a sufficient sample.

Thyroid carcinoma

No sonographic finding is characteristic of any type of thyroid carcinoma, and ultrasonography cannot differentiate benign from malignant nodules. Extrathyroidal extension of the tumour or lymphadenopathy may suggest thyroid carcinoma but it is not proof. The ultrasound appearance of thyroid carcinoma is highly variable. Generally, it is hypoechoic relative to normal thyroid and microcalcifications are often present. Since very small nodules of 2–3 mm can be detected, ultrasound examination is increasingly used in the follow-up of patients treated for thyroid carcinoma or at risk because of previous irradiation (e.g. post-Chernobyl). Characteristic sonolucent masses in the thyroid bed or adjacent tissues often suggest recurrent disease before this is clinically evident.

Computed tomography

CT offers excellent anatomical resolution by increasing the distinction of differences in density between soft tissues. Density differences as small as 0.5% can be detected compared to the 5–10% of conventional radiographic techniques. The accurate measurement of the absorption of X-rays by tissues (attenuation) enables individual tissues to be studied (2).

The technique is highly sensitive but just as nonspecific as ultrasonography in differentiating benign from malignant disease. It can distinguish solid from simple and complex cysts and enables the accurate determination of thyroid size. It is superior to ultrasonography when examining retroclavicular/intrathoracic goitre and it is not as observer dependent. The drawbacks are cost, limited availability for this purpose, length of the investigation, cooperability (claustrophobia), and exposure to ionizing irradiation (1–4 rads; 0.01–0.04 Gy). The image is not dynamic and although possible, CT-guided biopsy is more cumbersome than with ultrasonography. Intravenous contrast media, to visualize vascular relationships, pose a risk of allergic reactions (Table 3.1.6.1.1).

CT depends on the attenuation of an X-ray beam as it passes through tissues. The extent of attenuation depends on the tissue constituents, and the brightness of each portion (pixel) of the final image is proportional to the degree that it attenuates the X-rays passing through it. The image is usually depicted in shades of grey. Density values are expressed in CT numbers (Hounsfield units, HU), which are related to the attenuation value of water. The high endogenous iodine content of the thyroid enables its visualization. The CT density of the thyroid is closely correlated with its iodine content and can be used to estimate it.

Normal thyroid

The normal thyroid gland is easily visualized on CT and its density is always higher than surrounding tissues. Differences in density reported from various countries reflect differences in iodine intake. There is no sex difference in density but it decreases with age and as a consequence of L-thyroxine treatment.

Disease in the thyroid usually leads to decreased ability to concentrate iodine, therefore, reduced density on CT is the hallmark of thyroid disease. The exact density measurements have not proved useful in distinguishing between various thyroid disorders. Thus, the CT image may be compatible with a certain diagnosis but rarely specific for it.

Diffuse thyroid disease

Nonautoimmune nontoxic diffuse goitre appears to be homogeneously enlarged with various degrees of hypodensity. Graves' disease is characterized by a 50–70% decrease in density and may be slightly inhomogeneous. Hashimoto's thyroiditis typically demonstrates an inhomogeneous iodine distribution and a 50% decrease in CT density which is lowest in hypothyroid individuals. Increasing goitre size is characteristically associated with decreasing density. Asymmetrical hypodense areas should raise the suspicion of lymphoma or carcinoma.

Subacute thyroiditis is also characterized by hypodensity and is focal or diffuse depending on the extent of the disease. In the initial phases, acute suppurative thyroiditis has no characteristic CT image; however, as infection progresses, loculated abscesses with hypodensity may appear.

Multinodular goitre

Multinodular goitre is often an enlarged asymmetrical gland with multiple low density areas of varying degrees of discreteness. CT density is decreased but in an inhomogeneous way. After intravenous contrast, enhancement is obtained except for areas containing haemorrhage, necrosis, or cysts. Calcifications are seen in up to 50% of goitres. Compression of the trachea, oesophagus, and great vessels is easily ascertained and CT has found use especially in patients with monstrous and partly intrathoracic goitre, where it is ideal for the estimation of tracheal compression and quantitation of the intrathoracic extension of the goitre. Anatomical continuity with the cervical thyroid as well as a CT density greater than muscle, provides evidence of its thyroidal origin. Mediastinal lymphoma, lymphadenopathy, or thymus usually have markedly lower CT densities.

Thyroid cysts

Simple cysts are hypodense lesions, smooth-walled, and surrounded by normal thyroid tissue. The density of cyst fluid is always less than muscle and contrast injection does not lead to enhancement. Complex cysts are easily distinguished from simple cysts.

Benign thyroid nodules and carcinomas

Thyroid nodules are common, usually round or oval lesions of low density, and, as with ultrasonography, no CT characteristics will separate benign from malignant lesions (2). Invasive growth into surrounding structures and metastases to cervical lymph nodes are suggestive of carcinoma. Papillary and follicular carcinomas are usually irregular low-density lesions and calcifications are present in the majority. There may be slight enhancement after contrast injection. The CT feature of medullary thyroid carcinoma is a single or multiple low-density lesions of variable size in one or both lobes. Lesions of 1–2 mm in size can be detected. Calcification is less often seen than in papillary carcinoma. Patients with C-cell hyperplasia have normal CT scans.

Large irregular masses of low attenuation with central cystic or necrotic areas are suggestive of anaplastic carcinoma especially if calcification is pronounced. Again, these features may also be seen in benign multinodular goitre. Invasion of the trachea, cricoid, or thyroid cartilage, and growth into the tracheal lumen is highly suggestive of carcinoma. Both Hashimoto's thyroiditis and thyroid lymphoma appear as masses of reduced density with little enhancement after contrast injection, and CT alone cannot make a distinction between them.

CT is of value in the follow-up of patients with thyroid cancer. Recurrence is evident as discrete low-density lesions within or outside the thyroid bed. Lymph node metastases typically have a regular rim, a core of central lucency, and no enhancement after intravenous contrast. CT is highly sensitive in detecting extrathyroidal spread of disease and therefore complementary to whole-body scanning with radioactive iodine.

Combined CT and positron emission tomography (PET) with [^{18}F]2-fluoro-2-deoxy-D-glucose (FDG) is a novel multimodality technology that enables a more precise anatomical localization of an area with increased focal uptake (potentially malignant lesion). Its role in the initial evaluation of a thyroid nodule is limited, but can be of value in case of indeterminate cytology (10). It is increasingly used where there is suspicion of recurrence or spread of thyroid cancer (11).

Magnetic resonance imaging

MRI offers excellent anatomical resolution and generation of images in multiple planes. The technique is highly sensitive but just as nonspecific as ultrasonography and CT in differentiating benign from malignant lesions (2). It can distinguish solid from simple and complex cysts. It allows thyroid size determination and, as with CT and in contrast to ultrasonography, it can visualize the retrotracheal area and retroclavicular or intrathoracic goitre (12). Additionally, it is less operator dependent. The paramagnetic contrast agent gadolinium allows visualization of tumour vascularity. The drawbacks are cost, very limited availability for this purpose, length of the investigation, and cooperability (5% of patients cannot cooperate due to claustrophobia and some, especially children, need to be sedated). Patient and tissue movement (e.g. swallowing) decreases image quality and calcifications are better visualized with CT. MRI cannot be used in patients with cardiac pacemakers, implantable defibrillators, central nervous system aneurysmal clips, cochlear implants, and ferromagnetic ocular fragments. Small metal objects and orthopaedic devices decrease resolution and cause field inhomogeneity (Table 3.1.6.1.1).

MRI images depend on the magnetic properties of certain atomic nuclei. The MRI signal contains several variable components. T_1 relaxation time (longitudinal or spin-lattice relaxation time) reflects the time for protons to give up their energy to the surrounding environment (lattice) and return to their original alignment parallel to the magnetic field. The T_2 relaxation time (transverse or spin-spin relaxation time) is the time needed for synchronous transverse spinning to decay after excitation. Adjustment of the pulse sequence can favour one or the other of these magnetic properties.

Normal thyroid

On T_1-weighted images the normal thyroid gland is clearly seen on MRI and shows a nearly homogeneous signal with an intensity similar to that of the adjacent neck muscles. On T_2-weighted images, the normal thyroid has a much greater signal intensity than adjacent muscles. Blood vessels, lymph nodes, fat, and muscle are clearly identified and distinguished from the thyroid.

Diffuse thyroid disease

In Graves' disease the thyroid has slightly heterogeneous diffusely increased signal on both T_1- and T_2-weighted images. Hashimoto's thyroiditis causes a heterogeneous signal intensity on T_1-weighted images and a diffusely increased signal on T_2-weighted images.

Multinodular goitre

MRI can detect nodules as small as 3–5 mm (Fig. 3.1.6.1.3). Characteristically multinodular goitres have various degrees of heterogeneity and low to increased signal intensity on T_1-weighted images. T_2-weighted images show more pronounced heterogeneity and increased intensity. Nodules are better visualized on T_2-weighted images.

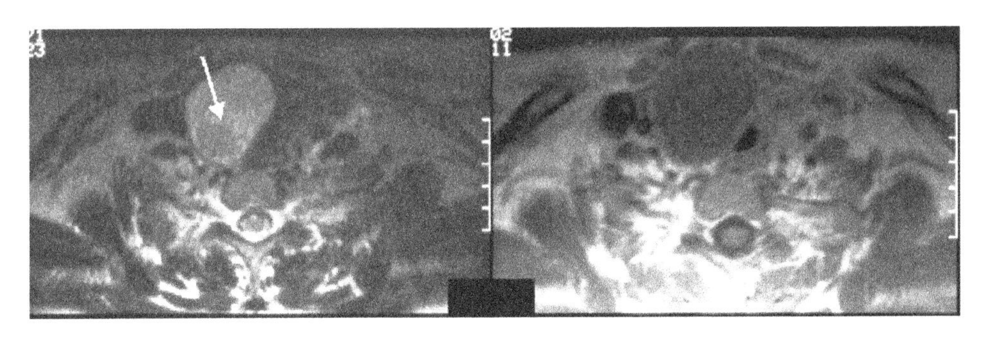

Fig. 3.1.6.1.3 Axial MRI with T_2- (left) and T_1-weighted (right) scans of a cystic–solid thyroid nodule in the right thyroid lobe. A hypointense solid component (arrow) can be seen in comparison with the relatively hyperintense fluid. In the T_1-weighted picture, the lesion cannot be recognized in the hypointense fluid.

Thyroid cysts

Simple cysts have a low-intensity signal on both T_1- and T_2-weighted imaging. The intensity on T_1-weighted images increases with increasing protein and lipid content.

Benign thyroid nodules and carcinomas

Follicular adenomas appear round or oval with a heterogeneous signal equal to or greater than that of normal tissue (2). On T_2-weighted images the nodules have increased signal intensity. No MRI characteristics will accurately separate benign from malignant lesions. Thyroid carcinomas appear as focal or nonfocal lesions of variable size; they are isointense or slightly hyperintense on T_1-weighted images and hyperintense on T_2-weighted images. The imaging characteristics of all types of thyroid carcinomas, including medullary carcinoma and lymphoma, are similar.

The extent of thyroid carcinoma can be determined preoperatively and may be useful in the planning of surgery. Extension into adjacent structures is usually evident. MRI cannot distinguish metastatic from inflammatory adenopathy, and both appear hyperintense on T_2-weighted images. Gadolinium may be useful since metastatic nodes are enhanced centrally after gadolinium injection. Furthermore, in the postoperative follow-up recurrent carcinoma enhance with gadolinium, whereas scarring generally does not.

Conclusions and recommendations

Although there is no absolute clinical indication for performing any of the imaging procedures and although none of them can accurately distinguish benign from malignant disease they are increasingly used (2–5). Thyroid ultrasonography is the most commonly used technique. This is explained partly by increased availability and reduced cost, and also because a growing number of endocrinologists and internists, including the authors, have found it of value in several outpatient situations. Even if ultrasonography cannot reliably diagnose or exclude malignancy, it is of value in providing superior morphological detail compared to scintigraphy and in allowing the accurate placing of needles for diagnostic and therapeutic purposes. Additionally, it provides an accurate size determination and evaluation of echogenicity and thereby aids in the classification and follow-up of various thyroid disorders. As more patients with thyroid nodular disease are offered nonsurgical treatment, mainly in the form of radioiodine and ultrasound-guided percutaneous therapy with ethanol or laser (6, 8, 9), thyroid ultrasonography should become an integral part of the evaluation of many thyroid patients in the outpatient clinics of endocrinological departments (2, 5, 6).

CT and MRI can provide much of the information that is obtained with ultrasonography (2). Their greater expense, limited availability, and other drawbacks argue against their use most of the time. CT is valuable in determining the extent of a substernal goitre or in the evaluation of a mediastinal mass. It can give valuable information in the evaluation of thyroid carcinoma and its spread. MRI may be useful in the same setting and is generally superior to CT in the evaluation of recurrent carcinoma, be it in the thyroid bed or in regional lymph nodes (2).

Recently, ultrasound elastography, which uses ultrasound to provide an estimation of tissue stiffness by measuring the degree of distortion applied with the transducer, was introduced. Malignant nodules are more firm, and elastography is currently being evaluated as an adjunctive tool for the preoperative selection of thyroid nodules (13). In the follow-up of thyroid cancer, especially in high-risk patients, aside from the use of ultrasonography for the detection of local recurrence and cervical lymph node metastases, radioiodine imaging and FDG PET/CT are the methods of choice for localizing metastatic disease (10, 11).

References

1. Jarlov AE, Nygaard B, Hegedüs L, Hartling SG, Hansen JM. Observer variation in the clinical and laboratory evaluation of patients with thyroid dysfunction and goiter. *Thyroid*, 1998; **8**: 393–8.
2. Hegedüs L, Bennedbæk FN. Nonisotopic techniques of thyroid imaging. In: Braverman LE, Utiger RD, eds. *Werner and Ingbar's The Thyroid*. Philadelphia: Lippincott, Williams and Wilkins, 2005: 373–83.
3. Bennedbæk FN, Perrild H, Hegedüs L. Diagnosis and treatment of the solitary thyroid nodule: results of a European survey. *Clin Endocrinol*, 1999; **50**: 357–63.
4. Bonnema SJ, Bennedbæk FN, Wiersinga WM, Hegedüs L. Management of the non-toxic multinodular goitre: a European questionnaire study. *Clin Endocinol*, 2000; **53**: 5–12.
5. Hegedüs L. Thyroid ultrasound. *Endocrinol Metab Clin North Am*, 2001; **30**: 339–60.
6. Hegedüs L. The thyroid nodule. *N Engl J Med*, 2004; **351**: 1064–71.
7. Delange F, Benker G, Caron P, Eber O, Ott W, Peter F, *et al.* Thyroid volume and urinary iodine in European school children: standardization of values for assessment of iodine deficiency. *Eur J Endocrinol*, 1997; **136**: 180–7.
8. Hegedüs L, Bonnema SJ, Bennedæk FN. Management of simple and nodular goiter: current status and future perspectives. *Endocr Rev*, 2003; **24**: 102–32.
9. Bennedbæk FN, Hegedüs L. Treatment of recurrent thyroid cysts with ethanol: a randomized double-blind controlled trial. *J Clin Endocrinol Metab*, 2003; **88**: 5773–7.
10. Sebastianes FM, Cerci JJ, Zanoni PH. Role of 18F-fluorodeoxyglucose positron emission tomography in preoperative assessment of cytologically indeterminate thyroid nodules. *J Clin Endocrinol Metab*, 2007; **92**: 4485–8.
11. Lind P, Kohlfurst S. Respective roles of thyroglobulin, radioiodine imaging, and positron emission tomography in the assessment of thyroid cancer. *Semin Nucl Med*, 2006; **36**: 194–205.
12. Jennings A. Evaluation of substernal goiters using computed tomography and MR imaging. *Endocrinol Metab Clin North Am*, 2001; **30**: 401–14.
13. Rago T, Santini F, Scutari M. Elastography: new developments in ultrasound for predicting malignancy in thyroid nodules. *J Clin Endocrinol Metab*, 2007; **92**: 2917–22.

3.1.7 Epidemiology of thyroid disease and swelling

Mark P.J. Vanderpump

Introduction

Thyroid disorders are among the most prevalent of medical conditions. Their manifestations vary considerably from area to area and are determined principally by the availability of iodine in the diet. The limitations of epidemiological studies of thyroid disorders should therefore be borne in mind when considering the purported frequency of thyroid diseases in different communities (1).

Almost one-third of the world's population live in areas of iodine deficiency and risk the consequences despite major national and international efforts to increase iodine intake, primarily through the voluntary or mandatory iodization of salt (2). The ideal dietary allowance of iodine recommended by the WHO is 150 μg iodine/day, which increases to 250 μg in pregnancy and 290 μg when lactating. The WHO estimates that two billion people, including 285 million school-age children still have iodine deficiency, defined as a urinary iodine excretion of less than 100 μg/l. This has substantial effects on growth and development and is the most common cause of preventable mental impairment worldwide. In areas where the daily iodine intake is below 50 μg, goitre is usually endemic, and when the daily intake falls below 25 μg, congenital hypothyroidism is seen. The prevalence of goitre in areas of severe iodine deficiency can be as high as 80%. Iodization programmes are of proven value in reducing goitre size and in preventing goitre development and cretinism in children. Goitrogens in the diet, such as thiocyanate in incompletely cooked cassava or thioglucosides in *Brassica* vegetables, can explain some of the differences in prevalence of endemic goitre in areas with similar degrees of iodine deficiency. Autonomy can develop in nodular goitres leading occasionally to hyperthyroidism, and iodization programmes can also induce hyperthyroidism, especially in those aged over 40 years with nodular goitres. Autoimmune thyroiditis or hypothyroidism has not been reported to complicate salt iodization programmes. Relatively little prevalence data exist for autoimmune thyroid disease in areas of iodine deficiency (3).

In iodine-replete areas, most people with thyroid disorders have autoimmune disease, ranging through primary atrophic hypothyroidism, Hashimoto's thyroiditis, to hyperthyroidism caused by Graves' disease. Cross-sectional studies in Europe, the USA, and Japan have determined the prevalence of hyperthyroidism, hypothyroidism, and the frequency and distribution of thyroid autoantibodies in different, mainly white, communities (1, 4–6). Recent US data have revealed differences in the frequency of thyroid dysfunction and serum antithyroid antibody concentrations in different ethnic groups (6), whereas studies from Europe have revealed the influence of dietary iodine intake on the epidemiology of thyroid dysfunction (7). Studies of incidence of autoimmune thyroid disease have only been conducted in a small number of developed countries (8–11). Following a review of the available epidemiological data, the value of screening adult populations for autoimmune thyroid disease will be considered.

Hyperthyroidism

In epidemiological studies, the clinical diagnosis of hyperthyroidism should be supported by measurements of serum thyroxine (T_4) (or triiodothyronine (T_3)) and thyrotropin (TSH) concentrations. Biochemical tests of thyroid function may reveal the diagnosis before it is clinically apparent. A rise in serum T_3 and fall in serum TSH are the earliest measures of thyroid overactivity, followed by a rise in serum T_4. The most common causes of hyperthyroidism are Graves' disease, followed by toxic multinodular goitre, while rarer causes include an autonomously functioning thyroid adenoma or thyroiditis. In epidemiological studies, however, the aetiology is rarely ascertained.

Prevalence of hyperthyroidism

The prevalence of hyperthyroidism in women is between 0.5 and 2%, and is 10 times more common in women than in men in iodine-replete communities. In the Whickham survey, between 1972 and 1974, of 2779 people aged over 18 years in north-east England closely matched to the UK population, the prevalence of undiagnosed hyperthyroidism, based on clinical features and elevated serum T_4 and free T_4 index values, was 4.7/1000 women (4). Hyperthyroidism had been previously diagnosed and treated in 20/1000 women, rising to 27/1000 women when possible but unproven cases were included, as compared with 1.6–2.3/1000 men, in whom no new cases were found at the survey. The mean age at diagnosis was 48 years. In the other available cross-sectional studies of the adult population the results are comparable to the Whickham data (Table 3.1.7.1). In the Third National Health and Nutrition Examination Survey (NHANES III) in the USA, serum TSH and total T_4 were measured in a representative sample of 16 533 people aged over 12 years (6). In those people who were neither taking thyroid medication nor reported histories of thyroid disease, 2/1000 had 'clinically significant' hyperthyroidism, defined as a serum TSH concentration less than 0.1 mU/l and a serum total T_4 concentration more than 170 nmol/l.

The prevalence data in older people show a wide range of results. In a survey of 1210 people aged over 60 years of age in a single general practice in Birmingham, UK, only one woman was found to be hyperthyroid. Other studies show prevalence rates between 0.4 and 2.0% (1) (see Table 3.1.7.1). A cross-sectional study of 2799 healthy community-dwelling adults aged 70–79 years in the USA found evidence of hyperthyroidism (defined biochemically as a serum TSH concentration less than 0.1 mU/l and a serum free T_4 concentration more than 23 pmol/l in only five people (one man and four women) (12). In a survey of 599 people aged between 85 and 89 years, only two people had newly diagnosed overt hyperthyroidism (13).

Several studies which assessed healthy volunteers found a prevalence of 0.3–0.9% depending on the age and sex distribution of the sample (1). The data available from these highly selected populations of presumably well-motivated individuals must be treated with caution before being applied to the general population. A cross-sectional survey of 25 862 people aged over 18 years attending a Health Fair in Colorado, USA found that overt hyperthyroidism, defined as serum TSH concentration less than 0.01 mU/l, was present in only 1/1000 of those not taking thyroid medication (5).

The prevalence of undiagnosed hyperthyroidism in Pescopagano, Italy, an area of mild iodine deficiency (median urinary iodine excretion 55 μg/l), was higher, at 2%, with a further 1% of adults there having a history of toxic nodular goitre (14). Approximately one-third had a diffuse goitre, and the frequency in men and women was similar. In a population sample of 2656 from Copenhagen, Denmark, another area of mild iodine deficiency (median urinary iodine excretion 70 μg/l), newly diagnosed hyperthyroidism was found in 1.2% of women and no men, and the prevalence of known hyperthyroidism was 1.4% (15).

Hospital inpatients and even those visiting outpatients are selected populations. Isolated alterations in serum TSH concentrations (either slightly low 0.1–0.5 mU/l or high 5–20 mU/l) occur in about 15% of such patients due to the lability of TSH secretion in

Table 3.1.7.1 Prevalence of previously undiagnosed overt hyperthyroidism and incidence of overt hyperthyroidism in epidemiological surveys of thyroid dysfunction

Study name[a]	Number	Age (years)	Test	Prevalence number/1000		Incidence number/1000 per year		
				Men	Women	Follow-up (years)	Men	Women
Whickham, UK (4,9)	2779	18	T_4, FT_4I	0	4.7	20	<0.1	0.8 (0.6–1.4)
Colorado, USA (5)	25 862	18+	TSH	1.0				
NHANES III, USA (6)	16 533	12+	TSH, TT_4	2.0				
Memphis/Pittsburgh, USA (12)	2799	70–79	TSH, FT_4	0.7		2.8		
Leiden, Netherlands (13)	599	85–89	TSH, FT_4	4.0				
Pescopagano, Italy (14)	922	15+	TSH, FT_4	20.0				
Mölnlycke, Sweden	2000	18+	TSH	0	2.5	–	–	–
Sapporo, Japan	4110	25+	TSH, TRAB	2.7	5.1	–	–	–
Hisayama, Japan	2421	40+	TSH	0	2.0	–	–	–
Kisa, Sweden	3885	39–60	TSH, FT_4I	–	5.1	–	–	–
Copenhagen, Denmark (15)	2656	41–71	TSH, FT_4	0	12.0			
Kisa, Sweden	1442	60+	TSH, FT_4I	–	19.4	–	–	–
Tayside, UK (1993–1997) (10)	390 000	0+	Treatment for hyperthyroidism	–	–	4	0.14 (0.11–0.17)	0.77 (0.70–0.84)
Tayside, UK (1997–2001) (11)	390 000	0+	As above	–	–	4	0.15 (0.10–0.22)	0.91 (0.78–1.05)
Göteborg, Sweden	1283	44–66	TSH	–	6.0	6	–	1.3
Oakland, USA	2704	18+	TSH, T_4, T_3	0	5.4	1	0.2	0.8
Johannesburg, South Africa	?	0+	T_4			1	0.007	0.09
Birmingham, UK	1210	60+	TSH	0.9		1	0	1.5
Gothenburg, Sweden	1148	70+	TSH	–	–	10	–	1.0
Olmstead Co., USA	?	0+	BMR, PBI	–	–	32	0.1	0.3
Funen, Denmark	450 000	0+	PBI, T_4, T_3	–	–	3	0.1	0.5
Iceland	230 000	0+	T_4, T_3	–	–	3	0.1	0.4
Malmö, Sweden	257 764	0+	PBI	–	–	5	0.1	0.4
Twelve towns in UK	1 641 949	0+	T_4	–	–	1	0.1	0.4

[a] See reference 1 unless stated.

BMR, basal metabolic rate; FT_4, free T_4; FT_4I, free T_4 index; PBI, protein-bound iodine; TRAB, TSHR antibody; TT_4, total T_4.

response to nonthyroidal illness or drugs. About 2–3% of hospitalized patients have serum TSH concentrations that are suppressed (less than 0.1 mU/l) or elevated (more than 20 mU/l), but less than one-half of these will have an underlying thyroid disorder. The reported point prevalence rates for previously undiagnosed hyperthyroidism, between 0.3 and 1%, are consistent with community surveys (1, 16).

Subclinical hyperthyroidism

The introduction of assays for serum TSH sensitive enough to distinguish between normal and low concentrations allowed people with subclinical hyperthyroidism to be identified. Subclinical hyperthyroidism is defined as a low serum TSH concentration and normal serum T_4 and T_3 concentrations, in the absence of hypothalamic or pituitary disease, nonthyroidal illness, or ingestion of drugs that inhibit TSH secretion such as glucocorticoids or dopamine. The available studies differ in the definition of a low serum TSH concentration and whether the people included were receiving thyroxine therapy (1, 17).

The reported overall prevalence ranges from 0.5 to 6.3%, with men and women over 65 years of age having the highest prevalence; approximately one-half of them are taking thyroxine (1, 17). Among these studies, the serum TSH cut-off value ranged from less than 0.1 mU/l to less than 0.5 mU/l and it is not clear how this difference affected the reported prevalence rates. In the Colorado study of 25 862 people (of whom 88% were white) and in which the serum TSH cut-off value was 0.3 mU/l, the overall prevalence of subclinical hyperthyroidism was 2.1% (5). In contrast, the NHANES III study, defining subclinical hyperthyroidism using a more stringent 0.1 mU/l as the serum TSH cut-off, reported an overall prevalence of 0.7% in the total population and 0.2% in the thyroid disease-free population (n = 13 344) (6). The rates were highest in those people aged 20–39 years and those more than age 79 years. In this study, the percentage of people with serum TSH concentrations less than 0.4 mU/l was significantly higher in women than men, and black people had significantly lower mean serum TSH concentrations, and therefore a higher prevalence of subclinical hyperthyroidism (0.4%) than white people (0.1%) or Mexican Americans (0.3%).

At the 20-year follow-up of the Whickham survey cohort, the thyroid status was documented in 91% of the 1877 survivors. Four per cent had serum TSH values less than 0.5 mU/l (reference range 0.5–5.2 mU/l), decreasing to 3% if those people taking thyroxine and those with newly diagnosed overt thyrotoxicosis were excluded (9). When serum TSH was measured in the same samples using a more sensitive TSH assay (detection limit of 0.01 mU/l, coefficient of variation of 10% at 0.08 mU/l, and a normal range of 0.17 to 2.89 mU/l), approximately 2% had subnormal serum TSH concentrations (more than 0.01 but less than 0.17 mU/l), and 1% had undetectable serum TSH concentrations (less than 0.01 mU/l). In people over 60 years of age in the Framingham Heart Study, 4% had a low serum TSH concentration (less than 0.1 mU/l), and one-half of these were taking thyroxine.

Among people with subclinical hyperthyroidism, those with low but detectable serum TSH values may recover spontaneously when retested. In the community survey of people aged over 65 years in Birmingham, UK, 6% had low serum TSH concentrations, and 2% of women and 1% of men had undetectable values (less than 0.05 mU/l) (1). One year later, 88% of those with subnormal serum TSH values (less than 0.05 mU/l) continued to have a subnormal value, and 76% with a value of 0.05–0.5 mU/l had normal values. In the US study of people aged 71–79 years the prevalence was 1.1% in women and 0.7% in men and there was no difference between black and white residents (12). In the Leiden study of people aged over 85 years, the prevalence was 3% (13).

The prevalence of subnormal serum TSH concentrations (detection limit 0.01 mU/l and excluding those people taking thyroxine) was higher in the iodine-deficient population of Pescopagano (6%), due to functional autonomy from nodular goitres (14). In Jutland, an area of mild iodine deficiency in Denmark, 10% of a random sample of 423 people had low serum TSH concentrations, as compared with 1% of 100 people of similar age in iodine-rich Iceland. Subclinical hyperthyroidism was not detected in a group of elderly nursing home residents in an iodine-rich region of Hungary (1) (See Table 3.1.7.2).

Table 3.1.7.2 Effect of environmental iodine intake on the prevalence of subclinical thyroid disease (1, 3, 7)

Iodine status	Subclinical hypothyroidism (%)	Subclinical hyperthyroidism (%)
Deficient	1–4	6–10
Replete	4–9	1–2
Excess	18–14	<1

Incidence of thyrotoxicosis

The incidence data available for overt hyperthyroidism in men and women from large population studies are comparable, at 0.4/1000 women and 0.1/1000 men, but the age-specific incidence varies considerably (see Table 3.1.7.1 and (1) for references). The peak age-specific incidence of Graves' disease was between 20 and 49 years in two studies, but increased with age in Iceland and peaked at 60–69 years in Malmö, Sweden. The peak age-specific incidence of hyperthyroidism caused by toxic nodular goitre and autonomously functioning thyroid adenomas in the Malmö study was over 80 years. The only available data in a black population from Johannesburg, South Africa suggest a 10-fold lower annual incidence of hyperthyroidism (0.09/1000 women and 0.007/1000 men) than in white people. In a prospective study of 12 towns in England and Wales, the annual incidence of antibody-negative hyperthyroidism was strongly correlated with the prevalence of endemic goitre among schoolchildren 60 years earlier. Subsequent to this survey, serum samples from 216 of the 290 cases identified were assayed for TSH receptor (TSHR) antibodies. The incidence of antibody-positive hyperthyroidism, an indicator of Graves' disease, did not correlate with goitre in the past.

In the survivors of the Whickham survey cohort, 11 women had been diagnosed and treated for hyperthyroidism after the first survey and five women were diagnosed at the second survey (9). The aetiology in these 16 new cases was Graves' disease in 10 people, multinodular goitre in three, an autonomously functioning thyroid adenoma in one, chronic autoimmune thyroiditis in one, and unknown in one. The mean annual incidence of hyperthyroidism in women was 0.8/1000 survivors (95% CI 0.5 to 1.4) (9). The incidence rate was similar in the deceased women. No new cases were detected in men. An estimate of the probability of the development of hyperthyroidism in women at a particular time averaged 1.4/1000 between the ages of 35 and 60 years (see Fig. 3.1.7.1). Serum antithyroid antibody status or goitre was not associated with the development of hyperthyroidism at follow-up. Other cohort studies provide comparable incidence data, which suggests that many cases of hyperthyroidism remain undiagnosed in the community unless routine testing is undertaken (1). In a large

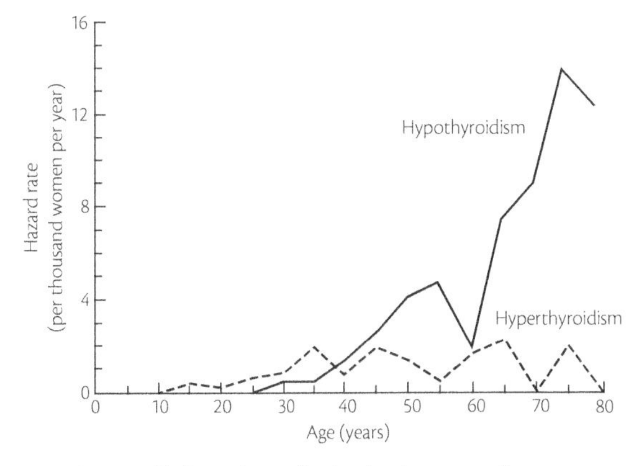

Fig. 3.1.7.1 Age-specific hazard rates for the development of overt hyperthyroidism and hypothyroidism in women at the 20-year follow-up of the Whickham survey. (From Vanderpump MPJ, Tunbridge WMG, French JM, Appleton D, Bates D, Clark F, *et al.* The incidence of thyroid disorders in the community: a twenty-year follow-up of the Whickham survey. *Clin Endocrinol*, 1995; 43: 60. Reproduced with permission, Blackwell Science.)

population study in Tayside, Scotland, 620 incident cases of hyperthyroidism were identified from medical records with an incidence rate of 0.77/1000 per year (95% CI 0.70 to 0.84) in women and 0.14/1000 per year (95% CI 0.12 to 0.18) in men (10). The incidence increased with age, and women were affected 2–8 times more than men across the age range. The incidence of hyperthyroidism increased in women but not in men between 1997 and 2001 (11). A prospective study of 790 healthy women aged 18–65 years with a family history of autoimmune thyroid disease in a first- or second-degree relative in the iodine-sufficient Netherlands found an annual incidence of 3.3/1000, which was 4.1–4.3 times higher than in the UK data (18).

Data on the risk of progression of subclinical hyperthyroidism to overt hyperthyroidism are limited. At the 1-year follow-up, of the 66 people aged over 60 years in Birmingham who initially had serum TSH values below normal, one man developed hyperthyroidism. Eighty-eight per cent of people with undetectable serum TSH values (less than 0.05 mU/l; n = 16) and 24% with a serum TSH of between 0.05 and 5 mU/l (n = 50) continued to have a subnormal value at 1 year. Only six people initially found to have a below normal serum TSH developed hyperthyroidism during 4 years of follow-up of the Framingham sample. Thus, in most people, a below normal serum TSH will eventually rise towards normal. In those people with an undetectable serum TSH and a confirmed aetiology due to Graves' disease or nodular disease, it has been calculated from short follow-up studies that the annual incidence is approximately 5% (1).

Hypothyroidism

The earliest biochemical abnormality in hypothyroidism is a rise in serum TSH associated with normal serum T_4 and T_3 concentrations (subclinical hypothyroidism or mild thyroid failure), followed by a fall in serum T_4, at which stage most patients have symptoms and benefit from treatment (overt hypothyroidism). In people living in iodine-replete areas, the cause is either chronic autoimmune disease (atrophic autoimmune thyroiditis or goitrous autoimmune thyroiditis (Hashimoto's thyroiditis)) or destructive treatment for thyrotoxicosis, but this is rarely discussed in the available studies.

Congenital hypothyroidism

Congenital hypothyroidism affects about one newborn in 3500–4000 births and is the most treatable cause of mental impairment. There is an inverse relationship between age at diagnosis and IQ in later life. In iodine-replete areas, 85% of the cases are due to sporadic developmental defects of the thyroid gland (thyroid dysgenesis), such as the arrested migration of the embryonic thyroid (ectopic thyroid) or a complete absence of thyroid tissue (athyreosis). The remaining 15% have thyroid dyshormonogenesis defects transmitted by an autosomal recessive mode of inheritance. Iodine deficiency (below 25 μg/day), particularly in preterm infants, accounts for many cases in Eastern Europe, Asia, and Africa. Clinical diagnosis occurs in less than 5% of newborns with hypothyroidism because symptoms and signs are often minimal. Without prompt diagnosis and treatment, most affected children gradually develop growth failure, irreversible mental impairment, and a variety of neuropsychological deficits.

Asymptomatic autoimmune thyroiditis

The presence of high serum concentrations of antithyroid antibodies (antithyroid peroxidase (microsomal) (TPO) and antithyroglobulin) correlates with the presence of focal thyroiditis in thyroid tissue obtained by biopsy and at autopsy from patients with no evidence of hypothyroidism during life. Early postmortem studies confirmed histological evidence of chronic autoimmune thyroiditis in 27% of adult women, with a rise in frequency over 50 years, and 7% of adult men, and diffuse changes in 5% of women and 1% of men (1). Patients with hypothyroidism caused by either atrophic or goitrous autoimmune thyroiditis usually have high serum concentrations of these same antibodies. These antibodies are often detected in serum of patients with Graves' disease and other thyroid diseases, but the concentrations are usually lower.

There is considerable variation in the frequency and distribution of antithyroid antibodies because of variations in techniques of detection, definition of abnormal titres, and inherent differences in the populations tested. In the Whickham survey, the mean serum TSH concentrations were significantly higher in both men and women with positive serum antithyroid antibody tests, and 3% of the people (5% of women, 1% of men) had both positive antibody tests and a serum TSH value more than 6 mU/l (4). Fifty per cent of those people who were antithyroid antibody positive had serum TSH more than 6 mU/l. Conversely, 60% of those with serum TSH more than 6 mU/l were antithyroid antibody positive, and 80% of those with serum TSH more than 10 mU/l were antithyroid antibody positive (see Fig. 3.1.7.2). In the NHANES III survey, the percentage of people with high serum TPO and antithyroglobulin antibody concentrations increased with age in both men and women, and high concentrations were more prevalent in women than in men and less prevalent in black people than in other ethnic groups (6). Using a competitive immunoassay procedure, the reported prevalence of detectable antithyroglobulin and TPO antibody levels were 10% and 12%, respectively, in the healthy population. A hypoechoic ultrasound pattern or an irregular echo pattern may precede TPO antibody positivity in autoimmune thyroid disease, and TPO antibody may not be detected in more than 20% of individuals with ultrasound evidence of thyroid autoimmunity (17).

At the 20-year follow-up of the Whickham survey, 19% of survivors had high serum TPO antibody concentrations and 5% had high serum antithyroglobulin antibody concentration (9).

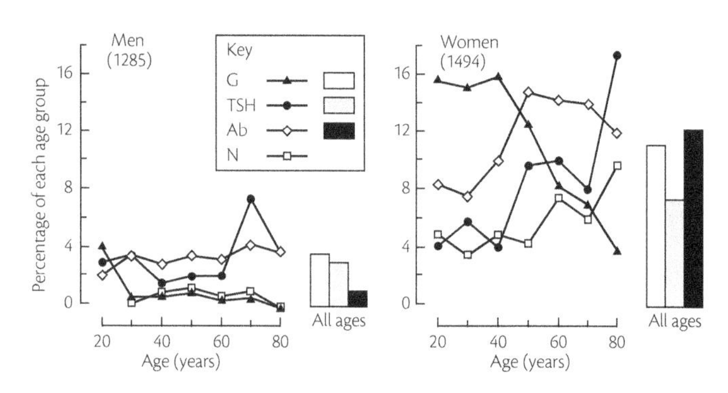

Fig. 3.1.7.2 Age and sex distribution of people with thyroid microsomal antibodies (Ab), raised serum TSH more than 6 mU/l (↑TSH), visible diffuse and multinodular goitre (G), and nodules (N) in the Whickham survey.
(From Tunbridge WMG, Evered DC, Hall R, Appleton D, Brewis M, Clark F, *et al.* The spectrum of thyroid disease in the community: the Whickham survey. *Clin Endocrinol*, 1977; 7: 485. Reproduced with permission, Blackwell Science.)

Seventeen per cent of women and 7% of men who initially had normal values now had high values, 9% of women and 2% of men had high values on both occasions, and 2% of women and 0.5% of men had high values initially but not at follow-up. The antithyroid antibodies were most often detected in women aged 55–65 years at follow-up (and who were therefore aged 35–45 years at the time of the first survey). Over 50% of the women in whom the serum antithyroid antibody concentrations changed from high to normal were receiving thyroxine treatment for hypothyroidism (1, 17). In summary, a significant proportion of people in the community have asymptomatic chronic autoimmune thyroiditis, and of these a substantial proportion have subclinical hypothyroidism.

Prevalence of hypothyroidism

In iodine-replete communities, the prevalence of spontaneous hypothyroidism is between 1 and 2%; it is more common in older women and 10 times more common in women than in men (1). In the Whickham survey, the prevalence of newly diagnosed overt hypothyroidism was 3/1000 women (4). The prevalence of previously diagnosed and treated hypothyroidism was 14/1000 women, increasing to 19/1000 women when possible, but unproven, cases were included. The overall prevalence in men was less than 1/1000. One-third had been previously treated by surgery or radio-iodine for thyrotoxicosis. Excluding iatrogenic causes, the prevalence of hypothyroidism was 10/1000 women, increasing to 15/1000 when possible, but unproven, cases were included. The mean age at diagnosis was 57 years. The diagnosis was based on clinical features and high serum TSH and low free T_4 index values in the new cases, and from the original records in the previously diagnosed and treated cases.

The Whickham data are comparable with other studies where the prevalence of newly diagnosed hypothyroidism ranged between 0.6 and 12/1000 women and between 1.3 and 4.0/1000 in men investigated in northern Europe, Japan, and the USA (see Table 3.1.7.3 and (1) for references). In the Colorado and NHANES III studies, the prevalence was 4/1000 and 3/1000, respectively (5, 6).

In iodine-deficient Pescopagano, the prevalence of newly diagnosed overt hypothyroidism was 0.3% of 573 women (autoimmune thyroiditis confirmed as aetiology); there were no cases among 419 men and no individual had been diagnosed and treated for hypothyroidism (14). In Copenhagen, 6/1000 of the women and

Table 3.1.7.3 Prevalence of previously undiagnosed overt hypothyroidism and incidence of overt hypothyroidism in epidemiological surveys of thyroid dysfunction

Study name[a]	Number	Age (years)	Test	Prevalence number/1000		Incidence number/1000 per year		
				Men	Women	Follow-up (years)	Men	Women
Whickham, UK (4, 9)	2779	18+	TSH, T_4	0	3.3	20	0.6 (0.3–1.2)	3.5 (2.8–4.5)
Colorado, USA (5)	25 862	18+	TSH	4.0				
NHANES III, USA (6)	16 533	12+	TSH	2.0				
Pescopagano, Italy (14)	992	15+	TSH, FT_4	0	3.0			
South Finland	3000	18+	TSH	2.0				
Mölnlycke, Sweden	2000	18+	TSH	1.3	12.0	–	–	–
Sapporo, Japan	4110	25+	TSH	2.4	8.5	–	–	–
Hisayama, Japan	2421	40+	TSH	4.0	7.0	–	–	–
Copenhagen, Denmark (15)	2656	41–71	TSH, FT_4	2.0	5.0			
Kisa, Sweden	3885	39–60	TSH, FT_4I	–	0	–	–	–
Memphis/Pitttsburgh, USA (12)	2799	70–79	TSH, FT_4	5.4	13.0			
Leiden, Netherlands (13)	599	85–89	TSH, FT_4	70				
Tayside, UK (1993–1997) (10)	390 000	0+	Treatment for hypothyroidism	–	–	4	0.88 (0.80–0.95)	4.98 (4.81–5.17)
Tayside, UK (1997–2001) (11)	390 000	0+	As above			4	1.09 (0.95–1.25	4.75 (4.46–5.07)
Göteborg, Sweden	1283	44–66	TSH	–	6.4	4	–	1–2
Oakland, USA	2704	18+	TSH, T_4, T_3	3.5	6.1	1	8.0	
Birmingham, UK	1210	60+	TSH	7.8	20.5	1	11.1	
Kisa, Sweden	1442	60+	TSH, FT_4I	–	5.5	–	–	–
Gothenburg, Sweden	1148	70+	TSH	–	–	10	–	2
Western Australia	1587	18+	TMA	–	–	6	3	
Barry, Wales	414	70+	TMA, TGA	4.8	5	4		

[a] See reference 1 unless stated.

FT_4, free T_4; FT_4I, free T_4 index; TGA, antithyroglobulin antibodies; TMA, antithyroid microsomal antibodies.

2/1000 men had overt but undiagnosed hypothyroidism, and 1% were taking thyroxine (15).

The prevalence is higher in surveys of older people in the community (1). The overall prevalence of hypothyroidism, including those already taking thyroxine, in Birmingham of 1210 people aged 60 and over was 4% of women and 0.8% of men. In people aged 60 years or more in Framingham, USA, 4% had a serum TSH concentration more than 10 mU/l, and, of these, one-third had low serum T_4 concentrations (1, 7). Overt hypothyroidism was found in 7% of those people aged 85 in Leiden, the Netherlands (13).

The testing of hospital inpatients, predominantly elderly women, might be expected to reveal a higher proportion of unsuspected hypothyroidism, but this is not supported by the available studies. Overt hypothyroidism, very rarely suspected clinically, was found in approximately 2% of patients admitted for treatment of an acute illness in studies of 98, 299, and 630 admissions. In another similar study, however, 6% of 364 patients admitted consecutively to an acute care teaching hospital had unrecognized or untreated thyroid failure. These people tended to be older and have more severe illnesses, but limiting testing to women over 50 years in this study would have missed 40% of those with significant hypothyroidism (1, 16).

Subclinical hypothyroidism

The term subclinical hypothyroidism is used to describe the finding of a raised serum TSH but a normal free T_4 in an asymptomatic patient. It represents a compensated state in which increased TSH output is required to maintain normal circulating thyroid hormone levels. An elevated serum TSH is a sensitive indicator of some degree of thyroid failure and, in contrast to below normal serum TSH levels, a clear inverse relationship is found with free T_4 levels. It is commonly found either following radio-iodine therapy or following surgery in up to 50% of apparently euthyroid patients. It may be evident for only a few months, but more often it represents a stage in the progression towards overt thyroid failure. Less frequent causes include external beam irradiation of malignant tumours of the head and neck, drugs including lithium, amiodarone, and interferon, and Addison's disease. In the community, the most common aetiology is chronic autoimmune thyroiditis (1, 17).

In the original Whickham survey, 8% of women (10% of women over 55 years of age) and 3% of men had subclinical hypothyroidism (4). Serum TSH concentrations did not change as a function of age among adult men, but in women over 40 years of age the concentrations increased. If, however, women with high serum antithyroid antibody concentrations were excluded, there was no age-related increase (see Fig. 3.1.7.2). In the Colorado study, 9.4% of the people had a high serum TSH concentration, of whom 9.0% had subclinical hypothyroidism (5). Among those with a high serum TSH concentration, 74% had a value between 5.1 and 10 mU/l and 26% had a value over 10 mU/l. The percentage of people with a high serum TSH concentration was higher for women than men in each decade of age, and ranged from 4 to 21% in women and 3 to 16% in men. An increase in serum TSH concentrations was also found in men in the NHANES III study. In the same study, serum TSH concentrations increased with age in both men and women and were higher in white people than black people, independent of serum antithyroid antibody concentrations (6).

Community studies of older people have confirmed the high prevalence of subclinical hypothyroidism in this age group, with approximately 10% of people over 60 years having serum TSH values above the normal range (1). A recent further analysis of the NHANES III data demonstrated that 11% of 20- to 29-year-olds had a serum TSH more than 2.5 mU/l, increasing to 40% in those aged 80 and over. The 97.5 percentile for those people aged 80 and over was 7.49 mU/l and 70% had a serum TSH above the population defined upper limit of the reference range of 4.5 mU/l; of these only 40% were antithyroid antibody positive (19). Data from a US cohort aged 70–79 years found that black people had a significantly lower prevalence of subclinical hypothyroidism (2% in men, 3% in women), as compared with white people (4% in men, 6% in women) (12). In iodine-deficient Pescopagano, there was a slightly lower prevalence of subclinical hypothyroidism (4% of women and 3% of men), but high serum antithyroid antibody concentrations were as prevalent, although at lower titres, as in iodine-replete communities (14). In borderline iodine-deficient Copenhagen, only 0.7% of people had subclinical hypothyroidism, and 83% of these had TPO antibody concentrations more than 200 kU/l (15). Other studies of older people in iodine-deficient areas have suggested a high prevalence of subclinical hypothyroidism with approximately 10% of people over 60 years having serum TSH values above the normal range. Subclinical hypothyroidism is found at higher frequency (18% in Iceland and 24% in Hungary) in areas where iodine intake is high, but most cases are not of autoimmune origin (1) (see Table 3.1.7.2). In surveys of hospital inpatients, the point prevalence rates were similar, being between 3 and 6%, with most people reverting to normal thyroid function 3 months following the acute illness (16).

Incidence of overt hypothyroidism

After destructive treatment of the thyroid for hyperthyroidism with either radio-iodine or by surgery, the incidence of overt hypothyroidism is greatest in the first year. The incidence of hypothyroidism in patients with Graves' disease was higher than that in patients with nodular goitre (55% versus 32%) and increased in those given higher doses of radio-iodine (7). If the patient had subclinical hypothyroidism 1 year or more after radio-iodine or surgical treatment, then the annual rate of progression to overt hypothyroidism after either treatment is 2–6%. Treatment of Graves' disease with antithyroid drugs alone is also associated with the eventual development of hypothyroidism in 5–20% of cases from either autoimmune thyroiditis or the presence of TSH-blocking antibodies. The incidence of hypothyroidism after surgery, external radiation therapy of the neck, or both in patients with head and neck cancer (including lymphoma) is as high as 50% within the first year after treatment, particularly in patients who underwent surgery and received high doses of radiation. The effect is dose-dependent, the onset is gradual, and subclinical hypothyroidism can be present for many years before the development of overt disease.

The 20-year follow-up of the Whickham cohort provided incidence data in a UK community sample and allowed the determination of risk factors for spontaneous hypothyroidism in this period (9). The mean annual incidence of spontaneous hypothyroidism in the surviving women during the 20-year follow-up period was 3.5/1000 (95% CI 2.8 to 4.5), increasing to 4.1/1000 (95% CI 3.3 to 5.0) if all cases including those who had received destructive treatment for thyrotoxicosis were included. The hazard rate, the estimate of the probability of a woman developing hypothyroidism at a particular time, increased with age to 13.7/1000 in women between 75 and 80 years of age (see Fig. 3.1.7.2). The mean annual incidence during the 20-year follow-up period in men (all spontaneous except for one case of lithium-induced hypothyroidism) was 0.6/1000 (95% CI 0.3 to 1.2). The risk of having developed hypothyroidism was examined with respect to risk factors identified in the first survey. The odds ratios (with 95% CI) of developing spontaneous hypothyroidism in surviving women are shown in Table 3.1.7.4. Either raised serum TSH or positive antithyroid antibodies alone or in combination are associated with a significantly increased risk of hypothyroidism. The odds are greatly increased when both risk factors are present and each had a similar effect. The smaller number of observed cases in men not only resulted in wide but highly significant confidence limits, but also did not allow the independent effects of these risk factors to be calculated. In the surviving women, the annual risk of spontaneous overt hypothyroidism was 4% in those who had both high serum TSH and antithyroid antibody concentrations, 3% if only their serum TSH concentration was high, and 2% if only their serum thyroid antibody concentration was high; at the time of follow-up the respective rates of hypothyroidism were 55%, 33%, and 27%. The probability of developing hypothyroidism was higher in those women who had serum TSH concentrations above 2.0 mU/l and high serum titres of antithyroid microsomal antibodies during the first survey (see Fig. 3.1.7.3). Neither a positive family history of any thyroid disease, nor the presence of a goitre at either the first or the follow-up survey, nor parity at first survey was associated with an increased risk of hypothyroidism.

Other incidence data for hypothyroidism are from short (and often small) follow-up studies (7). In a follow-up study of 437 healthy women 40–60 years of age in the Netherlands, 24% of those who initially had a positive test for antithyroid microsomal antibodies and normal serum TSH concentrations had a high serum TSH concentration (more than 4.2 mU/l) 10 years later, as compared with 3% in the women who had a negative test for the antibodies. As in the 20-year follow-up of the Whickham cohort, serum TSH concentrations in the upper part of the normal range

Table 3.1.7.4 Development of spontaneous hypothyroidism in surviving women and men at 20-year follow-up of Whickham survey

Risk factor	Women (odds ratios (95% CI))	Men (odds ratios (95% CI))
TSH raised, regardless of thyroid antibody status	14 (9–24)	44 (19–104)
Thyroid antibody +, regardless of TSH status	13 (8–19)	25 (10–63)
If thyroid antibody –, effect of raised TSH alone	8 (3–20)	
If thyroid antibody +, additional effect of raised TSH	5 (2–11)	
If TSH normal, effect of thyroid antibody + alone	8 (5–15)	
If TSH raised, additional effect of thyroid antibody +	5 (1–(15)	
TSH raised and thyroid antibody + combined	38 (22–65)	173 (81–370)

–, antithyroid antibody negative normal range; +, antithyroid antibody positive elevated.

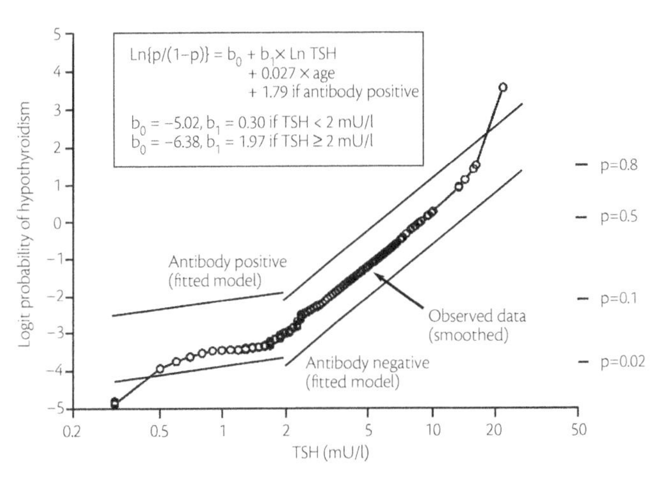

Fig. 3.1.7.3 Probability for development of hypothyroidism within 20 years with increasing values of serum TSH at first Whickham survey in 912 survivors. The coefficients for the fitted model are shown in the figure. (From Vanderpump MPJ, Tunbridge WMG, French JM, Appleton D, Bates D, Clark F, *et al.* The incidence of thyroid disorders in the community: a twenty-year follow-up of the Whickham survey. *Clin Endocrinol*, 1995; 43: 60. Reproduced with permission, Blackwell Science.)

in this study also appeared to have a predictive value. There was an annual incidence of hypothyroidism of 9.6/1000 in the 5-year follow-up study of 790 women with a family history of autoimmune thyroid disease in the Netherlands (18). Thus, in this cohort of at-risk women the incidence was 1.9–2.7 times higher than that seen in the general female population of the UK and was also higher in those with serum TSH more than 2.0 mU/l and high TPO antibody concentrations at baseline. In a 9-year follow-up of a cohort of 82 women with subclinical hypothyroidism, the cumulative incidence of overt hypothyroidism was 0% in those with serum TSH concentrations of 4–6 mU/l, 43% in those with serum TSH concentrations between 6 and 12 mU/l, and 77% in those with serum TSH concentrations more than 12 mU/l. In this study, the incidence of overt hypothyroidism was higher in those women with high serum antithyroid microsomal antibody concentrations at base line (59% versus 23%; p = 0.03), but a high serum antithyroid antibody concentration contributed much less to the risk of overt hypothyroidism than a high base-line serum TSH concentration, in contrast to the Whickham data (7, 17).

In older people, the annual incidence rate of hypothyroidism varies widely between 0.2 and 7% in the available studies (see Table 3.1.7.2 and (1) for references). In the survey of a Birmingham practice of 1210 people aged over 60 years, 18% of those with high serum TSH on initial testing had proceeded to overt hypothyroidism by 1 year. Over 50% of people with elevated serum TSH values were antithyroid microsomal antibody positive initially and they were the more likely to progress. Data from the large population study in Tayside, UK has demonstrated that the standardized incidence of primary hypothyroidism remained between 3.90 and 4.89/1000 women per year between 1993 and 2001. The incidence of hypothyroidism in men, however, significantly increased from 0.65 to 1.01/1000 per year (p = 0.0017). The mean age at diagnosis of primary hypothyroidism decreased in women from 1994 to 2001.

Spontaneous recovery has also been described in people with subclinical hypothyroidism, although the frequency of this phenomenon is unclear. In one study, 37% of patients normalized their serum TSH levels over a mean follow-up time of 31.7 months.

Normalization of serum TSH concentrations were more likely to occur in patients with negative antithyroid antibodies and serum TSH levels less than 10 mU/l, and within the first 2 years after diagnosis (17). However, all studies indicate that the higher the serum TSH value, the greater the likelihood of development of overt hypothyroidism in people with chronic autoimmune thyroiditis.

Thyroid disease in pregnancy

Pregnancy has variable effects on thyroid hormone concentrations throughout pregnancy as well as being associated with goitre (20). The latter is largely preventable by ensuring optimal iodine intake of at least 200µg/day. Hypothyroidism in pregnancy, usually characterized by a high serum TSH value, has been found to occur in around 2–3% of otherwise normal pregnancies with the prevalence of overt hypothyroidism estimated to be up to 0.5%. On a worldwide basis the most important cause of thyroid insufficiency remains iodine deficiency, while in iodine-replete communities the cause is usually chronic autoimmune thyroiditis. Untreated hypothyroidism may lead to obstetrical complications, such as preterm delivery and fetal loss. Women who are taking thyroxine at conception will require an increase in the dose during the pregnancy.

Epidemiological data suggest that the children of women with hypothyroxinaemia may have psychoneurological deficits. In classic areas of iodine deficiency, a similar range of deficits in children has been described where maternal hypothyroxinaemia rather than high serum TSH is the main biochemical abnormality. In these areas, maternal iodine intake is often substantially less than the 200 µg/day currently recommended. Even in areas previously thought to be iodine sufficient, there is now evidence of substantial gestational iodine deficiency, which may lead to low maternal circulating T_4 concentrations. In addition to the childhood neuropsychological problems relating to low T_4 values, there is evidence from a retrospective study that maternal TPO antibody may result in intellectual impairment even when there is normal thyroid function (20).

Hyperthyroidism is found in 0.1–0.4% of all pregnancies. It is usually caused by Graves' disease and is characterized by TSHR antibodies, which usually decrease in titre throughout pregnancy. Maternal complications include miscarriage, placental abruption, preeclampsia, and preterm delivery. High titres of TSHR antibodies if present at 36 weeks gestation predict a high risk of neonatal thyrotoxicosis. Postpartum Graves' disease also develops in predisposed women, although the prevalence of TSHR antibodies during gestation is much less than that of TPO antibodies (20).

Antithyroid antibodies, particularly TPO antibodies, occur in 10% of women at 14 weeks of gestation, which is compatible with the prevalence of antithyroid antibodies in community surveys (1, 20). A proportion of these women will have subclinical hypothyroidism with a high serum TSH, but most will be euthyroid. However, after delivery a transient, destructive autoimmune thyroiditis that occurs between the 12th and 16th week postpartum will develop in 50% of TPO antibody-positive women, as ascertained in early gestation, clinically apparent as postpartum thyroiditis (PPT). It presents as a temporary, usually painless, episode of hypothyroidism, occasionally preceded by a short episode of hyperthyroidism. Up to 25% of women progress to permanent hypothyroidism within approximately 5 years following an episode of PPT, particularly those with high antibody titres. It is not clear whether pregnancy actually alters the final incidence of autoimmune thyroid disease or merely brings forward the time that thyroid disease develops.

Goitre and thyroid nodules

The most common thyroid disease in the community is simple (diffuse) physiological goitre. The clinical grading of thyroid size is subjective and imprecise. The World Health Organization (WHO) grading system recognizes that an enlarged thyroid gland may be palpably but not visibly enlarged. Examiner variation is greatest in deciding whether a thyroid that is palpable but not visible is normal (WHO grade O-A) or enlarged (WHO grade O-B). Inter-examiner variation may also lead to differences in classification of the type of thyroid disease, whether a goitre is diffuse or multinodular goitre. There is also considerable overlap between the five WHO grades based on clinical criteria compared with thyroid volume estimated by ultrasonography. Ultrasonography has been used in epidemiological studies to assess thyroid size, leading to much higher estimates of goitre prevalence than in studies in which goitre size was assessed by physical examination (1).

Most studies define a thyroid that is visible as well as palpable as a goitre (WHO grade 1 or above). Considerable regional variations exist even in nonendemic goitre areas. In cross-sectional surveys, the prevalence of diffuse goitre declines with age, the greatest prevalence is in premenopausal women, and the ratio of women to men is at least 4:1 (1) (see Fig. 3.1.7.2). In the Whickham survey, 16% of the cohort had small but easily palpable diffuse or multinodular goitres (4). In men, the prevalence of goitre declined with age from 7% in those aged less than 25 years to 4% in those aged 65–74 years. No goitres were detected in men aged over 75 years. Among the women, 26% had a goitre; the frequency ranged from 31% in those aged less than 45 years (mostly diffuse) to 12% in those aged over 75 years (who had a higher proportion of multinodular goitre).

This decline in frequency of diffuse goitres with age is in contrast to the increase in frequency of thyroid nodules and thyroid antibodies with age. Fewer than 1% of the men but 5% of the women had thyroid nodules detected clinically, and this frequency increased to 9% in women aged over 75 years. In a study of 5234 people aged over 60 years in Framingham, USA, clinically apparent thyroid nodules were present in 6.4% of women and 1.5% of men (1). The prevalence of single thyroid nodules was 3% and multinodular goitre nodules was 1%.

In surveys of unselected people using ultrasonography, a significant proportion of women have at least one thyroid nodule. In Germany, an area of relative iodine deficiency, 96 278 working adults aged 18–65 years were screened by ultrasound scanning (21). Thyroid nodules or goitre were found in 33% of men and 32% of women and thyroid nodules over 1 cm were found in 12% of the population. The prevalence of nodular goitre increased with age from 3% and 2% in women and men aged 26–30 years, to 9% and 7% in women and men aged 36–40 years, to 14% and 12% in women and men aged 45–50 years, and to 18% and 15% in women and men over age 55 years. In several early autopsy surveys, up to 50% of patients had thyroid nodules. In patients with a single palpable nodule, 20–48% have additional nodules as detected by ultrasonography. Thus, while many nodules are detected because of their size or anterior position in the neck, or the skill of the physician performing the examination, most thyroid nodules are not clinically recognized. Ultrasonography as a screening tool is too sensitive and will result in unnecessary pursuit of findings which are so common that they rarely have pathological significance. However, it may have a place in investigating patients presenting with thyroid nodules to determine whether they are single or multiple.

Longitudinal studies confirm the decreasing frequency of diffuse goitre with age (1). In the 20-year follow-up of the Whickham cohort, 10% of women and 2% of men had a goitre, as compared to 23% and 5%, respectively, in the same people at the first survey (9). In a 20-year follow-up study of a sample of a south-western US population aged 11–18 years, spontaneous regression by the age of 30 years occurred in 60% of the people who initially had diffuse goitres (1). In the Whickham cohort, the presence of a diffuse goitre was not predictive of any clinical or biochemical evidence of thyroid dysfunction (9). In women, there was no association between goitre and thyroid antibody status in the initial survey, but at the 20-year follow-up there was a weak association. Although the order in which these events occurred is unknown, it would suggest an autoimmune aetiology for some goitres. In this iodine-replete population, thyroid function was similar in the goitrous and non-goitrous individuals. Serum TSH concentrations are noted to be raised only in areas with very severe iodine deficiency.

Thyroid cancer

The clinical presentation of thyroid cancer is usually as a solitary thyroid nodule or increasing goitre size. Although thyroid nodules are common, thyroid cancers are rare. Thyroid cancer is the most common malignant endocrine tumour and accounts for over 90% of the cancers of the endocrine glands, but constitutes less than 1% of all malignancies registered in the UK. The four major histological types are papillary, follicular, medullary, and anaplastic and each displays a different epidemiology.

The incidence of all thyroid cancer appears to be increasing slowly. In the period 1971–1995, the annual UK incidence was reported to be 2.4/100 000 women and 0.9/100 000 men, with approximately 900 new cases and 250 deaths recorded in England and Wales due to thyroid cancer every year. In 2001, data from Cancer Research UK showed 1200 new cases in England and Wales, with a reported annual incidence for the UK of 3.5/100 000 women and 1.3/100 000 men (22). In the USA, recent data obtained from the National Cancer Institutes' Surveillance, Epidemiology, and End Results (SEER) programme also indicate that the incidence of thyroid cancer has significantly increased from 3.6/100 000 in 1973 to 8.7/100 000 in 2002 (23). This represents a 2.4-fold increase (95% CI 2.2 to 2.6; $p < 0.001$ for trend). There was no significant change in the incidence of the less common histological types: follicular, medullary, and anaplastic ($p > 0.20$ for trend). Virtually the entire increase was attributable to an increase in the incidence of papillary thyroid cancer which increased from 2.7 to 7.7/100 000; this represented a 2.9-fold increase (95% CI 2.6 to 3.2; $p < 0.001$ for trend). Between 1998 (the first year SEER collected data on tumour size) and 2002, 49% (95% CI to 47–51%) of the increase consisted of papillary cancers measuring 1 cm or less and 87% (95% CI 85 to 89%) consisted of papillary cancers measuring 2 cm or less. There was no increase in mortality from all thyroid cancer between 1973 and 2002 (approximately 0.5 deaths/100 000).

Papillary and follicular tumours, which comprise 60–90% of the total, are among the most curable of cancers. They are rare in children and adolescents and their incidence increases with age in adults. Papillary thyroid carcinoma (PTC) is the most common thyroid malignancy and worldwide constitutes 50–90% of differentiated follicular cell-derived thyroid cancers. Papillary thyroid microcarcinomas (diameter less than 1 cm) are found in up to one-third of adults at postmortem in population-based studies. As diagnostic techniques for thyroid cancer have become more sensitive, particularly with the advent of ultrasonography and fine-needle aspiration, there has been an increased detection of subclinical papillary cancers. Most diagnoses of PTC occur in patients aged between 30 and 50 years (median age 44 years) and the majority (60–80%) occur in women. Follicular thyroid cancer occurs relatively infrequently compared to papillary cancer and accounts for approximately 15% of all thyroid cancer. In contrast, there is an increased frequency of follicular to papillary carcinoma (5:1) in iodine-deficient endemic goitre areas. It tends to be a malignancy of older people, with a mean age of 50 years in most studies.

In addition to female gender, advanced age, and low iodine intake, external radiation exposure, particularly in childhood, has been shown to be a major risk factor for papillary cancer, and some studies suggest that follicular cancer may also be affected. An increased incidence of thyroid cancer in the exposed children of Belarus and the Ukraine remains the most well-documented long-term effect of radioactive contamination after the Chernobyl nuclear accident in April 1986 (24). Multiple studies on approximately 4000 children and adolescents with thyroid cancer revealed that environmental exposure to radio-iodine during childhood carried an increased risk of thyroid cancer and that the risk was dependent on the radiation dose. The children aged less than 10 years were the most sensitive to radiation-induced carcinogenesis, and the minimal latent period for thyroid cancer development after exposure is as short as 4 years. The vast majority of these cancers are papillary carcinomas, many of which have characteristic solid or solid–follicular microscopic appearance. On the molecular level, post-Chernobyl tumours are characterized by frequent occurrence of chromosomal rearrangements, such as *RET/PTC*, whereas point mutations of *BRAF* and other genes are much less common in this population. There is no documented association between radio-iodine therapy for hyperthyroidism and subsequent development of thyroid cancer in adults.

Medullary thyroid cancer (MTC) is a rare calcitonin-secreting tumour of the C cells of the thyroid. It occurs in both sporadic and hereditary forms. The gender ratio in the sporadic form is 1 to 1.4 while both genders are equally affected in the familial variety. The highest incidence of sporadic disease occurs in the fifth decade. Hereditary MTC can be inherited as an autosomal dominant trait with a high degree of penetrance associated with multiple endocrine neoplasia type 2 syndrome or as familial MTC without any other endocrinopathies. It can be diagnosed before clinical presentation by genetic and biochemical screening.

Anaplastic thyroid cancer is very rare and is more frequent in populations with endemic goitre. It is speculated that dietary iodine supplementation explains why the reported incidence is declining. Anaplastic change can also rarely occur in a long-standing benign thyroid adenoma or differentiated carcinoma. The women-to-men ratio is less pronounced and the peak incidence is in patients in their seventies. Thyroid lymphoma is also uncommon constituting about 2% of extranodal lymphomas. It predominantly occurs in older women (median age of onset 60–70 years) which is consistent with its association with lymphocytic thyroiditis. Up to one-third of patients have a history of goitre while some have established autoimmune thyroiditis and may be taking thyroxine therapy.

Screening for thyroid disorders

Congenital hypothyroidism is the most treatable cause of mental impairment and the value of screening for congenital hypothyroidism in heel-prick blood specimens is unquestioned; it is now done routinely in many countries. Certain groups within the adult population who should have an assessment of thyroid function at least once to detect thyroid dysfunction include those with a goitre or thyroid nodule, atrial fibrillation, dyslipidaemia, subfertility, or osteoporosis. There is a high frequency of asymptomatic thyroid dysfunction in unselected patients with diabetes mellitus, and assessing thyroid function in the annual review of patients with diabetes appears cost-effective (16).

The value of screening for thyroid dysfunction in relation to pregnancy was considered in the recent Endocrine Society Guidelines (20). Case-finding of at-risk women is recommended, but ongoing studies may alter this recommendation. Further data are required to determine which screening tests should be used, their exact timing, and whether outcomes are improved following treatment. There is no consensus on whether healthy women should be screened for PPT. However, women with type 1 diabetes are 3 times more likely to develop postpartum thyroid dysfunction than are normal women, and therefore all should be tested. Any woman with a past history of PPT should be offered annual assessment of thyroid function, in view of their increased long-term risk of permanent hypothyroidism.

In view of the high prevalence of hypothyroidism in patients with Down's syndrome and Turner's syndrome, they also should have an annual assessment of thyroid function. Assessment of thyroid function is indicated every 6 months in patients receiving amiodarone and lithium, and every 12 months in those treated with external head and neck irradiation. All patients with hyperthyroidism who receive ablative treatment should be followed indefinitely for the development of hypothyroidism; this follow-up should begin 4–8 weeks after treatment, and then be done at 3-month intervals for 1 year and annually thereafter. Among patients hospitalized for acute illness, the occurrence of thyroid disease is no more common than in the general population. Therefore, testing should be limited but with a high index of clinical suspicion, particularly in elderly women, and with an awareness of the difficulties in interpreting thyroid function tests in the presence of acute illness (7, 16).

Controversy exists as to whether healthy adults living in an area of iodine sufficiency benefit from screening for thyroid disease. It is desirable to detect any disease in its early stage, particularly when treatment is available that will benefit the affected person and forestall or improve the natural history of the condition. The benefit from a screening programme must outweigh the physical and psychological harm caused by the test, diagnostic procedures, and treatment (25). Thyroid disorders secondary to autoimmune thyroid disease are among the most prevalent of medical conditions, and their symptoms and signs may be subtle and nonspecific and they can be mistakenly attributed to other illnesses, particularly in older people. The prevalence of unsuspected overt thyroid disease is low, but a substantial proportion of people tested will have evidence of thyroid dysfunction, with approximately 10% with subclinical hypothyroidism and 1% with subclinical hyperthyroidism. In the absence of the confounding effects of nonthyroidal illness or drugs, a normal serum TSH concentration has a high predictive value in ruling out thyroid disease in healthy people. In unselected populations, measurement of serum TSH has a sensitivity of 89–95% and a specificity of 90–96% for overt thyroid dysfunction, as compared to cases confirmed by history, examination, and additional testing. Normal serum TSH concentrations are found in some patients with hypothyroidism caused by pituitary or hypothalamic disease, but both these situations are rare. In nearly all populations screened, a serum TSH value of more than 5–6 mU/l is accepted as being raised.

Different recommendations and position papers have been reported by various physician organizations as to whether subclinical thyroid disease is of sufficient clinical importance to warrant screening and therapy. A cost–utility analysis using a computer decision model initially suggested that the cost-effectiveness of screening for subclinical hypothyroidism compared favourably with other preventive medical practices, such as screening for hypertension or breast cancer, in women in the same age group, while providing a similar increase in quality-adjusted life years (26). In 2004, US evidence-based consensus guidelines concluded that there were no adverse outcomes of subclinical hypothyroidism other than a risk of progression to overt hypothyroidism. In an observational cohort 10-year study, a low serum TSH concentration (less than 0.05 mU/l), but not a high serum TSH concentration, was associated with an increase in all-cause mortality and cardiovascular mortality (27). In addition, there were few data to justify thyroxine therapy in those people with a serum TSH between 5 and 10 mU/l, except in women who were preconception or pregnant. No consensus exists regarding the treatment of subclinical hyperthyroidism, although it has been strongly argued that therapy with antithyroid drugs or radio-iodine may be indicated in view of the long-term risk of atrial fibrillation and loss of bone density. Any potential benefits of therapy in subclinical hyperthyroidism must be weighed against the substantial morbidity associated with the treatment of hyperthyroidism.

Thyroxine therapy in mild thyroid failure may improve nonspecific symptoms, prevent progression to overt hypothyroidism, and potentially reduce the cardiovascular risk by improving the atherogenic lipid profile. However, normalization of serum TSH with thyroxine is often not achieved in clinical practice and detrimental effects on the skeleton, the cardiovascular system, and even mortality have been suggested by subclinical hyperthyroidism, which is often a consequence of overtreatment with thyroxine therapy (28). Since 2004, the controversial clinical issues in subclinical hypothyroidism remain unresolved. There is still debate as to what constitutes a normal TSH, particularly in older people. Although some of these people will progress to overt hypothyroidism, recent data suggest a significant proportion revert to normal or remain only mildly raised without treatment (18). There is even a suggestion in very elderly people that mild thyroid failure may even be associated with longevity (13). Two recent meta-analyses of selected population-based cohort studies have examined whether mild thyroid hormone failure or excess increase coronary heart disease (CHD) risk (29, 30). Ten studies reported risks associated with subclinical hypothyroidism and five examined risks associated with subclinical hyperthyroidism. For subclinical hyperthyroidism there is little evidence of an association with CHD events or mortality. For subclinical hypothyroidism, the relative risks for CHD events and cardiovascular and overall mortality were 1.2, 1.2, and 1.1 respectively. Limiting analyses to studies with the most rigorous methodologies slightly decreased the risk estimates. However, both analyses suggested the cardiovascular risks may be more significant in younger adults, approximately 1.5 versus 1.0 for populations with mean ages younger or older than 65 years, respectively. Other recent epidemiological data suggest that mild thyroid failure may be the only reversible cause of left ventricular diastolic dysfunction, particularly in those people with a serum TSH more than 10 mU/l (31). No appropriately powered prospective randomized controlled double-blinded interventional trial of thyroxine therapy for subclinical hypothyroidism exists. Adopting a 'wait and see' policy rather than intervention will avoid unnecessary treatment or the potential for harm. However, treatment in people less than 65 years old and those older people with evidence of heart failure may now be justified. There is an urgent need for long-term studies of the effects of identification and treatment of both subclinical hypothyroidism and subclinical hyperthyroidism to determine if there is indeed benefit from screening for thyroid dysfunction in adults.

References

1. Vanderpump MPJ. The epidemiology of thyroid diseases. In: Braverman LE, Utiger RD, eds. *Werner and Ingbar's The Thyroid*. 9th edn. Philadelphia: Lippincott-Raven, 2005: 398–406.
2. Zimmerman MB, Jooste PL, Pandav CS. Iodine-deficiency disorders. *Lancet*, 2008; **372**: 1251–62.
3. Laurberg P, Bulow Pedersen I, Knudsen N, Ovesen L, Andersen S. Environmental iodine intake affects the type of non-malignant thyroid disease. *Thyroid*, 2001; **11**: 457–69.
4. Tunbridge WMG, Evered DC, Hall R, Appleton D, Brewis M, Clark F, *et al.* The spectrum of thyroid disease in the community: the Whickham survey. *Clin Endocrinol*, 1977; **7**: 481–93.
5. Canaris GJ, Manowitz NR, Mayor G, Ridgway EC. The Colorado Thyroid Disease Prevalence Study. *Arch Intern Med*, 2000; **160**: 526–34.
6. Hollowell JG, Staehling NW, Flanders WD, Hannon WH, Gunter EW, Spencer CA, *et al.* Serum TSH, T_4, and thyroid antibodies in the United States population (1988 to 1994): National Health and Nutrition Examination Survey (NHANES III). *J Clin Endocrinol Metab*, 2002; **87**: 489–99.
7. Vanderpump MPJ, Tunbridge WMG. Epidemiology and prevention of clinical and subclinical hypothyroidism. *Thyroid*, 2002; **12**: 839–47.
8. McGrogan A, Seaman HE, Wright JW, de Vries CS. The incidence of autoimmune thyroid disease: a systematic review of the literature. *Clin Endocrinol*, 2008; **69**: 687–96.
9. Vanderpump MPJ, Tunbridge WMG, French JM, Appleton D, Bates D, Clark F, *et al.* The incidence of thyroid disorders in the community: a twenty-year follow-up of the Whickham survey. *Clin Endocrinol*, 1995; **43**: 55–69.
10. Flynn RV, MacDonald TM, Morris AD, Jung RT, Leese GP. The Thyroid Epidemiology, Audit and Research Study: thyroid dysfunction in the general population. *J Clin Endocrinol Metab*, 2004; **89**: 3879–84.
11. Leese GP, Flynn RV, Jung RT, MacDonald TM, Murphy MJ, Morris AD. Increasing prevalence and incidence of thyroid disease in Tayside, Scotland: the Thyroid Epidemiology, Audit and Research Study (TEARS). *Clin Endocrinol*, 2008; **68**: 311–16.
12. Kanaya AM, Harris F, Volpato S, Pérez-Stable EJ, Harris T, Bauer D. Association between thyroid dysfunction and total cholesterol level in an older biracial population. The Health, Aging and Body Composition Study. *Arch Intern Med*, 2002; **162**: 773–9.
13. Gussekloo J, van Exel E, de Craen AJM, Frölich M, Westendorp RGJ. Thyroid status, disability and cognitive function, and survival in old age. *JAMA*, 2004; **292**: 2591–9.
14. Aghini-Lombardi F, Antonangeli L, Martino E, Vitti P, Maccherini D, Leoli F, *et al.* The spectrum of thyroid disorders in an iodine-deficient community: the Pescopagano Survey. *J Clin Endocrinol Metab*, 1999; **84**: 561–6.
15. Knudsen N, J rgensen T, Rasmussen S, Christiansen, Perrild H. The prevalence of thyroid dysfunction in a population with borderline iodine deficiency. *Clin Endocrinol*, 1999; **51**: 361–7.
16. Association of Clinical Biochemistry, British Thyroid Association and British Thyroid Foundation. *UK guidelines for the use of thyroid function tests*. ACB and BTA, London. 2006. Available at: http://www.british-thyroid-association.org/info-for-patients/Docs/TFT_guideline_final_version_July_2006.pdf (accessed 23 May 2010).
17. Biondi B, Cooper DC. The clinical significance of subclinical thyroid dysfunction. *Endocr Rev*, 2008; **29**: 76–131.
18. Streider TGA, Tijssen JGP, Wenzel BE, Endert E, Wiersinga WM. Prediction of progression to overt hypothyroidism or hyperthyroidism in female relatives of patients with autoimmune thyroid disease using the Thyroid Events Amsterdam (THEA) score. *Arch Intern Med*, 2008; **168**: 1657–63.
19. Surks MI, Hollowell JG. Age-specific distribution of serum thyrotrophin and anti-thyroid antibodies in the US population: implications for the prevalence of subclinical hypothyroidism. *J Clin Endocrinol Metab*, 2007; **92**: 4575–82.
20. Abalovich M, Amino N, Barbour LA, Cobin RH, De Groot LJ, Glinoer D, *et al.* Management of thyroid dysfunction during pregnancy and postpartum: an Endocrine Society Clinical Practice Guideline. *J Clin Endocrinol Metab*, 2007; **92** (Suppl 8): S1–47.
21. Reiners C, Wegscheider K, Schicha H, Schicha H, Theissen P, Vaupel R, *et al.* Prevalence of thyroid disorders in the working population of Germany: ultrasonography screening in 96,278 unselected employees. *Thyroid*, 2004; **14**: 926–32.
22. British Thyroid Association and Royal College of Physicians. Guidelines for the management of thyroid cancer (Perros P. ed). *Report of the Thyroid Cancer Guidelines Update Group*. Royal College of Physicians, London. 2007. Available at: http://www.british-thyroid-association.org/news/Docs/Thyroid_cancer_guidelines_2007.pdf (accessed 23 May 2010).
23. Davies L, Welch HG. Increasing incidence of thyroid cancer in the United States, 1973–2002. *JAMA*, 2006; **295**: 2164–7.
24. Nikiforov YE. Radiation-induced thyroid cancer: what we have learned from Chernobyl. *Endocr Pathol*, 2006; **17**: 307–17.
25. Tunbridge WMG, Vanderpump MPJ. Population screening for autoimmune thyroid disease. *Endocrinol Metab*, 2000; **29**: 239–53.
26. Danese MD, Powe NR, Sawin CT, Ladenson PW. Screening for mild thyroid failure at the periodic health examination: a decision and cost-effectiveness analysis. *JAMA*, 1996; **276**: 285–92.
27. Surks MI, Ortiz E, Daniels GH, Sawin CT, Col NF, Cobin RH, *et al.* Subclinical thyroid disease: scientific review and guidelines for diagnosis and management. *JAMA*, 2004; **291**: 228–38.
28. Parle JV, Maisonneuve P, Sheppard MC, Boyle P, Franklyn JA. Prediction of all-cause and cardiovascular mortality in elderly

people from one thyrotropin result: a 10-year cohort study. *Lancet*, 2001; **358**: 861–5.

29. Ochs N, Auer R, Bauer DC, Nanchen D, Gussekloo J, Cornuz J, *et al.* Meta-analysis: subclinical thyroid dysfunction and the risk of coronary heart disease and mortality. *Ann Intern Med*, 2008; **148**: 832–45.
30. Razvi S, Shakoor A, Vanderpump M, Weaver J, Pearce S. The influence of age on the relationship between subclinical hypothyroidism and ischemic heart disease: a meta-analysis. *J Clin Endocrinol Metab*, 2008; **93**: 2969–71.
31. Rodondi N, Bauer DC, Cappola AR, Cornuz J, Robbins J, Fried LP, *et al.* Subclinical thyroid dysfunction, cardiac function, and the risk of heart failure. The Cardiovascular Health Study. *J Am Coll Cardiol*, 2008; **52**: 1152–9.

3.2

Aetiology of thyroid disorders

Contents

3.2.1 Genetic factors relating to the thyroid with emphasis on complex diseases

Francesca Menconi, Terry F. Davies, Yaron Tomer

Introduction: principles of genetics

Genes and chromosomes

The nucleus of each human cell encodes approximately 30 000 genes. A large fraction of the genes in each individual exist in a form that can vary between individuals. These variable genetic forms are termed polymorphisms, and they account for much of the normal variation in body traits, such as height and hair colour. The genetic information encoded in the DNA is stored on the chromosomes and each somatic cell contains 46 chromosomes (22 autosomes and two sex chromosomes), arranged in 23 pairs, one of each derived from each parent.

Since each individual inherits two copies of each chromosome (for autosomes), one from each parent, there are also two copies of each gene. The chromosomal location of a gene is termed the locus of the gene. When the gene in a certain locus exists in two or more forms, these variants of the gene are termed alleles. When an individual's two alleles at a locus are identical, that individual is said to be homozygous at that locus, and when the two alleles are different, the individual is a heterozygote.

Female somatic cells contain two X chromosomes, whereas male somatic cells contain only one X chromosome. Nevertheless, the activity of genes coded for by the X chromosome is no higher in females than in males. This is due to inactivation of most of the genes on one of the two X chromosomes. Thus, in female somatic cells only one X chromosome gene is expressed, and this process of suppression is called X-chromosome inactivation. X-chromosome inactivation occurs early in embryonic life and, thereafter, in each cell either the maternal or paternal chromosome is inactivated. This results in a tissue mosaic of paternally and maternally expressed X-chromosomal alleles, with an average of 1:1 distribution. As a result, a female who is heterozygous for an X-linked gene will show a mosaic-like distribution of cells expressing either one of the two alleles. Recently X-inactivation has been postulated to play a role in autoimmune diseases and may help explain the female preponderance of autoimmune diseases (see below).

Inheritance

When genetic information is transmitted from parent to offspring the process is called inheritance. Germ cells undergo meiosis, a process in which two gametes with 23 chromosomes are generated. During meiosis, paired chromosomes undergo recombination, a process in which paired chromosomes break at identical points along their length and switch genetic material on opposite sides of the breaking point. Recombination results in an exchange of matching segments of the chromosome between two homologous chromosomes (Fig. 3.2.1.1). Since recombination is a random event, the farther apart two genes are on the same chromosome, the greater the likelihood that a recombination will occur in the space between them. When two genes A and B are very far apart they are transmitted to the offspring independently, as if they were

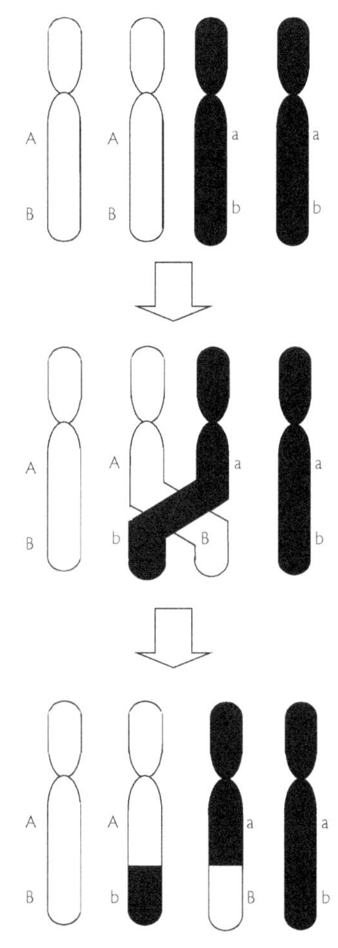

Fig. 3.2.1.1 Recombination. During meiosis, when homologous chromosomes pair, they often break at identical points along their length and switch the segments distal to the breaking point. This results in an exchange of identical segments of the chromosome between two homologous chromosomes. In the figure the crossing over results in two new recombinations of alleles of genes A and B.

located on different chromosomes. (i.e. the probability that a given parental allele of gene A will be transmitted to the offspring with the same parental allele of gene B is 50%, as would be expected to occur at random). On the other hand, if genes A and B are located close to each other, the probability that a given parental allele of gene A will be transmitted to the offspring with the same parent's allele of gene B is greater than 50%, and the genes are said to be linked (Fig. 3.2.1.1). In other words, if two gene loci are linked there is a greater than 50% probability that offspring will inherit the same combination of alleles that are present on the parental chromosome. This phenomenon is the basis for linkage analysis (see below).

Mutations and genetic diseases

A mutation is an alteration in DNA that once formed is inherited from one generation to another. Mutations in genes can change the structures and/or function of encoded proteins such as enzymes, receptors, structural proteins, or regulatory proteins. When several mutations in two or more genes produce a similar phenotype, genetic heterogeneity is said to exist. For example, in maturity onset diabetes of the young, similar phenotypes can be produced by mutations in the glucokinase gene or the hepatic nuclear factor 1α gene. In some diseases an individual may inherit the mutation but will not develop the disease phenotype. Such diseases are said to have reduced penetrance. The penetrance of the disease is defined as the probability that an individual inheriting the mutation will actually develop the disease phenotype. An example of a disease with reduced penetrance is multiple endocrine neoplasia type 2 (MEN 2) where not every individual inheriting the mutation in the RET proto-oncogene will develop the full phenotype of the disease.

Categories of genetic diseases

Genetic diseases can be divided into three broad categories: chromosomal disorders, mendelian disorders, and complex diseases. In chromosomal disorders the number of chromosomes in an individual (karyotype), or their structure, is altered producing excessive or deficient genetic material. Normally every individual has 22 pairs of autosomes and one pair of sex chromosome (XX in females and XY in males). In chromosomal disorders, the number of chromosomes may be altered (e.g. in Down's syndrome there are three copies of chromosome 21) or large segments of chromosomes may be deleted or exchanged with other chromosomes. Recently, it was found that changes in shorter segments of a chromosome can cause chromosomal, mendelian, and complex disorders. The most important of these changes are termed copy number variants, and they consist of deletions or duplications of DNA segments with a size of 1000 bases to several million bases. Other changes are also possible. Mendelian disorders are caused by a mutation in a single gene. They display specific patterns of inheritance that can be classified as dominant (inheritance of one mutant gene, from either parent, will cause disease), recessive (inheritance of both mutant genes, one from each parent will cause disease), or X-linked (see below). Complex diseases are disorders caused by interactions between multiple genes and, probably, epigenetic and environmental factors.

Inheritance of mendelian disorders

Dominant mendelian disorders

These disorders manifest in heterozygotes, i.e. when one mutant allele is present and the second allele of the same gene is normal. The mutant gene in this case is on one of the 22 autosomes. Examples of dominant mendelian disorders include thyroid hormone resistance syndrome and MEN 2.

Recessive mendelian disorders

These disorders are clinically apparent only in homozygotes, i.e. when both alleles at a particular genetic locus are mutant. The mutation in these disorders is on one of the 22 autosomes. Examples of recessive mendelian disorders include familial nonautoimmune hypothyroidism and Pendred's syndrome.

X-linked mendelian disorders

These disorders occur when the mutant gene is on the X chromosome. Most X-linked mendelian disorders are recessive. Therefore, females can be affected only if they inherit two mutant genes on both of their X chromosomes, while males are affected if they inherit only one mutant gene on their X chromosome. An example of an X-linked mendelian disorder is familial thyroxine-binding globulin deficiency.

Inheritance of complex diseases

The inheritance of complex diseases, such as Graves' disease and Hashimoto's thyroiditis, does not follow a simple mendelian pattern. These diseases are likely to be caused by several genes with additive

Table 3.2.1.1 Chromosomal disorders associated with autoimmune thyroid diseases

Disease	Chromosomal abnormality
Down's syndrome	Trisomy 21
Turner's syndrome	Female with one X chromosome (XO female)
Klinefelter's syndrome	Male with two X chromosomes (XXY male)

effects. Moreover, the penetrance of complex diseases is reduced, i.e. not all the individuals inheriting the mutation will actually develop the clinical phenotype. This results in nonmendelian transmission of the disease in pedigrees and makes mapping the susceptibility genes for complex diseases more challenging than mapping mendelian disorder genes.

A brief note on chromosomal and mendelian disorders of the thyroid

Chromosomal disorders associated with the thyroid

Several chromosomal disorders are known to be associated with an increased incidence of thyroid disease (Table 3.2.1.1). The association between Down's syndrome and autoimmune thyroid diseases (AITD) was especially intriguing because of the possibility that a gene conferring susceptibility to AITD was located on chromosome 21. However, this has been investigated extensively and to date there is no evidence of an AITD susceptibility gene on chromosome 21 (see below). Interestingly, on chromosome 21 is the autoimmune regulator (*AIRE*) gene and, when it is mutated, it causes autoimmune polyglandular syndrome type 1. However, the relevance of this to the increased incidence of AITD in Down's syndrome has not been studied.

Mendelian disorders involving the thyroid

Many mendelian disorders of thyroid hormonogenesis and regulation have been described (reviewed by Medeiros-Neto (1), Park and Chatterjee (2), and Refetoff and Dumitrescu (3); see also 4, 5). Advances in molecular biology since 1990 have helped unravel many of the mutations causing these disorders. Table 3.2.1.2 summarizes the main mendelian disorders affecting the thyroid, their pathophysiology, clinical characteristics, and their mode of inheritance. The major disorders are described elsewhere in this book.

Evidence for a genetic susceptibility to the AITD

The AITD are examples of complex genetic diseases affecting the thyroid. Classically, the AITD encompass two related disorders, Graves' disease and Hashimoto's thyroiditis, which are characterized by autoimmune responses to thyroid antigens. Additional variants of AITD include postpartum thyroiditis (reviewed by Roti and Uberti (6)), drug-induced thyroiditis, such as interferon-induced thyroiditis (7), thyroiditis associated with polyglandular autoimmune syndromes (reviewed by Obermayer-Straub and Manns (8)), and the presence of thyroid antibodies with no apparent clinical disease. The AITD are among the commonest human autoimmune disorders affecting up to 5% of the general population (9, 10). The AITD, including Graves' and Hashimoto's diseases, are categorized as complex diseases because they are believed to be caused by an interaction between several genes and environmental factors, and in recent years sound epidemiological evidence for a genetic susceptibility to AITD has been established. Box 3.2.1.1 summarizes the main epidemiological data pointing to a genetic susceptibility to AITD.

Geographical and longitudinal trends in the incidence of the AITD

The annual incidence of Graves' disease in populations from different geographical locations, excluding extremes of iodine intake, is similar and ranges from 0.22 to 0.27/1000 (reviewed by Tomer and Davies (11)). A similar pattern was observed for Hashimoto's thyroiditis. In the Whickham survey, the prevalence of spontaneous hypothyroidism was 15/1000 in women compared with less than 1/1000 in men (10). The mean annual incidence of spontaneous hypothyroidism in women was 3.5/1000 and in men was 0.6/1000 (12). Similar prevalence and incidence data of spontaneous hypothyroidism have also been reported in several geographical regions (reviewed by Tomer and Davies (11)). The comparable prevalence and incidence of the AITD in geographically different populations has suggested an important genetic contribution to the development of the AITD, because these populations are exposed to different environmental factors.

A longitudinal study from the Mayo clinic (1935–1967) showed no significant change in the incidence of Graves' disease over the 33 years of the study (13). The stable incidence of Graves' disease over time points to strong genetic effects because the genetic makeup of a population does not appear to change over several decades but environmental factors most probably do. The Mayo clinic observations were supported by a more recent study from Sweden (14). However, the Swedish study found an increased incidence of Graves' disease in a subset of the population, demonstrating that environmental effects do play a role in the aetiology of Graves' disease. In the Mayo survey (1935–1967) there was a significant increase in the incidence of Hashimoto's thyroiditis over the 33 years of the survey (13). This could reflect a stronger environmental influence on the development of Hashimoto's thyroiditis or change in the diagnostic criteria over time (15).

Familial clustering of the AITD

The familial occurrence of the AITD has been recognized by investigators for many years. By 1960 it had been recognized that a familial predisposition could be found in approximately 50% of patients with Graves' disease. Later studies have shown a high frequency of thyroid abnormalities in relatives of patients with AITD (reviewed by Tomer and Davies (11)), most commonly the presence of thyroid autoantibodies which were reported in up to 50% of the siblings of patients with Graves' disease (reviewed by Tomer and Davies (11)). A recent survey by our group revealed that 36% of Graves' disease patients with ophthalmopathy had a family history of AITD, while 32% had a first-degree relative with AITD (11). Moreover, a recent large study from Holland in which 790 healthy female relatives of AITD patients were followed for up to 5 years, showed that 7.5% of them developed overt hypothyroidism or hyperthyroidism (16).

Table 3.2.1.2 Mendelian disorders of the thyroid (reviewed by Medeiros-Neto (1), Park and Chatterjee (2), and Refetoff and Dumitrescu (3))

Gene	Locus/ chromosome	Disease	MOI	Gene mutation and pathogenesis	Clinical signs
TRH	3	Isolated TRH deficiency	AR	TRH deficiency leads to low TSH that increases with TRH administration	Central hypothyroidism
TSHB	1p13	Isolated TSH deficiency	AR	Mutations in the *TSHB* gene that lead to a mutated TSHβ protein that cannot associate with the α-subunit to produce a functional TSH heterodimer	Central hypothyroidism
PIT-1 (POU1F1)	3p11	Combined pituitary GH, PRL, TSH deficiency	AD/AR	Mutations in the transcription activating factor Pit-1 that regulates expression of GH, PRL, TSH and the development of somatotrophs, lactotrophs, and thyrotrophs	Central hypothyroidism and GH and PRL deficiencies
TSHR	14q31	Familial hypothyroidism/TSH resistance	AR	Inactivating mutations in the extracellular or transmembrane domains of the TSHR making it unresponsive to TSH	Congenital hypothyroidism, hypoplastic thyroid, or euthyroidism with high TSH
		Familial nonautoimmune hyperthyroidism	AD	Activating mutations in the transmembrane domain of the TSHR leading to constitutive activation of the TSHR	Hyperthyroidism, goitre, no signs of autoimmunity
		Familial gestational hyperthyroidism	AD	Mutation in the extracellular domain of the TSHR leading to hypersensitivity of the TSHR to chorionic gonadotropin	Gestational hyperthyroidism and hyperemesis gravidarum
TTF1	9q34	Congenital hypothyroidism	AD	Mutations (missense, nonsense) cause an alteration of the DNA-binding domain resulting in loss of functional activity and reduction in the production of TTF1 levels in heterozygotes (haploinsufficiency). The mechanism responsible for elevated TSH with normal thyroid gland, in several cases, is still unclear	Elevated TSH, normal or low T_4, neurological abnormalities, respiratory distress
TTF2	1q22	Congenital hypothyroidism	AR	Missense mutations of TTF2 lead to a protein with impaired DNA binding and total (homozygotes) or partial (heterozygotes) loss of transcriptional function	Congenital hypothyroidism with thyroid agenesis, cleft palate, spiky hair
PAX8	2q12-q14	Congenital hypothyroidism	AD	Mutations cause a markedly reduced DNA binding capacity with loss of transcriptional activation function	Congenital hypothyroidism, hypoplastic and sometimes ectopic thyroid, renal abnormalities
NIS (SLC5AS)	19p12	Congenital hypothyroidism	AR	Inactivating mutations of the Na/I symporter leading to defective or absent iodine uptake by thyroid cells	Congenital hypothyroidism, goitre, defective iodine uptake in the thyroid
TPO	2p25	Congenital hypothyroidism	AR	Inactivating mutations leading to inactive TPO, or to disturbed integration of TPO in the membrane thus causing defective or absent organification of iodide	Congenital hypothyroidism, goitre, abnormal perchlorate discharge test, sometimes mental impairment
Pendrin (*SLC26A4*)	7q22	Pendred's syndrome	AR	Inactivating mutations in the pendrin gene, which is a sulfate transporter, cause disruption of iodide transport from thyroid follicular cells to the follicular lumen	Goitre, congenital sensorineural deafness

TG	8q24	Congenital Tg deficiency	AR	Quantitative abnormalities in Tg, mutations in the *TG* gene, defects in glycosylation or transport of Tg cause impaired coupling of iodotyrosines	Goitre, hypothyroidism or euthyroidism, low or absent serum Tg, no colloid in the thyroid gland
DUOX2 (*THOX2*)	15q15.3	Congenital hypothyroidism	AD	Mutations (nonsense, missense) in the *DUOX2* gene result in insufficient or absent production of hydrogen peroxide, needed for TPO action	Permanent/transient congenital hypothyroidism, complete/partial iodide organification defect
DUOXA2	15q15.1	Congenital hypothyroidism	AR	Nonsense mutation of *DUOXA2* gene results in complete loss of function of the protein. Since DUOXA2 is essential for DUOX2 activity, it leads to a secondary deficit of DUOX2 (see above)	Congenital hypothyroidism, goitre, abnormal perchlorate discharge test
IYD (*DEHAL1*)	6q25	Goitrous hypothyroidism	AR	Missense mutations or deletion in *DEHAL1* gene lead to a protein with reduced capacity to deiodinate monoiodotyrosine and diiodotyrosine	Hypothyroidism in infancy or childhood, goitre, elevated serum diiodotyrosine. Mental and psychomotor impairment develop if hypothyroidism is not treated
SECISBP2	9q22.2	Reduced deiodinase activity	AR	Mutations in *SECISBP2* gene affect the synthesis of selenoproteins and lead to a reduction in deiodinase 2 activity	Short stature and delayed bone age. High T_4, low T_3, high reverse T_3, slightly elevated TSH
SERPINA7	Xq23	Congenital TBG deficiency	X-linked	Inactivating (deletions, missense, nonsense) mutations in the *SERPINA7* gene leading to partial or complete deficiency of TBG	Decreased total T_4, normal free T_4, euthyroidism
		Inherited TBG excess	?	Excess TBG of unknown cause results in elevated levels of TBG and total T_4	Increased total T_4, normal free T_4, euthyroidism
TTR	18	Familial euthyroid hyperthyroxinaemia due to TTR abnormalities	AD	Point mutations in the *TTR* gene cause increased affinity for T_4 and T_3	High total T_4, normal free T_4, euthyroidism, familial amyloidotic polyneuropathy
ALB	4q11	Familial dysalbuminaemic hyperthyroxinaemia	AD	Point mutations in the *ALB* gene lead to increased affinity for T_4 and T_3	High total T_4, normal free T_4, euthyroidism
MCT8 (*SLC16A2*)	Xq13.2	Allan–Herndon–Dudley syndrome	X-linked	Mutations (truncating, in-frame deletion, missense) in the *MCT8* gene alter the intracellular availability of thyroid hormones	Affected males present abnormal thyroid function tests (increased T_3 and decreased T_4 and reverse T_3) and severe psychomotor and developmental delay. Female carriers have only mild thyroid functions test abnormalities
THRB	3	Resistance to thyroid hormone	AD	Mutations in the *THRB* gene lead to a thyroid hormone receptor with reduced affinity for T_3 or abnormal interaction with a cofactor necessary for T_3 action	Goitre, tachycardia, hyperactivity, developmental delay. Elevated serum T_3 and T_4 with nonsuppressed TSH. Serum Tg is often elevated

AD, autosomal dominant; ALB, albumin; AR, autosomal recessive; DEHAL1, iodotyrosine deiodinase; DUOX2, dual oxidase 2; DUOXA2, dual oxidase maturation factor 2; GH, growth hormone; IYD, iodotyrosine deiodinase; MCT8, monocarboxylate transporter 8; MOI, mode of inheritance; Na/I symporter, sodium iodide symporter; PAX8, paired box 8; PRL, prolactin; SECISBP2, selenocysteine insertion sequence-binding protein 2; TBG, thyroxine-binding globulin; Tg, thyroglobulin; THOX2, thyroid oxidase 2; TPO, thyroid peroxidase; THRB, thyroid hormone receptor β; TRH, thyrotropin-releasing hormone; TSH, thyroid-stimulating hormone (thyrotropin); TSHR, thyroid-stimulating hormone receptor; TTF1, thyroid transcription factor 1; TTF2, thyroid transcription factor 2; TTR, transthyretin.

Box 3.2.1.1 Epidemiological evidence for a genetic susceptibility to Graves' disease (GD) and Hashimoto's thyroiditis (HT) (see text)

- Secular trends in the incidence of AITD
  - The incidence of GD/HT is similar in different ethnic populations
  - The incidence of GD has not changed over time in the past several decades
- Variations in the incidence of AITD with age
  - The incidence of GD/HT peaks in the fifth decade of life
  - After peaking, the incidence of GD/HT declines to zero (suggesting that all genetically susceptible individuals have developed the disease)
- Familial clustering of AITD
  - AITD develop in 20–30% of siblings of patients with AITD.
  - The sibling risk ratio (λ^s) for AITD is 16.9.
  - Thyroid antibodies are found in up to 50% of siblings of patients with AITD.
- Twin studies
  - Concordance rate in MZ twins for GD is 30–35% and in DZ twins it is 3–5%.
  - Concordance rate in MZ twins for HT is 55% and in DZ twins it is 0%.

AITD, autoimmune thyroid disease; DZ, dizygotic; MZ monozygotic.

Familial clustering of a disease can be due to nongenetic factors, such as the shared environmental exposures (e.g. infections, diet). Therefore, methods have been developed to determine whether familial clustering of a disease is the result of genetic susceptibility or nongenetic factors. One method is to calculate the sibling risk ratio (λ_s) which expresses the increased risk of developing the disease in an individual who has a sibling with the disease compared to the risk in the general population, and is a quantitative measure of the genetic contribution to the disease. A λ_s of more than 5 usually indicates a significant genetic contribution to the pathogenesis of a disease (reviewed by Tomer and Davies (11)). We have calculated the λ_s in AITD in a cohort of 155 AITD patients. The λ_s was 16.9 for AITD, 11.6 for Graves' disease, and 28.0 for Hashimoto's thyroiditis. These high λ_s values indicate a strong genetic influence on the development of AITD (11).

Twin studies

Twin studies can provide information concerning the inheritance of a disease and may yield certain quantitative evaluations on the role of heredity in relation to exogenous factors. Twin analysis is based upon comparison of the concordance (simultaneous occurrence) of a disease among monozygotic (MZ) twins versus dizygotic (DZ) twins. MZ twins have similar genetic makeup, whereas DZ twins share an average of 50% of their genes (like siblings). Therefore, if concordance is higher in the MZ twins when compared to the DZ twins it suggests that the disease has an inherited component. Any discordance among the MZ twin pairs is usually interpreted to mean that the gene or genes concerned show reduced penetrance, i.e. certain epigenetic or environmental factors must be present before the disease becomes manifest. The concordance rate in MZ twins is taken as an estimate of the penetrance of the disease but only up to the ages examined. For example, if the concordance rate among the MZ twins is 50%, this is taken to mean that the penetrance of the disease genes is approximately 50%. It must be emphasized that MZ twins are not identical in their immune repertoire due to somatic recombinations which T and B cells undergo throughout life, as well as individual immune experiences which influence the immune repertoire. Therefore, part of the observed discordance between MZ twins may also be due to the discordance in their immune repertoire.

The concordance rate for Graves' disease in MZ twins was found to be approximately 30–35% while the concordance rate in DZ twins was reported to be about 3–5% (reviewed by Tomer and Davies (11)). These data indicated that there is a substantial inherited susceptibility to Graves' disease, presumably related to both immune and nonimmune genes. For Hashimoto's thyroiditis the concordance rates were 55% and 0% for MZ and DZ twins, respectively (reviewed by Tomer and Davies (11)), again pointing to a strong genetic component in the aetiology of the disease. Finally, for thyroid antibodies, MZ twins had 80% concordance and DZ twins had 40% concordance (reviewed by Tomer and Davies (11)). Thus, the twin data support a substantial inherited susceptibility to AITD. Indeed, it has been estimated that 80% of the liability to the develop Graves' disease was due to genetic factors.

Thyroid autoantibodies

Autoantibodies to thyroglobulin and thyroid peroxidase (the microsomal antigen) have been widely used to show the population at most risk for the development of AITD. An increased prevalence of thyroid autoantibodies has been reported in relatives of patients with AITD. Antithyroid autoantibodies (antithyroglobulin and antithyroid peroxidase) have been found in up to 50% of the siblings of patients with AITD in contrast to a prevalence of 7–20% in the general population (reviewed by Tomer and Davies (11)). These findings are true in different populations such as the Japanese and British populations (reviewed by Tomer and Davies (11) and Huber *et al.* 17)). In one study, it was found that thyroid antibodies were almost always present in one of the parents of an individual affected with AITD (18). These data suggested an inherited influence on the production of antithyroid antibodies compatible with dominant inheritance. Indeed, segregation analyses in a panel of families with thyroid antibodies also suggested a mendelian dominant pattern of inheritance for the tendency to develop antithyroid antibodies. In keeping with these observations it was reported that recognition of particular thyroid peroxidase epitopes within the autoantibody immunodominant region may be transmitted within families (19).

Graves' ophthalmopathy

The milder forms of Graves' ophthalmopathy affect about 90% of patients with Graves' disease. However, the severe form of ophthalmopathy occurs in less than 10% of Graves' disease patients. Severe Graves' ophthalmopathy manifests by proptosis, conjunctival injection, eye muscle weakness to paralysis, and sometimes optic nerve damage. Graves' ophthalmopathy is considered pathognomonic of Graves' disease even when the individual is not thyrotoxic. It was speculated that the genetic influence on the development of Graves ophthalmopathy could be more pronounced because Graves' ophthalmopathy represents the most severe form of the disease. We therefore performed a segregation analysis in patients selected for severe Graves' ophthalmopathy. A segregation analysis is performed by studying the first-degree relatives of individuals with a certain disease (e.g. Graves' disease). If the disease is hereditary, the first-degree relatives are expected to be affected by the disease more often than individuals randomly selected from the general population. Our segregation analysis has shown that Graves' ophthalmopathy did not have a major genetic component (20). However, some genetic contribution to the susceptibility to develop Graves' ophthalmopathy does exist, as evidenced by the recent identification of interleukin (IL) 23 receptor gene as a possible susceptibility gene for Graves' ophthalmopathy (21). How such a nonspecific gene association could enhance susceptibility to Graves' ophthalmopathy remains to be explored and may simply be a marker of more severe disease.

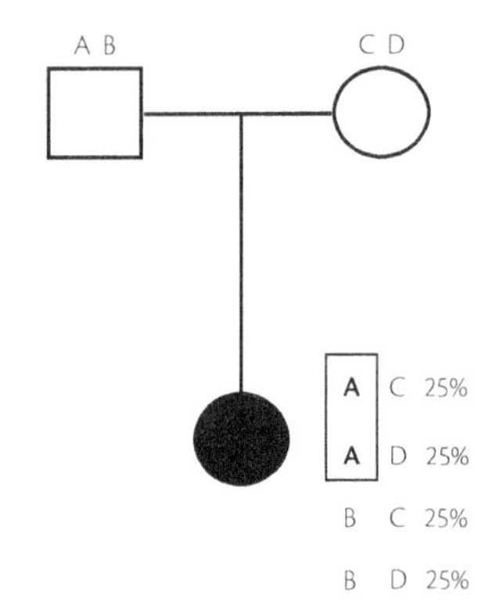

Fig. 3.2.1.2 Transmission disequilibrium test (TDT). This pedigree demonstrates the principles of the TDT. At the tested locus each parent is heterozygous and there are no shared alleles (A, B, C, and D). Allele A, e.g., is expected to be transmitted to affected individuals from their parents 50% of the time by chance alone. If, in a large number of pedigrees, allele A is transmitted to affected offspring more than 50% of the time (transmission distortion), then allele A is associated with the mutation in the disease gene.

Tools used to map genes of complex disease

Based on the abundant epidemiological evidence for a strong genetic effect on the development of AITD, searches for the susceptibility genes have been initiated. The basic strategies used for mapping complex disease genes include association and linkage studies of candidate genes, and whole genome screening (reviewed by Huber *et al.* (17)). These tools have proved successful in the mapping of many novel complex disease genes such as type 1 diabetes (17).

Association

Association analyses are very sensitive tests which can locate even minor susceptibility genes. Population-based association tests compare marker allele frequencies in unrelated patients and in unrelated, carefully matched, controls. Identification of a significant difference between patients and controls suggests that a genetic locus at, or near, the marker locus influences disease predisposition due to linkage disequilibrium. Linkage disequilibrium exists when chromosomes with the mutant allele at the disease locus carry certain marker alleles more often than expected by random chance. Association analysis is very sensitive and may detect genes contributing less than 5% of the total genetic contribution to a disease. Classically association studies were used for studying candidate genes, and for fine mapping linked loci. Recently, however, association studies have been utilized to screen the entire human genome (see below).

One of the weaknesses of the population-based methods is that they can produce spurious associations if the patients and controls are not accurately matched (population stratification). Therefore, family-based association tests have been developed which use an internal control group from within each family, thus avoiding the necessity to match patients and controls for ethnicity. The most widely used family-based association test is the transmission disequilibrium test (TDT). The TDT is based on the comparison of the parental marker alleles which are transmitted and those which are not transmitted to affected children (Fig. 3.2.1.2). Assuming two heterozygote parents for a certain tested marker, the four parental alleles in each family are categorized into two groups: those transmitted to a child with the disease (T alleles) and those not transmitted to any affected child (N alleles). The same allele may belong to the T group or the N group in different families. The frequency of the T alleles versus the N alleles is then compared by a Xx^2 test. An association between a certain allele and the disease exists if there is an excess occurrence of this allele in the T group compared to the N group.

Linkage

Genetic linkage techniques are powerful tools for analysing complex disease-related genes because they detect only genes that have a major effect (>5%) on the aetiology of a disease. The consequence is that linkage studies are less sensitive than association studies since they do not detect minor contributing genes. The principle of linkage analysis is based on the fact that if two genes are close together on a chromosome they will segregate together because the likelihood that a recombination will occur between them is low. Therefore, if a tested marker is close to a disease susceptibility gene, its alleles will cosegregate with the disease in families (Fig. 3.2.1.3). The logarithm of odds (LOD) score is the measure of the likelihood of linkage between a disease and a genetic marker. The LOD score is the base-10 logarithm of the odds ratio in favour of linkage.

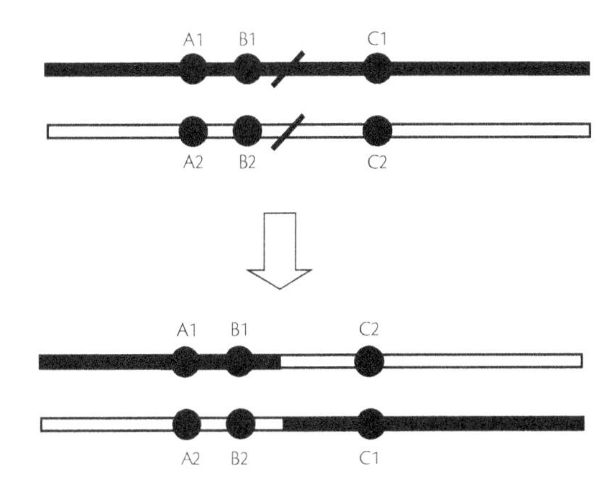

Fig. 3.2.1.3 Principle of linkage. The principle of linkage analysis is based on the fact that if two genes are close together on a chromosome they will segregate together. In the example shown, genes A and B will cosegregate more often with each other than with gene C which is more distant from them.

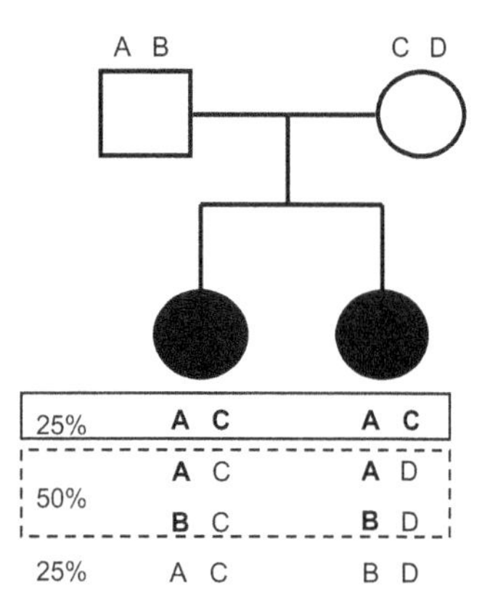

Fig. 3.2.1.4 Sib-pair analysis. This pedigree demonstrates the principles of sib-pair analysis. At the tested locus each parent is heterozygous and there are no shared alleles (A, B, C, and D). The two affected siblings are expected to share one allele 50% of the time and two alleles 25% of the time. If, in a large number of pedigrees, affected sib-pairs share at a certain locus one allele more than 50% of the time and/or two alleles more than 25% of the time, then the locus is assumed to be linked with the disease. The shared alleles are shown in bold.

An LOD score of greater than 3 (i.e. odds ratio greater than 1000) is considered strong evidence for linkage and an LOD score greater than 2 is suggestive of linkage. Linkage at a certain locus is established when at least two or more independent datasets give strong evidence for linkage at the same locus. Conversely, a LOD score lower than -2 is used to exclude linkage. The classic linkage tests are model based, i.e. a mode of inheritance and penetrance have to be assumed when calculating the likelihood of linkage. However, in complex diseases the mode of inheritance is often unknown and, therefore, model-independent methods have been advocated. One such method, which has become popular, is sib-pair analysis (Fig. 3.2.1.4). Here siblings, which are both affected by the disease being studied, are tested for sharing of alleles at a marker locus. By random chance alone the siblings would be expected to share one allele of the marker 50% of the time. If affected sib-pairs share a significantly higher than expected proportion of alleles at the marker locus, this suggests that the marker locus is in linkage disequilibrium with the disease gene. The observed to expected allele sharing can be converted to an LOD score equivalent.

Candidate gene analysis

Candidate genes are genes of known sequence and location that by virtue of their known functions may be involved in disease pathogenesis. For example, one can hypothesize that the thyroid-stimulating hormone receptor (*TSHR*) may be a candidate gene for Graves' disease because the hallmark of the disease is the presence of TSHR antibodies. If a candidate locus is indeed the cause of a disease, then markers in that locus should segregate with the disease within families giving high LOD scores. Since the basic abnormality in AITD is an immune response against thyroid antigens, possible candidate genes for AITD include genes that control immune responses (e.g. the major histocompatibility complex (MHC) genes and costimulatory molecule genes) and genes encoding the target autoantigens in AITD (thyroglobulin, thyroid peroxidase, iodide transporter, TSHR). Many of these genes have now been studied for their possible role in the genetic susceptibility to the AITD (see below).

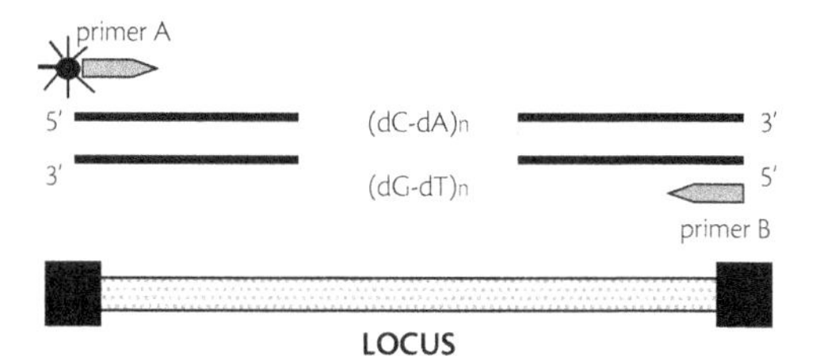

Fig. 3.2.1.5 Method for polymerase chain reaction (PCR) amplification of microsatellites. The locus is amplified by primers specific to the flanking regions of the dinucleotide repeat. One of the primers is labelled and, therefore, the PCR product will be labelled. The product size depends on the number of repeats each individual has for that particular microsatellite, and the size can be determined by separating the PCR products on a gel.

Whole genome screening

Another approach is to screen the whole human genome without any assumptions on disease pathogenesis. This method is called whole genome screening. Whole genome scans can be performed using linkage as well as association methods.

Linkage-based genome scans

The two requirements for performing a linkage-based whole genome screen in a complex disease are: (1) the availability of a sizeable and well-validated dataset of multiplex families (large families with more than one individual affected) and (2) the availability of a map of highly polymorphic markers covering the whole genome.

Microsatellite markers

The first useful polymorphic markers for whole genome screening were discovered in 1989 and were called microsatellites. Microsatellites are regions in the genome that are composed of short sequence repeats, most commonly two-base CA repeats (Fig. 3.2.1.5). Microsatellite loci are highly polymorphic (i.e. have many alleles) because the number of repeats in each individual is variable. Moreover, they are extremely abundant and uniformly distributed throughout the genome at distances of less than 1 million base pairs. Therefore, microsatellites serve as excellent markers in whole genome linkage studies.

Single nucleotide polymorphisms

Single nucleotide polymorphisms (SNPs) are single base pair positions in genomic DNA at which different sequence alternatives (alleles) exist in normal individuals. In humans, most SNPs are diallelic. SNPs are very abundant and current data suggest that their frequency is about one SNP for approximately every 500 base pairs. Since SNPs have only two alleles they are less informative than microsatellites, and a larger number of SNPs is required to screen the human genome by linkage. However, since SNPs are much more abundant and closely spaced than microsatellites, they are ideal for fine mapping genes, in linked regions, using association studies and for association-based genome scans (see below). The importance of SNPs stems from the fact that many have the potential to change the amino acid sequence of a gene product, or other regulatory sequences (e.g. promoter), and to be directly involved in the susceptibility to complex diseases because they cause changes in gene function. Thus, if a SNP allele inside a gene is found to be significantly associated with a disease it may be the actual causative allele, increasing susceptibility to the disease.

Using microsatellites or SNPs, linkage-based whole genome screens have been now completed for several complex diseases including the AITD (see below).

Genome-wide association studies

Genome-wide association studies also have two requirements: (1) the availability of a sizeable dataset of affected individuals and a sizable ethnically matched control group and (2) the availability of closely spaced polymorphic markers covering the whole genome. For genome-wide screening by association analysis one would need to employ more than 300 000 closely spaced markers. The completion of the HapMap project has made whole genome scanning by association studies feasible. The HapMap project genotyped more than one million SNPs spanning the entire human genome in four ethnically distinct human populations and tested these SNPs for linkage disequilibrium. This project discovered that the human genome is highly organized into discrete linkage disequilibrium blocks that are flanked by recombination hot spots, or areas at which recombinations are much more likely to occur. This enabled the utilization of tag SNPs (each SNP representing an entire linkage disequilibrium block) to test the entire human genome for association with disease. Moreover, microarray-based genotyping technology enabled the typing of up to 1000 000 SNPs in a single experiment. Thus, today it is possible to scan the entire human genome by association analysis using densely spaced SNPs on a chip.

Table 3.2.1.3 Some of the important HLA association studies in Graves' disease performed in white populations (reviewed by Huber *et al.* (17))

Country	Ethnic group	Number of patients	HLA allele	Relative risk of each allele
Canada	White	175	B8, DR3	3.1, 5.7
Belgium	White	101	DRB1*0301 DQA1*0501	–
UK	White	127	B8, DR3	2.8, 2.1
France	White	94	B8, DR3	3.4, 4.2
Hungary	White	256	B8, DR3	3.5, 4.8
Ireland	White	86	B8, DR3	2.5, 2.6
Canada	White	133	DR3	4.6
Sweden	White	78	B8, DR3	4.4, 3.9
USA	White	65	DR3	3.4
UK	White	120	DQA1*0501	3.8
UK[a]	White	228	DRB1*0304, DQB1*0301, DQA1*0501	2.7, 1.9, 3.2
USA	White	94	DQA1*0501	3.7

[a] In this study the transmission disequilibrium test also showed an association to the extended haplotype DRB1*0304-DQB1*02-DQA1*0501.

Genetic studies in the AITD

Role of HLA genes in the genetic susceptibility to AITD

The MHC region, encoding the HLA glycoproteins, consists of a complex of genes located on chromosome 6p21 (Fig. 3.2.1.6). The MHC region also encodes various additional proteins, most of which are associated with immune responsiveness. Since the HLA region is highly polymorphic and contains many immune response genes it was the first candidate genetic region to be studied for association and linkage with AITD.

Association of HLA with Graves' disease

Graves' disease was initially found to be associated with HLA-B8 in white people. This finding was then confirmed in a wide number of studies, mostly examining populations of white origin (Table 3.2.1.3). In these early studies HLA-B8 was associated with relative risks for Graves' disease ranging from 1.5 to 3.5. Subsequently, it was found that Graves' disease was more strongly associated with HLA-DR3, which is in linkage disequilibrium with HLA-B8. The frequency of DR3 in Graves' disease patients was 40–55% and in the general population 20–30% giving a relative risk for people with HLA-DR3 of 2 to 3 (reviewed by Huber *et al.* (17)).

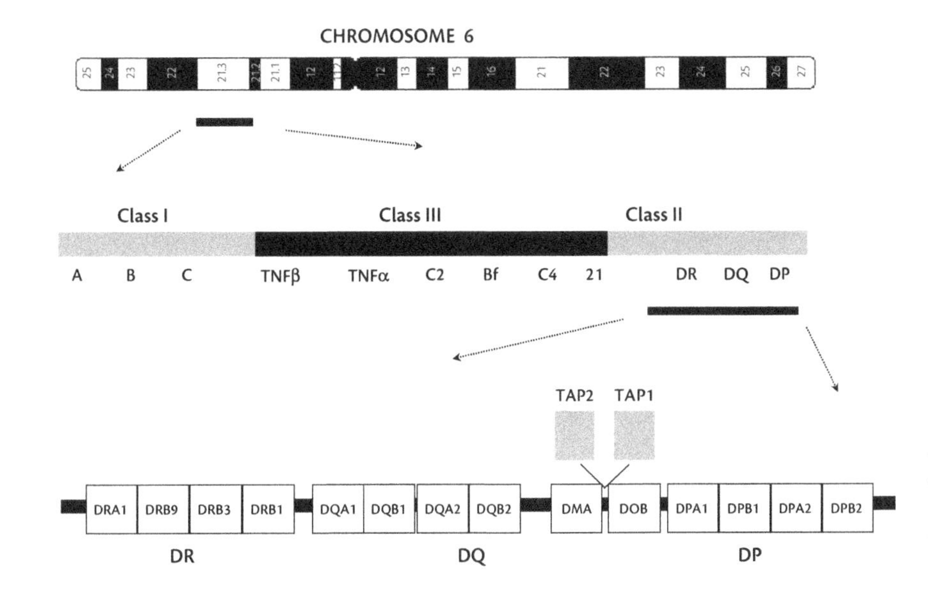

Fig. 3.2.1.6 The HLA region is located on chromosome 6p21. It is a complex genetic region which consists of several loci, all of which code for proteins which influence the different arms of the immune system. The major loci are shown.

Table 3.2.1.4 Some of the important HLA association studies in Graves' disease performed in nonwhite populations (reviewed by Jacobson *et al.* (22))

Country	Ethnic group	Number of patients	HLA allele(s)	Relative risk of each allele
Korea	Asian	128	B13, DR5, Drw8	3.8, 4.4, 2.3
India	Asian Indian	57	B8, Dqw2	4.1, 5.4
USA	Black	73	No association	–
South Africa	Black	103	DR1, DR3	3.5, 2.4
Japan	Japanese	30	DR5, Drw8	8.1, 3.1
Japan	Japanese	76	A2, DPB1*0501	2.9, 5.3
Hong Kong	Chinese	132	Bw46	4.8
Hong Kong	Chinese	67 (children)	DQB1*0303	4.2
Hong Kong	Chinese	97	B46, DR9, DQB1*0303	2.3, 2.2, 3.2

Table 3.2.1.5 Some of the important HLA association studies in Hashimoto's thyroiditis (reviewed by Jacobson *et al.* (22))

Country	Ethnic group	Number of patients	HLA allele	Relative risk of each allele
Canada + England	White	66	DR4 DR5 DQw7	2.9 3.8 4.7
Canada –Newfoundland	White	40	DRw3	3.5
Canada –Newfoundland	White	40	DR5	3.1
England	White	49	DQB1*0301 DQA1*0301/2	Not reported
England	White	36	DR5 DQ7	3.5
England	White	86	DR3	2.23
Japan	Japanese	99	DRw53	3.33

Even though the frequency of HLA-DR3 was increased in white people with Graves' disease, there were also HLA-DR3-negative associations with Graves' disease, and the HLA associations were found to be different in other ethnic groups (Table 3.2.1.4). In the Japanese population, Graves' disease was associated with HLA-B35, and in the Chinese population an increased frequency of HLA-Bw46 has been reported. In African-Americans no overall susceptibility could be associated with any DR allele, although subdivision of the patients revealed that DRw6 was associated with thyroid antibody formation (23). Among white populations, HLA-DQA1*0501 has also been associated with Graves' disease (Table 3.2.1.3), but it appears that the primary susceptibility allele in Graves' disease is indeed HLA-DR3 (HLA-DRB1*03) (reviewed by Tomer and Davies (11).

We have identified the exact amino acid sequence in the DRβ1 chain conferring susceptibility to Graves' disease by sequencing the HLA-DRB1 locus in a population of Graves' disease patients and controls. These studies identified arginine at position 74 of the HLA-DRβ1 chain (DRβ-Arg74) as the critical DR amino acid conferring susceptibility to Graves' disease (24). These data were replicated in an independent dataset (25). Further analysis showed that the presence of glutamine at position 74 was protective for Graves' disease. This suggests that position 74 of the DRβ1 chain is critical for Graves' disease development.

The role of HLA polymorphisms on the clinical expression of Graves' disease has also been explored. Some groups reported an association between the likelihood of relapse of Graves' disease and HLA-DR3 but others were unable to confirm this (reviewed by Huber *et al.* (17)). Studies of HLA associations in Graves' ophthalmopathy have also produced conflicting results with some workers reporting increased frequency of HLA-DR3 in patients with Graves' ophthalmopathy, and others reporting no difference in the distribution of HLA-DR alleles between Graves' disease patients with and without ophthalmopathy. Likewise, no difference in the DR3 frequency was found in Graves' disease patients with and without pretibial myxoedema (reviewed by Huber *et al.* (17)).

Association of HLA with Hashimoto's thyroiditis

Data on HLA haplotypes in Hashimoto's thyroiditis have been less definitive than in Graves' disease (Table 3.2.1.5). Earlier studies showed an association of goitrous Hashimoto's thyroiditis with HLA-DR5 (relative risk = 3.1) and of atrophic Hashimoto's thyroiditis with DR3 (relative risk = 5.1) in white populations. Later studies in white populations reported weak associations of Hashimoto's thyroiditis with HLA-DR3 and HLA-DR4 (reviewed by Huber *et al.* (17)). Associations of Hashimoto's thyroiditis with other HLA haplotypes have also been reported in different ethnic populations, e.g. HLA-DRw53 in Japanese and HLA-DR9 in Chinese (reviewed by Weetman (26)). Recently, we have also identified a pocket HLA-DR amino acid signature that conferred strong risk for Hashimoto's thyroiditis resulting in an odds ratio of 3.7 (27). This pocket amino acid signature resulted in a unique pocket structure that could have a strong influence on the binding of pathogenic peptides to HLA-DR pockets and their presentation to T cells.

Non-HLA genes in AITD

HLA genes account for only part of the genetic susceptibility to AITD. Therefore, non-HLA genes have been investigated. Five non-HLA genes have been found to confer risk for AITD. These include three immunoregulatory genes, *CTLA4*, *CD40*, and *PTPN22*, and two thyroid specific genes, *TG* and *TSHR*.

Cytotoxic T-lymphocyte-associated protein 4

CTLA4 is a costimulatory molecule that participates in the interaction between T cells and antigen-presenting cells. Antigen-presenting cells activate T cells by presenting to the T-cell receptor an antigenic peptide bound to an HLA class II protein on the cell surface. However, a second signal is also required for T-cell activation and the costimulatory signals are provided by a variety of proteins which are expressed on antigen-presenting cells (e.g. B7–1, B7–2, B7h, CD40) and interact with receptors (CD28, CTLA4, and CD40L) on the surface of CD4+ T lymphocytes during antigen presentation. Whereas, the binding of B7 to CD28 on T cells costimulates T-cell activation, the presence of CTLA4, which has a higher affinity for B7, down-regulates T-cell activation by competing for the binding of B7 to CD28. The suppressive effects of CTLA4 on T-cell activation have raised the possibility that polymorphisms altering CTLA4 expression and/or function could result in an exaggerated T-cell activation and lead to the development of autoimmunity. Indeed, CTLA4 has been consistently shown to be associated with many autoimmune conditions. CTLA4 is strongly associated with both Graves' disease and Hashimoto's thyroiditis, and the association between AITD and CTLA4 has been consistent across populations of different ethnic backgrounds (17).

Several CTLA4 variants are associated with AITD. Three CTLA4 variants have shown the most consistent associations with AITD, including an (AT)n microsatellite within the 3′UTR region of the *CTLA4* gene, a SNP at position 49 in the CTLA4 leader peptide (designated A/G49), resulting in an alanine/threonine substitution, and a SNP (designated CT60) located near the 3′UTR of the *CTLA4* gene (28). Interestingly the *CTLA4* gene also confers susceptibility to the production of thyroid antibodies without clinical disease, thus substantiating its role as a general autoimmunity gene.

CD40 molecule

CD40 is a member of the tumour necrosis factor receptor family of molecules and is expressed primarily on B cells and other antigen-presenting cells. CD40 plays a fundamental role in B-cell activation, inducing B-cell proliferation, immunoglobulin class switching, and antibody secretion (reviewed by Huber *et al.* (17)).

Recently, using a combination of linkage and association studies, we and others have identified *CD40* as a novel susceptibility gene for Graves' disease (reviewed by Huber *et al.* (17)). A C/T single nucleotide polymorphism (SNP) at the 5′UTR of *CD40* was associated with Graves' disease, with the CC genotype of this SNP conferring risk for disease. The association between the CC genotype and Graves' disease has been replicated in several studies. The association of the CC genotype was stronger in the subset of Graves' disease patients that had persistently high levels of thyroid antibodies after treatment.

Protein tyrosine phosphatase, non-receptor type 22 (*PTPN22*) gene

The lymphoid tyrosine phosphatase, encoded by the *PTPN22* gene, is a 110-kDa protein tyrosine phosphatase that, like CTLA4, is a powerful inhibitor of T-cell activation. A tryptophan/arginine substitution at codon 620 (R620W) of *PTPN22* was found to be associated with AITD, mostly with Graves' disease (29), as well as with other autoimmune diseases (reviewed by Huber *et al.* (17)).

Thyroglobulin

Thyroglobulin represents one of the major targets of the immune response in AITD. Recently, the *TG* gene was established as a major AITD susceptibility gene (reviewed by Huber *et al.* (17)). Four new *TG* SNPs were found to be significantly associated with AITD. Moreover, three of the associated *TG* SNPs were nonsynonymous, i.e. they caused amino acid changes in the thyroglobulin protein. The association between thyroglobulin and AITD has been replicated in other datasets, albeit the associated thyroglobulin polymorphism might be different in different populations (reviewed by Huber *et al.* (17)).

Thyrotropin receptor

The presence of stimulating TSHR autoantibodies is the hallmark of Graves' disease, and, therefore, the *TSHR* gene was always investigated and remains a strong candidate gene for Graves' disease (reviewed by Jacobson and Tomer (30)). Earlier studies examined three missense SNPs of the *TSHR* for association with Graves' disease, an aspartic acid to histidine substitution at position 36 (D36H), a proline to threonine substitution at position 52 (P52T), and a glutamic acid to aspartic acid substitution at position 727 (D727E). However, studies of these SNPs gave inconsistent results (reviewed by Huber *et al.* (17)). More recently it was found that noncoding SNPs of the *TSHR* were associated with Graves' disease. The most consistent association has been with an intron 1 SNP (31).

Whole genome screening in AITD

Several linkage-based whole genome screens were performed in AITD (reviewed by Huber *et al.* (17)). We performed a whole genome screening in Graves' disease and Hashimoto's thyroiditis in a dataset of 102 multiplex families (540 individuals). Our whole genome screening revealed seven new loci that showed evidence for linkage to AITD. Three loci, on chromosomes 6 (AITD1, distinct from the HLA region), 8 (thyroglobulin locus), and 10, showed evidence for linkage with both Graves' disease and Hashimoto's thyroiditis. One locus, on chromosome 12 (HT2), showed evidence for linkage to Hashimoto's thyroiditis. Three loci showed evidence for linkage with Graves' disease: GD1 on chromosome 14 (TSHR locus), GD2 on chromosome 20 (CD40 locus), and a locus on 7q. Another whole genome screen from Japan identified the same AITD locus on 8q, as well as a 5q locus. The same 5q locus was also identified in a genome scan performed in the Old Order Amish population in the USA (32). A recent large whole genome scan in 1119 European sib-pairs identified three novel loci on chromosomes 18p11, 2q36 (distinct from CTLA4), and 11p15 (33). These studies demonstrated that the genetic contribution to the development of AITD likely involves multiple genes with varying effects. In addition, these genome scans have shown that both distinct and shared genes contribute to the development of AITD. For example, the 8q locus (now known to be the *TG* gene) contributes both to Graves' disease and Hashimoto's thyroiditis, while the 14q locus (now known to be the *THSR* gene) is specific for Graves' disease.

Mechanisms of disease induction by susceptibility genes

Mapping susceptibility genes for complex diseases can improve our understanding of their pathogenesis. However, even when a complex disease gene is mapped, unravelling the mechanisms underlying its association with disease is not straightforward. In contrast to classic monogenic diseases where a genetic mutation usually inactivates a gene or causes unchecked activation of a gene, in complex diseases such as AITD the associated genetic variants may cause subtle changes in the function of one or more genes.

Therefore, even when a gene causing a complex disease is mapped, proving that a certain variant changes the function of the gene in a way that will promote the development of the disease can be challenging. Progress has been made in dissecting some of the mechanisms by which AITD genes predispose to disease. We will summarize here the known and postulated mechanisms by which the AITD genes identified so far, *HLA-DR*, *CTLA4*, *CD40*, *PTPN22*, *TG*, and *TSHR*, may confer risk for disease.

HLA-related susceptibility to AITD

The mechanisms by which HLA associations confer disease susceptibility in AITD are now beginning to be understood. For T cells to recognize and respond to an antigen requires the recognition of a complex between the antigenic peptide and an HLA class II molecule. It is thought that different HLA alleles have different affinities to autoantigens (e.g. thyroid antigens) which are recognized by T-cell receptors. Thus, certain alleles may permit the autoantigen to fit in the antigen-binding groove inside the HLA molecule and to be recognized by the T-cell receptor while others may not. This could determine if an autoimmune response to that antigen will develop.

Recent studies by our group have demonstrated that DRβ-Arg74 is the critical HLA-DR pocket amino acid associated with Graves' disease (reviewed by Huber *et al.* (17)). Position 74 of the DRβ chain is located in pocket 4 (P4) of the DR peptide-binding cleft. Structural modelling analysis demonstrated that the change at position 74, from the common neutral amino acids (Ala or Gln) to a positively charged hydrophilic amino acid (Arg), significantly modified the three-dimensional structure of the P4 peptide-binding pocket. This could alter the peptide-binding properties of the pocket favouring peptides which can induce Graves' disease. For Hashimoto's thyroiditis we have also identified a pocket HLA-DR amino acid signature that was strongly associated with disease (27). This pocket amino acid signature resulted in a unique pocket structure that could have a strong influence on the binding of pathogenic peptides to HLA-DR pockets and their presentation to T cells.

For thyroid autoantigens to be presented by HLA molecules to T cells, a mechanism of autoantigen presentation must exist within the target tissue. One potential mechanism not utilizing professional antigen-presenting cells may be through aberrant expression of HLA class II molecules on the target tissue cells. Indeed, thyroid epithelial cells from patients with AITD have been shown to express HLA class II antigen molecules which are normally expressed only on antigen-presenting cells such as macrophages and dendritic cells. This aberrant expression of HLA molecules on thyroid cells could initiate thyroid autoimmunity via direct thyroid autoantigen presentation (34).

CTLA4 participation in the development of AITD

In view of the function of CTLA4 as a negative regulator of T cells, one would expect a polymorphism that decreases CTLA4 function and/or cell surface expression to cause heightened T-cell activation and potentially lead to the development of an autoimmune condition. Several CTLA4 variants have been analysed in detail for their effect on CTLA4 function and/or expression (reviewed by Huber *et al.* (17)). The A/G49 SNP (rs57563726) causing a threonine to alanine substitution in the signal peptide, was reported to cause less efficient glycosylation and diminished surface expression of CTLA4 protein. However, this mechanism awaits confirmation. DeGroot and colleagues have shown an association between the G allele of the A/G49 SNP (associated with AITD) and reduced control of T-cell proliferation (35), results which were later replicated by us. This association could be due to a direct effect of the A/G49 SNP or due to the effects of another polymorphism in linkage disequilibrium with the A/G49 SNP. Studies by Davies and colleagues (36) in which they transiently transfected a T-cell line, devoid of endogenous CTLA4, with a CTLA4 construct harbouring either the G or the A allele of the A/G49 SNP showed no difference in CTLA4 expression and/or function. Therefore, it was concluded that the A/G49 SNP is, most likely, not the causative SNP, but rather is in linkage disequilibrium with the causative variant.

A recent comprehensive analysis of the *CTLA4* gene locus reported that the CT60 SNP of *CTLA4* (rs3087243) showed the strongest association with Graves' disease, suggesting that it might be the causative SNP (28). Further analysis in a small number of patients has shown that the GG (disease susceptible) genotype of CT60 was associated with reduced expression of the soluble form of CTLA4 (28). However, a recent large study could not replicate these data (37), and thus it is unclear whether CT60 is, indeed, the causative variant.

Another CTLA4 variant that was studied is the 3′UTR (AT)n microsatellite. The longer repeats of this microsatellite (associated with disease) are associated with reduced CTLA4 inhibitory function. However, as in the case of the A/G49 SNP, this could be due to linkage disequilibrium with another SNP which is the causative one. Interestingly, the 3′UTR region of CTLA4, harbouring the AT repeats, contains three AUUUA motifs which may affect mRNA stability (38). Indeed, it was shown that the 3′UTR microsatellite affected the half-life of the CTLA4 mRNA, with long repeats being correlated with shorter half-life compared to the short repeats (39). This could provide an attractive explanation for the association between the long alleles of the microsatellite and autoimmunity.

CD40 and Graves' disease

The CC genotype of the CD40 5′UTR SNP was shown to be associated with Graves' disease. By what mechanism can the CC genotype predispose to Graves' disease? The CD40 SNP resides in a region which can influence the initiation of translation and, therefore, the expression of CD40. Indeed, the C allele of the 5′UTR SNP was shown to increase the translation of CD40 mRNA transcripts, by 20–30% compared to the T allele (reviewed by Huber *et al.* (17)). At least two potential mechanisms can explain how the C allele of the CD40 5′UTR SNP increases the risk for Graves' disease: (1) the C allele may increase CD40 expression and function on B cells, thereby potentially lowering the threshold of activation of thyroid autoreactive B cell, and/or (2) the C allele may increase the expression of CD40 in the thyroid gland itself. CD40 signalling in thyrocytes can result in cytokine secretion (e.g. IL-6). Thus, Overexpression of CD40 on thyroid cells may, under certain conditions (e.g. infection), result in increased secretion of cytokines by thyroid cells causing local inflammation and activation of autoreactive T cells that were dormant or suppressed by peripheral regulatory mechanisms. This mechanism is known as a bystander mechanism of induction of autoimmunity and is seen in experimental thyroiditis.

PTPN22

The lymphoid tyrosine phosphatase (LYP) encoded by the *PTPN22* gene belongs to a family of protein tyrosine phosphatases that are expressed in both immature and mature B and T lymphocytes. LYP is a powerful inhibitor of the T-cell antigen receptor signalling pathway. LYP binds to the C-terminal of the protein kinase Csk restricting the response to antigens by disrupting protein tyrosine phosphorylation events that control cell activation and differentiation. This negative control mechanism prevents spontaneous T-cell activation (reviewed by Huber *et al.* (17)).

The exact mechanism by which the R620W variant of the *PTPN22* gene predisposes to autoimmunity is not known. The substitution of arginine with tryptophan at this position interferes with the interaction of LYP with Csk. *In vitro* experiments show that only LYP with arginine at position 620 forms a complex with Csk, whereas LYP with tryptophan at this position binds less efficiently (40). One study suggested that the tryptophan variant is a gain-of-function change that makes the protein an even stronger inhibitor of T cells (41). Thus, the disease-associated tryptophan variant would be expected to suppress T-cell activation and proliferation. How, can such a gain-of-function mutation in *PTPN22* promote the development of autoimmunity? One possible explanation for this enigma is that a lower T-cell receptor signalling could lead to a tendency for self-reactive T cells to escape thymic deletion and thus remain in the periphery.

Thyroglobulin

Thyroglobulin is a 660-kDa homodimeric protein that serves as a precursor and storehouse for thyroid hormones. Thyroglobulin is one of the main targets of the immune response in AITD, as well as in the mouse model of AITD, murine experimental autoimmune thyroiditis (EAT). EAT, like Hashimoto's thyroiditis, is characterized by a cellular infiltrate of the thyroid, antithyroglobulin T-cell responses, as well as high titres of antithyroglobulin autoantibodies. Thus, thyroglobulin is a critical thyroid-specific antigen in the aetiology of both AITD in humans and EAT in mice.

As mentioned above, the *TG* gene was established as a major AITD susceptibility gene. Three amino acid substitutions in *TG* were reported to be significantly associated with AITD, A734S, V1027M, and W1999R (reviewed by Huber *et al.* (17)).

Several mechanisms can be postulated to explain the association between thyroglobulin amino acid variants and AITD. One potential mechanism is by altering thyroglobulin peptide presentation by antigen-presenting cells to T cells. Since peptide antigens are presented within HLA class II molecules, this mechanism would imply that there exists an interaction between thyroglobulin variants and HLA-DR variants in predisposing to AITD. Indeed, we have shown that the W1999R variant had a strong statistical interaction with the Arg74 polymorphism of HLA-DR, resulting in a high odds ratio of 15 for Graves' disease (42). This statistical interaction may imply a biological interaction between thyroglobulin and HLA-DR. For example, the thyroglobulin peptide repertoire generated in individuals with the R allele of W1999R (associated with AITD) could be pathogenic, while DRβ-Arg74 could optimally present some of these pathogenic thyroglobulin peptides to T cells. Supporting this hypothesis is a recent study in which 'humanized' mice expressing HLA-DR3 and not mouse MHC II molecules, developed EAT when immunized with certain thyroglobulin peptides (43).

Thyroid-stimulating hormone receptor

As mentioned, all the TSHR SNPs which are consistently associated with Graves' disease are intronic (31). Therefore, the mechanism by which they predispose to Graves' disease is more challenging to dissect. It has been postulated that these intronic SNPs may influence the expression of the TSHR through regulatory elements. Alternatively, they may change the alternative splicing of the TSHR.

X chromosome and thyroid autoimmunity

There are a number of possible mechanisms whereby the X chromosome could influence the development of AITD. One mechanism is probabilistic. Females have two X chromosomes (one paternal and one maternal) while males have only one X chromosome (maternal). Therefore, females are twice as likely to inherit an X chromosome AITD susceptibility gene as males. Several immune regulatory genes are located on the X chromosome, and recently we have shown that one of them, the *FOXP3* gene, was associated with AITD in white populations (44). *FOXP3* is the master regulator gene of T-regulatory cell differentiation. It remains to be determined what functional effects the AITD-associated FOXP3 variants have. These data suggest one possible mechanism for the female preponderance of AITD.

Another possible mechanism involves X-inactivation. As described earlier, X-inactivation in females results in the production of two classes of cells that differ in the transcription of X-chromosome encoded genes, including genes coding for self-antigens. If these two cell classes extend to the thymic cells responsible for tolerizing T cells in embryonic life, some lymphocytes may not be tolerized to one of the two self-antigens encoded by the X chromosome. Such lymphocytes would be autoreactive to that antigen and could induce an autoimmune response. Supporting this hypothesis are recent data showing skewing of X-inactivation in females with AITD (reviewed by Huber *et al.* (17)).

Conclusions

Genetic susceptibility plays an important role in the development of AITD. Significant progress has been made in recent years in mapping the AITD susceptibility genes and understanding the

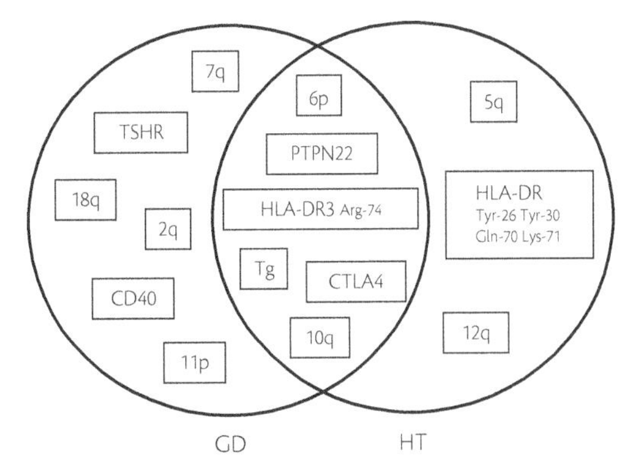

Fig. 3.2.1.7 The susceptibility genes for AITD identified so far include genes that are unique for Graves' disease or Hashimoto's thyroiditis and genes that are common to both diseases. In the case of *PTPN22*, strong association with Graves' disease has been shown, but the association with Hashimoto's thyroiditis is so far inconsistent.

mechanisms by which they confer risk for disease. Both candidate gene analysis and whole genome screening have been employed to identify AITD genes. Intriguingly, the AITD susceptibility genes identified so far participate in the immunological synapse and/or the signalling pathways activated by the immunological synapse. The immunological synapse is the interface between an antigen-presenting cell and a T cell formed during antigen presentation. This finding suggests that the genetic factors predisposing to AITD may lead to breakdown of tolerance by altering the immunological synapse.

Some of the AITD susceptibility genes identified so far are unique for Graves' disease or Hashimoto's thyroiditis, while others are common to both conditions (Fig. 3.2.1.7). Mechanistically, the AITD susceptibility genes can be divided into immune modulating genes (*HLA-DR*, *CD40*, *CTLA4*, and *PTPN22*), and thyroid-specific genes (*TG* and *TSHR*). Each of these genes appears to confer relatively small risks individually. However, interactions between these genes increase the risk significantly (reviewed by Huber *et al.* (17), as we have shown for *TG* and *HLA-DR* (42). In addition, some genes, while exerting small effects in all patients, have a much stronger effect in subsets of patients (45). It is clear that additional gene polymorphisms, deletions, insertions, or epigenetic changes must contribute to the genetic susceptibility to AITD, as well as to the different phenotypes of AITD. Identifying the AITD susceptibility genes and understanding the mechanisms by which they predispose to disease will hopefully lead to a better understanding of the molecular mechanisms causing thyroid autoimmunity.

References

1. Medeiros-Neto G. Clinical and molecular advances in inherited disorders of the thyroid system. *Thyroid Today*, 1996; **19**: 1–13.
2. Park SM, Chatterjee VK. Genetics of congenital hypothyroidism. *J Med Genet*, 2005; **42**: 379–89.
3. Refetoff S, Dumitrescu AM. Syndromes of reduced sensitivity to thyroid hormone: genetic defects in hormone receptors, cell transporters and deiodination. *Best Pract Res Clin Endocrinol Metab*, 2007; **21**: 277–305.
4. Zamproni I, Grasberger H, Cortinovis F, Vigone MC, Chiumello G, Mora S, *et al.* Biallelic inactivation of the dual oxidase maturation factor 2 (DUOXA2) gene as a novel cause of congenital hypothyroidism. *J Clin Endocrinol Metab*, 2008; **93**: 605–10.
5. Moreno JC, Klootwijk W, van Toor H, Pinto G, D'Alessandro M, Leger A, *et al.* Mutations in the iodotyrosine deiodinase gene and hypothyroidism. *N Engl J Med*, 2008; **358**: 1811–18.
6. Roti E, Uberti E. Post-partum thyroiditis: a clinical update. *Eur J Endocrinol*, 2002; **146**: 275–9.
7. Mandac JC, Chaudhry S, Sherman KE, Yaron Tomer. The clinical and physiological spectrum of interferon alpha induced thyroiditis: Towards a new classification. *Hepatology*, 2006; **43**: 661–72.
8. Obermayer-Straub P, Manns MP. Autoimmune polyglandular syndromes. *Baillieres Clin Gastroenterol*, 1998; **12**: 293–315.
9. Hollowell JG, Staehling NW, Flanders WD, Hannon WH, Gunter EW, Spencer CA, *et al.* Serum TSH, T(4), and thyroid antibodies in the United States population (1988 to 1994): National Health and Nutrition Examination Survey (NHANES III). *J Clin Endocrinol Metab*, 2002; **87**: 489–99.
10. Tunbridge WMG, Evered DC, Hall R, Appleton D, Brewis M, Clark F, *et al.* The spectrum of thyroid disease in a community: the Whickham survey. *Clin Endocrinol (Oxf)*, 1977; **7**: 481–93.
11. Tomer Y, Davies TF. Searching for the autoimmune thyroid disease susceptibility genes: from gene mapping to gene function. *Endocr Rev*, 2003; **24**: 694–717.
12. Vanderpump MPJ, Tunbridge WMG, French JM, Appleton D, Bates D, Clark F, *et al.* The incidence of thyroid disorders in the community: a twenty-year follow-up of the Whickham survey. *Clin Endocrinol (Oxf)*, 1995; **43**: 55–68.
13. Furszyfer J, Kurland LT, McConahey WM, Woolner LB, Elveback LR. Epidemiologic aspects of Hashimoto's thyroiditis and Graves' disease in Rochester, Minnesota (1935–1967), with special reference to temporal trends. *Metabolism*, 1972; **21**: 197–204.
14. Berglund J, Ericsson UB, Hallengren B. Increased incidence of thyrotoxicosis in Malmo during the years 1988–1990 as compared to the years 1970–1974. *J Intern Med*, 1996; **239**: 57–62.
15. Davies TF, Amino N. A new classification for human autoimmune thyroid disease. *Thyroid*, 1993; **3**: 331–3.
16. Strieder TG, Tijssen JG, Wenzel BE, Endert E, Wiersinga WM. Prediction of progression to overt hypothyroidism or hyperthyroidism in female relatives of patients with autoimmune thyroid disease using the Thyroid Events Amsterdam (THEA) score. *Arch Intern Med*, 2008; **168**: 1657–63.
17. Huber A, Menconi F, Corathers S, Jacobson EM, Tomer Y. Joint genetic susceptibility to type 1 diabetes and autoimmune thyroiditis: from epidemiology to mechanisms. *Endocr Rev*, 2008; **29**: 697–725.
18. Hall R, Stanbury JB. Familial studies of autoimmune thyroiditis. *Clin Exp Immunol*, 1967; **2**: 719–25.
19. Jaume JC, Guo J, Pauls DL, Zakarija M, McKenzie JM, Egeland JA, *et al.* Evidence for genetic transmission of thyroid peroxidase autoantibody epitopic "fingerprints". *J Clin Endocrinol Metab*, 1999; **84**: 1424–31.
20. Villanueva RB, Inzerillo AM, Tomer Y, Barbesino G, Meltzer M, Concepcion ES, *et al.* Limited genetic susceptibility to severe Graves' ophthalmopathy: no role for CTLA-4 and evidence for an environmental etiology. *Thyroid*, 2000; **10**: 791–8.
21. Huber AK, Jacobson EM, Jazdzewski K, Concepcion ES, Tomer Y. Interleukin (IL)-23 receptor is a major susceptibility gene for Graves' ophthalmopathy: the IL-23/T-helper 17 axis extends to thyroid autoimmunity. *J Clin Endocrinol Metab*, 2008; **93**: 1077–81.
22. Jacobson EM, Huber A, Tomer Y. The HLA gene complex in thyroid autoimmunity: from epidemiology to etiology. *J Autoimmun*, 2008; **30**: 58–62.
23. Sridama V, Hara Y, Fauchet R, DeGroot LJ. HLA immunogenetic heterogeneity in Black American patients with Graves' disease. *Arch Intern Med*, 1987; **147**: 229–31.
24. Ban Y, Davies TF, Greenberg DA, Concepcion ES, Osman R, Oashi T, *et al.* Arginine at position 74 of the HLA-DRb1 chain is associated with Graves' disease. *Genes Immun*, 2004; **5**: 203–8.
25. Simmonds MJ, Howson JM, Heward JM, Cordell HJ, Foxall H, Carr-Smith J, *et al.* Regression mapping of association between the human leukocyte antigen region and Graves' disease. *Am J Hum Genet*, 2005; **76**: 157–63.
26. Weetman AP. *Autoimmune Endocrine Disease.* Cambridge: Cambridge University Press, 1991.
27. Menconi F, Monti MC, Greenberg DA, Oashi T, Osman R, Davies TF, *et al.* Molecular amino acid signatures in the MHC class II peptide-binding pocket predispose to autoimmune thyroiditis in humans and in mice. *Proc Natl Acad Sci U S A*, 2008; **105**: 14034–9.
28. Ueda H, Howson JM, Esposito L, Heward J, Snook H, Chamberlain G, *et al.* Association of the T-cell regulatory gene CTLA4 with susceptibility to autoimmune disease. *Nature*, 2003; **423**: 506–11.
29. Velaga MR, Wilson V, Jennings CE, Owen CJ, Herington S, Donaldson PT, *et al.* The codon 620 tryptophan allele of the lymphoid tyrosine phosphatase (LYP) gene is a major determinant of Graves' disease. *J Clin Endocrinol Metab*, 2004; **89**: 5862–5.

30. Jacobson EM, Tomer Y. The CD40, CTLA-4, thyroglobulin, TSH receptor, and PTPN22 gene quintet and its contribution to thyroid autoimmunity: back to the future. *J Autoimmun*, 2007; **28**: 85–98.
31. Dechairo BM, Zabaneh D, Collins J, Brand O, Dawson GJ, Green AP, *et al.* Association of the TSHR gene with Graves' disease: the first disease specific locus. *Eur J Hum Genet*, 2005; **13**: 1223–30.
32. Allen EM, Hsueh WC, Sabra MM, Pollin TI, Ladenson PW, Silver KD, *et al.* A genome-wide scan for autoimmune thyroiditis in the Old Order Amish: replication of genetic linkage on chromosome 5q11.2-q14.3. *J Clin Endocrinol Metab*, 2003; **88**: 1292–6.
33. Taylor JC, Gough SC, Hunt PJ, Brix TH, Chatterjee K, Connell JM, *et al.* A genome-wide screen in 1119 relative pairs with autoimmune thyroid disease. *J Clin Endocrinol Metab*, 2006; **91**: 646–53.
34. Hanafusa T, Pujol Borrell R, Chiovato L, Russell RC, Doniach D, Bottazzo GF. Aberrant expression of HLA-DR antigen on thyrocytes in Graves' disease: relevance for autoimmunity. *Lancet*, 1983; **ii**: 1111–15.
35. Kouki T, Sawai Y, Gardine CA, Fisfalen ME, Alegre ML, DeGroot LJ. CTLA-4 gene polymorphism at position 49 in exon 1 reduces the inhibitory function of CTLA-4 and contributes to the pathogenesis of Graves' disease. *J Immunol*, 2000; **165**: 6606–11.
36. Xu Y, Graves P, Tomer Y, Davies T. CTLA-4 and autoimmune thyroid disease: lack of influence of the A49G signal peptide polymorphism on functional recombinant human CTLA-4. *Cell Immunol*, 2002; **215**: 133–40.
37. Mayans S, Lackovic K, Nyholm C, Lindgren P, Ruikka K, Eliasson M, *et al.* CT60 genotype does not affect CTLA-4 isoform expression despite association to T1D and AITD in northern Sweden. *BMC Med Genet*, 2007; **8**: 3.
38. Shaw G, Kamen R. A conserved AU sequence from the 3′ untranslated region of GM-CSF mRNA mediates selective mRNA degradation. *Cell*, 1986; **46**: 659–67.
39. Wang XB, Kakoulidou M, Giscombe R, Qiu Q, Huang D, Pirskanen R, *et al.* Abnormal expression of CTLA-4 by T cells from patients with myasthenia gravis: effect of an AT-rich gene sequence. *J Neuroimmunol*, 2002; **130**: 224–32.
40. Bottini N, Vang T, Cucca F, Mustelin T. Role of PTPN22 in type 1 diabetes and other autoimmune diseases. *Semin Immunol*, 2006; **18**: 207–13.
41. Vang T, Congia M, Macis MD, Musumeci L, Orru V, Zavattari P, *et al.* Autoimmune-associated lymphoid tyrosine phosphatase is a gain-of-function variant. *Nat Genet*, 2005; **37**: 1317–19.
42. Hodge SE, Ban Y, Strug LJ, Greenberg DA, Davies TF, Concepcion ES, *et al.* Possible interaction between HLA-DRbeta1 and thyroglobulin variants in Graves' disease. *Thyroid*, 2006; **16**: 351–5.
43. Flynn JC, McCormick DJ, Brusic V, Wan Q, Panos JC, Giraldo AA, *et al.* Pathogenic human thyroglobulin peptides in HLA-DR3 transgenic mouse model of autoimmune thyroiditis. *Cell Immunol*, 2004; **229**: 79–85.
44. Ban Y, Tozaki T, Tobe T, Ban Y, Jacobson EM, Concepcion ES, *et al.* The regulatory T cell gene FOXP3 and genetic susceptibility to thyroid autoimmunity: an association analysis in Caucasian and Japanese cohorts. *J Autoimmun*, 2007; **28**: 201–7.
45. Tomer Y, Menconi F, Davies TF, Barbesino G, Rocchi R, Pinchera A, *et al.* Dissecting genetic heterogeneity in autoimmune thyroid diseases by subset analysis. *J Autoimmun*, 2007; **29**: 69–77.

3.2.2 Environmental factors

Josef Köhrle

Introduction

The hypothalamus–pituitary–thyroid–periphery (HPTP) axis has been known to be a vulnerable target for environmental factors and nutritional agents for centuries. Goitrogenesis, hypo- and hyperthyroidism, tumorigenesis, and autoimmune diseases of this gland have been linked to single or combined deficiencies of several essential trace elements. Normal thyroid function depends on adequate and balanced availability of the essential trace elements iodine, selenium, iron, and the mineral zinc in the daily diet. It has been suggested that the evolution of humankind and Eve's route of migration out of Africa, to displace the Neanderthal people and to populate the other continents, closely followed coastlines and regions with high availability of iodine, the key element required for thyroid hormone synthesis (1, 2). Involuntary or voluntary environmental or nutritional exposure to adverse factors and agents impairing thyroid hormone synthesis, secretion, binding, transport, metabolism, and action ('goitrogens') contributes to the development and persistence of thyroid disorders (3). Iodine deficiency, still prevalent in many regions of our world, and iodine excess (4), both of which might occur during embryonal and fetal development as well as in newborns, adolescents, and adults, provide the platform for action of adverse agents, which might be well tolerated by a normally functioning 'quiescent' thyroid gland with adequate iodine supply (see Chapters 3.2.3, 3.2.4). Compounds adversely affecting the HPTP axis belong to several chemical classes of food ingredients and environmental contaminants, but might also represent pharmaceutical drugs acting either directly on biomolecules comprising the HPTP axis or after modification by phase I and/or II drug metabolism (see Table 3.2.2.1). Apart from by ingestion, several agents reach their targets after inhalation (e.g. occupational exposure or smoking) or by dermal application (e.g. UV screens).

Environmental factors such as temperature, light, altitude, and latitude of living, as well as physical, emotional, and acute mental stress, diseases, and adverse life events impinge on normal HPTP function (Box 3.2.2.1) (40). Very recently it has been suggested that the worldwide pandemic of diseases associated with changes in industrialized and developing countries, such as obesity, diabetes, and metabolic syndromes, is linked to inadequate iodine supply and altered thyroid hormone homeostasis by epigenetic mechanisms during development (15, 41). Current conditions in industrialized western-style countries are characterized by the permanent availability and overconsumption of energy-rich, fibre-poor, semiprocessed, manufactured, enhanced, fortified, or even 'novel' foods, a sedentary life style, and a lack of sufficient mobility and physical activity, all of which impinge on hormonal homeostasis that is mainly integrated at the hypothalamic level involving thyrotropin-releasing hormone-producing neurons. It is becoming apparent that not only starvation, fasting, and protein–calorie malnutrition in developing countries but also overfeeding with hypercaloric energy-dense food and obesity in western-style regions can lead to inadequate intake of micronutrients (minerals, vitamins, and secondary metabolites

Table 3.2.2.1 Agents and compounds interfering with the hypothalamus–pituitary–thyroid–periphery axis

Compound	Source and occurrence	Mechanism of action	Effects	Reference(s)
Environmental				
Perchlorate	Solid rocket and missile fuel; airbags	Inhibition of NIS	Goitrogenic	5–10
Phthalate esters	Daily life and medical products	?	?	11–13
Pyridines	Cigarette smoke, coal tar	Goitrogenic		14
Polychlorinated (PCB) and polybrominated (PBB) biphenyls	Chemicals, daily life products; flame retardants	TH transport, uptake, metabolism; T_3 receptor binding		11, 13, 15–17
Dioxins (TCDD) and furans	Unintentionally produced by-products, pyrolysis	TH transport, uptake, metabolism		12, 13, 16, 18
Polycyclic aromatic hydrocarbons (PAH)	Chemicals			19
(Poly-)phenols, e.g. bisphenol A (BPA)	Plasticizer in daily life products			20–23
Nitrate; nitrite	Fertilizers; food preservative	NIS inhibitors	Goitrogenic	24
UV screens (4-MBC, BP2)	Sun blockers in cosmetics, daily life products	NIS expression, TPO inhibitors	Goitrogenic	25
Tobacco and cigar smoke	Goitrogens, nicotine	Inhibition of TH synthesis, metabolism and action Perinatal programming for obesity in rodents	Goitrogenic Strongest risk factor for Graves' disease; might prevent Hashimoto's thyroiditis? Altered maternal and fetal thyroid function	26–29 30
Nutritional				
Various goitrogens	Staple food, vegetables, inappropriately processed food	TPO inhibitor	Goitrogenic	
Linamarin, goitrin, various glycosides	Staple food (cassava), vegetables (Cruciferaceae)	TPO inhibitor	Goitrogenic	31
Flavonoids (polyphenols)		TPO inhibitors, TTR competitors	Goitrogenic	3
Polyhydroxy phenols and phenol derivatives				12
Sulfurated organics, (iso-)thiocyanate, cyanide, thio-oxazolidone (goitrin)	Nutritional goitrogen Tobacco smoke	NIS inhibitor TPO inhibitor at higher concentration	Goitrogenic	5,6,32
Aliphatic disulphides	Onions, garlic Water contaminated from coal mining	TPO inhibitors	Goitrogenic	14
Humic acids	Ground and drinking water	Interference with TH synthesis	Goitrogenic?	33
Trans fatty acids	Thermally oxidized fats (French fries, fast food)	Altered TH serum levels	?	34
Deficiencies in trace elements and minerals				
Selenium deficiency	Seafood and red meat	Essential trace element for TH synthesis and metabolism	Goitrogenic	35
Iron deficiency	Protein malnutrition Genetic predisposition	Essential trace element for TH biosynthesis, inadequate function of the haemoprotein TPO for TH biosynthesis		36
Zinc deficiency				37
Pharmaceuticals				
Lithium	Antidepressant	Inhibition of TH secretion	Goitrogenic	38
Iodinated agents	Oral bile duct radiographic contrast agents (e.g. iopanoic acid); antiarrhythmic drug amiodarone	TR antagonist	Hypothyroidism	36,39

NIS, sodium-iodide symporter, TH, thyroid hormone; TPO, thyroid peroxidase; TR, T_3 receptor; TTR, transthyretin.

Box 3.2.2.1 Environmental agents and factors interfering with HTPT axis

- Light, day–night rhythm (shift workers)
- Latitude of living
- Ambient temperature
- Drinking water, food, nutritional components (voluntarily or involuntarily exposure)
- Inappropriately processed food: goitrogens, thermally oxidized fats (French fries, fast food)
- Diets:
  - Vegetarian, vegan, or macrobiotic diets with inadequate iodide, selenium, iron, zinc, and retinol content and inadequate micronutrients and vitamins
  - Diets containing constituents with goitrogenic effects under conditions of inadequate iodide intake
- Environmental emissions and exposure: inhalation of aerosol and particulate matter
- Industrial contaminants
- Agricultural environmental agents
- UV filters and UV screens

of plants). In addition, active and passive smoking, wellness-, life style-, fashion- and psychodrugs, and narcotics have a major impact on thyroid hormone synthesis, secretion, and action.

Impaired thyroid function has also been observed after consumption of protein-restricted diets, as recommended for patients with phenylketonuria or milder hyperphenylalaninaemias, where adequate iodide supply is essential to compensate for possible adverse effects on thyroid hormone synthesis and metabolism (51). Various staple foods, if inadequately processed or preserved, contain efficient goitrogens (e.g. linamarin, goitrin), which release (iso-)thiocyanate, potent inhibitors of NIS-mediated iodide uptake by thyrocytes and–at higher concentrations–also act as effective blockers of thyroperoxidase (TPO), if iodide supply is inadequate.

This chapter will summarize established data for humans, discuss recent findings and possible risk factors identified from exposure data of human subgroups, epidemiology, and findings in experimental animal models accepted as relevant for human risk analysis. Figure 3.2.2.1 illustrates currently identified targets of the HPTP axes for environmental agents. Issues of iodine deficiency and excess, pharmaceutical drugs, and radioactive isotopes interfering with the thyroid axis will be discussed elsewhere in this volume.

Various mechanisms for interference with the HPTP axis by environmental factors have been identified:

- Reversible and irreversible competition with ligand binding sites of the thyroid hormone axis
- Interference with or alterations to the feedback set points, which can already occur in the prenatal and early postnatal phase
- Classic 'goitrogenesis' by impaired hormone synthesis

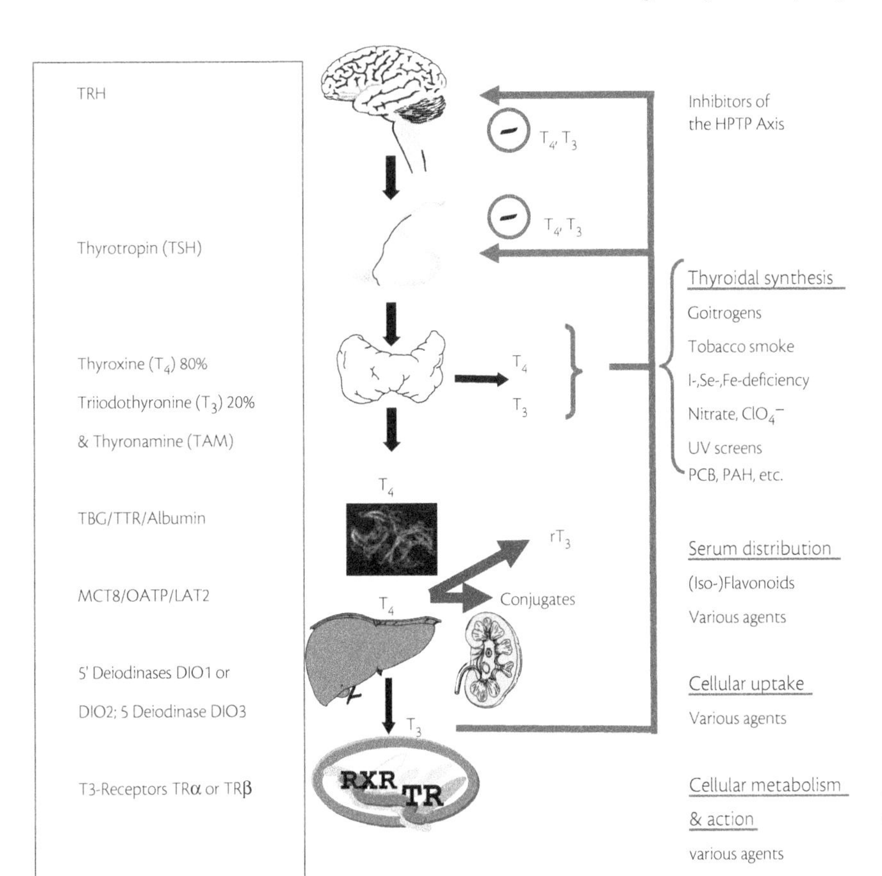

Fig. 3.2.2.1 Hypothalamus–pituitary–thyroid–periphery (HPTP) axis, hormonal feedback regulation, and interference by inhibitors. PAH, polycyclic aromatic hydrocarbons; PCB, polychlorinated biphenyls; RXR, retinoid X receptor; TR, T3 receptor.

- Disturbance of serum hormone binding, tissue distribution, cellular uptake, metabolism, and action

Many of these disturbances may be initially compensated by the complex regulatory network of the axis, which is characterized by multiply redundant and fail-safe feedback mechanisms and a high degree of plasticity and adaptation to the environment. However, long-term exposure to low-dose or acute challenge by adverse agents may overstrain the HPTP axis, especially under conditions of inadequate iodine supply or during vulnerable phases of the individual's life (development, pregnancy and lactation, nonthyroidal disease), and thus create harm or disease.

Adverse effects of various agents on the HPTP axis

Perchlorate

Perchlorate, similar to pertechnetate, perrhenate, astatinate, and (iso-)thiocyanate, is a voluminous anion and a relevant (electroneutral transport) substrate for the sodium-iodide symporter (NIS) (5), which is located not only in the basolateral membrane of thyrocytes but also in the lactating mammary gland, the salivary gland, and several internal epithelial structures (gastric mucosa, lung epithelium, etc.). These anions effectively compete for the essential iodide uptake (Table 3.2.2.2), but are not organified in thyroglobulin by the haemoprotein thyroid peroxidase (TPO). Thus, perchlorate has been used as an efficient pharmaceutical to treat hyperthyroidism and to block unwanted (radio-)iodide uptake into the gland or for the diagnostic perchlorate discharge test, performed to identify iodide organification defects. Hypothyroidism can be achieved by regular administration of perchlorate doses of 0.4 mg/kg body weight per day, while reference doses, where no appreciable risk can be observed for human populations, are in the order of 0.7 μg/kg per day. Thiocyanate or nitrate are less potent by a factor of 15 or 240, respectively (6). Recently, reports have been emerging on increasing contamination of surface land and water by potassium or ammonium perchlorate around areas close to civil or military plants as well as installations producing and handling rockets, missiles, ammunitions, and fireworks. Potassium and ammonium perchlorate are increasingly used and widely distributed over our planet as rocket and missile fuel waste; it is extremely stable and poorly degraded in the environment. Other perchlorate salts are used as oxidizers, electrolytes, and in various technical processes (7). Concerns have been raised and published whether this increasing contamination of surface soil and drinking water might negatively impact on thyroid function of exposed populations, especially babies, children, and adolescents who still have limited capacity and reserve to synthesize and store iodinated thyroglobulin. In contrast, adults, whose follicular colloid thyroglobulin stores might last for up to 3 months if adequately supplied with iodide before interference, might be less vulnerable, except during pregnancy or lactation where iodine demands are increased. This controversial issue is the subject of several ongoing surveys by environmental and regulatory authorities, but for the moment no clear evidence for risk assessment is available. However, concentrations in drinking water of exposed areas have been determined which are in the range or even exceed recommendations by regulatory authorities. Observations in workers regularly exposed to airborne perchlorate provided no evidence for adverse effects, but individuals with inadequate iodide intake, exposed to other environmental NIS inhibitors, or belonging to other susceptible risk groups might experience negative consequences of long-term perchlorate exposure by drinking water with perchlorate concentrations in the range of the discussed US reference doses (US Environmental Protection Agency reference dose 0.7 μg/kg body weight per day) (6).

Perchlorate exposure leads to increased urinary iodine excretion due to the blocking of thyroidal uptake (8) and perchlorate has been found in mothers' and cows' milk, generating a risk for babies and children with inadequate iodide supply. A longitudinal study in pregnant women exposed to different perchlorate concentrations in drinking water during pregnancy and lactation revealed no changes in thyroid status and function or adverse effects in mothers and newborns (9).

Exposure of tadpoles and adult African clawed frogs *Xenopus laevis* to perchlorate impairs amphibian metamorphosis and the thyroid function of these model organisms, which might serve as a very sensitive biomarker for monitoring purposes of several compensatory and also adverse effects caused by environmental exposure to goitrogens such as perchlorate and others; interspecies differences for adverse effects in amphibians, rodents, and humans have not been ruled out (10, 42). These studies indicate that aquatic life forms might already be affected by environmental agents, while humans and terrestrial animals might still be able to compensate or adapt to some extent as long as the concentrations of goitrogens are not excessive. Issues related to extrapolations of rodent studies with perchlorate to human iodide and thyroid

Table 3.2.2.2 Synthesis of thyroid hormones by follicular thyrocyte epithelial cells, storage of iodinated thyroglobulin in colloidal space, and secretion of thyroid hormones is affected by environmental and nutritional agents

Reaction contributing to thyroid hormone biosynthesis	Interfering compound
Basolateral iodide uptake by NIS	Perchlorate, (iso-) thiocyanate, 4-MBC
Apical export by pendrin (PDS)	?
Synthesis and apical secretion of Tg	?
Synthesis and apical insertion of TPO and DUOX	Iron,?
NADPH-dependent production of H_2O_2 by DUOX	?
Iodide oxidation, iodination of Tg tyrosyl residues	Goitrogens, goitrin;
Coupling of Tg iodotyrosine residues to iodothyronines is catalysed by TPO using H_2O_2 as cosubstrate	BP-2
Polymerization and deposition of iodinated Tg in colloid	?
Micropinocytosis, reduction, and proteolysis of Tg in secondary lysosomes	?
Release of thyroid hormones T_4 and T_3 into the blood by the transporter MCT8	?
Dehalogenation of DIT and MIT and reutilization of iodide for thyroid hormone biosynthesis	?
Secretion of pGPx (GPx-3) into the colloidal space for degradation of excess H_2O_2	Selenium,?

DIT, diiodotyrosine; DUOX, dual oxidase; MIT, monoiodotyrosine; NIS, sodium-iodide symporter; PDS, pendrin syndrome gene; Tg, thyroglobulin; TPO, thyroid peroxidase.

hormone kinetics and possible risk assessments have been extensively studied and discussed (43).

While another chloride compound, ClO_2, used for chlorination of drinking, sanitary, or swimming pool water, appears nontoxic, its by-product $NaClO_3$ is harmful to humans and might occur in water in concentrations of up to 2 mg/l (44). Bromate, BrO_3^-, the most prevalent water disinfection by-product generated during ozonation, is a carcinogen for the thyroid. For most of these adverse effects, which have been studied in the rat model, a dose-dependent increase in incidence and severity of follicular cell hyperplasia in a gender-specific manner has been observed, with male rats been more sensitive. The bromide anion cannot be efficiently utilized by the iodide-selective organification system of the thyroid follicle, but exposure to elevated bromide concentrations markedly impairs thyroid hormone synthesis and thyroid function (45) (for the effects of brominated organic compounds, see below).

Nitrate

A continuously increasing world population requires enhanced efforts for the production of sufficient food and this is achieved by a greater use of nitrogen-containing fertilizers in agricultural production. Nitrate and nitrite contamination of ground, surface, and drinking water as well as many food products, especially vegetables, is the downside of this development. Nitrite and nitrate are also widely used as preservatives for fish and meat. Nitrate efficiently interferes with NIS catalysed iodide uptake and represents a relevant goitrogen especially in children exposed to drinking water containing 100 mg/l or more nitrate (46). In highly contaminated or nutritionally exposed areas, the goitrogenic effects of nitrate/nitrite cannot be neglected, but adequate iodide supply might prevent this adverse effect and subchronic exposure (15 μg/kg body weight for 28 days in volunteers) appears to be tolerable in humans with respect to thyroid function (24). Whether nitrate also directly interferes with TPO or thyroid oxidase (DUOX) is unclear.

Nitric oxide, NO, identified as prostacyclin- and endothelium-derived hyperpolarizing factor, is a powerful signalling molecule activating guanylate cyclase and cGMP production in the vascular system and thyrocytes and acts as a potent inhibitor of thyroid hormone synthesis and function (47). Whether pharmaceuticals generating NO, which is also endogenously produced in the thyroid by NO synthase isoenzymes, have adverse or therapeutic effects on thyroid function in hyperthyroidism remains to be analysed (47).

Thiocyanate and smoking

This voluminous anion and its related structural isomer isothiocyanate are both potent iodide competitors for NIS, and at higher concentrations thiocyanate also inhibits TPO by acting as a pseudosubstrate. Thiocyanate and isothiocyanate are formed by metabolic pathways from cyanogenic glucosides or thioglucosides of plant origin, respectively. Plant and (bacterial) glucosidases in the gut cleave these glucosides and release cyanide, which is converted to thiocyanate or isothiocyanate. 'Goitrin' (L-5-vinyl-2-thio-oxazolidone), isolated from yellow turnips and from *Brassica* seeds, is a potent antithyroid compound and thiocyanate is also endogenously released from linamarin, a cyanogenic glucoside present particularly in the tuberous roots of the staple food cassava (31). Goitrin, a goitrogen as potent as 6-propyl-2-thiouracil, is not degraded like thioglycosides. Relevant sources for such goitrogens are the Brassicaceae (e.g. cabbage, broccoli, cauliflower, Brussels sprouts), Cruciferaceae, Compositae, and Umbelliferae, but the food content of these adverse metabolites largely depends on adequate processing by cooking, hydrolysis, and preservation. Exposure to these goitrogens, monitored by urinary excretion of (iso-)thiocyanate, is a major problem in developing countries, where inadequate economic and social life conditions or energy resources prevent correct processing of these staple foods such as cassava, sweet potatoes, lima beans, sorghum, pearl millet, and corn, which are the main source for carbohydrates. In addition, concomitant iodide deficiency and protein malnutrition leading to inadequate iron supply can exaggerate this problem for risk groups such as pregnant and lactating women, infants, children, and adolescents. In the thyroid, thiocyanate is metabolized to sulfate and thus does not accumulate.

Thiocyanate and isothiocyanate exposure is also of relevance in western countries, as recently documented (32) for nutritional sources; it is especially relevant for tobacco smokers, who inhale significant amounts of these goitrogens together with other adverse agents. Up to fourfold increases in thiocyanate concentrations were found in breast milk of breastfeeding mothers who smoked and this was associated with up to a twofold decrease in iodide content, the combination of which amplified the goitrogenic risk for the baby (48). Further adverse combinations might be observed if nutritional and environmental exposures to several of these goitrogens add to or amplify the risk and potential damage to thyroid hormone homeostasis. Altered maternal and fetal thyroid function has been reported for mothers who smoke (26) and smoking is one of the main risk factors for progress and severity of Graves' disease. Conversely, smoking reduces anti-TPO and antithyroglobulin antibodies and might reduce the incidence of Hashimoto's thyroiditis by mechanisms not understood so far (27, 28). Smoking is a also risk factor for goitrogenesis, even with an improved iodide supply (29).

Tolerable exposure limits recommended by environmental and health authorities and goitrogen contents of nutrients and foods vary greatly in different regions, countries, and continents of our globe. As several of these environmental or nutritional exposures cannot be modified by exposed individuals, it is more than necessary to ensure adequate iodide intake for the whole population, and especially for risk groups (6, 49).

Gaitan *et al.* have reported on the occurrence of small aliphatic disulphides (R-S-S-R; R = methyl-, ethyl-, *n*-propyl, phenyl-), which are goitrogens inhibiting iodide organification catalysed by TPO. These compounds occur in some vegetables (onion and garlic), well water, sedimentary rocks, and as water contaminants in aqueous effluents from coal-conversion processes (14). Humic acids, another coal or plant origin contaminant of well and drinking water, have also been identified as goitrogens, but again their effect is only observed when there is inadequate iodide supply, at least in animal experimental models (50).

Impaired thyroid function has also been observed after consumption of protein-restricted diets, as recommended for patients with phenylketonuria or milder hyperphenylalaninaemias, where adequate iodide supply is essential to compensate for possible adverse effects on thyroid hormone synthesis and metabolism (51).Various staple foods, if inadequately processed or preserved, contain efficient goitrogens (e.g. linamarin, goitrin), which release (iso-)thiocyanate, potent inhibitors of NIS-mediated iodide uptake by thyrocytes and–at higher concentrations–also act as effective blockers of TPO, if iodide supply is inadequate.

Table 3.2.2.3 Representative examples of nutritional and environmental agents interfering with the hypothalamus–pituitary–thyroid–periphery (HPTP) axis

Chemical structure	Compound name	IUPAC nomenclature	Molecular weight	Typical use
	Goitrin, DL-goitrin	5-Ethenyl-1,3-oxazolidine-2-thione	129	Contained in food, goitrogen
	Arochlor 1254	1,2,3-Trichloro-4-(2,3-dichlorophenyl)benzene	326	Antithyroid agent, pesticide
	Tetradioxin, dioxin	2,3,7,8-Tetrachlorooxanthrene	322	Insecticide, teratogen
	Minocycline	(2Z,4S,4aS,5aR,12aS)-2-[amino(hydroxy)methylidene]-4,7-bis(dimethylamino)-10,11,12a-trihydroxy-4a,5,5a,6-tetrahydro-4H-tetracene-1,3,12-trione	457	Antibacterial agent
	Bisphenol A, diphenylolpropane	4-[2-(4-hydroxyphenyl)propan-2-yl]phenol	228	Free radical scavenger
	Dibutyl phthalate	Dibutyl benzene-1,2-dicarboxylate	278	Plasticizer
	Benzophenone-2; Uvinol D-50	Bis(2,4-dihydroxyphenyl)methanone	246	UV screen
	Enzacamene; Neo Heliopan MBC; Eusolex 63	(3E)-1,7,7-trimethyl-3-[(4-methylphenyl)methylidene]bicyclo[2.2.1]heptan-2	254	UV screen

Box 3.2.2.2 Mechanisms of adverse action of environmental and nutritional agents interfering with the HPTP axis

- Known targets:
  - Thyroid: TSH receptor, NIS, TPO, DUOX
  - Serum: transthyretin, albumin, TBG
  - Target cells: uptake, deiodinases, conjugating enzymes, T3 receptors
- Possible targets:
  - TRH
  - TRH receptor
  - TRH-degrading ectoenzyme
  - TSH dehalogenase
  - Cathepsins
  - Cellular uptake systems: MCT8, MCT10, OATP14, LAT2
- Known mechanisms:
  - Direct competition (reversible, irreversible) for thyroid hormone protein binding sites
  - Inactivation of essential protein components of the HPTP axis (e.g. heavy metals, toxins)
- Probable mechanisms:
  - Epigenetic effects
- Age- and life phase-dependent actions:
  - Developmental
  - Teratogenic
  - In utero
  - Pregnancy
  - Lactation

Environmental chemicals

The remarkable progress of worldwide industrialization, expanded and intensified agricultural, (semi-)industrial production of nutrients and food, and the tremendous increase in quality of life associated with longevity, has had and continues to have a major impact on our environment, which raises several concerns. In particular, the synthesis, use, and dissemination of tens of thousands of new chemicals and compounds, some of which are produced at high tonnage worldwide, have introduced new agents into our environment, some of which interfere with the hormonal systems including the thyroid. Several candidate agents with relevance to the HPTP axis have been identified from effects in wildlife, including aquatic life forms, and for some compounds the adverse effects on thyroid morphology, structure, function, and thyroid hormone status have already been described. Among these are polychlorinated (polychlorinated biphenyls (PCBs), hexachlorobenzene (HCB), organochlorines) and polybrominated (polybrominated diphenyl ethers (PBDE)) aromatic and phenolic (resorcinol, bisphenol A (BPA)) compounds, chlorinated furans such as dioxin derivatives, polyphenolic hydrocarbons, phthalates, pyridines, and others (see Table 3.2.2.3 for selected compounds and their main characteristics).

The Seveso accident in 1976 releasing highly persistent 2,3,7,8-tetrachlorodibenzo-*p*-dioxin (TCDD) created a first indication, shortly followed by Bhopal, India in 1984, Basel 1986, and several other accidents, which raised awareness of the issue of endocrine disrupters which have not only immediate toxic effects but also might act in a transgenerational way including epigenetic mechanisms of action (Box 3.2.2.2).

Maternal exposure to TCDD and related compounds in the Seveso area has been linked to markedly elevated neonatal thyroid-stimulating hormone (TSH) blood levels in the inner versus the marginally affected and the control area (18) in the affected offspring after the accident. This still controversial data, although correlated with current plasma TCDD and coplanar dioxin-like compounds, suggests long-lasting impact of such contamination both for the immediately exposed population and for the subsequent generation. Elevated neonatal TSH is a well-accepted biomarker for fetal hypothyroidism and is used in the highly successful worldwide screening programmes for congenital hypothyroidism. Increased thyroid volume and elevated prevalence of antibodies against TPO and the TSH receptor associated with impaired fasting glucose were also reported for the young adult offspring of mothers exposed and living in a highly polluted area in eastern Slovakia, where a mix of organochlorines (PCBs, dichlorodiphenyldichloroethylene (DDE), HCB) can still be detected in the exposed inhabitants, albeit at lower levels in the young adults compared to their parents, but still higher than in a control region (16, 17). Again these data were discussed in the context of a transgenerational adverse effect on the HPTP and other endocrine axes, and convincing evidence for an altered HPTP axis seems obvious for the total exposed population of that region.

A major human biomonitoring programme was initiated in 2002 in a heavily industrialized and populated area in Flanders, Belgium. Results from this carefully conceived analysis, including internal exposure to various endocrine disrupters and agents, revealed, among other alterations of hormonal parameters, effects on the serum thyroid hormone levels (e.g. lowered TSH, and elevated free triiodothyronine (T_3) (52). Thyroid hormone serum profiles were also found to be altered in adolescents from the Akwesasne Mohawk Nation living in a PCB-exposed area (15). Different relationships were observed for different PCB congeners, HCB, and DDE versus TSH and free thyroxine (T_4) levels, with breastfeeding modulating these interactions. Although only a small group of adolescents had been analysed, the authors interpreted their findings as evidence for prenatal impact of exposure to these endocrine disrupters on long-lasting alterations of the set points of the HPTP axis, in agreement with several other recent studies in exposed regions. Apparently small amounts of selected persisting endocrine disrupters already present during fetal, postnatal, and pubertal development might lead to adverse effects on the HPTP axis via epigenetic mechanisms. Whether these mechanisms manifest only in certain subpopulations, susceptible or genetically predisposed subgroups or individuals, remains to be studied in more detail. Nevertheless, even subtle alterations of the HPTP axis will have a major impact on brain development, IQ, and long-term metabolic and age-related disease risks due to the pleiotropic nature of thyroid hormone action and feedback regulation (Box 3.2.2.3).

As there are trends for direct relationships between blood, tissue, adipose tissue, whole body, or breast milk contents for TCDD, polychlorinated dibenzofurans (PCDFs), PCB congeners, and other related endocrine disrupters to impaired thyroid function, especially in babies, children, and young adults (11), there is not only a need for monitoring and further research of potential long-term damage, but also the urgent necessity to implement adequate iodide intake in these areas. This precaution might reduce the risk of endocrine disrupter exposure and contamination of the HPTP axis. Even under such conditions breastfeeding should be considered, provided the mother adapts her iodine intake not only to pregnancy and lactation but also to her elevated endocrine disrupter contamination, transferred into the breast milk.

PCBs are environmentally persistent, and some of their more than 200 congeners show bioaccumulation in adipose tissue and exhibit high structural similarity to thyroid hormone. This is reflected by their significant competition of thyroid hormone binding to serum transthyretin but also significant competition for T_3 binding to T_3 receptor as demonstrated by *in vitro*, cellular, and intact animal experimental models. Whether these mechanistically plausible effects, which are however associated with divergent findings on serum thyroid hormone status of affected humans, will also have impact on functionally relevant readouts and biomarkers, remains to be analysed in long-term studies in larger cohorts.

Box 3.2.2.3 Current research concepts and paradigms for analysis of endocrine disrupter-like effects of HTPT axis

- Convergence of endocrine disrupter effects on neural and endocrine targets in hypothalamus
- Neuroendocrine regulation and organizational units of hypothalamus
- Timing of endocrine disrupter exposure is key to its ultimate effects, windows of susceptibility, life-course-specific effects
- Transgenerational effects of endocrine disrupters: both personal and parental exposure is relevant
- Analysis of subpopulations with high accidental or occupational exposure or (genetically) predisposed vulnerability
- Epidemiological analysis of consumer and occupationally exposed groups
- Impact of subtle thyroid axis alterations on pre- and postnatal development and long-term aging-associated risks

Recently several highly sensitive, powerful, and sophisticated high-throughput *in vitro* screening systems have been established, validated, and are currently used in research. They are also used for biomonitoring by environmental authorities and allow for detailed analysis of terrestrial and aquatic environment, food components, nutrition, and occupational exposure with respect to endpoints of interference of endocrine disrupters with thyroid hormone synthesis, metabolism, and action (12, 42, 53–55).

The 'xenoestrogen' BPA, recently receiving much scientific and public attention among the most controversial compounds, is a relevant antagonistic ligand for T_3 receptor and might affect modulation of T_3-responsive genes. BPA, an agent used as a plasticizer in daily life articles from polycarbonate baby bottles and food can inner linings to cosmetic and dental products, is currently intensively analysed as a potent endocrine disrupter not only for the thyroid but also the hypothalamus–pituitary–gonadal (HPG) axis (20–22). Some companies have already stopped using the compound in baby products. Animal experimental studies suggest immediate and also transgenerational BPA effects including alterations of sex differentiation. As long as only few accepted data exist on critical BPA leakage and human exposure levels during various life phases, caution should be taken in further expanding the use of this compound in human daily life. BPA has clear adverse effects on several components of the HPTP axis in experimental *in vitro* and *in vivo* models and is a powerful endocrine disrupter inhibiting several T_3-regulated pathways in vertebrate development, as analysed in the excellent premetamorphic *Xenopus laevis* model (23). These observations add complexity to the analysis of adverse effects and necessary risk assessment because BPA in scientific and public discussions has been mainly considered to be a 'xenoestrogenic' compound with impact on development, differentiation, and function of the HPG axis. Findings like this and related observations of endocrine disrupter agents affecting more than one endocrine axis with rather distinct developmental windows of susceptibility to even very low doses of the compounds led to new initiatives, paradigms, and approaches as to how to analyse such endocrine disrupter effects that will probably rarely be detected using the classic approaches of toxicology focusing on serum parameters, morphology, linear dose-response relationships, and toxicological endpoints (20). It should not be forgotten, that relevant species differences for the HPTP axis require careful analysis of potential human impact of finings in nonhuman *in vitro* and animal experimental models.

Similar considerations apply for the various phthalates in use, which have already created a worldwide significant exposure level in humans. Here only very few data have been collected related to their interference with the HPTP axis, but most studies indicate relevant interference with thyroid hormone levels in children, pregnant women, and adult individuals (13). The detailed mode of action remains unclear as the wide number of phthalate congeners and their metabolites poses major analytical problems for clear cause–effect analysis.

Also for another group of persistent organohalogen pollutants, the perfluorinated compounds, which are markedly enriched in the aquatic food chain, interference with the HPTP axis has been shown in environmental, nutritional, and occupational exposure analyses. Perfluorinated compounds are structurally related to free fatty acids and thus bind to albumin in the blood, thereby competing with thyroid hormone and interfering with thyroid hormone bioavailability to target tissues. While at high occupational exposures altered thyroid hormone serum parameters were reported, so far no clinical evidence for disturbed thyroid hormone status in humans is evident. However, as exposure to perfluorinated agents increases globally this issue will remain on the agenda.

Pharmaceuticals and drugs

Thyroid is a sensitive target for side effects of various drugs

Many drugs are known to interact with the thyroid gland or with components involved in the function and regulation of the HPTP axis. In toxicology departments of the pharmaceutical industry the thyroid gland is a well-known problematic target for adverse or toxic side effects of new pharmaceuticals. It is estimated that up to one-third of newly developed compounds, especially aromatic and polycyclic compounds, fail the acute or chronic toxicity screening test batteries due to their side effects leading to alterations of thyroid morphology, goitrogenesis, development of thyroid tumours, or merely changes of serum TSH and/or thyroid hormone levels. The reason for this is not completely understood, but the permanent lifelong H_2O_2 production by thyroid follicles catalysed by the NADPH-dependent DUOX and peroxide consumption by TPO for iodide oxidation, organification, and thyroid hormone synthesis on the thyroglobulin scaffold might be the major cause. Compounds accumulating in the thyroid and its luminal colloid might be exposed to H_2O_2, be chemically modified by oxidative processes, and be deposited there or damage the follicles. One illustrative example might be the rare observation of 'black thyroid' syndrome, which is a tetracycline (especially minocycline)-induced discolouration of the thyroid gland probably related to TPO-induced oxidation of the tetracycline (13).

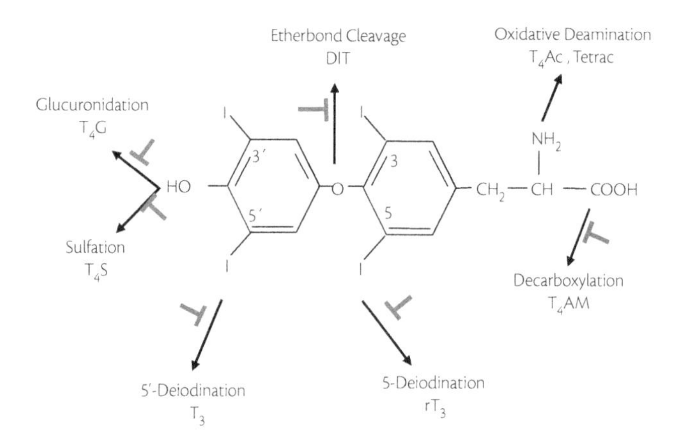

Fig. 3.2.2.2 Pathways of thyroxine (T_4) metabolism known to be affected by nutritional or environmental agents (⊣).

Benzofurans

The powerful benzofuran drugs amiodarone and dronedarone are widely used for treating resistant tachyarrhythmia. Apart from their target molecules in the heart, these drugs, the active metabolite desethylamiodarone, and other derivatives are potent antagonistic ligands for the T_3 receptor and inhibitors for the Dio enzymes (Fig. 3.2.2.2). However, debutyl dronedarone acts as a selective T_3 receptor $\alpha 1$ antagonist (see Chapter 3.3.12). Therefore, chronic administration leads to impaired thyroid function with a clear cumulative dose-associated increase in risk. The drugs are substantially accumulated in the thyroid, which in addition to the high iodine content of amiodarone (between 3 and 20 mg iodide are released per day into the blood) explains their prominent disturbance of thyroid function (39). Not only the iodide contamination associated with the administration of the drug but also the thyroid accumulation of the drug might lead to the severe structural defects of the gland and follicles seen in some patients treated with amiodarone (56). Therefore, the new iodine-free alternative dronedarone is of great interest as no comparable thyroid-related effects are reported, such as inhibition of deiodinase, binding to T_3 receptor, or thyroid accumulation. The adverse effects with respect to iodide contamination of other iodinated drugs, such as the iodinated oral bile radiographic contrast agent iopanoic acid and its congeners, will be discussed elsewhere in this volume.

UV screens in cosmetics and daily life products

A further representative example of a group of endocrine disrupters with relevance for the HPTP axis are widely used UV screens or absorbers. These are ubiquitous components of various plastic materials used in daily life which have to be protect from UV damage; also they are contained in sun screens and various cosmetics such as lip sticks or body lotions. UV screens may contain up to 10% (w/w) of typical compounds such as benzophenone 2 or 3, 4-methylbenzylidene camphor (4-MBC), and related products. Typical administration of the UV filters leads to measurable serum levels in the submicromolar to micromolar range (25). At these concentrations clear adverse effects have been observed in thyroid-related *in vitro* and *in vivo* animal models, such as rapid and dose-dependent goitrogenesis in rats after 4-MBC administration or efficient inhibition of TPO by benzophenone 2 (3). Some of these effects might be prevented or at least attenuated by adequate iodide supply which still is not warranted globally. Considering the increased application of these UV screens, not only for product protection but also for prevention of human skin cancer due to higher exposure to UV irradiation associated with ozone loss in the atmosphere, some of these UV filters might impose marked risks for the adequate function of the HPTP axis. This might apply especially to babies and children, whose skin is more sensitive to UV light and less protected by endogenous melanocytes, and therefore more frequently treated with these dermal UV lotions. Also these products might be even more easily absorbed by young skin. So far no clear evidence for a goitrogenic action of UV filter ingredients has been described in humans. Therefore, the advice might be to guarantee an adequate iodide supply and to protect skin from UV irradiation by avoiding too much sun and applying UV screens that have less risk for interference with the HPTP axis, especially in babies, children, and individuals with sensitive skin.

Heavy metals and thyroid

Environmental contamination by heavy metals and their ions has raised public concern based on their direct effects on several tissues and organs. Both accidentally and occupationally exposed subgroups are affected, and significant adverse effects might result in the CNS during development and with respect to the pathogenesis of neurodegenerative ageing-associated diseases. Whether the thyroid hormone system, known to have a major impact on proper brain development and function in children and adults, is directly involved in these processes remains unclear. As thyrocytes exhibit a highly active redox-regulated cellular metabolism (57), impairment of reactive redox centres of enzymes and other thyrocyte proteins such as metallothioneins by heavy metals will create problems for thyroid hormone synthesis and secretion. Therefore, environmental or occupational exposure to high mercury, lead, and cadmium concentrations has been associated with altered thyroid homeostasis. For example, a gender-specific effect on increased serum TSH, correlated with increased hair and blood mercury concentrations in males, has been reported in lakeside communities of Quebec and is associated with consumption of contaminated lake fish from the exposed environment (58, 59). Divergent reports have been published on the relationship between cadmium exposure and TSH, positively associated in several studies, but inversely related in a pilot study in cord blood of Japanese newborns (60). Animal experimental data clearly suggest adverse effects of cadmium exposure, which interferes with both thyroid hormone synthesis and peripheral Dio1 activity.

Adverse effects of lead on the thyroid axis have been reported. Previous environmental lead sources were lead-enhanced gasoline and lead-based paints, but both of these sources are of decreasing relevance due to bans that have been enforced in most countries, while contaminations by cadmium, mercury, and, recently, platinum leaking into environment from car exhaust catalytic converters are tending to further increase. Soldin and Aschner (61) reviewed the evidence that manganese, an essential constituent of several redox-relevant enzymes, such as manganese superoxide dismutase, may directly or indirectly affect thyroid function by injuring the thyroid gland or dysregulating dopaminergic modulation of thyroid hormone synthesis and thus contributing to altered thyroid hormone homeostasis and neurodegenerative diseases.

On the other hand, adequate selenium supply can efficiently counteract the adverse effects of several heavy metal cations such as cadmium, mercury, lead, and vanadium and thus avoid their age-related neurotoxicity (62, 63). Apparently selenium leads to their accumulation or deposition in a presumably nontoxic complex in the brain, kidney, and several other tissues.

Many nutritional and environmental contaminants exhibit their goitrogenic potential only under conditions of inadequate maternal, fetal, or neonatal iodide supply. Therefore, comprehensive nutritional iodide supplementation is one of the most efficient preventive measures to avoid impaired and delayed development of humans and other higher life forms.

Environmental temperature

Temperature, light, circadian and circannual rhythms, altitude, latitude, and extreme environmental life conditions are well known to influence thyroid hormone, energy, and thermoregulatory and metabolic homeostasis not only in free-living animals (homeotherms, hibernators, or aestivators such as bears) but also in humans and livestock adapted to modern housing conditions. Nevertheless, there exist clear circadian and circannual rhythms of TSH and, delayed in phase, of free T_3 in human serum, while T_4, tightly bound to its four serum distributor proteins (thyroxine-binding globulin (TBG), transthyretin, albumin, and lipoproteins) shows no significant circadian or circannual variation (64, 65).

Lowest TSH values are observed in spring and summer and increases of 25% are seen in autumn not reflected by T_4 variations and not related to iodine intake. It has to be kept in mind that the TSH response curve is exponentially related to linear changes in thyroid hormone serum concentration. Whether alterations in food intake, enhanced sympathetic tone and adrenergic stimulation of thermogenesis, altered contribution of thermogenesis by uncoupling protein 3 activation in skeletal muscles mediated by fatty acids and bile acid metabolites, or neuroendocrine hypothalamic adaptations are contributing to these changes remains to be studied. During a prolonged stay in arctic environments, enhanced thyroid hormone secretion by the thyroid has been documented, indicated by increased serum thyroglobulin and elevated T_3 production and turnover, reflected by decreased total and free T_3, but accompanied by unchanged total and free T_4 and TBG. This combination has been termed 'polar T_3 syndrome' and related combinations can be found under extreme physical exercise, endurance training, etc. Some of the changes might be prevented by increased calorie intake, sleep adaptation, or thyroid hormone treatment (66). As well as thyroid hormone changes, the melatonin system is altered under these unusual conditions, but direct relationships between these two hormones remain to be established for humans, although studies in pre- and postpubertal blind people (67) suggest an association, similar to clear evidence in various animal models.

Whether adaptations to altered ambient temperature reflect the situation of newborns after birth, characterized by a marked TSH elevation and enhanced synthesis and release of thyroid hormone, all of which can be blunted by elevated ambient temperature for the newborn, remains unclear until the mechanisms of hypothermia-induced activation of the HPTP axis have been elucidated. Recently, novel thyroid hormone metabolites, 3-T_1-thyronamine and related analogues, were shown to reversibly decrease body temperature in experimental animal models, but it is unclear whether they are involved in central hypothalamic and/or peripheral regulation of body temperature and activity of the thyroid hormone axis (68). Increased environmental temperature during summer time and also elevated body temperature during febrile conditions are associated with lower TSH and serum T_3 levels (69, 70).

Various short- and long-term adaptations of thyroid hormone secretion, turnover, serum levels, and feedback set points have been observed in studies examining the HPTP axis in people at high altitude, but results were controversial and might be confounded by other altered factors such as nutritional profiles, physical activity, light, sleep rhythm, and altered time zone adaptations. Animal experimental simulations could dissociate between distinct effects of high altitude and hypoxia and suggest powerful adaptations of the thyroid hormone axis, characterized by decreased thyroid hormone synthesis and secretion but elevated serum free thyroid hormone (40).

Acknowledgement

This work has been supported by grants of the Deutsche Forschungsgemeinschaft (DFG) to J. Köhrle (DFG GRK 1208 and DFG Ko 922/12–2).

References

1. Dobson JE. The iodine factor in health and evolution. *Geogr Rev*, 1998; **88**: 1–28.
2. Kraiem Z. Thoughts on the role of iodine in the emergence of modern humans. *Thyroid*, 2001; **11**: 807–8.
3. Kohrle J. Environment and endocrinology: the case of thyroidology. *Ann Endocrinol (Paris)*, 2008; **69**: 116–22.
4. Camargo R, Tomimori E, Neves S, Rubio I, Galrao A, Knobel M, *et al.* Thyroid and the environment: exposure to excessive nutritional iodine increases the prevalence of thyroid disorders in Sao Paulo, Brazil. *Eur J Endocrinol*, 2008; **159**: 293–9.
5. Dohan O, Portulano C, Basquin C, Reyna-Neyra A, Amzel LM, Carrasco N. The Na+/I- symporter (NIS) mediates electroneutral active transport of the environmental pollutant perchlorate. *Proc Natl Acad Sci U S A*, 2007; **104**: 20250–5.
6. De Groef B, Decallonne BR, Van der Geyten S, Darras VM, Bouillon R. Perchlorate versus other environmental sodium/iodide symporter inhibitors: potential thyroid-related health effects. *Eur J Endocrinol*, 2006; **155**: 17–25.
7. Srinivasan A, Viraraghavan T. Perchlorate: health effects and technologies for its removal from water resources. *Int J Environ Res Public Health*, 2009; **6**: 1418–42.
8. Braverman LE. Clinical studies of exposure to perchlorate in the United States. *Thyroid*, 2007; **17**: 819–22.
9. Téllez RT, Chacón PM, Abarca CR, Blount BC, Landingham CBV, Crump KS, *et al.* Long-term environmental exposure to perchlorate through drinking water and thyroid function during pregnancy and the neonatal period. *Thyroid*, 2005; **15**: 963–75.
10. Hu F, Sharma B, Mukhi S, Patino R, Carr JA. The colloidal thyroxine (T4) ring as a novel biomarker of perchlorate exposure in the African clawed frog Xenopus laevis. *Toxicol Sci*, 2006; **93**: 268–77.
11. Massart F, Meucci V. Environmental thyroid toxicants and child endocrine health. *Pediatr Endocrinol Rev*, 2007; **5**: 500–9.
12. Tanida T, Warita K, Ishihara K, Fukui S, Mitsuhashi T, Sugawara T, *et al.* Fetal and neonatal exposure to three typical environmental chemicals with different mechanisms of action: mixed exposure to phenol, phthalate, and dioxin cancels the effects of sole exposure on mouse midbrain dopaminergic nuclei. *Toxicol Lett*, 2009; **189**: 40–7.
13. Meeker JD, Altshul L, Hauser R. Serum PCBs, p,p′-DDE and HCB predict thyroid hormone levels in men. *Environ Res*, 2007; **104**: 296–304.
14. Gaitan E, Cooksey RC, Legan J, Cruse JM, Lindsay RH, Hill J. Antithyroid and goitrogenic effects of coal-water extracts from iodine-sufficient goiter areas. *Thyroid*, 1993; **3**: 49–53.
15. Schell LM, Gallo MV, Ravenscroft J, DeCaprio AP. Persistent organic pollutants and anti-thyroid peroxidase levels in Akwesasne Mohawk young adults. *Environ Res*, 2009; **109**: 86–92.
16. Langer P, Kocan A, Tajtakova M, Susienkova K, Radikova Z, Koska J, *et al.* Multiple adverse thyroid and metabolic health signs in the population from the area heavily polluted by organochlorine cocktail (PCB, DDE, HCB, dioxin). *Thyroid Res*, 2009; **2**: 3.
17. Langer P, Kocan A, Tajtakova M, Koska J, Radikova Z, Ksinantova L, *et al.* Increased thyroid volume, prevalence of thyroid antibodies and impaired fasting glucose in young adults from organochlorine cocktail polluted area: outcome of transgenerational transmission?. *Chemosphere*, 2008; **73**: 1145–50.
18. Baccarelli A, Giacomini SM, Corbetta C, Landi MT, Bonzini M, Consonni D, *et al.* Neonatal thyroid function in Seveso 25 years after maternal exposure to dioxin. *PLoS Med*, 2008; **5**: e161.
19. Builee TL, Hatherill JR. The role of polyhalogenated aromatic hydrocarbons on thyroid hormone disruption and cognitive function: a review. *Drug Chem Toxicol*, 2004; **27**: 405–24.
20. Myers JP, vom Saal FS, Akingbemi BT, Arizono K, Belcher S, Colborn T, *et al.* Why public health agencies cannot depend on good laboratory practices as a criterion for selecting data: the case of bisphenol A. *Environ Health Perspect*, 2009; **117**: 309–15.
21. Vandenberg LN, Maffini MV, Sonnenschein C, Rubin BS, Soto AM. Bisphenol-A and the great divide: a review of controversies in the field of endocrine disruption. *Endocr Rev*, 2009; **30**: 75–95.
22. Diamanti-Kandarakis E, Bourguignon JP, Giudice LC, Hauser R, Prins GS, Soto AM, *et al.* Endocrine-disrupting chemicals: an Endocrine Society scientific statement. *Endocr Rev*, 2009; **30**: 293–342.
23. Heimeier RA, Das B, Buchholz DR, Shi YB. The xenoestrogen bisphenol A inhibits postembryonic vertebrate development by antagonizing gene regulation by thyroid hormone. *Endocrinology*, 2009; **150**: 2964–73.
24. Hunault CC, Lambers AC, Mensinga TT, van Isselt JW, Koppeschaar HPF, Meulenbelt J. Effects of sub-chronic nitrate exposure on the thyroidal function in humans. *Toxicol Lett*, 2007; **175**: 64–70.
25. Janjua NR, Kongshoj B, Petersen JH, Wulf HC. Sunscreens and thyroid function in humans after short-term whole-body topical application: a single-blinded study. *Br J Dermatol*, 2007; **156**: 1080–2.
26. Shields B, Hill A, Bilous M, Knight B, Hattersley AT, Bilous RW, *et al.* Cigarette smoking during pregnancy is associated with alterations in maternal and fetal thyroid function. *J Clin Endocrinol Metab*, 2009; **94**: 570–4.
27. Effraimidis G, Tijssen JGP, Wiersinga WM. Discontinuation of smoking increases the risk for developing thyroid peroxidase antibodies and/or thyroglobulin antibodies: a prospective study. *J Clin Endocrinol Metab*, 2009; **94**: 1324–8.
28. Pedersen IB, Laurberg P, Knudsen N, Jorgensen T, Perrild H, Ovesen L, *et al.* Smoking is negatively associated with the presence of thyroglobulin autoantibody and to a lesser degree with thyroid peroxidase autoantibody in serum: a population study. *Eur J Endocrinol*, 2008; **158**: 367–73.
29. Ittermann T, Schmidt C, Kramer A, Below H, John U, Thamm M, *et al.* Smoking as a risk factor for thyroid volume progression and incident goiter in a region with improved iodine supply. *Eur J Endocrinol*, 2008; **159**: 761–6.
30. Oliveira E, Moura E, Santos-Silva A, Fagundes A, Rios A, Abreu-Villaca Y, *et al.* Short and long-term effects of maternal nicotine exposure during lactation on body adiposity, lipid profile and thyroid function of rat offspring. *J Endocrinol*, 2009; **202**: 397–405.
31. Ermans A-M, Bourdoux P. Antithyroid sulfurated compounds. In: Gaitan E, ed. *Environmental Goitrogenesis*. Boca Raton: CRC Press, 1989: 15–31.
32. Brauer VFH, Below H, Kramer A, Fuhrer D, Paschke R. The role of thiocyanate in the etiology of goiter in an industrial metropolitan area. *Eur J Endocrinol*, 2006; **154**: 229–35.

33. Andersen S, Pedersen KM, Iversen F, Terpling S, Gustenhoff P, Petersen SB, *et al.* Naturally occurring iodine in humic substances in drinking water in Denmark is bioavailable and determines population iodine intake. *Br J Nutr*, 2008; **99**: 319–25.
34. Luci S, Bettzieche A, Brandsch C, Eder K. Research paper effects of 13-HPODE on expression of genes involved in thyroid hormone synthesis, iodide uptake and formation of hydrogen peroxide in porcine thyrocytes. *Int J Vitam Nutr Res*, 2006; **76**: 398–406.
35. Schomburg L, Kohrle J. On the importance of selenium and iodine metabolism for thyroid hormone biosynthesis and human health. *Mol Nutr Food Res*, 2008; **52**: 1235–46.
36. Zimmermann MB, Köhrle J. The impact of iron and selenium deficiencies on iodine and thyroid metabolism: biochemistry and relevance to public health. *Thyroid*, 2002; **12**: 867–78.
37. Hess SY, Zimmermann MB. The effect of micronutrient deficiencies on iodine nutrition and thyroid metabolism. *Int J Vitam Nutr Res*, 2004; **74**: 103–15.
38. Johnston AM, Eagles JM. Lithium-associated clinical hypothyroidism: prevalence and risk factors. *Br J Psychiatry*, 1999; **175**:336–9.
39. Han TS, Williams GR, Vanderpump MP. Benzofuran derivatives and the thyroid. *Clin Endocrinol (Oxf)*, 2009; **70**: 2–13.
40. Sarne D. Effects of the environment, chemicals and drugs on thyroid function, in www.thyroidmanager.org, 26 May 2010. South Dartmouth MA: Endocrine Education Inc.
41. Verheesen RH, Schweitzer CM. Iodine deficiency, more than cretinism and goiter. *Med Hypotheses*, 2008; **71**: 645–8.
42. Opitz R, Schmidt F, Braunbeck T, Wuertz S, Kloas W. Perchlorate and ethylene thiourea induce different histological and molecular alterations in a non-mammalian vertebrate model of thyroid goitrogenesis. *Mol Cell Endocrinol*, 2009; **298**: 101–14.
43. Merrill EA, Clewell RA, Robinson PJ, Jarabek AM, Gearhart JM, Sterner TR, *et al.* PBPK model for radioactive iodide and perchlorate kinetics and perchlorate-induced inhibition of iodide uptake in humans. *Toxicol Sci*, 2005; **83**: 25–43.
44. Hooth MJ, Deangelo AB, George MH, Gaillard ET, Travlos GS, Boorman GA, *et al.* Subchronic sodium chlorate exposure in drinking water results in a concentration-dependent increase in rat thyroid follicular cell hyperplasia. *Toxicol Pathol*, 2001; **29**: 250–9.
45. Velicky J, Tilbach M, Lojda Z, Duskova J, Vobecky M, Strbak V, *et al.* Long-term action of potassium bromide on the rat thyroid gland. *Acta Histochem*, 1998; **100**: 11–23.
46. Radikova Z, Tajtakova M, Kocan A, Trnovec T, Sebokova E, Klimes I, *et al.* Possible effects of environmental nitrates and toxic organochlorines on human thyroid in highly polluted areas in Slovakia. *Thyroid*, 2008; **18**: 353–62.
47. Bazzara LG, Velez ML, Costamagna ME, Cabanillas AM, Fozzatti L, Lucero AM, *et al.* Nitric oxide/cGMP signaling inhibits TSH-stimulated iodide uptake and expression of thyroid peroxidase and thyroglobulin mRNA in FRTL-5 thyroid cells. *Thyroid*, 2007; **17**: 717–27.
48. Laurberg P, Nohr SB, Pedersen KM, Fuglsang E. Iodine nutrition in breast-fed infants is impaired by maternal smoking. *J Clin Endocrinol Metab*, 2004; **89**: 181–7.
49. Zimmermann MB, Jooste PL, Pandav CS. Iodine-deficiency disorders. *Lancet*, 2008; **372**: 1251–62.
50. Huang TS, Lu FJ, Tsai CW, Chopra IJ. Effect of humic acids on thyroidal function. *J Endocrinol Invest*, 1994; **17**: 787–91.
51. van Bakel MM, Printzen G, Wermuth B, Wiesmann UN. Antioxidant and thyroid hormone status in selenium-deficient phenylketonuric and hyperphenylalaninemic patients. *Am J Clin Nutr*, 2000; **72**: 976–81.
52. Croes K, Baeyens W, Bruckers L, Den Hond E, Koppen G, Nelen V, *et al.* Hormone levels and sexual development in Flemish adolescents residing in areas differing in pollution pressure. *Int J Hyg Environ Health*, 2009; **212**: 612–25.
53. Hofmann PJ, Schomburg L, Kohrle J. Interference of endocrine disrupters with thyroid hormone receptor-dependent transactivation. *Toxicol Sci*, 2009; **110**: 125–37.
54. Jugan ML, Oziol L, Bimbot M, Huteau V, Tamisier-Karolak S, Blondeau JP, *et al.* In vitro assessment of thyroid and estrogenic endocrine disruptors in wastewater treatment plants, rivers and drinking water supplies in the greater Paris area (France). *Sci Total Environ*, 2009; **407**: 3579–87.
55. Zoeller RT. Environmental chemicals impacting the thyroid: targets and consequences. *Thyroid*, 2007; **17**: 811–17.
56. Nakazawa T, Murata S, Kondo T, Nakamura N, Yamane T, Iwasa S, *et al.* Histopathology of the thyroid in amiodarone-induced hypothyroidism. *Pathol Int*, 2008; **58**: 55–8.
57. Schweizer U, Chiu J, Kohrle J. Peroxides and peroxide-degrading enzymes in the thyroid. *Antioxid Redox Signal*, 2008; **10**: 1577–92.
58. Abdelouahab N, Mergler D, Takser L, Vanier C, St Jean M, Baldwin M, *et al.* Gender differences in the effects of organochlorines, mercury, and lead on thyroid hormone levels in lakeside communities of Quebec (Canada). *Environ Res*, 2008; **107**: 380–92.
59. Jonklaas J, Soldin SJ. Tandem mass spectrometry as a novel tool for elucidating pituitary-thyroid relationships. *Thyroid*, 2008; **18**: 1303–11.
60. Iijima K, Otake T, Yoshinaga J, Ikegami M, Suzuki E, Naruse H, *et al.* Cadmium, lead, and selenium in cord blood and thyroid hormone status of newborns. *Biol Trace Elem Res*, 2007; **119**: 10–18.
61. Soldin OP, Aschner M. Effects of manganese on thyroid hormone homeostasis: potential links. *Neurotoxicology*, 2007; **28**: 951–6.
62. Whanger PD. Selenium and the brain: a review. *Nutr Neurosci*, 2001; **4**: 81–97.
63. Hammouda F, Messaoudi I, El Hani J, Baati T, Said K, Kerkeni A. Reversal of cadmium-induced thyroid dysfunction by selenium, zinc, or their combination in rat. *Biol Trace Elem Res*, 2008; **126**: 194–203.
64. Maes M, Mommen K, Hendrickx D, Peeters D, D'Hondt P, Ranjan R, *et al.* Components of biological variation, including seasonality, in blood concentrations of TSH, TT3, FT4, PRL, cortisol and testosterone in healthy volunteers. *Clin Endocrinol (Oxf)*, 1997; **46**: 587–98.
65. Russell W, Harrison RF, Smith N, Darzy K, Shalet S, Weetman AP, *et al.* Free triiodothyronine has a distinct circadian rhythm that is delayed but parallels thyrotropin levels. *J Clin Endocrinol Metab*, 2008; **93**:2300–6.
66. Do NV, Mino L, Merriam GR, LeMar H, Case HS, Palinkas LA, *et al.* Elevation in serum thyroglobulin during prolonged Antarctic residence: effect of thyroxine supplement in the polar 3,5,3′-triiodothyronine syndrome. *J Clin Endocrinol Metab*, 2004; **89**: 1529–33.
67. Bellastella A, Pisano G, Iorio S, Pasquali D, Orio F, Venditto T, *et al.* Endocrine secretions under abnormal light-dark cycles and in the blind. *Horm Res*, 1998; **49**: 153–7.
68. Scanlan TS. Minireview: 3-iodothyronamine (T1AM): a new player on the thyroid endocrine team?. *Endocrinology*, 2009; **150**: 1108–11.
69. Ljunggren JG, Kallner G, Tryselius M. The effect of body temperature on thyroid hormone levels in patients with non-thyroidal illness. *Acta Med Scand*, 1977; **202**: 459–62.
70. Epstein Y, Udassin R, Sack J. Serum 3,5,3'-triiodothyronine and 3,3',5'-triiodothyronine concentrations during acute heat load. *J Clin Endocrinol Metab*, 1979; **49**: 677–8.

3.2.3 Iodine deficiency disorders

Michael B. Zimmermann

Dietary sources and metabolism

Iodine (atomic weight 126.9 g/mol) is an essential component of the hormones produced by the thyroid gland. Thyroid hormones, and therefore iodine, are essential for mammalian life (1). The native iodine content of most foods and beverages is low, and the most commonly consumed foods provide 3–80 μg/serving (1). The major dietary sources of iodine in the United States of America and Europe are bread and milk (2). Boiling, baking, and canning of foods containing iodized salt cause only small losses (≤10%) of iodine content. The iodine content in foods is also influenced by iodine-containing compounds used in irrigation, fertilizers, livestock feed, dairy industry disinfectants, and bakery dough conditioners. The recommendations for iodine intake by age and population group (3) are shown in Table 3.2.3.1.

Iodide is rapidly and nearly completely absorbed (>90%) in the stomach and duodenum (4). Iodate, widely used in salt iodization, is reduced in the gut and absorbed as iodide. Thyroid clearance of circulating iodine varies with iodine intake; in conditions of adequate iodine supply, no more than 10% of absorbed iodine is taken up by the thyroid. In chronic iodine deficiency, this fraction can exceed 80% (1). Under normal circumstances, plasma iodine has a half-life of about 10 h, but this is reduced in iodine deficiency. During lactation, the mammary gland concentrates iodine and secretes it into breast milk to provide for the newborn. The body of a healthy adult contains 15–20 mg iodine, of which 70–80% is in the thyroid. In chronic iodine deficiency, the iodine content of the thyroid may fall to less than 20 μg. In iodine-sufficient areas, the adult thyroid traps about 60 μg iodine/day to balance losses and maintain thyroid hormone synthesis; the sodium-iodide symporter (NIS), transfers iodide into the thyroid at a concentration gradient 20–50 times that of plasma (5). Iodine comprises 65 and 59% of the weights of thyroxine (T_4) and triiodothyronine (T_3), respectively. Turnover is relatively slow; the half-life of T_4 is approximately 5 days and for T_3 it is 1.5–3 days. The released iodine enters the plasma iodine pool and can be taken up again by the thyroid or excreted by the kidney. More than 90% of ingested iodine is ultimately excreted in the urine.

Table 3.2.3.1 Recommendations for iodine intake (μg/day) by age or population group

Age or population group[a]	US Institute of Medicine (4)	Age or population group[c]	World Health Organization (3)
Infants 0–12 months[b]	110–130	Children 0–5 years	90
Children 1–8 years	90	Children 6–12 years	120
Children 9–13 years	120		
Adults ≥14 years	150	Adults >12 years	150
Pregnancy	220	Pregnancy	250
Lactation	290	Lactation	250

[a] Recommended daily allowance.
[b] Adequate intake.
[c] Recommended nutrient intake.

Historical perspective

In 1811, Courtois noted a violet vapour rising from burning seaweed ash, and Gay-Lussac subsequently identified the vapour as iodine, a new element. The Swiss physician Coindet, in 1813, hypothesized the traditional treatment of goitre with seaweed was effective because of its iodine content, and successfully treated goitrous patients with iodine (6). Two decades later, the French chemist Boussingault, working in the Andes Mountains, was the first to advocate prophylaxis with iodine-rich salt to prevent goitre. The French chemist Chatin was the first to publish, in 1851, the hypothesis that iodine deficiency was the cause of goitre. In 1883, Semon suggested myxoedema was due to thyroid insufficiency, and the link between goitre, myxoedema, and iodine was established when, in 1896, Baumann and Roos discovered iodine in the thyroid. In the first two decades of the 20th century, pioneering studies by Swiss and American physicians demonstrated the efficacy of iodine prophylaxis in the prevention of goitre and cretinism (6).

Epidemiology

Only a few countries—Switzerland, some of the Scandinavian countries, Australia, the United States of America, and Canada—were completely iodine sufficient before 1990. Since then, globally, the number of households using iodized salt has risen from less than 20% to over 70%, dramatically reducing iodine deficiency. This effort has been spurred on by a coalition of international organizations, including the International Council for the Control of Iodine Deficiency Disorders (ICCIDD), WHO, Micronutrient Initiative (MI), and Unicef, working closely with national iodine deficiency disorders (IDD) control committees and the salt industry; this informal partnership was established after the World Summit for Children in 1990.

In 2007, the WHO estimated nearly two billion individuals had an insufficient iodine intake, including one-third of all school-age children (7) (Table 3.2.3.2)). The lowest prevalence of iodine deficiency is in the Americas (10.6%), where the proportion of households consuming iodized salt is the highest in the world (*c.*90%). The highest prevalence of iodine deficiency is in Europe (52.0%), where the household coverage with iodized salt is the lowest (*c.*25%), and many of these countries have weak or nonexistent IDD control programmes. The number of countries where iodine deficiency remains a public health problem is 47. However, there has been progress since 2003; 12 countries have progressed to optimal iodine status and the percentage of school-age children at risk of iodine deficiency has decreased by 5%. However, iodine intake is more than adequate, or even excessive, in 34 countries, an increase from 27 in 2003. In Australia and the USA, two countries previously iodine sufficient, iodine intakes are falling. Much of Australia is now mildly iodine deficient, and in the USA the median urinary iodine is 160 μg/l, still adequate but one-half the median value of 321 μg/l found in the 1970s (8). These changes emphasize the

Table 3.2.3.2 Prevalence of iodine deficiency, as total number (millions) and percentages, in general population (all age groups) and in school-age children (6–12 years) in 2007

WHO regions[a]	Population with urinary iodine <100 μg/l[b]	
	General population	**School-age children**
Africa	312.9 (41.5)	57.7 (40.8)
Americas	98.6 (11.0)	11.6 (10.6)
Eastern Mediterranean	259.3 (47.2)	43.3 (48.8)
Europe	459.7 (52.0)	38.7 (52.4)
Southeast Asia	503.6 (30.0)	73.1 (30.3)
Western Pacific	374.7 (21.2)	41.6 (22.7)
Total	2000.0 (30.6)	263.7 (31.5)

[a] 193 WHO member states.
[b] Based on population estimates for 2006 (United Nations, Population Division, World Population Prospects: the 2004 revision).

importance of regular monitoring of iodine status in countries to detect both low and excessive intakes of iodine.

There are several limitations to these WHO prevalence data. First, extrapolation from a population indicator (median urinary iodine) to define the number of individuals affected is problematic, e.g. a country in which the children have a median urinary iodine of 100 μg/l would be classified as being iodine sufficient, yet at the same time 50% of children would be classified as having inadequate iodine intakes. Second, nationally representative surveys represent only 60% of the global population included in the WHO data, and subnational data may under- or overestimate the extent of iodine deficiency (7). Finally, there are insufficient data from nearly all countries to estimate the prevalence of iodine deficiency in pregnant women.

Pathogenesis and pathology

Iodine deficiency has multiple adverse effects on growth and development in animals and humans. These are collectively termed the IDD (Table 3.2.3.3) and they result from inadequate thyroid hormone production due to lack of sufficient iodine (1).

Goitre

Thyroid enlargement (goitre) is the classic sign of iodine deficiency and can occur at any age, even in the newborn. It is a physiological adaptation to chronic iodine deficiency. As iodine intake falls, secretion of thyroid-stimulating hormone (TSH) increases in an effort to maximize uptake of available iodine, and TSH stimulates thyroid hypertrophy and hyperplasia. Initially, goitres are characterized by diffuse homogeneous enlargement, but, over time, nodules often develop (Fig. 3.2.3.1). Many thyroid nodules derive from a somatic mutation and are of monoclonal origin; the mutations appear to be more likely to result in nodules under the influence of a growth promoter, such as iodine deficiency. Iodine deficiency is associated with a high occurrence of multinodular toxic goitre, mainly seen in women older than 50 years. Large goitres may be cosmetically unattractive, can obstruct the trachea and oesophagus, and may damage the recurrent laryngeal nerves and cause hoarseness. Surgery to reduce goitre has significant risks, including bleeding and nerve damage, and hypothyroidism may develop after removal of thyroid tissue.

Table 3.2.3.3 Iodine deficiency disorders, by age group (1)

Physiological groups	Health consequences of iodine deficiency
All ages	Goitre, including toxic nodular goitre
	Increased occurrence of hypothyroidism in moderate-to-severe iodine deficiency; decreased occurrence of hypothyroidism in mild-to-moderate iodine deficiency
	Increased susceptibility of the thyroid gland to nuclear radiation
Fetus	Abortion
	Stillbirth
	Congenital anomalies
	Perinatal mortality
Neonate	Infant mortality
	Endemic cretinism
Child and adolescent	Impaired mental function
	Delayed physical development
Adults	Impaired mental function
	Iodine-induced hyperthyroidism
	Overall, moderate-to-severe iodine deficiency causes subtle but widespread adverse effects in a population secondary to hypothyroidism, including decreased educability, apathy, and reduced work productivity, resulting in impaired social and economic development

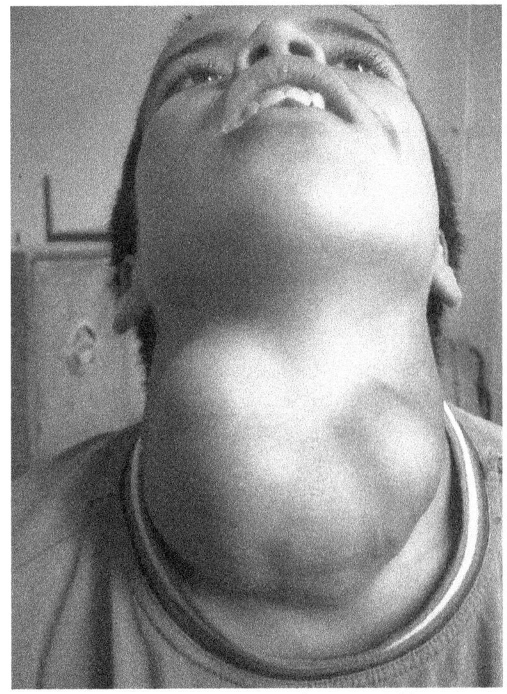

Photo: © MB Zimmermann

Fig. 3.2.3.1 Large nodular goitre in a 14-year-old boy photographed in 2004 in an area of severe IDD in northern Morocco, with tracheal and oesophageal compression and hoarseness, likely due to damage to the recurrent laryngeal nerves. (See also Plate 8)

(a)

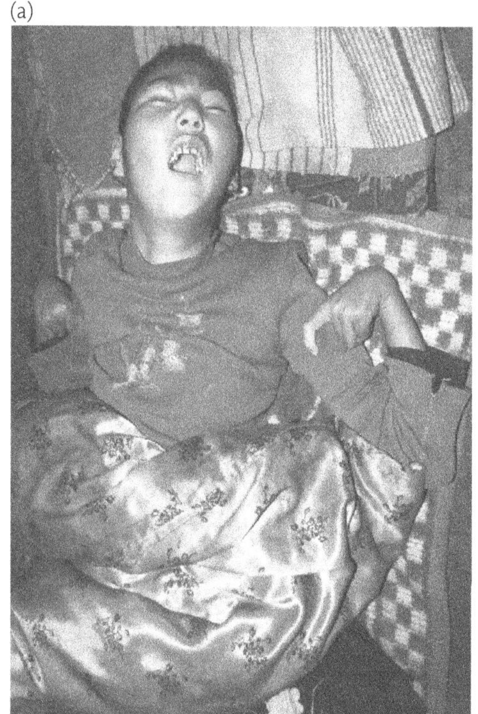

(b)

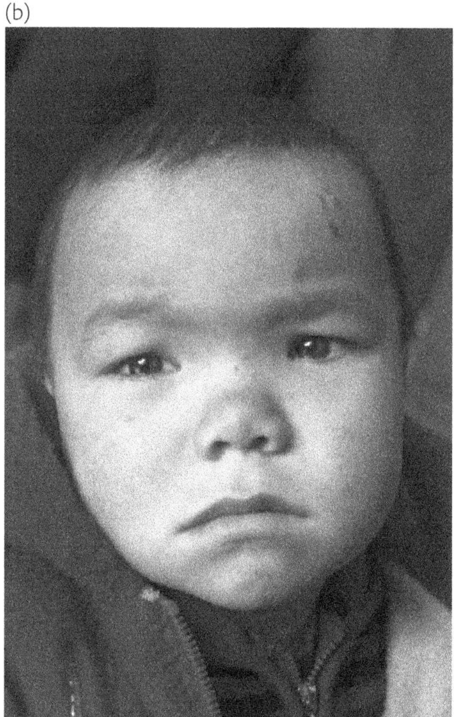

Photos: © MB Zimmermann

Fig. 3.2.3.2 (a) Neurological cretinism. This 2007 photograph of a 9-year-old girl from western China demonstrates the three characteristic features: severe mental deficiency together with squint, deaf–mutism, and motor spasticity of the arms and legs. The thyroid is present, and the frequency of goitre and thyroid dysfunction is similar to that observed in the general population. (b) Myxoedematous cretinism. This 2007 photograph of a 5-year-old boy from western China demonstrates the characteristic findings: profound hypothyroidism, severe growth impairment (height, 106cm), incomplete maturation of the features including the naso-orbital configuration, atrophy of the mandible, puffy features, myxoedematous thickened dry skin, and dry hair, eyelashes, and eyebrows. The thyroid typically shows atrophic fibrosis. (See also Plate 9)

Severe iodine deficiency in pregnancy: cretinism and increased fetal and perinatal mortality

The most serious adverse effect of iodine deficiency in pregnancy is damage to the fetus. Maternal thyroxine crosses the placenta before the onset of fetal thyroid function at 10–12 weeks and represents up to 20–40% of T_4 measured in cord blood at birth. Normal levels of thyroid hormones are required for neuronal migration and myelination of the fetal brain, and lack of iodine irreversibly impairs brain development (9). Severe iodine deficiency during pregnancy increases the risk for stillbirths, abortions, and congenital abnormalities (1). Iodine treatment of pregnant women in areas of severe deficiency reduces fetal and perinatal mortality and improves motor and cognitive performance of the offspring (10). Severe iodine deficiency *in utero* causes a condition characterized by gross mental impairment along with varying degrees of short stature, deaf-mutism, and spasticity that is termed cretinism (1). Two distinct types—neurological and myxoedematous—have been described, but it may also present as a mixed form (Figs. 3.2.3.2a, b). The more common neurological cretinism has specific neurological deficits that include spastic quadriplegia with sparing of the distal extremities. The myxoedematous form is seen most frequently in central Africa, and has the predominant finding of profound hypothyroidism with thyroid atrophy and fibrosis. In areas of severe iodine deficiency, cretinism can affect 5–15% of the population. Iodine prophylaxis has completely eliminated the appearance of new cases of cretinism in previously iodine-deficient Switzerland and many other countries, but it continues to occur in isolated areas of western China.

Mild-to-moderate deficiency in pregnancy

The potential adverse effects of mild-to-moderate iodine deficiency during pregnancy are unclear. Maternal subclinical hypothyroidism (an increased TSH in the second trimester) and maternal hypothyroxinaemia (a free T_4 concentration <10th percentile at 12 weeks gestation) are associated with impaired mental and psychomotor development of the offspring (12). However, in these studies, the maternal thyroid abnormalities were unlikely to have been due to iodine deficiency. In Europe, several randomized controlled trials of iodine supplementation in mild-to-moderately iodine-deficient pregnant women have been done (13). Iodine reduced maternal and newborn thyroid size, and, in some, decreased maternal TSH. However, none of the trials showed an effect on maternal and newborn total or free thyroid hormone concentrations, the most important outcome, and none measured long-term clinical outcomes, such as maternal goitre, thyroid autoimmunity, or child development (13).

Growth and cognition in childhood

Although iodine deficiency *in utero* impairs fetal growth and brain development, its postnatal effects on growth and cognition are less clear. Cross-sectional studies of moderate to severely iodine deficient children have generally reported impaired intellectual function and fine motor skills; meta-analyses suggest populations with chronic iodine deficiency experience a reduction in IQ of 12.5–13.5 points (14). However, observational studies are often confounded by other factors that affect child development, and these studies could not distinguish between the persistent effects of *in utero* iodine deficiency and the effects of current iodine status. In a controlled trial in 10- to 12-year-old moderately iodine deficient children who received oral iodized oil or placebo, iodine treatment significantly improved information processing, fine motor skills, and visual problem solving compared to placebo (15). Thus, in children born and raised in areas of iodine deficiency, cognitive impairment is at least partially reversible by iodine repletion (15).

Data from cross-sectional studies on iodine intake and child growth are mixed, with most studies finding modest positive correlations. In five Asian countries, household access to iodized salt was correlated with increased weight-for-age and mid-upper arm circumference in infancy (16). In iodine-deficient children, impaired thyroid function and goitre are inversely correlated with insulin-like growth factor (IGF)-1 and IGF binding protein 3 (IGFBP3) concentrations. Iodine repletion in school-age children increased IGF-1 and IGFBP3 and improved somatic growth (16).

Overall, iodine deficiency produces subtle but widespread adverse effects in a population, including decreased educability, apathy, and reduced work productivity, resulting in impaired social and economic development. Because mild-to-moderate iodine deficiency affects up to 30% of the global population (7) and can impair cognition, iodine deficiency is likely to be a common cause of preventable mental impairment worldwide. The International Child Development Steering Group identified iodine deficiency as one of four key global risk factors for impaired child development where the need for intervention is urgent (17).

Assessment and diagnosis

Four methods are generally recommended for assessment of iodine nutrition: (1) urinary iodine concentration, (2) the goitre rate, (3) serum TSH, and (4) serum thyroglobulin (3, 18). These indicators are complementary, in that urinary iodine is a sensitive indicator of recent iodine intake (days), thyroglobulin shows an intermediate response (weeks to months), while changes in the goitre rate reflect long-term iodine nutrition (months to years).

Thyroid size

Two methods are available for measuring goitre: (1) neck inspection and palpation and (2) thyroid ultrasonography. By palpation, a thyroid is considered goitrous when each lateral lobe has a volume greater than the terminal phalanx of the thumbs of the individual being examined (3). However, palpation of goitre in mild iodine deficiency has poor sensitivity and specificity, and measurement of thyroid volume by ultrasonography is preferable (18). Thyroid ultrasonography is noninvasive, quickly done (2–3 min/individual), and feasible even in remote areas using portable equipment. However, interpretation of thyroid volume data requires valid reference criteria and age- and gender-specific references are available for 6- to 12-year-old children (3), but there are no established reference values for adults. Goitre can be classified by thyroid ultrasonography only if thyroid volume is determined by a standard method. Thyroid ultrasound examination is subjective; differences in technique can produce interobserver errors in thyroid volume as high as 26% (18).

Urinary iodine concentration

Because more than 90% of ingested iodine is excreted in the urine, urinary iodine is an excellent indicator of recent iodine intake. Urinary iodine can be expressed as a concentration (micrograms/litre), in relation to creatinine excretion (micrograms iodine/gram creatinine), or as 24-h excretion (micrograms/day). For populations, because it is impractical to collect 24-h samples in field studies, urinary iodine can be measured in spot urine specimens from a representative sample of the target group and expressed as the median in micrograms/litre (3) (Table 3.2.3.4). However, the median urinary iodine is often misinterpreted. Individual iodine intakes and, therefore, spot urinary iodine concentrations are highly variable from day to day and a common mistake is to assume that all people with a spot urinary iodine of less than 100 μg/l are iodine deficient. To estimate iodine intakes in individuals, 24-h collections are preferable but difficult to obtain. An alternative is to use the age- and sex-adjusted iodine:creatinine ratio in adults, but this also has limitations (18). Creatinine may be unreliable for estimating daily iodine excretion from spot samples, especially in malnourished people where the creatinine concentration is low. Daily iodine intake can be extrapolated from the median urinary iodine in populations using estimates of mean 24-h urine volume and assuming an average iodine bioavailability of 92% using the following formula: urinary iodine (μg/l) × 0.0235 × body weight (kg) = daily iodine intake (4). Using this formula, a median urinary iodine of 100 μg/l in adults corresponds roughly to an average daily intake of 150 μg.

Table 3.2.3.4 Epidemiological criteria for assessing iodine nutrition in a population based on median and/or range of urinary iodine concentrations (3)

Median urinary iodine (μg/l)	Iodine intake	Iodine nutrition
School-age children		
<20	Insufficient	Severe iodine deficiency
20–49	Insufficient	Moderate iodine deficiency
50–99	Insufficient	Mild iodine deficiency
100–199	Adequate	Optimal
200–299	More than adequate	Risk of iodine-induced hyperthyroidism in susceptible groups
>300	Excessive	Risk of adverse health consequences (iodine-induced hyperthyroidism, autoimmune thyroid disease)
Pregnant women		
<150	Insufficient	
150–249	Adequate	
250–499	More than adequate	
≥500	Excessive[a]	
Lactating women[b]		
<100	Insufficient	
≥100	Adequate	
Children less than 2 years old		
<100	Insufficient	
≥100	Adequate	

[a] The term 'excessive' means in excess of the amount required to prevent and control iodine deficiency.

[b] In lactating women, the figures for median urinary iodine are lower than the iodine requirements because of the iodine excreted in breast milk.

Thyroid-stimulating hormone

Because serum TSH is determined mainly by the level of circulating thyroid hormone, which in turn reflects iodine intake, TSH can be used as an indicator of iodine nutrition. However, in older children and adults, although serum TSH may be slightly increased by iodine deficiency, values often remain within the normal range. TSH is therefore a relatively insensitive indicator of iodine nutrition in adults (3). In contrast, TSH is a sensitive indicator of iodine status in the neonatal period. Compared to the adult, the thyroid in the newborn contains less iodine but has higher rates of iodine turnover. Particularly when iodine supply is low, maintaining high iodine turnover requires increased TSH stimulation. Serum TSH concentrations are, therefore, increased in iodine-deficient infants for the first few weeks of life, a condition termed transient newborn hypothyroidism. In areas of iodine deficiency, an increase in transient newborn hypothyroidism, indicated by more than 3% of newborn TSH values above the threshold of 5 mU/l whole blood collected 3–4 days after birth, suggests iodine deficiency in the population (3). Newborn TSH is an important measure because it reflects iodine status during a period when the developing brain is particularly sensitive to iodine deficiency.

Thyroglobulin

Thyroglobulin is synthesized only in the thyroid, and is the most abundant intrathyroidal protein. In iodine sufficiency, small amounts of thyroglobulin are secreted into the circulation, and serum thyroglobulin is normally less than 10 μg/l (18). In iodine deficiency, serum thyroglobulin increases due to greater thyroid cell mass and TSH stimulation. Serum thyroglobulin is well correlated with the severity of iodine deficiency, as measured by urinary iodine. Thyroglobulin falls rapidly with iodine repletion, and is a more sensitive indicator of iodine repletion than TSH or T_4 (18).

A new assay for thyroglobulin has been developed for dried blood spots taken by a finger prick, thus simplifying collection and transport (19). In prospective studies, dried blood spot thyroglobulin has been shown to be a sensitive measure of iodine status and reflects improved thyroid function within several months after iodine repletion (19). However, several questions need to be resolved before thyroglobulin can be widely adopted as an indicator of iodine status, including the need for concurrent measurement of antithyroglobulin antibodies to avoid potential underestimation of thyroglobulin; it is unclear how prevalent antithyroglobulin antibodies are in iodine deficiency, or whether they are precipitated by iodine prophylaxis. Another limitation is large interassay variability and poor reproducibility, even with the use of standardization. This has made it difficult to establish normal ranges and/or cut-offs to distinguish severity of iodine deficiency. However, an international reference range and a reference standard for dried blood spot thyroglobulin in iodine-sufficient school-age children (4–40 μg/l) is now available (19).

Thyroid hormone concentrations

Thyroid hormone concentrations (T_4 and T_3) are poor indicators of iodine intake. In iodine-deficient individuals, serum T_3 increases or remains unchanged and serum T_4 usually decreases. However, these changes are often within the normal range and make thyroid hormone levels an insensitive measure of iodine nutrition, except in areas of severe IDD (3).

Prevention and treatment

Salt fortification with iodine

In nearly all regions affected by iodine deficiency, the most effective way to control iodine deficiency is through salt iodization (3). Universal salt iodization (USI) is a term used to describe the iodization of all salt for human (food industry and household) and livestock consumption. Although the ideal, USI is rarely achieved, even in countries with successful salt iodization programmes, as food industries are often reluctant to use iodized salt and many countries do not iodize salt for livestock.

WHO/UNICEF/ICCIDD recommend that iodine is added at a level of 20–40 mg iodine/kg salt, depending on local salt intake (3). Iodine can be added to salt in the form of potassium iodide (KI) or potassium iodate (KIO_3). Because KIO_3 has higher stability than KI in the presence of salt impurities, humidity, and porous packaging, it is the recommended form in tropical countries and those with low-grade salt. Iodine is usually added after the salt has been dried. Two techniques are used: (1) the wet method, where a solution of KIO_3 is dripped or sprayed at a regular rate onto salt passing by on a conveyor belt, or (2) the dry method, where KI or KIO_3 powder is sprinkled over the dry salt. Optimally, packaging should be in low-density polyethylene bags, as high humidity combined with porous packing may result in up to 90% loss of iodine after 1 year of storage in high-density polyethylene bags.

Health economics of salt iodization

Salt iodization remains the most cost-effective way of delivering iodine and of improving cognition in iodine-deficient populations (11, 20). Worldwide, the annual costs of salt iodization are estimated at US$0.02–0.05 per child covered, and the costs per child death averted are US$1000 and per disability-adjusted life year

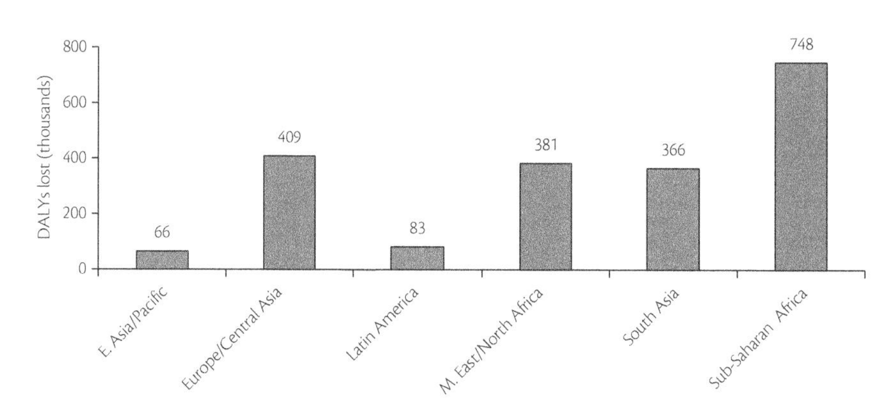

Fig. 3.2.3.3 Disability-adjusted life years (DALYs) (thousands) lost due to iodine deficiency among children under 5 years of age, by region. A DALY is calculated as the present value of the future years of disability-free life that are lost as a result of the premature deaths or cases of disability occurring in a particular year (data from Caulfield *et al.* (11)).

(DALY) gained are US$34–36 (Fig. 3.2.3.3) (11). Looked at in another way, before widespread salt iodization, the annual potential losses attributable to iodine deficiency in the developing world have been estimated to be US$35.7 billion as compared with an estimated US$0.5 billion annual cost for salt iodization, i.e. a 70:1 benefit:cost ratio (1). The World Bank (20) strongly recommends that governments invest in micronutrient programmes, including salt iodization, to promote development, and concludes: 'Probably no other technology offers as large an opportunity to improve lives at such low cost and in such a short time.'

Supplementation

In some regions, iodization of salt may not be practical for control of iodine deficiency, at least in the short term. This may occur in remote areas where communications are poor or where there are numerous small-scale salt producers. In these areas, iodized oil supplements can be used (3). Iodized oil is prepared by esterification of the unsaturated fatty acids in seed or vegetable oils and addition of iodine to the double bonds. It can be given orally or by intramuscular injection (3). The intramuscular route has a longer duration of action, but oral administration is more common because it is simpler. Usual dosages are 200–400 mg iodine/year and it is often targeted to women of child-bearing age, pregnant women, and children (3) (Table 3.2.3.5). Its disadvantages are an uneven level of iodine in the body over time and the need for direct contact with individuals with the accompanying increased programme costs.

Table 3.2.3.5 Recommendations for iodine supplementation in pregnancy and infancy in areas where less than 90% of households are using iodized salt and the median urinary iodine is less than 100 µg/l in school-age children (3)

Target group	Recommended dosage
Women of child-bearing age	A single annual oral dose of 400 mg iodine as iodized oil OR A daily oral dose of iodine as KI should be given so that the total iodine intake meets the RNI of 150 µg/day iodine
Women who are pregnant or lactating	A single annual oral dose of 400 mg iodine as iodized oil OR A daily oral dose of iodine as KI should be given so that the total iodine intake meets the new RNI of 250 µg/day iodine NB: Iodine supplements should not be given to a woman who has already been given iodized oil during her current pregnancy or up to 3 months before her current pregnancy started
Children aged 0–6 months	A single oral dose of 100 mg iodine as iodized oil OR A daily oral dose of iodine as KI should be given so that the total iodine intake meets the RNI of 90 µg/day iodine NB: These children should be given iodine supplements only if the mother was not supplemented during pregnancy or if the child is not being breastfed
Children aged 7–24 months	A single annual oral dose of 200 mg iodine as iodized oil as soon as possible after reaching 7 months of age OR A daily oral dose of iodine as KI should be given so that the total iodine intake meets the RNI of 90 µg/day iodine

RNI, recommended nutritional intake.

Iodine can also be given as KI or KIO_3 in drops or tablets. Single oral doses of KI monthly (30 mg) or biweekly (8 mg) can provide adequate iodine for school-age children (21). Lugol's iodine, containing approximately 6 mg iodine/drop, and similar preparations are often available as antiseptics in rural dispensaries in developing countries and offer another simple way to deliver iodine locally. In countries or regions where a salt iodization programme covers at least 90% of households, has been sustained for at least 2 years, and the median urinary iodine indicates iodine sufficiency (Table 3.2.3.4), pregnant and lactating women do not need iodine supplementation (3). In iodine-deficient countries or regions that have weak iodized salt distribution, supplements should be given to pregnant women, lactating women, and infants, according to the guidelines in Table 3.2.3.5 (3).

Clinical nutrition

Preterm infants

Balance studies in healthy preterm infants have suggested iodine intakes of at least 30 µg/kg body weight per day are required to maintain positive balance, and experts generally recommend iodine intakes of 30–60 µg/kg per day for this group (22, 23). Formula milks for preterm infants contain 20–170 µg iodine/l, and, depending on the dietary iodine intake of the mother, breast milk generally contains 50–150 µg/l. Thus, particularly during the first postnatal weeks when feed volumes are often low, enterally fed preterm infants may not achieve the recommended intake of iodine (23). US and European clinical nutrition societies recommend parenteral iodine intakes of 1 µg/kg body weight per day (24), far below fetal accretion rates. This conservative recommendation assumes parenterally fed preterm infants will absorb iodine through the skin from topical iodinated disinfectants, and also receive small amounts of adventitious iodine in other infusions. Frequent use of iodinated antiseptics in infants can result in transcutaneous absorption of at least 100 µg iodine/day, iodine excess, and neonatal hypothyroidism.

Because of concerns over possible iodine excess, use of iodinated antiseptics in infants may be decreasing, putting infants at risk of iodine deficiency (25). If parentally fed preterm infants are not exposed to adventitious sources of iodine, they may receive only 1–3 µg iodine/kg body weight per day, and be in negative iodine balance during the first few postnatal weeks (23). Several authors have argued that iodine deficiency should be avoided during this period because it may transiently lower thyroid hormone levels in the first weeks of life (23, 25), and transient hypothyroxinaemia in preterm infants has been linked to impaired neurodevelopment (26). However, a recent review concluded that the available data are insufficient to support supplementation of preterm infants with iodine (26).

Childhood

A daily dose of 1 µg iodine/kg body weight is recommended for children receiving parenteral nutrition (24), and parenteral trace element additives containing iodine are available for paediatric use. An example is Peditrace solution (Fresenius Kabi, Bad Homburg, Germany), which contains KI (1.3 µg/ml KI equivalent to 1 µg iodide/ml); the recommended dosage for infants and children weighing 15 kg or less, and 2 days old or older, is 1 ml/kg body weight per day, and the recommended daily dose is 15 ml to children weighing more than 15 kg.

Adults

Commercially available products for enteral nutrition generally supply 75–110 μg iodine/serving. A recent technical review recommended iodine intakes of 70–140 μg/day during parenteral nutrition (27). Although most parenteral nutrition formulations do not contain iodine, deficiency is not likely to occur because of cutaneous absorption from iodine-containing disinfectants and other adventitious sources of iodine. Iodine deficiency symptoms have not been reported with inhospital intravenous nutrition support. It is likely that thyroidal iodine stores are often adequate to meet the needs of patients requiring total parenteral nutrition for less than 3 months; in iodine-sufficient adults, thyroidal iodine content may be as high as 15–20 mg (1). For these reasons, supplemental iodine is not routinely recommended for patients receiving total parenteral nutrition (28). If needed, intravenous sodium iodide solutions are available. For example, Iodopen (APP Pharmaceuticals, Schaumberg, IL, USA) contains 100 μg iodine/ml, and the usual adult dosage for prophylaxis or treatment of iodine deficiency in adults is 1–2 μg iodine/kg body weight per day; for children and pregnant or lactating women, the recommended dosage is 2–3 μg iodine/kg per day.

Iodine intake and thyroid disorders in populations

Prospective data on the epidemiology of thyroid disorders caused by changes in iodine intake is scarce. In areas of iodine sufficiency, healthy individuals are remarkably tolerant to iodine intakes of up to 1 mg/day, as the thyroid is able to adjust to a wide range of intakes to regulate the synthesis and release of thyroid hormones. European (29) and US (4) expert committees have recommended tolerable upper intake levels for iodine, but caution that individuals with chronic iodine deficiency may respond adversely to intakes lower than these. In monitoring populations consuming iodized salt, the WHO/UNICEF/ICCIDD recommendations for the median urinary iodine that indicates more than adequate and excess iodine intake (3) are shown in Table 3.2.3.4.

To investigate the effects of iodine intake on thyroid disorders in China, a 5-year prospective community-based survey was carried out in three rural Chinese communities with mildly deficient, more than adequate (previously mild iodine deficiency corrected by iodized salt), and excessive iodine intake from environmental sources; the median urinary iodine was 88, 214, and 634 μg/l, respectively. For the three communities, the cumulative incidence of hyperthyroidism was 1.4, 0.9, and 0.8%; of overt hypothyroidism, 0.2, 0.5, and 0.3%; of subclinical hypothyroidism, 0.2, 2.6, and 2.9%; and of autoimmune thyroiditis, 0.2, 1.0, and 1.3%, respectively. In most individuals, these last two disorders were not sustained (30).

Denmark has documented the pattern of thyroid disease after careful introduction of iodized salt. New cases of overt hypothyroidism were identified in two areas of Denmark with previously moderate and mild iodine deficiency (Aalborg, median urinary iodine = 45 μg/l, and Copenhagen, median urinary iodine = 61 μg/l) before and for the first 7 years after introduction of a national programme of salt iodization. The overall incidence rate of hypothyroidism modestly increased during the study period: baseline 38.3/100 000 per year; after salt iodization 47.2/100 000 (versus baseline, relative risk = 1.23; 95% CI = 1.07 to 1.42). There was a geographical difference because hypothyroidism increased only in the area with previous moderate iodine deficiency. The increase occurred in young and middle-aged adults. Similarly, new cases of overt hyperthyroidism in these two areas of Denmark before and for the first 6 years after iodine fortification were identified. The overall incidence rate of hyperthyroidism increased (baseline 102.8/100 000 per year; after salt iodization 138.7/100 000). Hyperthyroidism increased in both sexes and in all age groups, but many of the new cases were observed in young people—the increase was highest in adults aged 20–39 years—and were presumably of autoimmune origin (30).

The overall incidence of differentiated thyroid carcinoma in populations does not appear to be influenced by iodine intake. The distribution of the subtypes of thyroid carcinoma is related to iodine intake (30); in areas of higher iodine intake, there appear to be fewer of the more aggressive follicular and anaplastic carcinomas, but more papillary carcinomas. When iodine prophylaxis is introduced in populations, there may be an increase in the ratio of papillary to follicular carcinoma, and this shift towards less malignant types of thyroid cancer, as well as a lower radiation dose to the thyroid in case of nuclear fallout, are benefits of the correction of mild-to-moderate iodine deficiency.

Summary

Globally, two billion individuals have inadequate iodine intake. Iodine deficiency has multiple adverse effects on growth and development due to inadequate thyroid hormone production; these effects are termed the IDD. The most serious adverse effect of iodine deficiency is damage to the fetus, and iodine deficiency remains one of the most common causes of preventable mental impairment worldwide. Four methods are generally recommended for assessment of iodine nutrition: (1) urinary iodine concentration, (2) the goitre rate, (3) blood concentration of TSH, and (4) blood concentration of thyroglobulin. Iodine repletion in pregnant women reduces fetal and perinatal mortality and improves motor and cognitive performance of the offspring. In children born and raised in areas of iodine deficiency, cognitive impairment is at least partially reversible by iodine repletion. Iodine repletion also increases circulating IGF and improves somatic growth in children. In nearly all countries, the best strategy to control iodine deficiency is salt iodization, one of the most cost-effective ways to contribute to economic and social development. When salt iodization is not possible, iodine supplements can be targeted to vulnerable groups. Daily iodine requirements in adult patients receiving total enteral or parenteral nutrition are estimated to be 70–150 μg. Although most parenteral nutrition formulations do not contain iodine, deficiency is not likely to occur because of cutaneous absorption from iodine-containing disinfectants and other adventitious sources of iodine. Because of concerns over possible iodine excess, use of iodinated antiseptics in infants may be decreasing, potentially increasing the risk of iodine deficiency in this group. However, the available data are insufficient to support supplementation of preterm infants with iodine. Iodine intakes up to 1 mg/day are well tolerated by most adults, as the thyroid is able to adjust to a wide range of intakes and to regulate the synthesis and release of thyroid hormones. The introduction of iodine to regions of chronic IDD may transiently increase the incidence of thyroid disorders, but overall, the relatively small risks of iodine excess are far outweighed by the substantial risks of iodine deficiency.

References

1. Zimmermann MB, Jooste PL, Pandav CS. The iodine deficiency disorders. *Lancet*, 2008; **372**: 1251–62.
2. Haldimann M, Alt A, Blanc A, K. Blondeau. Iodine content of food groups. *J Food Comp and Anal*, 2005; **18**: 461–71.
3. World Health Organization/International Council for the Control of the Iodine Deficiency Disorders/United Nations Children's Fund. *Assessment of the Iodine Deficiency Disorders and Monitoring their Elimination*. 2nd edn. Geneva: WHO, 2007.
4. Institute of Medicine (IOM), Academy of Sciences, USA. *Dietary Reference Intakes for Vitamin A, Vitamin K, Arsenic, Boron, Chromium, Copper, Iodine, Iron, Manganese, Molybdenum, Nickel, Silicon, Vanadium and Zinc*. Washington DC: National Academy Press, 2001.
5. Eskandari S, Loo DD, Dai G, Levy O, Wright EM, Carrasco N. Thyroid Na^+/I^- symporter. Mechanism, stoichiometry, and specificity. *J Biol Chem*, 1997; **272**: 27230–8.
6. Zimmermann MB. Research on iodine deficiency and goiter in the 19th and early 20th centuries. *J Nutr*, 2008; **138**: 2060–3.
7. de Benoist B, McLean E, Andersson M, Rogers L. Iodine deficiency in 2007: global progress since 2003. *Food Nutr Bull*, 2008; **29**: 195–202.
8. Caldwell KL, Miller GA, Wang RY, Jain RB, Jones RL. Iodine status of the U.S. population, National Health and Nutrition Examination Survey 2003–2004. *Thyroid*, 2008; **18**: 1207–14.
9. Morreale de Escobar G, Obregon MJ, Escobar del Rey F. Role of thyroid hormone during early brain development. *Eur J Endocrinol*, 2004; **151**: 25–37.
10. Cao XY, Jiang XM, Dou ZH, Rakeman MA, Zhang ML, O'Donnell K, *et al.* Timing of vulnerability of the brain to iodine deficiency in endemic cretinism. *N Engl J Med*, 1994; **331**: 1739–44.
11. Caulfield LE, Richard SA, Rivera JA, Musgrove P, Black RE. Stunting, wasting, and micronutrient deficiency disorders. In: Dean T, Jamison DT, Breman JG, Measham AR, Alleyne G, Claeson M, *et al.*, eds. *Disease Control Priorities in Developing Countries*. 2nd edn. New York: Oxford University Press, 2006: 551–68.
12. Haddow JE, Palomaki GE, Allan WC, Williams JR, Knight GJ, Gagnon J, *et al.* Maternal thyroid deficiency during pregnancy and subsequent neuropsychological development of the child. *N Engl J Med*, 1999; **341**: 549–55.
13. Zimmermann MB. The adverse effects of mild-to-moderate iodine deficiency during pregnancy and childhood: a review. *Thyroid*, 2007; **17**: 829–35.
14. Bleichrodt N, Garcia I, Rubio C, Morreale de Escobar G, Escobar del Rey F. Developmental disorders associated with severe iodine deficiency. In: Hetzel B, Dunn J, Stanbury J, eds. *The Prevention and Control of Iodine Deficiency Disorders*. Amsterdam: Elsevier, 1987: 65–84.
15. Zimmermann MB, Connolly K, Bozo M, Bridson J, Rohner F, Grimci L. Iodine supplementation improves cognition in iodine-deficient schoolchildren in Albania: a randomized, controlled, double-blind study. *Am J Clin Nutr*, 2006; **83**: 108–14.
16. Zimmermann MB, Jooste PL, Mabapa NS, Mbhenyane X, Schoeman S, Biebinger R, *et al.* Treatment of iodine deficiency in school-age children increases insulin-like growth factor (IGF)-I and IGF binding protein-3 concentrations and improves somatic growth. *J Clin Endocrinol Metab*, 2007; **92**: 437–42.
17. Walker SP, Wachs TD, Gardner JM, Lozoff B, Wasserman GA, Pollitt E, *et al.* Child development: risk factors for adverse outcomes in developing countries. *Lancet*, 2007; **369**: 145–57.
18. Zimmermann MB. Methods to assess iron and iodine status. *Br J Nutr*, 2008; **99**: 2–9.
19. Zimmermann MB, de Benoist B, Corigliano S, Jooste PL, Molinari L, Moosa K, *et al.* Assessment of iodine status using dried blood spot thyroglobulin: development of reference material and establishment of an international reference range in iodine-sufficient children. *J Clin Endocrinol Metab*, 2006; **91**: 4881–7.
20. McGuire J, Galloway R. *Enriching Lives. Overcoming Vitamin and Mineral Malnutrition in Developing Countries*. Washington, DC: World Bank, 1994.
21. Todd CH, Dunn JT. Intermittent oral administration of potassium iodide solution for the correction of iodine deficiency. *Am J Clin Nutr*, 1998; **67**: 1279–83.
22. Zimmermann MB, Crill CM. Iodine in enteral and parenteral nutrition. *Best Pract Res Clin Endocrinol Metab*, 2010; **24**(1):143–58.
23. Ares S, Escobar-Morreale HF, Quero J, Durán S, Presas MJ, Herruzo R, *et al.* Neonatal hypothyroxinemia: effects of iodine intake and premature birth. *J Clin Endocrinol Metab*, 1997; **82**: 1704–12.
24. Koletzko B, Goulet O, Hunt J, Krohn K, Shamir R; Parenteral Nutrition Guidelines Working Group; *et al.* Guidelines on paediatric parenteral nutrition of the European Society of Paediatric Gastroenterology, Hepatology and Nutrition (ESPGHAN) and the European Society for Clinical Nutrition and Metabolism (ESPEN), supported by the European Society of Paediatric Research (ESPR). *J Pediatr Gastroenterol Nutr*, 2005; **41** (Suppl 2): 1–87.
25. Rogahn J, Ryan S, Wells J, Fraser B, Squire C, Wild N, *et al.* Randomised trial of iodine intake and thyroid status in preterm infants. *Arch Dis Child Fetal Neonatal Ed*, 2000; **83**: F86–90.
26. Ibrahim M, Sinn J, McGuire W. Iodine supplementation for the prevention of mortality and adverse neurodevelopmental outcomes in preterm infants. *Cochrane Database of Syst Rev*, 2006; **2**: CD005253.
27. Koretz RL, Lipman TO, Klein S, American Gastroenterological Association. AGA technical review on parenteral nutrition. *Gastroenterology*, 2001; **121**: 970–1001.
28. Atkinson M, Worthley LI. Nutrition in the critically ill patient: part II. Parenteral nutrition. *Crit Care Resusc*, 2003; **5**: 121–36.
29. European Commission HaCPD-GSCoF. *Opinion of the Scientific Committee on Food on the Tolerable Upper Level of Intake Of iodine*. Brussels: European Commission, 2002.
30. Zimmermann MB. Iodine requirements and the risks and benefits of correcting iodine deficiency in populations. *J Trace Elem Med Biol*, 2008; **22**: 81–92.

3.2.4 Disorders of iodine excess

Shigenobu Nagataki, Misa Imaizumi, and Noboru Takamura

Introduction

Iodine is an essential substrate for the biosynthesis of thyroid hormone because both thyroxine (T_4) and triiodothyronine (T_3) contain iodine. An adequate supply of dietary iodine is therefore necessary for the maintenance of normal thyroid function. Dietary iodine intake is increasing in many regions, especially in developed countries, mainly due to iodization of salt or bread, and it is well known that various drugs and foods contain large quantities of iodine (1), e.g. seaweeds, such as konbu (*Laminaria japonica*), contain

0.3% of iodine dry weight. Furthermore, large doses of iodine are used for prophylaxis against exposure to ^{131}I. Excess iodine, as well as iodine deficiency, can induce thyroid dysfunction. The response of the thyroid gland to excess iodine and disorders due to excess iodine are the main subject of this chapter.

Thyroid autoregulation

The thyroid gland has intrinsic mechanisms responsive to variations in the quantity of iodine available and often to the resulting changes in thyroidal organic iodine content. Autoregulation was originally defined as a regulation of thyroidal iodine metabolism independent of thyroid-stimulating hormone (TSH) or other external stimulations, and the major autoregulating factor was considered to be excess iodide (2).

In the animal thyroid, acute inhibition of thyroidal organification of iodine by excess iodide, escape from the acute inhibitory effects, and changes of thyroid radio-iodine uptake in hypophysectomized animals in response to variations in dietary iodine intake are representative examples of autoregulation. The acute inhibitory effect of excess iodide is temporary and escape occurs despite continuous administration of iodide.

Mechanisms of autoregulation

Acute inhibitory effect (Wolff–Chaikoff effect)

Despite the numerous reports on the effects of excess iodide on the thyroid gland, little is known about the exact mechanism of autoregulation. A fundamental phenomenon of the acute inhibitory effect is an inhibition of organification of intrathyroidal iodide in response to a marked elevation of plasma iodide (3). Thyroid peroxidase-catalysed iodination requires thyroid peroxidase, an acceptor (protein or free tyrosine), iodide, and hydrogen peroxide. Preincubation of dog thyroid slices with excess iodide greatly inhibits iodide organification and hydrogen peroxide generation stimulated by TSH and carbamylcholine. When iodide supply is sufficient, hydrogen peroxide generation is the limiting step for iodide organification, and it is suggested that the inhibitory effect of iodide on hydrogen peroxide generation is associated with the acute inhibitory effect (4, 5). On the other hand, the effect of excess iodide on an acceptor (thyroglobulin or free tyrosine), which is also associated with organification of intrathyroidal iodide, has not been clarified.

Iodinate phospholipids and iodinated derivatives of arachidonic acid or iodolactone inhibit organification of iodide in both calf thyroid slices and homogenates (6). It is possible that iodinated arachidonic acid plays an important role in the acute inhibitory effect of excess iodide.

Escape from acute inhibitory effect

In animal experiments designed to test the duration of inhibition by excess iodide on organic binding of iodide in the thyroid, it was shown that this effect is transient despite the continued maintenance of a high level of plasma total iodine (7). Originally, this was the definition of 'escape from acute inhibitory effects'. However, the term 'escape' is now widely used, as described later.

The amounts of iodide taken up by the thyroid and incorporated in iodoamino acids and iodothyronines differ greatly according to dietary iodide intake, but the amounts of T_4 and T_3 released from the thyroid are remarkably constant in humans. Although, this is called 'adaptation to excess iodide', this adaptation is another concept of escape observed in experimental animals, since the acute inhibitory effect (Wolff–Chaikoff effect) is not observed in humans (see below).

Clinically, the term escape is also widely used. In patients with Graves' diseases, treatment with inorganic iodide decreases their serum T_4 and T_3 concentrations quickly, but subsequently, many patients escape from its inhibitory effects. Details of the mechanism of this escape are described in the following section.

As mentioned above, the term escape has wide-ranging concepts. In this section, the mechanism of escape from the acute inhibitory effect, which has been identified through *in vivo* experiments in rats, is mainly described. It is suggested that decreased iodide transport is an important mechanism in escape from the acute inhibitory effect of excess iodide. Braverman and Ingbar reported that adaptation to the acute Wolff–Chaikoff effects is caused by a decrease in iodide transport into the thyroid, which reduces the intrathyroidal iodide to concentrations that were insufficient to sustain the decreased organification of iodide (8). After cloning of the sodium-coupled iodide cotransporter or sodium-iodide symporter (NIS) (9), the role of this protein was re-examined, and it was suggested that a decrease of NIS protein resulting in a decrease in thyroidal iodine transport plays an important role in the escape phenomenon (10). In addition, other factors, such as iodinated arachidonic acid, are suggested to decrease iodide transport. However, high concentrations of iodide can enter into thyroid cells independently from active iodine transport. It is still unclear whether active transport can act as a 'main controller' of escape when thyroid is exposed to a huge amount of iodide.

Although several factors that are associated with acute blocking effects during organification of intrathyroidal iodide have been identified, the effects of these factors in the escape from the acute inhibitory effects phenomenon is still unknown. As described in the following section, factors other than iodide transport have been identified in adaptation in normal individuals and escape in patients with Graves' disease.

Autoregulation in humans

Autoregulation in normal individuals and patients with Graves' disease

When the iodide dose reaches over 1 mg/day in humans, thyroidal uptake of tracer doses of radio-iodine decreases, and the administration of perchlorate or thiocyanate results in discharge of radio-iodine from the thyroid, indicating a proportional decrease in organification of thyroidal iodide. There is no evidence, however, that overall organification is actually decreased by excess iodide; that is, there is no evidence for an acute Wolff–Chaikoff effect in humans. If a large dose is given, thyroid radio-iodine uptake is so low that the absolute iodine uptake cannot be calculated. Therefore, it is not possible to prove either the Wolff–Chaikoff effect or the escape from it in humans.

Acute administration of small or moderate doses of iodide does not change the percentage of thyroid uptake of concomitantly administered radio-iodine, leading to a linear increase in absolute iodine uptake. With progressively larger doses of iodide, thyroidal radio-iodine uptake decreases, but absolute iodine uptake calculated from thyroid radio-iodine and serum and urinary iodide concentrations increases (2). On the other hand, chronic iodide administration decreases thyroidal radio-iodine uptake, but absolute iodine

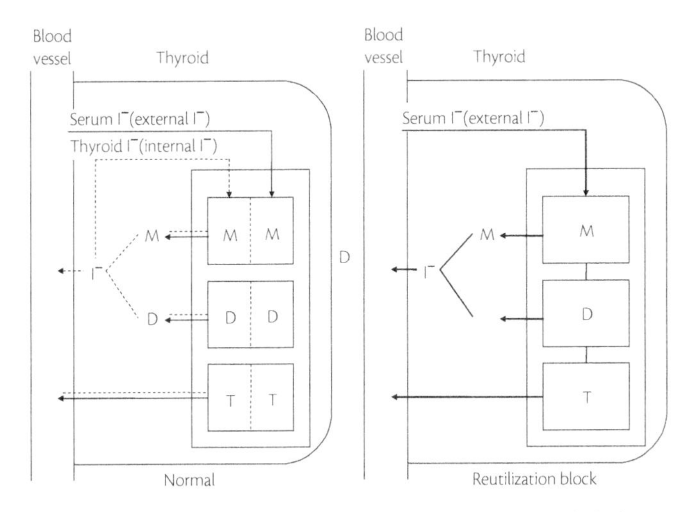

Fig. 3.2.4.1 Iodine metabolism in normal thyroid and in thyroid in which the reutilization of iodide is blocked. The blocking of the reutilization of iodide is the postulated result of iodide in excess given over a relatively long time. M, monoiodotyrosine; D, diiodotyrosine; T, triiodothyronine + thyroxine.

uptake increases as the intake of iodide increases. Serum levels of T_3 and T_4, and degradation of thyroid hormone are not affected (2). A recent study demonstrated that the administration of a large quantity of iodine (80 mg) for 2 weeks was accompanied by an increase of intrathyroidal total iodine, while intrathyroidal T_3 and T_4 contents and serum T_4 and T_3 remained unchanged (11).

The thyroid usually utilizes iodide from two routes to produce thyroid hormone (Fig. 3.2.4.1): transport iodide, which comes from serum iodide (external iodide), and iodide derived from the deiodination of iodotyrosine freed from thyroglobulin (internal iodide) (2). However, absolute iodine uptake or thyroidal organic iodine formation, which is calculated from the incorporation of serum radioactive iodide into thyroidal organic iodine, represents only organification of external iodide. If internal iodide is completely reutilized, organification of internal iodide should be from 2–4 times greater than that of external iodide, because the amount of iodotyrosine iodine freed from thyroglobulin is from 2 to 4 times greater than that transported from the blood, and release of iodotyrosine iodine should be roughly equal to the organification of external iodide in a steady state. If organification of internal iodide could be decreased when that of external iodide is increased, then the organification of external iodide could be increased from 2–4 times without changing total thyroidal iodination and hormone production. It should be noted that utilization of internal iodide is at the maximum in iodide-deficient individuals.

Acute administration of iodide decreases serum T_3 and T_4 levels and ameliorates thyrotoxicosis in patients with Graves' disease. However, the acute effect is due to inhibition of hormone release, and there is little evidence that the Wolff–Chaikoff effect occurs in Graves' patients. In patients, absolute iodine uptake increases several-fold during iodide treatment. Thyroidal organic iodine formation in Graves' disease is increased by iodide treatment despite a significant decrease in T_3 and T_4 secretion. In addition, thyroidal organic iodine formation did not change after escape from inhibition of hormone release when serum T_3 and T_4 levels increased to their pretreatment levels (12). The dissociation between thyroidal organic iodine formation and T_3 and T_4 release in Graves' patients is another unexplained feature of autoregulation.

Thyroid-stimulating hormone and autoregulation

Autoregulation was originally defined as regulation of thyroidal iodine metabolism that was independent of TSH. However, the development of sensitive assays of serum TSH and free T_4 concentration made it possible to determine significant changes in serum levels of these hormones even within the normal range (13). Serum free T_4 decreased and serum TSH increased significantly, mostly within the normal range, and the size of the thyroid gland increased in normal subjects given 27 mg iodine daily for 4 weeks (Fig. 3.2.4.2) (14). After iodide withdrawal, all values returned to baseline levels.

Serum TSH responses to thyrotropin-releasing hormone (TRH) are increased in normal subjects given moderate to large doses of iodides, indicating an antithyroid effect. In addition, administered iodide (as little as 0.75–1.5 mg daily) to normal subjects results in unsustained increases in serum TSH levels and TSH responses to TRH (Table 3.2.4.1) (13). These findings indicate that even moderate doses of iodide have antithyroid actions. Thus, several phenomena of autoregulation may, in fact, be dependent on TSH, and the definition of autoregulation may have to be reconsidered, because serum TSH levels are significantly increased by excess iodide at least in normal humans.

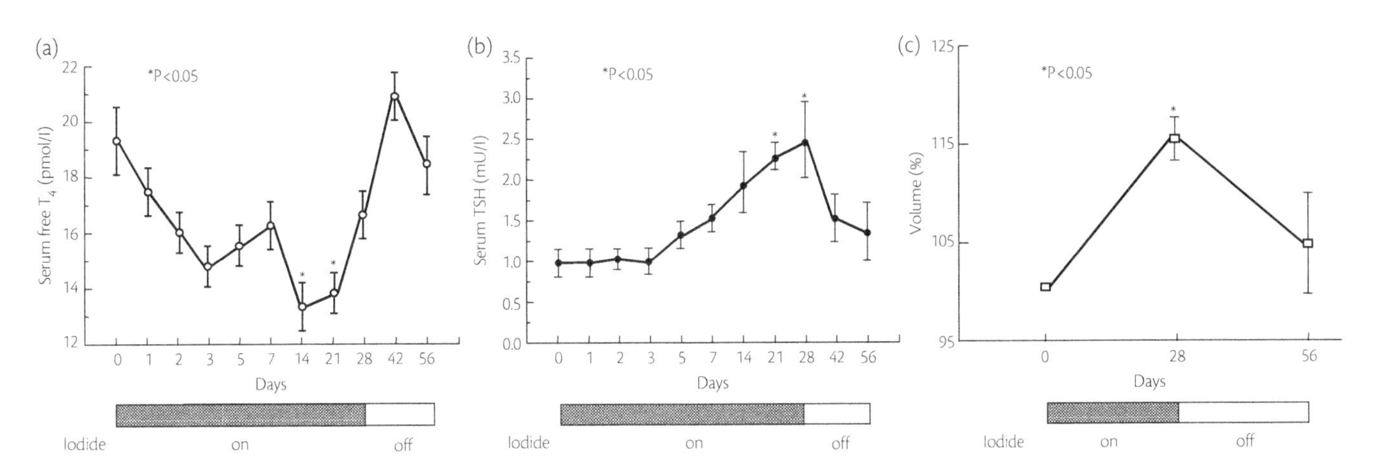

Fig. 3.2.4.2 Serum free T_4 (a) and TSH (b) concentration, and thyroid volume (c) calculated by ultrasonography before, during, and after administration of 27 mg iodine daily in 10 normal men. * $p < 0.05$ versus the value before iodine administration.

Table 3.2.4.1 Effects of iodide on serum TSH levels

Year	Iodide dose	Thyroxine (T_4)	Triiodothyronine (T_3)	Free T_4	Basal TSH	TSH-TRH
1974	190 mg/day, 10 days	↓	↓		↑	↑
1975	50 mg/day	→	↓		↑	↑
	250 mg/day, 13 days	↑	↓		↑	↑
1976	10 mg/day, 1 week	→	→		↑	↑
1988	(0.5), 1.5, 4.5 mg/day, 14 days	↓		↓	↑	↑
1991	0.75 mg/day, 28 days			↓	↑	
1993	27 mg/day, 28 days	→	→	↓	↑	
2007	80 mg/day, 15 days	→	→		↑	

Disorders of iodine excess

Disorders of iodine excess differ depending on the type and amount of iodide administered, the duration of exposure to iodide, and the background of individuals, i.e. whether they are in iodine-deficient or iodine-sufficient areas, or whether they are apparently euthyroid or have underlying thyroid diseases.

Iodide-induced goitre and hypothyroidism

General population and individuals with normal thyroid

Chronic intake of excess iodide

Excess intake of iodine, e.g. an iodine-rich diet (seaweed) or drinking water, in the long-term causes iodide-induced endemic goitre. It was detected in about 10% of the population of some areas on the coast of Hokkaido, Japan, so-called coast goitre. The inhabitants consume iodine-rich seaweed, konbu, and the mean urinary excretion of iodine in the endemic goitre areas was 23 mg/day. Despite the goitre, all patients were clinically euthyroid (15). About 90% of the inhabitants in these areas were free from clinical thyroid abnormalities.

In the prospective study among Japanese men (n = 10), oral administration of iodine tablets (27 mg daily total iodine dose) for 4 weeks caused an average 16% increase in thyroid volume. Serum TSH levels were significantly increased, but the values remained within the normal range, except for two men, and were accompanied by a small decline in serum free T_4 concentration within the normal range (14).

Smaller doses of iodide than those in the preceding report can increase the thyroid volume. Endemic iodide-induced goitre by the intake of iodine-rich (462 μg/l) drinking water was detected by echogram in 65% (n = 120) of children living in a village in central China. All children were clinically euthyroid except for two cases of overt hypothyroidism (16). Another study in China demonstrated that more than adequate (median urinary iodine excretion, 243 mg/L) or excessive iodine intake (median, 651 mg/L) was associated with elevated TSH but not with goitre (17). In an international sample of 6- to 12-year-old children from five continents with iodine intakes ranging from adequate to excessive, urinary concentrations of more than 500 μg/l are associated with increasing thyroid volume (18).

Overall, chronic loads of excess iodine for a period of time induce increasing thyroid volume but few individuals develop hypothyroidism. Although the mechanism remains unclear, failure to escape from the antithyroid effect may account for, or contribute to, iodide-induced hypothyroidism. Iodide-induced goitre and hypothyroidism disappear spontaneously within 2–6 weeks after iodide withdrawal (15). The thyroid radioactive iodine uptake rate in iodide-induced goitre varies with iodine intake. Histological examination of thyroid glands was performed in iodide-induced hypothyroid patients living in Kanazawa and Kurobe cities located on the west coast of Honshu Island in Japan. Hyperplastic changes in the follicle were observed and the change was reversible after iodine restriction. Lymphocytic infiltration was present in about one-half of them (19).

Occasional intake of excess iodide

In iodine-sufficient individuals without pre-existing thyroid diseases, occasional loads of excess iodide by iodine-rich foods or radiology contrast agents may induce subtle changes in thyroid function, including transient subclinical hypothyroidism, but iodide-induced hypothyroidism is exceedingly rare and the majority of individuals remain euthyroid. The average dietary iodine intake has been reported to be 1–3 mg in Japan (2) and iodine intake from seaweeds, especially Konbu, averaged 1.2 mg/day (20), but the amount of dietary iodine intake changes day by day from 0.1 to 30 mg even in the same person. The differences in the prevalence of thyroid abnormalities are not significant between Japan and other countries (Nagasaki and Whickham studies) (21, 22).

Graves' disease

The thyroid gland in Graves' disease is sensitive to iodide. Thyroid radioactive iodine uptake rate decreases with much smaller quantities of iodide in hyperthyroid patients than in euthyroid individuals. Thyroid function of hyperthyroid patients treated with iodide improves quickly. The inhibition of thyroid hormone secretion is usually evident sooner than that caused by antithyroid drugs. Subsequently, many patients escape from its inhibitory effects. Seventy per cent of patients treated by using 10 mg potassium iodine escape within a year (12, 13).

Hashimoto's thyroiditis and other thyroid diseases

Individuals with underlying Hashimoto's thyroiditis (23) or those with a previous history of postpartum thyroiditis are susceptible to the development of hypothyroidism upon exposure to iodine excess. Hypothyroidism is usually reversible after withdrawal of iodide (23). Individuals after an episode of subacute thyroiditis or patients who have undergone partial thyroidectomy are also prone to iodide-induced hypothyroidism.

Iodide-induced thyrotoxicosis

Iodine-deficient areas

Iodide-induced thyrotoxicosis has been observed when iodine is given as a prophylactic measure to prevent endemic goitre and hypothyroidism in iodine-deficient areas. The incidence of iodide-induced thyrotoxicosis in areas previously considered to be iodine deficient varied from 0% in Austria to 7% in Sweden after iodination programmes (24). Most patients with iodide-induced thyrotoxicosis have multinodular goitre. It appears that masked thyroid autonomy becomes evident by iodine repletion. The natural course of thyrotoxicosis is mild and restores spontaneously.

Iodine-sufficient areas

The frequency of iodide-induced thyrotoxicosis in individuals with an apparently normal thyroid living in iodine-sufficient areas is low. Iodide-induced thyrotoxicosis after coronary angiography with a contrast agent occurred only 0.25% of euthyroid not at-risk patients within 12 weeks (25).

Iodide-induced thyrotoxicosis sometimes occurs in patients with pre-existing euthyroid multinodular goitre. It was identified in 13 of 60 hospitalized thyrotoxic elderly patients with multinodular goitre in Australia and Germany who had undergone nonionic contrast radiography (26).

Patients previously treated for Graves' hyperthyroidism are also susceptible to iodide-induced thyrotoxicosis. Antithyroid drug therapy for Graves' disease reduces thyroidal iodide content. A small increase in dietary iodide increases thyroidal iodide content and, subsequently, leads the recurrence of thyrotoxicosis. Simultaneous administration of methimazole and ipodate may reduce the effectiveness of the antithyroid drug (27). The biochemical pattern is frequently that of T_4 toxicosis, and the thyroid radioactive iodine uptake is often undetectable. The thyrotoxic state is frequently, but not always, self-limiting (28).

Amiodarone-induced thyrotoxicosis

Amiodarone, a benzofuran-derived iodine-rich drug for the treatment of arrhythmia (a daily dose of 200 mg generates 6 mg iodine/day), induces thyrotoxicosis. The frequency of amiodarone-induced thyrotoxicosis is relatively high (9.6%) in iodine-deficient areas, but it is low (2%) in iodine-sufficient areas (29). Amiodarone-induced thyrotoxicosis is due to excess iodine (type 1) or to amiodarone-related destructive thyroiditis (type 2), although mixed forms often occur. In type 1, the administration of thionamides is used for the treatment, while steroids are the most useful therapeutic option in type 2 (30).

Iodide-induced thyrotoxicosis and iodine prophylaxis in iodine-deficient areas

It has been agreed that we should not hesitate to use iodine prophylaxis in iodine-deficient areas despite the possibility of iodide-induced thyrotoxicosis. The risk of iodide-induced thyrotoxicosis does not undermine the benefits of iodide supplements to prevent endemic goitre and hypothyroidism which are serious public health problems in iodine-deficient areas. Education to ensure the proper correction of iodide deficiency is needed.

References

1. Markou K, Georgopoulos N, Kyriazopoulou V, Vagenakis AG. Iodine-induced hypothyroidism. *Thyroid*, 2001; **11**: 501–10.
2. Nagataki S. Effect of excess quantities of iodide. In: Greer, MA, Solomon DH, eds. *Handbook of Physiology, section 7, Endocrinology 3*. Washington DC: American Physiological Society, 1974: 329–44.
3. Wolff J, Chaikoff IL. Plasma inorganic iodide as a homeostatic regulator of thyroid function. *J Biol Chem*, 1948; **174**: 555–64.
4. Corvilain B, Van Sande J, Dumont JE. Inhibition by iodide of iodide binding to proteins: the "Wolff-Chaikoff" effect is caused by inhibition of H2O2 generation. *Biochem Biophys Res Commun*, 1988; **154**: 1287–92.
5. Karbownik M, Lewinski A. The role of oxidative stress in physiological and pathological processes in the thyroid gland: possible involvement in pineal-thyroid interactions. *Neuro Endocrinol Lett*, 2003; **24**: 293–303.
6. Chazenbalk GD, Valsecchi RM, Krawiec L, Burton G, Juvenal GJ, Monteagudo E, *et al*. Thyroid autoregulation. Inhibitory effects of iodinated derivatives of arachidonic acid on iodine metabolism. *Prostaglandins*, 1988; **36**: 163–72.
7. Wolff J, Chaikoff IL, *et al*. The temporary nature of the inhibitory action of excess iodine on organic iodine synthesis in the normal thyroid. *Endocrinology*, 1949; **45**: 504–13.
8. Braverman LE, Ingbar SH. Changes in thyroidal function during adaptation to large doses of iodide. *J Clin Invest*, 1963; **42**: 1216–31.
9. Dai G, Levy O, Carrasco N. Cloning and characterization of the thyroid iodide transporter. *Nature*, 1996; **379**: 458–60.
10. Eng PH, Cardona GR, Fang SL, Previti M, Alex S, Carrasco N, *et al*. Escape from the acute Wolff-Chaikoff effect is associated with a decrease in thyroid sodium/iodide symporter messenger ribonucleic acid and protein. *Endocrinology*, 1999; **140**: 3404–10.
11. Theodoropoulou A, Vagenakis AG, Makri M, Markou KB. Thyroid hormone synthesis and secretion in humans after 80 milligrams of iodine for 15 days and subsequent withdrawal. *J Clin Endocrinol Metab*, 2007; **92**: 212–14.
12. Nagataki S, Shizume K, Nakao K. Effect of iodide on thyroidal iodine turnover in hyperthyroid subjects. *J Clin Endocrinol Metab*, 1970; **30**: 469–78.
13. Nagataki S. Autoregulation of thyroid function by iodine. In: Delange F, Dunn JT, Glinoer D, eds. *Iodine Deficiency in Europe: A Continuing Concern*. New York: Plenum Press, 1993: 43–8
14. Namba H, Yamashita S, Kimura H, Yokoyama N, Usa T, Otsuru A, *et al*. Evidence of thyroid volume increase in normal subjects receiving excess iodide. *J Clin Endocrinol Metab*, 1993; **76**: 605–8.
15. Suzuki H, Higuchi T, Sawa K, Ohtaki S, Horiuchi Y. 'Endemic coast goitre' in Hokkaido, Japan. *Acta Endocrinol (Copenh)*, 1965; **50**: 161–76.
16. Li M, Liu DR, Qu CY, Zhang PY, Qian QD, Zhang CD, *et al*. Endemic goitre in central China caused by excessive iodine intake. *Lancet*, 1987; **330**: 257–9.
17. Teng W, Shan Z, Teng X, *et al*. (2006). Effect of iodine intake on thyroid diseases in China. *N Engl J Med*, 2006; **354**: 2783–93.
18. Zimmermann MB, Ito Y, Hess SY, Fujieda K, Molinari L. High thyroid volume in children with excess dietary iodine intakes. *Am J Clin Nutr*, 2005; **81**: 840–4.
19. Mizukami Y, Michigishi T, Nonomura A, Hashimoto T, Tonami N, Matsubara F, *et al*. Iodine-induced hypothyroidism: a clinical and histological study of 28 patients. *J Clin Endocrinol Metab*, 1993; **76**: 466–71.
20. Nagataki S. The average of dietary iodine intake due to the ingestion of seaweeds is 1.2 mg/day in Japan. *Thyroid*, 2008; **18**: 667–8.
21. Nagataki S, Shibata Y, Inoue S, Yokoyama N, Izumi M, Shimaoka K. Thyroid diseases among atomic bomb survivors in Nagasaki. *JAMA*, 1994; **272**: 364–70.
22. Vanderpump MP, Tunbridge WM, French JM, Appleton D, Bates D, Clark F, *et al*. The incidence of thyroid disorders in the community: a twenty-year follow-up of the Whickham Survey. *Clin Endocrinol (Oxf)*, 1995; **43**: 55–68.
23. Tajiri J, Higashi K, Morita M, Umeda T, Sato T. Studies of hypothyroidism in patients with high iodine intake. *J Clin Endocrinol Metab*, 1986; **63**: 412–17.
24. Roti E, Uberti ED. Iodine excess and hyperthyroidism. *Thyroid*, 2001; **11**: 493–500.
25. Hintze G, Blombach O, Fink H, Burkhardt U, Kobberling J. Risk of iodine-induced thyrotoxicosis after coronary angiography: an

investigation in 788 unselected subjects. *Eur J Endocrinol*, 1999; **140**: 264–7.

26. Roti E, Vagenakis AG. Effect of excess iodide: clinical aspects. In: Braverman LE, Utiger RD, eds. *Werner & Ingbar's The Thyroid*. 9th edn. Philadelphia: Lippincott Williams & Wilkins, 2005: 288–305
27. Roti E, Gardini E, Minelli R, Bianconi L, Braverman LE. Sodium ipodate and methimazole in the long-term treatment of hyperthyroid Graves' disease. *Metabolism*, 1993; **42**: 403–8.
28. Fradkin JE, Wolff J. Iodide-induced thyrotoxicosis. *Medicine (Baltimore)*, 1983; **62**: 1–20.
29. Trip MD, Wiersinga W, Plomp TA. Incidence, predictability, and pathogenesis of amiodarone-induced thyrotoxicosis and hypothyroidism. *Am J Med*, 1991; **91**: 507–11.
30. Bogazzi F, Bartalena L, Gasperi M, Braverman LE, Martino E. The various effects of amiodarone on thyroid function. *Thyroid*, 2001; **11**: 511–19.

3.2.5 Radiation-induced thyroid disease

Furio Pacini, Rossella Elisei, Aldo Pinchera

Introduction

Radiation is a mitogen which may cause damage to the cell DNA. When sufficiently severe, the damage may result in cell death. When the damage is less severe, the consequences to the cell depend upon the gene and cell system that are affected. The thyroid gland is particularly sensitive to the effects of radiation and the evidence that radiation may damage the thyroid gland is overwhelming. Both external and internal radiation have been associated with thyroid diseases (cancer and hypothyroidism, with or without thyroid autoimmunity) both *in vitro* and *in vivo*. External radiation to the thyroid was first recognized as a cause of thyroid carcinoma in the 1950s, when cases were found in individuals who had been given radiotherapy during childhood for an enlarged thymus (1). Since then, numerous studies have confirmed and extended this initial observation.

Radioactive isotopes are used in several situations in humans. They are given in very large doses in the treatment of thyroid cancer, when the dose used is intended to kill all thyroid cancer cells, and in smaller doses in the treatment of thyrotoxicosis, with the intent to produce hypothyroidism. In these conditions the radiation doses are sufficiently high to kill the cells, thus no unwanted secondary thyroid disease occurs. Low doses of iodine isotopes are also used as tracers for diagnostic evaluation of the thyroid gland. In this situation, no cell killing is observed and there is the theoretical possibility for thyroid cell damage. However, no convincing evidence of subsequent thyroid disorders has so far been provided.

Many animal studies have shown that radio-iodine is carcinogenic to the thyroid. Some of the earlier data suggested that internal radiation by radio-iodine was less effective than external radiation, but according to one more recent study in rats (2), the carcinogenic potential of ^{131}I and X-rays appears to be the same. In both cases, the dose–response relationship seems to be linear, indicating that low doses also carry a risk. Iodine-131 is 20–30% as effective as external X- or χ-rays.

Thyroid carcinoma after external irradiation

Methodology in epidemiological studies

The relationship between radiation and thyroid carcinoma was first recognized in 1950 (1), and thyroid carcinoma was the first solid malignant tumour found to be increased among Japanese atomic bomb survivors (3). This relationship was confirmed subsequently by many epidemiological studies (4).

Two major limitations should be taken into account in studies of the relationship between radiation and thyroid carcinoma. One is due to the fact that many patients are unaware of, or uncertain about, prior radiation exposure, especially when therapeutic irradiation was administered at a young age (recall bias), taking into account that radiation-induced thyroid carcinoma occurs several years later. The second and perhaps more relevant limitation is related to the frequent occurrence of thyroid nodules in the general population (4–7% by palpation and up to 50% by ultrasonography in people over 60 years). Moreover, most thyroid tumours are indolent and frequently not recognized clinically. Thus, the diagnosis of thyroid tumours depends on the extent of the diagnostic procedures used (diagnostic bias).

In case-control studies, the cases are patients with thyroid cancer identified by entry into a tumour registry. The controls are matched subjects free from thyroid carcinoma. Information on risk factors, such as radiation exposure, is obtained and the distribution in the two groups is compared. In such studies diagnostic bias is minimized, but recall bias may be important. In cohort studies, exposure to radiation is generally well documented, and recall bias is minimized. The frequency of thyroid carcinoma in the radiation-exposed group is compared with a group of similar subjects not exposed to radiation. In this case, diagnostic bias may be important. A final additional caveat is due to the fact that retrospective estimates of doses delivered to the thyroid are necessary to prove the aetiological weight of radiation in thyroid cancer (dose–effect relationship). These estimates may be difficult to obtain and are subject to error.

Most epidemiological studies dealing with the risk of developing radiation-induced thyroid cancer use the relative risk (RR) as an index, i.e. the ratio between the observed (O) number of cancers in the radiation-exposed group and the expected (E) number of cancers in the nonexposed group (RR = O/E). When the expected number is obtained from a registry, the relative risk is called the standardized incidence ratio. The most frequently used indices of risk estimates are reported in Box 3.2.5.1.

Risk estimates for radiation-induced thyroid cancer have been calculated in people exposed to external radiation. According to the National Council of Radiation Protection (NCRP) (5), the excess absolute risk is 2.5×10^{-4}/Gy per year for persons exposed under the age of 18. For adults, the risk per year is assumed to be half this value. Because of their smaller number of years at risk, the lifetime risk for adults is about one-quarter the risk for children.

In a pooled analysis (6) the excess absolute risk was 4.4×10^{-4}/Gy per year for persons exposed before the age of 15, confirming that the relative risk is largely dependent upon age at exposure with young children carrying the highest risk. As shown in Tables 3.2.5.1

Box 3.2.5.1 Most common indices of cancer risk from radiation exposure

- RR (relative risk) = *O*/*E* (*n* observed in radiation exposed/*n* expected in non-exposed)
- SIR (standardized incidence ratio) = *O*/*E* when *E* is derived from a registry
- ERR (excess relative risk) = *O*/*E*–1
- ERR/gray = ERR/mean dose (Gy) in the group
- EAR (excess absolute risk)/gray = *O*–*E*/PYG (person-year-gray of exposure to the risk)

and 3.2.5.2, little risk is carried after the age of 20 and almost none after the age of 40, as demonstrated in the study of atomic bomb survivors in Hiroshima and Nagasaki (7).

External irradiation to the head and neck for benign diseases

Irradiation to the head and neck has been performed in children since 1920 for the treatment of benign conditions such as enlargement of the thymus, tonsils, adenoids, or neck lymph nodes, skin angioma, acne, otitis, or tinea capitis (4, 8–10). This modality of treatment was particularly popular in the USA, where in 1970 as many as 76% of children with thyroid carcinoma had a history of radiation exposure (11). In Europe, it was less frequently used: in two large referral centres for thyroid cancer, the Institut Gustave-Roussy in Villejuif, France and the Department of Endocrinology in Pisa, Italy, the incidence of radiation-induced thyroid carcinoma in children or adolescents was 10% and 7%, respectively.

Ron and colleagues (6) reported an analysis of radiation exposure and thyroid cancer from seven large studies of a total of 58 000 children exposed to external radiation, in whom individual doses to the thyroid were known. About 700 thyroid carcinomas were observed. The excess relative risk per gray (ERR/Gy) was 7.7 (95% CI 2.1 to 28.7). The authors concluded that 88% of thyroid carcinomas that were found in children exposed to 1 Gy were attributable to radiation. The excess absolute risk was 4.4/10 000 population-year-gray of exposure (95% CI 1.9 to 10.1). The risk of thyroid cancer significantly increased after a mean dose as low as 100 mGy to the thyroid. There was no evidence for a threshold dose below which the effect disappeared. At higher doses (up to 1500 cGy), there was a linear relationship between dose and risk of cancer.

Table 3.2.5.1 Thyroid cancer excess relative risk (ERR) from exposure to external radiation in adults

Study	Irradiated subjects	Mean does (cGy)	ERR/Gy
Atomic bomb	11 000	26	0.8
Neck cancer therapy	82 816	11	3.1
Tuberculous adenitis	124	820	1.2

Data taken from shore RE, *Radiation Research*, 1992; **131**: 98–111.
From Shore RE. Issues and epidemiological evidence regarding radiation-induced thyroid cancer. *Radiat Res*, 1992; **131**: 98–111.

Table 3.2.5.2 Thyroid cancer excess relative risk (ERR) from exposure to external radiation before the age of 20 years

Study	Irradiated subjects	Mean does (cGy)	ERR/Gy
Atomic bomb	13 000	23	4.7
Thymus	2475	136	9.1
Tinea capitis	10 384	9	32.5
Tonsils	2634	59	2.5
Skin haemangioma	14 351	26	4.9
Skin haemangioma	11 807	12	7.5
Lymphoid hyperplasia	1195	24	20
Childhood cancer	9170	1250	1.1

Data taken from shore RE, *Radiation Research*, 1992; **131**: 98–111.
From Shore RE. Issues and epidemiological evidence regarding radiation-induced thyroid cancer. *Radiat Res*, 1992; **131**: 98–111.

At doses higher than 1500 cGy, the risk per gray decreased, probably because of cell killing, but the overall risk remain elevated.

In a study of 2634 patients from the Michael Reese Hospital in Chicago (12), whose thyroids received a mean dose of 590 mGy for benign disorders during childhood, about 60% developed thyroid nodules and 15% developed thyroid carcinoma within 40 years after radiation. These studies indicate clearly that the risk of thyroid cancer after exposure to external radiation is indeed very high, suggesting that the thyroid gland is very sensitive to radiation, especially during childhood (Table 3.2.5.2).

In most studies, the latency period between the time of radiation exposure and the appearance of the thyroid nodule ranges between 5 and 15 years. In the pooled analysis of seven studies mentioned above (6), only two cases were observed within the first 5 years after exposure; the excess relative risk clearly increased between 5 and 9 years after exposure, with a peak at 15–19 years, an excess risk still being apparent at 40 years (12).

Since 1970, external radiation for benign disorders has been virtually abandoned in most countries.

External irradiation to the head and neck for malignant diseases

In case of external radiation to the head and neck for malignant disease, the dose delivered to the thyroid may be very high, and usually greater than that delivered for the treatment of benign conditions. Animal experiments have shown that for doses larger than 15–20 Gy, the risk of thyroid tumour is increased but the risk per gray decreases. This finding has been attributed to cell killing, which decreases the number of cells that may become neoplastic, and explains the high frequency of hypothyroidism observed in those animals.

In humans, high-dose radiation therapy to the neck (more than 20 Gy), as used for Hodgkin's disease, results in a high rate of hypothyroidism, but also in an increased risk of thyroid cancer (13). The final outcome of the thyroid damage is probably related to the distance between the thyroid gland and the radiation field. If this is far from the thyroid, as in case of thoracic or abdominal radiation fields in children, the thyroid gland may receive radiation doses of some hundred milligray, not enough to produce hypothyroidism but sufficient to trigger thyroid cancer (14, 15). Recently, it has been reported that all survivors of human cancer treated with craniospinal external radiotherapy during childhood require long-term observation, up to 25 years after the exposure, since their risk of developing thyroid cancer and other thyroid dysfunctions is increased with respect to the general population without a specific age-related plateau (16).

Atomic bombs in Hiroshima and Nagasaki

After the atomic bombing in Hiroshima and Nagasaki in 1945, the body dose was mainly due to external irradiation (X-rays and neutrons). Contamination by radioactive isotopes of iodine is poorly known. The health consequences were studied in a cohort of 94 000 survivors and of 26 000 individuals who resided in Hiroshima and Nagasaki shortly after the bombing. A total of 225 thyroid cancers were diagnosed between 1958 and 1987 among the 79 972 survivors who were alive and free of cancer as of January 1958 and who had radiation dose estimates (7). From a histological point of view, these tumors are very similar to conventional sporadic papillary thyroid cancer and, at variance with the post-Chernobyl thyroid tumors, the solid variant is very rare among atomic bomb survivors. However, molecular oncology analysis of 50 adult-onset papillary thyroid cancer exposed to A-bomb radiation showed that the prevalence of RET/PTC rearrangements was significantly correlated with the radiation dose and that other unknown gene alterations tended to be more frequent with increased radiation dose (17). These findings suggest that radiation-associated gene alterations, mainly chromosomal rearrangements, other than RET/PTC might be involved in the adult-onset thyroid cancer of subjects who were exposed to high radiation dose.

Factors affecting sensitivity to radiation-induced thyroid cancer

Age and sex

A major risk factor is a young age at the time of irradiation. The risk of thyroid cancer after external irradiation in children less than 5 years of age is 2 times higher than in children treated between 5 and 9 years and 5 times higher than in children treated between 10 and 14 years (6). From the Lifespan Study of atomic bomb survivors in Hiroshima and Nagasaki (16), it is known that little risk is carried for exposures after the age of 20 and almost none after the age of 40. The excess risk of thyroid cancer was 9.5, 3.0, 0.3, and 0.2 in the age categories 0–9, 10–19, 20–39, and over 40 years, respectively, at the time of bombing. The excess risk was not significant for subjects exposed above the age of 15–20 years. This increased risk of very young children to develop thyroid cancer after radiation exposure can be explained, at least in part, by the higher proliferative activity of thyroid cells during intrauterine development and childhood (18). The high susceptibility of young children to radiation has been confirmed in the thyroid cancer studies after the Chernobyl nuclear reactor accident (see below), supporting the concept that the radiation effect is maximal during periods of rapid cell proliferation, as in the case of the developing thyroid of very young children. Data on irradiation in adults are scarce, but estimates of the ERR/Gy are largely below those of individuals exposed during childhood, and probably the risk is negligible

Gender does not seem to influence the risk of developing radiation-induced thyroid cancer. Although females are 2–3 times more likely to develop both benign and malignant thyroid nodules after irradiation, this finding reflects the higher natural incidence of thyroid nodules and cancer in the female general population. Very recently a new study on the association between radiation dose and thyroid cancer incidence among Japanese survivors who were adults at the time of the atomic bombings of Hiroshima and Nagasaki has shown that the exposure to ionizing radiation in adults was positively associated with thyroid cancer among women atomic bomb survivors. However, this association was lower than that observed in those who were exposed during childhood (19).

Fractionation and dose rate

External radiation therapy for benign and malignant diseases is given at a high dose rate. Lower dose rates or fractionation of the dose may theoretically allow radiation-induced DNA lesions to be repaired, thus decreasing the carcinogenic effects of radiation. In the pooled analysis of seven studies, fractionation of the dose was associated with a 30% reduction of the ERR/Gy (6). However, in a recent update of thyroid cancer after radiation therapy for malignant disorders in childhood, no reduction in ERR/Gy was observed with fractionation.

The importance of the dose rate is suggested by several observations. In children treated for skin angioma of the neck, a dose–effect relationship was observed after external radiation at a high dose rate, but no such relation was found after brachytherapy at a low dose rate. The incidence of thyroid nodules is similar in two regions of China where natural radiation is different (i.e. 140 mGy and 50 mGy/lifetime, respectively) (20). In contrast, an increased relative risk (1.7) of thyroid cancer was found among 27 000 medical diagnostic radiographers in China, who probably received more than 1 Gy to the thyroid during their working life (21). No such increase was observed in similar workers in industrialized countries.

Genetic predisposition

Several clinical observations suggest that genetic predisposition, such as defects in the DNA repair mechanisms, may affect the risk of developing radiation-induced thyroid cancer (22, 23). Patients who experience one radiation-related cancer are more likely to develop a second radiation-related cancer. Sibling pairs, exposed to radiation, develop thyroid tumours more often than would be expected by chance (22, 23). The risk of thyroid cancer in patients treated with radiotherapy during childhood for a cancer (other than neuroblastoma) is 3–10 times higher than in children treated for benign conditions. Those treated for neuroblastoma have a fivefold risk of thyroid cancer with respect to patients treated for other cancers, suggesting a common predisposition for neuroblastoma and thyroid cancer.

The search for the gene(s) predisposing to radiation-induced thyroid cancer is currently in progress in pedigrees showing recurrence of thyroid cancer. No linkage has been found as yet with genes known to be involved in thyroid tumorigenesis, such as *ras*, *p53*, *BRaf*, or *RET/PTC*. A distinct genome-wide gene expression profiling has been reported in post-Chernobyl papillary thyroid cancer when compared with that occurring naturally, suggesting a greater susceptibility to thyroid cell radiation damage (24).

Thyroid carcinoma after exposure to radioactive iodine, and the Chernobyl experience

Iodine-131, being physiologically accumulated in the thyroid by an active mechanism, has been widely used for several decades in the diagnostic evaluation of the thyroid gland and in the treatment of patients with hyperthyroidism and differentiated thyroid cancer. The radiation dose delivered by ^{131}I to the thyroid is 1000- to 10 000-fold higher than that delivered to other tissues. Thus, even a relatively low amount of ^{131}I may deliver a significant, potentially carcinogenic radiation dose to the thyroid gland. Increasing the radiation dose beyond a few hundred megabecquerels, increases the likelihood of obtaining cell killing and decreases the possibility of tumoral changes.

The role of radioactive iodine for medical use in the development of thyroid cancer has been addressed in several studies, which showed no significant risk and led to the conclusion that ^{131}I is sufficiently safe both as a diagnostic and a therapeutic tool. However, most patients included in these studies were treated as adults, whereas the post-Chernobyl epidemic of thyroid cancer occurred mainly in children and adolescents, supporting evidence that the young thyroid is particularly sensitive to the effect of radiation. This event has renewed concern about the carcinogenic risk of medical use of ^{131}I, at least in young patients.

Exposure to ^{131}I for diagnostic purposes

The most informative analysis in this setting was performed in Sweden on 34 104 patients exposed to diagnostic doses of ^{131}I between 1950 and 1969, for a mean thyroid dose estimate of 110 cGy (25). A small increase in the number of observed thyroid cancers (n = 67) was found with respect to the expected number (n = 50). However, the increase was confined to patients undergoing thyroid scan for suspicion of thyroid cancer. When the analysis was limited to patients tested for reasons other than thyroid cancer, no increase was observed.

In the same Swedish cohort, the incidence of thyroid nodules was compared in a subset of 1005 women and 248 matched controls. The average length of follow-up was 26 years and the average age at exposure was 26 years. No difference was found in the two groups; the incidence of nodules was 10.6 and 11.7, respectively. Similar findings have been reported in other surveys in the USA and in Germany.

The conclusion drawn from this study is that diagnostic use of ^{131}I has no untoward health effect on the thyroid. However, a note of caution is needed because only a minority of the exposed patients were children. The excess relative risk of thyroid cancer after exposure to ^{131}I before age 20 and in adults is reported in Tables 3.2.5.3 and 3.2.5.4, respectively.

Table 3.2.5.3 Thyroid cancer excess relative risk (ERR)/Gy after exposure to ^{131}I before the age of 20 years

Study	Irradiated subjects	Mean does (cGy)	ERR/Gy
Swedish diagnostic ^{131}I	2408	150	0.25
Food and Drug Administration diagnostic ^{131}I	3503	80	0.10
Utah ^{131}I fallout	2473	17	7.9
Marshall Islanders	127	1240	0.32
Juvenile hyperthyroidism	602	8800	0.3

Data taken from shore RE, *Radiation Research*, 1992; **131**: 98–111.
From Shore RE. Issues and epidemiological evidence regarding radiation-induced thyroid cancer. *Radiat Res*, 1992; **131**: 98–111.

Table 3.2.5.4 Thyroid cancer excess relative risk (ERR)/Gy after exposure to ^{131}I in adult life

Study	Irradiated subjects	Mean does (cGy)	ERR/Gy
Swedish diagnostic ^{131}I	24200	42	<0
German diagnostic ^{131}I	13896	100	0.3
Marshall Islanders	126	466	0.5

Data taken from shore RE, *Radiation Research*, 1992; **131**: 98–111.
From Shore RE. Issues and epidemiological evidence regarding radiation-induced thyroid cancer. *Radiat Res*, 1992; **131**: 98–111.

Exposure to ^{131}I for therapeutic purposes

Radio-iodine is used widely to treat hyperthyroidism caused either by Graves' disease, toxic nodular goitre, or metastatic thyroid cancer. No evidence of an increased risk of thyroid cancer after treatment of hyperthyroidism with ^{131}I has been reported. In a Swedish study, including 10 552 adult patients (mean age 57 years) followed for a mean period of 15 years, the relative risk of thyroid cancer was not significantly increased (RR 1.29; 95% CI 0.76 to 2.03). The average estimated radiation dose to the thyroid was 100 Gy (26).

In a study carried out in the USA (27) in hyperthyroid patients, after a mean follow-up of 21 years, ^{131}I treatment was not found to be linked to total cancer deaths (standardized mortality ratio (SMR) 1.02), or to the development of any cancer other than thyroid cancer (SMR 3.94; 95% CI 2.52 to 5.86). The SMR was 2.08 in patients with Graves' disease and 6.53 in those with toxic nodular goitre. The excess number of deaths was small (observed/expected 27/10), and the underlying disease, rather than radiation, seemed to play the major role. This result is not surprising. The large dose delivered for the treatment of hyperthyroidism is frequently sufficient to produce hypothyroidism, through cell killing. Indeed, the risk of hypothyroidism at 2 years increases linearly with the thyroid dose, for radioactive concentrations ranging from 0.9 to 8.3 MBq/g.

As for the diagnostic use of ^{131}I, the hyperthyroid patients treated with radio-iodine were adults. In a few hundred children treated with ^{131}I, no significant increase in the incidence of thyroid cancer has been observed (26). However, in view of the high sensitivity of the young thyroid gland to radiation, it is probably advisable to avoid treating hyperthyroidism in young children and adolescents with ^{131}I.

As far as the treatment of differentiated thyroid cancer with ^{131}I is concerned, the only theoretical risk is the possibility that ^{131}I might act as an additional mutagen, inducing the progression of thyroid cancer to a more aggressive and less well-differentiated phenotype. At the present moment, no evidence supports this possibility. The other potential hazard of ^{131}I therapy of thyroid cancer is the occurrence of secondary effects on other organs when accumulating high radiation doses during several courses of treatment. Controversial data on this issue have been reported so far (28, 29).

Post-Chernobyl thyroid cancer

Circumstances of the accident

In April 1986, the explosion of one of the reactors at the nuclear power plant in Chernobyl, Ukraine released large amounts of radioactive particles into the atmosphere, including ^{131}I (32–46 MCi), ^{132}I (27 MCi; resulting from the decay of ^{132}Tc), and ^{133}I (68 MCi).

Most likely, radio-iodines were released intermittently over a period of 10 days or more after the explosion. The time and place of deposition varied, depending on the direction of the wind and other meteorological conditions. The most contaminated territories were southern Belarus, northern Ukraine, and to a lesser extent the Bryansk and Kaluga regions of southern Russia.

As a result of the accident, a tremendous increase in the number of childhood papillary thyroid cancers occurred in the following years (30) (Fig. 3.2.5.1). The magnitude of this increase and the geographical and temporal distribution of the cases, strongly suggest that thyroid cancer was due to the reactor explosion and, in particular, to the huge amount of iodine radioisotopes released. The initial scepticism, allowing the possibility that the increased incidence of thyroid cancer might be due to ascertainment bias following intensive screening, has been totally discouraged by subsequent compelling evidence. Many of the tumours diagnosed in the first years were relatively large, invasive, and associated with lymph node metastases, unlike those detected during screening programmes, which are minimal, limited to the thyroid, and not aggressive (31). The prevalence of childhood thyroid cancer exceeded that of any other country in the world and, very importantly, decreased dramatically in children conceived and born after the accident.

Being volatile, radioactive isotopes could be first inhaled and, after they were deposited on the ground, ingested. The time at which ingestion occurred varied considerably, but the milk chain, particularly in children, was the major route of ingestion: at this time, short-lived isotopes of iodine were no longer present. Several factors contributed to the high radiation exposure of the population. Immediate protective countermeasures, such as advising and evacuating the people at risk and distributing iodine prophylaxis, were not undertaken. Furthermore, the most contaminated regions were in a state of moderate iodine deficiency, which is responsible for increased iodine uptake. All these factors combined give enough explanation of why the most serious health consequence of the disaster was thyroid cancer, and why mostly children were affected (32).

In the case of radioactive contamination, the thyroid gland is a critical organ at risk. Its contamination depends upon the magnitude of contamination, the amount of radioactive iodine taken up by the gland, and the thyroid mass itself. Whatever the level of contamination, the thyroid dose is always higher in children than in adults. The thyroid dose is dependent on the final concentration, namely the ratio between radioiodine uptake and thyroid mass. In children, the uptake is similar to adults but, the thyroid mass being smaller, the dose per gram of tissue is greater, and extremely high in newborn and very young children.

In children who remained in the contaminated territories and drank locally produced milk, most of the radiation dose to the thyroid was due to ^{131}I and only a small amount to short-lived isotopes. The thyroid dose in children evacuated soon after the accident was lower, and mainly due to short-lived isotopes. Although dosimetric data are imprecise, the mean thyroid dose has been estimated to be nearly 700 mSv in Belarus. In Ukraine, 79% of the children received a thyroid dose below or equal to 300 mSv, 10.5% received from 300 mSv to 1 Sv, and 10.5% received more than 1 Sv (33). As a term of comparison, in children exposed to external irradiation (6) the risk of thyroid cancer was significant even for thyroid doses as low as 100 mSv.

In most of the children that developed thyroid cancer the estimated thyroid dose was equal to or less than 300 mGy. An excess thyroid cancer incidence has been observed even in areas where the mean thyroid dose in children was estimated at 50–100 mGy.

Clinical features of post-Chernobyl thyroid cancer

The increase in the number of thyroid carcinomas in children and adolescents has been observed since 1990, only 4 years after the Chernobyl accident, in southern Belarus and northern Ukraine, and from 1994 in southern Russia (34, 35). In the Gomel region, the most contaminated area of Belarus, the incidence between 1986 and 1996 was 13/100 000 children/year, compared to a baseline incidence of less than 1/year. To date, more than 5000 cases of thyroid cancer have been reported among those who were children or adolescents at the time of the accident and living in the three most contaminated countries, Belarus, Ukraine, and Russia (30).

As shown in Fig. 3.2.5.2, most of the cases were registered in children below age 10 at the time of the accident, and nearly two-thirds in those younger than 5 years. Thyroid cancer cases have also been registered up to 20 years after the nuclear accident in children who were already conceived but still *in utero*, at that time (36). With respect to the 12 years before the accident, in the 12 years after the accident the increase of thyroid cancer in Belarus was 75-fold in children aged 3–14 years at the time of diagnosis, 10.1-fold in adolescents (15–18 years at diagnosis), 3.7-fold in young adults (19–29 years), and 3.4-fold in adults (Table 3.2.5.5). This increase

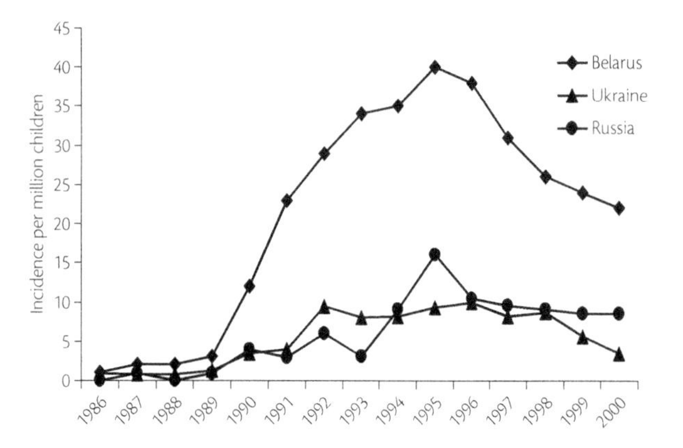

Fig. 3.2.5.1 New cases of thyroid carcinoma per year diagnosed in Belarus, Ukraine, and Russia in children and adolescents exposed to radiation fall out after the Chernobyl accident.

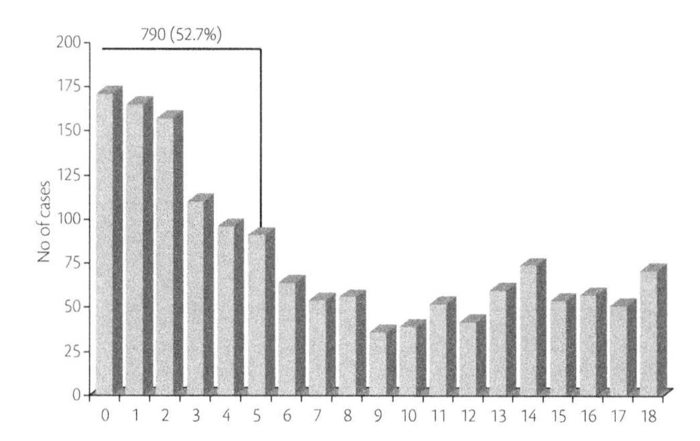

Fig. 3.2.5.2 Children and adolescents with post-Chernobyl thyroid cancer in Belarus (1500 cases diagnosed from 1986 to 2002).

Table 3.2.5.5 Thyroid cancer in Belarus before and after the Chernobyl accident

Age	1971–1985	1986–2000	Fold of increase
0–14	8	703	87.8
15–18	21	267	12.7
≥19	1465	6719	4.6
Total	1494	7689	5.1

in adults is much less important than that observed in children and it is likely to be due to greater attention to thyroid diseases after the nuclear accident.

Over 90% of the cancers were papillary. In the years following the accident most cancers were classified as a solid or follicular variant of papillary thyroid cancer (Fig. 3.2.5.3), i.e. the less frequently observed variant among naturally occurring papillary carcinomas. The clinical and pathological features were those of an aggressive tumour, as demonstrated by the histological appearance, the large size, the frequent multifocality and extracapsular invasion, and the frequency of node and lung metastases early in the course of the disease (31). However, later studies showed a decline over time in the proportion of the solid variant and an increase in the proportion of the classic variant. These changes correlated both with the increasing age and increasing latency period and it is not yet clear which of these two variables could be mostly responsible for these changing patterns, which are also associated with a change in the molecular features of these tumours (37).

The comparison between post-Chernobyl thyroid carcinomas diagnosed in Belarus and naturally occurring cases diagnosed in age-matched patients in Italy and France showed different clinical and epidemiological features (38). Post-Chernobyl tumours were much less influenced by gender (female:male ratio 1.6:1 versus 2.5:1 in Italy and France), were more advanced at presentation, were more frequently papillary, and were mainly diagnosed before age 15, while in Italy and France the majority were diagnosed after age 14.

As far as treatment and outcome are concerned, the available follow-up data indicate that post-Chernobyl thyroid carcinoma, when appropriately treated with a combination of total thyroidectomy, radio-iodine, and hormone suppressive therapy, has the same favourable outcome as naturally occurring papillary cancer. Definitive cure is achieved in many patients, even in those with node and lung involvement, the quality of life is good, and the death rate does not exceed the usual 1–2% reported in many series of paediatric thyroid cancer (39).

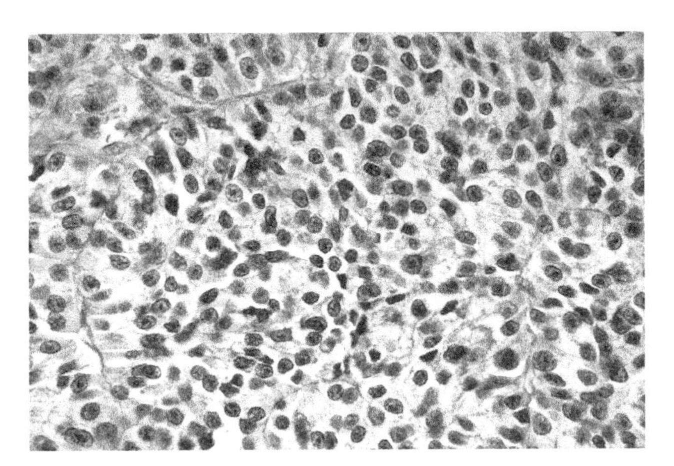

Fig. 3.2.5.3 Representative example of the solid variant of papillary thyroid cancer in a post Chernobyl thyroid cancer patient. (See also Plate 10)

A similar observation has been recently reported in a study focused on external radiation-induced thyroid carcinoma. Although these tumours showed generally more aggressive features, the similar prognostic factors for their outcome indicate that they should be treated and followed in the same way as naturally occurring thyroid cancer (40).

Genetics of post-Chernobyl thyroid cancer

Post-Chernobyl tumours show interesting genetic peculiarities when investigated by molecular biology. Molecular studies of the early post-Chernobyl thyroid cancer showed that a very high proportion harboured a RET/PTC rearrangement with a higher prevalence of RET/PTC3 (41–44). Also the subtype of *RET/PTC* rearrangement showed a peculiar pattern. Several authors reported that *RET/PTC3* (and more rare variants of *RET/PTC3*) was the form more frequently expressed in radiation-induced tumours, thus suggesting that RET/PTC3 might represent a marker for these tumours. A correlation was also established between the solid variant of papillary tumours and the activation of *RET/PTC3* (43). Interestingly, over the years and with the elongation of the latency period, the prevalence of RET/rearrangements became lower and more similar to that of naturally occurring thyroid carcinoma (Table 3.2.5.6). Also the relative prevalence of RET/PTC1 and 3 subtypes changed in favour of RET/PTC1 (37).

The presence of RET/PTC rearrangements in radiation-induced cancer is in keeping with the *in vitro* findings that RET/PTC rearrangements can be induced in human thyroid cells after exposure to 0.1–10 Gy γ-radiation (45) and that *RET* gene fragmentation induced by ionizing radiation exposure is significantly higher than fragmentation of any other DNA region (46). The generation of a RET/PTC3 rearrangement seems to be particularly facilitated by the alignment of ELE1 (i.e. the partner of RET/PTC3 rearrangement) and RET introns in opposite orientation (47). Since *RET/PTC* is also frequently found in paediatric papillary thyroid cancer without known exposure to radiation (43, 48), it is also possible that age *per se* may play an important role. Alternatively,

Table 3.2.5.6 RET activation in spontaneous and post-Chernobyl childhood papillary thyroid carcinoma

Spontaneous	Post-Chernobyl	References
12/17 (71%) USA	33/38 (87.0%) Belarus	(43)
n.d.	4/6 (66.6%) Belarus	(41)
n.d.	17/28 (60.7%) Ukraine	Thomas G.A *et al.* 1999
n.d.	20/39 (51.3%) Belarus	Thomas G.A *et al* 1999
n.d.	9/15 (60.0%) Belarus	(42)
n.d.	25/51 (49.0%) Belarus	Smida J. *et al.*, 1999
10/21 (48.0%) UK	n.d.	Williams G.H. *et al.*, 1996
6/9 (67.0%) Italy	n.d.	(48)
3/10 (30.0%) Japan	n.d.	Motomura T. *et al.*, 1998
10/25 (40%) Italy	19/25 (76%) Belarus	(44)
41/82 (50%)	127/202 (63%)	Meta-analysis (p = 0.045)

n.d., not determined.

one can speculate that virtually all paediatric papillary thyroid cancers are radiation-induced cancers, developing in children with an increased susceptibility to spontaneous background radiation.

It has been noted that no point mutations of BRAF oncogene have been found in post-Chernobyl childhood thyroid carcinomas (49). BRAF V600E activating mutation is present in about 40% of naturally occurring thyroid cancers in adults but is almost absent in children. The question of whether the very low frequency of BRAF mutations in post-Chernobyl childhood carcinoma is related to the young age of patients rather than the inability of ionizing radiation to induce oncogene point mutations is still not clarified. However, the finding of BRAF rearrangements in radiation-induced but not in naturally occurring thyroid cancer suggests that the oncogene alterations determined by ionizing radiations are mainly chromosomal rearrangements more than single point mutations (50). In recent years, studies on genomic profiling have suggested distinct patterns in radiation-induced and sporadic thyroid cancer and in particular the expression of seven genes was found to be completely different in the two groups (24, 51).

Radiation-induced thyroid diseases other than thyroid tumours

Thyroid cancer and benign thyroid nodules after thyroid radiation exposure occur as stochastic effects. Depending on the radiation dose, deterministic effects resulting in hypothyroidism and acute thyroiditis may also occur. Another documented consequence of radiation is the possibility of developing chronic autoimmune thyroid disorders.

Hypothyroidism is caused by radiation doses of the order of more than several gray to the thyroid. Such doses are used in the treatment of Graves' disease and toxic nodular goitre, and in these conditions hypothyroidism should be considered the aim rather than an untoward effect of treatment. Primary 'spontaneous' hypothyroidism (or subclinical hypothyroidism) was reported in survivors of the atomic bomb in Nagasaki (52). In a study of 2587 survivors, 43 were diagnosed with hypothyroidism, 27 of whom were thyroid antibody positive and 16 were thyroid antibody negative, with no gender differences. Since an association was observed between thyroid dose and prevalence of antibody positivity, but not antibody negativity, primary hypothyroidism could conceivably have stemmed from an underlying autoimmune thyroid disorder. However, more recently, the same group reported that 55–58 years after radiation exposure, autoimmune thyroid disorders were not found to be significantly associated with radiation exposure while, in the same study, the authors confirmed a significant linear dose-response relationship in the prevalence of both thyroid cancer and benign thyroid nodules and that the relationship was higher in individuals who were exposed at younger ages (53).

The occurrence of thyroid autoimmunity after external irradiation to the head and neck has been reported in several studies. An increased incidence of thyroid antibodies was found by De Groot *et al.* (54) in individuals who received radiation during childhood for benign disorders. Variable degrees of thyroid lymphocytic infiltration have been reported in more than two-thirds of individuals who received radiation several years before thyroidectomy for nodular thyroid lesions. In patients who received radiation of the neck for Hodgkin's disease, 3% or more developed Graves' disease (a 7- to 20-fold excess risk) and 1% thyroiditis.

Hypothyroidism has also been reported after exposure to internal radiation (radioactive iodine). In the people exposed to the fallout of the Marshall Islands accident (55), hypothyroidism was noted within 10 years after the accident. On this occasion most of the cases were not associated with an autoimmune thyroid reaction.

In contrast, an increased prevalence of antithyroid antibodies (19.5%), without hypothyroidism, has been reported in children living in a Belarus village heavily contaminated by the post-Chernobyl radioactive fallout, as opposed to children living in a noncontaminated village (3.8% prevalence) (56). The susceptibility to develop thyroid autoimmunity increased with age at the time of exposure and, in girls, reached its maximum at puberty, suggesting that puberty (oestrogen) and radiation have a cumulative effect in the development of thyroid antibodies in girls. However, a more recent study demonstrated that the increased prevalence of thyroid antibodies in exposed children was a real but transient phenomenon not accompanied by the development of 'overt' hypothyroidism or other thyroid dysfunction 13–15 years after the Chernobyl accident (57). A relationship between prevalence of subclinical hypothyroidism and individual ^{131}I thyroid doses due to environmental exposure has been reported in a very large cohort of people exposed to the post-Chernobyl radioactive fall out during childhood. However, the same authors suggest further prospective studies since the radiation increase in hypothyroidism was quite small (10% per gray) (58). In this regard it is worth noting that autoimmune hypothyroidism can naturally take place over decades (59) and, consequently, an unexposed age- and sex-matched control group should be analysed, especially as the cohort mean age increases. Furthermore, it should also be taken into account that differences in other environmental factors, such as iodine deficiency, may play some roles in favouring the development of autoimmune phenomena (60).

References

1. Duffy BJ, Fitzgerald PJ. Thyroid cancer in childhood and adolescents: a report on twenty-eight cases. *Cancer*, 1950; **3**: 1018–32.
2. Lee W, Chiacchierini RP, Shleien B, Telles NC. Thyroid tumors following 131I or localized X irradiation to the thyroid and pituitary glands in rats. *Radiat Res*, 1982; **92**: 307–19.
3. Socolow EL, Hashizume A, Neriishi S, Niitani R. Thyroid carcinoma in man after exposure to ionizing radiation. A summary of the findings in Hiroshima and Nagasaki. *N Engl J Med*, 1963; **268**: 406–10.
4. Shore RE. Issues and epidemiological evidence regarding radiation-induced thyroid cancer. *Radiat Res*, 1992; **131**: 98–111.
5. National Council of Radiation Protection and Measurements. *Induction of Thyroid Cancer by Ionizing Radiation*. Bethesda: NCRP Publications, 1985: (NCRP Report N. 80).
6. Ron E, Lubin JH, Shore RE, Mabuchi K, Modan B, Pottern LM, *et al.* Thyroid cancer after exposure to external radiation: a pooled analysis of seven studies. *Radiat Res*, 1995; **141**: 259–77.
7. Thompson DE, Mabuchi K, Ron E, Soda M, Tokunaga M, Ochikubo S, *et al.* Cancer incidence in atomic bomb survivors. Part II: solid tumors, 1958–1987. *Radiat Res*, 1994; **137** (Suppl 2): S17–67.
8. Lundell M, Hakulinen T, Holm LE. Thyroid cancer after radiotherapy for skin hemangioma in infancy. *Radiat Res*, 1994; **40**: 334–9.
9. Pottern LM, Kaplan MM, Larsen PR, Silva JE, Koenig RJ, Lubin JH, *et al.* Thyroid nodularity after childhood irradiation for lymphoid hyperplasia: a comparison of questionnaire and clinical findings. *J Clin Epidemiol*, 1990; **43**: 449–60.
10. Shore RE, Labert RE, Pasternack BS. Follow-up study of patients treated by X-ray epilation for tinea capitis. *Arch Environ Health*, 1976; **31**: 17–24.

11. Winship T, Rosvoll RV. Thyroid carcinoma in childhood: final report on a 20 year study. *Clin Proc Child Hosp Washington DC*, 1970; **26**: 327–48.
12. Schneider AB, Ron E, Lubin J, Stovall M, Gierlowski TC. Dose–response relationship for radiation-induced thyroid cancer and thyroid nodules: evidence for prolonged effects of radiation on the thyroid. *J Clin Endocrinol Metab*, 1993; **77**: 362–9.
13. Hancock SL, Cox RS, McDougall IR. Thyroid disease after treatment of Hodgkin's disease. *N Engl J Med*, 1991; **325**: 599–605.
14. Hawkins MM, Draper GJ, Kingston JE. Incidence of second primary tumours among childhood cancer survivors. *Br J Cancer*, 1987; **56**: 339–47.
15. Tucker MA, Jones PH, Boice JD Jr, Robison LL, Stone BJ, Stovall M, *et al.* Therapeutic radiation at a young age is linked to secondary thyroid cancer. *Cancer Res*, 1991; **51**: 2885–8.
16. Chow EJ, Friedman DL, Stovall M, Yasui Y, Whitton JA, Robison LL, *et al.* Risk of thyroid dysfunction and subsequent thyroid cancer among survivors of acute lymphoblastic leukemia: a report from the Childhood Cancer Survivor Study. *Pediatr Blood Cancer*. 2009; **53**: 432–7.
17. Nakachi K, Hayashi T, Hamatani K, Eguchi H, Kusunoki Y. Sixty years of follow-up of Hiroshima and Nagasaki survivors: current progress in molecular epidemiology studies. *Mutation Research*, 2008; **659**: 109–117.
18. Saad AG, Kumar S, Ron E, Lubin JH, Stanek J, Bove KE, *et al.* Proliferative activity of human thyroid cells in various age groups and its correlation with the risk of thyroid cancer after radiation exposure. *J Clin Endocrinol Metab*, 2006; **91**: 2672–7.
19. Richardson DB. Exposure to ionizing radiation in adulthood and thyroid cancer incidence. *Epidemiology*, 2009; **20**: 181–7.
20. Wang Z, Boice JD Jr, Wei LX, Beebe GW, Zha YR, Kaplan MM, *et al.* Thyroid nodularity and chromosome aberrations among women in areas of high background radiation in China. *J Natl Cancer Inst*, 1990; **82**: 478–85.
21. Wang JX, Inskip PD, Boice JD, Li BX, Zhang JY, Fraumeni JF. Cancer incidence among medical diagnostic X-ray workers in China, 1950 to 1985. *Int J Cancer*, 1990; **45**: 889–95.
22. Perkel VS, Gail MH, Lubin J, Pee DY, Weinstein R, Shore-Freedman E, *et al.* Radiation-induced thyroid neoplasms: evidence for familial susceptibility factors. *J Clin Endocrinol Metab*, 1988; **66**: 1316–22.
23. Schenider AB, Shore-Freedman E, Weinstein RA. Radiation-induced thyroid and other head and neck tumors: occurrence of multiple tumors and analysis of risk factors. *J Clin Endocrinol Metab*, 1986; **63**: 107–12.
24. Detours V, Delys L, Libert F, Weiss Solís D, Bogdanova T, Dumont JE, *et al.* Genome-wide gene expression profiling suggests distinct radiation susceptibilities in sporadic and post-Chernobyl papillary thyroid cancers. *Br J Cancer*, 2007; **97**: 818–25.
25. Hall P, Mattsson A, Boice JD. Thyroid cancer after diagnostic administration of iodine-131. *Radiat Res*, 1996; **145**: 86–92.
26. Holm LE, Hall P, Wiklund K, Lundell G, Berg G, Bjelkengren G, *et al.* Cancer risk after iodine-131 therapy for hyperthyroidism. *J Natl Cancer Inst*, 1991; **83**: 1072–7.
27. Dobyns BM, Sheline GE, Workman JB, Tompkins EA, McConahey WM, Becker DV. Malignant and benign neoplasms of the thyroid in patients treated for hyperthyroidism: a report of the cooperative thyrotoxicosis therapy follow-up study. *J Clin Endocrinol Metab*, 1974; **38**: 976–98.
28. Bhattacharyya N, Chien W. Risk of second primary malignancy after radioactive iodine treatment for differentiated thyroid carcinoma. *Ann Otol Rhinol Laryngol*, 2006; **115**: 607–10.
29. Rubino C, de Vathaire F, Dottorini ME, Hall P, Schvartz C, Couette JE, *et al.* Second primary malignancies in thyroid cancer patients. *Br J Cancer*, 2003; **89**: 1638–44.
30. Cardis E, Howe G, Ron E, Bebeshko V, Bogdanova T, Bouville A, *et al.* Cancer consequences of the Chernobyl accident: 20 years on. *J Radiol Prot*, 2006; **26**: 127–40.
31. Nikiforov YE, Heffess CS, Korzenko AV, Fagin JA, Gnepp DR. Characteristics of follicular tumors and nonneoplastic thyroid lesions in children and adolescents exposed to radiation as a result of the Chernobyl disaster. *Cancer*, 1995; **76**: 900–9.
32. Cardis E, Kesminiene A, Ivanov V, Malakhova I, Shibata Y, Khrouch V, *et al.* Risk of thyroid cancer after exposure to 131I in childhood. *J Natl Cancer Inst*, 2005; **97**: 724–32.
33. Karaoglou A, Desmet G, Kelly GN, Menzel HG. *The Radiological Consequences of the Chernobyl Accident.* Brussels-Luxembourg: Commission of the European Communities, 1996: (Publication EUR 16544 EN).
34. Baverstock K, Egloff B, Pinchera A, Ruchti C, Williams D. Thyroid cancer after Chernobyl. *Nature*, 1992; **359**: 21–2.
35. Kazakov VS, Demidchik EP, Astakhova LN. Thyroid cancer after Chernobyl. *Nature*, 1992; **359**: 21.
36. Hatch M, Brenner A, Bogdanova T, Derevyanko A, Kuptsova N, Likhtarev I, *et al.* A screening study of thyroid cancer and other thyroid diseases among individuals exposed in utero to iodine-131 from Chernobyl fallout. *J Clin Endocrinol Metab*, 2009; **94**: 899–906.
37. Williams D. Twenty years' experience with post-Chernobyl thyroid cancer. *Best Pract Res Clin Endocrinol Metab*, 2008; **22**: 1061–73.
38. Pacini F, Vorontsova T, Demidchik EP, Molinaro E, Agate L, Romei C, *et al.* Post-Chernobyl thyroid carcinoma in Belarus children and adolescents: comparison with naturally occurring thyroid carcinoma in Italy and France. *J Clin Endocrinol Metab*, 1997; **82**: 3563–9.
39. Ceccarelli C, Pacini F, Lippi F, Elisei R, Arganini M, Miccoli P, *et al.* Thyroid cancer in children and adolescents. *Surgery*, 1988; **104**: 1143–7.
40. Naing S, Collins BJ, Schneider AB. Clinical behavior of radiation-induced thyroid cancer: factors related to recurrence. *Thyroid*, 2009; **19**: 479–85.
41. Fugazzola L, Pilotti S, Pinchera A, Vorontsova TV, Mondellini P, Bongarzone I, *et al.* Oncogenic rearrangements of the RET proto-oncogene in papillary thyroid carcinomas from children exposed to the Chernobyl nuclear accident. *Cancer Res*, 1995; **55**: 5617–20.
42. Klugbauer S, Lengfelder E, Demidchik EP, Rabes HM. High prevalence of RET rearrangement in thyroid tumors of children from Belarus after the Chernobyl reactor accident. *Oncogene*, 1995; **11**: 2459–67.
43. Nikiforov YE, Rowland JM, Bove KE, Monforte-Munoz H, Fagin JA. Distinct pattern of RET oncogene rearrangements in morphological variants of radiation-induced and sporadic thyroid papillary carcinomas in children. *Cancer Res*, 1997; **57**: 1690–4.
44. Elisei R, Romei C, Vorontsova T, Cosci B, Veremeychik V, Kuchinskaya E, *et al.* RET/PTC rearrangements in thyroid nodules: studies in irradiated and not irradiated, malignant and benign thyroid lesions in children and adults. *J Clin Endocrinol Metab*, 2001; **86**: 3211–16.
45. Caudill CM, Zhu Z, Ciampi R, Stringer JR, Nikiforov YE. Dose-dependent generation of RET/PTC in human thyroid cells after in vitro exposure to gamma-radiation: a model of carcinogenic chromosomal rearrangement induced by ionizing radiation. *J Clin Endocrinol Metab*, 2005; **90**: 2364–9.
46. Volpato CB, Martínez-Alfaro M, Corvi R, Gabus C, Sauvaigo S, Ferrari P, *et al.* Enhanced sensitivity of the RET proto-oncogene to ionizing radiation in vitro. *Cancer Res*, 2008; **68**: 8986–92.
47. Nikiforov YE, Koshoffer A, Nikiforova M, Stringer J, Fagin JA. Chromosomal breakpoint positions suggest a direct role for radiation in inducing illegitimate recombination between the ELE1 and RET genes in radiation-induced thyroid carcinomas. *Oncogene*, 1999; **18**: 6330–4.
48. Bongarzone I, Fugazzola L, Vigneri P, Mariani L, Mondellini P, Pacini F, *et al.* Age-related activation of the tyrosine kinase receptor protooncogenes ret and NTRK1 in papillary thyroid carcinoma. *Journal of Clinical Endocrinology and Metabolism*, 1996; **81**: 2006–9.
49. Lima J, Trovisco V, Soares P, Máximo V, Magalhães J, Salvatore G, *et al.* BRAF mutations are not a major event in post-Chernobyl childhood thyroid carcinomas. *J Clin Endocrinol Metab*, 2004; **89**: 4267–71.
50. Ciampi R, Knauf JA, Kerler R, Gandhi M, Zhu Z, Nikiforova MN, *et al.* Oncogenic AKAP9-BRAF fusion is a novel mechanism of MAPK pathway activation in thyroid cancer. *J Clin Invest*, 2005; **115**: 94–101.

51. Port M, Boltze C, Wang Y, Röper B, Meineke V, Abend M. A radiation-induced gene signature distinguishes post-Chernobyl from sporadic papillary thyroid cancers. *Radiat Res*, 2007; **168**: 639–49.
52. Nagataki S, Shibata Y, Inoue S, Yokoyama N, Izumi M, Shimaoka K. Thyroid disease among atomic bomb survivors in Nagasaki. *JAMA*, 1994; **272**: 364–70.
53. Imaizumi M, Usa T, Tominaga T, Neriishi K, Akahoshi M, Nakashima E, *et al.* Radiation dose-response relationships for thyroid nodules and autoimmune thyroid diseases in Hiroshima and Nagasaki atomic bomb survivors 55-58 years after radiation exposure. *JAMA*, 2006; **295**: 1011–22.
54. De Groot LJ, Reilly M, Pinnamaneni K, Refetoff S. Retrospective and prospective study of radiation-induced thyroid disease. *Am J Med*, 1983; **74**: 852–6.
55. Larsen PR, Conard RA, Knudsen KD, Robbins J, Wolff J, Rall JE, *et al.* Thyroid hypofunction after exposure to fallout from a hydrogen bomb explosion. *JAMA*, 1982; **247**: 1571–5.
56. Pacini F, Vorontsova T, Molinaro E, Kuchinskaya E, Agate L, Shavrova E, *et al.* Prevalence of thyroid autoantibodies in children and adolescents from Belarus exposed to the Chernobyl radioactive fallout. *Lancet*, 1998; **352**: 763–6.
57. Agate L, Mariotti S, Elisei R, Mossa P, Pacini F, Molinaro E, *et al.* Thyroid autoantibodies and thyroid function in subjects exposed to Chernobyl fallout during childhood: evidence for a transient radiation-induced elevation of serum thyroid antibodies without an increase in thyroid autoimmune disease. *J Clin Endocrinol Metab*, 2008; **93**: 2729–36.
58. Ostroumova E, Brenner A, Oliynyk V, McConnell R, Robbins J, Terekhova G, *et al.* Subclinical hypothyroidism after radioiodine exposure: Ukrainian-American cohort study of thyroid cancer and other thyroid diseases after the Chernobyl accident (1998–2000). *Environ Health Perspect*, 2009; **117**: 745–50.
59. Vanderpump MP, Tunbridge WM, French JM, Appleton D, Bates D, Clark F, *et al.* The incidence of thyroid disorders in the community: a twenty-year follow-up of the Whickham Survey. *Clin Endocrinol (Oxf)*, 1995; **43**: 55–68.
60. Tronko MD, Brenner AV, Olijnyk VA, Robbins J, Epstein OV, McConnell RJ, *et al.* Autoimmune thyroiditis and exposure to iodine 131 in the Ukrainian cohort study of thyroid cancer and other thyroid diseases after the Chernobyl accident: results from the first screening cycle (1998-2000). *J Clin Endocrinol Metab*, 2006; **91**: 4344–51.

3.2.6 Autoimmune thyroid disease

Anthony P. Weetman

Introduction

Along with neoplasia, autoimmunity is the most common cause of endocrine disease and, of this group of disorders, thyroid autoimmunity is the most frequent. Conversely, the autoimmune thyroid diseases are the most common organ-specific or nonorgan-specific autoimmune conditions affecting any site.

This prevalence, the ease of access to the target organ, the often slow progression of disease, and the historical legacy of being the first distinctive autoimmune process to be defined, have ensured that there is now a reasonable understanding of the main factors involved in pathogenesis. This chapter assumes a basic knowledge of immunology; readers unfamiliar with this topic can obtain further details about the fundamental processes involved in self/non-self discrimination by the immune system elsewhere (1).

Spectrum of thyroid autoimmunity

The range of thyroid autoimmunity is shown in Table 3.2.6.1. The most frequent manifestation is probably the presence of focal thyroiditis, which can be found in around 40% of white women at autopsy, and is half as frequent in men (2). Focal thyroiditis is often accompanied by the formation of thyroid antibodies, discussed later, but it is presently unclear whether all examples of focal thyroiditis have a truly autoimmune basis, especially if negative for thyroid antibodies. Careful longitudinal community studies have shown that individuals with positive thyroid antibodies (and presumably an underlying focal thyroiditis) have an increased risk of developing overt or clinical autoimmune hypothyroidism, which in women might be expected to occur in 2.1% per year over a 20-year follow-up period (3). In men, the risk is three times greater. Individuals who have a sustained elevated thyroid-stimulating hormone (TSH) but normal free thyroxine (T_4) levels, a state termed subclinical hypothyroidism, have a similar risk of progression to clinical hypothyroidism, and it may be assumed that these patients initially had focal autoimmune thyroiditis which progressed, albeit without the autoimmune response giving rise to detectable thyroid antibodies. When individuals have both subclinical hypothyroidism and positive thyroid antibodies, the relative risk of progression to clinical hypothyroidism is 38 for women and 173 for men.

Postpartum thyroiditis, discussed in detail in Chapter 3.4.6, arises from subclinical autoimmune hypothyroidism. The underlying autoimmune process is enhanced 3–6 months postpartum, for reasons which remain obscure, and at this point biochemically or clinically evident thyroid dysfunction occurs, only to remit months later as the postpartum exacerbation subsides. The occurrence of permanent clinical hypothyroidism over the subsequent 5 years in 20–30% of women presumably results from a continued and worsening autoimmune injury, as found in any type of subclinical hypothyroidism. Like postpartum thyroiditis, silent (or painless) thyroiditis causes a transient disturbance of thyroid function, most often presenting with mild destructive thyrotoxicosis followed by hypothyroidism, and indeed in the early literature, postpartum and silent thyroiditis were not distinguished. Excess iodide is an inciting factor in some cases, and others are due to inadvertent exposure to thyroid hormone (e.g., thyroid contamination of meat products), but in many cases the condition seems to be a spontaneous exacerbation of an underlying autoimmune process and goitre, permanent hypothyroidism, or thyroid antibodies are present in one-half of such individuals several years after presentation.

The term 'Hashimoto's thyroiditis' is strictly a histological definition, with the features described below. Clinically, patients present with a painless, lymphocytic goitre of variable size, with or without hypothyroidism, hence the alternative name, goitrous thyroiditis. Thyroid antibodies are strongly positive in almost all cases. Primary myxoedema, or atrophic thyroiditis, presents with clinical hypothyroidism, because the thyroid has usually been severely damaged by the autoimmune process, as the name implies. There have been largely unsuccessful attempts to identify separate causes for atrophic and goitrous thyroiditis, but it seems more likely that there is a continuum from one to the other, with fibrosis and follicular destruction gradually dominating in a previously lymphocytic goitre.

At first sight, Graves' disease appears as a distinct autoimmune disorder, characterized by the presence of stimulating antibodies against the TSH receptor, but it is now clear that such antibodies

Table 3.2.6.1 Range of thyroid autoimmunity

	Goitre	Thyroid function	Features
Focal thyroiditis	No	Normal or subclinical hypothyroidism (elevated TSH; normal free T_4)	May progress to overt hypothyroidism; associated with positive thyroid antibodies[a]
Hashimoto's (or goitrous) thyroiditis	Variable size	Normal or hypothyroid (clinical or subclinical)	Almost always thyroid antibody positive
Atrophic thyroiditis (or primary myxoedema)	No	Hypothyroid	May evolve from goitrous thyroiditis; usually thyroid antibody positive
Silent thyroiditis	Small or absent	Transient thyrotoxicosis and/or hypothyroidism	May progress to permanent hypothyroidism; often thyroid antibody positive
Postpartum thyroiditis	Small	Transient thyrotoxicosis and/or hypothyroidism	May progress to permanent hypothyroidism; often thyroid antibody positive
Graves' disease	Variable size	Hyperthyroid	Associated with ophthalmopathy; positive for TSH-receptor stimulating antibodies and usually for other thyroid antibodies

[a] Thyroglobulin and/or thyroid peroxidase antibodies.

also occur in some patients with autoimmune hypothyroidism, in whom their effects are masked by a stronger autoimmune process leading to hypothyroidism. Moreover, up to 20% of Graves' patients treated successfully with antithyroid drugs develop spontaneous hypothyroidism over the subsequent 10–20 years, most likely due to the supervention of destructive autoimmunity (4). Infrequently in some patients fluctuation between hyper- and hypothyroidism occurs over weeks or months, and alterations in the relative levels of TSH-receptor antibodies with stimulating and blocking capabilities may explain this phenomenon. The term 'hashitoxicosis' is used to describe occasional patients with clinical Graves' disease but a histological picture of Hashimoto's thyroiditis, again demonstrating the close relationship between these disorders and their sharing of common pathogenetic features.

Pathological features

Autoimmune thyroiditis

In focal thyroiditis, the thyroid is usually normal in size and contains foci of lymphocytes which are predominantly T cells, although lymphoid follicles can also occur. Thyroid cells adjacent to these foci are usually atrophic and deficient in colloid, but away from the foci, thyroid follicular architecture is normal (5). Focal thyroiditis may also be prominent adjacent to a papillary carcinoma or other neoplasm. By contrast, the whole thyroid is usually involved in Hashimoto's thyroiditis. The lymphocytic infiltrate is more extensive, diffuse, and composed mainly of T cells, with prominent germinal centres containing B cells scattered through the gland (Fig. 3.2.6.1). Macrophages, dendritic cells, and sometimes giant cells may be prominent. The thyroid follicles go through variable degrees of destruction, depending largely on chronicity, and in the process undergo hyperplasia and oxyphil metaplasia, giving rise to so-called Hürthle or Askanazy cells. These cells are generally absent in juvenile autoimmune thyroiditis.

However, the relative proportion of lymphocytic infiltrate, thyroid follicular cell change, and fibrosis varies greatly, in keeping with the suggestion made previously that there is a broad spectrum of changes which may ultimately result in atrophic thyroiditis. In this condition, the thyroid is small, has extensive fibrosis mixed with a scattered lymphocytic infiltrate, and there is a marked reduction in thyroid follicular cells. Attempts have been made to subdivide these histological entities further, including a mixed variant of chronic thyroiditis, but the clinical value of this is limited. The pathology in postpartum and silent thyroiditis generally resembles mild to moderate Hashimoto's thyroiditis, although without the oxyphil metaplasia. Germinal centres are usually absent.

Graves' disease

It is now unusual to see the full histological picture of Graves' disease as patients are almost all treated with antithyroid drugs which diminish the lymphocytic infiltrate (5). Even after such treatment, however, there is often a diffuse or focal lymphocytic thyroiditis, predominantly of T cells, sometimes with germinal centre formation. As an aside, lymphoid hyperplasia may also involve the lymph nodes, thymus, and spleen in Graves' disease, once again being reversed by antithyroid drugs. The thyroid follicles are both hypertrophied and hyperplastic, with scalloping and reduction in colloid (Fig. 3.2.6.2). The epithelial cells are columnar and extend as papillae into the lumen. These changes are also attenuated by antithyroid drugs, so that after prolonged treatment, the colloid reaccumulates, the papillae regress, and the epithelium becomes cuboidal.

Factors determining susceptibility

A complex combination of genetic, environmental, and endogenous factors determines susceptibility (Fig. 3.2.6.3). These factors operate differently in individuals, so that the factors leading to disease in one patient will differ from the next, which makes analysis of the importance of each factor difficult with present tools. Genetic effects are seen most clearly in children and adolescents, with environmental factors having an increasing chance to operate with age.

Genetic factors

These are dealt with extensively in Chapter 3.2.1. However, a brief discussion is given here, in relation to genetic effects on the autoimmune process. It is obvious clinically that thyroid diseases cluster in families more often than expected by chance, although the association of Graves' disease and autoimmune hypothyroidism in such families, and their coassociation with autoimmune polyglandular syndrome type 2, indicates that at least some of the susceptibility is determined by genes that control a generalized tendency to organ-specific autoimmunity. One such determinant in white people is

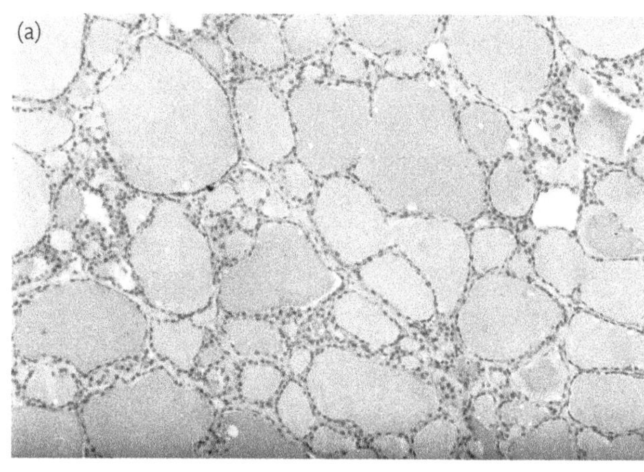

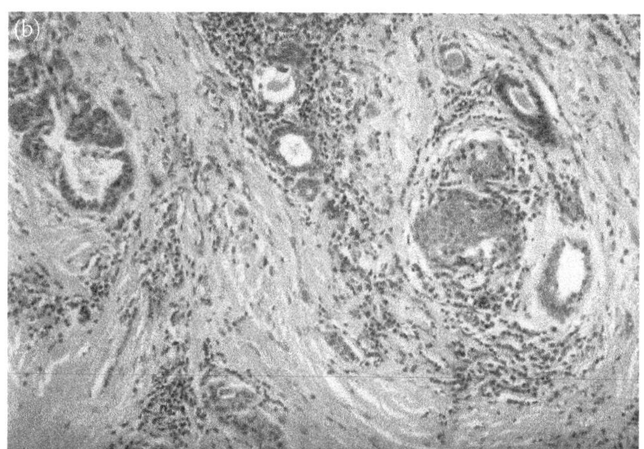

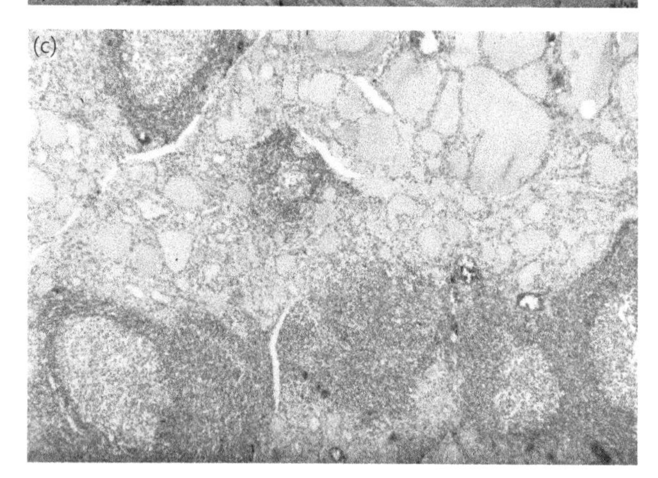

Fig. 3.2.6.1 Histological features of (a) normal thyroid, (b) atrophic thyroiditis, and (c) Hashimoto's thyroiditis (original magnification ×100; photomicrographs courtesy of Dr K. Suvarna).

the HLA-DR3 specificity, which is associated with all of the major autoimmune endocrinopathies (6, 7). As HLA-DR3-positive healthy individuals differ from those who are DR3 negative in a number of immunological measurements, such as immune complex clearance, circulating T-lymphocyte subsets, immune responses to particulate antigens, and production of the cytokine tumour necrosis factor, this association may simply reflect a heightened nonspecific immune responsiveness. Thus, if a DR3-positive individual develops thyroid autoimmunity for any reason, this will be more likely to progress to florid disease.

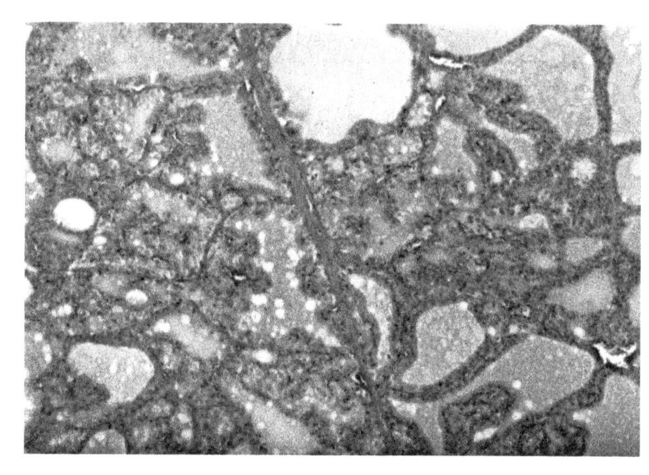

Fig. 3.2.6.2 Histological features of Graves' disease (original magnification ×100; photomicrograph courtesy of Dr K. Suvarna).

Another reason why the highly polymorphic alleles of HLA class II genes (also called major histocompatibility complex or MHC class II genes) are associated with autoimmunity is that their products are expressed by antigen-presenting cells and are crucial in initiating any immune response (Fig. 3.2.6.4). Autoimmune disease may arise because a certain class II allele is able to bind and present a crucial fragment of an autoantigen, called an epitope, to a CD4^{+} T cell. Alternatively, the effect of class II alleles in determining immune responsiveness may be exerted in the thymus during development, at which stage future autoreactive T cells may be deleted (negative selection) or allowed to develop (positive selection). Finally, some class II molecules may determine selection of regulatory T cells, and deficiencies in these cells have been postulated as a cause of autoimmunity. It still remains unclear whether other genes in linkage disequilibrium with HLA-D-region

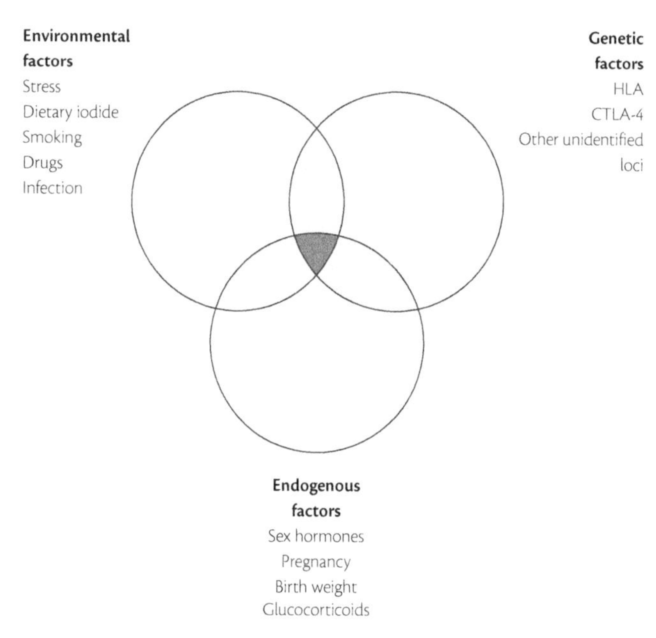

Fig. 3.2.6.3 Interaction of genetic, environmental, and endogenous factors in the susceptibility to autoimmune thyroid disease. Individual factors are frequent in the general population, but an appropriate combination, shown as the solid area, results in disease.

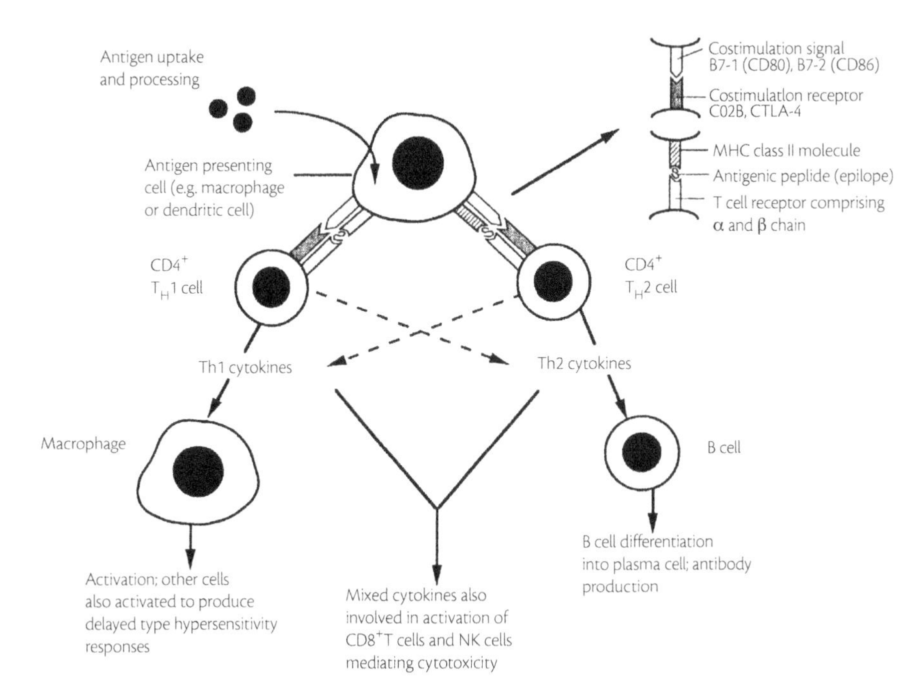

Fig. 3.2.6.4 Key steps in antigen presentation and T-cell activation. The dotted line represents an inhibitory pathway. (From Weetman AP. Recent progress in autoimmune thyroid disease: an overview for the clinician. *Thyroid Today*, 1996; **19**(2): 1–9, with permission).

genes confer additional susceptibility and it is possible that class I genes have a role independent of those in the class II region.

The existence of non-HLA susceptibility genes is shown by the higher frequency of thyroid autoimmunity in monozygotic twins than in HLA-identical siblings, which in turn is higher than non-HLA identical siblings. The critical role of CTLA4 in costimulation of T-cell responses is discussed below and this has made it an excellent candidate to test as a susceptibility gene. It is now clear that polymorphisms in this gene have a significant role in autoimmune thyroid disease as well as several other autoimmune disorders that are associated with thyroid disease clinically. More recently it has become clear that polymorphisms in other T-cell regulatory genes, including *PTPN22* and *interleukin-2 receptor/CD25*, can similarly increase susceptibility to autoimmune thyroid disease and related disorders. Overall it is now clear that many genes exerting small effects contribute to these diseases and their influence varies between individuals, which in turn may explain the diverse clinical presentations of thyroid autoimmunity.

Environmental factors

The lack of complete concordance for Graves' disease in monozygotic twins and the clinically obvious lack of a family history in many patients with autoimmune thyroid disease, point to a major role for environmental factors in determining susceptibility, as does temporal variability in incidence (8). Furthermore, at least part of the family clustering of disease could be the result of shared exposure to environmental triggers. Some of the best evidence for the involvement of the environmental factors shown in Fig. 3.2.6.3 comes from animal models of experimental autoimmune thyroiditis (Table 3.2.6.2) which resemble Hashimoto's thyroiditis (9). Excess dietary iodide exacerbates the severity of the lymphocytic thyroiditis in rats with experimental autoimmune thyroiditis, and

Table 3.2.6.2 Main experimental models of autoimmune thyroiditis

Model	Species	Antigen	
Immunization	Mouse, rat, rabbit, guinea pig	TG, TPO, TSHR	Strain-dependent, transient, and transferable using T cells
Thymectomy-induced	Mouse, rat	TG	May need additional sublethal irradiation
T-cell manipulation	Mouse	TG	Transfer of specific T cells to T-cell-depleted animals to induce thyroiditis
Spontaneous	Chicken, dog, rat	Mainly TG	Thyroiditis occurs in OS chickens, beagles, NOD mice, and BB and Buffalo strain rats (NOD and BB animals have autoimmune diabetes)
Transplantation	Severe combined immunodeficiency mouse or nude mouse	TG, TPO, TSHR	Transplanted thyroid tissues from patients with Graves' disease and Hashimoto' thyroiditis survive but the animal does not develop disease
cDNA immunization	Mouse	TSHR	TSHR antibodies produced
Immunization with fibroblasts transfected with TSHR and MHC class II	Mouse	TSHR	Closest animal model of Graves' disease

MHC, major histocompatibility complex; NOD, nonobese diabetic; OS, Obese strain; TG, thyroglobulin; TPO, thyroid peroxidase; TSHR, thyroid-stimulating hormone receptor.

leads to enhanced production of thyroglobulin antibodies; similar observations have been made in the Obese strain chicken which develops spontaneous autoimmune hypothyroidism. Indeed, rigorous depletion of iodide, starting at the stage of egg formation, virtually abolishes autoimmune thyroiditis in this strain of chicken. This observation neatly demonstrates the interaction possible between genetic and environmental factors. Excess iodide may have several effects, including an action directly on the immune system, the formation of an important part of a major T-cell epitope on the iodinated thyroid antigen thyroglobulin, and the generation of toxic metabolites within the thyroid which damage thyroid cells. There is epidemiological evidence to support a similar effect of excess iodide on human autoimmune thyroiditis (10), which is of some concern given the recent tendency for iodide intake to increase.

Infections could precipitate an autoimmune response by target-cell damage, leading to release of autoantigens, by altering target-cell expression of autoantigen or immunoregulatory molecules, such as HLA, or by molecular mimicry, in which an immune response against microorganism antigens that resemble host autoantigens triggers an autoimmune response. Despite the appeal of the notion and the success of animal models, there is surprisingly little evidence linking infection to human autoimmune disease. Autoimmune hypothyroidism occurs with increased frequency after congenital rubella infection, and epidemiological as well as serological studies have suggested a role for *Yersinia* infection in Graves' disease. On the other hand, studies showing a lower frequency of thyroid and other types of autoimmunity in areas with a poor standard of hygiene suggest that in some settings infections may enhance immune responses in a way that avoids the emergence of autoimmunity, perhaps through skewing of the cytokine secretion of T helper cells, discussed below, (11). Despite many attempts, no convincing role for retroviruses in autoimmune thyroid disease is proven. Taking the opposite view, subacute thyroiditis is caused by a wide variety of viruses, and gives rise to thyroid destruction, yet rarely (if ever) triggers autoimmune thyroid disease. Only low and infrequent levels of thyroid antibodies occur in the course of infection and then disappear, although subacute thyroiditis may lead to permanent hypothyroidism in individuals who have coincidental subclinical autoimmune thyroiditis.

Stress now appears to be an important precipitant of Graves' disease, based on analysis of preceding life events in newly diagnosed patients (12). A note of caution is necessary since retrospective recall and the influence of the evolving disease itself (both on recall and preceding interpersonal relationships) may have biased results, but reports are generally consistent and suggest an effect on susceptibility of roughly the same magnitude as HLA. The mechanism is presumed to be via the neuroendocrine effects of stress, in particular those mediated via the hypothalamus–pituitary–adrenal cortex axis. Interestingly, the Obese strain chicken, which develops spontaneous autoimmune thyroiditis, has an abnormal corticosteroid secretion profile that may be one of the genetic determinants of this disease (9).

As the therapeutic armamentarium expands, an increasing number of iatrogenic factors precipitate autoimmune thyroid disease. Mantle irradiation for lymphoma and other conditions is associated with an increased frequency of Graves' disease and autoimmune thyroiditis, and rare cases of Graves' disease have been reported following radio-iodine treatment of nodular thyroid disease. While these examples could be the result of thyroid injury, leading to autoantigen release, the lack of a parallel response in the wake of virally induced thyroid damage suggests additional mechanisms, such as a differentially suppressive effect of radiation on critical immunoregulatory T cells. An increased prevalence of thyroid autoantibodies has also been reported in children exposed to fallout form the Chernobyl nuclear reactor explosion (13). Lithium treatment is also associated with an increased prevalence of thyroid autoantibodies, hypothyroidism, and probably Graves' disease.

Therapeutic doses of cytokines precipitate autoimmune hypothyroidism, but rarely Graves' disease. The major culprit is α-interferon, probably because it is the most extensively used (14), but granulocyte-macrophage colony-stimulating factor, interleukin 2 (IL-2) and IL-4 have also been implicated. How these effects relate to the role of the same cytokines, at far lower endogenous concentrations, in untreated patients is unknown. However, an association exists between attacks of allergic rhinitis and the time of relapse of Graves' disease, which may well depend on the nonspecific enhancing effects of cytokines released during the allergic response.

Environmental pollutants and toxins are theoretically important factors but remain underinvestigated. Administration of anthracene derivatives to genetically predisposed rats can precipitate experimental autoimmune thyroiditis. The potential of pollutants to operate in this way in humans is illustrated by the association between cigarette smoking and thyroid-associated ophthalmopathy (Chapter 3.3.10) as well as, to a lesser extent, Graves' disease, whereas smoking appears to decrease the risk of Hashimoto's thyroiditis (15).

Endogenous factors

The most impressive effect is imposed by pregnancy, which can lead to postpartum thyroiditis in around 5% of ostensibly healthy women (Chapter 3.4.6). However, the frequency of Graves' disease is also increased in the 2 years postpartum and transient autoimmune hypothyroidism is frequently encountered after an episode of permanent hypothyroidism, indicating that pregnancy can produce a longer-lasting bias of the autoimmune response. Hyperprolactinaemia has only been inconsistently associated with an increased frequency of autoimmune thyroiditis, but clear evidence for a role of sex hormones has come from work on experimental autoimmune thyroiditis. Female animals given testosterone have a reduced frequency of thyroiditis, while castrated males, or those given oestrogen, have an increased frequency, which approaches that of females (9). These effects explain in large part the much higher rates of autoimmune thyroid disease in women, although it remains to be seen whether any other effects are encoded on the sex chromosomes to explain this dichotomy. Fetal microchimerism or skewed inactivation of the X chromosome are alternative possibilities (16). Low birthweight has only inconsistently been associated with an increased prevalence of thyroid autoimmunity in later life; presumably any such increase in risk depends on altered hormonal status determined *in utero*.

Autoantigens

There are three major autoantigens in autoimmune thyroid disease, detailed below, but there are also a number of specific and nonspecific autoantigens whose involvement is suggested by molecular cloning of candidates or by the demonstration of antibodies to cyto-skeletal or nuclear components. Thyroid hormones are occasionally the target of autoantibody formation. These antibodies have no physiological consequences but can interfere in some assays for thyroid hormones, although this is now less of a problem with improved methods.

Thyroglobulin

Thyroglobulin is a homodimeric 660-kDa glycosylated iodoprotein which is secreted by thyroid follicular cells and stored in the luminal colloid; thyroglobulin also circulates. There are around 100 tyrosine molecules in each molecule of thyroglobulin and around 25 are normally iodinated, but this varies greatly depending on iodine uptake and thyroid activity. The iodination reaction depends on thyroid peroxidase and occurs at the apical border of the thyroid cells. Four thyroglobulin domains, termed A to D, have been identified from analysis of internal homology, and contain between them four to eight hormonogenic sites, two of which, at residues 5 and 2746, correspond to sites of preferential T_4 and triiodothyronine (T_3) synthesis, respectively. When stimulated by TSH or thyroid-stimulating antibodies, thyroglobulin is endocytosed and hydrolysed in lysosomes to release T_3 and T_4.

Although iodination of thyroglobulin plays a major role in the antigenicity of the molecule in animal models of autoimmune thyroiditis, the place of iodination in human autoimmune thyroid disease is less clear, with continuing uncertainty over whether the hormonogenic sites are part of T- or B-cell epitopes. As the immune response diversifies with time, an increasing number of epitopes are recognized, especially by sera with high levels of thyroglobulin antibodies, but patients with autoimmune thyroid disease show greater restriction of epitope recognition by autoantibodies than those who have autoantibodies but remain clinically euthyroid (17). These epitopes are largely conformational, although certain Hashimoto sera recognize linear determinants; all thyroglobulin antibodies cloned from patients so far recognize native but not denatured thyroglobulin. The immunopathogenic nondominant nature of thyroid autoantibody epitopes suggests that the disease may arise from unmasking of cryptic epitopes, which leads to a loss of tolerance (18).

The antibody response to thyroglobulin is relatively restricted, with a predominance of IgG_1 and IgG_4 subclasses and over-representation of certain immunoglobulin variable (V) genes. However, thyroglobulin antibodies, even of the IgG_1 subclass, do not fix complement due to the wide spacing of epitopes, which prevents cross-linking. The potential role of these antibodies in pathogenesis is considered below. Less is known about T-cell epitopes on thyroglobulin, information about which could lead to important insights regarding molecular mimicry with other self-determinants or microbial antigens.

Thyroid peroxidase

Thyroid peroxidase is a glycosylated haemoprotein which exists in two alternatively spliced forms of 100–105 kDa. The predominant form, TPO1, is responsible for tyrosine iodination and coupling to form thyroid hormones and is predominantly located at the apical border of the thyroid cell, anchored by a transmembrane segment near the C-terminus, with the catalytic domain facing the follicular lumen. TPO2 has no enzymatic activity and is restricted to the endoplasmic reticulum: its role in autoimmunity is unknown.

Initial studies of B-cell epitopes on thyroid peroxidase found two sequences, C2 (amino acids 590–622) and C21 (amino acids 710–722), which are linear epitopes recognized by the majority of Hashimoto sera and a smaller proportion of Graves' sera (19). It is likely that these and other linear determinants identified subsequently are only the target of antibodies late in disease when degradation of thyroid peroxidase allows spreading of the immune response. In the initial stages, however, conformational epitopes are probably involved in antibody binding, and these have been identified by human and mouse monoclonal antibodies. There are two large overlapping domains, A and B, which are the target of more than 80% of thyroid peroxidase antibodies in Graves' disease and Hashimoto's thyroiditis and, in the absence of thyroid peroxidase crystals, modelling has allowed prediction of the structure of these. Furthermore the immunoglobulin V gene usage of thyroid peroxidase antibodies is remarkably restricted, with domain B-binding antibodies using a particular light-chain sequence (Vκ 012), irrespective of heavy chain, although heavy-chain V gene usage is also relatively restricted. Relative binding of thyroid peroxidase antibodies to the individual domains varies little over time, indicating a genetic component to the control of thyroid peroxidase antibody formation. Thyroid peroxidase antibodies in general show the same type of IgG subclass restriction as those against thyroglobulin but are able to fix complement.

T-cell epitopes are multiple and individual patients respond to different combinations of epitopes without any apparent correlation with disease type or chronicity (9). As the T-cell response is likely to have had many months to diversify or 'spread' by the time of diagnosis, this observation is not surprising, but it does emphasize how difficult identification of any dominant epitope (which might cross-react with a microbial epitope) will be.

Thyroid-stimulating hormone receptor

The TSH receptor is a typical G-protein-coupled receptor, with an extracellular domain of 398 amino acids, a transmembrane region of 266 amino acids organized in seven loops, and an intracellular domain of 93 amino acids (20). There are two subunits, A (55 kDa) and B (40 kDa), which correspond to the extracellular and transmembrane domains and are joined by disulphide bonds. The A subunit can be shed from the cell surface, which may have immunological consequences by allowing greater access of the autoantigen to the immune system. Polymorphisms in the gene encoding the TSH receptor have been associated with Graves' disease but not with autoimmune hypothyroidism (21), and elucidating the basis for this may be illuminating in understanding the differential expression of autoimmune thyroid diseases.

Although clearly highly expressed in the thyroid, where the receptor is fundamental for cell activation, there is now considerable evidence that the TSH receptor is expressed in fat, particularly preadipocytes, where it may make a contribution to thyroid-associated ophthalmopathy (see Chapter 3.3.10). The main physiological regulator of the TSH receptor is obviously TSH, which causes a rise in intracellular cAMP and, at high concentrations, activation of other signalling pathways, such as phospholipase C. These actions are mimicked by thyroid-stimulating antibodies in Graves' disease, with the possibility that activation of different signalling pathways leads to disease heterogeneity, including goitrogenesis.

The interaction of TSH-receptor antibodies with the receptor is even more complex, with additional antibodies blocking the effect of TSH (leading to hypothyroidism) and others appearing to bind without effects on function (neutral antibodies). The terminology of these antibodies has been obscure, and Table 3.2.6.3 gives an overview.

As would be predicted from the heterogeneous nature of TSH-receptor antibodies, multiple B-cell epitopes have been identified. In summary, the majority are conformational and comprise discontinuous sequences. Both stimulating and blocking antibodies bind to sites on the receptor which overlap with, but are distinct from, the TSH binding site (21, 22). The greatest separation between the binding of these three entities occurs at the N-terminal region of the receptor. Much is still to be determined, including whether the receptor dimerizes and how this could affect activation, and whether receptor desensitization might explain the poor correlation between circulating TSH-receptor stimulating antibody levels and the degree of abnormal thyroid function in patients. TSH-receptor stimulating antibodies show restriction immunoglobulin of heavy and light chain usage, implying oligoclonality of the B cell repertoire.

TSH-receptor T-cell epitopes have been identified and, as with thyroid peroxidase, there is considerable heterogeneity both within and between patients in the regions recognized, with no clear dominant epitope. Certain TSH-receptor sequences are recognized by 10–20% of healthy individuals, but it is not known whether these represent potentially pathogenic T cells kept in check by regulatory mechanisms or low-affinity nonspecific interactions of unlikely relevance to the initiation of Graves' disease.

T-cell function in autoimmune thyroid disease

Animal models

T cells play a vital role in the pathogenesis of experimental autoimmune thyroiditis. Disease is easily transferable with T cells, whereas attempts to transfer disease using serum or antibodies produce only weak or inconsistent effects at best. Full-blown disease requires the transfer of both $CD4^+$ and $CD8^+$ cells from an animal with experimental autoimmune thyroiditis to a naïve recipient (disease being established in the donor by immunization with thyroglobulin in adjuvant). However, a subpopulation within the $CD4^+$ cells also has an important regulatory function, being capable of preventing the action of thyroglobulin-specific, disease-inducing T cells (9). In essence, these findings are consistent with a model in which autoreactive T cells are largely, but not completely, deleted or rendered anergic in the thymus during development. These T cells are normally kept in check, either because they are controlled by a regulatory T-cell subset or through clonal ignorance in which the T cells fail to react to antigen in the absence of an appropriate costimulatory signal (Fig. 3.2.6.5). Animal strains particularly prone to experimental autoimmune thyroiditis have genetic defects either in positive/negative selection of T cells (which make it more likely that the adult animal has sufficient autoreactive T cells to develop disease) or in the regulatory T cell subsets, and these defects interact with environmental factors to result in disease (Table 3.2.6.4).

An appropriate balance of T helper cells (Th1 and Th2) (Table 3.2.6.5) is needed for full expression of disease, and the reciprocal inhibition between these two subsets (Fig. 3.2.6.4) may be one of the most important regulatory pathways controlling the activity of autoreactive T cells. For instance, blocking IL-2 receptor activation or removing γ-interferon leads to a granulomatous rather than lymphocytic thyroiditis, and the production of

Table 3.2.6.3 Nomenclature and assay of the major types of TSH-receptor antibodies

Antibody	Assay
Long-acting thyroid stimulator (LATS)	The original assay for TSAb which measured the effects of TSHR antibodies on radio-iodine release in the intact mouse
LATS-protector (LATS-P)	Assayed by measuring inhibition (protection) of LATS interaction with thyroid; now superseded by new assays
Thyroid-stimulating antibodies (TSAb)	Usually measurement of cAMP production by primary cultures of thyroid cells, thyroid cell lines (e.g. FRTL5) or Chinese hamster ovary cells transfected with TSHR. Other functions such as iodide uptake can be used as endpoints instead
Thyroid-blocking antibodies	Measurement of inhibition of cAMP production after TSH-mediated stimulation of thyroid cells or TSHR transfected cells
TSH-binding inhibiting immunoglobulins (TBII)	Measurement of inhibition of radiolabelled TSH binding to purified or recombinant TSHR by antibodies

TSHR, thyroid-stimulating hormone receptor.

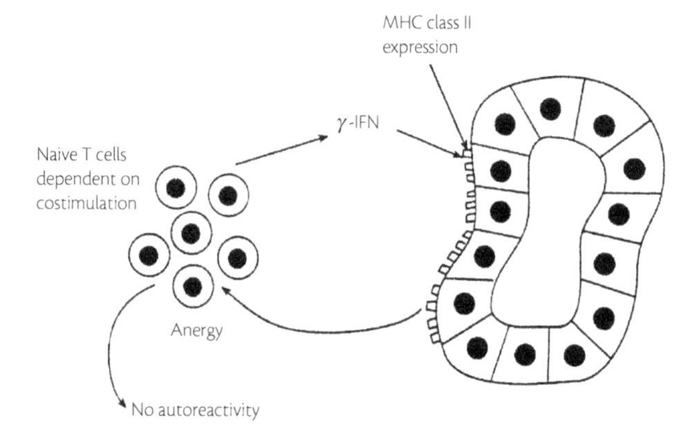

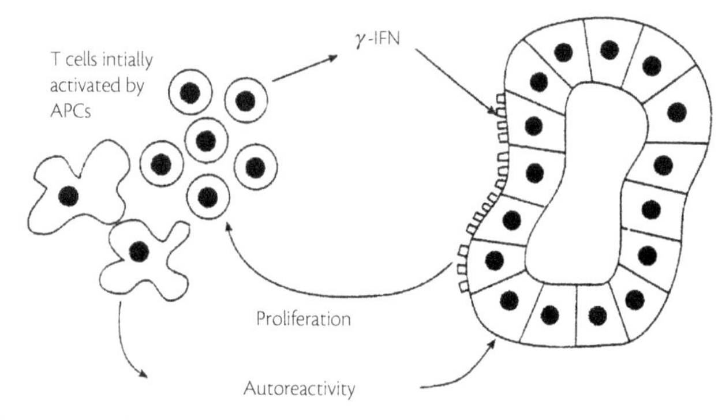

Fig. 3.2.6.5 Alternative outcomes of major histocompatibility complex (MHC) class II molecule expression by thyroid cells, depending on the provision of co-stimulatory signals from antigen-presenting cells (APCs).

Table 3.2.6.4 Interaction of experimental manipulations in animal models of autoimmune thyroiditis

Factor	Probable site of action
Genetic background Thymectomy (±irradiation) Intrathymic antigen	Thymic selection of T cells
Infection Sex hormones Adjuvant	Peripheral autoreactive T cells escaping intrathymic tolerance
Genetic background Cytokines	Peripheral tolerance
Genetic background Iodide uptake	Recognition of autoantigen
Genetic background Soluble autoantigen Thymectomy T-cell subset depletion Cytokines Toxins	Active suppression

high levels of thyroglobulin antibodies, due to preferential Th2 activation (23). Typical experimental autoimmune thyroiditis is most likely Th1 dependent through the action of thyroid-specific cytotoxic T cells.

Further support for this T-cell-dependent mode of pathogenesis comes from the induction of experimental autoimmune thyroiditis by modulation of the T-cell repertoire alone, without the need to immunize animals with thyroid antigen (Table 3.2.6.2). Certain strains of rat or mice develop experimental autoimmune thyroiditis after thymectomy, sometimes coupled with sublethal irradiation, when performed at a critical stage of postnatal development (9), and T-cell depletion/reconstitution or ciclosporin A can have similar effects. Disease is reversed by a subset of $CD4^+$

Table 3.2.6.5 Features of CD4+ T-cell helper (Th) cell subsets in the mouse; similar but not identical profiles are found in humans

	Th1	Th2
Cytokine profile IL-2	++	–
IL-3	++	++
IL-4	–	++
IL-5	–	++
IL-6	–	++
IL-10	–	++
γ-interferon (γ-IFN)	++	+
Tumour necrosis factor (TNF)	++	–
Lymphotoxin	++	+
Function Delayed-type hypersensitivity (for cell-mediated immunity)	++	+
B-cell help (for antibody synthesis)	+	++
Eosinophil/mast cell production	–	++

T cells from untreated donors. One major regulatory $CD4^+$ T-cell population can be identified because it expresses CD25 and Foxp3. Depletion of this T-cell subset causes severe thyroiditis in certain mouse strains and this subset also appears to be reduced when thymectomy is performed (24). From these studies it is clear that thyroid-reactive T cells are present early after birth and that preferential removal of a critical regulatory subset of $CD4^+$ T cells can induce organ-specific autoimmune disease. Transgenic mice have been used to confirm that tolerance, imposed in the thymus or periphery, is a major step in the production of thyroid reactivity; in contrast, B cells were not tolerized in animals overexpressing a membrane-bound antigen specifically on thyroid cells, presumably because the antigen is sequestered from B but not T cells (25). These B cells are harmless (or 'ignorant') unless specific T cells are available in a nontolerized state, in which case help in the form of B-cell stimulation might be provided, leading to thyroid antibody formation. The frequency of thyroid antibodies (and focal thyroiditis) in the healthy population may be due to the existence of such untolerized B cells, which can be partially activated if T cell tolerance is disrupted or bypassed, e.g. by the provision of B-cell-stimulatory cytokines by nonthyroid-specific T cells.

Human studies

The methods used to examine thyroid-reactive T cells in humans are shown in Table 3.2.6.6 and, despite their limitations, have provided important insights into the pathogenesis of autoimmune thyroid disease. A major problem has been the difficulty of access

Table 3.2.6.6 Methods used for examining T-cell responses to thyroid antigens

Assay	Comment
Phenotypic analysis	Measures expression of a huge array of T-cell surface molecules but provides only indirect evidence of function; may be extended to analysis of T-cell receptors or cytokines
Proliferation	Measures [^{3}H]thymidine incorporation after *in vitro* stimulation with antigen; most widely used measure of function
Migration inhibition factor (MIF) assay	Measures production of MIF, a poorly characterized cytokine, in response to antigen; no longer in widespread use
ELISpot assay	Measures production of cytokines (e.g. IL-1, γ-IFN) by individual T cells, usually after stimulation *in vitro*; very sensitive
Flow cytometry after activation by antigen *in vitro*	Measures cell surface expression of markers of activation (e.g. CD69)
Immunoglobulin or antibody production	An indirect assay of Th2-type responses by T cells cultured with autologous B cells
Cytotoxicity	Usually measures release of ^{51}Cr or ^{111}In from labelled target cells incubated with cytotoxic T cells

IFN, interferon; IL, interleukin, Th, T helper cell.

to thyroid-infiltrating T cells in untreated patients; blood-borne lymphocytes contain only a small proportion of thyroid-specific T cells which happen to be trafficking at the time of sampling, and although Graves' thyroid tissue is often available for study, such patients have usually received treatment with antithyroid drugs which reduce the severity of the lymphocytic infiltrate, making the remaining T cells unrepresentative. Furthermore, it is obvious that any immune response, initially directed against a single epitope on a single antigen, rapidly diversifies to involve other epitopes and antigens, and this phenomenon of determinant spreading makes any analysis of T-cell reactivity in autoimmune diseases as chronic as those affecting the thyroid very difficult to interpret.

T-cell phenotypes

Perhaps the simplest type of analysis, but giving the least easily understood information, is the definition of T-cell phenotypes using monoclonal antibodies against an array of surface molecules. From such studies on peripheral blood, it is now fairly clear that $CD8^+$ T-cell numbers are decreased in Graves' disease, active Hashimoto's thyroiditis, and postpartum thyroiditis, giving a rise in the ratio of CD4 to CD8 cells, and so-called activated T cells, expressing HLA-DR and other activation molecules, are also increased. However, the cause and meaning of these changes remain unclear, and their original interpretation as showing a defect in T-suppressor cells is naïve. It should also be noted that similar changes are found in many other autoimmune diseases.

Thyroid-infiltrating T cells are a mix of $CD4^+$ and $CD8^+$ cells, many expressing activation markers, and $CD4^+$ cells often predominate in Hashimoto's thyroiditis. Most of the T cells express the $\alpha\beta$ T-cell receptor, but a minor population of uncertain significance expresses the $\gamma\delta$ receptor. Analysis of clonality within the T-cell population expressing the $\alpha\beta$ receptor families by the unfractionated thyroid-infiltrating T-cell population in Hashimoto's thyroiditis and Graves' disease shows no evidence of restriction, even in the activated T-cell population which might be predicted to contain the most disease-specific cells (26). Although it is likely that the autoimmune response begins with a clonally restricted response, this response rapidly diversifies, particularly when multiple thyroid autoantigens are known to be involved. Detailed analysis of the T-cell infiltrate in autoimmune thyroiditis shows that there is an influx of recent thymic emigrants early on in the disease process, which in turn implies that there may be some disturbance of central tolerance, in addition to a problem with peripheral tolerance, in these patients (27).

Functional responses

Thyroglobulin-, thyroid peroxidase-, and TSH-receptor-reactive T cells can be identified in the circulating and thyroid lymphocyte populations of patients with thyroid autoimmunity using a number of assays, most commonly measuring T-cell proliferation (Table 3.2.6.6). However, such responses tend to be weak and, as already mentioned, epitope mapping studies with such assays have generally revealed a remarkably heterogeneous response. Another functional assay has measured production of a cytokine, migration inhibition factor, in response to stimulation with thyroid antigen, and this work has been extended to controversial attempts at demonstrating the existence of a thyroid-antigen-specific T-suppressor-cell defect in autoimmune thyroid disease (9). These putative cells are not the same as those recently identified as regulatory T cells; it is this group of T cells which is now known to have a central role in maintaining tolerance to autoantigens (28). Perhaps the clearest evidence for the importance of this mechanism comes from the rare, lethal disorder IPEX (immunodysregulation polyendocrinopathy enteropathy X-linked) syndrome in which there are mutations in the *FOXP3* gene that result in a defect in immunoregulatory T cells which express CD25 and Foxp3. Babies with this syndrome have very early onset autoimmune disorders including thyroid disease. A further possible example of thyroid autoimmunity appearing in the wake of a disturbance of T-cell-mediated immunoregulation occurs during reconstitution of the immune system after monoclonal antibody treatment directed against lymphocytes, or after antiretroviral treatment for HIV (29).

Other *in vitro* studies have yielded complex results, presumably because the number of thyroid antigen-specific T cells is low, even in full-blown disease. Analysis of cytokine production in thyroid autoimmunity, either *in situ* or by cultured T cells, has shown a complex picture, with both Th1 and Th2 cytokines being present (30). It is likely that the Th1 pattern predominates in autoimmune hypothyroidism, but the expected Th2 predominance in Graves' disease, shown by IL-4 production, is not apparent, either because the disease has been studied too late or because other cytokines known to be produced in the thyroid, such as IL-6, IL-10, and IL-13, are able to sustain antibody production. Besides $CD4^+$ T cells, $CD8^+$ T cells, macrophages, and the thyroid follicular cells all contribute to the intrathyroidal cytokine profile, and the pathogenic implications of such cytokines are discussed below.

Antigen presentation to T cells

Antigen presentation is the fundamental first step in any immune response (Fig. 3.2.6.4) and, in most cases, it is believed to be a function of specialized antigen-presenting cells, such as dendritic cells, macrophages, or B cells. These have the ability to take up antigen, process it into the form of epitopes, and present the epitope, bound to an MHC class II molecule, to a $CD4^+$ T cell which recognizes this bimolecular complex through a specific T-cell receptor. In addition, a number of other molecules on the antigen-presenting cell interact with the T cell, either to stabilize this interaction or deliver additional or costimulatory signals. T cells vary in their requirement for costimulatory signalling to achieve activation; broadly speaking, naïve T cells depend more on such signals than memory or activated T cells. Some antigen-presenting cell-derived signals may also mediate T-cell inhibition. For instance B7–1 and B7–2 (CD80 and CD86) cause T-cell activation when they bind to CD28 on a T cell, but if they bind instead to CTLA4, T-cell anergy ensues. Moreover, T cells dependent on B7 costimulatory signals are rendered anergic if antigen presentation occurs in the absence of the B7-mediated signal. This alternative outcome from antigen presentation is an important mechanism for determining peripheral tolerance, although much remains to be learned about what determines T-cell requirements for costimulatory signals.

Against this background, the identification of class II molecule expression by thyroid cells in Hashimoto's thyroiditis and Graves' disease, but not under normal conditions, was taken as evidence that such expression could initiate or perpetuate the autoimmune response through the presentation of thyroid antigens by thyrocytes which, in effect, had been converted to antigen-presenting cells (31). Such class II expression is not an intrinsic property of thyroid cells in the disease state, but depends instead on the cytokine γ-interferon released by the infiltrating T cells (6), and therefore it is highly unlikely to be the initiating step in thyroid autoimmunity. This is clearly the case in experimental autoimmune thyroiditis, in which the thyroid lymphocytic infiltrate precedes the appearance of class II molecules on thyroid cells. Moreover, when class II molecules are expressed *de novo* on thyroid cells in transgenic mice, thyroiditis does not appear (32).

Thyroid-specific T cells can be stimulated to proliferate in response to antigen presented by class II-positive thyroid cells, but using cloned T cells it is apparent that this is not a universal property, as T cells requiring B7 costimulation cannot be stimulated by thyroid cells which fail to express B7 (33). Moreover, the T cells that fail to respond are rendered anergic, as subsequent attempts at stimulation using conventional antigen-presenting cells fail, and this is achieved by at least two mechanisms, one partially reversible by addition of appropriate cytokines (especially IL-2) and the other dependent on Fas-mediated signalling (see below). Therefore, the peripheral tolerance induced by thyroid cells is complex and appears, teleologically, to be an appropriate mechanism for inducing peripheral tolerance in potentially autoreactive T cells, which could otherwise respond to released autoantigen, e.g., after viral thyroiditis (Fig. 3.2.6.5). The local production of γ-interferon during the infection may ensure sufficient MHC class II expression by thyroid cells to ensure that autoimmune responses are not initiated, but this backfires in the setting of an already ongoing autoimmune response. In this case, conventional antigen-presenting cells provide initial costimulatory signals and the resulting T cells, no longer dependent on costimulatory signals, will be further stimulated by class II-positive thyroid cells.

B-cell function in autoimmune thyroid disease

As already discussed, B cells specific for certain thyroid antigens are not deleted during development in transgenic animal models (25). Such ignorant but potentially autoaggressive populations of B cells may become activated nonspecifically in response to the right combination of cytokines, leading to autoantibody production. It is unknown in humans which thyroid autoantigens, if any, can actually induce B-cell tolerance, either through deletion or anergy mechanisms. Judging by the frequent appearance of low levels of low-affinity IgM class thyroglobulin antibodies in healthy individuals, B cells specific for thyroglobulin are frequently not tolerized, but whether such natural autoantibodies have a pathogenic role is uncertain. Maturation of the B-cell response, leading to the production of high levels of high-affinity IgG class thyroglobulin antibodies, requires $CD4^+$ T-cell help, and it is these antibodies that characterize autoimmune thyroid disease.

TSH receptor and thyroid peroxidase are much more localized to the thyroid than thyroglobulin and, therefore, might be expected to impose even less tolerance on B cells than thyroglobulin, which circulates at relatively high levels. However, little is known about the frequency of B cells with these specificities in normal individuals. *A priori*, it would seem that TSH-receptor-specific B cells are uncommon, particularly those capable of producing thyroid-stimulating antibodies, and there is even the possibility that such antibodies are the product of only a small number of B-cell clones.

Circulating B-cell numbers are largely normal in autoimmune thyroid disease, although increases in the $CD5^+$ B-cell subset, responsible for synthesis of polyreactive natural autoantibodies, can occur. Such increases in $CD5^+$ B cells occur in other autoimmune diseases and have no known pathogenic role in thyroiditis. B cells and plasma cells are found in varying numbers in the thyroid, and may be organized in germinal follicles, especially in Hashimoto's thyroiditis. Rarely, these follicles can show light-chain restriction, from which a single dominant clone may emerge to produce non-Hodgkin's lymphoma, a recognized complication of Hashimoto's thyroiditis.

Although both blood-borne and thyroid lymphocytes can produce thyroid antibodies *in vitro* after mitogen stimulation, only the thyroid lymphocytes produce antibody spontaneously, so that the thyroid seems likely to be a major source of antibodies *in vivo*. In addition, however, the bone marrow and lymph nodes draining the thyroid are sites of thyroid antibody production. The decline in thyroid antibody production which occurs after thyroid ablation is explicable as the result of either removal of thyroidal B cells or removal of thyroid antigen and thyroid-specific helper T cells (9). In simple terms of B-cell population size, it would seem that the thyroid is not the major site of antibody synthesis, but the real importance of this compartment may lie in the ability of B cells to take up specific autoantigen. B cells are uniquely able to amplify the T-cell response to any given autoantigen and may even break T-cell tolerance by presentation of cryptic self-epitopes generated by processing within the B cell. Thus, within the thyroid, the autoimmune response will be sustained and increased by B-cell-mediated presentation of locally derived thyroglobulin, thyroid peroxidase, and TSH receptor, and supported by the intrathyroidal production of cytokines which cause B-cell proliferation and differentiation (Fig. 3.2.6.6). This information has been central to attempts to treat Graves' disease and ophthalmopathy with rituximab, a monoclonal antibody that depletes B cells but not plasma cells. Initial results show that the there is a modest beneficial effect from this agent, which may not have a major clinical impact but does provide indirect evidence for the importance of B cells in autoimmune thyroid disease pathways (34).

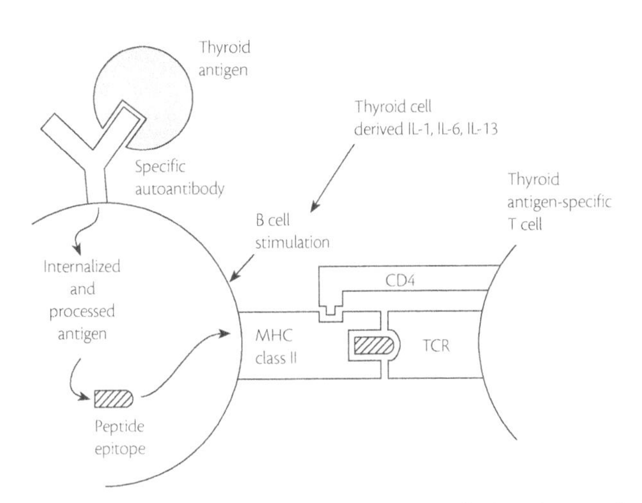

Fig. 3.2.6.6 Cognate interaction of B cells, capturing specific thyroid antigens by surface autoantibody, and T cells.

Mechanisms altering thyroid function

It is now clear that TSH-receptor stimulating antibodies cause Graves' disease, but there is no clear correlation between the circulating levels of these antibodies and the severity of hyperthyroidism. The most likely reason for this discrepancy is that humoral and cellular factors, identical to those operating in autoimmune hypothyroidism, are also active in Graves' disease, and it is the balance between the level of stimulatory antibodies and these conflicting processes, including antibodies which block the TSH receptor, that determines the degree of hyperthyroidism. As already noted, the natural history of Graves' disease tends to thyroid destruction over 10–15 years in a small proportion of patients (4). The mechanisms mediating hypothyroidism are less clear, in particular with regard to the relative importance of each in the pathogenesis of thyroid cell dysfunction and destruction, and these processes are considered next.

Humoral immunity

The role of thyroglobulin antibodies is uncertain, as they do not fix complement, but these antibodies may be involved in mediating antibody-dependent cell-mediated cytotoxicity. In this, the effector cell is a natural killer cell which binds to the antibody via Fc receptors on the natural killer cell surface. This allows the natural killer cell to destroy a specific target cell, in this case a thyroid cell, as otherwise natural killer cell-mediated destruction is not restricted by recognition of specific antigen. Antibody-dependent cell-mediated cytotoxicity is demonstrable *in vitro* with both thyroglobulin and thyroid peroxidase antibodies, small numbers of natural killer cells appear in the thyroid infiltrate, and monocytes may also be involved in this destructive pathway (35). However, transplacental transfer of thyroglobulin antibodies is not accompanied by thyroid dysfunction, and similar considerations apply to the frequent presence of thyroglobulin antibodies in euthyroid individuals. Thyroid peroxidase antibodies can fix complement but, for similar reasons, would seem to be of minor importance as primary mediators of thyroid cell destruction. Thyroid peroxidase may well be sequestered from access by autoantibodies until late in the disease process, when cell-mediated injury will permit antibody binding, although there is evidence for some internalization of thyroid peroxidase antibody by thyroid cells, the consequences of which are unknown.

A second reason for the failure of complement-fixing thyroid peroxidase antibodies to destroy thyroid cells is that, in common with all nucleated cells, thyroid cells express complement regulatory proteins which prevent lethal injury by interfering with C3 convertase activity or by impairing terminal complement component formation. The most important of these regulatory proteins functionally is CD59, and its expression is upregulated by IL-1, γ-interferon, and tumour necrosis factor, all of which are produced by the lymphocytic infiltrate, thus enhancing the ability of thyroid cells to defend themselves from complement attack (36). There is good evidence that complement is activated in thyroid autoimmunity, with elevated serum levels of terminal complement complexes, and local deposition of such complexes around the thyroid follicles in both Graves' disease and Hashimoto's thyroiditis. Unless formed in overwhelming amounts, complement membrane attack complexes do not overcome the thyroid cell's defences, but none the less, sublethal effects of complement attack are demonstrable *in vitro*, and include impaired responses to TSH stimulation and the release of cytokines, reactive oxygen metabolites, and prostaglandins, which will contribute to the local inflammatory response (36). Antithyroid drugs block this phlogistic response to complement attack, which may explain the selective immunomodulatory effects of these drugs.

A final mechanism by which antibodies can cause hypothyroidism is through their direct effects on cell function, most clearly illustrated by TSH-receptor antibodies. Although it is nearly certain that all patients with Graves' disease have TSH-receptor stimulating antibodies, these may be absent in the serum of around 5% of patients when measured using the currently available binding assays (37). As well as assay insensitivity as an explanation, it is possible in these cases that there is exclusively intrathyroidal production of autoantibody which is sufficient to sustain disease. Thyroid peroxidase antibodies can inhibit thyroid peroxidase enzymatic activity operating *in vitro*, which would contribute to hypothyroidism if also present *in vivo*, but the importance of this inhibition is questionable.

Cell-mediated immunity

Cytokines released locally by the infiltrating lymphocytes and macrophages may have a number of effects that exacerbate thyroid injury. Some of these effects are related to the metabolic activity of the thyroid cells, such as decreased synthesis of thyroglobulin or thyroid peroxidase, which will ultimately impair thyroid hormone production (Table 3.2.6.7), while others evoke responses by thyroid cells which have direct immunological relevance. One of these has already been discussed, namely the expression of MHC class II molecules induced by γ-interferon, but many other effects are being uncovered. Adhesion molecules allow cytotoxic T cells and natural killer cells to bind initially to their targets, and the up-regulation of thyroid cell adhesion molecule expression by cytokines will enhance the susceptibility of thyroid cells to such attack (9). Nitric oxide and reactive oxygen species may play a key role in thyroid injury and their production by thyroid cells is initiated by the intrathyroidal proinflammatory environment which exists in autoimmune thyroiditis (9, 38). Finally, certain cytokines, in particular IL-1, IL-6, IL-8, IL-12, IL-13, and IL-15, are produced by thyroid cells in response to inflammatory cytokines, especially

Table 3.2.6.7 Main functional effects of cytokines on human thyroid cells

Cytokine	Growth	Iodide uptake	cAMP production	Expression of TG or TPO
IL-1	↑ (but can also ↑ PGE_2, causing ↓ growth)	↓	↓	Biphasic: ↑ at low concentration and ↓ at high concentration
IL-6	↑ (with TSH)	0	↓/0	↓/0
	↓ (with EGF)			
γ-IFN	↓ (with TNF)/0	↓	Variable	↓
TNFα	0 (alone)	↓	↓/0	↓

↑, increase; ↓, decrease; 0, no effect; γ-IFN: *x*-interferon; EGF, epidermal growth factor; PGE_2, prostaglandin E_2; TG, thyroglobulin; TNFα: tumour necrosis factor-α; TPO, thyroid peroxidase.

IL-1 (30), and this may set up a mutually reinforcing pathway of cytokine interactions which results in escalation and perpetuation of the autoimmune process (Fig. 3.2.6.7).

As well as thyroid cells, vascular endothelial cells in the thyroid are exposed to cytokines which up-regulate expression of selectins and other molecules essential to the egress of inflammatory cells from the blood. Thyroid cells can also produce an array of chemokines, molecules which are able to enhance the recruitment of lymphocytes to the gland in disease. Chemokine synthesis may also be critical in the formation of lymphoid germinal centres in chronically affected thyroid tissue (39). Clearly, these processes of adhesion molecule expression and chemokine synthesis are essential to the recruitment of lymphocytes to the infiltrate, although it is unknown what proportion of these are blood-derived and what proportion result from local expansion.

Specific cytotoxic T cells have long been thought to be key mediators of thyroid cell destruction in autoimmune thyroiditis, but evidence for their existence is surprisingly sparse and best documented in experimental autoimmune thyroiditis (9). As well as releasing cytokines, cytotoxic T cells kill either by insertion of perforin into the target cell membrane, or by interaction of Fas ligand on the T-cell surface with the widely expressed Fas molecule on the target cell. Perforin-expressing T cells are present in the thyroid infiltrate in both Hashimoto's thyroiditis and Graves' disease, with slightly differing phenotypes in the two conditions (40). This certainly indicates the potential for perforin-mediated cell destruction, although recent attention has focused on Fas-mediated apoptosis as a major mechanism for thyroid cell death (41). This interest has been sparked by the demonstration of Fas ligand expression by thyroid cells in Hashimoto's thyroiditis, but not other conditions. Fas ligand expression was enhanced *in vitro* by IL-1β but not other cytokines, suggesting that, in addition to the classic pathway of apoptosis mediated by T cells, Fas and Fas ligand on thyroid cells could interact and lead to cell suicide. Normally Fas ligand expression is limited to sites of immunological privilege, such as the trophoblast and Sertoli cells, where it is clear that suicide is not an outcome; instead, Fas ligand expression at these sites ensures tolerance by deleting any autoaggressive Fas-expressing lymphocytes specific for these tissues. Thus a major effect of thyroid cell Fas ligand expression *in vivo* may be the evasion of thyroid cell recognition by T cells.

In summary, thyroid cell dysfunction and destruction result from a wide array of insults (Fig. 3.2.6.8) and, in the initial stage at least, seems dependent on cell-mediated autoimmune processes. It is likely that within the same clinically identified disease there are interindividual differences in the relative contributions from each type of injury. This variation would account for the diversity of pathological processes previously described, and because of this complexity, it is highly improbable that only two types of mechanism predominate, one resulting in atrophic thyroiditis and the other in goitrous thyroiditis.

Use of thyroid autoantibodies in diagnosis

Although thyroglobulin and thyroid peroxidase antibodies appear to have a secondary rather than a primary role in disease pathogenesis, nonetheless they are invaluable markers of the presence of autoimmune thyroid disease. After considering the assays available, this section will review the results from antibody testing and then consider the use of TSH-receptor antibodies in diagnosis.

Thyroglobulin and thyroid peroxidase antibodies

There are essentially four methods for assaying thyroglobulin and thyroid peroxidase antibodies. The two oldest are haemagglutination and indirect immunofluorescence, which depend on dilution of the test serum to determine the level of antibodies. Although robust and providing reasonably sensitive and specific results, the more modern methods of enzyme-linked immunosorbent assay (ELISA) and radioimmunoassay allow truly quantitative determination of antibodies and, in the case of assays for thyroid peroxidase antibodies, can use antigen of high purity, if necessary for research purposes. Thyroid peroxidase was previously called the microsomal antigen, and assays for these antibodies have relied on positive immunofluorescence staining with an appropriate pattern or, in the case of haemagglutination, have used an excess of

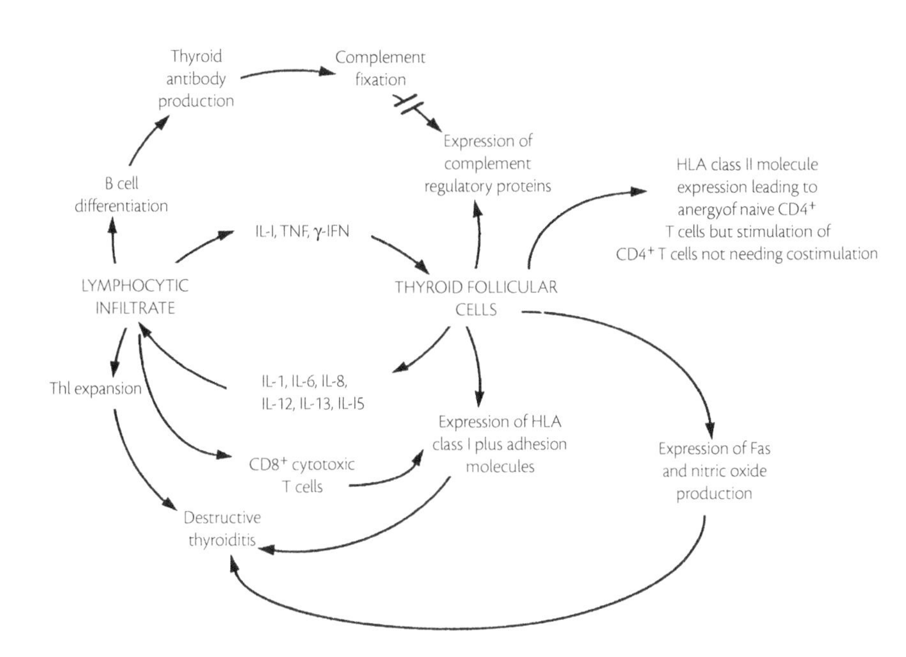

Fig. 3.2.6.7 Cytokine interactions between the immune system and thyroid cells in autoimmune thyroid disease. (From Weetman AP, Ajjan RA, Watson PF. Cytokines and Graves' disease. *Baillière's Clinical Endocrinology and Metabolism*, 1997; **11**: 481–97, with permission.)

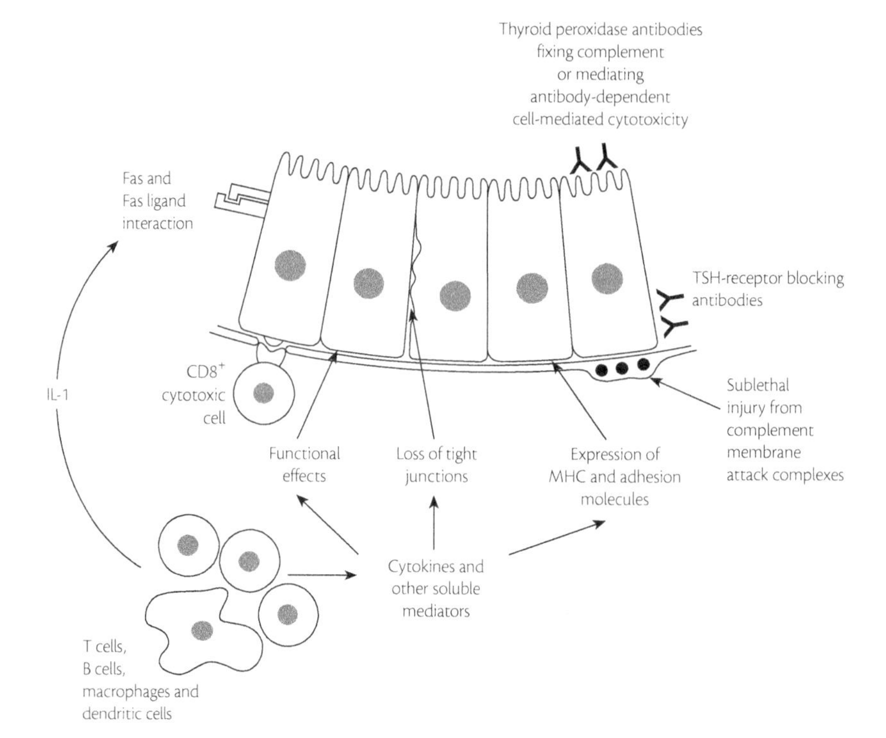

Fig. 3.2.6.8 Main mechanisms involved in thyroid-cell dysfunction in autoimmune hypothyroidism.

thyroglobulin to absorb out thyroglobulin antibody activity when testing crude microsomal extracts of thyroid homogenate. Comparison of assays based on haemagglutination with microsomal antigen and more modern methods with purified or even recombinant thyroid peroxidase has shown a good correlation between the two, although those assays based on thyroid peroxidase are more sensitive. Further improvement in assay standardization has come from the use of reference positive serum samples, such as those obtained from the National Institute of Biological Standards and Control, UK, and increased sensitivity is possible with the use of immunoradiometric assays.

With the most sensitive assays, up to 20% of healthy women have thyroglobulin and/or thyroid peroxidase antibodies, although in the majority the levels are very low. Using more conventional assays, 11% of women and 3% of men were positive in a large community-based survey in the UK (3) and similar results have been reported elsewhere. Antibodies are not entirely stable, appearing or disappearing in 17% and 2% of women, respectively, over a 20-year period (3). Moreover, although there is a rise in the frequency of thyroid antibodies with increasing age, healthy centenarians show a remarkably low frequency (Fig. 3.2.6.9), suggesting that thyroid autoimmunity is associated with senescence-related illnesses (42). Thyroid peroxidase antibodies are found in 80–90% of Graves' sera and 95–100% of Hashimoto sera, with thyroglobulin antibodies in up to 70% of Graves' sera and 90–100% of Hashimoto sera, using sensitive assays. Occasional patients with Hashimoto's thyroiditis are negative for serum thyroid antibodies, although synthesis can be detected locally within the thyroid, presumably at too low a level to be detectable in serum. In most patients, thyroglobulin antibodies are accompanied by thyroid peroxidase antibodies, but thyroid peroxidase antibodies frequently occur in the absence of thyroglobulin antibodies. This has led some centres to abandon routine testing for thyroglobulin antibodies in the diagnosis of autoimmune thyroid disease.

Thyroglobulin and thyroid peroxidase antibodies are found in a variety of other conditions at higher frequency than would be expected by chance (Box 3.2.6.1). As in healthy individuals, the presence of such antibodies is a marker of future thyroid dysfunction, especially if coupled with subclinical hypothyroidism, and all patients with positive thyroid antibodies should be offered annual screening to detect early thyroid failure, while patients with subclinical hypothyroidism should have antibodies measured to stratify their risk (3). Another situation where prospective thyroid antibody testing is particularly worthwhile is in patients starting amiodarone, as those with antibodies are more likely to develop amiodarone-induced hypothyroidism. Antibody testing is also useful in patients with Addison's disease, as around 25% may develop

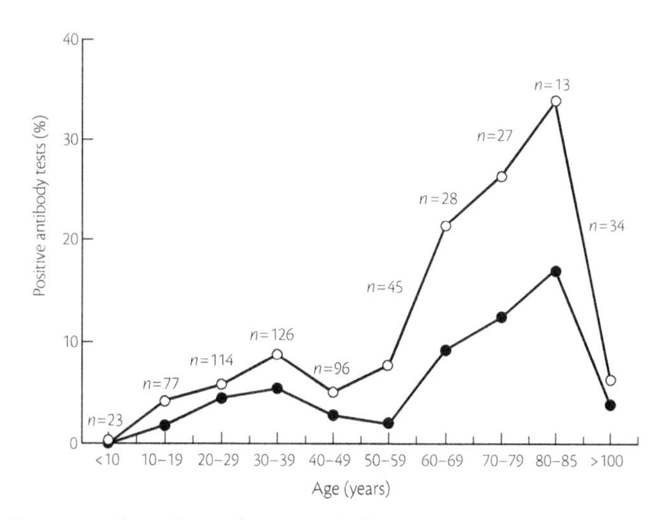

Fig. 3.2.6.9 Change in prevalence in antibodies to thyroglobulin (•) and thyroid peroxidase (o) in healthy subjects with age. (From Mariotti S *et al.* Thyroid and other organ-specific autoantibodies in healthy centenarians. *Lancet*, 1992; **339**: 1506–8, with permission.)

Box 3.2.6.1. Conditions associated with an increased prevalence of thyroglobulin and thyroid peroxidase antibodies

- Polyglandular disease
  - Insulin-dependent diabetes mellitus
  - Addison's disease
  - Premature ovarian failure
  - Lymphocytic hypophysitis
- Conditions associated with autoimmune polyglandular syndromes
  - Vitiligo
  - Pernicious anaemia
  - Alopecia
  - Myasthenia gravis
  - Coeliac disease and dermatitis herpetiformis
  - Autoimmune serositis
- Rheumatological disorders
  - Rheumatoid arthritis
  - Systemic lupus erythematosus
  - Sjögren's syndrome
  - Polymyalgia rheumatica/temporal arteritis
  - Relapsing polychondritis
  - Systemic sclerosis
- Other disorders
  - Chronic active hepatitis
  - Primary biliary cirrhosis

thyroid dysfunction due to associated autoimmune polyglandular syndrome type 2. Similar considerations apply to pernicious anaemia and other autoimmune disorders which are associated with a high frequency of thyroid autoimmunity (43).

On the other hand, thyroid antibodies can be misleading in goitre as 10–50% of patients with multinodular goitre have thyroid antibodies, although usually only at low or moderate levels. Similarly, 25–50% of patients with papillary or follicular thyroid cancer have thyroglobulin and/or thyroid peroxidase antibodies. Such patients have a somewhat better prognosis than those without thyroid antibodies, and the presence of antibodies is correlated with a coexistent thyroiditis, suggesting that this autoimmune response is beneficial.

Finally, research since 1980 has thrown up some new associations, the clinical importance of which is yet to be fully realized. Thyroid peroxidase antibody positivity is strongly related to postpartum thyroiditis, giving rise to the suggestion that it may be worthwhile screening all pregnant women antepartum, but the positive predictive value of thyroid peroxidase antibodies is quite low (about 40–60%) and some cases have been reported in women who are thyroid peroxidase antibody negative (44). Because of the high frequency of postpartum thyroiditis in type 1 diabetes mellitus, which is approximately 3 times normal, there is a strong case for thyroid peroxidase antibody screening of this group of women antepartum. Women with positive thyroid antibodies, even without clinical thyroid dysfunction, do seem at risk of postpartum depression (albeit mildly) and recurrent first-trimester miscarriage. There is also a threefold increase in the relative risk of depression in perimenopausal women with thyroid peroxidase antibodies (45). Whether the mental disorder is the cause or result of the autoimmune response is not yet known, but presumably some interaction between the neurological, endocrine, and immune systems is involved, akin to the adverse effects of stress described previously. An unexplained association also exists between thyroid autoantibody positivity and breast cancer, with an improved prognosis in those women who have positive thyroid peroxidase (46). Most recently, an association between the presence of thyroid antibodies and miscarriage has been identified (47), which in turn has led to the concept that thyroxine treatment should be considered even in euthyroid individuals with thyroid antibodies and a history of such an adverse outcome in pregnancy.

Thyroid-stimulating hormone-receptor antibodies

The terminology of TSH-receptor antibodies (Table 3.2.6.3) has evolved from the methods used for their measurement. In essence there are two current methods: (1) the binding assay, which measures the capacity of immunoglobulins to inhibit the binding of radiolabelled TSH to purified or recombinant TSH receptor and (2) bioassays which measure the stimulatory or inhibitory effects of immunoglobulins on some aspect of thyroid cell function (48). Generally, cAMP production is used as the endpoint in bioassays, but there has been an irreversible move away from using primary cultures of animal or human thyroid cells in these assays, with their attendant problems of supply and standardization, to using either cell lines, such as rat FRTL5 cells, or Chinese hamster ovary cells transfected with TSH receptor, such as JPO9 cells. With the most sensitive bioassays for TSH-receptor stimulating antibodies almost all patients with Graves' disease are positive, but these antibodies are rarely found in its absence, and then would be associated with a greatly increased risk of future hyperthyroidism. This is shown most clearly by the finding that 30–50% of euthyroid patients with thyroid-associated ophthalmopathy have TSH-receptor antibodies, and this proportion increases if the most sensitive assays are used.

As would be predicted, there is only a weak or absent correlation between levels of TSH-receptor antibodies measured in the binding and stimulatory bioassays. Up to 95% of patients with Graves' disease are positive using modern binding assays, as are 10–20% of patients with autoimmune hypothyroidism. In the latter, the binding activity is mostly due to TSH-receptor blocking antibodies, but neutral antibodies with binding but not biological activity could theoretically also be detected. Antibodies against the TSH receptor are present at much lower concentrations than thyroid peroxidase antibodies and this makes the development of robust and simple solid-phase assays very difficult, compounded by problems in expressing the TSH receptor in its native form.

TSH-receptor antibody testing is not recommended for routine use in the diagnosis of Graves' disease when the diagnosis is clinically obvious, such as when there is coincident ophthalmopathy, or when such information will not influence management, for instance if the decision has already been made to proceed with radio-iodine treatment (49). Measurement of thyroid peroxidase antibodies, coupled with clinical examination and, if necessary, a thyroid scan to confirm a diffuse goitre, are also reasonable alternatives to TSH-receptor antibody testing for diagnostic purposes, if the latter are not readily available. When it is necessary to test for these antibodies, second-generation binding assays give information which is essentially comparable to bioassays, providing the results are interpreted in the light of the patient's clinical and biochemical status. Prediction of outcome after antithyroid drugs has been another suggested use for these assays, but although there is no doubt that the presence of detectable TSH-receptor antibodies after treatment is associated with a higher rate of relapse, the sensitivity and specificity of this measurement is too poor to be used in clinical prognosis. The one situation where TSH-receptor antibody measurement is definitely indicated is during pregnancy in Graves' disease; a high level of maternal antibodies at the beginning of the third trimester is a strong predictor of neonatal thyrotoxicosis (50).

References

1. Jiang H, Chess L. Regulation of immune responses by T cells. *N Engl J Med*, 2006; **354**: 1166–76.
2. Pearce EN, Farwell AP, Braverman LE. Thyroiditis. *N Engl J Med*, 2003; **348**: 2646–55.
3. Vanderpump MPJ, Tunbridge WM, French JM, Appleton D, Bates D, Clark F, *et al.* The incidence of thyroid disorders in the community: a twenty-year follow-up of the Whickham survey. *Clin Endocrinol*, 1995; **43**: 55–68.
4. Okayasu I, Hara Y, Nakamura K, Rose NR. Racial and age-related differences in incidence and severity of focal autoimmune thyroiditis. *Am J Pathol*, 1994; **101**: 698–702.
5. LiVolsi VA. The pathology of autoimmune disease: a review. *Thyroid*, 1994; **4**: 333–9.
6. Zeitlin AA, Simmonds MJ, Gough SC. Genetic developments in autoimmune thyroid disease: an evolutionary process. *Clin Endocrinol*, 2008; **68**: 671–82.
7. Anderson MS. Update in endocrine autoimmunity. *J Clin Endocrinol Metab*, 2008; **93**: 3663–70.
8. Benvenga S, Trimarchi F. Changed presentation of Hashimoto's thyroiditis in North-Eastern Sicily and Calabria (Southern Italy) based on a 31-year experience. *Thyroid*, 2008; **18**: 429–41.
9. Weetman AP, DeGroot L. *Autoimmunity to the thyroid gland*, in http://www.thyroidmanager.org, 29 May 2010. South Dartmouth MA: Endocrine Education Inc.
10. Zois C, Stavrou I, Svarna E, Seferiadis K, Tsatsoulis A. Natural course of autoimmune thyroiditis after elimination of iodine deficiency in northwestern Greece. *Thyroid*, 2006; **16**: 289–93.
11. Kondrashova A, Viskari H, Haapala AM, Seiskari T, Kulmala P, Ilonen J, *et al.* Serological evidence of thyroid autoimmunity among schoolchildren in two different socioeconomic environments. *J Clin Endocrinol Metab*, 2008; **93**: 729–34.
12. Mizokami T, Wu Li A, El-Kaissi S, Wall JR. Stress and thyroid autoimmunity. *Thyroid*, 2004; **14**: 1047–55.
13. Agate I, Mariotti S, Elisei R, Mossa P, Pacini F, Molinaro E, *et al.* Thyroid autoantibodies and thyroid function in subjects exposed to Chernobyl fallout during childhood: evidence for a transient radiation-induced elevation of serum thyroid antibodies without an increase in thyroid autoimmune disease. *J Clin Endocrinol Metab*, 2008; **93**: 2729–36.
14. Carella C, Mazziotti G, Amato G, Braverman LE, Roti E. Clinical review 169: Interferon-alpha-related thyroid disease: pathophysiological, epidemiological, and clinical aspects. *J Clin Endocrinol Metab*, 2004; **89**: 3656–61.
15. Krassas GE, Wiersinga W. Smoking and autoimmune thyroid disease: the plot thickens. *Eur J Endocrinol*, 2006; **154**: 777–80.
16. Brix TH, Knudsen GP, Kristiansen M, Kyvik KO, Orstavik KH, Hegedüs L. High frequency of skewed X-chromosome inactivation in females with autoimmune thyroid disease: a possible explanation for the female predisposition to thyroid autoimmunity. *J Clin Endocrinol Metab*, 2005; **90**: 5949–53.
17. Latrofa F, Ricci D, Grasso L, Vitti P, Masserini L, Basolo F, *et al.* Characterization of thyroglobulin epitopes in patients with autoimmune and non-autoimmune thyroid diseases using recombinant human monoclonal thyroglobulin autoantibodies. *J Clin Endocrinol Metab*, 2008; **93**: 591–6.
18. Gentile F, Conte M, Formisano S. Thyroglobulin as an autoantigen: what can we learn about immunopathogenicity from the correlation of antigenic properties with protein structure?. *Immunology*, 2004; **112**: 13–25.
19. McLachlan SM, Rapoport B. Thyroid peroxidase as an autoantigen. *Thyroid*, 2007; **17**: 939–48.
20. Rapoport B, McLachlan SM. The thyrotropin receptor in Graves' disease. *Thyroid*, 2007; **17**: 911–22.
21. Dechairo BM, Zabaneh D, Collins J, Brand O, Dawson GJ, Green AP, *et al.* Association of the TSHR gene with Graves' disease: the first disease specific locus. *Eur J Hum Genet*, 2005; **13**: 1223–30.
22. Smith BR, Sanders J, Furmaniak J. TSH receptor antibodies. *Thyroid*, 2007; **17**: 923–38.
23. Tang H, Sharp GC, Peterson KP, Braley-Mullen H. IFN-γ-deficient mice develop severe granulomatous experimental autoimmune thyroiditis in eosinophil infiltration in thyroids. *J Immunol*, 1998; **160**: 5105–12.
24. Yu S, Maiti PK, Dyson M, Jain R, Braley-Mullen H. B cell-deficient NOD.H-2h4 mice have CD4+CD25+ T regulatory cells that inhibit the development of spontaneous autoimmune thyroiditis. *J Exp Med*, 2006; **203**: 349–58.
25. Akkaraju S, Canaan K, Goodnow CC. Self-reactive B cells are not eliminated or inactivated by autoantigen expressed on thyroid epithelial cells. *J Exp Med*, 1997; **186**: 2005–12.
26. McIntosh RS, Tandon N, Pickerill AP, Davies R, Barnett D, Weetman AP. IL-2 receptor positive intrathyroidal lymphocytes in Graves' disease: analysis of Vα transcript microheterogeneity. *J Immunol*, 1993; **151**: 3884–93.
27. Armengol MP, Sabater L, Fernández M, Ruíz M, Alonso N, Otero MJ, *et al.* Influx of recent thymic emigrants into autoimmune thyroid disease glands in humans. *Clin Exp Immunol*, 2008; **153**: 338–50.
28. Sakaguchi S, Yamaguchi T, Nomura T, Ono M. Regulatory T cells and immune tolerance. *Cell*, 2008; **133**: 775–87.
29. Coles AJ, Wing M, Smith S, Coraddu F, Greer S, Taylor C, *et al.* Pulsed monoclonal antibody treatment and autoimmune thyroid disease in multiple sclerosis. *Lancet*, 1999; **354**: 1691–5.
30. Bottazzo GF, Pujol-Borrell R, Hanafusa T, Feldmann M. Role of aberrant HLA-DR expression and antigen presentation in induction of endocrine autoimmunity. *Lancet*, 1983; **ii**: 1115–19.
31. Ajjan RA, Weetman AP. Cytokines in thyroid autoimmunity. *Autoimmunity*, 2003; **36**: 351–9.
32. Marelli-Berg F, Weetman A, Frasca L, Deacock SJ, Imami N, Lombardi G, *et al.* Antigen presentation by epithelial cells induces anergic immunoregulatory CD45R0+ T cells and deletion of CD45RA+ T cells. *J Immunol*, 1997; **159**: 5853–61.
33. Kimura H, Kimura M, Tzou SC, Chen YC, Suzuki K, Rose NR, *et al.* Expression of class II major histocompatibility complex molecules on thyrocytes does not cause spontaneous thyroiditis but mildly increases its severity after immunization. *Endocrinology*, 2005; **146**: 1154–62.
34. El Fassi D, Nielsen CH, Bonnema SJ, Hasselbalch HC, Hegedüs L. B lymphocyte depletion with the monoclonal antibody rituximab in Graves' disease: a controlled pilot study. *J Clin Endocrinol Metab*, 2007; **92**: 1769–72.

35. Rebuffat SA, Nguyen B, Robert B, Castex F, Peraldi-Roux S. Antithyroperoxidase antibody-dependent cytotoxicity in autoimmune thyroid disease. *J Clin Endocrinol Metab*, 2008; **93**: 929–34.
36. Weetman AP, Tandon N, Morgan BP. Antithyroid drugs and release of inflammatory mediators by complement-attacked thyroid cells. *Lancet*, 1992; **340**: 633–6.
37. Vos XG, Smit N, Endert E, Tijssen JG, Wiersinga WM. Frequency and characteristics of TBII-seronegative patients in a population with untreated Graves' hyperthyroidism: a prospective study. *Clin Endocrinol*, 2008; **69**: 311–17.
38. Burek CL, Rose NR. Autoimmune thyroiditis and ROS. *Autoimmun Rev*, 2008; **7**: 530–7.
39. Marinkovic T, Garin A, Yokota Y, Fu YX, Ruddle NH, Furtado GC, *et al.* Interaction of mature $CD3^+CD4^+$ T cells with dendritic cells triggers the development of tertiary lymphoid structures in the thyroid. *J Clin Invest*, 2006; **116**: 2622–32.
40. Wu Z, Podack ER, McKenzie JM, Olsen KJ, Zakarija M. Perforin expression by thyroid-infiltrating T cells in autoimmune thyroid disease. *Clin Exp Immunol*, 1994; **98**: 470–7.
41. Stassi G, De Maria R. Autoimmune thyroid disease: new models of cell death in autoimmunity. *Nat Rev Immunol*, 2002; **2**: 195–204.
42. Mariotti S, Sansoni P, Barbesino G, Caturegli P, Monti D, Cossarizza A, *et al.* Thyroid and other organ-specific autoantibodies in healthy centenarians. *Lancet*, 1992; **339**: 1506–8.
43. Weetman AP. Non-thyroid autoantibodies in autoimmune thyroid disease. *Best Pract Res Clin Endocrinol Metab*, 2005; **19**: 17–32.
44. Amino N, Tada H, Hidaka Y, Crapo LM, Stagnaro-Green A. Screening for postpartum thyroiditis. *J Clin Endocrinol Metab*, 1999; **84**: 1813–21.
45. Pop VJ, Maartens LH, Leusink G, van Son MJ, Knottnerus AA, Ward AM, *et al.* Are autoimmune thyroid dysfunction and depression related? *J Clin Endocrinol Metab*, 1998; **83**: 3194–7.
46. Smyth PPA, Shering SG, Kilbane MT, Murray MJ, McDermott EW, Smith DF, *et al.* Serum thyroid peroxidase autoantibodies, thyroid volume, and outcome in breast carcinoma. *J Clin Endocrinol Metab*, 1998; **83**: 2711–16.
47. Prummel MF, Wiersinga WM. Thyroid autoimmunity and miscarriage. *Eur J Endocrinol*, 2004; **150**: 751–5.
48. Schott M, Scherbaum WA, Morgenthaler NG. Thyrotropin receptor autoantibodies in Graves' disease. *Trends Endocrinol Metab*, 2005; **16**: 243–8.
49. Ajjan RA, Weetman AP. Techniques to quantify TSH receptor antibodies. *Nat Clin Pract Endocrinol Metab*, 2008; **4**: 461–8.
50. Laurberg P, Nygaard B, Glinoer D, Grussendorf M, Orgiazzi J. Guidelines for TSH-receptor antibody measurements in pregnancy: results of an evidence-based symposium organized by the European Thyroid Association. *Eur J Endocrinol*, 1998; **139**: 584–6.

3.2.7 Thyroiditis

Beth Kaplan, Elizabeth N. Pearce, Alan P. Farwell

Introduction

Thyroiditis comprises a diverse group of disorders that are among the most common endocrine abnormalities encountered in clinical practice. These disorders range from the extremely common chronic lymphocytic thyroiditis (Hashimoto's thyroiditis) to the extremely rare invasive fibrous thyroiditis (Riedel's thyroiditis) (Box 3.2.7.1). Clinical presentations are also diverse, ranging from an incidental finding of a goitre to potentially life-threatening illness, from hypothyroidism to thyrotoxicosis. The term 'thyroiditis' implies that the disorders described in this section are inflammatory processes involving the thyroid gland. However, some of the lesions are not inflammatory, but are included in the thyroiditis category largely for convenience. A rational approach to such patients, including history, physical examination, laboratory evaluation, radionuclide or ultrasonographic imaging, and fine-needle aspiration biopsy, will allow the appropriate diagnosis to be made in the vast majority of cases.

This chapter will review the following forms of thyroiditis: Hashimoto's, subacute, infectious, and Riedel's. Other forms of thyroiditis are discussed within other chapters, as follows: postpartum thyroiditis (Chapter 3.4.6), radiation thyroiditis (Chapter 3.2.5), drug-induced thyroiditis (Chapter 3.1.4), thyroiditis associated with neoplasms (Chapter 3.5.5), and focal thyroiditis associated with nontoxic nodular goitre (Chapter 3.5.1).

Autoimmune thyroiditis (Hashimoto's, chronic)

Autoimmune thyroiditis, also known as struma lymphomatosa, chronic lymphocytic thyroiditis, and Hashimoto's thyroiditis, was first described by Hashimoto in 1912 (Table 3.2.7.1). He described four patients with goitres, the thyroid histology of which were all characterized by diffuse lymphocytic infiltration, atrophy of parenchymal cells, fibrosis, and eosinophilic change in some of the parenchymal cells. While this condition is common, there are several variants that differ somewhat from the one initially described by Hashimoto (1). Classically, the disorder occurs as a painless diffuse goitre (goitrous form) in a young or middle-aged woman and often presents as an incidental finding during a routine physical examination. The atrophic form of Hashimoto's thyroiditis is less common and is usually diagnosed by serology in the hypothyroid

Box 3.2.7.1 Types of thyroiditis (most common to least common)

- Chronic lymphocytic thyroiditis (Hashimoto's thyroiditis)
- Subacute lymphocytic thyroiditis
- Postpartum thyroiditis
- Sporadic silent thyroiditis
- Subacute granulomatous thyroiditis (De Quervain's thyroiditis)
- Radiation thyroiditis
- Acute suppurative thyroiditis
- Bacterial, fungal, parasitic
- Invasive fibrous thyroiditis (Riedel's thyroiditis)
- Miscellaneous
  - Sarcoid
  - Amyloid
  - Drug-associated
  - Traumatic
  - Palpation-induced

Table 3.2.7.1 Comparison between the syndromes of thyroiditis

	Hashimoto's thyroiditis	Painless/postpartum thyroiditis	Subacute thyroiditis	Infectious thyroiditis	Riedel's thyroiditis
Age of onset (years)	All ages, peak 30–50	Painless: all ages, peak 30–40 Postpartum: childbearing years	20–60	Children, 20–40	30–60
Sex ratio (F:M)	8–9:1	Silent–2:1	5:1	1:1	3–4:1
Incidence	General population 10%, elderly women 25%	Postpartum: 2–21% Silent: unknown	Common	Rare	Extremely rare
Aetiology	Autoimmune	Autoimmune	Viral (?)	Infectious organisms	Unknown
Genetic predisposition	Moderate, HLA-DR3, -DR5, -B8	Low	Moderate, HLA-Bw35, -DRw8	Low	Low
Pathology	Lymphocytic infiltration, germinal centres, fibrosis	Lymphocytic infiltration	Giant cells, granulomas	Abscess formation	Dense fibrosis
Prodrome	None	Pregnancy	Viral illness	Viral illness	None
Goitre	Nonpainful, persistent	Nonpainful, persistent	Painful, transient	Painful, transient	Nonpainful, persistent
Fever and malaise	No	No	Yes	Yes	No
Thyroid antibodies	High titre, persistent	High titre, persistent	Low titre/absent, transient	Absent	Present in most patients
Thyroid function	Hypothyroid	Thyrotoxicosis followed by hypothyroidism	Thyrotoxicosis followed by hypothyroidism	Usually euthyroid	Usually euthyroid
ESR	Normal	Normal	High	High	Normal
Radioactive iodine uptake (24–h)	Variable	<5%	<5%	Normal	Low/normal
Relapse	Persistent	Common with subsequent pregnancies	Rare	Common only with pyriform sinus fistula	Persistent
Permanent hypothyroidism	Frequent	Common	Occasionally	Rare	Occasionally

With permission from the Massachusetts Medical Society © 2003. All rights reserved.

patient with a normal-sized or atrophic thyroid. The hallmarks of this disorder are high circulating titres of antibodies to thyroid peroxidase (primarily) and thyroglobulin (less often).

In iodine-sufficient countries, the most common cause of goitre, hypothyroidism, and elevated thyroid antibody levels is Hashimoto's thyroiditis. The incidence of autoimmune thyroiditis has increased over the past three generations, perhaps due to the increase in iodine intake that has occurred in the Western world (1). Elevated serum thyroid antibody concentrations are found in approximately 10% of the US population and in up to 25% of US women over the age of 60 (1). About 45% of older women will have lymphocytic infiltration within the thyroid gland. Autoimmune thyroiditis has a female predominance with reported female to male ratios ranging between 5:1 and 9:1.

Aetiology and pathogenesis

While it is clear that Hashimoto's thyroiditis is an autoimmune disease, the nature of the autoimmune process is still debated. These disorders tend to aggregate in families, and a genetic link has been suggested. There have been associations between HLA-DR3, HLA-DR4, and HLA-DR5 and Hashimoto's thyroiditis; however, this was demonstrated only in a cohort of white individuals (1). While HLA genes may be critical to the development of Hashimoto's thyroiditis, this weak association makes it clear that there are other genes that have not been identified yet and that play a role in this multigenic disease (see Chapter 3.2.1). Smoking has also been identified both as a risk factor for hypothyroidism (2) and to protect against hypothyroidism (3).

The defect in immunoregulation is also still a matter for debate (see Chapter 3.2.6). Human T-lymphotropic virus type 1 (HTLV1) has been found to be associated with autoimmune diseases and carriers of the virus have been shown to have a higher frequency of thyroid antibody positivity as well as a higher incidence of Hashimoto's thyroiditis compared to controls (4). Other theories hold that thyrocyte expression of class I and class II genes allows the thyrocyte to present antigen, and thus induce autoimmune thyroid disease; however, in contrast, available evidence indicates that thyrocyte expression of these genes promotes anergy, and thus may protect against autoimmune thyroid disease (5). The prime defect probably lies in antigen-presenting genes in professional antigen-presenting cells, e.g. macrophages, such that specific regulatory T lymphocytes, normally necessary for tolerance, are not fully activated (6). This, together with environmental factors that may serve to down-regulate the immune system, might act together to disturb immunoregulation, and allow for the development of autoimmune thyroid disease.

Many antibodies are often present in patients with Hashimoto's thyroiditis. Antithyroid peroxidase antibodies are complement fixing and are detectable in about 90% of patients with Hashimoto's thyroiditis. Antithyroglobulin antibody, a noncomplement-fixing antibody, is found in about 20–50% of patients with Hashimoto's thyroiditis (7). Thyroid-stimulating hormone (TSH) receptor antibodies that block TSH binding but do not stimulate the thyroid cell function may play a role in the clinical presentation of Hashimoto's thyroiditis, producing or exacerbating hypothyroidism in the absence of significant thyroid gland destruction (8). Such antibodies have been reported to bind to epitopes near the carboxyl end of the TSH-receptor extracellular domain, in contrast to thyroid-stimulating antibodies, which bind to epitopes near the N-terminus (9). The prevalence of TSH-receptor blocking antibodies in adult hypothyroid patients has been reported to be as high as 10% (10) and a decrease in the titre of these antibodies is likely to be responsible for 'remission' of hypothyroidism in some patients with Hashimoto's thyroiditis (11). Antibodies to colloid antigen, other thyroid autoantigens, thyroxine (T_4) and triiodothyronine (T_3), as well as other growth promoting and inhibiting antibodies may also be present.

Pathologically, there is lymphocytic infiltration of equal proportions of T and B cells and the formation of germinal centres (Fig. 3.2.7.1a). The follicular cells undergo metaplasia into larger, eosinophilic cells known as Hürthle or Askanazy cells which are packed with mitochondria. These cells exhibit high metabolic activity but ineffective hormonogenesis. There is progressive fibrosis, which may be extensive. The quantity of parenchymal tissue left in the thyroid is variable, as the pathological involvement ranges from focal regions to an entire lobe to the entire gland.

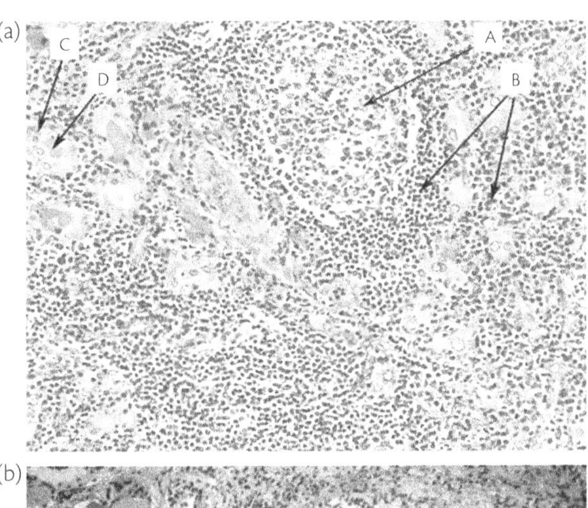

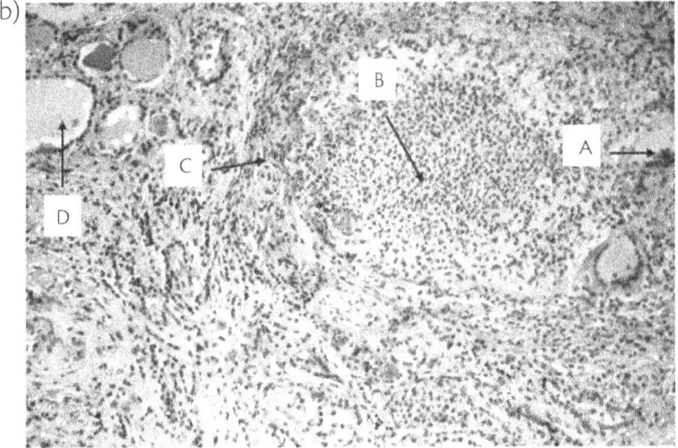

Fig. 3.2.7.1 Typical pathological changes of Hashimoto's thyroiditis and subacute thyroiditis. (a) Hashimoto's thyroiditis. A, lymphoid follicle with germinal centres; B, small lymphocytes and plasma cells; C, thyroid follicles with Hürthle cell metaplasia; D, minimal colloid material. (b) Subacute thyroiditis. A, multinucleate giant cell; B, mixed inflammatory infiltrate; C, fibrous band; D, residual follicles. Haematoxylin and eosin, ×200. (With permission from the Massachusetts Medical Society © 2003. All rights reserved.) (See also Plate 11)

Clinical features

Hashimoto's thyroiditis occurs most frequently in middle-aged women but can occur at any age. The usual presentation is as an incidental finding of a goitre during routine physical examination. While usually asymptomatic, some patients may complain of an awareness of fullness in the neck. The usual course is for slow enlargement of the thyroid over years; however, the thyroid occasionally may enlarge rapidly and can produce compressive symptoms of dyspnoea and/or dysphagia. Rarely, Hashimoto's thyroiditis may be painful (1, 12) and must be distinguished from subacute thyroiditis (see below). Systemic symptoms of hypothyroidism will be present in up to 20% of patients at the time of diagnosis (13), although this incidence is a little higher with the atrophic form of the disorder. Conversely, Hashimoto's thyroiditis is found to be the aetiology in the vast majority of patients in the USA with hypothyroidism.

Physical examination typically reveals a firm bumpy non-tender goitre, which is generally symmetrical and often has a palpable pyramidal lobe. Regional lymph node enlargement may be observed. While nodular thyroid disease can, and frequently does, occur in Hashimoto's thyroiditis, single nodules and dominant nodules in a multinodular gland should be evaluated with a fine-needle aspiration biopsy to rule out a coexistent malignancy. Ophthalmopathy is present in a small subset of patients with Hashimoto's thyroiditis (14). Furthermore, there is evidence of chronic autoimmune thyroiditis in many patients with euthyroid Graves' ophthalmopathy.

Laboratory evaluation and diagnosis

The hallmark of Hashimoto's thyroiditis is elevated thyroid antibody levels. The majority of individuals with elevated thyroid antibody levels are biochemically euthyroid. Up to 10% of postmenopausal women with an elevated thyroid antibody level will have an increased TSH but a minority of these (*c.*0.5%) will have overt hypothyroidism (1). Women with elevated thyroid antibody levels have been reported to develop overt hypothyroidism at a rate of 2–4% per year (1, 13, 15) (see Chapter 3.1.7). Mild thyrotoxicosis ('Hashitoxicosis') has been reported to be the initial manifestation in some patient's with Hashimoto's thyroiditis (16). The clinical course in these patients follows a pattern similar to that observed in sporadic silent or postpartum thyroiditis (Chapter 3.4.6), suggesting that differentiation between these disorders may be largely semantic.

The diagnosis of Hashimoto's thyroiditis is confirmed by the presence of antithyroid antibodies. Serum T_4 and TSH concentrations depend on the level of thyroidal dysfunction that is present and are not specific to hypothyroidism due to Hashimoto's thyroiditis. Serum T_3 concentrations are often preserved in all but the most severely hypothyroid patient and, thus, are of little clinical value. Similarly, the radioactive iodine uptake is usually not helpful, as it may be elevated, normal, or depressed. Thyroid isotope scanning usually reveals patchy uptake and, in general, provides little useful information unless a dominant thyroid nodule is present. Ultrasound examination of the thyroid frequently reveals marked hypoechogenicity with pseudonodules (17).

When imaged, an enlarged thymus gland is frequently found in Hashimoto's thyroiditis and may be important in the pathogenesis of the condition. In both affected patients and their relatives, there is an association with other autoimmune diseases including insulin-dependent diabetes mellitus, pernicious anaemia, Addison's disease, and vitiligo. Thyroid lymphoma is rare; however, the risk is increased in those individuals with Hashimoto's thyroiditis by a factor of 67 (1, 18). In patients in whom a fine-needle aspiration biopsy is performed, lymphocyte subsets should be determined on the biopsy specimen if the more typical pathological features of Hashimoto's thyroiditis are not present.

Treatment

Treatment of Hashimoto's thyroiditis consists of thyroid hormone replacement if hypothyroidism is present. L-thyroxine is the hormone of choice for thyroid hormone replacement therapy because of its consistent potency and prolonged duration of action. The average daily adult replacement dose of L-thyroxine sodium in a 68-kg person is 112 µg. Institution of therapy in healthy younger individuals can begin at full replacement doses. Because of the prolonged half-life of thyroxine (7 days), new steady-state concentrations of the hormone will not be achieved until 4–6 weeks after a change in dose. Thus, re-evaluation with determination of serum TSH concentration need not be performed at intervals of less than 4–6 weeks. The goal of thyroxine replacement therapy is to achieve a TSH value in the normal range, as over-replacement of thyroxine suppressing TSH values to the subnormal range may induce osteoporosis and cause cardiac dysfunction (19). In noncompliant young patients, the cumulative weekly doses of L-thyroxine may be given as a single weekly dose which is safe, effective, and well tolerated. In individuals over the age of 60, institution of therapy at a lower daily dose of L-thyroxine sodium (25 µg/day) is indicated to avoid exacerbation of underlying and undiagnosed cardiac disease. Daily doses of thyroxine may be interrupted periodically because of intercurrent medical or surgical illnesses that prohibit taking medications by mouth. A lapse of several days of hormone replacement is unlikely to have any significant metabolic consequences. However, if more prolonged interruption in oral therapy is necessary, L-thyroxine may be given intravenously at a dose 25–50% less than the patient's daily oral requirements. The treatment of euthyroid asymptomatic patients is not so clear-cut, and the recommendations for treatment of increased TSH without a corresponding low T_4 concentration are divided (19, 20).

In addition to replacement therapy, thyroid hormone therapy may be considered in patients with a serum TSH in the normal range in an attempt to decrease the size of a goitre or as a preventative measure to preclude the development of overt hypothyroidism. While goitre suppression with L-thyroxine is frequently not fruitful, in the subset of patients with Hashimoto's thyroiditis early in the course of the disease and before fibrosis develops such therapy may be useful. However, goitre suppression with L-thyroxine is unlikely to be successful if the initial TSH is less than 1 mU/l. The goal of L-thyroxine suppression therapy is to decrease the serum TSH into the subnormal range. Patients on L-thyroxine suppression therapy should be re-evaluated periodically and the suppressive hormone dose should be reduced or discontinued if significant goitre reduction is not achieved. In the absence of cancer, surgery is indicated for compressive goitres with local obstructive symptoms.

Subacute thyroiditis

Subacute thyroiditis, like painless sporadic and postpartum thyroiditis, is a spontaneously remitting inflammatory disorder of the thyroid that may last for weeks to months (1, 21) (Table 3.2.7.1). This disorder has a number of eponyms, including De Quervain's thyroiditis, giant cell thyroiditis, pseudogranulomatous thyroiditis, subacute painful thyroiditis, subacute granulomatous thyroiditis, acute simple thyroiditis, noninfectious thyroiditis, acute diffuse thyroiditis, migratory 'creeping' thyroiditis, pseudotuberculous thyroiditis, and viral thyroiditis. The first description of subacute thyroiditis was in 1895 by Mygind, who reported 18 cases of 'thyroiditis akuta simplex' (21). However, the pathology of subacute thyroiditis was first described in 1904 by Fritz De Quervain, whose name is associated with the disorder, when he showed giant cells and granulomatous-type changes in the thyroids of affected patients. Subacute thyroiditis is the most common cause of the painful thyroid and may account for up to 5% of clinical thyroid abnormalities (1, 21). As with other thyroid disorders, women are more frequently affected than men, with a peak incidence in the fourth and fifth decades. This disorder is rarely observed in children and older people. While the term 'subacute thyroiditis' connotes a temporal quality that could apply to any thyroidal inflammatory process of intermediate duration and severity, it is actually referring specifically to the granulomatous appearance of the thyroid found on pathological examination. This pathological appearance of the thyroid is specific for the disease.

Aetiology and pathogenesis

Infectious association

Although there is no clear evidence for a specific aetiology, indirect evidence suggests that subacute thyroiditis may be caused by a viral infection of the thyroid (22, 23). The condition is often preceded by a prodromal phase of myalgias, malaise, low-grade fevers, fatigue, and frequently by an upper respiratory tract infection. It has been reported most frequently in the temperate zone, and only rarely from other parts of the world. It has been found to occur seasonally; the highest incidence is in the summer months (July through September) which coincide with the peak of enterovirus (echovirus, Coxsackie virus A and B) infection (24). The incidence rate has been shown to vary directly with viral epidemics; during certain viral epidemics, specifically mumps, the incidence of subacute thyroiditis has been found to be higher. Interestingly, antibodies to the mumps virus have even been detected in individuals with subacute thyroiditis who do not have clinical evidence of mumps. Subacute thyroiditis has also been associated with measles, influenza, the common cold, adenovirus, infectious mononucleosis, Coxsackie virus, myocarditis, cat-scratch fever, St Louis encephalitis, hepatitis A, and the parvovirus B19 infection. Antibodies to Coxsackie virus, adenovirus, influenza, and mumps have been detected in the convalescent phase of this disease (25). Coxsackie virus is most commonly associated with subacute thyroiditis and, in fact, Coxsackie virus antibody titres have been shown to directly follow the course of the thyroid disease (24). Isolation of a cytopathic virus of possible pathogenic significance from the thyroids of 5 of 28 patients with subacute thyroiditis was reported in 1976 (26).

Certain nonviral infections including Q fever and malaria, have been associated with a clinical syndrome similar to subacute thyroiditis. In addition, a case of subacute thyroiditis occurring simultaneously with giant cell arteritis has been reported. Another case of subacute thyroiditis developed during α-interferon treatment for hepatitis C.

Autoimmune association

Unlike painless or postpartum thyroiditis, there is no clear association between subacute thyroiditis and autoimmune thyroid disease. Serum thyroid peroxidase and thyroglobulin antibody levels are usually normal. When described, the levels of thyroid peroxidase and thyroglobulin antibodies correlated with the phase of transient hypothyroidism. Antibodies to an unpurified thyroid preparation can be detected for up to 4 years after a bout of subacute thyroiditis.

Antibodies to the thyrotropin (TSH) receptor have been detected only in some patients during the course of subacute thyroiditis (27). In most studies, there was no correlation between the presence of thyrotropin-receptor-binding inhibitory immunoglobulin or of thyrotropin-receptor stimulating immunoglobulin and the thyrotoxic phase of the thyroiditis. On the other hand, there has been some correlation between thyroid-blocking antibodies and the development of hypothyroidism. It is thought that the appearance of the TSH-receptor antibodies results from an immune response that occurs after there is damage to the thyrocytes, specifically membrane desquamation (22, 23). Following recovery from the inflammatory process of subacute thyroiditis, all immunological phenomena disappear (27). The transitory immunological markers that are observed during the course of subacute thyroiditis appear to occur in response to the release of antigenic material from the thyroid, and thus the inflammatory destruction of the gland appears to be a normal physiological response.

Genetic association

There is an apparent genetic predisposition for subacute thyroiditis, with HLA-Bw35 reported in all ethnic groups (21). The relative risk of HLA-Bw35 in subacute thyroiditis is high, ranging from 8.0 to 56 (21). Additional evidence for genetic susceptibility is the simultaneous development of subacute thyroiditis in identical twins heterozygous for the HLA-Bw35 haplotype (28). However, an epidemic of 'atypical' subacute thyroiditis was described in a town in the Netherlands where HLA-B15/62 was found in five of 11 patients tested while only one patient tested positive for HLA-Bw35 (29). Finally, a weak association of subacute thyroiditis with HLA-DRw8 has been reported in Japanese patients (30).

Pathology

The primary events in the pathology of subacute thyroiditis are destruction of the follicular epithelium and loss of follicular integrity; however, the histopathological changes are distinct from those found with Hashimoto's thyroiditis (Fig. 3.2.7.1b). The lesions are patchy in distribution and are of varying stages of development, with infiltration of mononuclear cells in affected regions and partial or complete loss of colloid and fragmentation and duplication of the basement membrane. Histiocytes congregate around masses of colloid, both within the follicles and in the interstitial tissues, producing 'giant cells'; often these giant cells consist of masses of colloid surrounded by large numbers of individual histiocytes, and so they more accurately should be termed 'pseudogiant cells'. The term 'granulomatous' thyroiditis, a synonym for subacute thyroiditis, should likewise be changed to 'pseudogranulomatous' thyroiditis. However, true giant cells and granulomas do appear in this disease as well.

During recovery, the inflammation recedes and there is a variable amount of fibrosis and fibrotic band formation. In addition, follicular regeneration occurs without caseation, haemorrhage, or calcification. Recovery is generally complete. Only in rare instances is there complete destruction of the thyroid parenchyma that leads to permanent hypothyroidism. In the few electron microscope studies reported, viral inclusion bodies have not been demonstrated. Fine-needle aspiration biopsies often show large numbers of histiocytes, epithelioid granulomas, multinucleated giant cells, and follicular cells with intravacuolar granules (31).

Clinical features

The manifestations may be preceded by an upper respiratory tract infection, or a prodromal phase of malaise, generalized myalgias, pharyngitis, and low-grade fevers. Pain or swelling in the thyroid region develops later accompanied by higher fevers; up to 50% of patients have symptoms of thyrotoxicosis (1). Pain may be moderate or severe but in a few cases symptoms are entirely lacking. Similarly, tenderness may be moderate or severe (or even exquisite), or, conversely, may also be lacking. One of the lobes may be involved initially, and later spread to the opposite lobe (creeping thyroiditis) or it may involve both lobes from the outset. The systemic reaction may be minimal or severe, and fevers may reach 40 °C. Rarely, subacute thyroiditis may present as a nontender solitary nodule. In these cases, the diagnosis has been made after fine-needle aspiration biopsy. Atypical presentations are often misdiagnosed as papillary cancer.

Patients can generally localize the pain to the thyroid region over one or both lobes. They may refer to their symptoms as a 'sore throat', but upon specific questioning, it becomes apparent that pain is in the neck, not within the pharynx. Typically, pain radiates from the thyroid region up to the angle of the jaw or to the ear on the affected side(s). The pain may also radiate to the anterior chest or may be centred over the thyroid only. Moving the head, swallowing, or coughing may aggravate the pain. Although some patients have no systemic symptoms, most complain of myalgias, fatigue, and fevers. Malaise can be extreme and can be associated with arthralgias.

On physical examination, most patients appear uncomfortable and flushed on inspection, with variable elevations in temperature. Palpation usually reveals an exquisitely tender hard ill-defined nodular thyroid. The tender region may encompass an entire lobe and mild tenderness may be present in the contralateral lobe. The overlying skin is occasionally warm and erythematous. Cervical lymphadenopathy is rarely present. While the vast majority of patients are only mildly to moderately ill, subacute thyroiditis may have a dramatic presentation, with marked fever, severe thyrotoxicosis, and obstructive symptoms due to pronounced thyroid inflammation and oedema.

Laboratory evaluation

During the active/painful phase of subacute thyroiditis, the ESR is usually markedly elevated. In fact, a normal ESR essentially rules out subacute thyroiditis as a tenable diagnosis. The white blood cell count is normal to mildly increased and there is often a normochromic normocytic anaemia. There are also increases in serum ferritin, soluble intercellular adhesion molecule-1, selectin, interleukin-6 levels, and C-reactive protein during the inflammatory phase (4, 22). Alkaline phosphatase and other hepatic enzymes may be elevated in the early phase. It has been suggested that subacute thyroiditis may actually represent a multisystem disease also affecting the thyroid.

In the thyrotoxic phase, the serum T_4 concentration is disproportionately elevated relative to the serum T_3 concentration, reflecting the intrathyroidal T_4:T_3 ratio. In addition, the acute illness decreases the peripheral deiodination of T_4 to T_3, resulting in lower serum T_3 concentrations than expected. Serum TSH concentrations are low to undetectable. Antibodies directed against thyroglobulin and thyroid peroxidase are either absent or present in low titre; these develop several weeks after disease onset and tend to disappear thereafter.

The radioactive iodine uptake during the thyrotoxic phase is low, most often below 2% at 24 h. As with the ESR discussed above, a normal radioactive iodine uptake essentially rules out subacute thyroiditis as a tenable diagnosis. Ultrasound examination may show generalized, multiple, or single regions of hypoechogenicity (32).

Diagnosis

Subacute thyroiditis must be differentiated from the other causes of anterior neck pain. The diagnosis should present no difficulties in patients with typical manifestations. However, because 'sore throat' is a frequent complaint, many patients are initially misdiagnosed with pharyngitis. Acute haemorrhage into a nodule or cyst and nonthyroidal aetiologies can be differentiated with radioiodine scanning, as there will be normal function in the nonaffected areas of the gland. Painful Hashimoto's thyroiditis usually involves the entire gland and antibodies directed against thyroglobulin and thyroid peroxidase are usually present in high titre. Acute suppurative thyroiditis is distinguished by a much greater leucocytosis and febrile response, a greater inflammatory reaction in surrounding tissues, and often a septic focus is evident elsewhere, such as in the urinary or respiratory tracts. The radioactive iodine uptake is usually normal in acute suppurative thyroiditis and the scan will reveal decreased uptake in the region of suppuration.

Rarely, infiltrating cancer of the thyroid can present with a clinical and laboratory picture indistinguishable from subacute thyroiditis, requiring fine-needle aspiration biopsy for the diagnosis. Amiodarone, an iodine-rich antiarrhythmic drug, may cause iodine-induced thyrotoxicosis (Jod-Basedow disease) and, less commonly, thyroiditis, which may occasionally be painful. Both sporadic silent and postpartum thyroiditis follow a similar clinical course as subacute thyroiditis but lack the clinical feature of a painful goitre. In addition, patients with painless or postpartum thyroiditis often exhibit high titres of antithyroglobulin and antithyroid peroxidase antibodies and the ESR is normal to only slightly elevated. Fine-needle aspiration biopsies may be useful, but may show large numbers of histiocytes and thus may be misleading.

Course and management

Despite the differing aetiologies, the clinical course of subacute thyroiditis is similar to that of painless and postpartum thyroiditis (see Chapter 3.4.6). The initial phase is characterized by pain and thyrotoxicosis in most patients and may last up to 3–4 months. The thyrotoxicosis may not be clinically apparent in some instances, and it is usually mild when it is clinically evident. As noted above, the thyrotoxicosis is due to a disruptive process within the thyroid causing leakage of colloid material into the interstices, where it liberates thyroid hormones, thyroglobulin, and other iodoamino acids into the circulation. If present, β-adrenergic blocking drugs such as propranolol are useful. Antithyroid drugs have no role in the management of subacute thyroiditis as the gland is not hyperfunctioning.

Salicylates and nonsteroidal anti-inflammatory drugs are often adequate to decrease thyroidal pain in mild to moderate cases. In more severe cases, oral glucocorticoids (prednisone up to 40 mg/day) may provide dramatic relief of pain and swelling, often within a few hours of administration and in most cases within 24–48 h. In fact, if thyroidal/neck pain fails to begin to improve after 24 h of corticosteroid therapy, the diagnosis of subacute thyroiditis should be questioned. Despite the clinical response to corticosteroids, the underlying inflammatory process may persist, and symptoms may recur if the dose is tapered too rapidly. Up to one-third of patients will have a recurrence of thyroidal pain upon discontinuation of prednisone, which responds to restarting the corticosteroid. In general, full-dose corticosteroids are given for a week, followed by tapering of the dose over at least 2–4 weeks.

Determination of the radioactive iodine uptake before discontinuing prednisone may be helpful in identifying those patients at high risk for relapse. If the radioactive iodine uptake is still low, the inflammatory process is ongoing and corticosteroids should not be discontinued. If the radioactive iodine uptake has returned to normal, then the corticosteroid can be safely withdrawn. Patients with recurrent exacerbations of symptoms after withdrawal of corticosteroids usually respond to reinstitution or continuation of the corticosteroids for an additional month. While subacute thyroiditis is a self-limited disease and the vast majority of patients respond to the measures discussed above, there are occasional patients who have repeated exacerbations of pain and inflammation. In these patients, therapy with L-thyroxine or L-triiodothyronine has been helpful in preventing exacerbations, suggesting that endogenous TSH may contribute to their occurrence. Rarely, thyroidectomy or thyroid ablation with radioactive iodine may be necessary for management of patients with protracted courses of severe neck pain and malaise.

After the acute phase, a period of transient (1–2 months) asymptomatic euthyroidism follows. Hypothyroidism may occur after several more weeks and may last for 6–9 months. The final recovery phase follows, when all aspects of thyroid function return to normal, including morphology. Hypothyroidism may be permanent in up to 5% of patients and relapse of subacute thyroiditis is rare, occurring in less than 2% of patients (33). However, some patients with a history of subacute thyroiditis were found to be particularly sensitive to the inhibitory effects of exogenously administered iodides, suggesting a persistent thyroid abnormality. Thus, long-term follow-up of patients after an episode of subacute thyroiditis is recommended.

Infectious thyroiditis

Infectious thyroiditis is also known as acute thyroiditis, suppurative thyroiditis, bacterial thyroiditis, and pyogenic thyroiditis (Table 3.2.7.1). Bacterial infections of the thyroid are rare, with only 224 cases having been reported in the literature from 1900 to 1980 (34) and only 60 cases reported in the paediatric literature (35). Bacterial infections are the aetiology of most cases of infectious thyroiditis and the infections are generally suppurative and acute. Infectious thyroiditis caused by fungal and parasitic infections are more frequently chronic and indolent. In this section, emphasis will be placed on bacterial infections. The reader is referred to other reviews for further information on the less frequent causes of infectious thyroiditis (21).

Aetiology and pathogenesis

The thyroid gland's high iodine content, significant vascularity, lymphatic drainage, as well as its protective capsule provide the thyroid gland with notable resistance to infection (21). The most common predisposing factor to infections of the thyroid appears to be pre-existing thyroid disease. Simple goitre, nodular goitre, Hashimoto's thyroiditis, or thyroid carcinoma has been observed in up to two-thirds of women and one-half of men with infectious thyroiditis (34). Patients with AIDS are a population particularly at risk for bacterial thyroiditis. As with other opportunistic infections in AIDS patients, infections of the thyroid gland are often chronic and insidious in onset.

In the adult, *Staphylococcus aureus* and *Streptococcus pyogenes* are the offending pathogens in more than 80% of patients and are the sole pathogen in over 70% of cases (21) (Table 3.2.7.2). In children, α- and β-haemolytic streptococcus and a variety of anaerobes account for about 70% of cases, while mixed pathogens are identified in over 50% of cases (35). Other thyroidal bacterial pathogens that have been shown to cause infectious thyroiditis include *Salmonella brandenburg*, *Salmonella enteritidis*, *Actinomyces naeslundii*, *Actinobacillus actinomycetemcomitans*, *Brucella melitensis*, *Clostridium septicum*, *Eikenella corrodens*, *Enterobacter*, *Escherichia coli*, *Haemophilus influenzae*, *Klebsiella* sp., *Pseudomonas aeruginosa*, *Serratia marcescens*, *Acinetobacter baumannii*, and *Staphylococcus non-aureus* (21).

Infection and suppuration may result from direct spread from a nearby infection, or via the bloodstream or lymphatics. The seminal observation regarding the pathogenesis of bacterial thyroiditis was made in 1979 when Takai *et al.* reported seven cases of infectious thyroiditis due to a fistula originating from the left pyriform sinus (36). Subsequently, studies involving over 100 patients with infectious thyroiditis have identified pyriform sinus fistulae, primarily left-sided, in up to 90% of these patients, especially in those with recurrent episodes (21). Additional reports identified infected embryonic cysts from the third and fourth brachial pouches and thyroglossal duct cysts as routes of thyroidal infection. On pathological examination, the characteristic changes of acute bacterial inflammation, including necrosis and abscess formation, are commonly found.

Clinical manifestations

Bacterial thyroiditis is often preceded by an upper respiratory tract infection, which may induce inflammation of the fistula and promote the transmission of pathogens to the thyroid. Consistent with these observations, bacterial thyroiditis is more common in the late autumn and late spring. Over 90% of patients will present with thyroidal pain, tenderness, fever, and local compression resulting in dysphagia and dysphonia; the pain is often referred diffusely to adjacent structures. Systemic symptoms such as fever, chills, tachycardia, and malaise are seen frequently.

Table 3.2.7.2 Pathogenesis of acute suppurative thyroiditis

Organism	Frequency (%)
Bacterial	68
Parasitic	15
Mycobacterial	9
Fungal	5
Syphilitic	3

Laboratory findings

Thyroid function tests are usually normal; however, cases of hypothyroidism and thyrotoxicosis have been reported (21). A nuclear medicine thyroid scan may show the suppurative region as a 'cold' area, whereas an ultrasound examination may reveal a cystic or 'complex' nodule. The polymorphonuclear leucocyte count and the sedimentation rate are usually elevated. The organism frequently can be identified by Gram's stain and culture, although sterile cultures are seen in approximately 8% of cases (21).

Diagnosis

The diagnosis is made with a fine-needle aspiration, Gram's stain, and culture. Symptomatically, infective thyroiditis may be difficult to differentiate from subacute thyroiditis in the early phases, although the characteristic thyroid function changes in the latter disease should be helpful in discriminating the two (23). Leucocytosis and an elevated ESR are not discriminatory tests as they are commonly observed in both subacute thyroiditis and infectious thyroiditis. In general, patients with bacterial thyroiditis have a greater febrile response than those with subacute thyroiditis. Once abscess formation has occurred, the local redness, lymphadenopathy, hyperpyrexia, and leucocytosis should lead to the correct diagnosis. Malignant neoplasms and haemorrhages into cysts may sometimes present with manifestations that mimic this disorder.

Course and management

The prognosis of bacterial thyroiditis is often dependent on the prompt recognition and treatment of this disorder, as mortality may approach 100% if the diagnosis is delayed and appropriate antimicrobial therapy is not instituted. Much depends upon the identification of the microorganism either from needle aspirate, incision, and drainage, or occasionally from blood culture. If no organisms are seen on the Gram's stain, nafcillin and gentamicin or a third-generation cephalosporin is appropriate initial therapy in adults while a second-generation cephalosporin or clindamycin is reasonable in children. If an abscess develops and prompt response to antibiotics does not occur, incision and drainage is necessary. Sometimes partial lobectomy must be performed, especially if the disease is recurrent. Usually the lesions heal with reasonable speed after initiation of the correct antimicrobial agent, and recurrences are uncommon. Mortality from acute bacterial thyroiditis has markedly improved from the 20–25% reported in the early 1900s, with the extensive review by Berger estimating an overall mortality of 8.6% (34). Recent reviews involving over 100 patients failed to list mortality as a complication of acute bacterial thyroiditis (37).

Sclerosing thyroiditis (Riedel's thyroiditis)

Sclerosing thyroiditis, also known as invasive fibrous thyroiditis, Riedel's struma, Riedel's thyroiditis, struma fibrosa, ligneous

(Eisenharte) struma, chronic fibrous thyroiditis, and chronic productive thyroiditis, is a rare disorder of unknown cause, characterized pathologically by dense fibrous tissue which replaces the normal thyroid parenchyma and extends into adjacent tissues, such as muscles, parathyroid glands, blood vessels, and nerves (22) (Table 3.2.7.1). The first report by Riedel in 1896 described cases of chronic sclerosing thyroiditis, primarily affecting women, which frequently caused pressure symptoms in the neck and tended to progress ultimately to complete destruction of the thyroid gland. Riedel's interesting description was that of a 'specific inflammation of mysterious nature producing an iron-hard tumefaction of the thyroid'.

This condition is quite rare (1, 22, 38). In thyroidectomies performed for all disorders, an incidence between 0.03 and 0.98% has been reported. At the Mayo Clinic, the operative incidence over 64 years was 0.06%, and the incidence in outpatients was 1.06/100 000. Because the manifestations are likely to lead to surgery, the incidence of invasive fibrous thyroiditis among patients undergoing thyroidectomy is much greater than the incidence in patients with goitres in general.

Aetiology

The cause of this disorder remains unknown. Thyroid antibodies have been reported in up to 67% of patients (39). This observation, in addition to the presence of both B and T cells in the inflammatory infiltrate, suggests a possible autoimmune mechanism, although no direct relationship has been shown. It is not uncommon for those with invasive fibrous thyroiditis to have other autoimmune diseases, such as insulin-dependent diabetes mellitus and Addison's disease (40–42). One patient was reported to have both invasive fibrous thyroiditis and pernicious anaemia, which is another autoimmune disease. The expression of HLA-DR, heat-shock protein (HSP72), and soluble intercell adhesion molecule-1 (ICAM-1) receptor in invasive fibrous thyroiditis tissue suggests a role for an active cell-mediated immune response early in the evolution of this condition (40–43).

Marked tissue eosinophilia and eosinophil degranulation have been observed in Riedel's struma (44). These findings may suggest that the release of eosinophil-derived products may play a role in the fibrogenic stimulus. The nature of these products is not yet known.

Whatever the ultimate aetiology is, it will have to account for the extrathyroidal fibrosclerosis as well. This was first noted as early as 1885 and was described as a common accompaniment of invasive fibrous thyroiditis (22). These areas of extrathyroidal fibrosclerosis include salivary gland fibrosis, sclerosing cholangitis, pseudotumours of the orbits, fibrous mediastinitis, retroperitoneal fibrosis, and lachrymal gland fibrosis. Long-term follow-up of patients with invasive fibrous thyroiditis (follow-up time 10 years) has shown that one-third develop fibrosing disorders of the retroperitoneal space (often with ureteral obstruction), chest, or orbit, almost always with a single extracervical site involved. Conversely, less than 1% of patients with retroperitoneal fibrosis have invasive fibrous thyroiditis. The association of certain drugs with retroperitoneal fibrosis has not been observed with invasive fibrous thyroiditis. There does not seem to be a genetic predisposition for this condition.

Clinical features

The age of onset varies between 23 and 78 years, although most cases are diagnosed in the fourth to sixth decades. The female to male ratio varies between 2:1 and 4:1.

The clinical presentation is of a painless goitre that is gradually or rapidly enlarging; constitutional symptoms of inflammation are rare. The extensive fibrosis is progressive and may eventually cause compression of adjacent structures, particularly the trachea and oesophagus. Local compressive symptoms include a marked sense of pressure or severe dyspnoea, with symptoms out of proportion to the size of the goitre. In some patients, the fibrotic process affects the entire gland causing hypothyroidism; the prevalence of hypothyroidism in this population is between 25 and 40%. Hypoparathyroidism can develop when parathyroid gland infiltration occurs and tetany associated with this process has been described.

On examination, the thyroid gland is stony hard, often described as 'woody' in texture, densely adherent to adjacent cervical structures (such as muscles, blood vessels, and nerves), and may move poorly on swallowing. The lesion may be limited to one lobe. It has a harder consistency than a carcinoma and is usually nontender. Although adjacent lymph nodes are only occasionally enlarged, when they are present a diagnosis of carcinoma is often suspected.

Laboratory findings

At presentation, most patients with Riedel's thyroiditis are euthyroid; however, as mentioned earlier, some patients do develop hypothyroidism. Thyroid antibodies may be detected in the majority of these patients. Calcium and phosphorus levels should be evaluated at presentation to identify those patients who also have concurrent hypoparathyroidism. Thyroid radionuclide imaging can show either a heterogeneous pattern or low isotope uptake; the 'cold' areas reflect the fibrosis. The extent of the fibrosis can best be determined on either CT or MRI; the affected regions appear homogeneous and hypointense on T_1- and T_2-weighted MRI images. Ultrasound examinations can be helpful as the areas affected appear hypoechoic; on colour flow Doppler, the fibrotic areas are avascular. The white blood cell count and sedimentation rate are usually normal, but can be elevated.

Pathology consists of an exuberant fibrosis involving part of or the entire thyroid. Fibrotic extension beyond the capsule of the thyroid into adjacent structures such as nerves, blood vessels, muscles, parathyroid glands, trachea, and oesophagus is characteristic. Pathological diagnostic criteria for this condition includes complete destruction of involved thyroid tissue with absence of normal lobulation, lack of a granulomatous reaction, and extension of the fibrosis beyond the thyroid into adjacent muscle, nerves, blood vessels, and adipose. Histological examination reveals almost no thyroid follicles and few plasma cells, eosinophils, and Hürthle cells. Lymphocytes are also sparse, in contrast to the findings in Hashimoto's thyroiditis, although occasionally a few foci of lymphocytes may be observed. An associated arteritis and phlebitis with intimal proliferation, medial destruction, adventitial inflammation, and thrombosis may also occur. Similar features are observed in the extracervical fibrosclerotic lesions, retroperitoneal and mediastinal regions, orbit, and lachrymal glands, and in sclerosing cholangitis.

Diagnosis and treatment

The diagnosis is made by biopsy of the goitre in order to differentiate this disorder from carcinoma. However, a fine-needle aspiration biopsy is usually inadequate due to the extreme hardness of the gland and, thus, an open biopsy is often required.

Treatment of Riedel's thyroiditis is surgical to relieve compressive symptoms. Extensive resection is often impossible due to fibrosis of surrounding structures, but wedge resection, especially over the isthmus to relieve tracheal compression, is often extremely effective. Despite its invasive nature, recurrences of obstruction after resection are rare. Thyroid hormone therapy is indicated only if hypothyroidism is present, as suppression therapy is ineffective. Calcium and vitamin D therapy is indicated in those patients with associated hypoparathyroidism. There have been several reports of disease improvement with glucocorticoid therapy, and relapses have reversed with the reinstitution of steroids; however, it has not been helpful in all instances. Tamoxifen has been reported to cause disease regression in a few case reports. Its mechanism of action is unclear; however, it may play a role in fibroblastic proliferation inhibition (45).

Prognosis

Riedel's thyroiditis is usually progressive; however, it may stabilize or remit spontaneously. Following surgery, the disease can remit or be self-limiting. Repeat surgery is only rarely required. Mortality rates range from 6 to 10%, with deaths usually attributed to asphyxia secondary to tracheal compression or laryngospasm. However, these mortality rates are derived from older literature, and may not reflect (the presumably lower) current rates. In many instances, the condition is self-limiting, and improvement often persists after isthmic wedge resection.

References

1. Pearce EN, Farwell AP, Braverman LE. Thyroiditis. *N Engl J Med*, 2003; **348**: 2646–55.
2. Nystrom E, Bengtsson C, Lapidus L, Petersen K, Lindstedt G. Smoking: a risk factor for hypothyroidism. *J Endocrinol Invest*, 1993; **16**: 129–31.
3. Asvold BO, Bjoro T, Nilsen TI, Gunnell D, Vatten LJ. Thyrotropin levels and risk of fatal coronary heart disease: the HUNT study. *Arch Intern Med*, 2008; **168**: 855–60.
4. Pearce EN, Bogazzi F, Martino E, Brogioni S, Pardini E, Pellegrini G, *et al*. The prevalence of elevated serum C-reactive protein levels in inflammatory and noninflammatory thyroid disease. *Thyroid*, 2003; **13**: 643–8.
5. Yue SJ, Enomoto T, Matsumoto Y, Kawai K, Volpe R. Thyrocyte class I and class II upregulation is a secondary phenomenon and does not contribute to the pathogenesis of autoimmune thyroid disease. *Thyroid*, 1998; **8**: 755–63.
6. Volpe R. The immunology of human autoimmune thyroid disease. In: Volpe R, ed. *The Autoimmune Endocrinopathies. Contemporary Endocrinology Series*. Totowa: Humana Press, 1999: 217–44
7. Furmaniak J SJ, Rees-Smith, B. Autoantigens in the autoimmune endocrinopathies. In: Volpe R, ed. *The Autoimmune Endocrinopathies. Contemporary Endocrinology Series*. Totowa: Humana Press, 1999: 183–216
8. Botero D, Brown RS. Bioassay of thyrotropin receptor antibodies with Chinese hamster ovary cells transfected with recombinant human thyrotropin receptor: clinical utility in children and adolescents with Graves' disease. *J Pediatr*, 1998; **132**: 612–18.
9. Kosugi S, Ban T, Akamizu T, Kohn LD. Identification of separate determinants on the thyrotropin receptor reactive with Graves' thyroid-stimulating antibodies and with thyroid-stimulating blocking antibodies in idiopathic myxedema: these determinants have no homologous sequence on gonadotropin receptors. *Mol Endocrinol*, 1992; **6**: 168–80.
10. Tamaki H, Amino N, Kimura M, Hidaka Y, Takeoka K, Miyai K. Low prevalence of thyrotropin receptor antibody in primary hypothyroidism in Japan. *J Clin Endocrinol Metab*, 1990; **71**: 1382–6.
11. Takasu N, Yamada T, Takasu M, Komiya I, Nagasawa Y, Asawa T, *et al*. Disappearance of thyrotropin-blocking antibodies and spontaneous recovery from hypothyroidism in autoimmune thyroiditis. *N Engl J Med*, 1992; **326**: 513–18.
12. Leung AK, Hegde K. Hashimoto's thyroiditis simulating De Quervain's thyroiditis. *J Adolesc Health Care*, 1988; **9**: 434–5.
13. Tunbridge WMG, Brewis M, French JM, Appleton D, Bird T, Clark F, *et al*. Natural history of autoimmune thyroiditis. *Br Med J*, 1981; **282**: 258–62.
14. Bartalena L, Baldeschi L, Dickinson AJ, Eckstein A, Kendall-Taylor P, Marcocci C, *et al*. Consensus statement of the European group on Graves' orbitopathy (EUGOGO) on management of Graves' orbitopathy. *Thyroid*, 2008; **18**: 333–46.
15. Vanderpump MP, Tunbridge WM, French JM, Appleton D, Bates D, Clark F, *et al*. The incidence of thyroid disorders in the community: a twenty-year follow-up of the Whickham Survey. *Clin Endocrinol (Oxf)*, 1995; **43**: 55–68.
16. Nabhan ZM, Kreher NC, Eugster EA. Hashitoxicosis in children: clinical features and natural history. *J Pediatr*, 2005; **146**: 533–6.
17. Rago T, Chiovato L, Grasso L, Pinchera A, Vitti P. Thyroid ultrasonography as a tool for detecting thyroid autoimmune diseases and predicting thyroid dysfunction in apparently healthy subjects. *J Endocrinol Invest*, 2001; **24**: 763–9.
18. Matsubayashi S, Kawai K, Matsumoto Y, Mukuta T, Morita T, Hirai K, *et al*. The correlation between papillary thyroid carcinoma and lymphocytic infiltration in the thyroid gland. *J Clin Endocrinol Metab*, 1995; **80**: 3421–4.
19. Biondi B, Cooper DS. The clinical significance of subclinical thyroid dysfunction. *Endocr Rev*, 2008; **29**: 76–131.
20. Papi G, Uberti ED, Betterle C, Carani C, Pearce EN, Braverman LE, *et al*. Subclinical hypothyroidism. *Curr Opin Endocrinol Diabetes Obes*, 2007; **14**: 197–208.
21. Farwell AP. Infectious and subacute thyroiditis. In: Braverman LE, Utiger RD, eds. *The Thyroid*. Philadelphia: Lippincott-William & Wilkins, 2005: 536–48.
22. Volpe R. Subacute and sclerosing thyroiditis. In: DeGroot L, ed. *Endocrinology*. 4th edn. Philadelphia: Saunders, 2001.
23. Volpe R. Subacute thyroiditis. In: Burron GNOJ, Volpe R, eds. *Thyroid Function and Disease*. Philadelphia: Saunders, 1989: 179–90.
24. Desailloud R, Hober D. Viruses and thyroiditis: an update. *Virol J*, 2009; **6**: 5.
25. Volpe R, Row VV, Ezrin C. Circulating viral and thyroid antibodies in subacute thyroiditis. *J Clin Endocrinol Metab*, 1967; **27**: 1275–84.
26. Stancek D, Ciampor F, Mucha V, Hnilica P, Stancekova M. Morphological, cytological and biological observations on viruses isolated from patients with subacute thyroiditis de Quervain. *Acta Virol*, 1976; **20**: 183–8.
27. Volpe R. Immunology of the thyroid. In: Volpe R, ed. *Autoimmune Diseases of the Endocrine System*. Boca Raton: CRC Press, 1990: 73–240.
28. Hamaguchi E, Nishimura Y, Kaneko S, Takamura T. Subacute thyroiditis developed in identical twins two years apart. *Endocr J*, 2005; **52**: 559–62.
29. de Bruin TW, Riekhoff FP, de Boer JJ. An outbreak of thyrotoxicosis due to atypical subacute thyroiditis. *J Clin Endocrinol Metab*, 1990; **70**: 396–402.

30. Goto H, Uno H, Tamai H, Kuma K, Hayashi Y, Matsubayashi S, *et al.* Genetic analysis of subacute (de Quervain's) thyroiditis. *Tissue Antigens*, 1985; **26**: 110–13.
31. Lu CP, Chang TC, Wang CY, Hsiao YL. Serial changes in ultrasound-guided fine needle aspiration cytology in subacute thyroiditis. *Acta Cytol*, 1997; **41**: 238–43.
32. Omori N, Omori K, Takano K. Association of the ultrasonographic findings of subacute thyroiditis with thyroid pain and laboratory findings. *Endocr J*, 2008; **55**: 583–8.
33. Iitaka M, Momotani N, Ishii J, Ito K. Incidence of subacute thyroiditis recurrences after a prolonged latency: 24-year survey. *J Clin Endocrinol Metab*, 1996; **81**: 466–9.
34. Berger SA, Zonszein J, Villamena P, Mittman N. Infectious diseases of the thyroid gland. [Review]. *Rev Infect Dis*, 1983; **5**: 108–22.
35. Rich EJ, Mendelman PM. Acute suppurative thyroiditis in pediatric patients. [Review]. *Pediatr Infect Dis J*, 1987; **6**: 936–40.
36. Takai S-I, Miyauchi A, Matsuzuka F, Kuma K, Kosaki G. Internal fistula as a route of infection in acute suppurative thyroiditis. *Lancet*, 1979; **i**: 751–2.
37. Jeng LB, Lin JD, Chen MF. Acute suppurative thyroiditis: a ten-year review in a Taiwanese hospital. *Scand J Infect Dis*, 1994; **26**: 297–300.
38. Papi G, LiVolsi VA. Current concepts on Riedel thyroiditis. *Am J Clin Pathol*, 2004: **121** (Suppl): S50–63.
39. Schwaegerle SM, Bauer TW, Esselstyn C, Jr. Riedel's thyroiditis. [Review]. *Am J Clin Pathol*, 1988; **90**: 715–22.
40. Heufelder AE HI, Carney JA, Gorman CA. Coexistence of Graves' disease and Riedel's (invasive fibrous) thyroiditis: further evidence of a link between Riedel's thyroiditis and organ-specific autoimmunity. *Clin Invest*, 1994; **72**: 788–93.
41. Zimmermann-Belsing T, Feldt-Rasmussen U. Riedel's thyroiditis: an autoimmune or primary fibrotic disease? *J Intern Med*, 1994; **235**: 271–4.
42. Heufelder AE, Hay ID. Further evidence for autoimmune mechanisms in the pathogenesis of Riedel's invasive fibrous thyroiditis. *J Intern Med*, 1995; **238**: 85–6.
43. Heufelder AE, Bahn RS. Soluble intercellular adhesion molecule-1 (sICAM-1) in sera of patients with Graves' ophthalmopathy and thyroid diseases. *Clin Exp Immunol*, 1993; **92**: 296–302.
44. Heufelder AE, Goellner JR, Bahn RS, Gleich GJ, Hay ID. Tissue eosinophilia and eosinophil degranulation in Riedel's invasive fibrous thyroiditis. *J Clin Endocrinol Metab*, 1996; **81**: 977–84.
45. Few J, Thompson NW, Angelos P, Simeone D, Giordano T, Reeve T. Riedel's thyroiditis: treatment with tamoxifen. *Surgery*, 1996; **120**: 993–9.

3.3

Thyrotoxicosis and related disorders

Contents

3.3.1 Clinical assessment and systemic manifestations of thyrotoxicosis

Claudio Marcocci, Filomena Cetani, Aldo Pinchera

Introduction

The term thyrotoxicosis refers to the clinical syndrome that results when the serum concentrations of free thyroxine, free triiodothyronine, or both, are high. The term hyperthyroidism is used to mean sustained increases in thyroid hormone biosynthesis and secretion by the thyroid gland; Graves' disease is the most common example of this. Occasionally, thyrotoxicosis may be due to other causes such as destructive thyroiditis, excessive ingestion of thyroid hormones, or excessive secretion of thyroid hormones from ectopic sites; in these cases there is no overproduction of hormone by thyrocytes and, strictly speaking, no hyperthyroidism. The various causes of thyrotoxicosis are listed in Chapter 3.3.5. The clinical features depend on the severity and the duration of the disease, the age of the patient, the presence or absence of extrathyroidal manifestations, and the specific disorder producing the thyrotoxicosis. Older patients have fewer symptoms and signs of sympathetic activation, such as tremor, hyperactivity, and anxiety, and more symptoms and signs of cardiovascular dysfunction, such as atrial fibrillation and dyspnoea. Rarely a patient with 'apathetic' hyperthyroidism will lack almost all of the usual clinical manifestations of thyrotoxicosis (1).

Almost all organ systems in the body are affected by thyroid hormone excess, and the high levels of circulating thyroid hormones are responsible for most of the systemic effects observed in these patients (Table 3.3.1.1). However, some of the signs and symptoms prominent in Graves' disease reflect extrathyroidal immunological processes rather than the excessive levels of thyroid hormones produced by the thyroid gland (Table 3.3.1.2).

Table 3.3.1.1 Systemic effects of thyrotoxicosis

System	Effects
General	Heat intolerance, weight loss, fatigue, insomnia, nervousness, tremulousness
Skin	Fine, warm and moist, hyperpigmentation, hyperhidrosis, onycholysis, fine and often straight hair, urticaria, pruritus
Eye	Exophthalmos, lid oedema, lid lag, globe lag, chemosis, ophthalmoplegia, optic nerve involvement
Mental	Irritability, restlessness, anxiety, inability to concentrate, lability, depression, psychiatric reactions
Neurological	Syncope, delirium, stupor, coma, choreoathetosis
Cardiovascular	Tachycardia, overactive heart, widened pulse pressure, and bounding pulse. Occasionally cardiomegaly, signs of congestive heart failure, angina pectoris, and paroxysmal tachycardia or atrial fibrillation
Respiratory	Dyspnoea
Gastrointestinal	Hyperphagia, increased thirst, diarrhoea or increased frequency of stools, elevated liver function tests, hepatomegaly
Neuromuscular	Tremulousness, quickened and hypermetric reflexes, weakness of proximal muscles, muscle atrophy, myopathy, periodic paralysis
Metabolic	Elevated serum calcium, decreased serum magnesium, increased bone alkaline phosphatase, hypercalciuria
Osseous	Osteopenia or osteoporosis
Reproductive	Irregular menses or amenorrhoea, gynaecomastia, decreased fertility
Haematopoietic	Anaemia (usually normochromic, normocytic), lymphocytosis, splenomegaly, lymphadenopathy, enlarged thymus

Skin, hair, and nails

Thyrotoxicosis is accompanied by cutaneous alterations that reflect the basic pathophysiological process and by various manifestations that may have practical diagnostic significance. Cutaneous changes occur whenever there is an increase in the metabolic rate and heat production. The skin has a smooth and silky texture. The typical thyrotoxic patient's skin is usually moist and warm because of vasodilatation, which represents a homeostatic mechanism for dissipating the heat being generated in the body (2). Temperature elevation and erythema are consequences of increased dermal blood flow. The patient may complain of cutaneous flushing, perspiration at rest, and sweaty palms. As a consequence of excessive perspiration found in about one-half of thyrotoxic patients, miliaria, caused by poral occlusion and intracutaneous sweat retention, may be present. Pigmentation may be increased and is often diffuse, although a spectrum of abnormalities may be seen ranging from localized to diffuse hyperpigmentation particularly in such areas as the knuckles and skin creases. Vitiligo of variable extent occurs in a substantial number of patients with Graves' disease and Hashimoto's thyroiditis as a marker of autoimmune disease (3, 4). Among the less frequently reported cutaneous changes in thyrotoxicosis are dermographism, urticaria, purpura, and ill-defined generalized erythematous eruptions. Pruritus may be the chief complaint in a few cases. The epidermal changes are rapidly reversed after restoration of euthyroidism.

The hair may be fine and soft, and hair loss can be excessive. Alopecia areata and loss of axillary, pubic, body, and eyebrow hairs have been noted since the initial description by von Basedow, but are uncommon. The severity of hair loss is not directly related to the severity of the endocrine abnormality.

Localizing nonpitting oedema is a clinical finding that can be the tip-off to establish the diagnosis of Graves' disease. Although this manifestation occurs along the shins (so-called pretibial myxoedema), it can occur elsewhere, generally on extensor surfaces (Fig. 3.3.1.1) (4). The lesion reflects the deposition of increased amounts of glycosaminoglycans in the subcutaneous connective tissue. The lesion is elevated above the surrounding tissue and is often finely dimpled and hyperpigmented, or pruritic and red.

The nails become shiny and may be soft and friable. The rate of nail growth is increased, and longitudinal striations associated with a flattening of the surface contour result in a scoop-shovel appearance. In many patients the nail is separated prematurely from the nail bed (onycholysis). Onycholysis is not specific to thyrotoxicosis, but when it occurs in this setting it usually begins under the distal central portion of the fourth fingernail. Such nail changes are less common in thyrotoxic patients over 60 years of age.

Eyes

Retraction of the upper eyelid, evident as the presence of a rim of sclera between the lid and the limbus, is frequent in all forms of thyrotoxicosis, and is responsible for the bright-eyed 'stare' or 'fish eyes' of the patient with thyrotoxicosis (Fig. 3.3.1.2). Lid lag is caused by the fact that the upper lid lags behind the globe when the patient is asked to gaze downward; globe lag occurs when the globe lags behind the upper lid when the patient gazes slowly upward. In severe cases the movements of the lids are jerky and spasmodic, and a fine tremor of the lightly closed lids can be observed. These ocular manifestations appear to be the result of increased adrenergic activity. It is important to differentiate these ocular manifestations from those of infiltrative ophthalmopathy, characteristic of Graves' disease (5, 6) (see Chapter 3.3.10).

Thyroid gland

Thyrotoxicosis due to nodular goitre or Graves' disease is usually associated with an enlargement of the thyroid (Fig. 3.3.1.3a); excessive ingestion of thyroid hormones is not associated with goitre unless superimposed on a pre-existing thyroid enlargement. An asymmetrical thyroid gland is generally found in patients with toxic adenoma or multinodular goitre (Fig. 3.3.1.3b), but such a gland can also be observed in Graves' disease. The thyroid gland in a typical patient with Graves' disease is diffusely enlarged and visible, although a retrosternal gland or a low-lying nodule may be clinically inapparent. The size is related, but not closely, to the severity of the disease. The pyramidal lobe should always be searched for, since enlargement indicates the presence of diffuse disease of the thyroid. The marked increase in the blood flow to the thyroid gland in Graves' disease is reflected clinically by the presence of a bruit or a thrill. The bruit is usually continuous but sometimes heard only in systole and is most readily detected at the upper or lower poles. Either the bruit or a thrill is highly suggestive,

Table 3.3.1.2 Clinical findings in patients with Graves' hyperthyroidism and controls[a]

	Hyperthyroid				Controls			
	Total	Age decades			Total	Age decades		
		2nd	3rd to 5th	6th to 8th		2nd	3rd to 5th	6th to 8th
Number	880	74	635	171	880	79	636	165
Symptoms (%)								
Palpitations	65	58	57	56	13	6	14	10
Increased perspiration	45	39	49	30	7	1	9	3
Heat intolerance	55	49	60	36	8	6	8	8
Weight loss	61	29	60	74	13	6	13	13
Weight gain	12	29	12	5	21	26	21	16
Increased appetite	42	61	12	5	5	9	21	16
Decreased appetite	11	5	10	16	6	6	7	4
Increased number of bowel movements	22	19	22	21	2	6	2	1
Increased appetite with weight loss	24	19	24	20	0	0	0	0
Tiredness	69	62	70	69	41	32	43	37
Irritability	45	47	35	33	18	16	21	10
Nervousness	69	59	71	64	15	11	17	12
Signs (%)								
Fine finger tremor	69	69	70	59	6	5	5	4
Pulse rate ≥90 beats/min	80	84	80	78	18	21	18	19
Atrial fibrillation[b]	3	0	1	9	–	–	–	–
Thyroid size (× normal)	1.9±0.6	2.4±0.6	2.0±0.6	1.4±0.4	1.3±0.4	1.4±0.6	1.3±0.4	1.3±0.4

[a] Modified from Nordyke RA, Gilbert FI Jr, Harada AS. Graves' disease. Influence of age on clinical findings. *Arch Int Med*, 1988; **148**: 626–31.

[b] The presence of atrial fibrillation was not assessed in control subjects.

but not pathognomonic, of thyrotoxicosis. If local examination of a goitre discloses either of these signs, even though other evidence of hyperfunction may be lacking, a careful investigation of thyroid function is indicated. Both thrill and bruits decrease in intensity as thyrotoxicosis subsides. Colour flow Doppler sonography shows hypervascularity and increased peak systolic velocity (7). Dysphagia and the sensation of a lump in the neck may be produced by goitre.

Respiratory system

Respiratory changes occurring in thyrotoxicosis are reported in Box 3.3.1.1. There are not many detailed studies of the effects of thyrotoxicosis on the lung. The frequency and the relative relevance of these changes is uncertain because available data are scarce and often conflicting. The increased metabolic rate stresses the lung, requiring a more rapid net rate of gas exchange to accommodate the increased oxygen consumption and carbon dioxide production. Dyspnoea is present in a large majority of severely affected thyrotoxic patients (8) and several factors may contribute to this condition, such as respiratory muscle weakness, reduction of vital capacity, decreased pulmonary compliance, and increase in respiratory dead space ventilation.

Lung volumes and flow rates

A decrease of residual volume, vital capacity, and total lung capacity have been reported in early studies in one-quarter of patients (8). In more recent studies no significant differences in the mean baseline vital capacity, total lung capacity, residual volume, static compliance, or pressure–volume curves between patients and controls have been observed (9). In some studies, the residual volume is increased and the total lung capacity is decreased, suggesting muscle weakness, but in other reports the results are contradictory. These heterogeneous findings may reflect either inclusion of patients with underlying lung diseases or the fact that thyrotoxicosis may cause several types of changes in the lungs, which may variably occur in different patients. For example, the weakness of respiratory muscles resulting from chronic thyrotoxic myopathy probably occurs only in some patients. Arterial blood gas partial pressures and oxygen–haemoglobin and carbon dioxide–haemoglobin dissociation curves are usually normal. Although the total amount of oxygen extracted by the peripheral tissues is increased, the efficiency of oxygen extraction is decreased.

Lung compliance and respiratory muscle weakness

Lung compliance may be altered by changes in the elastic properties or by vascular engorgement. It is calculated from the static pressure–volume curve of the lung, with measurement of the intrathoracic pressure using an oesophageal balloon manometer. In some cases it is difficult to separate patients with pure respiratory muscle weakness from patients who have only decreased lung compliance. Manifestations of respiratory muscle dysfunction include rapid, shallow respirations, respiratory dyskinesis, hypoventilation, respiratory acidosis, and easy fatigability (10). Most thyrotoxic

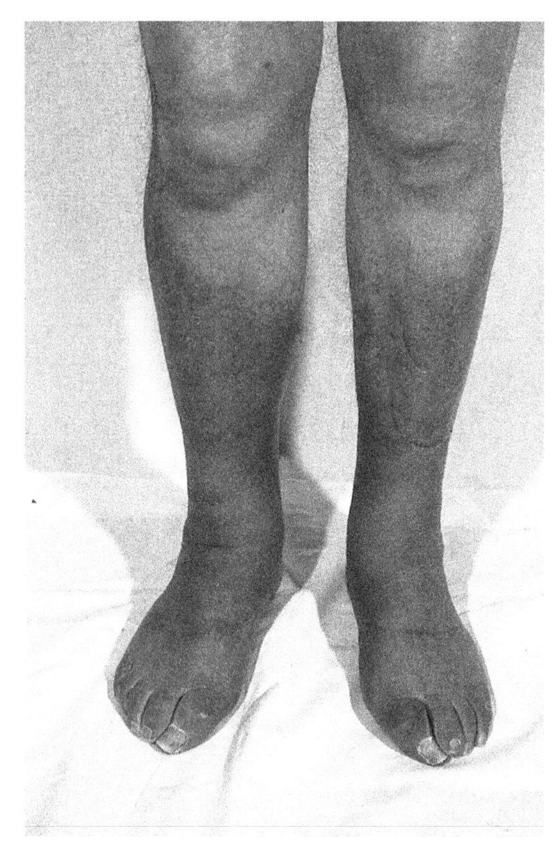

Fig. 3.3.1.1 Dermopathy of Graves' disease. Marked thickening of the skin is noted, usually over the pretibial area. Thickening will occasionally extend downwards over the ankle and the dorsal aspect of the foot, but almost never above the knee. (See also Plate 12)

patients with overt thyrotoxicosis have diminished proximal muscle strength. Chronic thyrotoxic myopathy affects the diaphragm and other respiratory muscles in up to one-half of severely affected thyrotoxic patients, causing loss of maximal respiratory muscle power.

Ventilatory control

Thyrotoxicosis may affect the central regulatory response to a blood gas perturbation, which can be assessed by evaluating the increase of ventilation while breathing either a hyperoxic hypercapnic or a hypoxic isocapnic gas mixture. Both these responses are increased in most thyrotoxic patients. These changes are independent of the β-adrenergic effects of catecholamines, and their mechanisms are not completely understood. Thyrotoxicosis, by increasing the ventilatory drive superimposed on underlying lung disease, may worsen dyspnoea and cause respiratory failure.

Exercise

Resting heart rate, cardiac output, respiratory rate, and minute ventilation are increased (9). The amount of oxygen required to perform any work load is increased. Both minute ventilation and cardiac output for a given level of oxygen consumption are elevated at all levels of oxygen consumption. Pulmonary artery pressures of thyrotoxic patients may rise more than usual with exercise, but this has not been evaluated carefully. Exercise normally decreases the mixed venous oxygen saturation and the dead space/tidal volume ratio; the converse occurs in thyrotoxicosis.

Effects of cardiac changes on the lungs

Cardiac changes of thyrotoxicosis may affect the lungs in two ways, either by pulmonary artery dilatation or by high-output cardiac failure (11). The pulmonary artery may appear dilated on plain chest radiographs. The findings of an accentuated pulmonary second heart sound and a right ventricular heave suggest pulmonary hypertension. Mild increases of resting pulmonary artery pressure are common with thyrotoxicosis, and the pressure frequently rises significantly during exercise. A physical sign of thyrotoxicosis is the Means–Lerman sign, a scratchy coarse systolic ejection rub or murmur that is heard best along the left sternal border at the base of the heart. This sign has been attributed to rubbing of the dilated aorta or pulmonary artery against other mediastinal structures or to turbulent pulmonary artery blood flow. The precise origin and the physiological significance of this sign are unknown.

Renal system

Most of the renal effects in thyrotoxic patients produce no symptoms except mild polyuria (12).

Renal haemodynamics and tubular function

Thyrotoxicosis is associated with an increase in renal plasma flow and glomerular filtration rate, probably because of the increase in cardiac output and decrease in peripheral resistance. Intrarenal vasodilatation also occurs. The mean 24-h urine creatinine excretion is significantly lower in thyrotoxic patients as compared to normal subjects. The latter finding has been attributed to loss of muscle mass and it occurs despite an increase in urea clearance (12). These changes are normalized when the eumetabolic state is restored. Renal tubular mass is increased, and the morphological changes that occur in renal tubules are accompanied by an increased renal tubular capacity for transport. An activation of the renin–angiotensin system contributes to cardiac hypertrophy in patients with thyrotoxicosis (13).

Water and electrolyte metabolism

Thyrotoxic patients rarely have abnormalities in water metabolism. Serum electrolytes are usually normal. Some thyrotoxic patients have polydipsia, with 24-h urine volumes up to 3–4 litres. Polyuria in these patients is due to increased thirst, as in primary polydipsia, and could be secondary to an increase of plasma angiotensin II concentration. Polydipsia and polyuria revert to normal after treatment of thyrotoxicosis.

Plasma atrial natriuretic hormone levels and plasma renin activity are increased in thyrotoxicosis; these changes seem to have no clinical consequences except for mild oedema. The total amount of exchangeable potassium is decreased, but the amount of exchangeable sodium tends to be increased. Despite these changes, serum sodium, potassium, and chloride concentrations are normal. The level of exchangeable magnesium concentration is often decreased, and urinary magnesium excretion is increased.

Renal tubular acidosis

Renal tubular acidosis occasionally occurs in association with thyrotoxicosis. In this condition there is a failure to achieve maximal urinary acidification. This rarely results from hypercalcaemia and hypercalciuria, which can cause nephrocalcinosis, tubular damage, and impairment of renal acidification. Renal tubular acidosis may

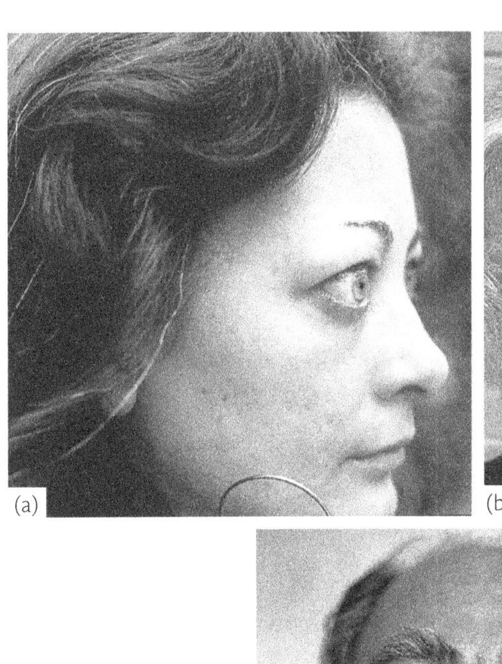

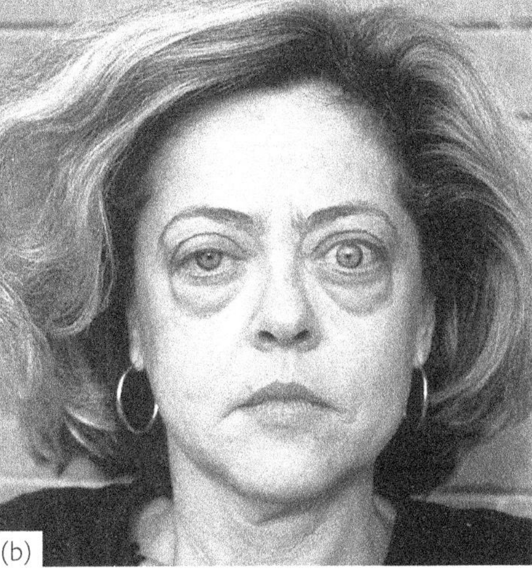

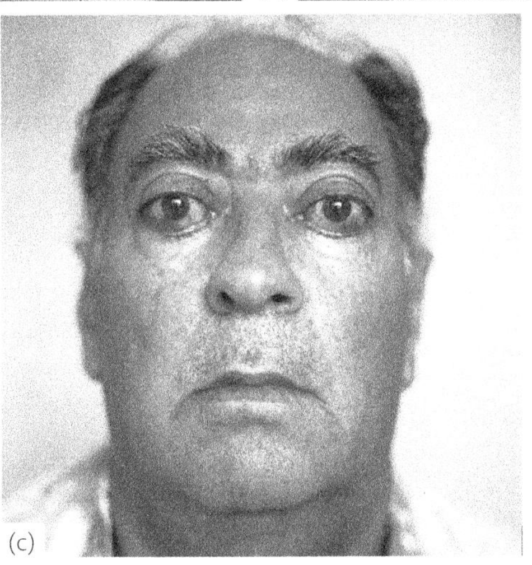

Fig. 3.3.1.2 Clinical presentation of Graves' ophthalmopathy.
(a) Retraction of both upper eyelids.
(b) Severe periorbital oedema and retraction of both upper eyelids.
(c) Marked conjunctival infection and chemosis, together with retraction of both lower eyelids. (See also Plate 13)

occur in association with thyrotoxicosis caused by Graves' disease, also in the absence of nephrocalcinosis, and may persist after restoration of the euthyroid state. This condition may have an autoimmune basis (14).

Oedema

Patients with thyrotoxicosis may develop pitting oedema involving the legs, hands, ankles, and sacrum. Oedema results from renal salt and water retention in response to the reduction in effective arterial volume, and this retention contributes to an increase in blood volume and venous pressure. The oedema that develops under these circumstances does not necessarily imply the presence of congestive heart failure. Severe thyrotoxic patients also may have protein-calorie malnutrition and hypoalbuminaemia leading to an expansion of plasma volume and oedema.

Gastrointestinal system

The classic gastrointestinal manifestations of thyrotoxicosis are rapid intestinal transit, increased frequency of semiformed stools, and weight loss from increased caloric requirement or malabsorption (15). These changes are not necessarily frequent. An increase in appetite, both at mealtimes and between meals, is a common symptom, but it is usually not seen in patients with mild disease. In severe disease, the increased intake of food is usually inadequate to meet the increased caloric requirements, and weight is lost at a variable rate. Anorexia, rather than hyperphagia, sometimes accompanies severe thyrotoxicosis. It occurs in about one-third of elderly patients and contributes to the picture of 'apathetic' thyrotoxicosis.

Gut motility

Frequent bowel movements are significantly more common in patients with thyrotoxicosis than in normal controls. Diarrhoea is rare (16). When constipation was present before the development of thyrotoxicosis, bowel function may become normal. More often stools are less well formed, and the frequency of bowel movements is increased. Anorexia, nausea, and vomiting are rare, but may occur with severe disease. Gastric emptying and intestinal motility are increased, and these changes appear to be responsible for slight malabsorption of fat. Steatorrhoea is common in severe thyrotoxicosis. The mechanism underlying the gastrointestinal hypermotility has not been elucidated, but hypermotility disappears when euthyroidism is restored. Coeliac disease and Graves' disease may coexist more frequently than can be accounted for by chance; both have an autoimmune origin.

Hepatic function

Hepatic function may be altered, particularly when the disease is severe (17); hypoproteinaemia and increased serum alkaline

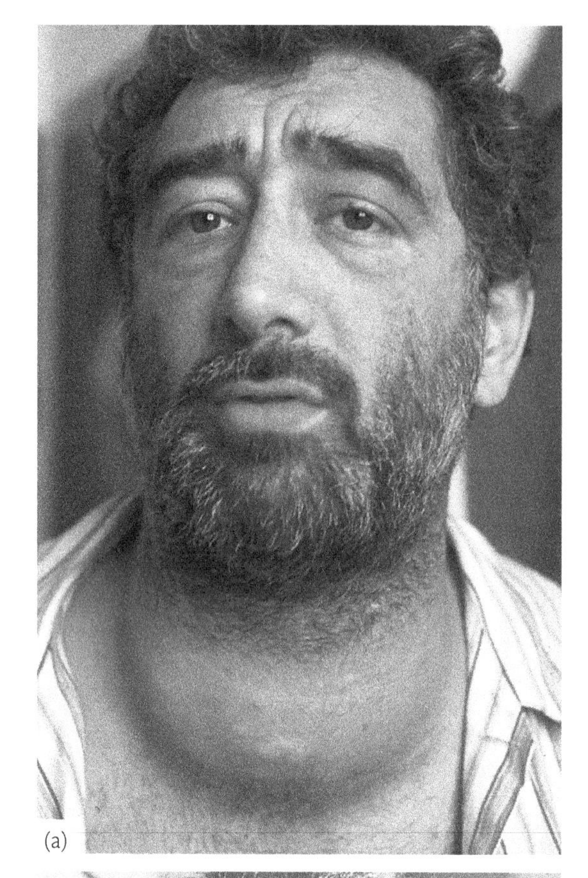
(a)

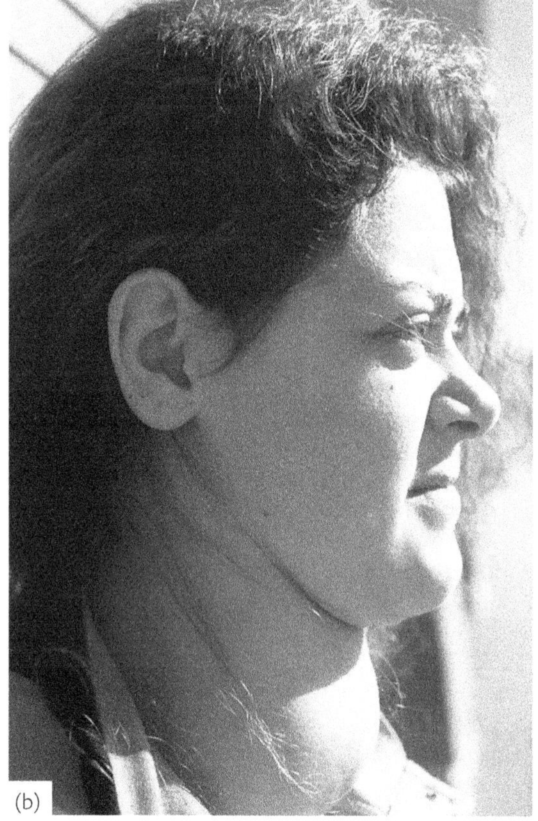
(b)

Fig. 3.3.1.3 (a) Massive thyroid enlargement related to diffuse toxic goitre. (b) An asymmetrical thyroid enlargement related to multinodular goitre. (See also Plate 14).

Box 3.3.1.1 Respiratory changes in thyrotoxicosis

- Dyspnoea
- Respiratory muscle weakness
- Decreased vital capacity
- Decreased pulmonary compliance
- Increased ventilation
- Increased oxygen uptake
- Pulmonary artery dilatation and hypertension
- Increased carbon dioxide production
- Increased ventilatory response to hypercapnia

phosphatase and transaminase levels may be present. In severe cases hepatomegaly and jaundice may be found. Graves' disease and autoimmune hepatitis coexist more often than can be expected by chance. Because of the alterations in hepatic function, the metabolism of various drugs may be affected.

Nervous system

Neuropsychiatric syndromes

Hyperactivity, emotional lability, distractibility, and anxiety observed in thyrotoxicosis may reflect changes in the nervous system, but the pathogenetic mechanisms remain obscure (18). The hyperactivity is characteristic: movements are quick, jerky, and exaggerated. Examination reveals a fine rhythmic tremor of the hands, tongue, or slightly closed eyelids. Emotional lability causes patients to lose their tempers easily and to have episodes of crying without apparent reason. Crying may be evoked by merely questioning the patient about the symptom. In rare cases mental disturbance may be severe. Anxiety is characterized by restlessness, shortness of attention span, and a compulsion to be moving around, despite a feeling of fatigue. Fatigue is due both to muscle weakness or to insomnia which is frequently present.

Neurological syndromes

Persistent fine tremor is the most prominent finding. It most commonly involves the hands, but may also affect the feet, chin, lips, and tongue. The tremor may sometimes mimic that of parkinsonism, and a pre-existing parkinsonian tremor can be accentuated. Chorea seldom appears as a manifestation of thyrotoxicosis (19). Chronic atrial fibrillation is associated with an increased risk of embolic stroke. The neurological manifestation of thyrotoxic crisis (20) may rarely include coma and status epilepticus (21). In patients with convulsive disorders, the frequency of seizures is increased.

The electroencephalogram of most thyrotoxic patients reveals increased fast-wave activity. The basal metabolic rate tends to correlate with the frequency of brain waves, but at the extremes of thyroid abnormality the correlation is frequently poor.

Muscle

Muscle weakness and fatigue are frequent (22). In most instances they are not accompanied by objective evidence of local disease of muscle except for the generalized wasting associated with weight loss. Weakness is often most prominent in the proximal muscles of the limbs, causing difficulties in climbing stairs or in maintaining the leg in an extended position. Occasionally, in severe untreated cases, muscle wasting occurs as a predominant symptom (thyrotoxic myopathy). In extreme forms, the patient may be unable to rise from a sitting or lying position and may be virtually unable to walk.

Muscle manifestations affect men with thyrotoxicosis more commonly than women and may overshadow other manifestations of the syndrome. In severe forms, the myopathy involves mainly distal muscles and extremities and the muscles of the trunk and face. The involvement of ocular muscles may mimic myasthenia gravis. Graves' disease occurs in about 3–5% of patients with myasthenia gravis, and about 1% of patients with Graves' disease develop myasthenia gravis (23). Myasthenia gravis associated with Graves' disease has a mild expression characterized by preferential involvement of the eye muscles (23). Another myopathy sometimes observed in association with thyrotoxicosis is hypokalaemic periodic paralysis (24). It is characterized by sporadic attacks (which may last from minutes to many hours), most commonly involving flaccidity and paralysis of either legs, arms, or trunk, even though any muscle can be involved. Episodes can occur spontaneously, after carbohydrate ingestion, or after exercise. Hypokalaemic periodic paralysis is most frequent in Asian populations (see Chapter 3.3.2).

Skeletal system: calcium and phosphorus metabolism

Thyrotoxicosis is associated with an increase of bone turnover and eventually bone loss, especially in postmenopausal women (25). Patients with a longstanding history of thyrotoxicosis may have overt osteoporosis and an increased risk of fractures (26).

Alterations in mineral metabolism

Bone turnover is increased, but the increase in bone resorption is relatively greater than that of bone formation, so the urinary excretion of calcium, phosphorus, and hydroxyproline is increased (26, 27). As a consequence of this acceleration in bone resorption, hypercalcaemia may occur in a significant proportion of patients with thyrotoxicosis. Total serum calcium may be slightly increased in as many as 27% of patients and ionized serum calcium level in 47%. However, patients are rarely symptomatic due to hypercalcaemia. The concentrations of alkaline phosphatase and osteocalcin are also frequently increased (28). These findings are reminiscent of those of primary hyperparathyroidism. Parathyroid hormone and 1,25-dihydroxyvitamin D_3 levels tend to be low as a result of the increased calcium released from bone. True primary hyperparathyroidism and thyrotoxicosis may sometimes coexist. The alterations in bone metabolism in thyrotoxicosis are reversed when the eumetabolic state is restored (28, 29).

Excretion of calcium in the faeces is also increased in thyrotoxic patients. The secretions of the gastrointestinal tract are altered in thyrotoxicosis and the transit time of calcium in the intestine is shortened.

Alteration in skeletal metabolism

Thyrotoxicosis is one of the well-known risk factors for osteoporosis (26). In thyrotoxicosis there is an increase in osteoid, the unmineralized bone matrix. The microscopic appearance of the bone is similar to that of osteomalacia. The direct effect of thyroid hormone on osteoblasts accounts for the increased circulating levels of alkaline phosphatase and osteocalcin frequently present in thyrotoxic patients. Despite the increased mineralization rate and osteoblastic activity, the increased bone formation cannot compensate for increments in bone resorption, and bone mass may be decreased. The pathological changes are variable and may include osteoporosis, osteomalacia, and osteitis fibrosa. Individuals with a history of thyrotoxicosis have a slightly increased risk of fracture, and sustain fractures at an earlier age than individuals who have never been thyrotoxic. As the thyrotoxicosis is treated, bone density may return to predisease levels in premenopausal patients (29, 30). Postmenopausal women, however, may have a permanent reduction in bone density that may require treatment with agents that increase bone mass.

The skeletal effects of thyroid hormone replacement are unclear. Recently, some reports suggested that patients receiving chronic L-thyroxine treatment, particularly those treated with doses that suppress thyroid-stimulating hormone (TSH) secretion (suppressive doses), may have a reduced bone mass (31). Recently, other studies (32, 33) suggested that L-thyroxine suppressive therapy, if carried out carefully and monitored, using the smallest dose necessary to suppress TSH secretion, has no significant effect on bone metabolism or bone mass, at least in premenopausal women and in men, whereas in postmenopausal women some degree of bone loss can be observed.

Arthropathies

Thyroid acropachy occurs in approximately 1% of patients with Graves' disease, and is always associated with exophthalmos and pretibial myxoedema (34). It frequently develops after treatment of thyrotoxicosis. This condition affects the peripheral skeleton and consist of clubbing, periostitis, and swelling.

Haematopoietic system

In most patients with thyrotoxicosis, red blood cells are usually normal, but the red blood cell mass is increased. The increase in erythropoiesis appears to be due both to a direct effect of thyroid hormones on the erythroid marrow and to an increased production of erythropoietin. A parallel increase in plasma volume also occurs, and therefore the haematocrit value is normal.

The most common red blood cell morphological abnormality is microcytosis, which is found in at least 37% of patients. The cause of this change is unclear. Iron deficiency is occasionally reported in thyrotoxic states. Microcytosis usually resolves with the restoration of euthyroidism. Some patients with severe thyrotoxicosis may develop a normocytic anaemia. Defective iron use has been shown to occur in thyrotoxic patients and may be responsible for the development of anaemia.

Approximately 3% of patients with Graves' disease have pernicious anaemia, and a further 3% have antibodies to intrinsic factor but normal absorption of vitamin B_{12}. Autoantibodies against gastric parietal cells are present in about one-third of the patients with Graves' disease, and the requirements for vitamin B_{12} and folic acid appear to be increased.

The total white blood cell count is often low because of a decrease in the number of neutrophils. The absolute lymphocyte count is normal or increased, leading to a relative lymphocytosis. The numbers of monocytes and eosinophils may also be increased. A generalized lymphadenopathy may be present, and the spleen, although not often palpable on physical examination, has been shown to be enlarged in 10% of patients with thyrotoxicosis due to Graves' disease.

Blood platelets and the intrinsic clotting mechanism are normal. However, the concentration of factor VIII is often increased and returns to normal when thyrotoxicosis is treated. Furthermore, there is an enhanced sensitivity to coumarin anticoagulants because of an accelerated clearance of vitamin K-dependent clotting factors. A hypercoagulable state has been described in hyperthyroid patients (35).

Cardiovascular system

The cardiovascular manifestations of thyrotoxicosis constitute some of the most profound and characteristic symptoms and signs of the disorder (Box 3.3.1.2) (36, 37). Tissue blood flow is increased in response to accelerated metabolism and increased oxygen consumption. Haemodynamic changes in thyrotoxic patients are characterized by an elevated cardiac output and a decreased peripheral vascular resistance. The mechanism responsible for the reduced vascular resistance is unclear. Thyroid hormone itself may be involved directly through its action on the smooth muscle of blood vessels (38). Moreover, the finding in thyrotoxic patients of elevated levels of plasma adrenomedullin and proadrenomedullin-N-terminal 20-peptide, which have a potent vasodilatory activity, raises the possibility that these substances might also be involved in the decrease of vascular resistance in these patients (39).

Clinically, nearly all patients have tachycardia and a bounding pulse; the widened pulse pressure reflects both the increase in cardiac output and the decrease in peripheral vascular resistance. The common complaint of palpitations usually indicates a resting tachycardia. The heart rate is also elevated during sleep; this helps to distinguish tachycardia of thyrotoxic origin from that of psychogenic origin. Other common cardiovascular symptoms include exercise intolerance and dyspnoea on exertion. The latter is usually present with sustained activity, but may also arise with activity as limited as climbing a flight of stairs. Because of the diffuse and forceful nature of the apex beat, the heart may be enlarged, but echocardiography is usually normal. In elderly thyrotoxic patients the cardiovascular manifestations of thyrotoxicosis may be limited to resting tachycardia; (40) other classic thyrotoxic symptoms may be absent, possibly due to the relative paucity of adrenergic activity (41).

Box 3.3.1.2 Cardiovascular symptoms and signs of thyrotoxicosis

- Palpitations
- Paroxysmal tachycardia
- Orthopnoea
- Exercise intolerance
- Hyperdynamic precordium
- Third heart sound
- Atrial fibrillation
- Widened pulse pressure
- Cardiac flow murmurs

Thyrotoxic patients may have chest pain similar in almost all respects to angina pectoris, probably caused by either relative myocardial ischaemia or coronary artery spasm. In elderly patients, however, the increased myocardial oxygen demand due to thyrotoxicosis may unmask coronary artery disease. The plasma level of homocysteine, an independent risk factor for cardiovascular disease, in thyrotoxic patients did not differ significantly from that of controls (42). On the contrary, hyperhomocysteinaemia has been found in hypothyroid patients and, in association with lipid abnormalities, may contribute to the increased risk of coronary artery disease (43).

Physical examination

In patients with thyrotoxicosis, tachycardia is the most common of all abnormal findings. The heart rate is increased, with bounding pulses in the larger arteries due to widened pulse pressure. Systolic blood pressure is elevated and diastolic blood pressure is decreased (44); the mean blood pressure is usually normal. An exaggerated increase in systolic blood pressure may be present in older patients due to the loss of elasticity of the larger arteries (44); the mean blood pressure in these patients may also be high. The first heart sound may be sharp and audible. Auscultation may reveal a systolic ejection murmur and a gallop rhythm caused by rapid flow of blood through the aortic outflow tract. Systolic murmurs may arise from valve prolapse, left ventricular dilatation, or dysfunction of the mitral valve apparatus. A systolic 'scratch' is heard in the pulmonary area corresponding to contact between the pleural and pericardial surfaces during cardiac contraction. Mild oedema not uncommonly occurs in the absence of heart failure. Heart failure rarely occurs in thyrotoxic patients, unless an underlying cardiac disease is also present (41).

Cardiac rhythm disturbances

Sinus tachycardia is present on routine electrocardiographic tracings in the majority of thyrotoxic patients (37). Cardiac arrhythmias are almost invariably supraventricular. Approximately 10% of patients with thyrotoxicosis have atrial fibrillation, and a similar percentage of patients with otherwise unexplained atrial fibrillation are thyrotoxic (41). This manifestation may be the presenting symptom of thyrotoxicosis, particularly in older people. Most patients with atrial fibrillation have arrhythmia for less than 4–8 weeks before the diagnosis of thyrotoxicosis, and a spontaneous reversion often occurs. In elderly patients with subclinical thyrotoxicosis the risk of developing persistent atrial fibrillation is approximately 3 times that of normal subjects (41, 45). Paroxysmal supraventricular tachycardia may be demonstrable or may be suggested by the history. Ventricular premature contractions are rare. Angina pectoris and myocardial infarction may rarely occur in the absence of coronary artery disease. Nonspecific electrocardiographic changes may occur in thyrotoxicosis. A shortening of the P–R interval is common, secondary to the increased rate of conduction through the atrioventricular node.

Heart failure

Thyrotoxicosis alone may determine heart failure in elderly and, much less often, in young patients (44). In large clinical studies of thyrotoxic patients with heart failure, patients were generally old and, therefore, at risk of underlying heart disease, and had chronic thyrotoxicosis. Elderly patients with rhythm disturbances, including atrial fibrillation, have the greatest risk of heart failure (40, 46); in the absence of atrial fibrillation, heart failure is rare. In young patients, or in the absence of underlying heart disease, the heart failure is thought to be 'high output'. High-output heart failure may not be a true heart failure but a circulatory congestion caused by fluid retention. In thyrotoxicosis, cardiac output is potentially near to maximal at rest and cannot increase in response to exercise, stress, surgery, or pregnancy (36, 47). As a consequence, atrial filling pressures rise, leading to pulmonary and peripheral oedema. This situation may be worse if atrial fibrillation is present. Left ventricular function is impaired because the persistent tachyarrhythmia alters this function. Sustained tachycardia causes abnormal ventricular systolic and diastolic function, which resolves when arrhythmia is treated. β-adrenergic receptor blockade-mediated slowing of the heart rate can rapidly reverse even severe degrees of left ventricular dysfunction in thyrotoxic patients.

Endocrine system

Pituitary

Thyrotoxicosis affects the secretion of most pituitary hormones, in particular the secretion of growth hormone, prolactin, adrenocorticotropin (ACTH), follicle-stimulating hormone, and luteinizing hormone. Children with thyrotoxicosis grow more rapidly than normal children (48). The height and bone ages are accelerated, but their relationship remains normal. Growth acceleration in thyrotoxicosis suggests that growth hormone secretion might be greater than normal. Serum growth hormone concentrations, however, are lower in thyrotoxic patients than normal subjects. This decrease is probably due to the increased metabolic clearance rate. Serum insulin-like growth factor-1 concentration is higher in thyrotoxic patients and returns to normal values after restoration of the euthyroid state. Basal secretion of prolactin and its response to thyrotropin-releasing hormone may also be decreased. No physiological or clinical consequences of these abnormalities are known.

Adrenal cortex

Thyrotoxicosis has several effects on adrenocortical function and adrenocortical hormone metabolism, with an increased clearance of the latter (49). The half-life of cortisol is shortened, but both the number of bursts of ACTH and the resulting burst of cortisol secretion are increased and maintain serum cortisol levels (50). A subtle impairment of adrenocortical reserve has been reported in thyrotoxicosis (50). The plasma concentration of corticosteroid-binding globulin is normal. The urinary excretion of the free cortisol and 17-hydroxycorticosteroids is normal or slightly increased, whereas the urinary excretion of 17-ketosteroids may be reduced (51). The turnover rate of aldosterone is increased, but its plasma concentration is normal. Plasma renin activity is increased, and sensitivity to angiotensin II is reduced.

Catecholamines and the sympathoadrenal system

β-adrenergic receptor blockade ameliorates most of the cardiovascular manifestations of thyrotoxicosis. This suggests that catecholamines play a role in their genesis, but the secretion rate and plasma levels of adrenaline and noradrenaline are normal in thyrotoxic patients (52). Indeed, the apparent sympathetic hyperactivity appears to be the consequence of a direct effect of thyroid hormones on peripheral tissues. Some effects induced by thyroid hormones are also reminiscent of those of the carcinoid syndrome, but plasma serotonin levels, urinary 5-hydroxyindoleacetic acid excretion, and platelet monoamine oxidase activity are normal. Thyrotoxicosis in early life may cause delayed sexual maturation, although physical development is normal and skeletal growth may be accelerated.

Female reproductive system

Thyrotoxicosis, after puberty, influences the reproductive function (53), especially in women. An increase in libido occurs in both genders. The intermenstrual interval may be prolonged or shortened, and menstrual flow initially diminishes and ultimately ceases. Fertility may be reduced. In some women, menstrual cycles are predominantly anovulatory with oligomenorrhoea, but in most, ovulation occurs. It is unclear whether these changes are due to a direct action of thyroid hormones on the ovary and uterus, or on the pituitary and hypothalamus, or both. The effects of thyroid hormones on fertility are less well established, although the disturbances in menstrual cycles will obviously disturb fertility. With treatment, menstrual cycles return to their regular pattern. Thyrotoxicosis in prepubertal girls may result in slightly delayed menarche. In premenopausal women with thyrotoxicosis, basal plasma concentrations of luteinizing hormone and follicle-stimulating hormone are normal but may display an enhanced responsiveness to luteinizing hormone-releasing hormone (54).

Male reproductive system

An increase in libido has also been reported in men (54), An increase in sex hormone-binding globulin is a prominent feature of thyrotoxicosis and is responsible for many of the alterations in steroid metabolism (55). Because of the increase in sex hormone-binding globulin, the metabolic clearance rates of testosterone and, to some extent, of oestradiol are decreased. Testosterone levels are elevated because of the increased concentration of sex hormone-binding globulin. Free testosterone levels tend to be normal. The metabolic clearance rate of oestradiol is normal, suggesting that tissue metabolism of the hormone is increased. Conversion rates of androstenedione to testosterone, oestrone, and oestradiol, and of testosterone to dihydrotestosterone are increased. Extragonadal conversion of androgens to oestrogens is increased and this could be the mechanism responsible for gynaecomastia observed in a consistent minority of thyrotoxic men. Abnormalities in sperm motility which are reversible after restoration of euthyroidism have been described in male hyperthyroid patients (56).

Energy metabolism: protein, carbohydrate, and lipid metabolism

One of the most prominent symptoms in the hyperthyroid patient is heat intolerance. The symptom reflects an increase in the basal metabolism of many substrates (57). The increase in metabolic activity results in increased consumption of ATP and oxygen. The consequent thermogenesis is responsible for heat intolerance. Despite the increased food intake, a state of chronic caloric inadequacy often ensues, depending on the degree of increased metabolism, and becomes more pronounced with age. In addition to losing fat stores, there is often a loss of muscle mass as well, making weakness a common complaint. Both synthesis and degradation of proteins are increased, the latter to a greater extent than the former, so that there is a net decrease in tissue protein content.

Both glucose absorption and glucose production are increased (58). The oral glucose tolerance test is often abnormal. The most common abnormality is a faster rise in plasma glucose after glucose ingestion, but some patients have a delayed peak plasma glucose or a peak value that is higher than in normal subjects (59). These abnormalities may reflect changes in glucose absorption rather than metabolism (60), since many patients who have abnormal oral glucose tolerance have normal responses to intravenous glucose administration. Pre-existing diabetes mellitus is aggravated by thyrotoxicosis, one cause being increased degradation of insulin.

Both synthesis and clearance of cholesterol and triglycerides are increased, but the latter effect predominates, so that serum levels are generally low (60). Plasma phospholipid and low-density lipoprotein (LDL) cholesterol concentrations fall, while high-density lipoprotein (HDL) cholesterol levels increase. Malnutrition and weight loss, commonly present in thyrotoxic patients, may account for part of the cholesterol-lowering action of thyroid hormones. In addition, hypermetabolism may also lower serum lipid levels. Finally, thyroid hormones may influence cholesterol metabolism by increasing its conversion to bile acid and its clearance through the membrane surface LDL receptors (61). In this regard, experimental evidence using HepG2 cells indicates that triiodothyronine increases LDL receptor promoter activity and surface LDL receptor protein (61).

Although fatty acid synthesis is increased in both adipose tissue and liver, degradation of most lipids appears to be stimulated out of proportion to synthesis; body lipid deposits consequently become depleted and plasma concentrations of various lipid components fall. Rates of fatty acid oxidation and free fatty acid release from adipose tissue are increased in both human and experimental thyrotoxicosis, and the enhanced rate of cholesterol synthesis is counterbalanced by a concomitant increase in the rate of cholesterol degradation and excretion (62).

Several studies have investigated the relationship between leptin level and thyroid status. With the exception of two reports suggesting a relative hypoleptinaemia, most clinical studies have found no effect of thyrotoxicosis on leptin levels (63).

Vitamin metabolism in thyrotoxicosis

Thyrotoxicosis can influence the metabolism of vitamin A in different ways. Vitamin A concentrations tend to be low and a minor impairment of dark adaptation has been detected in some patients. Alterations in calcium metabolism and vitamin D are also present in thyrotoxicosis. Serum parathyroid hormone levels are low and the conversion of 25-hydroxyvitamin D to 1,25-hydroxyvitamin D is diminished, resulting in lowered serum concentrations of the latter (64). Calcium balance is negative as a result of decreased intestinal absorption and increased urinary calcium loss. The serum concentration of vitamin E tends to be reduced in thyrotoxicosis. This reduction may be secondary to generalized disturbances in lipid metabolism, because serum concentrations of HDL and LDL, in which vitamin E is incorporated, are decreased (65).

Differential diagnosis of thyrotoxicosis

Several features of thyrotoxicosis are common to other disorders and may confuse the diagnosis. The condition that most frequently simulates thyrotoxicosis is an anxiety state characterized by nervous irritability, fatigue, and insomnia. Fatigue is pronounced and differs from that in thyrotoxicosis because it is not accompanied by a desire to be active. Tachycardia is common during examination but, in contrast to thyrotoxicosis, the sleeping pulse rate is normal. Hyperreflexia is present in both disorders.

Phaeochromocytoma may closely resemble thyrotoxicosis. Tachycardia and hypermetabolism are common to both conditions. The patient may have weight loss despite a good appetite and may have hyperglycaemia with glycosuria. In the patient with phaeochromocytoma, goitre is absent and serum thyroid hormones are normal.

Myeloproliferative disorders may mimic thyrotoxicosis because patients with these diseases have increased sweating, weight loss, and tachycardia, especially if anaemia is present. Goitre is absent and the laboratory indices are normal. In diabetes mellitus, weight loss despite a good appetite, muscle wasting, and occasionally diarrhoea may suggest thyrotoxicosis.

References

1. Chiovato L, Mariotti S, Pinchera A. Thyroid disease in the elderly. *Baillieres Clin Endocrinol Metab*, 1997; **11**: 251–70.
2. Rosen T, Kleman WR. Cutaneous manifestations of thyroid disease. *J Am Acad Dermatol*, 1992; **26**: 885–7.
3. Ortonne J-P, Mosher DB, Fitzpatrick TB. *Vitiligo and Other Hypomelanoses of Hair and Skin*. New York: Plenum, 1983: 182.
4. Farourechi V, Pajouhi M, Fransway A. Dermopathy of Graves' disease (pretibial myxedema): review of 150 cases. *Medicine (Baltimore)*, 1994; **73**: 1–7.
5. Dickinson AJ, Perros P. Controversies in the clinical evaluation of active thyroid-associated orbitopathy: use of detailed protocol with comparative photographs for objective assessment. *Clin Endocrinol*, 2001; **55**: 283–303.
6. European Group on Graves' Orbitopathy (EUGOGO), Wiersinga WM, Perros P, Kahaly GJ, Mourits MP, Baldeschi L, *et al.* Clinical assessment of patients with Graves' orbitopathy: the European Group on Graves' Orbitopathy recommendations to generalists, specialists and clinical researchers. *Eur J Endocrinol*, 2006; **55**: 387–9.
7. Vitti P, Rago T, Mazzeo S, Brogioni S, Lampis M, De Liperi A, *et al.* Thyroid blood flow evaluation by color-flow Doppler sonography distinguishes Graves' disease from Hashimoto's thyroiditis. *J Endocrinol Invest*, 1995; **18**: 857–61.
8. Kendric AH, O'Reilly JR, Laszlo G. Lung function and exercise performance in hyperthyroidism before and after treatment. *QJM*, 1988; **68**: 615–18.
9. Small D, Gibbons W, Levy RD, de Lucas P, Gregory W, Cosio MG. Exertional dyspnea and ventilation in hyperthyroidism. *Chest*, 1992; **101**: 1268–73.
10. Siafakas NM, Alexopoulou C, Bouros D. Respiratory muscle function in endocrine disease. *Monaldi Arch Chest Dis*, 1999; **54**: 154–9.
11. Kahaly GJ, Kampann C, Mohr-Kahaly S. Cardiovascular hemodynamics and exercise tolerance in thyroid diseases. *Thyroid*, 2002; **12**: 473–781.
12. Bradley SE, Stephan F, Coehlo JB, Reville P. The thyroid and the kidney. *Kidney Int*, 1974; **6**: 346–8.
13. Basset A, Blanc J, Messas E, Hagège A, Elgozi JL. Renin-angiotensin system contribution to cardiac hypertrophy in experimental hyperthyroidism: en echocardiographic study. *J Cardiovasc Pharmacol*, 2001; **37**: 163–72.
14. Konishi K, Hayashi M, Saruta T. Renal tubular acidosis with autoantibody directed to renal collecting-duct cells. *N Engl J Med*, 1994; **331**: 1593–6.

15. Baker JT, Harvey RF. Bowel habits in thyrotoxicosis and hyperthyroidism. *BMJ*, 1971; **1**: 322–4.
16. Culp KS, Piiak VK. Thyrotoxicosis presenting with secretory diarrhea. *Ann Int Med*, 1986; **105**: 216–19.
17. Huang MJ, Li KL, Wei JS, Wu SS, Fan KD, Liaw YF. Sequential liver and bone biochemical changes in hyperthyroidism: prospective controlled follow-up study. *Am J Gastroenterol*, 1994; **89**: 1071–6.
18. Jandresic DP. Psychiatric aspects of hyperthyroidism. *J Psychosom Res*, 1990; **34**: 603–15.
19. Javaid A, Hilton DD. Persistent chorea as a manifestation of thyrotoxicosis. *Postgrad Med J*, 1988; **64**: 789–92.
20. Tonner DR, Schlecheter JA. Neurologic complications of thyroid and parathyroid disease. *Med Clin North Am*, 1993; **77**: 251–63.
21. Safe AF, Griffiths KD, Maxwell RT. Thyrotoxic crisis presenting as status epilepticus. *Postgrad Med*, 1990; **66**: 150–3.
22. Cakir M, Samanchi N, Balci N, Balci MK. Musculoskeletal manifestations in patients with thyroid disease. *Clin Endocrinol (Oxf)*, 2003; **59**: 162–7.
23. Marinó M, Ricciardi R, Pinchera A, Barbesino G, Manetti L, Chiovato L, *et al.* Mild clinical expression of myasthenia gravis associated with autoimmune thyroid diseases. *J Clin Endocrinol Metab*, 1997; **82**: 438–43.
24. Akhter J, Weide LG. Thyrotoxic periodic paralysis, a reversible cause of paralysis to remember. *S D J Med*, 1997; **50**: 357–8.
25. Mundy GR, Shapiro JL, Bandelin JG, Canalis EM, Raisz LG. Direct stimulation of bone resorption by thyroid hormones. *J Clin Invest*, 1976; **58**: 529–32.
26. Cummings SR, Nevitt MC, Browner WS, Stone K, Fox KM, Ensrud KE, *et al.* Risk factors for hip fractures in white women. Study of Osteoporotic fractures research group. *N Engl J Med*, 1995; **332**: 767–73.
27. Eriksen EF, Mosekilde L, Melsen F. Trabecular bone remodeling and bone balance in hyperthyroidism. *Bone*, 1985; **6**: 421–5.
28. Garnero P, Vassy V, Bertholin A, Riou JP, Delmas PD. Markers of bone turnover in hyperthyroidism and the effects of treatment. *J Clin Endocrinol Metab*, 1994; **78**: 955–9.
29. Diamond T, Vine J, Smart R, Butler P. Thyrotoxic bone disease in women: a potentially reversible disorder. *Ann Intern Med*, 1994; **120**: 8–12.
30. Rosen C, Adler RA. Longitudinal changes in lumbar bone density among thyrotoxic patients after attainment of euthyroidism. *J Clin Endocrinol Metab*, 1992; **75**: 1531–4.
31. Taeelman P, Kaufman JM, Janssens X, Vandecauter H, Vermeulen A. Reduced forearm bone mineral content and biochemical evidence of increased bone turnover in women with euthyroid goiter treated with thyroid hormone. *Clin Endocrinol*, 1990; **33**: 107–17.
32. Marcocci C, Golia F, Bruno-Bossio G, Vignali E, Pinchera A. Carefully monitored levothyroxine suppressive therapy is not associated with bone loss in premenopausal women. *J Clin Endocrinol Metab*, 1994; **78**: 818–23.
33. Marcocci C, Golia F, Vignali E, Pinchera A. Skeletal integrity in men chronically treated with suppressive doses of L-thyroxine. *J Bone Miner Res*, 1997; **12**: 72–7.
34. Fatourechi V, Ahmed D.F, Swartz KM. Thyroid acropachy: report of 40 patients treated at a single institution in a 26-year period. *J Clin Endocrinol Metab*, 2002; **87**: 5435–41.
35. Franchini M. Hemostatic changes in thyroid diseases: haemostasis and thrombosis. *Hematology*, 2006; **11**: 203–8.
36. Klein I, Ojamaa K. Thyrotoxicosis and the heart. *Endocrinol Metab Clin North Am*, 1998; **27**: 57–62.
37. Fadel BM, Ellahham S, Ringel MD, Lindsay J Jr, Wartofsky L, Burman KD. Hyperthyroid heart disease. *Clin Cardiol*, 2000; **23**: 402–8.
38. Ojamaa K, Balkman C, Klein IL. Acute effects of triiodothyronine on arterial smooth muscle cells. *Ann Thorac Surg*, 1993; **56**: S61–7.
39. Tuniyama M, Kitamura K, Ban Y, Sugita E, Ito K, Katagiri T. Elevation of circulating proadrenomedullin-N terminal 20-peptide in thyrotoxicosis. *Clin Endocrinol*, 1997; **46**: 271–4.
40. Kahaly GJ, Nieswandt J, Mohr-Kahays S. Cardiac risk of hyperthyroidism in the elderly. *Thyroid*, 1998; **8**: 1165–9.
41. Dahl P, Dansi S, Klein I. Thyrotoxic cardiac disease. *Curr Heart Fail Rep*, 2008; **5**: 170–6.
42. Nedrebø BG, Ericsson UB, Nygård O, Refsum H, Ueland PM, Aakvaag A, *et al.* Plasma total homocysteine levels in hyperthyroid and hypothyroid patients. *Metabolism*, 1998; **47**: 89–93.
43. Catargi B, Parrot-Roulard F, Cochet C, Ducassou D, Roger P, Tabarin A. Homocysteine, hypothyroidism, and effect of thyroid hormone replacement. *Thyroid*, 1999; **9**: 1163–6.
44. Dansi S, Klein I. Thyroid hormone and blood pressure regulation. *Curr Hypertens Rep*, 2003; **5**: 513–20.
45. von Olshausen KV, Bischoff S, Kahaly G, Mohr-Kahaly S, Erbel R, Beyer J, *et al.* Cardiac arrhythmias and heart rate in hyperthyroidism. *Am J Cardiol*, 1989; **63**: 290–4.
46. Sawin CT, Geller A, Wolf PA, Belanger AJ, Baker E, Bacharach P, *et al.* Low serum thyrotropin levels as a risk factor for atrial fibrillation in older persons. *N Engl J Med*, 1994; **33**: 1249–52.
47. Biondi B, Palmieri EA, Lombardi G, Fazio S. Effects of thyroid hormone on cardiac function: the relative importance of heart rate, loading conditions, and myocardial contractility in the regulation of cardiac performance in human hyperthyroidism. *J Clin Endocrinol Metabol*, 2002; **87**: 986–74.
48. Wong GW, Lai J, Cheng PS. Growth in childhood thyrotoxicosis. *Eur J Pediatr*, 1999; **158**: 776–9.
49. Gallagher TF, Hellman L, Finkelstein J, Yoshida K, Weitzman ED, Roffwarg HD, *et al.* Hyperthyroidism and cortisol secretion in man. *J Clin Endocrinol Metab*, 1972; **34**: 919–22.
50. Tsotsoulis A, Johnson EO, Kalogera CH, Seferiadis K, Tsolas O. The effect of thyrotoxicosis on adrenocortical reserve. *Eur J Endocrinol*, 2000; **142**: 231–5.
51. Gordon GG, Southren AL. Thyroid hormone effects on steroid hormone metabolism. *Bull N Y Acad Med*, 1977; **53**: 241–4.
52. Coulombe P, Dussault JH, Walker P. Catecholamine metabolism in thyroid disease. II. Norepinephrine secretion rate in hyperthyroidism and hypothyroidism. *J Clin Endocrinol Metab*, 1977; **44**: 1185–9.
53. Krassas GE. Thyroid disease and female reproduction. *Fertil Steril*, 2000; **74**: 1063–70.
54. Ridgway EC, Maloof F, Longcope C. Androgen and oestrogen dynamics in hyperthyroidism. *J Clin Endocrinol Metab*, 1990; **20**: 250–4.
55. Rosner W. The functions of corticosteroid-binding globulin and sex hormone-binding globulin: recent advances. *Endocr Rev*, 1990; **11**: 80–4.
56. Krassas GR, Pontikides N, Deligianni V, Miras K. A prospective controlled study of the impact of hyperthyroidism on reproductive function in males. *J Clin Endocrinol Metab*, 2002; **87**: 3667–71.
57. Silva JE. The thermogenic effect of thyroid hormone and its clinical implications. *Ann Intern Med*, 2003; **139**: 205–13.
58. Møller N, Nielsen S, Nyholm B, P rksen N, Alberti KG, Weeke J. Glucose turnover, fuel oxidation and forearm substrate exchange in patients with thyrotoxicosis before and after medical treatment. *Clin Endocrinol*, 1996; **44**: 453–9.
59. Woeber KA, Arky R, Braverman LE. Reversal by guanethidine of abnormal oral glucose tolerance in thyrotoxicosis. *J Clin Endocrinol Metab*, 1998; **80**: 102–5.
60. Bech K, Damsbo P, Eldrup E, Beck-Nielsen H, R der ME, Hartling SG, *et al.* Beta-cell function and glucose and lipid oxidation in Graves' disease. *Clin Endocrinol*, 1996; **44**: 59–66.
61. Bakker O, Hudig F, Meijessen S, Wiersinga WM. Effects of triiodothyronine and amiodarone on the promoter of the human LDL receptor gene. *Biochem Biophys Res Commun*, 1998; **249**: 517–21.

62. Beylot M, Martin C, Laville M, Riou JP, Cohen R, Mornex R. Lipolytic and ketogenic fluxes in human hyperthyroidism. *J Clin Endocrinol Metab*, 1991; **73**: 242–6.
63. Korbonits M. Leptin and the thyroid: a puzzle with missing pieces. *Clin Endocrinol*, 1998; **49**: 569–72.
64. Bouillon R, Muls E, DeMoor P. Influence of thyroid function on the serum concentrations of 1,25-dihydroxyvitamin D. *J Clin Endocrinol Metab*, 1980; **51**: 793–5.
65. Krishnamurthy S, Prasanna D. Serum vitamin E and lipid peroxides in malnutrition, hyper-and hypothyroidism. *Acta Vitaminol Enzymol*, 1984; **6**: 17–20.

3.3.2 Thyrotoxic periodic paralysis

Annie W.C. Kung

Epidemiology

The association of thyrotoxicosis and periodic paralysis was first described in 1902 in a white patient. However, it soon became evident that thyrotoxic periodic paralysis (TPP) affects mainly Asian populations, in particular Chinese and Japanese, although isolated cases have also been reported in other ethnic groups such as white, Hispanic, African-American, and American Indian populations. The incidence of TPP in non-Asian thyrotoxic patients is around 0.1%, whereas in Chinese and Japanese thyrotoxic patients, TPP affects 1.8% and 1.9%, respectively (1–3). Despite a higher incidence of thyrotoxicosis in women, TPP affects mainly men, with a male to female ratio ranging from 17:1 to 70:1, according to different series. In the Chinese population, TPP affects 13% of male and 0.17% of female thyrotoxic patients. In the Japanese population, TPP was reported to occur in 8.2% of male and 0.4% of female thyrotoxic patients in the 1970s, but in 1991 the reported incidence had decreased to 4.3% and 0.04%, respectively (4).

Clinical features

TPP patients are usually between 20 and 40 years of age, similar to the age distribution for thyrotoxicosis. The paralytic attacks are characterized by transient recurrent episodes of muscle weakness. Attacks involve proximal more than the distal muscles, with an initial involvement of the lower limbs and subsequently the truncal muscles, and finally all four limbs. The degree of weakness varies from mild weakness to total flaccid paralysis and hyporeflexia. Some patients may experience prodromal symptoms of aches, cramps, or stiffness in the affected muscles. Weakness usually affects skeletal muscles only. However, total paralysis of respiratory, bulbar, and ocular muscles has been reported in severe cases (5–7). Recovery is usually complete, but the duration of paralysis can vary from a few hours in a mild attack to 36–72 h in a severe attack. Electromyographic studies have confirmed the myopathic changes with intact peripheral nerve function. The presentation of TPP may be confused with Guillain–Barré syndrome, acute spinal cord compression, myelitis, and hysteria. The attacks of weakness are similar to those of familial hypokalaemic periodic paralysis (FHPP) except for the presence of hyperthyroidism. While FHPP is an autosomal dominant condition affecting mainly white people, TPP is a sporadic disease found mainly in Asian men, and familial cases of TPP are extremely rare.

High carbohydrate loads and strenuous exercise are well-recognized precipitating factors for TPP (8). The paralytic attacks do not occur during exercise but occur during the resting period that follows strenuous exercise, and the attacks may be aborted by continuation of exercise. In subtropical cities such as Hong Kong, attacks are most common during the summer season. This seasonal variation is probably associated with an increased intake of sugary drinks as well as outdoor activities and exercise in summer. In tropical cities, such as Singapore, seasonal variation is not seen. Attacks usually occur in the middle of the night or early morning, which coincides with a period of rest following a heavy meal or exercise. Paralysis can be induced in these patients with high carbohydrate loads with or without insulin infusion, strenuous exercise, or even thyroxine therapy. However, attacks cannot be induced once the patient has become euthyroid.

Hypokalaemia is the hallmark of TPP. Plasma potassium concentrations have been reported to be as low as 1.1 mmol/l. Some patients may have a near to normal plasma potassium concentration if they are admitted during the recovery phase of the attack. Mortality due to cardiac arrhythmia associated with the hypokalaemia has been reported. The complication of rhabdomyolysis may occur in a severe attack. Potassium concentration returns to normal when the patient recovers spontaneously from the weakness. The degree of hypokalaemia and the severity of weakness have no correlation with the severity of hyperthyroidism and the serum thyroid hormone concentration. Indeed, many patients have relatively few symptoms of hyperthyroidism and TPP may be their only manifestation of thyrotoxicosis. Apart from hypokalaemia, patients may also experience mild to moderate hypophosphataemia and hypomagnesaemia. These are also a result of intracellular shift as these electrolyte abnormalities would return to normal spontaneously when the patient recovers from the paralysis.

The underlying cause of hyperthyroidism in the majority of TPP patients is Graves' disease. However, TPP can also be associated with thyroiditis (either spontaneous or induced by interferon therapy), toxic nodular goitre, toxic adenoma, thyroid-stimulating hormone (TSH)-secreting pituitary tumour, and even overdosage of thyroid hormone. TPP is usually the early presentation of the underlying thyroid disease. In the case of Graves' disease, TPP can also be a presenting feature of relapse of the disease. Paralysis only occurs when the patient is thyrotoxic and not when euthyroid.

Muscle biopsies from patients with TPP have revealed a variety of abnormalities. The most consistent finding is proliferation and focal dilation of the sarcoplasmic reticulum and transverse tubular system, with prominent vacuoles arising from the sarcoplasmic reticulum (9). It is uncertain whether these vacuoles represent coalescence of dilated sarcoplasmic reticulum or sequestrated areas of focal myofibrillar necrosis.

Pathogenesis

The pathogenesis of TPP remains unclear. Hypokalaemia is due to a rapid and massive shift of plasma potassium from the extracellular into the intracellular compartment, mainly into the muscles, and is not due to depletion through losses in urine or faeces. This massive shift of potassium is believed to be due to increased Na^+,K^+-ATPase pump activity in these patients. It is known that thyroid hormone can increase Na^+,K^+-ATPase activity in skeletal muscle, liver, and kidney, and also induce influx of plasma potassium into the intracellular space (10). A thyroid hormone responsive element has been described in the promoter region of the α1- and β1-subunits of the Na^+,K^+-ATPase pump. The action of thyroid hormone on Na^+,K^+-ATPase activity is believed to be mediated through both transcriptional and post-transcriptional levels. Thyroid hormone also increases the number and sensitivity of β-adrenergic receptors. The increased β-adrenergic stimulation further increases Na^+,K^+-ATPase activity, which may explain why nonselective β-blockers can prevent attacks of TPP. The finding that selective β_1 antagonists do not protect patients from paralytic attacks is consistent with the specific role of the β_2 receptor in mediating the catecholamine-induced increase in Na^+,K^+-ATPase activity in skeletal muscle (11).

As it is difficult to determine potassium transport in intact skeletal muscles during TPP and in between attacks, most studies have resorted to measurement of the potassium flux and sodium pump activity in peripheral tissues such as the red blood cells, leucocytes, and platelets. Various groups have shown that the number of Na^+,K^+-ATPase pumps, as well as Na^+,K^+-ATPase-mediated cation influx, were increased in leucocytes (12) and platelets (13) in thyrotoxic patients with or without TPP when compared to healthy controls. However, TPP patients have significantly higher pump capacity and activity than those with plain thyrotoxicosis. When thyrotoxicosis is controlled, the Na^+,K^+-ATPase activity in TPP patients returns to levels similar to those of healthy individuals.

Insulin stimulates Na^+,K^+-ATPase and plays a permissive role for the potassium shift in TPP. Serum insulin levels vary widely in spontaneous attacks or during induction of paralysis, but hyperinsulinaemia during the attack or after glucose challenge has been reported in TPP (14). The hyperinsulinaemic response may explain the association of the paralysis with heavy meals or sweet snacks. Exercise releases potassium from muscle while rest promotes influx of potassium, which may explain why mild exercise may abort an attack. It would thus appear that TPP patients have an underlying predisposition for activation of Na^+,K^+-ATPase activity, and that thyroid hormone and insulin enhance the exaggerated response of the pump activity in these people. It is of interest to note that Na^+,K^+-ATPase activity is possibly increased by androgens and inhibited by oestrogens, and this may explain the male predilection for TPP (15).

A number of genetic association studies on TPP have been reported. Associations with the HLA genotypes HLA-B46, HLA-DR9, and HLA-DQBl*0303 were reported in Hong Kong Chinese, HLA-A2, HLA-Bw22, HLA-AW19, and HLA-B17 in Singapore Chinese, and HLA-DRW8 in Japanese populations (16). However, it is uncertain whether these associations were related to the genetic predisposition to Graves' disease rather than to TPP, especially when the majority of these TPP patients had an underlying autoimmune thyroid disease.

In view of the similar presentations between TPP and FHPP, the role of the voltage-dependent calcium channel or dihydropyridine-sensitive L-type calcium channel receptor ($Ca_v1.1$), which is associated with FHPP 1, was studied in TPP patients. None of the few mutation hot spots associated with FHPP was present in Asian or non-Asian patients with TPP (17, 18). However, certain single nucleotide polymorphisms (SNPs) of $Ca_v1.1$, including nucleotide (nt) 476, intron 2 nt 57, and intron 26 nt 67, were associated with TPP in southern Chinese (18). The location of these SNPs lies at or close to the thyroid hormone responsive element (TRE) of the gene, and it is likely that they affect the binding affinity of thyroid hormone responsive element (TRE) and modulate the stimulation of thyroid hormone on the $Ca_v1.1$ gene. Similarly, isolated case reports with mutations in other skeletal muscle ionic channels were reported in white individuals but were not identified in other populations.

In view of the insulin resistance and increased Na^+,K^+-ATPase activity and increased adrenergic response observed in TPP patients, the genes encoding for the α1-, α2-, β1-, β2-, and β4-subunits of Na^+,K^+-ATPase and β-adrenergic receptor were examined. Ryan *et al.* (19) have recently reported that one in three patients with TPP carries a mutation of a gene encoding an inwardly rectifying potassium (Kir) channel Kir 2.6, suggesting that TPP might be a channelopathy like FHPP.

Treatment

Treatment of TPP consists of two components: (1) the acute management of the paralytic attack and (2) the definitive treatment of hyperthyroidism. During the paralysis associated with marked hypokalaemia, treatment with intravenous potassium can hasten the recovery of muscle function and prevent cardiac arrhythmia. However, the serum potassium level has to be monitored closely, as rebound hyperkalaemia may occur when the potassium is being shifted back into the extracellular compartment. The use of oral potassium supplements during the early phase of weakness can sometimes help to prevent further progression to complete paralysis. Whereas potassium replacement is most effective during paralysis, regular potassium supplements are not effective for prophylaxis against further paralytic attack. Further attacks of paralysis can be prevented by the administration of spironolactone or propranolol. The most effective agent is propranolol, a nonselective β-blocker. At a dosage of 40 mg 4 times a day, propranolol can prevent paralysis induced by high carbohydrate load in about two-thirds of those with a history of TPP (20). The selective β_1 antagonist metoprolol does not protect patients from paralytic attacks. Thyroxine and acetazolamide have been reported to reduce the frequency of attacks in FHPP, whereas the reverse is the case with TPP.

Patients should be advised to avoid the factors that may precipitate the attack, including heavy carbohydrate intake, alcohol ingestion, and excessive exertion. However, since patients will not have further paralytic attacks when they are euthyroid, adequate control of hyperthyroidism is necessary. Definitive treatment of the hyperthyroidism with radioactive iodine or thyroidectomy is indicated. It has to be noted that TPP may occur after radioactive iodine therapy when the patient is still thyrotoxic, and addition of antithyroid drugs for several weeks after radioactive iodine therapy may be necessary to establish a euthyroid state. When treatment leads to hypothyroidism, careful monitoring of the thyroxine replacement therapy is essential to avoid overtreatment, which may lead to a recurrence of paralytic attacks.

References

1. Kelley DE, Gharib H, Kennedy FP, Duda RJ, McManis MB. Thyrotoxic periodic paralysis. Report of 10 cases and review of electromyographic findings. *Arch Int Med*, 1989; **149**: 2597–600.
2. McFadzean AJS, Yeung R. Periodic paralysis complicating thyrotoxicosis in Chinese. *BMJ*, 1967; **1**: 451–5.
3. Tinker TD, Vannatta JB. Thyrotoxic hypokalemic periodic paralysis. Report four cases and review of the literature. *J Okla State Med Assoc*, 1987; **80**: 76–83.

4. Shizume K, Shishiba Y, Kuma K, Noguchi S, Tajiri J, Ito K, *et al.* Comparison of the incidence of association of periodic paralysis and hyperthyroidism in Japan in 1957 and 1991. *Endocrinol Jpn*, 1992; **39**: 315–18.
5. Liu YC, Tsai WS, Chau T, Lin SH. Acute hypercapnic respiratory failure due to thyrotoxic periodic paralysis. *Am J Med Sci*, 2004; **327**: 264–7.
6. Ahlawat SK, Sachdev A. Hypokalemic paralysis. *Postgrad Med J*, 1999; **75**: 193–7.
7. Crane MG. Periodic paralysis associated with hyperthyroidism. *Calif Med*, 1960; **92**: 285–8.
8. Yeo PPB, Lee KO, Cheah JS. Hyperthyroidism and periodic paralysis. In: Imura H, Shizume K, Yoshida S, eds. *Progress in Endocrinology*. Vol 2. Amsterdam: Excerpta Medica, 1988: 1341–6.
9. Cheah JS, Tock EPC, Kan SP. The light and electron microscopic changes in the skeletal muscles during paralysis in thyrotoxic periodic paralysis. *Am J Med Sci*, 1975; **269**: 365–74.
10. Curfman GD, Crowley TJ, Smith TW. Thyroid-induced alterations in myocardial sodium-potassium-activated adenosine triphosphatase, monovalent cation active transport, and cardiac glycoside binding. *J Clin Invest*, 1977; **59**: 586–90.
11. Layzer RB. Periodic paralysis and the sodium-potassium pump. *Ann Neurol*, 1982; **11**: 547–52.
12. Khan FA, Baron DN. Ion flux and Na^+,K^+-ATPase activity of erythrocytes and leucocytes in thyroid disease. *Clin Sci*, 1987; **72**: 171–9.
13. Chan A, Shinde R, Chow CC, Cockram CS, Swaminathan R. In vivo and in vitro sodium pump activity in subjects with thyrotoxic periodic paralysis. *BMJ*, 1991; **303**: 1096–9.
14. Lee KO, Taylor EA, Oh VMS, Cheah JS, Aw SE. Hyperinsulinaemia in thyrotoxic hypokalaemic periodic paralysis. *Lancet*, 1991; **337**: 1063–4.
15. Fraser CL, Sarnacki P. Na^+-K^+-ATPase pump function in rat brain synaptosomes is different in males and females. *Am J Physiol*, 1989; **257**: E284–9.
16. Ober KP. Thyrotoxic periodic paralysis in the United States. Report of 7 cases and review of the literature. *Medicine*, 1992; **71**: 109–20.
17. Dias de Silva MR, Cerutti JM, Tengan CH, Furuzawa GK, Vieira TCA, Gabbai AA, *et al.* Mutations linked to familial hypokalemic periodic paralysis in the calcium channel α1 subunit gene ($Ca_v1.1$) are not associated with thyrotoxic hypokalaemic periodic paralysis. *Clin Endocrinol (Oxf)*, 2002; **56**; 367–75.
18. Kung AWC, Lau KS, Fong GCY, Chan V. Association of novel single nucleotide polymorphisms in the calcium channel α1 subunit gene ($Ca_v1.1$) and thyrotoxic periodic paralysis. *J Clin Endocrinol Metab*, 2004; **89**: 1340–5.
19. Ryan DP, da Silva MR, Soong TW, Fontaine B, Donaldson MR, Kung AWC *et al.* Mutations in potassium channel Kir2.6 cause susceptibility to thyrotoxic hypokalemic periodic paralysis. *Cell*, 2010; **140**: 88–98.
20. Young RTT, Tse TF. Thyrotoxic periodic paralysis. Effect of propranolol. *Am J Med*, 1974; **57**: 584–90.

3.3.3 Thyrotoxic storm

Joanna Klubo-Gwiezdzinska, Leonard Wartofsky

Introduction

Although a rare presentation of the exaggerated manifestations of thyrotoxicosis, thyrotoxic storm is arguably the most serious complication of hyperthyroidism because of its high mortality rate. An accurate estimation of its incidence is impossible to determine because of considerable variability in the criteria for its diagnosis. The syndrome does appear to be significantly less common today than in the past, perhaps because of earlier diagnosis and treatment of thyrotoxicosis, thereby precluding its progression to the stage of crisis. Nevertheless, the syndrome may occur in 1–2% of hospital admissions for thyrotoxicosis. In such patients, it is not usually possible to distinguish those with thyrotoxic storm from those with uncomplicated thyrotoxicosis simply on the basis of routine function tests. Rather, the clinical diagnosis is based on the identification of signs and symptoms which are seen typically in thyrotoxic storm and which suggest decompensation of a number of organ systems. Some of these typical or cardinal manifestations include fever (temperature usually above 38.5°C), tachycardia out of proportion to the fever, central nervous system signs varying from confusion to apathy and even coma, and gastrointestinal dysfunction, which can include nausea, vomiting, diarrhoea, and, in severe cases, jaundice. A semiquantitative scale (Table 3.3.3.1) has been developed to aid in diagnosis (1). The earliest possible diagnosis and subsequent implementation of treatment are required to avoid a fatal outcome. Even with early diagnosis, death can occur, and reported mortality rates have ranged from 10% to 75% in hospitalized patients (1–3).

Clinical features

The patient's history may include a previously partially treated thyrotoxicosis, but the initiation of the decompensation into thyrotoxic crisis usually follows some specific precipitating event, as indicated in Box 3.3.3.1. Most patients will have obvious signs and symptoms of thyrotoxicosis, including goitre and perhaps Graves' ophthalmopathy. Rarely, thyrotoxic storm may occur with subacute thyroiditis or factitious thyrotoxicosis due to intentional thyroxine overdose (4, 5). In older patients, particularly those who may have an underlying toxic multinodular goitre rather than Graves' disease, the thyrotoxic storm may present as so-called masked or apathetic thyrotoxicosis (6).

Thyrotoxic storm seen in the immediate postoperative setting after thyroidectomy has been termed 'surgical storm' and was seen more frequently several decades ago before the routine preparation of patients for elective thyroidectomy by treatment with antithyroid drugs. Such a presentation, although rare today, may still occur in spite of improvements in medical therapy. However, several types of surgery (non-thyroidal) or other trauma have precipitated crisis in patients with previously undiagnosed thyrotoxicosis. Indeed, thyrotoxic storm has occurred as a result of vigorous repetitive examination of a large Graves' gland, and the mechanism in surgical storm may be at least in part on the same basis, i.e. the result of trauma to the thyroid with discharge of thyroxine (T_4) and triiodothyronine (T_3) into the blood. Thyroid storm has been seen in pregnancy, during labour, and in complications such as placenta praevia. Other aspects of perioperative events, such as anaesthesia, stress, and volume depletion, may also play a role. This is so because these conditions are associated with increases in free thyroid hormone concentration that can be seen as part of the 'euthyroid sick' syndrome and the hormonal changes would be exaggerated in a hyperthyroid individual. Other clinical circumstances in which storm may be seen include crisis induced by cytotoxic chemotherapy for acute leukaemia, aspirin overdose (7–9), or organophosphate intoxication (10).

In hospitalized patients, the most common precipitating event associated with thyrotoxic storm is some form of infection. The

Table 3.3.3.1 Diagnostic criteria for thyroid storm (1)

Criteria		Score
Thermoregulatory dysfunction		
Temperature:	99–99.9 °F (37.2–37.7 °C)	5
	100–100.9 °F (37.8–38.2 °C)	10
	101–101.9 °F (38.3–38.8 °C)	15
	102–102.9 °F (38.9–39.3 °C)	20
	103–103.9 °F (39.4–39.9 °C)	25
	≥104 °F (40°C) or higher	30
Central nervous system effects		
Absent		0
Mild agitation		10
Delirium, psychosis, lethargy		20
Seizure or coma		30
Gastrointestinal dysfunction		
Absent		0
Diarrhoea, nausea, vomiting, or abdominal pain		10
Unexplained jaundice		20
Cardiovascular dysfunction		
Tachycardia:	90–109 beats/min	5
	110–119 beats/min	10
	120–129 beats/min	15
	130–139 beats/min	20
	≥140 beats/min	25
Congestive heart failure:	Absent	0
	Mild (oedema)	5
	Moderate (bibasilar rales)	10
	Severe (pulmonary oedema)	15
Atrial fibrillation:	Absent	0
	Present	10
History of precipitating event (surgery, infection, etc.)		
Absent		0
Present		10

Points are assigned as applicable and the scores totalled. When it is not possible to distinguish a finding due to an intercurrent illness from that of thyrotoxicosis, the higher point score is given so as to favour empiric therapy. Based upon the total score, the likelihood of the diagnosis of thyrotoxic storm is: unlikely <25; impending 25–44; highly likely >45.

differential diagnosis between true storm and uncomplicated infection in a thyrotoxic patient may be quite difficult, because of the likely presence of signs of tachycardia and fever in both. In this regard, very high fever seemingly out of proportion to an apparent infection along with dramatic diaphoresis could be a strong clinical clue to impending thyrotoxic storm. This is the time to consider initiation of a vigorous treatment plan, for no other clear-cut signal of the presence of thyrotoxic crisis may present itself before the inexorable decline of vital functions in the patient. As the storm progresses, symptoms of central nervous system dysfunction simulating an encephalopathic picture will appear, which may include increasing agitation and emotional lability, confusion, paranoia, psychosis, and finally even coma (11). Patients have been reported who presented with thyroid storm associated with status epilepticus and stroke and with bilateral basal ganglia infarction (12). The longer a patient remains untreated, the greater the likelihood of irreversible progression and ultimate demise. Hence, when the diagnosis is likely but indefinite, prudent management dictates that treatment for thyrotoxic storm should be initiated; it can always be discontinued if the patient improves rapidly, e.g. after antibiotic treatment for an infection.

Box 3.3.3.1 Events associated with precipitation of thyrotoxic storm

- More common:
  - Withdrawal of antithyroid drug treatment
  - Iodine-131 treatment
  - Sepsis, infection
  - Surgery, trauma
  - Iodinated contrast dyes
  - Parturition
  - Vigorous palpation of thyroid
  - Burn injury
  - Diabetic ketoacidosis
  - Pulmonary thromboembolism
- Less common
  - Hypoglycaemia
  - Emotional stress
  - Subacute thyroiditis
  - Thyroxine overdosage
  - Cytotoxic chemotherapy
  - Aspirin overdosage
  - Organophosphates
  - Seizure disorder

Cardiovascular manifestations

Cardiovascular manifestations are typically present in storm due to the direct and indirect influence of thyroid hormones on the heart, arteries, and veins. Rhythm disturbances commonly seen include sinus tachycardia, atrial fibrillation or other supraventricular tachyarrhythmias, and rarely ventricular tachyarrhythmias, which can be observed even in patients without previous heart disease (13). The signs and symptoms of congestive heart failure may be present. Although elderly patients are more likely to have symptoms of heart failure due to underlying rheumatic or arteriosclerotic heart disease, cardiac decompensation also may be seen in relatively young or middle-aged patients without known antecedent cardiac disease because functional reserve of the cardiovascular system is decreased. Most patients will have systolic hypertension with widened pulse pressure, at least initially. A high output state is present due to the increased preload secondary to activation of the renin–angiotensin–aldosterone axis and to decreased afterload secondary to a direct effect of thyroid hormone causing relaxation of vascular muscle cells. Another presentation of heart failure in thyrotoxic storm may be as a reversible dilated cardiomyopathy (14). Due to high oxygen demand and coronary artery spasm induced by the elevated catecholamines associated with excessive thyroid hormones, myocardial infarction can be observed, even in young patients (15, 16). A relatively rare complication of severe hyperthyroidism is pulmonary hypertension, which is presumed to be on an autoimmune basis when associated with Graves' disease but which also may be secondary to an augmented blood volume, cardiac output, and sympathetic tone, leading to pulmonary vasoconstriction and increased pulmonary arterial pressure. This condition is usually reversible after treatment with antithyroid drugs. The other possible reason for pulmonary hypertension is pulmonary embolism due to the thrombotic or hypercoagulable state that has been observed in severe hyperthyroidism.

Respiratory manifestations

The main symptom is tachypnoea related to an increased oxygen demand. The increased work of breathing, augmented ventilatory response to hypercapnia, and hypoxia may lead to the diaphragmatic dysfunction. As a consequence of coexistent decreased lung compliance and hyperdynamic cardiomyopathy, acute respiratory failure is not unusual in thyrotoxic crisis (17). Respiratory failure may be seen when severe thyrotoxicosis presents in a patient with known pulmonary disease. For example, asthma may be exacerbated in hyperthyroid patients due to enhanced free radical production by neutrophils and alveolar macrophages (18, 19).

Gastrointestinal manifestations

The most common symptoms are diffuse abdominal pain, vomiting, or diarrhoea which can cause volume depletion, postural hypotension, and shock with vascular collapse. When this occurs, death is virtually inevitable. The pathophysiological mechanisms underlying these symptoms are complex, but impaired neurohormonal regulation of gastric myoelectrical activity with delayed gastric emptying plays an important role (20). Other gastrointestinal manifestations could include presentation as an acute abdomen (21), intestinal obstruction (22), hepatomegaly, splenomegaly, and various abnormalities in liver function tests. Congestive failure or hepatic necrosis may cause the liver to be tender to palpation. The presence of jaundice is another poor prognostic sign and warrants immediate and vigorous therapy. Although the majority of presentations of an acute abdomen in thyrotoxicosis are medical in nature, surgical conditions may also occur (23).

Acid–base balance and renal and electrolyte manifestations

Due to augmented lipolysis and ketogenesis, ketoacidosis may occur with lactic acidosis in extreme cases of thyrotoxicosis such as thyroid storm. The cause of increased lactate production may be due to basal metabolic demands that exceed oxygen delivery and/or reduced hepatic clearance of lactic acid. Although hyperthyroidism is often associated with an accelerated glomerular filtration rate, renal failure is not uncommon and can progress due to glomerulosclerosis, proteinuria, and oxidative stress, or rarely to rhabdomyolysis (24). Renal failure may have a postrenal basis as well, with urinary retention due to dyssynergy of the detrusor muscle, leading to bladder dysfunction (25). Moreover, the most common cause of thyrotoxicosis, Graves' disease, can be accompanied by autoimmune complex-mediated nephritis (26).

Neuropsychiatric manifestations

Presentation of a wide range of central nervous system signs and symptoms in the hyperthyroid patient was described above as a key component for the diagnosis of thyrotoxic crisis. In patients with neurological symptoms, a high index of suspicion for cerebral sinus thrombosis should be considered, because of the higher prevalence of this condition in severe hyperthyroidism (27). Paralysis observed in thyroid crisis might be the result of a cerebrovascular accident, but thyrotoxic periodic paralysis with hypokalaemia should be considered, especially in Asian men (28). The factors predisposing to this condition are high carbohydrate diet, strenuous physical activity followed by rest, trauma, surgery, cold exposure, or infection. Another uncommon condition in patients with severe thyrotoxicosis is an acute peripheral neuropathy, as first described by Charcot in 1889 (29).

Hyperthermia

Hyperthermia in thyroid crisis can represent both defective thermoregulation by the hypothalamus and/or increased basal metabolic rate. Oxidation of lipids is responsible for more than 60% of the resting energy expenditure (30). Sometimes pyrexia is not observed in elderly patients as part of the complex of so-called apathetic thyrotoxicosis with storm (6).

Haematological manifestations

Hyperthyroidism may be associated with hypercoagulability due to increased concentrations of fibrinogen, factors VIII and IX, tissue plasminogen activator inhibitor 1, and von Willebrand's factor, and a tendency to augmented platelet plug formation (31). High oxygen demand tends to up-regulate erythropoietin secretion resulting in an increase in red blood cell mass, which also compounds the hypercoagulability. Major thromboembolic complications are responsible for 18% of deaths caused by thyrotoxicosis (31–36). Evidence suggests that the rate of central nervous system embolism in thyrotoxic atrial fibrillation exceeds that of nonthyrotoxic atrial fibrillation (34). As a consequence, therapeutic initiatives should be undertaken in thyroid storm to prevent thromboembolic complications. Optimal treatment requires a balance between anticoagulant dosage and the effect of vitamin K antagonists that can be potentiated by thyrotoxicosis (35).

Laboratory findings

Relatively similar estimates of serum total T_4 and T_3, T_3 resin uptake, and the 24-h radio-iodine uptake will be found in thyrotoxic storm as in uncomplicated thyrotoxicosis. Indeed, serum total T_3 levels may be within normal limits, as these patients may have some underlying illness which precipitated the storm and which is responsible for altering their thyroid function tests in the direction of the sick patient that is congruent with the 'euthyroid sick syndrome'. Thus, a low serum T_3 may be seen in diabetic ketoacidosis and other patients with coexistent thyrotoxic storm and underlying systemic illness (37, 38), but the decreased (or misleadingly normal) serum T_3 may serve to obscure the diagnosis of thyrotoxicosis until thyrotoxic storm becomes clinically apparent. Perhaps the most rapid confirmation of the diagnosis in a patient with previously undiagnosed thyrotoxicosis may be obtained from a 2-h radio-iodine uptake, although it should be feasible to obtain the result of serum T_4 and thyroid-stimulating hormone (TSH) determinations within a few hours on an emergency basis in most hospitals. Initiation of treatment should not be delayed if there is a high index of suspicion, merely because one is awaiting laboratory confirmation of the diagnosis. Given the mortality rate of untreated thyrotoxic storm, the presence of goitre with a thrill and bruit or ophthalmopathy in the clinical setting described above should be considered as sufficient support for the diagnosis of thyrotoxic crisis to warrant treatment. Other settings in which thyroid storm has been seen include a patient with thermal burn injury and metastatic thyroid carcinoma (39), pregnancy (40), and after relatively mild trauma (41).

Other laboratory abnormalities may include a modest hyperglycaemia in the absence of diabetes mellitus, probably as a result of augmented glycogenolysis and catecholamine-mediated inhibition of insulin release as well as increased insulin clearance and insulin resistance. When thyrotoxicosis is prolonged leading to the depletion of glycogen deposits, hypoglycaemia may occur, particularly in older people when aggravated by malnutrition secondary to emesis or abdominal pain (42). Although most haematology values tend to be normal, a moderate leucocytosis with a mild shift to the left is common even in the absence of infection. Increased serum calcium levels may be seen perhaps due to both haemoconcentration and the known effects of thyroid hormone on bone resorption, but serum sodium, potassium, and chloride are usually normal. Hepatic dysfunction in thyroid storm will result in elevated levels of serum lactate dehydrogenase, glutamic oxaloacetate transaminase (aspartate aminotransferase), and bilirubin. The origin of increases in serum alkaline phosphatase levels is due mainly to increased osteoblastic bone activity in response to the augmentation of bone resorption. Because serum cortisol levels should be elevated in thyrotoxic storm, as in any other acute stressful situation, a normal value may be interpreted as being inappropriately low. In view of the known coincidence of adrenal insufficiency with Graves' disease, one should maintain a reasonably high index of suspicion for this disorder, particularly if there is hypotension and suggestive electrolyte abnormalities. This diagnosis may be identified by obtaining a serum sample for cortisol determination before the administration of corticosteroid. Even in the absence of adrenal insufficiency, adrenal reserve may be exceeded in thyrotoxic crisis because of the inability of the adrenal gland to meet the demand placed on it as a result of the accelerated turnover and disposal of glucocorticoids that occur in thyrotoxicosis.

Pathogenesis

The precise pathogenesis underlying the precipitation of thyroid storm may not be the same in all cases and remains incompletely understood. Several factors could be important. Because there may be higher levels of total serum T_4 or T_3 in uncomplicated thyrotoxicosis than are seen in many instances of thyrotoxic crisis, the serum hormone levels themselves do not appear to be critical. One illustrative model is that provided by children with astronomically high serum T_4 and T_3 concentrations after accidental ingestion of T_4 in whom storm is not seen. For this reason, an acute increase in release of T_4 or T_3 from the thyroid is probably not critical to the pathogenesis of storm. However, an acute discharge of hormone in the appropriate clinical setting certainly might trigger a crisis, and cases have been reported following vigorous palpation of the thyroid, ^{131}I therapy (43), withdrawal of propylthiouracil therapy, or after administration of lithium, stable iodine, or iodinated contrast dyes. Indeed, the dramatic clinical improvement seen after an abrupt decrease in serum T_4 or T_3 by peritoneal dialysis or plasmapheresis suggests that hormone elevation does play a role (44, 45). But in general, serum total T_4 and T_3 values do not differ significantly from those in uncomplicated thyrotoxicosis, although the levels in an affected person could be higher than the values before the precipitating event.

We believe that the critical factor relates to the actual 'free' concentration of thyroid hormone and not the 'total' measured hormone in blood. This former concentration is directly associated with the relationship of the hormone to its circulating binding proteins (thyroxine binding globulin, transthyretin, and albumin). The absolute concentration of free T_4 or T_3 is the product of the total concentration and the fraction that is unbound. Thus, any perturbation of hormone binding which might alter the fraction that is free could increase the absolute concentration of free hormone. Conditions known to be associated with inhibition of binding of hormone to its circulating binding proteins, which thereby increase the fraction that is free, include surgery and anaesthesia, stress, infection, burns (39), and ketoacidosis (46). Such decreases in binding affinity may be due to circulating inhibitors (37) which reduce protein binding of hormone. That this phenomenon may apply in thyroid storm is indicated by the observed increases in both the percentage of dialysable or free T_4 and the absolute free hormone concentration often seen during the early presentation of thyroid storm (47, 48). But the pathogenesis may involve more than one factor. For example, storm has been reported after radio-iodine ablation of the thyroid in Graves' disease patients, and a review of the clinical circumstances and characteristics of these patients indicated that it was the oldest and the most ill patients, often with cardiorespiratory conditions, who appeared to be predisposed to develop this complication (43). Patients with a systemic illness would have decreased binding and higher free T_4 due to the illness and to circulating inhibitors to hormone binding. McDermott *et al.* recommended a more cautious approach to radio-iodine therapy in such patients to avoid thyrotoxic crisis (43).

A possible interaction between the effects of thyroid hormone and the catecholamines has been a subject of both research and clinical interest for decades, particularly because many of the signs and symptoms of severe thyrotoxicosis could be due to catecholamines or their interaction with the excessive levels of circulating thyroid hormone. Although normal serum catecholamine levels and urinary excretion rates mitigate against the idea of augmented adrenergic activity, there remains some likelihood for an important role of the sympathetic nervous system in the pathogenesis of thyrotoxic storm. Dramatic clinical improvement follows the use of agents that either deplete tissue catecholamines, such as reserpine, or block β-adrenergic receptors, such as propranolol. Indeed, the availability and use of propranolol may be responsible for the improvement in survival statistics reported in patients with thyrotoxic storm. On the other hand, we should avoid being lulled into a false sense of security in patients receiving β-adrenergic blockers, because the customarily used doses of these agents may not prevent the occurrence of storm (49). In patients who are either refractory or overly sensitive to propranolol (50), a trial of reserpine may be attempted.

Treatment of thyroid storm

To avoid a disastrous outcome, a four-part approach to management is recommended. The relative importance of each part of treatment will vary in a given patient. First, specific antithyroid drugs must be used to reduce the increased thyroid production and release of T_4 and T_3. The second approach comprises treatment intended to block the effects of the remaining but excessive circulating concentrations of free T_4 and T_3. The third arm involves treatments directed against the underlying systemic decompensation which may be characterized, e.g. by fever, congestive failure, and shock. The final component addresses any underlying precipitating illness such as infection or ketoacidosis. In view of the poor prognosis associated with incompletely treated thyroid storm, no one component should be neglected.

Therapy directed to the thyroid gland

Inhibition of new synthesis of the thyroid hormones is achieved by administration of thionamide antithyroid drugs, such as carbimazole, propylthiouracil, or methimazole (tapazole). These drugs are given by mouth or by nasogastric tube, if necessary in the comatose or uncooperative patient, because there are no available parenteral preparations of these compounds in the USA. There is an intravenous form of thiamazole used in European countries. Either methimazole (and presumably carbimazole) or propylthiouracil may also be administered per rectum if necessary (51, 52). In view of the gravity of thyroid storm, thionamide doses are higher than for otherwise uncomplicated thyrotoxicosis. For example, propylthiouracil can be started in a dose of 1200–1500 mg/day, given as 200–250 mg every 4 h. In the case of methimazole, the daily dose is approximately one-tenth of that of propylthiouracil or 120 mg (given as 20 mg every 4 h). Some experienced clinicians believe that propylthiouracil will provide more rapid clinical improvement because it has the additional advantage of inhibiting conversion of T_4 to T_3, a property not shared by methimazole. Because thionamides reduce new hormone synthesis but not thyroidal secretion of preformed glandular stores of hormone, separate treatment must be administered to inhibit proteolysis of colloid and the continuing release of T_4 and T_3 into the blood. Either inorganic iodine or lithium carbonate may be used for this purpose. Iodides may be given either orally as Lugol's solution or as a saturated solution of potassium iodide (8 drops every 6 h). An earlier mainstay of treatment, the use of an intravenous infusion of sodium iodide (0.5–1 g every 12 h) has not been feasible recently as sterile sodium iodide has not been available for intravenous use, at least not in the USA. However, a sterile intravenous preparation could be prepared by a hospital pharmacy. The sequence of administration of iodine and antithyroid drugs to thyrotoxic patients is very important. Use of iodine without prior thionamide dosage is to be avoided because the iodine will enhance thyroid hormone synthesis, enrich hormone stores within the gland, and thereby permit further exaggeration of thyrotoxicosis. Sole therapy with stable iodine will also complicate future management by any treatment method because ultimate efficacy of antithyroid drugs will be delayed, surgical risk will be increased, and the use of radio-iodine will be substantially delayed, pending clearance of the stable iodine load. Thyrotoxic storm has occurred in patients who were treated with iodine alone and who deteriorated weeks to months after their initial improvement. Patients may present with exaggerated thyrotoxicosis (or thyroid storm) when iodine has been used as a sole agent to prepare patients for thyroidectomy and the surgery then was postponed for some reason. However, when iodine is administered in conjunction with full doses of antithyroid drugs, dramatic rapid decreases in serum T_4 are seen, with values approaching the normal range within 4 or 5 days (53).

Other agents that may be used in this manner are the radiographic contrast dyes ipodate (Oragrafin) and iopanoic acid (Telepaque), although they are no longer available in the USA. These drugs decrease hepatic uptake of T_4 and the percentage of free T_4 and T_3 in serum, and their use can be associated with remarkable clinical improvement. These agents act by decreasing peripheral conversion of T_4 to T_3 and decreasing thyroid hormone release, as well as possibly blocking binding of both T_3 and T_4 to their cellular receptors. After a loading dose of 3 g, ipodate may be administered as 1 g orally on a daily basis and, like iodine, should only be employed with simultaneous thionamide. Amiodarone, an antiarrhythmic and antianginal drug which is also rich in iodine, may cause either an iodine-induced thyrotoxicosis (type 1) or a destructive thyroiditis (type 2); the latter has been reported as a cause of thyroid storm refractory to the usual treatment with thionamides as well as corticosteroids and plasmapheresis (54).

In patients who may be allergic to iodine, lithium carbonate may be used as an alternative agent to inhibit hormonal release (55), although some caution has been raised in regard to its use in the setting of storm (56). This drug also may be used in thyrotoxic patients who are known to have serious toxic reactions to the thionamides. Lithium should be administered initially as 300 mg every 6 h, with subsequent adjustment of dosage as necessary to maintain serum lithium levels at about 1 mmol/l.

Therapy directed at the continuing effects of thyroid hormone in the periphery

Given high levels of circulating T_4 and T_3 in a large vascular pool and tissue distribution space, the practical question is how to enhance their reduction or disposal. Peritoneal dialysis or plasmapheresis (44, 45) have been used, as has experimental haemoperfusion through a resin bed (57) or charcoal columns (58). Such aggressive management should be considered in a severe case. Oral administration of cholestyramine resin (59) provides a less aggressive means of removing T_4 and T_3, by binding thyroid hormone entering the gut via enterohepatic recirculation; the resin–hormone complex is then excreted. A highly aggressive approach has been employed where plasmapheresis for rapid lowering of serum T_3 and T_4 was followed by immediate total thyroidectomy. Early thyroidectomy has been reported to reduce the mortality rate from 20–40% under standard treatment to less then 10% (60).

Hughes (61) was the first to treat a patient with thyrotoxic storm using a β-adrenergic blocker to ameliorate the manifestations of thyroid hormone excess, and other reports soon followed. Propranolol is the most commonly used agent in the USA. The oral dosage of 20–40 mg every 6 h generally given in uncomplicated thyrotoxicosis may have to be increased to 60–120 mg every

6 h in crisis or impending crisis (62, 63). Indeed, because of the more rapid metabolism of the drug in severe thyrotoxicosis, even larger oral doses, or preferably intravenous doses, should be given. A plasma propranolol level in excess of 50 ng/ml may have to be maintained to establish clinical response (62). Initial intravenous doses of 0.5–1 mg should be given cautiously while the patient's cardiac rhythm is continuously monitored, with subsequent doses of 2–3 mg given intravenously over 10–15 min every several hours, while awaiting clinical improvement from the effect of orally administered drug.

Clinically dramatic improvement in the cardiovascular system may be attributed to β-adrenergic blockade, with rapid onset of reduction in heart rate, cardiac work, and cardiac output. One caution in patients with significant underlying intrinsic cardiac disease relates to the adverse effect of adrenergic blockade in neutralizing the little remaining sympathetic drive to the myocardium. Although use of propranolol might be contraindicated in patients with moderate to severe congestive heart failure, it may be used judiciously in patients with minor cardiac compromise related to their thyrotoxicosis (64). There may be a theoretical benefit derived from the inhibitory effect of propranolol on the conversion of T_4 to T_3 (65), but a significant effect is seen only with doses higher then 160 mg/day.

Given the poor prognosis in storm and the complexities inherent in management, patients with thyrotoxic storm, particularly those with cardiac decompensation, should be managed in an intensive care setting. Careful monitoring of fluids, volume status, and central haemodynamics is essential in these patients because they are likely to be receiving high-dose propranolol, pressors, digoxin, diuretics, and intravenous fluids. Added benefits of β-adrenergic blockade in these patients include improvement in agitation, convulsions, psychotic behaviour, tremor, diarrhoea, fever, and diaphoresis. In some patients, there may be relative risks or contraindications to the use of these agents. In patients with a history of bronchospasm or asthma, either treatment with reserpine, guanethidine, or selective β1-blocking agents should be considered instead. A very short acting β-adrenergic blocker, esmolol, has also been used in thyroid storm with success. An initial loading dose of 0.25–0.5 mg/kg is followed by continuous infusion of 0.05–0.1 mg/kg per min (66, 67).

Some authors have suggested that in situations such as thyroid storm with potential benefit from rapid normalization of thyroid hormones, the supplemental administration of 1α(OH) vitamin D_3 will accelerate the reduction of serum T_4 and T_3. In spite of a theoretical risk of hypercalcaemia in thyrotoxicosis, supplementation with vitamin D_3 may actually suppress calcium release from bones (68). In a recent study, the administration of L-carnitine 2 g/day in thyrotoxic storm facilitated a dose reduction of methimazole. The mechanism appears to be related to an inhibition by L-carnitine of T_3 and T_4 entry into cell nuclei (69, 70). Advocates for this therapy claim that carnitine has no toxicity, teratogenicity, contraindications, or important side effects (70). While these preliminary findings are of interest, the utility of this adjunct to therapy requires confirmation.

Therapy directed at systemic decompensation

Fluid depletion caused by the hyperpyrexia and diaphoresis, as well as by vomiting or diarrhoea if present, must be vigorously replaced to avoid vascular collapse. Vigorous fluid therapy will usually correct hypercalcaemia when present. Shock may be refractory to cautious fluid resuscitation in younger patients, whereas judicious replacement of fluids is necessary in elderly patients with congestive heart failure or other cardiac compromise. Intravenous fluids containing 10% dextrose in addition to electrolytes will better restore depleted hepatic glycogen. For fever, acetaminophen rather than salicylates is the preferred antipyretic, because salicylates inhibit thyroid hormone binding and could increase free hormone, thereby transiently worsening the thyrotoxic crisis. External cooling with alcohol sponging, ice packs, or a hypothermia blanket also may be used. Vitamin supplements may be added to the intravenous fluids to replace probable coexistent deficiency. Use of the skeletal muscle relaxant dantrolene was associated with clinical improvement in one case (71), but significant risk associated with its use precludes routine recommendation. When present, congestive heart failure should be treated with the usual measures, including digoxin and diuretics, although somewhat greater than usual doses of digoxin may be required.

Hypotension not readily reversed by adequate hydration may temporarily require pressor therapy, and glucocorticoids have been given on the basis of postulated relative adrenal insufficiency. The ability of steroids to inhibit conversion of T_4 to T_3 is additional justification for their use. An initial dose of 300 mg hydrocortisone followed by 100 mg every 8 h during the first 24–36 h should be adequate. Thyroid storm has been reported to recur when steroids had been discontinued after initial clinical improvement (72).

Therapy directed at the precipitating illness

Untreated or incompletely treated thyrotoxicosis may have existed in many patients presenting in thyroid storm until some precipitating event, such as infection, led to increments in free T_4 and signs and symptoms of exaggerated thyrotoxicosis. Thus, therapy is not complete unless a diagnosis of the possible precipitating event is made, and early treatment as indicated for that underlying illness is implemented. This is not a problem in obvious cases, such as trauma, surgery, or labour, all of which are known precipitants of thyrotoxic crisis, but which require no additional management. However, patients with enhanced thyroid secretion caused by withdrawal of thiourea treatment or the administration of iodine, iodinated contrast dyes, or ^{131}I may require some specific attention. Since the premature withdrawal of treatment could result in an exacerbation of thyrotoxicosis, an effective blockade of hormone biosynthesis and release must be continued beyond the period of immediate improvement.

Conditions such as ketoacidosis, pulmonary thromboembolism, or stroke may underlie thyrotoxic crisis, particularly in the obtunded or psychotic patient, and require the same vigorous management ordinarily indicated. In the patient with thyrotoxic crisis in whom none of the latter precipitating factors is apparent, a diligent search for some focus of infection must be carried out. Routine cultures of urine, blood, and sputum should be obtained in the febrile thyrotoxic patient, and cultures of other sites may be warranted on clinical grounds. Broad-spectrum antibiotic coverage on an empirical basis may be required initially while awaiting results of cultures. In most patients who survive thyrotoxic crisis, clinical improvement is dramatic and demonstrable within 12 or 24 h. The subsequent 72–96 h will be marked by defervescence and improvement in agitation or coma, heralding continued progressive recovery. During this recovery period, supportive therapy such as corticosteroids, antipyretics, and intravenous fluids, may be tapered and gradually withdrawn on the basis of patient status, oral intake of calories and fluids, vasomotor stability, and their continuing improvement.

After the crisis has been resolved, attention may be turned to consideration of future short- and long-term management of the patient's thyrotoxicosis. Radio-iodine treatment is often precluded by the recent use of inorganic iodine in virtually all cases of storm, but it could be considered at a later date, in which case antithyroid thionamide drug therapy is continued to restore and maintain euthyroidism until such time as ablative therapy could be administered. Continuing treatment with antithyroid drugs alone in the hope of the patient's sustaining a spontaneous remission is also possible. Surgery may be chosen, as many physicians favour a more definitive form of therapy in a patient with a recent history of thyrotoxic storm. Should thyroidectomy be considered, thyrotoxicosis must have been adequately treated beforehand, to obviate any likelihood of another episode of crisis during the surgery. Although routine perioperative management with β-blockers alone is not recommended, it is possible to operate successfully on some thyrotoxic patients with no preparation other than propranolol. When a surgical approach is selected, a total thyroidectomy is the procedure of choice in view of reports of recurrent severe thyrotoxicosis and thyroid crisis after subtotal thyroidectomy (73).

References

1. Burch HB, Wartofsky L. Life-threatening thyrotoxicosis. Thyroid storm. *Endocrinol Metab Clin North Am*, 1993; **22**: 263–77.
2. Dillman WH. Thyroid storm. *Curr Ther Endocrinol Metab*, 1997; **6**: 81–5.
3. Tietgens ST, Leinung MC. Thyroid storm. *Med Clin North Am*, 1995; **79**: 169–84.
4. Swinburne JL, Kreisman SH. A rare case of subacute thyroiditis causing thyroid storm. *Thyroid*, 2007; **17**: 73–6.
5. Yoon SJ, Kim DM, Kim JU, Kim KW, Ahn CW, Cha BS, *et al.* A case of thyroid storm due to thyrotoxicosis factitia. *Yonsei Med J*, 2003; **44**: 351–4.
6. Feroze M, May H. Apathetic thyrotoxicosis. *Int J Clin Pract*, 1997; **51**: 332–3.
7. Al-Anazi KA, Inam S, Jeha MT, Judzewitch R. Thyrotoxic crisis induced by cytotoxic chemotherapy. *Support Care Cancer*, 2005; **13**: 196–8.
8. Sebe A, Satar S, Sari A. Thyroid storm induced by aspirin intoxication and the effect of hemodialysis: a case report. *Adv Ther*, 2004; **21**: 173–7.
9. Hirvonen EA, Niskanen LK, Niskanen MM. Thyroid storm prior to induction of anaesthesia. *Anaesthesia*, 2004; **59**: 1020–2.
10. Yuan YD, Seak CJ, Lin CC, Lin LJ. Thyroid storm precipitated by organophosphate intoxication. *Am J Emerg Med*, 2007; **25**: 861.
11. Aiello DP, DuPlessis AJ, Pattishall EG III, Kulin HE. Thyroid storm presenting with coma and seizures. *Clin Pediatr (Phila)*, 1989; **28**: 571–4.
12. Lee TG, Ha CK, Lim BH. Thyroid storm presenting as status epilepticus and stroke. *Postgrad Med J*, 1997; **73**: 61.
13. Jao YT, Chen Y, Lee WH, Tai FT. Thyroid storm and ventricular tachycardia. *South Med J*, 2004; **976**: 604–7.
14. Daly MJ, Wilson CM, Dolan SJ, Kennedy A, McCance DR. Reversible dilated cardiomyopathy associated with post-partum thyrotoxic storm. *QJM*, 2009; **102**: 217–19.
15. Opdahl H, Eritsland J, Sovik E. Acute myocardial infarction and thyrotoxic storm—a difficult and dangerous combination. *ACTA Anaesthesiol Scand*, 2005; **49**: 707–11.
16. Lee SM, Jung TS, Hahm JR, Im SI, Kim SK, Lee KJ, *et al.* Thyrotoxicosis with coronary spasm that required coronary artery bypass surgery. *Intern Med*, 2007; **46**: 1915–18.
17. Liu YC, Tsai WS, Chau T, Lin SH. Acute hypercapnic respiratory failure due to thyrotoxic periodic paralysis. *Am J Med Sci*, 2004; **327**: 264–7.
18. Mezosi E, Szabo J, Nagy EV, Borbely A, Varga E, Paragh G, *et al.* Nongenomic effect of thyroid hormone on free-radical production in human polymorphonuclear leukocytes. *J Endocrinol*, 2005; **185**: 121–9.
19. Luong KV, Nguyen LT. Hyperthyroidism and asthma. *J Asthma*, 2000; **37**: 125–30.
20. Barczynski M, Thor P. Reversible autonomic dysfunction in hyperthyroid patients affects gastric myoelectrical activity and emptying. *Clin Auton Res*, 2001; **114**: 243–9.
21. Bhattacharyya A, Wiles PG. Thyrotoxic crisis presenting as acute abdomen. *J R Soc Med*, 1997; **90**: 681–2.
22. Cansler CL, Latham JA, Brown PM Jr, Chapman WH, Magner JA. Duodenal obstruction in thyroid storm. *South Med J*, 1997; **90**: 1143–6.
23. Leow MK, Chew DE, Zhu M, Soon PC. Thyrotoxicosis and acute abdomen: still as defying and misunderstood today? Brief observations over the recent decade. *QJM*, 2008; **101**: 943–7.
24. van Hoek I, Daminet S. Interactions between thyroid and kidney function in pathological conditions of these organ systems: A review. *Gen Comp Endocrinol*, 2009; **160**: 205–15.
25. Goswami R, Seth A, Goswami AK, Kochupillai N. Prevalence of enuresis and other bladder symptoms in patients with active Graves' disease. *Br J Urol*, 1997; **804**: 563–6.
26. Kahara T, Yoshizawa M, Nakaya I, Uchiyama A, Miwa A, Iwata Y, *et al.* Thyroid crisis following interstitial nephritis. *Intern Med*, 2008; **47**: 1237–40.
27. Dai A, Wasay M, Dubey N, Giglio P, Bakshi R. Superior sagittal sinus thrombosis secondary to hyperthyroidism. *J Stroke Cerebrovasc Dis*, 2000; **9**: 89–90.
28. Lu KC, Hsu YJ, Chiu JS, Hsu YD, Lin SH. Effects of potassium supplementation on the recovery of thyrotoxic periodic paralysis. *Am J Emerg Med*, 2004; **22**: 544–7.
29. Pandit L, Shankar SH, Gayathri N, Pandit A. Acute thyrotoxic neuropathy: Basedow's paraplegia revisited. *J Neurol Sci*, 1998; **155**: 211–14.
30. Riis AL, Gravholt CH, Djurhuus CB, N rrelund H, J rgensen JO, Weeke J, *et al.* Elevated regional lipolysis in hyperthyroidism. *J Clin Endocrinol Metab*, 2002; **87**: 4747–53.
31. Homoncik M, Gessl A, Ferlitsch A, Jilma B, Vierhapper H. Altered platelet plug formation in hyperthyroidism and hypothyroidism. *J Clin Endocrinol Metab*, 2007; **92**: 3006–12.
32. Romualdi E, Squizzato A, Ageno W. Venous thrombosis: a possible complication of overt hyperthyroidism. *Eur J Intern Med*, 2008; **19**: 386–7.
33. Pekdemir M, Yilmaz S, Ersel M, Sarisoy HT. A rare cause of headache; cerebral venous sinus thrombosis due to hyperthyroidism. *Am J Emerg Med*, 2008; **26**: 383.
34. Osman F, Gamma MD, Sheppard MC, Franklyn JA. Clinical review 142: cardiac dysrhythmias and thyroid dysfunction: the hidden menace? *J Clin Endocrinol Metab*, 2002; **87**: 963–7.
35. Squizzato A, Gerdes VE. Thyroid disease and haemostasis: a relationship with clinical implications? *Thromb Haemost*, 2008; **100**: 727–8.
36. Lippi G, Franchini M, Targher G, Montagnana M, Salvagno GL, Guidi GC, *et al.* Hyperthyroidism is associated with shortened APTT and increased fibrinogen values in a general population of unselected outpatients. *J Thromb Thrombolysis*, 2008; **28**: 362–5.
37. Wartofsky L, Burman KD. Alterations in thyroid function in patients with systemic illness: the 'euthyroid sick syndrome'. *Endocr Rev*, 1982; **3**: 164–217.
38. Wartofsky L. The low T_3 or 'sick euthyroid syndrome': update 1994. In: Braverman LE, Refetoff S, eds. *Endocrine Reviews Monographs. 3. Clinical and Molecular Aspects of Diseases of the Thyroid*. Bethesda: The Endocrine Society, 1994: 248–51.

39. Naito Y, Sone T, Kataoka K, Sawada M, Yamazaki K. Thyroid storm due to functioning metastatic thyroid carcinoma in a burn patient. *Anesthesiology*, 1997; **87**: 433–5.
40. Tewari K, Balderston KD, Carpenter SE, Major CA. Papillary thyroid carcinoma manifesting as thyroid storm of pregnancy: case report. *Am J Obstet Gynecol*, 1998; **179**: 818–19.
41. Yoshida D. Thyroid storm precipitated by trauma. *J Emerg Med*, 1996; **14**: 697–701.
42. Kobayashi C, Sasaki H, Kosuge K, Miyakita Y, Hayakawa M, Suzuki A, *et al.* Severe starvation hypoglycemia and congestive heart failure induced by thyroid crisis, with accidentally induced severe liver dysfunction and disseminated intravascular coagulation. *Intern Med*, 2005; **44**: 234–9.
43. McDermott MT, Kidd GS, Dodson LE, Hofeldt FD. Radioiodine-induced thyroid storm. *Am J Med*, 1983; **75**: 353–9.
44. Ashkar FS, Katims RB, Smoak WM, Gilson AJ. Thyroid storm treatment with blood exchange and plasmapheresis. *JAMA*, 1970; **214**: 1275–9.
45. Herrmann J, Hilger P, Kruskemper HL. Plasmapheresis in the treatment of thyrotoxic crisis (measurement of half-concentration tissues for free and total T_3 and T_4). *Acta Endocrinol Suppl (Copenh)*, 1973; **173**: 22.
46. Ahmad N, Conen MP. Thyroid storm with normal serum triiodothyronine level during diabetic ketoacidosis. *JAMA*, 1981; **245**: 2516–17.
47. Colebunders R, Bordoux P, Bekaert J, Mahler C, Parizel G. Determination of free thyroid hormones and their binding proteins in a patient with severe hyperthyroidism (thyroid storm?) and thyroid encephalopathy. *J Endocrinol Invest*, 1984; **7**: 379–81.
48. Brooks MH, Waldstein SS. Free thyroxine concentrations in thyroid storm. *Ann Intern Med*, 1980; **93**: 694–7.
49. Eriksson MA, Rubenfeld S, Garber AJ, Kohler PO. Propranolol does not prevent thyroid storm. *N Engl J Med*, 1977; **296**: 263–4.
50. Anaissie E, Tohme JF. Reserpine in propranolol resistant thyroid storm. *Arch Intern Med*, 1985; **145**: 2248–9.
51. Nareem N, Miner DJ, Amatruda JM. Methimazole: an alternative route of administration. *J Clin Endocrinol Metab*, 1982; **54**: 180–1.
52. Yeung SC, Go R, Balasubramanyam A. Rectal administration of iodide and propylthiouracil in the treatment of thyroid storm. *Thyroid*, 1995; **5**: 403–5.
53. Wartofsky L, Ransil BJ, Ingbar SH. Inhibition by iodine of the release of thyroxine from the thyroid glands of patients with thyrotoxicosis. *J Clin Invest*, 1970; **49**: 78–86.
54. Samaras K, Marel GM. Failure of plasmapheresis, corticosteroids and thionamides to ameliorate a case of protracted amiodarone-induced thyroiditis. *Clin Endocrinol*, 1996; **45**: 365–8.
55. Boehm TM, Burman KD, Barnes S, Wartofsky L. Lithium and iodine combination therapy for thyrotoxicosis. *Acta Endocrinol (Copenh)*, 1980; **94**: 174–83.
56. Reed J, Bradley EL III. Postoperative thyroid storm after lithium preparation. *Surgery*, 1985; **98**: 983–6.
57. Burman KD, Yeager HC, Briggs WA, Earll JM, Wartofsky L. Resin hemoperfusion: a method of removing circulating thyroid hormones. *J Clin Endocrinol Metab*, 1976; **42**: 70–8.
58. Candrina R, DiStefano O, Spandrio S, Giustina G. Treatment of thyrotoxic storm by charcoal plasmaperfusion. *J Endocrinol Invest*, 1989; **12**: 133–4.
59. Solomon BL, Wartofsky L, Burman KD. Adjunctive cholestyramine therapy for thyrotoxicosis. *Clin Endocrinol (Oxf)*, 1993; **38**: 39–43.
60. Enghofer M, Badenhoop K, Zeuzem S, Schmidt-Matthiesen A, Betz C, Encke A, *et al.* Fulminant hepatitis A in a patient with severe hyperthyroidism; rapid recovery from hepatic coma after plasmapheresis and total thyroidectomy. *J Clin Endocrinol Metab*, 2000; **85**: 1765–9.
61. Hughes G. Management of thyrotoxic crisis with a beta-adrenergic blocking agent (pronethalol). *Br J Clin Pract*, 1966; **20**: 579–81.
62. Feely J, Forrest A, Gunn A, Hamilton W, Stevenson I, Crooks J. Propranolol dosage in thyrotoxicosis. *J Clin Endocrinol Metab*, 1980; **51**: 658–61.
63. Rubenfeld S, Silverman VE, Welch KMA, Mallette LE, Kohler PO. Variable plasma propranolol levels in thyrotoxicosis. *N Engl J Med*, 1979; **300**: 353–4.
64. Ikram H. Haemodynamic effects of beta-adrenergic blockade in hyperthyroid patients with and without heart failure. *BMJ*, 1977; **1**: 1505–7.
65. Wiersinga WM. Propranolol and thyroid hormone metabolism. *Thyroid*, 1991; **1**: 273–7.
66. Brunette DD, Rothong C. Emergency department management of thyrotoxic crisis with esmolol. *Am J Emerg Med*, 1991; **9**: 232–4.
67. Knighton JD, Crosse MM. Anaesthetic management of childhood thyrotoxicosis and the use of esmolol. *Anaesthesia*, 1997; **52**: 67–70.
68. Kawakami-Tani T, Fukawa E, Tanaka H, Abe Y, Makino I. Effect of alpha-hydroxyvitamin D_3 on serum levels of thyroid hormones in hyperthyroid patients with untreated Graves' disease. *Metabolism*, 1997; **46**: 1184–8.
69. Benvenga S, Lapa D, Cannavo S, Trimarchi F. Successive thyroid storms treated with L-carnitine and low doses of methimazole. *Am J Med*, 2003; **115**: 417–18.
70. Benvenga S, Ruggeri RM, Russo A, Lapa D, Campenni A, Trimarchi F. Usefulness of L-carnitine, a naturally occurring peripheral antagonist of thyroid hormone action, in iatrogenic hyperthyroidism: a randomized, double-blind, placebo-controlled clinical trial. *J Clin Endocrinol Metab*, 2001; **86**: 3579–94.
71. Bennett MH, Wainwright AP. Acute thyroid crisis on induction of anesthesia. *Anaesthesia*, 1989; **44**: 28–30.
72. Kidess AJ, Caplan RH, Reynertson MD, Wickus G. Recurrence of ^{131}I induced thyroid storm after discontinuing glucocorticoid therapy. *Wis Med J*, 1991; **90**: 463–5.
73. Leow MK, Loh KC. Fatal thyroid crisis years after two thyroidectomies for Graves' disease: is thyroid tissue auto transplantation for postthyroidectomy hypothyroidism worthwhile? *J Am Coll Surg*, 2002; **195**: 434–5.

3.3.4 Subclinical hyperthyroidism

Jayne A. Franklyn

Definition

Subclinical hyperthyroidism is defined biochemically as the association of a low serum thyroid-stimulating hormone (TSH) value with normal circulating concentrations of free thyroxine (T_4) and free triiodothyronine (T_3). The biochemical diagnosis of subclinical hyperthyroidism is dependent upon the use of sensitive assays for TSH able to distinguish normal values found in euthyroid people from reduced values, so our understanding of this topic has accumulated in recent years since such assays became widely available. An expert panel has recently classified patients with subclinical hyperthyroidism into two groups (1): (1) those with low but detectable serum TSH (0.1–0.4 mU/l) and (2) those with undetectable serum TSH (<0.1 mU/l) reflecting the fact that studies of this condition largely divide people into these categories and that the likely consequences reflect the biochemical severity of the condition.

Causes, prevalence, and natural history of subclinical hyperthyroidism

The biochemical finding of low serum TSH in association with normal serum thyroid hormone concentrations may reflect an underlying thyroid disorder (Box 3.3.4.1) but low serum TSH often reflects other nonthyroidal illnesses or their treatment. Furthermore, in those with underlying thyroid disease, the cause of TSH suppression may be exogenous, i.e. reflecting thyroid hormone therapy, or endogenous, i.e. reflecting a degree of autonomous thyroid function.

People who have been treated for Graves' hyperthyroidism with antithyroid drugs, partial thyroidectomy, or radio-iodine may have suppression of serum TSH concentrations for months or occasionally years after restoration of a clinically euthyroid state and return of serum T_4 and T_3 concentrations to the reference range. In those who have received drug therapy alone for Graves' hyperthyroidism, suppression of TSH may serve as an early marker for relapse. The finding of persistent suppression of TSH may reflect the long period of recovery of pituitary thyrotrophs after removal of thyroid hormone excess, or may reflect a degree of persistent thyroid autonomy since suppression of serum TSH may be more common in those with persistent thyroid-stimulating autoantibodies and such individuals have higher circulating thyroid hormone concentrations, albeit within the reference range. Suppression of serum TSH is also common in those with Graves' ophthalmopathy but absent clinical and biochemical features of overt hyperthyroidism. In individuals with symptoms or signs suggestive of thyroid eye disease, the presence of suppression of serum TSH, together with the presence of thyroid autoantibodies, lends supporting evidence to the diagnosis of Graves' ophthalmopathy. A further group with a high prevalence of subclinical hyperthyroidism is that with thyroid enlargement. Up to 75% of patients with a nodular goitre have suppression of TSH (with normal serum T_4 and T_3) reflecting autonomous function of one or more thyroid nodules. Imaging studies, typically with ^{99m}Tc, reveal the presence of one or more 'hot' nodules with suppression of uptake of isotope into surrounding areas of the thyroid.

Box 3.3.4.1 Causes of subclinical hyperthyroidism

- Causes or associations related to thyroid disease and its treatment
  - Thyroxine therapy
  - Previous Graves' hyperthyroidism
  - Graves' ophthalmopathy
  - Nodular goitre
- Causes or associations related to nonthyroidal illnesses and drug therapy
  - Any significant illness, e.g. myocardial infarct, liver or renal failure, diabetes mellitus
  - Therapy with drugs such as glucocorticoids, dopamine, anticonvulsants
  - Iodine-containing compounds, e.g. amiodarone, radiographic contrast agents
  - Pregnancy, especially first trimester

The most common group with circulating TSH concentrations below the normal range is that prescribed thyroxine replacement therapy. One study of patients treated in primary care for hypothyroidism revealed reduction in TSH in 25%, this finding being most common in those prescribed thyroxine in doses of 150 μg/day or more (2). Similar findings have been reported in a large population-based study in the USA (3).

Nonthyroidal illness and therapy with a variety of drugs represent the other major associations with a biochemical diagnosis of subclinical hyperthyroidism. Illness itself may be associated with suppression of TSH through ill-defined effects upon the hypothalamic–pituitary axis, the inflammatory cytokine interleukin-6 being one factor implicated in the pathogenesis of the changes in tests of thyroid function found in hospital inpatients. A variety of pharmacological agents, particularly glucocorticoids and dopamine, are associated with low circulating concentrations of TSH, probably through direct inhibitory effects of these drugs on hypothalamic secretion of thyrotropin-releasing hormone and/or pituitary secretion of TSH. Iodine-containing compounds, most notably the antiarrhythmic drug amiodarone, may cause TSH suppression, as may anticonvulsants such as phenytoin. Suppression of TSH is also common in the first trimester of pregnancy, probably due to a rise in circulating human chorionic gonadotropin (which itself has a thyroid-stimulating effect). In nonthyroidal illness, the serum TSH value is typically low but detectable.

There have been several large population-based studies of the prevalence of subclinical hyperthyroidism and results vary depending upon the demographic features of the group examined, as well as the inclusion or exclusion of those with known thyroid disease or taking thyroid hormone therapy and the assay for TSH employed (see Chapter 3.1.7). The large NHANES III study in the USA (4) showed that endogenous subclinical hyperthyroidism is more common in women, in older people, and in black people compared with white people, with an overall prevalence in adults of 3.2% (cut-off serum TSH <0.4 mU/l) or 0.7% with undetectable TSH (TSH <0.1 mU/l). We recently conducted a prevalence study of almost 6000 community-dwelling people in the UK without known thyroid disease and aged more than 65 years. We found subclinical hyperthyroidism with low but detectable serum TSH in 2.1% and undetectable TSH in 0.7% (5). Exogenous subclinical hyperthyroidism is found in 10–30% of those prescribed thyroid hormones. In the Colorado study of more than 25 000 people, a serum TSH of <0.3 mU/l was found in 0.9% of those not taking thyroid hormones but 20.7% of those taking such medications (3).

The natural history of subclinical hyperthyroidism depends upon its cause and severity (in terms of the degree of reduction of serum TSH below the reference range). Some patients with TSH suppression associated with Graves' hyperthyroidism or nodular goitre will progress to overt hyperthyroidism, although the incidence is relatively low at around 1–3% per year. Most of these patients with an underlying thyroid disorder demonstrate complete suppression of serum TSH concentrations to below the limit of assay sensitivity (rather than TSH values below normal but still detectable) and when compared as a group with normal controls display higher mean circulating concentrations of T_4 and T_3, consistent with a minor degree of thyroid hormone excess. In contrast, those in whom low serum TSH values reflect nonthyroidal illness or drug therapy often have low but detectable serum TSH concentrations, as well as serum T_3 (and less frequently T_4 values) below the reference range, and in these patients the biochemical abnormality often disappears after recovery from illness or cessation of drug therapy. A recent large study demonstrated that serum TSH below 0.35 mU/l returns to normal in more than one-half of patients after a follow-up period of 5 years (6). We screened an ambulatory population of people aged over 60 years recruited in primary care and found that TSH values below normal were present in 6.3% of women and 5.5% of men (undetectable TSH in 1.5% of women and 1.4% of men). The follow-up of those patients with low serum TSH showed that of those with low but detectable TSH at initial testing, TSH had returned to normal in 76% of them at 1 year, compared with the group with undetectable TSH in whom 88% still had undetectable TSH at 1 year (7). A 10-year follow-up of the same group showed that only 4.3% of those with low serum TSH developed overt hyperthyroidism (8).

Consequences of subclinical hyperthyroidism

The often transient nature of the biochemical abnormality in those in whom reduction in TSH is associated with illness or drug therapy suggests that in this group the diagnosis of subclinical hyperthyroidism is of little consequence in terms of long-term effects. The potential consequences of subclinical hyperthyroidism are therefore probably confined to those in whom suppression of TSH reflects a minor degree of thyroid hormone excess, the major patient groups being those with thyroid autonomy due to the presence of a nodular goitre or Graves' disease and those receiving thyroxine replacement therapy. Unsurprisingly, any association with specific symptoms and signs is weak, although palpitation may be more frequent. We have reported a lack of association with cognitive dysfunction or symptoms of depression (9). Research has largely focused upon the effects of subclinical hyperthyroidism on bone metabolism and upon the heart, findings highlighting possible adverse effects upon these tissues and leading to debate about treatment of this biochemically defined condition.

Subclinical hyperthyroidism and bone metabolism

Overt hyperthyroidism is associated with an increase in bone turnover and a net loss of bone, while effective treatment is associated with restoration of bone metabolism to normal and an increase in bone mineral density (BMD). The increasing recognition of subclinical hyperthyroidism as a frequent biochemical finding has prompted many studies of the effect of more minor degrees of thyroid hormone excess upon bone metabolism and hence upon risk of osteoporotic fracture. The results of these studies have proved conflicting and their interpretation difficult because of the relatively small numbers of patients investigated, their heterogeneous nature (including those with previous goitre or hyperthyroidism), and relatively poor matching with controls in terms of factors which may modify BMD. Our own early studies of patients with thyroid disease and carefully matched controls suggested that subclinical hyperthyroidism secondary to T_4 therapy (even when administered in TSH-suppressive doses long-term) is not associated with significant reductions in BMD, in contrast to the situation in those with a past history of overt hyperthyroidism (especially postmenopausal women) in whom small reductions in BMD compared with controls are evident (regardless of the need for subsequent T_4 replacement therapy) (10, 11). Two meta-analyses of cross-sectional studies of BMD in those with subclinical hyperthyroidism secondary to long-term therapy with thyroxine have demonstrated small but significant effects upon BMD of T_4 given in doses associated with reduction in TSH, but only in postmenopausal women (12, 13).

Evidence that such changes in BMD are translated into an increase in risk of osteoporotic fracture, especially fracture of the femur, is so far relatively poor. T_4 usage was not associated with fracture in a case–control study of patients admitted to hospital with hip fracture (14). An important population-based study has examined prospectively risk factors for the later incidence of fracture of the femur in postmenopausal women. Thyroxine prescription was identified as a risk factor for fracture (RR 1.6; 95% CI 1.1 to 2.3) but this relative risk was no longer significant when a previous history of overt hyperthyroidism was taken into account, previous hyperthyroidism itself being associated with a relative risk of 1.8 (95% CI 1.2 to 2.6) (15). Even fewer studies have evaluated endogenous subclinical hyperthyroidism and fracture risk. In a study of 686 women aged over 65 years with low serum TSH levels, a three- to fourfold increased risk of hip or vertebral fracture was found after adjustment for previous hyperthyroidism and thyroxine prescription when compared with individuals with normal TSH levels (16).

While more large-scale prospective studies of the effects of T_4 treatment upon BMD and upon fracture risk are required to clarify the situation, it seems likely that subclinical hyperthyroidism secondary to mild thyroid hormone excess does result in a minor increase in bone loss and fracture risk. This risk is probably clinically significant only in postmenopausal women, reflecting an associated deleterious effect of oestrogen deficiency. Preliminary evidence suggests that adverse effects of thyroid hormone excess upon BMD can be reversed in this group by oestrogen replacement therapy, and perhaps by other agents such as bisphosphonates, but the role of such interventions in patients with subclinical hyperthyroidism has yet to be defined. One small study of postmenopausal women treated with methimazole to normalize serum TSH levels found that forearm BMD was increased after 2 years of treatment; however, another small prospective study in premenopausal women found no difference.

Effects of subclinical hyperthyroidism on the cardiovascular system

Subclinical hyperthyroidism has clear effects upon the cardiovascular system similar to overt hyperthyroidism, although these are less marked. These effects include an increase in nocturnal heart rate, shortening of the systolic time interval (a marker of left systolic ventricular function), and an increase in frequency of atrial premature beats. Left ventricular mass is typically increased. While the significance of these findings is unclear, more convincing evidence of harm has accrued from epidemiological studies examining atrial fibrillation and death from vascular diseases. In the Framingham cohort, a 3.1-fold increased relative risk for atrial fibrillation was evident after 10 years in elderly individuals (>60 years) with TSH levels of not more than 0.1 mU/l, whereas a relative risk of 1.6 was observed in those with low but detectable TSH (0.1–0.4 mU/l) (17). A large retrospective study demonstrated an adjusted relative risk of 2.8 for the finding of atrial fibrillation in individuals with low TSH levels when compared with those with normal TSH (18). The association between endogenous subclinical hyperthyroidism and atrial fibrillation is further supported by an important study showing an increased incidence of atrial fibrillation (approximately twofold) in elderly individuals followed for 13 years, which included evidence for an increased incidence in those with low, but detectable, TSH values (19). Furthermore, we performed a cross-sectional study of 5860 people aged 65 years and over and observed a higher prevalence of atrial fibrillation in participants with subclinical hyperthyroidism than in those with normal serum TSH (20). We also found that serum free T_4 was independently associated with the finding of atrial fibrillation by electrocardiogram, even in euthyroid individuals with normal free T_4 and TSH values (Fig. 3.3.4.1).

There is also evidence linking subclinical hyperthyroidism and mortality. We reported increased deaths from circulatory diseases (both cardiovascular and cerebrovascular) in association with low TSH in a 10-year study of 1191 individuals aged more than 60 years (8) (Fig. 3.3.4.2). This increased mortality occurred in the absence of increased deaths from other common causes. In very elderly people (>85 years), a Dutch study reported increased cardiovascular mortality during a 4-year follow-up in those with low levels (21). By contrast, another study of elderly people did not find increased mortality after adjustment for age and sex, despite positive findings for atrial fibrillation (19). Taken together, the evidence for an association of subclinical hyperthyroidism with mortality is less strong than for atrial fibrillation.

Again, preliminary evidence suggests that antithyroid treatment in those with endogenous subclinical hyperthyroidism may reverse adverse effects. A study of 10 patients examined the effect of 6 months of treatment with methimazole (median dose 20 mg daily) to restore TSH to normal and reported reduced heart rate and ectopic beats, and restoration of left ventricular mass index to that of euthyroid individuals (22). Another study of six women with subclinical hyperthyroidism and nodular goitre treated with radio-iodine to normalize serum TSH resulted in reduced heart rate and cardiac output. Unfortunately, no long-term studies have examined the effect of antithyroid drugs or radio-iodine treatment

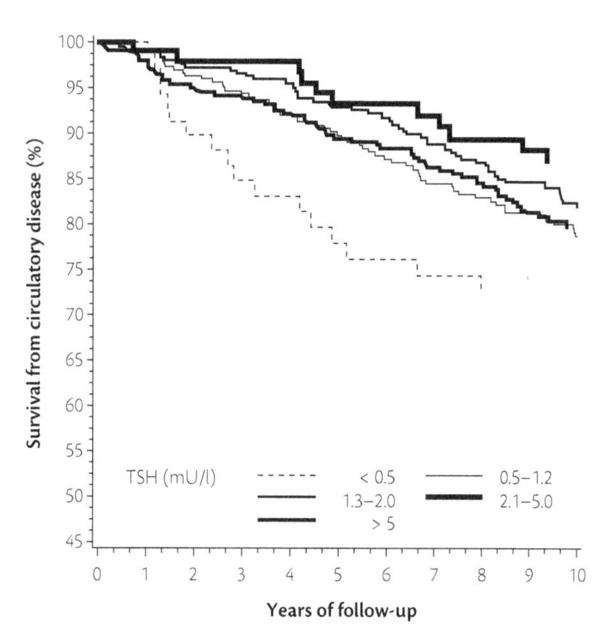

Fig. 3.3.4.2 Kaplan-Meier survival curves showing the relation between survival from circulatory disease and serum thyrotropin (TSH) concentration. (Reproduced from Parle JV, Maisonneuve P, Sheppard MC, Boyle P, Franklyn JA. Prediction of all-cause and cardiovascular mortality in elderly people from one low serum thyrotropin result: a 10-year cohort study. *Lancet*, 2001; **358**: 861–5.)

on the risk of atrial fibrillation or other clinically relevant endpoints such as mortality.

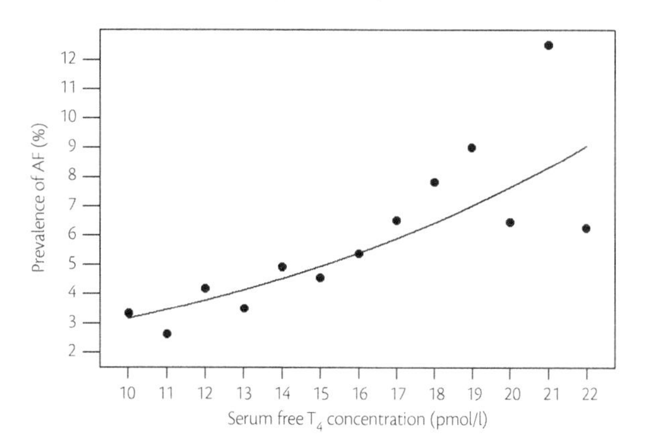

Fig. 3.3.4.1 Prevalence of atrial fibrillation (AF) on resting 12-lead electrocardiogram plotted against serum free thyroxine (T_4) concentrations in 5860 people aged 65 years and older. The plotted points were obtained by rounding each free T_4 measurement to the nearest integer; the superimposed curve is that given by a logistic regression on the actual values of free T_4 versus the presence/absence of atrial fibrillation. (Reproduced with permission from Gammage MD, Parle JV, Holder RL, Roberts LM, Hobbs FD, Wilson S, *et al.* Association between serum free thyroxine concentration and atrial fibrillation. *Arch Intern Med*, 2007; **167**: 928–34. Copyright © 2007 American Medical Association. All rights reserved.)

To treat or not to treat?

In patients taking thyroxine therapy, intervention is relatively simple, i.e. dose reduction followed by further biochemical testing to ensure that TSH has returned to the reference range. Whether this is a cost-effective exercise given the marked prevalence of T_4 prescription in the general population and so far inconclusive evidence for harm in the long term (with the possible exception of occurrence of atrial fibrillation) remains unclear. In patients starting T_4 therapy it appears appropriate to aim for biochemical as well as clinical euthyroidism, in line with both UK and US guidelines.

The question of intervention is even more complicated in those in whom suppression of TSH reflects autonomous thyroid function. Given the lack of substantive evidence that treatment of endogenous subclinical hyperthyroidism is beneficial, it is perhaps surprising that surveys of thyroid specialists in the USA and UK indicate that treatment is now regularly undertaken, typically with radio-iodine. Some clinicians argue that the evidence for harm associated with subclinical hyperthyroidism is sufficient to drive the need for treatment. As radio-iodine can induce hypothyroidism (with potential associated adverse outcomes) it would be preferable to await results of cost–benefit analyses before treatment is routinely offered. Meanwhile, treatment decisions might be tailored according to biochemistry or clinical factors. In light of the limited evidence linking low but detectable TSH concentrations with adverse outcomes, a consensus statement suggested that treatment should be considered only for patients with undetectable TSH (1). More contentious is the question of whether treatment should be confined to older people or those with atrial fibrillation, given the associations of subclinical hyperthyroidism with poor outcomes in these groups. This approach might be correct but it could be argued that young patients might eventually accrue the greatest benefit in terms of atrial fibrillation and fracture prevention and long-term survival. Further evidence is required to determine which is the correct approach.

Key points

- Subclinical hyperthyroidism is a biochemical diagnosis defined as reduced serum TSH with normal circulating thyroid hormone concentrations.
- Low serum TSH is very common and may reflect autonomous thyroid function (endogenous), subclinical hyperthyroidism, ingestion of thyroid hormones (exogenous), or a nonspecific influence of nonthyroidal illnesses or drug therapies.
- The pathophysiological consequences are different for these categories of subclinical hyperthyroidism and are more significant if TSH is fully suppressed (i.e. <0.1 mU/l) and reflects underlying thyroid disease.
- Subclinical hyperthyroidism is associated with reduced bone mineral density particularly in postmenopausal women. Evidence that this translates into fracture risk is limited.
- Subclinical hyperthyroidism is associated with increased risk of atrial fibrillation and a lesser degree of evidence supports association with cardiac failure and vascular mortality.
- Evidence that intervention (e.g. radio-iodine or antithyroid drug treatment) in endogenous subclinical hyperthyroidism results in improved outcome is lacking.
- There is an increasing trend to treat subclinical hyperthyroidism if it reflects underlying thyroid disease. Guidelines suggest that treatment should be considered in those at particular risk of adverse outcomes, e.g. older people and those with atrial fibrillation.

References

1. Surks MI, Ortiz E, Daniels GH, Sawin CT, Col NF, Cobin RH, *et al.* Subclinical thyroid disease: scientific review and guidelines for diagnosis and management. *JAMA*, 2004; **291**: 228–38.
2. Parle JV, Franklyn JA, Cross KW, Jones SR, Sheppard MC. Thyroxine prescription in the community: serum thyroid stimulating hormone level assays as an indicator of undertreatment or overtreatment. *Br J Gen Pract*, 1993; **43**: 107–9.
3. Canaris GJ, Manowitz NR, Mayor G, Ridgway EC. The Colorado thyroid disease prevalence study. *Arch Intern Med*, 2000; **160**: 526–34.
4. Hollowell JG, Staehling NW, Flanders WD, Hannon WH, Gunter EW, Spencer CA, *et al.* Serum TSH, T(4), and thyroid antibodies in the United States population (1988 to 1994): National Health and Nutrition Examination Survey (NHANES III). *J Clin Endocrinol Metab*, 2002; **87**: 489–99.
5. Wilson S, Parle JV, Roberts LM, Roalfe AK, Hobbs FD, Clark P, *et al.* Prevalence of subclinical thyroid dysfunction and its relation to socioeconomic deprivation in the elderly: a community-based cross-sectional survey. *J Clin Endocrinol Metab*, 2006; **91**: 4809–16.
6. Meyerovitch J, Rotman-Pikielny P, Sherf M, Battat E, Levy Y, Surks MI. Serum thyrotropin measurements in the community: five-year follow-up in a large network of primary care physicians. *Arch Intern Med*, 2007; **167**: 1533–8.
7. Parle JV, Franklyn JA, Cross KW, Jones SC, Sheppard MC. Prevalence and follow-up of abnormal thyrotrophin (TSH) concentrations in the elderly in the United Kingdom. *Clin Endocrinol (Oxf)*, 1991; **34**: 77–83.
8. Parle JV, Maisonneuve P, Sheppard MC, Boyle P, Franklyn JA. Prediction of all-cause and cardiovascular mortality in elderly people from one low serum thyrotropin result: a 10-year cohort study. *Lancet*, 2001; **358**: 861–5.
9. Roberts LM, Pattison H, Roalfe A, Franklyn J, Wilson S, Hobbs FD, *et al.* Is subclinical thyroid dysfunction in the elderly associated with depression or cognitive dysfunction? *Ann Intern Med*, 2006; **145**: 573–81.
10. Franklyn J, Betteridge J, Holder R, Daykin J, Lilley J, Sheppard M. Bone mineral density in thyroxine treated females with or without a previous history of thyrotoxicosis. *Clin Endocrinol (Oxf)*, 1994; **41**: 425–32.
11. Franklyn JA, Daykin J, Drolc Z, Farmer M, Sheppard MC. Long-term follow-up of treatment of thyrotoxicosis by three different methods. *Clin Endocrinol (Oxf)*, 1991; **34**: 71–6.
12. Faber J, Galloe AM. Changes in bone mass during prolonged subclinical hyperthyroidism due to L-thyroxine treatment: a meta-analysis. *Eur J Endocrinol*, 1994; **130**: 350–6.
13. Uzzan B, Campos J, Cucherat M, Nony P, Boissel JP, Perret GY. Effects on bone mass of long term treatment with thyroid hormones: a meta-analysis. *J Clin Endocrinol Metab*, 1996; **81**: 4278–89.
14. Wejda B, Hintze G, Katschinski B, Olbricht T, Benker G. Hip fractures and the thyroid: a case-control study. *J Intern Med*, 1995; **237**: 241–7.
15. Cummings SR, Nevitt MC, Browner WS, Stone K, Fox KM, Ensrud KE, *et al.* Risk factors for hip fracture in white women. Study of Osteoporotic Fractures Research Group. *N Engl J Med*, 1995; **332**: 767–73.
16. Bauer DC, Ettinger B, Nevitt MC, Stone KL. Risk for fracture in women with low serum levels of thyroid-stimulating hormone. *Ann Intern Med*, 2001; **134**: 561–8.
17. Sawin CT, Geller A, Wolf PA, Belanger AJ, Baker E, Bacharach P, *et al.* Low serum thyrotropin concentrations as a risk factor for atrial fibrillation in older persons. *N Engl J Med*, 1994; **331**: 1249–52.
18. Auer J, Scheibner P, Mische T, Langsteger W, Eber O, Eber B. Subclinical hyperthyroidism as a risk factor for atrial fibrillation. *Am Heart J*, 2001; **142**: 838–42.
19. Cappola AR, Fried LP, Arnold AM, Danese MD, Kuller LH, Burke GL, *et al.* Thyroid status, cardiovascular risk, and mortality in older adults. *JAMA*, 2006; **295**: 1033–41.
20. Gammage MD, Parle JV, Holder RL, Roberts LM, Hobbs FD, Wilson S, *et al.* Association between serum free thyroxine concentration and atrial fibrillation. *Arch Intern Med*, 2007; **167**: 928–34.
21. Gussekloo J, van Exel E, de Craen AJ, Meinders AE, Frolich M, Westendorp RG. Thyroid status, disability and cognitive function, and survival in old age. *JAMA*, 2004; **292**: 2591–9.
22. Sgarbi JA, Villaca FG, Garbeline B, Villar HE, Romaldini JH. The effects of early antithyroid therapy for endogenous subclinical hyperthyroidism in clinical and heart abnormalities. *J Clin Endocrinol Metab*, 2003; **88**: 1672–7.

3.3.5 Causes and laboratory investigations of thyrotoxicosis

Francesco Latrofa, Paolo Vitti, Aldo Pinchera

Introduction

The term thyrotoxicosis identifies the clinical syndrome caused by elevated circulating thyroid hormones of all sources, while the term hyperthyroidism includes only the disorders due to an increased secretion of hormones by the thyroid gland. Hyperthyroidism is the most frequent cause of thyrotoxicosis. Destructive processes involving the thyroid gland that induce unregulated discharge of preformed thyroid hormones (destructive thyrotoxicosis) and circulating thyroid hormone of extrathyroidal origin (exogenous or extrathyroidal thyrotoxicosis) are less common causes of thyrotoxicosis. Although careful history taking and physical examination often allows a diagnosis of thyrotoxicosis to be made, laboratory confirmation by measurement of thyroid-stimulating hormone (TSH) and thyroid hormone is always needed. Once thyrotoxicosis is confirmed, laboratory testing and thyroid imaging are required to identify the cause of thyrotoxicosis.

Causes of thyrotoxicosis

Classification

From a clinical standpoint it is useful to classify the different causes of thyrotoxicosis according to their pathogenic mechanisms. A practical classification is outlined in Table 3.3.5.1 and distinguishes the forms of thyrotoxicosis in two broad syndromes of thyroidal and of nonthyroidal origin. The first group, generally the most frequent, can be further divided into forms associated with thyroid hormone hypersecretion (hyperthyroidism) and forms characterized by the release of preformed hormones, secondary to destructive processes (destructive thyrotoxicosis). The second group includes a heterogeneous group of rare disorders in which the thyroid gland is not the primary source of thyroid hormone. The most useful test in differentiating hyperthyroidism from the other causes of thyrotoxicosis is thyroidal radioactive iodine uptake (RAIU), which is elevated or high to normal in hyperthyroidism and very low in destructive thyrotoxicosis and in thyrotoxicosis of nonthyroidal origin.

Table 3.3.5.1 Classification of known causes of thyrotoxicosis, with their distinctive diagnostic features and radioactive iodine uptake (RAIU) findings

Disease	Distinctive features	Neck RAIU
Thyrotoxicosis of thyroidal origin, associated with hyperthyroidism		
Graves' disease	Diffuse goitre Ophthalmopathy Positive TSHR autoantibodies	High
Toxic adenoma	Single 'hot' nodule at thyroid scan	High
Multinodular toxic goitre	Multiple 'hot' nodules at thyroid scan	High
Iodine-induced thyrotoxicosis	High urinary iodine	Low to high
TSH-secreting adenomas	Inappropriately high TSH level	High
Familial gestational hyperthyroidism	Pregnancy-associated DNA analysis	Presumably high
Trophoblastic tumours	High chorionic gonadotropin	High
Neonatal transfer thyrotoxicosis	Positive TSHR autoantibodies	High
Nonautoimmune congenital and familial hyperthyroidism	TSH receptor gene mutations by DNA analysis	High
Thyrotoxicosis of thyroidal origin, associated with thyroid destruction		
Subacute thyroiditis	Neck pain High ESR	Low
Silent thyroiditis	Positive thyroid autoantibodies	Low
Type 2 amiodarone-induced thyrotoxicosis	High urinary iodine High serum interleukin-6	Low
Thyrotoxicosis of nonthyroidal origin		
Factitious thyrotoxicosis	History Low serum thyroglobulin	Low
Thyroid hormone intoxication	History Low serum thyroglobulin	Low
Dermoid tumours (struma ovarii)	Abdominal RAIU	Low
Metastatic differentiated thyroid cancer	Bone RAIU	Low

TSH, thyroid-stimulating hormone; TSHR, thyroid-stimulating hormone receptor.

Causes of hyperthyroidism

Graves' disease

Graves' disease is the most frequent cause of hyperthyroidism, accounting for more than 70% of cases in iodine-sufficient countries, where its prevalence may be as high as 2% in women (1). In Graves' disease, hyperthyroidism is caused by an autoimmune reaction to the thyroid, leading to the production of autoantibodies to the TSH receptor (TSHR autoantibodies) (2). These antibodies mimic the action of TSH in stimulating the TSH receptor on thyroid follicular cells (TSHR-S autoantibodies). Since there is no feedback of thyroid hormone on the production of TSHR autoantibodies, uncontrolled stimulation of the receptor causes growth of the thyroid gland and excessive production and release of thyroid hormone, ultimately leading to hyperthyroidism.

TSHR autoantibody epitopes comprise discontinuous sequences of the polypeptide chain that are contiguous in the folded protein under native conditions (reviewed by Rapoport *et al.* (2)). Evidence that the shed TSHR ectodomain (primarily the A subunit) is the primary antigen driving affinity maturation of TSHR-S autoantibodies is mounting (3). TSHR autoantibodies with TSH binding inhibiting but not TSHR stimulating activity have been demonstrated in serum of individuals with no evidence of autoimmune thyroid diseases (4).

As the effect of TSHR-S autoantibodies is exerted on all follicular cells, a diffusely enlarged thyroid is the hallmark of the disease, but in some cases thyroid nodules can develop as a consequence of either a long-standing disease or of a pre-existing nodular goitre. Graves' ophthalmopathy and, rarely, pretibial myxoedema are other typical physical findings. The clinical manifestations of Graves' ophthalmopathy have been described elsewhere in this text. On careful physical examination, 30–45% of patients with Graves' disease have some signs of Graves' ophthalmopathy (5) and, when studied with refined imaging techniques, suggestive findings can be observed in up to 70% of cases. When obviously present, Graves' ophthalmopathy is extremely useful in supporting Graves' disease as the cause of thyrotoxicosis. Pretibial myxoedema is a peculiar skin manifestation of Graves' disease characterized by oedema, inflammation, and lymphocytic infiltration localized to the pretibial dermis. It is only rarely observed in Graves' disease, but almost never observed without it. Therefore, while its presence can confirm the diagnosis, its absence is by no means an exclusion criterion.

Toxic adenoma and multinodular toxic goitre

Toxic adenoma and multinodular toxic goitre are frequent causes of hyperthyroidism, especially in iodine-deficient areas. Toxic adenomas are benign isolated follicular tumours that synthesize thyroid hormones independently of TSH stimulation. One or more autonomous adenomas may develop in an otherwise normal thyroid. Unregulated thyroid hormone secretion first suppresses pituitary TSH secretion and eventually leads to overt hyperthyroidism. Because of TSH suppression, the extranodular thyroid tissue becomes functionally quiescent and may undergo some degree of atrophy. The incidence of toxic adenoma has been estimated at about 5/100 000 per year in Sweden (6). Toxic adenomas account for about 10% of the cases of thyrotoxicosis and are more common in areas of mild or overt iodine deficiency than in iodine-sufficient areas (7). Toxic adenomas tend to occur in the aged population and are more frequent in women than in men. The natural history of toxic adenoma is characterized by a slow growth over many years and a change, through different stages, of its functional properties. In the early phases, the amount of secreted thyroid hormones is not sufficient to completely suppress TSH secretion (partial autonomy) and the function of the extranodular tissue. With further growth of the nodule, TSH suppression becomes complete, while circulating thyroid hormones are in the upper range of normal values (complete autonomy). Eventually, overt thyrotoxicosis ensues, with frankly elevated thyroid hormone levels. The rate of progression is quite slow and in a large follow-up study, only 14 out of 159 autonomous nodules developed overt hyperthyroidism in 6 years, the risk being higher for adenomas more than 3 cm in size. Somatic mutations of the TSHR gene, which cause amino acid changes leading to constitutive activation of the TSHR, are the cause of 20–80% of toxic adenomas, while the rate of mutations of the Gsα-protein range from 8% to 75% (8). Both kinds of mutations cause permanent activation of the TSHR intracellular signalling pathway in the absence of TSH.

Multinodular toxic goitre is also often detected in iodine-deficient countries, in which accounts for up to 60% of cases of thyrotoxicosis (7). Epidemiological studies have clearly shown that multinodular toxic goitre represents the long-term outcome of many long-standing endemic goitres and is more common in older people and in women (7). The prevalence of multinodular toxic goitre in iodine-deficient areas has been reduced by iodine prophylaxis. The same somatic activating mutations of the TSHR demonstrated in toxic adenoma have been observed in toxic multinodular goitre (9, 10). However, in many nodules neither TSHR nor Gsα-protein mutations have been observed (8). The natural history of multinodular toxic goitre is similar to that of toxic adenoma, with the slow formation of multiple autonomously functioning nodular areas in the setting of an overall nodular goitre. The only known mechanism inducing subclinical hyperthyroidism and overt thyrotoxicosis is the administration of excessive amounts of iodine (11). Because of the slow progression through several degrees of thyrotoxicosis and because of their advanced age, patients with multinodular toxic goitre may report few symptoms.

Thyroid-stimulating hormone-secreting adenoma

TSH secretion by a benign pituitary adenoma, which is characterized by a partial or complete loss of the feedback regulation by thyroid hormones (central hyperthyroidism), causes a sustained stimulation of the thyroid gland, with the subsequent development of goitre and hyperthyroidism. TSH-secreting adenomas are rare, account for less than 1% of all pituitary adenomas, and have an estimated prevalence of about one case per million. However, its prevalence seems to have increased, probably as a consequence of the introduction of ultrasensitive assays for TSH measurement that enable an earlier detection of an inappropriate secretion of TSH (caused by a TSH-secreting adenoma or by resistance to thyroid hormones) (see below). TSH-secreting adenoma has a similar frequency in the two sexes and can be an expression of the multiple endocrine neoplasia type 1 syndrome (MEN 1). Most of the TSH-secreting tumours are macroadenomas (>10 mm), present with extrasellar extension, and show invasiveness into the surrounding tissues. Cosecretion of growth hormone and/or prolactin occurs in 25% of cases. TSH-secreting pituitary carcinomas and ectopic TSH-secreting adenomas are exceedingly rare.

The severity of thyrotoxicosis is extremely variable, ranging from slight to very high elevations of thyroid hormones. As a consequence, the patients may report no or few symptoms, or present as overtly thyrotoxic. On physical examination, a diffuse goitre is often felt, but multinodular goitres can also be observed, especially in long-standing diseases. Visual field defects can be rarely observed with large adenomas. When growth hormone and prolactin are cosecreted, acromegaly and galactorrhoea are present. Since most TSH-secreting adenomas are macroadenomas, involvement of other pituitary hormones and/or of the optic chiasm are common.

Human chorionic gonadotropin-dependent hyperthyroidism

Human chorionic gonadotropin (hCG) is secreted in large amounts by placental tissue in normal pregnancy and also by trophoblastic tumours (hydatidiform mole and choriocarcinoma). Due to its partial homology with TSH, hCG can act as a weak TSH agonist and, when present in large amounts in the bloodstream, can overstimulate the thyroid gland and induce hyperthyroidism.

Trophoblastic tumours

Hyperthyroidism may ensue in patients with a hydatidiform mole or a choriocarcinoma as a consequence of the large quantities of hCG produced by the tumour. Although thyrotoxicosis is common in trophoblastic tumours, clinically overt thyrotoxicosis is observed in a minority (10%) of patients in whom extraordinarily high levels of hCG (>3 000 000 IU/l) are found. The routine use of ultrasonography during pregnancy has led to earlier diagnosis of hydatidiform mole, when the tumour mass is smaller and the thyrotoxicosis less likely.

Hyperemesis gravidarum

Hyperemesis gravidarum is a poorly understood complication of early pregnancy, characterized by prominent nausea and vomiting, weight loss, ketosis, and electrolyte abnormalities. It occurs in 1.5% of pregnancies. In 25–75% of pregnancies, increased levels of thyroid hormones have been reported, which correlate with serum hCG concentrations. A clinically evident thyrotoxicosis (termed gestational hyperthyroidism) is rare (12).

Familial gestational hyperthyroidism

One family with an inherited hyperthyroidism that is exclusively associated with pregnancy has been reported (13). Hyperthyroidism was caused by a mutation in the *TSHR* gene causing increased responsiveness to hCG. Hyperthyroidism only manifests during pregnancy and recurs every time an affected woman becomes pregnant. The genetic defect does not have an effect in nonpregnant women and in men.

Fetal and neonatal transfer hyperthyroidism

TSHR-S autoantibodies in the serum of mothers with Graves' disease can cross the placenta and cause fetal and neonatal hyperthyroidism through direct stimulation of the fetal thyroid. The disease can be very severe and is characterized by tachycardia, jaundice, heart failure, and failure to thrive. A goitre is usually present. The disease is transient and resolves within 3 months after birth, when TSHR-S autoantibodies disappear.

Nonautoimmune congenital and familial hyperthyroidism

After the first report of congenital hyperthyroidism caused by a germline *de novo* activating mutation of the *TSHR* gene (14), only a few cases of nonautoimmune neonatal hyperthyroidism, resulting from mutations of the TSHR, inherited as an autosomal dominant trait or arisen *de novo*, have been described (15, 16). The diagnosis should be suspected when a neonate presents with severe hyperthyroidism and goitre and the mother has no history of Graves' disease.

Familial hyperthyroidism was described in 1994 (17). Autosomal dominant activating germline mutations of the *TSHR* gene are the cause of hyperthyroidism in this case, but since the effect of the mutation is mild, hyperthyroidism and goitre only develops in adults. Patients with the same mutation of the *TSHR* gene may present with wide phenotypic variability, with respect to the age of onset, severity of hyperthyroidism, and goitre (18). However, germline mutations of the *TSHR* gene have been reported to be uncommon in juvenile thyrotoxicosis (19). Cases of congenital hyperthyroidism from mutations of the Gsα-protein have also been reported and are associated with the McCune–Albright syndrome.

Causes of destructive (low RAIU) thyrotoxicosis

Subacute thyroiditis

Subacute thyroiditis (also called granulomatous, giant cell, or de Quervain's thyroiditis) is an inflammatory disorder of the thyroid, most probably of viral origin, which may last for weeks or months, predominates in females, and peaks in the fourth and fifth decades (see Chapter 3.2.7).

Painless thyroiditis

Painless thyroiditis (sporadic or silent thyroiditis), an autoimmune thyroid disorder, is characterized by a transient phase of thyrotoxicosis, similar to subacute thyroiditis, in the absence of neck pain and general symptoms. A goitre can develop or a pre-existing goitre can enlarge. At histology, a lymphocytic chronic infiltration closely resembling that of Hashimoto's thyroiditis is usually found. The incidence of painless thyroiditis has been reported to vary from less than 5% to 23% of all cases of thyrotoxicosis and is more prevalent in the third to the sixth decades of life. The female to male ratio is 2:1. In some cases, painless thyroiditis is precipitated by radiotherapy, iodine, and treatments with lithium, interleukin-2, interferon-α, and granulocyte colony stimulating factor. HLA-DR3 and HLA-DR5 are more common in patients with painless thyroiditis. Circulating thyroid autoantibodies are detected in the vast majority of cases. The thyrotoxicosis is usually mild and self-limited and can be followed by transient hypothyroidism. Progression to spontaneous permanent hypothyroidism is observed in as many as 20% of patients in the long-term follow-up. Sometimes clinical findings suggestive of painless thyroiditis are found in the presence of positive TSHR autoantibodies and high uptake, with goitre and rapid evolution in hypothyroidism. These cases may be classified as a variant of Graves' disease with predominant cytotoxic aspects, quickly leading to a clinical picture of Hashimoto's thyroiditis. Painless thyroiditis is seldom associated with Graves' ophthalmopathy.

Postpartum thyroiditis

Postpartum thyroiditis (PPT) is the painless thyroiditis that occurs in susceptible women within 12 months after delivery. It develops in 5–10% of pregnancies and is more common in women with type 1 diabetes. The presence of serum thyroid peroxidase (TPO) and thyroglobulin autoantibodies before or during the onset of the disease and the association with some HLA haplotypes (HLA-A26, -BW46, -DR3, -DR4, and -DR5) support the autoimmune pathogenesis of PPT (see Chapter 3.4.6).

Other forms of destructive thyrotoxicosis

Rarely, destructive thyrotoxicosis can be precipitated by anterior neck injuries. Thyrotoxic crises following thyroid surgery, a frequent complication in the early days of thyroid surgery, have now become extremely rare with the optimal use of antithyroid drugs and with the refinement of surgical procedures. Thyrotoxicosis may transiently worsen or recur in patients with Graves' disease, toxic adenomas, and multinodular toxic goitre who are treated with radio-iodine. Two mechanisms are responsible for this phenomenon: (1) ongoing thyroid hyperfunction before radio-iodine fully takes effect and (2) radiation-induced thyroid destruction.

Iodine-induced thyrotoxicosis and amiodarone

Iodine deficiency increases thyrocyte proliferation and mutation rates, inducing the development of multifocal autonomous growth and cell clones harbouring activating mutations of the TSHR. Some of these nodules maintain the ability to store iodine and can become autonomous causing thyrotoxicosis after iodine excess or even iodine supplementation. Because a pre-existing thyroid autonomy is required for the development of these disorders,

Box 3.3.5.1 Thyroid disorders predisposing to iodine-induced thyrotoxicosis

- Autonomous or pretoxic thyroid adenoma
- Nontoxic, autonomous, or pretoxic endemic multinodular goitre
- Euthyroid or 'latent' Graves' disease
- Graves' disease, in remission after or during antithyroid drug treatment

iodine-induced thyrotoxicosis is far more prevalent in elderly patients and in areas of iodine deficiency (Box 3.3.5.1). A transient, unavoidable increase in the prevalence of mild thyrotoxicosis has been well documented in iodine-deficient countries soon after carrying out iodine supplementation programmes with physiological doses of iodine. Another predisposing condition is euthyroid or latent Graves' disease or Graves' disease in remission. In individual thyrotoxic patients, iodine contamination may be caused by a variety of medications and diagnostics, including lipid-soluble contrast media, disinfectants, and drugs, and some foods containing large amounts of iodine (Box 3.3.5.2).

Among drugs, the antiarrhythmic amiodarone deserves a special mention because of the dual mechanism by which it can cause thyrotoxicosis. One tablet of 200 mg amiodarone contains approximately 75 mg organic iodide and will release about 8 mg free iodine, a tremendous amount when compared with the daily recommended dose of 200 μg. In iodine-deficient regions, where some elderly people have nodular thyroid autonomy, and in patients with euthyroid Graves' disease, this amount of iodine can precipitate hyperthyroidism (type 1 amiodarone-induced thyrotoxicosis) (20). However, in patients with no underlying thyroid disease, amiodarone can be directly cytotoxic to thyroid follicular cells *in vitro* (21) and can cause a form of subacute thyroiditis *in vivo* with the release of preformed hormones (type 2 amiodarone-induced thyrotoxicosis). Distinction between the two forms is useful for the appropriate treatment (20). Unfortunately, many patients present with a mixed form of thyrotoxicosis. The incidence of amiodarone-induced thyrotoxicosis ranges from 1% to 32%, being higher in regions with low iodine intake than in iodine-sufficient areas (20).

Box 3.3.5.2 Common sources of iodine contamination

- Foods
  - Seaweed and seaweed-containing foods (Japanese cuisine)
- Food supplements
  - Kelp and other seaweed derivatives
  - Vitamin supplements
- Radiological contrast agents
  - Intravenous and oral (diatrizoate, iopanoic acid, sodium ipodate)
- Antiseptics
  - Povidone-iodine
  - Iodoform gauze
- Drugs
  - Amiodarone
  - Expectorants
- Iodine solutions
  - Lugol's solution, SSKI, KI

Thyrotoxicosis of extrathyroidal origin

Thyrotoxicosis factitia

The term thyrotoxicosis factitia describes the voluntary excessive ingestion of thyroid hormone preparations with the purpose of mimicking thyrotoxicosis (Latin *factitius* = fake). However, the term has been widely applied to all forms of thyrotoxicosis due to the ingestion of thyroid hormones. True thyrotoxicosis factitia is most often observed in women with psychiatric disturbances who have access to thyroid medication, e.g. health professionals or people with relatives treated with thyroid hormones. Very often thyroid hormone is taken for weight reduction or to receive medical attention. Denial of thyroid hormone consumption may be extreme in these patients and the diagnosis is rarely obtained at history taking. Accidental or suicidal ingestion of large amounts of thyroid hormone has been also described, but this can usually be diagnosed by history alone. Sometimes, thyroid hormone is inadvertently taken as a component of 'herbal' or 'alternative' medications, usually for weight reduction. Finally, accidental grinding of cattle thyroids in hamburger meat has been reported as the cause of an outbreak of thyrotoxicosis among hamburger consumers in the USA (22).

Struma ovarii

Struma ovarii is a teratoma of the ovary that differentiates into thyroid cells. It comprises about 3% of ovarian teratomas, is bilateral in 10% of cases, and malignant in 10%. Thyrotoxicosis occurs in 10% of cases.

Functional metastatic thyroid carcinoma

Differentiated thyroid carcinoma, even when metastatic and with large tumour burdens, does not usually produce relevant amounts of thyroid hormones. Very rarely, however, thyroid carcinomas of the follicular histotype, extensively metastatic to bone, may cause thyrotoxicosis. Coexistent TSHR-S autoantibodies are an extremely rare cause of thyrotoxicosis in patients with metastatic thyroid cancer.

Laboratory diagnosis of thyrotoxicosis

Thyroid-stimulating hormone measurements

The mainstay of the diagnosis of thyrotoxicosis is measurement of serum thyroid hormones and TSH. Because of its high correlation with free thyroxine (T_4), TSH is the single most useful test in confirming the presence of thyrotoxicosis (23). The current immunoassays are very sensitive and can measure TSH levels well below the normal range, with a functional sensitivity (TSH concentration at which the response of the assay has a coefficient of variation of 20%) of less than 0.02 mU/l. Since pituitary TSH secretion is tightly down-regulated by thyroid hormone level, TSH is undetectable in most cases of thyrotoxicosis. The only remarkable exceptions are TSH-secreting adenomas, in which a high or inappropriately normal TSH level is found in spite of overt thyrotoxicosis. Because of the sensitivity of the assay, low (less than 0.4 mU/l) but detectable TSH levels can be found. These levels are encountered in subclinical thyrotoxicosis and in other conditions, such as nonthyroidal illnesses and endogenous or exogenous corticosteroid excess (Box 3.3.5.3). TSH is a heterogeneous molecule and different TSH isoforms circulate in the blood and are present in pituitary extracts used for assay standardization (24). Although current methods have eliminated cross-reactivity with other glycoprotein hormones, they may detect different epitopes of abnormal TSH isoforms secreted by some euthyroid individuals and some patients with pituitary diseases. Very rarely, the presence in the serum of antimouse immunoglobulin antibodies may interfere in the TSH assay, causing falsely elevated TSH levels.

Thyroid hormone measurements

Measurement of serum thyroid hormone levels is mandatory in all patients with suspected thyrotoxicosis for a proper evaluation of a low TSH level and for an estimation of the severity of the disease. The active form of the hormones in serum is the very small amount of freely circulating T_4 and triiodothyronine (T_3), which can enter cells, interacting with the specific receptors. Total T_4 and total T_3 can be easily and inexpensively measured by radioimmunoassay, but their levels are influenced by the levels of binding protein levels, which vary in healthy people and may change in several conditions (25). Thus total thyroid hormone levels may not parallel those of free thyroid hormones, and their measurement is nowadays considered less useful in the evaluation of thyrotoxicosis (24, 26). Measurements of free thyroid hormone levels, although not completely exempt from flaws, are more satisfactory, since they provide a more accurate measurement of the active hormone (27).

In iodine-sufficient countries a single measurement of free T_4 is sufficient to confirm or reject the suspicion of thyrotoxicosis and, after TSH measurement, this is the test most often used in North America for thyroid function screening (28). In contrast, in iodine-deficient countries, a significant proportion of hyperthyroid patients (up to 12%) may have elevated free T_3 and normal free T_4 levels, a condition termed T_3 toxicosis. Conversely, free T_4 can be falsely elevated in conditions causing reduced peripheral conversion of T_4 to T_3, such as amiodarone treatment. In our practice, when thyrotoxicosis is suspected, we initially assess both free T_4 and free T_3 levels together with TSH, with little additional expense, in order to obtain a complete assessment of the thyroid function status.

Subclinical thyrotoxicosis

Occasionally, a low or undetectable TSH level and normal free thyroid hormone levels are detected at routine thyroid function testing or in patients complaining of mild thyrotoxic symptoms. This condition is termed 'subclinical thyrotoxicosis' or 'subclinical hyperthyroidism' (29). This name is based on the recognition that even subtle variations in thyroid hormone levels can have a large effect on TSH secretion. In this respect, a low TSH level would be the first manifestation of a pending or subtle hyperthyroidism. However, the definition is somewhat unsatisfactory, since a subnormal TSH level can also be found in many nonthyroidal conditions, in the absence of true thyrotoxicosis, e.g. corticosteroid treatment, psychiatric and severe nonthyroidal illnesses, pregnancy, and others (Box 3.3.5.3). When biochemical findings suggest subclinical thyrotoxicosis, all of these conditions should be ruled out. Because of their high sensitivity, TSH tests now available can distinguish between partially (0.1–0.4 mU/l) and completely suppressed (<0.1 mU/l) TSH values.

Box 3.3.5.3 Causes of low serum TSH levels in the absence of thyrotoxicosis

- Nonthyroidal chronic or acute illness
- Starvation and malnutrition
- Pituitary diseases
- Hypercortisolism
- Endogenous depression
- Anorexia nervosa
- Early pregnancy
- Drugs
  - Dopamine agonists
  - Somatostatin
  - Glucocorticoids
  - Triiodoacetic acid

Laboratory investigations in the differential diagnosis of thyrotoxicosis

In many cases, history and physical examination can readily identify the cause of thyrotoxicosis. However, in many other situations, a careful differential diagnosis is needed in order to establish an aetiological diagnosis. Classically, RAIU has represented a mainstay of the differential diagnosis of thyrotoxicosis. RAIU is easily performed by administering a minimal (tracer) dose of radioactive iodine and then measuring the per cent of administered radioactivity accumulated in the neck. In iodine-sufficient countries the upper limit of RAIU, 24 h after the administration of the tracer, is around 25%, while it may reach 40% in areas with mild to moderate iodine deficiency (30). Whenever excessive active formation of thyroid hormone takes place in the thyroid gland, RAIU is increased, since the thyroidal machinery for iodine trapping and organification is activated. Therefore, a high RAIU readily identifies true hyperthyroidism (i.e. with thyroid hyperfunction). In contrast, thyrotoxicosis with a low RAIU indicates either thyroidal destruction, with release of preformed hormone, or an extrathyroidal source of thyroid hormone. In thyroid destruction, the damaged follicular cells transiently lose their capability of iodine trapping, while when exogenous hormones are administered in excess, the suppression of the pituitary secretion of TSH causes shutting-off of the trapping capacity of follicular cells. The only exception to this rule is iodine-induced thyrotoxicosis, in which a low RAIU can be observed because of dilution of the tracer dose in the large body pool of iodine, in spite of true hyperthyroidism.

Nowadays, RAIU is not universally performed in the initial assessment of a thyrotoxic patient and a vast array of laboratory and imaging techniques have provided excellent tools for accurately identifying the cause of thyrotoxicosis without the information provided by RAIU. RAIU is still useful in difficult cases to broadly define forms of thyrotoxicosis according to their pathogenesis in order to proceed methodically with adjunctive diagnostic tools.

Graves' disease

Thyroid-stimulating hormone receptor autoantibodies

Since the cause of Graves' disease hyperthyroidism is uncontrolled thyroid gland stimulation by circulating TSHR autoantibodies, their detection in the serum of thyrotoxic patients is particularly useful in establishing the diagnosis of Graves' disease. Serum TSHR-S autoantibodies can be measured by different methods (2, 31). They were originally detected with *in vivo* bioassays, and later by *in vitro* systems. The most common tests assess the displacement of labelled TSH or TSHR autoantibodies from the TSHR by the immunoglobulin fraction of patients' sera. These methods are termed TSH-binding inhibition (TBI) tests and do not distinguish between TSHR-S autoantibodies and TSHR blocking (TSHR-B) autoantibodies, which can also be detected in thyroid autoimmune disorders (2). TSHR-S autoantibodies can be tested in cellular systems carrying a functional TSH receptor, detecting the release of cAMP in the culture medium upon challenge with serum or purified immunoglobulins (TSHR-S autoantibodies assay) (2, 32). In a modification of the assay, TSHR-B autoantibodies can be detected as well (33). Since TSHR-S autoantibodies are properly the cause of hyperthyroidism in Graves' disease, their assay should be considered the gold standard in the diagnosis of Graves' disease. Unfortunately, the assay is quite expensive and requires cell-culture capabilities, making it available only to research centres. For clinical purposes, the TBI assays are most often used. By using the latest generation of assays, positive TBI tests are found in 75–95% of patients, with a high specificity (99%) (34). A TBI test is strictly needed in a minority of cases of Graves' disease in which the clinical picture is unclear, e.g. in the differential diagnosis of hyperemesis gravidarum, in the nodular variants of Graves' disease that must be differentiated from toxic nodular goitre, in patients with exophthalmos without thyrotoxicosis (euthyroid Graves' disease) (5), and in pregnant women with Graves' disease. The presence of high levels of TSHR autoantibodies at the end of antithyroid drug therapy has a high positive predictive value and specificity for relapse of hyperthyroidism but a low negative predictive value and sensitivity (35).

Whereas TSHR-S autoantibodies interact mainly with the N-terminal components of the ectodomain, TSHR-B autoantibodies interact to a greater extent with the C-terminus and to a lesser extent with the N-terminus and the midregion of the TSHR (2, 36). Accordingly, immunization of mice with the N-terminal component of the TSHR or with the TSHR holoreceptor generated preferentially TSHR-S and TSHR-B autoantibodies, respectively (37). Whereas the epitope(s) for TSHR-S autoantibodies are partially sterically hindered on the holoreceptor by the plasma membrane, those for TSHR-B autoantibodies are fully accessible (38).

Thyroid peroxidase and thyroglobulin autoantibodies

TPO autoantibodies can be found by commercial radioimmunoassays in up to 90% of patients with untreated Graves' disease (39), while Tg autoantibodies are less frequently positive, in about 50–80% of patients. Both autoantibodies, however, are also present in other forms of thyroid autoimmune disorders, some of which may cause thyrotoxicosis, such as postpartum thyroiditis and silent thyroiditis. A relatively high percentage (up to 25%) of positive thyroid autoantibodies tests is also found in normal individuals, especially women (40). Thus, TPO and Tg autoantibody tests do not establish the diagnosis of Graves' disease as the cause of thyrotoxicosis, but may be useful as complementary tests in confirming the presence of thyroid autoimmunity. The view that the binding of Tg autoantibodies from patients with autoimmune thyroid diseases is restricted to a few epitopic regions on Tg has been recently confirmed (41, 42).

The finding of autoantibodies cross-reacting with thyroglobulin and TPO in patients with autoimmune thyroid diseases, which suggested a role for cross-reactivity of the B-cell response to Tg and TPO (43), has not been confirmed (44). Thyroid autoantibody production requires the presence of thyroid autoantigens, as indicated by their disappearance after total thyroid ablation obtained by thyroidectomy plus ^{131}I treatment (45).

Other thyroid autoantibodies

Megalin (gp330) binds Tg with high affinity and participates in its transcytosis across thyroid cells (46). Autoantibodies to megalin were detected in 50% of patients with chronic autoimmune thyroiditis and in some patients with Graves' disease and thyroid carcinoma, but not in normal individuals (47). A role of the sodium-iodide symporter as autoantigen in thyroid autoimmunity has been proposed by some authors but excluded by others (48, 49).

Thyroid RAIU and scan

In untreated hyperthyroid Graves' disease patients, a high value of RAIU at 24 h is always found. As a distinctive feature, in some cases the 3- or 6-h value can be even higher than the 24-h value, as an expression of an extremely high iodine turnover. The test is very useful for ruling out transient thyrotoxicosis due to Hashitoxicosis or painless or subacute thyroiditis, factitious thyrotoxicosis, and type 2 amiodarone-induced thyrotoxicosis (20).

Thyroid imaging with radioisotopes can be performed with radio-iodine at the time RAIU is carried out or by using ^{99m}Tc pertechnetate. Thyroid scanning in Graves' disease is useful only when coexisting nodules are detected by palpation and their functional status needs to be evaluated.

Thyroid ultrasonography

The ultrasonographic appearance of the thyroid gland undergoes typical changes during Graves' disease hyperthyroidism. Because of the reduction in the colloid content and of the lymphocytic infiltrate, the gland becomes diffusely hypoechoic (50). A similar pattern is also observed in chronic goitrous thyroiditis and, when diffuse, indicates the presence of thyroid autoimmunity (51). Therefore thyroid ultrasound scanning can be useful in confirming the suspicion of thyroid autoimmunity, during the evaluation of thyrotoxicosis. Marked hypoechogenicity at the end of antithyroid drug therapy may predict recurrence of thyrotoxicosis (52). As an adjunctive value, thyroid ultrasound scanning also allows an accurate measurement of the goitre size (53), information that is important in the choice of the most appropriate treatment. Finally thyroid ultrasound scanning accurately distinguishes true thyroid nodules from the lobulations that can be occasionally felt at palpation in Graves' disease glands. The information provided by thyroid ultrasound examination is therefore quite useful in the initial evaluation of the Graves' disease patients, although not strictly needed from a diagnostic standpoint.

The measurement of blood flow to the thyroid gland by colour flow Doppler ultrasonography has been also used in Graves' disease patients. In untreated Graves' disease, the colour flow Doppler pattern is characterized by markedly increased signals with a patchy distribution (54, 55). Colour flow Doppler studies of the thyroid gland can therefore be used in the same way as RAIU in distinguishing Graves' disease from other forms of thyrotoxicosis, e.g. amiodarone-induced destructive thyrotoxicosis (56) or subacute thyroiditis and, possibly, painless thyroiditis.

Toxic adenoma

When a single nodule is palpated in the thyroid of a patient being evaluated for thyrotoxicosis, the presence of a toxic adenoma must always be suspected. In confirming the diagnosis of thyrotoxicosis, it is important to measure both free T_4 and free T_3 levels, since T_3 toxicosis is distinctly frequent in toxic adenomas (26). A blunted nocturnal TSH surge may be an early indicator of progression to hyperthyroidism in patients who are still euthyroid on baseline testing (57). ^{99m}Tc or radio-iodine thyroid scanning is extremely helpful in confirming the diagnosis, yielding typical findings. The nodule will appear 'warm', with the extranodular thyroid tissue clearly visible, when partial autonomy is present. In this case, parallel thyroid function tests will show a low but detectable TSH, and thyroid hormone levels in the upper part of the normal range. Only the nodule is visible on the scan when TSH is completely suppressed, e.g. in case of complete autonomy or of overt thyrotoxicosis. Ultrasound scanning of the neck provides no direct diagnostic information on the functional property of the nodule, but it is useful in detecting coexisting cold nodules and accurately defining the size of the nodule. Preliminary reports have shown a distinctive colour flow Doppler pattern in autonomously functioning thyroid nodules, characterized by an increased blood flow in the nodular tissue, in good correlation with radionuclide scans. However, the technique is not able to distinguish benign from malignant nodules (58) and is therefore of limited value. Ultrasound elastography has showed high sensitivity and specificity in differentiating benign from malignant thyroid nodules (59). Fine-needle aspiration biopsy is recommended in the initial evaluation of every solitary thyroid nodule, but often provides undetermined (follicular) neoplasm in hot nodules. The risk of malignancy in hot nodules is extremely low, although occasionally reported. Therefore, in the presence of a low TSH, fine-needle aspiration is only needed when coexisting nodules detected by palpation or ultrasonography are cold at radionuclide scanning.

Further imaging, such as neck radiographs, barium swallow, and CT scans, may be needed in selected patients with large nodules in order to evaluate the presence of significant tracheal and/or oesophageal compression. It is important to remember that CT scan, when done with this purpose, should always be performed without the administration of iodinated contrast media, since these may worsen thyrotoxicosis or precipitate it in the presence of partially autonomous nodules.

Toxic multinodular goitre

The same range of thyroid function test alterations described in toxic adenomas can be observed in toxic multinodular goitre, from a subnormal TSH level to an undetectable TSH level with frankly elevated thyroid hormone levels. The diagnosis of toxic multinodular goitre can often be suspected on history and physical findings. Thyroid radionuclide scanning is quite useful in identifying and mapping autonomous nodules and distinguishing them from other coexistent cold nodules. Scanning is also useful as an adjunct to TSHR autoantibody measurement in distinguishing true toxic multinodular goitre from Graves' disease hyperthyroidism which develops on a pre-existing nontoxic multinodular goitre. RAIU is always elevated, unless iodine overload is present, but sometimes is not necessary for establishing the diagnosis. Thyroid ultrasonography is also useful to measure goitre size and, in association with radionuclide scanning images, to identify cold nodules amenable to fine-needle aspiration biopsy. Fine-needle biopsy should be performed in any palpable dominant nodule that is cold at scan.

Thyroid-stimulating hormone-secreting adenoma

The presence of a TSH-secreting adenoma should be suspected when a detectable TSH level in the presence of clearly elevated circulating thyroid hormone levels (inappropriate secretion of TSH) is found. The first step in the evaluation of inappropriate secretion of TSH is making sure that artefacts in the measurement of TSH or thyroid hormone levels are not the cause of the laboratory findings. Falsely elevated TSH levels can be observed occasionally when heterophilic antibodies are present in the patient's serum. These antibodies are antimouse immunoglobulins that bind both the solid-phase and the labelled mouse antibodies employed in most TSH immunoradiometric assays, causing bridging between the two and therefore mimicking the presence of TSH (24). The problem can be overcome by incubating the patient's serum with mouse immunoglobulins before TSH testing, thus precipitating the heterophilic antibody (60). The most recent TSH commercial assays contain these antibodies in their incubation buffers, making this problem quite rare nowadays. Falsely elevated free T_4 and free T_3 levels must also be excluded in the preliminary evaluation of suspected inappropriate secretion of TSH. Mild spurious elevations of free T_4 and free T_3 can occasionally be found in the presence of thyroid hormone autoantibodies, genetic or drug-induced alterations of thyroxine-binding globulin, and in nonthyroidal illnesses (27). The two-step methods for measurement of free thyroid hormones may be useful to rule out these conditions. Once these artefacts have been excluded, extensive laboratory testing is required to clarify the cause of inappropriate secretion of TSH. True inappropriate secretion of TSH is observed in two conditions: (1) TSH-secreting pituitary adenoma and (2) resistance to thyroid hormone. In theory, only TSH-secreting adenomas cause true and symptomatic hyperthyroidism and therefore should be considered in the differential diagnosis (see below).

The syndrome of resistance to thyroid hormone is caused by a relative insensitivity of the thyroid hormone receptor to the action of its ligand. Therefore, higher thyroid hormone concentrations are needed to down-regulate TSH secretion. In most patients, the defect is due to mutations of thyroid hormone β-receptor gene and is inherited in a dominant autosomal fashion (61). Less common are *de novo* mutations of thyroid hormone β-receptor gene (22%) or resistance in the absence of thyroid hormone β-receptor gene mutations (7%). As a consequence of the defect, the pituitary set point for TSH suppression is set at a higher level of circulating thyroid hormone, i.e. a higher level of thyroid hormone is required for TSH suppression. Since the same abnormality is present at the tissue level, higher thyroid hormone levels are also required to exert normal peripheral thyroid hormone actions and the patient is therefore only biochemically hyperthyroid. The clinical picture is, however, more complex because some patients with resistance to thyroid hormone present with mild symptoms suggestive of thyrotoxicosis, especially tachycardia. As an explanation, the existence of a distinct syndrome of selective pituitary resistance to thyroid hormone has been proposed, in which normal tissue effects of thyroid hormone are present, in spite of insufficient TSH suppression, causing true peripheral thyrotoxicosis (62). The observation that similar thyroid hormone receptor abnormalities have been found in patients with the generalized and pituitary form of the disease and the absence of clinical features clearly distinguishing the two disorders, however, challenges this view and rather suggests that resistance to thyroid hormone encompasses a spectrum of manifestations, due to variable expression of the defect in different tissues (62). As in TSH-secreting adenomas, sustained TSH stimulation leads to the development of goitre, mostly diffuse, but some distinctive clinical features can be found, such as skeletal abnormalities and hearing defects (61).

Differential diagnosis

When the suspicion of inappropriate secretion of TSH is confirmed, the presence of a TSH-secreting adenoma must be differentiated from resistance to thyroid hormone. Because of the overlapping clinical presentation and because no single test accurately allows clear-cut differentiation between the two conditions, extensive baseline and dynamic laboratory testing is usually required.

A number of tests have been used to confirm the presence of thyrotoxicosis at the tissue level. Nocturnal heart rate, Achilles reflexometry, and other indirect measures of peripheral thyroid hormone actions have been used for this purpose (63), but are cumbersome and not sensitive enough, especially when only mild elevations of thyroid hormones are present. The presence of thyrotoxicosis at the tissue level can be documented by measuring a variety of biochemical markers of thyrotoxicosis such as sex hormone-binding globulin, alkaline phosphatase, cholesterol, and creatine phosphokinase (63). Unfortunately, these parameters are quite nonspecific and may be elevated (or reduced) in a number of other conditions. At variance with normal pituitary, TSH-secreting adenomas secrete the α-subunit of TSH in molar excess with respect to TSH. A serum α-subunit/TSH ratio of more than 1 is observed in approximately 90% of patients with TSH-secreting adenoma (64). High ratios can also be observed in postmenopausal women and even in normal individuals, making this test alone unable to establish the diagnosis. Growth hormone, insulin growth factor-I, and prolactin serum measurements are useful, since about 30% of TSH-secreting adenomas cosecrete growth hormone and prolactin.

Dynamic testing aims at the demonstration of the unresponsiveness of TSH-secreting adenomas to normal stimuli. In most (92%) TSH-secreting tumours, the TSH level fails to increase in response to a standard thyrotropin-releasing hormone (TRH) stimulation test, while a normal or increased response is observed in resistance to thyroid hormone (64). A diagnostic protocol to test the response of pituitary TSH to exogenous T_3 is also used. T_3 is administered orally and the dose is increased every 3 days, starting from 50 μg/daily and increasing to 200 μg/daily (65). Before every increase, basal and TRH-stimulated TSH is measured, together with peripheral markers of thyroid hormone action (65). In TSH-secreting adenomas, only partial or no suppression of TSH secretion is observed, while complete or partial suppression is observed in resistance to thyroid hormone. Alternatively, 80–100 μg T_3 can be administered for 8–10 days. Using this protocol, complete TSH suppression is obtained in normal individuals, while no changes or slight reduction in TSH levels are observed in all patients with TSH-secreting adenomas. In contrast, clear-cut reductions of TSH levels are observed in resistance to thyroid hormone patients (64). The test is contraindicated in elderly patients and in patients with arrhythmias and/or coronary artery disease. Available tests for the differential diagnosis of the syndrome of inappropriate secretion of TSH are given in Table 3.3.5.2.

Pituitary imaging is very important in confirming the diagnosis. Ninety per cent of TSH-secreting adenomas are more than 1 cm in diameter at diagnosis and therefore easily detected at pituitary MRI scanning (64). In addition, radiolabelled-octreotide pituitary scintigraphy can be useful in detecting small tumours (66), although it can be positive in other types of pituitary tumours.

Human chorionic gonadotropin-dependent thyrotoxicosis

The presence of a trophoblastic tumour should be suspected when thyrotoxicosis is found in an amenorrhoeic woman, especially when a palpable abdominal mass is found. The diagnosis is readily confirmed by the finding of extremely high circulating hCG levels and of a pelvic mass at ultrasonography. In trophoblastic tumours, serum hCG levels usually exceed 200 U/ml, whereas the peak concentration for normal pregnant women is 100 U/ml.

The diagnosis of thyrotoxicosis during hyperemesis gravidarum can be particularly challenging and it is one of exclusion. Because of weight loss and malnutrition, free T_3 levels may be disproportionately low or even normal in comparison with free T_4 levels, due to a reduced peripheral conversion of T_4 to T_3. The TSH level is often low during early normal pregnancy, but seldom undetectable, as it is in true thyrotoxicosis. The only distinctive laboratory feature is an inappropriately high hCG level, but large overlap with normal pregnancies exists. Therefore, the diagnosis of thyrotoxicosis in hyperemesis gravidarum relies mainly on the clinical picture and

Table 3.3.5.2 Laboratory investigations in the differential diagnosis of the syndrome of inappropriate secretion of TSH

Test	TSH-secreting adenomas	Resistance to thyroid hormone	Comment
Peripheral markers of thyroid hormone action	High	Normal to high	Nonspecific
α-subunit/TSH molar ratio	>1	1	High in menopause
TSH after T_3 suppression test	Unchanged or slightly reduced	Frankly reduced or suppressed	Hazardous in elderly and cardiopathic patients
TSH after TRH	Unchanged	Increased	
Pituitary imaging	Positive	Negative	Confirmatory

TRH, thyrotropin-releasing hormone; TSH, thyroid-stimulating hormone.

on appropriate exclusion of other more common forms of hyperthyroidism by appropriate testing. It is important to remember that RAIU is absolutely contraindicated in pregnancy, as is any other *in vivo* radioisotopic procedure.

Fetal and neonatal hyperthyroidism

Mothers with a past or present history of Graves' disease should be carefully monitored throughout pregnancy. Fetuses of mothers who have been previously treated with radio-iodine or surgery are at high risk because they lack the protective effect of antithyroid drugs administered to the mother. The presence of a fetal heart rate above 160 beats/min, in the absence of other fetal abnormalities, is suggestive of fetal hyperthyroidism. The persistence of high levels of TSHR autoantibodies in the maternal serum by the end of pregnancy, when the transplacental passage is maximal, is a predictor of hyperthyroidism in the neonate. Fetal cord blood sampling has been performed to diagnose fetal hyperthyroidism, but it is a risky procedure and is not generally recommended. In contrast, it is very useful to test neonatal cord blood at the time of delivery for thyroid function tests and TSHR autoantibodies. When the mother has been treated with high-dose antithyroid drugs, the neonate should be retested 10 days after birth, since transplacental passage of methimazole or propylthiouracil may initially mask hyperthyroidism.

Neonatal hyperthyroidism in the absence of a maternal history of Graves' disease and with negative TSHR autoantibodies should raise the suspicion of nonautoimmune congenital hyperthyroidism. Familiar hyperthyroidism should be suspected when relatives are affected and serum TSHR autoantibodies are absent. In both types of hyperthyroidism, sequencing of the TSHR gene is required to confirm the diagnosis.

Iodine-induced thyrotoxicosis

Excessive iodine consumption should be always suspected when hyperthyroidism abruptly appears in a patient with a history of nodular thyroid disease. A careful history often identifies the source of iodine and all patients should be asked about recent consumption of any of the compounds listed in Box 3.3.5.2. With the exception of type 2 amiodarone-induced thyrotoxicosis, RAIU is usually low in thyrotoxic patients with heavy iodine contamination, but it is almost never suppressed, a feature that allows distinction from subacute and painless thyroiditis. The iodine/creatinine urinary ratio is, however, the gold standard in confirming iodine contamination and will be high in all cases.

Amiodarone-induced thyrotoxicosis

When a history of taking amiodarone is elicited in a thyrotoxic patient, further testing is required to distinguish between the type 1 and type 2 forms of amiodarone-induced thyrotoxicosis, since treatment may be radically different (20). Type 1 (nondestructive) amiodarone-induced thyrotoxicosis differs little from other forms of iodine-induced thyrotoxicosis and an underlying thyroid disease such as Graves' disease or nodular thyroid disease is usually detected with the appropriate diagnostic tools. Accordingly, RAIU is usually low, but not suppressed and may be normal or increased. In contrast, in type 2 (destructive) amiodarone-induced thyrotoxicosis, RAIU is always low or suppressed and often no clear underlying thyroid disorder can be identified. High circulating interleukin-6 levels have been proposed as a useful marker of thyroid tissue destruction. In type 2 amiodarone-induced thyrotoxicosis, colour flow Doppler ultrasonography shows a distinctive absence of vascularization in the gland (56).

Subacute, painless, and postpartum thyroiditis

Classically, subacute, painless, and postpartum thyroiditis are characterized by a low (<1%) RAIU during the thyrotoxic phase. This test alone, in the presence of a suggestive clinical presentation allows the diagnosis in almost all cases. Serum T_4 concentration is disproportionately elevated compared with T_3 concentration, reflecting the preferential release of T_4 from the injured thyroid. In subacute thyroiditis, a very high (always >50 mm/h and often >100 mm/h) ESR is a distinctive diagnostic feature. C-reactive protein is also elevated and a mild leucocytosis is often observed. High titres of TPO and Tg autoantibodies are usually found in postpartum and painless thyroiditis, as a marker of prominent thyroid autoimmunity, while only weakly and transiently positive tests are occasionally found in subacute thyroiditis. Ultrasonographic findings are generally characterized by patchy areas of hypoechogenicity in subacute thyroiditis, while a more diffuse hypoechoic pattern, closely resembling Hashimoto's thyroiditis is found in postpartum and painless thyroiditis. The colour flow Doppler pattern shows reduced vascularity in the three disorders. Occasionally, and especially when patients are first seen in the recovery or hypothyroid phase, a more subtle picture can emerge from testing with a low but not nil RAIU, and with only mild elevations of ESR, making the differential diagnosis more difficult.

Thyrotoxicosis of extrathyroidal origin

An extrathyroidal source of thyroid hormone should be suspected when more frequent causes of low RAIU thyrotoxicosis have been ruled out. When factitia thyrotoxicosis is suspected, a serum Tg measurement can be extremely useful in confirming the diagnosis, since this disorder represents the only condition in which thyrotoxicosis is associated with an undetectable Tg level (67). At the time of Tg measurement, however, it is important to test the patient's serum for Tg autoantibodies, since these may cause falsely low Tg levels. Given the high prevalence of thyroid nodularities in the general population, especially in iodine-deficient areas, it is also useful to perform ultrasound scanning of the neck, since, in the presence of thyroid nodules, Tg may be elevated in spite of the ingestion of exogenous thyroid hormone. Colour flow Doppler ultrasonography shows hypervascularity of the thyroid in Graves' disease and in toxic nodular goitre, and hypovascularity in factitious thyrotoxicosis.

The suspicion of struma ovarii can be confirmed at the time of RAIU, simply by scanning the pelvic area with the probe. The presence of functional thyroid tissue is demonstrated by a significantly increased uptake of iodine in the ovarian region. Further imaging (CT or ultrasound scan) will confirm the presence of an ovarian mass. The levels of CA 125 are elevated in both malignant and benign tumours.

When the source of thyroid hormone is metastatic thyroid follicular cancer, the presence of the latter is usually evident from the history. Since all patients with differentiated thyroid cancer after thyroidectomy take L-thyroxine in TSH-suppressive doses, thyroid function tests should be repeated after withdrawal of the medication in order to rule out iatrogenic thyrotoxicosis. Confirmation is obtained with whole body radio-iodine scanning that will show multiple foci of uptake in several skeletal regions.

References

1. Hollowell JG, Staehling NW, Flanders WD, Hannon WH, Gunter EW, Spencer CA, *et al.* Serum TSH, T(4), and thyroid antibodies in the United States population (1988 to 1994): National Health and Nutrition Examination Survey (NHANES III). *J Clin Endocrinol Metab*, 2002; **87**: 489–99.
2. Rapoport B, Chazenbalk GD, Jaume JC, McLachlan SM. The thyrotropin (TSH) receptor: interaction with TSH and autoantibodies. *Endocr Rev*, 1998; **19**: 673–716.
3. Mizutori Y, Chen CR, Latrofa F, McLachlan SM, Rapoport B. Evidence that shed thyrotropin receptor A subunits drive affinity maturation of autoantibodies causing Graves' disease. *J Clin Endocrinol Metab*, 2009; **94**: 927–35.
4. Latrofa F, Chazenbalk GD, Pichurin P, Chen CR, McLachlan SM, Rapoport B. Affinity-enrichment of thyrotropin receptor autoantibodies from Graves' patients and normal individuals provides insight into their properties and possible origin from natural antibodies. *J Clin Endocrinol Metab*, 2004; **89**: 4734–45.
5. Bartalena L, Pinchera A, Marcocci C. Management of Graves' ophthalmopathy: reality and perspectives. *Endocr Rev*, 2000; **21**: 168–99.
6. Berglund J, Christensen SB, Hallengren B. Total and age-specific incidence of Graves' thyrotoxicosis, toxic nodular goiter and solitary toxic adenoma in Malmo 1970–74. *J Intern Med*, 1990; **227**: 137–41.
7. Laurberg P, Pedersen KM, Vestergaard H, Sigurdsson G. High incidence of multinodular toxic goiter in the elderly population in a low iodine intake area vs. high incidence of Graves' disease in the young in a high iodine intake area: comparative surveys of thyrotoxicosis epidemiology in East-Jutland Denmark and Iceland. *J Intern Med*, 1991; **229**: 415–20.
8. Krohn K, Fuhrer D, Bayer Y, Eszlinger M, Brauer V, Neumann S, *et al.* Molecular pathogenesis of euthyroid and toxic multinodular goiter. *Endocr Rev*, 2005; **26**: 504–24.
9. Tonacchera M, Chiovato L, Pinchera A, Agretti P, Fiore E, Cetani F, *et al.* Hyperfunctioning thyroid nodules in toxic multinodular goiter share activating thyrotropin receptor mutations with solitary toxic adenoma. *J Clin Endocrinol Metab*, 1998; **83**: 492–8.
10. Tonacchera M, Agretti P, Chiovato L, Rosellini V, Ceccarini G, Perri A, *et al.* Activating thyrotropin receptor mutations are present in nonadenomatous hyperfunctioning nodules of toxic or autonomous multinodular goiter. *J Clin Endocrinol Metab*, 2000; **85**: 2270–4.
11. Aghini-Lombardi F, Antonangeli L, Martino E, Vitti P, Maccherini D, Leoli F, *et al.* The spectrum of thyroid disorders in an iodine-deficient community: the Pescopagano survey. *J Clin Endocrinol Metab*, 1999; **84**: 561–6.
12. Goodwin TM, Montoro M, Mestman JH, Pekary AE, Hershman JM. The role of chorionic gonadotropin in transient hyperthyroidism of hyperemesis gravidarum. *J Clin Endocrinol Metab*, 1992; **75**: 1333–7.
13. Rodien P, Bremont C, Sanson ML, Parma J, Van Sande J, Costagliola S, *et al.* Familial gestational hyperthyroidism caused by a mutant thyrotropin receptor hypersensitive to human chorionic gonadotropin. *N Engl J Med*, 1998; **339**: 1823–6.
14. Kopp P, Van Sande J, Parma J, Duprez L, Gerber H, Joss E, *et al.* Brief report: congenital hyperthyroidism caused by a mutation in the thyrotropin-receptor gene. *N Engl J Med*, 1995; **332**: 150–4.
15. Tonacchera M, Agretti P, Rosellini V, Ceccarini G, Perri A, Zampolli M, *et al.* Sporadic nonautoimmune congenital hyperthyroidism due to a strong activating mutation of the thyrotropin receptor gene. *Thyroid*, 2000; **10**: 859–63.
16. Chester J, Rotenstein D, Ringkananont U, Steuer G, Carlin B, Stewart L, *et al.* Congenital neonatal hyperthyroidism caused by germline mutations in the TSH receptor gene. *J Pediatr Endocrinol Metab*, 2008; **21**: 479–86.
17. Duprez L, Parma J, Van Sande J, Allgeier A, Leclere J, Schvartz C, *et al.* Germline mutations in the thyrotropin receptor gene cause non-autoimmune autosomal dominant hyperthyroidism. *Nat Genet*, 1994; **7**: 396–401.
18. Akcurin S, Turkkahraman D, Tysoe C, Ellard S, De Leener A, Vassart G, *et al.* A family with a novel TSH receptor activating germline mutation (p.Ala485Val). *Eur J Pediatr*, 2008; **167**: 1231–7.
19. Tonacchera M, Perri A, De Marco G, Agretti P, Banco ME, Di Cosmo C, *et al.* Low prevalence of thyrotropin receptor mutations in a large series of subjects with sporadic and familial nonautoimmune subclinical hypothyroidism. *J Clin Endocrinol Metab*, 2004; **89**: 5787–93.
20. Martino E, Bartalena L, Bogazzi F, Braverman LE. The effects of amiodarone on the thyroid. *Endocr Rev*, 2001; **22**: 240–54.
21. Chiovato L, Martino E, Tonacchera M, Santini F, Lapi P, Mammoli C, *et al.* Studies on the in vitro cytotoxic effect of amiodarone. *Endocrinology*, 1994; **134**: 2277–82.
22. Hedberg CW, Fishbein DB, Janssen RS, Meyers B, McMillen JM, MacDonald KL, *et al.* An outbreak of thyrotoxicosis caused by the consumption of bovine thyroid gland in ground beef. *N Engl J Med*, 1987; **316**: 993–8.
23. Spencer CA, LoPresti JS, Patel A, Guttler RB, Eigen A, Shen D, *et al.* Applications of a new chemiluminometric thyrotropin assay to subnormal measurement. *J Clin Endocrinol Metab*, 1990; **70**: 453–60.
24. Baloch Z, Carayon P, Conte-Devolx B, Demers LM, Feldt-Rasmussen U, Henry JF, *et al.* Laboratory medicine practice guidelines. Laboratory support for the diagnosis and monitoring of thyroid disease. *Thyroid*, 2003; **13**: 3–126.
25. Refetoff S. Inherited thyroxine-binding globulin abnormalities in man. *Endocr Rev*, 1989; **10**: 275–93.
26. Bartalena L, Bogazzi F, Brogioni S, Burelli A, Scarcello G, Martino E. Measurement of serum free thyroid hormone concentrations: an essential tool for the diagnosis of thyroid dysfunction. *Horm Res*, 1996; **45**: 142–7.
27. Ekins R. Measurement of free hormones in blood. *Endocr Rev*, 1990; **11**: 5–46.
28. Singer PA, Cooper DS, Levy EG, Ladenson PW, Braverman LE, Daniels G, *et al.* Treatment guidelines for patients with hyperthyroidism and hypothyroidism. Standards of Care Committee, American Thyroid Association. *JAMA*, 1995; **273**: 808–12.
29. Pinchera A. Subclinical thyroid disease: to treat or not to treat?. *Thyroid*, 2005; **15**: 1–2.
30. O'Hare NJ, Murphy D, Malone JF. Thyroid dosimetry of adult European populations. *Br J Radiol*, 1998; **71**: 535–43.
31. Vitti P, Elisei R, Tonacchera M, Chiovato L, Mancusi F, Rago T, *et al.* Detection of thyroid-stimulating antibody using Chinese hamster ovary cells transfected with cloned human thyrotropin receptor. *J Clin Endocrinol Metab*, 1993; **76**: 499–503.
32. Vitti P, Chiovato L, Fiore E, Mammoli C, Rocchi R, Pinchera A. Use of cells expressing the human thyrotropin (TSH) receptor for the measurement of thyroid stimulating and TSH-blocking antibodies. *Acta Med Austriaca*, 1996; **23**: 52–6.
33. Chiovato L, Vitti P, Bendinelli G, Santini F, Fiore E, Capaccioli A, *et al.* Detection of antibodies blocking thyrotropin effect using Chinese hamster ovary cells transfected with the cloned human TSH receptor. *J Endocrinol Invest*, 1994; **17**: 809–16.
34. Costagliola S, Morgenthaler NG, Hoermann R, Badenhoop K, Struck J, Freitag D, *et al.* Second generation assay for thyrotropin receptor antibodies has superior diagnostic sensitivity for Graves' disease. *J Clin Endocrinol Metab*, 1999; **84**: 90–7.
35. Vitti P, Rago T, Chiovato L, Pallini S, Santini F, Fiore E, *et al.* Clinical features of patients with Graves' disease undergoing remission after antithyroid drug treatment. *Thyroid*, 1997; **7**: 369–75.
36. Schwarz-Lauer L, Chazenbalk GD, McLachlan SM, Ochi Y, Nagayama Y, Rapoport B. Evidence for a simplified view of autoantibody interactions with the thyrotropin receptor. *Thyroid*, 2002; **12**: 115–20.
37. Chen CR, Pichurin P, Nagayama Y, Latrofa F, Rapoport B, McLachlan SM. The thyrotropin receptor autoantigen in Graves' disease is the culprit as well as the victim. *J Clin Invest*, 2003; **111**: 1897–904.

38. Chazenbalk GD, Pichurin P, Chen CR, Latrofa F, Johnstone AP, McLachlan SM, *et al.* Thyroid-stimulating autoantibodies in Graves' disease preferentially recognize the free A subunit, not the thyrotropin holoreceptor. *J Clin Invest*, 2002; **110**: 209–17.
39. Mariotti S, Caturegli P, Piccolo P, Barbesino G, Pinchera A. Antithyroid peroxidase autoantibodies in thyroid diseases. *J Clin Endocrinol Metab*, 1990; **71**: 661–9.
40. Mariotti S, Sansoni P, Barbesino G, Caturegli P, Monti D, Cossarizza A, *et al.* Thyroid and other organ-specific autoantibodies in healthy centenarians. *Lancet*, 1992; **339**: 1506–8.
41. Latrofa F, Phillips M, Rapoport B, McLachlan SM. Human monoclonal thyroglobulin autoantibodies: epitopes and immunoglobulin genes. *J Clin Endocrinol Metab*, 2004; **89**: 5116–23.
42. Latrofa F, Ricci D, Grasso L, Vitti P, Masserini L, Basolo F, *et al.* Characterization of thyroglobulin epitopes in patients with autoimmune and non-autoimmune thyroid diseases using recombinant human monoclonal thyroglobulin autoantibodies. *J Clin Endocrinol Metab*, 2008; **93**: 591–6.
43. Ruf J, Carayon P. The molecular recognition theory applied to bispecific antibodies. *Nat Med*, 1995; **1**: 1222.
44. Latrofa F, Pichurin P, Guo J, Rapoport B, McLachlan SM. Thyroglobulin-thyroperoxidase autoantibodies are polyreactive, not bispecific: analysis using human monoclonal autoantibodies. *J Clin Endocrinol Metab*, 2003; **88**: 371–8.
45. Chiovato L, Latrofa F, Braverman LE, Pacini F, Capezzone M, Masserini L, *et al.* Disappearance of humoral thyroid autoimmunity after complete removal of thyroid antigens. *Ann Intern Med*, 2003; **139**: 346–51.
46. Lisi S, Pinchera A, McCluskey RT, Willnow TE, Refetoff S, Marcocci C, *et al.* Preferential megalin-mediated transcytosis of low-hormonogenic thyroglobulin: a control mechanism for thyroid hormone release. *Proc Natl Acad Sci U S A*, 2003; **100**: 14858–63.
47. Marino M, Chiovato L, Friedlander JA, Latrofa F, Pinchera A, McCluskey RT. Serum antibodies against megalin (GP330) in patients with autoimmune thyroiditis. *J Clin Endocrinol Metab*, 1999; **84**: 2468–74.
48. Chin HS, Chin DK, Morgenthaler NG, Vassart G, Costagliola S. Rarity of anti- Na^+/I^- symporter (NIS) antibody with iodide uptake inhibiting activity in autoimmune thyroid diseases (AITD). *J Clin Endocrinol Metab*, 2000; **85**: 3937–40.
49. Tonacchera M, Agretti P, Ceccarini G, Lenza R, Refetoff S, Santini F, *et al.* Autoantibodies from patients with autoimmune thyroid disease do not interfere with the activity of the human iodide symporter gene stably transfected in CHO cells. *Eur J Endocrinol*, 2001; **144**: 611–18.
50. Gutekunst R, Hafermann W, Mansky T, Scriba PC. Ultrasonography related to clinical and laboratory findings in lymphocytic thyroiditis. *Acta Endocrinol (Copenh)*, 1989; **121**: 129–35.
51. Vitti P, Lampis M, Piga M, Loviselli A, Brogioni S, Rago T, *et al.* Diagnostic usefulness of thyroid ultrasonography in atrophic thyroiditis. *J Clin Ultrasound*, 1994; **22**: 375–9.
52. Vitti P, Rago T, Mancusi F, Pallini S, Tonacchera M, Santini F, *et al.* Thyroid hypoechogenic pattern at ultrasonography as a tool for predicting recurrence of hyperthyroidism after medical treatment in patients with Graves' disease. *Acta Endocrinol (Copenh)*, 1992; **126**: 128–31.
53. Vitti P, Martino E, Aghini-Lombardi F, Rago T, Antonangeli L, Maccherini D, *et al.* Thyroid volume measurement by ultrasound in children as a tool for the assessment of mild iodine deficiency. *J Clin Endocrinol Metab*, 1994; **79**: 600–3.
54. Ralls PW, Mayekawa DS, Lee KP, Colletti PM, Radin DR, Boswell WD, *et al.* Color-flow Doppler sonography in Graves' disease: 'thyroid inferno'. *AJR Am J Roentgenol*, 1988; **150**: 781–4.
55. Vitti P, Rago T, Mazzeo S, Brogioni S, Lampis M, De Liperi A, *et al.* Thyroid blood flow evaluation by color-flow Doppler sonography distinguishes Graves' disease from Hashimoto's thyroiditis. *J Endocrinol Invest*, 1995; **18**: 857–61.
56. Bogazzi F, Bartalena L, Brogioni S, Mazzeo S, Vitti P, Burelli A, *et al.* Color flow Doppler sonography rapidly differentiates type I and type II amiodarone-induced thyrotoxicosis. *Thyroid*, 1997; **7**: 541–5.
57. Bartalena L, Martino E, Velluzzi F, Piga M, Petrini L, Loviselli A, *et al.* The lack of nocturnal serum thyrotropin surge in patients with nontoxic nodular goiter may predict the subsequent occurrence of hyperthyroidism. *J Clin Endocrinol Metab*, 1991; **73**: 604–8.
58. Becker D, Bair HJ, Becker W, Gunter E, Lohner W, Lerch S, *et al.* Thyroid autonomy with color-coded image-directed Doppler sonography: internal hypervascularization for the recognition of autonomous adenomas. *J Clin Ultrasound*, 1997; **25**: 63–9.
59. Rago T, Santini F, Scutari M, Pinchera A, Vitti P. Elastography: new developments in ultrasound for predicting malignancy in thyroid nodules. *J Clin Endocrinol Metab*, 2007; **92**: 2917–22.
60. Zweig MH, Csako G, Spero M. Escape from blockade of interfering heterophile antibodies in a two-site immunoradiometric assay for thyrotropin. *Clin Chem*, 1988; **34**: 2589–91.
61. Refetoff S, Weiss RE, Usala SJ. The syndromes of resistance to thyroid hormone. *Endocr Rev*, 1993; **14**: 348–99.
62. Beck-Peccoz P, Forloni F, Cortelazzi D, Persani L, Papandreou MJ, Asteria C, *et al.* Pituitary resistance to thyroid hormones. *Horm Res*, 1992; **38**: 66–72.
63. Beck-Peccoz P, Roncoroni R, Mariotti S, Medri G, Marcocci C, Brabant G, *et al.* Sex hormone-binding globulin measurement in patients with inappropriate secretion of thyrotropin (IST): evidence against selective pituitary thyroid hormone resistance in nonneoplastic IST. *J Clin Endocrinol Metab*, 1990; **71**: 19–25.
64. Beck-Peccoz P, Brucker-Davis F, Persani L, Smallridge RC, Weintraub BD. Thyrotropin-secreting pituitary tumors. *Endocr Rev*, 1996; **17**: 610–38.
65. Sarne DH, Sobieszczyk S, Ain KB, Refetoff S. Serum thyrotropin and prolactin in the syndrome of generalized resistance to thyroid hormone: responses to thyrotropin-releasing hormone stimulation and short term triiodothyronine suppression. *J Clin Endocrinol Metab*, 1990; **70**: 1305–11.
66. Lamberts SW, Krenning EP, Reubi JC. The role of somatostatin and its analogs in the diagnosis and treatment of tumors. *Endocr Rev*, 1991; **12**: 450–82.
67. Mariotti S, Martino E, Cupini C, Lari R, Giani C, Baschieri L, *et al.* Low serum thyroglobulin as a clue to the diagnosis of thyrotoxicosis factitia. *N Engl J Med*, 1982; **307**: 410–12.

3.3.6 Antithyroid drug treatment for thyrotoxicosis

Anthony Toft

Introduction

The most effective and commonly used antithyroid drugs are the thionamides, including carbimazole and its active metabolite methimazole (not available in the UK). These act by inhibiting the synthesis of thyroid hormones, principally by interfering with the iodination of tyrosine by serving as preferential substrates for the iodinating intermediate of thyroid peroxidase. Oxidized iodine is thus diverted from potential iodination sites in thyroglobulin. The iodinated antithyroid drugs are desulfurated and further oxidized to inactive metabolites. There is also some evidence for an immunosuppressive action which is of doubtful clinical significance as most patients relapse after drug withdrawal. Another thionamide, propylthiouracil, is, in addition, a potent inhibitor of type 1 outer ring deiodinase and acutely inhibits thyroxine (T_4) to triiodothyronine (T_3) conversion, but there is no good evidence to suggest that this effect is of any clinical relevance. Propylthiouracil tends to be reserved for those patients who have developed an adverse reaction to carbimazole or methimazole.

Selection of patients

The natural history of the hyperthyroidism of Graves' disease is shown in Fig. 3.3.6.1. A course of antithyroid drugs is appropriate for the minority (30–50%) of patients in whom a single episode of hyperthyroidism is followed by prolonged remission. The majority of patients have a relapsing and remitting course over many years and despite efforts to predict the natural history of the hyperthyroidism, using markers such as HLA status, the presence of thyrotropin (TSH)-receptor antibody (TRAb), goitre size, serum thyroid-stimulating hormone (TSH) response to thyrotropin-releasing hormone, and thyroid suppressibility (alone or in combination), it has not proved possible to categorize individual patients with Graves' disease in respect of outcome with any degree of accuracy (1). On a group basis, small goitre, low serum concentration of TRAb, and increasing age favour remission after a course of antithyroid drugs, whereas the risk of relapse in a young male with severe hyperthyroidism and a large vascular goitre is so great that most would advocate surgery as the primary treatment. Standard practice in Europe has been that the initial treatment in most patients under 40–45 years of age is with an antithyroid drug, with a recommendation for surgery should relapse occur. In the USA, however, ^{131}I therapy is not restricted to older patients and the use of antithyroid drugs is relatively uncommon. Antithyroid drugs are not normally indicated in the treatment of toxic nodular goitre, unless to render the patient euthyroid before surgery, as recurrence of hyperthyroidism is invariable after drug withdrawal. There is no role for antithyroid drugs in subacute or postpartum thyroiditis in which the thyrotoxicosis is caused by the release of preformed thyroid hormones.

Duration of therapy

The most consistent observation in patients with Graves' hyperthyroidism has been that the longer the duration of therapy, the

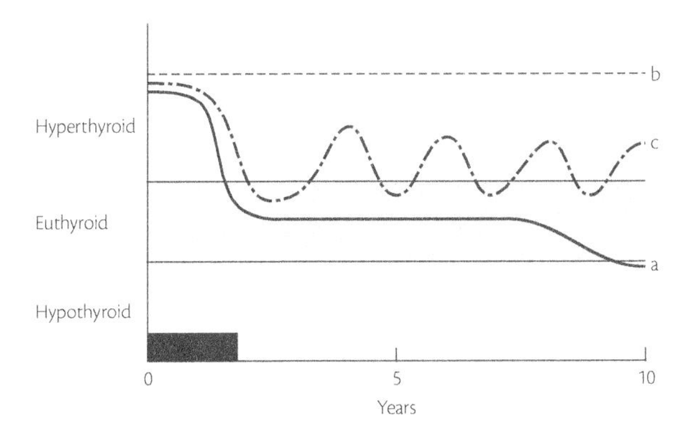

Fig. 3.3.6.1 The natural history of the hyperthyroidism of Graves' disease. The minority (a) have a single episode of hyperthyroidism, lasting a few months only. The rest (b+c) either have prolonged continuous episodes or follow a relapsing and remitting course over many years. In some there is the eventual spontaneous development of hypothyroidism. The use of an antithyroid drug (solid black area) will only be successful in patients in group a.

better the remission rate. In a study in children with Graves' disease, and there is no reason to believe that the results in adults would be different, when antithyroid drug withdrawal was attempted regularly, the mean duration of hyperthyroidism was 4.5 years; this is probably an underestimate as remission was defined as euthyroidism for 12 months (2). The conventional period of antithyroid drug therapy of 12–24 months is best viewed as a compromise by which those destined to have a single short-lived episode of hyperthyroidism are identified and primary destructive therapy by surgery or with ^{131}I avoided. Most patients (50–70%), however, usually relapse within the first 2 years.

Long-term treatment with antithyroid drugs

Although radio-iodine is increasingly the treatment of choice in patients with hyperthyroidism due to Graves' disease, there perhaps needs to be more caution about a therapy that almost always results in hypothyroidism. This is especially so when there is no consensus on what constitutes correct thyroid hormone replacement (3) and when there is anxiety about the bioequivalence of branded versus generic L-thyroxine and between the various generic preparations (4). Some patients abhor the idea of irradiation of any kind and patients worry that they will gain excessive weight if rendered hypothyroid and this may be true if serum concentrations of TSH are simply restored to the reference range with thyroxine (5). Of some concern are the recent reports that ^{131}I treatment itself may cause increased morbidity and mortality from cardiovascular disease in the long term (6, 7). There is no reason why patients with relapsing and remitting hyperthyroidism cannot be treated with successive doses of antithyroid drugs. Indeed, continuing methimazole uninterruptedly for 10 years after the first relapse has been shown to be safe and cheaper than ^{131}I (8).

Dosage

Carbimazole is available as 5 and 20 mg tablets. The initial dosage is 40–45 mg daily for 3–4 weeks, reducing to 30 mg daily for a further 3–4 weeks, with further adjustments on the basis of measurement of serum concentrations of T_3, T_4, and TSH, until a maintenance dose of 5–15 mg daily is achieved, usually within 3–4 months. Patients begin to feel an improvement at 10–14 days. Once-daily dosage is appropriate for all but the most severely thyrotoxic, who benefit from being given carbimazole as 20 mg twice daily or 15 mg three times daily. Initial changes in drug dosage should be based on thyroid hormone concentrations, as delayed recovery of thyrotrophs, previously exposed to high levels of T_3 and T_4, may result in inappropriately low serum TSH concentrations. After 10–12 weeks of treatment, serum TSH is the best guide as to whether the dosage of carbimazole is appropriate, high and low concentrations indicating excessive and inadequate therapy, respectively. A daily dose of 20 mg carbimazole is almost as effective in restoring euthyroidism by the 10th week as 40 mg daily in mild to moderate hyperthyroidism (9). However, in the absence of overwhelming evidence that the major adverse reaction, agranulocytosis, is dose-related, there would seem little point in delaying the restoration of thyroid function to normal from 4 to 10 weeks, particularly in patients with troublesome symptoms or serious complications such as atrial fibrillation. The appropriate dose of propylthiouracil is 10 times that of carbimazole, and 30 mg methimazole is approximately equivalent to 40 mg carbimazole.

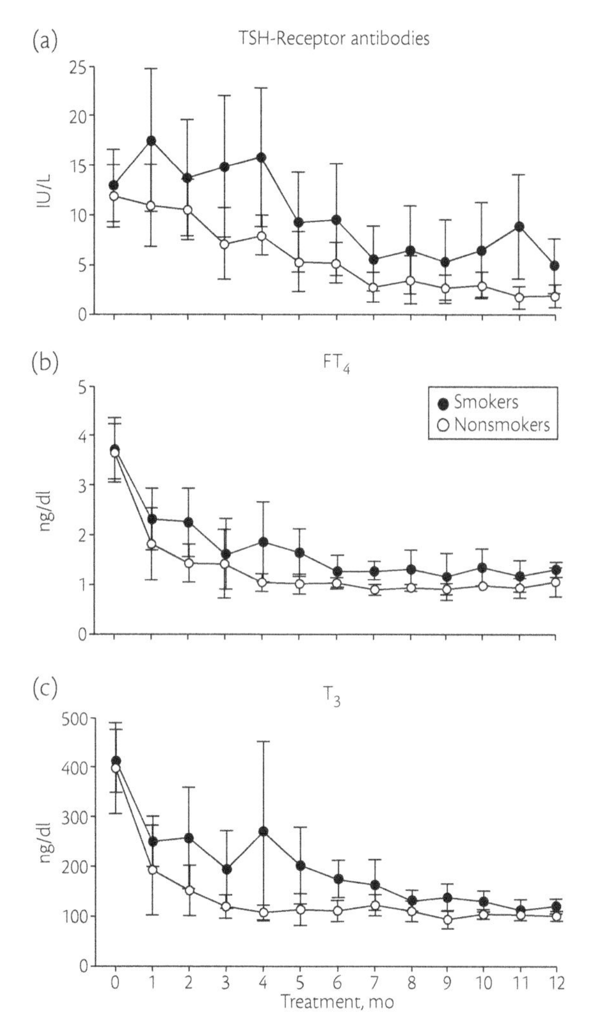

Fig. 3.3.6.2 Thyroid-Stimulating Hormone (TSH)–Receptor Antibody and Thyroid Hormone Concentrations in Smokers and Nonsmokers With Graves Disease During Treatment With Carbimazole.

The rate of reduction in the serum concentrations of TRAb, T_3, and T_4 is slower and the dose of carbimazole required to achieve euthyroidism greater in patients with Graves' disease who smoke. Smoking is also associated with a greater chance of relapse after a standard course of antithyroid drugs (Fig. 3.3.6.2) (10).

'Block and replace' therapy

In this regime, carbimazole is continued at the high dosage of 30–45 mg daily after the patient is euthyroid, and hypothyroidism avoided in the long term by adding thyroxine at a dosage of 100–150 µg daily. The dose of thyroxine, but not carbimazole, is adjusted to maintain serum TSH within the lower part of the reference range. This combination therapy has long been thought to be beneficial in patients with significant ophthalmopathy, presumably as a result of avoiding hypothyroidism, and in those with brittle 'hyperthyroidism', fluctuating between over- and undertreatment with antithyroid drugs despite good compliance and supervision, and now known to be due to changing concentrations and activities of TRAb (Table 3.3.6.1). Remission rates are not improved by standard block and replace therapy. Claims for a regime in which, after 18 months of combined therapy, thyroxine alone was continued for a further 3 years, during which time the relapse rate was less than 2% have not been substantiated (11).

Adverse reactions

The adverse effects of antithyroid drugs can occur at any time but almost always within 3–6 weeks of starting treatment. There is some cross-sensitivity between carbimazole (methimazole) and propylthiouracil. Although it is common practice to change to the alternative antithyroid drug in the event of a minor adverse reaction, such as a skin rash, opinion is divided over whether the development of agranulocytosis is an absolute contraindication to further drug therapy.

Life-threatening reactions

The most serious adverse reaction is agranulocytosis, which develops in 0.2–0.5% of patients. Agranulocytosis is characterized by fever, systemic upset, oropharyngeal bacterial infection, and a granulocyte count of less than 0.25×10^9/l. The onset is sudden and the consensus is that there is no purpose in routine monitoring of the white blood cell count (12). Patients should simply be instructed to contact their medical practitioner immediately in the event of developing a sore throat or mouth ulceration. After stopping antithyroid drug therapy, the white blood cell count returns to normal within 1–3 weeks, during which time the affected patient should be isolated and treated with broad-spectrum antibiotics. Recovery of the white blood cell count may be hastened by the use of granulocyte colony stimulating factor, but its value in those with the most profound reduction in granulocyte count (less than 0.1 ×

Table 3.3.6.1 Sequential thyroid function test results and serum thyrotropin-receptor antibody (TRAb) concentrations in a patient with 'brittle' hyperthyroidism treated initially with carbimazole. More satisfactory control was achieved by using a 'block and replace' regime

Time (weeks)	Free thyroxine (pmol/l)	T_3 (nmol/l)	TSH (mU/l)	TRAb (U/l)	Daily dose of carbimazole (mg)
Presentation	98	6.2	<0.01	70	–
4	21	2.7	<0.01	55	45
8	7	1.4	18.2	15	30
12	32	3.4	<0.01	35	20
18	10	1.6	4.6	40	30
24	21	2.2	<0.01	20	30 mg thyroxine
30	24	2.1	<0.01	11	30 mg thyroxine
36	22	2.2	<0.01	9	30 mg thyroxine

Reference ranges: free thyroxine, 10–25 pmol/l; T_3, 1.1–2.6 nmol/l; TSH, 0.15–3.5 mU/l; TRAb, 0–7 U/l.

10^9/l) is unclear (13). Mild leucopenia with a relative lymphocytosis is common in Graves' disease and is not a contraindication to the use of antithyroid drugs.

Other reactions

The most common reactions are nausea, loss of taste, headache, and hair loss, which may be self-limiting and do not necessarily require drug withdrawal. The most troublesome in this category is a skin rash, which is usually urticarial and affects between 1% and 2% of patients. A migratory polyarthritis may occur alone or in association with the rash and resolves within 4 weeks of stopping treatment. Much rarer adverse effects include cholestatic jaundice (14), vasculitis which may be associated with antineutrophil cytoplasmic antibody (15), a lupus-like syndrome, and the nephrotic syndrome.

Adjunct to treatment with ^{131}I

Iodine-131 takes some 6–8 weeks to be effective, and during this latent period hyperthyroidism may be exacerbated, with an increase in morbidity and even mortality in those with severe thyrotoxicosis and associated cardiovascular disease. For this reason it is not uncommon to render the patient euthyroid before radio-iodine treatment and to continue the antithyroid drug for 6 weeks thereafter. In order not to interfere with the efficacy of the ^{131}I, carbimazole should not be given for 48 h before and after treatment. If this course of action is not taken, the thyroid gland is more resistant to the effects of ^{131}I and larger doses should be used (16). An added advantage of pretreatment with an antithyroid drug is that the patient is more likely to comprehend the various aspects of treatment when not in the agitated and unreceptive state of hyperthyroidism.

Antithyroid drugs in pregnancy

Maternal hyperthyroidism in pregnancy is usually due to Graves' disease. TRAb crosses the placenta and, if the mother is thyrotoxic, it must be assumed that the fetus is similarly affected. Before effective treatment was available the fetal death rate could be as high as 50%. Fortunately, antithyroid drugs also cross the placenta and, by careful monitoring of maternal thyroid function, normal fetal development can be achieved, even though cord blood may show evidence of overtreatment. Like other organ-specific autoimmune diseases, Graves' hyperthyroidism tends to improve or even remit during pregnancy. A small daily dose of antithyroid drug, such as 5–10 mg carbimazole, will maintain free T_4 and TSH concentrations in the reference ranges (Fig. 3.3.6.3). It is good clinical practice to review the mother every 4 weeks during pregnancy and to stop the antithyroid drug 4 weeks before the expected date of delivery to avoid any possibility of fetal hypothyroidism when brain development is at a maximum. Measurement of TRAb concentration in maternal serum at the last review before delivery may be helpful, as a high level is a predictor of neonatal thyrotoxicosis. Since thyroid hormones cross the placenta relatively poorly, the 'block and replace' regime is not recommended in pregnancy.

Carbimazole (methimazole) or propylthiouracil?

Aplasia cutis congenita is a rare disorder of the skin, usually affecting the scalp and less than 3 cm in diameter, which has been reported in a small number of neonates whose mothers received methimazole during pregnancy. Aplasia cutis congenita has not been reported in association with propylthiouracil, which is widely used

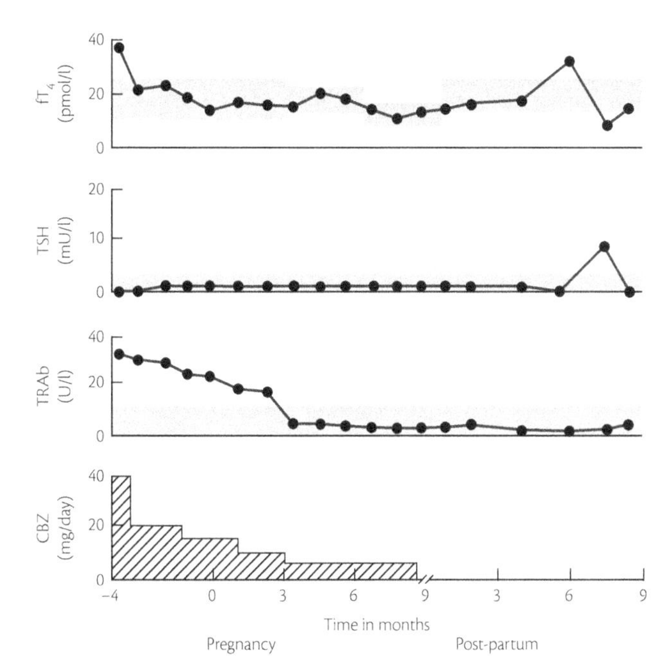

Fig. 3.3.6.3 Carbimazole dosage and sequential measurements of fT_4, TSH, and TRAb in a 25-year-old woman discovered to have hyperthyroidism due to Graves' disease while attending an infertility clinic. Within weeks of control of the hyperthyroidism she became pregnant. Note (1) the trimester-adjustedreference range for fT_4; (2) the fall in TRAb concentration during treatment with carbimazole, and the further fall during pregnancy; (3) the low dose of carbimazole required to maintain euthyroidism during pregnancy and the withdrawal of the antithyroid drug 4 weeks before the expected date of delivery; (4) the development of post-partum thyroiditis, characterized by transient hyperthyroidism followed by an equally short-lived episode of hypothyroidism in the absence of TRAb. Normal ranges are indicated by the shaded areas. CBZ: carbimazole.

in North America, and there are those who take the view that propylthiouracil is the drug of choice in pregnancy or in those planning pregnancy. The consensus, however, is that there is insufficient evidence to establish a direct causal relationship between aplasia cutis congenita and methimazole. Since both carbimazole (methimazole) and propylthiouracil are equally effective in controlling Graves' hyperthyroidism during pregnancy, it makes sense to use the preparation with which one has most experience.

If hyperthyroidism recurs after delivery, is due to Graves' disease and not post-partum thyroiditis, and the mother wishes to breastfeed, propylthiouracil is the drug of choice as it is transferred to the milk one-tenth as well as carbimazole (methimazole). Carbimazole will not affect thyroid function in the infant if a dosage of less than 15 mg daily is employed (17), and daily doses of 5–10 mg methimazole given for 1 year to breastfeeding mothers had no deleterious effect on infant thyroid function or subsequent intellectual development (18).

Other drugs used in the treatment of hyperthyroidism

β-adrenoceptor antagonists (β-blockers)

Many of the clinical features of hyperthyroidism, such as palpitations, tremor, and heat intolerance, are ameliorated, but not abolished, by the use of nonselective β-blockers. For example, the resting heart rate may fall from 120 to 90 beats/min. Although β-blockers also inhibit the extrathyroidal conversion of T_4 to T_3, the fall in serum T_3 concentrations is small and is not thought to contribute to their efficacy. The principle use of β-blockers is in relieving troublesome symptoms before investigation and treatment, during the latent period of 10–14 days or 6–8 weeks before antithyroid drugs or ^{131}I begin to be effective, and during the transient hyperthyroid phase of subacute or postpartum thyroiditis.

The most commonly used β-blocker is propranolol. The usual dosage is 80–160 mg daily as a long-acting preparation. Clearance of propranolol may be variably accelerated in patients with thyrotoxicosis and dosages as high as 480 mg daily may be necessary to control heart rate. Nadolol in a single daily dose of 80–160 mg is an alternative nonselective β-blocker.

These drugs are contraindicated in patients with thyrotoxicosis and obstructive airways disease, as they may precipitate worsening bronchospasm; insulin-dependent diabetes mellitus, as they may slow the recovery from and mask the symptoms of hypoglycaemia; and cardiac failure, unless this is associated with atrial fibrillation and is primarily due to the hyperthyroidism.

Potassium iodide, sodium ipodate, and sodium iopanoate

Iodide, as potassium iodide, is normally used only in the preparation of patients with hyperthyroidism for surgery. When euthyroid, the antithyroid drug is stopped 10–14 days before surgery and potassium iodide (60 mg 3 times daily) is substituted. This maintains thyroid status principally by inhibiting thyroid hormone release and reduces the vascularity of the gland, making surgery technically easier. Potassium iodide has also been used successfully in combination with propranolol in preparing patients for surgery over a period of 10 days (19). Although this regime cannot be universally recommended, it is valuable in patients with mild to moderate hyperthyroidism in whom domestic or business pressures make urgent surgical treatment necessary.

The oral cholecystographic agents sodium ipodate (Oragraphin) and sodium iopanoate (Telepaque) as well as having an iodide effect, also reduce T_4 to T_3 conversion by inhibiting outer ring deiodinase. Serum T_3 concentrations fall dramatically within 24 h compared with the 5–7 days for potassium iodide. The dosage of these agents is 0.5–1.0 g daily. As cholecystography has been superseded by ultrasound examination of the gallbladder these agents are, unfortunately, no longer widely available.

Potassium perchlorate

Perchlorate competitively inhibits iodine transport and was used successfully in the treatment of hyperthyroidism. Unfortunately it was associated with the development of aplastic anaemia and gastric ulceration and should only be considered in the management of severe hyperthyroidism induced by amiodarone therapy, which is difficult to control with thionamides alone in areas of iodine deficiency.

Lithium carbonate

Lithium has an iodide-like action and has been used in the management of hyperthyroidism. Patients may escape, however, from the effects of lithium, and, indeed, long-term therapy in patients with manic depressive illness is associated with an increased risk of thyrotoxicosis. In addition, the therapeutic window for lithium is narrow and the current consensus is that the drug has no place in the treatment of hyperthyroidism (20).

References

1. Schleusner H, Schwander J, Fischer C, Holle R, Holl G, Badenhoop K, *et al.* Prospective multicentre study on the prediction of relapse after antithyroid drug treatment in patients with Graves' disease. *Acta Endocrinol*, 1989; **120**: 689–701.
2. Lippe BM, Landau EM, Kaplan SA. Hyperthyroidism in children treated with long-term medical therapy: twenty-five per cent remission every two years. *J Clin Endocrinol Metab*, 1987; **64**: 1241–5.
3. Toft A. Which thyroxine. *Thyroid*, 2005; **15**: 124–6.
4. Eisenberg M, Di Stefano III J. TSH-based protocol, tablet instability and absorption effects on L-T_4 bioequivalence. *Thyroid*, 2009; **19**: 103–10.
5. Tigas S, Idiculla J, Beckett G, Toft A. Is excessive weight gain after ablative treatment of hyperthyroidism due to inadequate thyroid hormone therapy. *Thyroid*, 2000; **10**: 1107–11.
6. Nyirenda MJ, Clark DN, Finlayson AR, Read J, Elders A, Bain M, *et al.* Thyroid disease and increased cardiovascular risk. *Thyroid*, 2005; **15**: 718–24.
7. Metso S, Auvinen A, Salmi J, Huhtala H, Jaatinen P. Increased long-term cardiovascular morbidity among patients treated with radioactive iodine for hyperthyroidism. *Clin Endocrinol*, 2008; **68**: 450–7.
8. Azizi F, Esmaillzadeh A, Mirmiran P, Ainy E. Effect of long-term continuous methimazole treatment of hyperthyroidism: comparison with radioiodine. *Eur J Endocrinol*, 2005; **152**: 695–701.
9. Page SR, Sheard CE, Herbert M, Hopton M, Jeffcoate WJ. A comparison of 20 or 40 mg per day of carbimazole in the initial treatment of hyperthyroidism. *Clin Endocrinol*, 1996; **45**: 511–15.
10. Nyirenda MJ, Taylor PN, Stoddart M, Beckett GJ, Toft AD. Thyroid-stimulating hormone-receptor antibody and thyroid hormone concentrations in smokers vs non-smokers with Graves' disease treated with carbimazole. *JAMA*, 2009; **301**: 162–4.
11. McIver B, Rae P, Beckett G, Wilkinson E, Gold A, Toft A. Lack of effect of thyroxine in patients with Graves' hyperthyroidism who are treated with an antithyroid drug. *N Engl J Med*, 1996; **334**: 220–4.
12. Toft AD, Weetman AP. Screening for agranulocytosis in patients treated with antithyroid drugs. *Clin Endocrinol*, 1998; **49**: 271.
13. Hirsch D, Luboschitz J, Blum L. Treatment of antithyroid drug-induced agranulocytosis by granulocyte colony-stimulating factor: a case of primum non nocere. *Thyroid*, 1999; **9**: 1033–5.
14. Kim HJ, Kim BH, Han YS, Yang I, Kim KJ, Dong SH, *et al.* The incidence and clinical characteristics of symptomatic propylthiouracil-induced hepatic injury in patients with hyperthyroidism: a single-center retrospective study. *Am J Gastroenterol*, 2001; **96**: 165–9.
15. Miller RM, Savige J, Nassis L, Cominos BI. Antineutrophil cytoplasmic antibody (ANCA)-positive cutaneous leucocytoclastic vasculitis associated with antithyroid therapy in Graves' disease. *Australas J Dermatol*, 1998; **39**: 96–9.
16. Bonnema SJ, Bartalena L, Toft AD, Hegedus L. Controversies in radioiodine therapy: relation to ophthalmopathy, the possible radioprotective effect of antithyroid drugs, and use in large goiters. *Eur J Endocrinol*, 2002; **147**. 1–11.
17. Lamberg BA, Ikonen E, Osterlund K, Teramo K, Pekonen F, Peltola J, *et al.* Antithyroid treatment of maternal hyperthyroidism during lactation. *Clin Endocrinol*, 1984; **21**: 81–7.
18. Azizi F, Khoshniat M, Bahrainian M, Hedayati M. Thyroid function and intellectual development of infants nursed by mothers taking methimazole. *J Clin Endocrinol Metab*, 2000; **85**: 3233–8.
19. Feek CM, Sawers JSA, Irvine WJ, Beckett JG, Ratcliffe WA, Toft AD. Combination of potassium iodide and propranolol in preparation of patients with Graves' disease for thyroid surgery. *N Engl J Med*, 1980; **302**: 883–5.
20. Lazarus JH. Effect of lithium on the thyroid gland. In: Weetman AP, Grossman A, eds. *Pharmacotherapeutics of the Thyroid Gland*. Berlin: Springer, 1997: 207–23.

Further reading

Brent GA. Graves' disease. *N Engl J Med*, 2008; **358**: 2594–605.
Cooper DS. Drug therapy: antithyroid drugs. *N Engl J Med*, 2005; **352**: 905–17.

3.3.7 Radio-iodine treatment of hyperthyroidism

Markus Luster, Michael Lassmann

Introduction

Radioactive iodine has been used successfully for almost 70 years since the first treatment took place at the Massachusetts General Hospital in Boston in 1941. However, it was not until after the Second World War that ^{131}I became generally available for clinical applications (1). The radioactive iodine isotope is chemically identical to 'stable' iodine (^{127}I) and thus becomes a part of the intrathyroidal metabolism. Its principle of action is based on the emission of β-rays with a range of 0.5–2 mm in the tissue leading to high local radiation absorbed doses while sparing surrounding structures. The additional γ-ray component of ^{131}I allows for scintigraphic imaging of the distribution in the gland and can also be used for pre- and post-therapeutic individual dosimetry (see below).

Several therapeutic options are available for the treatment of benign thyroid disorders, namely hyperthyroidism: surgical resection (hemithyroidectomy, near-total, or total thyroidectomy), long-term antithyroid drug medication (ATD), and radio-iodine therapy (RAIT) (2, 3). These different treatment modalities are used in varying frequencies depending on geographical location, e.g. iodine supply, availability and logistics, cultural background, and patient-specific features, e.g. goitre size, presence of local symptoms, age, and hormonal status. The diversity of approaches on an international scale still remains impressive and is reflected by a great heterogeneity throughout Europe and also when compared to the USA where radio-iodine therapy is still being applied more frequently than in most European countries (4–8).

Radio-iodine therapy was originally aimed at eliminating hyperthyroidism and thus leaving the patient euthyroid. Up-to-date strategies, however, established postradio-iodine induction of hypothyroidism as the treatment objective and, thus, it is included in the category of 'cure'. This definition holds especially true for the management of Graves' disease when long-term hypothyroidism was the rule and stabilization of euthyroidism failed in the majority of cases. In fact, the term 'ablation', meaning removal or destruction, has been increasingly used to characterize radio-iodine therapy and administration of larger amounts of radio-iodine have tended to make this a self-fulfilling prophecy. Although many clinicians prefer that the end result of treatment be the more easily managed hypothyroidism, others are still reluctant to give up the therapeutic ideal of euthyroidism as the preferred result of radio-iodine therapy and continue their efforts to solve the enigma of thyroid radiosensitivity.

Indications

The causes of hyperthyroidism include the following: (1) autoimmune hyperthyroidism, previously called toxic diffuse goitre (Graves' disease), (2) toxic adenoma, (3) toxic multinodular goitre (Plummer's disease), (4) silent thyroiditis, and (5) painful subacute thyroiditis. The first three entities constitute a clear indication for radio-iodine treatment, while silent thyroiditis and subacute thyroiditis are never treated with radio-iodine.

Recently, there has been an emerging role for ^{131}I in the treatment of subclinical hyperthyroidism caused by any of the three first entities (5). Another potential category that is frequently regarded as a new entity for this kind of treatment are patients with non-toxic goitre (NTG). They are a group of patients who are euthyroid but may benefit from reduction of thyroid volume (9–11). The available treatment options in NTG patients in whom the risk of malignancy is considered low are a 'wait-and-see' policy, surgery, L-thyroxine, and radio-iodine treatment. The main indications for radio-iodine treatment of NTG are to reduce the size of a goitre to relieve compressive signs or symptoms and secondly to alleviate potential cosmetic problems for the patient. Surgery is the fastest way to reduce goitre size and relieve any acute compressive symptoms and is mandatory if there are any doubts about malignancy. Prestimulation with recombinant human thyroid-stimulating hormone may represent a future option for this condition by augmenting the effectiveness of radio-iodine (11, 12).

Radio-iodine is, in most cases, the first-line treatment for Graves' disease and toxic adenoma, or it can be administered if hyperthyroidism is not controlled or recurs after antithyroid drug treatment (13). Surgery should only be considered if there are contraindications to radio-iodine therapy.

Contraindications

Pregnancy and breastfeeding are absolute contraindications to radio-iodine treatment; all females of reproductive age should have a pregnancy test immediately before administration. It is generally recommended that women should not attempt conception for 6–12 months after radio-iodine treatment. Iodine-131 is not indicated for patients who have urinary incontinence, whereas concomitant haemodialysis for renal failure is not an exclusion criterion and is routinely performed in experienced centres.

Technical aspects and response to radio-iodine

The effect of radio-iodine therapy is gradual and varies substantially among individuals, resulting in the necessity for repeated testing after the treatment to rule out persistent hyperthyroidism or short-term development of a hypothyroid state. After 8–12 weeks, a follow-up visit may scheduled to evaluate the effect of the procedure. In case of pre-existing marked hyperthyroidism, symptom relief should be achieved peritherapeutically by the administration of β-blocking agents, and resumption of antithyroid drugs should be considered when tachycardia and palpitations are present. The influence of antithyroid drugs on the efficiency of radio-iodine therapy is a permanent matter of controversy, but there is growing evidence that coadministration of methimazole and propylthiouracil during radio-iodine therapy has a negative influence on the therapeutic outcome (14–17). If tolerated, restarting antithyroid drugs should preferably be initiated 1 week after the radio-iodine has been administered to avoid altering radio-iodine kinetics in the thyroid.

Potential side effects

Acute side effects

Clinical exacerbation of hyperthyroidism after radio-iodine treatment appears to be relatively uncommon and is usually of minor clinical significance. It presumably is related to radiation thyroiditis, with destruction of thyroid follicles and release of thyroglobulin and stored hormone into the circulation. There may be a transient rise in free thyroxine and free triiodothyronine levels several days following administration, and patients with poorly controlled symptoms before radio-iodine therapy may encounter an exacerbation of cardiac arrhythmia and heart failure. In some patients a 'thyroid storm' may develop. Intravenous infusion of antithyroid drugs, corticosteroids, and β-blockers is the treatment of choice, but prophylactic measures and a thorough initial work-up are crucial.

Patients with large goitres may notice transient swelling and dyspnoea. Thyroid enlargement may last until approximately 1 week following therapy and some discomfort may be associated with it. Slight irritation of the salivary gland function may be noted, but in contrast to thyroid cancer, the risk of permanent injury is negligible due to the much lower activities applied for therapy of thyrotoxicosis.

Hypothyroidism

The main side effect of radio-iodine treatment is permanent hypothyroidism. The rate of hypothyroidism varies and incidence continues to increase over time, so that lifelong follow-up is essential. Pretreatment prediction is not possible using current variables; however, the incidence is higher in Graves' disease than in toxic nodular goitre and relatively uncommon in solitary hyperfunctioning nodules. The most prominent radiobiological factor for the determination of overall outcome, besides radiation sensitivity of the thyroid follicular cells, remains the radiation absorbed dose to the thyroid tissue; however, its exact calculation is one of the obstacles in therapeutic nuclear medicine.

Ophthalmopathy

Graves' disease is frequently accompanied by ophthalmopathy; the reported incidences largely depend on the diagnostic criteria employed (18–20). Prospective randomized controlled trials have shown that radio-iodine treatment is associated with a greater risk of the appearance or worsening of ophthalmopathy in patients with Graves' disease than antithyroid drug treatment. The risk is especially increased in patients who smoke cigarettes, in keeping with the importance of smoking as a susceptibility factor in the development of ophthalmopathy, so patients should be strongly advised to quit smoking. Oral or intravenous administration of steroids with ^{131}I helps prevent exacerbation of ophthalmopathy, and this approach has to be considered the standard of care in patients who have clinically active ophthalmopathy at the time of treatment (21–25). A radiation absorbed dose below 200 Gy, a thyroid volume of more than 55 ml, and the use of radio-iodine without steroid medication have been shown to be associated with a higher risk of worsening of eye symptoms. Despite the controversy regarding adequate management of patients with Graves' hyperthyroidism and thyroid eye disease, most authors agree that in the presence of predisposing risk factors, such as large goitres or heavy smoking, ablative therapy should be recommended (16) (see Chapter 3.3.10).

Radiation-induced cancers

A small excess of mortality from malignancy was reported in one investigation but the study was biased by the increased surveillance. In other large series, no effects of radio-iodine therapy on survival have been observed, whereas some reports suggested an increased relative risk for the development of certain types of cancer (thyroid, stomach, bladder, kidney, and haematological malignancies). However, these observations still remain to be confirmed by monitoring larger patient samples, so that currently no definite conclusion with respect to risk for subsequent malignancies can be drawn (26–30).

Dosimetry

For the treatment of Graves' disease or Plummer's disease (toxic nodular goitre), ^{131}I is normally administered orally using activities between 100 and 1500 MBq. The rationale behind dosimetry for this kind of treatment is that the incidence of long-term hypothyroidism is higher with an earlier onset for patients treated with higher activities (31) resulting in an attempt to individualize and thus optimize therapy. A large variation exists in the literature on the value of target absorbed dose to be delivered to the hyperthyroid tissue to become euthyroid. Most authors indicate 70 Gy but absorbed doses as high as 200 Gy are reported (32).

For a pretherapeutic dosimetric assessment of the activity needed to achieve a certain prescribed absorbed dose to the target volume in general, an adapted version of the Quimby–Marinelli formula is recommended for use:

$$A\,[\mathrm{MBq}] = \frac{F}{\ln 2} \cdot \frac{M\,[\mathrm{g}] \cdot D\,[\mathrm{Gy}]}{\int_0^{\infty} \mathrm{RIU}(t)\,dt}$$

The activity A to be administered is calculated from:

M: Mass of the target volume

D: Absorbed dose to be achieved in the target volume

RIU(t): Relative radio-iodine uptake (unit: %) as a function of time

F: Constant which contains conversion factors and the mean absorbed energy in the target volume per decay for a target volume of 20 ml (5% γ-ray contribution)

$F = 24.7\ \mathrm{MBq \cdot d \cdot \% \cdot g^{-1} \cdot Gy^{-1}}$ (33).

A guide to the assessment and details of the calculation procedures can be found in the guidelines of the German Society of Nuclear Medicine (34). In short, a determination of the mass of the target volume and of the pretherapeutic iodine biokinetics are needed. For measuring the biokinetics either serial scans of the patient's neck or probe measurements of the patient's thyroid for at least 4–8 days are needed. Care with the appropriate calibration of the measuring system should be taken.

The thyroid or the target volume mass is generally determined by ultrasonography (35), pretherapeutic scintigraphy (36), CT (37), MRI (38), or ^{124}I-PET (39). A change in the thyroid mass during therapy might be considered in the calculation but the data published up to now are still under evaluation (40).

This dosimetric approach assumes that the iodine kinetics of a tracer and of a therapeutic amount of administered activity are similar. For a confirmation of the absorbed dose achieved after therapy, a post-therapeutic dose assessment is recommended as, according to some authors, a pretherapeutic tracer dose may induce 'stunning'. This effect might limit the uptake of the therapeutic activity in the thyroid gland (41). Due to the uncertainties related to all of these procedures described above, an overall systematic uncertainty of the dose assessment process of 30–50% must be assumed (42).

Special considerations in children

Hyperthyroidism in children is mostly caused by Graves' disease and the risk of relapse in this age group is much higher than in adults. There is good evidence that the fetal and young thyroid is particularly sensitive to radiation and it is therefore appropriate to avoid treating hyperthyroid children with radio-iodine if reasonable and safe alternatives are available. This can be a difficult decision since surgical thyroidectomy in young children has been accompanied by a relatively high morbidity and antithyroid drugs have a certain incidence of compliance problems and drug complications (43–45). At the very least, an extended trial of antithyroid drugs is advisable, although occasionally drug toxicity makes this strategy impractical. However, reports of radio-iodine therapy in young children have shown that it is effective and late follow-up has shown no deleterious effects (26, 46).

References

1. Becker DV, Sawin CT. Radioiodine and thyroid disease: the beginning. *Semin Nucl Med*, 1996; **26**: 155–64.
2. Hegedüs L. Treatment of Graves' hyperthyroidism: evidence-based and emerging modalities. *Endocrinol Metab Clin North Am*, 2009; **38**: 355–71.
3. Brent GA. Clinical practice. Graves' disease. *N Engl J Med*, 2008; **358**: 2594–605.
4. Meier DA, Brill DR, Becker DV, Clarke SE, Silberstein EB, Royal HD, *et al.* Procedure guideline for therapy of thyroid disease with (131) iodine. *J Nucl Med*, 2002; **43**: 856–61.
5. Surks MI, Ortiz E, Daniels GH, Sawin CT, Col NF, Cobin RH, *et al.* Subclinical thyroid disease: scientific review and guidelines for diagnosis and management. *JAMA*, 2004; **291**: 228–38.
6. Stokkel MP, Handkiewicz Junak D, Lassmann M, Dietlein M, Luster M. EANM procedure guidelines for therapy of benign thyroid disease. *Eur J Nucl Med Mol Imaging*, 2010; **37**(11): 2218–28. Epub 13 Jul 2010.
7. Weetman A, Armitage M, Clarke S, Frank J, Franklyn J, Lapsley P, *et al. Radioiodine in the Management of Benign Thyroid Disease: Clinical Guidelines: Report of a Working Party*. London: Royal College of Physicians, 2007.
8. Vaidya B, Williams GR, Abraham P, Pearce SH. Radioiodine treatment for benign thyroid disorders: results of a nationwide survey of UK endocrinologists. *Clin Endocrinol (Oxf)*, 2008; **68**: 814–20.
9. Bonnema SJ, Bennedbaek FN, Ladenson PW, Hegedüs L. Management of the nontoxic multinodular goiter: a North American survey. *J Clin Endocrinol Metab*, 2002; **87**: 112–17.
10. Bachmann J, Kobe C, Bor S, Rahlff I, Dietlein M, Schicha H, *et al.* Radioiodine therapy for thyroid volume reduction of large goiters. *Nucl Med Commun*, 2009; **30**: 466–71.
11. Fast S, Nielsen VE, Bonnema SJ, Hegedüs L. Time to reconsider nonsurgical therapy of benign non-toxic multinodular goiter: focus on recombinant human TSH augmented radioiodine therapy. *Eur J Endocrinol*, 2009; **160**: 517–28.
12. Fast S, Nielsen VE, Grupe P, Bonnema SJ, Hegedüs L. Optimizing ^{131}I uptake after rhTSH stimulation in patients with nontoxic multinodular goiter: evidence from a prospective, randomized, double-blind study. *J Nucl Med*, 2009; **50**: 732–7.
13. Weetman AP. Radioiodine treatment for benign thyroid diseases. *Clin Endocrinol (Oxf)*, 2007; **66**: 757–64.
14. Walter MA, Briel M, Christ-Crain M, Bonnema SJ, Connell J, Cooper DS, *et al.* Effects of antithyroid drugs on radioiodine treatment: systematic review and meta-analysis of randomised controlled trials. *BMJ*, 2007; **334**: 514–17.
15. Lind P. Strategies of radioiodine therapy for Graves' disease. *Eur J Nucl Med Mol Imaging*, 2002; **29** (Suppl 2): S453–7.
16. Sabri O, Zimny M, Schulz G, Schreckenberger M, Reinartz P, Willmes K, *et al.* Success rate of radioiodine therapy in Graves' disease: the influence of thyrostatic medication. *J Clin Endocrinol Metab*, 1999; **84**: 1229–33.
17. Imseis RE, Vanmiddlesworth L, Massie JD, Bush AJ, Vanmiddlesworth NR. Pretreatment with propylthiouracil but not methimazole reduces the therapeutic efficacy of iodine-131 in hyperthyroidism. *J Clin Endocrinol Metab*, 1998; **83**: 685–7.
18. Acharya SH, Avenell A, Philip S, Burr J, Beva JS, Abraham P. Radioiodine therapy for Graves' disease and the effect on ophthalmopathy: a systematic review. *Clin Endocrinol*, 2008; **69**: 943–50.
19. Sisson JC, Schipper MJ, Nelson CC, Freitas JE, Frueh BR. Radioiodine therapy and Graves' ophthalmopathy. *J Nucl Med*, 2008; **49**: 923–30.
20. Tanda ML, Lai A, Bartalena L. Relation between Graves' orbitopathy and radioiodine therapy for hyperthyroidism: facts and unsolved questions. *Clin Endocrinol (Oxf)*, 2008; **69**: 845–7.
21. Laurberg P, Wallin G, Tallstedt L, Abraham-Nordling M, Lundell G, Tørring O. TSH receptor autoimmunity in Graves' disease after therapy with anti-thyroid drugs' surgery, or radioiodine: a 5-year prospective randomized study. *Eur J Endocrinol*, 2008; **158**: 69–75.
22. Bartalena L, Baldeschi L, Dickinson AJ, Eckstein A, Kendall-Taylor P, Marcocci C, *et al.* Consensus statement of the European Group on Graves' orbitopathy (EUGOGO) on management of GO. *Eur J Endocrinol*, 2008; **158**: 273–85.
23. Perros P, Kendall-Taylor P, Neoh C, Frewin S, Dickinson J. A prospective study of the effects of radioiodine therapy for hyperthyroidism in patients with minimally active Graves' ophthalmopathy. *J Clin Endocrinol Metab*, 2005; **90**: 5321–3.
24. Bartalena L, Marcocci C, Bogazzi F, Manetti L, Tanda ML, Dell'Unto E, *et al.* Relation between therapy for hyperthyroidism and the course of Graves' ophthalmopathy. *N Engl J Med*, 1998; **338**: 73–8.
25. Wiersinga WM. Preventing Graves' ophthalmopathy. *N Engl J Med*, 1998; **338**: 121–2.
26. Read CH Jr, Tansey MJ, Menda Y. A 36-year retrospective analysis of the efficacy and safety of radioactive iodine in treating young Graves' patients. *J Clin Endocrinol Metab*, 2004; **89**: 4229–33.
27. Hall P, Holm LE. Late consequences of radioiodine for diagnosis and therapy in Sweden. *Thyroid*, 1997; **7**: 205–8.
28. Saenger EL, Thoma GE, Tompkins EA. Incidence of leukemia following treatment of hyperthyroidism. Preliminary report of the Cooperative Thyrotoxicosis Therapy Follow-Up Study. *JAMA*, 1968; **205**: 855–62.
29. Ron E, Doody MM, Becker DV, Brill AB, Curtis RE, Goldman MB, *et al.* Cancer mortality following treatment of adult hyperthyroidism. *JAMA*, 1998; **280**: 347–55.
30. Holm LE, Hall P, Wiklund K, Lundell G, Berg G, Bjelkengren G, *et al.* Cancer risk after iodine-131 therapy for hyperthyroidism. *J Natl Cancer Inst*, 1991; **83**: 1072–7.
31. Clarke SEM. Radionuclide therapy of the thyroid. *Eur J Nucl Med*, 1991; **18**: 984–91.

32. Bockisch A, Jamitzky T, Derwanz R, Biersack HJ. Optimized dose planning of radioiodine therapy of benign thyroidal diseases. *J Nucl Med*, 1993; **34**: 1632–8.
33. Snyder WS, Ford MR, Warner GGS. Absorbed Dose per Unit Cumulated Activity for Selected Radionuclides and Organs. MIRD Pamphlet 11. New York: Society of Nuclear Medicine, 1975.
34. Dietlein M, Dressler J, Eschner W, Lassmann M, Leisner B, Reiners *et al.* [Procedure guideline for radioiodine test (Version 3)]. *Nuklearmedizin*, 2007; **46**: 198–202.
35. Hegedüs L, Perrild H, Poulsen LR, Andersen JR, Holm B, Schnohr P, *et al.* The determination of thyroid volume by ultrasound and its relation to body weight, age, and sex in normal subjects. *J Clin Endocrinol Metab*, 1983; **56**: 260–3.
36. van Isselt JW, de Klerk JMH, van Rijk PP, van Gils APG, Polman LJ, Kamphuis C, *et al.* Comparison of methods for thyroid volume estimation in patients with Graves' disease. *Eur J Nucl Med*, 2003; **30**: 525–31.
37. Hermans R, Bouillon R, Laga K, Delaere PR, Foer BD, Marchal G, *et al.* Estimation of thyroid gland volume by spiral computed tomography. *Eur Radiol*, 1997; **7**: 214–16.
38. Bonnema SJ, Andersen PB, Knudsen DU, Hegedüs L. MR imaging of large multinodular goiters: observer agreement on volume versus observer disagreement on dimensions of the involved trachea. *Am J Roentgenol*, 2002; **179**: 259–66.
39. Crawford DC, Flower MA, Pratt BE, Hill C, Zweit J, McCready VR, *et al.* Thyroid volume measurement in thyrotoxic patients: comparison between ultrasonography and iodine-124 positron emission tomography. *Eur J Nucl Med*, 1997; **24**: 1470–8.
40. Traino AC, Di Martino F, Grosso M, Monzani F, Dardano A, Caraccio N, *et al.* A predictive mathematical model for the calculation of the final mass of Graves' disease thyroids treated with ^{131}I. *Phys Med Biol*, 2005; **50**: 2181–91.
41. Sabri O, Zimny M, Schreckenberger M, Meyer-Oelmann A, Reinartz P, Buell U. Does thyroid stunning exist? A model with benign thyroid disease. *Eur J Nucl Med*, 2000; **27**: 1591–7.
42. Traino AC, Xhafa B. Accuracy of two simple methods for estimation of thyroidal ^{131}I kinetics for dosimetry-based treatment of Graves' disease. *Med Phys*, 2009; **36**: 1212–18.
43. Rivkees SA, Dinauer C. An optimal treatment for pediatric Graves' disease is radioiodine. *J Clin Endocrinol Metab*, 2007; **92**: 797–800.
44. Lee JA, Grumbach MM, Clark OH. The optimal treatment for pediatric Graves' disease is surgery. *J Clin Endocrinol Metab*, 2007; **92**: 801–3.
45. Becker DV. The role of radioiodine treatment in childhood hyperthyroidism. *J Nucl Med*, 1979; **20**: 890–4.
46. MacDougal IR. Which therapy for Graves' hyperthyroidism in children. *Nucl Med Commun*, 1989; **10**: 855–57.

3.3.8 Surgery for thyrotoxicosis

Mauricio Moreno, Nancy D. Perrier, Orlo Clark

Introduction

Surgical intervention plays a critical role in the management of thyrotoxicosis. Despite this, radioactive iodine is still the most popular treatment modality in the USA. Thyrotoxicosis, the condition of hyperthyroidism, is due to the increased secretion of thyroid hormone, and may be caused by toxic solitary nodules, toxic multinodular goitre (Plummer's disease), or diffuse toxic goitre (Graves' disease). Graves' disease is the condition of goitre and associated clinical features of tachycardia and bulging eyes described by Dr Robert James Graves (1797–1853) in 1835 (1). Understanding the pathophysiology of the condition of thyrotoxicosis is essential in the appropriate selection of surgical candidates and planning the most suitable technique. Generally, accepted indications for thyroidectomy for thyrotoxicosis include: suspicion of malignancy by physical examination (firmness, irregularity, or attachment to local structures) or by fine-needle aspiration cytology of nodules; pregnancy; women desiring pregnancy within 6–12 months of treatment; lactation; medical necessity for rapid control of symptoms (patients with cardiac morbidity); local compression (pain, dysphagia); recurrence after antithyroid drug treatment; fear of radioactive iodine treatment; resistance to ^{131}I or antithyroid drugs; or thyroid storm unresponsive to medical therapy. Other more relative indications for thyroidectomy also include: large goitres greater than 100 g that are less likely to respond to radioactive treatment and require a large treatment dose of ^{131}I; severe Graves' ophthalmopathy; poor compliance with antithyroid drugs; children and adolescents; a large, bothersome, and unsightly goitre; amiodarone-induced thyrotoxicosis, in cases when medical treatment is ineffective and amiodarone is necessary to treat cardiac disease; or hypersensitivity to iodine.

There are multiple advantages of thyroidectomy compared to other treatment modalities. Thyroidectomy is the fastest alternative for controlling hyperthyroidism. In most cases the medical preparation for the procedure can be achieved in 4–6 weeks (2), whereas antithyroid drugs require continuous therapy for 6–12 months with close medical surveillance. Radioactive iodine usually takes 2–6 months to become effective. Additionally thyroidectomy avoids the severe side effects of prolonged thionamide and/or radioactive iodine treatment (3). Decisions about such management strategies include issues that may have future consequences. For example, for women of childbearing age, most experts recommend avoiding pregnancy for 4–6 months after radioactive iodine treatment (4). Planning for such a decision should be discussed with the patient and family. Additionally, patients treated with radio-iodine have an increased mortality from multiple causes (5).

Surgical treatment of thyrotoxicosis is highly successful and provides a reliable cure with a recurrence of hyperthyroidism of 0.7–9.8% depending upon the size of the thyroid remnant (6). When weighing options, radioactive iodine treatment has a comparable efficacy but at 6 months only 50% of the patients are euthyroid and eventually all patients become hypothyroid. For patients treated with antithyroid drugs, the overall relapse rate exceeds 80% after treatment is discontinued (7).

Hypothyroidism is a common complication of ablative treatments and is found in 36% of the patients at 8.5 years and 50% of the patients at 12 years. Following the first year of treatment, patients have about a 3% risk per year of developing hypothyroidism. Radioactive iodine is of limited success in clinical ablation of the toxic nodule (64% remain palpable at 8.5 years). Comparatively, the rate of hypothyroidism after surgery depends on the remnant size, but is less frequent in patients who undergo a subtotal thyroidectomy than in those treated with radioactive iodine (8).

Thyroidectomy removes coexisting occult thyroid nodules. Approximately 13% of patients with Graves' disease have nodules that are suspicious for carcinoma (9) and small thyroid carcinomas are found in up to 9.8% of the patients (2). This risk is slightly increased in patients treated with radioactive iodine. A cooperative study encompassing 36 000 patients demonstrated a prevalence of thyroid cancer twice as high in patients with Graves' disease versus euthyroid patients (10). An increased aggressiveness has been reported for thyroid cancers arising in patients with Graves' disease, as some thyroid cancers are thought to be stimulated by the thyroid-stimulating antibodies (11).

For the paediatric population, Graves' disease is associated with poor school performance, decreased attention, and frequent mood changes (12). Adverse effects of antithyroid drugs are higher than in the adult population and long-term compliance is poor. Such factors lead to a higher relapse rate. Thyroidectomy is beneficial because it has an immediate effect in controlling symptoms and effects of hyperthyroidism in thyrotoxic children. The relapse rate is below 4% (12). Most importantly, the risks of thyroidectomy in children are comparable to adults when the procedure is performed in a specialized centre (12).

From the North American perspective, surgical management is the most cost-effective strategy across a wide range of ages, with the exception of those patients with significant comorbidities that would increase surgical mortality (13). The specific advantage is age-related and, for patients older than 60 years, radioactive iodine appears to be a more cost-effective alternative.

Graves' ophthalmopathy is present in approximately 50% of patients with Graves' disease and in up to 8% of cases may lead to malignant exophthalmos. Radioactive iodine therapy is associated with a small but definitive risk of progression or development of ophthalmopathy (14). It is well documented that a course of steroids can prevent the exacerbation of Graves' ophthalmopathy in virtually every case, but the side effects of steroid treatment for Graves' ophthalmopathy include the appearance of cushingoid features (14), osteopenia, cerebral haemorrhage, atrial fibrillation, and heart failure (15). Controlled trials comparing the effect of subtotal versus total thyroidectomy on Graves' ophthalmopathy found no significant differences (16, 17). In a recent trial, near-total thyroidectomy followed by radioactive iodine therapy was superior to total thyroidectomy alone for controlling progression of Graves' ophthalmopathy (0% versus 25% of Graves' ophthalmopathy progression at 9 months) (18). Considering these results, total thyroid ablation, when it can be done safely, is recommended for patients with severe ophthalmopathy to decrease the risk of progression.

Choices of thyroid surgery

The surgical management of goitre was greatly advanced by Theodor Kocher, whose techniques significantly reduced the morbidity and mortality of thyroidectomy; he was awarded the Nobel Prize for his work in 1909. He advocated subtotal thyroidectomy as the surgical treatment for Graves' disease and this became the standard therapy until the introduction of radioactive iodine in the 1940s (19). The various operative approaches for patients are total or near-total thyroidectomy, subtotal thyroidectomy which leaves bilateral remnants of about 2.5 g, and total lobectomy and contralateral subtotal lobectomy (Hartley–Dunhill procedure) which leaves thyroid remnant of about 4–5 g on one side. The Hartley–Dunhill operation results in leaving a larger unilateral remnant on only one side. The advantage of this procedure over bilateral subtotal thyroidectomy is that it decreases the small risk of nerve injury on the remnant side and is easier to tailor the precise size of the thyroid remnant. It also decreases the risk of injury to the recurrent laryngeal nerve to one side of the neck in the event of a recurrence requiring reoperation. There are no differences in mortality, recurrent laryngeal nerve palsy, hypocalcaemia, wound complications, or recurrence rate between the two techniques (bilateral versus unilateral remnant) of subtotal thyroidectomy (20, 21).

In the cases of subtotal thyroidectomy, remnant size is directly related to the risk of developing postoperative hypothyroidism or recurrent hyperthyroidism. There are other factors associated with a higher risk of recurrent hyperthyroidism including young age, high iodine intake, Graves' ophthalmopathy, high thyroid-stimulating immunoglobulin (TSI) titres, and lymphocytic infiltration of the thyroid gland. The coexistence of Hashimoto's disease may decrease the risk of recurrence so that a larger thyroid remnant can be left in such patients.

A meta-analysis of 7241 patients on 35 studies compared the results after total thyroidectomy (TT) and subtotal thyroidectomy (ST) for Graves' disease (22). In this study there was no difference in recurrent laryngeal nerve palsy (0.9% for TT versus 0.7% for ST), transient hypocalcaemia (9.6% for TT versus 7.4% for ST), or permanent hypoparathyroidism (0.9% for TT versus 1.0% for ST). Sixty per cent of the patients in the subtotal thyroidectomy group achieved euthyroidism and 29% developed hypothyroidism; the recurrence rate for this group was 7.9% (versus 0% for the TT group). In contrast with these findings, other controlled trials have described a lower risk of permanent hypoparathyroidism for patients treated with subtotal thyroidectomy (17).

The rationale for recommending total or near-total thyroidectomy for patients with Graves' disease is based on a significantly reduced risk for recurrence, reduced risk of requiring ^{131}I ablative therapy or reoperation, comparable morbidity, and removal of coexisting pathology. The surgeon should be completely confident of the viability of the parathyroid glands and function of the recurrent laryngeal nerve on the initial side when planning a total thyroidectomy; if this is not the case, a Hartley–Dunhill procedure should be considered.

Preoperative patient preparation

Before surgical intervention, the patient should be rendered euthyroid using thionamides coupled with a β-blocker (Table 3.3.8.1). Thionamides can induce granulocytopenia or agranulocytosis. Because of this, baseline white blood cell counts should be obtained before use. In young patients with hyperthyroidism, an increased alkaline phosphatase suggests an increased 'bone turnover'; it usually takes about 8 weeks of treatment with thionamides before the alkaline phosphatase level returns to normal.

Preoperative β-blockade is recommended to control symptoms of tachycardia, tremor, restlessness, and anxiety and to decrease gland vascularity, which usually makes for a technically easier operation. β-blockade is continued up to the time of surgical intervention. If necessary, intravenous β-blockade with esmolol or propranolol can be titrated to control tachycardia or arrhythmia during the operation, although this should not be necessary for a properly prepared patient. β-blockade is contraindicated for patients who have a history of asthma, obstructive airway disease,

Table 3.3.8.1 Recommended preoperative medications

Name	Family	Preoperative dosage	Initiation
Propylthiouracil	Thionamide	150–300 mg every 6 h, orally	Begin at least 2 weeks before surgery
Methimazole	Thionamide	15–30 mg every 8 h, orally	Begin at least 2 weeks before surgery
Propranolol	β-blocker	15–40 mg every 6–8 h, orally 0.5–1 mg titrated IV	Titrated to keep resting heart rate below 90 beats/min
Nadolol	β-blocker	120–160 mg every day orally	Begin at least 2 weeks before surgery
SSKI	Potassium iodide	500 mg twice daily, orally	Begin 3–4 days before surgery
Lugol's solution	Iodine with potassium iodide	Three drops twice daily, orally	Begin 1–2 weeks before surgery

SSKI, saturated solution of potassium iodide.

bradycardia, or symptoms mimicking congestive heart failure. In any of these cases, the use of thionamides should be extended to 4–6 weeks preoperatively.

Iodides, in addition to reducing the uptake of iodide and inhibiting the release of thyroid hormone, also decrease the vascularity of the thyroid gland. For this reason, Lugol's solution or a saturated solution of potassium iodide (SSKI) is recommended for about 10 days preoperatively. Although serum triiodothyronine (T_3) and thyroxine (T_4) levels fall initially in all patients, this occurrence is incomplete and transient; therefore iodine should not be used alone or beyond 2 weeks. Both iodides and β-blockers should be given together or with a thionamide in preparation for an operation. In patients with intolerance to thionamides, noncompliance, or the necessity of emergency thyroidectomy, β-blockade plus iodide or steroids may be used.

Sodium ipodate is an oral cholecystographic agent that has several effects on thyroid hormone metabolism. Sodium ipodate releases iodine after it is metabolized, thereby inhibiting the synthesis and secretion of thyroid hormones and it is also a potent inhibitor of the peripheral conversion of T_4 to T_3. Usually, a total dose of 3 g is utilized and this can be administered starting 3 or 4 days before surgery with similar effectiveness (23). Steroids such as prednisone are added to prevent adrenal exhaustion and to decrease the extrathyroidal conversion of T_4 to T_3 in patients with severe hyperthyroidism or thyroid storm (24). In patients who report voice changes or those with previous neck surgery, preoperative vocal cord examination should be routinely performed.

Surgical procedure

The ideal surgical therapy depends on the aetiology of the disease. In Graves' disease and/or in toxic multinodular goitre, a subtotal thyroidectomy leaving approximately 5 g of thyroid is the procedure of choice. A toxic adenoma confirmed by radionuclide scan can be treated by excision or a unilateral lobectomy. If coexisting thyroid pathology is present, such as thyroid carcinoma, a total thyroidectomy is recommended (25). Thyroid operations are associated with minimal morbidity and almost negligible mortality when performed by experienced surgeons.

The patient is placed in the supine position with the neck hyperextended. A rolled drape is placed longitudinally along the patient's spine to mobilize the thyroid gland anteriorly and cephalad. The site of the incision is marked approximately 1 cm below the cricoid cartilage, which places the incision directly over the isthmus of the thyroid gland. Superior and inferior skin flaps are raised in the subplatysmal plane and the midline raphe is opened. The strap muscles are dissected from the anterior surface of the gland and retracted laterally. The carotid sheath is retracted laterally, tensing the middle thyroid veins which are transected close to the gland. Careful inspection for the parathyroid glands and recurrent laryngeal nerve begins once the middle thyroid vein is divided. The gland is rotated medially creating tension on the inferior thyroid artery and usually bringing the recurrent laryngeal nerve into view (Fig. 3.3.8.1). If the nerve is not identified at this point, it can be recognized with careful dissection along the capsule of the gland at the level of the cricoid cartilage, where it enters the larynx posterior to the cricothyroid muscle. The right recurrent laryngeal nerve courses obliquely after travelling around the subclavian artery and the left recurrent laryngeal nerve travels almost vertically after traversing around the ligamentum arteriosum.

At this point, the surgeon must choose between controlling the superior or inferior thyroid pedicle based on his/her personal preference. If the superior pedicle is addressed first, the superior thyroid artery and vein should be ligated individually as low as possible on the thyroid parenchyma to avoid possible injury to the external laryngeal nerve. No thyroid tissue should remain cephalad to the point of ligation. The external laryngeal nerve is responsible for high-pitched sounds and is referred to as the 'Amelita Galli-Curci nerve'. Care is taken to avoid injury to this nerve by dissecting lateral to the cricothyroid muscle, where the external laryngeal nerve can often be identified.

The upper parathyroid glands are more consistent in position and can usually be identified at the level of the cricoid cartilage. The thyroid lobe is retracted anteriorly and medially and the tissues on the undersurface carefully dissected. The lower parathyroid glands are almost always anterior to the recurrent nerve and 80% of the time are within 1 cm of the junction of the inferior thyroid artery and the nerve. A broad vascular pedicle is left around the parathyroid glands to minimize the risk of devascularization. In the rare event that this cannot be accomplished, the parathyroid should be excised, its identity confirmed by frozen section analysis, and 1-mm sections autotransplanted into separate pockets in the sternocleidomastoid muscle. Once the thyroid is separated from the parathyroid glands and the recurrent nerve, the inferior thyroid veins can be safely ligated. The gland is then dissected from the anterior surface of the trachea. A dense posterior suspensory ligament (Berry's ligament) firmly attaches the thyroid to the first two tracheal rings. This is the most common site of nerve injury and special care must be taken when bleeding occurs at this site. There is a small artery and vein that are situated in this ligament,

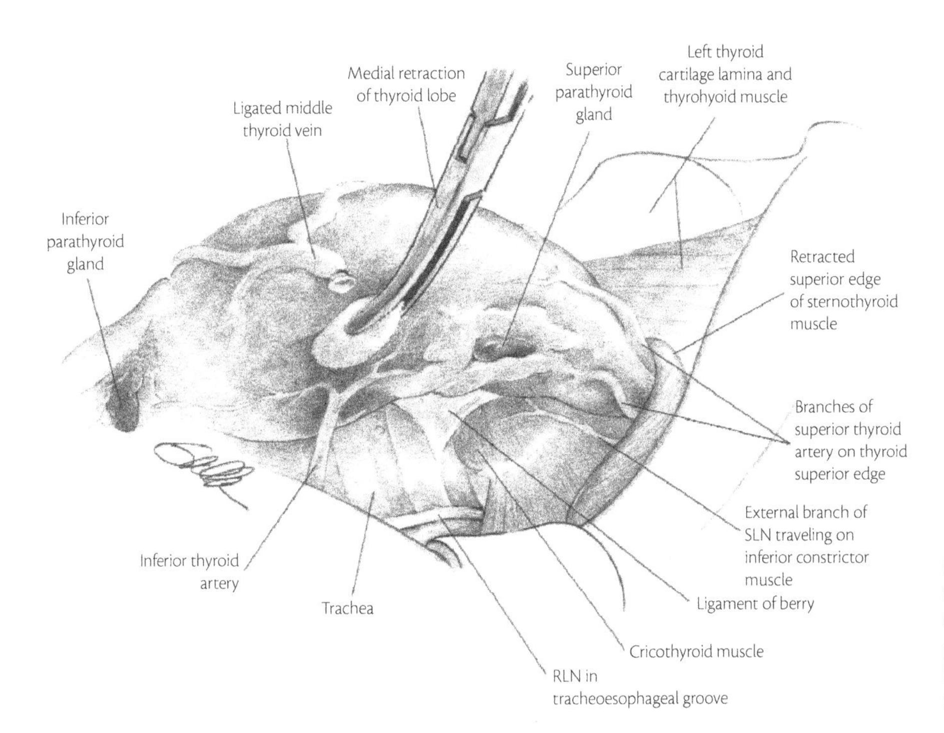

Fig. 3.3.8.1 Surgical anatomy of the recurrent laryngeal nerve in relation to the inferior thyroid artery and parathyroid glands (2). RLN, recurrent laryngeal nerve; SLN, superior laryngeal nerve.

but no vessels should be clamped in this area until the recurrent laryngeal nerve is fully visualized. The bleeding can be controlled by gentle pressure with a peanut sponge.

For subtotal resection a similar process is repeated on the opposite side, except that a thyroid remnant should be left in the area of the intersection of the recurrent nerve and cricothyroid muscle. The inferior thyroid artery is also usually kept intact to provide a blood supply to the remnant. Remnant size can be approximated by matching it to a measured and weighed tissue sample taken from the previously removed contralateral lobe. If the indications call for total thyroidectomy, no remnant is left in the neck. For patients with Graves' disease, we prefer the Hartley–Dunhill operation, which is a total lobectomy on one side and a subtotal or near-total lobectomy on the other, leaving 2–6 g depending on the desired outcome. For children, a smaller thyroid remnant is necessary because recurrence is more likely.

Perfect haemostasis is achieved. The sternothyroid muscles are approximated leaving a small opening in the midline at the suprasternal notch to enable blood to escape and to make bleeding more evident if it were to occur postoperatively. The platysma muscle is aligned and approximated, and the skin is closed with a subcutaneous suture or winged clips. Dressings are applied and the patient is wakened, extubated, and transported to the postoperative recovery area. Most patients are ready for discharge on the following morning.

There are several schools of thought on how much thyroid remnant to leave. Some surgeons aim to create hypothyroidism and not achieve a euthyroid state in order to avoid recurrence, while others aim for euthyroidism by leaving an appropriate amount of thyroid tissue (26). In a range of 2–8 g, increasing the remnant size by 1 g decreases the rate of postoperative hypothyroidism by about 10%. This calculation is based on a 70% rate of hypofunction if 2 g are left intact. However, increasing the remnant size to above 10 g does not further decrease hypothyroidism but rather increases the risk of recurrence.

Some surgeons leave 3–5 g of tissue on both sides of the neck. This procedure is associated with a recurrence rate of about 10% and a hypothyroid rate of 10% (27). We generally aim to leave between 4 to 7 g of thyroid remnant on one side of the neck when we wish to render the patient euthyroid. A smaller remnant or no remnant is left in children because recurrence is more likely; the same applies to patients in whom radioactive iodine therapy is undesirable or those with severe complications following antithyroid drugs.

Postoperative complications

Specific complications after thyroid surgery for thyrotoxicosis include the following in order of importance: bleeding, recurrent laryngeal nerve injury, hypocalcaemia due to parathyroid hypofunction or hungry bone disease, as well as infection, thyroid storm, keloid formation, and seroma. Luckily, these complications are rare and 99% of patients can be discharged on the first postoperative day. Patients rendered euthyroid with antithyroid drugs or Lugol's solution before surgery do not require these medications postoperatively. If β-blockade was used preoperatively it should be continued for 3–5 days postoperatively because the half-life of thyroid hormone is about 1 week and the half-life of propranolol is 2–4 h.

Thyroid storm is exceedingly rare today. Treatment for such patients includes intravenous β-blockers, oxygen, cooling, sedation, intravenous steroids, sodium ipodate, hydrocortisone, and propylthiouracil in an intensive care setting. Aspirin should be avoided in the management of hyperthermia because it increases free thyroid hormone levels and may exacerbate the condition (28). The primary cause of thyroid storm is probably the marked increase in β-adrenergic effects rather than an acute increase in thyroid hormone concentration.

All patients after a thyroid operation should be carefully evaluated for postoperative bleeding. If any patient develops respiratory distress within 24 h of the thyroid operation, it is due to a neck hematoma until proven otherwise. Injury to the external laryngeal nerve may not be noticeable in some patients but can be a major disability in others who enjoy singing or speaking publicly. Unilateral recurrent laryngeal nerve injury occurs in 1–2% of patients and results in hoarseness and aspiration. Bilateral injury manifests as respiratory distress although patients may be able to speak, which is often confusing to the caring clinician. Bilateral vocal cord paralysis is exceptionally rare but when present often requires prolonged intubation (2–7 days) or tracheotomy.

Temporary hypocalcaemia (serum calcium <8.0 mg/dl or 2 mmol/L) occurs relatively frequently after thyroidectomy for hyperthyroidism. The incidence is as high as 46%, although less than one-half of these patients are symptomatic. Causes can be attributed to hungry bone syndrome due to postoperative reversal of thyrotoxic osteodystrophy, release of calcitonin during operative manipulation, or damage, devascularization, or inadvertent removal of the parathyroid glands during the surgery. Permanent hypoparathyroidism is a serious and potentially life-threatening complication that requires the patients to be on calcium and vitamin D permanently. Patients who undergo a total thyroidectomy for Graves' disease are considered by some to be at high risk for developing permanent hypoparathyroidism. However, in a recent series of 4426 patients, there was no difference in the incidence of hypoparathyroidism after total thyroidectomy in patients operated on for Graves' disease (1.5%) versus other conditions (1.7%) (29).

We recommend monitoring serum calcium levels at 5 and 20 h after thyroidectomy, and repeat measurements if low. Treatment is not usually necessary unless the value drops below 7.5 mg/dl or 1.875 mmol/L, or symptoms develop. Symptoms may be subtle, including tingling or numbness of the perioral area or fingertips, anxiety, paraesthesias, muscle cramps, and, if untreated, convulsions. For acute symptoms, oral calcium 1–2 g every 4–8 h is given. If the calcium level falls despite this treatment, calcium gluconate or chloride, 1–2 g every 4 h, is given intravenously. It is essential to be certain that no extravasation occurs as it can cause tissue necrosis. Calcitriol (0.25–0.75 μg twice daily) is useful for profound hypocalcaemia and phosphate binders should be reserved for patients with hyperphosphataemia.

Postoperative thyroid function

Thyroid function following thyroidectomy depends on the size and function of the thyroid remnant. Postoperative hypothyroidism ranges from 2% to 48% and recurrent hyperthyroidism ranges from 0% to 15%. Comparison among studies is difficult because of: (1) variations in patient selection, comparing those with toxic diffuse goitres, toxic multinodular goitres, and toxic adenomas; (2) different definitions of euthyroidism; and (3) inaccurate estimation of the size of the thyroid remnant. Thyroid function should be initially assessed with measurements of T_3, T_4, and thyroid-stimulating hormone (TSH) levels. The best time to judge whether a patient is hypothyroid is at least 3–6 months post-thyroidectomy. At 6 months, 20% of those patients with initial postoperative hypothyroidism will be euthyroid and most of the patients with permanent hypothyroidism will be documented.

For most patients, TSH is the only thyroid function test that is necessary, but T_3 and free T_4 are helpful in patients who have been treated for possible postoperative hypothyroidism because TSH levels may not accurately reflect the clinical state in patients who have been treated for hyperthyroidism. Most patients who develop permanent hypothyroidism after subtotal thyroid resection do so within 2 years of surgery. Every year thereafter the rate is 0.7% or lower, which compares to a 3% increase each year thereafter with radioactive iodine treatment. All patients should be monitored with a yearly serum TSH level.

References

1. Graves RJ. New observed affection of the thyroid gland in females (clinical lectures). *London Med Surg J*, 1835; **7**: 516–17.
2. Randolph G. *Surgery of the Thyroid and Parathyroid Glands*. 1st edn. Philadelphia: Saunders, 2002: 495.
3. Edmonds CJ, Smith T. The long-term hazards of the treatment of thyroid cancer with radioiodine. *Br J Radiol*, 1986; **59**: 45–51.
4. Kaplan MM, Meier DA, Dworkin HJ. Treatment of hyperthyroidism with radioactive iodine. *Endocrinol Metab Clin North Am*, 1998; **27**: 205–23.
5. Franklyn JA, Maisonneuve P, Sheppard MC, Betteridge J, Boyle P. Mortality after the treatment of hyperthyroidism with radioactive iodine. *N Engl J Med*, 1998; **338**: 712–18.
6. Erickson D, Gharib H, Li H, van Heerden JA. Treatment of patients with toxic multinodular goiter. *Thyroid*, 1998; **8**: 277–82.
7. Bouma DJ, Kammer H, Greer MA. Follow-up comparison of short-term versus 1-year antithyroid drug therapy for the thyrotoxicosis of Graves' disease. *J Clin Endocrinol Metab*, 1982; **55**: 1138–42.
8. Patwardhan NA, Moront M, Rao S, Rossi S, Braverman LE. Surgery still has a role in Graves' hyperthyroidism. *Surgery*, 1993; **114**: 1108–13.
9. Carnell NE, Valente WA. Thyroid nodules in Graves' disease: classification, characterization, and response to treatment. *Thyroid*, 1998; **8**: 571–6.
10. Dobyns BM, Sheline GE, Workman JB, Tompkins EA, McConahey WM, Becker DV. Malignant and benign neoplasms of the thyroid in patients treated for hyperthyroidism: a report of the cooperative thyrotoxicosis therapy follow-up study. *J Clin Endocrinol Metab*, 1974; **38**: 976–98.
11. Belfiore A, Garofalo MR, Giuffrida D, Runello F, Filetti S, Fiumara A, *et al.* Increased aggressiveness of thyroid cancer in patients with Graves' disease. *J Clin Endocrinol Metab*, 1990; **70**: 830–5.
12. Sherman J, Thompson GB, Lteif A, Schwenk WF 2nd, van Heerden J, Farley DR, *et al.* Surgical management of Graves' disease in childhood and adolescence: an institutional experience. *Surgery*, 2006; **140**: 1056–62.
13. Vidal-Trecan GM, Stahl JE, Eckman MH. Radioiodine or surgery for toxic thyroid adenoma: dissecting an important decision. A cost-effectiveness analysis. *Thyroid*, 2004; **14**: 933–45.
14. Bartalena L, Marcocci C, Bogazzi F, Manetti L, Tanda ML, Dell'Unto E, *et al.* Relation between therapy for hyperthyroidism and the course of Graves' ophthalmopathy. *N Engl J Med*, 1998; **338**: 73–8.
15. Acharya SH, Avenell A, Philip S, Burr J, Bevan JS, Abraham P. Radioiodine therapy (RAI) for Graves' disease (GD) and the effect on ophthalmopathy: a systematic review. *Clin Endocrinol (Oxf)*, 2008; **69**: 943–50.
16. Järhult J, Rudberg C, Larsson E, Selvander H, Sjövall K, Winsa B, *et al.* Graves' disease with moderate-severe endocrine ophthalmopathy: long term results of a prospective, randomized study of total or subtotal thyroid resection. *Thyroid*, 2005; **15**: 1157–64.
17. Witte J, Goretzki PE, Dotzenrath C, Simon D, Felis P, Neubauer M, *et al.* Surgery for Graves' disease: total versus subtotal thyroidectomy-results of a prospective randomized trial. *World J Surg*, 2000; **24**: 1303–11.
18. Menconi F, Marinò M, Pinchera A, Rocchi R, Mazzi B, Nardi M, *et al.* Effects of total thyroid ablation versus near-total thyroidectomy alone on mild to moderate Graves' orbitopathy treated with intravenous glucocorticoids. *J Clin Endocrinol Metab*, 2007; **92**: 1653–8.

19. Schussler-Fiorenza CM, Bruns CM, Chen H. The surgical management of Graves' disease. *J Surg Res*, 2006; **133**: 207–14.
20. Andåker L, Johansson K, Smeds S, Lennquist S. Surgery for hyperthyroidism: hemithyroidectomy plus contralateral resection or bilateral resection? A prospective randomized study of postoperative complications and long-term results. *World J Surg*, 1992; **16**: 765–9.
21. Muller PE, Bein B, Robens E, Bein HS, Spelsberg F. Thyroid surgery according to Enderlen-Hotz or Dunhill: a comparison of two surgical methods for the treatment of Graves' disease. *Int Surg*, 2001; **86**: 112–16.
22. Palit TK, Miller CC 3rd, Miltenburg DM. The efficacy of thyroidectomy for Graves' disease: a meta-analysis. *J Surg Res*, 2000; **90**: 161–5.
23. Tomaski SM, Mahoney EM, Burgess LP, Raines KB, Bornemann M. Sodium ipodate (oragrafin) in the preoperative preparation of Graves' hyperthyroidism. *Laryngoscope*, 1997; **107**: 1066–70.
24. Cesareo R, De Meo M, Agostino A, Reda G. [Pre-surgical medical therapy of hyperthyroidism]. *Recenti Prog Med*, 1997; **88**: 277–80.
25. Abe Y, Sato H, Noguchi M, Mimura T, Sugino K, Ozaki O, *et al.* Effect of subtotal thyroidectomy on natural history of ophthalmopathy in Graves' disease. *World J Surg*, 1998; **22**: 714–17.
26. van Heerden JA. *Common Problems in Endocrine Surgery*. Chicago: Year Book Medical Publishers, 1998.
27. Jörtsö E, Lennquist S, Lundström B, Norrby K, Smeds S. The influence of remnant size, antithyroid antibodies, thyroid morphology, and lymphocyte infiltration on thyroid function after subtotal resection for hyperthyroidism. *World J Surg*, 1987; **11**: 365–71.
28. Larsen PR. Salicylate-induced increases in free triiodothyronine in human serum. Evidence of inhibition of triiodothyronine binding to thyroxine-binding globulin and thyroxine-binding prealbumin. *J Clin Invest*, 1972; **51**: 1125–34.
29. Gaujoux S, Leenhardt L, Trésallet C, Rouxel A, Hoang C, Jublanc C, *et al.* Extensive thyroidectomy in Graves' disease. *J Am Coll Surg*, 2006; **202**: 868–73.

3.3.9 Management of Graves' hyperthyroidism

Jacques Orgiazzi, Claire Bournaud

Introduction

The treatment strategy for the hyperthyroidism of Graves' disease remains a matter of controversy for several reasons. Treatment modalities available so far are symptomatic rather than pathophysiological, patients are heterogeneous in the severity and prognosis of the disease, and, in many patients, the disease is lifelong. Even symptomatic treatment should be adapted to the severity of the disease, both in terms of intensity of hyperthyroidism and degree of immunological derangement, an elusive goal so far. Current treatment modalities are medical/conservative with antithyroid drugs, often marred by relapse, and radical/destructive with radioiodine or surgery with subsequent hypothyroidism. Being controversial, the selection of the treatment strategy also requires the patient's informed cooperation. Finally, another peculiarity of the management of Graves' disease is the frequent requirement of a multidisciplinary approach. This chapter will discuss general and specific therapeutic approaches of hyperthyroid Graves' disease.

Variability of therapeutic strategies

In 1985, a survey of the therapeutic indications in Graves' disease was initiated within the European Thyroid Association. Subsequently, similar national surveys were carried out in several European countries and then, on a worldwide basis, among members of the American and Japanese Thyroid Associations. A common report appeared in 1991 (1). Within Europe, despite regional variations, a consensus existed in favour of antithyroid drugs as the first-line treatment for the 'typical' patient with Graves' disease (i.e. a 43-year-old female patient with moderate hyperthyroidism and diffuse goitre without severe ophthalmopathy). Radio-iodine therapy was employed only in limited circumstances. Surgery had little or no place as the first-line treatment. Treatment policies vary widely in different areas of the world. In the USA, the first choice of treatment (69%) for an average patient is radioactive iodine; only 30% of thyroidologists select antithyroid drugs and 1% surgery. Only for younger patients (<19 years) would thyroidologists prefer antithyroid drugs (60%) over radioactive iodine (30%). In contrast, the radioactive option is less favoured in Europe (22%) and Japan (11%), except for recurrences after surgery for which the respective figures are 80% and more than 50%; for recurrences after antithyroid drug treatment the proportions are 65% and 25%, respectively. European and Japanese thyroidologists much prefer antithyroid drugs as the first-line treatment for the average patient, whatever the gender of the patient or the severity of the disease. These surveys also demonstrate that US thyroidologists are very reluctant to use thyroid surgery, even for large goitres, in contrast to their European (50%) and Japanese (24%) counterparts.

The results of these questionnaires have not been actualized. They do, however, confirm significant regional bias in the management of Graves' disease, which can be related to cultural and educational, epidemiological, genetic and epigenetic, and even administrative causes. For instance, ambulatory use of ^{131}I is limited to activities of 74 MBq in Germany, 185 MBq in Austria and Switzerland, 370 MBq in the Netherlands, 555 MBq in Greece, Poland, Hungary, and Belgium, 740 MBq in the UK and France, and 1110 MBq in Italy and the USA.

Advantages and disadvantages of the various treatment modalities of Graves' disease

Table 3.3.9.1 summarizes the main characteristics of each type of treatment. Several treatment options are available for Graves' disease and, in the absence of specific guidelines, treatment may be adapted to meet a patient's preference. Iatrogenic hypothyroidism is no longer considered as a complication of the radical treatment options but is the ultimate goal in order to ensure the prevention of relapse of the disease.

Comparison of the three treatment methods

In a prospective randomized study performed between 1983 and 1990 by Törring *et al.* and the Swedish Thyroid Study Group, 179 patients were allocated randomly to an 18-month 'block and replace' antithyroid drug treatment (71 patients), near-total thyroidectomy (67 patients), or radioactive iodine (120 Gy; 41 patients) (2).

Table 3.3.9.1 Advantages and disadvantages of the various modalities of treatment of Graves' hyperthyroidism

Treatment modality	Advantages	Disadvantages
Antithyroid drug	◆ Theoretical possibility of long-term remission	◆ Long duration (1–2 years) of treatment and repeated consultations ◆ High relapse rate
Radio-iodine[a]	◆ Simplicity (depending on local regulation) ◆ Low cost ◆ Rarity of recurrence (depending in the dose)	◆ Delay of action ◆ Transient expansion of anti-TSHR autoimmunity
Surgery[b]	◆ Highest restoration rate of euthyroidism ◆ Recurrence uncommon	◆ Highly experienced surgical/medical team mandatory ◆ Low but unavoidable morbidity ◆ High cost

[a] Prior restoration of euthyroidism with antithyroid drugs is appropriate in severe cases.
[b] Prior restoration of euthyroidism requires several weeks antithyroid drugs treatment.
TSHR, thyroid-stimulating hormone receptor.

Only patients over 35 years of age were randomized to radioactive iodine; the proportion of 'young' (20–34) and 'old' (35–55) patients allocated to medical or surgical treatment was comparable; cigarette smoking was similar in each group. Patients with large goitres were excluded from the study. Patients were followed up for 4 years after treatment. The main results from this study are listed below.

- The risk of relapse was higher in the medically treated 'young' (42%) than 'old' (34%) patients; relapse was 21% after radio-iodine treatment and 3–8% after surgery.
- Patients' satisfaction with the randomly allocated treatment was excellent (95–98%); only 8–11% feared adverse effects from their treatment while 14% were concerned about receiving radioactivity; 68%, 74%, and 84% allocated to medical, surgical, or ^{131}I treatment, respectively, would recommend it to a friend.
- Occurrence of relapse was considered a point of major disappointment by 57% of the patients treated medically, by 75% surgically, and by only 40% of those who received ^{131}I.
- Another point of major interest was the time taken to return to a state of wellbeing; 48% of those operated on felt they had recovered in less than 3 months as compared with 24% for the other two treatment groups. At 1 year, 61% of those treated surgically, and 39% and 48% of the patients in the medical and radioactive groups, respectively, felt well.
- Interestingly, sick leave was comparable (62–74 days) in the three groups.
- Occurrence or worsening of ophthalmopathy during or after treatment was observed exclusively in patients in the radioactive group, mainly in those who had received more than one dose of ^{131}I.

The study raises some interesting points regarding selection of treatment.

- There was no difference in satisfaction related to the choice of treatment.
- There was a feeling of strong disappointment associated with relapse.
- There was concern about receiving radioactive iodine.
- The delay before full recovery was longer for the medical and radiation treatments than for the surgical option.

Also, longer follow-up (14–21 years) of the same cohort of patients showed that it was Graves' disease itself, and not the treatment modality, which has negative consequences on the health-related quality of life, especially with regard to mental performance and vitality (3).

The cost-effectiveness of the various modalities of treatment has been evaluated according to different models (4), but individually studied only in two publications (5, 6). Both conclude that the cost-effective primary treatment modality for hyperthyroidism is radio-iodine. In all the studies the surgical modality cost is the highest. The cost of the medical treatment modality is intermediate. However, inclusion of the relapse costs tends to level off the differences between the three modalities (4).

Treatment modalities

Therapeutic modalities are discussed according to the various clinical presentations, including the usual ones, the presence of a large goitre, children and adolescents, pregnancy, and presence of ophthalmopathy. Severe or acute forms (thyrotoxic storm) are examined in Chapter 3.3.3.

Typical form of hyperthyroid Graves' disease

This corresponds to the average 40- to 50-year-old female patient referred to in the surveys described above.

Antithyroid drug treatment

Since the main drawback of antithyroid drugs as the sole treatment is the overall 50% relapse rate, many investigations have been performed to optimize either the indications or the modality of the treatment. Many studies have tried to identify, at the time of diagnosis, factors, clinical or biological, which could predict the outcome of the disease after the end of the antithyroid drug course. Male gender, young age, as well as severity of hyperthyroidism, thyroid volume, and level of antithyroid-stimulating hormone-receptor antibodies (TRAb), which are interdependent factors, are statistically correlated with a greater risk of relapse. However, for a given patient there is no marker, either initially or during antithyroid treatment, which is really predictive of the subsequent outcome. The dose of antithyroid drugs and the duration of treatment, as well as the addition of L-thyroxine, have been thoroughly evaluated to define the regimen with the highest remission/relapse ratio. Four results have emerged from these studies (7–10).

- Remissions are more frequent after prolonged (12–18 months) antithyroid drug treatment than after shorter courses (62% versus 42%).
- A high daily dose of antithyroid drug (60 mg carbimazole), as compared to the usual one (30 mg), has no advantage; on the contrary, untoward effects appear to be dose-dependent.
- The combination of L-thyroxine with a fixed dose of antithyroid drugs (the block and replace regimen) does not improve the post-treatment outcome as compared to the titration of antithyroid

drugs to euthyroidism; however, the block and replace regimen may be simpler to monitor, at least during the first months of treatment, since iatrogenic hypothyroidism is prevented.

- There is no single good marker to determine, on an individual basis, when to stop the treatment and hence, the fixed duration of treatment; however, lack of goitre volume reduction, persistence of thyroid hypervascularity, and, in those with the titration regimen—the more appropriate at this stage—noncorrection of the suppressed thyroid-stimulating hormone (TSH) and the persistent requirement for a full dose of antithyroid drugs are indicative of disease activity and of recurrence at drug withdrawal. Similar information is provided by persistently elevated titres of TRAb.

In practical terms, antithyroid drug treatment is usually started at 30–40 mg/day for carbimazole, 30 mg/day for methimazole, or 300 mg/day for propylthiouracil (PTU). After 4–8 weeks of treatment, the dose of the drug is progressively decreased to avoid hypothyroidism (titration regimen), or maintained at the same dose and L-thyroxine introduced (block and replace regimen) at a progressive dosage to reach 100–125 μg/day after 6–10 weeks. Regular clinical and biological control is mandatory. Except in cases of noncompliance or of the occurrence of untoward effects that the patient should be instructed to report without delay, the course of the treatment is usually uneventful, and in most cases correction of hyperthyroidism is sufficient to allow resumption of a near-normal life within a few weeks. At the start, alleviation of symptoms is accelerated by β-blocker treatment. After about 18 months of treatment, antithyroid drugs are usually withdrawn, or progressively decreased until cessation. Continuation of L-thyroxine treatment has no beneficial effect. In the case of the block and replace modality it is advisable to shift to the titration modality after 10–14 months of treatment so that functional thyroid status can be better assessed. Close follow-up is necessary to avoid misinterpreting the period of euthyroidism that follows drug withdrawal as a true remission. Most relapses occur within months of cessation of antithyroid drugs and 90% within 3 years. In more than 50% of the patients, relapse cannot be predicted.

There is no specific treatment strategy for relapsing Graves' disease; however, a radical approach appears more appropriate and acceptable to patients. No study demonstrates that relapse risk is greater after a second antithyroid drugs course. In some patients, continuation of antithyroid drug treatment for 2–3 years, or even longer, appears an appropriate option. The necessary conditions for this are: (1) a low antithyroid drug dosage requirement (carbimazole 5 mg/day, PTU 50 mg/day, or less), (2) patient dependability and drug tolerance, and (3) moderate intensity of the disease, with absent or small goitre and absence of extrathyroidal manifestation. That such a low-dose maintenance treatment is efficient is suggested by the possible occurrence of a relapse at drug withdrawal or after iodine contamination.

Radioactive iodine

The risk of hypothyroidism after treatment with ^{131}I is generally taken, at least in Europe, as a justification for an initial trial with medical treatment. In addition, the patients' concern about potential radiation danger to themselves and others, apparently encouraged in some countries by local legislation, may be difficult to overcome. In many places radioactive iodine is not administered to patients under 30–35 years of age.

Using thyroid irradiation, restoration of euthyroidism is an unrealistic target because of the inaccuracy of intrathyroidal ^{131}I dosimetry. Therefore, as for thyroidectomy, hypothyroidism is the price to pay for the definitive eradication of hyperthyroidism. In addition, aiming at hypothyroidism will decrease the risk of post-irradiation subclinical hyperthyroidism, a potentially deleterious condition (11). Patients should be prepared for life-long thyroxine treatment and follow-up. Evaluation of the dose of ^{131}I to be administered has been discussed in Chapter 3.3.7. In order to eradicate hyperthyroidism, ablative ^{131}I doses range from 5.9 to 6.5 MBq/g (160–176 μCi/g) of thyroid tissue for adjusted doses, or from 400 to 600 MBq (10.8–16.2 mCi) when fixed doses are administered. Whether routine measurement of the effective half-life of intrathyroidal ^{131}I is cost-effective has to be evaluated according to local iodine intake status. This range of doses eradicates hyperthyroidism in around two-thirds of patients (12). Failure can be treated 6 months after initial irradiation with a second dose of ^{131}I. Radioiodine as the first-line treatment is more appropriate for patients in whom a relapse is more likely to occur after an antithyroid drug course, if monitoring of antithyroid drug treatment appears impractical, or at relapse after a first antithyroid drug course.

The issue of whether or not antithyroid drug treatment should be recommended before ^{131}I administration remains unsettled. To prevent a possible destructive exacerbation of hyperthyroidism and to shorten the delay to euthyroidism, 20–40% of thyroidologists would prescribe antithyroid drugs before or after radioactive iodine. In typical patients, the risk of aggravation of hyperthyroidism is small or absent. Adjunctive antithyroid drugs reduce biochemical and clinical hyperthyroidism in the weeks after radioiodine treatment (13). But antithyroid drugs increase the rate of failure and reduce the rate of hypothyroidism when they are given the week before or after radio-iodine, which can be overcome by increasing the dose of ^{131}I. There are no data on the optimal interruption period of antithyroid drugs before radio-iodine administration in order not to interfere with efficiency of irradiation. According to some studies, PTU appears to interfere more, and for a longer period, with radio-iodine efficiency than methimazole (13, 14). Administration of antithyroid drugs after ^{131}I treatment, starting 10–15 days later and for a limited period of 4–8 weeks, is a reasonable option which, however, may precipitate the occurrence of hypothyroidism when ablative doses of ^{131}I are used. In order to avoid hypothyroidism, close follow-up is mandatory. In some centres with a rather high ^{131}I dose policy, L-thyroxine, 100 μg/day, is systematically started 15 days after isotope administration. In any case, plasma thyroid hormone concentration should be tested 4–6 weeks after irradiation and then monthly. The effect of the radioactive treatment can be evaluated at 4 months.

Following ^{131}I treatment hypothyroidism may be transient, and hyperthyroidism may even recur subsequently. Reversibility of hypothyroidism is to be suspected in case of early occurrence, moderation of clinical and biological abnormalities, and the lack of reduction of the volume of the thyroid. TSH suppression may outlast normalization of thyroid hormone levels. The routine measurement of TRAb has no practical indication.

Radio-iodine therapy increases thyroid autoimmune activity presumably through the release of thyroid antigens. Serum TRAb and other antithyroid autoantibodies increase transiently, peaking 3–5 months after irradiation. In prospective studies, this rise could be prevented by antithyroid drugs or glucocorticoids (15). This effect of ^{131}I should not be overlooked in women of childbearing age as well as in adolescents, since blood TRAb may remain elevated for several years with the subsequent risk, during pregnancy, of transplacental fetal thyroid disease (16). Finally, every patient treated with ^{131}I should be included in a long-term follow-up programme with systematic recall to avoid overlooking subsequent subclinical hyperthyroidism, as well as late-onset hypothyroidism.

Thyroid surgery

In the typical patient with Graves' disease, there is almost no place for surgery. Subtotal thyroidectomy is to be considered in the case of agranulocytosis or severe intolerance to antithyroid drugs and if radio-iodine treatment is inadvisable because of the severity of hyperthyroidism or iodine contamination. In this condition, preparation for surgery requires a β-blocker either by mouth (40 mg/6 h) or intravenously (infusion rate 5–10 mg/h) to lower the resting pulse to less than 80 beats/min. In severe cases, high-dose glucocorticoid (betamethasone 0.5 mg/6 h) may be useful (17).

Other clinical conditions including presence of a large goitre

As mentioned previously, subtotal or near-total thyroidectomy is the treatment preferred by thyroidologists in Europe and Japan but not in the USA. An experienced surgical team is mandatory. The schedule of the therapeutic management programme must be precisely defined. It includes: (1) an antithyroid drug course of 6–12 weeks, with close monitoring of the thyroid status and prevention of iatrogenic hypothyroidism and goitrogenesis; (2) if required by the surgical team, preoperative iodine (50–120 mg/day: Lugol's solution or saturated solution of potassium iodide (SSKI)), the duration of which should not exceed 10 days; (3) the operation itself; (4) postoperative management. Alternative preoperative programmes have been advocated using only β-blockers with or without iodide. They require tight monitoring and highly trained medical and surgical teams. Whatever the preparation, surgery on patients with hypervascular goitre has to be carefully planned and is best performed in selected centres.

Children and adolescents

Incidence of Graves' disease in this age group is 0.8/100 000 per year. All the treatment difficulties—controversies over the choice of therapy, advantages and disadvantages of each type of treatment, patient compliance, and feasibility of extended follow-up—are exaggerated in this age group.

Medical treatment

On the whole, antithyroid drugs treatment was the first choice of 99% of professionals in a recent European questionnaire study (18). Carbimazole is given at a median initial dose of 0.8 mg/kg per day, titrated to euthyroidism in 39% or according to the block and replace regimen in 56%, and for a fixed period (1–2 years or longer for 44% of the respondents). Surgery is selected only in case of large goitre (16%) or of recurrence after antithyroid drugs (4%). Radioactive iodine is restricted to recurrences after subtotal thyroidectomy (18% of the respondents) or after antithyroid drugs treatment (7%). Antithyroid drugs may cause untoward effects in 20–30% of the patients in this age group (19). They are usually benign but serious complications appear as frequently as in adults (e.g. incidence of agranulocytosis is 0.4%). In some children and adolescents, antithyroid drugs may fail to control the thyrotoxic status effectively, with consequent irritability, tiredness, and behavioural, psychological, and school difficulties. This apparent resistance to antithyroid drugs may develop after several months of uneventful and efficient treatment, and despite good compliance. Goitre often enlarges, with vascular bruit, and there is a marked increase in serum triiodothyronine (T_3). Increasing the dose of antithyroid drugs is not always efficient and radical treatment is usually mandatory. Thyroid cancer in children and adolescents with Graves' disease appears to be exceptional. However, it is appropriate to mention that, at least in adults, the incidence of thyroid carcinoma is greater in those treated with antithyroid drugs than with the other treatments.

In this age group, the remission rate after antithyroid drugs treatment is very low, 19–38%, even after treatments of long duration ranging from 1 to 8 years. It is lower in prepubertal than pubertal individuals. It has been shown that older age (12.5 versus 10.9 years), higher body mass index (19.0 versus 16.6), lower heart rate (110 versus 121 beats/min) and thyroid size, lower platelet count (272 versus 339 × 10^9/l), lower serum thyroxine T_4 and T_3 concentrations (T_4 18.3 versus 22.5 μg/dl; T_3 439 versus 613 ng/dl), and lower thyroid-stimulating antibody positivity (50% versus 93%) at presentation were significantly correlated with early remission (20). In a recent French multicentre study of 154 children with Graves' disease treated with antithyroid drugs for 24 months, the relapse rate was 59%. The risk of relapse was higher for nonwhite patients and patients with high serum TRAb and free T_4 levels at diagnosis. Relapse risk decreased with increasing age at onset and duration of the first course of antithyroid drug. Three different risk groups were identified with 2-year relapse rates of 46%, 77%, and 98% (21).

In practical terms, it is suitable that antithyroid drugs remain the first-line therapy, with the block and replace regimen achieving better control and requiring fewer hospital visits. However, it is advisable to consider radical treatments when antithyroid drug therapy no longer appears appropriate for whatever reason: poor compliance or erratic follow-up, excessive interference with daily life, apparent inefficacy, untoward effects, growth of thyroid volume, or persistence or resumption of signs of disease activity.

Radical treatment

In the face of the many drawbacks and indirect inconvenience of prolonged or iterative antithyroid drug treatments in this age group, radical treatment is often inescapable. The choice between surgical and radioactive treatments does not rely on well-established guidelines. Convincing data (18, 22) indicate that neither excess thyroid malignancy nor adverse events could be attributed to radio-iodine therapy in children and adolescents. Radio-iodine should be properly administered, i.e. not below 5 years of age, when risk of radiation-induced thyroid carcinogenesis and the total body radiation doses appear to be greatest, and with a larger (of the order of 120–160 μCi/g) rather than a lower dose, the latter being more likely to be potentially carcinogenic as it does not interfere with the replication potential of residual cells. The immediate advantages of radioactive iodine appear to outweigh its theoretically low later risks. Strict and prolonged follow-up is mandatory to detect subclinical hypothyroidism.

Surgical treatment is less controversial, especially in the case of a significant goitre, provided an experienced surgeon is available. The complication rate for subtotal or total thyroidectomy used to be considered greater than in adults. However, in recent series, prevalence of definitive vocal cord paralysis has been less than

0.5% and that of definitive hypocalcaemia less than 5% (23). There are no data on the complication rates of thyroidectomy for Graves' disease in children. Recurrence of hyperthyroidism (6–7%) is to be treated with radioactive iodine.

Graves' disease and pregnancy

The incidence of thyrotoxicosis during pregnancy, usually due to Graves' disease (24), is lower than in the general population and approximates 0.1%. Hyperthyroidism may cause maternal congestive heart failure, impair the normal evolution of pregnancy, with increased risk of spontaneous abortion, premature labour, low-birthweight babies, and fetal death, and also cause malformation in the infants. Graves' disease, after a transient exacerbation of clinical symptoms likely related to the first-trimester peak of human chorionic gonadotropin, usually tends to spontaneously improve or even remit in the second half of pregnancy. The primary therapeutic objectives are: (1) restoration of maternal euthyroidism, (2) avoidance of fetal hypothyroidism, and (3) evaluation of the risk of fetal hyperthyroidism due to the transplacental transfer of maternal stimulating TRAb. Antithyroid drugs at a dose sufficient to maintain maternal T_4 levels within the normal range may induce mild hypothyroidism in the fetus. Maternal doses of 10 mg methimazole or 30 mg carbimazole, or 100–300 mg PTU, may cause an elevation of cord blood TSH values. Since the transfer of T_4 from mother to fetus is limited, the block and replace regimen is contraindicated. Therefore, management of thionamide therapy during pregnancy, in addition to the general rules of utilization of the drugs, should aim at maintaining the maternal free T_4 in the upper normal range through periodic titration. Antithyroid treatment can be withdrawn in most cases near midpregnancy. In contrast, in rare cases, usually with large hypervascular goitre and very high T_3 and TRAb concentrations, restoration of euthyroidism requires prolonged full-dose antithyroid drug treatment. Tight management is mandatory in these difficult cases to ensure treatment compliance. This usually allows avoiding thyroidectomy during pregnancy, an option which does not protect the fetus from the risk of hyperthyroidism (25). In these cases there is a risk of fetal hyperthyroidism or, on the contrary, of iatrogenic fetal hypothyroidism (see below).

The teratogenicity of antithyroid drugs is a matter of controversy. Multiple case reports associating aplasia cutis and carbimazole or methimazole have been reported. Also, some instances of choanal or oesophageal atresia have been associated with exposure to carbimazole or methimazole in the first trimester of pregnancy. Although epidemiological data are not conclusive, it is recommended to use PTU rather than carbimazole or methimazole during the first trimester of pregnancy (24).

Hyperthyroidism occurs in 2–10% of babies born to women with active Graves' disease. It may also occur in women previously treated with radioactive iodine or thyroidectomy who are euthyroid on L-thyroxine treatment. In more than 95% of the cases, fetal or neonatal hyperthyroidism can be predicted by determining maternal TRAb at the beginning of the third trimester. Women who must be screened for TRAb include: (1) patients with ongoing Graves' disease, (2) patients previously treated for Graves' disease either by surgery or radio-iodine whatever their current thyroid status, and (3) patients with a previous child with neonatal transient hyper- or hypothyroidism (24). If the test is positive for TRAb activity, a biological assay could be performed to assess the stimulating potency of the autoantibody. Fetal thyroid status may be assessed indirectly through clinical signs of hyperthyroidism (tachycardia above 160 beats/min, agitation, intrauterine growth retardation), but these are of low sensitivity and specificity. Fetal thyroid is enlarged at ultrasonography performed after the 23rd to 25th week of pregnancy (26). However, depending on the serum concentration of stimulating TRAb or on the dose of antithyroid drug in the mother, fetal thyroid enlargement may reflect either fetal hyperthyroidism or fetal hypothyroidism, the differentiation of which may require, especially when the goitre is large, TSH and thyroid hormone determination in fetal blood through cordocentesis (24). A team approach, including obstetrician, neonatologist, and endocrinologist, is mandatory to monitor properly fetal development in the last trimester, parturition, the thyroid status of the neonate, and breastfeeding, as well as the risk of postpartum maternal exacerbation of hyperthyroidism. Neonatal hyperthyroidism, although self-limited, may be immediately fatal if unrecognized or poorly managed. Antithyroid drugs, β-blocker, and supportive measures should be started even before the exacerbation of thyrotoxicosis that follows clearance of the maternally transferred antithyroid drugs.

Ophthalmopathy

Occurrence of significant or severe ophthalmopathy is one of the most troublesome manifestations of Graves' disease. In many cases, clinical ophthalmopathy begins or grows worse during or after the treatment of hyperthyroidism. Therefore, it is tempting to ascribe the orbital complications to the treatment. It has been shown that radio-iodine treatment might favour the development of ophthalmopathy more than antithyroid drugs or thyroid surgery, especially in the more severely hyperthyroid patients (27–29). In addition to cigarette smoking, a well-demonstrated triggering factor, iatrogenic hypothyroidism appears to be a significant risk factor of orbitopathy. Administration of radio-iodine can be considered in cases of moderate ophthalmopathy since glucocorticoid treatment (0.4–0.5 mg prednisone/kg per day, starting 2–3 days following the dose of ^{131}I for 1 month and then tapered over 2 months) prevents the potentially deleterious effect of radio-iodine treatment on the orbit (27). It should be stressed that noninflammatory orbitopathy, with a clinical activity score of less than 3 is unaffected by radio-iodine therapy which then does not require concomitant glucocorticoid treatment (30). Whether medical or radical treatment of hyperthyroidism is more appropriate in cases of severe or malignant ophthalmopathy remains unresolved (28). Antithyroid drug treatment is appropriate when management of ophthalmopathy is urgent. In any case, prevention of the least degree of iatrogenic hypothyroidism is of the utmost importance (see Chapter 3.3.10).

Conclusion

It may seem that no significant improvement has been achieved in recent years in the treatment of Graves' disease. Currently, however, optimization of existing therapeutic strategies may offer every patient the most appropriate management strategy. The cost-effectiveness of the treatment and the socioprofessional and psychological aspects of the disease are of increasing importance and must also be taken into account. Ongoing clinical investigations, as well as immunological research, aim at improving the understanding and management efficiency of Graves' disease. There is no doubt that, in the future, new immunospecific therapeutic approaches will become available.

The risk of PTU-induced liver failure leading to transplantation was estimated to be about 1 in 10,000 adults. The number of adults developing PTU-induced liver injury that was reversible was estimated to be about 1 in 100 individuals. The risk of PTU-induced liver failure leading to transplantation was estimated to be about 1 in 2000 children. The number of children developing PTU-induced liver injury that was reversible was estimated to be about 1 in 200. The risk of PTU-induced liver failure leading to transplantation was estimated to be about 1 in 2000 children. The number of children developing PTU-induced liver injury that was reversible was estimated to be about 1 in 200. Therefore, long-term PTU therapy, especially in children, is not justifiable. Hence, the use of PTU in children (and adults) should now be limited to exceptional circumstances and pregnancy (Rivkees, SA. 63 years and 75 days to the 'boxed warning': unmasking of the propylthiouracil problem. Int J Pediatr Endocrinol. Epub 2010 Jul 12).

References

1. Wartofsky L, Glinoer D, Solomon B, Nagataki S, Lagasse R, Nagayama Y, *et al.* Differences and similarities in the diagnosis and treatment of Graves' disease in Europe, Japan and the United States. *Thyroid*, 1991; **1**: 129–35.
2. Törring O, Tallstedt L, Wallin G, Lundell G, Ljunggren JG, Taube A, *et al.* Graves' hyperthyroidism: treatment with antithyroid drugs, surgery, or radioiodine. A prospective, randomized study. *J Clin Endocrinol Metab*, 1996; **81**: 2986–93.
3. Abraham-Nordling M, Wallin G, Lundell G, Törring O. Thyroid hormone state and quality of life at long-term follow-up after randomized treatment of Graves' disease. *Eur J Endocrinol*, 2007; **156**: 173–9.
4. Ljunggren JG, Törring O, Wallin G, Taube A, Tallstedt L, Hamberger B, *et al.* Quality of life aspects and costs in treatment of Graves' hyperthyroidism with antithyroid drugs, surgery, or radioiodine: results from a prospective, randomized study. *Thyroid*, 1998; **8**: 653–9.
5. Patel NN, Abraham P, Buscombe J, Vanderpump MP. The cost effectiveness of treatment modalities for thyrotoxicosis in a U.K. center. *Thyroid*, 2006; **16**: 593–8.
6. Cruz Júnior AF, Takahashi MH, Albino CC. Clinical treatment with anti-thyroid drugs or iodine-131 therapy to control the hyperthyroidism of Graves' disease: a cost-effectiveness analysis. *Arq Bras Endocrinol Metabol*, 2006; **50**: 1096–101.
7. Allannic H, Fauchet R, Orgiazzi J, Madec AM, Genetet B, Lorcy Y, *et al.* Antithyroid drugs and Graves' disease: a prospective randomized evaluation of the efficacy of treatment duration. *J Clin Endocrinol Metab*, 1990; **70**: 675–9.
8. Reinwein D, Benker G, Lazarus JH, Alexander WD. A prospective randomized trial of antithyroid drug dose in Graves' disease therapy. European Multicenter Study Group on antithyroid drug treatment. *J Clin Endocrinol Metab*, 1993; **76**: 1516–21.
9. Rittmaster RS, Zwicker H, Abbott EC, Douglas R, Givner ML, Gupta MK, *et al.* Effect of methimazole with or without exogenous L-thyroxine on serum concentrations of thyrotropin (TSH) receptor antibodies in patients with Graves' disease. *J Clin Endocrinol Metab*, 1996; **81**: 3283–8.
10. McIver B, Rae P, Beckett G, Wilkinson E, Gold A, Toft A. Lack of effect of thyroxine in patients with Graves' hyperthyroidism who are treated with an antithyroid drug (see comments). *N Engl J Med*, 1996; **334**: 220–4.
11. Franklyn JA, Maisonneuve P, Sheppard MC, Betteridge J, Boyle P. Mortality after the treatment of hyperthyroidism with radioactive iodine. *N Engl J Med*, 1998; **338**: 712–18.
12. Boelaert K, Syed AA, Manji N, Sheppard MC, Holder RL, Gough SC, *et al.* Prediction of cure and risk of hypothyroidism in patients receiving ^{131}I for hyperthyroidism. *Clin Endocrinol (Oxf)*, 2009; **70**: 129–38.
13. Walter MA, Briel M, Christ-Crain M, Bonnema SJ, Connell J, Cooper DS, *et al.* Effects of antithyroid drugs on radioiodine treatment: systematic review and meta-analysis of randomised controlled trials. *BMJ*, 2007; **334**: 514.
14. Imseis RE, VanMiddlesworth L, Massie JD, Bush AJ, VanMiddlesworth NR. Pretreatment with propylthiouracil but not methimazole reduces the therapeutic efficacy of iodine-131 in hyperthyroidism. *J Clin Endocrinol Metab*, 1998; **83**: 685–7.
15. Gamstedt A, Karlsson A. Pretreatment with betamethasone of patients with Graves' disease given radioiodine therapy: thyroid autoantibody responses and outcome of therapy. *J Clin Endocrinol Metab*, 1991; **73**: 125–31.
16. Laurberg P, Wallin G, Tallstedt L, Abraham-Nordling M, Lundell G, Tørring O. TSH-receptor autoimmunity in Graves' disease after therapy with anti-thyroid drugs, surgery, or radioiodine: a 5-year prospective randomized study. *Eur J Endocrinol*, 2008; **158**: 69–75.
17. Hermann M, Richter B, Roka R, Freissmuth M. Thyroid surgery in untreated severe hyperthyroidism: perioperative kinetics of free thyroid hormones in the glandular venous effluent and peripheral blood. *Surgery*, 1994; **115**: 240–5.
18. Perrild H, Grüters-Kieslich A, Feldt-Rasmussen U, Grant D, Martino E, Kayser L, *et al.* Diagnosis and treatment of thyrotoxicosis in childhood. A European questionnaire study. *Eur J Endocrinol*, 1994; **131**: 467–73.
19. Rivkees SA, Sklar C, Freemark M. The management of Graves' disease in children, with special emphasis on radioiodine treatment. *J Clin Endocrinol Metab*, 1998; **83**: 3767–76.
20. Glaser NS, Styne DM. Predictors of early remission of hyperthyroidism in children. *J Clin Endocrinol Metab*, 1997; **82**: 1719–26.
21. Kaguelidou F, Alberti C, Castanet M, Guitteny MA, Czernichow P, Léger J, *et al.* Predictors of autoimmune hyperthyroidism relapse in children after discontinuation of antithyroid drug treatment. *J Clin Endocrinol Metab*, 2008; **93**: 3817–26.
22. Rivkees SA, Dinauer C. An optimal treatment for pediatric Graves' disease is radioiodine. *J Clin Endocrinol Metab*, 2007; **92**: 797–800.
23. Lal G, Ituarte P, Kebebew E, Siperstein A, Duh QY, Clark OH. Should total thyroidectomy become the preferred procedure for surgical management of Graves' disease? *Thyroid*, 2005; **15**: 569–74.
24. Abalovich M, Amino N, Barbour LA, Cobin RH, De Groot LJ, Glinoer D, *et al.* Management of thyroid dysfunction during pregnancy and postpartum: an Endocrine Society Clinical Practice Guideline. *J Clin Endocrinol Metab*, 2007; **92** (Suppl): S1–47.
25. Laurberg P, Bournaud C, Karmisholt J, Orgiazzi J. Management of Graves' hyperthyroidism in pregnancy: focus on both maternal and foetal thyroid function, and caution against surgical thyroidectomy in pregnancy. *Eur J Endocrinol*, 2009; **160**: 1–8.
26. Luton D, Le Gac I, Vuillard E, Castanet M, Guibourdenche J, Noel M, *et al.* Management of Graves' disease during pregnancy: the key role of fetal thyroid gland monitoring. *J Clin Endocrinol Metab*, 2005; **90**: 6093–8.
27. Tanda ML, Lai A, Bartalena L. Relation between Graves' orbitopathy and radioiodine therapy for hyperthyroidism: facts and unsolved questions. *Clin Endocrinol (Oxf)*, 2008; **69**: 845–7.
28. Bartalena L, Tanda ML. Clinical practice. Graves' ophthalmopathy. *N Engl J Med*, 2009; **360**: 994–1001.
29. Acharya SH, Avenell A, Philip S, Burr J, Bevan JS, Abraham P. Radioiodine therapy (RAI) for Graves' disease (GD) and the effect on ophthalmopathy: a systematic review. *Clin Endocrinol (Oxf)*, 2008; **69**: 943–50.
30. Perros P, Kendall-Taylor P, Neoh C, Frewin S, Dickinson J. A prospective study of the effects of radioiodine therapy for hyperthyroidism in patients with minimally active Graves' ophthalmopathy. *J Clin Endocrinol Metab*, 2005; **90**: 5321–3.

3.3.10 Graves' ophthalmopathy and dermopathy

Wilmar M. Wiersinga

Clinical presentation

The many and often disfiguring features of a typical patient with Graves' ophthalmopathy are obvious at first glance (Fig. 3.3.10.1). The changed appearance of the patient has a profound effect on their emotional and social status. The various signs and symptoms can be described according to the NO SPECS classification (1) (Box 3.3.10.1). Class 1 signs can be present in any patient with thyrotoxicosis regardless of its cause. Upper eyelid retraction causes stare and lid lag on downward gaze (the latter is the well-known von Graefe's sign). Soft tissue involvement (class 2) comprises swelling and redness of eyelids, conjunctiva, and caruncle. Symptoms are a gritty sandy sensation in the eyes, retrobulbar pressure, lacrimation, photophobia, and blurring of vision. Proptosis (class 3) can be quite marked. Upper eyelid retraction by itself may already give the impression of exophthalmos. Extraocular muscle involvement (class 4) may result in aberrant position of the globe, or fixation of the globe in extreme cases. More common is limitation of eye muscle movements in certain directions of gaze, especially in upward gaze; it is usually associated with diplopia.

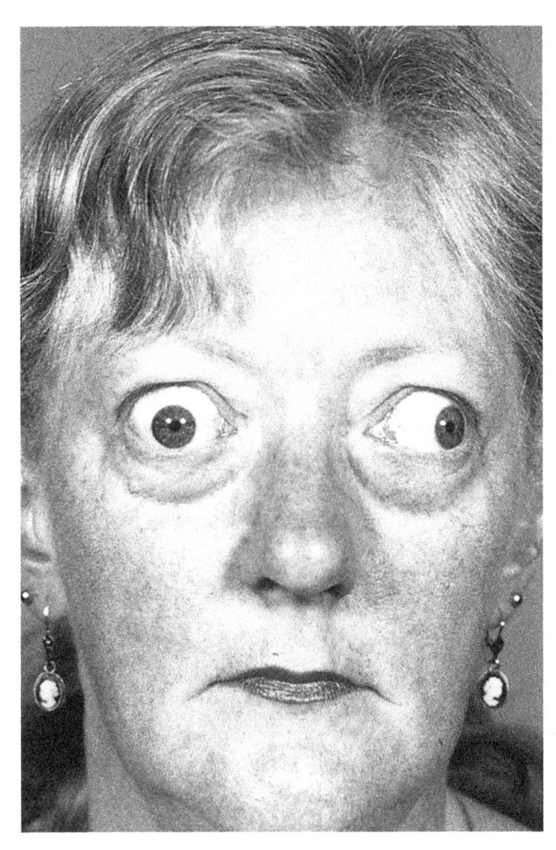

Fig. 3.3.10.1 Bilateral eye disease due to Graves' ophthalmopathy. Note lid retraction, stare, periorbital swelling, marked proptosis, and exotropia of the left globe. (See also Plate 15)

Diplopia will not occur if the vision of one eye is very low (e.g. in amblyopia), or if the impairment of eye muscle motility is strictly symmetrical. Patients may correct for double vision by tilting the head, usually backwards and sideways; the ocular torticollis often leads to neck pain and headache. Corneal involvement (class 5) occurs through overexposure of the cornea due to lid lag, lid retraction, and exophthalmos, easily leading to dry eyes and keratitis. Lagophthalmos is often noted first by the patient's partner because of incomplete closure of the eyelids during sleep. Sight loss (class 6) due to optic nerve involvement is the most serious feature, often referred to as dysthyroid optic neuropathy (DON). Besides the decrease of visual acuity, there may be loss of colour vision and visual field defects. Visual blurring may disappear after blinking (caused by alteration of the tear film on the surface of the cornea due to lacrimation or dry eyes) or after closing one eye (attributable to eye muscle imbalance). Visual blurring that persists is of great concern as it may indicate optic neuropathy (2).

The frequency of the various eye changes among patients with Graves' ophthalmopathy is as follows (3): von Graefe's sign 59%, upper eyelid swelling 75%, proptosis of 21 mm or higher 63%, diplopia 49%, impairment of elevation 49%, impairment of abduction 32%, impairment of depression 17%, corneal involvement 16%, and optic nerve involvement 21%. Predisposing factors for DON are male sex, old age, smoking, and diabetes mellitus (4, 5) (Fig. 3.3.10.2). Diabetes is present in 9%, and glaucoma or cataract in 14%. Unilateral eye disease is observed in about 10% of patients. Eye changes are similar to those of patients with bilateral eye disease, but unilateral cases are more often euthyroid. Eye muscle enlargement of the fellow eye can be detected by imaging in about one-half of cases. Progression to bilateral eye disease is common (6). Unilateral Graves' ophthalmopathy may thus represent an early stage of the disease that already is or will develop shortly into a bilateral disease. Unknown local factors must be involved in the unilateral expression of Graves' ophthalmopathy, which essentially is a bilateral and fairly symmetrical eye disease.

Epidemiology

A population-based cohort study in Olmsted County, Minnesota, USA reports an overall age-adjusted incidence rate of Graves' ophthalmopathy of 16.0 women and 2.9 men/100 000 inhabitants per year (7). The incidence rate exhibits an apparent bimodal peak in the fifth and seventh decades of life. Male sex and older age are

Box 3.3.10.1 The NO SPECS classification of eye changes in Graves' disease

- Class 0: No physical signs or symptoms
- Class 1: Only signs (limited to upper lid retraction, stare, and lid lag)
- Class 2: Soft tissue involvement (swollen eyelids, chemosis, etc.)
- Class 3: Proptosis
- Class 4: Eye muscle involvement (usually with diplopia)
- Class 5: Corneal involvement
- Class 6: Sight loss (due to optic nerve involvement)

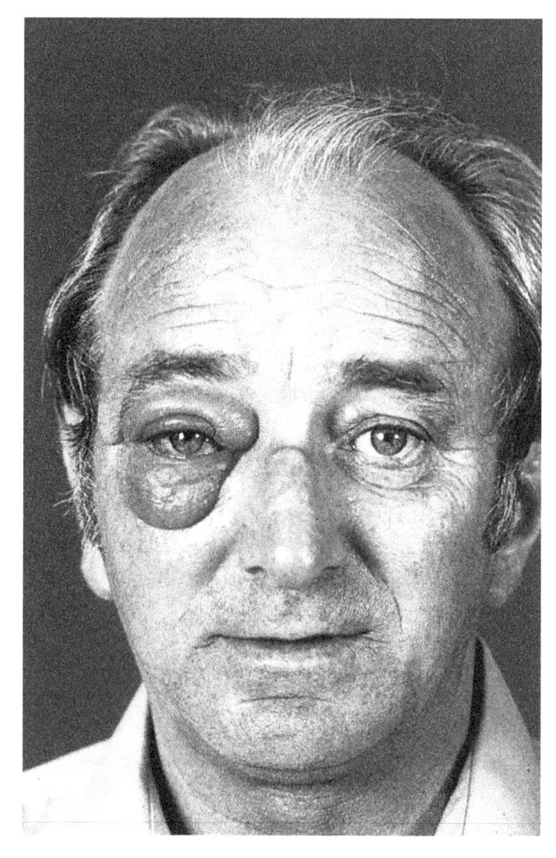

Fig. 3.3.10.2 Unusual presentation of Graves' ophthalmopathy as unilateral eye disease. Male sex, advanced age, and heavy smoking all predisposed this patient to the development of severe eye disease; note the absence of exophthalmos in this case of dysthyroid optic neuropathy. (See also Plate 16)

associated with more severe ophthalmopathy (4, 5). Childhood Graves' ophthalmopathy is rare (8, 9). Clinical manifestations are less severe in paediatric patients: exophthalmos is seen in 75%, but impaired muscle motility only in 11%.

Smoking greatly increases the risk for Graves' ophthalmopathy (odds ratio 7.7, 95% CI 4.3 to 13.7) (10). Smokers have more severe eye disease than nonsmokers (Fig. 3.3.10.3). A trend to a lower incidence rate of Graves' ophthalmopathy is reported. In a single centre in the UK, the proportion of patients with Graves' ophthalmopathy among all referred patients with Graves' hyperthyroidism decreased from 57% in 1960 to 35% in 1990; there was also a decline in the prevalence of severe Graves' ophthalmopathy

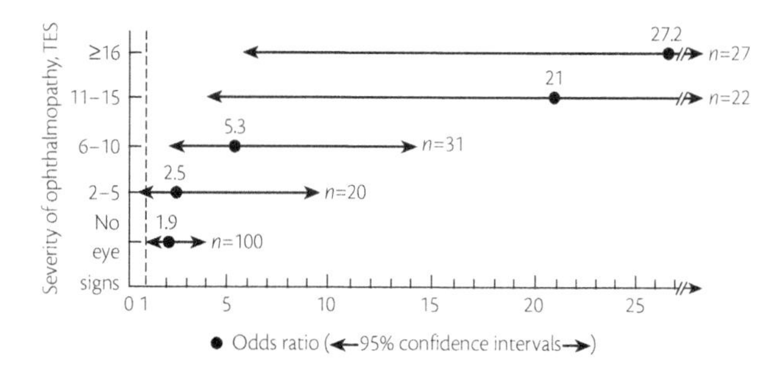

Fig. 3.3.10.3 Increase in the prevalence of smokers (represented by the odds ratio with 95% CI) in relation to the severity of eye changes (assessed by the total eye score, TES) in patients with Graves' hyperthyroidism. (Reproduced with permission from Prummel MF, Wiersinga WM. Smoking and risk of Graves' disease. *JAMA*, 1993; **269**: 479–82.)

(diplopia or DON) from 30% to 21% (11). In a European questionnaire study in 1998, 43% of respondents thought Graves' ophthalmopathy was decreasing in frequency, 42% thought it unchanged, and 12% thought it to be increasing (12). In this respect it is noteworthy that all responders from Hungary and Poland, where the prevalence of smoking had increased since 1990, indicated an increased incidence of Graves' ophthalmopathy. The trend to a lower incidence rate of Graves' ophthalmopathy might therefore be causally linked to a secular decrease in the prevalence of smoking. Alternatively, earlier diagnosis and treatment of Graves' hyperthyroidism could be involved in view of the introduction of sensitive thyroid-stimulating hormone (TSH) assays in the late 1980s.

Relationship with thyroidal Graves' disease

Graves' ophthalmopathy is usually but not invariably associated with Graves' hyperthyroidism. Graves' hyperthyroidism is present in about 90% of patients with Graves' ophthalmopathy, autoimmune hypothyroidism in 3%, and euthyroidism in 7% (3). The euthyroid and primarily hypothyroid patients have milder and more asymmetrical Graves' ophthalmopathy than the hyperthyroid Graves' ophthalmopathy patients (13). It is not unusual that hypothyroid Graves' ophthalmopathy patients proceed to Graves' hyperthyroidism, linked to a shift from TSH-receptor blocking to stimulating antibodies. Euthyroid Graves' ophthalmopathy patients develop hyperthyroidism in due time in about 20%, but it is unknown why others remain euthyroid although TSH-receptor stimulating antibodies can be detected in almost everyone (14).

Among patients with both Graves' ophthalmopathy and Graves' hyperthyroidism, the eye disease becomes manifest before the onset of hyperthyroidism in about 20% (the interval can be months to years), concurrent with hyperthyroidism in 40%, and after the onset of hyperthyroidism in 40% (2). Autoimmune thyroid disease is therefore present in most if not all patients with Graves' ophthalmopathy. Conversely, Graves' ophthalmopathy is present in the majority if not all patients with Graves' hyperthyroidism, although over one-half of patients with Graves' hyperthyroidism have no clinically appreciable ophthalmopathy. Evidence for subclinical ophthalmopathy is, however, found in most patients with Graves' hyperthyroidism without apparent eye changes, encompassing a shift to higher proptosis values in this group as compared with healthy controls, an abnormal increase in intraocular pressure on upgaze in 61%, and enlarged extraocular muscles on ultrasound or CT scan in 70–100% (2).

The available data strongly support the view that the eye and thyroid manifestations belong to the same disease entity, Graves' disease, a multiorgan autoimmune disorder. Factors determining the differential expression of the disease remain largely unknown, but smoking is definitely involved.

Pathogenesis

Mechanistic explanation of eye changes

Graves' ophthalmopathy is characterized by enlargement of extraocular muscles and retro-ocular connective/adipose tissue. The increase in tissue volume and the associated rise of retrobulbar pressure can explain the various signs and symptoms (2). The swollen retrobulbar tissues will impair the venous drainage of the eyelids and conjunctiva, resulting in oedematous swelling of the eyelids and chemosis. Upper and lower eyelid swelling can also

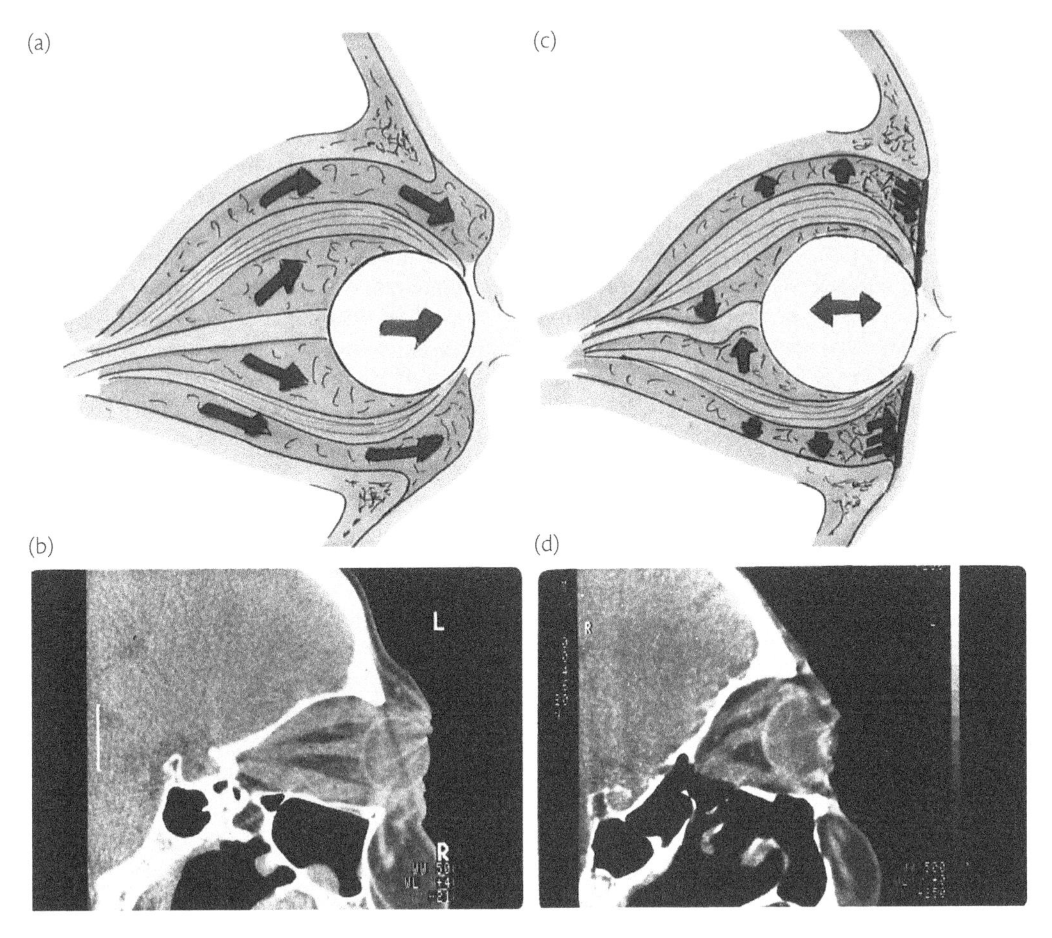

Fig. 3.3.10.4 Swelling of extraocular muscles raises retrobulbar pressure, by which the globe is pushed forwards and exophthalmos develops (a, b). A tight connective tissue system might prevent forward displacement of the globe and 'nature's own decompression' does not occur; retrobulbar pressure rises further and may cause optic neuropathy (c, d). (Reproduced with permission from Koornneef L, Schmidt ED, van der Gaag R. The orbit: structure, autoantigens, and pathology. In: Wall J, How J, eds. *Graves' Ophthalmopathy*. Oxford: Blackwell Scientific Publications, 1990: 1–16.)

be caused by herniation of retrobulbar fat through openings in the orbital septum (Fig. 3.3.10.4a, b). The only other outlet for the increased orbital content, in view of the confinement within the bony walls of the orbit, is pushing forward the eyeball, resulting in exophthalmos (Fig. 3.3.10.4a, b). The volume of the orbital cavity is approximately 26 ml, and of the combined extraocular muscles about 3.3 ml. A three- to fourfold increase in size of extraocular muscles is observed in severe cases, and an increase of 4 ml in muscle volume will cause a proptosis of 6 mm (15).

The enlargement of extraocular muscles impairs muscle relaxation, not the ability for muscle contraction. Limited motion of eye muscles is due to impaired relaxation of the antagonist upon contraction of the agonist. Impaired elevation is thus primarily the result of insufficient relaxation of the rectus inferior muscle. This can be appreciated by the forced duction test: by actually grasping the globe and attempting to move it in the affected direction, mechanical resistance is felt. Restricted eye muscle motility may cause diplopia. Upper eyelid retraction (due either to an increased adrenergic activity in hyperthyroidism or to swelling of the levator muscle) and proptosis contribute to overexposure of the cornea, which may become dry and inflamed.

Marked swelling of the extraocular muscles in the apex of the orbit (known as apical crowding), close to the entrance of the optic nerve in the optic canal, may damage the optic nerve either via direct pressure or via impairment of the blood supply to the nerve. The resulting optic neuropathy causes loss of visual functions. The degree of proptosis in patients with optic neuropathy, despite a greater mass of extraocular muscles, is less than in patients without optic neuropathy (16). This is remarkable because the retrobulbar pressure (in the normal orbit 3.0–4.5 mmHg) is greatly elevated in patients with DON up to values between 17 and 40 mmHg, much higher than the pressure of 9–11 mmHg measured in orbits of patients with exophthalmos but no optic neuropathy (17). A well-developed tight orbital septum might preclude proptosis, resulting in a very high retrobulbar pressure and optic neuropathy (Fig. 3.3.10.4c,d).

Immunopathogenesis

The macroscopic appearance of the orbital content in Graves' ophthalmopathy is dominated by enlargement of extraocular muscles and to a lesser extent of retrobulbar fat and connective tissue. Microscopy demonstrates lymphocytic infiltration, oedema, and fibrosis. The swelling of tissues is largely caused by an increase of ground substance consisting of collagen and glycosaminoglycans. Glycosaminoglycans, because of their hydrophilic nature, attract water, resulting in oedematous swelling. The ground substance accumulates in the endomysial space between the muscle fibres. There is no increase in the number of muscle fibres and no ultrastructural damage to the muscle cells themselves (except in very advanced cases when some damage may be seen). An increased number of fibroblasts is found in the endomysial space and in the connective and adipose tissues. The fibroblasts are responsible for the excessive production of glycosaminoglycans.

The lymphocytic infiltrate is often focal, and consists of T helper cells, suppressor/cytotoxic T cells, many macrophages, and relatively few B cells (18). There is abundant expression of HLA-DR.

Many of these cells are activated memory cells ($CD45RO^+$), frequently located adjacent to blood vessels. The lymphocytic infiltration diminishes in the late inactive stage of the disease. The infiltrating immunocompetent cells produce cytokines capable of remodelling orbital tissues. The cytokine profile in the early stages is predominantly derived from T helper 1 cells, whereas, in patients with a duration of Graves' ophthalmopathy longer than 2 years, cytokines are mostly derived from T helper 2 cells (19). The data suggest Graves' ophthalmopathy is primarily a T-cell mediated disease. In keeping with this notion is the observation that, in contrast to neonatal Graves' hyperthyroidism, no single convincing case of neonatal Graves' ophthalmopathy has been reported (whereas immunoglobulins cross the placenta, T cells do not). The cytokines induce expression of immunomodulatory proteins on orbital endothelial cells and fibroblasts, such as HLA-DR, heat shock protein 72, and several adhesion molecules. Cytokine-activated orbital fibroblasts synthesize chemoattractants IL-16 and RANTES, generating T-cell migration. More T cells migrate to the orbit, perpetuating the immune attack. Macrophages may present antigen to T cells (CD40L) through provision of costimulatory signals and proinflammatory cytokines. Activated T cells may bind to $CD40^+$ fibroblasts inducing hyaluronan synthesis, cytokines, COX2, and PGE2. Orbital fibroblasts are considered the target cells of the autoimmune attack. Retrobulbar T cells from patients with Graves' ophthalmopathy recognize autologous orbital fibroblasts (but not eye muscle extracts) in a major histocompatibility complex (MHC) class I restricted manner, and proliferate in response to autologous proteins from orbital fibroblasts (but not from orbital myoblasts). Conversely, orbital fibroblasts proliferate in response to autologous T cells dependent on MHC class II and CD40-CD40L signalling (18).

Orbital fibroblasts have site-specific characteristics. Orbital fibroblasts expressing Thy-1 (present in orbital fat and muscles) produce more PGE2, whereas fibroblasts not expressing Thy-1 (present only in orbital fat) may differentiate into mature adipocytes (e.g. when incubated with IL-1 or PPARγ agonists). The process of adipogenesis contributes to volume expansion, but interestingly is also associated with increased TSH-receptor expression (20). This brings us to the nature of the autoantigen in the orbit.

The TSH receptor is presently viewed as the major autoantigen in Graves' ophthalmopathy. Orbital fibroblasts express full-length functional TSH receptors; the expression is more abundant in active than in inactive disease and is directly related to IL-1β (21). Graves' immunoglobulins recognize TSH receptors on orbital fibroblasts as evident from increased cAMP and hyaluronan production in cell cultures of differentiated orbital fibroblasts (18). Clinical studies support the role of TSH receptors. The serum concentrations of TSH-receptor antibodies are higher in patients with Graves' ophthalmopathy than in Graves' patients without eye changes (22), and are related to the severity and activity of the ophthalmopathy (whereas thyroid peroxidase and thyroglobulin antibodies are not) (23, 24). The higher the level of TSH-receptor antibodies, the higher the risk for an unfavourable course of the eye changes (25). However, experimental studies in which animals were immunized against the TSH receptor, observed hyperthyroidism in some animals but so far never ophthalmopathy. Another candidate is the IGF-1 receptor. Older studies reported inhibition of [^{125}I] IGF-1 binding to orbital fibroblasts by Graves' IgG, and more recent studies indicate Graves' IgG recognize and activate IGF-1 receptors on orbital fibroblasts inducing synthesis of IL-1β and hyaluronan (26). Further studies propose colocalization of TSH and IGF-1 receptors to cell membranes (27). Expression of IGF-1 receptors is increased in orbital fibroblasts and peripheral blood T cells of patients with Graves' disease (28). These intriguing data remain to be confirmed, but may well indicate involvement of fibrocytes in the extrathyroidal manifestations of Graves' disease. Antibodies against eye muscle antigens (such as calsequestrin) are likely secondary responses to tissue destruction and release of sequestered proteins (29, 30).

Taken together, Graves' ophthalmopathy starts with the accumulation of immune cells in the orbit, giving rise to cytokine release and up-regulation of TSH receptors on orbital fibroblasts, the target cells of the autoimmune attack. The cellular response of fibroblasts includes glycosaminoglycan production and differentiation of preadipocytes into mature adipocytes (adipogenesis). Consequently, the intraorbital pressure rises due to volume expansion, and mechanical trauma by itself will further attract immune cells (Fig. 3.3.10.5). This sequence of events has aptly been called the cycle of disease (31).

Many questions, however, remain unanswered. It is difficult to explain why many patients with Graves' hyperthyroidism, despite high titres of TSH-receptor antibodies, do not develop Graves' ophthalmopathy. The different phenotypes of Graves' disease might be related to genetic and environmental factors. Graves' ophthalmopathy is more prevalent in white patients than in Asian patients (32). Whereas several susceptibility genes for Graves' disease have been identified, there is no difference in the frequency of particular polymorphisms in these genes (*HLA*, *CTLA4*, *PTPN22*, *CD40*, *FRCL3*, *TSHR*) between Graves' hyperthyroid patients with and without ophthalmopathy (33). Some polymorphisms in genes encoding for intercellular adhesion molecule 1, interferon-γ, and tumour necrosis factor are more

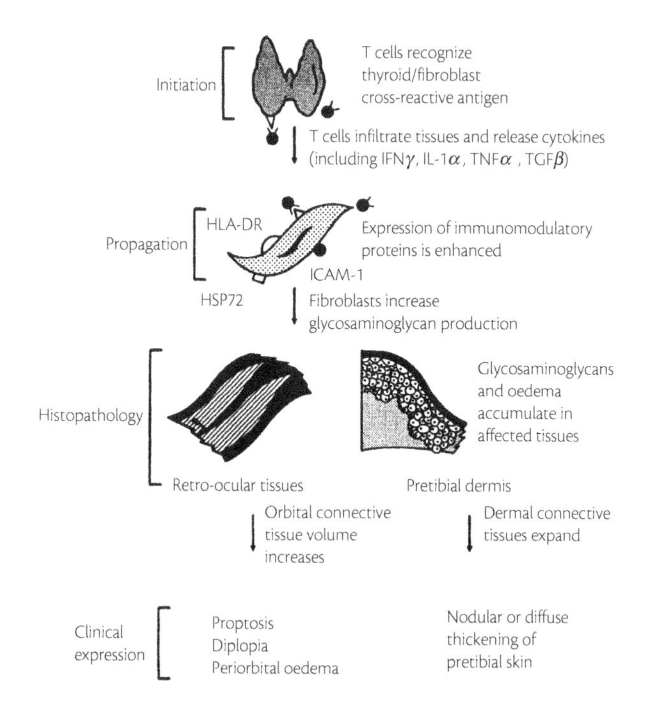

Fig. 3.3.10.5 Proposed sequence of events in the pathogenesis of Graves' ophthalmopathy and dermopathy (localized myxoedema). (Reproduced with permission from Bahn RS, Heufelder AE. Pathogenesis of Graves' ophthalmopathy. *N Engl J Med*, 1993; **329**: 1468–75.)

prevalent in Graves' ophthalmopathy, enhancing slightly the risk for eye changes. In contrast, smoking increases greatly the risk of Graves' ophthalmopathy by incompletely understood mechanisms. Orbital fibroblasts when cultured under hypoxic conditions produce more glycosaminoglycans (34). Exposure of orbital fibroblasts *in vitro* to cigarette smoke extract dose-dependently increases adipogenesis and hyaluronan production (35).

Natural history

Graves' ophthalmopathy has a tendency towards spontaneous improvement. There have been few studies on the natural history of the eye disease. The most extensive ones were carried out in the 1940s and 1950s by Rundle (36) (Fig. 3.3.10.6). He described a stage of ingravescence, characterized by the development of exophthalmos (by 0.5 mm monthly, up to an average extent of 2–5 mm) and limitation of elevation; 4–5 degrees elevation is lost for each millimetre of protrusion. Thereafter a stage of remission occurs, which is slower and less complete than ingravescence. Recovery from restricted eye muscle motility precedes that from proptosis. This dynamic phase is succeeded by a static phase, in which exophthalmos and eye muscle disturbance remain unchanged in 75% of patients. The time period in which the stable endstage is reached varies considerably between patients, ranging from several months up to 5 years. Despite spontaneous improvement, the eye changes do not completely disappear in about 60% of patients (37). Recent studies confirm these earlier observations: during a 1-year follow-up in patients whose ophthalmopathy did not require immediate treatment, substantial improvement occurred in 22%, slight improvement occurred in 42%, the disease remained stable in 22%, and the disease progressed in 14% (38).

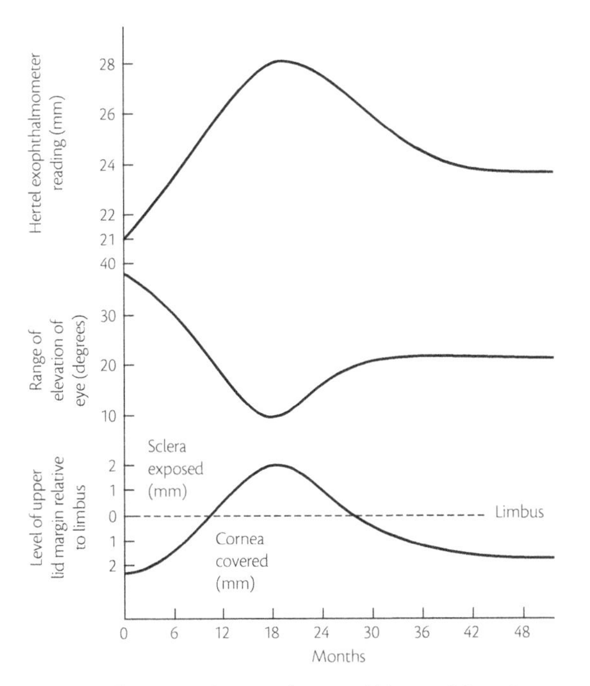

Fig. 3.3.10.6 Rundle's curves depicting the natural history of Graves' ophthalmopathy, characterized by an initial dynamic phase of ingravescence and remission, followed by the static endstage. (Reproduced with permission from Rundle FF. Management of exophthalmos and related ocular changes in Graves' disease. *Metabolism*, 1957; **6**: 36–47.)

The few histological studies support Rundle's observations. In the early active stage of the disease there is usually a lymphocytic infiltrate, oedema, and activated fibroblasts; in the endstages there is only fibrosis. The data imply that the natural history of Graves' ophthalmopathy can also be described according to the activity of the eye disease, as well as Rundle's curves depicting the severity of the eye disease (39) (Fig. 3.3.10.7). Assessment of the activity of the eye disease may influence the treatment plan. Immunosuppression is unlikely to be effective when given in the fibrotic inactive endstage of the disease, but might be of much benefit in the early active stage with ongoing inflammation. Likewise, the results of eye muscle and lid surgery might be lost when performed in the active stage.

Investigation of the patient

The initial work-up is aimed at delineating the optimal treatment plan (40). Treatment will depend on the severity and activity of the eye disease and its influence on the quality of life of the patient. Timing of a particular treatment option may depend on thyroid function. If the diagnosis of Graves' ophthalmopathy is uncertain, several other conditions must be considered.

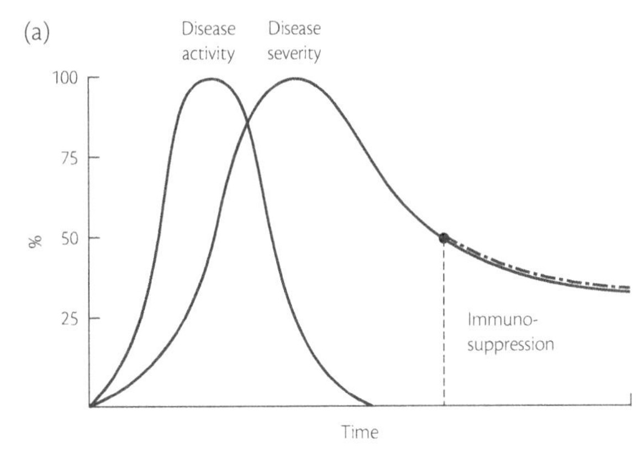

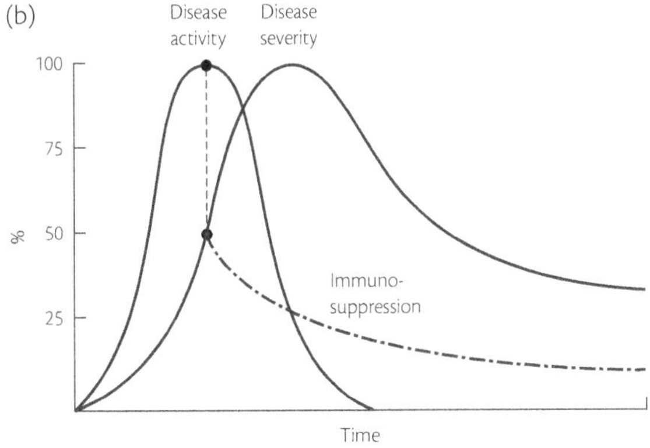

Fig. 3.3.10.7 Outcome of immunosuppressive treatment of Graves' ophthalmopathy as a function of disease activity. The natural history of the activity and the severity of the eye disease are depicted by two separate curves. Immunosuppression is given at one-half maximal disease severity: the response to treatment is negligible when given at zero activity (a) but substantial when applied at peak disease activity (b). (Reproduced with permission from Wiersinga WM. Advances in medical therapy of thyroid-associated ophthalmopathy. *Orbit*, 1996; **15**: 177–86.)

Assessment of thyroid function

Close monitoring of thyroid function is relevant because the eye changes are more severe in patients who still have an abnormal thyroid function (41). Serum concentrations of TSH-receptor antibodies are usually high in Graves' ophthalmopathy, and their presence may support the diagnosis of Graves' ophthalmopathy in euthyroid patients.

Assessment of disease severity

The patient is usually reluctant to voice cosmetic complaints and will at first focus on symptoms such as gritty feeling, photophobia, excessive lacrimation, and blurred vision. Diplopia may be present only when fatigued. Typically, the patient will report difficulty in reading or watching television (subtitles) in the evening. Diplopia can be present only in certain directions of gaze, e.g. hampering driving because of double vision when looking in the rear-view mirror. When diplopia is present in the primary position of gaze, it will severely affect daily activities. Severe asymmetrical motility disorders can be masked by a ocular torticollis. Typically, the head is tilted backwards, which often results in headaches originating from tense neck muscles. Positioning of the head in the default position will unmask diplopia.

The NO SPECS system is a useful memory aid in the physical examination of eye signs (Table 3.3.10.1). Quantitative measurements are preferred whenever possible. Lid aperture is measured with the ruler centred on the pupil while the facial muscles are relaxed and gaze is directed straight ahead. The degree of soft tissue swelling is difficult to assess objectively, but using a comparative photographic colour atlas is very helpful in this respect (42). Proptosis is readily quantified with an exophthalmometer. The normal range in white people is 12–20 mm, in African-Caribbean people is 14–22 mm, and in Asian people is 10–18 mm. Significant exophthalmos may develop without proptosis readings exceeding the upper normal limit; consequently, a normal reading does not always exclude exophthalmos. Comparison with pictures of the patient before the onset of disease can be helpful in this respect.

Motility disturbances are recognized by asking the patient to move the eyes upwards, downwards, and from side to side. Ductions in the four directions of gaze (elevation, depression, abduction, and adduction) are age dependent, and can be measured by a Goldman or modified hand perimeter (43). Diplopia can be graded subjectively. A more objective description of diplopia in the various positions of gaze is obtained by the Hess chart or Lancaster red–green test and by measuring the field of single binocular vision on a Goldman perimeter.

The cornea is investigated by split lamp and application of dyes. Stippling of the cornea may be seen, and in more severe cases ulceration, clouding, necrosis, and perforation.

Visual acuity can be measured using the Snellen chart; the use of a pinhole may correct for refraction disorders and sight loss due to keratitis. Not all patients with optic neuropathy have decreased visual acuity. Further investigation is warranted if optic nerve involvement is suspected, e.g. in patients complaining of persistent blurred vision or greyish vision. In patients with DON, decreased visual acuity is present in 80%, reduced colour vision in 77%, visual field defects in 71%, afferent pupillary defect (Marcus Gunn's phenomenon) in 45%, optic disc oedema in 56%, and disc pallor in 4% (44). Choroidal folds, caused by impression of the globe by retrobulbar tissues, are rare.

Table 3.3.10.1 Methods to assess the severity of Graves' ophthalmopathy

NO SPECS class	Item	Method
1	Lid aperture	Maximum lid fissure in millimetres, using a ruler
2	Lid swelling	Subjective grading; photographs
3	Proptosis	In millimetres using a Hertel exophthalmometer
4	Motility	Range of motion in various directions of gaze
		Goldmann or modified hand perimeter
	Diplopia	Subjective grading as follows: ◆ No diplopia ◆ Intermittent diplopia (at awakening or when tired) ◆ Inconstant diplopia (only at extremes of gaze) ◆ Constant diplopia (in primary gaze or reading position)
		Hess or Lancaster red–green screens
		Field of single binocular vision
5	Cornea	Assessment of keratitis with rose Bengal or fluorescein
6	Optic nerve	Visual acuity
		Visual fields
		Colour vision
		Pupillary function
		Fundoscopy

Assessment of disease activity

In some patients, such as the one depicted in Fig. 3.3.10.2, one glance is sufficient to conclude that the eye disease is in the active phase. However, if it is not self-evident whether the eye disease is active or inactive, an assessment of disease activity provides guidance in selecting the most appropriate treatment (Fig. 3.3.10.7). The gold standard for activity could be histological examination of retrobulbar tissues, but retrobulbar biopsies are not feasible in daily practice. Consequently, the response to immunosuppression has been introduced as a surrogate standard. Any parameter proposed to indicate disease activity should accordingly be validated by its predictive value for the outcome of immunosuppression, thereby serving its clinical purpose.

Clinical parameters

No change of the eye signs over a period of 6 months is generally considered proof that the eye disease is inactive. A duration of the ophthalmopathy of less than 18 months (as obtained from the history of the patient) is likely to be associated with active disease (45). A clinical activity score of 4 or above, based on the classic signs of inflammation, indicates active disease (46) (Table 3.3.10.2, Fig. 3.3.10.8).

Imaging techniques

Tissue oedema prolongs the T_2 relaxation time of MRI. A prolonged T_2 relaxation time in extraocular muscles (>130 ms) is

Table 3.3.10.2 Clinical activity score (CAS) for the assessment of disease activity in Graves' ophthalmopathy. For each item present, one point is given; the sum represents the CAS with a maximum value of 10. Excluding changes over time in proptosis, motility and visual acuity allow immediate assessment of CAS with a maximum value of 7

Item	Description
Pain (*dolor*)	Painful, oppressive feeling on or behind the globe, during the last 4 weeks
	Pain on attempted up-, side-, or down-gaze
Redness (*rubor*)	Redness of the eyelids
	Redness of the conjunctiva, covering at least one quadrant
Swelling (*tumor*)	Swelling of the eyelids
	Chemosis
	Swelling of the caruncle
	Increase in proptosis of >2 mm over 1–3 months
Impaired function (*functio laesa*)	Decrease in eye muscle motility in any direction of >8 degrees in 1–3 months
	Decrease in visual acuity of >1 line on the Snellen chart (using a pinhole) in 1–3 months

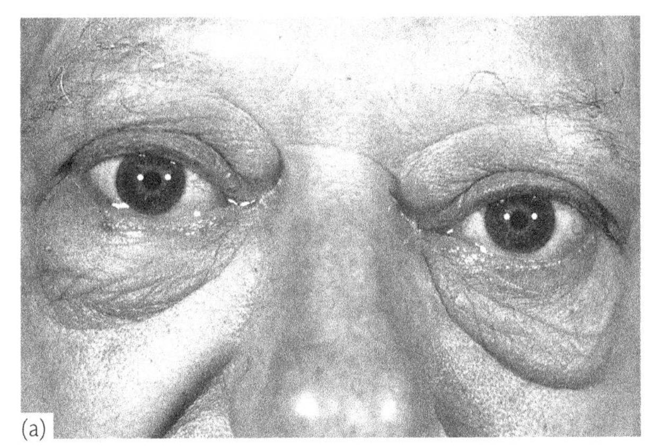

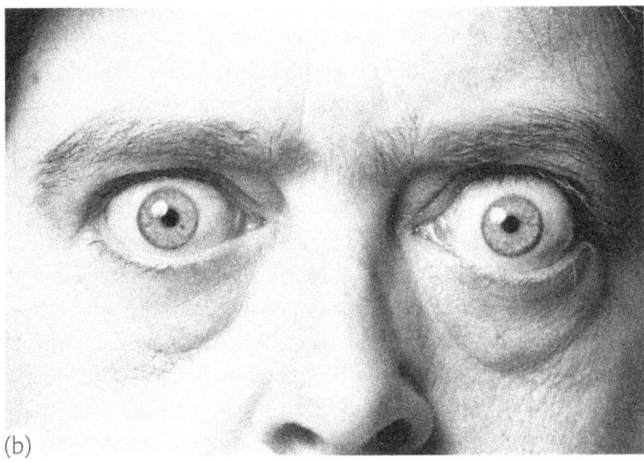

Fig. 3.3.10.8 Active versus inactive Graves' ophthalmopathy. (a) Note periorbital swelling caused by oedema, redness of eyelids, redness of conjunctiva, and chemosis in a patient with active eye disease. (b) Periorbital swelling in a patient with inactive eye disease is due to fat prolapse through the orbital septum and/or fibrotic degeneration; redness and chemosis are absent.

associated with a favourable response to immunosuppression (47). A-mode echography depicts the internal echogenicity of eye muscles, which may be low in oedematous and high in fibrotic muscles. A value below 30% in the muscle with the lowest reflectivity has modest predictive value (45). ^{111}In-labelled octreotide scintigraphy may reveal significant uptake in the orbital region. It may be explained by the binding of octreotide to somatostatin receptors expressed on activated lymphocytes and fibroblasts. A positive orbital octreotide scan would thus indicate active eye disease. An orbital/occipital skull uptake ratio of more than 1.85 is associated with a favourable response to immunosuppression (48, 49).

Laboratory investigations

Serum TSH-receptor antibodies interpreted in relation to the duration of eye changes, help to predict a favourable or unfavourable course of Graves' ophthalmopathy (25). Serum concentrations of particular cytokines, cytokine receptors, and adhesion molecules differ between Graves' ophthalmopathy patients and controls, and between patients with active and inactive eye disease. However, the overlap between the groups is too large for meaningful application in individual patients. The same holds true for urinary glycosaminoglycans.

None of the clinical and radiological parameters can be used on their own to make therapeutic decisions about the value of administering immunosuppression. Most parameters have a good positive but rather low negative predictive value for the outcome of immunosuppression, except MRI which has a high negative but low positive predictive value. A combination of tests might optimize distinction between active and inactive eye disease. The drawback of orbital Octreoscan (besides being very expensive) and ultrasonography is the high operator dependency of these methods. For the time being, the combination of duration of the eye disease, clinical activity score, and T_2 relaxation time on orbital MRI seems to be the most reliable and cost-effective manner for assessing disease activity.

Orbital imaging

The degree of swelling of extraocular muscles and orbital fat can be evaluated using CT scans or MRI. Coronal sections are preferred in view of the pear-shaped orbit with its axis directing backwards and medially. The bony structures are best evaluated by CT scan and are of relevance in case of surgical decompression. MRI has the advantage of providing an activity parameter in addition to imaging. The muscles are swollen typically at the belly, leaving the tendons uninvolved (Fig. 3.3.10.4). For unknown reasons the inferior and medial rectal muscles are most frequently enlarged, followed by the superior rectus; the lateral rectus muscle is least affected (2). The extraocular muscles originate in Zinn's annulus, which surrounds the optic canal and thus the optic nerve. Muscle swelling at this location (apical crowding) and intracranial fat prolapse are risk factors for optic neuropathy (44, 50) (Figs. 3.3.10.4 and 3.3.10.9).

Assessment of quality of life

Eye changes adversely affect a patient's self-image and daily functioning. The overall health-related quality of life of patients with moderately severe Graves' ophthalmopathy is lower than for patients with other chronic conditions such as diabetes mellitus, emphysema, or heart failure (51). Because the goal of treatment in

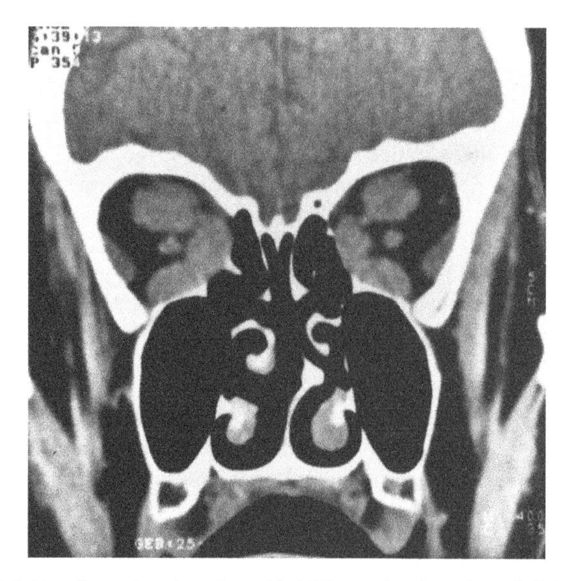

Fig. 3.3.10.9 Coronal section of an orbital CT scan, showing enlarged inferior, medial, and superior rectus muscles but no apical crowding. Effacement of the perineural fat surrounding the optic nerve over more than 50% of its circumference puts the patient at risk for optic neuropathy (50).

Graves' ophthalmopathy is to improve daily life and to make patients feel better rather than to prolong life, clinical measures are often surrogate outcomes for what we really want to measure, the effect of treatment on patients' lives. Consequently, self-assessment of the eye condition is recommended. A disease-specific Graves' ophthalmopathy quality of life questionnaire has been developed, the GO-QOL (52, 53). It contains eight questions about problems with visual functioning and eight questions about the psychosocial consequences of changed appearance. The answers are summarized to one score for visual functioning and one score for appearance. The GO-QOL might be useful not only in evaluation of treatment, but also in reconciling priorities of the patient and of the physician in delineating a management plan. The psychosocial burden imposed by Graves' ophthalmopathy is considerable, and support by mental health care professionals might be needed (54).

Differential diagnosis

The diagnosis of Graves' ophthalmopathy can be quite easy in patients with typical bilateral eye signs and, past or present, Graves' hyperthyroidism. However, it can be difficult in euthyroid patients or in unilateral eye disease. The finding of thyroid autoantibodies may provide circumstantial evidence for the autoimmune nature of the ophthalmopathy. Orbital imaging in unilateral eye disease is mandatory to exclude other conditions, although Graves' ophthalmopathy is the single most common cause of unilateral proptosis representing 15% of cases.

None of the eye signs is pathognomonic for Graves' ophthalmopathy. Lid retraction can be due to non-Graves' thyrotoxicosis, contralateral ptosis, or cocaine use. Diplopia is common in myasthenia gravis, and bilateral proptosis can be caused by orbital fat accumulation (Cushing's syndrome, obesity), lithium therapy, liver cirrhosis, Wegner's granulomatosis, arteriovenous malformations, lymphoma, metastatic tumours, or severe myopia (pseudoproptosis).

Proptosis, motility disturbances, and optic nerve compression can be caused by the ill-defined disease entity of orbital pseudotumour, an idiopathic unilateral focal or diffuse fibroinflammatory orbital lesion (55). The clinical presentation is characterized by acute or subacute signs of inflammation (pain, redness, oedema) and mass effects; CT shows a focal or diffuse mass which is poorly demarcated. Orbital myositis is, after Graves' ophthalmopathy, the second most common cause of extraocular muscle enlargement, due to nonspecific inflammation perhaps of autoimmune aetiology. The cardinal clinical feature is acute orbital pain exacerbating on eye movements. The disease is bilateral in 50% of patients. One or more muscles may be enlarged and, in contrast to Graves' ophthalmopathy, involve the anterior muscle tendons, as evident from CT scans. Orbital pseudotumour and orbital myositis respond quickly to corticosteroids, but recurrences occur in 50% of patients.

Management

Management of Graves' ophthalmopathy requires close consultation between the patient, the endocrinologist, and the eye physician, but in this respect notable differences in the delivery of care exist (56). Combined thyroid–eye clinics are most appropriate to delineate the treatment plan best suited for a particular patient. The timing and mode of thyroid treatment, immunosuppressive treatment, and surgical treatment should be coordinated in a multidisciplinary approach. The patient should be reassured of the possibilities for improvement of eye changes, both functionally and cosmetically, but at the same time be informed that it may require 1–2 years before full rehabilitation is reached. In this respect the experience of other patients with Graves' ophthalmopathy can be quite informative, and contact with patient self-help groups is very useful. The European Group on Graves' Orbitopathy (EUGOGO) has published a consensus statement on management (57). An overview is given in Box 3.3.10.2.

Stop smoking

The advice to stop smoking should be given repeatedly. Progression of eye changes after ^{131}I therapy is more frequent in smokers than in nonsmokers (58, 59). Improvement of eye changes after prednisone or retrobulbar irradiation is less frequent in smokers (60, 61). Smoking increases the risk of recurrence in Graves' hyperthyroidism (62). Some evidence exists that passive smoking is also a risk for developing Graves' ophthalmopathy (63).

Thyroid treatment

The ophthalmopathy is more severe in patients who still have an abnormal thyroid function despite antithyroid treatment; it improves slightly after thyroid function has returned to normal (41, 64). Restoration and maintenance of euthyroidism is thus relevant for the eyes. Prolonged treatment with antithyroid drugs (preferably in combination with thyroxine, the so-called block and replace regimen) until full rehabilitation of the ophthalmopathy is obtained is a feasible option. When the eye disease has become inactive and needs no further treatment, antithyroid drugs can be discontinued; if Graves' hyperthyroidism recurs, it can be treated with ^{131}I without adverse effects on the eyes (65).

Iodine-131 therapy is associated with a risk of about 20% for developing or worsening of eye changes in patients with no or

Box 3.3.10.2 Management of Graves' ophthalmopathy: an integrated approach

1 STOP SMOKING

2 THYROID TREATMENT

- Antithyroid drugs and thyroidectomy are safe
- ^{131}I therapy is feasible but should be combined with oral steroids in high-risk patients

3 EYE TREATMENT

- In any stage
  - Liberal use of artificial tears
  - Occlusive eye pads and eye ointments at night for corneal exposure
  - Dark glasses and prisms as required
- In mild Graves' ophthalmopathy
  - Wait-and-see policy
- In moderately severe Graves' ophthalmopathy
  - In case of active eye disease immunosuppression:
    Intravenous pulses of methylprednisolone
  - Retrobulbar irradiation
  - In case of inactive eye disease, rehabilitative surgery
  - Orbital decompression (for disfiguring proptosis)
  - Eye muscle surgery (for diplopia)
  - Eyelid surgery (for lid positioning and appearance)
- In very severe Graves' ophthalmopathy (optic neuropathy)
  - Intravenous pulses of methylprednisolone for 2 weeks, thereafter oral prednisone
  - Urgent orbital decompression in case of steroid failure

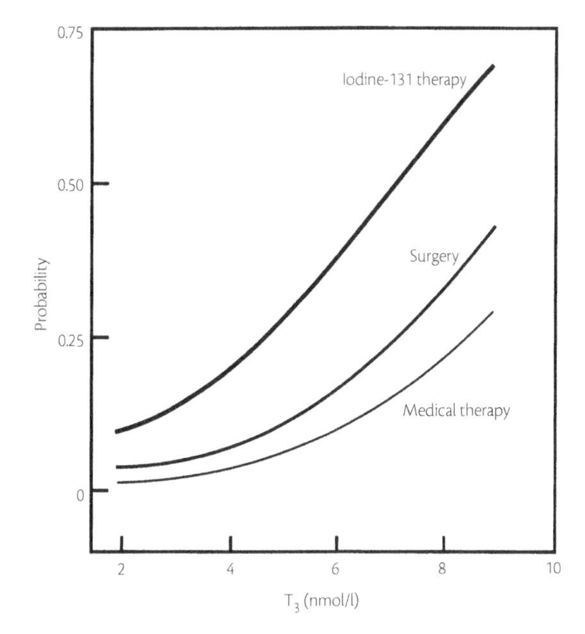

Fig. 3.3.10.10 Probability of developing or worsening of ophthalmopathy in Graves' hyperthyroidism as a function of pretreatment plasma triiodothyronine. Patients with no or mild eye changes before treatment were randomized to receive ^{131}I therapy, subtotal thyroidectomy, or antithyroid drugs. (Reproduced with permission from Tallstedt L, Lundell G, Tørring O, Wallin G, Ljunggren JG, Blomgren H, *et al.* Occurrence of ophthalmopathy after treatment for Graves' hyperthyroidism. *N Engl J Med*, 1992; **326**: 1733–8.)

minimal ophthalmopathy before treatment. This conclusion is based on three large randomized clinical trials (58, 59, 66) and a systematic review (67). Risk factors for developing or worsening of Graves' ophthalmopathy after ^{131}I therapy are a pretreatment triiodothyronine value above 5 nmol/l (Fig. 3.3.10.10), pre-existent active ophthalmopathy, high TSH-binding inhibiting immunoglobulin (TBII) values, and smoking. High TSH levels after ^{131}I therapy also constitute a risk for ophthalmopathy and should be avoided (68, 69). The eye changes after ^{131}I therapy usually occur within 6 months and are mostly transient and mild in nature. They can be prevented by steroids (Table 3.3.10.3), but to expose all patients selected for radio-iodine to the side effects of prednisone to prevent persistent eye changes in 5% is not warranted. It might be better to restrict steroids to patients with one or more risk factors (70). Preventive steroids do not interfere with the efficacy of ^{131}I therapy (71), but uncertainty exists about the most appropriate dosage schedule: oral prednisone 0.2 mg/kg per day given for 6 weeks might be as effective as 0.3–0.5 mg/kg per day given for 3 months. A causal relationship between ^{131}I therapy and the eye changes is plausible in view of the release of thyroid antigens following radiation injury. The resulting T-cell activation and prolonged increase in serum TBII (which lasts for 5 years, in sharp contrast to the fall in serum TBII observed after treatment with antithyroid drugs or thyroidectomy) (72) may trigger autoimmune reactions in the orbit. A similar mechanism would explain the occurrence of ophthalmopathy after neck irradiation for nonthyroidal neoplastic disease (73).

Total thyroidectomy has been recommended in Graves' ophthalmopathy in order to remove all thyroid antigens and thyroid-directed T lymphocytes. This approach is logical assuming cross-reactivity between thyroid and orbital antigens is involved in the immunopathogenesis of Graves' ophthalmopathy, although orbital autoimmunity may proceed independently once the eye disease is well established. In a case–control study, however, development or worsening of eye changes after near-total thyroidectomy occurred in 3.3%, exactly the same as in carefully matched patients treated with methimazole (74). Another study found no difference in the course of ophthalmopathy between subtotal and total thyroidectomy (75). A recent randomized trial in Graves' ophthalmopathy

Table 3.3.10.3 Randomized clinical trial on eye changes upon ^{131}I treatment of Graves' hyperthyroidism in patients with no or previously mild ophthalmopathy (58)

Eye changes		
Improvement (%)	**No change (%)**	**Development or worsening (%)**
2	95	3
0	85	15
35	65	0

found total thyroid ablation (total thyroidectomy + ^{131}I ablation) associated with a slightly better outcome at 9 months than total thyroidectomy alone, but improvement was limited to lid aperture and proptosis and was of minor clinical relevance (76).

In summary, how hyperthyroidism should be treated in the presence of Graves' ophthalmopathy needs to be judged on an individual basis. Antithyroid drugs and thyroidectomy seem to be neutral with respect to the course of the eye changes. If ^{131}I therapy is chosen, preventive steroids should be given in high-risk patients, particularly in patients who smoke and still have active eye disease.

Eye treatment

General recommendations are aimed at protecting the cornea and relieving symptoms such as photophobia and diplopia (Box 3.3.10.2). Prisms can be helpful when the angle of strabismus is constant and not too large. While awaiting definitive treatment, botulinum toxin injections can be given into the upper eye lid to relieve exposure problems, or into the glabellar muscles to alleviate frowning. Further specific recommendations depend on the severity and activity of the ophthalmopathy (57).

Treatment of very severe (sight-threatening) ophthalmopathy

Patients with DON require immediate intervention. The effect of retrobulbar irradiation develops slowly, and consequently radiotherapy is not the treatment of choice in DON. The effect of surgical decompression is observed within days, and that of glucocorticoids within weeks. There is only one randomized controlled trial in DON, which, although its sample size is limited, indicates that intravenous pulses of methylprednisolone are associated with better outcome than immediate surgical decompression (77). Our current scheme therefore is to start with methylprednisolone pulses (1000 mg daily, given as a 60-min intravenous infusion, on three successive days in week 1 and repeated in week 2). If visual functions have not improved after 2 weeks, we do an urgent surgical decompression. Otherwise we continue with oral prednisone (40 mg/day for 2 weeks, 30 mg/day for 4 weeks, 20 mg/day for 4 weeks, and then tapering to zero dose by 2.5 mg/week).

Treatment of mild ophthalmopathy

Mild Graves' ophthalmopathy is defined as having only one or more of the following features: lid retraction less than 2 mm, mild soft tissue involvement, exophthalmos less than 3 mm above normal, and intermittent or no diplopia. The impact on daily life is minor and insufficient to justify immunosuppressive or surgical treatment (57). Spontaneous improvement can be expected in about 30% of patients after 1 year. Therefore, in general, a 'wait-and-see' policy is recommended. Sometimes the mild eye changes have such a negative impact on a patient's life that intervention is warranted. Retrobulbar irradiation in mild ophthalmopathy has a response rate of 50–60%, twice as high as that of sham irradiation, but it does not prevent progress to the more severe ophthalmopathy that occurs in about 15% of patients (78, 79). Recent data suggest selenium treatment improves the outcome of mild ophthalmopathy.

Treatment of moderately severe ophthalmopathy

Immunosuppressive treatment modalities in moderately severe Graves' ophthalmopathy are listed in Table 3.3.10.4. Immunosuppression, in general, is effective for the relief of pain and restoring visual acuity; its effectiveness is moderate for improvement of soft tissue involvement and extraocular muscle dysfunction, and poor for reduction of proptosis. Immunosuppression consequently seldom cures the ophthalmopathy, and most patients still require rehabilitative surgery afterwards. The main accomplishment of immunosuppression seems to be inactivation of the eye disease, thereby permitting earlier corrective surgery.

Table 3.3.10.4 Immunosuppressive treatment modalities in moderately severe Graves' ophthalmopathy

Treatment	Dose
Oral prednisone	60 mg daily for 2 weeks, followed by 40 mg for 2 weeks, 30 mg for 4 weeks, 20 mg for 4 weeks, and then tapered by 2.5 mg/week
Intravenous methylprednisolone	500 mg (infused in 1 h) once weekly for 6 weeks, followed by 250 mg once weekly for another 6 weeks; cumulative dose 4.5 g
Retrobulbar irradiation	20 Gy in 2 weeks: 10 daily sessions of 2 Gy each

Glucocorticoids

Glucocorticoids are better than placebo (80) and generally considered to be the mainstay of immunosuppression in Graves' ophthalmopathy. Intravenous pulses of methylprednisolone have a higher response rate than oral prednisone (74–88% vs 51–63%), and have fewer side effects (17–56% vs 51–85%) (81, 82). Intravenous pulsed methylprednisolone is thus presently the treatment of choice (57, 83). However, four deaths due to acute liver failure occurred in patients receiving large cumulative doses (8–15 g) of intravenous methylprednisolone with an estimated incidence of 0.04%. This has not been observed at a lower cumulative dose of 4.5 g which is currently recommended and can be considered relatively safe as long as liver function tests and hepatitis serology are checked (84). Whereas the combination of oral prednisone and radiotherapy is more effective than oral prednisone alone (83), addition of radiotherapy to intravenous pulsed methylprednisolone may have no extra benefit (85). If the eye changes worsen after discontinuation of glucocorticoids, a combination of low-dose oral prednisone (20 mg/day) with either orbital irradiation or ciclosporin can be tried.

Retrobulbar irradiation

The rationale of orbital radiotherapy is the radiosensitivity of lymphocytes and fibroblasts. Improvement is seen in about 50–60% of patients, predominantly in soft tissue swelling and eye muscle ductions (57, 83, 86). The efficacy of orbital radiotherapy administered in 20 divided fractions of 1 Gy weekly over 20 weeks is slightly better than that of 10 fractions of 1 or 2 Gy daily over 2 weeks (87). Even lower doses than 20 or 10 Gy may be effective. Side effects of retrobulbar irradiation are few. A transient increase of conjunctival irritation is seen in 15% of patients. Radiation-induced retinopathy is extremely rare; the reported cases are, with few exceptions, associated with errors in dosage calculation and radiation technique, or diabetes (86). Although long-term follow-up studies did not detect serious complications after 21 years (88, 89), there exists a theoretical risk of about 0.5% for radiation-induced cancer. The attributable life-time risk from small radiation doses is considerably larger at a younger age than later in life. It is prudent to avoid radiotherapy in patients under 35 years of age, as well as in patients with diabetes or undergoing chemotherapy.

Ciclosporin A

Improvement after ciclosporin monotherapy occurs in 22% of patients, probably reflecting the natural course of the disease (90). The combination of ciclosporin with a low dose of prednisone (20 mg/day) can be effective in patients not responding to steroids or in whom radiotherapy is contraindicated (90, 91). For other modalities, randomized controlled trials have shown no benefit of azathioprine, ciamexone, or acupuncture, but intravenous immunoglobulins can be effective. Somatostatin analogues such as octreotide and lanreotide decrease slightly the clinical activity score but otherwise have little effect (83). The new analogue pareotide is promising because it binds with higher affinity to somatostatin receptor subtypes 1, 2, 3, and 5, all expressed on orbital fibroblasts. Antibodies against tumour necrosis factor (etanercept and infliximab) or against CD20 (rituximab) have shown some beneficial effects but so far have not been tested in randomized controlled trials (92, 93).

Rehabilitative surgery

Once Graves' ophthalmopathy has become inactive, rehabilitative surgery can be carried out to improve visual functions and appearance. If surgery is performed while the disease is still active, the benefits might be lost because of ongoing disease. Most orbital surgeons therefore require stable eye disease for 6 months before surgery.

Orbital decompression, achieved by removal of part of the bony orbital wall, is very effective in reducing exophthalmos. The more orbital wall that is removed, the greater the reduction in proptosis. Careful fat removal during bony decompression is increasingly done. Photographs of how the patient looked before the onset of Graves' ophthalmopathy are helpful in determining the required extent of proptosis reduction. Transeyelid or transconjunctival incisions leave a barely visible scar. Postoperative *de novo* or worsening of diplopia occurs in 10–30% of patients; corrective eye muscle surgery for diplopia should therefore not be done before decompressive surgery. Single binocular vision can be obtained in about 80% of patients, but more than one surgical session is often required to reach this goal. Lastly, eyelid surgery can be performed in order to correct upper or lower eyelid retraction; blepharoplasty can reduce any remaining eyelid swelling.

Graves' dermopathy

Graves' dermopathy or localized myxoedema occurs usually in the pretibial area, but can occasionally occur at other sites associated with a history of trauma. The most frequent form (49%) is nonpitting oedema with violet discolouration and induration of the skin and prominent hair follicles, so that the lesions have the appearance and texture of orange peel (*peau d'orange*). Other clinical forms are plaques (27%), nodules (18%), and elephantiasis (5%) (94). Graves' dermopathy occurs almost always in conjunction with Graves' ophthalmopathy and high serum concentrations of TSH-receptor antibodies. It is observed in 4% of patients with clinically evident ophthalmopathy, and develops mostly about 1 year after the onset of ophthalmopathy (94). The postulated pathogenesis of dermopathy is remarkably similar to that of ophthalmopathy (Fig. 3.3.10.5): cytokine-induced glycosaminoglycan production by dermal fibroblasts, up-regulated TSH receptor expression on dermal fibroblasts, and a contributory role of local mechanical pressure (95).

The natural course of Graves' dermopathy is not well known. One-half of the patients do not require any therapy, and in such cases 50% have complete remission within 17 years. If treatment is necessary because of functional or cosmetic complaints, night-time occlusive dressings of 0.05–0.1% triamcinolone acetonide in a cream base induce partial remissions in 38% of patients. Usually a trial of 4–10 weeks is needed, followed by intermittent maintenance therapy. The use of compressive bandages or stockings during the day provides additional benefit. Treatment of the coexistent ophthalmopathy with systemic glucocorticoids may cause regression of the skin lesions as well.

References

1. Werner SC. Modification of the classification of the eye changes of Graves' disease: recommendations of the ad hoc committee of the American Thyroid Association. *J Clin Endocrinol Metab*, 1997; **44**: 203–4.
2. Burch HB, Wartofsky L. Graves' ophthalmopathy: current concepts regarding pathogenesis and management. *Endocr Rev*, 1993; **14**: 747–93.
3. Prummel MF, Bakker A, Wiersinga WM, Baldeschi L, Mourits MP, Kendall-Taylor P, *et al.* Multi-center study on the characteristics and treatment strategies of patients with Graves' orbitopathy: the first European Group on Graves' Orbitopathy experience. *Eur J Endocrinol*, 2003; **148**: 491–5.
4. Perros P, Crombie AL, Matthews JNS, Kendall-Taylor P. Age and gender influence the severity of thyroid-associated ophthalmopathy: a study of 101 patients attending a combined thyroid-eye clinic. *Clin Endocrinol*, 1993; **38**: 367–72.
5. Neigel JM, Rootman J, Belkin RI, Nugent RA, Drance SM, Beattie CW, *et al.* Dysthyroid optic neuropathy. The crowded orbital apex syndrome. *Ophthalmology*, 1988; **95**: 1515–21.
6. Daumerie Ch, Duprez Th, Boschi A. Long-term multidisciplinary follow-up of unilateral thyroid-associated orbitopathy. *Eur J Intern Med*, 2008; **19**: 531–6.
7. Bartley GB, Fatourechi V, Kadrmas EF, Jacobsen SJ, Ilstrup DM, Garrity JA, *et al.* The incidence of Graves' ophthalmopathy in Olmsted County, Minnesota. *Am J Ophthalmol*, 1995; **120**: 511–17.
8. Krassas GE, Segni M, Wiersinga WM. Childhood Graves' ophthalmopathy: results of a European questionnaire study. *Eur J Endocrinol*, 2005; **153**: 515–20.
9. Durairaj VD, Bartley GB, Garrity JA. Clinical features and treatment of Graves' ophthalmopathy in pediatric patients. *Ophthal Plast Reconstr Surg*, 2006; **22**: 7–12.
10. Prummel MF, Wiersinga WM. Smoking and risk of Graves' disease. *JAMA*, 1993; **269**:479–82.
11. Perros P, Kendall-Taylor P. Natural history of thyroid eye disease. *Thyroid*, 1998; **8**: 423–5.
12. Weetman AP, Wiersinga WM. Current management of thyroid-associated ophthalmopathy in Europe: results of an international survey. *Clin Endocrinol*, 1998; **49**: 21–8.
13. Eckstein AK, Lösch C, Glowacka D, Schott M, Mann K, Esser J, *et al.* Euthyroid and primarily hypothyroid patients develop milder and significantly more asymmetrical Graves' ophthalmopathy. *Br J Ophthalmol*, 2009; **93**: 1052–6.
14. Khoo DH, Eng PH, Ho SC, Tai ES, Morgenthaler NG, Seah LL, *et al.* Graves' ophthalmopathy in the absence of elevated free thyroxine and triiodothyronine levels: prevalence, natural history, and thyrotropin receptor antibody levels. *Thyroid*, 2000; **10**: 1093–100.
15. Rundle FF, Pochin EE. The orbital tissues in thyrotoxicosis: a quantitative analysis relating to exophthalmos. *Clin Sci*, 1944; **5**: 51–74.
16. Feldon SE, Lee CP, Muramatsu K, Weiner JM. Quantitative computed tomography of Graves' ophthalmopathy. *Arch Ophthalmol*, 1985; **103**: 213–15.

17. Otto AJ, Koornneef L, Mourits MP, Deen-van Leeuwen L. Retrobulbar pressures measured during surgical decompression of the orbit. *Br J Ophthalmol*, 1996; **80**: 1042–5.
18. Prabhakar BS, Bahn RS, Smith TJ. Current perspective on the pathogenesis of Graves' disease and ophthalmopathy. *Endocr Rev*, 2003; **24**: 802–35.
19. Aniszewski JP, Valyasevi RW, Bahn RS. Relationship between disease duration and predominant orbital T cell subset in Graves' ophthalmopathy. *J Clin Endocrinol Metab*, 2000; **85**: 776–80.
20. Valyasevi RW, Erickson DZ, Harteneck DA, Dutton CM, Heufelder AE, Jyonouchi SC, *et al.* Differentiation of human orbital preadipocyte fibroblasts induces expression of functional thyrotropin receptor. *J Clin Endocrinol Metab*, 1999; **84**: 2257–62.
21. Wakellamp IMMJ, Bakker O, Baldeschi L, Wiersinga WM, Prummel MF. TSH-R expression and cytokine profile in orbital tissue of active vs. inactive Graves' ophthalmopathy patients. *Clin Endocrinol*, 2003; **58**: 280–7.
22. Vos XG, Smit N, Endert E, Tijssen JG, Wiersinga WM. Frequency and characteristics of TBII-seronegative patients in a population with untreated Graves' hyperthyroidism: a prospective study. *Clin Endocrinol*, 2008; **69**: 311–17.
23. Gerding MN, van der Meer JWC, Broenink M, Bakker O, Wiersinga WM, Prummel MF. Association of thyrotropin receptor antibodies with the clinical features of Graves' ophthalmopathy. *Clin Endocrinol*, 2000; **52**: 267–71.
24. Eckstein AK, Plicht M, Lax H, Hirche H, Quadbeck B, Mann K, *et al.* Clinical results of anti-inflammatory therapy in Graves' ophthalmopathy and association with thyroidal autoantibodies. *Clin Endocrinol*, 2004; **61**: 612–18.
25. Eckstein AK, Plicht M, Lax H, Neuhäuser M, Mann K, Lederbogen S, *et al.* Thyrotropin receptor autoantibodies are independent risk factors for Graves' ophthalmopathy and help to predict severity and outcome of the disease. *J Clin Endocrinol Metab*, 2006; **91**: 3464–70.
26. Pritchard J, Han R, Horst N, Cruikshank WW, Smith TJ. Immunoglobulin activation of T cell chemoattractant expression in fibroblasts from patients with Graves' disease is mediated through the insulin-like growth factor-1 receptor pathway. *J Immunol*, 2003; **170**: 6348–54.
27. Tsui S, Naik V, Hoa N, Hwang CJ, Afifiyan NF, Sinha Hikim A, *et al.* Evidence for an association between thyroid-stimulating hormone and insulin-like growth factor 1 receptors: a tale of two antigens implicated in Graves' disease. *J Immunol*, 2008; **181**: 4397–405.
28. Douglas RS, Gianoukakis AG, Kamat S, Smith TJ. Aberrant expression of the insulin-like growth factor-1 receptor by T cells from patients with Graves' disease may carry functional consequences for disease pathogenesis. *J Immunol*, 2007; **178**: 3281–7.
29. McGregor AM. Has the autoantigen for Graves' ophthalmopathy been found? *Lancet*, 1998; **352**: 595–6.
30. Gopinath B, Musselman R, Adams CL, Tani J, Beard N, Wall JR. Study of serum antibodies against three eye muscles antigens and the connective tissue antigen collagen XIII in patients with Graves' disease with and without ophthalmopathy: correlation with clinical features. *Thyroid*, 2006; **16**: 967–74.
31. Bahn RS. Pathophysiology of Graves' ophthalmopathy: the cycle of disease. *J Clin Endocrinol Metab*, 2003; **88**: 1939–46.
32. Tellez M, Cooper J, Edmonds C. Graves' ophthalmopathy in relation to cigarette smoking and ethnic origin. *Clin Endocrinol*, 1992; **36**: 291–4.
33. Bednarczuk T, Gopinath B, Ploski R, Wall JR. Susceptibility genes in Graves' ophthalmopathy: searching for a needle in a haystack? *Clin Endocrinol*, 2007; **67**: 3–19.
34. Metcalfe RA, Weetman AP. Stimulation of extraocular muscle fibroblasts by cytokines and hypoxia: possible role in thyroid-associated ophthalmopathy. *Clin Endocrinol*, 1994; **40**: 67–72.
35. Cawood TJ, Moriarty P, O'Farrelly C, O'Shea D. Smoking and thyroid-associated ophthalmopathy: a novel explanation of the biological link. *J Clin Endocrinol Metab*, 2007; **92**: 59–64.
36. Rundle FF. Management of exophthalmos and related ocular changes in Graves' disease. *Metabolism*, 1957; **6**: 36–47.
37. Bartley GB, Fatourechi V, Kadrmas EF, Jacobsen SJ, Ilstrup DM, Garrity JA, *et al.* Long-term follow-up of Graves' ophthalmopathy in an incidence cohort. *Ophthalmology*, 1996; **103**: 958–62.
38. Perros P, Crombie AL, Kendall-Taylor P. Natural history of thyroid associated ophthalmopathy. *Clin Endocrinol*, 1995; **42**: 45–50.
39. Wiersinga WM. Advances in medical therapy of thyroid-associated ophthalmopathy. *Orbit*, 1996; **15**: 177–86.
40. European Group on Graves' Orbitopathy (EUGOGO), Wiersinga WM, Perros P, Kahaly GJ, Mourits MP, Baldeschi L, *et al.* Clinical assessment of patients with Graves' orbitopathy: the European Group on Graves' Orbitopathy recommendations to generalists, specialists and clinical researchers. *Eur J Endocrinol*, 2006; **155**: 387–9.
41. Prummel MF, Wiersinga WM, Mourits MP, Koornneef L, Berghout A, van der Gaag RD. Effect of abnormal thyroid function on the severity of Graves' ophthalmopathy. *Arch Intern Med*, 1990; **150**: 1098–101.
42. Dickinson AJ, Perros P. Controversies in the clinical evaluation of active thyroid-associated orbitopathy: use of a detailed protocol with comparative photographs for objective assessment. *Clin Endocrinol*, 2001; **55**: 283–303.
43. Mourits MP, Prummel MF, Wiersinga WM, Koornneef L. Measuring eye movements in Graves' ophthalmopathy. *Ophthalmology*, 1994; **101**: 1341–6.
44. McKeag D, Lane C, Lazarus JH, Baldeschi L, Boboridis K, Dickinson AJ, *et al.* Clinical features of dysthyroid optic neuropathy: a European Group on Graves' Orbitopathy (EUGOGO) survey. *Br J Ophthalmol*, 2007; **91**: 455–8.
45. Gerding MN, Prummel MF, Wiersinga WM. Assessment of disease activity in Graves' ophthalmopathy by orbital ultrasonography and clinical parameters. *Clin Endocrinol*, 2000; **52**: 641–6.
46. Mourits MP, Prummel MF, Wiersinga WM, Koornneef L. Clinical activity score as a guide in the management of patients with Graves' ophthalmopathy. *Clin Endocrinol*, 1997; **47**: 9–14.
47. Hiromatsu Y, Kojima K, Ishisaka N, Tanaka K, Sato M, Nonaka K, *et al.* Role of magnetic resonance imaging in thyroid-associated ophthalmopathy: its predictive value for therapeutic outcome of immunosuppressive therapy. *Thyroid*, 1992; **2**: 299–305.
48. Gerding MN, van der Zant FM, van Royen EA, Koornneef L, Krenning EP, Wiersinga WM, *et al.* Octreotide-scintigraphy is a disease-activity parameter in Graves' ophthalmopathy. *Clin Endocrinol*, 1999; **50**: 373–9.
49. Colao A, Lastoria S, Ferone D, Pivonello R, Macchia PE, Vassallo P, *et al.* Orbital scintigraphy with [^{111}In-diethylenetriamine pentaacetic acid-D-phe^{1}]-octreotide predicts the clinical response to corticosteroid therapy in patients with Graves' ophthalmopathy. *J Clin Endocrinol Metab*, 1998; **83**: 3790–4.
50. Birchall D, Goodall KL, Noble JL, Jackson AJ. Graves' ophthalmopathy: intracranial fat prolapse on CT images as an indicator of optic nerve compression. *Radiology*, 1996; **200**: 123–7.
51. Gerding MN, Terwee CB, Dekker FW, Koornneef L, Prummel MF, Wiersinga WM. Quality of life in patients with Graves' ophthalmopathy is markedly decreased: measurement by the Medical Outcomes Study instrument. *Thyroid*, 1997; **7**: 885–9.
52. Terwee CB, Gerding MN, Dekker FW, Prummel MF, Wiersinga WM. Development of a disease-specific quality of life questionnaire for patients with Graves' ophthalmopathy: the GO-QOL. *Br J Ophthalmol*, 1998; **82**: 773–9.
53. Terwee CB, Gerding MN, Dekker FW, Prummel MF, van der Poll JP, Wiersinga WM. Test-retest reliability of the GO-QOL: a disease-specific quality of life questionnaire for patients with Graves' ophthalmopathy. *J Clin Epidemiol*, 1999; **52**: 875–84.
54. Kahaly GJ, Petrak F, Hardt J, Pitz S, Egle UT. Psychosocial morbidity of Graves' orbitopathy. *Clin Endocrinol*, 2005; **63**: 395–402.

55. Mombaerts I, Goldschmeding R, Schlingemann RO, Koornneef L. What is orbital pseudotumor? A clinical pathological review. *Surv Ophthalmol*, 1996; **41**: 66–78.
56. European Group of Graves' Orbitopathy, Perros P, Baldeschi L, Boboridis K, Dickinson AJ, Hullo A, *et al.* A questionnaire survey on the management of Graves' orbitopathy in Europe. *Eur J Endocrinol*, 2006; **155**: 207–11.
57. Bartalena L, Baldeschi L, Dickinson A, Eckstein A, Kendall-Taylor P, Marcocci C, *et al.* Consensus statement of the European Group on Graves' Orbitopathy (EUGOGO) on management of GO. *Eur J Endocrinol*, 2008; **158**: 273–85.
58. Bartalena L, Marcocci C, Bogazzi F, Manetti L, Tanda ML, Dell'Unto E, *et al.* Relation between therapy for hyperthyroidism and the course of Graves' ophthalmopathy. *N Engl J Med*, 1998; **338**: 73–8.
59. Träisk F, Tallstedt L, Abraham-Nordling M, Andersson T, Berg G, Calissendorff J, *et al.* Thyroid-associated ophthalmopathy after treatment for Graves' hyperthyroidism with antithyroid drugs or iodine-131. *J Clin Endocrinol Metab*, 2009; **94**: 3700–7.
60. Bartalena L, Marcocci C, Tanda ML, Manetti L, Dell'Unto E, Bartolomei MP, *et al.* Cigarette smoking and treatment outcomes in Graves' ophthalmopathy. *Ann Intern Med*, 1998; **129**: 632–5.
61. Eckstein A, Quadbeck B, Mueller G, Rettenmeier AW, Hoermann R, Mann K, *et al.* Impact of smoking on the response to treatment of thyroid associated ophthalmopathy. *Br J Ophthalmol*, 2003; **87**: 773–6.
62. Glinoer D, de Nayer P, Bex M. Effects of L-thyroxine administration, TSH-receptor antibodies and smoking on the risk of recurrence in Graves' hyperthyroidism treated with antithyroid drugs: a double-blind prospective randomized study. *Eur J Endocrinol*, 2001; **144**: 475–83.
63. Krassas GE, Wiersinga WM. Smoking and autoimmune thyroid disease: the plot thickens. *Eur J Endocrinol*, 2006; **154**: 777–80.
64. Prummel MF, Wiersinga WM, Mourits MPh, Koornneef L, Berghout A, van der Gaag RD. Amelioration of eye changes of Graves' ophthalmopathy by achieving euthyroidism. *Acta Endocrinol*, 1989; **121**(Suppl 2): 185–9.
65. Perros P, Kendall-Taylor P, Neoh C, Frewin S, Dickinson J. A prospective study of the effects of radioiodine therapy for hyperthyroidism in patients with minimally active Graves' ophthalmopathy. *J Clin Endocrinol Metab*, 2005; **90**: 5321–3.
66. Tallstedt L, Lundell G, T rring O, Wallin G, Ljunggren JG, Blomgren H, *et al.* Occurrence of ophthalmopathy after treatment for Graves' hyperthyroidism. *N Engl J Med*, 1992; **326**: 1733–8.
67. Acharya SH, Avenell A, Philip S, Burr J, Bevan JS, Abraham P. Radioiodine therapy (RAI) for Graves' disease (GD) and the effect on ophthalmopathy: a systematic review. *Clin Endocrinol*, 2008; **69**: 943–50.
68. Tallstedt L, Lundell G, Blomgren H, Bring J. Does early administration of thyroxine reduce the development of Graves' ophthalmopathy after radioiodine treatment? *Eur J Endocrinol*, 1994; **130**: 494–7.
69. Kung AWC, Yau CC, Cheng A. The incidence of ophthalmopathy after radioiodine therapy for Graves' disease: prognostic factors and the role of methimazole. *J Clin Endocrinol Metab*, 1994; **79**: 542–6.
70. Wiersinga WM. Preventing Graves' ophthalmopathy. *N Engl J Med*, 1998; **338**: 121–2.
71. Jansen BE, Bonnema SJ, Hegedus L. Glucocorticoids do not influence the effect of radioiodine therapy in Graves' disease. *Eur J Endocrinol*, 2005; **153**: 15–21.
72. Laurberg P, Wallin G, Tallstedt L, Abraham-Nordling M, Lundell G, Torring O. TSH-receptor autoimmunity in Graves' disease after therapy with anti-thyroid drugs, surgery, or radioiodine: a 5-year prospective randomized study. *Eur J Endocrinol*, 2008; **158**: 69–75.
73. Wasnich RD, Grumet FC, Payne RO, Kriss JP. Graves' ophthalmopathy following external neck irradiation for nonthyroidal neoplastic disease. *J Clin Endocrinol Metab*, 1973; **37**: 703–13.
74. Marcocci C, Bruno-Bossio G, Manetti L, Tanda ML, Miccoli P, Iacconi P, *et al.* The course of Graves' ophthalmopathy is not influenced by near-total thyroidectomy: a case-control study. *Clin Endocrinol*, 1999; **51**: 503–8.
75. Jarhult J, Rudberg C, Larsson E, Selvander H, Sjövall K, Winsa B, *et al.* Graves' disease with moderate-severe endocrine ophthalmopathy: long term results of a prospective, randomized study of total or subtotal thyroid resection. *Thyroid*, 2005; **15**: 1157–64.
76. Menconi F, Marinò M, Pinchera A, Rocchi R, Mazzi B, Nardi M, *et al.* Effects of total thyroid ablation versus near-total thyroidectomy alone on mild to moderate Graves' orbitopathy treated with intravenous glucocorticoids. *J Clin Endocrinol Metab*, 2007; **92**: 1653–8.
77. Wakelkamp IMMJ, Baldeschi L, Saeed P, Mourits MP, Prummel MF, Wiersinga WM. Surgical or medical decompression as a first-line treatment of optic neuropathy in Graves' ophthalmopathy? A randomized controlled trial. *Clin Endocrinol*, 2005; **63**: 323–8.
78. Prummel MF, Terwee CB, Gerding MN, Baldeschi L, Mourits MP, Blank L, *et al.* A randomized controlled trial of orbital radiotherapy versus sham irradiation in patients with mild Graves' ophthalmopathy. *J Clin Endocrinol Metab*, 2004; **89**: 15–20.
79. Mourits MP, Van Kempen-Harteveld ML, Begonia Garcia M, Koppeschaar HPF, Tick L, Terwee CB. Randomized placebo-controlled study of radiotherapy for Graves' orbitopathy. *Lancet*, 2000; **355**: 1505–9.
80. van Geest RJ, Sasim IV, Koppeschaar HP, Kalmann R, Stravers SN, Bijlsma WR, *et al.* Methylprednisolone pulse therapy for patients with moderately severe Graves' orbitopathy: a prospective, randomized, placebo-controlled study. *Eur J Endocrinol*, 2008; **158**: 229–37.
81. Marcocci C, Bartalena L, Tanda ML, Manetti L, Dell'Unto E, Rocchi R, *et al.* Comparison of the effectiveness and tolerability of intravenous or oral glucocorticoids associated with orbital radiotherapy in the management of severe Graves' ophthalmopathy: results of a prospective, single-blind, randomized study. *J Clin Endocrinol Metab*, 2001; **86**: 3562–7.
82. Kahaly GJ, Pitz S, Hommel G, Dittmar M. Randomized, single blind trial of intravenous versus oral steroid monotherapy in Graves' orbitopathy. *J Clin Endocrinol Metab*, 2005; **90**: 5234–40.
83. Stiebel-Kalish H, Robenshtok E, Hasanreisoglu M, Ezrachi D, Shimon I, Leibovici L. Treatment modalities for Graves' ophthalmopathy: systematic review and metaanalysis. *J Clin Endocrinol Metab*, 2009; **94**: 2708–16.
84. Le Moli R, Baldeschi L, Saeed P, Regensburg N, Mourits MP, Wiersinga WM. Determinants of liver damage associated with intravenous methylprednisolone pulse therapy in Graves' ophthalmopathy. *Thyroid*, 2007; **17**: 357–62.
85. Ohtsuka K, Sato A, Kawaguchi S, Hashimoto M, Suzuki Y. Effect of steroid pulse therapy with and without orbital radiotherapy on Graves' ophthalmopathy. *Am J Ophthalmol*, 2003; **135**: 285–90.
86. Bradley EA, Gower EW, Bradley DJ, Meyer DR, Cahill KV, Custer PL, *et al.* Orbital radiation for Graves' ophthalmopathy. A report by the American Academy of Ophthalmology. *Ophthalmology*, 2008; **115**: 398–409.
87. Kahaly GJ, Rösler HP, Pitz S, Hommel G. Low- versus high-dose radiotherapy for Graves' ophthalmopathy: a randomized, single blind trial. *J Clin Endocrinol Metab*, 2000; **85**: 102–8.
88. Marcocci C, Bartalena L, Rocchi R, Marinò M, Menconi F, Morabito E, *et al.* Long-term safety of orbital radiotherapy for Graves' ophthalmopathy. *J Clin Endocrinol Metab*, 2003; **88**: 3561–6.
89. Wakelkamp IM, Tan H, Saeed P, Schlingemann RO, Verbraak FD, Blank LE, *et al.* Orbital irradiation for Graves' ophthalmopathy. Is it safe? A long-term follow-up study. *Ophthalmology*, 2004; **111**: 1557–62.
90. Prummel MF, Mourits MP, Berghout A, Krenning EP, van der Gaag R, Koornneef L, *et al.* Prednisone and cyclosporine in the treatment of severe Graves' ophthalmopathy. *N Engl J Med*, 1989; **321**: 949–54.
91. Kahaly G, Schrezenmeir J, Krause U, Schweikert B, Meuer S, Muller W. Cyclosporin and prednisone versus prednisone in treatment of Graves' ophthalmopathy: a controlled, randomized and prospective study. *Eur J Clin Invest*, 1986; **16**: 415–22.

92. Paridaens D, van den Bosch WA, van der Loos TL, Krenning EP, v an Hagen PM. The effect of etanercept on Graves' ophthalmopathy: a pilot study. *Eye*, 2005; **19**: 1286–9.
93. Salvi M, Vannucchi G, Campi I, Currò N, Dazzi D, Simonetta S, *et al.* Treatment of Graves' disease and associated ophthalmopathy with the anti-CD20 monoclonal antibody rituximab: an open study. *Eur J Endocrinol*, 2007; **156**: 33–40.
94. Fatourechi V. Pretibial myxedema. Pathophysiology and treatment options. *Am J Clin Dermatol*, 2005; **6**: 295–309.
95. Rapoport B, Alsabeh R, Aftergood D, McLachlan SM. Elephantiasic pretibial myxedema: insight into and a hypothesis regarding the pathogenesis of the extrathyroidal manifestations of Graves' disease. *Thyroid*, 2000; **10**: 685–92.

Further reading

Wiersinga WM, Kahaly GJ (eds). *Graves' Orbitopathy. A Multidisciplinary Approach*. Basel: Karger, 2010 (2nd edition).

Kuriyan AE, Phipps RP, Feldon SE. The eye and thyroid disease. *Curr Opin Ophthalmol*, 2008; **19**: 499–506.

Dickinson J, Perros P. Thyroid-associated orbitopathy: who and how to treat. *Endocrinol Metab Clin North Am*, 2009; **38**: 373–8.

Bartalena L, Tanda ML. Clinical practice. Graves' ophthalmopathy. *N Engl J Med*, 2009; **360**: 994–1001.

3.3.11 Management of toxic multinodular goitre and toxic adenoma

Dagmar Führer, John H. Lazarus

Definition

Toxic adenoma and toxic multinodular goitre represent the clinically important presentations of thyroid autonomy. Thyroid autonomy is a condition where thyrocytes produce thyroid hormones independently of thyrotropin (TSH) and in the absence of TSH-receptor stimulating antibodies (TSAB).

Toxic adenoma (TA) is a clinical term referring to a solitary autonomously functioning thyroid nodule. The autonomous properties of TA are best shown by radio-iodine or ^{99m}Tc imaging. The classic appearance of TA is that of circumscribed increased uptake with suppression of uptake in the surrounding extranodular thyroid tissue ('hot' nodule, Fig. 3.3.11.1).

Toxic multinodular goitre (TMNG) is a heterogeneous disorder characterized by the presence of autonomously functioning thyroid nodules in a goitre with or without additional nodules. These additional nodules can show normal or decreased uptake (cold nodules) on scintiscan. TMNG constitutes the most frequent form of thyroid autonomy.

Epidemiology and pathogenesis

The prevalence of thyroid autonomy is inversely correlated with iodine intake. Thus, thyroid autonomy is a common finding in iodine-deficient areas, where it accounts for up to 60% of cases of thyrotoxicosis (TMNG *c.*50%; TA *c.*10%), but is rare (5–10%) in regions with iodine sufficiency (1, 2). Several studies have suggested that TMNG originates from euthyroid goitres and microscopic autonomous foci have been demonstrated in up to 40% of euthyroid goitres in iodine-deficient areas. Moreover, the prevalence of thyroid autonomy correlates with thyroid nodularity and increases with age. Correction of iodine deficiency in a population results in decrease of thyroid autonomy and this has been impressively shown, e.g. in Switzerland where a doubling in iodine salt content resulted in a 73% reduction of TMNG.

Somatic mutations of the G-protein-coupled TSH receptor or less frequently the Gsα-protein subunit (GSP; 5–10%) have been identified in TA and TMNG and represent the predominant molecular cause of thyroid autonomy. These mutations cause constitutive activation of the cAMP pathway, which stimulates thyroid hormone production and thyroid growth (2–4).

Clinical features and diagnosis

Clinical features of thyroid autonomy may be related to hyperthyroidism and/or compression signs due to the nodule and TMNG (4, 5). Clinical presentation of overt hyperthyroidism, defined by suppressed TSH with elevated free thyroxine (T_4) and/or free triiodothyronine (T_3) varies with age. While classic hyperthyroid features such as tremor, sweating, and hyperkinesis can be found in younger patients, thyrotoxicosis is often oligosymptomatic in older people. In this population, atrial fibrillation, congestive heart failure, and anorexia may prevail. Subclinical hyperthyroidism, defined by low or suppressed TSH with normal free T_4 and free T_3 levels, is also more commonly observed in older patients and is more than 'just' a low TSH status, since it confers increased risk for atrial fibrillation and in postmenopausal women contributes to reduced bone density (6).

In addition, a history of possible iodine contamination (contrast media, amiodarone) should be obtained. In the European Study Group of Hyperthyroidism, iodine contamination was found in 36.8% of patients from iodine-deficient areas with first diagnosis of hyperthyroidism. Severity of iodine deficiency, autonomous thyroid cell mass, and older age have been proposed as risk factors for the development of iodine-induced hyperthyroidism, which responds less well to antithyroid drug treatment and puts the patient at risk for a life-threatening thyroid storm (7, 8). Alternatively, a patient may present with a lump or disfigurement of the neck, intolerance of tight necklaces, or increase in collar size. Moreover, dysphagia or breathing difficulties due to local oesophageal or tracheal compression may be present, particularly with TMNG.

Unusually, in some patients there may be a family history of thyroid autonomy and a characteristic course of frequent relapses of hyperthyroidism following thyrostatic therapy or partial thyroidectomy. Depending on the age of onset (neonatal to adulthood) these patients may present with a diffusely enlarged goitre or a TMNG. The underlying cause of this condition is an activating germline mutation in the TSH-receptor gene, which can be confirmed through molecular diagnostics from a peripheral blood sample. Patients with an activating TSH-receptor germline mutation require definitive treatment in the form of a total thyroidectomy or an ablative dose of radio-iodine to prevent further relapses. Genetic counselling is also mandatory as the condition is autosomal dominantly inherited (3, 4).

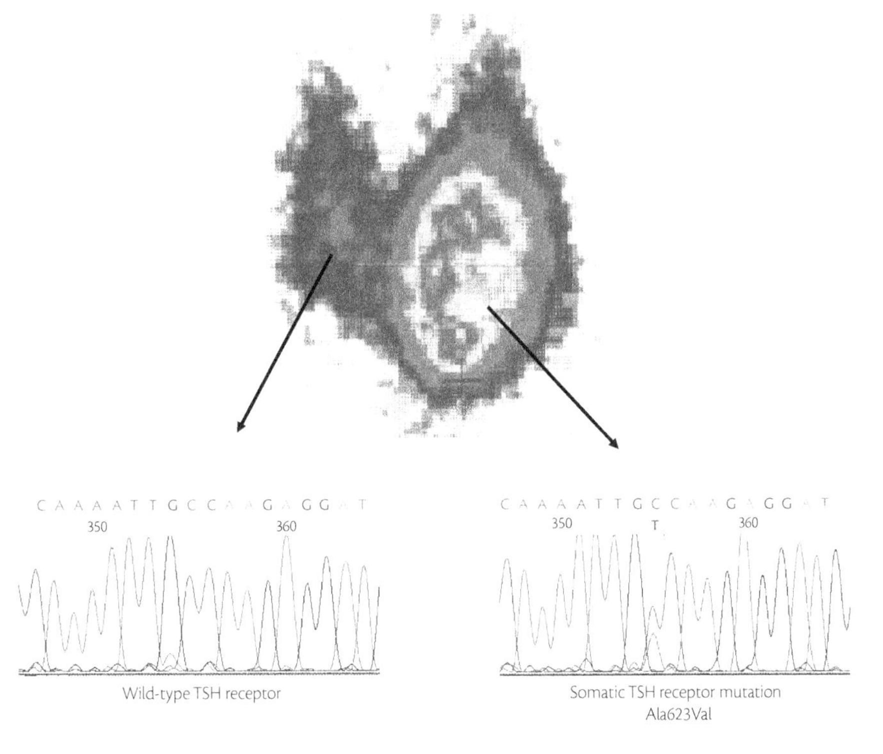

Fig. 3.3.11.1 Scintiscan of a uninodular goitre showing a circumscribed area of increased technetium uptake in the left lobe ('hot' nodule). DNA was extracted from the toxic adenoma and surrounding normal thyroid tissue and exon 10 of the TSH receptor was amplified by polymerase chain reaction (PCR). Sequencing of the PCR products showed the presence of a heterozygous point mutation (GCC→GTC) resulting in an amino acid exchange (Ala→Val) in the toxic adenoma (right) whereas only the wild-type TSH receptor was present in the normal thyroid tissue (left). The mutation causes a constitutive activation of the TSH receptor which leads to thyrotoxicosis and thyroid growth. (See also Plate 17)

The diagnosis of TA and TMNG is based on clinical examination, thyroid function tests, thyroid ultrasonography, and scintiscanning (4, 5). Examination of the neck will reveal the degree of thyroid enlargement and nodularity of the gland. A history of a recently enlarging nodule and cervical lymph node enlargement should be noted because of the concern for a developing malignancy at this site. In addition, clinical evidence of lymph node enlargement and tracheal deviation and/or compression should be sought. Standard thyroid function tests (TSH, free T_4, and free T_3) will confirm overt or subclinical hyperthyroidism, but depending on the autonomous cell mass, euthyroidism may still prevail. Localization, size, and number of thyroid nodule(s) as well as goitre volume can be determined by ultrasound scanning using a 7.5- or 9-MHz linear scanner. In addition, the presence or absence of cervical lymph node enlargement should be noted. Increased ^{99m}Tc or ^{123}I radionucleotide uptake in the nodule(s) concomitant with a decreased uptake in the surrounding extranodular thyroid tissue is the typical finding on scintiscanning (Fig. 3.3.11.1). If thyroid autonomy is suspected in a patient with a (still) euthyroid nodule, a 'suppression' scan can be performed after administration of thyroid hormones (e.g. 75 µg/day L-thyroxine for 2 weeks followed by 150 µg/day for 2 weeks). Thereby nonautonomous tissue will be suppressed and thyroid autonomy unmasked.

Measurement of thyroid autoantibodies is not routinely performed in thyroid autonomy. However, in iodine-deficient areas distinction between Graves' disease and TMNG can be difficult if extrathyroidal manifestations of autoimmune thyroid disease are absent and ultrasound scanning shows the presence of thyroid nodules (*c.*27–34%). In this scenario, measurement of TSAB is helpful to establish the correct diagnosis. Urinary iodine excretion can be measured in cases of suspected iodine contamination. CT or MRI are not routinely indicated for diagnosis of thyroid autonomy but may be used for presurgical planning in cases of large and partly intrathoracic TMNG.

Treatment of toxic multinodular goitre and toxic adenoma

The management of patients with thyroid autonomy (TMNG and TA) will to some extent depend on the patient's age, the severity of hyperthyroidism, the size of the thyroid gland, and concomitant medical illness (4, 5, 9). Antithyroid medication (ATD) is the first-line treatment in all patients with overt hyperthyroidism. Depending on the type of antithyroid drug, an initial dosage of 30 mg/day methimazole, 40–60 mg/day carbimazole, or 3 × 50 mg/day propylthiouracil is recommended. Higher dosages are associated with more frequent adverse effects and will only result in marginally faster resolution of thyrotoxicosis. ATDs are usually combined with β-blockers (preferably nonselective propranolol) for symptom relief, until the patient is euthyroid. A trial of low-dose antithyroid medication (5–10 mg methimazole/day) may be justified in selected patients with symptomatic subclinical hyperthyroidism, i.e. atrial fibrillation; alternatively, β-blocking agents can be used (6). Monitoring of thyroid function and ATD side effects, in particular full blood count and liver function tests, are mandatory.

Due to the underlying molecular defect there is no spontaneous resolution of thyroid autonomy and definitive treatment is indicated once thyroid autonomy becomes clinically manifest. Elderly patients with severe nonthyroidal illness may be an exception to this rule. However, benefits and risks of such long-term ATD have to be considered against the nowadays very low risk of definitive treatment.

Three different ablative treatment options are available for TA and TMNG: thyroid surgery, radio-iodine treatment, and percutaneous ethanol injection. The purpose of thyroid surgery is to cure hyperthyroidism by removing all autonomously functioning thyroid tissue and other macroscopically visible nodular thyroid tissue (5, 10). Thus the extent of surgery will vary depending on preoperative ultrasound findings and intraoperative morphological inspection.

For TA, hemithyroidectomy is usually adequate, if no further nodules are detectable, while in the case of TMNG a subtotal, near-total, or total thyroidectomy is performed. The advantages of surgery are a fast ablation of hyperthyroidism and the immediate relief of compression symptoms. The disadvantages of surgery are thyroid-specific side effects, i.e. vocal cord paralysis and permanent hypoparathyroidism, which should be less than 1% with an experienced endocrine surgeon. Clearly, the rate of postoperative hypothyroidism will vary with the extent of thyroid resection, and cases of near-total or total thyroidectomy require the start of efficient thyroid hormone replacement therapy (1.6–1.8 µg/kg body weight L-thyroxine), aiming for a TSH value of approximately 1 mU/l shortly after surgery. Surgery is usually recommended in large TMNG (>100 ml) and is indicated in case of suspicion of thyroid cancer. In addition, surgery is also advocated in patients with overt hyperthyroidism and adverse side effects of ATD, or as an early emergency procedure in patients with thyroid storm (7, 8).

Radio-iodine therapy is also highly effective for ablation of hyperthyroidism and reduction of TA or TMNG volume (5, 9, 11). Different protocols have been suggested for ^{131}I therapy in benign thyroid disease. Some investigators prefer to administer a standard dose, e.g. 370–740 MBq/thyroid gland, while others apply a certain ^{131}I activity/g thyroid tissue. The success rate of an individually dosed ^{131}I therapy has been reported to range between 85% and 100% in TA and reaches up to 90% in TMNG. An average thyroid and/or nodule volume reduction of about 40% can be anticipated. The advantages of radio-iodine therapy are its simple and outpatient-based applicability. The disadvantages are the 'time to euthyroidism' period (6 weeks to more than 3 months), during which time ATD has to be continued and thyroid function monitored at 3- to 6-week intervals. Radio-iodine treatment is contraindicated in pregnancy, and contraception is advocated for at least 6 months after receiving ^{131}I therapy. Population-based studies comprising more than 35 000 patients treated with ^{131}I have not shown increased risk of thyroid cancer, leukaemia, other malignancies, reproductive abnormalities, or congenital defects in the offspring, so that ^{131}I therapy can be considered a very safe treatment. Postradio-iodine hypothyroidism in TMNG and TA usually develops insidiously and depends on the extent of TSH suppression before ^{131}I therapy and the protocol applied. In one study, the incidence of hypothyroidism was 3% at 1 year, 31% at 8 years, and 64% at 24 years follow-up after radio-iodine treatment. These data emphasize the requirement for long-term monitoring of thyroid function in all patients receiving ^{131}I therapy.

The principle of percutaneous ethanol injection treatment (PEIT) is the induction of a coagulative necrosis of the autonomous tissue by ultrasound-guided injection of 95% ethanol, usually accompanied by thrombosis of small vessels (5, 9). PEIT has been studied predominantly in specialized centres in Italy and has been demonstrated to be a cost-effective treatment of thyroid autonomy with reported overall cure rates of 68–90%. Between 1 and 9 ml ethanol (usually 1 or 2 ml) is injected into the nodule under ultrasound control. Three to eight treatment sessions over 2–4 weeks are required to destroy an average autonomously functioning nodule. The total amount of alcohol delivered is about 1.5 times the nodular volume. The limited follow-up time and lack of evaluation of PEIT in comparison to standard treatment of thyroid autonomy, however, makes this modality an alternative treatment for patients with contraindications to surgery or radio-iodine (e.g. old age, patients on dialysis, severe nonthyroidal illness). Side effects include transient vocal cord paralysis (3% within 1 week to 3 months) and transient thyroid pain (30% at the time of treatment). A summary of the advantages and disadvantages of the different treatment modalities for TA and TMNG is shown in Table 3.3.11.1.

Table 3.3.11.1 Treatment of toxic multinodular goitre and toxic adenoma

Modality	Advantages	Disadvantages
Surgery	Effective Simple operation Rapid euthyroidism	Hospitalization Anaesthesia Side effects (vocal cord paralysis, hypoparathyroidism)
Radio-iodine therapy	Outpatient therapy	Time to cure Possible hypothyroidism in the long term
Antithyroid drugs	Rapid euthyroidism Not destructive	Relapse on stopping Side effects (skin, liver, bone marrow)
Percutaneous ethanol treatment	Outpatient procedure Effective	Limited long-term experience Several treatment sessions required Side effects (vocal cord paralysis, pain)

Follow-up

The long-term management of patients with TA and TMNG is directed at the detection and adequate treatment of thyroid dysfunction (TSH level), detection of novel nodular thyroid disease (palpation and ultrasonography), and, in case of surgery, detection and treatment of postsurgical hypoparathyroidism (serum calcium). In case of ^{131}I therapy, long-term follow-up for development of hypothyroidism is mandatory, e.g. annually. Thyroxine with or without iodine is often administered after thyroid surgery to prevent recurrent goitre/thyroid nodules. Although large randomized trials are lacking to provide definite evidence that postoperative thyroxine administration is beneficial, unless the patient is hypothyroid, this treatment strategy is inferred by studies treating goitre/nodules with L-thyroxine. In addition, in iodine-deficient areas iodine supplementation may be appropriate to prevent further nodular thyroid disease.

References

1. Delange F, de Benoist B, Pretell E, Dunn JT. Iodine deficiency in the world: where do we stand at the turn of the century? *Thyroid*, 2001; **11**: 437–47.
2. Krohn K, Führer D, Bayer Y, Eszlinger M, Brauer V, Neumann S, *et al.* Molecular pathogenesis of euthyroid and toxic multinodular goiter. *Endocr Rev 2005*, 2005; **26**: 504–24.
3. Parma J, Duprez L, Van Sande J, Cochaux P, Gervy C, Mockel J, *et al.* Somatic mutations in the thyrotropin receptor gene cause hyperfunctioning thyroid adenomas. *Nature*, 1993; **365**: 649–51.
4. Führer D, Krohn K, Paschke R. Toxic adenoma and toxic multinodular goiter. In: Braverman LE, Utiger RD, eds. *Werner and Ingbar's The Thyroid*. 9th edn. Philadelphia: Lippincott-Raven, 2005.
5. Hegedus L. Clinical practice. The thyroid nodule. *N Engl J Med*, 2004; **351**: 1764–71.
6. Biondi B, Cooper DS. The clinical significance of subclinical thyroid dysfunction. *Endocr Rev*, 2008; **29**: 76–131.
7. Roti E, Uberti ED. Iodine excess and hyperthyroidism. *Thyroid*, 2001; **11**: 493–500.

8. Sarlis NJ, Gourgiotis L. Thyroid emergencies. *Rev Endocr Metab Disord*, 2003; **4**: 129–36.
9. Hegedus L, Bonnema SJ, Bennedbaek FN. Management of simple nodular goiter: current status and future perspectives. *Endocr Rev*, 2003; **24**: 102–32.
10. Porterfield JR Jr, Geoffrey B, Thompson AE, Grant CS, Richards ML. Evidence-based management of toxic multinodular goiter (Plummer's disease). *World J Surg*, 2008; **32**: 1278–84.
11. Reiners C, Schneider P. Radioiodine therapy of thyroid autonomy. *Eur J Nucl Med Mol Imaging*, 2002; **29** (Suppl 2): S471–8.

3.3.12 Management of thyrotoxicosis without hyperthyroidism

Wilmar M. Wiersinga

Introduction

Thyrotoxicosis without hyperthyroidism is a condition of thyroid hormone excess not caused by increased biosynthesis of thyroid hormones in the thyroid gland. The thyroid hormone excess in such cases originates either from the thyroid gland as a result of destructive lesions or from extrathyroidal sources. The hallmark of thyrotoxicosis without hyperthyroidism is a low uptake of radio-iodine in the neck (see Chapter 3.3.5). Cytokine-, iodine-, and amiodarone-induced thyrotoxicosis manifest themselves either as thyrotoxicosis without hyperthyroidism, or as thyrotoxicosis with hyperthyroidism in which thyroidal radio-iodine uptake is preserved. Both types are discussed in this chapter.

Thyrotoxicosis due to destructive thyroiditis

The inflammatory reaction in these conditions disrupts the normal architecture of the thyroid gland, causing release of thyroxine (T_4) and triiodothyronine (T_3) from the colloid. The colloid contains more T_4 than T_3, explaining the lower serum T_3/T_4 ratio in thyrotoxic patients without hyperthyroidism as compared to thyrotoxic patients with hyperthyroidism (1). Leakage of the iodine-rich contents of the colloid into the bloodstream expands the iodide pool in the circulation; administered radio-iodine will be diluted in the expanded iodide pool, which in conjunction with damage to the thyrocytes causes a low thyroidal radio-iodine uptake. The efficacy of treatment with radio-iodine or antithyroid drugs is consequently very low.

Subacute, painless, and postpartum thyroiditis run a self-limited course, in which the inflammation gradually subsides under restoration of the normal thyroid architecture. Thyrotoxicosis associated with thyroiditis is usually mild, lasting for only a few weeks, and either no treatment or treatment with a β-adrenoceptor antagonist is sufficient. Short-term salicylates, or glucocorticoids in more resistant cases, may be required to relieve neck pain in subacute thyroiditis (see Chapter 3.2.7). The thyrotoxic phase may be followed by a hypothyroid phase in any type of thyroiditis and can last for 1–4 months. Thyroxine treatment may be warranted in symptomatic patients, but should be withdrawn after 6 months because most patients will spontaneously regain euthyroidism. Postpartum thyroiditis is very likely to recur after a subsequent pregnancy. Permanent hypothyroidism develops in about one-third of patients with silent or postpartum thyroiditis (see Chapter 3.4.6).

Radiation-induced thyroiditis occurs most often in patients given large doses of ^{131}I. It develops in the first 2 weeks after ^{131}I therapy, and is characterized by neck and ear pain, painful swallowing, thyroid swelling and tenderness, and mild transient thyrotoxicosis. It resolves spontaneously within a week or two, and requires no specific treatment besides salicylates for mild pain; glucocorticoids (e.g. 30 mg prednisone daily) may be given for severe pain or swelling, tapering the dose when the complaints have disappeared (see also Chapters 3.2.5 and 3.5.2).

Cytokine-induced thyroiditis has been observed after the administration of interleukin-2, interferon-α (IFNα), or granulocyte-macrophage colony stimulating factor (2). The clinical picture may resemble that of destructive thyroiditis: transient thyrotoxicosis developing after a few weeks to months, followed by a hypothyroid phase which may be transient as well. Radio-iodine thyroid uptake is low and a small nontender goitre is sometimes present. However, it is not uncommon that the hypothyroid phase is permanent, or develops much later without preceding thyrotoxicosis.

In patients treated with IFNα for viral hepatitis, *de novo* occurrence of thyroid antibodies is observed in 10–14% (3). Thyroid dysfunction develops in 6% of such patients due to autoimmune hypothyroidism (*c.*50%), Graves' hyperthyroidism (*c.*25%), or destructive thyroiditis (*c.*25%) (4). These abnormalities have a median date of onset 17 weeks after starting treatment, but can occur at any time (from 4 weeks until 23 months). IFNα-induced thyroid dysfunction is related to female sex (RR 4.4) and pre-existent thyroid antibodies (RR 3.9) (4), but not to dosage or efficacy of IFNα treatment (5). It is therefore recommended to measure thyroid-stimulating hormone (TSH) and thyroid peroxidase (TPO) antibodies before treatment, and to monitor thyroid function during treatment, e.g. by TSH every 3 months (3). IFNα-induced Graves' disease does not resolve spontaneously after discontinuation of IFNα (6), and thyroid ablation with ^{131}I or surgery is preferred; antithyroid drugs are not favoured since they can worsen liver function. In contrast, IFNα-induced destructive thyroiditis is mostly mild or subclinical and resolves spontaneously, although permanent hypothyroidism develops in less than 5% of cases. IFNα treatment can usually be continued, except in very severe cases. Corticosteroids are generally contraindicated in patients with hepatitis C. Rechallenge with IFNα may result in recurrent destructive thyroiditis.

Trauma of the thyroid gland may result in transient thyrotoxicosis associated with a low radio-iodine thyroid uptake. It occurs rarely in patients with a previously normal thyroid gland: the few described cases developed after parathyroid surgery or after massive haemorrhage in the thyroid due to neck trauma under treatment with oral anticoagulants (7, 8). The thyrotoxicosis spontaneously resolves in about 4 weeks, and requires no treatment or merely symptomatic treatment.

Infections of the thyroid gland are uncommon. It can be difficult to differentiate between infectious thyroiditis and subacute thyroiditis as fever, sore throat, a small tender goitre, and an elevated ESR are found in both conditions (see Chapter 3.2.7).

Radio-iodine uptake may be low in infectious thyroiditis. Thyrotoxicosis or hypothyroidism can be present, but thyroid function remains normal in most patients. Treatment is primarily directed against the infectious agent.

Infiltration of the thyroid gland with malignant lymphoma or cancer metastases may cause thyrotoxicosis associated with low radio-iodine thyroid uptake in exceptional cases and is due to invasion and disruption of thyroid follicles (9, 10).

Iodide-induced thyrotoxicosis

Iodide-induced thyrotoxicosis (IIT) is commonly related to mutational or epigenetic events in thyroid follicular cells that lead to autonomous thyroid function. When the mass of thyrocytes with such an event becomes sufficient and iodine supply is increased, the patient may become hyperthyroid (11). The proposed pathogenesis is in line with the observed (transient) increase in the incidence of hyperthyroidism in iodine-deficient regions after the introduction of iodine prophylaxis (see Chapter 3.2.3), and also with known risk factors for the development of IIT in iodine-sufficient regions, such as multinodular goitre, a suppressed TSH, and old age (12) (see Chapter 3.2.4). In these cases of IIT the thyrotoxicosis is associated with hyperthyroidism because the thyrocytes synthesize large amounts of thyroid hormone, and thyroidal radio-iodine uptake may be normal or even high. IIT resolves spontaneously in one-half of the patients on average after 6 months. The duration of the disease is similar in treated and untreated cases, making it difficult to attribute improvement seen after antithyroid drugs to therapy. β-blockade or no treatment at all may suffice in mild cases (13, 14).

In contrast to the above, IIT may also develop in people without any pre-existent thyroid disease. In this type of IIT the sex ratio is about equal and thyroid radio-iodine uptake is low (13, 14). The disease resolves spontaneously within 6 months, often after a hypothyroid phase. It is uncertain if antithyroid drugs shorten the interval to restoration of the euthyroid state. These patients may well have thyrotoxicosis without hyperthyroidism due to cytotoxic effects of high doses of iodide.

A common source of iodine excess is exposure to iodine-containing contrast agents (15). The risk for developing IIT is 0.3% in unselected people after coronary angiography in iodine-deficient areas (16). In selected patients who had thyroid autonomy before coronary angiography, treatment with 20 mg thiamazole and/or 900 mg sodium perchlorate, starting the day before angiography and continued for 2 weeks, was not very effective in preventing IIT (17, 18). Close monitoring of high-risk patients rather than prophylaxis is thus recommended, with institution of β-adrenoceptor antagonists if thyrotoxicosis occurs (15, 19).

Amiodarone-induced thyrotoxicosis

One tablet of 200 mg amiodarone contains 74.4 mg iodine of which 10% is released *in vivo* during biotransformation of the drug. A maintenance dose of 300 mg amiodarone daily results in a 40-fold rise of plasma inorganic iodide and urinary iodide excretion (20). The iodine excess may induce thyrotoxicosis in patients with underlying thyroid disease, referred to as amiodarone-induced thyrotoxicosis (AIT) type 1 (Table 3.3.12.1). Amiodarone and especially its main metabolite desethylamiodarone have a potent cytotoxic effect on thyrocytes causing destructive thyroiditis (21, 22); it may give rise to a destructive type of thyrotoxicosis, referred to as AIT type 2 (see also Chapter 3.3.5). The analogy with iodide-induced thyrotoxicosis is obvious, but the molar concentrations required for the cytotoxic effect are about 3 times lower for amiodarone than for potassium iodide (21).

Monitoring of thyroid function

Whereas amiodarone-induced hypothyroidism (AIH) is most prevalent in iodine-sufficient regions, AIT is more prevalent in iodine-deficient areas. Among patients with amiodarone-induced thyroid dysfunction residing in the Americas (by now a largely iodine-replete continent), 66% have AIH and 34% AIT; in Europe (with still many iodine-deficient regions) 25% have AIH and 75% AIT (23). The incidence rate/100 person-years in France is 4.61 for AIH and 1.62 for AIT (24). The high incidence and the potential danger of worsening of heart disease upon occurrence of AIH or AIT (25) call for thyroid monitoring. Baseline assessment by TSH and TPO antibodies is recommended, and follow-up assessment every 6 months by TSH only (26, 27). A normal serum TSH during follow-up, however, does not guarantee that AIT will not develop in the interval to the next visit in view of the often sudden onset of

Table 3.3.12.1 Characteristics of amiodarone-induced thyrotoxicosis types 1 and 2

	Type 1	Type 2
Underlying thyroid abnormality	Yes	No
Pathogenesis	Iodide-induced thyrotoxicosis	Destructive thyrotoxicosis
Physical examination	Usually nodular or diffuse goitre	Occasionally small diffuse firm goitre
Thyroid antibodies	Can be present	Mostly absent
Thyroid ultrasound	Diffuse or nodular goitre	Heterogeneous pattern
Doppler sonography	Normal or increased flow	Decreased flow
Thyroidal radio-iodine uptake	Low or normal	Low or absent
^{99m}Tc-sestamibi scan	Clear thyroid retention	No thyroid uptake
Spontaneous remission	Unlikely	Likely
Preferred drug treatment	$KClO_4$ + methimazole	Glucocorticoids
Subsequent hypothyroidism	Unlikely	Possible

AIT (28). Furthermore, the finding of a suppressed TSH during follow-up does not necessarily mean AIT that has to be treated, because in one-half of these cases TSH returns spontaneously to normal values (28). AIT can develop up to 12 months after discontinuation of treatment, related to the very long terminal half-life of the drug.

Diagnosis

AIT can be asymptomatic. Recurrence of cardiac arrhythmias, which previously had been controlled, may suggest the diagnosis. Symptoms at diagnosis are unexplained weight loss (50%), heavy sweating (42%), palpitations (37%), hyperkinesia (29%), muscle weakness (27%), heat intolerance (24%), overall weakness (12%), and diarrhoea (12%) (29). The biochemical diagnosis of AIT is based on a suppressed TSH in combination with an elevated free T_4. T_3 can be elevated or normal, and cases of T_4 toxicosis do occur. The free T_4 to free T_3 ratio in AIT (as in IIT and subacute thyroiditis) is much higher than in Graves' hyperthyroidism.

Distinction between AIT subtypes is considered to be useful because management of types 1 and 2 is different (Table 3.3.12.1). However, none of the proposed methods accurately discriminates between both subtypes. Serum interleukin-6 was originally advocated as a good discriminator (being much higher in type 2 than in type 1), but subsequent studies have been unable to confirm its value. Thyroidal radio-iodine uptake is low or absent in type 2, but can also be low in type 1, and in one study did not differ at all between both types (30).Colour flow Doppler sonography can be useful, revealing a patchy pattern of thyroid vascularity to a markedly increased blood flow in type 1 and an absent blood flow in type 2 (27, 31). The latest tool has been the ^{99m}Tc-sestamibi scan, showing mostly increased MIBI retention in type 1 and no uptake in type 2 (32).

Treatment

The available treatment options are listed below.

- Wait-and-see policy. After discontinuation of amiodarone, most patients with AIT type 1 are still thyrotoxic after 6–9 months, whereas many patients with AIT type 2 will be cured in 3–5 months (27).
- Antithyroid drugs. As in IIT and in subacute thyroiditis, the efficacy of antithyroid drugs is decreased in AIT.
- Prednisone. There are no good data for AIT type 1. In AIT type 2, prednisone (starting dose 30 mg for 2 weeks, gradually tapered and withdrawn after 3 months) restored euthyroidism more rapidly than iopanoic acid (after 43 ± 34 days and 221 ± 111 days, respectively) (33). In another Italian study, the median time to normalize free T_4 upon prednisone treatment was 30 days (95% CI 23 to 37) and to normalize TSH 90 days (95% CI 77 to 103) (34). An American study did not observe a difference in the time to normalize free T_4 and TSH between patients treated with or without prednisone, but baseline free T_4 was higher in the prednisone group (29).
- Potassium perchlorate. $KClO_4$ by acutely inhibiting thyroidal iodide uptake reduces intrathyroidal iodine content, thereby rendering the thyroid gland more sensitive to thionamides. The combination of $KClO_4$ with thionamides has become the preferred treatment of AIT type 1. Its usefulness in AIT type 2 has been less appreciated, although $KClO_4$ inhibits the *in vitro* cytotoxic effect of amiodarone on thyrocytes albeit to a lesser extent than steroids (22). No serious side effects of $KClO_4$ (e.g. agranulocytosis) have been reported so far in AIT, provided the daily dose is limited to 1000 mg (twice daily 500 mg) and restricted to 4–6 months.
- *Lithium.* Propylthiouracil (PTU) + lithium normalized thyroid function faster than PTU alone, but the number of patients (mainly AIT type 2) in this open study was very low (35).
- *Thyroidectomy.* In patients resistant to medical therapy, total thyroidectomy is an option with, despite compromised cardiac function, rather low mortality and morbidity (36, 37).
- *Radioactive iodine.* Recent studies indicate ^{131}I therapy is feasible in AIT types 1 and 2, despite the low radioactive iodine uptake, by applying either high doses of ^{131}I or recombinant human TSH (38, 39).

To select the most appropriate treatment option in a particular patient, try to answer the following questions (27).

1. Is it necessary to stop amiodarone? It seems logical to discontinue amiodarone, and this is generally recommended. However, many cardiologists will favour continuation of amiodarone treatment. In recent questionnaire studies, continuation of amiodarone was thought feasible by 11% of respondents in type 1 and by 20% in type 2 (23). In the absence of controlled trials, our own preference is to stop amiodarone in AIT type 1 (in view of its protracted course) but to continue amiodarone in AIT type 2 (in view of its mostly self-limiting course) (Fig. 3.3.12.1).
2. Is it necessary to treat AIT? The severity of AIT ranges from very mild to very severe, and fatal outcomes do happen. Patients with mild AIT and stable cardiovascular condition may not need treatment, especially type 2 cases in view of its self-limiting nature. In this context one should be reminded that slightly increased free T_4 levels up to 25 pmol/l are not unusual during amiodarone treatment, occurring in the presence of a normal TSH. Smaller thyroid volumes and modest increases of free T_4 are predictors of a fast response to steroids in AIT type 2 (34), and may help in choosing an expectant or active policy.
3. What is the preferred treatment algorithm? There are no controlled trials to support any of the published treatment algorithms. In Turkey it is proposed to stop amiodarone and start with $KClO_4$ + methimazole; if after 1 month free T_4 has not normalized or decreased by more than 50%, prednisone is added (30). In contrast, in the UK it is proposed to continue amiodarone and to start with prednisone + carbimazole; if after 2 weeks T3 levels have not decreased, $KClO_4$ is considered (40). The differences between both algorithms may have to do with differences in ambient iodine intake between both countries. We think it is worthwhile to try to distinguish between AIT type 1 and 2 in order to select a treatment modality that is appropriate from a pathophysiological point of view. An accurate distinction may not always be possible, and mixed forms of AIT do occur (23, 41). Still, a stepwise approach seems preferable as the alternative (treat all AIT patients with $KClO_4$, methimazole, and prednisone) exposes all patients to possible side effects of three drugs, whereas most patients can be cured with less than three different drugs. The proposed Amsterdam algorithm (Fig. 3.3.12.1) does not specify the time interval between decision points, which depend on AIT severity and cardiovascular stability. One may

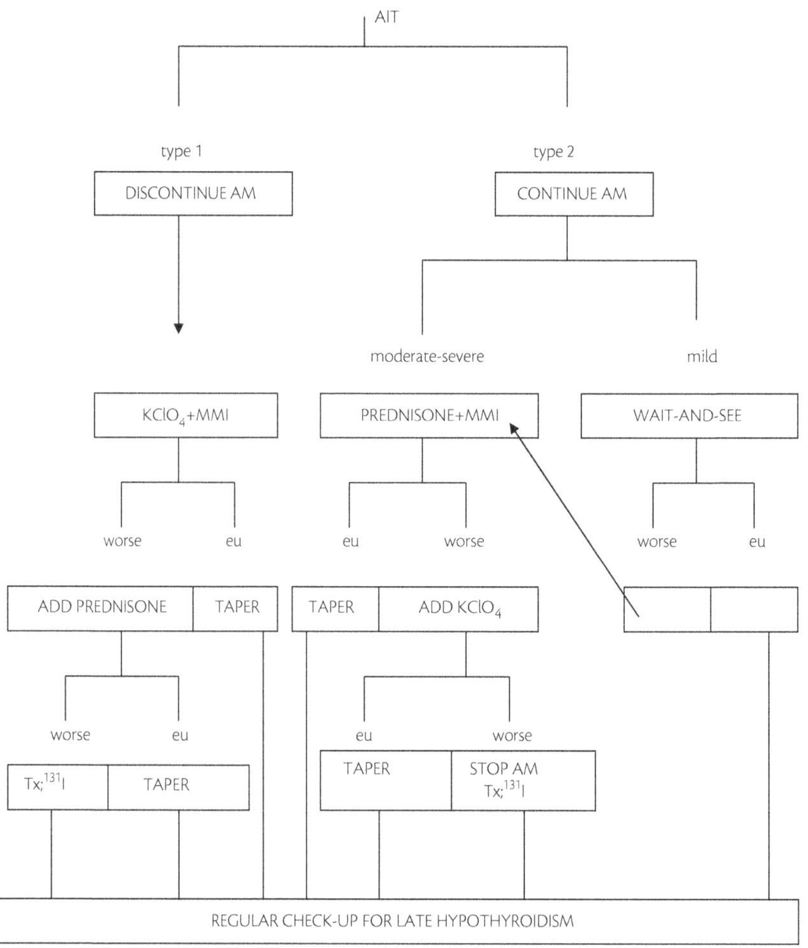

Fig. 3.3.12.1 Amsterdam algorithm for the management of amiodarone-induced thyrotoxicosis (AIT). AM, amiodarone; eu, euthyroid; ^{131}I, high therapeutic dose ± recombinant human TSH; $KClO_4$, twice daily 500 mg potassium or sodium perchlorate; MMI, once daily 30 mg methimazole; PREDNISONE, once daily 30 mg; Tx, total thyroidectomy. (Reproduced with permission from Eskes SA, Wiersinga WM. Amiodarone and thyroid. *Best Pract Res Clin Endocrinol Metab*, 2009; **23**: 735–51.)

monitor thyroid function every 2 weeks in the first month, and every 4 weeks thereafter.

4 What to do when euthyroidism has been restored? After discontinuation of amiodarone and restoration of the euthyroid state, 22–38% of questionnaire respondents would ablate the thyroid in case of type 1, but only 8–16% would do so in case of type 2 (23, 27). Periodic assessment of thyroid function is indicated: in AIT type 2, 17% developed permanent hypothyroidism occurring 10 months (range 6–24 months) after reaching euthyroidism (42). In case amiodarone needs to be restarted, prophylactic ^{131}I or thyroidectomy is recommended by most physicians for type 1 but not for type 2 (23). Few data are available to support this policy. When AIT type 2 has been cured under continuation of amiodarone, there is a risk of recurrent AIT. The risk seems to be low: recurrences were observed in 3 out of 50 patients at 5, 6, and 8 years after the first episode, and were less severe than the initial event (43).

Prognosis

Although AIT treatment is often difficult, euthyroidism can be restored in most patients. However, fatalities do happen. Mortality is associated with higher age and a low ejection fraction (not with sex, free T_4, or cumulative dose of amiodarone) (29, 44). AIT itself contributes to adverse outcomes. In a study among 354 patients treated with amiodarone for 48 months, patients who developed AIT had more major adverse cardiovascular events (mostly ventricular arrhythmias) than patients remaining euthyroid (31.6% vs 10.7%); AIT and an ejection fraction less than 45% were independent predictors of these adverse events (25). Patients who developed AIH had a higher rate of myocardial infarction (4.1% vs 0.4%). All-cause mortality was no different between groups.

Thyrotoxicosis of extrathyroidal origin

Factitious thyrotoxicosis is due to ingestion of excess thyroid hormone (45). The hormone can be ingested unintentionally in diet pills and in ground beef contaminated with bovine thyroid tissue, or intentionally by people (mostly women) with psychiatric disturbances and by children as an accident (46). Characteristic features are thyrotoxicosis associated with a low thyroidal radioiodine uptake, normal urinary iodine excretion, no goitre, and no thyroid antibodies. Strong evidence for the existence of factitious thyrotoxicosis is the finding of a low serum thyroglobulin.

The disease will resolve spontaneously after the ingestion of excess thyroid hormone is stopped, but patients with underlying psychiatric disease may continue the use of thyroid hormone.

Thyrotoxicosis due to the ingestion of a well-cooked 227-g hamburger prepared from contaminated ground beef disappears within 1 month (47). Symptomatic treatment with propranolol may be necessary. Acute thyroxine intoxication may benefit from gastric lavage; plasmapheresis has been recommended only in life-threatening situations (45). Discrepancy is often noted between modest clinical toxicity and very high thyroid hormone concentrations in serum.

Struma ovarii is an ovarian tumour with thyroid tissue as an important constituent. It is mostly unilateral, and occurs in less than 1% of all ovarian tumours. The highest incidence is in the fourth to sixth decade. Thyrotoxicosis develops in 5–15%, especially in tumours more than 30 mm in size. Radio-iodine uptake is low in the neck and high in the abdomen at the side of the lesion in classic cases, but the presence of a goitre (with some uptake) is not uncommon (48, 49). Treatment is by surgical removal of the tumour.

Metastases of differentiated thyroid cancer are a rare cause of thyrotoxicosis due to a large bulk of tumour. Treatment is primarily by radio-iodine. Percutaneous interstitial laser photocoagulation may enhance the safety and efficacy of ^{131}I treatment (50).

References

1. Yoshida K, Sakurada T, Kaise N, Kaise K, Kitaoka H, Fukazawa H, *et al.* Serum free thyroxine and triiodothyronine concentrations in subacute thyroiditis. *J Clin Endocrinol Metab*, 1982; **55**: 185–8.
2. Hoekman K, von Blomberg-van der Flier BME, Wagstaff J, Drexhage HA, Pinedo HM. Reversible thyroid dysfunction during treatment with GM-CSF. *Lancet*, 1991; **338**: 541–2.
3. Mandac JC, Chaudhry S, Sherman KE, Tomer Y. The clinical and physiological spectrum of interferon-alpha induced thyroiditis. *Hepatology*, 2006; **43**: 661–72.
4. Prummel MF, Laurberg P. Interferon-alpha and autoimmune thyroid disease. *Thyroid*, 2003; **13**: 547–51.
5. Dalgard O, Bjøro K, Hellum K, Myrvang B, Bjøro T, Haug E, *et al.* Thyroid dysfunction during treatment of chronic hepatitis C with interferon-alpha: no association with either interferon dosage or efficacy of therapy. *J Intern Med*, 2002; **251**: 400–6.
6. Wong V, Fu AX, George J, Cheung NW. Thyrotoxicosis induced by alpha-interferon therapy in chronic viral hepatitis. *Clin Endocrinol*, 2002; **56**: 793–8.
7. Walfish PG, Caplan D, Rosen IB. Postparathyroidectomy transient thyrotoxicosis. *J Clin Endocrinol Metab*, 1992; **75**: 224–7.
8. Skowsky WR. Toxic hematoma: an unusual and previously undescribed type of thyrotoxicosis. *Thyroid*, 1995; **5**: 129–32.
9. Shimaoka K, Van Herle AJ, Dindogru A. Thyrotoxicosis secondary to involvement of the thyroid with malignant lymphoma. *J Clin Endocrinol Metab*, 1976; **43**: 64–8.
10. Eriksson M, Ajmani S, Mallette LE. Hyperthyroidism from thyroid metastasis of pancreatic adenocarcinoma. *JAMA*, 1977; **238**: 1276–8.
11. Stanbury JB, Ermans AE, Bourdoux P, Todd C, Oken E, Tonglet R, *et al.* Iodine-induced hyperthyroidism: occurrence and epidemiology. *Thyroid*, 1998; **8**: 83–100.
12. Martin FJR, Tress BW, Colman PG, Dean DR. Iodine-induced hyperthyroidism due to nonionic contrast radiography in the elderly. *Am J Med*, 1993; **95**: 78–82.
13. Fradkin JE, Wolff J. Iodide-induced thyrotoxicosis. *Medicine*, 1983; **62**: 1–20.
14. Leger AF, Massin JP, Laurent MF, Vincens M, Auriol M, Helal OB, *et al.* Iodine-induced thyrotoxicosis: analysis of eighty-five consecutive cases. *Eur J Clin Invest*, 1984; **14**: 449–55.
15. Wiersinga WM. The effect of iodine-containing contrast media on the thyroid. *Eur J Hosp Pharm Pract*, 2005; **11**: 50–2.
16. Hintze G, Blombach O, Fink H, Burkhardt U, Köbberling J. Risk of iodine-induced thyrotoxicosis after coronary angiography: an investigation in 788 unselected subjects. *Eur J Endocrinol*, 1999; **140**: 264–7.
17. Nolte W, Müller R, Siggelkow H, Emrich D, Hüfner M. Prophylactic application of thyrostatic drugs during excessive iodine exposure in euthyroid patients with thyroid autonomy: a randomized study. *Eur J Endocrinol*, 1996; **134**: 337–41.
18. Fricke E, Fricke H, Esdorn E, Kammeier A, Lindner O, Kleesiek K, *et al.* Scintigraphy for risk stratification of iodine-induced thyrotoxicosis in patients receiving contrast agent for coronary angiography: a prospective study of patients with low thyrotropin. *J Clin Endocrinol Metab*, 2004; **89**: 6092–6.
19. van der Molen AJ, Thomsen HS, Morcos SK. Effect of iodinated contrast media on thyroid function in adults. *Eur Radiol*, 2004; **14**: 902–7.
20. Rao RH, McReady VR, Spathis GS. Iodine kinetic studies during amiodarone treatment. *J Endocrinol Metab*, 1986; **62**: 563–7.
21. Chiovato L, Martino E, Tonacchera M, Santini F, Lapi P, Mammoli C, *et al.* Studies on the in vitro cytotoxic effect of amiodarone. *Endocrinology*, 1994; **134**: 2277–82.
22. Brennan MD, Erickson DR, Carney JA, Bahn RS. Nongoitrous (type I) amiodarone-associated thyrotoxicosis: evidence of follicular disruption in vitro and in vivo. *Thyroid*, 1995; **5**: 177–83.
23. Tanda ML, Piantanida E, Lai A, Liparulo L, Sassi L, Bogazzi F, *et al.* Diagnosis and management of amiodarone-induced thyrotoxicosis: similarities and differences between North American and European thyroidologists. *Clin Endocrinol*, 2008; **69**: 612–18.
24. Bongard V, Marc D, Philippe V, Jean-Louis M, Maryse LM. Incidence rate of adverse drug reactions during long-term follow-up of patients newly treated with amiodarone. *Am J Ther*, 2006; **13**: 315–19.
25. Yiu KH, Jim MH, Siu C-W, Lee CH, Yuen M, Mok M, *et al.* Amiodarone-induced thyrotoxicosis is a predictor of adverse cardiovascular outcome. *J Clin Endocrinol Metab*, 2009; **94**: 109–14.
26. Basaria S, Cooper DS. Amiodarone and the thyroid. *Am J Med*, 2005; **118**: 706–14.
27. Eskes SA, Wiersinga WM. Amiodarone and thyroid. *Best Pract Res Clin Endocrinol Metab*, 2009; **23**: 735–51.
28. Trip MD, Wiersinga WM, Plomp TA. Incidence, predictability, and pathogenesis of amiodarone-induced thyrotoxicosis and hypothyroidism. *Am J Med*, 1991; **91**: 507–11.
29. Conen D, Melly L, Kaufmann C, Bilz S, Ammann P, Schaer B, *et al.* Amiodarone-induced thyrotoxicosis: clinical course and predictors of outcome. *J Am Coll Cardiol*, 2007; **49**: 2350–5.
30. Erdogan MF, Gulec S, Tutar E, Baskal N, Erdogan C. A stepwise approach to the treatment of amiodarone-induced thyrotoxicosis. *Thyroid*, 2003; **13**: 205–9.
31. Bogazzi F, Bartalena L, Brogioni S, Mazzeo S, Vitti P, Burelli A, *et al.* Color flow Doppler sonography rapidly differentiates type I and type II amiodarone-induced thyrotoxicosis. *Thyroid*, 1997; **7**: 541–5.
32. Piga M, Cocco MC, Serra A, Boi F, Loy M, Mariotti S. The usefulness of 99mTc-sestaMIBI thyroid scan in the differential diagnosis and management of amiodarone-induced thyrotoxicosis. *Eur J Endocrinol*, 2008; **159**: 423–9.
33. Bogazzi F, Bartalena L, Cosci C, Brogioni S, Dell'Unto E, Grasso L, *et al.* Treatment of type II amiodarone-induced thyrotoxicosis by either iopanoic acid or glucocorticoids: a prospective, randomized study. *J Clin Endocrinol Metab*, 2003; **88**: 1999–2002.
34. Bogazzi F, Bartalena L, Tomisti L, Rossi G, Tanda ML, Dell'Unto E, *et al.* Glucocorticoid response in amiodarone-induced thyrotoxicosis resulting from destructive thyroiditis is predicted by thyroid volume and serum free thyroid hormone concentrations. *J Clin Endocrinol Metabol*, 2007; **92**: 556–62.

35. Dickstein G, Shechner C, Adawi F, Kaplan J, Baron E, Ish-Shalom S. Lithium treatment in amiodarone-induced thyrotoxicosis. *Am J Med*, 1997; **102**: 454–8.
36. Houghton SG, Farley DR, Brennan MD, van Heerden JA, Thompson GB, Grant CS. Surgical management of amiodarone-induced thyrotoxicosis: Mayo Clinic experience. *World J Surg*, 2004; **24**: 1083–7.
37. Gough J, Gough IR. Total thyroidectomy for amiodarone-associated thyrotoxicosis in patients with severe cardiac disease. *World J Surg*, 2006; **30**: 1957–61.
38. Albino CC, Paz-Filho G, Graf H. Recombinant human TSH as an adjuvant to radioiodine for the treatment of type 1 amiodarone-induced thyrotoxicosis (AIT). *Clin Endocrinol*, 2009; **70**: 810–11.
39. Gursoy A, Tutuncu NB, Gencoglu A, Anil C, Demirer AN, Demirag NG. Radioactive iodine in the treatment of type 2 amiodarone-induced thyrotoxicosis. *J Natl Med Assoc*, 2008; **100**: 706–19.
40. Han TS, Williams GR, Vanderpump MPJ. Benzofuran derivatives and the thyroid. *Clin Endocrinol*, 2009; **70**: 2–13.
41. Franklyn JA, Gammage MD. Treatment of amiodarone-associated thyrotoxicosis. *Nat Clin Pract Endocrinol Metab*, 2007; **3**: 662–6.
42. Bogazzi F, Dell'Unto E, Tanda MI, Tomisti L, Cosci C, Aghini-Lombardi F, *et al.* Long-term outcome of thyroid function after amiodarone-induced thyrotoxicosis, as compared to subacute thyroiditis. *J Endocrinol Invest*, 2006; **29**: 694–9.
43. Uzan L, Guignat L, Meune C, Mouly S, Weber S, Bertagna X, *et al.* Continuation of amiodarone therapy despite type II amiodarone-induced thyrotoxicosis. *Drug Saf*, 2006; **29**: 231–6.
44. O'Sullivan AJ, Lewis M, Diamond T. Amiodarone-induced thyrotoxicosis: left ventricular dysfunction is associated with increased mortality. *Eur J Endocrinol*, 2006; **154**: 533–6.
45. Cohen JH, Ingbar SH, Braverman LE. Thyrotoxicosis due to ingestion of excess thyroid hormone. *Endocr Rev*, 1989; **10**: 113–24.
46. Kaiserman I, Avni M, Sack J. Kinetics of the pituitary–thyroid axis and the peripheral thyroid hormones in 2 children with thyroxine intoxication. *Horm Res*, 1995; **44**: 229–3.
47. Hedberg CW, Fishbein DB, Janssen RS, Meyers B, McMillen JM, MacDonald KL, *et al.* An outbreak of thyrotoxicosis caused by the consumption of bovine thyroid gland in ground beef. *N Engl J Med*, 1987; **316**: 993–8.
48. Bayot MR, Chopra IJ. Coexistence of struma ovarii and Graves' disease. *Thyroid*, 1995; **5**: 469–71.
49. Rotman-Pikielny P, Reynolds JC, Barker WC, Yen PM, Skarulis MC, Sarlis NJ. Recombinant human thyrotropin for the diagnosis and treatment of a highly functional metastatic struma ovarii. *J Clin Endocrinol Metab*, 2000; **85**: 237–44.
50. Guglielmi R, Pacella CM, Dottorini ME, Bizzarri GC, Todino V, Crescenzi A, *et al.* Severe thyrotoxicosis due to hyperfunctioning liver metastasis from follicular carcinoma: treatment with ^{131}I and interstitial laser ablation. *Thyroid*, 1999; **9**: 173–7.

3.4

Hypothyroidism and pregnancy- and growth-related thyroid disorders

Contents

3.4.1 Clinical assessment and systemic manifestations of hypothyroidism

Massimo Tonacchera, Luca Chiovato, Aldo Pinchera

Introduction

Hypothyroidism may affect people of both sexes and all ages. The clinical expression of thyroid hormone deficiency varies considerably between individuals. It is influenced mainly by the age of the patient and the rate at which hypothyroidism develops although being largely independent of its cause. Most adult patients complain of a slowing of physical and mental activity.

Hypothyroidism is a graded phenomenon, ranging from very mild cases, in which biochemical abnormalities (subclinical hypothyroidism; see Chapter 3.4.4) are present but the individual hardly notices symptoms and signs of thyroid hormone deficiency, to very severe cases in which the danger exists of sliding down into a life-threatening myxoedema coma.

Organ system manifestations of hypothyroidism

Cutaneous manifestations and changes in the connective tissues

The cutaneous changes observed in hypothyroidism belong to the most classic and frequent findings of the disease (Table 3.4.1.1) (1). Although other important symptoms and signs of hypothyroidism may be present, changes in the skin may be the most important factor for seeking medical attention (1). In over 80% of patients

Table 3.4.1.1 Cutaneous signs and symptoms of hypothyroidism

Cutaneous manifestation	Frequency (%)
Cold intolerance	50–95
Nail abnormality	90
Thickening and dryness of hair and skin	80–90
Oedema of hands, face, and eyelids	70–85
Change in shape of face	70
Malar flush	50
Nonpitting oedema	30
Alopecia	30–40
Pallor	25–60
Decreased sweat secretion	10–70

with primary hypothyroidism, the epidermis is dry, rough, cool, and covered with fine superficial scales. This is an expression of decreased cutaneous metabolism, reduced secretion of sweat and sebaceous glands, vasoconstriction, thinning of the epidermis, and hyperkeratosis of the stratum corneum. The skin may have a finely wrinkled, parchment-like character. Unusual coldness of the arms and legs is sometimes a subject of complaint. The palms are cool and dry. Subcutaneous fat may be increased, with the formation of definite fat pads, especially above the clavicles, but is conspicuously absent in the more advanced form of the disease (myxoedematous cachexia). The hands and feet have a broad appearance, due to thickening of subcutaneous tissue.

The diffuse pallor and pale waxy surface colour can be attributed to two mechanisms. First vasoconstriction occurs and second the excess fluid and mucopolysaccharides in the dermis may compress small vessels to create blanching as well as interference with the transmission of colour from the deeper vessels. Anaemia may also contribute to pallor. Yellowish discolouration of the skin, most notably of the palms, soles, and nasolabial folds, occurs in patients with long-standing hypothyroidism and is caused by elevation of serum and tissue carotene concentrations. The face is puffy, pale, and expressionless at rest (Fig. 3.4.1.1). The skin of the face is also parchment-like. In spite of the swelling, it may be traced with fine wrinkles, particularly

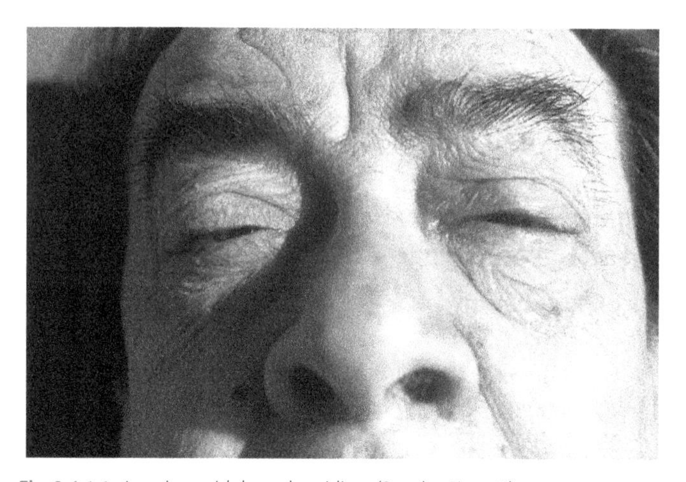

Fig. 3.4.1.1 A patient with hypothyroidism. (See also Plate 18)

in pituitary myxoedema. The swelling sometimes gives it a round or moonlike appearance. The palpebral fissure maybe narrowed because of blepharoptosis, due to diminished tone of the sympathetic nervous fibres to Müller's elevator palpebral superior muscle. The modest measurable exophthalmos seen in some patients with myxoedema is presumably related to accumulation of the same mucous oedema in the orbit as is seen elsewhere.

The tongue is usually large, and some patients will complain of this problem. The tongue is smooth if pernicious anaemia coexists. The voice is husky, low-pitched, and coarse due to the enlargement of the tongue and thickening of the pharyngeal and laryngeal mucous membranes. The speech is deliberate and slow, and there may be difficulty in articulation.

There are other, less common, cutaneous findings seen in adult hypothyroid patients. Six patients have been reported in literature of an acquired palmoplantar keratoderma, verrucous in character, and predominantly affecting the plantar surface (2). An additional reported cutaneous finding specifically linked to atrophic thyroiditis is dermatitis herpetiformis, a gluten-sensitive skin disease characterized by blisters on the elbows, buttock, and knees (3).

Hair follicles and nails

The hair is dry, dull, and coarse, growing slowly, becoming sparse, and falling out readily. Loss of scalp, genital, and beard hair may also occur. Hair may be lost from the temporal aspects of the eyebrows (Queen Anne's sign). However, this sign is not uncommon in elderly euthyroid women and occurs in association with several types of cutaneous disease, including atopic dermatitis, seborrhoeic dermatitis, and lupus erythematosus. In men, the beard becomes sparse and its rate of growth becomes greatly retarded. The scalp is dry and scaly. The nails, through retardation of growth, become thickened and brittle, striated both in transverse and longitudinal grooves, and show frequent deformities.

Dermal changes

The dermal pathological findings in patients with hypothyroidism are clinically manifested by the nonpitting swelling, most marked around the eyes and hands, that is myxoedema. This is due to an abnormal accumulation of salts, mucopolysaccharides, and protein in the interstitial spaces of the skin (4). Histopathological examination of the skin reveals that the connective tissue fibres are separated by an increased amount of metachromatically staining, periodic acid-Schiff-positive mucinous material (1). This material consists of protein complexed with two mucopolysaccharides, hyaluronic acid and chondroitin sulfate B (1). An increase in the synthesis and accumulation of glycosaminoglycans leads to an excess of these normal intercellular substances.

The glycosaminoglycans are polymers of D-glucuronic acid and *N*-acetyl-D-glucosamine, forming hyaluronic acid, or of L-hyaluronic acid and *N*-acetyl-D-galactosamine sulfate, forming chondroitin sulfate B. They exist free and in ionic or covalent linkage to proteins. These mucoproteins comprise part of the normal nonfibrillar intercellular matrix, the ground substance holding cells together. Due to its strong water binding capacity, accumulated hyaluronic acid may also contribute to the peculiar nonpitting quality of myxoedema. Capillary permeability is augmented in hypothyroidism with increased accumulation of sodium, water, and proteins.

Cardiovascular changes

Lack of thyroid hormones causes multiple alterations in the cardiovascular system (5). The most frequent changes in hypothyroid patients are increased systemic vascular resistance, diastolic dysfunction, reduced systolic function, and decreased cardiac preload (5). Bradycardia, cardiomegaly, and low voltage complexes on the ECG are well-known features (Box 3.4.1.1). The decrease in pulse rate approximately parallels the decrease in the body's metabolic rate. Myocardial contractility is reduced. The cardiac output at rest is decreased because of reduction in both stroke volume and heart rate, reflecting loss of the inotropic and chronotropic effects of thyroid hormones (5). The mechanism responsible for the impaired ventricular performance is multifactorial. In animal models, low thyroid hormone concentrations alter the expression of myocyte-specific genes and the distribution of the heavy-chain isoforms of sarcomeric myosin and of the calcium-regulating proteins (6). Alterations in myocyte calcium uptake and release are responsible for the change in the inotropic state (6). Peripheral vascular resistance at rest is increased, and blood volume is reduced. These haemodynamic alterations cause narrowing of pulse pressure, prolongation of circulation time, and decreased blood flow to the tissues. In most tissues the decrease in blood flow is proportional to the decrease in oxygen consumption, so the arteriovenous oxygen difference remains normal or may be slightly increased. Slow peripheral circulation, and therefore more complete extraction of oxygen, as well as anaemia, may be responsible for the increased arteriovenous oxygen difference. Myocardial oxygen consumption is decreased, usually more than blood supply to the myocardium, so that angina is infrequent (5). In some patients a reduction in cardiac output greater than the decline in oxygen consumption indicates specific cardiac damage from the myxoedema (5).

The haemodynamic alterations at rest resemble those of congestive heart failure, but cardiac output increases and peripheral vascular resistance decreases normally in response to exercise unless the hypothyroid state is severe (5). The nonpitting oedema observed in hypothyroid patients is due to an increase in protein distribution in the extravascular extracellular space resulting from increased capillary permeability.

Box 3.4.1.1 Cardiovascular signs and symptoms in hypothyroidism

- Symptoms
  - Dyspnoea
  - Decreased exercise tolerance
  - Angina
- Signs
  - Low pulse rate
  - Increased systemic vascular resistance
  - Diastolic hypertension
  - Cadiomegaly
  - Pericardial effusion
  - Peripheral non-pitting oedema
  - Low voltage ECG, non specific ST-T changes

Venous pressure is normal, but peripheral resistance is increased. The mechanism responsible for the increase in systemic vascular resistance is not known. Triiodothyronine (T_3) may act as a vasodilator and in its absence vascular resistance may rise (5, 7). Arterial blood pressure is often mildly increased. Hypertension is present in 10–20% of patients with hypothyroidism (5, 7). Diastolic hypertension is usually restored to normal after treatment (7). Three factors can contribute to systemic hypertension, increased peripheral resistance, increased arterial stiffness, and endothelial dysfunction (7–9).

Few symptoms referable to the cardiovascular system are referred in patients with hypothyroidism. Exertional dyspnoea and exercise intolerance are probably due to skeletal muscle dysfunction. There has been much discussion as to whether the hypercholesterolaemia that accompanies primary hypothyroidism accelerates the development of coronary atherosclerosis. An increased risk for atherosclerosis is supported by autopsy and epidemiological studies in patients with thyroid hormone deficiency and may be, in part, explained by the hypercholesterolaemia and marked increase in low-density lipoprotein (LDL) (8). Moreover diastolic hypertension, increased arterial stiffness and endothelial dysfunction, altered coagulability, and increased levels of C-reactive protein may further contribute to the increased cardiovascular risk (8, 9). Most autopsied myxoedematous individuals have severe atherosclerosis, but they are also usually 60 years of age or more. Occasionally angina pectoris is encountered in myxoedema (5). Sometimes angina or angina-like pain is present before treatment. This generally indicates the presence of significant coronary artery disease since there is inadequate myocardial oxygenation despite reduced cardiac output and oxygen utilization. Angina may also appear for the first time after treatment has been initiated, indicating that coronary flow is inadequate for resumption of normal cardiac function (7). The presence of a structural lesion must be strongly suspected.

On physical examination certain findings can suggest hypothyroidism. The heart rate is lowered, the pulse pressure is narrowed, and the carotid upstroke and left ventricular apical impulse are diminished (5). The heart sounds are diminished in intensity; this finding is due largely to effusion into the pericardial sac of fluid rich in protein and glycosaminoglycans.

The combination of a large heart, associated with typical haemodynamic and electrocardiographic alterations, and the serum enzyme changes (creatine kinase, aspartate aminotransferase, and lactate dehydrogenase may be increased) has been termed myxoedema heart. This term was introduced by Zondek in 1918 (10). It embraced dilatation of the left and right sides of the heart, a slow indolent heart action with normal blood pressure, and lowering of the P and T waves of the electrocardiogram. Zondek found that after treatment with thyroid hormone there was a return of the dilated heart to near normal size, a more rapid pulse without change in blood pressure, and gradual return of the P and T waves to normal. Microscopic examination discloses myxoedematous changes of the myocardial fibres. The myocardium is pale and flabby. Histopathological examination of the myocardium reveals interstitial oedema and swelling of the muscle fibres with loss of striations. The cause of the cardiac enlargement has been disputed. It is not due to hypertrophy alone, since it would not disappear so rapidly with treatment. One factor may be a decrease in contractility of the heart muscle; this would require a lengthening of muscle fibres in order to perform the required work.

In myxoedema, when the heart does not return to a normal size under thyroid hormone administration, hypertrophy due to some other disease is present as a complication. The slow and progressive return to normal size under treatment requires between 3 weeks and 10 months for completion. This decrease in size, like the progressive elevation of the T waves, is of diagnostic value.

Electrocardiographic changes

Electrocardiographic changes include sinus bradycardia, prolongation of the P–R interval, low amplitude of the P wave and QRS complex, alterations of the ST segment, and flattened or inverted T waves. Although suggestive of myocardial ischaemia, these waveform changes often disappear during thyroxine (T_4) treatment. Pericardial effusion is probably responsible for the low amplitude. Rarely, complete heart block may be present, but this disappears when the hypothyroidism is treated. In hypothyroidism, the atrial pacemaker function is normal and atrial ectopy is rare, but ventricular premature beats and occasionally ventricular tachycardia may occur. The syndrome of *torsades de pointes* with a long Q–T interval and ventricular tachycardia can occur with hypothyroidism, and resolve with T_4 treatment alone.

Systolic time intervals and echographic findings

Systolic time intervals are altered, the pre-ejection period is prolonged, and the ratio of pre-ejection period to left ventricular ejection time is increased. Some patients have been reported to have asymmetrical hypertrophy of the intraventricular septum by echocardiography that resolves with T_4 treatment (11), but a recent study failed to show septal hypertrophy in any hypothyroid patient studied. Pericardial effusion occurs in one-third to one-half of patients with overt hypothyroidism. The effusion is more common and their volume is greater in patients with long-standing severe disease. Cardiac tamponade is very rare. More sophisticated techniques have recently been used to assess systolic and diastolic function and myocardial texture, such as cardiac MRI, tissue Doppler imaging (12), and ultrasonic myocardial textural analysis (12).

Laboratory tests

The serum levels of creatine kinase, aspartate aminotransferase, and lactate dehydrogenase may be increased. Serum creatine kinase activity is high in as many as 30% of patients. Whereas the increase may reflect myocardial necrosis, in most patients the isoenzyme distribution indicates its origin from the skeletal rather than cardiac muscle. Prolongation of the half-life of creatine kinase in the circulation contributes to the elevated serum concentration.

Respiratory changes

Respiratory troubles are rarely a serious complaint in hypothyroid patients. However, hypothyroidism may cause respiratory problems through: (1) depression of the respiratory centre in the brain; (2) disturbed neural conduction and/or neuromuscular transmission to the respiratory muscles (due to hypothyroid neuropathy); (3) diseased respiratory muscle function (due to hypothyroid myopathy); and (4) changes in the alveolar-capillary membranes and the surfactant lining the alveoli, leading to impaired gas exchange. Fatigue and dyspnoea on exertion are frequent symptoms. Dyspnoea is a frequent complaint of myxoedematous patients, but is also a common symptom among well people. Congestive heart failure of separate origin, pleural effusion, anaemia, obesity, or pulmonary disease may be responsible.

Some information on pulmonary function in hypothyroidism is available (13). Wilson and Bedell (13) found a normal vital capacity and arterial $P\text{co}_2$ and $_\text{P}\text{o}_2$ in 16 hypothyroid patients. They also found a decreased maximal breathing capacity, decreased diffusion capacity, and decreased ventilatory response to carbon dioxide. Decreased ventilatory drive is present in about one-third of hypothyroid patients, and the response to hypoxia returns rapidly within a week after beginning therapy. Summarizing the few studies, there is little abnormality of resting pulmonary function in most nonobese patients with hypothyroidism (14). Some patients may exhibit a decreased vital capacity, probably due to muscular weakness. Overall oxygen transfer may be slightly decreased, as evidenced by a decreased $_\text{P}\text{o}_2$, possibly due to a decreased diffusing capacity for carbon monoxide. An increase in ventilation perfusion mismatching or an opening of anatomical shunts may also contribute to these modifications.

The severity of hypothyroidism parallels the incidence of impaired ventilatory drive (15, 16) Patients with myxoedema may develop carbon dioxide retention, and carbon dioxide narcosis may be a cause of myxoedema coma. Hypothyroidism-induced breathing disorders during sleep, particularly sleep apnoea syndromes, have been described (17). Obstructive sleep apnoea has been documented in hypothyroidism in about 7% of patients and is reversible with treatment (17). Hypothyroidism may predispose to upper airway obstruction by several mechanisms: increased size of the tongue and other pharyngeal skeletal muscles; a slow and sustained pharyngeal muscle contraction pattern; or diminished neural output of the respiratory centre. Myxoedematous patients are more subject to respiratory infections. Pleural effusions usually are evident only on radiological examination.

Gastrointestinal changes

The gastrointestinal manifestations of hypothyroidism are listed in Box 3.4.1.2. Poor appetite can be a leading symptom in hypothyroid patients. Anorexia can be interpreted as the reflection of a lowered food requirement. Although two-thirds of patients have reported weight gain, it is of modest degree and due largely to retention of fluid by hydrophilic glycoprotein deposits in the tissues. True obesity is not a feature of hypothyroidism. Younger patients with iatrogenic hypothyroidism secondary to treatment for thyrotoxicosis commonly gain weight because of decreased physical activity coupled with unchanged food intake.

Constipation is commonly present and is the result of a lowered food intake and decreased peristaltic activity. The latter may lead to faecal impaction and may mimic mechanical ileus when accompanied by colicky pains. Spontaneous hypothyroidism most often afflicts older people, who may discount the significance of an insidious decrease of bowel movements (18). Severe constipation that is unresponsive to treatment may, therefore, be a prominent finding at the time of diagnosis. Gastric emptying and intestinal transit time are prolonged (18). Gaseous distension may be a troublesome symptom; it responds slowly to thyroid treatment. In most patients

Box 3.4.1.2 Gastrointestinal manifestations of hypothyroidism

- Symptoms
  - Anorexia
  - Gaseous distension
  - Constipation
  - Prolonged gastric emptying
- Signs
  - Prolonged intestinal transit time
  - Aseites
  - Elevated liver enzymes
  - Gallbladder hypotonia

intestinal absorption is normal. Although the rates of absorption for many substances are decreased (18), the total amount absorbed may be normal or even increased because the decreased bowel motility may allow more time for absorption. Occasional malabsorption has been attributed to myxoedema of the intestinal mucosa or altered intestinal motility. Galactose and glucose tolerance curves show a delayed rise to a lower peak than normal and a delayed return to baseline.

Ascites in the absence of another cause is unusual in hypothyroidism, but it can occur in association with pleural and pericardial effusion (19). Myxoedema ascites consists of a yellow and gelatinous peritoneal exudate. It has been related to congestive heart failure, enhanced capillary permeability, or inappropriate secretion of antidiuretic hormone.

Atrophy of the gastric (20) and intestinal mucosa and myxoedematous infiltration of the bowel wall may be present at histological examination. Immune gastritis is often observed in hypothyroid patients (20) with autoimmune thyroiditis. As many as 50% of patients with autoimmune hypothyroidism have achlorhydria, 25% have circulating antibodies directed against the gastric parietal cells or intrinsic factor, and 10% have pernicious anaemia caused by impaired absorption of vitamin B_{12}.

A history of overt hypothyroidism has been associated with small intestinal bacterial overgrowth (SIBO), which is a clinical condition caused by an increased level of microorganisms exceeding the presence of more than 106 colony-forming units/ml within the small intestine. SIBO is considered a malabsorption syndrome (21).

Symptoms or signs of disturbed liver or exocrine pancreatic function are usually not encountered, but biochemical tests may suggest disease. The association of liver disease and hypothyroidism is suggestive of a multisystem autoimmune disease affecting both the liver (e.g. chronic active hepatitis or primary biliary cirrhosis) and the thyroid. Structural liver damage is unusual in hypothyroidism. Serum glutamic-oxaloacetic transaminase, lactate dehydrogenase, and creatine phosphokinase levels are elevated in patients with hypothyroidism (22). The enzymes return to normal over 2–4 weeks during treatment. Urinary amylase levels may be increased. Gallbladder motility is decreased, and the gallbladder may appear distended on radiographic examination.

Cerebral and neurological changes

Thyroid hormone is essential for the development of the central nervous system. Deficiency in fetal life or at birth causes hypoplasia of cortical neurons with poor development of cellular processes, retarded myelination, and reduced vascularity. Deficiency of thyroid hormone beginning in adult life causes less severe manifestations that usually respond to treatment with thyroid hormone. Recent studies using ^{32}P nuclear magnetic resonance spectroscopy of the frontal lobe of adult hypothyroid patients report reversible alterations in phosphate metabolism, suggesting impairment of mitochondrial metabolism (23). Cerebral blood flow is reduced in hypothyroidism, but cerebral oxygen consumption is usually normal (24). This finding is in accord with the observation that the oxygen consumption of isolated brain tissue *in vitro*, unlike that of most other tissues, is not stimulated by the administration of thyroid hormones. In severe cases, decreased cerebral blood flow may lead to cerebral hypoxia. These and other findings indicate that the adult human brain is a thyroid hormone responsive organ.

Box 3.4.1.3 lists the numerous symptoms suggesting either neurological or psychiatric disorders in patients with moderate to severe hypothyroidism. In adult and elderly patients, mental changes may go unrecognized because of their slow development and because they may mimic cerebral atherosclerosis. However, an unusual complacency, fatigue, and pronounced somnolence or even lethargy together with a prolonged reaction time should suggest the possibility of hypothyroidism. Special attention is required for patients who need an increasing amount of sleep (over 12–14 h/day). They may lapse into stupor or even coma, and develop convulsions. This may be the beginning of myxoedema coma, a rare but very serious condition, the extreme expression of severe hypothyroidism. All intellectual functions, including speech, are slowed. There is loss of initiative, and slow wittedness and memory defects are common; in a study (25) working memory was impaired in hypothyroidism. Dementia in elderly patients may be mistaken for senile dementia. Memory is undoubtedly impaired,

Box 3.4.1.3 Neurologic and psychiatric manifestations in hypothyrodism

- Neurologic symptoms or signs
  - Somnolence, lethargy
  - Slow speech
  - Impaired cognitive functions
  - Headache
  - Paraesthesias
  - Cerebellar ataxia
  - Deafness
  - Vertigo
  - Delayed relaxation of deep tendon reflexes
- Psychiatric syndromes
  - Depression
  - Bipolar disorders
  - Affective psychosis

and attention and the desire to think are reduced. The emotional level seems definitely low, and irritability is decreased. Except in the terminal stage, reasoning power is preserved. Cognitive tests of patients with moderate to severe hypothyroidism indicate difficulties in performing calculations, recent memory loss, reduced attention span, and slow reaction time (26). Headaches are frequent.

In a minority of patients, nervousness and apprehension are present. Psychiatric disorders are common and are usually of the paranoid or depressive type and may induce agitation (myxoedema madness). Depression is so often associated with hypothyroidism (26) that thyroid function tests should be performed in the evaluation of any patient presenting with this symptom (27). Central 5-hydroxytryptamine activity is reduced in hypothyroid patients, and T_3 supplementation might increase the efficacy of antidepressant drugs. At times, this manifestation of hypothyroidism is more severe than are many of the other clinical manifestations of the disease. Because hypothyroidism is so readily treated, it is an especially important cause to eliminate.

In rare cases of long-standing hypothyroidism cerebellar ataxia with or without intention tremor has been found. Jellinek and Kelly (28) described a series of myxoedematous patients with ataxia, intention tremor, nystagmus, and dysdiadochokinesia. Ataxia has been noted in 8% of a large series of hypothyroid patients (29). Patients may have intention tremor, nystagmus, and an inability to make rapid alternating movements. The cause of this syndrome is not apparent, but myxoedematous infiltrates of glycogen and mucinous material have been found in the cerebellum. There may be foci of degeneration and an increase in glial tissue. These symptoms show a prompt and definite decrease after replacement therapy with thyroid hormone.

Sensory phenomena are common. Numbness and tingling of the extremities are frequent. Mononeuropathies occur in hypothyroidism, as attested to by the high incidence of carpal tunnel syndrome (compression of the median nerve at the wrist) (30). Nocturnal paraesthesia and pain in the median nerve distribution in one or both hands is a common manifestation of this condition. Paraesthesia or lancing pain in the legs are manifestations of lower extremity peripheral neuropathy. A study of 39 patients with primary hypothyroidism found complaints of polyneuropathy in 64%, findings of polyneuropathy in 33%, and a definite diagnosis by electrophysiological criteria in 72% (30). A metachromatic infiltrate has been found in the lateral femoral cutaneous nerve and sural nerve, together with axon cylinder degeneration.

The tendon reflexes are slow, especially during the relaxation phase, producing the characteristic 'hung-up' reflexes: this phenomenon is due to a decrease in the rate of muscle contraction and relaxation, rather than a delay in nerve conduction. The presence of extensor plantar responses or diminished vibration sense should alert the physician to the possibility of coexisting pernicious anaemia with combined system disease.

Electroencephalographic changes include slow α-wave activity and general loss of amplitude. The concentration of protein in the cerebrospinal fluid is often increased, but cerebrospinal pressure is normal.

Deafness is a very characteristic and troublesome symptom of hypothyroidism. It may be due to both conduction or nerve impairment and usually responds very well to treatment. Vestibular abnormalities have also been demonstrated. Serous otitis media is not uncommon. Two-thirds of patients complain of dizziness, vertigo, or occasionally tinnitus: these problems suggest damage to the eighth nerve or labyrinth, or possibly to the cerebellum. Whatever type of deafness is present, there is marked improvement after thyroid treatment. Acquired hearing loss in association with adult-onset hypothyroidism should be distinguished from the sensorineural deafness of Pendred's syndrome. In the latter, treatment of hypothyroidism does not correct the hearing defect.

Night blindness is not uncommon. It is caused by a deficiency in the pigment retinene, which is required for the adaptation to dark.

Musculoskeletal changes

Muscles

In patients with hypothyroidism, disordered muscle function often is the predominating feature of the clinical syndrome. Generalized muscular hypertrophy, accompanied by easy fatigue and slowness of movements, occurs in some myxoedematous children or adults. It has been referred to as the Kocher–Debré–Sémélaigne syndrome in children (31) and as Hoffmann's syndrome in adults. These patients do not have the classic electromyography findings of myotonia. The myopathy of hypothyroidism in some patients is associated with weakness even though the muscles are hypertrophied. The typical patient presents with firm large well-developed muscles, like those of an athlete. The entire musculature is affected to some extent, but the most obvious enlargement is in the arms and legs.

Muscle symptoms such as myalgia, muscle weakness, stiffness, cramps, and easy fatigability are very prevalent in hypothyroid patients (32, 33). The symptoms are aggravated by exposure to cold. They are also prominent during the rapid onset of hypothyroidism after surgery or ^{131}I treatment. Impairment of mitochondrial oxidative metabolism provides a biochemical substrate for these complaints.

Reflex contraction and relaxation time is prolonged mainly because of the intrinsic alterations in muscle contractility. Nerve conduction time may also be prolonged. Delayed reflex relaxation is characteristic and has been developed into a diagnostic test of thyroid function. The rate-limiting step in muscle relaxation is the reuptake of calcium by the sarcoplasmic reticulum. In skeletal muscle, this process is dependent on the content of Ca^{2+}-ATPase. Recent studies have indicated that Ca^{2+}-ATPase activity of the fast twitch variety (SERCA1) is markedly reduced in hypothyroidism (34) with impairment of calcium reuptake as a consequence. This occurs at a transcriptional level, since thyroid hormone response elements have been identified in the 5′ flanking region of the SERCA1 Ca^{2+}-ATPase gene. The reduction in Ca^{2+}-ATPase would explain the delayed relaxation of the deep tendon reflexes. On histopathological examination the muscles appear pale and swollen. The muscle fibres may show swelling, loss of normal striation, and mucinous deposits.

Skeletal system: calcium and phosphorus metabolism

In the adult skeleton, thyroid hormone deficiency decreases recruitment, maturation, and activity of bone cells, leading to decreased remodelling, which is especially reflected in the impaired function of the osteoclasts (35). Despite this decrease in osteoclastic activity, trabecular bone volume and bone mineral density appear to be comparable to age-matched normals, presumably because of the corresponding decrease in osteoblastic activity (36). Urinary excretion of calcium is decreased as is the glomerular filtration rate, whereas faecal excretion of calcium and both urinary and faecal excretion of phosphorus are variable. The concentrations of calcium and phosphorus in serum are usually normal, but calcium may be slightly elevated. Serum alkaline phosphatase levels are often decreased, as are serum osteocalcin levels. Because the levels of parathyroid hormone are often slightly increased, some degree of resistance to its action may be present. Serum concentrations of 1,25-dihydroxycholecalciferol are also increased.

Joints

At the clinical level, patients with hypothyroidism often complain of articular and muscular pain and stiffness of the extremities. These symptoms may suggest rheumatoid arthritis or also polymyalgia rheumatica or primary myositis. Patients may exhibit joint effusions involving the knees and small joints of the hands and feet. In 5–10% of patients with carpal tunnel syndrome, primary hypothyroidism may be the cause due to the accumulation of the hygroscopic glycosaminoglycan in the interstitial space with compression of the median nerve.

Changes in kidney function

Clinically significant disturbances of kidney function, and hence of water and electrolyte metabolism, are uncommon in hypothyroidism. Renal blood flow and glomerular filtration rate can be reduced (37, 38). Because of the moderate extent of these reductions and the hypothyroidism-induced decreased metabolism, renal failure does not usually occur. Factors contributing to the decrease in renal blood flow are a decrease in cardiac output, a decrease in plasma volume, and a narrowing of renal blood vessels through enlargement of endothelial and mesangial cells and thickening of the glomerular basement membrane.

Laboratory examinations may reveal a slight increase of serum creatinine and uric acid (37). Urine flow is reduced, and delay in the excretion of a water load may result in reversal of the normal diurnal pattern of urine excretion. The delay in water excretion appears to be due to decreased volume delivery to the distal diluting segment of the nephron resulting from diminished renal perfusion and inappropriate secretion of vasopressin (37). Since urinary hydroxycorticoid excretion is decreased, the adrenals might be responsible for delayed water excretion. Other evidence suggests that the tissue supply of adrenal cortical hormones is usually normal in myxoedema. The ability to concentrate urine may be slightly impaired. Occasionally, minimal proteinuria is seen. This condition could be due to congestive heart failure or to the increased capillary transudation of protein typical of hypothyroidism.

The total body sodium content is increased (39). The excessive sodium is presumably bound to extracellular mucopolysaccharides. In spite of reduced renal blood flow and blood volume, the sodium retention is probably not a reflection of altered renal function. In fact, salt loads are usually excreted readily and serum sodium concentrations tend to be low (39), in contrast to other clinical situations associated with sodium retention, such as congestive heart failure. No consistent changes in plasma potassium levels have been reported. Total magnesium levels may be elevated and the bound fraction and urinary excretion are reduced. Plasma homocysteine concentrations are increased in hypothyroidism, related to lower folate levels and a lower creatinine clearance in thyroid hormone deficiency (40).

Haematological changes

Erythrocytes

Anaemia is present in up to two-thirds of hypothyroid children and adolescents, and in about one-third of adults with hypothyroidism (41). Anaemia is usually mild. In two reports on a large series of patients with hypothyroidism from various causes, the incidence of anaemia ranged from 32% to as high as 84% (41). Anaemia in hypothyroidism may be a normochromic and normocytic anaemia due to the diminished oxygen requirements and decreased production of erythropoietin (41) or may result from a specific depression of marrow that lacks thyroid hormone (41). The bone marrow generally shows mild hypoplasia with an increase in fatty marrow. The anaemia may be macrocytic, sometimes from deficiency of vitamin B_{12}. Folate deficiency from malabsorption or dietary inadequacy may also cause macrocytic anaemia. The frequent menorrhagia and the defective absorption of iron resulting from achlorhydria may contribute to a microcytic hypochromic anaemia.

Leucocytes and thrombocytes

Granulocyte, lymphocyte, and platelet counts are usually normal in hypothyroidism. Leucopenia might indicate associated vitamin B_{12} or folic acid deficiency. Mean platelet volume can be decreased. The ESR may be elevated in uncomplicated hypothyroidism.

Haemostasis

Hypothyroid patients may have bleeding symptoms such as easy bruising, menorrhagia, or prolonged bleeding after tooth extraction. The most frequent defects in haemostasis are prolonged bleeding time, decreased platelet adhesiveness, and low plasma concentrations of factor VIII and von Willebrand's factor (42). Desmopressin rapidly reduces these abnormalities, and may be useful for the acute treatment of bleeding or as cover for surgery. Fibrinolytic activity in hypothyroidism is increased. Usually the clinical relevance of these abnormalities is limited, as illustrated by no excess blood loss or bleeding complications during and after surgery in many hypothyroid patients.

Changes in the reproductive tract

In both sexes thyroid hormone influences sexual development and reproductive function. Infantile hypothyroidism leads to sexual immaturity and juvenile hypothyroidism causes a delay in the onset of puberty followed by anovulatory cycles. Paradoxically, primary hypothyroidism may also cause precocious sexual development and galactorrhoea (43).

In adult men, hypothyroidism may lead to impotence, lack of libido, and, rarely, to testicular tubular involution. The testicles are histologically immature if hypothyroidism preceded puberty and show tubular involution if its onset was after puberty (44). In adult hypothyroid men, semen analysis is usually normal. In a recent study (45), delayed ejaculation, hypoactive sexual desire, and erectile dysfunction have been described. In adult women, severe hypothyroidism may be associated with diminished libido and failure of ovulation (46, 47). In general, hypothyroid women complain of menorrhagia and, occasionally, oligo- and amenorrhoea.

Plasma gonadotropins are usually in the normal range in primary hypothyroidism and the pulsatile gonadotropin release in the follicular phase is normal (46), but the ovulatory surge may not happen. Secretion of progesterone is inadequate, and endometrial proliferation persists, resulting in excessive and irregular breakthrough menstrual bleeding. The anovulation is reflected in the frequent finding of a proliferative endometrium. These changes may be due to a deficient secretion of luteinizing hormone. Mild to moderate hyperprolactinaemia is a frequent finding in hypothyroid women, with or without galactorrhoea. It is attributed to the stimulatory effect of increased thyrotropin-releasing hormone on prolactin secretion. Fertility is reduced, and spontaneous abortion may result, although many pregnancies are successful.

The total concentrations of both testosterone and oestradiol in serum are decreased, predominantly due to a diminution in the concentration of the carrier sex hormone-binding globulin. Because of the concomitant increase in the unbound fraction of sex steroids, their absolute free concentration remains normal. The metabolism of testosterone is shifted towards aetiocholanolone rather than androsterone. With respect to oestradiol and oestrone, hypothyroidism favours metabolism of these steroids via 16α-hydroxylation with the result that formation of oestriol is increased.

The literature contains many reports of pregnancy in untreated hypothyroid women (47, 48). Euthyroid neonates born to hypothyroid mothers during pregnancy have been reported to achieve a lower IQ later in life (49). When treatment has been started during pregnancy, generally a normal child is produced (47), but abortion is frequent in women with myxoedema. Pregnancy-induced hypertension is 2–3 times more common in hypothyroid women. Low birthweight is secondary to premature delivery for gestational hypertension. The incidence of various congenital abnormalities may be increased, but recent studies do not report an increased risk of fetal death or congenital anomalies with proper treatment (47, 50).

Other endocrine glands

Pituitary function

Hypothyroidism can affect the secretion of all pituitary hormones. The effect of hypothyroidism on the secretion of vasopressin, follicle-stimulating hormone, and luteinizing hormone are discussed in other sections. Hypothyroidism decreases growth hormone secretion and hypothyroid children have a dramatic retardation of growth (51). Retarded growth caused by hypothyroidism appears to result from deficient secretion of growth hormone as well as from impaired action of growth hormone. Many hypothyroid children have subnormal serum growth hormone response to insulin-induced hypoglycaemia. Growth hormone secretion is decreased in hypothyroidism related to an increase in hypothalamic somatostatinergic tone (51), and results in low serum insulin-like growth factor (IGF)-1 concentrations (51). Serum IGF-2, IGFBP1, and IGFBP3 also fall, whereas IGFBP2 rises; these changes are reversible upon treatment (51).

Thyrotroph hyperplasia caused by primary hypothyroidism may result in sellar enlargement, particularly when the condition has remained untreated for a long time (52). Rarely, such hyperplasia may give rise to a pituitary macroadenoma that shrinks after thyroxine replacement (53). Patients with severe hypothyroidism may have an increase in serum prolactin level that correlates with the level of serum thyroid-stimulating hormone (TSH), and some patients develop galactorrhoea. Since thyroid hormone decreases the mRNA for preprothyrotropin-releasing hormone in the paraventricular nuclei, hypothyroidism may lead to increased thyrotropin-releasing hormone secretion, unopposed by thyroid hormones, with consequent hyperprolactinaemia.

Adrenal cortex

Patients with primary hypothyroidism have subtle abnormalities of pituitary–adrenal function that may be correlated with the severity and duration of hypothyroidism (54). Cortisol secretion and the rate of turnover are decreased in patients with hypothyroidism. The net result is that serum cortisol concentrations and urinary cortisol excretion are normal. Hepatic clearance of cortisol and adrenal androgens 17-hydroxycorticosteroids and 17-ketosteroids are decreased. This slowing is principally due to a decrease in the rate of cortisol oxidation as a result of reduced 11-hydroxysteroid dehydrogenase activity (54). Conjugation with glucuronic acid in the liver is normal. The turnover rate of aldosterone is also decreased in hypothyroidism (55). The decrease in hepatic clearance causes an increase in its plasma half-life. The reduced rate of clearance of aldosterone is balanced by a lower secretion rate. The serum concentration of aldosterone is normal and there is no clinical evidence of hyperaldosteronism. Angiotensinogen production in the liver is reduced, as is plasma renin activity. These subtle modifications are not responsible for alterations in sodium and potassium homeostasis.

The adrenal response to adrenocorticotropic hormone (ACTH) is normal or reduced. Pituitary–adrenal responses to the metyrapone test have been variable. Normal but delayed peak response, impaired response, or even lack of response has been reported. Grossly impaired responses to the stimulation with lysine-8-vasopressin and a delayed increase in serum cortisol levels after insulin-induced hypoglycaemia have also been observed. Whether steroid production can be augmented sufficiently in times of stress is not clear, but the provocative test results suggest that these patients usually have a mildly impaired hypothalamic–pituitary–adrenal axis.

Metabolic changes

Energy metabolism

The decrease in energy metabolism and heat production is reflected in the low basal metabolic rate, decreased appetite, cold intolerance, and slightly low basal body temperature. Measurement of the resting energy expenditure is rarely performed nowadays. In patients with complete athyreosis it falls to between 35% and 45% below normal. In Addison's disease, the basal metabolic rate may fall to 25% or 30% below normal, and in hypopituitarism to 50% below normal.

The effect of hypothyroidism on appetite and energy intake is not precisely known, but energy expenditure decreases leading to a slight net gain in energy stores. An increase in adipose tissue mass results in an increase of serum leptin, which mediates a decrease in energy intake while energy disposal increases, eventually leading to a reduction in adipose tissue mass. In hypothyroid patients an increase, no change, or a decrease in plasma leptin has been reported. Thyroid hormone apparently modulates serum leptin to a small extent (56).

Protein metabolism

Both the synthesis and the degradation of proteins are decreased, the latter especially so, with the result that nitrogen balance is usually slightly positive. Despite both a decrease in the rate of albumin synthesis and degradation, the total exchangeable albumin pool increases in myxoedema (57). The albumin is distributed in a much larger volume, suggesting enhanced permeability of capillary walls. The synthesis of thyroid hormone-responsive proteins is clearly reduced in the hypothyroid state, whereas that of proteins such as TSH or glycosaminoglycans may be increased under the same circumstances.

Comparative studies of protein translation by hepatic ribosomes from T_3-treated hypothyroid rats show that the mRNAs from some proteins are increased and others are decreased. Most of these proteins have not been identified. Treatment of myxoedema is accompanied by a marked but temporary negative nitrogen balance, reflecting the mobilization of extracellular protein (57). In a later phase there is an increase in urinary potassium and phosphorus together with nitrogen in amounts suggesting that cellular protein is also being metabolized.

Carbohydrate metabolism

In hypothyroidism, absorption of glucose from the gastrointestinal tract is slowed and peripheral glucose assimilation is retarded. At the same time, glycerol release from adipose tissue is slowed, and the availability of amino acids and glycerol for gluconeogenesis is decreased. The oral glucose tolerance curve is characteristically flat, and the insulin response to glucose is delayed. Degradation of insulin is slow, so the sensitivity to exogenous insulin may be increased. Despite the easily demonstrable abnormalities in carbohydrate metabolism in hypothyroidism, clinical manifestations of these abnormalities are seldom conspicuous. Although hypoglycaemia is sometimes listed as a manifestation of hypothyroidism, it is rarely a sign of isolated hormone deficiency, and the presence of hypoglycaemia in a patient with hypothyroidism should suggest the presence of hypopituitarism. The occurrence of hypothyroidism in a patient with insulin-dependent diabetes mellitus may result in a diminution in exogenous insulin requirement and a greater risk of developing hypoglycaemia.

Lipid metabolism

A variety of abnormalities in plasma lipid concentrations occur in hypothyroidism (Box 3.4.1.4). Plasma free fatty acid concentrations are normal, plasma concentrations of triglycerides, phospholipids, and LDL cholesterol are well elevated (58). Biosynthesis of fatty acids and lipolysis are reduced. The changes bear, in general, a reciprocal relationship to the level of thyroid activity.

The increased serum cholesterol may represent an alteration in the substrate steady-state level caused by a transient proportionally greater retardation in degradation than in synthesis (58). The increase of serum cholesterol is largely accounted for by an increase of LDL cholesterol, which is cleared less efficiently from the circulation due to a decreased T_3-dependent gene expressing the hepatic LDL receptor (58). Interestingly, the LDL particles of hypothyroid patients are also susceptible to increased oxidizability (58). The increase of high-density lipoprotein (HDL) 2 but not of HDL3 cholesterol is due to a diminished activity of cholesterol ester transfer protein (59) and hepatic lipase (which is involved in the conversion of HDL2 to HDL3). The modest increase of serum triglycerides seen in certain cases has been related to a decreased lipoprotein lipase activity in postheparin plasma. Lipoprotein(a) is increased in hypothyroidism in some but not all studies.

Box 3.4.1.4 Changes in serum lipids in hypothyroidism

- Total cholesterol-increase
- LDL-cholesterol-increase
- HDL2-cholesterol-modest increase
- HDL3-cholesterol-no change
- Triglycerides-no change or modest increase

Clinical aspects of hypothyroidism at different ages

Infantile and juvenile hypothyroidism

Hypothyroidism in newborn infants results in mental and physical impairment unless treatment is initiated within weeks after birth (see Chapter 3.4.7). Hypothyroidism in children is mainly characterized by retarded growth and impaired mental performances. Infantile hypothyroidism leads to sexual immaturity; juvenile hypothyroidism causes a delay in the onset of puberty followed by anovulatory cycles in girls. Rarely precocious puberty may occur (43).

Thyroid hormone is essential for normal growth and maturation of the skeleton (36). Deficient thyroid hormone production *in utero* and in the neonate retards growth and delays skeletal maturation. Deficiency in early life leads both to a delay in the development of and an abnormal stippled appearance of the epiphyseal centres of ossification (epiphyseal dysgenesis). Before puberty, thyroid hormones also play an important role in the maturation of bone. Impairment of linear growth leads to dwarfism in which the limbs are disproportionately short in relation to the trunk (36). Bone age is retarded in hypothyroid children (36).

Hypothyroidism in adults

In adults, the clinical manifestations of hypothyroidism, though they may be profound, are reversible (19). The development of spontaneous hypothyroidism is usually slow and many patients seek medical attention for variable and nonspecific symptoms (19). In contrast, patients who develop hypothyroidism rapidly (when replacement therapy is discontinued in a patient with primary hypothyroidism, or after surgical removal of the gland) have more symptoms. In such patients, manifestations of overt hypothyroidism are present by 6 weeks. Older patients tend to have fewer symptoms and signs of hypothyroidism than do young adults.

In adults, common features of hypothyroidism include easy fatigability, tiredness, coldness, weight gain, constipation, menstrual irregularities, and muscle cramps. Drowsiness and slowing of intellectual and motor activity is often referred. Sensitivity to cold is suggested by the use of more blankets on the bed. Women frequently complain of hair loss, brittle nails, and dry skin. Periorbital puffiness may be present. Stiffness and aching of muscles may be attributed to rheumatism. Constipation may occur. Numbness and tingling of the extremities are frequent. Physical findings include a cool, dry skin, puffy face and hands, hoarse husky voice, and slow reflexes.

Hypothyroidism in older people

Hypothyroidism in older people is often atypical and elusive and lacks the classic clinical features present in younger patients (60). This is due to a combination of factors including the insidious onset, the ambiguity of several signs and symptoms (fatigue, weakness, cold intolerance, dry skin, hair loss, constipation, poor appetite, depression and/or mental deterioration, hearing loss, cardiomegaly, congestive heart failure) which may be attributed to normal ageing, and to the frequent coexistence of several age-associated diseases.

The most relevant clinical findings that lead one to suspect hypothyroidism in older people are an unexplained increase in serum cholesterol, constipation, congestive heart failure (particularly when it presents as restrictive cardiomyopathy), and macrocytic anaemia (as a consequence of folate deficiency or coexistent autoimmune gastritis and pernicious anaemia). Other common clinical features encountered in elderly hypothyroid patients include neurological signs (syncope, seizures, impaired cerebellar function, carpal tunnel syndrome) and vague arthritic complaints. Due to the frequent involvement of the cardiovascular system, the presenting symptoms of hypothyroidism in elderly patients include dyspnoea in more than 50% and chest pain in up to one-quarter. A significant minority of elderly hypothyroid patients may paradoxically lose weight as a consequence of reduced appetite. Neuropsychiatric symptoms are often prominent and depression occurs in up to 60% of patients; psychoses are rare. Dementia may be found in elderly hypothyroid patients but it is rarely the direct consequence of thyroid failure, although a few patients show marked improvement of intellectual function after correction of hypothyroidism.

Elderly patients are more susceptible to myxoedema coma, a rare but serious complication of hypothyroidism. It generally occurs in the winter months, in hospitalized patients, and can be precipitated by intercurrent nonthyroidal illness, use of drugs, exposure to cold, and stress. Progressive deterioration of mental status to stupor and coma, localized neurological signs, marked hypothermia (which may not be present in patients with systemic infections), hyponatraemia, and hypoglycaemia are the hallmarks of myxoedema coma. The mortality of clearly hypothermic myxoedema coma is very high (over 80%), unless vigorous supportive therapy and thyroid hormone replacement are given immediately.

Clinical aspects of hypothyroidism due to different aetiologies

Primary hypothyroidism

Primary hypothyroidism in adults results mainly from autoimmune thyroiditis, it is more common in women than in men, and occurs between the ages of 40 and 60 years (61). In these patients, clinical features of hypothyroidism may be accompanied by the typical goiter of Hashimoto's thyroiditis. When present, the goiter is usually firm in consistency, generally moderate in size, and often lobulated; well-defined nodules are unusual. Both lobes are enlarged, but the gland may be asymmetrical. Adjacent structures, such as the trachea, oesophagus, and recurrent laryngeal nerves may be compressed but this is a rare occurrence. Goiter develops gradually over many years. Rarely, the thyroid enlarges rapidly and may be accompanied by pain and tenderness. In other cases of hypothyroidism due to autoimmune thyroiditis the gland is atrophied. Infiltrative ophthalmopathy similar to that of Graves' disease occurs in a small proportion of patients.

Other organ-specific autoimmune diseases such as insulin-dependent diabetes mellitus, Addison's disease, premature ovarian failure, hypoparathyroidism, myasthenia gravis, and coeliac disease may coexist (62). Patients with primary hypothyroidism may also complain of vitiligo and alopecia. Primary autoimmune hypothyroidism may be present as a component of either the type I or type II polyglandular autoimmune syndrome. The specific association of primary hypothyroidism and primary adrenal cortical insufficiency is known as Schmidt's syndrome (62). The type I syndrome consists of at least two of the triad of Addison's disease, hypoparathyroidism, and chronic mucocutaneous candidiasis; other autoimmune disorders, such as alopecia, chronic autoimmune thyroiditis, and malabsorption syndrome, may also be present. Autoimmune thyroid disease is reported in 10–12% of these patients. Type I polyglandular autoimmune syndrome generally presents in childhood, whereas the type II syndrome is more common and usually presents in adult life. Addison's disease, Hashimoto's thyroiditis, and type 1 diabetes are the most common endocrine deficiencies found in these patients, although gonadal failure, pernicious anaemia, and vitiligo are observed in a significant percentage.

Rarely a combination of primary and pituitary hypothyroidism with or without ACTH deficiency occurs, presumably also on an autoimmune basis. Thus, other glands may be affected with increased frequency in patients with autoimmune hypothyroidism.

Postablative hypothyroidism

A common cause of hypothyroidism in adults is the type following total thyroidectomy for thyroid carcinoma or near-total thyroidectomy for euthyroid or toxic multinodular goiter or Graves' disease. Hypothyroidism following radio-iodine treatment for Graves' hyperthyroidism is also frequent, and is currently regarded as a common outcome of ^{131}I treatment rather than a complication (63).

Overt hypothyroidism in patients who have received ^{131}I is often preceded by subclinical hypothyroidism, which may become apparent within 2–4 months after ^{131}I therapy. The early onset of hypothyroidism may cause distinct symptoms in the previously thyrotoxic patient who received ^{131}I or surgery. These patients may develop muscle cramps, often in large muscle groups (trapezius, latissimus dorsi, or the proximal muscles of the extremities).

Central hypothyroidism

The clinical picture of central hypothyroidism varies depending on the severity of thyroid failure, the extent of the associated hormone deficiencies, the age of the patients, and the nature of the underlying lesion. Central hypothyroidism is due to TSH deficiency caused by either hypothalamic or pituitary disease (64). The differentiation of secondary from primary hypothyroidism is important for the institution of the proper therapy. The clinical features of central hypothyroidism are similar to those of primary hypothyroidism, although generally less pronounced. The skin is pale and cool, but not as coarse and dry as in primary hypothyroidism. Periorbital and peripheral oedema are uncommon in patients with central hypothyroidism. Loss of axillary, pubic, and facial hair and thinning of the lateral eyebrows are more pronounced. The tongue is not enlarged, and hoarseness of the voice is not prominent as in primary hypothyroidism. The heart tends to be small, and blood pressure is low. Atrophic breasts and amenorrhoea are found in women. Body weight is more likely to be reduced than increased. Defects in growth hormone and gonadotropin secretion usually precede TSH insufficiency, and in most cases ACTH secretion is the last to be affected. Growth failure with delayed skeletal maturation results from growth hormone deficiency in children. Hypoglycaemia may occur. Gonadotropin insufficiency results in impotence, loss of libido, diminished beard growth, amenorrhoea, infertility, and atrophy of the breasts in women. ACTH deficiency leads to weakness, postural hypotension, and depigmentation of the areole and of other normally pigmented areas of the skin. Symptoms and signs that arise directly from the hypothalamic or pituitary lesion may precede, accompany, and even obscure manifestations of pituitary failure. The manifestations of a sellar mass include headache and symptoms secondary to compression of adjacent structures with visual field disturbances and ophthalmoplegia.

Diagnostic accuracy

Several attempts have been made to develop a clinical score system, based on the most frequent symptoms and signs of hypothyroidism, that could accurately predict the diagnosis of thyroid failure in individual patients. In the 1960s, Billewicz *et al.* (65) described a diagnostic index that scored the presence or absence of various signs and symptoms of hypothyroidism. However, at that time, modern laboratory thyroid function tests were not available to validate the diagnostic accuracy of such a score (65). Recently a convenient clinical score has been proposed by Zulewski *et al.* (66) that is both easy to perform and sensitive for individual assessment of the severity of thyroid failure. The frequencies of the 14 more common symptoms and signs of overt hypothyroidism are shown in Table 3.4.1.2. The most common features in hypothyroid patients were prolonged ankle reflex (77%) and complaints about dry skin (76%). A reduced pulse rate and cold intolerance were recorded with a high frequency in euthyroid controls and were, therefore, excluded from this score. The sensitivity and specificity of each symptom and sign of hypothyroidism and the analysis of their positive and negative predictive values are shown in Table 3.4.1.2. Table 3.4.1.3 shows the scoring system of symptoms and signs of hypothyroidism. Because a correlation analysis revealed a significant correlation of these scores with age, a simple age correcting factor was defined by adding 1 point to the sum of symptoms and signs in women younger than 55 years. According to this analysis, the following diagnostic ranges for the clinical judgement with the age-corrected score were defined: hypothyroid, more than 5 points; euthyroid, 0–2; intermediate, 3–5 points (66).

References

1. Rosen T, Kleman GA. Thyroid and skin. In: Callen JP, Jorizzo J, Bolognia J, Piette W, eds. *Dermatological Signs of Internal Disease*. 2nd edn. Philadelphia: WB Saunders, 1994: 189–204.
2. Miller J, Roling D, Spiers E, Davies A, Rawlings A, Leyden J. Palmoplantar keratoderma associated with hypothyroidism. *Br J Dermatol*, 1998; **139**: 738–59.
3. Zetting G, Weissel M, Flores J, Dudczak R, Volgensang H. Dermatitis herpetiformis is associated with atrophic but not with goitrous variant of Hashimoto's thyroiditis. *Eur J Clin Invest*, 2000; **30**: 53–7.
4. Smith TJ, Horwitz AL, Refetoff S. The effect of thyroid hormone on glycosaminoglycan accumulation in human skin fibroblasts. *Endocrinology*, 1981; **108**: 2397–9.

Table 3.4.1.2 Sensitivity and specificity of the 14 symptoms and signs of hypothyroidism and analysis of their positive and negative predictive values

Symptoms and signs	Sensitivity (%)	Specificity (%)	Positive predictive value (%)	Negative predictive value (%)
Ankle reflex	77	93	92	80
Dry skin	76	64	68	73
Cold intolerance	64	65	65	64
Coarse skin	60	81	76	67
Puffiness	60	96	94	71
Pulse rate	58	42	50	50
Sweating	54	86	79	65
Weight increase	54	77	70	63
Paraesthesia	52	82	75	63
Cold skin	50	80	71	61
Constipation	48	85	76	62
Slow movements	36	99	96	61
Hoarseness	34	87	73	57
Hearing	22	97	90	53

Table 3.4.1.3 Scoring of symptoms and signs of hypothyroidism

	On the basis of	Score	
		Present	Absent
Symptoms			
Diminished sweating	Sweating in a warm room or on a hot summer day	1	0
Hoarseness	Speaking voice, singing voice	1	0
Paraesthesia	Subjective sensation	1	0
Dry skin	Dryness of skin, noticed spontaneously, requiring treatment	1	0
Constipation	Bowel habit, use of laxative	1	
Impairment of hearing	Progressive impairment of hearing	1	0
Weight increase	Recorded weight increase, tightness of clothes	1	0
Physical signs			
Slow movements	Observe patient removing his/her clothes	1	0
Delayed ankle reflex	Observe the relaxation of the reflex	1	0
Coarse skin	Examine hands, forearms, elbows for roughness and thickening of skin	1	0
Periorbital puffiness	This should obscure the curve of the malar bone	1	0
Cold skin	Compare temperature of patient's hands with examiner's	1	0

For clinical judgement, add 1 point to the sum of symptoms and signs present in women younger than 55 years. Hypothyroid, more than 5 points; euthyroid, less than 3 points; intermediate, 3–5 points.

5. Biondi B, Klein I. Hypothyroidism as a risk factor for cardiovascular disease. *Endocrine*, 2004; **24**: 1–13.
6. Ojamaa K, Klein I. In vivo regulation of recombinant cardiac myosin heavy chain gene expression by thyroid hormone. *Endocrinology*, 1993; **132**: 1002–6.
7. Kahly GJ, Dillmann WH. Thyroid hormone action in the heart. *Endocr Rev*, 2005; **26**: 704–28.
8. Coppola AR, Landenson PW. Hypothyroidism and atherosclerosis. *J Clin Endocrinol Metab*, 2003; **88**: 2438–44.
9. Mattace-Raso SU, van der Cammen TJ, Hofman A, van Popele NM, Bos ML, Schalekamp MA, *et al.* Arterial stiffness and risk of coronary heart disease and stroke: the Rotterdam study. *Circulation*, 2006; **113**: 657–63.
10. Zondek H. Das Myxödemherz. *Muench Med Wochenschr*, 1918; **65**: 1180–3.
11. Santos AD, Miller RP, Mathew PK, Wallace WA, Cave WT Jr, Hinojosa L. Echocardiographic characterization of the reversible cardiomyopathy of hypothyroidism. *Am J Med*, 1980; **68**: 675–9.
12. Galderisi M, Vitale G, D'Errico A, Lupoli GA, Ciccarelli A, Cicala S. Usefulness of pulsed tissue Doppler for the assessment of left ventricular myocardial function in overt hypothyroidism. *Ital Heart J*, 2004; **5**: 257–64.
13. Wilson WR, Bedell GN. The pulmonary abnormalities in myxedema. *J Clin Invest*, 1960; **39**: 42–5.
14. Duranti R, Gheri RG, Gorini M, Gigliotti F, Spinelli A, Fanelli A, *et al.* Control of breathing in patients with severe hypothyroidism. *Am J Med*, 1993; **95**: 29–33.
15. Ambrosino N, Pacini F, Paggiaro PL, Martino E, Contini V, Turini L, *et al.* Impaired ventilatory drive in short-term primary hypothyroidism and its reversal by L-triiodothyronine. *J Endocrinol Invest*, 1985; **8**: 533–8.
16. Ladenson PW, Goldenheim PD, Ridgway EC. Prediction and reversal of blunted ventilatory responsiveness in patients with hypothyroidism. *Am J Med*, 1988; **84**: 877–83.
17. Pelttari L, Rauhala E, Polo O, Hyyppä MT, Kronholm E, Viikari J, *et al.* Upper airway obstruction in hypothyroidism. *J Intern Med*, 1994; **236**: 177–81.
18. Shafer RB, Prentiss RA, Bond JH. Gastrointestinal transit in thyroid disease. *Gastroenterology*, 1994; **86**: 852–6.
19. Tachman ML, Guthrie GP Jr. Hypothyroidism: diversity of presentation. *Endocr Rev*, 1984; **5**: 456–64.
20. Counsell CE, Taha A, Rudell WJJ. Coeliac disease and autoimmune thyroid disease. *Gut*, 1994; **35**: 844–50.
21. Lauritano EC, Bilotta AL, Gabrielli M, Scarpellini E, Lupascu A, Laginestra A, *et al.* Association between hypothyroidism and small intestinal bacterial overgrowth. *J Clin Endocrinol Metab*, 2007; **92**: 4180–4.
22. Saha B, Maity C. Alterations of serum enzymes in primary hypothyroidism. *Clin Chem Lab Med*, 2002; **40**: 609–11.
23. Smith CD, Ain KB. Brain metabolism in hypothyroidism studied with **31**P magnetic-resonance spectroscopy. *Lancet*, 1995; **345**: 619–20.
24. Constant EL, Volder AG, Ivanoiu A, Bol A, Labar D, Seghers A, *et al.* Cerebral blood flow and glucose metabolism in hypothyroidism: a positron emission tomography study. *J Clin Endocrinol Metab*, 2001; **86**: 3864–70.
25. Zhu DF, Wang ZX, Zhang DR, Pan ZL, He S, Hu XP, *et al.* fMRI revealed neural substrate for reversible working memory dysfunction in subclinical hypothyroidism. *Brain*, 2006; **129**: 2923–30.
26. Grabe HI, Völzke H, Lüdemann J, Wolff B, Schwahn C, John U, *et al.* Mental and physical complaints in thyroid disorders in the general population. *Acta Psychiatr Scand*, 2005; **112**: 286–93.
27. Bartalena L, Placidi GF, Martino E, Falcone M, Pellegrini L, Dell'Osso L, *et al.* Nocturnal serum thyrotropin (TSH) surge and the TSH response to TSH-releasing hormone: dissociated behavior in untreated depressives. *J Clin Endocrinol Metab*, 1990; **71**: 650–5.
28. Jellinek EH, Kelly RE. Cerebellar syndrome in myxoedema. *Lancet*, 1960; **ii**: 225–8.

29. Sanders V. Neurological manifestations of myxedema. *N Engl J Med*, 1962; **266**: 599–604.
30. Torres CF, Moxley RT. Hypothyroid neuropathy and myopathy: clinical and electrodiagnostic longitudinal findings. *J Neurol*, 1990; **237**: 271–5.
31. Debré R, Sémélaigne G. Syndrome of diffuse muscular hypertrophy in infants causing athletic appearance: its connection with congenital myxedema. *Am J Dis Child*, 1935; **50**: 1351–4.
32. Duyff RF, Bosch J, Laman DF, van Loon BJ, Linssen WH. Neuromuscular findings in thyroid dysfunction: a prospective clinical and electrodiagnostic study. *J Neurol Neurosurg Psychiatry*, 2000; **68**: 750–55.
33. Cakir M, Samanci N, Balci N, Balci MK. Musculoskeletal manifestations in patients with thyroid disease. *Clin Endocrinol*, 2003; **59**: 162–7.
34. Famulski KS, Pilarska M, Wrzosek A, Sarzala MG. ATPase activity and protein phosphorylation in rabbit fast skeletal muscle sarcolemma. *Eur J Biochem*, 1988; **171**: 363–7.
35. Eriksen EF. Normal and pathological remodeling of human trabecular bone. Three dimensional reconstruction of the remodeling sequence in normals and in metabolic bone disease. *Endocr Rev*, 1986; **7**: 379–84.
36. Levenson D, Bialik GM, Ochberg Z. Differential effects of hypothyroidism on the cartilage and the osteogenic process in the mandibular condyle: recovery by growth hormone and thyroxine. *Endocrinology*, 1994; **135**: 1504–9.
37. Montenegro J, González O, Saracho R, Aguirre R, González O, Martínez I. Changes in renal function in primary hypothyroidism. *Am J Kidney Dis*, 1996; **27**: 195–8.
38. Karanikas G, Schtz M, Szabo M, Becherer A, Wiesner K, Dudczac R, *et al.* Isotopic renal function studies in severe hypothyroidism and after thyroid hormone replacement therapy. *Am J Nephrol*, 2004; **24**: 41–5.
39. Hanna FWF, Scanlon MF. Hyponatraemia, hypothyroidism and role of arginine-vasopressin. *Lancet*, 1997; **350**: 755–6.
40. Diekman MJM, Put NM, Blom HJ, Tijssen JGP, Wiersinga WM. Determinants of changes in plasma homocysteine in hyperthyroidism and hypothyroidism. *Clin Endocrinol*, 2001; **54**: 197–204.
41. Erslev AJ. Anemia of endocrine disorders. In: Williams WJ, Beutler E, Erslev AJ, Lichtman MA, eds. *Hematology*. 4th edn. New York: McGraw-Hill, 1990: 408–15.
42. Squizzato A, Romualdi E, Buller HR, Gerdes VE. Clinical review: thyroid dysfunction and effects on coagulation and fibrinolysis: a systematic review. *J Clin Endocrinol Metab*, 2007; **92**: 2415–20.
43. Anasti JN, Flack MR, Froehlich J, Nelson LM, Nisula BC. A potential novel mechanism for precocious puberty in juvenile hypothyroidism. *J Clin Endocrinol Metab*, 1995; **80**: 276–9.
44. Van Haaster LH, de Jong FH, Docter R, de Rooij DG. The effect of hypothyroidism on Sertoli cell proliferation and differentiation and hormone levels during testicular development in the rat. *Endocrinology*, 1992; **131**: 1574–81.
45. Carani C, Isidori MI, Granata A, Carosa E, Maggi M, Lenzi A, *et al.* Multicenter study on the prevalence of sexual symptoms in male hypo- and hyperthyroid patients. *J Clin Endocrinol Metab*, 2005; **90**: 6472–9.
46. Tomasi PA, Fanciulli G, Zini M, Demontis MA, Dettori A, Delitala G. Pulsatile gonadotropin secretion in hypothyroid women of reproductive age. *Eur J Endocrinol*, 1997; **136**: 406–9.
47. Chiovato L, Lapi P, Fiore E, Tonacchera M, Pinchera A. Thyroid autoimmunity and female gender. *J Endocrinol Invest*, 1993; **16**: 384–91.
48. Burrow GN, Fisher DA, Larsen PR. Maternal and fetal thyroid function. *N Engl J Med*, 1994; **331**: 1072–9.
49. Haddow JE, Palomaki GE, Allan WC, Williams JR, Knight GJ, Gagnon J, *et al.* Maternal thyroid deficiency during pregnancy and subsequent neuropsychological development of the child. *N Engl J Med*, 1999; **341**: 549–55.
50. Liu H, Momotani N, Noh JY, Ishikawa N, Takebe K, Ito K. Maternal hypothyroidism during early pregnancy and intellectual development of progeny. *Arch Intern Med*, 1994; **154**: 785–9.
51. Miell JP, Taylor AM, Zini M, Maheshwari HG, Ross RJ, Valcavi R. Effects of hypothyroidism and hyperthyroidism on insulin-like growth factors and growth hormone and IGF-binding proteins. *J Clin Endocrinol Metab*, 1993; **76**: 950–5.
52. Yamamoto K, Saito K, Takai T, Naito M, Yoshida S. Visual field defects and pituitary enlargement in primary hypothyroidism. *J Clin Endocrinol Metab*, 1983; **57**: 283–6.
53. Sarlis NJ, Brucker-Davis F, Doppman JL, Skarulis MC. MRI-demonstrable regression of a pituitary mass in a case of primary hypothyroidism after a week of acute thyroid hormone therapy. *J Clin Endocrinol Metab*, 1997; **82**: 808–11.
54. Iranmanesh A, Lizarralde G, Johnson ML, Veldhuis JD. Dynamics of 24 hour endogenous cortisol secretion and clearance in primary hypothyroidism assessed before and after partial hormone replacement. *J Clin Endocrinol Metab*, 1990; **70**: 155–60.
55. Deschepper CF, Hong-Brown LQ. Hormonal regulation of the angiotensinogen gene in liver and other tissues. In: Raizada MK, Phillips MI, Sumners C, eds. *Cellular and Molecular Biology of Renin-Angiotensin System*. Boca Raton: CRC Press, 1993: 152–65.
56. Diekman MJM, Romin JA, Endert E, Sauerwein H, Wiersinga WM. Thyroid hormones modulate serum leptin levels: observations in thyrotoxic and hypothyroid women. *Thyroid*, 1998; **8**: 1081–6.
57. Marchesini G, Fabbri A, Bianchi GP, Motta E, Bugianesi E, Urbini D, *et al.* Hepatic conversion of amino nitrogen to urea nitrogen in hypothyroid patients and upon L-thyroxine therapy. *Metabolism*, 1993; **42**: 1263–8.
58. Martinez-Triguero ML, Hernández-Mijares A, Nguyen TT, Muñoz ML, Peña H, Morillas C, *et al.* Effect of thyroid hormone replacement on lipoprotein (a), lipids, and apolipoproteins in subjects with hypothyroidism. *Mayo Clin Proc*, 1998; **73**: 837–41.
59. Tan KCB, Shiu SWM, Kung AWC. Plasma cholesteryl ester transfer protein activity in hyper- and hypothyroidism. *J Clin Endocrinol Metab*, 1998; **83**: 140–3.
60. Mariotti S, Franceschi C, Cossarizza A, Pinchera A. The aging thyroid. *Endocr Rev*, 1995; **16**: 686–715.
61. Mariotti S, Sansoni P, Barbesino G, Caturegli P, Monti D, Cossarizza A, *et al.* Thyroid and other organ-specific autoantibodies in healthy centenarians. *Lancet*, 1992; **339**: 1506–8.
62. Ahonen P, Myllaruiemi DDS, Sipila I, Perheentupa J. Clinical variation of autoimmune polyendocrinopathy-candidiasis-ectodermal dystrophy in a series of 68 patients. *N Engl J Med*, 1990; **322**: 1829–32.
63. Bartalena L, Marcocci C, Bogazzi F, Panicucci M, Lepri A, Pinchera A. Use of corticosteroids to prevent progression of Graves' ophthalmopathy after radioiodine therapy for hyperthyroidism. *N Engl J Med*, 1989; **321**: 1349–52.
64. Martino E, Bartalena L, Pinchera A. Central hypothyroidism. In: Braverman LE, Utiger RD, eds. *Werner & Ingbar's, The Thyroid*. 8th edn. Philadelphia: Lippincott Raven, 2000: 762–73.
65. Billewicz WZ, Chapman RS, Crooks J, Day ME, Gossage J, Wayne E, *et al.* Statistical methods applied to the diagnosis of hypothyroidism. *QJM*, 1969; **38**: 255–66.
66. Zulewski H, Muller B, Exer P, Miserez AR, Staub JJ. Estimation of tissue hypothyroidism by a new clinical score: evaluation of patients with various grades of hypothyroidism and controls. *J Clin Endocrinol Metab*, 1997; **82**: 771–6.

3.4.2 Causes and laboratory investigation of hypothyroidism

Ferruccio Santini, Aldo Pinchera

Introduction

Hypothyroidism is the clinical state that develops as a result of the lack of action of thyroid hormones on target tissues (1). Hypothyroidism is usually due to impaired hormone secretion by the thyroid, resulting in reduced concentrations of serum thyroxine (T_4) and triiodothyronine (T_3). The term primary hypothyroidism is applied to define the thyroid failure deriving from inherited or acquired causes that act directly on the thyroid gland by reducing the amount of functioning thyroid tissue or by inhibiting thyroid hormone production. The term central hypothyroidism is used when pituitary or hypothalamic abnormalities result in an insufficient stimulation of an otherwise normal thyroid gland. Both primary and central hypothyroidism may be transient, depending on the nature and the extent of the causal agent. Hypothyroidism following a minor loss of thyroid tissue can be recovered by compensatory hyperplasia of the residual gland. Similarly, hypothyroidism subsides when an exogenous inhibitor of thyroid function is removed.

Peripheral hypothyroidism may also arise as a consequence of tissue resistance to thyroid hormones due to a mutation in the thyroid hormone receptor. Resistance to thyroid hormones is a heterogeneous clinical entity with most patients appearing to be clinically euthyroid while some of them have symptoms of thyrotoxicosis and others display selected signs of hypothyroidism. The common feature is represented by pituitary resistance to thyroid hormones, leading to increased secretion of thyrotropin that in turn stimulates thyroid growth and function. The variability in clinical manifestations depends on the severity of the hormonal resistance, the relative degree of tissue hyposensitivity, and the coexistence of associated genetic defects (see Chapter 3.4.8).

Primary hypothyroidism

A list of the causes of primary hypothyroidism is given in Box 3.4.2.1. Autoimmune thyroiditis is the most common cause of spontaneous hypothyroidism in areas with adequate iodine intake. Iatrogenic hypothyroidism is responsible for many hypothyroid patients in these regions and inborn errors of thyroid hormone synthesis, goitrogens, and other destructive processes of the thyroid gland account for a few cases. Iodine deficiency is crucial in the pathogenesis of endemic cretinism and of adult hypothyroidism in areas in which an efficient iodine prophylaxis has not been undertaken.

Autoimmune thyroiditis

Autoimmune thyroiditis includes a spectrum of diseases that are distinguished for their clinical course, the degree of thyroid dysfunction, and the changes of thyroid size. All these variants recognize an

Box 3.4.2.1 Causes of primary hypothyroidism

- Autoimmune thyroiditis
  - Chronic thyroiditis
    - Hashimoto's thyroiditis
    - Atrophic thyroiditis
  - Postpartum thyroiditis
  - Graves' disease (spontaneous late evolution)
- Subacute thyroiditis
- Riedel's thyroiditis
- Iatrogenic
  - Thyroidectomy
  - ^{131}I therapy for hyperthyroidism
  - External radiotherapy
  - Excessive iodine
  - Drugs
    - Thionamides
    - Amiodarone
    - Lithium
    - Tyrosine kinase inhibitors
    - Others
- Severe iodine deficiency
- Natural goitrogens
- Thalassaemia major
- Congenital abnormalities
  - Thyroid dysgenesis
    - Agenesis
    - Ectopic gland
    - Hypoplasia
- Inherited defects in thyroid hormone biosynthesis
  - Iodide transport defect
  - Organification defect
  - Pendred's syndrome
  - Iodotyrosine deiodinase defect
  - Thyroglobulin defect
  - TSH-receptor defect
  - Gs-protein defects
- Transient neonatal hypothyroidism
  - Iodine deficiency or excess
  - Administration of antithyroid agents to the mother
  - Maternal TSH-blocking antibody.

immune-mediated pathogenesis and usually present with high titres of circulating antithyroid antibodies. As in most organ-specific autoimmune reactions, the aetiology of autoimmune thyroiditis is still unknown but is somehow linked to genetic and environmental factors, and is influenced by the gender and the age (see Chapter 3.2.6).

Chronic thyroiditis

Chronic thyroiditis is the most common among the autoimmune thyroidites. Historically, two clinical variants of the disease are described. A goitrous variant (Hashimoto's thyroiditis), characterized by heavy lymphocytic infiltration and thyroid enlargement, and an atrophic variant (primary myxoedema) with progressive fibrosis and reduction of thyroid size. In clinical practice, a clear distinction between the two forms is not always possible. In the initial stage of the disease the two variants commonly do not present distinctive features. Moreover, atrophy may be a destructive end result of goitrous thyroiditis with the thyroid gland showing near complete replacement with fibrosis. When overt hypothyroidism has occurred, thyroid volume shows a unimodal distribution, with thyroid atrophy and goiter being extremes within the distribution (2). Overall, these observations suggests that the two variants do not represent separate disorders.

Thyroid failure usually develops very slowly and, as thyroid function fades, the resulting increase in serum thyroid-stimulating hormone (TSH) limits the decline in thyroid secretion. Thus overt hypothyroidism is commonly preceded by a variable period of time in which elevated TSH is the only hormonal abnormality (subclinical hypothyroidism) (3, 4). The transition from euthyroidism to hypothyroidism may pass unrecognized and initial symptoms may be attributed to ageing, menopause, or other chronic concomitant diseases (5). Thus, it is not uncommon that chronic thyroiditis is diagnosed when clinical manifestations of thyroid failure become severe or complications of hypothyroidism have occurred. The circumstances leading to early diagnosis of the disease include family history for autoimmune thyroid diseases, appearance of goiter, blood testing for screening of autoimmune diseases in patients with polyglandular autoimmunity, routine diagnostic protocols for patients with menstrual dysfunction, or hyperlipidaemia. Occasionally hypothyroidism may be due to TSH-receptor blocking antibodies preventing thyroid cell stimulation by TSH. TSH-receptor blocking antibodies are more frequent in atrophic thyroiditis than in goitrous thyroiditis (6). Hypothyroidism may be reversible if the TSH-receptor blocking antibody titre declines and enough thyroid tissue remains for thyroid hormone synthesis. Graves' hyperthyroidism may develop in hypothyroid patients with chronic thyroiditis because of a change in the nature of TSH-receptor antibodies from blocking to stimulating (7).

In some instances the disease may be preceded by a transient phase of thyrotoxicosis (hashitoxicosis) due to the discharge of preformed thyroid hormones, as a result of an unusually intense inflammatory process. The gland is tender and sometimes painful, resembling subacute thyroiditis. Hypothyroidism usually develops in a short time and may be permanent, especially in patients with elevated thyroid peroxidase antibody.

Features of thyroid-associated ophthalmopathy may occur in patients with chronic thyroiditis and hypothyroidism. This condition is termed 'hypothyroid Graves' disease' and may represent a distinct entity with pathogenetic mechanisms common to Graves' disease, or may be the endstage of Graves' disease after spontaneous remission of hyperthyroidism.

Focal thyroiditis is characterized by spotty collections of mononuclear cells within thyroid tissue, and minimal changes in follicular epithelium or stromal fibrosis. Most patients with focal thyroiditis are euthyroid and only 10–20% have subclinical hypothyroidism (8). The disease may be suspected at ultrasound examination in patients with circulating thyroid autoantibodies, or may be a histological occurrence in surgical or autopsy specimens. In the presence of circulating thyroid autoantibodies, focal thyroiditis may represent the earliest stage of chronic autoimmune thyroiditis, whereas the clinical significance of nonspecific isolated lymphocytic infiltration in patients without circulating autoantibodies has still to be clarified.

Juvenile thyroiditis (autoimmune thyroiditis in childhood and adolescence) is described as a separate entity because follicular oxyphilia is usually mild or absent, goiter is soft, and thyroid antibody titres are not as high as in adults. Fine-needle aspiration biopsy is sometimes required to establish the diagnosis. Spontaneous resolution is relatively common but hypothyroidism may develop during the course of the disease (9).

Postpartum thyroiditis

Pregnancy is known to influence the clinical course of various autoimmune disorders, including autoimmune thyroid disease. Typically, amelioration during pregnancy is followed by aggravation after delivery. This phenomenon is thought to depend on the physiological need of inhibiting maternal immune reactions that might cause rejection of the fetus. Thus, thyroid peroxidase antibodies, thyroglobulin antibodies, and TSH-receptor antibody titres decrease or may even disappear during pregnancy. Following delivery, a rebound of autoimmune processes occurs and may result in destructive thyroiditis with release of preformed thyroid hormones and transient thyrotoxicosis. This clinical entity is named postpartum thyroiditis and occurs in 5–9% of unselected postpartum women (10). (see Chapter 3.4.6).

Graves' disease

Spontaneous hypothyroidism may develop during the course of Graves' disease whenever destructive processes of thyroiditis predominate over thyroid-stimulating events (burnt out Graves' disease). This may occur after long-term remission of hyperthyroidism associated with disappearance of TSH-receptor stimulating antibodies, or following prolonged therapy with antithyroid drugs (11). TSH-receptor blocking antibodies may also appear and neutralize TSH-receptor stimulating antibodies, leading to hypothyroidism.

Subacute thyroiditis

Subacute thyroiditis is an inflammatory disease of viral origin (12). Although the disease is relatively uncommon it must be suspected any time a patient presents with anterior neck pain. Recovery is complete in most patients but in rare cases (1–5%) epithelial loss is severe, resulting in permanent hypothyroidism (see Chapter 3.2.7).

Riedel's thyroiditis

Riedel's thyroiditis is an extremely rare chronic disease of unknown aetiology, characterized by progressive fibrosis of the thyroid and surrounding tissues (13). Hypothyroidism develops when fibrosclerosis has involved most of the gland (see Chapter 3.2.7).

Iatrogenic hypothyroidism

Thyroid ablation for therapeutic purposes is a common cause of primary hypothyroidism in the adult. Thyroid failure is an obvious consequence of total or subtotal thyroidectomy for thyroid cancer, goiter, or Graves' disease, but clinical hypothyroidism does not develop as long as substitutive therapy is started shortly after surgery. Similarly, ^{131}I therapy for Graves' disease is directed to destroy thyroid tissue. However, the success rate of radio-iodine therapy and the time of onset of hypothyroidism are not fully predictable; they depend on several factors including the dose of radiation delivered, the size of the goiter, and the underlying autoimmune phenomena (14, 15). Drug-induced hypothyroidism is also common. Excessive inhibition of thyroid hormone synthesis commonly occurs during therapy for hyperthyroidism with antithyroid agents. Furthermore, primary hypothyroidism may develop as a side effect of several drugs administered for different purposes.

Postoperative hypothyroidism

Total thyroidectomy is performed for thyroid cancer, Graves' disease, and large diffuse or multinodular goiters, occasionally also harbouring Hashimoto's thyroiditis. However, hypothyroidism does not develop as long as L-thyroxine replacement therapy is started soon after thyroidectomy. In patients with thyroid cancer, thyroid hormone therapy must be discontinued at an appropriate time before ^{131}I scanning and therapy. Thus, patients develop transient, and usually not severe, clinical hypothyroidism. The availability of recombinant human TSH for clinical use will avoid hypothyroidism due to thyroid hormone withdrawal in thyroid cancer patients (see Chapter 3.5.6).

The frequency of hypothyroidism after subtotal thyroidectomy varies depending on the mass of remaining tissue and the degree of its autonomous function. A small thyroid residue may be sufficient for maintenance of the euthyroid state in Graves' disease. On the other hand, a large residue of a multinodular or Hashimoto's goiter may not be enough for adequate thyroid hormone secretion. Partial thyroidectomy or lobectomy for multinodular goiters or solitary nodules are usually not associated with permanent hypothyroidism.

Postirradiation hypothyroidism

Among different radioactive isotopes of iodine, ^{131}I is the agent of choice in the treatment of thyroid hyperfunction. After oral administration, radio-iodine is completely absorbed, rapidly concentrated, oxidized, and organified by thyroid follicular cells. The biological effects of radio-iodine include necrosis of follicular cells, shorter survival and impaired replication of undestroyed cells, and vascular occlusion, leading to atrophy and fibrosis of thyroidal tissue.

The goal of radio-iodine therapy for hyperthyroidism is to destroy sufficient thyroid tissue to cure the hyperthyroidism with one dose of ^{131}I. This dose is calculated on the basis of thyroid size and uptake of ^{131}I. Because of radiation safety restrictions, in some centres small repeated doses of radio-iodine are administered. In other centres standard fixed doses are given. Small glands are destroyed more readily by radio-iodine than larger ones, and toxic adenoma or toxic multinodular goiter are usually more radioresistant than Graves' glands. Radio-iodine has a delayed effect and several months may be required for the complete control of hyperthyroidism.

In the case of Graves' disease, the goal of radio-iodine should be to destroy as much thyroid tissue as possible (15). This strategy has been adopted because residual tissue, necessary to ensure euthyroidism, is responsible for the relapse of hyperthyroidism in a large proportion of patients. A strict control of thyroid function is required during the first 6–12 months following ^{131}I therapy for Graves' disease to avoid the appearance of symptoms of hypothyroidism, which may be rapidly progressive and severe. Early postradio-iodine hypothyroidism may be transient, and hyperthyroidism may relapse during L-thyroxine replacement therapy.

Radio-iodine-induced hypothyroidism is less frequent after treatment for toxic adenoma or multinodular goiter because non-functioning thyroid tissue should not receive the radioisotope. Yet, hypothyroidism may develop whenever TSH is not completely suppressed at the time ^{131}I is administered. Furthermore, a small degree of iodine uptake is maintained in normal thyroid cells even in the absence of TSH stimulation, and this may be the cause of hypothyroidism many years after radio-iodine administration.

External irradiation to the neck for nonthyroidal neoplasias (lymphomas, tumours of the head and neck, spinal tumours, or metastases) may produce hypothyroidism in up to 50% of patients (16). Thyroid failure may develop after a variable interval, depending on the dose of radiation that has been administered. Hypothyroidism after total body irradiation for acute leukaemia or aplastic anaemia has also been reported (17). An increased risk of hypothyroidism has been found in older breast cancer patients treated with radiation, since a portion of the thyroid gland may be included in the treatment fields (18).

Drug-induced hypothyroidism

Transient hypothyroidism is common in the course of medical treatment for hyperthyroidism with thionamides, and quickly subsides with adjustment of the dose. Excess iodide, such as in disinfectants, radiographic contrast agents, and seaweed-containing preparations, may precipitate hypothyroidism in autoimmune chronic thyroiditis, due to failure of the thyroid to escape from the Wolff–Chaikoff effect. Animal studies suggest that excessive iodide increases the incidence of thyroid autoimmunity but evidence in humans is controversial. Amiodarone is an antiarrhythmic agent containing about 37 mg iodine per 100 mg drug. Amiodarone may produce hypothyroidism by the excess iodine released with metabolism of the drug. As in other cases of excess iodine administration, an underlying autoimmune thyroid disease is a prerequisite (19). Amiodarone may also induce destructive thyroiditis in an otherwise normal thyroid gland. The pathogenetic mechanisms of this phenomenon are not clear, and hypothyroidism follows a transient thyrotoxic phase. Distinction of the two forms of amiodarone-induced hypothyroidism is important for choosing the right treatment measures and method of follow-up.

Lithium inhibits thyroid hormone synthesis and secretion, and long-term lithium therapy for psychiatric disorders may result in subclinical (up to 23%) or overt (up to 19%) hypothyroidism (20). The risk of development of hypothyroidism is increased in patients with positive antithyroid antibodies or with minor thyroid abnormalities, which reduce the ability of the thyroid gland to override the inhibitory effects of lithium. Goiter is also common in lithium-treated patients, even when serum thyroid hormones and TSH are within normal limits.

Tyrosine kinase inhibitors are newly developed drugs approved for the treatment of several tumours. The first observation of hypothyroidism after sunitinib treatment has been reported in 2006 (21). Since then several studies have been published and have confirmed that various tyrosine kinase inhibitors can affect thyroid function tests through different physiopathological mechanisms impairing thyroid function or thyroid hormone metabolism (22).

Several other drugs have been reported to be capable of inducing primary hypothyroidism (23). Treatment with interferon-α or interleukin-2 may produce hypothyroidism, thyrotoxicosis, or the biphasic pattern of silent thyroiditis. Pre-existent thyroid autoimmunity increases the risk of thyroid dysfunction during treatment with these agents. Other medications occasionally reported to induce hypothyroidism include sulfonamides, sulfonylureas, ethionamide, *p*-aminosalicylic acid, phenylbutazone, and nicardipine, but the antithyroid potential of these drugs is weak and an underlying thyroid abnormality or concurrent iodine deficiency are usually associated.

Severe iodine deficiency and natural goitrogens

Environmental iodine deficiency is common in many areas throughout the world, particularly in inland mountainous areas. Goiter is the most common disorder due to iodine deficiency and its prevalence is inversely related to the median iodine intake of the population. Endemic goiter is usually not associated with hypothyroidism. However, the pattern of circulating thyroid hormones in the population from areas of severe iodine deficiency differs from that found in iodine-sufficient areas (24). The mean serum T_4 is reduced while serum T_3 is unchanged or increased and an inverse correlation between serum TSH and T_4 is found. The low iodine content within the thyroid gland and the increased TSH stimulation lead to preferential secretion of T_3, which is far more potent than T_4 in terms of metabolic responses. Thus, the relative increase in T_3 secretion enables a patient to maintain the euthyroid status in spite of reduced availability of iodide.

Cretinism is the result of an insufficient supply of thyroid hormones to fetal tissues and is due to severe iodine deficiency in both the mother and the fetus during early stages of gestation (25). Fetal hypothyroidism is not compensated by transplacental passage of maternal T_4 and is responsible for severe physical and neurological damage.

Adult hypothyroidism may occur in rural populations living in areas of severe iodine deficiency where isolation prevents access to iodine-rich foodstuff. In this case, hypothyroidism is rapidly reversed by iodine supplementation. Consumption of food containing antithyroid agents, such as thiocyanate in cassava meal and flavonoids in a variety of plants, may aggravate the effects of dietary iodine deficiency and add to the development of goiter and hypothyroidism. Phloroglucinol, a potent antithyroid compound contained in some species of seaweeds, may play an additional role to that of iodine excess in the development of iodine-induced hypothyroidism. More recently, attention has been focused on environmental endocrine disrupters (pesticides and industrial pollutants) as a possible cause of thyroid imbalance, but their effects on human thyroid function have not been fully elucidated (see also Chapter 3.2.2) (26).

Thalassaemia major

A high prevalence of primary hypothyroidism has been described in patients with thalassaemia major. The incidence and severity of thyroidal dysfunction appears related to the degree of iron overload. Hypothyroidism may contribute to deterioration of heart function, and regular iron chelation therapy should be advised for these patients (27, 28).

Congenital abnormalities

Congenital hypothyroidism occurs in 1/3000–4000 neonates worldwide, and may be classified as permanent or transient. Primary congenital hypothyroidism accounts for most affected children, whereas central congenital hypothyroidism is rare (29) (see Chapter 3.4.7).

Both the fetus and the neonate are particularly sensitive to the block of thyroid function induced by excess iodide since the immature gland is not able to escape from the Wolff–Chaikoff effect (30). Iodide-induced transient hypothyroidism is most common in premature infants and in low-birthweight babies, and has occurred more in relatively iodine-deficient areas of Europe (31), than in iodine-sufficient North America.

Transient fetal–neonatal hypothyroidism and goiter may develop in babies born to hyperthyroid mothers with Graves' disease treated with excessive doses of propylthiouracil or methimazole. Both hypothyroidism and goiter resolve spontaneously with the clearance of the drug from the circulation of the neonate. TSH-receptor blocking antibodies may be present in patients with autoimmune hypothyroidism; the antibodies compete with TSH and inhibit the biological effects of TSH on thyroid cell function and growth (6). These antibodies have been found mainly in patients with autoimmune atrophic thyroiditis, and contribute to the development of thyroid failure and atrophy. The maternal TSH-receptor antibody responsible for thyroid failure in the neonate inhibits TSH binding to its receptor and therefore blocks the effect of TSH on adenylate cyclase stimulation, iodine uptake, and thyroid cell growth (32). TSH-receptor blocking antibodies may also occur in women with Graves' disease and be transmitted to the fetus. Although thyroid-stimulating antibodies usually predominate in these patients, transient hypothyroidism is possible in the offspring of women with Graves' disease due to very high TSH-blocking antibody titres and relatively low concentrations of thyroid-stimulating antibody. Because TSH-induced growth is blocked, these infants do not have a goiter.

Central hypothyroidism

Central hypothyroidism is the consequence of anatomical or functional disorders of the pituitary or the hypothalamus. Several of the causes reported in Box 3.4.2.2 may affect both the pituitary and the hypothalamus, and in many instances the main anatomical site of the dysfunction cannot be identified. Thus, the former terms of secondary hypothyroidism (of pituitary origin) and tertiary hypothyroidism (of hypothalamic origin) are no longer recommended (33). Central hypothyroidism is rarely isolated, being part of a generalized disorder involving the secretion of other pituitary hormones. Permanent central hypothyroidism is rare, its prevalence being about 0.005% of the general population. However, transient functional abnormalities of TSH secretion are relatively common, and often pass unrecognized due to rapid recovery of the normal thyroid hormone balance.

Box 3.4.2.2 Causes of central hypothyroidism

- Tumours
  - Pituitary adenomas
  - Craniopharyngioma
  - Meningioma
  - Dysgerminoma
  - Other brain tumours
  - Metastatic tumours
- Ischaemic necrosis
  - Postpartum (Sheehan's syndrome)
  - Severe shock
  - Diabetes mellitus
- Aneurysm of internal carotid artery
- Iatrogenic
  - External radiation
  - Surgery
- Infectious diseases
  - Abscesses
  - Tuberculosis
  - Syphilis
  - Toxoplasmosis
- Sarcoidosis
- Histiocytosis
- Haemosiderosis
- Chronic lymphocytic hypophysitis
- Empty sella
- Traumatic brain injury
- Subarachnoid haemorrhage
- Pituitary dysplasia
- Congenital malformations of the hypothalamus
- Genetic abnormalities in TSH or TRH synthesis
- Transient central hypothyroidism
  - Drugs
  - Glucocorticoids
  - Dopamine
  - Bexarotene

Maternal thyroid-stimulating hormone-blocking antibodies

Pituitary adenomas represent the most common cause of central hypothyroidism. Reduced secretion of TSH is usually a consequence of mechanical compression of nontumorous cells and of adenohypophyseal blood vessels by the adenoma (33). The pituitary stalk and the hypothalamus may also be involved by suprasellar extension of the tumour. The tumour may be nonfunctioning or secrete other hormones. Thus, the resulting syndrome will depend on the extent of hypopituitarism and on the particular hormone secreted by the adenoma. A sudden enlargement of pituitary adenomas may occur as a result of haemorrhage within the tumour, leading to pituitary apoplexy. Several other causes may produce central hypothyroidism, by acting at the hypothalamic or pituitary level. Primary extrasellar brain tumours or metastatic tumours originating from other sites may produce a variable degree of hypopituitarism, depending on the location and the extension of their mass. Among brain tumours, craniopharyngiomas should be suspected when central hypothyroidism is diagnosed in young people. Craniopharyngiomas are usually extrasellar but they may extend inferiorly causing destruction of the bony margins of the sella. Pituitary infarction may develop postpartum following excessive blood loss during delivery (Sheehan's syndrome), or in patients with severe shock or during systemic anticoagulation therapy. Various degrees of pituitary insufficiency may be observed in these cases. Traumatic head injuries can lead to central hypothyroidism because of hypothalamic or pituitary infarction or haemorrhage. Iatrogenic causes of central hypothyroidism include external radiation and surgery for pituitary or brain tumours. The empty sella syndrome is caused by a defect of the sellar diaphragm leading to cisternal herniation within the pituitary fossa and flattening of the pituitary. Hypopituitarism develops slowly along with expansion of the cisternal herniation caused by transmission of cerebrospinal fluid pressure.

Hypothalamic or pituitary lesions may derive from any of the infectious or granulomatous diseases listed in Box 3.4.2.2. Chronic lymphocytic hypophysitis may be responsible for pituitary insufficiency, and has been described in association with autoimmune thyroiditis or adrenalitis. Recent studies have demonstrated a high prevalence of hypothyroidism following traumatic brain injury or subarachnoid haemorrhage, although TSH deficiency is less common than growth hormone, luteinizing hormone/follicle-stimulating hormone, and adrenocorticotropic hormone deficiencies (34). Bexarotene, a selective ligand for the retinoid X receptor which has been approved for the treatment of cutaneous T-cell lymphoma, may cause central hypothyroidism, with marked reductions in serum TSH and thyroid hormone levels in a significant proportion of treated patients (35). Pituitary aplasia or hypoplasia is a rare congenital defect, usually associated with other severe malformations. In most instances these patients die shortly after birth. Genetic abnormalities in TSH synthesis may cause central hypothyroidism characterized by inherited isolated TSH deficiency. Mutations in the TSH β-subunit gene or in a pituitary-specific transcription factor (Pit1/GHF-1) have been described in a few families (36, 37). Inactivating mutations in the thyrotropin-releasing hormone (TRH) receptor gene have also been reported (38, 39). In some patients no demonstrable pathology can be found to explain TSH deficiency, and the term idiopathic central hypothyroidism is therefore applied. Impairment of TRH secretion, TSH synthesis, or TSH release have been hypothesized in the pathogenesis of this disorder.

Transient impairment of TSH secretion is commonly observed and may depend on a variety of causes (see Box 3.4.2.2). The recognition of these conditions is essential to avoid unnecessary and expensive diagnostic procedures. In most instances replacement therapy is not necessary or is contraindicated.

Table 3.4.2.1 Differential diagnosis of hypothyroidism

	Primary	Central	Resistance to thyroid hormone	Nonthyroidal illness
Symptoms of hypothyroidism	Present	Present	Occasionally present	Absent
Thyroid volume	↑, N, ↓	N, ↓	↑	N
TSH	↑	N, ↓, (↑)	N, ↑	N, ↓, (↑)
Free T_4	↓	↓	↑	N, ↓, (↑)
Free T_3	N, ↓	N, ↓	↑	↓
Radio-iodine uptake	↑, N, ↓	↓	↑	N, ↓
TSH response to TRH	↑	N, ↓	↑	N, ↓, (↑)

↑, increased; N, normal; ↓, decreased; (·), slight changes.

Laboratory investigation of hypothyroidism

The diagnosis of hypothyroidism and of its cause requires the evaluation of several clinical, laboratory, and instrumental parameters to manage the patient properly (Table 3.4.2.1).

Hormonal evaluation

A small decrease in thyroid secretion may produce only minor changes in serum concentrations of thyroid hormones that remain within the normal range. The most sensitive index of a reduction in serum thyroid hormone concentration is serum TSH because of a decrease in feedback inhibition of pituitary TSH secretion. Thus, elevated serum TSH is the earliest laboratory abnormality in patients with primary hypothyroidism. The combination of normal thyroid hormones and elevated TSH is defined as subclinical hypothyroidism (3). With the progression of thyroid dysfunction, serum levels of T_4 fall below the normal limit while serum T_3 may still be normal. This is because high TSH levels induce preferential secretion of T_3 by residual thyroid tissue.

The lack of TSH response to reduced thyroid hormone levels complicates the diagnosis of central hypothyroidism, and the finding of low serum T_4 is a prerequisite for the diagnosis of this condition. Usually in central hypothyroidism, basal serum TSH concentrations are inappropriately low with respect to reduced serum thyroid hormones. Yet, in some instances serum TSH may be slightly elevated due to secretion of immunoreactive but biologically inactive TSH (40).

Assays for measurement of total thyroid hormones in serum are gradually being replaced by methods that determine the free (unbound) fraction of T_4 and T_3 (41). Although measurement of free T_4 and free T_3 concentrations is more cumbersome as compared to that for total T_4 and T_3, free T_4 and free T_3 determinations are preferred because free thyroid hormones are those capable of entering the cell and therefore represent the biologically active hormone. Indeed, the concentrations of total thyroid hormones may be elevated or reduced in spite of normal free fractions, due to changes in the concentrations of serum transport protein (see Chapter 3.1.2) (42).

Measurement of the serum TSH response to TRH (200–500 μg intravenously) may be useful in selected patients with a borderline to low value of T_4 and borderline to high or borderline to low values of basal TSH, to identify subclinical primary or central hypothyroidism, respectively. An exaggerated response will be observed in primary hypothyroidism whereas in central hypothyroidism the serum response of TSH may be reduced or abnormally prolonged. The TRH test may be useful also to measure the increase in serum T_3 levels following the rise in serum TSH. In people with normal thyroid function, serum T_3 increases 30–100% above the baseline value 120–180 min after the injection of 200 μg TRH. In central hypothyroidism, the T_3 response may be impaired or absent in spite of a normal peak of TSH, indicating secretion of biologically inactive TSH (43). Evaluation of the nocturnal surge of TSH in samples taken every 30 min from 11.00 p.m. to 2.00 a.m. may be useful to confirm the diagnosis of central hypothyroidism. At variance with people with normal thyroid function, the TSH surge is blunted or absent in central hypothyroid patients (44).

A transient phase of central hypothyroidism may occur in patients with nonthyroidal illness, particularly hospitalized patients with medical or psychiatric illnesses. In these cases repeated hormonal measurements are useful since values usually become normal as patients recover from that illness.

Other *in vitro* tests

Antithyroglobulin and antithyroperoxidase antibodies are sensitive markers of thyroid autoimmunity. Thus, if present, they may contribute to the diagnosis of autoimmune thyroiditis, represent a prognostic index for the development of postpartum thyroiditis, and help to predict the outcome of iodine- or drug-induced hypothyroidism. Antithyroglobulin antibodies are found in up to 70% of patients and antithyroperoxidase antibodies in 80–95% of patients with chronic autoimmune thyroiditis. Low titres can be found in 20–35% of patients with other nonautoimmune thyroid diseases and sometimes also in people with normal thyroid function (45). L-thyroxine therapy has been shown to reduce serum levels of antithyroglobulin antibodies and antithyroperoxidase antibodies in patients with autoimmune chronic thyroiditis. TSH-receptor antibodies can either have stimulating activity (thyroid-stimulating antibody), as in Graves' disease, or block the receptor (TSH-receptor blocking antibody) preventing TSH stimulation of the follicular cell. TSH-receptor blocking antibodies are highly specific for autoimmune thyroiditis. They are found in up to 30% of patients with chronic autoimmune thyroiditis and can produce or add to the development of hypothyroidism by blocking the thyroid response to TSH (6). Hypothyroidism produced by TSH-receptor blocking antibodies can spontaneously remit following disappearance of antibody from serum. Assays for TSH-receptor antibodies measure the ability of a patient's IgG to inhibit the binding of ^{125}I-TSH to its receptor in thyroid membrane preparations. Radioreceptor assays are now easy to perform, inexpensive, and provide reliable results but do not distinguish thyroid-stimulating antibodies from

TSH-receptor blocking antibodies. For this purpose methods that assess the capacity of IgG to stimulate or to prevent TSH-induced cAMP production in thyroid preparations are necessary.

Endogenous antibodies against thyroid hormones may develop in patients with autoimmune thyroiditis (46). These antibodies usually have no clinical relevance, but may interfere on assays for serum total and free T_4 and T_3, producing artefactual results depending on the technique used to measure the hormones. The presence of T_4 or T_3 antibodies should always be suspected in autoimmune patients with unexpected results of thyroid hormone assays. These antibodies can be detected easily by immunoprecipitation of radiolabelled T_4 or T_3 with the patient's serum.

Thyroglobulin is present at low concentrations in serum of people with normal thyroid function, and is elevated in all states associated with enlargement, hyperfunction, or injury of the thyroid gland (47). Measurement of serum thyroglobulin has no meaning for the diagnosis or the management of hypothyroidism, but may be useful to estimate the amount of residual thyroid tissue after surgery or other thyroid destructive events. Furthermore, detectable serum thyroglobulin in congenital hypothyroidism excludes thyroid agenesis. Antithyroglobulin antibodies in serum interfere with measurement of thyroglobulin and therefore this test should not be performed in such patients.

Measurement of urinary iodide provides information about the daily iodide intake in epidemiological studies (48). The demonstration of elevated concentrations of urinary iodide in a hypothyroid patient may be useful if exposure to excessive iodide is suspected.

Thyroid imaging in hypothyroidism

Ultrasonography

Thyroid ultrasonography may be helpful in determining the cause of hypothyroidism by providing important information on location, size, structure, and vascularity of the gland. In autoimmune thyroiditis a gross inhomogeneity and low echogenicity characterize the echo pattern of the gland. Areas of apparently normal tissue of variable size may be observed, whereas true nodules reflect a different aetiology and should raise the possibility of coexisting nodular goiter, adenomas, or malignancies. A diffuse low thyroid echogenicity is indicative of diffuse autoimmune involvement of the gland and is associated with or may predict the development of hypothyroidism (49). Studies using colour flow Doppler show a variable degree of vascularity in goitrous autoimmune thyroiditis, whereas vascularity is decreased in the atrophic variant of the disease. In subacute thyroiditis the gland is usually enlarged and presents large hypoechoic areas with poorly defined boundaries, mainly within the painful lobe. A large diffuse or multinodular goiter can be documented by ultrasonography in hypothyroidism with inherited defects in thyroid hormone biosynthesis. No evidence of thyroidal tissue in its appropriate location and the demonstration of an ectopic gland are helpful in the diagnosis of congenital hypothyroidism due to thyroid dysgenesis.

In vivo isotopic tests

Thyroid scintiscan may be helpful in the evaluation of hypothyroid patients to indicate the location of functioning thyroid tissue and to provide an estimation of overall thyroid size, although in this regard better evidence is usually obtained by thyroid ultrasonography. Occasionally scintiscan may reveal ectopic thyroid tissue not discernible by other means (e.g. lingual thyroid). Thyroid scintiscan can also be used to reveal substernal thyroid tissue when hypothyroidism is associated with a large goiter.

Radio-iodine uptake is expressed as the percentage of radioactivity that is trapped by the thyroid at a given time after administration of a tracer quantity of inorganic radio-iodine. Early radio-iodine uptake measurements (3–6 h) provide information on the rates of transport and organification of iodide within the gland, whereas 24- and 48-h radio-iodine uptake measurement reflects the rate of release of radio-iodine from thyroidal tissue. It is also a way of estimating the extrathyroidal pool of iodide, being low to absent after intake of excess iodide but increased in iodine deficiency. An exception is represented by amiodarone-induced hypothyroidism in which radio-iodine uptake is preserved despite iodine excess (50). Radio-iodine uptake is increased if hypothyroidism is caused by defective synthesis of thyroid hormones since TSH stimulates all steps in hormone synthesis capable of response. In chronic autoimmune thyroiditis values of the radio-iodine uptake depend on the amount of residual functioning thyroid tissue and the serum concentration of TSH. Radio-iodine uptake may be normal or even increased during the initial phase of chronic thyroiditis, whereas it tends to decrease as the disease progresses. Very low values of the radio-iodine uptake are characteristic of the early phase of destructive thyroiditis (e.g. subacute thyroiditis) which is usually associated with thyrotoxicosis caused by follicular disruption. In these cases, return of radio-iodine uptake to within the normal range may be helpful to indicate recovery of thyroid function. Radio-iodine uptake measurement, which is obviously reduced in postablative hypothyroidism, may be used occasionally to estimate the amount of residual thyroid tissue after thyroidectomy or radioactive treatment.

References

1. Devdhar M, Ousman YH, Burman KD. Hypothyroidism. *Endocrinol Metab Clin North Am*, 2007; **36**: 595–615.
2. Carlè A, Pedersen IB, Knudsen N, Perrild H, Oversen L, Jorgensen T, *et al.* Thyroid volume in hypothyroidism due to autoimmune disease follows a unimodal distribution: evidence against primary thyroid atrophy and autoimmune thyroiditis being distinct diseases. *J Clin Endocrinol Metab*, 2009; **94**: 833–9.
3. Tunbridge WM, Brewis M, French JM, Appleton D, Bird T, Clark F, *et al.* Natural history of autoimmune thyroiditis. *BMJ*, 1981; **282**: 258–62.
4. Wiersinga WM. Subclinical hypothyroidism and hyperthyroidism. I. Prevalence and clinical relevance. *Neth J Med*, 1995; **46**: 197–204.
5. Mariotti S, Chiovato L, Franceschi C, Pinchera A. Thyroid autoimmunity and aging. *Exp Gerontol*, 1998; **33**: 535–41.
6. Chiovato L, Vitti P, Santini F, Lopez G, Mammoli C, Bassi P, *et al.* Incidence of antibodies blocking thyrotropin effect *in vitro* in patients with euthyroid or hypothyroid autoimmune thyroiditis. *J Clin Endocrinol Metab*, 1990; **71**: 40–5.
7. Ludgate M, Emerson CH. Metamorphic thyroid autoimmunity. *Thyroid*, 2008; **18**: 1035–7.
8. Mizukami Y, Michigishi T, Nonomura A, Nakamura S, Ishizaki T. Pathology of chronic thyroiditis: a new clinically relevant classification. *Pathol Annu*, 1994; **29**: 135–58.
9. Bachrach LK, Foley TP Jr. Thyroiditis in children. *Pediatr Rev*, 1989; **11**: 184–91.
10. Lazarus JH. Clinical manifestations of postpartum thyroid disease. *Thyroid*, 1999; **9**: 685–9.
11. Wood LC, Ingbar SH. Hypothyroidism as a late sequela in patient with Graves' disease treated with antithyroid agents. *J Clin Invest*, 1979; **64**: 1429–36.
12. Volpe R. The management of subacute (DeQuervain's) thyroiditis. *Thyroid*, 1993; **3**: 253–5.

13. Schwaegerle SM, Bauer TW, Esselstyn CB Jr. Riedel's thyroiditis. *Am J Clin Pathol*, 1988; **90**: 715–22.
14. Cunnien AJ, Hay ID, Gorman CA, Offord KP, Scanlon PW. Radioiodine-induced hypothyroidism in Graves' disease: factors associated. *J Nucl Med*, 1982; **23**: 978–83.
15. Chiovato L, Santini F, Pinchera A. Treatment of hyperthyroidism. *Thyroid Int*, 1995; **2**: 1–16.
16. DeGroot LJ. Effects of irradiation on the thyroid gland. *Endocrinol Metab Clin North Am*, 1993; **22**: 607–15.
17. Carlson K, Lonnerholm G, Smedmyr B, Oberg G, Simonsson B. Thyroid function after autologous bone marrow transplantation. *Bone Marrow Transplant*, 1992; **10**: 123–7.
18. Smith GL, Smith BD, Giordano SH, Shih YC, Woodward WA, Strom EA, *et al.* Risk of hypothyroidism in older breast cancer patients treated with radiation. *Cancer*, 2008; **112**: 1371–9.
19. Martino E, Aghini-Lombardi F, Bartalena L, Grasso L, Loviselli A, Velluzzi F, *et al.* Enhanced susceptibility to amiodarone-induced hypothyroidism in patients with thyroid autoimmune disease. *Arch Intern Med*, 1994; **154**: 2722–6.
20. Kleiner J, Altshuler L, Hendrick V, Hershman JM. Lithium-induced subclinical hypothyroidism: review of the literature and guidelines for treatment. *J Clin Psychiatry*, 1999; **60**: 249–55.
21. Desai J, Yassa L, Marqusee E, George S, Frates MC, Chen MH, *et al.* Hypothyroidism after sunitinib treatment for patients with gastrointestinal stromal tumors. *Ann Intern Med*, 2006; **145**: 660–4.
22. Illouz F, Laboureau-Soares S, Dubois S, Rohmer V, Rodien P. Tyrosine kinase inhibitors and modifications of thyroid function tests: a review. *Eur J Endocrinol*, 2009; **160**: 331–6.
23. Kaplan MM. Interaction between drugs and thyroid hormones. *Thyroid Today*, 1981; **4**: 5.
24. Delange F, Camus M, Ermans AM. Circulating thyroid hormones in endemic goiter. *J Clin Endocrinol Metab*, 1972; **34**: 891–5.
25. Utiger RD. Maternal hypothyroidism and fetal development. *N Engl J Med*, 1999; **341**: 601–2.
26. Brucker-Davis F. Effects of environmental synthetic chemicals on thyroid function. *Thyroid*, 1998; **8**: 827–56.
27. Tiosano D, Hochberg Z. Endocrine complications of thalassemia. *J Endocrinol Invest*, 2001; **24**: 716–23.
28. De Sanctis V, De Sanctis E, Ricchieri P, Gubellini E, Gilli G, Gamberini MR. Mild subclinical hypothyroidism in thalassemia major: prevalence, multigated radionuclide test, clinical and laboratory long-term follow-up study. *Pediatr Endocrinol Rev*, 2008; **6** (Suppl 1): 174–80.
29. LaFranchi S. Congenital hypothyroidism: etiologies, diagnosis, and management. *Thyroid*, 1999; **9**: 735–40.
30. Burrow GN, Fisher DA, Larsen PR. Maternal and fetal thyroid function. *N Engl J Med*, 1994; **331**: 1072–8.
31. Montanelli L, Pinchera A, Santini F, Cavaliere R, Vitti P, Chiovato L. Transient congenital hypothyroidism: physiopathology and clinica. *Ann Ist Super Sanita*, 1998; **34**: 321–9.
32. van der Gaag RD, Drexhage HA, Dussault JH. Role of maternal immunoglobulins blocking TSH-induced thyroid growth in sporadic forms of congenital hypothyroidism. *Lancet*, 1985; **i**: 246–50.
33. Martino E, Pinchera A. Central hypothyroidism. In: Braverman LE, Utiger Rd, eds. *Werner & Ingbar's The Thyroid*. Philadelphia: Lippincott-Raven, 2005: 754–67.
34. Yamada M, Mori M. Mechanisms related to the pathophysiology and management of central hypothyroidism. *Nat Clin Pract Endocrinol Metab*, 2008; **4**: 683–94.
35. Golden WM, Weber KB, Hernandez TL, Sherman SI, Woodmansee WW, Haugen BR. Single-dose rexinoid rapidly and specifically suppresses serum thyrotropin in normal subjects. *J Clin Endocrinol Metab*, 2007; **92**: 124–30.
36. Hayashizaki Y, Hiraoka Y, Tatsumi K, Hashimoto T, Furuyama J, Miyai K, *et al.* Deoxyribonucleic acid analyses of five families with familial inherited thyroid stimulating hormone deficiency. *J Clin Endocrinol Metab*, 1990; **71**: 792–6.
37. Pfaffle RW, Martinez R, Kim C, Frisch H, Lebl J, Otten B, *et al.* GH and TSH deficiency. *Exp Clin Endocrinol Diabetes*, 1997; **105** (Suppl 4): 1–5.
38. Collu R, Tang J, Castagné J, Lagacé G, Masson N, Huot C, *et al.* A novel mechanism for isolated central hypothyroidism: inactivating mutations in the thyrotropin-releasing hormone receptor gene. *J Clin Endocrinol Metab*, 1997; **82**: 1561–5.
39. Bonomi M, Busnelli M, Beck-Peccoz P, Costanzo D, Antonica F, Dolci C, *et al.* A family with complete resistance to thyrotropin-releasing hormone. *N Engl J Med*, 2009; **360**: 731–4.
40. Beck-Peccoz P, Persani L. Variable biological activity of thyroid-stimulating hormone. *Eur J Endocrinol*, 1994; **131**: 331–40.
41. Bartalena L, Bogazzi F, Brogioni S, Burelli A, Scarcello G, Martino E. Measurement of serum free thyroid hormone concentrations: an essential tool for the diagnosis of thyroid dysfunction. *Horm Res*, 1996; **45**: 142–7.
42. Bartalena L. Recent achievements in studies on thyroid hormone-binding proteins. *Endocr Rev*, 1990; **11**: 47–64.
43. Faglia G, Ferrari C, Paracchi A, Spada A, Beck-Peccoz P. Triiodothyronine response to thyrotropin releasing hormone in patients with hypothalamic-pituitary disorders. *Clin Endocrinol*, 1975; **4**: 585–90.
44. Bartalena L, Martino E, Falcone M, Buratti L, Grasso L, Mammoli C, *et al.* Evaluation of the nocturnal serum thyrotropin (TSH) surge, as assessed by TSH ultrasensitive assay, in patients receiving long term L-thyroxine suppression therapy and in patients with various thyroid disorders. *J Clin Endocrinol Metab*, 1987; **65**: 1265–71.
45. Drexhage HA. The spectrum of thyroid autoimmune diseases. Pathogenetic mechanisms. *Thyroid Int*, 1994; **4**: 3–16.
46. Pietras SM, Safer JD. Diagnostic confusion attributable to spurious elevation of both total thyroid hormone and thyroid hormone uptake measurements in the setting of autoantibodies: case report and review of related literature. *Endocr Pract*, 2008; **14**: 738–42.
47. Spencer CA. Thyroglobulin. In: Braverman LE, Utiger RD, eds. *Werner & Ingbar's The Thyroid*. Philadelphia: Lippincott-Raven, 2005: 345–59.
48. Rendl J, Bier D, Reiners C. Methods for measuring iodine in urine and serum. *Exp Clin Endocrinol Diabetes*, 1998; **106** (Suppl 4): S34–41.
49. Marcocci C, Vitti P, Cetani F, Catalano F, Concetti R, Pinchera A. Thyroid ultrasonography helps to identify patients with diffuse lymphocytic thyroiditis who are prone to develop hypothyroidism. *J Clin Endocrinol Metab*, 1991; **72**: 209–13.
50. Wiersinga WM, Touber JL, Trip MD, van Royen EA. Uninhibited thyroidal uptake of radioiodine despite iodine excess in amiodarone-induced hypothyroidism. *J Clin Endocrinol Metab*, 1986; **63**: 485–91.

3.4.3 Myxoedema coma

Joanna Klubo-Gwiezdzinska, Leonard Wartofsky

Introduction

Myxoedema coma is the extreme expression of severe hypothyroidism and fortunately is quite rare. The first reported case appears to have been in 1879 by Ord from St Thomas's Hospital, London. Two other patients who died in a hypothyroid coma were reported in 1888 in the proceedings of the Clinical Society of London (1). The next cases in the literature appeared in 1953 (2, 3), and some

300 cases have since been reported. Epidemiological data indicate an incidence rate of 0.22/1 000 000 per year (4). The most common presentation of the syndrome is in hospitalized elderly women with long-standing hypothyroidism, with 80% of cases occurring in women over 60 years of age. However, myxoedema coma occurs in younger patients as well, with 36 documented cases occurring during pregnancy (5, 6). In spite of early diagnosis and treatment, the mortality rate may be as high as 40–60%.

Clinical presentation and precipitating events

Patients with myxoedema coma generally present in the winter months, suggesting that external cold may be an aggravating factor. Other precipitating events include pulmonary infections, congestive heart failure, and cerebrovascular accidents (Box 3.4.3.1). The comatose and hypoventilating patient is also at risk for pulmonary infection or aspiration pneumonia as a secondary event. Similarly, other abnormalities frequently accompanying myxoedema coma, such as hypoglycaemia, hypercalcaemia, hyponatraemia, hypercapnia, and hypoxaemia, may be either precipitating factors or secondary consequences. In hospitalized patients, drugs such as anaesthetics, narcotics, sedatives, antidepressants, and tranquillizers may depress respiratory drive and thereby either cause or compound the deterioration of the hypothyroid patient into coma.

Hypothermia (often profound to 80 °F (26.7 °C)) and unconsciousness constitute two of the cardinal features of myxoedema coma. The syndrome will typically present in a patient who develops an infection or other systemic disease superimposed upon previously undiagnosed hypothyroidism. Sometimes a history of antecedent thyroid disease, thyroidectomy, treatment with radioactive iodine, or thyroxine (T_4) replacement therapy that was discontinued for no apparent reason can be elicited. Other clues to the presence of underlying thyroid disease may be seen on examination of the neck, such as a surgical thyroidectomy scar, goiter, or even the absence of palpable thyroid tissue as may be seen in chronic Hashimoto's thyroiditis. A pituitary or hypothalamic basis for hypothyroidism is encountered in less than 10–15% of patients. In one large series (7) that identified 12 patients with myxoedema coma, the findings on presentation included hypoxaemia in 80%, hypercapnia in 54%, and hypothermia with a temperature below 94 °F (34.4 °C) in 88%. Six patients died despite treatment with thyroid hormone. A dreaded aspect of the usual clinical course is progression into respiratory failure and CO_2 retention which is heralded by hypoventilation with lethargy progressing to stupor and then coma. Because of the delayed metabolism of drugs in hypothyroidism, the deterioration may be hastened by the use of sedative hypnotics or narcotics.

Box 3.4.3.1 Myxoedema coma: precipitating factors

- Cerebrovascular accidents
  - Drugs
  - Anaesthetics
  - Sedatives
  - Tranquillizers
  - Narcotics
  - Amiodarone
  - Lithium carbonate
- Hypothermia
- Congestive heart failure
- Infections
- Trauma
- Gastrointestinal bleeding
- Metabolic disturbances compounding obtundation
  - Acidosis
  - Hypoglycaemia
  - Hyponatraemia
  - Hypercapnia

Cardiovascular manifestations

In myxoedema coma, typical findings of hypothyroid heart disease may include bradycardia, decreased quality and intensity of the heart sounds, enlarged cardiac silhouette, and minor ECG abnormalities such as varying degrees of block, low voltage, flattened or inverted T waves, and prolonged Q–T interval which can result in *torsades de pointe* ventricular tachycardia (8). Myocardial infarction should be ruled out by the usual diagnostic procedures. The lactate dehydrogenase isoenzyme pattern in severe hypothyroidism may mimic that of myocardial infarction (9), and creatine kinase levels also are elevated (10, 11). Moreover, aggressive or injudicious T_4 replacement may increase the risk of myocardial infarction (see below). The enlarged cardiac silhouette may be due, in part, to ventricular dilatation or a pericardial effusion which can be confirmed by echocardiography. This fluid is rich in mucopolysaccharide and tends to accumulate slowly over time, only rarely causing cardiac tamponade.

Cardiac contractility is impaired, leading to reduced stroke volume and cardiac output, but congestive heart failure is rare. T_4 replacement therapy will slowly reverse the abnormalities in left ventricular function; although the pericardial effusion may also gradually diminish, reduced cardiac output with hypotension secondary to the effusion must be borne in mind. Patients should be admitted to an intensive care unit because of the propensity for shock and potentially fatal arrhythmias. Hypotension may occur in spite of increases in total body water and extracellular fluid volume because of reduction in intravascular volume. Although blood pressure may be normalized with T_4 replacement, severe hypotension or shock may supervene acutely before the T_4 effect is seen, necessitating the use of pressor drugs.

Respiratory system

The mechanism for hypoventilation in profound myxoedema is a combination of a depressed hypoxic respiratory drive and a depressed ventilatory response to hypercapnia (12). CO_2 narcosis results from the reduction in alveolar ventilation with the hypoventilation compounded by impairment in respiratory muscle function ultimately leading to coma. The central factor in the pathophysiology of coma appears to be a depressed ventilatory response to CO_2 (13–15). When present, obesity may impair the bellows action of the chest. Improvement in the response to CO_2

after T_4 therapy has been seen in some (13, 15, 16) but not all (12) studies. Irrespective of the underlying pathophysiology, the mechanical function of the chest in myxoedema coma usually is reduced sufficiently to require mechanically assisted ventilation. Tidal volume may be reduced by other factors such as pleural effusion or ascites. Upper airway partial obstruction may also play a role, caused by oedema or swelling of the tongue, or laryngeal obstruction due to marked oedema of the vocal cords. Hypothyroid patients may be predisposed to increased airway hyper-responsiveness and chronic inflammation (17). Even with appropriate and adequate therapy, the complexity of the pathophysiology of respiratory failure means that ultimate recovery may be prolonged.

Gastrointestinal manifestations

The gastrointestinal tract in myxoedema may be marked by mucopolysaccharide infiltration and oedema of the muscularis and neuropathic changes leading to impaired peristalsis, obstipation, and potential paralytic ileus. Given the risks of anaesthesia in the profoundly hypothyroid patient, surgical intervention should be temporized for apparent obstruction by conservative management with decompression until the therapeutic response to thyroid hormone might occur. Initially, parenteral administration of T_4 or triiodothyronine (T_3) may be preferable because absorption of oral medications could be impaired due to the gastric atony often present in myxoedema coma. Ascites has been documented in 51 cases (18) and gastrointestinal bleeding can occur secondary to a coagulopathy.

Renal and electrolyte manifestations

Alterations in mineral metabolism and renal clearance in severe hypothyroidism may include decreases in plasma volume, serum sodium and osmolality, glomerular filtration rate, and renal plasma flow, and increases in total body water, urine sodium, and urine osmolality. Atony of the urinary bladder with retention of large residual urine volumes is commonly seen. High creatine kinase levels are typical of hypothyroidism, but unusually high values may be a clue to underlying rhabdomyolysis. Increased serum antidiuretic hormone levels (19) and impaired water diuresis caused by reduced delivery of water to the distal nephron (20) are likely to account for the hyponatraemia. Depending upon its duration and severity, hyponatraemia will add to altered mental status, and when severe may be largely responsible for precipitating the comatose state. T_4 treatment promotes water diuresis resulting in an increase in serum sodium and a decrease in oedema and total body water.

Neuropsychiatric manifestations

Although coma is the predominant clinical presentation in myxoedema coma, a history of disorientation, depression, paranoia, or hallucinations ('myxoedema madness') may often be elicited. Other findings present either just before entering the comatose state or early during recovery include cerebellar signs, such as poorly coordinated purposeful movements of the hands and feet, ataxia, adiadochokinesia, poor memory and recall, or even frank amnesia. Abnormal findings on electroencephalography are few and include low amplitude and a decreased rate of α-wave activity. Status epilepticus has been described (21) and up to 25% of patients with myxoedema coma may experience minor to major seizures possibly related to hyponatraemia, hypoglycaemia, or hypoxaemia due to reduced cerebrovascular perfusion from low cardiac output and atherosclerotic vessels in elderly patients. T_4 treatment will generally lead to improved perfusion.

Haematological manifestations

A microcytic anaemia may be seen secondary to gastrointestinal haemorrhage, or a macrocytic anaemia due to vitamin B_{12} deficiency which may also worsen the neurological state. Granulocytopenia with a decreased cell-mediated immunological response may contribute to a higher risk of severe infection. In contrast to the tendency to thrombosis seen in mild hypothyroidism, severe hypothyroidism is associated with a higher risk of bleeding due to coagulopathy related to an acquired von Willebrand's syndrome (type 1) and decreases in factors V, VII, VIII, IX, and X (22). The von Willebrand syndrome is reversible with T_4 therapy (23). Another cause of bleeding may be disseminated intravascular coagulation associated with sepsis.

Hypothermia

The first clinical clue to the diagnosis of myxoedema coma may be hypothermia which occurs in approximately 75% of patients and may be dramatic (below 80°F (26.7°C)), with temperatures of less than 90°F (32.2°C) being associated with the worst prognosis. Because patients with myxoedema and infection may not mount a febrile response, a diagnosis of profound hypothyroidism should be entertained in any unconscious patient with a known infection but no fever. In view of the latter and because undiscovered infection might lead inexorably to vascular collapse and death, some authors have advocated the routine use of antibiotics in patients with myxoedema coma. Underlying hypoglycaemia may further compound the decrement in body temperature. With T_4 therapy, the hypothermia gradually improves in parallel with the fall in serum thyroid-stimulating hormone (TSH) and increments in serum T_4 and T_3 levels.

Diagnosis

The typical patient presenting with myxoedema coma is a woman in the later decades of her life who may have a history of thyroid disease and who is admitted to hospital during the winter months, possibly with pneumonitis. Physical findings could include bradycardia, macroglossia, hoarseness, delayed reflexes, dry skin, general cachexia, hypoventilation, and hypothermia, commonly without shivering. Laboratory evaluation may indicate anaemia, hyponatraemia, hypercholesterolaemia, and increased serum lactate dehydrogenase and creatine kinase. On lumbar puncture there is increased pressure and the cerebrospinal fluid will have a high protein content. The electrocardiogram and chest radiograph may demonstrate the characteristic findings described above. If hypothyroidism is suspected in a comatose patient, blood should be obtained for thyroid function testing but treatment should not be delayed to await laboratory confirmation of the diagnosis. On the other hand, a correct diagnosis is particularly important because the unnecessary administration of large doses of T_4 or T_3 to an elderly euthyroid patient could induce a fatal arrhythmia or coronary event. In addition to routine thyroid function tests, ancillary studies should be performed to determine whether CO_2 retention, hypoxia, hyponatraemia, or infection are present. Indeed, in many patients the clinical features may be so notable as to render the measurement of thyroid function tests necessary only for confirmation of the diagnosis. The urgency of the diagnosis should be stressed to the laboratory, which often can perform a serum T_4 and TSH determination in 3–4 h. Although an elevated serum TSH concentration is the most important laboratory evidence of the diagnosis, the presence of severe complicating systemic illness or treatment with drugs such as dopamine, dobutamine, or corticosteroids may serve to reduce the elevation in TSH levels (24, 25). There may also be a pituitary cause for the hypothyroidism, in which case an increased TSH would not be found. Until the presence of pituitary disease is ruled out, corticosteroid therapy is recommended in addition to T_4.

Treatment

Myxoedema coma is a true medical emergency, and treatment must be instituted in a critical care setting with modern electronic monitoring equipment as soon as the diagnosis is made in view of the extremely high mortality anticipated in these patients when treatment is delayed. As outlined below, a multifaceted approach is required because of the multiple metabolic derangements derived from, or affecting, several organ systems which may be contributing to the comatose state.

Ventilatory support

The patient's comatose state is perpetuated by hypoventilation with CO_2 retention and respiratory acidosis. Appropriate diagnostic and therapeutic measures must be instituted for any suspicious infiltrate seen on chest radiographs. The high mortality rate is often related to inexorable respiratory failure, and hence maintenance of an adequate airway and prevention of hypoxaemia is the single most important supportive measure required to avoid a disastrous outcome. Mechanical ventilation is usually required during the first 36–48 h, particularly if the hypoventilation is related in part to drug-related respiratory depression. Although the patient may become alert by the second or third day of treatment, it may be necessary to continue assisted ventilation for as long as 2–3 weeks in some patients.

Intubation may be necessary initially or with worsening of hypoxaemia or hypercarbia, and arterial blood gases need to be monitored regularly until the patient is fully recovered. The hypercapnia may be rapidly relieved with mechanical ventilation, but the hypoxia may tend to persist possibly due to shunting in nonaerated lung areas (26). Moreover, the physician should guard against extubating the patient prematurely; some case reports have cited the danger of relapse, and it should not be attempted until the patient is fully conscious.

Hyponatraemia

Total body sodium is believed to be normal to increased, but it is the impaired excretion of water that causes hyponatraemia. Low serum sodium may cause a semicomatose state or seizures even in euthyroid patients, and the very severe hyponatraemia (105–120 mmol/l) in profound myxoedema is likely to contribute substantially to the coma in these patients. With such severe hyponatraemia, it may be appropriate to administer a small amount of hypertonic saline (50–100 ml 3% sodium chloride), enough to increase sodium concentration by about 2 mmol/l early in the course of treatment, and this can be followed by an intravenous bolus dose of 40–120 mg furosemide to promote a water diuresis (27).

A small quick increase in the serum sodium concentration (2–4 mmol/l) is effective in acute hyponatraemia because even a slight reduction in brain swelling results in a substantial decrease in intracerebral pressure (28). On the other hand, too rapid correction of hyponatraemia can cause a very dangerous complication, the osmotic demyelination syndrome. In patients with chronic hyponatraemia this complication is avoided by limiting the sodium correction to less than 10–12 mmol/l in 24 h and to less than 18 mmol/l in 48 h.

After achieving a sodium level of more than 120 mmol/l, no further hypertonic saline infusion should be required, and restriction of fluids may be all that is necessary to correct hyponatraemia, especially if it is mild (120–130 mmol/l). Because of the likelihood of decreased cardiac reserve, therapy with saline or other intravenous fluids must be approached cautiously. If hypoglycaemia is present, dextrose in 0.5 N sodium chloride may be used to correct the low blood glucose. With regard to fluid or saline therapy, careful monitoring of volume status based on clinical parameters and central venous pressure measurements is essential in patients with significant cardiovascular decompensation.

A new vasopressin antagonist, intravenous conivaptan, has been approved by the FDA for the treatment of hospitalized patients with euvolaemic and hypervolaemic hyponatraemia. This treatment could be attempted in this clinical setting in view of the high vasopressin levels observed in myxoedema coma. Current dosing recommendations are for a 20-mg loading dose to be infused over 30 min followed by 20 mg/day continuous infusion for up to 4 days. No data are available on the use of conivaptan in severe hyponatraemia (<115 mmol/L) in hypothyroid patients, or whether sole therapy with conivaptan without hypertonic saline would be effective (29).

Hypothermia

Restoration of body temperature to normal will require administration of T_4 or T_3. Blankets or increasing room temperature can be used to keep the patient warm until the thyroid hormone effect is achieved, but caution must be exercised in the use of more vigorous electric warming blankets. Too aggressive warming may cause peripheral vasodilatation, a precipitous fall in peripheral vascular resistance with increased peripheral blood flow, and increased oxygen consumption, which may then lead to hypotension or shock.

Hypotension

Hypotension should also be correctable by treatment with T_4; this may take several days and the hypotensive patient may require additional therapy. Fluids may be administered cautiously as 5–10% glucose in 0.5 N sodium chloride initially, or as isotonic normal saline if hyponatraemia is present. It is wise to administer hydrocortisone (100 mg intravenously every 8 h) until the hypotension is corrected. Pressors are only very rarely required, and the possibility of an adverse cardiac event needs to be kept in mind, especially in patients with suspected underlying ischaemic heart disease. An agent such as dopamine might be employed to maintain coronary blood flow, but patients should be weaned off the pressor as soon as possible. The physician must weigh the risk of a pressor-induced ischaemic event against the known high mortality of poorly managed hypotension in myxoedema coma.

Corticosteroids

A rising urea nitrogen, hypotension, hypothermia, hypoglycaemia, hyponatraemia, and hyperkalaemia may signal the coexistence of adrenal insufficiency. Indeed, decreased adrenal reserve has been found in 5–10% of patients on the basis of either hypopituitarism or primary adrenal failure accompanying Hashimoto's disease (Schmidt's syndrome). Otherwise, plasma total and free cortisol levels and the adrenal response to adrenocorticotropic hormone (ACTH) infusion should be normal in hypothyroidism or myxoedema coma. However, ACTH reserve or the ACTH response to stress may be impaired in myxoedema coma. There should be no reluctance to administer short-term corticosteroids until the patient is stable and the integrity of the pituitary–adrenal axis can be determined. On theoretical grounds, one should also administer corticosteroids when first instituting thyroid hormone therapy, in view of the potential risk of precipitating acute adrenal insufficiency due to the accelerated metabolism of cortisol that follows T_4 therapy. The typical dosage of hydrocortisone is 50–100 mg every 6–8 h during the first 7–10 days with tapering of the dosage thereafter based upon clinical response and any plans for further diagnostic evaluation.

Thyroid hormone therapy

One of the most controversial aspects of the management of myxoedema coma is which thyroid hormone medication to give and how to give it (dose, frequency, and route of administration). Because of the relative rarity of this condition, the paucity of reported treatment results, and the difficulties inherent in performing a controlled investigation, the optimum treatment remains uncertain, and several approaches will be discussed. Some of the differences of opinion relate to whether to administer T_4 and rely on the patient to convert it to the more active T_3, or to give T_3 itself. One must balance the need for quickly attaining physiologically effective thyroid hormone levels against the risk of precipitating a fatal tachyarrhythmia or myocardial infarction. T_4 provides a steady smooth onset of action with a lower risk of adverse effects.

Parenteral preparations of either T_4 or T_3 are available for intravenous administration. Although oral forms of either T_3 or T_4 can be given by nasogastric tube in the comatose patient, this route is fraught with risks of aspiration and uncertain absorption, particularly in the presence of gastric atony or ileus. Parenteral preparations of T_4 are available in ampoules of 100 and 500 µg. The latter dose, as a single intravenous bolus, was popularized by reports (30) suggesting that replacement of the entire estimated pool of extrathyroidal T_4 (usually 300–600 µg) was desirable to restore near-normal hormonal status. After this initial 'loading' dose, a maintenance dose of 50–100 µg is given daily (either intravenously or by mouth if the patient is adequately alert). This method may be attended by increases in serum T_4 to within the normal range within 24 h and by significant decrements in serum TSH. Larger doses of T_4 probably have no advantage and may, in fact, be more dangerous (31). Due to its conversion from T_4, a progressive increase in serum T_3 is seen after 300- to 600-µg doses of T_4, as has been described by Ridgway *et al.* (31).

The approach to therapy employing an initial large intravenous bolus dose of T_4 followed by maintenance therapy has been considered optimal (30, 31), but other evidence suggests improved outcomes with lower doses of thyroid hormone (32). This was also indicated in a prospective trial in which patients were randomized to receive either a 500-µg loading dose of intravenous T_4 followed by a 100-µg daily maintenance dose, or only the maintenance dose (34). The overall mortality rate was 36.4% with a lower mortality rate in the high dose group (17%) versus the low dose group (60%). Although suggestive, the difference was not statistically significant. Factors associated with a worse outcome included a decreased level of consciousness, lower Glasgow coma score, and increased severity of illness on entry as determined by an APACHE II score of more than 20.

T_4 treatment has been generally considered effective, but there is one important drawback to total reliance on T_3 generation from T_4. The rate of conversion of T_4 to T_3 is reduced in many systemic illnesses (the euthyroid sick or low T_3 syndrome) (25) and hence T_3 generation may be reduced in myxoedema coma as a consequence of any associated illness (27). Theoretically then, one might administer T_4, see increases in serum T_4 levels confirming adequate absorption, but fail to witness any significant fall in TSH or dramatic clinical improvement. As a consequence, small supplements of T_3 should be given along with T_4 during the initial few days of treatment, especially if obvious associated illness is present. Irrespective of the type of treatment selected, all patients should have continuous ECG monitoring with reduction in thyroid hormone dosage should arrhythmias or ischaemic changes be detected.

T_3 is available for intravenous use (Triostat) in 1 ml vials containing 10 µg/ml. When therapy is approached with T_3 alone, it may be given as a 10- to 20-µg bolus followed by 10 µg every 4 h for the first 24 h, dropping to 10 µg every 6 h for days 2–3, by which time oral administration should be feasible. T_3 has a much quicker onset of action than T_4 and increases in body temperature and oxygen consumption may occur 2–3 h after intravenous T_3, compared to 8–14 h after intravenous T_4. A patient with profound secondary myxoedema believed due to postpartum pituitary necrosis has been reported who presented with cardiogenic shock which responded to T_3 but not T_4 therapy (33). Because of the high mortality rate in myxoedema coma, advocates for T_3 therapy argue that the more rapid onset of action could make the difference between life and death. But the benefits of the more rapid onset of action need to be weighed against the greater risk of complications. As a consequence, it is difficult to justify the high risk/benefit ratio of a regimen that uses rapid replacement with relatively large doses of intravenous T_3 alone. Such treatment would be marked by large and unpredictable fluctuations in serum T_3 levels, and high serum T_3 levels during treatment with thyroid hormone have been associated with fatal outcomes (34).

A more conservative but seemingly rational course of management is to provide combined therapy with both T_4 and T_3. Rather than administer 300–500 µg T_4 intravenously initially, a dose of 4 µg/kg lean body weight (or about 200–300 µg) is given, and an additional 100 µg is given 24 h later. By the third day, the dose is reduced to a daily maintenance dose of 50 µg, which can be given by mouth as soon as the patient is conscious. Simultaneously with the initial dose of T_4, a bolus of 10 µg T_3 is given and intravenous T_3 is continued at a dosage of 10 µg every 8–12 h until the patient is conscious and taking maintenance T_4. Sensitivity to thyroid hormone in terms of cardiac risk varies, depending on age, cardiac medications, and the presence of underlying hypoxaemia, coronary artery disease, congestive failure, and electrolyte imbalance. Clinical improvement has been seen with even a single dose of only 2.5 μg T_3 (35). It is wise to monitor the patient for any untoward effects of therapy before administering each dose of thyroid hormone.

Myxoedema coma and emergent surgery

Clearly, given their fragile clinical state, nonemergent surgery should be deferred in a patient with myxoedema coma. However, in the patient with myxoedema coma requiring emergent surgery, the same general management principles prevail (36) with particular attention to careful monitoring of intraoperative and postoperative respiratory and cardiovascular status. Postoperatively, close monitoring for maintenance of the airway is essential.

General supportive measures

In addition to the specific therapies outlined, other treatments will be indicated as in the management of any other elderly patient with multisystemic problems. This might include the treatment of underlying problems such as infectious processes, congestive heart failure, diabetes, or hypertension. The dosage of specific medications (e.g. digoxin for congestive heart failure) may need to be modified based on their altered distribution and slowed metabolism in myxoedema. Even with this vigorous therapy, the prognosis for myxoedema coma remains grim, and patients with severe hypothermia and hypotension seem to do the worst. Several prognostic factors may be associated with a fatal outcome (32, 34, 37, 38) and include: older age, persistent hypothermia or bradycardia, lower degree of consciousness by Glasgow Coma Scale, multiorgan impairment indicated by an APACHE II score of more than 20, or SOFA score ≥6. The most common causes of death are respiratory failure, sepsis, and gastrointestinal bleeding. Early diagnosis and prompt treatment, with meticulous attention to the details of management during the first 48 h, remain critical for the avoidance of a fatal outcome.

References

1. Report of a committee of the Clinical Society of London to investigate the subject of myxedema. *Trans Clin Soc (Lond) (Suppl)*, 1888: **21**.
2. LeMarquand HS, Hausmann W, Hemstead EH. Myxedema as a cause of death. *BMJ (Clin Res)*, 1953; **1**: 704–6.
3. Summers VK. Myxedema coma. *BMJ (Clin Res)*, 1953; **2**: 336–8.
4. Rodríguez I, Fluiters E, Pérez-Méndez LF, Luna R, Páramo C, García-Mayor RV. Factors associated with mortality of patients with myxoedema coma: prospective study in 11 cases treated in a single institution. *J Endocrinol*, 2004; **180**: 347–50.
5. Blignault EJ. Advanced pregnancy in severely myxedematous patient. A case report and review of the literature. *S Afr Med J*, 1980; **57**: 1050–1.
6. Patel S, Robinson S, Bidgood RJ, Edmonds CJ. A pre-eclamptic-like syndrome associated with hypothyroidism during pregnancy. *Q J Med*, 1991; **79**: 435–41.
7. Reinhardt W, Mann K. Incidence, clinical picture and treatment of hypothyroid coma. Results of a survey. *Med Klin*, 1997; **92**: 521–4.
8. Schenck JB, Rizvi AA, Lin T. Severe primary hypothyroidism manifesting with torsades de pointes. *Am J Med Sci*, 2006; **331**: 154–6.
9. Aber CP, Noble RL, Thomson GS, Jones EW. Serum lactic dehydrogenase isoenzymes in 'myxedema heart disease'. *Br Heart J*, 1966; **28**: 663–73.
10. Nee PA, Scane SC, Lavelle PH, Fellows IW, Hill PG. Hypothermic myxedema coma erroneously diagnosed as myocardial infarction because of increased creatine kinase MB. *Clin Chem*, 1987; **33**: 1083–4.
11. Hickman PE, Silvester W, Musk AA, McLellan GH, Harris A. Cardiac enzyme change in myxedema coma. *Clin Chem*, 1987; **33**: 622–4.
12. Zwillich CW, Pierson DJ, Hofeldt FD, Lufkin EG, Weil JV. Ventilatory control in myxedema and hypothyroidism. *N Engl J Med*, 1975; **292**: 662–5.
13. Massumi RA, Winnacker JL. Severe depression of the respiratory center in myxedema. *Am J Med*, 1964; **36**: 876–82.
14. Ladenson PW, Goldenheim PD, Ridgway EC. Prediction of reversal of blunted respiratory responsiveness in patients with hypothyroidism. *Am J Med*, 1988; **84**: 877–83.
15. Domm BB, Vassallo CL. Myxedema coma with respiratory failure. *Am Rev Respir Dis*, 1973; **107**: 842–5.
16. Wilson WR, Bedell GN. The pulmonary abnormalities in myxedema. *J Clin Invest*, 1960; **39**: 42–55.
17. Birring SS, Patel RB, Parker D, McKenna S, Hargadon B, Monteiro WR, *et al.* Airway function and markers of airway inflammation in patients with treated hypothyroidism. *Thorax*, 2005; **60**: 249–53.
18. Ji JS, Chae HS, Cho YS, Kim HK, Kim SS, Kim CW, *et al.* Myxedema ascites: case report and literature review. *J Korean Med Sci*, 2006; **21**: 761–4.
19. Skowsky WR, Kikuchi TA. The role of vasopressin in the impaired water excretion of myxedema. *Am J Med*, 1978; **64**: 613–21.
20. DeRubertis FR Jr, Michelis MF, Bloom ME, Mintz DH, Field JB, Davis BB. Impaired water excretion in myxedema. *Am J Med*, 1971; **51**: 41–53.
21. Jansen HJ, Doebé SR, Louwerse ES, van der Linden JC, Netten PM. Status epilepticus caused by a myxoedema coma. *Neth J Med*, 2006; **64**: 202–5.
22. Manfredi E, van Zaane B, Gerdes VE, Brandjes DP, Squizzato A. Hypothyroidism and acquired von Willebrand's syndrome: a systematic review. *Haemophilia*, 2008; **14**: 423–33.
23. Michiels JJ, Schroyens W, Berneman Z, van der Planken M. Acquired von Willebrand syndrome type 1 in hypothyroidism: reversal after treatment with thyroxine. *Clin Appl Thromb Hemost*, 2001; **7**: 113–15.
24. Hooper MJ. Diminished TSH secretion during acute non-thyroidal illness in untreated primary hypothyroidism. *Lancet*, 1976; **i**: 48–9.
25. Wartofsky L, Burman KD. Alterations in thyroid function in patients with systemic illness: the 'euthyroid sick syndrome'. *Endocr Rev*, 1982; **3**: 164–217.
26. Nicoloff JT. Thyroid storm and myxedema coma. *Med Clin North Am*, 1985; **69**: 1005–17.
27. Pereira VG, Haron ES, Lima-Neto N, Medeiros-Neto GA. Management of myxedema coma: report on three successfully treated cases with nasogastric or intravenous administration of triiodothyronine. *J Endocrinol Invest*, 1982; **5**: 331–4.
28. Verbalis JG, Goldsmith SR, Greenberg A, Schrier RW, Sterns RH. Hyponatremia treatment guidelines 2007: expert panel recommendations. *Am J Med*, 2007; **120**: S1–21.
29. Hline SS, Pham PT, Pham PT, Aung MH, Pham PM, Pham PC. Conivaptan: a step forward in the treatment of hyponatremia. *Ther Clin Risk Manag*, 2008; **4**: 315–26.
30. Holvey DN, Goodner CJ, Nicoloff JT, Dowling JT. Treatment of myxedema coma with intravenous thyroxine. *Arch Intern Med*, 1964; **113**: 139–46.
31. Ridgway EC, McCammon JA, Benotti J, Maloof F. Acute metabolic responses in myxedema to large doses of intravenous L-thyroxine. *Ann Intern Med*, 1972; **77**: 549–55.
32. Yamamoto T, Fukuyama J, Fujiyoshi A. Factors associated with mortality of myxedema coma: report of eight cases and literature survey. *Thyroid*, 1999; **9**: 1167–74.

33. McKerrow SD, Osborn LA, Levy H, Eaton RP, Economou P. Myxedema-associated cardiogenic shock treated with triiodothyronine. *Ann Intern Med*, 1992; **117**: 1014–15.
34. Hylander B, Rosenqvist U. Treatment of myxoedema coma: factors associated with fatal outcome. *Acta Endocrinol (Copenh)*, 1985; **108**: 65–71.
35. McCulloch W, Price P, Hinds CJ, Wass JA. Effects of low dose oral triiodothyronine in myxoedema coma. *Intensive Care Med*, 1985; **11**: 259–62.
36. Mathes DD. Treatment of myxedema coma for emergency surgery. *Anesth Analg*, 1998; **86**: 450–1.
37. Jordan RM. Myxedema coma. Pathophysiology, therapy, and factors affecting prognosis. *Med Clin North Am*, 1995; **79**: 185–94.
38. Dutta P, Bhansali A, Masoodi SR, Bhadada S, Sharma N, Rajput R. Predictors of outcome in myxoedema coma: a study from a tertiary care centre. *Crit Care*, 2008; **12**: 1–8.

Further reading

Sanders V. Neurologic manifestations of myxedema. *N Engl J Med*, 1962; **266**: 547–52.
Kwaku MP, Burman KD. Myxedema coma. *J Intensive Care Med*, 2007; **22**: 224–31.
Fliers E, Wiersinga WM. Myxedema coma. *Rev Endocr Metab Disord*, 2003; **4**: 137–41.
Ringel MD. Management of hypothyroidism and hyperthyroidism in the intensive Care unit. *Crit Care Clin*, 2001; **17**: 59–74.

3.4.4 Subclinical hypothyroidism

Jayne A. Franklyn

Definition

Subclinical hypothyroidism is defined biochemically as the association of a raised serum thyroid-stimulating hormone (TSH) concentration with normal circulating concentrations of free thyroxine (T_4) and free triiodothyronine (T_3). The term subclinical hypothyroidism implies that patients should be asymptomatic, although symptoms are difficult to assess, especially in patients in whom thyroid function tests have been checked because of nonspecific complaints such as tiredness. An expert panel has recently classified individuals with subclinical hypothyroidism into two groups (1): (1) those with mildly elevated serum TSH (typically TSH in the range 4.5–10.0 mU/l) and (2) those with more marked TSH elevation (serum TSH >10.0 mU/l).

Prevalence, causes, and natural history of subclinical hypothyroidism

Several population-based studies have examined the prevalence of subclinical hypothyroidism. Variation in results reflects the demographic characteristics of the populations studied, as well as the upper limit set for TSH measurements. Considerable debate has surrounded the setting of the upper limit of the reference range for TSH, with some arguing in favour of reduction in this upper limit to a value which would include a large proportion of the adult population. Meticulous studies in the USA and elsewhere have addressed this question, taking into account the influence of inclusion or exclusion of individuals with a personal or family history of thyroid disease or those with positive antithyroid antibodies. Evidence from one such study (NHANES III) of a very large 'reference' population without evidence of thyroid disease has suggested that 95% of adults have a serum TSH within the range 0.45–4.12 mU/l (2), determining that the widely applied upper limit of normal for serum TSH measurements of approximately 4.5–5.0 mU/l remains appropriate.

Using this biochemical definition for TSH elevation, most studies including all ages and both sexes have revealed a prevalence of subclinical hypothyroidism of around 5–10%, the diagnosis being more common in women and increasing with increasing age (see Chapter 3.1.7). The NHANES III study in the USA found subclinical hypothyroidism (TSH >4.6 mU/l) in 4.3% (2), while the Whickham survey in the UK reported TSH of more than 6.0 mU/l in 7.5% of females and 2.8% of males (3). TSH did not vary with age in males but increased markedly in women aged more than 45 years. In the large Colorado study of people attending health fairs, 9.5% had raised TSH, 75% of whom had mildly elevated TSH in the range 5.0–10.0 mU/l and 25% of them were taking thyroid hormones (4). Our own study of 1210 patients aged over 60 years who were recruited in primary care revealed a prevalence of subclinical hypothyroidism of 11.6% in women and 2.9% in men in that age group (5). Significant titres of antithyroid antibodies were found in 46% of those with a serum TSH between 5 and 10 mU/l, and in 81% of those with a serum TSH greater than 10 mU/l, providing supporting evidence for underlying autoimmune thyroid disease in the majority. However, a recent community screening study of older people in the same area revealed a lower population prevalence of subclinical hypothyroidism of 2.9%, perhaps reflecting more frequent testing of thyroid function and earlier treatment of raised TSH in the intervening years (6).

The commonest cause of subclinical hypothyroidism is autoimmune thyroiditis. Another major cause is previous treatment for hyperthyroidism (Box 3.4.4.1). It is well known that treatment of hyperthyroidism with radio-iodine results in thyroid failure in at least 50% of patients (depending upon the dose administered) (7), a rise in TSH being the earliest biochemical indicator. Partial thyroidectomy for hyperthyroidism or nodular goiter is associated with a similar risk of development of hypothyroidism, which is again first identified by a rise in serum TSH. In the early months after both radio-iodine treatment and partial thyroidectomy, subclinical hypothyroidism may be a transient phenomenon not always indicative of progressive or permanent thyroid failure. Graves' disease is itself associated with the eventual development of hypothyroidism in 5–20% of patients (even in the absence of ablative thyroid treatment).

A further major category of patients with a biochemical diagnosis of subclinical hypothyroidism is that already treated with thyroxine for thyroid failure, a high serum TSH indicating that the dose prescribed is inadequate or compliance is poor. We found a raised serum TSH in approximately 25% of patients on T_4 identified in the community, with a close relationship evident between prescribed dose and TSH results, indicating that, at least in some patients (especially those prescribed T_4 in doses of 75 μg/day or

Box 3.4.4.1 Causes of subclinical hypothyroidism

- Causes or associations related to thyroid disease and its treatment
  - Autoimmune (Hashimoto's thyroiditis)
  - Previous radio-iodine therapy
  - Previous thyroid surgery
  - Graves' hyperthyroidism
  - Postpartum thyroiditis
  - Thyroxine therapy—poor compliance or inadequate dose prescription
- Other causes or associations
  - Radiotherapy to head or neck
  - Other autoimmune diseases, e.g. type 1 diabetes, Addison's disease, pernicious anaemia
  - Down's syndrome
  - Therapy with iodine-containing drugs, e.g. amiodarone
  - Other causes of iodine excess (kelp ingestion, radiographic contrast agents)
  - Lithium therapy
  - Nonthyroidal illness—especially recovery phase
  - Previous Graves' hyperthyroidism

less), the cause of subclinical hypothyroidism was inadequate dose prescription (8).

As well as those with a history of treatment for hyperthyroidism, other groups at particular risk of subclinical hypothyroidism include those with other autoimmune diseases such as type 1 diabetes mellitus and Addison's disease. (Glucocorticoid deficiency may itself be associated with a rise in serum TSH which is corrected by steroid replacement alone and is not necessarily indicative of underlying thyroid disease.) Down's syndrome is also associated with the development of both subclinical and overt thyroid failure of autoimmune aetiology. The risk of subclinical hypothyroidism during pregnancy is considerable in women identified in the first trimester as having positive antithyroid antibodies. This antibody status also represents a risk factor for the development of postpartum thyroiditis, subclinical or overt hypothyroidism being a feature of postpartum thyroiditis in about 75% of cases (9). While hypothyroidism may be a transient feature of postpartum thyroiditis, there is good evidence that the majority of affected women go on to develop permanent hypothyroidism after a period of months or years of follow-up (9). Subclinical hypothyroidism may also be a feature of thyroiditis which follows pregnancy loss, even of short duration.

A further well-documented cause of subclinical hypothyroidism is radiotherapy to the head and neck (which is itself associated with the development of positive antithyroid antibodies). Nonthyroidal illness may be associated with a transient and typically modest increase in serum TSH, especially in the recovery phase from illness, although in most instances, even in patients with subclinical hypothyroidism diagnosed in hospital, an underlying 'thyroid' cause can be identified. Therapy with drugs such as lithium can induce subclinical hypothyroidism, as can administration of iodine-containing compounds such as radiographic contrast agents. Treatment with the iodine-containing antiarrhythmic drug amiodarone frequently leads to a modest elevation in serum TSH early in treatment, reflecting inhibition of thyroid hormone release, as well as a later increased risk of overt thyroid failure which is first identified by a sustained and progressive rise in serum TSH. Even the use of topical iodine-containing antiseptics can result in thyroid dysfunction, subclinical hypothyroidism being identified in one study in 20.8% of iodine-exposed infants (10).

The natural history of subclinical hypothyroidism depends upon the underlying cause of the biochemical disturbance and the population studied. One large follow-up study has shown that in those with modest elevation of serum TSH (5.5–10.0 mU/l) the TSH measurement returns spontaneously to the reference range in more than 60% of cases during 5 years of follow-up (11). Transient cases may occur in the early weeks or months after recovery from nonthyroidal illness, in the first 6 months after partial thyroidectomy or radio-iodine, or after iodine exposure (e.g. after starting amiodarone). Our own study of people over the age of 60 in the community revealed that the finding of a raised serum TSH identified on screening disappeared in 5.5% after a period of 12 months, while the biochemical abnormality remained stable in 76.7% and relatively few (17.8%) progressed to overt hypothyroidism (the latter defined biochemically as elevation in serum TSH in association with a serum free T_4 below the reference range) (5). Follow-up for 20 years of the Whickham cohort in the north-east of England revealed an annual rate of progression of subclinical to overt hypothyroidism of 2.6% if thyroid antibodies were negative, but a rate of progression of 4.3% if antibodies to thyroid peroxidase were present (12). The risk of development of hypothyroidism in that population was greater if serum TSH was within the upper half rather than the lower half of the typical reference range, fuelling debate regarding the 'true' upper limit of normal for TSH.

Consequences of subclinical hypothyroidism

Given the prevalence of this biochemical diagnosis, much attention has focused upon the effects of mild thyroid hormone deficiency upon symptoms, quality of life, and cognitive function. Because of possible effects on the lipid profile, recent studies have focused on the cardiovascular system and effects on vascular morbidity and mortality. Epidemiological studies are beginning to provide insight into the question of whether subclinical hypothyroidism is associated with adverse outcomes and therefore should be treated with thyroxine replacement.

Subclinical hypothyroidism and symptoms, quality of life, and cognitive function

Studies addressing the relationship between symptoms suggestive of thyroid hormone deficiency and the finding of subclinical hypothyroidism have produced conflicting results. The Colorado health fair study revealed a slight increase in the mean number of reported symptoms in those with high TSH compared with euthyroid controls (13.8% vs 12.1%, $p < 0.05$) (4); however, in another study, a combination of symptoms and signs was not predictive of subclinical hypothyroidism in a geriatric population. Similarly, in a cross-sectional study of women aged 18–75 years, subclinical hypothyroidism was not associated with poorer wellbeing or quality of life (13). Results are also conflicting with regard to any association with depression or decline in cognitive function. Nearly all large studies have failed to find an association with symptoms of depression or impaired cognitive function. For example, in our own study of 5865 subjects aged over 65 years, of whom 168 had subclinical hypothyroidism, we found no association with tests of cognitive function, anxiety, or depression (14).

Several placebo-controlled trials have examined the question of whether T_4 replacement leads to improvement in such measures. Once more results are conflicting, probably reflecting small sample sizes and sometimes short duration of therapy and failure to achieve stable euthyroidism in the treatment group. One of the larger studies of 66 women with a mean TSH of 11.7 mU/l demonstrated no difference between T_4-treated and placebo groups after 48 weeks therapy, although some improvement in symptoms was seen in those with TSH of more than 12.0 mU/l (15). Other studies of 89 subjects (mean TSH 5.57 mU/l) (16) and 100 subjects (17), found no significant effects of T_4 treatment on various tests of cognitive function, quality of life, and depression scores.

Effects of subclinical hypothyroidism on the lipid profile and cardiovascular system

Overt hypothyroidism results in reductions in the synthesis and degradation of lipids, but the latter effect predominates so that hypothyroidism results in increases in total and low-density lipoprotein (LDL) cholesterol, as well as marked changes in other lipoprotein and apolipoprotein concentrations. Lipid changes in subclinical hypothyroidism are considerably less marked. Cross-sectional studies comparing subjects with subclinical hypothyroidism and euthyroid controls have shown that subclinical hypothyroidism is associated with variable and inconsistent increases in total cholesterol, LDL cholesterol, and an inconsistent decrease in high-density lipoprotein cholesterol, findings compatible with an increase in atherogenic risk. For example, in the NHANES III cohort, mean total cholesterol (but not LDL) levels were higher in subclinical hypothyroid subjects than euthyroid controls, a finding lost in terms of statistical significance when adjusted for factors such as age and use of lipid-lowering agents (18). Overall, it has been estimated that 0.5 mmol/l total cholesterol might be accounted for by subclinical hypothyroidism. Unsurprisingly, meta-analyses of intervention studies with T_4 have shown only minor effects on the lipid profile, and the most recent meta-analysis revealed reductions of 0.2–0.3 mmol/l in total and LDL cholesterol values after T_4 treatment, with no associated change in triglycerides (19). Generally, more marked changes in cholesterol are seen in those with higher baseline values and in those with higher TSH.

Influences of subclinical hypothyroidism upon the vascular system have been studied in some detail, the most consistent findings being left ventricular diastolic dysfunction in association with an increase in systemic vascular resistance and arterial thickness. Generally, these haemodynamic changes are thought to be corrected by T_4 replacement. These, together with lipid findings, have prompted epidemiological studies of vascular morbidity and mortality, with inconsistent results. In the 20-year follow-up of the Whickham cohort from the north-east of England, there was no association with a diagnosis of autoimmune thyroid disease and a diagnosis of ischaemic heart disease (12). In contrast, in the Rotterdam cohort of women over 55 years there was an association between subclinical hypothyroidism and atherosclerosis (defined as aortic calcification on lateral radiograph) and with a history of myocardial infarction, although no association with incident ischaemic heart disease (20). In our own study of 1200 subjects aged more than 60 years followed for 10 years, we found no association of subclinical hypothyroidism with circulatory mortality (although 40% had commenced T_4 therapy during follow-up) (21). Intriguingly, in the Leiden study of those aged more than 85 years, raised TSH was associated with increased longevity and decreased risk of death from cardiovascular disease (22). The longitudinal Cardiovascular Health Study in the USA found no association between subclinical hypothyroidism and the incidences of cardiovascular or cerebrovascular diseases, nor all-cause mortality (23); however, an association between a serum TSH of more than 10.0 mU/l and heart failure events has recently been described in the same cohort (24). A recent meta-analysis has examined the possible association between subclinical hypothyroidism and vascular or all-cause mortality. It was concluded that, at present, the evidence for association is weak (25).

Should we screen for and treat subclinical hypothyroidism?

Subclinical hypothyroidism is a common condition, especially among specific patient groups including elderly patients, those with a past or family history of thyroid disease, those with other autoimmune diseases such as type 1 diabetes, and those receiving therapy with drugs such as amiodarone and lithium. The marked prevalence of this disorder has led to debate regarding the appropriateness of population screening (i.e. routine testing of asymptomatic individuals). This debate centres on the lack of evidence that treatment of subclinical (as opposed to overt) hypothyroidism has a beneficial effect in terms of patient wellbeing and/or long-term morbidity, e.g. due to cardiovascular disease, and takes into account the variable natural history of the disorder in different patient groups and the potential influence upon patient wellbeing of the knowledge that they have an abnormal test result. While opposing views have been expressed, a consensus statement from UK experts in thyroid disease has suggested that general testing of the population is at present unjustified, even in those aged over 60 years and those with a family history of thyroid disease; these views are in accord with a US consensus panel (1) and the US Preventative Task Force. Groups in whom screening is considered appropriate include those with a past history of treatment for hyperthyroidism with radio-iodine or surgery and, perhaps, those with type 1 diabetes (especially in pregnancy), as well as those receiving lithium or amiodarone (see also Chapter 3.1.7).

Once the diagnosis of subclinical hypothyroidism has been made, either as a result of routine testing of a particular patient group or prompted by nonspecific symptoms such as tiredness or weight gain, the question arises as to if and when to treat with thyroxine replacement therapy. Given the relative paucity of evidence that treatment of subclinical hypothyroidism results in benefit in terms of symptoms or long-term outcome, the debate continues. The association between serum TSH values of more than 10 mU/l and 'adverse' findings, such as faster progression to overt hypothyroidism, hyperlipidaemia, and perhaps vascular morbidity, leads many experts to treat with thyroxine in this group. It is much less clear that those with modestly elevated serum TSH (<10 mU/l) should be treated. The US consensus panel of experts concluded that there was insufficient evidence to warrant treatment of those with mildly elevated TSH (who should have repeat testing at 6–12 monthly intervals) but that those with TSH of more than 10 mU/l should be considered for treatment (1). An exception is in pregnancy where most experts would recommend thyroxine treatment for even modest elevations of serum TSH in view of possible adverse outcomes, such as pregnancy loss and slightly impaired neurodevelopment in offspring (see Chapter 3.4.5).

Key points

- Subclinical hypothyroidism is a biochemical diagnosis defined as raised serum TSH in association with normal circulating free T_4.
- Subclinical hypothyroidism is a common biochemical finding, especially in women and in older people. It is especially common in those prescribed thyroid hormones, reflecting either poor compliance or inadequate dose prescription.
- The pathophysiological consequences are different if the TSH is more markedly elevated (serum TSH >10.0 mU/l) than if there is only minor elevation of TSH (4.5–10 mU/l).
- There is a paucity of evidence associating mild subclinical hypothyroidism with symptoms or adverse outcomes such as vascular disease or mortality.
- More marked subclinical hypothyroidism progresses more rapidly to overt hypothyroidism and may be associated with symptoms, with hyperlipidaemia, and possibly with heart failure events.
- Most experts recommend treatment with thyroxine if serum TSH is persistently above 10.0 mU/l.
- Evidence is lacking that treatment of more minor degrees of hypothyroidism is beneficial although those with this biochemistry should have occasional testing to detect deterioration in thyroid function.
- Population screening for subclinical hypothyroidism is not warranted although targeted screening of some groups, such as those taking lithium, those with a previous history of treatment for hyperthyroidism, and those with other autoimmune conditions such as type 1 diabetes, is warranted.

References

1. Surks MI, Ortiz E, Daniels GH, Sawin CT, Col NF, Cobin RH, *et al.* Subclinical thyroid disease: scientific review and guidelines for diagnosis and management. *JAMA*, 2004; **291**: 228–38.
2. Hollowell JG, Staehling NW, Flanders WD, Hannon WH, Gunter EW, Spencer CA, *et al.* Serum TSH, T(4), and thyroid antibodies in the United States population (1988 to 1994): National Health and Nutrition Examination Survey (NHANES III). *J Clin Endocrinol Metab*, 2002; **87**: 489–9.
3. Tunbridge WM, Evered DC, Hall R, Appleton D, Brewis M, Clark F, *et al.* The spectrum of thyroid disease in a community: the Whickham survey. *Clin Endocrinol (Oxf)*, 1977; **7**: 481–93.
4. Canaris GJ, Manowitz NR, Mayor G, Ridgway EC. The Colorado thyroid disease prevalence study. *Arch Intern Med*, 2000; **160**: 526–34.
5. Parle JV, Franklyn JA, Cross KW, Jones SC, Sheppard MC. Prevalence and follow-up of abnormal thyrotrophin (TSH) concentrations in the elderly in the United Kingdom. *Clin Endocrinol (Oxf)*, 1991; **34**: 77–83.
6. Wilson S, Parle JV, Roberts LM, Roalfe AK, Hobbs FD, Clark P, *et al.* Prevalence of subclinical thyroid dysfunction and its relation to socioeconomic deprivation in the elderly: a community-based cross-sectional survey. *J Clin Endocrinol Metab*, 2006; **91**: 4809–16.
7. Boelaert K, Syed AA, Manji N, Sheppard MC, Holder RL, Gough SC, *et al.* Prediction of cure and risk of hypothyroidism in patients receiving (131)I for hyperthyroidism. *Clin Endocrinol (Oxf)*, 2009; **70**: 129–38.
8. Parle JV, Franklyn JA, Cross KW, Jones SR, Sheppard MC. Thyroxine prescription in the community: serum thyroid stimulating hormone level assays as an indicator of undertreatment or overtreatment. *Br J Gen Pract*, 1993; **43**: 107–9.
9. Lazarus JH. Epidemiology and prevention of thyroid disease in pregnancy. *Thyroid*, 2002; **12**: 861–5.
10. Linder N, Davidovitch N, Reichman B, Kuint J, Lubin D, Meyerovitch J, *et al.* Topical iodine-containing antiseptics and subclinical hypothyroidism in preterm infants. *J Pediatr*, 1997; **131**: 434–9.
11. Meyerovitch J, Rotman-Pikielny P, Sherf M, Battat E, Levy Y, Surks MI. Serum thyrotropin measurements in the community: five-year follow-up in a large network of primary care physicians. *Arch Intern Med*, 2007; **167**: 1533–8.
12. Vanderpump MP, Tunbridge WM, French JM, Appleton D, Bates D, Clark F, *et al.* The incidence of thyroid disorders in the community: a twenty-year follow-up of the Whickham Survey. *Clin Endocrinol (Oxf)*, 1995; **43**: 55–68.
13. Bell RJ, Rivera-Woll L, Davison SL, Topliss DJ, Donath S, Davis SR. Well-being, health-related quality of life and cardiovascular disease risk profile in women with subclinical thyroid disease: a community-based study. *Clin Endocrinol (Oxf)*, 2007; **66**: 548–56.
14. Roberts LM, Pattison H, Roalfe A, Franklyn J, Wilson S, Hobbs FD, *et al.* Is subclinical thyroid dysfunction in the elderly associated with depression or cognitive dysfunction. *Ann Intern Med*, 2006; **145**: 573–81.
15. Meier C, Staub JJ, Roth CB, Guglielmetti M, Kunz M, Miserez AR, *et al.* TSH-controlled L-thyroxine therapy reduces cholesterol levels and clinical symptoms in subclinical hypothyroidism: a double blind, placebo-controlled trial (Basel Thyroid Study). *J Clin Endocrinol Metab*, 2001; **86**: 4860–6.
16. Jorde R, Waterloo K, Storhaug H, Nyrnes A, Sundsfjord J, Jenssen TG. Neuropsychological function and symptoms in subjects with subclinical hypothyroidism and the effect of thyroxine treatment. *J Clin Endocrinol Metab*, 2006; **91**: 145–53.
17. Razvi S, Ingoe L, Keeka G, Oates C, McMillan C, Weaver JU. The beneficial effect of L-thyroxine on cardiovascular risk factors, endothelial function, and quality of life in subclinical hypothyroidism: randomized, crossover trial. *J Clin Endocrinol Metab*, 2007; **92**: 1715–23.
18. Hueston WJ, Pearson WS. Subclinical hypothyroidism and the risk of hypercholesterolemia. *Ann Fam Med*, 2004; **2**: 351–5.
19. Danese MD, Ladenson PW, Meinert CL, Powe NR. Clinical review 115: effect of thyroxine therapy on serum lipoproteins in patients with mild thyroid failure: a quantitative review of the literature. *J Clin Endocrinol Metab*, 2000; **85**: 2993–3001.
20. Hak AE, Pols HA, Visser TJ, Drexhage HA, Hofman A, Witteman JC. Subclinical hypothyroidism is an independent risk factor for atherosclerosis and myocardial infarction in elderly women: the Rotterdam Study. *Ann Intern Med*, 2000; **132**: 270–8.
21. Parle JV, Maisonneuve P, Sheppard MC, Boyle P, Franklyn JA. Prediction of all-cause and cardiovascular mortality in elderly people from one low serum thyrotropin result: a 10-year cohort study. *Lancet*, 2001; **358**: 861–5.
22. Gussekloo J, van Exel E, de Craen AJ, Meinders AE, Frolich M, Westendorp RG. Thyroid status, disability and cognitive function, and survival in old age. *JAMA*, 2004; **292**: 2591–9.

23. Cappola AR, Fried LP, Arnold AM, Danese MD, Kuller LH, Burke GL, *et al.* Thyroid status, cardiovascular risk, and mortality in older adults. *JAMA*, 2006; **295**: 1033–41.
24. Rodondi N, Bauer DC, Cappola AR, Cornuz J, Robbins J, Fried LP, *et al.* Subclinical thyroid dysfunction, cardiac function, and the risk of heart failure. The Cardiovascular Health study. *J Am Coll Cardiol*, 2008; **52**: 1152–9.
25. Volzke H, Schwahn C, Wallaschofski H, Dorr M. Review: the association of thyroid dysfunction with all-cause and circulatory mortality: is there a causal relationship. *J Clin Endocrinol Metab*, 2007; **92**: 2421–9.

3.4.5 Thyroid disease during pregnancy

John H. Lazarus, L.D. Kuvera, E. Premawardhana

Introduction

Thyroid disorders are common. The prevalence of hyperthyroidism is around 5/1000 in women and overt hypothyroidism about 3/1000 in women. Subclinical hypothyroidism has a prevalence in women of childbearing age in iodine-sufficient areas of between 4% and 8%. As these conditions are generally much more common in females, it is to be expected that they will appear during pregnancy. Developments in our understanding of thyroid physiology (1) and immunology (2) in pregnancy, as well as improvements in thyroid function testing (3), have highlighted the importance of recognizing and providing appropriate therapy to women with gestational thyroid disorders. Before considering the clinical entities occurring during and after pregnancy it is useful to briefly review thyroid physiology and immunology in relation to pregnancy.

Iodine and pregnancy

The recommended daily iodine intake in pregnancy has been increased to 250 µg/day which implies a urinary iodine excretion of 150–250 µg/day as being adequate (4) Urinary iodine excretion in pregnancy is maximal in the first trimester followed by a decline in the second and third trimesters. Often there is an increase in urinary iodine in the first trimester compared to control nonpregnant women, but where the population has a high median iodine concentration this difference may not occur.

Iodine deficiency during pregnancy is associated with maternal goiter due to the imbalance between the intake and increased requirements for iodine during gestation and results eventually in a reduced circulating maternal thyroxine (T_4) concentration. This gestational goitrogenesis is preventable by iodine supplementation (5) not only in areas of severe iodine deficiency (24-h urinary iodine less than 50 µg) but also in areas where trials have shown clear beneficial effects on maternal thyroid size. Clinical studies of children born to mothers with known iodine deficiency clearly showed impaired neurointellectual development, sometimes to the extreme of cretinism in severely deficient states. These defects can be corrected by iodine administration before and even during gestation and this should be performed in areas of moderate to severe iodine deficiency.

Thyroid function and pregnancy

Pregnancy is associated with significant, but reversible changes in thyroid function (Table 3.4.5.1). Thyroid hormone transport proteins, particularly thyroxine-binding globulin, increase due to enhanced hepatic synthesis and a reduced degradation rate due to oligosaccharide modification. Serum concentrations of free thyroid hormones are decreased, increased, or unchanged during gestation depending on the assays used. Nevertheless, there is a transient rise in free T_4 in the first trimester due to the relatively high circulating human chorionic gonadotropin (hCG) concentration and a decrease of free T_4 in the second and third trimester. Because of these variations (Fig. 3.4.5.1) there is a need for normative trimester-specific reference ranges for thyroid hormones (6). In iodine-deficient areas (including marginal iodine deficiency seen in many European countries), pregnant woman may become significantly hypothyroxinaemic with preferential triiodothyronine (T_3) secretion. The thyroidal 'stress' is also evidenced by a rise in the median thyroid-stimulating hormone (TSH) and serum thyroglobulin.

Thyroid supply to the fetus

The fetal thyroid begins concentrating iodine at 10–12 weeks gestation and is under the control of fetal pituitary TSH by about 20 weeks gestation. Although there is no functioning fetal thyroid in early pregnancy, thyroid hormone is important in the development of many organs including the brain. Maternal circulating T_4 crosses the placenta into the fetus at all stages of pregnancy by incompletely understood mechanisms but involving both the type 2 and type 3 deiodinase enzymes, both expressed in the placenta. Type 3 deiodinase (D3), which degrades thyroid hormones (7), is also expressed in pregnant uterus, placenta, and fetal and neonatal tissues, and may act as a 'gatekeeper' to prevent too much thyroid hormone transport. Type 2 deiodinase, also located in the uterus and other parts of the genital tract, degrades T_4 in the fetus to provide T_3 for tissue growth and differentiation and may have a role in fetal implantation.

Table 3.4.5.1 Physiological changes in pregnancy that influence thyroid function tests

Physiological change	Thyroid function test change
↑ Thyroxine-binding globulin	↑ Serum total T_4 and T_3 concentration
First trimester human chorionic gonadotropin elevation	↑ Free T_4 and ↓ TSH
↑ Plasma volume	↑ T_4 and T_3 pool size
Type 3 5-deiodinase (inner ring deiodination) due to increased placental mass	↑ T_4 and T_3 degradation resulting in requirement for increased hormone production
Thyroid enlargement (in some women)	↑ Serum thyroglobulin
↑ Iodine clearance	↓ Hormone production in iodine-deficient areas

From Brent GA. Maternal thyroid function: interpretation of thyroid function tests in pregnancy. *Clin Obstet Gynecol*, 1997; **40**: 3–15.

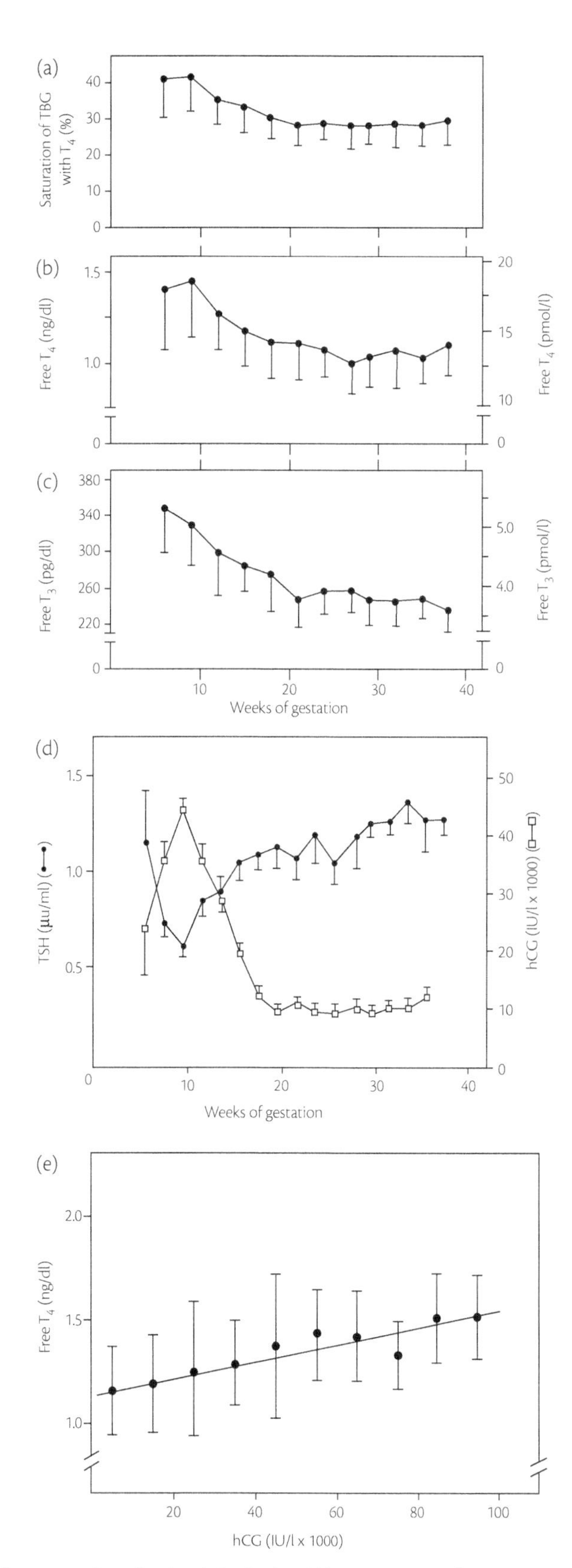

Fig. 3.4.5.1 Gestational variation in thyroid function in normal women Data from 606 normal pregnancies showing the rise in thyroxine-binding globulin (TBG) (a) accompanied by the changes in free T_4 (b) and free T_3 (c) concentrations throughout gestation in a mildly iodine-deficient area (Brussels). Relationship between serum TSH and human chorionic gonadotropin (hCG) as a function of gestational age (d) and the relationship between free T_4 and hCG in the first half of gestation (e). (Adapted with permission from Glinoer DG. The regulation of thyroid function in pregnancy: pathways of endocrine adaptation from physiology to pathology. *Endocr Rev*, 1997; **18**: 404–33.)

Pregnancy and the immune system

Human immune regulation involves homeostasis between T helper 1 (Th1) and T helper 2 (Th2) activity, with Th1 cells driving cellular immunity and Th2 cells humoral immunity (2). In pregnancy there is a bias towards a Th2 lymphocyte response evidenced by the fetal/placental unit producing Th2 cytokines, which inhibit Th1. Th1 cytokines are potentially harmful to the fetus as, e.g. interferon-α is a known abortifacient.

Pregnancy also has a significant effect on the immune system in order to maintain the fetal–maternal allograft and prevent rejection (Box 3.4.5.1). The trophoblast does not express the classic major histocompatibility complex (MHC) class Ia or II which are needed to present antigenic peptides to cytotoxic cells and T helper cells, respectively. Instead HLA-G, a nonclassic MHC Ib molecule is expressed which may be a ligand for the natural killer (NK) cell receptor so protecting the fetus from NK cell damage; it may also activate $CD8^+$ T cells that may have a suppressor function. Human trophoblasts also express abundant Fas ligand, thereby contributing to the immune privilege by mediating apoptosis of activated Fas-expressing lymphocytes of maternal origin (8).

Pregnancy and thyroid antibodies

Antithyroid peroxidase antibodies (TPOAbs) are found in around 10% of otherwise normal pregnant women when measured at the end of the first trimester. The presence of TPOAbs before and during gestation have several implications. Fertility is impaired in hypothyroid women with autoimmune thyroid disease and, if such patients do achieve pregnancy, the hypothyroid state is associated with a higher incidence of miscarriage early in pregnancy. Thyroid autoimmunity, with positive TPOAbs present during early pregnancy even in the euthyroid situation, is associated with an increased risk of subsequent miscarriage (9). TPOAb-positive women miscarry at a rate of between 13% and 22% compared to 3.3–8.4% in control euthyroid antibody-negative women. One controlled trial has shown that thyroxine administration reduced the miscarriage rate in TPOAb-positive women. The association between TPOAbs and recurrent abortion is less strong than for miscarriage but one uncontrolled study reported a significant success rate with thyroxine administration (10).

Box 3.4.5.1 Immunological and hormonal features of pregnancy

- Clinical improvement in:
  - Graves' hyperthyroidism
  - Rheumatoid arthritis
  - Psoriatic arthritis and other autoimmune diseases
- Trophoblast: HLA-G expression
- Fas ligand expression
- Lymphocytes:
  - Th2 response
  - Th2 cytokines produced by the fetal/placental unit
- Hormones:
  - Progesterone increase; reduction in B-cell activity
  - Oestrogen increase; fall in autoantibody levels
  - Cortisol, 1,25 vitamin D, and norepinephrine all affect the immune response

Box 3.4.5.2 Causes of hyperthyroidism in pregnancy

- Graves' disease
- Transient gestational hyperthyroidism
- Toxic multinodular goiter
- Single toxic adenoma
- Subacute thyroiditis
- Trophoblastic tumour
- Iodide-induced hyperthyroidism
- Struma ovarii
- TSH-receptor activation

Hyperthyroidism and pregnancy

Hyperthyroidism occurs in 2/1000 pregnancies, the commonest cause (85%) being Graves' hyperthyroidism, due to thyroid stimulation by thyrotropin receptor stimulating antibodies (TRAb) (Box 3.4.5.2). Transient gestational thyrotoxicosis (due to thyroid stimulation by hCG) is seen in the first trimester and is more common in Asian women than European women. A deterioration in previously diagnosed Graves' disease is not infrequent during the first trimester of pregnancy, and may be due to an increase in the titre of TRAb or high levels of hCG acting as a thyroid stimulator. Relapse may also be caused by impaired absorption of antithyroid medication secondary to pregnancy-associated vomiting or by reluctance to continue medication in the first trimester.

The immune status of pregnancy is a Th2 state, which allows tolerance of the fetus during pregnancy, and this is thought to be the reason why there is usually an amelioration of the severity of Graves' hyperthyroidism (and other autoimmune diseases) after the first trimester. Graves' hyperthyroidism before pregnancy may remit during pregnancy but will exacerbate in the postpartum period as the immune status reverts to a Th1 state.

Maternal complications of hyperthyroidism include miscarriage, placental abruption, and preterm delivery. Congestive heart failure and thyroid storm may also occur, the risk of pre-eclampsia is significantly higher in women with poorly controlled hyperthyroidism, and a low-birthweight infant may be up to nine times more likely (11). Neonatal hyperthyroidism, prematurity, and intrauterine growth retardation may be observed. There are no increased risks of subclinical hyperthyroidism. Women with thyroid hormone resistance (where thyroid hormone levels and TSH are inappropriately high not due to autoimmunity) also have a high miscarriage rate, indicating a direct toxic effect of thyroid hormones on the fetus.

There is no doubt that overt clinical and biochemical hyperthyroidism should be treated to lessen the rate of complications described above. Gestational amelioration of Graves' disease is usually associated with a reduction in titre of TSH-receptor antibodies and sometimes a change from stimulatory to blocking antibody activity. Of neonates of mothers with Graves' disease, 1–5% have hyperthyroidism due to the transplacental passage of maternal stimulating TRAb (even though the mother may be euthyroid and has received previous treatment for Graves' disease). Neonatal hyperthyroidism may also be due to an activating mutation of the TSH receptor dominantly inherited from the mother. Transient neonatal central hypothyroidism is due to poorly controlled Graves' disease leading to suppression of the fetal pituitary–thyroid axis due to placental transfer of T_4.

Clinical features and diagnosis

Undiagnosed Graves' hyperthyroidism is present in approximately 0.15% and others will already be known to have the disease before gestation. Features such as tachycardia, palpitations, systolic murmur, bowel disturbance, emotional upset, and heat intolerance may be seen in normal pregnancy but should alert the clinician to the possibility of hyperthyroidism, particularly if goiter or more specific features of thyroid disease (weight loss, eye signs, tremor, or pretibial myxoedema) are observed.

Management

Ideally a woman who is known to have hyperthyroidism should seek prepregnancy advice; appropriate education should allay fears that are commonly present in these women. She should be referred for specialist care for frequent checking of her thyroid status, thyroid antibody evaluation, and close monitoring of her medication needs (12).

At all stages of pregnancy, the use of antithyroid drugs (ATDs) is the preferred treatment option. Radio-iodine is contraindicated and surgery requires pretreatment with ATDs to render the patient euthyroid. The thionamides carbimazole (CMI), methimazole (MMI), and propylthiouracil (PTU) are all effective in inhibiting thyroidal biosynthesis of thyroxine during pregnancy. PTU is the preferred drug in pregnancy due to the possibility (albeit rare) of teratogenic effects of CMI and MMI (aplasia cutis and MMI embryopathy). There are no long-term adverse effects of ATD exposure *in utero*, in particular on IQ scores or psychomotor development in MMI- and PTU-exposed individuals. The starting dosage of PTU is 300–450 mg/day, up to 600 mg daily if necessary, given in two or three divided doses. Some improvement is usually seen after 1 week of treatment with ATDs but 4–6 weeks may be needed for a full effect. Once the thyrotoxicosis has been controlled, the dose needs to be gradually reduced by one-quarter to one-third every 3–4 weeks, typically to 50–100 mg twice daily. The main principle of therapy is to administer the lowest ATD dose needed for controlling clinical symptoms, with the aim of restoring normal maternal thyroid function but ensuring that fetal thyroid function is minimally affected. Maternal free T_4 levels should be kept in the upper one-third of the normal nonpregnant reference range to avoid fetal hypothyroidism, as with this management serum free T_4 levels are normal in more than 90% of neonates. The administration of L-thyroxine together with PTU as a 'block and replace' regimen is not advisable in pregnancy as the amount of ATD may be excessive in proportion to the amount of thyroxine which crosses the placenta, resulting in fetal goiter and hypothyroidism. Recently there has been concern expressed relating to the hepatic side effects of PTU. The current recommendation is therefore to use PTU only in the first trimester.

β-adrenergic blocking agents such as propranolol may be used for a few weeks to ameliorate the peripheral sympathomimetic actions of excess thyroid hormone but prolonged use can result in restricted fetal growth, impaired response to hypoxic stress, together with postnatal bradycardia and hypoglycaemia. If a woman is already receiving CMI, a change to PTU is recommended. Although these patients may have received ATDs, surgery, or radio-iodine therapy and be euthyroid on or off thyroxine therapy, neonatal hyperthyroidism may still occur.

TRAb should be measured early in pregnancy in a euthyroid pregnant women previously treated by either surgery or radio-iodine (13). If the TRAb level is high at this time the fetus should be evaluated carefully during gestation by serial ultrasonography (14). Ultrasonographic evidence of fetal thyroid disease includes intrauterine growth restriction, tachycardia, cardiac failure, hydrops, advanced bone age, and goiter. In the presence of a fetal goiter, it may not be possible to distinguish fetal hyper- from hypothyroid disease on clinical grounds; fetal blood sampling may then be necessary to enable a diagnosis to be made. If fetal hyperthyroidism is diagnosed, treatment involves modulation of maternal ATDs. If fetal hypothyroidism has resulted from administration of ATDs to the mother, maternal treatment should be decreased or stopped and administration of intra-amniotic thyroxine considered. Early delivery may need to be considered in the case of fetal thyroid dysfunction, depending on the gestation at diagnosis and the severity of fetal symptoms. TRAb should be measured again in the last trimester (at about 32 weeks) and if positive the neonate needs to be checked for hyperthyroidism following delivery.

Thyroid surgery (in the second trimester) is indicated if control of the hyperthyroidism is poorly controlled on account of poor compliance, inability to take drugs, or pressure symptoms due to goiter size. The administration of radioactive iodine (^{131}I) is contraindicated during pregnancy. Because fetal thyroid uptake of ^{131}I commences after 12 weeks gestation, exposure before 12 weeks is not associated with fetal thyroid dysfunction and the irradiation dose is not considered sufficient to justify termination of pregnancy. However, the fetal thyroid does concentrate iodine after 13–15 weeks gestation and the fetal tissues are more radiosensitive. ^{131}I given after this gestational age therefore potentially leads to significant radiation to the fetal thyroid, resulting in biochemical hypothyroidism and even cretinism in the neonate.

Hypothyroidism and pregnancy

The incidence of hypothyroidism during pregnancy is around 2.5% (15) and is nearly always subclinical, which is equally as important in its adverse effects affecting mother and neonate as the full expression of the disease. The aetiology is usually autoimmune thyroiditis (TPOAb positive), but it may also be due to postoperative thyroid failure and noncompliance with existing thyroxine therapy. The symptoms of hypothyroidism, such as tiredness, are also seen in pregnancy. Many patients with subclinical hypothyroidism are asymptomatic but then notice an improvement after taking thyroid hormone therapy. Classic clinical features of hypothyroidism are described in Chapter 3.4.1. Maternal hypothyroxinaemia (without increased TSH) is also being increasingly accepted as deleterious to the neuropsychological development of the child (16). Care should be taken in the interpretation of TSH concentrations in early gestation due to the thyrotrophic effects of hCG.

Previous studies have documented the effects of hypothyroidism on maternal and fetal wellbeing, drawing attention to increased incidence of abortion, obstetrical complications, and fetal abnormalities in untreated women (Box 3.4.5.3). Women already receiving thyroxine for hypothyroidism require an increased dose during gestation (17). This is critical to ensure adequate maternal thyroxine levels for delivery to the fetus especially during the first trimester. The dose should normally be increased by 50–100 μg/day as soon as pregnancy is diagnosed; subsequent monitoring of TSH and free T_4 is then necessary to ensure correct replacement dosage.

Box 3.4.5.3 Pregnancy complications in women with untreated hypothyroidism

- Maternal
  - Gestational hypertension
  - Anaemia
  - Postpartum haemorrhage
  - Placental abruption
- Fetal
  - Spontaneous abortion
  - Small for gestational age
  - Fetal distress in labour
  - Fetal death
  - Transient congenital hypothyroidism (transplacental passage of maternal TSH-binding inhibitory immunoglobulins)
  - Impairment in cognitive function (at least up to 7 years old)

Thyroid hormones are major factors for the normal development of the brain. The mechanisms of actions of thyroid hormones in the developing brain are mainly mediated through two ligand-activated thyroid hormone receptor isoforms. It is known that thyroid hormone deficiency may cause severe neurological disorders resulting from the deficit of neuronal cell differentiation and migration, axonal and dendritic outgrowth, myelin formation, and synaptogenesis (18). This is the situation well documented in iodine-deficient areas where the maternal circulating T_4 concentrations are too low to provide adequate fetal levels particularly in the first trimester. There is also evidence that in an iodine-sufficient area maternal thyroid dysfunction (hypothyroidism, subclinical hypothyroidism, or hypothyroxinaemia) during pregnancy results in neurointellectual impairment of the child. Haddow *et al.* (19) found that the full IQ scores of children whose mothers had a high TSH during gestation were 7 points lower than controls ($p < 0.005$) and that 19% of them had scores of less than 85 compared to 5% of controls ($p < 0.007$). Maternal hypothyroxinaemia during early gestation was shown to be an independent determinant of neurodevelopmental delay, but when free T_4 concentrations increased during gestation in women who had low free T_4 in early pregnancy, infant development was not adversely affected (20). Pop *et al.* (21) have also shown a significant decrement in IQ in children aged 5 years whose mothers were known to have circulating anti-TPO-Abs at 32 weeks gestation and were biochemically euthyroid. The neurodevelopmental impairment is similar to that seen in iodine-deficient areas and implies that iodine status should be normalized in regions of deficiency. However, much of the USA and parts of Europe are not iodine deficient, which raises the question of routine screening of thyroid function during early pregnancy or even at preconception.

Nodular thyroid disease

Thyroid nodules are claimed to be detected in up to 10% of pregnant women. Fine-needle aspiration biopsy is the first investigation of choice which may yield a malignancy/suspicious result in 35% (22). When malignancy is diagnosed it is usually a differentiated tumour which may be surgically resected in the second trimester or in some cases safely left until the postpartum period before therapy is started. The impact of pregnancy on thyroid cancer seems to be minimal in that there is no difference in rates of metastases or recurrence compared to nonpregnant women with the same disease. Whether women already treated for thyroid malignancy should become pregnant is of concern but current evidence suggests that differentiated thyroid cancer should not inhibit an intended pregnancy. Previous ^{131}I therapy does not result in demonstrable adverse events in subsequent pregnancies, although miscarriage appears to be more frequent during the year preceding conception.

Screening for thyroid dysfunction in pregnancy

It is clear from the information already discussed relating to the effects of thyroid dysfunction in pregnancy on both mother and fetus together with the high prevalence of thyroid abnormalities that consideration be given to screening thyroid function in pregnancy with the aim of interventional therapy (with L-thyroxine) if necessary. The development of normative reference ranges for thyroid hormone during pregnancy would assist this process considerably. Screening is a strategy to detect a disease in asymptomatic individuals in order to improve health outcomes by early diagnosis and treatment. The current recommendation of the clinical practice guideline published under the auspices of the Endocrine Society (23) is that targeted screening should be performed in those women at high risk for thyroid disease (Box 3.4.5.4). A study to validate this strategy found that restricting screening to these groups of women would miss about one-third of women with significant thyroid dysfunction (23). A cost-effective analysis of screening pregnant women for autoimmune thyroid disease concluded that screening pregnant women in the first trimester for TSH was cost effective compared with no screening (24, 25).

Box 3.4.5.4 Selected high-risk pregnant women in whom the Endocrine Society Clinical Practice Guidelines recommend targeted case-finding

- Women with a history of thyroid disease (including hyperthyroidism, hypothyroidism, and postpartum thyroiditis) or thyroid surgery
- Women with a goiter
- Women with symptoms or signs suggestive of hypothyroidism or hyperthyroidism
- Women with a family history of thyroid disease
- Women with thyroid antibodies (when known)
- Women with type 1 diabetes or other autoimmune disorders
- Women with a history of infertility (as part of their infertility work-up), miscarriage, or preterm delivery
- Women with a history of head or neck irradiation

Adapted from Abalovich M, Amino N, Barbour LA, Cobin RH, De Groot LJ, Glinoer D, *et al.* Management of thyroid dysfunction during pregnancy and postpartum: an Endocrine Society Clinical Practice Guideline. *J Clin Endocrinol Metab*, 2007; **92** (Suppl 8): S1–47.

Screening using anti-TPOAbs was also cost effective. Until the results of carefully controlled randomized prospective outcome studies are available, the screening controversy will continue.

References

1. Glinoer D. The regulation of thyroid function in pregnancy: pathways of endocrine adaptation from physiology to pathology. *Endocr Rev*, 1997; **18**: 404–33.
2. Weetman AP. The immunology of pregnancy. *Thyroid*, 1999; **9**: 643–6.
3. Brent GA. Maternal thyroid function: interpretation of thyroid function tests in pregnancy. *Clin Obstet Gynecol*, 1997; **40**: 3–15.
4. de Benoist B, Delange F, eds. Report of a WHO technical consultation on prevention and control of iodine deficiency in pregnancy, lactation, and in children less than 2 years of age. *Public Health Nutr*, 2007; **12**: 1527–1611.
5. Zimmerman MB. Iodine deficiency in pregnancy and the effects of maternal iodine supplementation on the offspring: a review. *Am J Clin Nutr*, 2009; **89** (Suppl): S1–5.
6. Stricker R, Echenard M, Eberhart R, Chevailler MC, Perez V, Quinn FA, *et al.* Evaluation of maternal thyroid function during pregnancy: the importance of using gestational age-specific reference intervals. *Eur J Endocrinol*, 2007; **157**: 509–14.
7. Hernandez A, Martinez ME, Fiering S, Galton VA, St Germain D. Type 3 deiodinase is critical for the maturation and function of the thyroid axis. *J Clin Invest*, 2006; **116**: 476–84.
8. Szekeres-Bartho J. Immunological relationship between the mother and the fetus. *Int Rev Immunol*, 2002; **21**: 471–95.
9. Stagnaro-Green A, Glinoer D. Thyroid autoimmunity and the risk of miscarriage. *Best Pract Res Clin Endocrinol Metab*, 2004; **18**: 127–49.
10. Negro R, Formoso G, Mangieri T, Pezzarossa A, Dazzi D, Hassan H. (2006). Levothyroxine treatment in euthyroid pregnant women with autoimmune thyroid disease: effects on obstetrical complications. *J Clin Endocrinol Metab*, **91**: 2587–91.
11. Mestman JH. Hyperthyroidism in pregnancy. *Best Prac Res Clin Endocrinol Metab*, 2004; **18**: 267–88.
12. Marx H, Amin P, Lazarus JH. Pregnancy plus: hyperthyroidism and pregnancy. *BMJ*, 2008; **336**: 663–7.
13. Laurberg P, Nygaard B, Glinoer D, Grussendorf M, Orgiazzi J. Guidelines for TSH-receptor antibody measurements in pregnancy: results of an evidence based symposium organized by the European Thyroid Association. *Eur J Endocrinol*, 1998; **139**: 584–6.
14. Luton D, Le Gac I, Vuillard E, Castanet M, Guibourdenche J, Noel M, *et al.* Management of Graves' disease during pregnancy: the key role of fetal thyroid gland monitoring. *J Clin Endocrinol Metab*, 2005; **90**: 6093–8.
15. Klein RZ, Haddow JE, Faixt JD, Brown RS, Hermos RJ, Pulkkinen A, *et al.* Prevalence of thyroid deficiency in pregnant women. *Clin Endocrinol*, 1991; **35**: 41–6.
16. Morreale de Escobar G, Obregon MJ, Escobar del Rey F. Is neuropsychological development related to maternal hypothyroidism or to maternal hypothyroxinemia. *J Clin Endocrinol Metab*, 2000; **85**: 3975–87.
17. Alexander EK, Marqusee E, Lawrence J, *et al.* Timing and magnitude of increases in levothyroxine requirements during pregnancy in women with hypothyroidism. *N Engl J Med*, 2004; **351**: 241–9.
18. Williams GR. Neurodevelopmental and neurophysiological actions of thyroid hormone. *J Neuroendocrinol*, 2008; **20**: 784–94.
19. Haddow JE, Palomaki GE, Allan WC, Williams JR, Knight GJ, Gagnon J, *et al.* Maternal thyroid deficiency during pregnancy and subsequent neuropsychological development of the child. *N Engl J Med*, 1999; **341**: 549–55.
20. Pop VJ, Brouwers EP, Vadert HL, Vulsma T, van Baar AL, de Vijlder JJ. Maternal hypothyroxinaemia during early pregnancy and subsequent child development: a 3-year follow-up study. *Clin Endocrinol*, 2003; **59**: 282–8.

21. Pop VJ, de Vries E, Van Baar Al, Waelkens JJ, de Rooy HA, Horsten M, *et al.* Maternal thyroid peroxidase antibodies during pregnancy: a marker of impaired child development. *J Clin Endocrinol Metab*, 1995; **80**: 3561–6.
22. Hay I. Nodular thyroid disease diagnosed during pregnancy: how and when to treat. *Thyroid*, 1999; **9**: 667–70.
23. Abalovich M, Amino N, Barbour LA, Cobin RH, De Groot LJ, Glinoer D, *et al.* Management of thyroid dysfunction during pregnancy and postpartum: an Endocrine Society Clinical Practice Guideline. *J Clin Endocrinol Metab*, 2007; **92** (Suppl 8): S1–47.
24. Vaidya B, Anthony S, Bilous M, Shields B, Drury J, Hutchison S, *et al.* Detection of thyroid dysfunction in early pregnancy: universal screening or targeted high-risk case finding. *J Clin Endocrinol Metab*, 2007; **92**: 203–7.
25. Dosiou C, Sanders GD, Araki SS, Crapo LM. Screening pregnant women for autoimmune thyroid disease: a cost-effectiveness analysis. *Eur J Endocrinol*, 2008; **158**: 841–51.

Further Reading

Anselmo J, Cao D, Karrison T, Weiss RE, Refetoff S. Fetal loss associated with excess thyroid hormone exposure. *JAMA*, 2004; **292**: 691–5.

Glinoer D. *Thyroid regulation and dysfunction in the pregnant patient*, in www.thyroidmanager.org, (accessed 19 June 2010). South Dartmouth MA: Endocrine Education Inc.

Lazarus JH. Thyroid disease in pregnancy and childhood. *Minerva Endocrinol*, 2005; **30**: 71–87.

Lazarus JH. Thyroid disease during pregnancy. In: Krassas GE, Rivkees SA, Kiess W, eds. *Diseases of the Thyroid in Childhood and Adolescence*. Basel: Karger, 2007: 25–43.

3.4.6 Thyroid disease after pregnancy: postpartum thyroiditis

Nobuyuki Amino, Sumihisa Kubota

Definition of postpartum thyroiditis

Postpartum thyroiditis is defined as an exacerbation of autoimmune thyroiditis during the postpartum period (1). Patients do not develop thyroid autoimmunity at the onset of postpartum thyroiditis, but have 'subclinical autoimmune thyroiditis' beforehand which is exacerbated after delivery. Typically an exacerbation induces destructive thyrotoxicosis followed by transient hypothyroidism. However, various types of thyroid dysfunction may occur, including Graves' disease. Therefore, any kind of thyroid dysfunction observed during the postpartum period, is referred to as 'postpartum thyroid dysfunction'.

Pathogenesis

The pathogenesis of postpartum thyroiditis is similar to that of postpartum exacerbation of Graves' disease or Hashimoto's thyroiditis, which occurs by the enhancement of immune activities after parturition. The difference is only their stage of autoimmune disease. In postpartum thyroiditis, immune activation causes the transition of subclinical into overt autoimmune thyroid disease, whereas in previously manifest Graves' or Hashimoto's disease, immune activation results in exacerbation or relapse after parturition. During pregnancy, maternal immune activities are suppressed in order to prevent rejection of the fetus. Sudden release from the immune suppression at the time of delivery intensifies immune activities above the normal level, just as the sudden cessation of immunosuppressive drugs gives rise to the exacerbation of autoimmune diseases (2). The serial changes in titres of microsomal (thyroid peroxidase) antibodies in pregnant women with Graves' disease and Hashimoto's disease (Fig. 3.4.6.1) support this view (3). The immune rebound seems to be a general phenomenon observed in the postpartum period, since serum levels of immunoglobulins, and counts of lymphocytes and natural killer (NK)/K cell activity decrease in late pregnancy and increase after delivery even in normal pregnant women (2, 4). As immunological situations after abortion are similar to those during the postpartum period, postabortional thyroid dysfunction may occur in some cases (5, 6). The postpartum rebound of immune activities comprises two phases. Cytotoxic T cells and NK cells increase from 1 to 4 months postpartum (Fig. 3.4.6.2) (7, 8). The enhancement of cellular immunity may exacerbate tissue injury in Hashimoto's thyroiditis. In contrast, CD5 B cells, which produce autoantibodies, increase from 7 to 10 months postpartum (Fig. 3.4.6.2) (7). The enhancement of humoral immunity may cause postpartum Graves' disease by an increase of antithyroid-stimulating hormone (TSH)-receptor autoantibodies. Indeed, Hashimoto's thyroiditis is commonly aggravated from 1 to 4 months postpartum and Graves' disease may develop or relapse from 4 to 12 months postpartum (Fig. 3.4.6.3).

A recent study on the production of cytokines revealed that T helper 1 (Th1)-type and T helper 2 (Th2)-type cytokines decreased during pregnancy, Th1-type cytokines increased during the early postpartum period and Th2-type cytokines increased during the later postpartum period (9). These data also strongly support the immune rebound hypothesis (2). A possible role of fetal microchimerism was proposed as the mechanism of postpartum exacerbation of autoimmune thyroid disease (10), but it is necessary to accumulate more evidence to prove this hypothesis.

Prevalence

Postpartum thyroid dysfunction is a very common phenomenon (2, 11) with an incidence of about 5% (1.1–16.7%; Table 3.4.6.1) in mothers in the general population, i.e. one in 20 pregnant women develop postpartum thyroid dysfunction (11). Postpartum thyroid dysfunctions are classified into five groups by their clinical features, hyperthyroid and/or hypothyroid, transient or persistent (Fig. 3.4.6.4):

1 persistent thyrotoxicosis
2 transient thyrotoxicosis
3 destructive thyrotoxicosis followed by transient hypothyroidism
4 transient hypothyroidism
5 persistent hypothyroidism

Patients with persistent thyrotoxicosis (group 1) and some with transient thyrotoxicosis (group 2) reveal a high radio-iodine uptake due to Graves' disease. Transient thyrotoxicosis with a high radio-iodine uptake is common in postpartum Graves' disease; the overproduction of thyroid hormones ceases spontaneously within a year. The prevalence of postpartum Graves' disease (both persistent and transient) is estimated at 11% of those with postpartum thyroid dysfunction and 0.54% of the general population (12). Thyrotoxicosis due to postpartum Graves' disease occurs between 3 and 10 months postpartum.

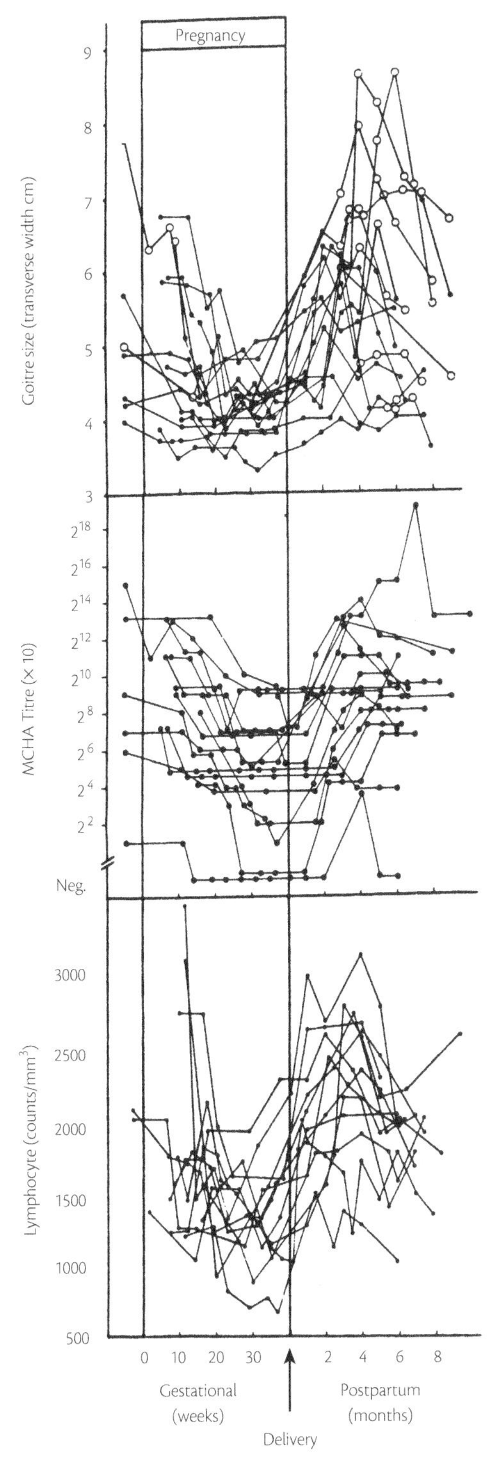

Fig. 3.4.6.1 Serial changes in goiter size, titres of antithyroid microsomal antibody, and the counts of peripheral lymphocytes during pregnancy and the postpartum period in patients with Hashimoto's thyroiditis. Open circles denote that TSH was more than 10 mU/l at time of measurement. MCHA, microsomal haemagglutination antibody.

The other three types of postpartum thyroid dysfunction are associated with thyroid tissue damage due to an exacerbation of autoimmune thyroiditis. They often manifest themselves as transient thyrotoxicosis (destructive thyrotoxicosis) developing at 1–3 months postpartum. Depending on the extent of the destruction, transient hypothyroidism may follow (group 3) or not (group 2, with a low radio-iodine uptake).

Occasionally, Graves' disease occurs closely following, or concomitantly with destructive thyrotoxicosis (13). When cellular damage occurs slowly, hypothyroidism alone, rather than destructive thyrotoxicosis, may be observed after delivery. In many cases, it is transient (group 4). However, it may be persistent in a few cases (group 5). Destructive transient thyrotoxicosis (group 2, with a low radio-iodine uptake, and group 3) is the most common form of postpartum thyroid dysfunction, accounting for 50–60% of all postpartum thyroid dysfunction. The rest (groups 4 and 5) show only the hypothyroid phase, however, persistent hypothyroidism is very rare (<0.1%).

Symptoms and signs

Thyroid dysfunction is most often subclinical: the patient has no complaints of hyper- or hypothyroidism, and thyroid function tests reveal only mild changes in serum TSH and thyroid hormones. Symptoms and signs in overt postpartum thyroid dysfunction are no different from those in nonpostpartum cases. Hypermetabolic and hyperdynamic symptoms, such as palpitation, sweating, and finger tremor, can be observed in any type of postpartum thyrotoxicosis. In postpartum Graves' disease, eye signs and/or pretibial myxoedema may be present. In postpartum hypothyroidism, symptoms such as weakness, fatigue, dry skin, constipation, and cold intolerance, and signs such as cold skin, bradycardia, and thyroid enlargement are common. Since the hypothyroidism is of short duration, there is little risk of myxoedema. Postpartum depression, sometimes found with postpartum thyroid dysfunction, is an

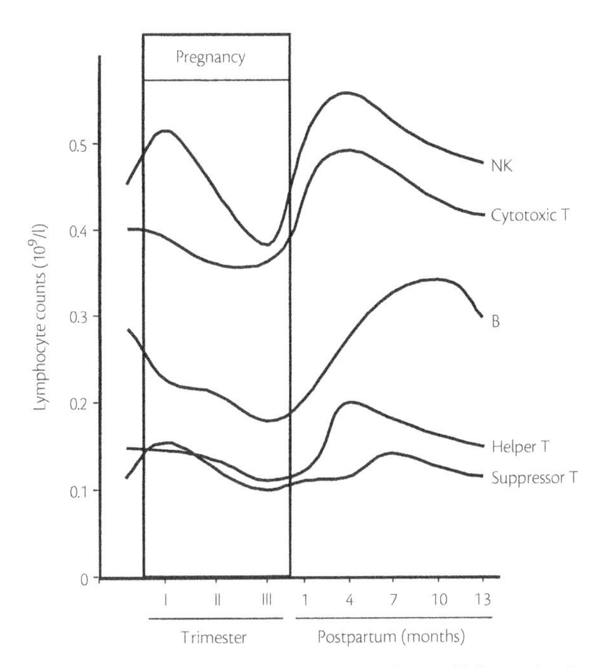

Fig. 3.4.6.2 Changes in peripheral T cells, B cells, and natural killer (NK) cells during pregnancy and the postpartum period in normal women.

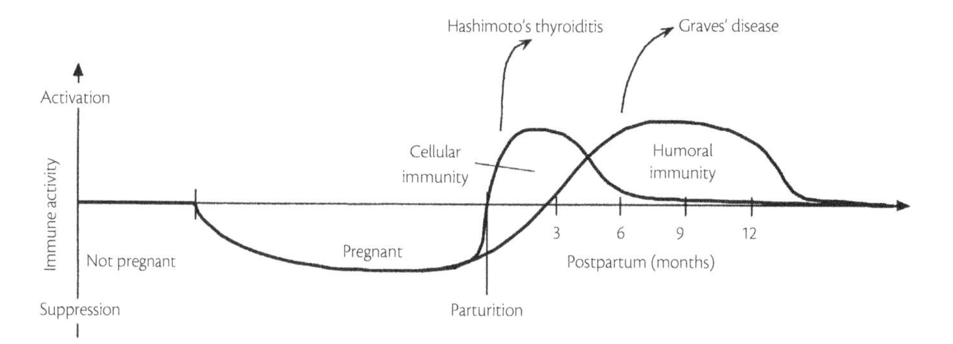

Fig. 3.4.6.3 Immune rebound hypothesis of postpartum autoimmune thyroid diseases. One to 3 months after delivery cellular immunity dominates, and development or exacerbation of autoimmune thyroiditis is observed. Three to 6 months after delivery humoral immunity dominates, and development or exacerbation of Graves' disease is observed.

important problem. Depression was found to be associated with antithyroid autoantibodies rather than hypothyroidism (14).

Diagnosis

Diagnosis of postpartum thyroid dysfunction is simple when the patient shows abnormal thyroid function tests during the postpartum period and positive thyroid autoantibodies. Thyroid dysfunction, however, is most often subclinical. For patients with overt thyrotoxicosis, it is essential to differentiate between postpartum Graves' disease and destructive thyrotoxicosis. Usually an educated guess can be made from the time of onset (4–8 months after parturition in Graves' disease versus 1–3 months in destructive thyrotoxicosis). Anti-TSH-receptor antibody and other markers helpful for the differential diagnosis are summarized in Table 3.4.6.2 (15, 16). Blood tests, however, are not conclusive since anti-TSH-receptor autoantibodies are sometimes found in Hashimoto's thyroiditis and other tests do not have distinct cut-off values. The quantitative measurement of thyroid blood flow using Doppler ultrasonography is useful for differentiation and it is high in Graves' disease and low in destructive thyrotoxicosis (17). The measurement of radioactive iodine uptake gives a definitive clue in the differential diagnosis between Graves' disease (high uptake) and destructive thyrotoxicosis (low uptake). However, it should not be performed in mothers who are breastfeeding. There is no reliable way to differentiate between transient and persistent Graves' disease.

Table 3.4.6.1 Incidence of postpartum thyroid dysfunction

Year	First author	Country	Prevalence (%)
1982	Amino	Japan	5.5
1984	Jansson	Sweden	6.5
1985	Walfish	Canada	7.1
1986	Freeman	USA	1.9
1987	Nikolai	USA	6.7
1987	Lervang	Denmark	3.9
1988	Fung	UK	16.7
1990	Rasmussen	Denmark	3.3
1990	Rajatanavin	Thailand	1.1
1991	Roti	Italy	8.7
1991	Lobig	Germany	2.0
1992	Walfish	Canada	6.0
1992	StagnaroGreen	USA	8.8
1998	Kuijpens	The Netherlands	12.4
2000	Lucas	Spain	7.8
2000	Barca	Brazil	13.3
2001	Shahbazian	Iran	11.4
2001	Bagis	Turkey	5.5

For hypothyroidism, most cases are transient and due to an exacerbation of autoimmune thyroiditis. The finding of positive antithyroid microsomal antibody and/or antithyroglobulin antibody supports the existence of autoimmune thyroiditis, but negative results are obtained in 5–30% of patients. Cases of iodine-deficient hypothyroidism may occur in areas where iodine intake is marginal or mildly deficient, such as Europe (18), although it is likely that mothers already had hypothyroidism during pregnancy. Once the diagnosis is established, patients should be followed up for 1 year since Graves' disease may occur shortly after destructive thyrotoxicosis.

In postpartum thyroid dysfunction some immunological abnormalities are observed before the onset of thyroid dysfunction (and, therefore, before and during pregnancy). Among these, the measurement of thyroid peroxidase antibodies or microsomal antibodies (MCAb) is the most useful marker for the prediction of the occurrence of postpartum thyroid dysfunction (19). If thyroid peroxidase antibodies are present, there is always lymphocytic infiltration into the thyroid and, therefore, 'subclinical autoimmune thyroiditis'(20), which may be exacerbated after delivery. Of women with a positive measurement of thyroid peroxidase antibodies in early pregnancy, 60–70% develop postpartum thyroid dysfunction (2), whereas the risk of developing postpartum thyroid dysfunction in women with negative thyroid peroxidase antibody is estimated to be 0.6%. Mothers with a high thyroid peroxidase antibody titre (MCAb more than 5000–10 000 reciprocal dilution) always develop postpartum thyroid dysfunction. However, the measurement of thyroid peroxidase antibodies does not provide any information on the type of dysfunction that will occur. Although the measurement of thyroid peroxidase antibodies with semiquantitative antimicrosomal particle agglutination (MCPA) tests is simple and cheap, the value of screening for postpartum autoimmune thyroid syndrome remains unresolved (see also Chapter 3.1.7), probably depending on each country's national health system (21). Antithyroid peroxidase antibody is as useful as semiquantitative particle agglutination tests for predicting postpartum thyroid dysfunction (22).

Graves' disease is aggravated in early pregnancy, ameliorates in the latter half of pregnancy, but often relapses postpartum (23).

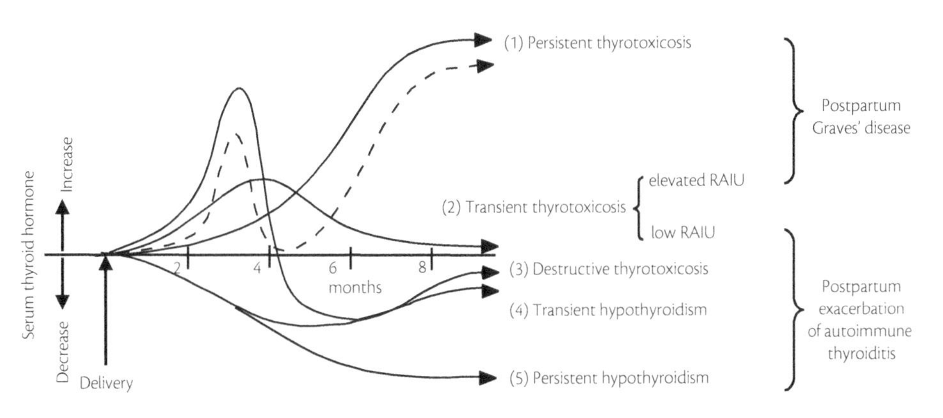

Fig. 3.4.6.4 Various types of postpartum thyroid dysfunction. RAIU, radioactive iodine uptake.

Human chorionic gonadotropin (hCG) plays a crucial role in the aggravation of Graves' thyrotoxicosis in early pregnancy (24). The relapse of Graves' thyrotoxicosis after parturition may occur even in patients in remission before pregnancy. The new onset of Graves' disease in the postpartum period is of great interest, since early diagnosis and treatment at the onset of the disease can lead to early remission (12). It is also an important period of Graves' onset, since 40% of Graves' patients who have had one or more deliveries developed their disease postpartum (25). TSH-receptor stimulating antibodies can be taken as a marker for postpartum development of Graves' disease, since TSH-receptor stimulating antibodies are positive before the onset of Graves' disease (26) when measured with a sensitive bioassay. Pregnant women with positive TSH-receptor stimulating antibodies in early pregnancy have a high-risk of developing postpartum Graves' disease. Seventy-one pregnant women with positive thyroid peroxidase antibodies in early pregnancy were prospectively observed from early pregnancy to the postpartum period (12). Among them, seven showed positive TSH-receptor stimulating antibodies, five (70%) of whom developed postpartum Graves' disease. Thyrotoxicosis in three of those five was transient and spontaneously improved within a year. Graves' disease did not occur in the TSH-receptor stimulating antibody-negative patients (Fig. 3.4.6.5). The conventional radioreceptor assay for anti-TSH-receptor antibodies was not able to discriminate postpartum Graves' disease.

Table 3.4.6.2 Differences between postpartum Graves' disease and postpartum destructive thyrotoxicosis

	Graves' disease	Destructive thyrotoxicosis
Onset	3–6 months postpartum	1–3 months postpartum
Anti-TSH-receptor antibody	Positive	Negative in most cases
Eye signs	Yes	No
Total T_3/total T_4 ratio (ng/µg)	>20 in 80% of cases	<20
Thyroid blood flow	High	Low
Radioactive iodine uptake[a]	High	Low
Serial change in serum thyroglobulin	<50% increase from a month before the onset	>50% increase from a month before the onset

[a] this test is not used for lactating women.

Treatment

In postpartum Graves' disease, treatment options are antithyroid agents, radioactive iodine, or subtotal thyroidectomy, as in 'typical' Graves' disease. Antithyroid drug treatment is a good initial choice because: (1) postpartum Graves' hyperthyroidism is often transient, (2) even in persistent Graves' disease the early diagnosed patients are easily controlled with antithyroid drugs (12), and (3) mothers may not want breastfeeding to be interrupted by radioiodine therapy (see also Chapters 3.3.6 and 3.3.9). Radioactive iodine treatment can still be applied when hyperthyroidism persists after 1 year and has not gone into remission during antithyroid drug treatment.

In destructive thyrotoxicosis, the thyrotoxic phase is always transient and spontaneously ceases in 1–3 months. Treatments should be symptomatic, mainly with β-adrenergic antagonists for cardiovascular hyperdynamic symptoms. Because breastfeeding should be discontinued, β-adrenergic antagonists are indicated only in severe cases. Antithyroid therapy is not indicated. The treatment of hypothyroidism is required only when the patient has symptoms of hypothyroidism. Usually thyroxine (T_4) therapy with a gradual reduction in dose may go well, but recovery of patient's thyroid function cannot be followed explicitly. Alternatively, replacement with a submaximal dose of triiodothyronine (15–50 µg T_3 daily by mouth in one to three divided doses) is useful in most transient cases, since spontaneous recovery of thyroid function can be monitored by an increase of serum T_4. In permanent hypothyroidism, when serum T_4 does not recover after several months of T_3 treatment, T_4 replacement is indicated. Recently successful prevention for postpartum development of thyroid dysfunction was achieved by short-term immunosuppressive therapy in patients who were predicted to develop postpartum hypothyroidism (27). It is also reported that selenium supplementation during pregnancy and in the postpartum period reduced thyroid inflammatory activity and the incidence of hypothyroidism (28).

Prognosis

Little is known about the long-term prognosis of postpartum Graves' hyperthyroidism, although a better outcome than in 'typical' Graves' disease might be expected in view of early diagnosis just after the onset of disease. In destructive thyrotoxicosis and/or hypothyroidism due to exacerbation of autoimmune thyroiditis,

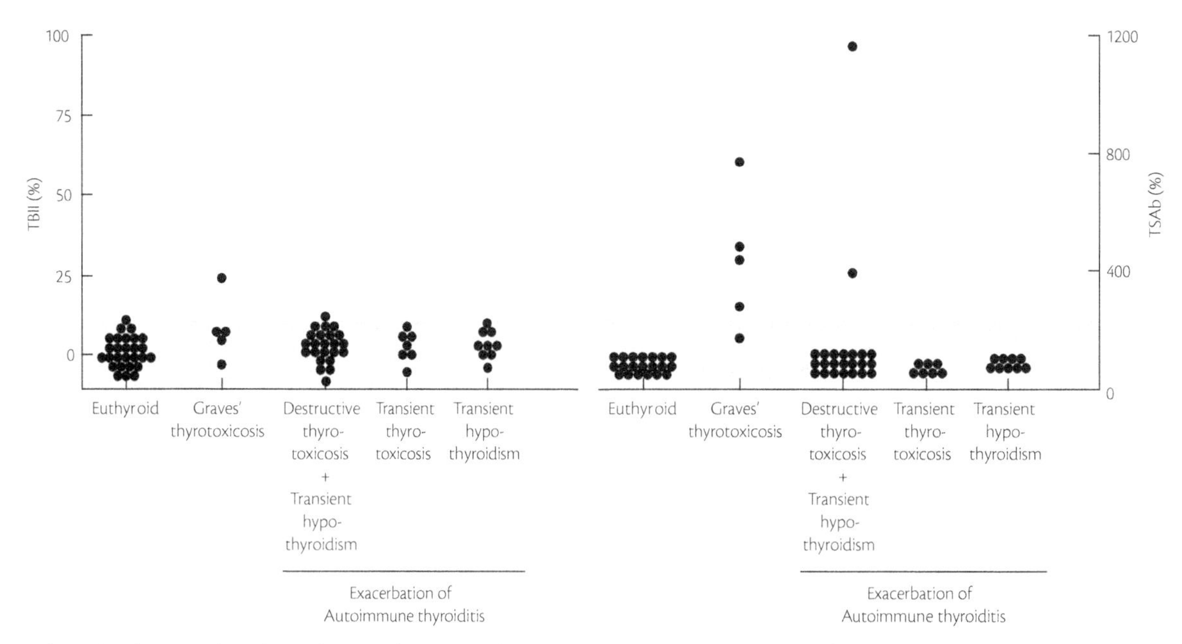

Fig. 3.4.6.5 Relationships between thyroid-stimulating antibodies in early pregnancy and postpartum thyroid dysfunctions. TBII, anti-TSH-receptor antibody detected by radioreceptor assay (left); TSAb: TSH-receptor stimulating antibody (right).

thyroid dysfunction is transient and most patients recover spontaneously to euthyroidism. Only in a few cases, hypothyroidism may persist. High titres of thyroglobulin antibodies and/or thyroid peroxidase antibodies are risk factors of persistent hypothyroidism. Even after recovery from hypothyroidism, abnormalities in ultrasonography and/or iodide perchlorate discharge tests may persist for a long time (29, 30), reflecting underlying chronic autoimmune thyroiditis. The patients almost certainly will develop postpartum thyroid dysfunction after the next parturition, with similar time of onset, type of thyroid dysfunction, and duration of dysfunction as in the previous episode.

Late development (after 5 years or more) of permanent hypothyroidism is found in 25–60% of the patients with postpartum thyroiditis (31–33) and, therefore, these patients should be followed up at appropriate intervals (once every 1–2 years) (34). Othman *et al.* reported that high titres of anti-MCAb and the severity of the hypothyroid phase of postpartum thyroiditis are risk factors for the late development of permanent hypothyroidism, but there was no association with HLA haplotype or family history of thyroid disease (31). In contrast, in Japanese women, high titres of thyroglobulin antibodies and HLA-DRw9 and/or B51 genotype were risk factors of permanent hypothyroidism (32).

References

1. Amino N, Mori H, Iwatani Y, Tanizawa O, Kawashima M, Tsuge I, *et al.* High prevalence of transient post-partum thyrotoxicosis and hypothyroidism. *N Engl J Med*, 1982; **306**: 849–52.
2. Amino N, Tada H, Hidaka Y. Postpartum autoimmune thyroid syndrome: a model of aggravation of autoimmune disease. *Thyroid*, 1999; **9**: 705–13.
3. Amino N, Kuro R, Tanizawa O, Tanaka F, Hayashi C, Kotani K, *et al.* Changes of serum anti-thyroid antibodies during and after pregnancy in autoimmune thyroid disease. *Clin Exp Immunol*, 1978; **31**: 30–7.
4. Hidaka Y, Amino N, Iwatani Y, Kaneda T, Nasu M, Mitsuda N, *et al.* Increase in peripheral natural killer cell activity in patients with autoimmune thyroid disease. *Autoimmunity*, 1992; **11**: 239–46.
5. Amino N, Miyai K, Kuro R, Tanizawa O, Azukizawa M, Takai S, *et al.* Transient post-partum hypothyroidism: Fourteen cases with autoimmune thyroiditis. *Ann Intern Med*, 1977; **87**: 155–9.
6. Stagnaro-Green A. Post-miscarriage thyroid dysfunction. *Obstet Gynaecol*, 1992; **80**: 490–2.
7. Watanabe M, Iwatani Y, Kaneda T, Hidaka Y, Mitsuda N, Morimoto Y, *et al.* Changes in T, B, and NK lymphocyte subsets during and after normal pregnancy. *Am J Reprod Immunol*, 1997; **37**: 368–77.
8. Stagnaro-Green A, Roman S, Cobin R, El-Harazy H, Wallenstein S, Davies T. A prospective study of lymphocyte-initiated immunosuppression in normal pregnancy: evidence of a T-cell etiology for post-partum thyroid dysfunction. *J Clin Endocrinol Metab*, 1992; **74**: 645–53.
9. Shimaoka Y, Hidaka Y, Tada H, Nakamura T, Mitsuda N, Morimoto Y, *et al.* Changes in cytokine production during and after normal pregnancy. *Am J Reprod Immunol*, 2000; **44**: 143–7.
10. Ando T, Davies TF. Postpartum autoimmune thyroid disease: the potential role of fetal microchimerism. *J Clin Endocrinol Metab*, 2003; **88**: 2965–71.
11. Nicholson WK, Robinson KA, Smallridge RC, Ladenson PW, Powe NR. Prevalence of postpartum thyroid dysfunction: a quantitative review. *Thyroid*, 2006; **16**: 573–82.
12. Hidaka Y, Tamaki H, Iwatani Y, Tada H, Mitsuda N, Amino N. Prediction of post-partum onset of Graves' thyrotoxicosis by measurement of thyroid stimulating antibody in early pregnancy. *Clin Endocrinol (Oxf)*, 1994; **41**: 15–20.
13. Momotani N, Noh J, Ishikawa N, Ito K. Relationship between silent thyroiditis and recurrent Graves' disease in the post-partum period. *J Clin Endocrinol Metab*, 1994; **79**: 285–9.
14. Kuijpens JL, Vader HL, Drexhage HA, Wiersinga WM, van Son MJ, Pop VJ. Thyroid peroxidase antibodies during gestation are a marker for subsequent depression postpartum. *Eur J Endocrinol*, 2001; **145**: 579–84.
15. Amino N, Yabu Y, Miyai K, Fujie T, Azukizawa M, Onishi T, *et al.* Differentiation of thyrotoxicosis induced by thyroid destruction from Graves' disease. *Lancet*, 1978; **ii**: 344–6.
16. Hidaka Y, Nishi I, Tamaki H, Takeoka K, Tada H, Mitsuda N, *et al.* Differentiation of the postpartum thyrotoxicosis by serum thyroglobulin: usefulness of the new multisite immunoradiometric assay. *Thyroid*, 1994; **4**: 275–8.

17. Ota H, Amino N, Morita S, Kobayashi K, Kubota S, Fukata S, *et al.* Quantitative measurement of thyroid blood flow for differentiation of painless thyroiditis from Graves' disease. *Clin Endocrinol (Oxf)*, 2007; **67**: 41–5.
18. Glinoer D, Delange F, Laboureur I, de Nayer P, Lejeune B, Kinthaert J, *et al.* Maternal and neonatal thyroid function at birth in an area of marginally low iodine intake. *J Clin Endocrinol Metab*, 1992; **75**: 800–5.
19. Amino N, Tada H, Hidaka Y, Izumi Y. Postpartum autoimmune thyroid syndrome. *Endocr J*, 2000; **47**: 645–55.
20. Yoshida H, Amino N, Yagawa K, Uemura K, Satoh M, Miyai K, *et al.* Association of serum antithyroid antibodies with lymphocytic infiltration of the thyroid gland: studies of seventy autopsied cases. *J Clin Endocrinol Metab*, 1978; **46**: 859–62.
21. Hayslip CC, Fein HG, O'Donnell VM, Friedman DS, Klein TA, Smallridge RC. The value of serum antimicrosomal antibody testing in screening for symptomatic post-partum thyroid dysfunction. *Am J Obstet Gynaecol*, 1988; **159**: 203–9.
22. Feldt-Rasmussen U, Hoier MM, Rasmussen NG, Hegedus L, Hornnes P. Anti-thyroid peroxidase antibodies during pregnancy and postpartum. Relation to post-partum thyroiditis. *Autoimmunity*, 1990; **6**: 211–14.
23. Amino N, Tanizawa O, Mori H, Iwatani Y, Yamada T, Kurachi K, *et al.* Aggravation of thyrotoxicosis in early pregnancy and after delivery in Graves' disease. *J Clin Endocrinol Metab*, 1982; **55**: 108–12.
24. Tamaki H, Itoh E, Kaneda T, Asahi K, Mitsuda N, Tanizawa O, *et al.* Crucial role of serum human chorionic gonadotropin for the aggravation of thyrotoxicosis in early pregnancy in Graves' disease. *Thyroid*, 1993; **3**: 189–93.
25. Tada H, Hidaka Y, Tsuruta E, Kashiwai T, Tamaki H, Iwatani Y, *et al.* Prevalence of post-partum onset of disease within patients with Graves' disease of child-bearing age. *Endocr J*, 1994; **41**: 325–7.
26. Kasagi K, Hatabu H, Tokuda Y, Iida Y, Endo K, Konishi J. Studies on thyrotrophin receptor antibodies in patients with euthyroid Graves' disease. *Clin Endocrinol (Oxf)*, 1988; **29**: 357–66.
27. Tada H, Hidaka Y, Izumi Y, Takano T, Nakata Y, Tatsumi K, *et al.* A preventive trial of short-term immunosuppressive therapy in postpartum thyroid dysfunction. *Int J Endocrinol Metab*, 2003; **2**: 48–54.
28. Negro R, Greco G, Mangieri T, Pezzarossa A, Dazzi D, Hassan H. The influence of selenium supplementation on postpartum thyroid status in pregnant women with thyroid peroxidase autoantibodies. *J Clin Endocrinol Metab*, 2007; **92**: 1263–8.
29. Adams H, Jones MC, Othman S, Lazarus JH, Parkes AB, Hall R, *et al.* The sonographic appearances in postpartum thyroiditis. *Clin Radiol*, 1992; **45**: 311–15.
30. Creagh FM, Parkes AB, Lee A, Adams H, Hall R, Richards CJ, *et al.* The iodide perchlorate discharge test in women with previous post-partum thyroiditis: relationship to sonographic appearance and thyroid function. *Clin Endocrinol (Oxf)*, 1994; **40**: 765–8.
31. Othman S, Phillips DI, Parkes AB, Richards CJ, Harris B, Fung H, *et al.* A long-term follow-up of postpartum thyroiditis. *Clin Endocrinol (Oxf)*, 1990; **32**: 559–64.
32. Tachi J, Amino N, Tamaki H, Aozasa M, Iwatani Y, Miyai K. Long term follow-up and HLA association in patients with post-partum hypothyroidism. *J Clin Endocrinol Metab*, 1988; **66**: 480–4.
33. Azizi F. The occurrence of permanent thyroid failure in patients with subclinical postpartum thyroiditis. *Eur J Endocrinol*, 2005; **153**: 367–71.
34. Abalovich M, Amino N, Barbour LA, Cobin RH, De Groot LJ, Glinoer D, *et al.* Management of thyroid dysfunction during pregnancy and postpartum: an Endocrine Society Clinical Practice Guideline. *J Clin Endocrinol Metab*, 2007; **92** (Suppl 8): S1–47.

3.4.7 Thyroid disease in newborns, infants, and children

A.S. Paul van Trotsenburg, Thomas Vulsma

Congenital thyroid disease

Thyroid hormone and brain development

There are good reasons to describe congenital hypothyroidism and hyperthyroidism separately from acquired thyroid diseases because the risks of a disturbed thyroid hormone supply in young children are clearly different from the risks in older children or adults. For adequate metabolism, vertebrates with a higher degree of development, or a more complex ontogeny, are highly dependent on thyroid hormone. Nevertheless, humans appear to be able to 'vegetate' for years in the absence of this hormone. After resumption of hormone supply the metabolism normalizes again. However, brain development in young children does not. With the exception of the development of the neural tube, thyroid hormone is involved in regulation of later events, such as cell migration and the formation of cortical layers, and in neuronal and glial cell differentiation. Thyroid hormone also controls differentiation of not only neurons and oligodendrocytes, but also astrocytes and microglia (1).

The important role of the thyroid in brain development had already been recognized by 1850 when the British surgeon Curlings reported two mentally impaired children with large tongues, who appeared to have no thyroid gland at obduction. Later, more detailed publications about congenital hypothyroidism patients appeared and, in 1871, the British internist Fagge described some of his patients as extremely small (adult height less than 100 cm), with short broad hands and feet, a broad face with a flat root of the nose, thick nostrils, a large open mouth and thick lips, swollen skin, mental impairment, and often deaf. Osler, in 1897, called these patients 'pariahs of nature'. Although at that time a relation was suggested between this striking disease and the absence of the thyroid, the function of this organ was still completely unknown. Remarkably, by the 1890s it was known that administration of (animal) thyroid preparations to children with congenital hypothyroidism improved their clinical condition markedly.

The belief that endemic cretinism, characterized by neurological problems such as mental impairment, deafness, pareses, spasticity, and squint, and endemic goiter might be caused by lack of iodine dates back to the 1850s. In the following century awareness gradually developed that the aforementioned cretinoid features in the offspring are the result of impaired thyroid hormone synthesis during pregnancy. In the event of long-standing iodine deficiency, neither the pregnant woman nor her fetus are able to make sufficient thyroxine (T_4) to prevent cerebral damage. Since 1989 it has been clear that the amount of T_4 that the healthy pregnant woman donates to her baby is usually sufficient to secure fetal brain development, even if the fetus itself is unable to produce T_4 (2). The fundamental value of an adequate maternal thyroid function during pregnancy is well illustrated by case histories of both severely impaired maternal and fetal T_4 production due to a dominant *POU1F1* mutation (see section on disturbances in thyrotropin synthesis and regulation) and due to thyrotropin binding inhibiting immunoglobulins; in both instances children developed severe cognitive and motor disability, in spite of immediate postnatal T_4 therapy (3). Moreover, recent cohort studies have demonstrated that when women have a moderately impaired thyroid function, or just low to normal plasma free T_4 levels during early pregnancy, the mean IQ in the offspring is slightly impaired (4, 5).

The major problem in congenital hypothyroidism, disturbance of brain development resulting in life-long cognitive and motor problems, appears to be dependent on the severity and duration of the hypothyroid condition in the postnatal phase. Administration of T_4 to the affected neonate as soon as possible will largely prevent this problem (6). Because clinical signals are often lacking or are not recognized at that time, neonatal screening has been introduced in many countries. Diagnosis by means of such a mass-screening programme demands an essentially different approach to that used in individual symptomatic thyroid problems. Knowledge about the cause of congenital hypothyroidism is not only scientifically important, but also gives indispensable support to the treatment, (genetic) counselling, and knowledge about the long-term prognosis of the patient.

Fetal and neonatal thyroid hormone supply

Throughout gestation the thyroid hormone supply of the fetal tissues is a subtle interplay between the fetal thyroid and its regulatory system, the maternal thyroid and its regulatory system, the various deiodinating enzymes and thyroid hormone receptors in the placenta, and the fetal target organs. This interplay brings about correct thyroid hormone status (optimal thyroid hormone receptor occupancy) in the different tissues, including the brain, in the different phases of development.

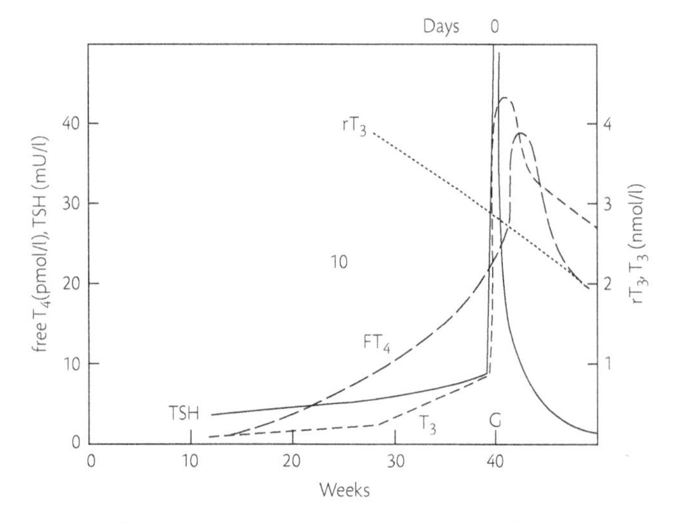

Fig. 3.4.7.1 Fetal and neonatal plasma concentrations of free thyroxine (FT_4), triiodothyronine (T_3), reverse T_3, and thyroid-stimulating hormone (TSH). (Adapted from Thorpe-Beeston JG, Nicolaides KH, Felton CV, Butler J, McGregor AM. Maturation of the secretion of thyroid hormone and thyroid-stimulating hormone in the fetus. *N Engl J Med*, 1991; **324**: 532–6 and Brown RS, Huang SA, Fisher DA. The maturation of thyroid function in the perinatal period and during childhood. In: Braverman LE, Utiger RD, eds. *The Thyroid. A Fundamental and Clinical Text*. 9th edn. Philadelphia: Lippincott Williams & Wilkins, 2005: 1013–28.)

Ontogeny of the thyroid gland

The thyroid develops primarily as a ventral bulge of the endoderm, located between the first and second branchial arches. Sometimes, in later life, a remnant of this median anlage is recognizable as the foramen caecum of the tongue. About 17 days after conception the human primordial thyroid can be detected close to the developing heart, and around day 30 a hollow bilobate structure is formed. Both lobes then fuse with the ultimobranchial bodies (lateral anlagen), developed from the fourth branchial pouches. The calcitonin-secreting cells (C cells) of the thyroid originate from these ultimobranchial bodies.

The thyrocytes are organized into tubes 8 weeks after conception, and 2 weeks later intercellular follicles form and iodine can be bound, indicating that the thyrocytes are able to synthesize thyroperoxidase and thyroglobulin, and to transport these thyroid-specific proteins into the follicular lumen by exocytosis. For some time, the number of follicles is increased by budding from the primary follicles; later on, the thyroid growth is mainly due to the increasing volume of existing follicles (7).

Development of thyroid hormone synthesis during gestation

Near the end of the first trimester (free) T_4 and thyroxine-binding globulin become detectable in the fetal circulation, in very low concentrations compared to normal values for infants and adults (Fig. 3.4.7.1). Subsequently, the concentrations of thyroid-stimulating hormone (TSH), thyroxine-binding globulin, and T_4 increase more or less arithmetically, while free T_4 increases geometrically; all reach adult values at about 36 weeks. Until about 30 weeks gestation, fetal plasma triiodothyronine (T_3) is hardly detectable. It then increases geometrically, although the concentration at term is still very low compared to the normal values for infants and adults (Fig. 3.4.7.1) (8). In contrast, the prenatal levels of reverse T_3 are high (9). The fetus cannot produce its own T_4 until about midgestation and so is completely dependent on the maternal hormone supply. Thyroid hormone synthesis presumably increases gradually in the second half of gestation, since at term the infant provides its own T_4 supply completely.

Birth induces a number of changes in thyroid hormone production and metabolism within a short period (Fig. 3.4.7.1). This adaptation process starts with an acute surge of TSH into the circulation. About 30 min after birth, plasma TSH reaches its maximum level. Thereafter, it gradually decreases and stabilizes within 1–2 days at slightly higher values than those in adults (10). Immediately after birth a rapid and substantial surge of the plasma T_3 concentration takes place. The TSH surge significantly increases the thyroid production of T_4 and thyroglobulin. Plasma T_4 and T_3 reach maximum levels approximately 24 h after birth, while plasma thyroglobulin level peaks about 3 days after birth. In the first week after birth, plasma reverse T_3 concentration decreases rapidly, caused by the loss of placental and hepatic type deiodinase activity (T_4 to reverse T_3 conversion) (9).

The functional maturation of the thyroid in preterm infants at birth is incomplete. Timing of the TSH surge is similar to that of term neonates, but quantitatively lower, especially in preterm infants with respiratory distress syndrome. During the first day following the TSH surge, increasing plasma T_4 and T_3 concentrations can indeed be observed, but the T_4 and T_3 peak levels are lower as the pregnancy is shorter and in the case of complications, such as intrauterine growth retardation and respiratory distress syndrome, a nadir is observed at about 1 week after birth, followed by a second TSH increase. On average the plasma thyroglobulin concentrations in preterm infants are higher than in term infants and are highest in preterm infants with respiratory distress syndrome, in spite of the lower TSH surge (11). Although premature neonates temporarily have lower postpartum free T_4 levels than would be normal for intrauterine life at the same age, administration of T_4 immediately after birth has no significant influence on mortality and morbidity, except for extremely preterm infants (less than 27 weeks gestation) in whom such a bridging T_4 supplement may be beneficial for brain development (12).

Maternal–fetal transfer of thyroid hormone

Maternal–fetal T_4 transfer has been described from the second month of pregnancy. Initially the transfer takes place via the coelomic cavity and yolk sac. After approximately 8–10 weeks gestation nuclear T_3 receptors are detectable in the embryonic tissues. Thereafter, the T_3-receptor concentrations increase strongly (13). In children who are unable to produce any thyroid hormone by themselves, T_4 concentrations in term cord plasma are 30–70 nmol/l, which is 25–50% of the normal cord plasma concentrations (2). This can only be of maternal origin. These thyroid hormone concentrations appear to be high enough to prevent cerebral damage (almost) completely (6, 14).

Although the maternal contribution to the fetal thyroid hormone provision is indispensable, a free placental transfer of T_4 and T_3 may have disadvantages. As far as can be deduced from the course of the fetal plasma (free) T_4 concentration during the first trimester, and of the (free) T_3 concentration throughout the whole gestation, a partial barrier to T_4 and T_3 between the maternal and fetal circulations is maintained.

Newborns of women with untreated hyperthyroidism during pregnancy have been found to have inappropriately low free T_4 concentrations during the first weeks to months of life, without a concomitant increase in the secretion of TSH (fulfilling the criteria of central hypothyroidism) (15). Since this phenomenon is not reported to occur in the offspring of treated euthyroid pregnant women with Graves' disease, it is less likely that maternal antibodies are primarily responsible. Apparently, the severely hyperthyroxinaemic environment of the fetus, during at least the third trimester, may override the placental barrier and inhibit the maturation of thyrotropic cells in the fetal pituitary, or alter the set point for thyroid hormone homeostasis.

Detection and diagnosis of congenital hypothyroidism

Signs and symptoms

The clinically detectable consequences of congenital hypothyroidism are mainly dependent on the severity and duration of the hypothyroid state. Furthermore, the variability in expression between individuals is considerable. At early ages the external signs are only recognizable in cases of severe congenital hypothyroidism (Box 3.4.7.1); milder types may remain undetected for years. Questioning of the parents of neonates with congenital hypothyroidism, detected by screening, showed that subtle signs of hypothyroidism had been observed in the first weeks of life (16).

In only a minority of cases with thyroid dyshormonogenesis is the neonate's thyroid clearly visible or palpable. There is no clearly observable correlation between severity of the defect and neonatal goiter size. Goitrogenesis rarely leads to airway obstruction. Depending on the aetiology of the congenital hypothyroidism, there may be other subtle signs and symptoms (Box 3.4.7.1) (7, 17).

Transient congenital hypothyroidism, usually of short duration and often accompanied by other paediatric problems, usually escapes clinical detection. In such cases the hypothyroid state forms a complicating factor and will be an extra threat to the sick newborn. Data from the (maternal) medical history dealing with, for instance, maternal thyroid disease, use of thyroid-influencing medication, iodine-containing radiographic contrast agents, and disinfectants should draw attention to the neonate's thyroid function.

Neonatal screening

Starting administration of T_4 to congenital hypothyroidism patients shortly after birth will prevent (postnatal) cerebral damage. Unfortunately, congenital hypothyroidism in neonates is difficult to recognize. In 1974 it became possible, on a large scale, to determine T_4 and TSH in just a few drops of blood, obtained by a heel puncture, and absorbed in filter paper. Since then many countries have introduced neonatal mass-screening procedures.

While most European countries have chosen to determine TSH, the Netherlands opted for the North American method of screening based on determination of T_4. Later, the procedure was modified to reduce the number of false-positives: TSH is determined in the 20% of samples with the lowest T_4 concentrations, and thyroxine-binding globulin in the samples with the 5% lowest T_4 levels from which T_4/thyroxine-binding globulin can be calculated. The long-term results of the Dutch screening method are that probably all cases with permanent primary congenital hypothyroidism are diagnosed at an early stage (incidence in Dutch newborns between 1 April 2002 and 31 May 2004 is 1:2 400) and probably more than 90% of cases with permanent secondary/tertiary congenital hypothyroidism (incidence 1:21 000 to 1:16 400) (Table 3.4.7.1) (18–20).

Estimates from a number of international screening reports in areas without endemic iodine deficiency give the mean incidence of permanent primary congenital hypothyroidism as roughly 1:3500 newborns, with considerable ethnic differences (extremes are 1:30 000 among African-Americans in the USA and 1:900 among Asian groups in the UK).

Aetiological classification of congenital hypothyroidism

A clear diagnosis is required to decide upon the optimal treatment and to evaluate the risk of other (endocrine) defects or complications, the risk of recurrence in the family, and the possibilities of prenatal diagnosis and treatment (21). It may also be possible to judge the longer term consequences of congenital hypothyroidism for the patient, especially the risk of a delay in cognitive and motor development.

A clinicopathological approach is the main method used, so that diagnosis is as efficient as possible. The starting point is to produce an aetiological description ('clinicopathological entity'), that is as detailed as possible, for every case of congenital hypothyroidism (22). The gene structures and coding sequences of several proteins involved in T_4 synthesis have been explained in recent years.

Box 3.4.7.1 Signs and symptoms of hypothyroidism in neonates with (severe) congenital hypothyroidism

- Signs and symptoms as a result of hypothyroidism
  - Common
    - Feeding problems
    - Prolonged jaundice
    - Mottled dry skin
    - Open posterior fontanelle
    - Typical (puffy) face
    - Enlarged tongue
    - Umbilical hernia
    - Muscular hypotonia
  - Rare
    - Obstipation
    - Respiratory distress
    - Bradycardia
    - Hypothermia
    - Low-pitched voice
    - Hypoactivity
- Signs and symptoms pointing to a specific cause of the congenital hypothyroidism
  - Rare
    - Cleft palate, choanal atresia, and spiky hair: Bamfort-Lazarus syndrome[a]
    - Respiratory and neurological problems[b]
    - Goiter[c]
    - Sensorineural hearing loss[d]
    - Hypoglycaemia, micropenis, or midline defects[e]

[a]Thyroid dysgenesis due to *FOXE1* gene mutation.
[b]Thyroid dysgenesis due to *TITF1/NKX2-1* gene mutation.
[c]Thyroid dyshormonogenesis.
[d]Thyroid dyshormonogenesis due to Pendrin's gene mutation.
[e]Congenital hypothyroidism of central origin.
Modified from De Felice M, Di LR. Thyroid development and its disorders: genetics and molecular mechanisms. *Endocr Rev*, 2004; **25**: 722–46; Gruters A. Screening for congenital hypothyroidism: effectiveness and clinical outcome. In: Kelnar CJH, ed. *Pediatric Endocrinology (Baillières Clinical Pediatrics)*. London: Bailliere Tindall, 1996: 259–76; and Bizhanova A, Kopp P. Minireview: the sodium-iodide symporter NIS and pendrin in iodide homeostasis of the thyroid. *Endocrinology*, 2009; **150**: 1084–90.

Nevertheless, cDNA containing a novel mutation usually has to be expressed and its function tested before the mutation can be established as the primary cause. At present it is possible to establish this in only a minority of patients with congenital hypothyroidism. This implies that the 'classic' diagnostic methods, such as plasma TSH, free T_4, thyroglobulin, and thyroid autoantibody determination, ultrasound imaging, radio-iodide uptake with a perchlorate test, measurement of the urinary excretion of iodine and iodotyrosines, radio-iodide saliva/blood ratio, and the mode of inheritance will still be needed in the foreseeable future. For the list of known clinicopathological entities, we have developed a set of diagnostic profiles, each representing the combined data of this series of determinants (Table 3.4.7.2) (22). By combining the measurements for series of determinants, each of which alone yields little specific data, the most likely aetiology can be established.

The actual stimulatory activity of TSH is of great importance to the determinants representing the thyroid's action. For instance, generally the plasma thyroglobulin concentration and the radio-iodide uptake are related to plasma TSH concentration, TSH bioactivity, TSH-receptor responsiveness, and the amount of thyroid tissue present, but in the case of a thyroglobulin synthesis defect the plasma thyroglobulin concentration is unusually low. Ultrasound imaging is a useful, fast, and noninvasive diagnostic technique for localizing the thyroid and measuring its volume, but it does not detect small remnants. These, however, are easily visualized with ^{123}I (23). The most sensitive determinant for detecting traces of thyroid tissue is the plasma thyroglobulin concentration (24).

Permanent congenital hypothyroidism of thyroidal (primary) origin

Congenital hypothyroidism resulting from thyroid disorders are due to two main causes: disturbances in the thyroid's ontogeny, making up the major portion of defects, and inborn errors in the thyroid's hormonogenesis (extensively reviewed elsewhere) (22).

Disturbances in thyroid ontogeny

Congenital hypothyroidism caused by disturbances in the development of the thyroid gland may result in mild to very severe hypothyroidism. The thyroid gland may be completely absent (agenesis) or remnants of variable size may be present along the tract of the thyroglossal duct (Fig. 3.4.7.2). These structures, called dystopic (synonym: ectopic) remnants, are often localized in the sublingual area. Agenesis is characterized by complete absence of any thyroid tissue (indicated by ^{123}I and ultrasound imaging), and complete inability to produce thyroid hormone and thyroglobulin (2, 22). However, patients with a negative ^{123}I scintigram and (almost) complete absence of circulating thyroid hormone, but with clearly measurable plasma thyroglobulin levels, have been described (24). As the thyrocytes are the only cells able to produce thyroglobulin, this cell type has to be present, although it cannot be localized. We introduce the term 'cryptic thyroid remnant' to describe this type of disorder.

Why the migration and development of the thyroid becomes disturbed is still unexplained. Studies in mice showed the involvement of the four transcription factors TITF1/NKX2-1, PAX8, FOXE1 (formerly called TTF2), and NKX2-5 (7, 25). Mice missing the *TTF1/NKX2-1* gene were stillborn, lacked thyroid, pituitary, and lung parenchyma, and had extensive defects in brain development; the heterozygous animals were phenotypically normal. Mice lacking *PAX8* only had a rudimentary thyroid gland, almost completely composed of calcitonin-producing C cells. Mice missing the *FOXE1* gene had dystopic thyroid tissue and cleft palate, and their pituitary responded normally to the decreased plasma free T_4 levels, whereas with *TITF1/NKX2-1*, heterozygous mice showed normal thyroid function. Mouse embryos missing the *NKX2-5* gene appeared to have a smaller thyroid bud.

Table 3.4.7.1 Incidence and aetiological classification of congenital hypothyroidism in the 288 patients born in 1981 and 1982, and the 234 patients born between 1 April 2002 and 31 May 2004, detected by the Dutch neonatal screening

	1981–1982 (346 335 neonates screened)		From April 2002 to May 2004[a] (430 764 neonates screened)	
	Number	Incidence	Number	Incidence
CH, total	288	1:1200	234	1:1800
Permanent CH	134	1:2600	200	1:2200
CH-T	118[b]	1:2900	179	1:2400
Thyroid dysgenesis	95[b]	1:3600		
◆ Agenesis	26			
◆ Cryptic remnant	10			
◆ Dystopic remnant	59			
Thyroid dyshormonogenesis	21[b]	1:15 100		
◆ Thyroglobulin synthesis defect	6			
◆ Total iodide organification defect	5			
◆ Partial iodide organification defect	3			
◆ Pendred's syndrome (pendrin deficiency)	1			
◆ Albright's syndrome (Gsα deficiency)	1			
◆ TSH hyporesponsiveness	2			
◆ Down's syndrome (thyroid defect unknown)	3			
CH-T, not specified	2			
CH-C	16	1:21 600	21	1:20 500
Transient CH	154	1:2200	34	1:12 700
CH-T	153	1:2200	24	1:17 900[c]
CH-C	1	1:346 000	10	1:43 000

[a]A 26-month period.

[b]Within the group of children with CH-T approximately 80% have thyroid dysgenesis and 20% thyroid dyshormonogenesis.

[c]The fall in the incidence of transient CH-T in the Netherlands can be explained by the decreased use of iodine as an antiseptic in the perinatal period.

CH, congenital hypothyroidism; CH-C, congenital hypothyroidism of central origin; CH-T, congenital hypothyroidism of thyroidal origin.

From Vulsma T. *Etiology and Pathogenesis of Congenital Hypothyroidism: Evaluation and Examination of Patients Detected by Neonatal Screening in the Netherlands*. Amsterdam: Rodopi, 1991 and Kempers MJ, Lanting CI, van Heijst AF, van Trotsenburg AS, Wiedijk BM, De Vijlder JJ, *et al.* Neonatal screening for congenital hypothyroidism based on thyroxine, thyrotropin, and thyroxine-binding globulin measurement: potentials and pitfalls. *J Clin Endocrinol Metab*, 2006; **91**: 3370–6.

In contrast to the findings in knockout mice, in patients with thyroid dysgenesis only monoallelic inactivating mutations in *PAX8* have been found. In humans homozygous missense mutations in the forkhead domain of *FOXE1* were shown to be associated with congenital hypothyroidism, cleft palate, and choanal atresia (7). Missense mutations in *NKX2-5* have been found in three patients with dystopic thyroid remnants (thyroid ectopy) and in one patient with thyroid agenesis (25).

Although there are strong indications that transcription factors encoded by *TITF1/NKX2-1*, *PAX8*, *FOXE1*, *NKX2-5*, and the TSH receptor play a role in the ontogeny of the human thyroid, only a small minority of the patients with thyroid dysgenesis mutations in these transcription factors has been found (7). This accords with the observations worldwide that familial occurrence of thyroid dysgenesis is rare. It is puzzling, too, why a dysgenic thyroid remnant hardly develops after the embryonic phase, while its hormone production seems to be adequate for the amount of tissue, especially in view of the impressive growth capacity of normally developed thyroids under similar TSH stimulation. Because the more caudally located remnants are usually the larger ones, it is likely that common factors are responsible for both the impaired growth potential, the insufficient 'descendance', and the absence of bifurcation into two lobes.

Disturbances in thyroid hormonogenesis

Inborn errors can occur in all regulatory and metabolic steps involved in the synthesis of thyroid hormone.

Thyroid-stimulating hormone hyporesponsiveness

This refers to defects in the various components of the TSH stimulation pathway. In general, a defect in TSH action is characterized by the presence of a eutopic, often somewhat undersized, thyroid gland, low to very low plasma free T_4 and thyroglobulin concentrations (especially when related to the (very) high TSH concentration), and low thyroidal radio-iodide uptake with a slow iodine turnover. Several loss-of-function mutations in the TSH-receptor gene have been described, that produce congenital hypothyroidism

Table 3.4.7.2 Classification of disorders causing permanent congenital hypothyroidism according to the clinicopathological characteristics

Aetiological entity	Diagnostic determinant						Responsible gene(s) (and mode of inheritance[e])	Remarks
	Plasma free T_4 concentration[a]	Plasma TSH concentration[b]	Plasma thyroglobulin concentration	Thyroid imaging: location and size	Radio-iodide uptake in the thyroid[c]	Radio-iodide release after $NaClO_4$[d]		
Hypothalamic/pituitary CH (secondary and tertiary CH)[f]								
Hypothalamic and/or pituitary dysgenesis	Low	Low to (slightly) increased	Low	Normal to hypoplastic	NI	NI	*HESX1* (AR/AD), *LHX3* (AR), *LHX4* (AD), *SOX3* (XL), *POU1F1* (AR/AD), *PROP1* (AR)	Septo-optic dysplasia
Hypothalamic/pituitary dyshormonogenesis								
TRH hyporesponsiveness	Low	Low	Low	Normal to hypoplastic	NI	NI	*TRHR* (AR)	
TSH deficiency	Low	Low	Low	Normal to hypoplastic	NI	NI	*TSH* (AR)	
Thyroidal CH (primary CH)								
Thyroid dysgenesis								
Thyroid agenesis	Absent[g]	Very high	Absent	Absent	Absent	Absent	*FOXE1* (AD)	Agenesis
Cryptic thyroid remnant	Absent[g]	Very high	Low to normal	Absent	Absent	Absent	*PAX8* (AD)	Mild hypoplasia to agenesis
Dystopic thyroid remnant	Low to normal	(Very) high	Low to high	(Sub)lingual	Low to normal	Absent	*TITF1/NKX2-1* (AR)	Normal thyroid gland, hypoplasia, and hemiagenesis
Eutopic thyroid remnant	Low to normal	(Very) high	Unknown	Hypoplastic	Low to normal	Absent	*NKX2-5*	Dystopic thyroid remnant and agenesis
Thyroid dyshormonogenesis								
TSH hyporesponsiveness								
TSH receptor deficiency	Low to normal	High	Low to normal	Normal to hypoplastic	Low	Absent	*TSHR* (AR)	
Gsα deficiency	Normal to low	Normal to high	Low to normal	Normal	Low	Absent	*GNAS1* (AD)	
Total iodide transport defect	(Very) low	Very high	Very high	Normal to hyperplastic	Absent[h]	Absent	*NIS* (AR)	Saliva/serum ratio of radio-iodide

Total iodide organification defect	Absent[g]	Very high	Very high	Normal to hyperplastic	Rapid and high	Total	*TPO* (AR), *DUOX2* (AR), *DUOXA2* (AR)	
Partial iodide organification defect	Low to normal	High	(Very) high	Normal to hyperplastic	High	Partial		
Pendrin deficiency (Pendred's syndrome)[i]	Normal to low	Normal to low	Normal to high	Normal to hyperplastic	Normal to high	Partial	*SLC26A4* (AR)	
Thyroglobulin synthesis defect	Low to normal	High	Absent to normal	Normal to hyperplastic	Rapid and high	Absent	*TG* (AR)	Urinary excretion of iodopeptides
Iodide recycling defect (synonym: dehalogenase defect)	Low to normal	High	(Very) high	Normal to hyperplastic	High	Absent	*DEHAL1* (AR)	Urinary excretion of MIT and DIT

[a] Lower limit of the free T_4 reference interval: 2nd to 4th week of life is *c.*12 pmol/l; 2nd and 3rd month of life is *c.*11 pmol/l.

[b] Upper limit of the TSH reference interval: 2nd to 4th week of life is *c.*10 mU/l; 2nd and 3rd month of life is *c.*6 mU/l.

[c] $Na^{123}I$ is administered intravenously (1 MBq (27 μCi) for infants younger than 1 year and 2 MBq (54 μCi) for older children). In general, the radio-iodide uptake is a function of the amount of thyroid tissue and the degree of stimulation by TSH.

[d] $NaClO_4$ is administered intravenously 2 h after $Na^{123}I$ (10 mg/kg body mass, maximum 400 mg). Discharge of thyroidal radio-iodide after 1 h: less than 10% is normal; 10–20% is borderline; more than 20% is abnormal.

[e] When the full-blown disease has an autosomal recessive pattern of inheritance, some heterozygous relatives have mild abnormalities in the relevant tests.

[f] The most significant determinant for central hypothyroidism is MRI of the cerebral midline structures; the TSH response to intravenously administered TRH may discriminate newborns with congenital hypothyroidism of central origin as part of multiple pituitary hormone deficiency from newborns with isolated TSH deficiency.

[g] When a newborn infant cannot produce any T_4, maternal–fetal transfer is responsible for T_4 concentrations of 2.7–5.4 μg/dl (35–70 nmol/l) in cord serum, which disappear with a half-life of 2.7–5.3 days.

[h] Most characteristic determinant for the diagnosis of (total) iodide transport defect is the (very) low saliva/serum ratio of radio-iodide: for neonates, more than 10 is normal, 3–10 is borderline, and less than 3 is abnormal. The saliva/blood ratio is 1.17 times the saliva/serum ratio (95% CI 1.15 to 1.19). Partial iodide transport defect is an ill-defined condition; if it exists, the diagnostic determinants depend entirely on the iodine intake, which varies greatly worldwide.

[i] The most significant determinant for Pendred's syndrome is the sensorineural hearing defect.

AD, autosomal dominant; AR, autosomal recessive; CH, congenital hypothyroidism; DIT, diiodotyrosine; MIT, monoiodotyrosine; NI, no indication for this test; XL, X-linked.

Adapted from Vulsma T, De Vijlder JJM. Genetic defects causing hypothyroidism. In: Braverman LE, Utiger RD, eds. *The Thyroid. A Fundamental and Clinical Text*. 9th edn. Philadelphia: Lippincott Williams & Wilkins, 2005: 714–30; Afink G, Kulik W, Overmars H, de Randamie J, Veenboer T, van Cruchten A, *et al.* Molecular characterization of iodotyrosine dehalogenase deficiency in patients with hypothyroidism. *J Clin Endocrinol Metab*, 2008; **93**: 4894–901; van Tijn DA, De Vijlder JJ, Verbeeten B Jr, Verkerk PH, Vulsma T. Neonatal detection of congenital hypothyroidism of central origin. *J Clin Endocrinol Metab*, 2005; **90**: 3350–9; Mehta A, Dattani MT. Developmental disorders of the hypothalamus and pituitary gland associated with congenital hypopituitarism. *Best Pract Res Clin Endocrinol Metab*, 2008; **22**: 191–206; and Yamada M, Mori M. Mechanisms related to the pathophysiology and management of central hypothyroidism. *Nat Clin Pract Endocrinol Metab*, 2008; **4**: 683–94.

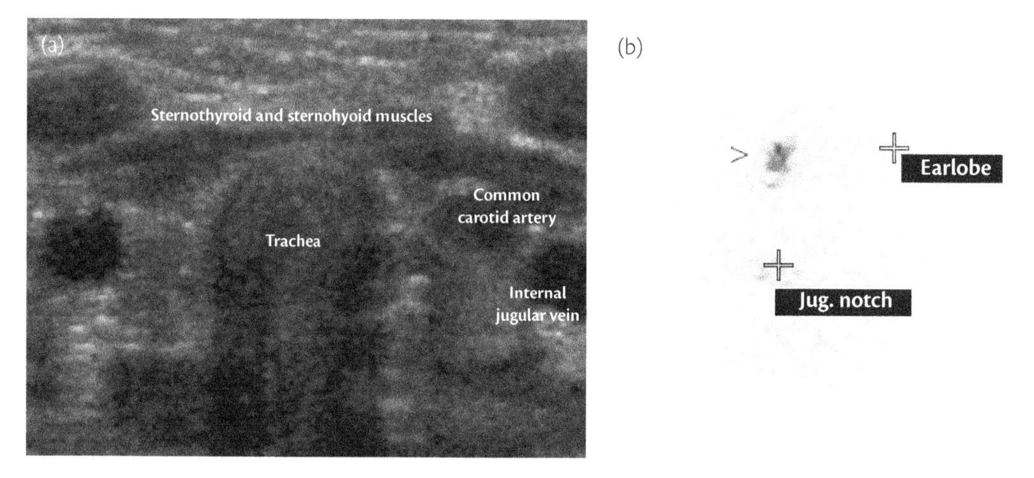

Fig. 3.4.7.2 Ultrasonography (a) and thyroid ^{123}I scintigraphy (b) of the neck and head/neck, respectively, of a 14-day-old boy whose abnormal neonatal screening result was suggestive of congenital hypothyroidism of thyroidal origin, which was confirmed by finding a plasma TSH concentration of 186 mU/l (normal <10 mU/l) and a free T_4 concentration just below the reference interval. Ultrasonography showed no thyroid tissue in the trachea–'muscles'–carotid artery triangle. Scintigraphy showed a dystopic thyroid remnant (>).

with strongly variable expression, ranging from subclinical to overt hypothyroidism (26, 27). A related type of TSH hyporesponsiveness has been described in patients with pseudohypoparathyroidism type 1A (Albright's hereditary osteodystrophy). The cause of this autosomal dominant inherited disease is a mutation in the *GNAS* gene, coding for the α-subunit of the Gs-protein (28). Some of the patients become hypothyroid; only a minority is detected by the neonatal congenital hypothyroidism screening. In some patients with the clinicopathological characteristics of TSH hyporesponsiveness, inherited in an autosomal dominant way, no mutations in TSH-receptor or *GNAS* genes could be found, suggesting the presence of mutations in more distal components of the TSH signalling pathway.

Defects in iodide transport

The first step in thyroid hormonogenesis is the active transport of iodide into the thyrocytes. Iodide transport across the basal membrane is mediated by the sodium-iodide symporter (NIS). Currently, at least 12 iodide transport defect-causing mutations of the *NIS* gene have been identified. Patients are hypothyroid from birth, show gradual goitrogenesis, low or very low plasma T_4 concentrations, high plasma thyroglobulin concentrations, undetectable thyroidal radio-iodide uptake, and a radio-iodide saliva/blood ratio of about unity. Heredity is autosomal recessive (17). Both the severity of hypothyroidism and the neurodevelopmental impairment vary considerably, probably due to variations in dietary iodine intake. Treatment with large doses of iodine is possible, but therapy with T_4 is preferred, especially in young children.

Defects in iodination of thyroglobulin

Oxidation of trapped iodide and binding to tyrosine residues in proteins, particularly thyroglobulin, is commonly referred to as iodide organification. Both steps take place at the apical brush border of the thyrocyte, mainly in the follicular lumen. Oxidative coupling of iodothyronine residues requires a proper thyroglobulin structure, normal peroxidase activity, and a regulated presence of hydrogen peroxide (H_2O_2). H_2O_2 is generated by (thyroid) dual oxidase 2. Defects in any of these compounds will impair thyroid hormonogenesis, resulting in primary congenital hypothyroidism. When left untreated goitrogenesis will occur.

In patients with iodination defects, the T_4 synthesis is decreased or absent depending on whether the trapped iodide is only partially or not at all organified. As a consequence of the low plasma thyroid hormone concentrations, the TSH level is enhanced, resulting in a high (radio)iodide uptake and an elevated plasma thyroglobulin concentration. The delayed or absent iodide oxidation and organification causes a high intracellular (inorganic) iodide content, which is rapidly released after the administration of sodium perchlorate (Fig. 3.4.7.3) (see notes to Table 3.4.7.2) (29).

In (almost) all cases, total iodide organification defects are caused by mutations in the gene coding for thyroperoxidase. The defect is transmitted in an autosomally recessive way. Inactivation of thyroperoxidase is caused by several types of mutations, such as deletions, insertions, missense and nonsense mutations, and splicing defects. The most frequent mutation is a duplication of a GGCC sequence in exon 8 (30). Partial organification defects are not only caused by (heterozygous) mutations in the thyroperoxidase gene, but also by mutations in the genes encoding dual oxidase 2 and dual oxidase maturation factor 2. Biallelic as well as heterozygous mutations in the *DUOX2* gene appear to result in transient congenital hypothyroidism (31, 32) The single patient with a homozygous mutation in the *DUOXA2* gene had relatively mild but permanent congenital hypothyroidism (33).

A remarkable subtype of partial organification defect is Pendred's syndrome, with an estimated prevalence of 1 in 40 000. Pendrin, encoded by the *SLC26A4* gene, is a highly hydrophobic membrane protein located at the apical membrane of thyrocytes, where it could function as an iodide transporter. In the inner ear, pendrin is important for generation of the endocochlear potential. Currently, more than 150 mutations of the *SLC26A4* gene have been reported (17). Most patients have a moderate to severe sensorineural hearing loss from infancy. Hypothyroidism (usually mild) and goiter may be present at birth or may develop later in life. Only a few patients with Pendred's syndrome are detected by neonatal screening.

Defects in the synthesis of thyroglobulin

Thyroglobulin plays a central role in thyroid hormone synthesis. Thyroglobulin synthesis occurs exclusively in the thyrocyte. The protein is very large and is encoded by a thyroglobulin mRNA

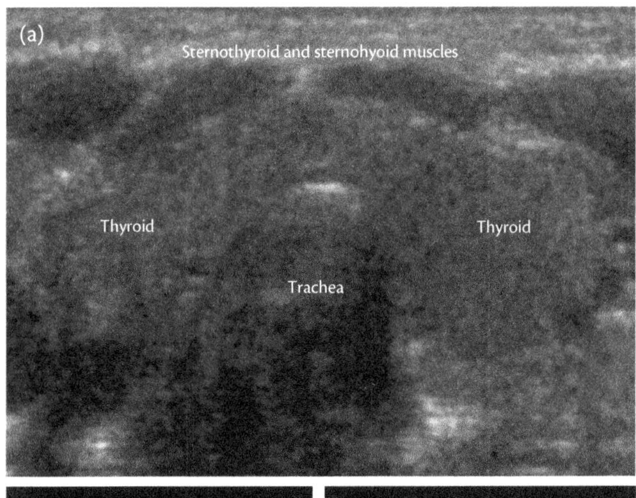

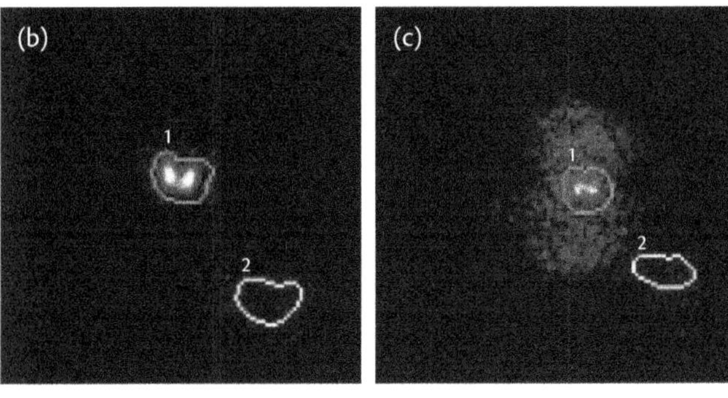

Fig. 3.4.7.3 Ultrasonography of the neck (a) and thyroid ^{123}I scintigraphy before (b) and after (c) perchlorate administration in a 14-day-old boy whose abnormal neonatal screening result was suggestive of congenital hypothyroidism of thyroidal origin and which was confirmed by laboratory testing. Ultrasonography and scintigraphy showed a normally localized thyroid. However, ^{123}I uptake decreased from 20.7% before to 4.3% after the administration of perchlorate, confirming the diagnosis 'iodide organification defect'.

containing 8307 nucleotides. Thyroglobulin is a homodimer with subunits of 330 000 Da, each containing 60 disulfide bridges and 10% carbohydrates (34).

For maximal production of iodothyronines, mainly T_4, an optimal stereospecific configuration of thyroglobulin is required. This configuration is dependent on the primary structure, disulfide bridges, the extent of glycosylation, and possibly other processes such as phosphorylation. A distorted configuration will result in an impaired formation of iodothyronines. Patients classified under the entity 'thyroglobulin synthesis defects' are moderately to severely hypothyroid. In relation to the TSH concentration, the plasma thyroglobulin concentration is usually low, but there are exceptions. The processes of iodide uptake, oxidation, and organification are intact. A clinicopathological evaluation, however, cannot distinguish whether disorders in the synthesis of thyroglobulin are caused by defects in transcription, translation, or post-translational processes and transport. Therefore this entity comprises all these types of defects.

The exceptional size of the gene coding for thyroglobulin makes it difficult to identify mutations in the coding regions. In four human families and three animal strains, various mutations have been described: deletions, nonsense and missense mutations, and acceptor splice-site mutations that cause alternative splicing. The mutations are all homozygous in character; the inheritance is autosomal recessive (34).

Defects in the recycling of iodide

Thyroglobulin, internalized by endocytosis from the follicular lumen into the thyrocyte, is incorporated into early and late endosomes. These organelles, containing proteolytic enzymes, hydrolyse thyroglobulin to its constituent amino acids, including the iodotyrosines monoiodotyrosine and diiodotyrosine, as well as T_4 and T_3. Subsequently, the iodotyrosines are deiodinated by specific deiodinase(s) in the thyroid and other tissues.

Iodotyrosine deiodinase defects, hereditary disorders in this deiodinating system, lead to loss of the iodotyrosines from the thyroid, and rapid excretion by the kidneys. The excessive loss of iodine results in postnatal hypothyroidism and mimics hypothyroidism due to iodine deficiency. Only recently, the first homozygous missense mutations and deletion in the gene encoding iodotyrosine deiodinase (*DEHAL1*) were described in four patients who presented with severe goitrous hypothyroidism diagnosed in infancy and childhood. The two patients who underwent neonatal screening were not detected, and one of these two patients was found to be mentally impaired. This implies that infants with *DEHAL1* defects may have normal thyroid function at birth and they may be missed by neonatal screening programmes for congenital hypothyroidism (35). Elevated urine di- and monoiodotyrosine concentrations are suggestive of the diagnosis (36). Although the heredity is autosomal recessive, one recently described heterozygous carrier of an inactivating mutation presented with overt hypothyroidism suggesting dominant inheritance with incomplete penetration (36).

Permanent congenital hypothyroidism of central (secondary/tertiary) origin

While a clear distinction can be made between thyroid dysgenesis and dyshormonogenesis in the case of congenital hypothyroidism of thyroidal origin, such a distinction is less straightforward in secondary/tertiary congenital hypothyroidism. Moreover, it is difficult to discriminate, using clinicopathological criteria, between secondary (synonym: pituitary) and tertiary (synonym: hypothalamic) disorders. For that reason the entity 'congenital hypothyroidism of central origin' is introduced, a term that does not exclude simultaneous occurrence of other pituitary hormone deficiencies.

Disturbances in the ontogeny of the thyroid's regulatory system

Most cases of congenital hypothyroidism of central origin concern developmental disturbances of the pituitary and/or hypothalamus and are easy to visualize with MRI (Fig. 3.4.7.4). In these cases the endocrine problem is not restricted to the thyrotropic axis. As in congenital hypothyroidism of thyroidal origin, there are sporadic and hereditary types of central congenital hypothyroidism, but the developmental problems that cause central congenital hypothyroidism are not just 'sporadic'. In a recent series of patients with central congenital hypothyroidism detected through the Dutch neonatal screening programme, 53% of these patients had a so-called posterior pituitary ectopia. All of these patients had multiple pituitary hormone deficiencies, with cortisol deficiency as the most (life-)threatening problem (37). Posterior pituitary ectopia may be accompanied by other (minor) malformations, often of other cerebral structures. The underlying cause is unknown. Currently, only a small percentage of the cases of multiple pituitary hormone deficiency can be explained by mutations in genes encoding transcription

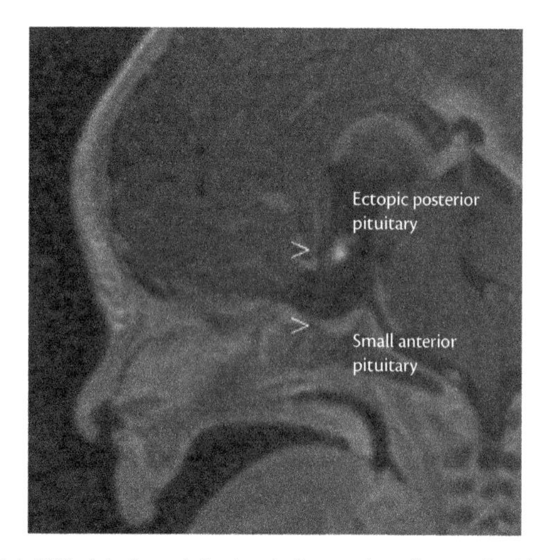

Fig. 3.4.7.4 MRI of the hypothalamic–pituitary region of a 4-week-old girl, showing a somewhat small anterior pituitary (lower >) and 'posterior pituitary ectopia' (upper >). The girl had an abnormal neonatal screening result suggestive of congenital hypothyroidism of central origin, which was confirmed by finding a free T_4 concentration below the reference interval and a delayed TSH rise after thyrotropin-releasing hormone administration at the age of 19 days. In addition, the girl turned out to have central adrenal insufficiency, and growth hormone and gonadotropin deficiency.

factors involved in hypothalamus and pituitary development (Table 3.4.7.2) (38, 39).

Disturbances in thyrotropin synthesis and regulation

Inborn errors may occur in all regulatory and metabolic steps involved in the synthesis of TSH. These may be located in the hypothalamus or pituitary gland.

Thyrotropin-releasing hormone deficiency

Knowledge about the mechanism of thyrotropin-releasing hormone (TRH) production in the hypothalamus is limited. The tripeptide TRH is also present elsewhere in the central nervous system, indicating that neither synthesis nor action is restricted to the thyrotropic axis. Isolated TRH deficiency in humans has not yet been reported.

Thyrotropin-releasing hormone hyporesponsiveness

Diminished TRH responsiveness is only a partially explained entity. Based on the analogy of TSH hyporesponsiveness, it might be assumed that mutations in TRH receptor and defects in postreceptor processes (G-protein deficiency, etc.) may result in secondary congenital hypothyroidism. Homozygous mutations in the TRH receptor gene are found which result in the formation of receptors that are unable to bind TRH. The patients are mildly hypothyroid with complete absence of TSH and prolactin responses to TRH (40).

In another group of patients with central hypothyroidism, missense and nonsense mutations, and deletions in the genes encoding the transcription factors POU1F1 and PROP1, have been described. POU1F1 regulates the expression of the *TSHβ*, growth hormone, and prolactin genes. Mutation of the *POU1F1* gene results in combined pituitary hormone deficiencies, including complete growth hormone and prolactin deficiency as well as central congenital hypothyroidism. Most cases show autosomal recessive inheritance, but some show an autosomal dominant inheritance pattern. PROP1 is involved in the early development of several lineages of anterior pituitary cells. Mutations in the *PROP1* gene cause multiple pituitary hormone deficiency that is autosomal recessive and is, in addition to central congenital hypothyroidism, associated with deficiency of luteinizing hormone/follicle-stimulating hormone, growth hormone, prolactin, and, less frequently, adrenocorticotropic hormone (39). Patients with hereditary defects in the *TSHβ* gene are rare. The hypothyroidism may be severe, and plasma TSH may vary from undetectable to slightly raised. In the latter case the circulating TSH is biologically inactive (39).

Permanent congenital hypothyroidism of peripheral origin

Congenital hypothyroidism or hypothyroidism originating during the first weeks to months of life can also result from increased inactivation (infantile haemangioma expressing type 3 deiodinase) or loss of T_4 (congenital nephrotic syndrome) (41, 42). Affected patients may need a rather high T_4 dose to correct the hypothyroidism. Since the cause of the hypothyroidism is not in the thyroid gland, pituitary, or hypothalamus, the entity 'congenital hypothyroidism of peripheral origin' is introduced. Other forms of congenital hypothyroidism of peripheral origin are resistance to thyroid hormone (due to thyroid hormone receptor β (*TRβ*) gene mutations), and the recently discovered thyroid hormone transporter and thyroid hormone metabolism defects (due to monocarboxylate transporter 8 (*MCT8*) gene and to 'selenocysteine insertion sequence-binding protein 2' (*SBP2*) gene mutations, respectively). In all of these conditions, of which the clinical and biochemical features are extensively reviewed in Chapter 3.4.8, there is reduced sensitivity to thyroid hormone (43). T_4 treatment is probably not beneficial in these conditions.

Transient congenital hypothyroidism of thyroidal origin

Transient primary congenital hypothyroidism is often due to exposure of the neonate (or the fetus) to excessive quantities of iodine, e.g. iodine-containing radiographic contrast agents and disinfectants. These agents are mostly used in premature or very ill infants. Detection by the neonatal congenital hypothyroidism screening depends on the timing of the exposure. There are no data available from systematic psychological or neurological investigations to estimate the risk of brain damage in children who are perinatally exposed to iodine excess. Yet, prevention of this type of thyroid dyshormonogenesis is indicated, preferably by avoiding unnecessary use of excessive quantities of iodine, or by timely administration of T_4.

Incidentally, maternal thyroid-inhibiting antibodies may cause transient congenital hypothyroidism for several weeks or months, depending on the initial concentration of circulating antibodies (44). Rarely the use of antithyroid drugs by the mother leads to abnormal congenital hypothyroidism screening results.

Transient congenital hypothyroidism of central origin

Transient congenital hypothyroidism of central origin has been reported in a number of newborns of women with untreated Graves' hyperthyroidism during pregnancy. It may be caused by exposure of the fetal hypothalamic–pituitary–thyroid system to higher than normal thyroid hormone concentrations, impairing its physiological maturation during intrauterine life (45).

Treatment, control of treatment, and psychological follow-up of congenital hypothyroidism

The main treatment goal in congenital hypothyroidism is prevention of cerebral damage due to lack of thyroid hormone. This implies that the period with decreased levels of circulating free T_4

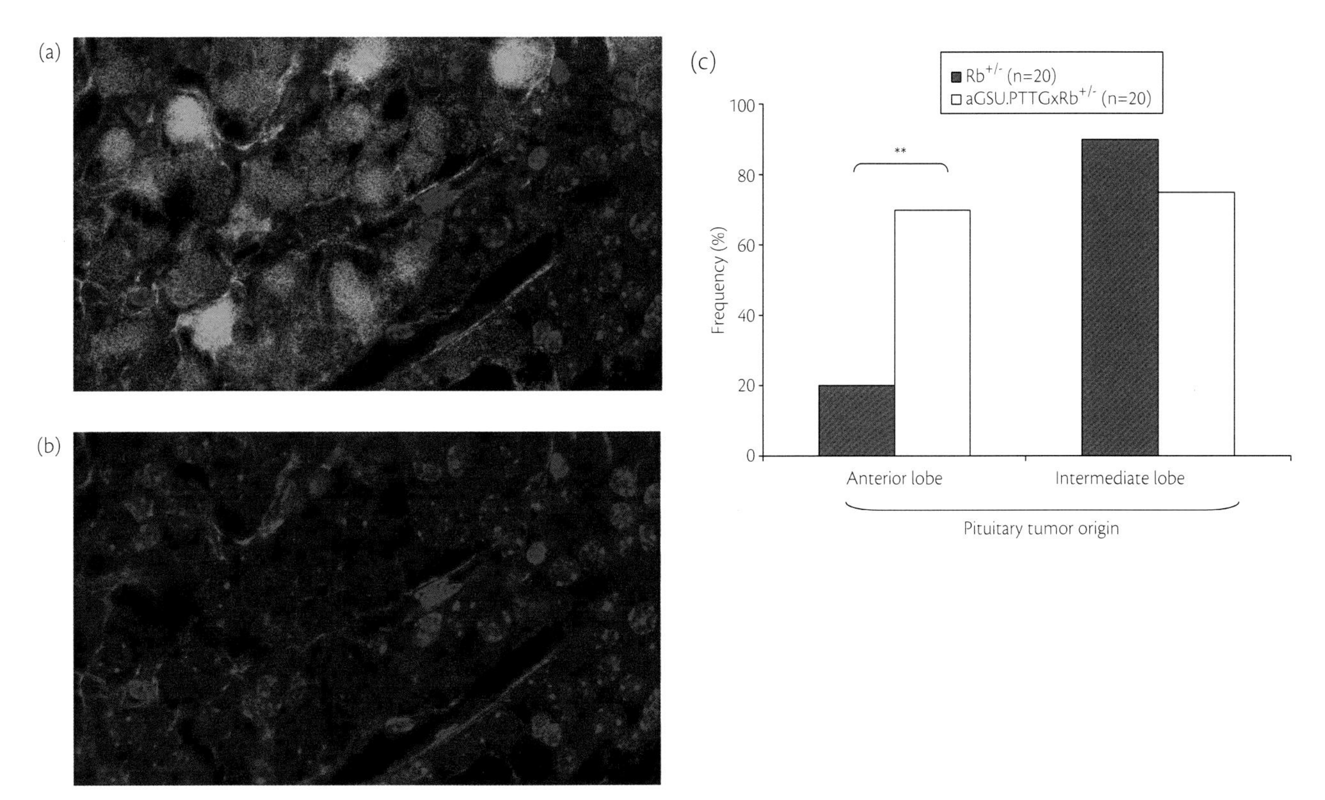

Plate 1 Targeted *PTTG* overexpression to anterior lobe pituitary cells results in cell hyperplasia and increased tumour formation. Fig. 2.3.2.4(a) and (b) are duplicates of the same image, overview of pituitary cells expressing a*GSU.PTTG1.IRESeGFP* transgene. (a) is the untouched image, and in (b) the green layer (eGFP) has been hidden for better visualization of nuclear morphology. Contrast between eGFP positive (overexpressing PTTG) and eGFP negative (normal PTTG content) can be appreciated, notably presence of macronuclei and reorganization of chromatin suggestive of hyperplastic cells. (See also Plate 1) Fig. 2.3.2.4(c) depicts that bitransgenic a*GSU.PTTG;Rb*$^{+/-}$ mice exhibit higher prevalence of anterior lobe and similar prevalence of intermediate lobe pituitary tumours when compared with *Rb*$^{+/-}$ mice. Pathological analysis of pituitary tumours reveals that frequency of tumours arising from anterior lobe is higher in a*GSU.PTTG;Rb*$^{+/-}$ (white bars) than in *Rb*$^{+/-}$ (black bars) pituitary tumours (**, $p = 0.0036$), but frequency of tumours arising from the intermediate lobe (where there was no *PTTG* overexpression) is similar. n, total number of pituitary tumours analyzed. (From Donangelo I, Gutman S, Horvath E, Kovacs K, Wawrowsky K, Mount M, *et al.* Pituitary tumor transforming gene overexpression facilitates pituitary tumor development. *Endocrinology*, 2006; **147**: 4781–91 (6), with permission. (See also Fig. 2.3.2.4))

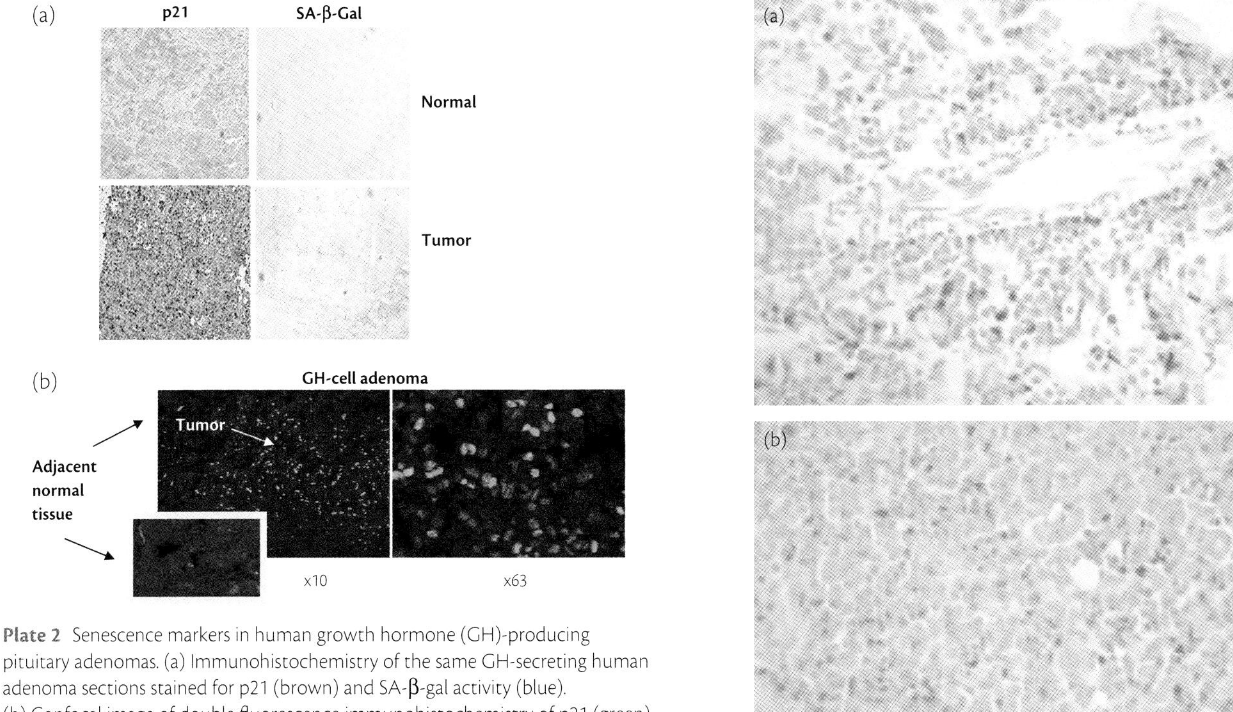

Plate 2 Senescence markers in human growth hormone (GH)-producing pituitary adenomas. (a) Immunohistochemistry of the same GH-secreting human adenoma sections stained for p21 (brown) and SA-β-gal activity (blue). (b) Confocal image of double fluorescence immunohistochemistry of p21 (green) and β-galactosidase (red) proteins coexpression in human pituitary adenoma but not in normal adjacent tissue (left panel). High resolution (×63) image of the same slide (right panel). (From Chesnokova V, Zonis S, Kovacs K, Ben-Shlomo A, Wawrowsky K, Bannykh S, et al p21(Cip1) restrains pituitary tumor growth. *Proc Natl Acad Sci U S A*, 2008; **105**: 17498–503 (30), with permission.) (See also Fig. 2.3.2.5)

Plate 3 (a) Pituitary tumour and (b) cervical metastasis excised 4 years later, both showing positive (brown) immunostaining for prolactin (6). (See also Fig. 2.3.14.2)

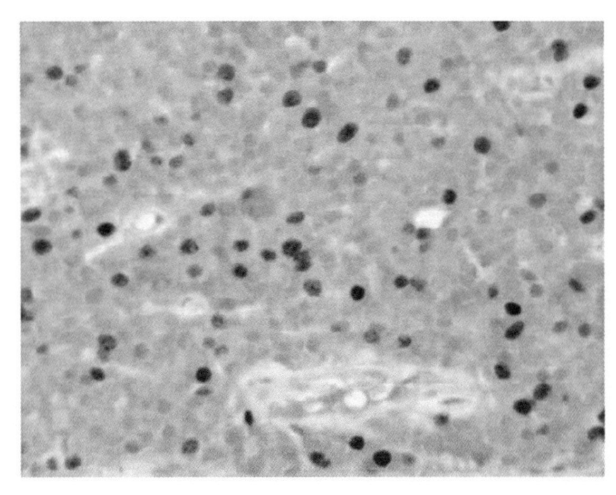

Plate 4 Ki-67 staining using MIB1 antibody in a cervical metastasis from a pituitary carcinoma; the MIB1 proliferation index is around 10% (6). (See also Fig. 2.3.14.3)

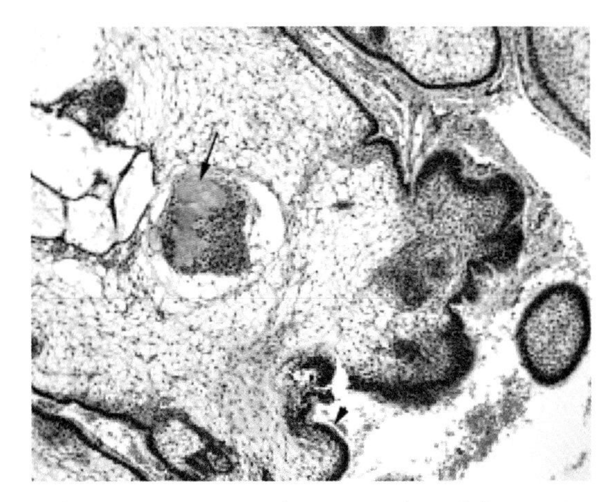

Plate 5 Adamantinomatous craniopharyngioma. The epithelium consists of a palisade basal layer of cells (arrowhead), an intermediate stellate reticulum, and a layer of flattened, keratinized squamous cells. Nodules of 'wet' keratin (arrow) are also shown. (Reprinted from Karavitaki N, Cudlip S, Adams CBT, Wass JAH. Craniopharyngiomas. *Endocr Rev*, 2006; **27**: 371–97 (1) with permission. Copyright 2006, The Endocrine Society.) (See also Fig. 2.4.2.1)

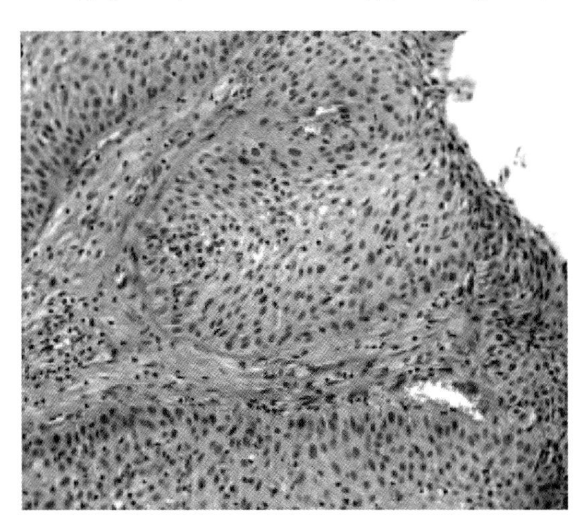

Plate 6 Papillary craniopharyngioma. The epithelium is mature squamous forming pseudopapillae downward into the underlying tissues. (Reprinted from Karavitaki N, Cudlip S, Adams CBT, Wass JAH. Craniopharyngiomas. *Endocr Rev*, 2006; **27**: 371–97 (1) with permission. Copyright 2006, The Endocrine Society.) (See also Fig. 2.4.2.2)

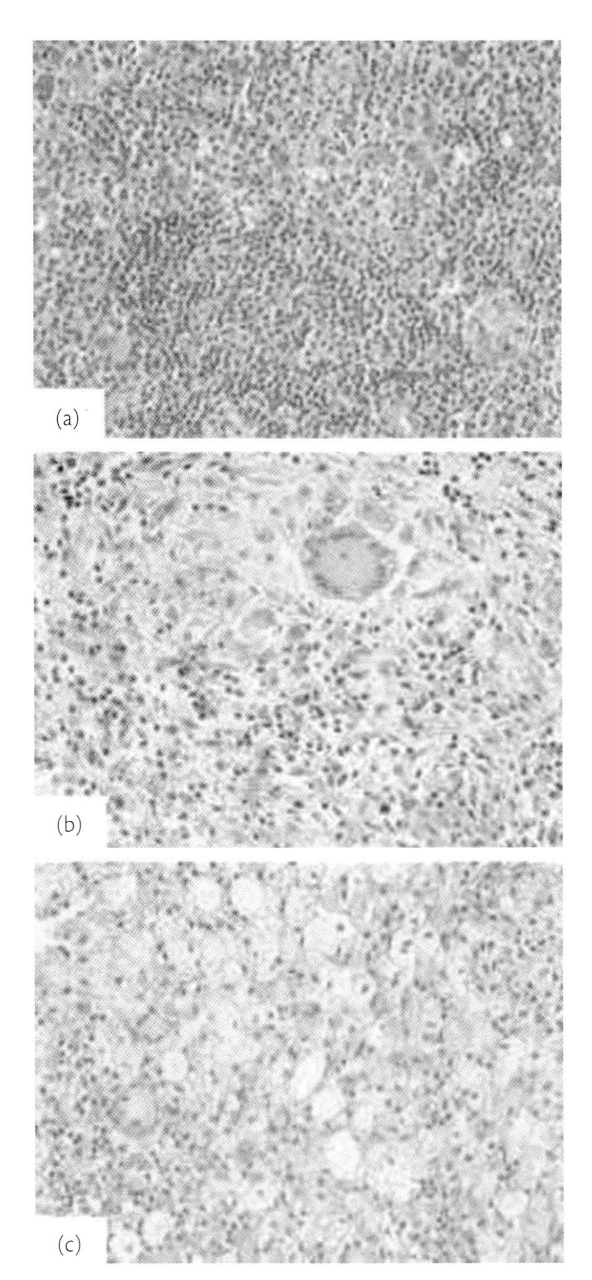

Plate 7 Histological subtypes of primary hypophysitis. (a) Lymphocytic hypophysitis. Note massive lymphocytic infiltration of pituitary with scattered islands of preserved pituitary cells. (b) Idiopathic granulomatous hypophysitis. Characteristic multinucleated giant cells and granuloma surrounded by fibrosis; there is sparse infiltration of plasma cells. (c) Xanthomatous hypophysitis. Predominance of foamy macrophages, a few lymphocytes, and single plasma cells. Haematoxylin and eosin, original magnification ×40. (10). (See also Fig. 2.4.4.1)

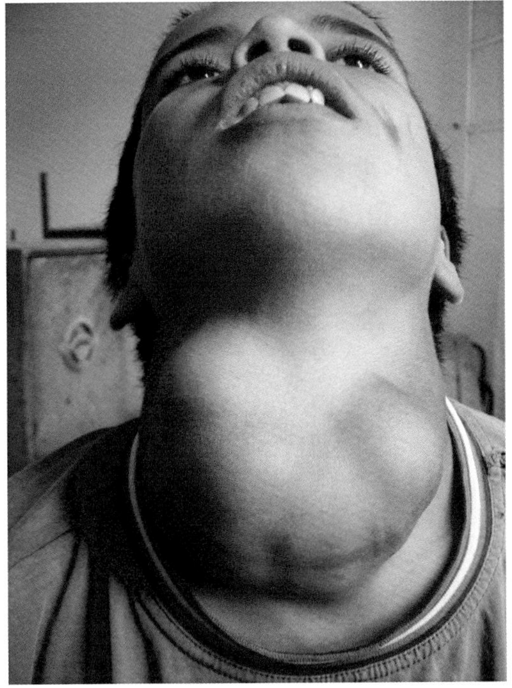

Photo: © MB Zimmermann

Plate 8 Large nodular goitre in a 14-year-old boy photographed in 2004 in an area of severe IDD in northern Morocco, with tracheal and oesophageal compression and hoarseness, likely due to damage to the recurrent laryngeal nerves. (See also Fig. 3.2.3.1)

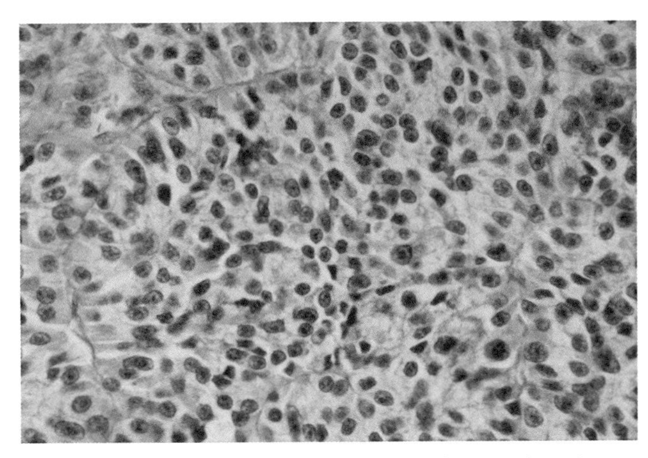

Plate 10 Representative example of the solid variant of papillary thyroid cancer in a post Chernobyl thyroid cancer patient. (See also Fig. 3.2.5.3)

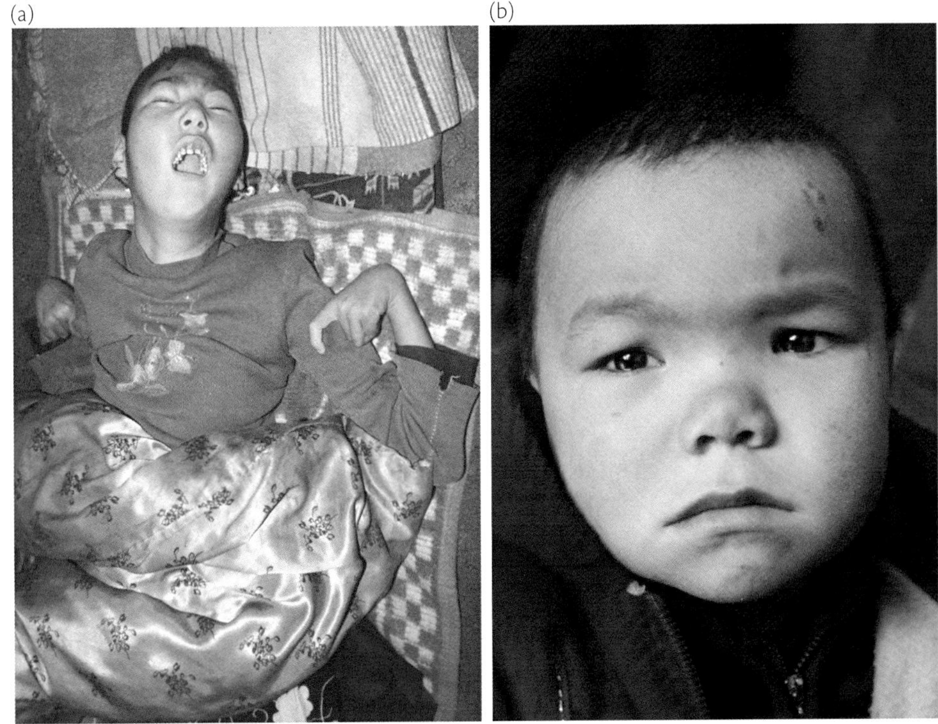

Photos: © MB Zimmermann

Plate 9 (a) Neurological cretinism. This 2007 photograph of a 9-year-old girl from western China demonstrates the three characteristic features: severe mental deficiency together with squint, deaf–mutism, and motor spasticity of the arms and legs. The thyroid is present, and the frequency of goitre and thyroid dysfunction is similar to that observed in the general population. (b) Myxoedematous cretinism. This 2007 photograph of a 5-year-old boy from western China demonstrates the characteristic findings: profound hypothyroidism, severe growth impairment (height, 106 cm), incomplete maturation of the features including the naso-orbital configuration, atrophy of the mandible, puffy features, umbilical hernia, myxoedematous thickened dry skin, and dry hair, eyelashes, and eyebrows. The thyroid typically shows atrophic fibrosis. (See also Fig. 3.2.3.2)

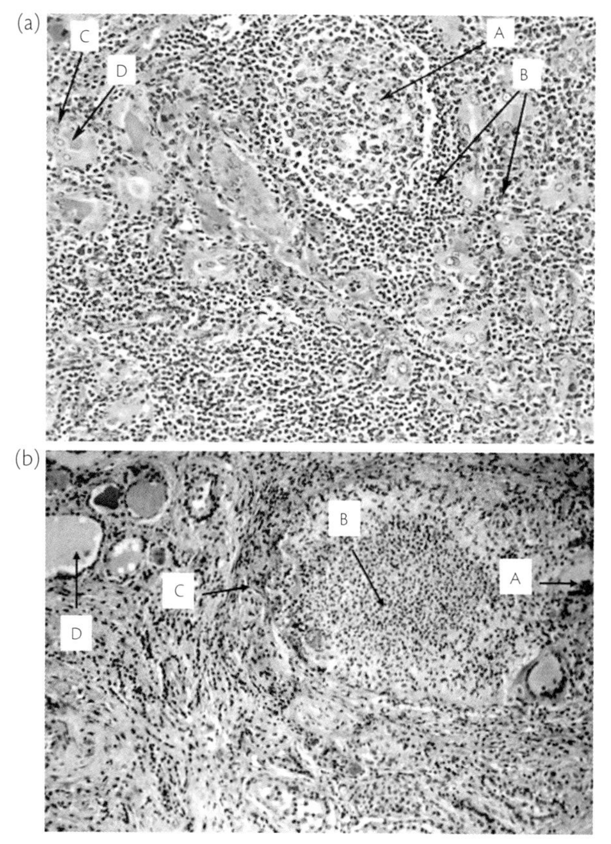

Plate 11 Typical pathological changes of Hashimoto's thyroiditis and subacute thyroiditis. (a) Hashimoto's thyroiditis. A, lymphoid follicle with germinal centres; B, small lymphocytes and plasma cells; C, thyroid follicles with Hürthle cell metaplasia; D, minimal colloid material. (b) Subacute thyroiditis. A, multinucleate giant cell; B, mixed inflammatory infiltrate; C, fibrous band; D, residual follicles. Haematoxylin and eosin, ×200. (With permission from the Massachusetts Medical Society © 2003. All rights reserved.) (See also Fig. 3.2.7.1)

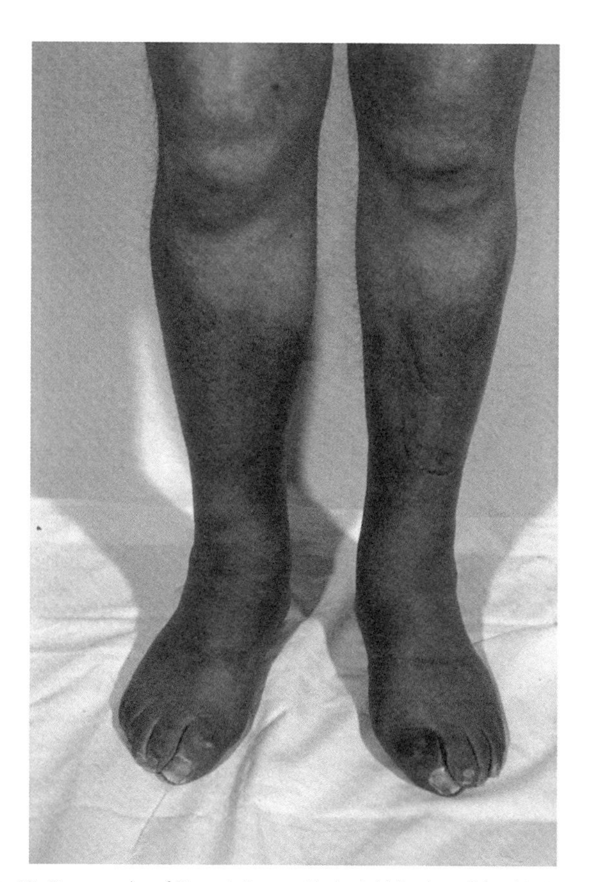

Plate 12 Dermopathy of Graves' disease. Marked thickening of the skin is noted, usually over the pretibial area. Thickening will occasionally extend downwards over the ankle and the dorsal aspect of the foot, but almost never above the knee. (See also Fig. 3.3.1.1)

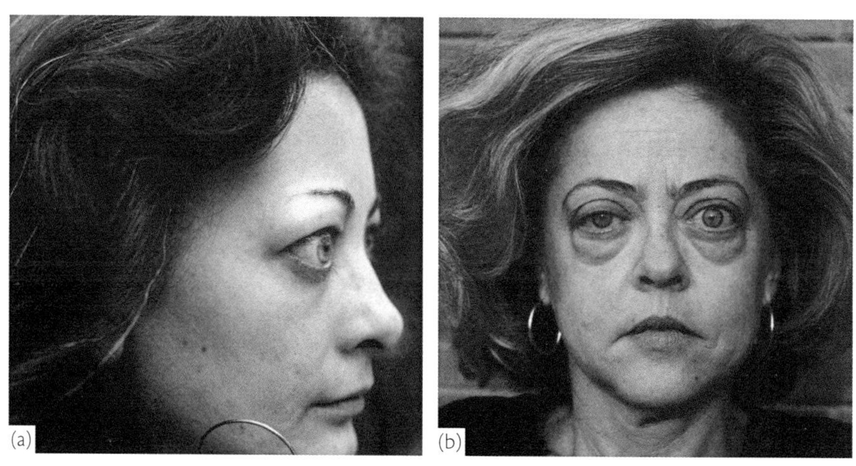

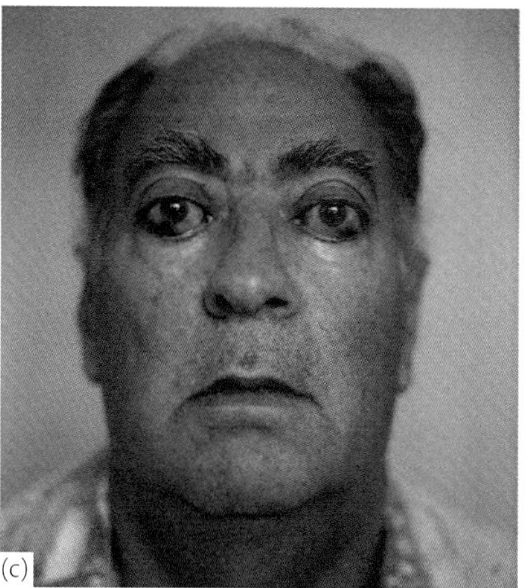

Plate 13 Clinical presentation of Graves' ophthalmopathy. (a) Retraction of both upper eyelids. (b) Severe periorbital oedema and retraction of both upper eyelids. (c) Marked conjunctival infection and chemosis, together with retraction of both lower eyelids. (See also Fig. 3.3.1.2)

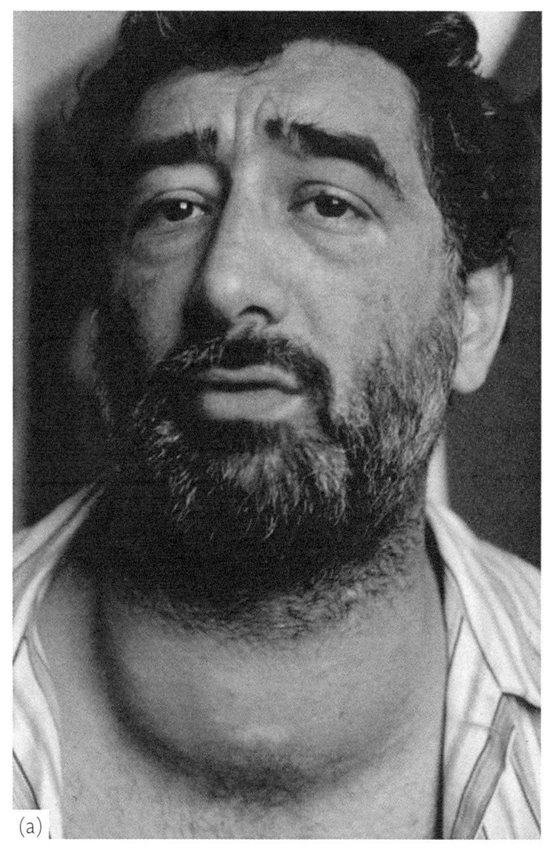

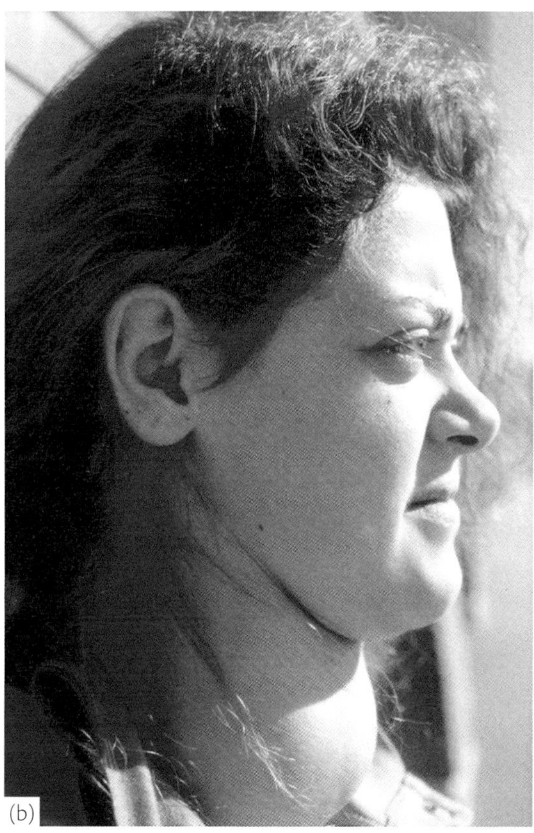

Plate 14 (a) Massive thyroid enlargement related to diffuse toxic goitre. (b) An asymmetrical thyroid enlargement related to multinodular goitre. (See also Fig. 3.3.1.3).

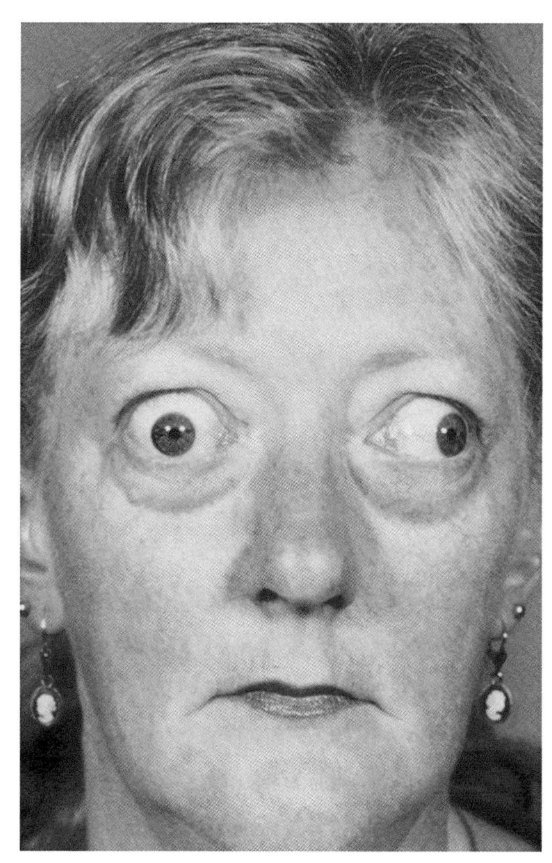

Plate 15 Bilateral eye disease due to Graves' ophthalmopathy. Note lid retraction, stare, periorbital swelling, marked proptosis, and exotropia of the left globe. (See also Fig. 3.3.10.1)

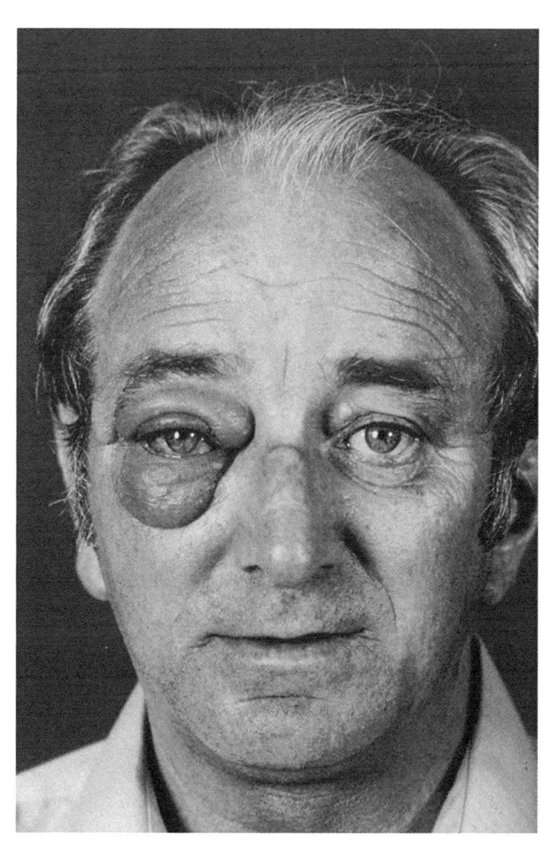

Plate 16 Unusual presentation of Graves' ophthalmopathy as unilateral eye disease. Male sex, advanced age, and heavy smoking all predisposed this patient to the development of severe eye disease; note the absence of exophthalmos in this case of dysthyroid optic neuropathy. (See also Fig. 3.3.10.2)

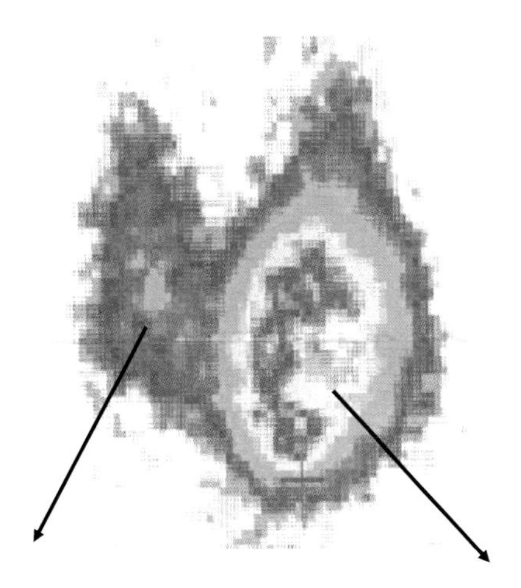

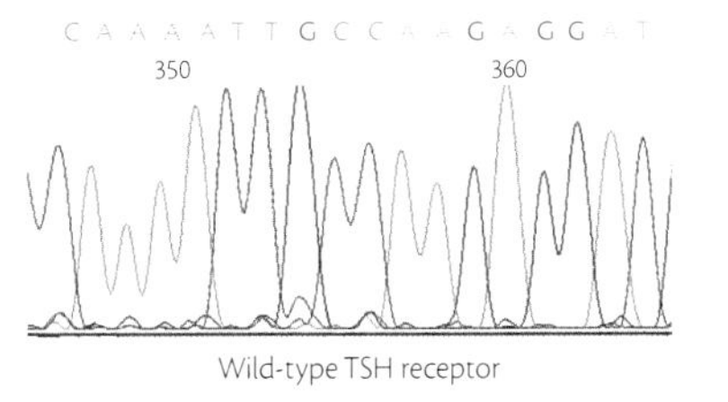

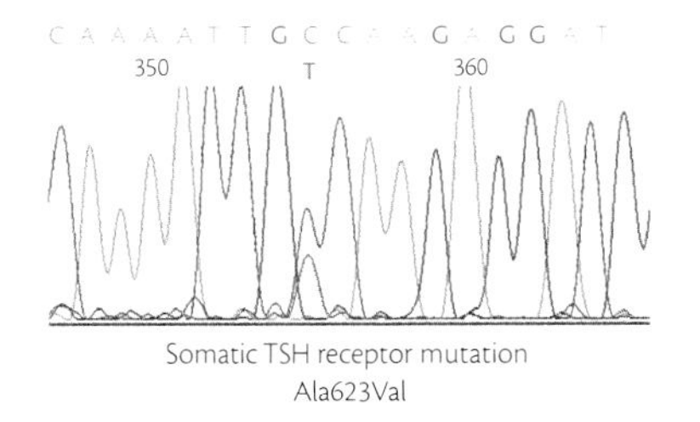

Plate 17 Scintiscan of a uninodular goitre showing a circumscribed area of increased technetium uptake in the left lobe ('hot' nodule). DNA was extracted from the toxic adenoma and surrounding normal thyroid tissue and exon 10 of the TSH receptor was amplified by polymerase chain reaction (PCR). Sequencing of the PCR products showed the presence of a heterozygous point mutation (GCC→GTC) resulting in an amino acid exchange (Ala→Val) in the toxic adenoma (right) whereas only the wild-type TSH receptor was present in the normal thyroid tissue (left). The mutation causes a constitutive activation of the TSH receptor which leads to thyrotoxicosis and thyroid growth. (See also Fig. 3.3.11.1)

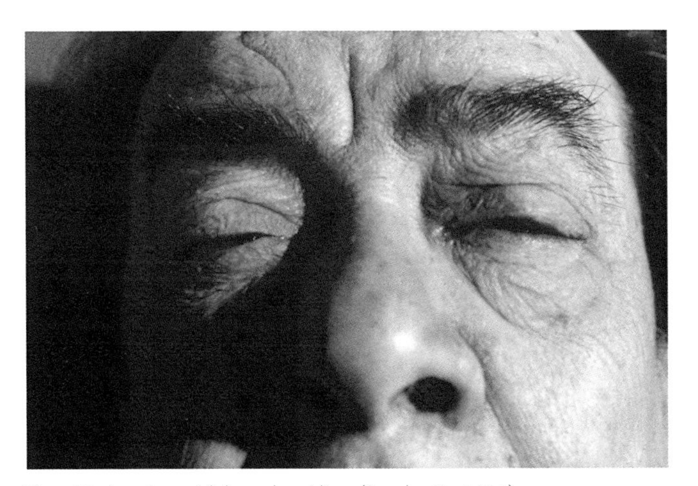

Plate 18 A patient with hypothyroidism. (See also Fig. 3.4.1.1)

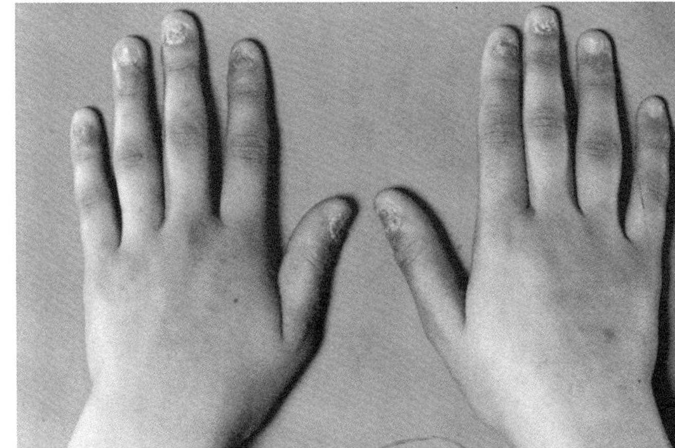

Plate 19 Moniliasis and hyperpigmentation of the hands, particularly over the knuckles, is seen in this 8-year-old patient with hypoparathyroidism and Addison's disease. The patient also had vitiligo, and thus had some of the features of the polyglandular autoimmune syndrome type 1. (Reproduced with permission from Thakker RV. Hypocalcaemic disorders. In: Thakker RV, Wass JAH, ed. *Medicine. Vol* 25. Abingdon, Oxon, UK: The Medicine Group (Journals), 1997; 68–70.) (See also Fig. 4.5.2)

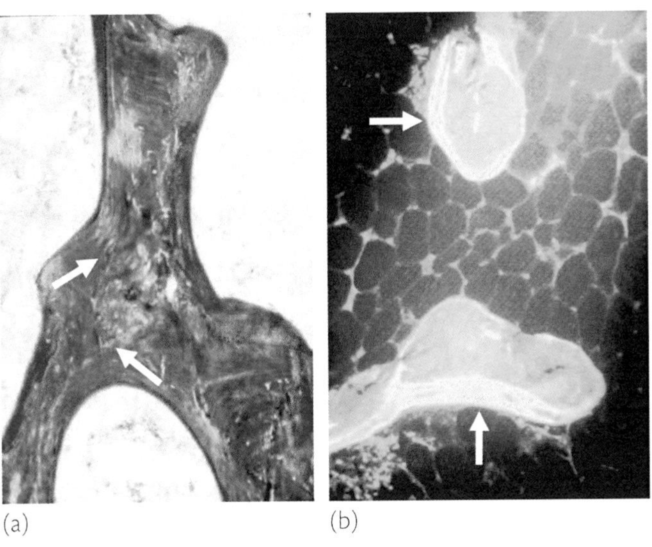

Plate 20 (a) Osteomalacia: Undecalcified bone shows excessive red-staining osteoid covering all surfaces of blue-staining, mineralized trabeculae. Osteoid also forms 'halos' (arrows) surrounding osteocytes indicative of X-linked hypophosphataemia (Masson stain; × 250). (b) Normal bone formation: Two discrete yellow bands at the surface of trabeculae (arrows) indicate that bone mineralization is ongoing. In osteomalacia, such fluorescent 'labels' are absent or smeared (x 250). (See also Fig. 4.10.4)

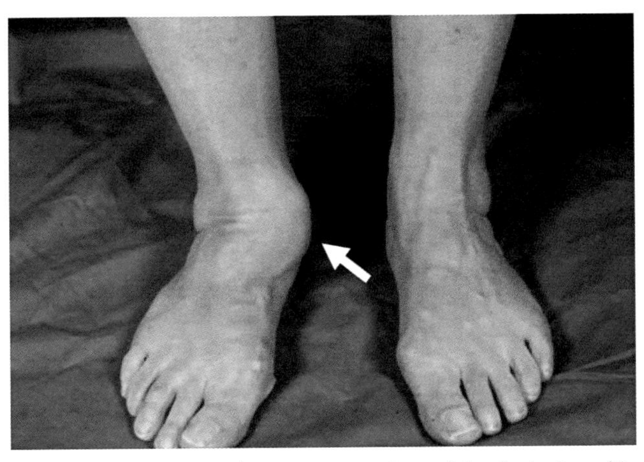

Plate 21 Oncogenic osteomalacia: A mass over the medial malleolus (arrow) had been present for 7 years in this 57-year-old woman. She was cured by resection of this mixed mesenchymal tumour. (See also Fig. 4.10.5)

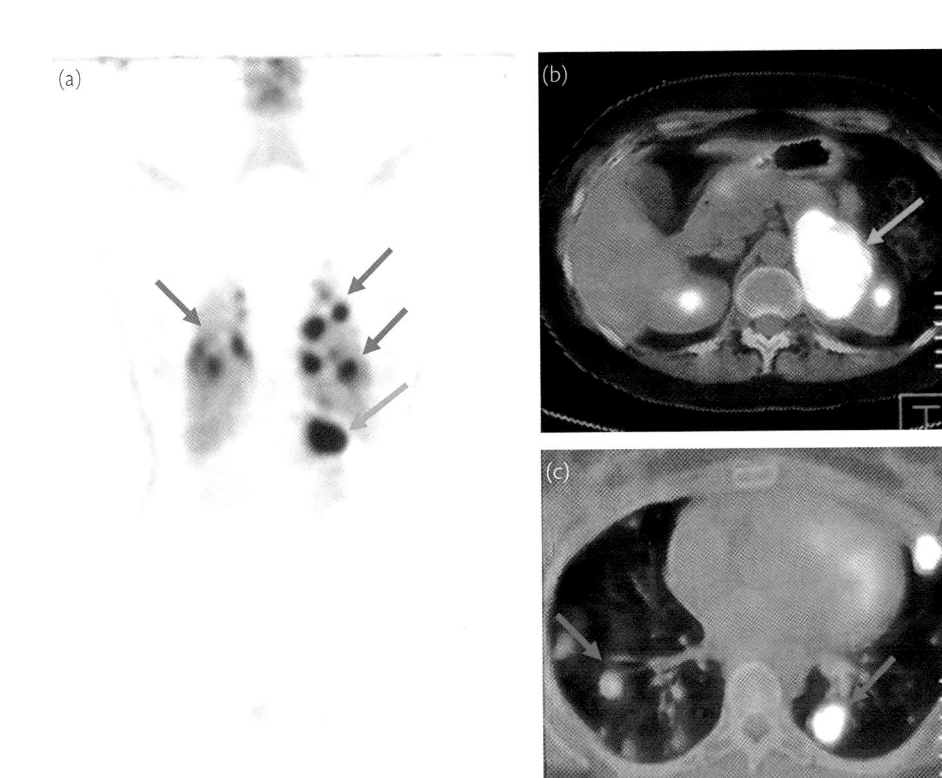

Plate 22 ^{18}F-fluorodeoxyglucose positron emission tomography (FDG-PET) of a metastatic adrenocortical cancer. (a) The left adrenal tumour presents a high uptake on the FDG-PET scan (green arrow) and pulmonary metastasis are detected at diagnosis (blue arrows) in this patient with a Stage 4 tumour. Combination of the PET imaging with a CT-scan (PET/CT) shows the adrenal primary tumour (b) and the pulmonary metastases (c). (See also Fig. 5.4.4)

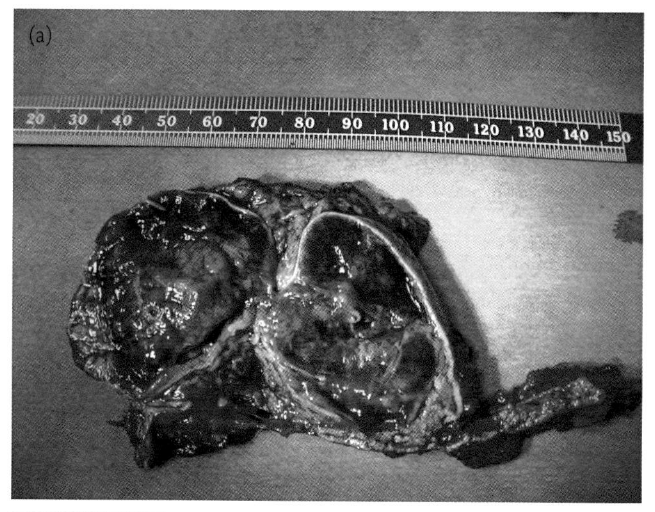

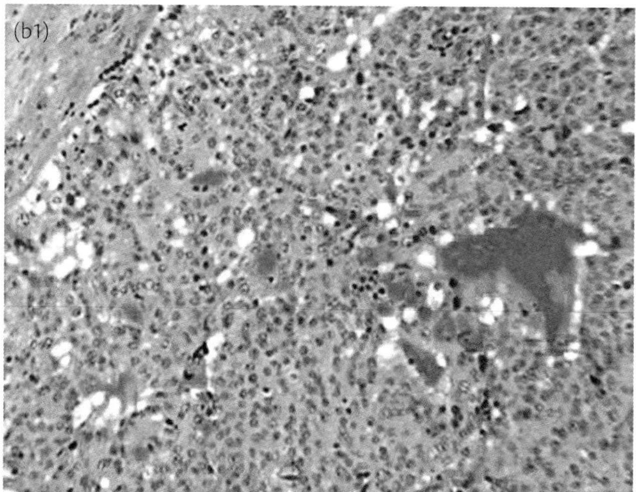

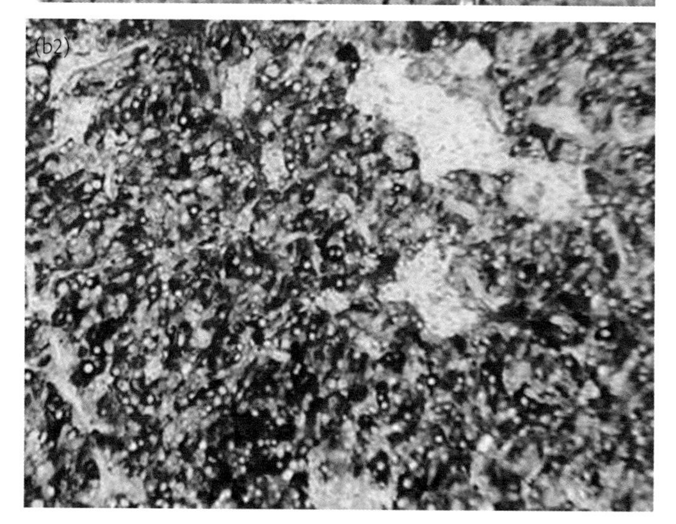

Plate 23 Pathological appearances of phaeochromocytoma.
(a) Macroscopically, phaeochromocytomas are often greyish or haemorrhagic in appearance and there may be areas of necrosis. A capsule may be present around the tumour and a rim of normal adrenal cortex is sometimes seen.
(b) Microscopically, phaeochromocytomas consist of clusters of cells with variable degrees of mitotic figures and containing catecholamine secretory granules. (b1) The cells have amphophilic granular cytoplasm and eccentric nucleoli. (b2) Phaeochromocytomas usually stain positively for neuroendocrine and neural tissue markers including chromogranin, synaptophysin, neurospecific enolase, and S-100. (See also Fig. 5.5.1)

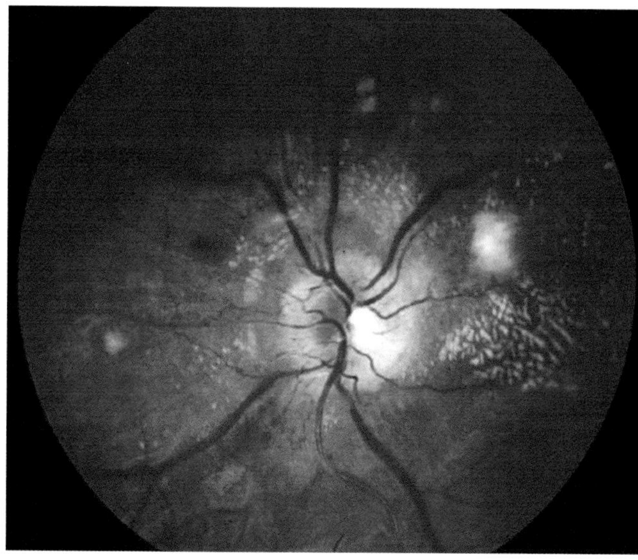

Plate 24 Accelerated hypertension—retinal changes. This 23-year-old woman presented with accelerated hypertension. She had a history of several years of treated hypertension, headaches, and sweating. Retinal changes seen in accelerated hypertension include flame-shaped haemorrhages, papilloedema, and macular exudates (macular star). She was found to have an adrenal phaeochromocytoma. (See also Fig. 5.5.3)

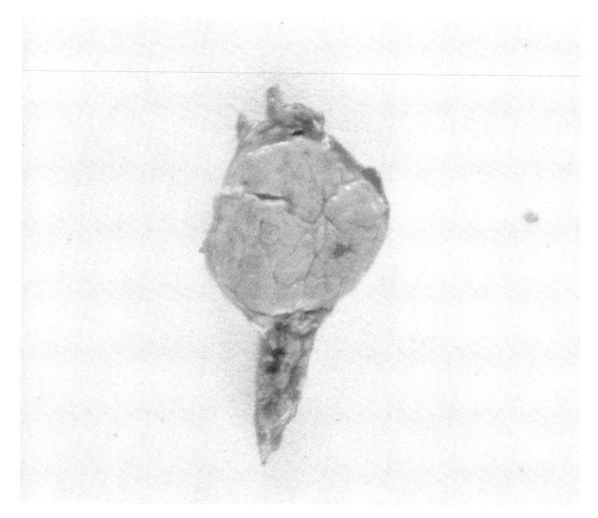

Plate 25 Typical Conn's adenoma: note the typical yellow appearance of the cut surface. (See also Fig. 5.6.4)

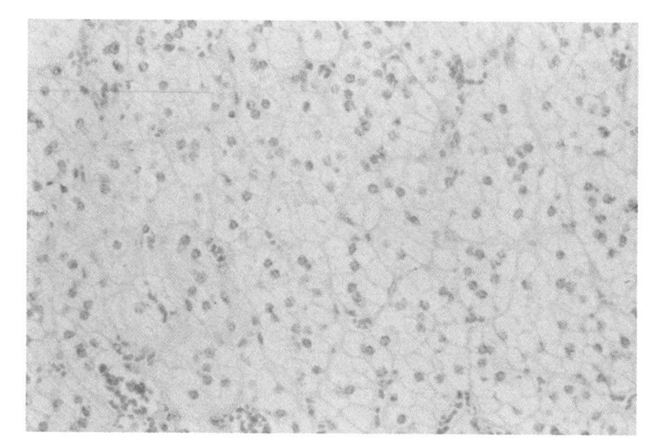

Plate 26 Histological appearance of a typical Conn's adenoma (H and E: ×200). Typical lipid-laden cells with zona fasciculata type morphology are seen. (See also Fig. 5.6.5)

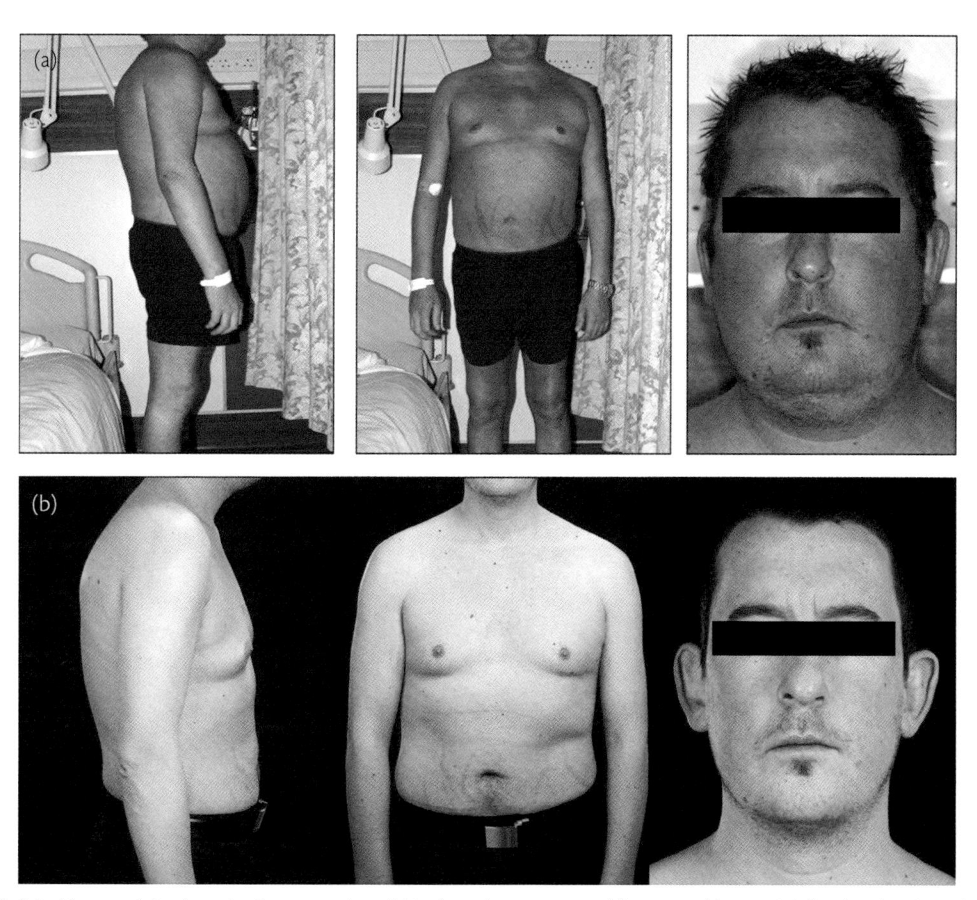

Plate 27 Resolution of clinical features following selective trans-sphenoidal microadenomectomy. (a) 33-year-old man with florid Cushing's syndrome; note truncal obesity, striae, proximal muscle wasting, and facial plethora. (b) Dramatic resolution of clinical features 4 months after selective removal of ACTH-secreting microadenoma. Patient underwent bilateral inferior petrosal sinus sampling to confirm pituitary source of ACTH. (See also Fig. 5.7.4)

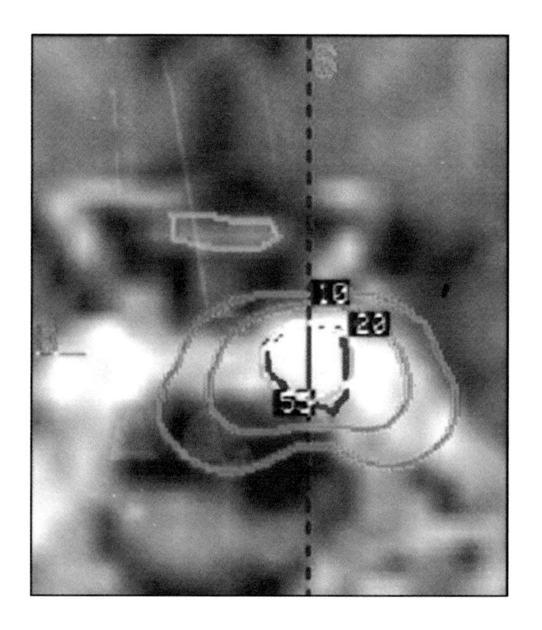

Plate 28 Gamma knife stereotactic radiosurgery for Cushing's disease. Figure shows diagnostic and planning MRI images of a patient with severe Cushing's disease treated by gamma knife radiosurgery as the primary and only definitive therapy at our institution, and who remains in remission with no pituitary deficit 10 years later.
Tumour targeting with gammaknife—50% isodose to the tumour margin is shown; note the margin of safety from the 10% isodose to optic chiasm (outlined). (See also Fig. 5.7.6b)

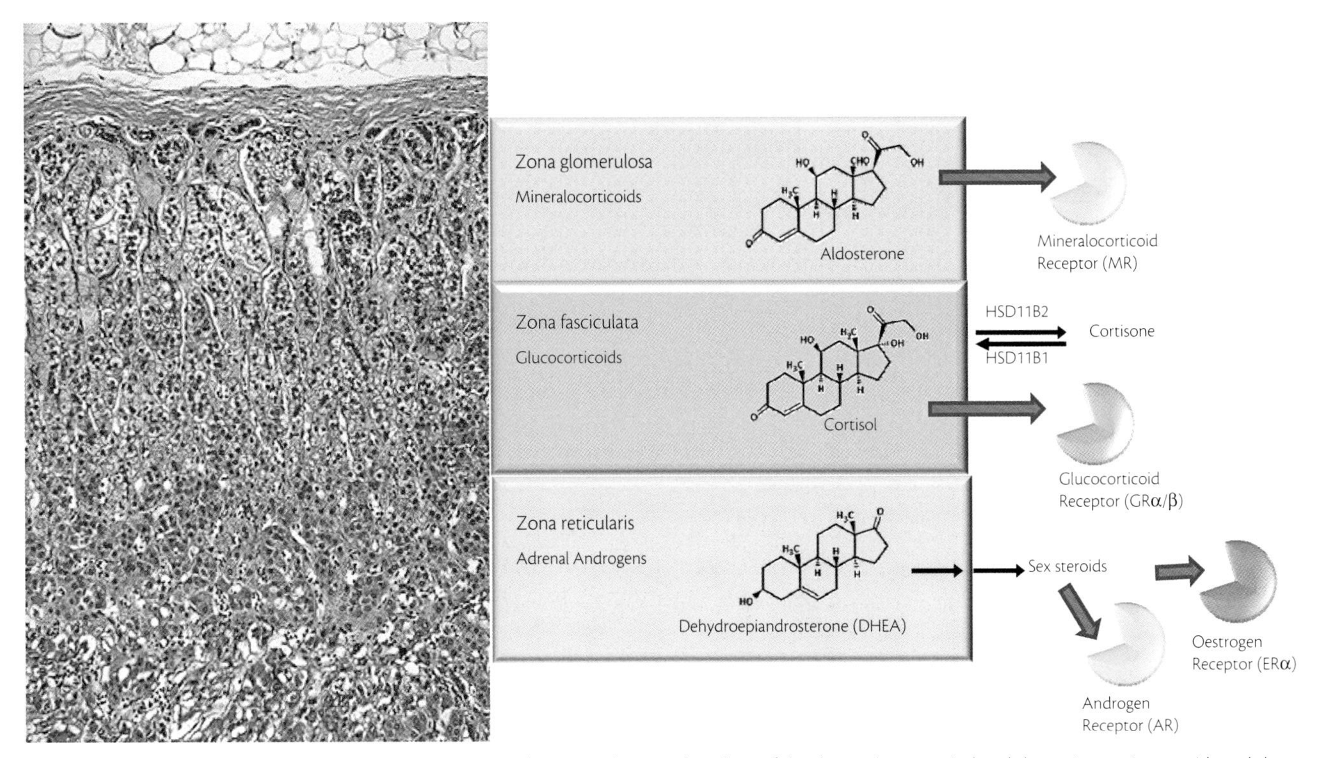

Plate 29 Schematic representation of adrenal zonation and steroidogenesis, depicting histology of the three adrenocortical and the major corticosteroids and the receptors mediating their action. While cortisol and aldosterone can bind and activate the glucocorticoid and mineralocorticoid receptor, respectively, DHEA requires conversion to active androgens and further aromatization to oestrogens prior to exerting sex steroid action. (See also Fig. 5.9.1)

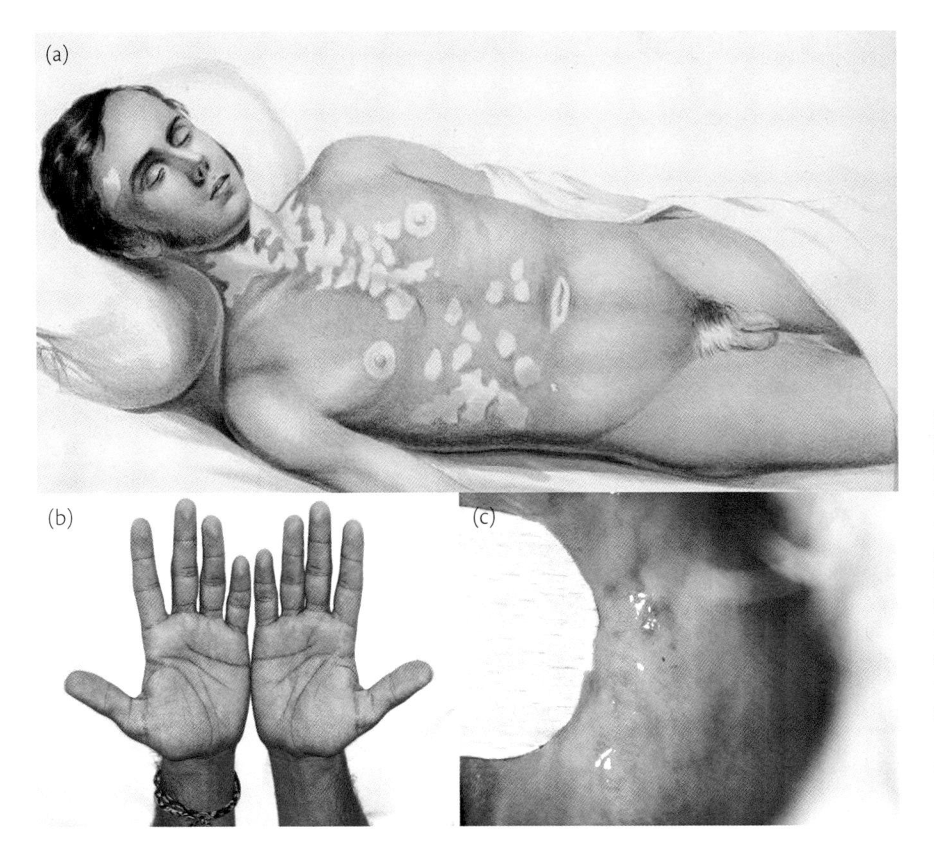

Plate 30 Skin changes observed in primary adrenal insufficiency (Addison's disease). (a) Panel drawn by Thomas Addison (1855) of a patient with Addison's disease, depicting generalized hyperpigmentation, in particular in areas of increased friction, and patchy vitiligo, indicative of autoimmune polyglandular syndrome. (b) Hyperpigmentation of the palmar creases in a patient with acute primary adrenal insufficiency. (c) Patchy hyperpigmentation of the oral mucosa in a patient with acute primary adrenal insufficiency. (See also Fig. 5.9.3)

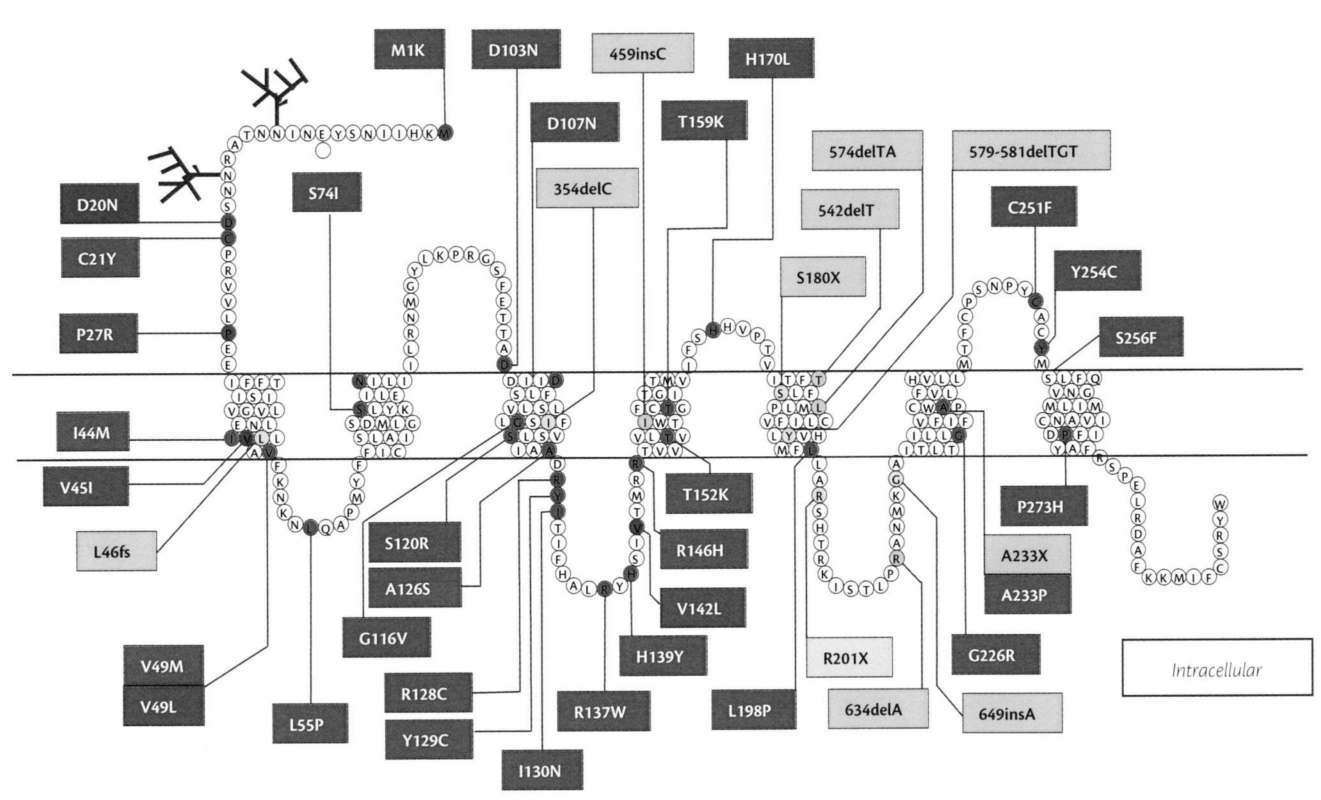

Plate 31 Schematic diagram showing the locations of all MC2R mutations that are known to be associated with FGD type 1. Those shown in red are missense mutations, those in blue are probable benign polymorphisms, and those in green are nonsense or frameshift mutations. (Reprinted from Clark AJ, Metherell LA, Cheetham ME, Huebner A. Inherited ACTH insensitivity illuminates the mechanisms of ACTH action. *Trends Endocrinol Metab*, 2005; **16**: 451–7 (10) with permission.) (See also Fig. 5.10.1)

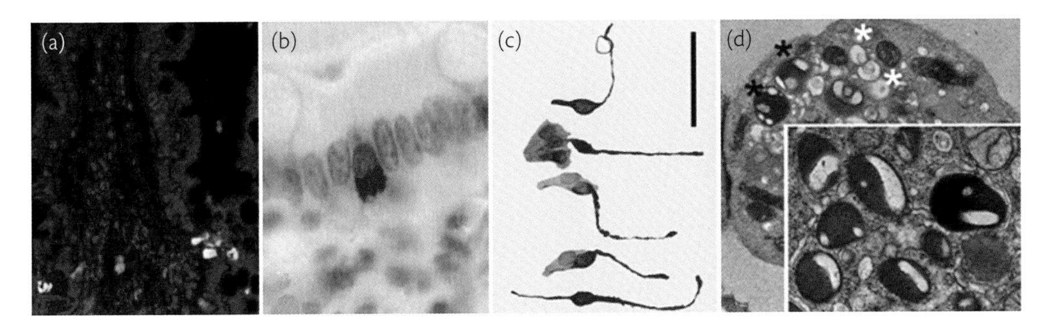

Plate 32 Neuroendocrine cell morphology. (a) Confocal immunofluorescence micrograph of normal human intestine. Enterochromaffin cells (yellow fluorescence; colocalization of Cy5 (red-labelled), CgA, and Fluorescein isothiocyanate (FITC) (green-labelled) Tryptophan hydroxylase (TPH) are located at the base of the crypt. (b) Serotonin immunostaining (brown) of an enterochromaffin cell demonstrating localization of serotonin in vesicles. (c) Microdissected rat rectal enterochromaffin cells immunostained with serotonin demonstrating lengthy dendritic-like basal extensions consistent with a neural and endocrine phenotype. (d) Electron micrograph (7200 × magnification) of rodent small intestinal enterochromaffin cells demonstrating a typical admixture of large dense granules and electroluscent (empty) vesicles (inset shows the characteristic dense content and pear or ovoid shape of the vesicles). (See also Fig. 6.1.3)

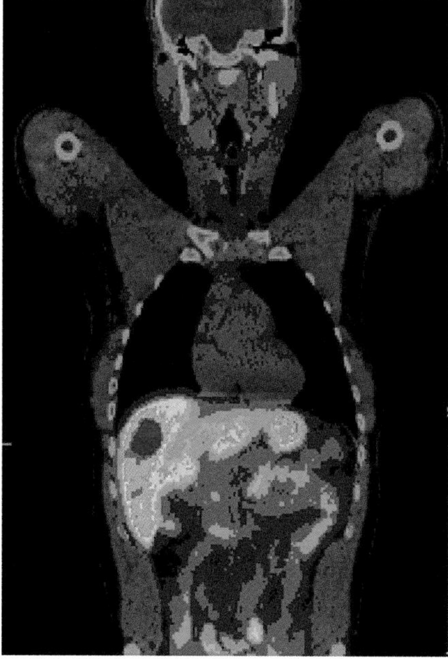

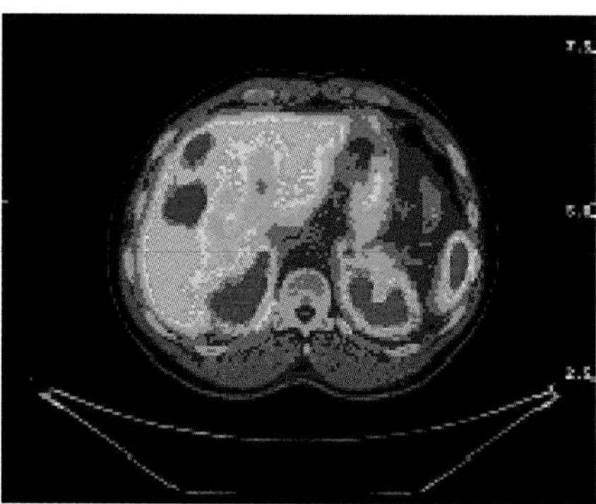

Plate 33 Ga-68 DOTATATE PET images from patient with metastatic neuroendocrine tumour. Images show Ga-68 DOTATATE-avid liver metastases. (See also Fig. 6.3.1)

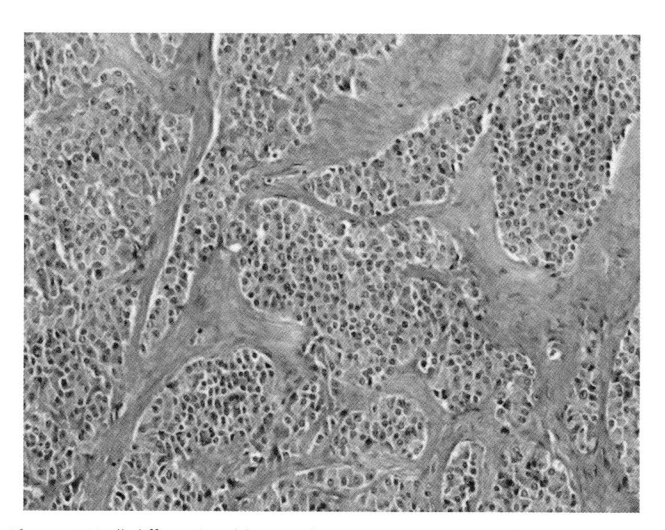

Plate 34 Well-differentiated, low-grade pancreatic gastrinoma. (See also Fig. 6.4.1)

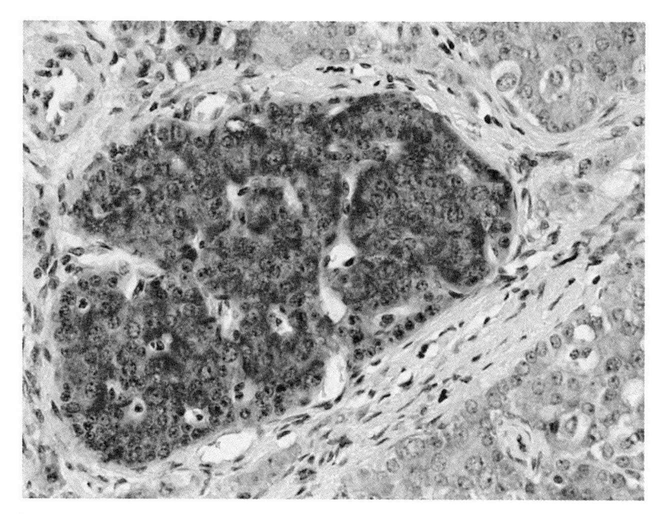

Plate 35 Gastrin immunostaining in the same patient as in Plate 34 with pancreatic gastrinoma. (See also Fig. 6.4.2)

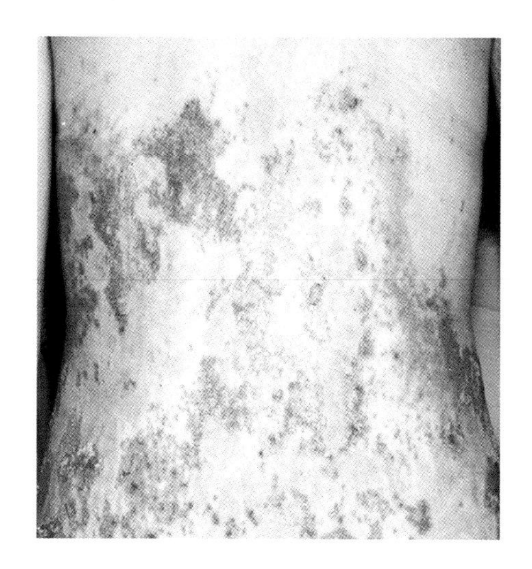

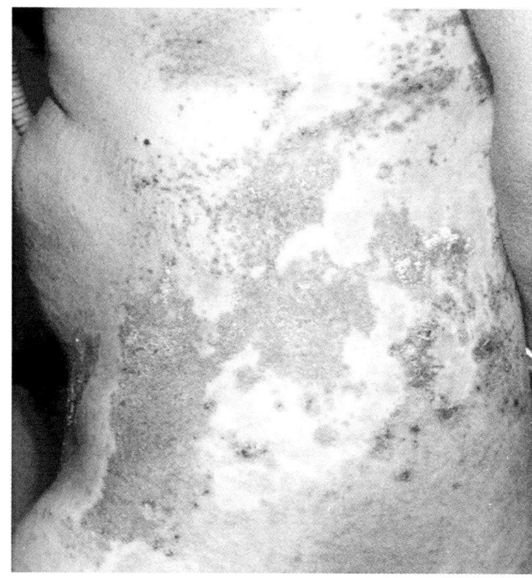

Plate 36 Necrolytic migratory erythema on the back and trunk of patient with malignant glucagonoma. (See also Fig. 6.6.1)

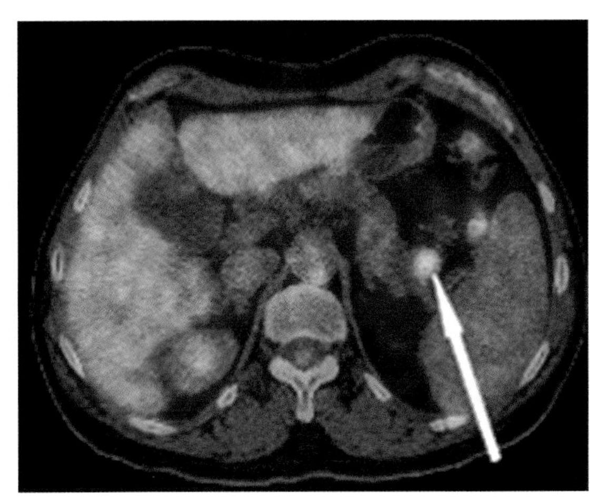

Plate 37 Man with Zollinger–Ellison syndrome. Fused FDG-PET/CT image demonstrates localization of the radiopharmaceutical to the tumour. No other lesions were identified on this study and only this single tumour was found at subsequent surgery. (See also Fig. 6.9.4b)

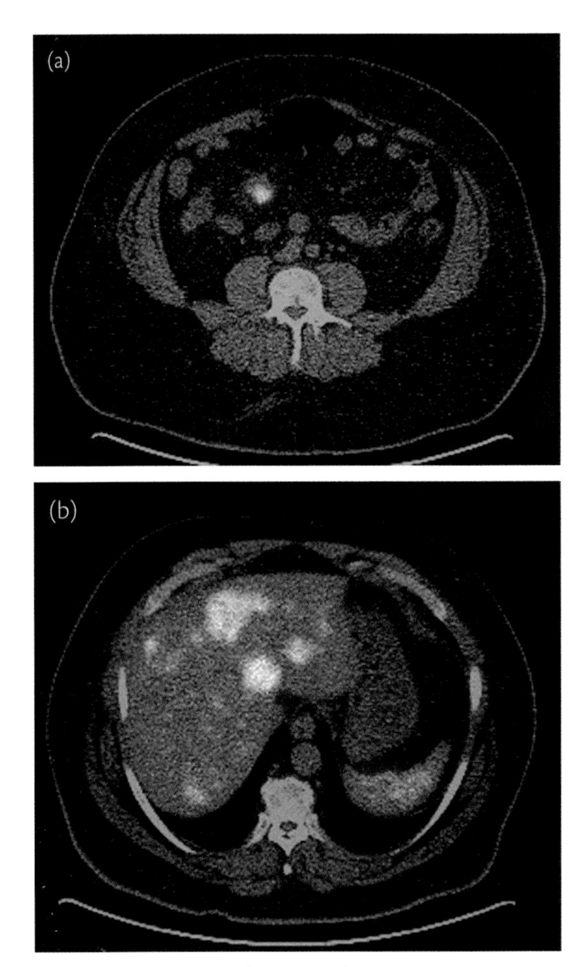

Plate 38 Man with carcinoid syndrome. Fused Ga-68 PET-CT images demonstrate intense localization of the radiopharmaceutical to the primary tumour and liver metastases. (See also Fig. 6.9.7a,b)

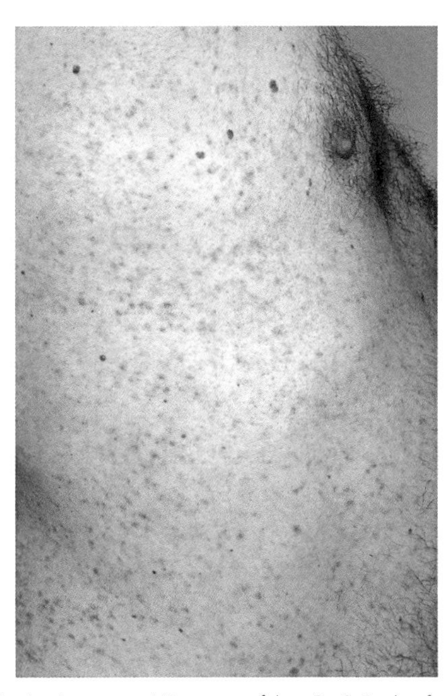

Plate 39 Urticaria pigmentosa. We are grateful to Dr C. Bunker for providing this figure. (See also Fig. 6.10.1)

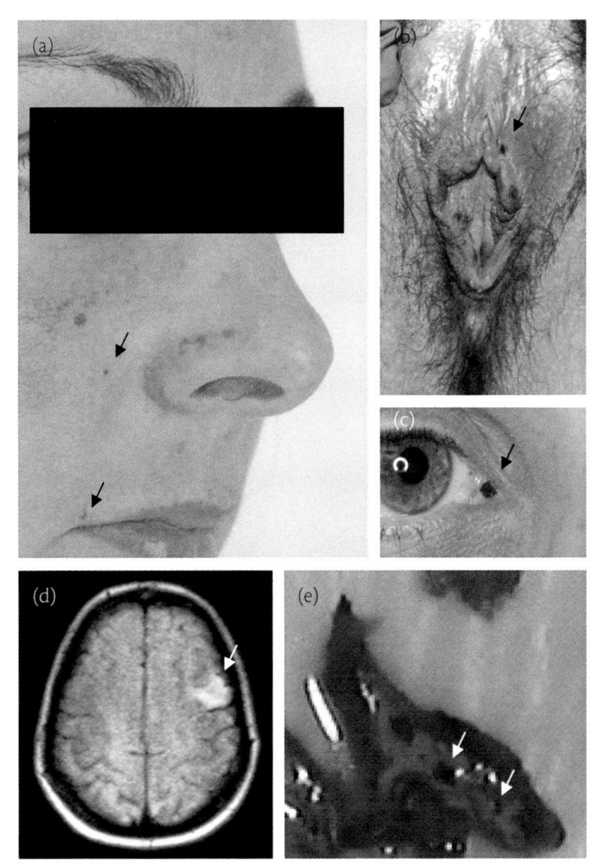

Plate 40 A patient with Carney's complex (CAR47.01) with the germline IVS2+1 G>A *PRKAR1A* mutation. (a) Since childhood the patient had freckling on the vermillion border of the upper lip (lower arrow) and blue nevi on the face (upper arrow) and elsewhere. (b) Extensive genital pigmented nevi and lentigines (arrow). (c) Pigmentation of the inner canthus that is pathognomonic for Carney's complex. (d) The patient first presented with a stroke (arrow) and right-sided paralysis due to dislodged right atrial cardiac myxoma. (e) She developed Cushing's syndrome due to primary pigmented nodular adrenocortical disease, which is characterized by the many brown micronodules (arrows) present throughout the adrenal cortex. (See also Fig. 6.15.1)

must be kept as short as possible by administering a T_4 dose that restores euthyroidism as soon as possible. Nowadays, after an abnormal congenital hypothyroidism screening result it should be feasible to start treatment before the age of 14 days. The short-term goals of T_4 treatment in the neonatal period are to normalize the plasma (free) T_4 and TSH concentrations within 2 and 4 weeks, respectively. Higher T_4 starting doses (i.e. more than 10 μg/kg per day) result in more rapid normalization of the plasma hormone concentrations than lower doses (46).

Long-term effect evaluation of the cognitive and motor development of patients with congenital hypothyroidism has demonstrated that timely and adequate T_4 treatment results in psychological test scores within the normal range for most children (14, 47, 48). However, even with a treatment start before the age of 14 days, patients with congenital hypothyroidism have an approximately 0.5 SD deficit in their (full-scale) IQ, with the difference being somewhat greater in patients with severe congenital hypothyroidism (e.g. caused by thyroid agenesis) (14, 49).

Over recent years it has been suggested that a high T_4 starting dose may further improve the developmental outcome, especially in patients with severe congenital hypothyroidism (50). However, in a recent Cochrane review addressing this issue it was concluded that there is inadequate evidence to suggest that a high dose is more beneficial compared to a low dose for initial thyroid hormone replacement in the treatment of congenital hypothyroidism (51). Furthermore, a relatively high T_4 starting dose (more than 10 μg/kg per day) has been associated with behavioural problems later in life (52).

With this in mind, our recommendations are:

1 Start T_4 administration as soon as possible.
2 Achieve euthyroidism quickly by using an appropriate initial T_4 dose, but prevent overshoot by frequent control of the plasma (free) T_4 and TSH concentrations, and, if necessary, dose adjustments.
3 Prevent large (free) T_4 fluctuations as much as practicable.
4 Prevent goitrogenesis when applicable.

Usually an initial T_4 dose of about 10–12 μg/kg once a day will do. In the case of a severely hypothyroid neonate, the body's T_4 deficit can be corrected by one additional T_4 dose, 12 h after the initial dose. The supplementary dose of T_4 is mainly dependent on body mass, age, and intestinal resorption, and less so on aetiology or severity of the disease. In milder forms of congenital hypothyroidism the residual thyroid function is almost completely suppressed under treatment. Whereas adults in general are adequately supplied with a daily T_4 dose of about 1.6 μg/kg, neonates require about five to six times this dose. However, a large interindividual variability exists, which cannot be predicted when treatment starts.

In general, when treated with T_4, moderately increased free T_4 levels are necessary to suppress plasma TSH levels to values within the normal range. It may sometimes take up to 1 month to return the usually extremely high initial TSH values to normal. To prevent under- or overtreatment, the plasma free T_4 concentration should be measured weekly for the first 4 weeks. Further controls can be done once every 2 weeks, later monthly, and after the age of 6 months the frequency of controls can be gradually lowered to once every 3 months between the ages of 1 and 3 years. Because a healthy thyroid produces, besides the prohormone T_4, substantial amounts of bioactive T_3, it is debatable whether the optimal preparation would be a mixture of T_4 and T_3. However, there is no evidence of benefit of adding T_3 to the T_4 treatment.

In cases of congenital hypothyroidism of central origin plasma TSH levels are useless for therapy control, and one has to rely on free T_4 concentrations. Usually the need for T_4 per kilogram of body mass is somewhat lower than in cases of congenital hypothyroidism of thyroidal origin. Obviously, a normally developed thyroid, even in the absence of TSH stimulation, is able to produce some T_4. As a rule of thumb, a T_4 starting dose of approximately 6–8 μg/kg per day is suitable. In cases of accompanying ACTH deficiency, it is important to start cortisol supplements as soon as possible, preferably before beginning T_4 therapy. Under normal conditions, young infants need 10–12 mg/m^2 per day of cortisol orally in three or four divided doses. The cortisol dose must be increased immediately in case of stress (illness, pain, etc.).

Treatment of transient congenital hypothyroidism is rarely necessary because the hypothyroid phase is usually short. Finally, even in doubtful cases, adequate treatment is mandatory and should not be delayed, regardless of whether the aetiology is known.

Congenital hyperthyroidism

The prevailing view is that congenital hyperthyroidism is usually caused by thyroid-stimulating antibodies of maternal origin crossing the placenta from early in gestation and stimulating the (fetal) thyroid from midgestation (21). Remarkably, only a small percentage (estimated at 2%) of the children of mothers with Graves' disease develop congenital or neonatal hyperthyroidism, indicating that what appears to stimulate the maternal thyroid does not automatically stimulate the fetal or neonatal thyroid. Yet, in the case of very high maternal levels of thyroid-stimulating antibodies during pregnancy, the child becomes hyperthyroid. Onset and severity not only depend on the level of stimulating antibodies, but also on the presence of blocking antibodies and antithyroid drugs that may mitigate, postpone, or even overrun the excessive thyroid hormone production by the fetal/neonatal gland. The suppressive effect of the antithyroid drug taken by the mother stops within a day after birth; blocking antibodies have a longer plasma half-life and may counteract the stimulating antibodies for several weeks. Breastfeeding does not influence the child's condition significantly (53). In summary, it is difficult to predict which child is really at risk, whereas the consequences are important.

Fetal and neonatal hyperthyroidism are severe life-threatening conditions. The prenatal signs may be intrauterine growth retardation, microcephaly, goitrogenesis, tachycardia, and premature birth. After birth the infant may be extremely restless, irritable, with an exophthalmus-like appearance, and signs of hypermetabolism and multiple organ failure. The infant may die if treatment is not instituted immediately.

If a neonate has clinical and/or clinicochemical manifestations of hyperthyroidism, the child's thyroid must be inhibited as soon as possible. Postnatal treatment consists of methimazole (0.5–1.0 mg/kg per day, orally in two or three divided doses) and, depending on the severity of the condition, propranolol (1–2 mg/kg per day, orally in three or four divided doses), iodide (1 drop of Lugol's solution every 8 h after the start of antithyroid drug therapy; Lugol's solution contains 126 mg iodine/ml), and, if necessary, corticosteroids. If heart failure is imminent, digitalization is indicated (54). After the critical condition is stabilized and the euthyroid state reached, only the antithyroid drug therapy should be continued for several months, and T_4 must be added to prevent hypothyroidism ('block and replace'). Most infants remit by 3–4 months of age. If the fetus is found to have hyperthyroidism, the mother should be treated with an antithyroid drug, preferably propylthiouracil, while keeping her euthyroid by T_4 administration.

In cases of congenital hyperthyroidism due to a gain-of-function mutation of the TSH-receptor gene, remission will not occur. On the contrary, due to the ongoing growth of the gland the inhibiting action of the antithyroid drug tends to become less effective over time, and the only reliable long-term treatment is removal of the whole gland. Mental impairment, microcephaly, and growth problems may occur when treatment is delayed.

Acquired thyroid disease

Autoimmune thyroid diseases in children

The prevalence of autoimmune thyroid disease(s) in children is low. Since the great majority of the paediatric patients are (post) pubertal at diagnosis there is little or no risk that brain growth and development are threatened by hypo- or hyperthyroidism caused by this disease. As in adults, autoimmune thyroid disease in children occurs predominantly in girls. Apart from consequences for growth and pubertal development, all features of autoimmune thyroid disease in childhood are similar to those in adults.

In young children the presence of thyroid autoantibodies without thyroid dysfunction or goiter is rare. In older children and adolescents the prevalence of detectable serum autoantibodies may be as high as 480 in 10 000, approximately one-third of the prevalence in adults (55).

Autoimmune hypothyroidism

By far the most common cause of acquired hypothyroidism in children is chronic lymphocytic thyroiditis due to autoimmune disease (Hashimoto's disease). The incidence in children is much lower than in adults, but gradually increases with age. Recently reported incidences from Denmark are 0.08 in 10 000 in 0- to 9-year-olds and 0.4 in 10 000 in 9- to 19-year-old children and teenagers (56). Autoimmune hypothyroidism is 4–7 times more frequent in girls than in boys. The severity of the hypothyroidism varies from the inability to produce any thyroid hormone (atrophic thyroiditis) to subclinical hypothyroidism (with or without palpable goiter). As long as there is sufficient functioning, thyroid tissue remission may occur (57). It is even possible that after long-standing hypothyroidism the patient becomes euthyroid.

The most common clinical manifestations of acquired hypothyroidism in children are growth retardation and pubertal delay, accompanied by goiter. Especially in milder cases there is a poor correlation between clinical expression and plasma thyroid hormone levels. Although very rare, in infants acquired autoimmune hypothyroidism may manifest itself as a progressive delay in development (58).

The risk of developing autoimmune hypothyroidism is increased in children and adolescents with Down's syndrome. Published prevalences vary between 0 and 660 in 10 000 (59). This high prevalence is ascribed to a greater tendency to develop autoimmunity and might be caused by overexpression of one or more chromosome 21 genes directly or indirectly influencing the immune system (60). Because the symptoms and signs of overt hypothyroidism are not always easy to recognize in Down's syndrome, and acquired hypothyroidism occurs more frequently in infancy compared with non-Down's syndrome children, the Committee on Genetics of the American Academy of Pediatrics recently recommended thyroid function screening at the age of 6 months, again at age 12 months, and then annually during childhood (61). In adults with Down's syndrome, yearly to 2-yearly testing is recommended. Several other syndromes and disorders (e.g. Klinefelter's syndrome, Turner's syndrome, type 1 diabetes mellitus, type 1 autoimmune polyendocrinopathy, juvenile idiopathic arthritis, and coeliac disease) are also associated with a substantially higher risk of developing chronic autoimmune thyroiditis.

The only (necessary) treatment is administration of T_4. Any goiter usually shrinks somewhat (the result of decreased TSH stimulation) but often does not disappear (indicating that inflammation persists). Because autoimmune hypothyroidism may be self-limited, periodic re-evaluation of the thyroid's hormone-producing capacity is necessary. Untreated, euthyroid patients with autoimmune goiter should have periodic measurement of their free T_4 and TSH concentrations and ultrasound imaging of the thyroid. If nodules develop, these should be examined cytologically to exclude malignant degeneration. Very rarely Hashimoto's goiter may be painful. Prednisolone treatment is often successful in controlling this symptom, but thyroidectomy may be necessary in some patients, e.g. because of unacceptable steroid side effects.

Autoimmune hyperthyroidism

Acquired juvenile hyperthyroidism (synonym: thyrotoxicosis) is, with very few exceptions, due to Graves' disease. It is a rare disease with incidence figures between 0.079 and 0.65 in 10 000 children/year (62, 63). It affects mainly girls, although this predominance is less than in adult women (5:1 vs 10:1). The prevalence of Graves' disease in children with Down's syndrome is higher than in the general population (59).

While it is assumed that all patients with Graves' disease have thyroid-stimulating antibodies, they are not always detected by the available assays. The aetiological diagnosis is then made on clinical grounds, usually supplemented by tests for other antibodies. In the great majority of affected children a small firm symmetrical goiter is present. Ophthalmopathy is mostly absent or very mild.

Full-blown Graves' disease in children is easily recognized by the abundance of signs and symptoms, but sometimes the disease develops insidiously. One has to keep in mind that the clinical expression is extremely variable, and that there are patients with clearly elevated free T_4 levels and plasma TSH concentrations below the detection limit (usually less than 0.01 mU/l), who have hardly any complaint. The various clinical manifestations (see Chapter 3.3.1) are mostly aspecific and quite common in childhood and adolescence. For example, signs of hyperthyroidism during puberty can easily be interpreted as pubertal behavioural problems. Sometimes the clinical condition even resembles hypothyroidism. In such cases the plasma TSH level discriminates from thyroid hormone hyporesponsiveness.

Differential diagnosis in juvenile hyperthyroidism is very similar to that in adults (see Chapter 3.3.5). It is usually simple to demonstrate that Graves' disease is the cause. However, especially in young children it may not be easy to conclude that the disorder is an acquired one, because congenital disorders such as hereditary hyperthyroidism (due to activating TSH-receptor gene mutations) and McCune–Albright syndrome may become clinically manifest several years after birth.

Although the spectrum of therapeutic possibilities for juvenile hyperthyroidism is the same as in adults, the choice may be different and depend on the patient's age. Because of the possibility of long-term remissions, most paediatric endocrinologists recommend antithyroid drugs as the initial treatment rather than radio-iodide destruction or subtotal thyroidectomy. Given the risk of propylthiouracil-related acute liver failure (possibly 1 in 2000 in children), methimazole is the drug of first choice (64). Since it is difficult to realize permanent euthyroidism by titrating the drug on plasma free T_4 and/or TSH levels, we prefer to administer the combination of a suppressive dose of methimazole (0.5 mg/kg per day, in two divided doses) and a dose of T_4 that is adjusted primarily on plasma free T_4 concentrations. TSH secretion may remain suppressed for several months, making it an unsuitable determinant for the control of initial treatment. Unfortunately, the chance of permanent remission in children after antithyroid drug treatment is probably not much higher than 20–30%, even after treatment for longer than 1–2 years (65). When there is need for a more definitive form of treatment, radio-iodide destruction seems a safe alternative to subtotal thyroidectomy (65, 66).

Malignant thyroid diseases in children

Differentiated thyroid carcinoma is not uncommon in children and adolescents. It accounts for 1% of paediatric cancer cases in prepubertal children, and 7% in adolescents aged 15–19 years old (67). The overall incidence of thyroid carcinoma in children is approximately 17.5 in 10 000 with a higher incidence in girls than in boys and an approximately 5 times higher incidence in 15- to 19-year-old teenagers than in 0- to 14-year-old children (67). Differentiated thyroid carcinoma shows mostly a papillary histological pattern and usually has a good prognosis despite the clinical characteristic of rather aggressive behaviour. It is important to realize that a child with a single thyroid nodule has a 20% chance of having thyroid cancer, which is higher than in adults. Because the long-term survival of children with malignant diseases has improved impressively since the 1980s, differentiated thyroid carcinoma is becoming a rather common (second) malignancy after external radiation of the neck (malignant tumours in the cervical region, before bone marrow transplantation).

Malignant thyroid tumours tend to develop more rapidly in young children than in adolescents and adults. This has been shown clearly in the populations exposed to the radio-iodine in the fall-out after the Chernobyl disaster (see Chapter 3.2.5). Also, thyroid cancer recurrences usually occur earlier in young children. Nevertheless, long-term monitoring is required because recurrence may even arise several decades after the initial diagnosis and treatment.

In general, patients are effectively treated by surgery, (often) followed by radio-iodine therapy and suppression of TSH secretion. The surgical treatment in children is similar to that in adults (see Chapter 3.5.6). Treatment with T_4 aiming at TSH suppression, however, should not interfere with the child's growth and pubertal development. Furthermore, it is not always possible to suppress the plasma TSH concentration permanently below the detection limit (less than 0.01 mU/l), because children continuously 'grow out of their T_4 dosage' unless an overdose is given. A recent T_4 treatment scheme that gives in to these 'objections' initially suppresses TSH levels to less than 0.1 mU/l and then allows the TSH concentration to rise to 0.5 mU/l once the child enters remission (67). The most sensitive indicators of thyroid cancer recurrence are TSH-stimulated radio-iodide whole body scanning and measurement of the plasma thyroglobulin concentration, after withdrawal of T_4 therapy or administration of recombinant human TSH.

Medullary thyroid carcinoma is an uncommon but highly malignant disease (see Chapter 3.5.7). It is, however, relevant to paediatric endocrinologists because in about 20% of cases it is part of the autosomal dominant inherited multiple endocrine neoplasia type 2 (MEN 2) syndromes: MEN 2A with medullary thyroid carcinoma, phaeochromocytoma, and hyperparathyroidism; MEN 2B with medullary thyroid carcinoma, phaeochromocytoma, multiple mucosal neuromas, and a marfanoid body habitus; and familial medullary thyroid carcinoma (FMTC) without other endocrine or neural abnormalities. In MEN 2B the medullary thyroid carcinoma can sometimes be so aggressive that widespread metastases have already occurred in childhood. All three of these syndromes stem from characteristic mutations in the *RET* proto-oncogene on chromosome 10, and it has become clear that most mutation carriers will develop disease sooner or later. It has also become clear that some mutations result in earlier development of medullary thyroid carcinoma than others (68). The prognosis of medullary thyroid carcinoma is much worse than that of differentiated thyroid carcinoma, especially once metastases have developed. However, prophylactic thyroidectomy before the development of medullary thyroid carcinoma probably prevents disease (69). Therefore, it is advisable to screen the offspring of patients with these syndromes at a very young age, and to thyroidectomize the children that carry the mutant allele. Nowadays, a prophylactic thyroidectomy between the ages of 1 and 6 months is recommended in case of MEN 2B, before the age of 5 years in MEN 2A, and between the ages of 5 and 10 years in FMTC (70).

References

1. Bernal J, Guadano-Ferraz A, Morte B. Perspectives in the study of thyroid hormone action on brain development, function. *Thyroid*, 2003; **13**: 1005–12.
2. Vulsma T, Gons MH, De Vijlder JJ. Maternal-fetal transfer of thyroxine in congenital hypothyroidism due to a total organification defect or thyroid agenesis. *N Engl J Med*, 1989; **321**: 13–16.
3. De Zegher F, Pernasetti F, Vanhole C, Devlieger H, Van den Berghe G, Martial JA. The prenatal role of thyroid hormone evidenced by fetomaternal Pit-1 deficiency. *J Clin Endocrinol Metab*, 1995; **80**: 3127–30.
4. Haddow JE, Palomaki GE, Allan WC, Williams JR, Knight GJ, Gagnon J, *et al.* Maternal thyroid deficiency during pregnancy and subsequent neuropsychological development of the child. *N Engl J Med*, 1999; **341**: 549–55.
5. Pop VJ, Kuijpens JL, van Baar AL, Verkerk G, van Son MM, De Vijlder JJ, *et al.* Low maternal free thyroxine concentrations during early pregnancy are associated with impaired psychomotor development in infancy. *Clin Endocrinol (Oxf)*, 1999; **50**: 149–55.
6. Derksen-Lubsen G, Verkerk PH. Neuropsychologic development in early treated congenital hypothyroidism: analysis of literature data. *Pediatr Res*, 1996; **39**: 561–6.
7. De Felice M, Di LR. Thyroid development and its disorders: genetics and molecular mechanisms. *Endocr Rev*, 2004; **25**: 722–46.
8. Thorpe-Beeston JG, Nicolaides KH, Felton CV, Butler J, McGregor AM. Maturation of the secretion of thyroid hormone and thyroid-stimulating hormone in the fetus. *N Engl J Med*, 1991; **324**: 532–6.

9. Brown RS, Huang SA, Fisher DA. The maturation of thyroid function in the perinatal period and during childhood. In: Braverman LE, Utiger RD, eds. *The Thyroid. A Fundamental and Clinical Text*. 9th edn. Philadelphia: Lippincott Williams & Wilkins, 2005: 1013–28.
10. Nelson JC, Clark SJ, Borut DL, Tomei RT, Carlton EI. Age-related changes in serum free thyroxine during childhood and adolescence. *J Pediatr*, 1993; **123**: 899–905.
11. Kok JH, Tegelaers WH, De Vijlder JJ. Serum thyroglobulin levels in preterm infants with and without respiratory distress syndrome. II. A longitudinal study during the first 3 weeks of life. *Pediatr Res*, 1986; **20**: 1001–3.
12. van Wassenaer AG, Westera J, Houtzager BA, Kok JH. Ten-year follow-up of children born at <30 weeks' gestational age supplemented with thyroxine in the neonatal period in a randomized, controlled trial. *Pediatrics*, 2005; **116**: e613–18.
13. Bernal J. Thyroid hormone receptors in brain development and function. *Nat Clin Pract Endocrinol Metab*, 2007; **3**: 249–59.
14. Heyerdahl S, Oerbeck B. Congenital hypothyroidism: developmental outcome in relation to levothyroxine treatment variables. *Thyroid*, 2003; **13**: 1029–38.
15. Kempers MJ, van Tijn DA, van Trotsenburg AS, De Vijlder JJ, Wiedijk BM, Vulsma T. Central congenital hypothyroidism due to gestational hyperthyroidism: detection where prevention failed. *J Clin Endocrinol Metab*, 2003; **88**: 5851–7.
16. Gruters A. Screening for congenital hypothyroidism: effectiveness and clinical outcome. In: Kelnar CJH, ed. *Pediatric Endocrinology (Baillière's Clinical Pediatrics)*. London: Baillieve Tindall, 1996: 259–76.
17. Bizhanova A, Kopp P. Minireview: the sodium-iodide symporter NIS and pendrin in iodide homeostasis of the thyroid. *Endocrinology*, 2009; **150**: 1084–90.
18. Vulsma T. *Etiology and Pathogenesis of Congenital Hypothyroidism: Evaluation and Examination of Patients Detected by Neonatal Screening in the Netherlands*. Amsterdam: Rodopi, 1991.
19. Lanting CI, van Tijn DA, Loeber JG, Vulsma T, De Vijlder JJ, Verkerk PH. Clinical effectiveness and cost-effectiveness of the use of the thyroxine/thyroxine-binding globulin ratio to detect congenital hypothyroidism of thyroidal and central origin in a neonatal screening program. *Pediatrics*, 2005; **116**: 168–73.
20. Kempers MJ, Lanting CI, van Heijst AF, van Trotsenburg AS, Wiedijk BM, De Vijlder JJ, *et al.* Neonatal screening for congenital hypothyroidism based on thyroxine, thyrotropin, and thyroxine-binding globulin measurement: potentials and pitfalls. *J Clin Endocrinol Metab*, 2006; **91**: 3370–6.
21. Van VG, Polak M, Ritzen EM. Treating fetal thyroid and adrenal disorders through the mother. *Nat Clin Pract Endocrinol Metab*, 2008; **4**: 675–82.
22. Vulsma T, De Vijlder JJM. Genetic defects causing hypothyroidism. In: Braverman LE, Utiger RD, eds. *The Thyroid. A Fundamental and Clinical Text*. 9th edn. Philadelphia: Lippincott Williams & Wilkins, 2005: 714–30.
23. Perry RJ, Maroo S, Maclennan AC, Jones JH, Donaldson MD. Combined ultrasound and isotope scanning is more informative in the diagnosis of congenital hypothyroidism than single scanning. *Arch Dis Child*, 2006; **91**: 972–6.
24. Djemli A, Fillion M, Belgoudi J, Lambert R, Delvin EE, Schneider W, *et al.* Twenty years later: a reevaluation of the contribution of plasma thyroglobulin to the diagnosis of thyroid dysgenesis in infants with congenital hypothyroidism. *Clin Biochem*, 2004; **37**: 818–22.
25. Dentice M, Cordeddu V, Rosica A, Ferrara AM, Santarpia L, Salvatore D, *et al.* Missense mutation in the transcription factor NKX2–5: a novel molecular event in the pathogenesis of thyroid dysgenesis. *J Clin Endocrinol Metab*, 2006; **91**: 1428–33.
26. Davies TF, Ando T, Lin RY, Tomer Y, Latif R. Thyrotropin receptor-associated diseases: from adenomata to Graves' disease. *J Clin Invest*, 2005; **115**: 1972–83.
27. Narumi S, Muroya K, Abe Y, Yasui M, Asakura Y, Adachi M, *et al.* TSHR mutations as a cause of congenital hypothyroidism in Japan: a population-based genetic epidemiology study. *J Clin Endocrinol Metab*, 2009; **94**: 1317–23.
28. Fernandez-Rebollo E, Barrio R, Perez-Nanclares G, Carcavilla A, Garin I, Castano L, *et al.* New mutation type in pseudohypoparathyroidism type Ia. *Clin Endocrinol (Oxf)*, 2008; **69**: 705–12.
29. Cavarzere P, Castanet M, Polak M, Raux-Demay MC, Cabrol S, Carel JC, *et al.* Clinical description of infants with congenital hypothyroidism and iodide organification defects. *Horm Res*, 2008; **70**: 240–8.
30. Bakker B, Bikker H, Vulsma T, de Randamie JS, Wiedijk BM, De Vijlder JJ. Two decades of screening for congenital hypothyroidism in the Netherlands: TPO gene mutations in total iodide organification defects (an update). *J Clin Endocrinol Metab*, 2000; **85**: 3708–12.
31. Moreno JC, Bikker H, Kempers MJ, van Trotsenburg AS, Baas F, De Vijlder JJ, *et al.* Inactivating mutations in the gene for thyroid oxidase 2 (THOX2) and congenital hypothyroidism. *N Engl J Med*, 2002; **347**: 95–102.
32. Maruo Y, Takahashi H, Soeda I, Nishikura N, Matsui K, Ota Y, *et al.* Transient congenital hypothyroidism caused by biallelic mutations of the dual oxidase 2 gene in Japanese patients detected by a neonatal screening program. *J Clin Endocrinol Metab*, 2008; **93**: 4261–7.
33. Zamproni I, Grasberger H, Cortinovis F, Vigone MC, Chiumello G, Mora S, *et al.* Biallelic inactivation of the dual oxidase maturation factor 2 (DUOXA2) gene as a novel cause of congenital hypothyroidism. *J Clin Endocrinol Metab*, 2008; **93**: 605–10.
34. van de Graaf SA, Ris-Stalpers C, Pauws E, Mendive FM, Targovnik HM, De Vijlder JJ. Up to date with human thyroglobulin. *J Endocrinol*, 2001; **170**: 307–21.
35. Moreno JC, Klootwijk W, van Toor H, Pinto G, D'Alessandro M, Leger A, *et al.* Mutations in the iodotyrosine deiodinase gene and hypothyroidism. *N Engl J Med*, 2008; **358**: 1811–18.
36. Afink G, Kulik W, Overmars H, de Randamie J, Veenboer T, van Cruchten A, *et al.* Molecular characterization of iodotyrosine dehalogenase deficiency in patients with hypothyroidism. *J Clin Endocrinol Metab*, 2008; **93**: 4894–901.
37. van Tijn DA, De Vijlder JJ, Verbeeten B Jr, Verkerk PH, Vulsma T. Neonatal detection of congenital hypothyroidism of central origin. *J Clin Endocrinol Metab*, 2005; **90**: 3350–9.
38. Mehta A, Dattani MT. Developmental disorders of the hypothalamus and pituitary gland associated with congenital hypopituitarism. *Best Pract Res Clin Endocrinol Metab*, 2008; **22**: 191–206.
39. Yamada M, Mori M. Mechanisms related to the pathophysiology and management of central hypothyroidism. *Nat Clin Pract Endocrinol Metab*, 2008; **4**: 683–94.
40. Collu R, Tang J, Castagne J, Lagace G, Masson N, Huot C, *et al.* A novel mechanism for isolated central hypothyroidism: inactivating mutations in the thyrotropin-releasing hormone receptor gene. *J Clin Endocrinol Metab*, 1997; **82**: 1561–5.
41. Huang SA, Tu HM, Harney JW, Venihaki M, Butte AJ, Kozakewich HP, *et al.* Severe hypothyroidism caused by type 3 iodothyronine deiodinase in infantile hemangiomas. *N Engl J Med*, 2000; **343**: 185–9.
42. Finnegan JT, Slosberg EJ, Postellon DC, Primack WA. Congenital nephrotic syndrome detected by hypothyroid screening. *Acta Paediatr Scand*, 1980; **69**: 705–6.
43. Refetoff S, Dumitrescu AM. Syndromes of reduced sensitivity to thyroid hormone: genetic defects in hormone receptors, cell transporters and deiodination. *Best Pract Res Clin Endocrinol Metab*, 2007; **21**: 277–305.
44. Brown RS, Bellisario RL, Botero D, Fournier L, Abrams CA, Cowger ML, *et al.* Incidence of transient congenital hypothyroidism due to maternal thyrotropin receptor-blocking antibodies in over one million babies. *J Clin Endocrinol Metab*, 1996; **81**: 1147–51.
45. Kempers MJ, van Trotsenburg AS, van Rijn RR, Smets AM, Smit BJ, De Vijlder JJ, *et al.* Loss of integrity of thyroid morphology and

function in children born to mothers with inadequately treated Graves' disease. *J Clin Endocrinol Metab*, 2007; **92**: 2984–91.
46. Selva KA, Mandel SH, Rien L, Sesser D, Miyahira R, Skeels M, *et al.* Initial treatment dose of L-thyroxine in congenital hypothyroidism. *J Pediatr*, 2002; **141**: 786–92.
47. Gruters A, Liesenkotter KP, Zapico M, Jenner A, Dutting C, Pfeiffer E, *et al.* Results of the screening program for congenital hypothyroidism in Berlin (1978–1995). *Exp Clin Endocrinol Diabetes*, 1997; **105** (Suppl 4): 28–31.
48. Kempers MJ, van der Sluijs Veer L, Nijhuis-van der Sanden RW, Lanting CI, Kooistra L, Wiedijk BM, *et al.* Neonatal screening for congenital hypothyroidism in the Netherlands: cognitive and motor outcome at 10 years of age. *J Clin Endocrinol Metab*, 2007; **92**: 919–24.
49. Dimitropoulos A, Molinari L, Etter K, Torresani T, Lang-Muritano M, Jenni OG, *et al.* Children with congenital hypothyroidism: long-term intellectual outcome after early high-dose treatment. *Pediatr Res*, 2009; **65**: 242–8.
50. Bongers-Schokking JJ, de Muinck Keizer-Schrama SM. Influence of timing and dose of thyroid hormone replacement on mental, psychomotor, and behavioral development in children with congenital hypothyroidism. *J Pediatr*, 2005; **147**: 768–4.
51. Ng SM, Anand D, Weindling AM. High versus low dose of initial thyroid hormone replacement for congenital hypothyroidism. *Cochrane Database Syst Rev*, 2009; **1**: CD006972.
52. Rovet JF, Ehrlich RM. Long-term effects of L-thyroxine therapy for congenital hypothyroidism. *J Pediatr*, 1995; **126**: 380–6.
53. Momotani N, Yamashita R, Makino F, Noh JY, Ishikawa N, Ito K. Thyroid function in wholly breast-feeding infants whose mothers take high doses of propylthiouracil. *Clin Endocrinol (Oxf)*, 2000; **53**: 177–81.
54. Peters CJ, Hindmarsh PC. Management of neonatal endocrinopathies: best practice guidelines. *Early Hum Dev*, 2007; **83**: 553–61.
55. Hollowell JG, Staehling NW, Flanders WD, Hannon WH, Gunter EW, Spencer CA, *et al.* Serum TSH, T(4), and thyroid antibodies in the United States population (1988 to 1994): National Health and Nutrition Examination Survey (NHANES III). *J Clin Endocrinol Metab*, 2002; **87**: 489–99.
56. Carle A, Laurberg P, Pedersen IB, Knudsen N, Perrild H, Ovesen L, *et al.* Epidemiology of subtypes of hypothyroidism in Denmark. *Eur J Endocrinol*, 2006; **154**: 21–8.
57. Rallison ML, Dobyns BM, Meikle AW, Bishop M, Lyon JL, Stevens W. Natural history of thyroid abnormalities: prevalence, incidence, and regression of thyroid diseases in adolescents and young adults. *Am J Med*, 1991; **91**: 363–70.
58. Foley TP Jr, Abbassi V, Copeland KC, Draznin MB. Brief report: hypothyroidism caused by chronic autoimmune thyroiditis in very young infants. *N Engl J Med*, 1994; **330**: 466–8.
59. van Trotsenburg AS. *Early Development and the Thyroid Hormone State in Down Syndrome.* The Netherlands: University of Amsterdam, 2006.
60. van Trotsenburg AS, Kempers MJ, Endert E, Tijssen JG, De Vijlder JJ, Vulsma T. Trisomy 21 causes persistent congenital hypothyroidism presumably of thyroidal origin. *Thyroid*, 2006; **16**: 671–80.
61. American Academy of Pediatrics. Health supervision for children with Down syndrome. *Pediatrics*, 2001; **107**: 442–9.
62. Lavard L, Ranlov I, Perrild H, Andersen O, Jacobsen BB. Incidence of juvenile thyrotoxicosis in Denmark, 1982–1988. A nationwide study. *Eur J Endocrinol*, 1994; **130**: 565–8.
63. Wong GW, Cheng PS. Increasing incidence of childhood Graves' disease in Hong Kong: a follow-up study. *Clin Endocrinol (Oxf)*, 2001; **54**: 547–50.
64. Rivkees SA, Mattison DR. Ending propylthiouracil-induced liver failure in children. *N Engl J Med*, 2009; **360**: 1574–5.
65. Rivkees S. Radioactive iodine use in childhood Graves' disease: time to wake up and smell the I-131. *J Clin Endocrinol Metab*, 2004; **89**: 4227–8.
66. Read CH Jr, Tansey MJ, Menda Y. A 36-year retrospective analysis of the efficacy and safety of radioactive iodine in treating young Graves' patients. *J Clin Endocrinol Metab*, 2004; **89**: 4229–33.
67. Dinauer CA, Breuer C, Rivkees SA. Differentiated thyroid cancer in children: diagnosis and management. *Curr Opin Oncol*, 2008; **20**: 59–65.
68. Brandi ML, Gagel RF, Angeli A, Bilezikian JP, Beck-Peccoz P, Bordi C, *et al.* Guidelines for diagnosis and therapy of MEN type 1 and type 2. *J Clin Endocrinol Metab*, 2001; **86**: 5658–71.
69. Skinner MA, Moley JA, Dilley WG, Owzar K, Debenedetti MK, Wells SA Jr. Prophylactic thyroidectomy in multiple endocrine neoplasia type 2A. *N Engl J Med*, 2005; **353**: 1105–13.
70. Kouvaraki MA, Shapiro SE, Perrier ND, Cote GJ, Gagel RF, Hoff AO, *et al.* RET proto-oncogene: a review and update of genotype-phenotype correlations in hereditary medullary thyroid cancer and associated endocrine tumors. *Thyroid*, 2005; **15**: 531–44.

3.4.8 Thyroid hormone resistance syndrome

Mark Gurnell and V. Krishna Chatterjee

Introduction

Thyroid hormones (thyroxine **T4** and triiodothyronine **T3**) regulate many cellular processes in virtually every type of tissue. The diverse effects of thyroid hormone include regulation of growth, control of basal metabolic rate, enhanced myocardial contractility, and functional differentiation of the central nervous system. The synthesis of thyroid hormones is controlled by hypothalamic thyrotrophin-releasing hormone (**TRH**) and pituitary thyroid-stimulating hormone (**TSH**), and in turn, T4 and T3 regulate TRH and TSH production as part of a negative feedback loop.

The regulation of such physiological processes by thyroid hormones are mediated by changes in expression of specific target genes in different tissues. Thus, the feedback effects of thyroid hormones on TSH production are mediated by inhibition of hypothalamic TRH and pituitary TSHα and β subunit gene expression. Conversely, target genes which are induced by thyroid hormone include malic enzyme and sex-hormone binding globulin (**SHBG**) in the liver, myosin heavy chain and sodium-calcium ATPase in myocardium, myelin basic protein in brain and sodium-potassium ATPase in skeletal muscle. The regulation of target genes by thyroid hormone is mediated by a nuclear thyroid receptor (**TR**), which is a member of the steroid nuclear receptor superfamily of proteins. Via a central zinc finger domain, the receptor binds to specific regulatory DNA sequences (so-called thyroid response elements – **TREs**), usually located in the promoter regions of target genes. Although the nuclear receptor can bind these sequences as a monomer or homodimer, it usually interacts preferentially as a heterodimer with another nuclear receptor partner – the retinoid X receptor (**RXR**). In the absence of hormone, many promoters are repressed or 'silenced' by unliganded receptor. Hormone binding to the carboxyterminal domain of TR results in relief of repression followed by ligand-dependent activation of gene transcription

(Fig. 3.4.8.1). Specific cofactor complexes which mediate silencing and transcription activation functions, have been isolated: a family of corepressor proteins (e.g. nuclear receptor corepressor, **N-CoR**; silencing mediator for retinoic acid and thyroid receptors, **SMRT**) interact with unliganded TR, but dissociate following T3 binding; conversely, a number of coactivator proteins (e.g. steroid receptor coactivator 1 (**SRC-1**), cAMP response element-binding protein (**CREB**)-binding protein (**CBP**), CBP-associated factor (**pCAF**)) that are recruited by TR and other nuclear receptors in a hormone-dependent manner have also been identified. Some of these cofactors have been shown to possess intrinsic enzymatic activity. Thus, the corepressors recruit a factor (histone deacetylase, **HDAC**), which can deacetylate histones; conversely, SRC-1, CBP, and pCAF exhibit histone acetylase activity. Enzymatic modification of core histones within nucleosomes by cofactor complexes modulates the accessibility or binding of general transcription factors to DNA, thereby regulating levels of target gene transcription (Fig. 3.4.8.1).

In humans, two highly homologous thyroid hormone receptors, denoted TRα and TRβ, are encoded by separate genes on chromosomes 17 and 3 respectively. Alternate splicing generates three main receptor isoforms (TRα1, TRβ1, TRβ2), which are widely expressed, but with differing tissue distributions: TRα1 is most abundant in the central nervous system, myocardium, and skeletal muscle; TRβ1 is predominant in liver and kidney; the TRβ2 isoform is most highly expressed in the pituitary and hypothalamus, but is also found in the inner ear and retina. A fourth splice variant, TRα2, which is unable to bind thyroid hormone due to modification of its carboxyterminal region, is expressed in a variety of tissues (e.g. brain, testis), where it may act as a functional antagonist of TR signalling pathways.

Thyroid hormone action is also regulated at several other levels. For example, it is now recognised that entry of thyroid hormones into cells is not simply a passive process. Monocarboxylate transporter 8 (MCT8), a membrane protein, has been shown to mediate cellular thyroid hormone uptake, particularly in the central nervous system (CNS). Intracellularly, a family of deiodinase enzymes (DIOs) mediate hormone metabolism: type 1 deiodinase (DIO1) in peripheral tissues is responsible for T3 generation; type 2 deiodinase (DIO2) mediates T4 to T3 conversion in the CNS, including pituitary and hypothalamus; type 3 deiodinase (DIO3) catabolises T4 and T3 to inactive metabolites (Fig. 3.4.8.1).

Resistance to thyroid hormone

The syndrome of resistance to thyroid hormone (**RTH**) is characterized by reduced responsiveness of target tissues to circulating thyroid hormones. Thus, resistance to thyroid hormone action in the hypothalamic–pituitary–thyroid axis gives rise to the biochemical hallmark of this disorder, with inappropriate pituitary TSH secretion driving T4 and T3 production, to establish a new equilibrium with high serum levels of thyroid hormones together with a non-suppressed TSH.

Resistance to thyroid hormone was first described in 1967 in two siblings with high circulating thyroid hormone levels who were clinically euthyroid and exhibited several other abnormalities including deaf-mutism, delayed bone maturation with stippled femoral epiphyses, and short stature as well as dysmorphic facies, winging of the scapulae and pectus carinatum(1). Some of these features are unique to this kindred in which the disorder was recessively inherited.

The estimated prevalence of resistance to thyroid hormone is approximately 1 in 50 000 live births and over 700 cases (from more than 250 families) have been described to date. The disorder is usually dominantly inherited and associated with variable clinical

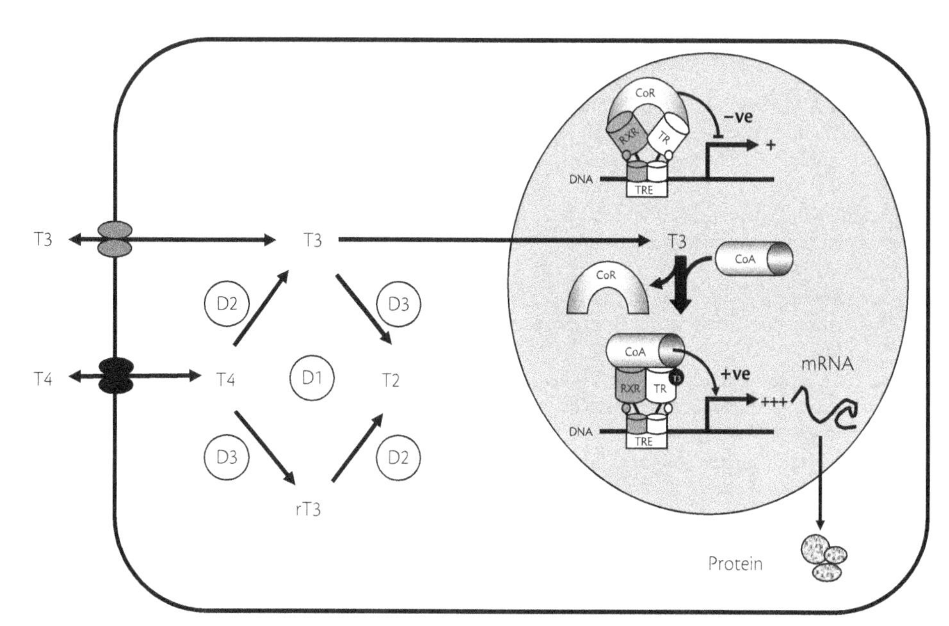

Fig. 3.4.8.1 Schematic outline of thyroid hormone uptake, metabolism and regulation of target gene transcription via binding to the nuclear receptor TR (positively-regulated target gene shown). Transporters are required for the passage of T3 and T4 across the plasma membrane. The deiodinases (D1-3) catalyse conversion of T4 to T3 (D1, D2) or inactivation of T4 to reverse T3 (rT3) and T3 to T2 (D3). In the absence of ligand, TR binds to target gene response elements (TREs) as either a homodimer (not shown) or heterodimer with the retinoid X receptor (RXR). Basal gene transcription is inhibited by recruitment of a corepressor complex (CoR). The deacetylation of core histones in chromatin reduces access to general transcription factors resulting in transcriptional repression. Following addition of T3, TR homodimers dissociate, whereas the heterodimer-DNA complex is stable. The corepressor complex is released, enabling recruitment of coactivator proteins (CoA). The intrinsic histone acetylase activity of the latter results in remodelling of chromatin leading to transcriptional activation.

features (2). Many patients are either asymptomatic or have nonspecific symptoms and may have a goiter, prompting testing of thyroid function, which suggests the diagnosis. In these individuals, classified as exhibiting generalized resistance (GRTH), the high thyroid hormone levels are thought to compensate for ubiquitous tissue resistance, resulting in a euthyroid state. In contrast, a subset of individuals with the same biochemical abnormalities exhibit thyrotoxic clinical features: in adults these can include weight loss, tremor, palpitations, insomnia, and heat intolerance; in children failure to thrive, accelerated growth, and hyperkinetic behaviour have also been noted. When the latter clinical entity was first described, patients were thought to have 'selective' or predominant pituitary resistance to thyroid hormone action (PRTH), with preservation of normal hormonal responses in peripheral tissues (3).

However, a careful comparison of the clinical and biochemical characteristics of individuals classified clinically with either generalized or pituitary resistance to thyroid hormone indicates that there is significant overlap between these entities. For example, there are no differences in age, sex ratio, frequency of goiter, or levels of free T4, free T3 or TSH between patients with the two types of disorder. Significantly, features such as tachycardia, hyperkinetic behaviour, and anxiety have been documented in individuals with generalized resistance to thyroid hormone. Conversely, serum SHBG – a hepatic marker of thyroid hormone action – is normal in patients with pituitary resistance to thyroid hormone, suggesting that tissue resistance is not solely confined to the pituitary–thyroid axis in this group (4). Indeed, in some cases, hypothyroid features such as growth retardation, delayed dentition or bone age in children, or fatigue and hypercholesterolaemia in adults may coexist with thyrotoxic symptoms in the same individual. Nevertheless, the absence or presence of overt thyrotoxic symptoms, signifying either generalized or pituitary resistance to thyroid hormone, is a clinical distinction which will probably remain useful as a guide to the most appropriate form of treatment (see below).

Clinical features

Goiter:

A palpable goiter is the commonest presenting feature, being present in up to 65% of individuals – especially adult women. Although the enlargement is generally diffuse, following inappropriate surgical attempts to correct the biochemical abnormality, which tend to be unsuccessful, recrudescence of multinodular gland enlargement and thyroid dysfunction occurs. Interestingly, fewer children with resistance to thyroid hormone born to affected mothers exhibit thyroid enlargement (35%) compared to offspring born of unaffected mothers (87%), suggesting that maternal hyperthyroxinaemia may protect against goiter formation (5). The biological activity of circulating TSH has been shown to be significantly enhanced in resistance to thyroid hormone, and this may explain the occurrence of marked goiter and very elevated serum thyroid hormones with normal levels of immunoreactive TSH in some cases (6).

Cardiovascular system:

The combination of palpitations and a resting tachycardia (75% of generalized, nearly all pituitary resistance to thyroid hormone), with goiter has often led to a misdiagnosis of Graves' disease in subjects with RTH, particularly before the availability of sensitive TSH assays. In a prospective study of cardiovascular involvement in a large cohort of children and adults with RTH, resting heart rate was significantly raised and some indices of cardiac systolic and diastolic function (e.g. stroke volume, cardiac output) were intermediate between values in normal and hyperthyroid subjects (7). However, other parameters were not different, suggesting a 'partially hyperthyroid' cardiac phenotype in this condition. Atrial fibrillation is commoner in older people with resistance to thyroid hormone, but we (7) have not documented more frequent mitral valve prolapse as suggested by others (5).

Musculoskeletal system:

Childhood short stature (height less than the fifth centile) has been noted in 18% and delayed bone age (more than two standard deviations) in 29% in both generalized and pituitary resistance to thyroid hormone, but final adult height is not usually affected (5). In adults, we have measured bone mineral density in approximately 80 subjects with RTH and documented a reduction in both the femoral neck (mean Z score −0.71) and lumbar spine (mean Z score −0.73), but with normal bone turnover markers (Gurnell, Chatterjee and Beck-Peccoz, unpublished observations).

Basal metabolic rate:

The basal metabolic rate (BMR) is variably altered in resistance to thyroid hormone, being normal in some cases (2) but elevated in others, particularly in childhood. This may account for the abnormally low body mass index seen in approximately one third of children. Recently, we have shown that resting energy expenditure (REE) is substantially increased in adults and children with RTH, which appears to be related to mitochondrial uncoupling in skeletal muscle due to tissue selective retention of TRα sensitivity (8). Interestingly, this increase in REE was accompanied by a substantial (approximately 40%) increase in energy intake in RTH subjects who exhibited marked hyperphagia, particularly in childhood (8).

Central nervous system:

Two studies have documented neuropsychological abnormalities in patients with resistance to thyroid hormone. Firstly, a history of attention-deficit hyperactivity disorder (ADHD) in childhood was elicited more frequently (75%) in patients with resistance to thyroid hormone compared to their unaffected relatives (15%) (9). A second study showed that both children and adults with resistance to thyroid hormone exhibited problems with language development, manifested by poor reading skills and problems with articulation (10). Frank mental retardation (IQ less than 60) is quite uncommon but 30 per cent of patients show mild learning disability (IQ less than 85) (2). A direct comparison of individuals with attention-deficit hyperactivity disorder and resistance to thyroid hormone versus attention-deficit hyperactivity disorder alone indicated an association with lower nonverbal intelligence and academic achievement in the former group (11). Indeed, in detailed analyses of one family, resistance to thyroid hormone cosegregated with lower IQ rather than attention-deficit hyperactivity disorder (12). In addition, when cohorts of unselected children with attention-deficit hyperactivity disorder were screened biochemically using thyroid function tests no cases of resistance to thyroid hormone were found, suggesting that the latter disorder is unlikely to be a common cause of hyperactivity (13). Magnetic resonance imaging shows anomalies of the Sylvian fissure or

Heschl's gyri more frequently in resistance to thyroid hormone, but these features do not correlate with attention-deficit hyperactivity disorder (14).

Hearing and vision:

Significant hearing loss has been documented in 21% of resistance to thyroid hormone cases (5): in most, audiometry indicated a conductive defect, probably related to an increased incidence of recurrent ear infections in childhood; abnormal otoacoustic emissions, suggestive of cochlear dysfunction, were also documented in those with hearing deficit (5,15) and cochlear expression of TRβ has been demonstrated (16).

Although deletion of the TRβ2 isoform in mice is associated with selective loss of M-cone photoreceptors and abnormal colour vision (17), detailed assessment of 10 subjects with TRβ mutations and dominantly inherited RTH showed no common colour vision disturbancies (Gurnell and Chatterjee, unpublished observations).

Other associated disorders:

Cases of RTH have been described where coexistent autoimmune thyroid disease has also been documented, and Refetoff and colleagues have recently reported an increased prevalence of thyroglobulin and thyroid peroxidise antibodies in a large cohort of individuals with RTH (18). Pituitary enlargement has also been reported in the context of RTH: in one patient, who had undergone inappropriate thyroid ablation, marked thyrotroph hyperplasia only regressed once thyroxine replacement sufficient to normalise TSH levels was administered (19); a small number of cases of RTH associated with pituitary adenomas have also been described. Recurrent pulmonary and upper respiratory tract infections occur more often in resistance to thyroid hormone and affected individuals have reduced circulating immunoglobulin levels. Pubertal development and overall survival are not adversely affected by the disorder. Retrospective analyses in a single large kindred showed a higher miscarriage rate and growth retardation in unaffected offspring of mothers with RTH, suggesting that intrauterine exposure to elevated thyroid hormones could be detrimental (20). The main clinical features that are recognized in association with resistance to thyroid hormone are summarized in Box 3.4.8.1.

Box 3.4.8.1 Clinical and biochemical features

- Elevated serum free thyroid hormones
- Non-suppressed TSH with enhanced bioactivity
- Goiter
- Growth retardation, short stature
- Low body mass index in childhood
- Increased resting energy expenditure
- Attention-deficit hyperactivity disorder, reduced IQ
- Tachycardia, atrial fibrillation, heart failure
- Ear, nose, and throat infections and hearing loss
- Osteopenia

Box 3.4.8.2 Causes of elevated thyroid hormone levels with non-suppressed TSH

- Raised serum binding proteins
- Familial dysalbuminaemic hyperthyroxinaemia
- Anti-iodothyronine antibodies
- Heterophile and anti-TSH antibodies
- Non-thyroidal illness (including acute psychiatric disorders)
- Neonatal period
- Thyroxine replacement therapy (including non-compliance)
- Drugs (e.g. amiodarone, heparin)
- TSH-secreting pituitary tumour
- Resistance to thyroid hormone
- Disorder of thyroid hormone transport
- Disorder of thyroid hormone metabolism

Differential diagnosis

The biochemical hallmark of resistance to thyroid hormone is elevated serum thyroid hormones together with non-suppressed TSH levels. However, as shown in Box 3.4.8.2, a variety of different conditions can be associated with this pattern of results. Careful clinical assessment combined with a systematic approach to laboratory investigation is therefore required to distinguish the different causes. The first step in making a diagnosis is to verify the validity of hormone measurements.

Confirmation of elevated free thyroid hormone levels (FT4, FT3) in direct 'two-step' or equilibrium dialysis assays excludes abnormal circulating binding proteins or the presence of anti-iodothyronine (anti-T4, anti-T3) antibodies. If the measured TSH falls linearly with serial dilution of serum, a spurious result due to heterophilic antibodies is unlikely. Other causes (neonatal period, systemic illness, drugs) are excluded by recognition of the abnormal clinical context or documenting subsequent normalization of thyroid function following recovery or drug withdrawal. Genetic disorders associated with elevated thyroid hormone levels can also be distinguished on the basis of different patterns of abnormal thyroid function (e.g. raised FT3 but normal/low FT4 and low reverse T3 levels are characteristic of the rare Allan-Herndon-Dudley syndrome due to loss-of-function mutations in the thyroid hormone transporter *MCT8* (21,22); elevated FT4 but normal/low FT3 levels are found in subjects with defective biosynthesis of selenoproteins, which include the deiodinase enzymes (23).

The main differential diagnosis of resistance to thyroid hormone is from a TSH-secreting pituitary tumour (Fig. 3.4.8.2) and this distinction can be difficult – particularly when the former is associated with hyperthyroid features. There are no significant differences in age, sex, FT4, FT3, or TSH levels between the two groups of patients. Pituitary imaging may show an obvious macroadenoma, but the occurrence of pituitary 'incidentalomas' or thyrotroph hyperplasia following inappropriate thyroid ablation in RTH can lead to diagnostic difficulties. Dynamic tests of the pituitary-thyroid axis can be helpful. Circulating TSH shows a normal or exaggerated response to TRH that is suppressed following T3 administration

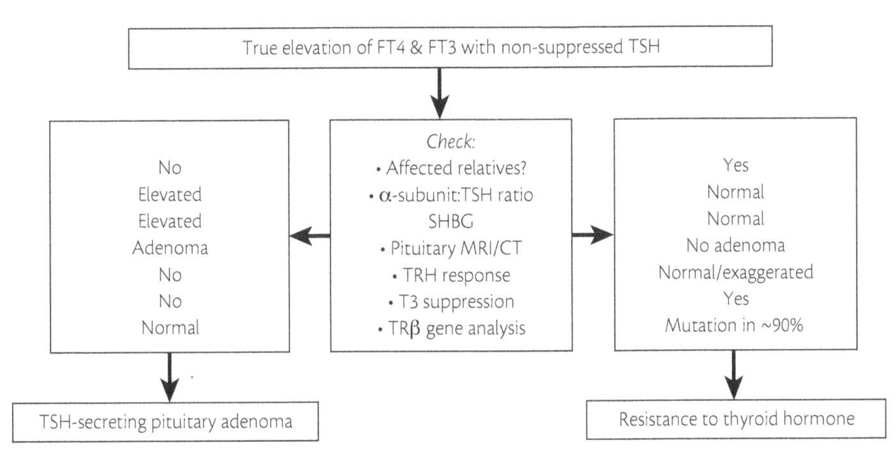

Fig. 3.4.8.2 An algorithm to differentiate RTH from a TSH-secreting pituitary adenoma.

(Werner test: 80–100 μg orally for 8–10 days) in patients with resistance to thyroid hormone, whereas TSH secretion from autonomous tumours is unresponsive. However, the specificity of such dynamic testing is not absolute. Likewise, the molar ratio of serum glycoprotein hormone α-subunit to TSH is normal in resistance to thyroid hormone and elevated with most (but not all) TSH-omas. In our experience, two additional investigations are of value: (1) serum SHBG is almost invariably normal in RTH, but often elevated into the thyrotoxic range with TSH-secreting tumours; (2) similar thyroid function test abnormalities in first-degree relatives are virtually diagnostic of resistance to thyroid hormone as the disorder is familial in 90 per cent of cases. In addition to clinical signs and symptoms, the measurement of indices of thyroid hormone action are of use in evaluating the differing responses of various target organs and tissues to elevated circulating thyroid hormones in this syndrome (Box 3.4.8.3). Although these measurements are most useful in assessing the effects of marked thyroid hormone excess states such as overt hyperthyroidism, they may be less discriminatory in individuals with borderline thyroid dysfunction or in hypothyroidism. In order to improve the sensitivity and specificity of these parameters, resistance to thyroid hormone syndrome patients should be assessed following the administration of graded supraphysiological doses of T3 (50, 100, and 200 μg/day, each given for a period of 3 days) with comparison of any change in indices to baseline values and responses in normal subjects. A protocol that can be used to make such measurements is shown in Fig. 3.4.8.3.

Box 3.4.8.3 Useful indices in assessing tissue resistance

Central
- Pituitary
  - TSH

Peripheral
- General
  - Basal metabolic rate
- Hepatic
  - Sex hormone binding globulin (SHBG), ferritin, cholesterol
- Muscle
  - Creatine kinase, ankle jerk relaxation time
- Cardiac
  - Sleeping pulse rate, systolic time interval, diastolic isovolumic relaxation time
- Bone
  - Height, bone age, bone density, alkaline phosphatase, osteocalcin, collagen-1-telopeptide (ICTP), pyridinium crosslinks
- Haematological
  - Soluble interleukin-2 receptor (sIL-2R)
- Lung
  - Angiotensin converting enzyme (ACE)

Molecular genetics

Following cloning of the thyroid hormone receptors, resistance to thyroid hormone syndrome was shown to be tightly linked to the TRβ gene locus in a single family (24). This prompted analysis of the gene in other cases and a growing number of receptor mutations have since been associated with the disorder. In keeping with the dominant inheritance of RTH, affected individuals are heterozygous for mutations in the TRβ gene, which occur afresh in approximately 10% of sporadic cases. Over 100 different defects, including point mutations, in-frame deletions, and frame-shift insertions have been documented to date, which localize to three mutation clusters within the hormone-binding domain of the receptor (Fig. 3.4.8.4). Within each cluster, some codon changes (for example, R243W, R338W, R438H) are particularly frequent and represent transitions in CpG dinucleotides, which are known to be mutated frequently in many other genes.

Based on the supposition that pituitary resistance to thyroid hormone was associated with selective pituitary resistance, it had been hypothesised that this disorder might be associated with defects in the pituitary DIO2 enzyme or the TRβ2 receptor isoform. However, TRβ gene mutations have also been documented in pituitary resistance to thyroid hormone (25). Receptor mutations occurring in individuals with pituitary resistance to thyroid hormone have also been documented in cases of generalized resistance to thyroid hormone in unrelated kindreds. Furthermore, even within a single family, the same receptor mutation can be associated with abnormal thyroid function and thyrotoxic features consistent with pituitary resistance to thyroid hormone in some individuals, but similar biochemical abnormalities and a lack of symptoms indicative of generalized resistance to thyroid hormone in other members.

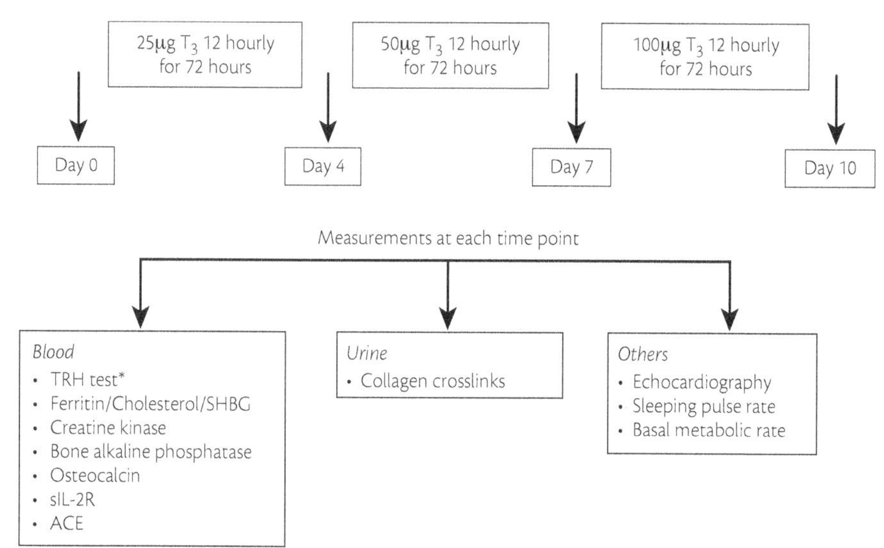

Fig. 3.4.8.3 Protocol for dynamic assessment of tissue resistance in RTH. Physiological and biochemical measurements are carried out at baseline and following incremental doses of T3 as indicated. Useful indices which can be measured at each time point are listed.

Overall, these findings indicate that generalized and pituitary resistance to thyroid hormone represent differing phenotypic manifestations of a single genetic entity.

In a small but significant number of cases, clear-cut biochemical evidence of resistance to thyroid hormone is not associated with a mutation in the coding region of TRβ – so-called 'non-TRβ RTH'. Several explanations have been postulated to account for such cases, including the existence of somatic TRβ mutations whose expression is limited so as to be undetectable in peripheral blood leucocyte DNA. In some families or sporadic cases, mutations in

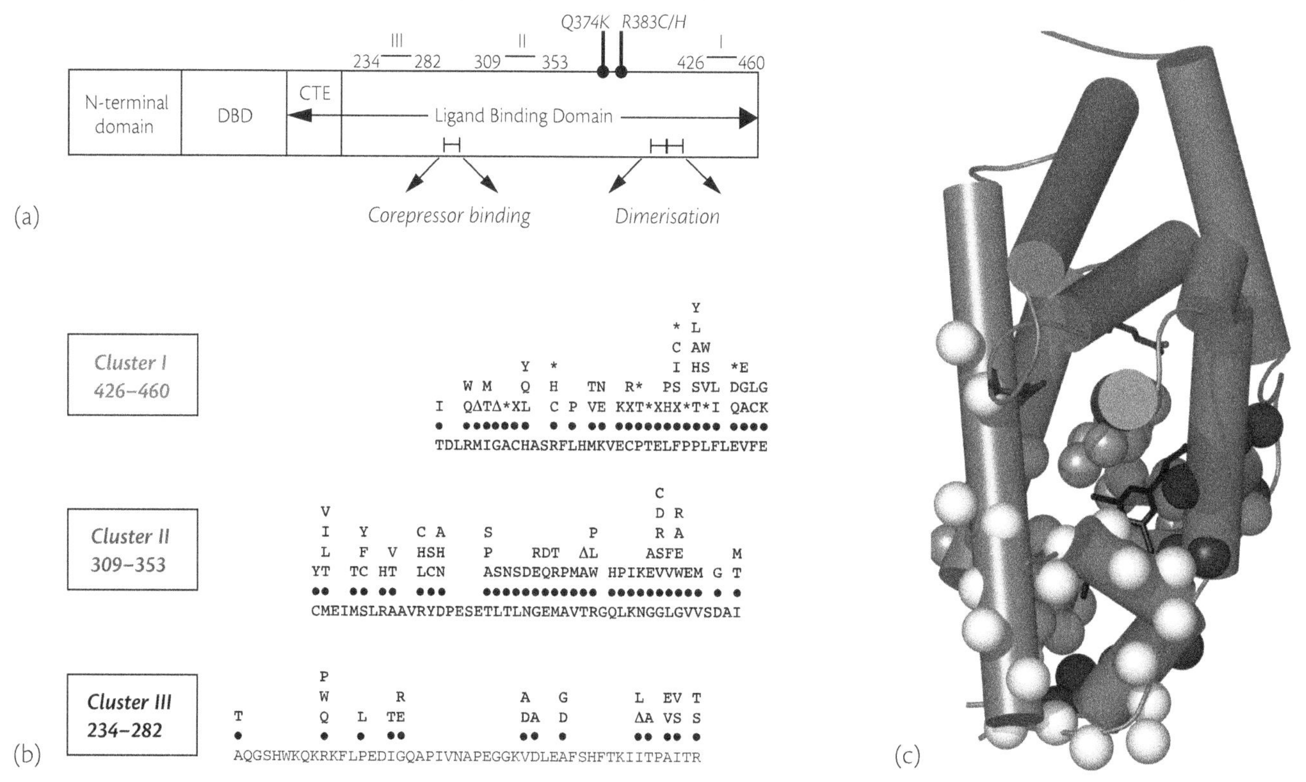

Fig. 3.4.8.4 (a) Schematic representation of the domains of TRβ, showing that with two exceptions (Q374K, R383C/H), RTH mutations localize to three clusters within the ligand binding domain (LBD). (b) The receptor defects in each cluster are shown and include missense mutations, in-frame codon deletions (Δ), premature termination codons (X), and frame-shift (*) mutations. The mutations shown include those listed in a public database (HGMD) together with our unpublished data. No mutations have been identified in the DNA binding domain (DBD) or regions in the LBD which are important for dimerization or corepressor binding.
(c) The crystal structure of the TRβ ligand-binding domain (LBD) composed of 12α-helices is shown, with the location of missense mutations associated with resistance to thyroid hormone superimposed. As anticipated from their functional properties, most mutations involve residues which surround the hydrophobic ligand-binding cavity. The upper part of the structure contains helices which mediate DNA binding, corepressor interaction or dimerization, which are devoid of natural receptor mutations.

TRβ2 and defects at the TRβ locus have also been excluded. This suggests the existence of novel non-receptor mechanisms by which thyroid hormone action is disrupted to produce the resistance to thyroid hormone phenotype. Although mutations in several different molecules involved in the TR signalling pathway could conceivably give rise to an RTH phenotype, evidence exists to favour some candidate genes over others, including RXR and the cofactors. For example, in one case, TRβ bound aberrantly to an 84 kD protein from patient fibroblast nuclear extracts, raising the possibility of abnormal receptor interaction with a cofactor (26). Patients with Rubinstein-Taybi syndrome, a disorder associated with defects in the nuclear receptor coactivator CREB-binding protein (CBP), exhibit a number of somatic abnormalities (broad thumbs, mental retardation, short stature), yet have normal thyroid function. However, disruption of the steroid receptor coactivator 1 (SRC-1) gene in mice, results in resistance to thyroid and steroid hormones, raising the possible existence of a homologous human defect (27). Finally, it is tempting to speculate that a combination of 'less functionally deleterious' mutations or even polymorphisms in several genes involved in thyroid hormone action could result in an RTH phenotype, in keeping with an oligogenic basis for the disorder.

Properties of mutant receptors

In keeping with their location in the hormone-binding domain, the ability of mutant receptors to bind T3 is moderately or markedly reduced and their ability to activate or repress target gene expression is impaired. A subset of receptor mutations, which exhibit normal hormone binding but markedly reduced transcriptional function, involve residues that are critical for mediating TR interaction with coactivators.

In the first documented family with resistance to thyroid hormone, in which the disorder was recessively inherited, both affected siblings were found to be homozygous for a complete deletion of the TR receptor gene (28). Significantly, their heterozygous parents harbouring a deletion of one TR allele, were completely normal with no evidence of thyroid dysfunction. Thus, a simple lack of functional receptor, as a consequence of the single deleted TR allele, is insufficient to generate the resistance phenotype; and mutant receptors in dominantly inherited resistance to thyroid hormone may not be simply functionally impaired, but may also be capable of inhibiting wild type receptor action. Indeed, experiments indicate that when co-expressed, the mutant proteins are able to inhibit the function of their wild type counterparts in a 'dominant negative' manner (29). Further clinical and genetic evidence to support this hypothesis is provided by a unique childhood case in which severe biochemical resistance with marked developmental delay, growth retardation, and cardiac hyperthyroidism proved fatal due to heart failure following septicaemia. This individual was homozygous for a point mutation in both alleles of the TR gene and the extreme phenotype presumably reflects the compound effect of two dominant negative mutant receptors (30).

Studies of mutant receptors indicate that although they are transcriptionally impaired and dominant negative inhibitors, their ability to bind DNA and form heterodimers with RXR is preserved. Indeed, the introduction of additional artificial mutations which abolish DNA binding or heterodimer formation, abrogates the dominant negative activity of mutant receptors (29,31). The ability of mutant receptors in resistance to thyroid hormone to repress or 'silence' basal gene transcription is also likely to be an important attribute contributing to their dominant negative activity. Non T3-binding mutants exhibit constitutive silencing function, particularly when bound to DNA as homodimers, which cannot be relieved by hormone. Conversely, resistance to thyroid hormone receptor mutants with impaired homodimerization properties are weaker dominant negative inhibitors. When tested directly, some RTH receptor mutants either bind corepressor more avidly or fail to dissociate from corepressor following receptor occupancy by hormone. Furthermore, artificial mutations that abolish corepressor binding abrogate the dominant negative activity of natural receptor mutants (32). Finally, an unusual RTH receptor mutant (R383H), exhibits both delayed corepressor release and impaired negative regulation of TRH and TSHα and β subunit genes. Given the pivotal role of these genes in the pathogenesis of resistance to thyroid hormone, aberrantly enhanced corepressor binding may well prove to be the critical derangement of receptor function in this disorder (33).

Taken together, these observations suggest that mutant receptor–corepressor complexes occupy thyroid response elements in target gene promoters to mediate dominant negative inhibition (Fig. 3.4.8.5). This model may provide an explanation for the clustering of receptor mutations associated with resistance to thyroid hormone syndrome. When mapped on the crystal structure of the TRβ ligand-binding domain, most resistance to thyroid hormone mutations are located around the hydrophobic hormone-binding pocket. Helices which correspond to receptor regions mediating DNA binding, dimerization, and corepressor interaction are devoid of naturally occurring mutations (Fig. 3.4.8.4), perhaps because such mutations elude discovery by lacking dominant negative activity – therefore being clinically and biochemically silent.

Pathogenesis of variable tissue resistance

The ability to exert a dominant negative effect within the hypothalamic-pituitary-thyroid axis is a key property of RTH mutant receptors, which generates the characteristically abnormal thyroid function tests leading to the identification of the disorder. For a subset of resistance to thyroid hormone mutants, there is a correlation between their functional impairment *in vitro* and the degree of central pituitary resistance as quantified by the degree of elevation in serum free T4 *in vivo* (8). On this biochemical background, the variable clinical phenotypes may be due to variable degrees of peripheral resistance in different individuals, as well as variable resistance in different tissues within a single subject. A number of factors might contribute to such variable tissue resistance.

One factor may be the differing tissue distributions of receptor isoforms. The hypothalamus/pituitary and liver express predominantly TRβ2 and TRβ1 receptors respectively, whereas TRα is the main species expressed in myocardium. Therefore, mutations in the TRβ gene are likely to be associated with pituitary and liver resistance, as exemplified by normal SHBG and non-suppressed TSH levels, whereas the tachycardia and cardiac hyperthyroidism often seen in resistance to thyroid hormone may represent retention of myocardial sensitivity to thyroid hormones mediated by a normal alpha receptor function (Fig. 3.4.8.6). Another factor which may regulate the degree of tissue resistance is the relative expression of mutant versus wild type TRβ alleles. Although one study has suggested that both alleles are expressed equally, another showed marked differences in the relative levels of wild type and mutant receptor messenger RNA in skin fibroblasts and a temporal

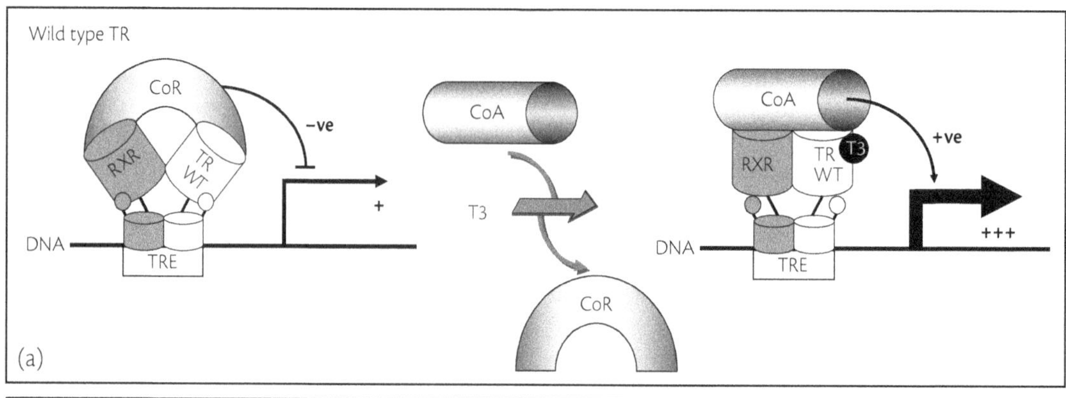

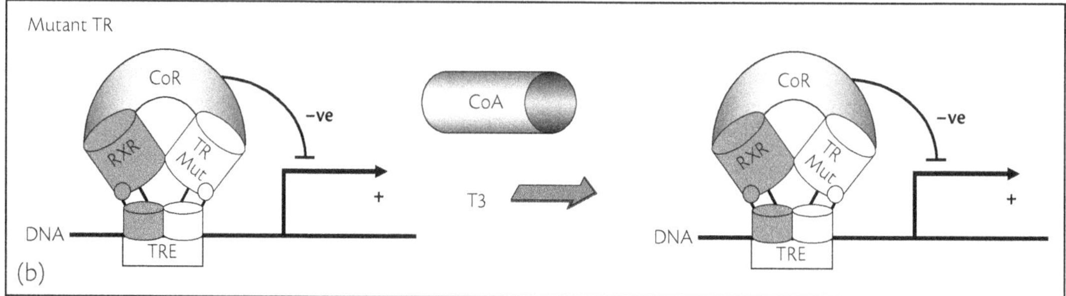

Fig. 3.4.8.5 Possible mechanism for dominant negative inhibition by resistance to thyroid hormone mutants. The upper panel (a) depicts wild type (WT) TR action on target genes. The unliganded RXR-TR heterodimer recruits a corepressor complex (CoR) to silence basal gene transcription. Receptor occupancy by ligand (T3), promotes corepressor dissociation followed by binding of a coactivator complex (CoA) which leads to target gene activation. The lower panel (b) shows mutant receptor action. In comparison to wild type TR, the primary defect in mutant receptors is impaired hormone-dependent corepressor release or coactivator recruitment. For most mutants, this functional alteration is a consequence of reduced ligand binding. However, a subset exhibit enhanced corepressor binding and delayed corepressor release with preserved hormone binding. Occupancy of promoter thyroid response elements (TREs) by mutant receptor-corepressor complexes results in inhibition of target gene expression.

variation in expression of the mutant allele appeared to correlate with the degree of skeletal tissue resistance (34). The dominant negative inhibitory potency of mutant receptors has been shown to differ with target gene promoter context and is a further variable which may influence the degree of resistance.

Attempts to correlate the clinical phenotype of resistance to thyroid hormone with the nature of the underlying receptor mutation have been confounded by three factors: first, the imprecision of clinical criteria used to define generalized and pituitary resistance to thyroid hormone; second, the apparently spontaneous temporal variation in thyrotoxic features in some cases of resistance to thyroid hormone; third, the relatively small number of individuals with any given mutation that have been identified so far. Nevertheless, some interesting associations have emerged from the published literature. The first patient described with pituitary resistance to thyroid hormone was found to harbour an R338W receptor mutation and the same phenotype has been associated with most cases having substitutions at this codon (25). When tested *in vitro*, this mutant exhibits dominant negative activity with the negatively regulated pituitary TSHα subunit gene promoter, but is a relatively poor inhibitor of wild-type receptor action in other thyroid response element contexts. Furthermore, when introduced into other resistance to thyroid hormone receptor mutant backgrounds, this mutation weakens their dominant negative potency on positively regulated reporter genes. A patient harbouring the R383H receptor mutation, which is impaired mainly in the regulation of the TRH and TSH genes, exhibited predominantly central resistance following T3 administration. For similar reasons, another mutation (R429Q) may also occur more frequently in pituitary resistance to thyroid hormone. Some resistance to thyroid hormone receptor mutants (R338W or L, V349M, R429Q, I431T) associated with pituitary resistance to thyroid hormone exert a greater dominant negative effect in a TRβ2 than TRβ1 context. A receptor mutation that selectively fails to bind NCoR but not SMRT is also associated with pituitary resistance (35).

Finally, non-receptor-mutation related factors may influence the phenotype. For example, a deleterious R316H mutation was associated with normal thyroid function in some members of one kindred, but abnormal thyroid hormone levels in an unrelated family, suggesting that other genetic variables can modulate the effect of mutant receptors on the pituitary–thyroid axis.

Murine models of resistance to thyroid hormone

An animal model involving targeted disruption of the mouse TRβ locus recapitulates many of the features found in individuals with the recessively-inherited form of resistance to thyroid hormone associated with a TRβ gene deletion. Homozygous TRβ null mice exhibit elevated serum thyroid hormones and an inappropriately elevated TSH analogous to resistance to thyroid hormone, and importantly heterozygous animals are biochemically normal, corroborating the findings in their human counterparts. The homozygous animals also exhibit profound sensorineural deafness without obvious cochlear malformation, indicating that the deaf-mutism in recessive human resistance to thyroid hormone syndrome is also related to a defect in TR, rather than deletion of a contiguous gene (36). Together with the hearing abnormalities

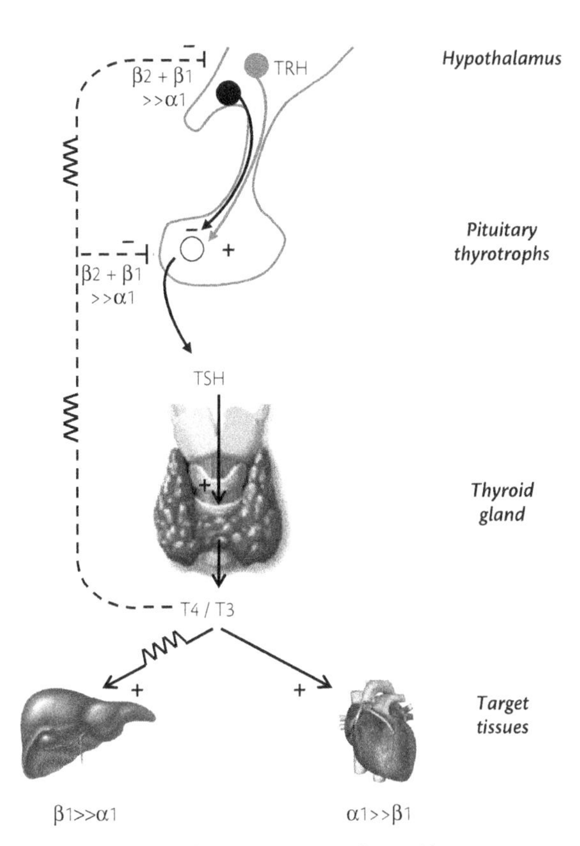

Fig. 3.4.8.6 The influence of tissue distribution of thyroid hormone receptor isoforms on the phenotype of RTH. TRβ2 and TRβ1 are the predominant isoforms in pituitary and hypothalamus, generating resistance in the feedback axis and the characteristic pattern of abnormal thyroid function tests. The abundance of TRβ1 in liver is associated with hepatic resistance, whereas the predominance of TRα1 in myocardium is associated with retention of cardiac sensitivity to thyroid hormones.

found in patients with dominantly-inherited resistance to thyroid hormone syndrome, these findings underscore the importance of TRβ in auditory development and function.

To explore the properties of mutant TRβs in RTH *in vivo*, transgenic mice in which dominant-negative mutant TRβ has been overexpressed ubiquitously (37) have been generated, resulting in an animal model with generalized tissue resistance, decreased body weight, hyperactivity, and learning deficit, which are recognized features of the human syndrome (37). However, an important limitation of this animal model is that expression of the mutant receptor transgene is not controlled by the TRβ gene promoter, such that the pattern of mutant receptor expression or the resulting phenotype might not correspond with that of human RTH. Mice in which either a frame-shift mutation involving 14 carboxy-terminal amino acids (TRβ PV) (38) or an in-frame deletion of a threonine residue (Δ337T) (39) have been introduced into the TR-β gene locus have also been generated with both mutations having been previously associated with human RTH. Extensive characterization of the phenotype of TRβ PV (38,40) and Δ337T (39) mice has indicated that these animal models fully recapitulate the human RTH phenotype, with heterozygous mice exhibiting mild-to-moderate resistance, and homozygous littermates severe resistance, in the HPT axis. Interestingly, when compared with TR-β KO mice, thyroid hormone and TSH levels were significantly more elevated in the Δ337T knock-in animals, supporting the notion that dominant- negative inhibition by the mutant receptor antagonizes residual TRβ1 activity in the HPT axis. The interplay of receptor isoform predominance (e.g. TRβ1 in liver, TRα1 in heart), together with the promoter context of target gene TREs influences the degree of dominant-negative inhibition observed in different tissues (40).

Finally, it is appropriate to include a brief description of mice harboring mutations in the TRα gene locus: Mice with heterozygous point mutations in TRα that correspond to naturally occurring TRβ mutations in RTH, have either normal or mildly reduced thyroid hormone levels (41–44) with additional features including bradycardia, growth retardation, central nervous system abnormalities (41,44) and insulin resistance (42). These phenotypes are quite dissimilar to RTH and suggests the existence of a distinct homologous human disorder (43).

Management

The management of resistance to thyroid hormone syndrome is complex, as variable resistance makes it difficult to maintain euthyroidism in all tissues. In general, the presence or absence of overt thyrotoxic or hypothyroid features is a useful guide to the need for treatment. In most individuals, the receptor defect is compensated by high circulating thyroid hormone levels, leading to a clinically euthyroid state not associated with abnormalities other than a goiter. Inappropriate thyroid ablation with surgery or radioiodine to correct the biochemical abnormality is commonly unsuccessful, with recrudescence of the goiter and disruption of the pituitary-thyroid axis, which renders the resistance to thyroid hormone patient hypothyroid. This is one context in which levo-thyroxine (L-T4) replacement in supraphysiologic dosage is indicated. Other circumstances, such as hypercholesterolaemia in adults or developmental delay and growth retardation in children, may also warrant the administration of supraphysiological doses of L-T4 to overcome a higher degree of resistance in certain tissues. Although successful in some cases, such treatment needs careful monitoring of other peripheral indices of thyroid hormone action (for example, heart rate, basal metabolic rate, bone markers), to avoid the adverse cardiac effects or excess catabolism associated with overtreatment.

On the other hand, a reduction in thyroid hormone levels may be of benefit in the management of patients with thyrotoxic symptoms. However, the administration of conventional antithyroid drugs usually causes a further rise in serum TSH with consequent thyroid enlargement and may also induce pituitary thyrotroph hyperplasia, with a theoretical risk of inducing autonomous tumours in either organ. Accordingly, agents which inhibit pituitary TSH secretion, yet are devoid of peripheral thyromimetic effects, are used to reduce thyroid hormone levels. The most widely used agent is 3,5,3'-triiodothyroacetic acid (**TRIAC**), a thyroid hormone analogue which has been shown to be beneficial in both childhood and adult cases (45,46). This compound has two interesting properties which make it an attractive therapeutic option in resistance to thyroid hormone: first, it exerts predominantly pituitary and hepatic thyromimetic effects *in vivo* – target tissues which are relatively refractory to thyroid hormones in resistance to thyroid hormone; second, it exhibits a higher affinity for TRβ than TRα *in vitro*. A daily dose of 1.4 to 2.8 mg is used and one study suggested that twice-daily administration might inhibit TSH secretion more effectively (47). The use of TRIAC in one pregnancy controlled maternal thyrotoxic symptoms but may have induced fetal goiter. However, TRIAC treatment is not always successful and dextro-thyroxine (D-T4) is another agent which has been shown to be effective in some cases (48). The dopaminergic agent bromocriptine, or the somatostatin analogue octreotide have been used but, unlike TSH-omas, pituitary TSH secretion escapes from their inhibitory effects (49,50). In view of the spontaneous variation in thyrotoxic symptoms in resistance to thyroid hormone syndrome, periodic cessation of thyroid hormone lowering therapy and re-evaluation of the clinical status of the patient is advisable. Thyroid ablation followed by subphysiological thyroxine replacement can be used in rare circumstances such as resistance to thyroid hormone associated with life-threatening thyrotoxic cardiac failure.

The treatment of resistance to thyroid hormone syndrome with thyrotoxic manifestations (for example, failure to thrive) in childhood also requires careful monitoring to ensure that any reduction in thyroid hormone levels is not associated with growth retardation or adverse neurological sequelae. Indeed, control of cardiac and sympathetic overactivity with β-blockade may be the safest course in this context. One study showed that L-T3 therapy improved hyperactivity in nine children with attention-deficit hyperactivity disorder and resistance to thyroid hormone syndrome, including three individuals who were unresponsive to methylphenidate (51). In the future, TRβ selective thyromimetics (e.g., Eprotirome) may have utility in treating some abnormalities (e.g., dyslipidaemia) in RTH (52). Rational drug design has also led to the development of TR isoforms selective antagonists, which may be useful in controlling TRα-mediated hyperthyroid features of RTH (53).

References

1. Refetoff S, De Wind LT, De Groot LJ. Familial syndrome combining deaf-mutism, stippled epiphyses, goiter and abnormally high PBI: possible target organ refractoriness to thyroid hormone. *J Clin Endocrinol Metab*, 1967; **27**: 279–94.
2. Refetoff S, Weiss RE, Usala SJ. The syndromes of resistance to thyroid hormone. *Endocr Rev*, 1993; **14**: 348–99.
3. Gershengorn MC, Weintraub BD. Thyrotropin-induced hyperthyroidism caused by selective pituitary resistance to thyroid hormone. A new syndrome of inappropriate secretion of TSH. *J Clin Invest*, 1975; **56**: 633–42.
4. Beck Peccoz P, Chatterjee VKK. The variable clinical phenotype in thyroid hormone resistance syndrome. *Thyroid*, 1994; **4**: 225–32.
5. Brucker-Davis F *et al.* Genetic and clinical features of 42 kindreds with resistance to thyroid hormone. *Ann Intern Med*, 1995; **123**: 572–83.
6. Persani L, Asteria C, Tonacchera M, Vitti P, Chatterjee VKK, Beck Peccoz P. Evidence for the secretion of thyrotropin with enhanced bioactivity in syndromes of thyroid hormone resistance. *J Clin Endocrinol Metab*, 1994; **78**: 1034–9.
7. Kahaly JG *et al.* Cardiac involvement in thyroid hormone resistance. *J Clin Endocrinol Metab*, 2002; **87**: 204–12.
8. Mitchell CS *et al.* Resistance to thyroid hormone is associated with raised energy expenditure, muscle mitochondrial uncoupling, and hyperphagia. *J Clin Invest*, 2010; **120**: 1345–54.
9. Hauser P *et al.* Attention deficit-hyperactivity disorder in people with generalized resistance to thyroid hormone. *N Engl J Med*, 1993; **328**: 997–1001.
10. Mixson AJ *et al.* Correlation of language abnormalities with localization of mutations in the -thyroid hormone receptor in 13 kindreds with generalized resistance to thyroid hormone: identification of four new mutations. *J Clin Endocrinol Metab*, 1992; **75**: 1039–45.
11. Stein MA, Weiss RE, Refetoff S. Neurocognitive characteristics of individuals with resistance to thyroid hormone: comparisons with individuals with attention-deficit hyperactivity disorder. *J Dev Behav Paediatr*, 1995; **16**: 406–11.
12. Weiss RE *et al.* Low intelligence but not attention deficit hyperactivity disorder is associated with resistance to thyroid hormone caused by mutation R316H in the thyroid hormone receptor β gene. *J Clin Endocrinol Metab*, 1994; **78**: 1525–28.
13. Valentine J, Rossi E, O'Leary P, Parry TS, Kurinczuk JJ, Sly P. Thyroid function in a population of children with attention deficit hyperactivity disorder. *J Paediatr Child Health*, 1997; **33**: 117–20.
14. Leonard CM, Martinez P, Weintraub BD, Hauser P. Magnetic resonance imaging of cerebral anomalies in subjects with resistance to thyroid hormone. *Am J Med Genet*, 1995; **60**: 238–43.
15. Brucker-Davis F *et al.* Prevalence and mechanisms of hearing loss in patients with resistance to thyroid hormone. *J Clin Endocrinol Metab*, 1996; **81**: 2768–72.
16. Bradley DJ, Twole HC, Young WS. α and β thyroid hormone receptor (TR) gene expression during auditory neurogenesis: Evidence for TR isoform specific transcriptional regulation in vivo. *Proc Nat Acad Sci USA*, 1994; **91**: 439–443.
17. Ng L *et al.* A thyroid hormone receptor that is required for the development of green cone photoreceptors. *Nat Genet*, 2001; **27**: 94–98.
18. Barkoff MS, Kocherginsky M, Anselmo J, Weiss RE, Refetoff S. Autoimmunity in patients with resistance to thyroid hormone. *J Clin Endocrinol Metab*, 2010; **95**: 3189–93.
19. Gurnell M *et al.* Reversible pituitary enlargement in the syndrome of resistance to thyroid hormone. *Thyroid*, 1998; **8**: 679–682.
20. Anselmo J *et al.* Fetal loss associated with excess thyroid hormone exposure. *JAMA*, 2004; **292**: 691–695.
21. Dumitrescu AM *et al.* A novel syndrome combining thyroid and neurological abnormalities is associated with mutations in a monocarboxylate transporter gene. *Am J Hum Genet*, 2004; **74**: 168–75.
22. Friesema EC *et al.* Association between mutations in a thyroid hormone transporter and severe X-linked psychomotor retardation. *Lancet*, 2004; **364**: 1435–37.
23. Dumitrescu AM *et al.* Mutations in SECISBP2 result in abnormal thyroid hormone metabolism. *Nat Genet*, 2005; **37**: 1247–1252.
24. Usala SJ *et al.* Tight linkage between the syndrome of generalized thyroid hormone resistance and the human c-erbA gene. *Molecular Endocrinology*, 1988; **2**: 1217–20.
25. Adams M, Matthews CH, Collingwood TN, Tone Y, Beck Peccoz P, Chatterjee VK K. Genetic analysis of twenty-nine kindreds with generalised and pituitary resistance to thyroid hormone. *J Clin Invest*, 1994; **94**: 506–15.
26. Weiss RE *et al.* Dominant inheritance of resistance to thyroid hormone not linked to defects in the thyroid hormone receptor or genes may be due to a defective cofactor. *J Clin Endocrinol Metab*, 1996; **81**: 4196–203.
27. Weiss RE, Xu J, Ning G, Pohlenz J, O'Malley BW, Refetoff S. Mice deficient in the steroid receptor coactivator 1 (SRC-1) are resistant to thyroid hormone. *EMBO J*, 1999; **18**: 1900–4.
28. Takeda K, Sakurai A, De Groot LJ, Refetoff S. Recessive inheritance of thyroid hormone resistance caused by complete deletion of the protein-coding region of the thyroid hormone receptor- gene. *J Clin Endocrinol Metab*, 1992; **74**: 49–55.
29. Collingwood TN, Adams M, Tone Y, Chatterjee VKK. Spectrum of transcriptional dimerization and dominant negative properties of twenty different mutant thyroid hormone receptors in thyroid hormone resistance syndrome. *Mol Endocrinol*, 1994; **8**: 1262–77.
30. Ono S, Schwartz ID, Mueller OT, Root AW, Usala SJ, Bercu BB. Homozygosity for a dominant negative thyroid hormone receptor gene responsible for generalized resistance to thyroid hormone. *J Clin Endocrinol Metab*, 1991; **73**: 990–4.
31. Nagaya T, Jameson JL. Thyroid hormone receptor dimerization is required for dominant negative inhibition by mutations that cause thyroid hormone resistance. *J Biol Chem*, 1993; **268**: 15766–71.

32. Yoh SM, Chatterjee VKK, Privalsky ML. Thyroid hormone resistance syndrome manifests as an aberrant interaction between mutant T3 receptors and transcriptional corepressors. *Mol Endocrinol*, 1997; **11**: 470–80.
33. Clifton-Bligh RJ *et al.* A novel TR mutation (R383H) in resistance to thyroid hormone predominantly impairs corepressor release and negative transcriptional regulation. *Mol Endocrinol*, 1998; **12**: 609–21.
34. Mixson AJ, Hauser P, Tennyson G, Renault JC, Bodenner DL, Weintraub BD. Differential expression of mutant and normal T3 receptor alleles in kindreds with generalized resistance to thyroid hormone. *J Clin Invest*, 1993; **91**: 2296–300.
35. Wu SY *et al.* A novel thyroid hormone receptor-beta mutation that fails to bind nuclear receptor corepressor in a patient as an apparent cause of severe, predominantly pituitary resistance to thyroid hormone. *J Clin Endocrinol Metab*, 2006; **91**: 1887–95.
36. Forrest D *et al.* Recessive resistance to thyroid hormone in mice lacking thyroid hormone receptor: evidence for tissue-specific modulation of receptor function. *EMBO J*, 1996; **15**: 3006–15.
37. Wong R *et al.* Transgenic mice bearing a human mutant thyroid hormone b1 receptor manifest thyroid function anomalies, weight reduction and hyperactivity. *Mol Med*, 1997; **3**: 303–14.
38. Kaneshige M *et al.* Mice with a targeted mutation in the thyroid hormone beta receptor gene exhibit impaired growth and resistance to thyroid hormone. *Proc Nat Acad Sci USA*, 2000; **97**: 13209–214.
39. Hashimoto K *et al.* An unliganded thyroid hormone receptor causes severe neurological dysfunction. *Proc Nat Acad Sci USA*, 2001; **98**: 3998–4003.
40. Cheng S-Y. Multi-factorial regulation of in vivo action of TRb mutants. Lessons learned from RTH mice with a targeted mutation in the TRb gene. In Beck-Peccoz P (ed): Syndromes of Hormone Resistance on the Hypothalamic-Pituitary-Thyroid Axis, 1st ed, Boston, Kluwer Academic Publishers, 2004, p 137–148.
41. Kaneshige M *et al.* A targeted dominant negative mutation of the thyroid hormone a1 receptor causes increased mortality, infertility, and dwarfism in mice. *Proc Nat Acad Sci USA*, 2001; **98**: 15095–100.
42. Liu YY *et al.* A thyroid hormone receptor alpha gene mutation (P398H) is associated with visceral adiposity and impaired catecholamine-stimulated lipolysis in mice. *J Biol Chem*, 2003; **278**: 38913–20.
43. Vennstrom B, Mittag J, Wallis K. Severe psychomotor and metabolic damages caused by a mutant thyroid hormone receptor alpha 1 in mice: can patients with a similar mutation be found and treated? *Acta Paediatr*, 2008; **97**: 1605–10.
44. Tinnikov A *et al.* Retardation of post-natal development caused by a negatively acting thyroid hormone receptor alpha1. *EMBO J*, 2002; **21**: 5079–87.
45. Beck Peccoz P, Piscitelli G, Cattaneo MG, Faglia G. Successful treatment of hyperthyroidism due to nonneoplastic pituitary TSH hypersecretion with 3,5,3'-triiodothyroacetic acid (TRIAC). *J Endocrinol Invest*, 1983; **6**: 217–23.
46. Radetti G *et al.* Clinical and hormonal outcome after two years of TRIAC treatment in a child with thyroid hormone resistance. *Thyroid*, 1997; **7**: 775–8.
47. Ueda S *et al.* Differences in response of thyrotropin to 3,5,3'triiodothyronine and 3,5,3'-triiodothyroacetic acid in patients with resistance to thyroid hormone. *Thyroid*, 1996; **6**: 563–70.
48. Hamon P, Bovier-LaPierre M, Robert M, Peynaud D, Pugeat M, Orgiazzi J. Hyperthyroidism due to selective pituitary resistance to thyroid hormones in 15-month-old boy: efficacy of D-thyroxine therapy. *J Clin Endocrinol Metab*, 1988; **67**: 1089–93.
49. Dulgeroff AJ, Geffner ME, Koyal SN, Wong M, Hershman JM. Bromocriptine and TRIAC therapy for hyperthyroidism due to pituitary resistance to thyroid hormone. *J Clin Endocrinol Metab*, 1992; **75**: 1071–5.
50. Beck Peccoz P *et al.* Treatment of hyperthyroidism due to inappropriate secretion of thyrotropin with the somatostatin analog SMS 201–995. *J Clin Endocrinol Metab*, 1989; **68**: 208–14.
51. Weiss RE, Stein MA, Refetoff S. Behavioral effects of liothyronine (L-T3) in children with attention deficit hyperactivity disorder in the presence and absence of resistance to thyroid hormone. *Thyroid*, 1997; **7**: 389–93.
52. Ladenson P *et al.* Use of the thyroid hormone analogue eprotirome in statin-treated dyslipidaemia. *N Engl J Med*, 2010; **362**: 906–16.
53. Schapira M *et al.* Discovery of diverse thyroid hormone receptor antagonists by high-throughput docking. *Proc Natl Acad Sci USA*, 2003; **100**: 7354–59.

3.4.9 Treatment of hypothyroidism

Anthony Toft

Introduction

Treatment of primary hypothyroidism is usually both gratifying and simple and, in most cases, lifelong. Thyroxine, as L-thyroxine sodium, is the therapy of choice and is available in the UK as tablets of 25, 50, and 100 μg. A greater variety of tablet strength is marketed in other parts of Europe and North America. Thyroxine has a half-life of some 7 days and should be given as a single daily dose which improves compliance. Thyroxine, taken at bedtime, is associated with higher thyroid hormone concentrations and lower thyroid-stimulating hormone (TSH) concentrations compared to the same dose taken in the morning, probably due to greater gastrointestinal uptake of thyroxine during the night (1). Omitting the occasional tablet is of no consequence and those who forget to take their medication, e.g. on vacation, will experience little in the way of symptoms for the first 2 weeks.

Dosage

Before the availability of sensitive assays for TSH the recommended dose of thyroxine in most major textbooks of medicine was 200–400 μg daily. These doses were associated with high serum thyroxine (T_4) concentrations, e.g. total T_4 180–200 nmol/l (normal 60–150 nmol/l), thought to be needed before it was recognized that thyroxine was converted to the metabolically active triiodothyronine (T_3) by widespread peripheral monodeiodination, and with serum TSH concentrations that were unresponsive to thyrotropin-releasing hormone. Subsequently, it was shown that doses of thyroxine of as little as 100–150 μg daily were adequate in restoring TSH secretion to normal. The consensus, however, was that the pituitary thyrotrophs were uniquely sensitive to changes in serum thyroid hormone concentrations within their respective reference ranges (2), and that these cells derived proportionately more of their triiodothyronine than other organs from local deiodination of thyroxine (3). Suppression of thyrotropin secretion was not, therefore, necessarily regarded as a sign of overtreatment with thyroxine.

Opinion changed, however, with the advent of thyrotropin assays with a functional limit of detection of 0.1 mU/l or less, which were capable of distinguishing normal from low concentrations. Doses of thyroxine sufficient to suppress thyrotropin secretion without necessarily increasing serum thyroid hormone concentrations into the thyrotoxic range appeared to have more widespread effects. These included changes in nocturnal heart rate, left ventricular wall thickness, systolic time intervals, urinary sodium excretion, liver and muscle enzyme activity, red cell sodium concentrations, and serum lipid concentrations, similar to, but less marked than, those present in overt thyrotoxicosis (4). These changes may not only resolve with prolonged treatment, as there is evidence of tissue adaptation to thyroid hormone excess (5), but also depend upon the cause of the hypothyroidism (6). It was the concern that a low serum TSH concentration might be associated with reduced bone mineral density (7) that prompted the American Thyroid Association to make its landmark statement (8), since reinforced (9), that 'the goal of therapy [with thyroxine] is to restore patients to the euthyroid state and to normalize serum T_4 and TSH concentrations'. This advice was strengthened by the report that a low serum TSH was a risk factor for the development of atrial fibrillation in older people (10), even although the patients in the study were a heterogeneous group only some of whom were taking thyroxine. The pharmaceutical industry reacted by producing a variety of strengths and colours of thyroxine tablets in an attempt to ensure the recommended biochemical control in patients taking replacement therapy. There is, however, no consensus about what constitutes the most appropriate dose or form of thyroid hormone replacement (11). Most hypothyroid patients treated according to the above guidelines have no complaints and feel returned to normal health. However, a substantial minority claim only to achieve a sense of wellbeing if thyroxine is given in a dose of 50 μg greater than that needed to restore normal TSH secretion (12). There is no convincing evidence that this degree of 'overtreatment' is a risk factor for osteoporosis (13), or is associated with increased morbidity or mortality (14). Furthermore, studies of weight gain following destructive therapy for Graves' disease suggest that restoration of serum TSH to normal by thyroxine alone may not constitute adequate hormone replacement (15). It makes sense, therefore, to allow hypothyroid patients who are dissatisfied with the outcome of restoring serum T_4 and TSH concentrations to normal to increase the dose of thyroxine such that serum TSH is suppressed, in which case serum free T_4 is likely to be between 20 and 25 pmol/l. In this circumstance it is essential, however, that the serum T_3 concentration is unequivocally normal.

Initiating therapy

Practice varies slightly from centre to centre and between countries, but a reasonable starting daily dose of thyroxine in a middle-aged patient with no history of cardiac disease is 50 μg, increasing to 100 μg, and then to 125–150 μg at intervals of 2–3 weeks. After 3 months or so of therapy any minor adjustment to the dose can be made such that the serum concentrations of T_4 (free or total) and TSH are at the upper and lower parts of their respective reference ranges. The reason for the stepwise increment in the dose of thyroxine is the fear that a sudden increase in metabolic rate in a patient with long-standing severe hypothyroidism may unmask previously unrecognized ischaemic heart disease and precipitate angina, myocardial infarction, dysrhythmia, or even sudden death, although the evidence for such a cautious approach is anecdotal. On the other hand, it is quite appropriate to prescribe what is thought to be a full replacement dose with immediate effect in a young patient in whom the thyroid failure is known to have been of short duration, such as following total thyroidectomy for differentiated thyroid carcinoma. In contrast, in older patients in whom thyroxine requirements are reduced, and in those with concurrent symptomatic ischaemic heart disease, it is customary to begin with a dose of thyroxine of 25 μg daily with increments of 25 μg daily every 3–4 weeks. Worsening angina is no longer a reason for suboptimal replacement therapy, as coronary artery bypass surgery or angioplasty is safe and effective before clinical and biochemical euthyroidism has been established.

Patients begin to feel better within 10–14 days of starting thyroxine, even in doses as little as 25 μg daily. Reduction in body weight, which is rarely more than 10% and largely due to fluid loss, and improvements in periorbital puffiness are among the early responses, whereas maximum improvement in hair and skin texture may take up to 3 months, and reversal of the rare feature of cerebellar ataxia, considerably longer.

Ensuring compliance

Once the correct dose of thyroxine has been established it is good practice to evaluate the patient and measure serum T_4 and TSH concentrations annually to improve compliance, as long-term medication is often not taken regularly or in the recommended dose, and thyroxine is no exception. Weekly administration of 7 times the daily dose of thyroxine may be of benefit in poorly compliant patients (16), but there is little or no experience of its efficacy and safety. The most common reason for a raised serum TSH concentration in a patient taking 150 μg or more of thyroxine daily is poor compliance. The seemingly anomalous combination of raised serum T_4 and TSH concentrations is most likely due to overzealous tablet-taking for a few days before a clinic visit by a patient who was previously taking thyroxine sporadically. Whereas computerized follow-up schemes are the most effective method of ensuring that thyroid function tests are performed regularly, there is an unfortunate tendency for advice about changing dosage of thyroxine to be based solely on biochemical results without considering the clinical status of the patient.

Variation in dosage

Even in conscientious patients, regular review of dosage is advisable as requirements may change for a variety of reasons (Box 3.4.9.1). The concurrent administration of any of several drugs may necessitate an increase in thyroxine dosage to maintain a normal serum TSH concentration, the most recently recognized being omeprazole (17) and the antidepressant sertraline (18). Ingestion of dietary fibre supplements may reduce bioavailability of thyroxine by its adsorption on to wheat bran (19).

The mean dose of thyroxine required by patients developing hypothyroidism during the first 1–2 years after surgery or ^{131}I therapy for hyperthyroidism due to Graves' disease is lower than in those with spontaneous primary hypothyroidism, but a higher dose may be required in later years. The explanation is the continued presence of stimulating TSH-receptor antibodies in the early stages after ablative therapy for Graves' disease, resulting in nonsuppressible secretion of thyroid hormones by the thyroid remnant. As the production of the antibodies declines, this autonomous secretion declines as well (Fig. 3.4.9.1). Rarely, patients with long-standing primary hypothyroidism develop Graves'

Box 3.4.9.1 Situations in which an adjustment of the dose of thyroxine may be necessary

- Increased dose required
  - Use of other medication
    - Phenobarbital
    - Phenytoin
    - Carbamazepine
    - Rifampicin
    - Sertraline[a]

      } Increased thyroxine clearance
    - Chloroquine[a]
    - Omeprazole
    - Cholestyramine
    - Sucralfate
    - Aluminium hydroxide

      } Interference with intestinal absorption
    - Ferrous sulfate
    - Dietary fibre supplements
    - Tyrosine kinase inhibitors
  - Pregnancy (increased concentration of serum thyroxine-binding globulin; increased body mass)
  - After surgical or iodine-131 ablation of Graves' disease (reduced thyroidal secretion with time)
  - Malabsorption, e.g. coeliac disease
- Decreased dose required
  - Ageing (decreased thyroxine clearance)
  - Graves' disease developing in patient with long-standing primary hypothyroidism (switch from production of blocking to stimulating TSH-receptor antibodies)

[a]Mechanism not fully established.

disease due to a switch in production from blocking to stimulating TSH-receptor antibodies.

Most patients require an increase in thyroxine dosage during pregnancy, as serum TSH concentrations rise into the hypothyroid range if the prepregnancy dose of thyroxine is maintained. The average increase in thyroxine dosage required is 50 µg daily, and this may be evident within 6 weeks of conception. The principal reason for this change in thyroxine requirement is the increase in the serum concentration of thyroxine-binding globulin in pregnancy, which results in decreased serum concentrations of free T_3 and T_4. These decreases cannot be compensated for by increased thyroidal secretion because of lack of functioning thyroid tissue (20).

Finally, there are numerous manufacturers of thyroxine preparations and, from time to time, there is divergence in bioequivalence. This possibility should be entertained in any patient in whom serum TSH concentrations rise when no new medication has been prescribed and the dose of thyroxine has been stable for many years. It is important that the same preparation of thyroxine is dispensed at each prescription refill (11).

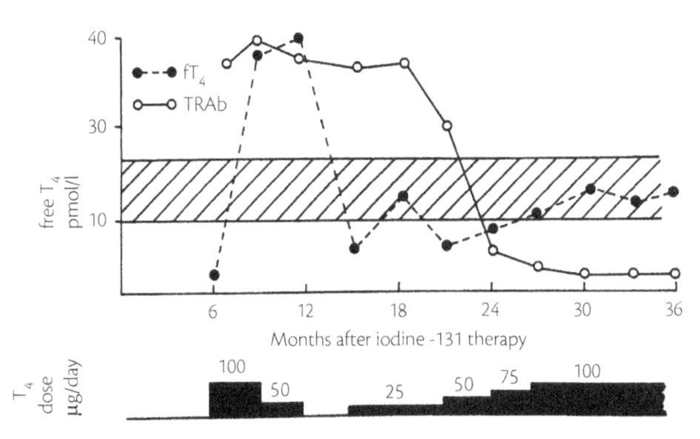

Fig. 3.4.9.1 Difficulty in controlling hypothyroidism with thyroxine in the early stages after ^{131}I therapy for Graves' disease due to high concentrations of TSH-receptor antibodies (TRAb) stimulating the thyroid remnant. As the antibody concentration declines, the dose of thyroxine necessary to maintain normal serum T_4 concentrations increases. The initial phase of hypothyroidism proved temporary. Reference range for free T_4 (fT_4) is indicated by the cross-hatched area.

Temporary hypothyroidism

Most patients with primary hypothyroidism require lifelong thyroxine therapy. However, hypothyroidism may be transient and even short-term treatment with thyroxine may be unnecessary. This is the case for the thyroid failure developing within the first 6 months after surgery for Graves' disease and failure to appreciate such a phenomenon has led to spuriously high estimates of postoperative hypothyroidism. Raised serum TSH concentrations, as high as 200 mU/l, and low or undetectable serum T_4 concentrations may be recorded in 30% of patients at 3 months after surgery, with or without symptoms of mild hypothyroidism. By the sixth month, however, without thyroxine substitution, serum T_4 and usually TSH concentrations have returned to normal (Table 3.4.9.1)(21). A similar pattern of thyroid function occurs after ^{131}I therapy for Graves' disease, and a rise in the concentration of blocking TSH-receptor antibodies has been implicated in the thyroid failure (22). It follows that permanent hypothyroidism should not be diagnosed before 6 months have elapsed following treatment of Graves' disease by surgery or [131]I. If, because of symptoms at 2–4 months, thyroxine treatment is deemed necessary, a suboptimal dose of 50–75 µg daily should be prescribed, which allows meaningful assessment of thyroid function at 6 months. If at that stage the serum TSH concentration is elevated, the thyroid failure should be considered permanent and the dose of thyroxine increased appropriately, but if serum TSH is normal or low, the thyroxine should be stopped and the thyroid function reassessed 4–6 weeks later. An exception to this policy should be made in patients with significant orbitopathy, as raised serum TSH concentrations are a risk factor for worsening of thyroid eye disease. In such patients it is important to avoid any degree of thyroid failure following ^{131}I or surgical treatment of Graves' disease by early treatment with adequate doses of thyroxine, accepting that the question of permanent or temporary hypothyroidism can be resolved at some stage in the future.

Other examples of transient hypothyroidism include the recovery phase of subacute (De Quervain's), painless, and postpartum thyroiditis; Hashimoto's thyroiditis, particularly if excess iodine or iodine-containing drugs, such as amiodarone, have been implicated in the development of the thyroid failure; in the

Table 3.4.9.1 Temporary hypothyroidism following subtotal thyroidectomy for Graves' disease

Time (months)	1	2	3	4	5	6	7	12
Free T_4 (pmol/l)	8	6	6	15	16	20	20	19
TSH (mU/l)	<0.05	23	60	21	5.6	1.2	1.6	1.1
Thyroxine (μg/day)	–	–	75	75	75	–	–	–

Thyroxine in a dose of 75 μg daily was started at 3 months because of symptoms, but because of normal concentrations of serum T_4 and TSH at 6 months treatment was stopped with no deterioration in thyroid function.

neonatal period in children born to a minority of mothers with autoimmune hypothyroidism due to the transplacental passage of TSH-receptor blocking antibodies; and in 5% of patients with chronic autoimmune thyroiditis as a result of the disappearance of these same antibodies from the serum. In addition, the use of iodine-containing antiseptics applied vaginally during labour and topically to the skin of the newborn infant may also result in transient hypothyroidism. Temporary thyroid failure may occur 2 months to 2 years after starting treatment with interferon-α for hepatitis C. Raised serum TSH concentrations of greater than 15 U/l are often recorded in patients with untreated or inadequately treated Addison's disease, but usually fall to normal with glucocorticoid replacement. Similarly, raised serum TSH concentrations may be found during the recovery phase of nonthyroidal illness.

Other treatments of hypothyroidism

Animal thyroid extract

This was first used successfully by mouth in the treatment of hypothyroidism in 1892 and for the next 50 years or so was the only therapy. These extracts from oxen, sheep, and pigs contain, among other iodinated amino acids and proteins, thyroxine and triiodothyronine in variable amounts. They lost favour among endocrinologists in the 1960s due to problems with standardization, and because synthetic L-thyroxine became readily available. From time to time thyroid extract has enjoyed a renaissance, usually among practitioners on the fringes of medicine, because of its effectiveness in weight reduction, but only as a consequence of inducing mild hyperthyroidism which is not in the best interests of the patient.

Combinations of thyroxine and triiodothyronine

These combinations, e.g. Liotrix and Novothyral, are not widely used as most, if not all, contain molar ratios of T_4 to T_3 significantly less than the molar ratio for secretion by the human thyroid gland of 14:1, thereby providing an excess of triiodothyronine. Administration of triiodothyronine as a bolus, alone or in combination with thyroxine, coupled with its rapid intestinal absorption, contributes to the appearance of peaks of elevated serum T_3. These are often associated with undesirable cardiac effects, such as palpitations, as the heart derives most of its triiodothyronine from plasma. It has been assumed that all the necessary triiodothyronine is derived from peripheral monodeiodination of orally administered thyroxine, a view for which there is recent support in respect of concentrations of T_3 in the serum (23). However, there is evidence from the thyroidectomized, and therefore hypothyroid, rat that it is only possible to restore normal concentrations of T_3 in all tissues, while maintaining normal serum concentrations of T_3, T_4, and TSH, by giving a combination of thyroxine and triiodothyronine, and not thyroxine alone, unless in supraphysiological doses (24). That a similar situation might exist in humans was suggested when a combination of thyroxine and triiodothyronine, approximating the ratio normally secreted by the thyroid gland, resulted in significant improvements in mood and neuropsychological function, when compared to a higher dose of thyroxine alone, and without suppressing serum TSH (25). This claim has not been substantiated (26) but some patients prefer the combination therapy despite the absence of any objective benefit. There is also emerging evidence that patients who do respond to the addition of triiodothyronine to thyroxine therapy possess an inherited variant of the type II deiodinase gene, present in 16% of the population (27). The pragmatic approach in patients who fail to achieve the desired sense of wellbeing, despite a dose of thyroxine which suppresses serum TSH to less than 0.05 mU/l, albeit with an unequivocally normal serum T_3 concentration, is to reduce the dose of thyroxine by 50 μg daily and add triiodothyronine in a dose of 10 μg daily. If the patient remains symptomatic it is clear that thyroid dysfunction is not responsible. This most commonly occurs in female patients and they should be encouraged to address outstanding issues at home and in the workplace which may be the cause of the nonspecific symptoms of weight gain, tiredness, and low mood. Many of these patients are menopausal and oestrogen replacement is likely to be more effective than tinkering with the dose or form of thyroid hormone replacement.

Unnecessary thyroxine therapy

Occasionally, patients may have been started on treatment with thyroxine for nonspecific symptoms such as tiredness and weight gain, without confirmatory tests of thyroid function, on the basis of equivocal results, or in a situation when the thyroid failure may have been temporary, such as in the first year postpartum. In order to assess the continued need for thyroxine, treatment should be stopped for 4 weeks if the serum TSH concentration is normal, or for 6 weeks if it is undetectable, in order to allow recovery of the suppressed pituitary thyrotrophs. Measurement of serum T_4 and TSH concentrations at this stage will determine whether the patient is truly hypothyroid.

References

1. Bolk N, Visser TJ, Kalsbeck A, van Domburg RT, Berghout A. Effects of evening vs morning thyroxine ingestion on serum thyroid hormone profiles in hypothyroid patients. *Clin Endocrinol*, 2007; **66**: 43–8.
2. Snyder PJ, Utiger RD. Inhibition of thyrotropin response to thyrotropin-releasing hormone by small quantities of thyroid hormones. *J Clin Invest*, 1972; **51**: 2077–84.

3. Visser TJ, Kaplan MM, Leonard JL, Larsen PR. Evidence for two pathways of iodothyronine 5′-deiodination in rat pituitary that differs in kinetics, propylthiouracil sensitivity, and response to hypothyroidism. *J Clin Invest*, 1983; **71**: 992–1002.
4. Leslie PJ, Toft AD. The replacement therapy problem in hypothyroidism. *Baillieres Clin Endocrinol Metab*, 1988; **2**: 653–69.
5. Nyström E, Lundberg P-A, Petersen K, Bengtsson C, Lindstedt G. Evidence for a slow tissue adaptation to circulating thyroxine in patients with chronic L-thyroxine treatment. *Clin Endocrinol*, 1989; **31**: 143–50.
6. Gow SM, Caldwell G, Toft AD, Beckett GJ. Different hepatic responses to thyroxine replacement in spontaneous and ^{131}I-induced primary hypothyroidism. *Clin Endocrinol*, 1989; **30**: 505–12.
7. Ross DS, Neer RM, Ridgway EC, Daniels GH. Subclinical hyperthyroidism and reduced bone density as a possible result of prolonged suppression of the pituitary-thyroid axis with L-thyroxine. *Am J Med*, 1987; **82**: 1167–70.
8. Surks MI, Chopra IJ, Mariash CN, Nicoloff JT, Solomon DH. American Thyroid Association guidelines for the use of laboratory tests in thyroid disorders. *JAMA*, 1990; **263**: 1529–32.
9. Surks MI, Ortiz E, Daniels GH, Sawin CT, Col NF, Cobin RH, *et al.* Subclinical thyroid disease: scientific review and guidelines for diagnosis and management. *JAMA*, 2004; **291**: 228–38.
10. Sawin CT, Geller A, Wolf PA, Belanger AJ, Baker E, Bacharach P, *et al.* Low serum thyrotropin concentrations as a risk factor for atrial fibrillation in older persons. *N Engl J Med*, 1994; **331**: 1249–52.
11. Toft A. Which thyroxine. *Thyroid*, 2005; **15**: 124–6.
12. Carr D, McLeod DT, Parry G, Thorner HM. Fine adjustment to thyroxine replacement dosage: comparison of the thyrotrophin releasing hormone test using a sensitive thyrotrophin assay with measurement of free thyroid hormones and clinical assessment. *Clin Endocrinol*, 1988; **28**: 325–33.
13. Bower DC, Nevitt MC, Ettinger B, Stone K. Low thyrotropin levels are not associated with bone loss in older women: a prospective study. *J Clin Endocrinol Metab*, 1997; **82**: 2931–6.
14. Leese GP, Jung RT, Guthrie C, Waugh N, Browning MC, *et al.* Morbidity in patients on L-thyroxine: comparison of those with a normal TSH to those with a suppressed TSH. *Clin Endocrinol*, 1992; **37**: 500–3.
15. Tigas S, Idiculla J, Beckett GJ, Toft A. Is excessive weight gain after ablative treatment of hyperthyroidism due to inadequate thyroid hormone therapy. *Thyroid*, 2000; **10**: 1107–11.
16. Grebe SK, Cooke RR, Ford HC, Fagerström JN, Cordwell DP, Lever NA, *et al.* Treatment of hypothyroidism with once weekly thyroxine. *J Clin Endocrinol Metab*, 1997; **82**: 870–5.
17. Centanni M, Gargano L, Canettieri G, Viceconti N, Franchi A, Delle Fave G, *et al.* Thyroxine in goiter, *Helicobacter pylori* infection, and chronic gastritis. *N Engl J Med*, 2006; **354**: 1787–95.
18. McCowen KC, Garber JR, Spark R. Elevated serum thyrotropin in thyroxine-treated patients with hypothyroidism given sertraline. *N Engl J Med*, 1997; **337**: 1010–11.
19. Liel Y, Harman-Boehm I, Shany S. Evidence for a clinically important adverse effect of fiber-enriched diet on the availability of levothyroxine in adult hypothyroid patients. *J Clin Endocrinol Metab*, 1996; **81**: 857–9.
20. Alexander EK, Marqusee E, Lawrence J, Jarobin P, Fischer GA, Larsen PR. Timing and magnitude of increase in levothyroxine requirements during pregnancy in women with hypothyroidism. *N Engl J Med*, 2004; **351**: 241–9.
21. Toft AD, Irvine WJ, Sinclair I, McIntosh D, Seth J, Cameron EHD. Thyroid function after surgical treatment of thyrotoxicosis: a report of 100 cases treated with propranolol before operation. *N Engl J Med*, 1978; **298**: 643–7.
22. Yoshida K, Aizawa Y, Kaise N, Fukazawa H, Kiso Y, Sayama N, *et al.* Role of thyroid-stimulating blocking antibody in patients who developed hypothyroidism within one year after ^{131}I treatment for Graves' disease. *Clin Endocrinol*, 1998; **48**: 17–22.
23. Jonklass J, Davidson B, Bhagat S, Soldin SJ. Triiodothyronine levels in athyreotic individuals during levothyroxine therapy. *JAMA*, 2008; **299**: 817–19.
24. Escobar-Morreale HF, Escobar del Ray F, Obregon MJ, Morreale de Escobar G. Only the combined treatment with thyroxine and triiodothyronine ensures euthyroidism in all tissues of the thyroidectomized rat. *Endocrinology*, 1996; **137**: 2490–502.
25. Bunevicius R, Kazanavicius G, Zalinkevicius R, Prange AJ. Comparative effects of thyroxine versus thyroxine plus triiodothyronine in patients with hypothyroidism. *N Engl J Med*, 1999; **340**: 424–9.
26. Escobar-Morreale HF, Botella-Carretero JI, Escobar del Rey F, Morreale de Escobar G. Treatment of hypothyroidism with combination of levothyroxine plus liothyronine. *J Clin Endocrinol Metab*, 2005; **90**: 4946–54.
27. Panicker V, Saravanan P, Vaidya B, Evans J, Hattersley AT, Frayling TM, *et al.* Common variation in the DI02 gene predicts baseline psychological well-being and response to combination thyroxine plus triiodothyronine therapy in hypothyroid patients. *J Clin Endocrinol Metab*, 2009; **94**: 1623–9.

3.5

Thyroid lumps

Contents

3.5.1 Pathogenesis of nontoxic goitre

Dagmar Führer

Definition

'Goitre' is a clinical term defined by a thyroid enlargement above the gender- and age-specific reference range (Table 3.5.1.1). Goitre may arise from very different pathological conditions (Table 3.5.1.2) and may present with euthyroid, hyperthyroid, or hypothyroid function. On morphological grounds, a goitre may be diffuse or nodular. This chapter will focus on the pathogenesis of nontoxic goitre, also called simple or dysplastic goitre in the older literature.

Nodular goitre can be divided into solitary nodular and multinodular thyroid disease and constitutes a complex thyroid disorder with heterogeneous morphological functional and pathogenetic properties (1). Histologically, thyroid nodules are distinguished by morphological criteria according to the World Health Organization classification (2). On functional grounds, nodules are classified as either 'cold', 'normal', or 'hot' depending on whether they show decreased, normal, or increased uptake on scintiscan. In contrast to solitary nodular thyroid disease, which has a more uniform clinical, pathological, and molecular picture, multinodular goitre (MNG) usually comprises a mixed group of nodular entities, i.e. one usually finds a combination of hyperfunctional, hypofunctional, or normally functioning thyroid lesions within the same thyroid gland. The overall balance of functional properties of individual thyroid nodules within an MNG ultimately determines the functional status in the individual patient, which may be euthyroidism, subclinical hyperthyroidism, or overt hyperthyroidism. On the molecular level, thyroid nodules within a nodular goitre may represent polyclonal lesions or true monoclonal thyroid neoplasia.

Role of environmental factors

The development of nodular goitre is influenced by extrinsic factors interacting with constitutional parameters of gender and age (1–6). The most important trigger for nodular (and diffuse) goitre is iodine deficiency (3). There is a direct correlation between goitre prevalence and iodine deficiency and vice versa between correction of iodine deficiency and regression of goitre incidence. For instance, iodine deficiency was common in Germany until the early 1990s, when iodized salt was introduced into food industries leading to a marked improvement in nutritional iodine supply as reflected in increased urinary iodine excretion (median 72 μg iodine/l urine in 1994 to 125 μg iodine/l urine in 2003). The use of iodized salt is currently estimated to be above 80% in private households, 70–80% in restaurants, and 35–40% in food industries. In 1994, the prevalence of diffuse goitre was 21% in the age group 18–30 years and 33% in the age group 46–65 years, while in 2002, an impressive reduction in goitre frequency was found with a goitre prevalence of 6% in the 18- to 30-year-olds and of 26% in the 46- to 65-year-olds, in the Papillon study, in which 96 000 German employees were investigated (4). Another recent epidemiological study (SHIP) has underscored this decrease in overall goitre prevalence due to improved iodine supply; thyroid nodules now tend to occur in normal-sized rather than enlarged thyroid glands (5). This may be explained by the thyroid's inherent disposition to develop focal hyperplasia, discussed below.

Table 3.5.1.1 Gender- and age-dependent upper reference values for normal thyroid volume

Gender and age	Upper reference value (ml)
Men	25
Women	18
13–14 years	8–10
3–4 years	3
Newborn	0.8–1.5

Various other goitrogenic factors are known and are relevant to thyroid disease in situations with co-existing iodine deficiency. First, metabolites of various nutrients (e.g. cabbage, cauliflower, and broccoli) may interfere with iodine uptake. Second, industrial pollutants, including resorcinol and phthalic acid, are known to be goitrogenic. Third, deficiencies of selenium, iron, and vitamin A may exacerbate the pathogenic effects of iodine deficiency (3).

Other risk factors for nodular goitre have been suggested, but their putative impact on the prevalence of thyroid nodules occurring in a normal-sized or enlarged thyroid gland is less clear (1, 6). Smoking has been proposed as a risk factor for goitre, and nodules were also found with higher prevalence in goitres of smokers compared with nonsmokers. The impact of smoking on thyroid disease is most likely due to increased thiocyanate levels in smokers exerting a competitive inhibitory effect on iodide uptake. In line with this, the association is more pronounced in areas with iodine deficiency. Radiation is another environmental risk factor not only for thyroid malignancy but also for benign nodular thyroid disease. An increased prevalence of thyroid nodule disease has been associated with exposure to radionuclear fallouts and therapeutic external radiation.

Nodular thyroid disease and goitre are more frequent (2.5-fold to sevenfold) in women but the reasons for this still remain to be clarified. A growth-promoting effect of oestrogens has been described *in vitro* and oestradiol has been suggested to amplify growth factor-dependent signalling in normal thyroid cells and thyroid tumours. However, pregnancy-related thyroid enlargement appears to be mostly related to iodine deficiency, and in one German study increased MNG prevalence with parity was only observed in women who had not taken iodine supplementation during an earlier pregnancy. Several studies suggest that thyroid volume is also significantly correlated with body mass index. In agreement with this, a recent study has shown that in obese women, weight loss of more than 10% may result in a significant decrease in thyroid volume.

Lastly, because of the cumulative impact of external risk factors on the thyroid gland, the prevalence of thyroid nodular disease increases with age. For example, in a borderline iodine deficiency area, multinodular goitre was present in 23% of the studied population of 2656 Danish people aged 41–71 years and increased with age in women (from 20% to 46%) as well as men (from 7% to 23%) (1).

Genetic disposition

Thyroid nodules (and goitre) also occur in individuals without exposure to iodine deficiency, and not all individuals in an iodine-deficient region develop goitre. A familial clustering for nodular goitre is well documented and family and twin pair studies in endemic and nonendemic goitre regions have underscored a genetic predisposition for goitre development (1, 5). For example, twin studies show a concordance rate of 80% for monozygotic twins and of 42% for dizygotic twins in endemic regions and of 40–50% and 13% in nonendemic regions, respectively, strongly suggesting interplay between genetic and environmental factors. On the basis of twin studies, the contribution of genetic susceptibility to goitre development has been calculated to be 39% in endemic regions and 82% in a nonendemic area (7).

Genetic defects in enzymes involved in thyroid hormone synthesis (e.g. thyroglobulin (TG), thyroperoxidase (TPO), sodium-iodide symporter (NIS)) typically result in hypothyroid goitres but in some rare cases genetic variations in the *TG*, *TPO*, and *NIS* genes have also been reported in association with a (diffuse or) nodular euthyroid goitre. Furthermore, alterations in the pendrin gene account for the syndromic occurrence of euthyroid nodular goitre and congenital sensorineural hearing loss.

Since these monogenetic defects are exceptionally rare, linkage studies have been performed to identify susceptibility loci for nontoxic goitre on a broader scale (8). A locus on chromosome 14 (termed MNG1 locus) has been identified in a Canadian and a German study and was found to cosegregate with familial nontoxic goitre. In an Italian pedigree with euthyroid goitre, an X-linked autosomal pattern of inheritance with a putative genetic defect in the Xp22 region was suggested. Moreover, in a study by the European Thyroid Association working group on the 'Genetics of euthyroid goiter', 18 extended Danish, German, and Slovakian families were analysed in a genome-wide scan. Further putative candidate loci for nontoxic goitre were identified on chromosomes 3p, 2q, 7q, and 8p emphasizing the genetic heterogeneity of euthyroid goitre. However, no germline mutation that cosegregates with

Table 3.5.1.2 Differential diagnosis of goitre

Disease entity	Thyroid function	Goitre	Cause
Simple goitre	Eu-/hyperthyroid	Diffuse or nodular	Iodine deficiency, goitrogens, external irradiation
Thyroid cancer	Euthyroid	Nodular	Mutations in oncogenes
Hashimoto's disease, Graves' disease	Hypo-/eu-/hyperthyroid	Diffuse	Thyroid autoimmunity
Thyroiditis	Hypo-/eu-/hyperthyroid	Diffuse or nodular	Infections, autoimmunity (acute, subacute, chronic)
Thyroid hormone biosynthesis defects	Hypo-/euthyroid	Diffuse or nodular	Mutations in *NIS*, *TG*, *TPO*, *THOX*
Thyroid hormone resistance	Euthyroid		Mutations in *TRβ1*
TSHoma	Hyperthyroid	Diffuse	TSH dependent
Acromegaly	Euthyroid	Diffuse	IGF-1 dependent
Drugs	Hypo-/eu-/hyperthyroid	Diffuse	See Chapters 3.3.5 and 3.4.2

goitre in the affected families has been identified to date. Thus, for the majority of euthyroid goitres, a complex multifactorial pathogenesis including interactions between various environmental factors, gender-specific components, and the genetic background has to be assumed.

Molecular processes involved in nodule formation

Development of nodular goitre most likely proceeds in two phases that involve global activation of thyroid epithelial cell proliferation (e.g. as the result of iodine deficiency or other goitrogenic stimuli) leading to hyperplasia and a focal increase of thyroid epithelial cell proliferation causing thyroid nodules. So far, the most common stimulus for focal proliferation is a somatic mutation.

Two driving pathogenetic events have to be considered (Fig. 3.5.1.1): first, iodine deficiency causing an increase in thyroid cell numbers (true hyperplasia), as observed in animal models, and second, H_2O_2 production and free radical formation, which occurs physiologically during thyroid hormone synthesis and may damage genomic DNA. Thus in a mouse model, the spontaneous mutation rate in the naïve thyroid gland has been found to be almost 10 times higher than in other organs (9, 10).

Both processes provide a mutagenic milieu, in which the likelihood of somatic mutations is increased. Whether these somatic mutations lead to thyroid nodular disease critically depends on the affected gene and most likely the environmental selection factors (e.g. iodine deficiency; Fig. 3.5.1.2). A proof of principle for this concept is the evolution of a toxic adenoma from a somatic TSH-receptor mutation (1, see Chapter 3.3.5). Other examples include the origin of papillary thyroid cancer based on *BRAF* mutations or *RET/PTC* rearrangements. These somatic mutations have been found already in microscopic lesions of thyroid autonomy and papillary microcarcinoma, respectively. Besides the driving mutation, increased growth factor production and auto- and paracrine action of secreted growth factors (e.g. IGF-1) has been found in monoclonal thyroid tumours and may further propel nodule development. The development of polyclonal thyroid lesions in a nontoxic goitre is less clear and putatively is linked to exogenous

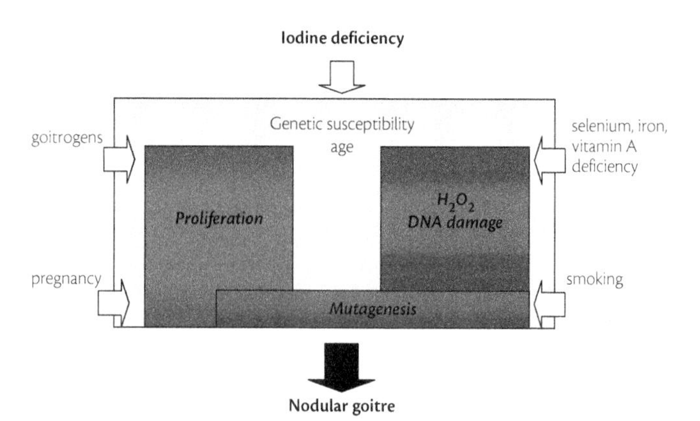

Fig. 3.5.1.1 Interaction of extrinsic and intrinsic factors contributing to the development of nodular goitre. Note that the pathogenetic influence of several goitrogenic components (e.g. selenium deficiency, pregnancy) will be aggravated with coexisting iodine deficiency. The two elementary molecular pathological mechanisms are increased cell proliferation, leading to hyperplasia/goitre, and oxidative stress, leading to increased mutagenesis and nodule formation (1).

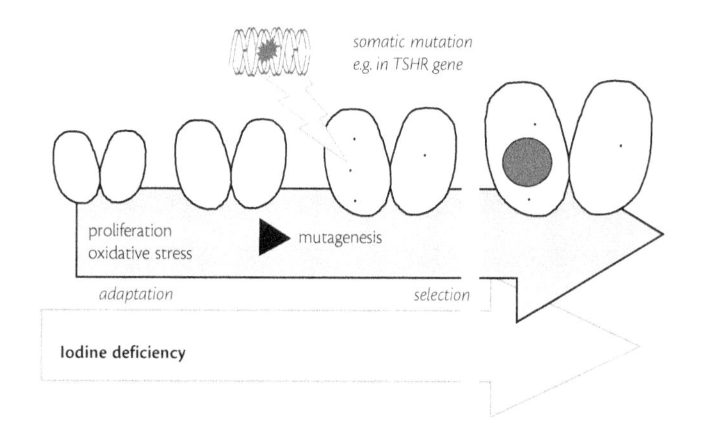

Fig. 3.5.1.2 Pathogenesis of nodular goitre in an iodide-deficient environment. According to current concepts the development of nodular goitre proceeds in two phases that involve: (1) adaptive increase in thyroid epithelial cell proliferation and function, providing a mutagenic milieu with increased likelihood for occurrence of somatic mutations, and (2) clone expansion to a macroscopic thyroid nodule by growth advantage of cell clone with somatic mutation and propagation in persisting iodine deficiency.

factors, e.g. intrathyroidal production of growth factors such as IGF-1, which act on the naturally functional and morphological heterogeneous thyroid follicles (11).

Natural course of disease

From the epidemiological data discussed above, one might expect an inherent progressive course of nodular thyroid disease. Studies aimed at accurate assessment of the nodules by ultrasonography differ in terms of follow-up period, definition of growth, type of thyroid lesion, and the background in which they are conducted. Moreover, the interobserver variability of long-term studies of nodule volumes is not known. With these caveats in mind, the following observations have been reported (1, 6). In iodine-sufficient areas, nodule 'growth' has been reported in 35% of US patients over a follow-up period of 4.9–5.6 years. On long-term follow-up over 15 years in an area of iodine sufficiency, only one-third of benign nodules showed growth as assessed by palpation and ultrasonography, compared with the majority of nodules which remained unchanged or even showed a decrease in size. In Germany, a mean 3-year follow-up of 109 consecutive patients showed a steady and significant (30% volume) increase in nodular size in 50% of patients. In a Danish study, only four (8%) of 45 cold nodules in an area of borderline iodine deficiency showed a change in size (5 mm in diameter), of which only one nodule actually increased and three nodules shrank over a follow-up period of 2 years. Thus, in iodine-deficient and iodine-sufficient settings a varying proportion of nodules will grow, and the speed of growth is highly heterogeneous.

References

1. Krohn K, Führer D, Bayer Y, Eszlinger M, Brauer V, Neumann S, *et al.* Molecular pathogenesis of euthyroid and toxic multinodular goiter. *Endocr Rev*, 2005; **26**: 504–24.
2. DeLellis R, Lloyd RV, Heitz H, Eng C. *World Health Organization Classification of Tumors. Pathology and Genetics of Tumors of Endocrine Organs.* Lyon: IARC Press, 2004.
3. Reiners C, Wegscheider K, Schicha H, Theissen P, Vaupel R, Wrbitzky R, *et al.* Prevalence of thyroid disorders in the working population of

Germany: ultrasonography screening in 96 278 unselected employees. *Thyroid*, 2004; **14**: 926–32.
4. Völzke H, Lüdemann J, Robinson DM, Spieker KW, Schwahn C, Kramer A, *et al.* The prevalence of undiagnosed thyroid disorders in a previously iodine-deficient area. *Thyroid*, 2003; **13**: 803–10.
5. Zimmermann MB. Iodine deficiency. *Endocr Rev*, 2009; **30**: 376–408.
6. Hegedüs L, Bonnema SJ, Bennedbaek FN. Management of simple nodular goiter: current status and future perspectives. *Endocr Rev*, 2003; **24**: 102–32.
7. Hansen PS, Brix TH, Bennedbaek FN, Bonnema SJ, Kyvik KO, Hegedüs L. Genetic and environmental causes of individual differences in thyroid size: a study of healthy Danish twins. *J Clin Endocrinol Metab*, 2004; **89**: 2071–7.
8. Bayer Y, Neumann S, Meyer B, Rüschendorf F, Reske A, Brix T, *et al.* Genome-wide linkage analysis reveals evidence for four new susceptibility loci for familial euthyroid goiter. *J Clin Endocrinol Metab*, 2004; **89**: 4044–52.
9. Krohn K, Maier J, Paschke R. Mechanisms of disease: hydrogen peroxide, DNA damage and mutagenesis in the development of thyroid tumors. *Nat Clin Pract Endocrinol Metab*, 2007; **3**: 713–20.
10. Song S, Driessens N, Costa M. Roles of hydrogen peroxide in thyroid physiology and disease. *J Clin Endocrinol Metab*, 2007; **92**: 3764–73.
11. Studer H, Derwahl M. Mechanisms of nonneoplastic endocrine hyperplasia—a changing concept: a review focused on the thyroid gland. *Endocr Rev*, 1995; **16**: 411–26.

3.5.2 Management of nontoxic multinodular goitre

Wilmar M. Wiersinga

Introduction

Goitres can be classified according to thyroid function into toxic goitres, hypothyroid goitres, and euthyroid or nontoxic goitres (see Chapter 3.5.1). The most prevalent causes of nontoxic goitre are endemic (iodine-deficient) goitre and sporadic nontoxic goitre (diffuse or nodular). The disease entity of sporadic nontoxic goitre is defined as a benign enlargement of the thyroid gland of unknown cause, in euthyroid patients (normal serum free thyroxine (T_4) and free triiodothyronine (T_3) concentrations) living in an area without endemic goitre. The diagnosis is by exclusion. The prevalence of sporadic nontoxic goitre (also called simple goitre) in the adult population is high, 3.2% in the UK (see Chapter 3.1.7), and it is more common in women (5.3%) than in men (0.8%). This chapter deals predominantly with sporadic nontoxic multinodular goitre.

Natural history

In a cross-sectional survey of 102 consecutive patients referred because of sporadic nontoxic goitre, goitre size is positively related to age and to duration of goitre (1) (Fig. 3.5.2.1). Patients with a multinodular goitre are older and have a larger goitre than patients with a diffuse or uninodular goitre. Plasma thyroid-stimulating hormone (TSH) is negatively related to goitre size (Fig. 3.5.2.2). Patients with a multinodular goitre and a suppressed TSH are older and have higher plasma free T_4 concentrations and larger goitres than those with a multinodular goitre and a normal TSH. The data suggest a continuous growth of nontoxic goitre and provide

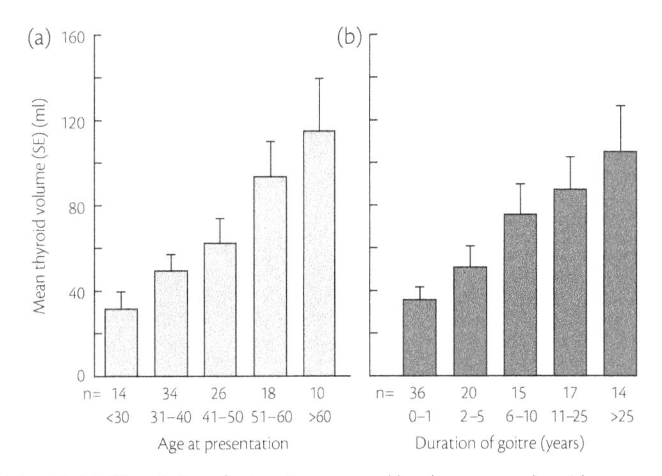

Fig. 3.5.2.1 The relation of goitre size measured by ultrasonography with age at presentation (panel a) and with duration of goitre (panel b) in 102 consecutive patients with sporadic non-toxic goitre. Reproduced from Berghout A, Wiersinga WM, Smits NJ, Touber JL. Interrelationships between age, thyroid volume, thyroid nodularity, and thyroid function in patients with sporadic non-toxic goiter. *American Journal of Medicine*, 1990; **89**: 602–8, with permission.

support for the concept of increasing thyroid nodularity and autonomy of thyroid function, related to increasing goitre size, during the natural history of the disease (see Chapter 3.5.1).

Clinical examination

Several nontoxic goitre patients have no symptoms at all, or just complaints of cosmetic disfigurement (Box 3.5.2.1). Local discomfort in the neck is very common. Obstructive symptoms range from very slight to severe, caused by compression of neighbouring structures such as the upper airways, the recurrent laryngeal nerve, the oesophagus, and the great veins in the thoracic inlet. Not all compressive goitres, however, are symptomatic. Upper airway compression may cause dyspnoea, cough, and a mild choking sensation aggravated by recumbency, but these complaints occur only in one-half of the patients in whom tracheal compression is noted (2). The trachea presumably needs to lose 75% of its cross-sectional area before a stridor is clearly recognizable (3). The inspiratory stridor may be noticed on deep inspiration but not on ordinary breathing, and is frequently related to recumbency. In patients with

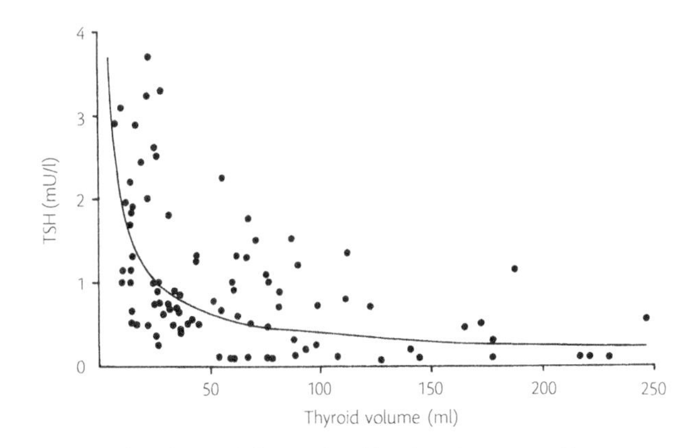

Fig. 3.5.2.2 The relation of plasma TSH with goitre size measured by ultrasonography ($y=\delta 2x^{-0.667}$, r=0.58, $p<0.001$) in 102 consecutive patients with sporadic non-toxic goitre. Reproduced From Berghout A, Wiersinga WM, Smits NJ, Touber JL. Interrelationships between age, thyroid volume, thyroid nodularity, and thyroid function in patients with sporadic non-toxic goiter. *American Journal of Medicine*, 1990; **89**: 602–8, with permission.

Box 3.5.2.1 History of 102 consecutive patients presenting with sporadic non-toxic goitre[1]

- Detection of goitre (by patient, physician, or relatives)
  - 48%/25%/27%
- Recent goitre growth
  - 50%
- Complaints of goiter
  - 70%
- Neck discomfort
  - 61%
- Cosmetic complaints
  - 19%
- Fear of malignancy
  - 17%
- Shortness of breath
  - 17%
- Family history of thyroid disease
  - 60%

substernal goitre, 8–13% complain about hoarseness. Vocal cord paresis occurs in 3–4% of substernal goitres, apparently due to stretching and ischaemia of the recurrent laryngeal nerve; it is not by itself indicative of malignant growth (4). Extrinsic pressure on the oesophagus produces dysphagia in about 20% of patients (2).

The presence of a goitre is usually ascertained by inspection and palpation of the neck. Agreement between observers on the presence of a goitre and on the diffuse or nodular nature of a goitre is low (5). Haemorrhage in a nodule may cause local neck pain for a few weeks. Some retrosternal extension of the goitre is quite common, but intrathoracic or substernal goitres (defined as having its greater mass inferior to the thoracic inlet) occur only in 3–5%, especially in elderly women with long-standing compressive goitres. The thyroid gland is not palpable in 10–30% of substernal goitres (4). Rarely, a 'goitre *plongeant*' or plunging goitre is observed: the goitre disappears into the thoracic cavity and reappears in the neck on swallowing or coughing. Clinical clues to the presence of a substernal goitre (in the absence of a cervical mass) are facial plethora, dilated veins over the thoracic inlet, and nocturnal dyspnoea when the patient sleeps on the side of the goitre. In this respect Pemberton's sign is helpful too: the patient is asked to elevate both arms until they touch the sides of the face, and the presence of a substernal goitre narrowing the thoracic inlet and obstructing the great veins may reveal itself after a few moments by congestion of the face, some cyanosis, and distress. A goitre occluding the thoracic inlet has been named appropriately 'the thyroid cork' (3). Downhill oesophageal varices secondary to obstruction of the superior caval vein is rarely reported in substernal goitre.

Laboratory investigations

Having completed the history and physical examination of the patient, determination of plasma TSH and thyroid ultrasonography and scintigraphy usually suffice for assessing the functional and anatomical characteristics of the goitre.

Thyroid function tests

Subclinical hyperthyroidism (i.e. a suppressed TSH in the presence of a normal free T_4 and free T_3) is present in about 20% of patients, especially in the older age group with large multinodular goitres (1). It is prudent to determine plasma T_3 in these cases in order not to overlook T_3 toxicosis, which is not uncommon in multinodular goitres and requires treatment (see Chapter 3.3.11). Plasma thyroglobulin can be markedly elevated as it is positively related to goitre size (1), but its determination serves no useful purpose. Serum thyroid peroxidase antibodies are found in 15–20% of patients; if present, the patient is at risk of developing Graves'-like hyperthyroidism or hypothyroidism after ^{131}I therapy (see below).

Imaging techniques

Radionuclide scintigraphy with ^{123}I or ^{99m}Tc pertechnetate usually visualizes the goitre. Typically, an inhomogeneous uptake of the radionuclide will be seen with relatively cold and hot areas in an enlarged thyroid gland, compatible with multinodular goitre (see Chapter 3.1.6). Ultrasonography accurately assesses the size of a goitre in the neck, but is of no use in substernal goitres. CT scans have diagnostic value for substernal goitres and characteristic features are: (1) anatomical continuity with the cervical thyroid, (2) focal calcifications, (3) precontrast attenuation of about 15 Hounsfield units greater than muscle due to the high iodine content of thyroid tissue, and (4) prolonged contrast enhancement after the administration of iodinated contrast material (6). Iodine-containing contrast agents in this setting, however, carry a risk of inducing thyrotoxicosis (see Chapters 3.2.4 and 3.3.1). MRI scans may provide similar valuable information on the extension of the goitre in relation to neighbouring structures. Chest radiographs may reveal an intrathoracic goitre by a smooth or nodular superior mediastinal paratracheal mass. Displacement and/or compression of the trachea is a frequent finding on radiographs, and tracheal compression is noted in 25–33% of patients (2).

Functional evaluation of obstructive symptoms

Spirometric pulmonary function tests can be helpful. Visual inspection of the flow volume loop is a sensitive method for detecting upper airway obstruction (7) (Fig. 3.5.2.3). After reduction of goitre size, a significant increase in peak inspiratory and expiratory flow occurs. Inspiratory airflow is more severely affected than expiratory flow because of the tendency of the extrathoracic trachea to collapse on inspiration. Large goitres may contribute to obstructive sleep apnoea syndrome (8). Laryngoscopy can be performed to assess vocal cord mobility; rarely, acute angulation of the larynx is observed, making intubation hazardous. Barium oesophagograms and cine films are seldom useful in the diagnosis or management of compressive goitre.

Malignancy

Thyroid cancer is found in 4–17% of multinodular goitres depending on how carefully the surgical specimens are examined. Of 107 patients operated on for a benign multinodular goitre without suspicion of malignancy before surgery, 7.5% harboured incidental carcinomas, with papillary carcinoma being the most common variety (9). Substernal goitres also harbour malignant (mostly occult) cancer in 7% (4). It is

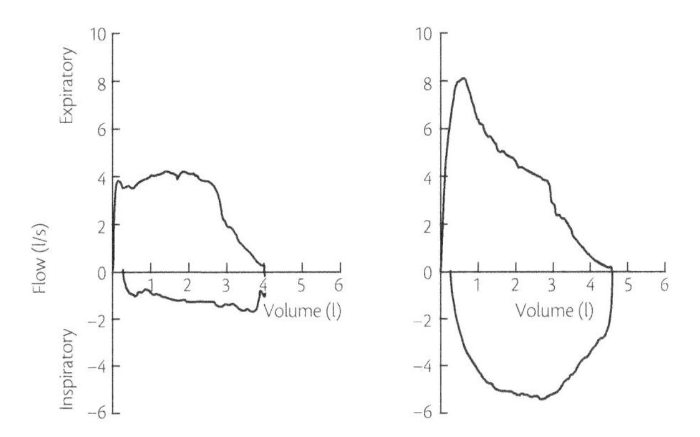

Fig. 3.5.2.3 Flow volume loops (plotting the instantaneous flow rate against the lung volume at which that flow rate occurs) of a woman with upper airway obstruction due to goitre: before surgery on the left, after subtotal thyroidectomy on the right. Reproduced from Miller MR, Pincock AC, Ontes GD, Wilkinson R, Skene-Smith H. Upper airway obstruction due to goitre: detection, prevalence and results of surgical management. *Quarterly Journal of Medicine*, 1990; **74**: 177-88, with permission.

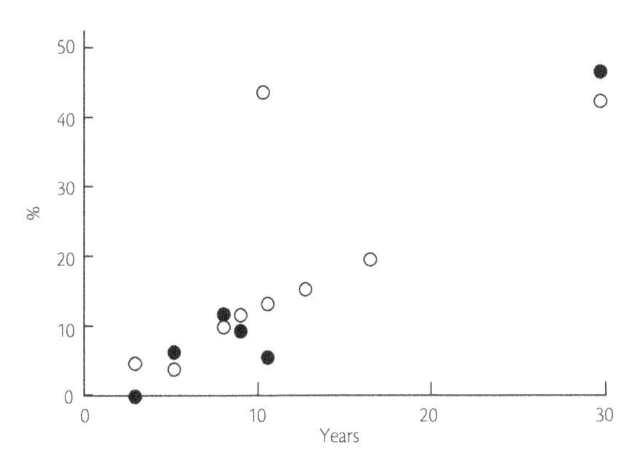

Fig. 3.5.2.4 Recurrence of non-toxic nodular goitre after subtotal thyroidectomy in patients with (•) and without (○) postoperative thyroxine medication. Reproduced from Röjdmark J, Järhult J. High long-term recurrence rate after subtotal thyroidectomy for nodular goitre. *European Journal of Surgery*, 1995; **161**: 725–7, with permission.

doubtful, however, if these incidental cancers adversely affect life expectancy. Fear of malignancy is in general not warranted for women with a history of long-standing slowly growing multinodular goitre and family members with the same condition. However, in patients with a dominant cold nodule, a fast-growing nodule, or a nodule with a very firm texture, fine-needle aspiration cytology is indicated to exclude malignancy (10). Ultrasonographic characteristics of nodules may help in selecting nodules which should be biopsied.

Treatment options

Options in the management of patients with nontoxic multinodular goitre are simple observation, surgery, L-thyroxine, and radioactive iodine (11).

Observation

Data on the natural history of the disease indicates a gradual increase in goitre size by about 4.5% per year, under simultaneous development of increasing thyroid nodularity and thyroid autonomy (1). Long-term outcome studies report development of thyrotoxicosis (toxic multinodular goitre or Plummer's disease) in 10% after a mean follow-up period of 4–5 years. (12, 13).

Thyroidectomy

The big advantage of thyroidectomy is that it rapidly and effectively removes the goitre, albeit at the expense of a low but unavoidable morbidity. Surgical complications include postoperative haemorrhage in 0.5%, vocal cord paresis in 1–2%, and hypoparathyroidism in 2–4%, dependent upon surgical skill and experience. Persistent voice disabilities (dysphonia, hoarseness, fatigue, or reduction of voice range) are not uncommon (15%), and late hypothyroidism occurs in 5–8%.

The reported incidence of recurrent goitre after surgery varies widely, ranging from 4% to 20%, and even 40% after 30 years. In general, the recurrence rate increases with longer follow-up (14) (Fig. 3.5.2.4). The determinants of postoperative recurrences remain largely unknown. Most studies find no difference in postoperative plasma TSH and T_4 concentrations between recurrent goitre patients and those without, the presence of thyroglobulin antibodies and thyroid peroxidase antibodies, the type of surgery (unilateral or bilateral resection), the extent of lymphocytic infiltration in the surgical specimen, or thyroid remnant size (15–17), although a larger thyroid remnant size in the recurrent group is sometimes observed (18). One study indicates a higher frequency of a family history of thyroid disease in the recurrent goitre patients, implying a role of still unknown genetic factors (16). The relatively high recurrence rate has led some surgeons to advocate removal of all nodules found at intraoperative digital palpation, or even total thyroidectomy (19).

Whether or not postoperative treatment with thyroxine prevents recurrent goitre, remains controversial. Most open uncontrolled studies find that the recurrence rate is not lowered by T_4 medication (14, 16) (Fig. 3.5.2.4), and the same conclusion is reached in the few randomized but not placebo-controlled studies (17). Although these results are compatible with the finding that postoperative growth of the thyroid remnant is to a certain extent independent of TSH (20), serum TSH was not really suppressed in these studies. Italian studies (in iodine-deficient areas) observed a lower recurrence rate with TSH-suppressive doses of T_4 than with TSH-nonsuppressive doses (21), and additional benefit of adding iodine to T_4 treatment (22). In contrast, another large study found no preventive effect of T_4 despite suppressed TSH values (18). The available data do not support the routine use of T_4 in order to prevent postoperative recurrent goitre.

Thyroxine

The rationale of T_4 treatment is to suppress TSH. TSH as a stimulus of thyroid growth is thought to play a permissive role in the pathogenesis of sporadic nontoxic goitre (see Chapter 3.5.1). In addition, administration of T_4 significantly inhibits growth of human multinodular goitre tissue transplanted to nude mice (23). The effect varies, however, in different specimens of nontoxic goitre, indicating a varying degree of autonomous replicating activity. Older observational studies report reduction of goitre size upon thyroid hormone medication in about two-thirds of cases; the response was better in diffuse than in nodular goitres (11).

In a placebo-controlled double-blind randomized clinical trial in patients with sporadic nontoxic multinodular goitre, the T_4 dose (initially 2.5 μg/kg per day) was aimed at TSH suppression and adjusted accordingly, resulting in a mean daily dose of 175 μg. A response was defined as a decrease of goitre size of more than 13% (the mean plus two standard deviations of the coefficient of variation of thyroid volume measurements by ultrasonography)

(24). There were 5% responders in the placebo group and 58% responders in the T_4-treated group. After 9 months of treatment, goitre size had increased by 20% in the placebo group, remained almost the same in T_4 nonresponders, and decreased by 25% in T_4 responders; after discontinuation of T_4 treatment, the goitre grew again (Fig. 3.5.2.5). Thus, T_4 treatment in the so-called T_4 nonresponders arrested goitre growth, and continuous T_4 treatment is necessary to maintain its therapeutic effect. Goitre reduction by T_4 treatment was not related to pretreatment characteristics such as age, family history of thyroid disease, duration and size of the goitre, or radio-iodine uptake (24, 25). Only a pretreatment plasma TSH lower than 0.4 mU/l or insufficient TSH suppression during T_4 treatment seems to be related to a less favourable outcome. The reduction in the size of multinodular goitres is largely accounted for by a decrease in the combined nodular volumes (26).

The optimal degree of TSH suppression is not well established, but it seems reasonable to aim at TSH values of 0.1 mU/l. This means the induction of subclinical hyperthyroidism, which is poorly tolerated by some patients, requiring reduction of the T_4 dose in about 25% (24, 25). Subclinical hyperthyroidism carries a risk of atrial fibrillation and bone loss (see also Chapter 3.3.4).

Radioactive iodine

There is renewed interest in ^{131}I treatment of nontoxic multinodular goitre. The median ^{131}I dose reported in the literature, is 1416 MBq or 4.6 MBq/g thyroid (125 μCi/g) corrected for 100% 24-h uptake (25, 27–30). The relatively low thyroidal radio-iodine uptake necessitates the use of high doses of ^{131}I. An estimate of goitre size is required for dose calculation, preferably by ultrasonography (31). A large dose of ^{131}I may require hospital admission for a few days; however, fractionation of the total radio-iodine dose over several months is feasible without jeopardizing outcome, allowing for treatment as an outpatient (32).

Iodine-131 therapy is very effective. The goitre (mean initial size of 126 g), shrinks in 94% of patients; the mean reduction in goitre size is 45%. The greatest fall in goitre size is observed in the first year after treatment; no further reduction is seen after 2 years (Fig. 3.5.2.6). Obstructive symptoms and signs are also favourably affected: in patients with large compressive goitres (including some with intrathoracic goitres), 1 year after ^{131}I therapy the maximal tracheal deviation had decreased by 20%, the smallest cross-sectional area of the tracheal lumen had increased by 36%, dyspnoea and inspiratory stridor had improved in 8 of 12 patients, and compression of the superior vena cava had disappeared in 2 of 2 patients (28).

Independent variables determining the effect of ^{131}I therapy are the administered ^{131}I dose and initial goitre size; age and goitre duration are dependent variables, both being directly related to initial goitre size (30). The ^{131}I dose required for a 50% reduction of goitre size is 4.8 MBq/g thyroid (29, 30). The larger the goitre, the lower the reduction in goitre size (30). Nonresponders and those with late recurrence of goitre growth (8% at 3–5 years after ^{131}I therapy) have larger goitres and more often dominant nodules than responders (30). A second dose of ^{131}I seems to be as beneficial as the first treatment (30).

An increase of obstructive symptoms after ^{131}I treatment is often warned about but rarely seen, even in patients with large compressive goitres (28). Serial measurements of goitre size for 5 weeks after ^{131}I therapy did not demonstrate a significant increase of thyroid volume, the maximum increase in the median volume being 4% on day 7 (33). Routine administration of prednisone as a preventive measure is thus not warranted.

Serum free T_3 and free T_4 indices increase transiently by 20% at day 7, reducing to 13% at day 14, and returning to baseline values at 3 weeks (33). Radiation thyroiditis with tenderness of the neck and slight thyrotoxic symptoms develops in the first few weeks after ^{131}I treatment in 4% of patients. In view of its self-limiting and mostly mild nature, treatment is usually not necessary but salicylates (or, rarely, corticosteroids) can be applied successfully.

Graves'-like hyperthyroidism occurs in 4% of patients, usually developing 3–6 months after ^{131}I therapy, and is related to the new appearance of TSH-receptor antibodies triggered by radiation-induced release of antigens from the thyroid (34, 35). The hyperthyroidism may be severe and may require treatment with antithyroid drugs for several months. The presence of thyroid peroxidase antibodies before treatment increases the risk of developing this complication (34).

The incidence of postradio-iodine hypothyroidism varies widely between studies. A cumulative 5-year risk of 22% is reported in one study (27), in good agreement with 25% hypothyroidism after 2–9.5 years reported in the literature. Determinants are the presence of thyroid peroxidase antibodies, a family history of thyroid disease, and a relatively small goitre (30, 34).

Large doses of ^{131}I carry a theoretical risk of cancer development. A dose of 1.9 GBq (51 mCi) has a calculated 1.6% life-time

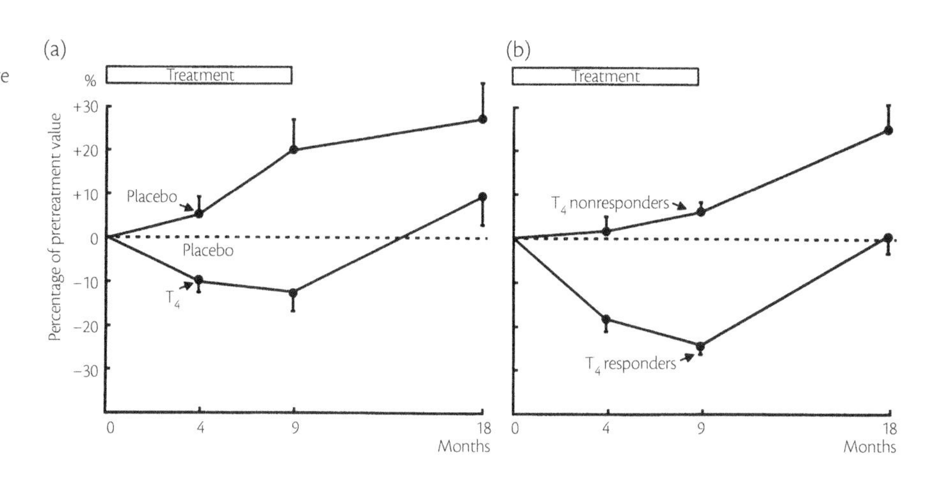

Fig. 3.5.2.5 Relative changes of goitre size measured by ultrasonography in patients with sporadic non-toxic goitre randomized to receive placebo or TSH-suppressive doses of L-thyroxine (panel a), and in responders and non-responders of the T4 treatment group (panel b). Reproduced from Berghout A, Wiersinga WM, Drexhage HA, Smits NJ, Touber JL. Comparison of placebo with L-thyroxine alone or with carbimazole for treatment of sporadic non-toxic goitre. *Lancet*, 1990; **336**: 193–7, with permission.

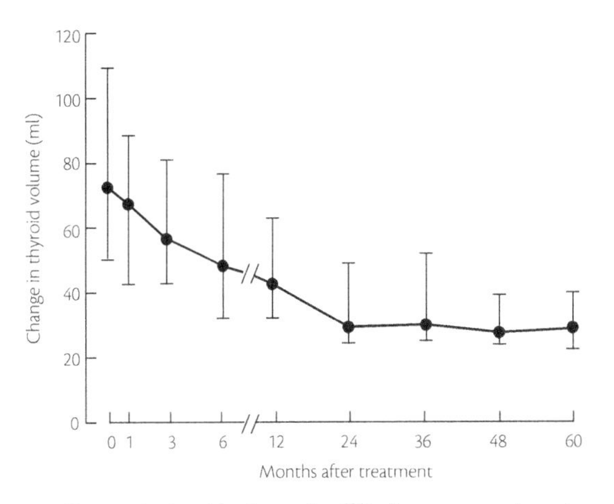

Fig. 3.5.2.6 Changes in thyroid volume after ^{131}iodine treatment in patients with non-toxic multinodular goitre. Bars are quartiles. Reproduced from Nygaard B, Hegedüs L, Gervil M, Hjalgrim H, Søe-Jensen P, Mølholm Hansen J. Radioiodine treatment of multinodular non-toxic goitre. *British Medical Journal*, 1993; **307**: 828-32, with permission.

risk of development of cancer outside the thyroid gland (36). When applied to people of 65 years and older the estimated risk is approximately 0.5% (36, 37).

Recent experimental studies have investigated whether the outcome of ^{131}I therapy could be improved by prior administration of recombinant human TSH (rhTSH). The use of rhTSH overcomes the problems of a low radioactive iodine uptake (RAIU) (rhTSH significantly enhances the absorbed thyroid ^{131}I dose) (38) and of an irregular RAIU (rhTSH gives a more homogeneous distribution of RAIU) (39). One could use rhTSH aiming at lowering the radiation dose of absorbed ^{131}I; indeed, a single low dose of 0.01 or 0.03 mg rhTSH intramuscularly allows for a 50–60% reduction of the usual therapeutic ^{131}I dose without compromising the effect on goitre reduction (39). Alternatively, one could use rhTSH to enhance the efficacy of ^{131}I. Indeed, a number of placebo-controlled randomized clinical trials have demonstrated a larger reduction in goitre size after a single relatively high dose of 0.30 or 0.45 mg rhTSH intramuscularly (40–42). However, this is obtained at the expense of more adverse events, a higher rate of transient thyrotoxicosis in the first 3–4 weeks, and late hypothyroidism (40–43). Thus, the most appropriate schedule taking full advantage of rhTSH has not yet been established, and the results of a new formulation of modified-release rhTSH for use in nontoxic goitre is eagerly awaited.

Box 3.5.2.2 Indications for treatment of sporadic non-toxic multinodular goiter

- Obstructive symptoms
- Cosmetic complaints
- Suspicion of malignancy
- Suppressed TSH
- Prevention of progression to compressive and/or toxic goitre

Management of the individual patient

Indications for treatment are listed in Box 3.5.2.2. The preferred treatment in a particular case requires much deliberation between patient and physician, taking into account the efficacy and side effects of each type of treatment (Table 3.5.2.1).

Surgery is the treatment of choice if malignant growth is suspected. It can also be considered the standard therapy in the case of large compressive or substernal goitres, but radio-iodine is a suitable alternative to surgery in elderly patients and those with cardiopulmonary disease (37). Radio-iodine is a perfect choice for patients who already have a suppressed TSH, a condition which precludes the use of thyroxine, but the efficacy of radio-iodine is smaller if a dominant nodule or a very large goitre is present.

In symptomatic patients who are younger and have smaller goitres, an alternative to surgery is thyroxine. The efficacy of thyroxine in reducing the size of multinodular goitre is low, and requires the continuous administration of TSH-suppressive doses raising concern about its long-term safety. Radio-iodine, although not devoid of side effects, has been offered as an alternative in view of its greater efficacy and better tolerance than thyroxine (25); it should probably be restricted to patients older than 40 years. Future developments may decrease the theoretical risk of radiation-induced cancer by the use of rhTSH in conjunction with radio-iodine, hopefully allowing a lower dose of ^{131}I.

In the asymptomatic patient, a wait-and-see policy seems to be prudent. Although the natural history is characterized by continuous growth, large variation exists in the growth rate between individuals. If progressive goitre growth is observed during follow-up, intervention to prevent development of compressive and/or toxic goitres should be considered. In this respect, early rather than late intervention is advantageous when choosing radio-iodine, in view of the greater efficacy and lower radiation burden of ^{131}I if the goitre is still relatively small.

Table 3.5.2.1 Efficacy and side-effects of treatment options in the management of patients with sporadic non-toxic multinodular goiter

	Efficacy – goiter reduction	**Side-effects**
Observation	0% responders Goitre size increases by 4.5% per year	Large, often compressive goitres Hyperthyroidism in 10%
Thyroidectomy	100% responders (goitre size decreases by 100%) 4–20% goiter recurrences	Low, but unavoidable morbidity (recurrent laryngeal nerve palsy in 1–2%, hypoparathyroidism in 2–4%) Hypothyroidism in 5–8%
L-thyroxine	51% responders (goitre size decreases by 25%) Goitre regrowth after discontinuation of L-T_4	Induction of subclinical hyperthyroidism with risk on atrial fibrillation and bone loss
^{131}Iodine	94% responders (goitre size decreases by 45%) 8% goitre recurrences	Radiation thyroiditis in 4% Graves'-like hyperthyroidism in 4% Hypothyroidism in 25% Theoretical risk of radiation-induced cancer

The management of nontoxic multinodular goitre should be tailored according to the individual patient's need, taking into account sex, age, symptoms, goitre size and texture, and serum TSH. However, no consensus exists on the most appropriate treatment for a particular patient, as was evident from a recent questionnaire among thyroidologists worldwide asking how they would treat a 42-year-old women with a multinodular nontoxic goitre of 50–80 g causing moderate local neck discomfort in the absence of clinical suspicion on malignancy (44). Of the respondents, 35% opted for no treatment at all, 42% for thyroxine, 15% for surgery, 5% for radio-iodine, and 3% for stable iodine. Marked differences in preferences existed between countries.

References

1. Berghout A, Wiersinga WM, Smits NJ, Touber JL. Interrelationships between age, thyroid volume, thyroid nodularity, and thyroid function in patients with sporadic non-toxic goiter. *Am J Med*, 1990; **89**: 602–8.
2. Alfonso A, Christoudias G, Amaruddia Q, Herbsman H, Gardner B. Tracheal or esophageal compression due to benign thyroid disease. *Am J Surg*, 1981; **142**: 350–4.
3. Editorial. The thyroid cork. *Lancet*, 1990; **ii**: 1374–5.
4. Singh B, Lucente FE, Shahn AR. Substernal goiter: a clinical review. *Am J Otolaryngol*, 1994; **15**: 409–16.
5. Jarlov AE, Hegedüs L, Gjørup T, Hansen JM. Observer variation in the clinical assessment of the thyroid gland. *J Intern Med*, 1991; **229**: 159–61.
6. Glazer GM, Axel L, Moss AA. CT diagnosis of mediastinal thyroid. *Am J Radiol*, 1982; **138**: 495–8.
7. Miller MR, Pincock AC, Ontes GD, Wilkinson R, Skene-Smith H. Upper airway obstruction due to goitre: detection, prevalence and results of surgical management. *QJM*, 1990; **74**: 177–88.
8. Deegan PC, McNamara VM, Morgan WE. Goitre: a cause of obstructive sleep apnoea in euthyroid patients. *Eur Respir J*, 1997; **10**: 500–2.
9. Koh KBH, Chang KW. Carcinoma in multinodular goitre. *Br J Surg*, 1992; **79**: 266–7.
10. Rios A, Rodriguez JM, Galindo PJ, Montoya M, Tebar FJ, Sola J, *et al.* Utility of fine-needle aspiration for diagnosis of carcinoma associated with multinodular goitre. *Clin Endocrinol*, 2004; **61**: 732–7.
11. Hegedus L, Bonnema SJ, Bennedbaek FN. Management of nodular goiter: current status and future perspectives. *Endocr Rev*, 2003; **24**: 102–32.
12. Wiener JD, de Vries AA. On the natural history of Plummer's disease. *Clin Nucl Med*, 1979; **4**: 181–90.
13. Elte JW, Bussemaker JK, Haak A. The natural history of euthyroid multinodular goitre. *Postgrad Med J*, 1990; **66**: 186–90.
14. Röjdmark J, Järhult J. High long-term recurrence rate after subtotal thyroidectomy for nodular goitre. *Eur J Surg*, 1995; **161**: 725–7.
15. Husby S, Blichert-Toft M, Bang U, Nielsen B. Investigation of TSH dependency, circulating thyroid autoantibody, and morphological features of recurrent non-toxic goitre. *Acta Med Scand*, 1985; **217**: 61–5.
16. Berghout A, Wiersinga WM, Drexhage HA, van Trotsenburg P, Smits NJ, van der Gaag RD, *et al.* The long-term outcome of thyroidectomy for sporadic non-toxic goitre. *Clin Endocrinol*, 1989; **31**: 193–9.
17. Bistrup C, Nielsen JD, Gregersen G, Franch P. Preventive effect of levothyroxine in patients operated for non-toxic goitre: a randomized trial of one hundred patients with nine years follow-up. *Clin Endocrinol*, 1994; **40**: 323–7.
18. Hegedüs L, Nygaard B, Mølholm Hansen J. Is routine thyroxine treatment to hinder postoperative recurrence of non-toxic goiter justified?. *J Clin Endocrinol Metab*, 1999; **84**: 756–60.
19. Wheeler MH. Total thyroidectomy for benign thyroid disease. *Lancet*, 1998; **351**: 1526–7.
20. Berglund J, Aspelin P, Bondeson AG, Bondeson L, Christensen SB, Ekberg O, *et al.* Rapid increase in volume of the remnant after hemithyroidectomy does not correlate with serum concentration of thyroid stimulating hormone. A randomised evaluation by ultrasound. *Eur J Surg*, 1998; **164**: 257–62.
21. Miccoli P, Antonelli A, Iacconi P, Alberti B, Gambuzza C, Baschieri L. Prospective, randomized, double-blind study about effectiveness of levothyroxine therapy in prevention of recurrence after operation: result at the third year of follow-up. *Surgery*, 1993; **114**: 1097–102.
22. Carella C, Mazziotti G, Rotondi M, Del Buono A, Zito G, Sorvillo F, *et al.* Iodized salt improves the effectiveness of L-thyroxine therapy after surgery for nontoxic goitre: a prospective and randomized study. *Clin Endocrinol*, 2002; **57**: 507–13.
23. Smeds S, Peter HJ, Gerber H, Jörtsö E, Lennquist S, Studer H. Effects of thyroxine on cell proliferation in human multinodular goiter: a study on growth of thyroid tissue transplanted to nude mice. *World J Surg*, 1988; **12**: 241–5.
24. Berghout A, Wiersinga WM, Drexhage HA, Smits NJ, Touber JL. Comparison of placebo with L-thyroxine alone or with carbimazole for treatment of sporadic non-toxic goitre. *Lancet*, 1990; **336**: 193–7.
25. Wesche MFT, Tiel-van Buul MMC, Lips P, Smits NJ, Wiersinga WM. A randomized trial comparing L-thyroxine with radioactive iodine in the treatment of sporadic non-toxic goiter. *J Clin Endocrinol Metab*, 2001; **86**: 998–1005.
26. Lima N, Knobel M, Cavaliere H, Sztejnsznajd C, Tomimori E, Medeiros-Neto G. Levothyroxine suppressive therapy is partially effective in treating patients with benign, solid thyroid nodules and multinodular goiters. *Thyroid*, 1997; **7**: 691–7.
27. Nygaard B, Hegedüs L, Gervil M, Hjalgrim H, Søe-Jensen P, Mølholm Hansen J. Radioiodine treatment of multinodular non-toxic goitre. *BMJ*, 1993; **307**: 828–32.
28. Huysmans DAKC, Hermus ARMM, Corstens FHM, Barentse JO, Kloppenborg PWC. Large, compressive goiters treated with radioiodine. *Ann Intern Med*, 1994; **121**: 757–62.
29. de Klerk JMH, van Isselt JW, van Dijk A, Hakman ME, Pameijer FA, Koppeschaar HP, *et al.* Iodine-131 therapy in sporadic non-toxic goiter. *J Nucl Med*, 1997; **38**: 372–6.
30. le Moli R, Wesche MFT, Tiel-van Buul MMC, Wiersinga WM. Determinants of longterm outcome of radioiodine therapy of sporadic non-toxic goiter. *Clin Endocrinol*, 1999; **50**: 783–9.
31. Wesche MFT, Tiel-van Buul MM, Smits NJ, Wiersinga WM. Ultrasonographic versus scintigraphic measurement of thyroid volume in patients referred for ^{131}I therapy. *Nucl Med Commun*, 1998; **19**: 341–6.
32. Howarth DM, Epstein M, Thomas PA, Allen LW, Akerman R, Lan L. Outpatient management of patients with large multinodular goitres treated with fractionated radioiodine. *Eur J Nucl Med*, 1997; **24**: 1465–9.
33. Nygaard B, Faber J, Hegedüs L. Acute changes in thyroid volume and function following ^{131}I therapy of multinodular goitre. *Clin Endocrinol*, 1994; **41**: 715–18.
34. Nygaard B, Knudsen JH, Hegedüs L, Veje A, Mølholm Hansen JE. Thyrotropin receptor antibodies and Graves' disease, a side-effect of ^{131}I treatment in patients with non-toxic goiter. *J Clin Endocrinol Metab*, 1997; **82**: 2926–30.
35. Huysmans AK, Hermus RM, Edelbroek MA, Tjabbes T, Oostdijk, Ross HA, *et al.* Autoimmune hyperthyroidism occurring late after radioiodine treatment for volume reduction of large multinodular goiters. *Thyroid*, 1997; **7**: 535–9.
36. Huysmans DA, Buijs WC, van de Ven MT, van den Broek WJ, Kloppenborg PW, Hermus AR, *et al.* Dosimetry and risk estimates of radioiodine therapy for large, multinodular goiters. *J Nucl Med*, 1996; **37**: 2072–9.
37. Hermus AR, Huysmans DA. Treatment of benign nodular thyroid disease. *N Engl J Med*, 1998; **338**: 1438–47.
38. Nielsen VE, Bonnema SJ, Boel-Jorgensen H, Veje A, Hegedus L. Recombinant human thyrotropin markedly changes the ^{131}I kinetics during ^{131}I therapy of patients with nodular goiter: an evaluation by a randomized double-blinded trial. *J Clin Endocrinol Metab*, 2005; **90**: 79–83.
39. Nieuwlaat WA, Huysmans DA, van den Bosch HC, Sweep CG, Ross HA, Corstens FH, *et al.* Pretreatment with a single, low dose of recombinant human thyrotropin allows dose reduction of radioiodine therapy in patients with nodular goiter. *J Clin Endocrinol Metab*, 2003; **88**: 3121–9.

40. Silva MN, Rubio IG, Romão R, Gebrin EM, Buchpiguel C, Tomimori E, *et al.* Administration of a single dose of recombinant human thyrotrophin enhances the efficacy of radioiodine treatment of large compressive multinodular goitres. *Clin Endocrinol*, 2004; **60**: 300–8.
41. Nielsen VE, Bonnema SJ, Boel-Jorgensen H, Grupe P, Hegedus L. Stimulation with 0.3-mg recombinant human thyrotropin prior to iodine 131 therapy to improve the size reduction of benign nontoxic nodular goiter. A prospective randomized double-blind trial. *Arch Intern Med*, 2006; **166**: 1476–82.
42. Bonnema SJ, Nielsen VE, Boel-Jørgensen H, Grupe P, Andersen PB, Bastholt L, *et al.* Improvement of goiter volume reduction after 0.3 mg recombinant human thyrotropin stimulated radioiodine therapy in patients with a very large goiter: a double-blinded, randomized trial. *J Clin Endocrinol Metab*, 2007; **92**: 3424–8.
43. Nielsen VE, Bonnema SJ, Hegedus L. Transient goiter enlargement after administration of 0.3 mg of recombinant human thyrotropin in patients with benign nontoxic nodular goiter: a randomized, double-blind, crossover trial. *J Clin Endocrinol Metab*, 2006; **91**: 1317–22.
44. Diehl LA, Garcia V, Bonnema SJ, Hegedüs L, Albino CC, Graf H, *et al.* Management of nontoxic multinodular goiter in Latin America: comparison with North America and Europe, an electronic survey. *J Clin Endocrinol Metab*, 2005; **90**: 117–23.

3.5.3 Management of the single thyroid nodule

Laszlo Hegedüs, Finn N. Bennedbæk

Introduction

The main concern of patients and physicians alike, when dealing with the solitary thyroid nodule, is to diagnose the few cancers (approximately 5%) as rapidly and cost-effectively as possible, and to reduce superfluous thyroid surgery. Management has changed in recent years, but differences prevail as shown by an investigation among European thyroidologists (1). This chapter focuses on the palpably discrete swelling within an otherwise normal gland in the clinically and biochemically euthyroid patient (2, 3). The toxic nodule is dealt with in Chapter 3.3.11, and thyroid malignancy in Chapters 3.5.4–3.5.7.

Occurrence

The estimated life-time risk of developing a thyroid nodule is between 5% and 10% (2, 3), but factors such as sex (4 times more common in women), age (frequency increases with age), regional iodine intake (more prevalent in iodine-deficient areas), and whether the diagnosis is made clinically (palpation), by ultrasonography, or at autopsy (5–10 times more prevalent using the last two) are of importance when estimating prevalence (2, 3). The incidence of clinical disease has been estimated at 0.1% by palpation (2, 3).

Natural history

Very little is known regarding the natural history of thyroid nodules since data are highly selective and generally concern patients with small nodules without suspicion of malignancy and not causing pressure symptoms or cosmetic complaints. With these restrictions, most nodules appear not to change appreciably over time. The nodules that increase in size are predominantly solid and carry a higher risk of harbouring thyroid carcinoma than those predominantly cystic, being more prone to decrease in size or even disappear.

In most patients, ultrasonography will identify nodules not evident clinically and, given time, most of these patients will be classified as having multinodular goitre. Therefore, the risk of thyroid malignancy is independent of whether the nodule is solitary or the dominant nodule in an otherwise multinodular gland (2–4).

Diagnosis

Clinical examination

Almost any thyroid disease can appear as a clinically solitary nodule. The differential diagnostic spectrum is given in Box 3.5.3.1. Although 42–77% of surgically removed nodules are colloid nodules, 15–40% are adenomas, and 8–17% are carcinomas, few patients undergo surgery. Therefore, the risk of a solitary nodule harbouring a thyroid carcinoma is no higher than 5–10% (2, 3).

History and physical examination are important and patients with a risk of thyroid carcinoma can be identified (Box 3.5.3.2). A positive family history of benign goitre suggests a benign disorder, whereas medullary thyroid carcinoma or even papillary or follicular thyroid carcinoma in the family should raise suspicion. Nodules occurring in the young or in the old are especially likely to be cancerous, the risk being higher in men than in women. Head or neck irradiation in childhood leads to clinically evident thyroid abnormality in 10–40% of patients 5–40 years later. Thyroid carcinomas, mainly papillary carcinomas, are seen in 30% of those with thyroid abnormality. Rapid tumour growth (weeks to months) and symptoms of local invasion, such as pain, dysphagia, hoarseness, or dyspnoea, suggests a carcinoma, but only a minority of patients have these symptoms. Furthermore, these symptoms can occur in patients with large multinodular benign goitres. Growth during L-thyroxine treatment should raise concern as to possible malignancy.

The physical examination is important in the work-up and certain signs and symptoms are highly suspicious of thyroid malignancy (Box 3.5.3.2), but inter- and intraobserver variation is alarmingly high (5) and the specificity and sensitivity of the diagnosis of a solitary thyroid nodule is low. Thus, nodules of 10 mm or more can usually be palpated depending on their localization in the neck. However, one-half of the nodules found by ultrasound examination escape clinical detection, one-third of which are more than 20 mm in diameter. A hard nodule is not necessarily a carcinoma (chronic thyroiditis), whereas a soft nodule may well be a cystic papillary cancer. Although generally believed to carry a higher risk of thyroid malignancy, the solitary thyroid nodule probably does not imply a higher risk of malignancy than that of a dominant nodule in a multinodular goitre (2–5). In view of this, fine-needle aspiration biopsy (FNAB) is mandatory but should be interpreted in the light of the history and the physical examination. As a consequence, several patients are operated on in spite of a benign cytology (1).

Laboratory investigation

The only relevant biochemical test that is routinely needed is serum thyroid-stimulating hormone (TSH) measured with a sensitive assay. Subnormal serum TSH values should lead to determination of free thyroxine (T_4) and free triiodothyronine (T_3). In the presence of normal thyroid hormone levels, a suppressed serum TSH

Box 3.5.3.1 Causes of thyroid nodules and the relative distribution of fine-needle aspiration biopsy results

- Benign (no evidence of malignancy); 69% (range 53–90%)
  - Colloid nodule
  - Thyroiditis (chronic, acute, or subacute)
  - Cyst
- Suspicious; 10% (range 5–23%)
  - Follicular neoplasm
  - Normofollicular (simple)
  - Macrofollicular
  - Microfollicular (fetal)
  - Trabecular and solid (embryonal)
  - Oxyphilic cell type (Hürtle cell)
- Malignant; 4% (range 1–10%)
  - Follicular carcinoma
  - Papillary carcinoma
  - Medullary carcinoma (C-cell carcinoma)
  - Undifferentiated (anaplastic) carcinoma
  - Lymphoma
  - Metastasis (rare)
- Nondiagnostic (insufficient); 17% (range 15–20%)

on repeat examination should lead to treatment, especially in older patients (Chapter 3.3.4). Scintigraphy is advised and will most likely demonstrate a hot or a toxic nodule (Chapters 3.1.6 and 3.3.11) in such patients. Most patients are euthyroid, including those with thyroid malignancy. It seems that the risk of malignancy in a thyroid nodule increases with serum TSH concentration, within the normal range, at presentation, and thus serves as an adjunctive and independent predictor of malignancy (6). Hypothyroidism suggests that the patient has Hashimoto's thyroiditis.

Box 3.5.3.2 Clinical factors increasing the likelihood of thyroid malignancy in a euthyroid patient with a solitary nodule

- Family history of thyroid malignancy
- Age less than 20 or more than 60 years
- Male sex
- History of head and neck irradiation in infancy, childhood, or adolescence
- Large nodule (greater than 4 cm in diameter) and partially cystic
- Rapid nodule growth
- Pain
- Firm or hard nodule
- Fixation to adjacent structures
- Compression symptoms: dysphagia, dyspnoea, vocal cord paralysis
- Regional lymphadenopathy
- Growth during L-thyroxine therapy

Thyroglobulin in serum is positively correlated with thyroid size but has no place in the routine investigation or in the follow-up of benign nodules. Calcitonin is the only clinically relevant biochemical marker of medullary thyroid carcinoma. Routine determination has been suggested by European guidelines (7). It allows the detection of unsuspected medullary thyroid carcinoma with a frequency of 1 in 200–300 thyroid nodules, with better sensitivity than FNAB (7). However, there remains unresolved issues of sensitivity, specificity, assay performance, and cost-effectiveness. Thyroid autoantibodies against thyroid peroxidase cannot differentiate between malignant and benign disease. In our opinion, they should be determined routinely in the work-up to identify patients with possible Hashimoto's thyroiditis. These antibodies are markers of an increased risk of developing hypo- or hyperthyroidism (Graves' disease) spontaneously or secondary to surgery or radioiodine treatment (8). TSH-receptor antibodies are rarely present and should not be determined routinely.

Diagnostic imaging

No method of imaging can differentiate benign and malignant nodules accurately. However, 88% of European thyroidologists use either scintigraphy (66%), ultrasonography (80%), or both (58%) in the evaluation of patients with a clinically solitary thyroid nodule, illustrating that the diagnosis is not always straightforward and that they believe diagnostic imaging gives valuable information (see also Chapters 3.1.6 and 3.1.6.1) (1).

There is no consensus on the use of scintigraphy in the euthyroid patient. Since most have a cold nodule—increasing the risk of thyroid malignancy at least 10-fold—many investigators, mainly in the USA, advocate the use of FNAB as the first step (2, 3). Imaging, if performed, can be with ^{123}I, ^{131}I, or ^{99m}Tc pertechnetate, the last being preferred (86%) among European thyroidologists (1), although iodine should be used if the aim is also to reduce the risk of overlooking malignancy. A clinically dominant nodule that is cold on scintigraphy, should be treated as a solitary cold nodule, the risk of malignancy being the same (2–5), and FNAB should be performed. In case of suppressed serum TSH or overt hyperthyroidism, the risk of malignancy is thought to be much lower as is the need for FNAB.

Ultrasonography, often used in Europe (80%) and less so in the USA, allows determination of total thyroid volume, individual nodule size and echogenicity, morphology of extranodular tissue, and investigation of regional lymph nodes (1). Supplemental colour flow Doppler adds information regarding regional blood flow and nodule vascularity. Ultrasonography aids in performing accurate biopsies and cyst punctures, as well as therapeutic procedures such as percutaneous ethanol injection and laser therapy of solid as well as cystic nodules (2, 9, 10). There is no ultrasound pattern, alone or in combination with other techniques, that may be considered specific for thyroid cancer. For the objective determination of thyroid or nodule size, whether initially or during follow-up, it is the technique of choice. CT and MRI are generally of little value except in the evaluation of the intrathoracic goitre or in the evaluation and follow-up of malignant thyroid disease.

Fine-needle aspiration biopsy

FNAB provides the most direct and specific information about a thyroid nodule, and it is used by 99% of European Thyroid Association members on an outpatient basis (1). As the cornerstone in the evaluation it is virtually without complications, inexpensive, and easy to learn to perform. Its use reduces the number of thyroidectomies by approximately 50% (2, 3), roughly doubles the surgical yield of carcinoma, and reduces the overall cost of medical care in these patients by 25% (2, 3).

The technique involves the use of a 5- to 20-ml plastic syringe with a 22- to 27-gauge needle. The skin is cleaned with alcohol and may be infiltrated with 1–2 ml 1% lidocaine, but, in general, local anaesthesia is not needed for FNAB of palpable nodules. The needle, attached to the syringe, is quickly inserted perpendicularly to the anterior surface of the neck (Fig. 3.5.3.1). Rapid (three excursions per second) sampling motions with brief dwell time within the nodule may diminish bloody dilution (11). Negative pressure is only applied if no fluid appears in the hub of the needle. Production of one or two slides per biopsy reflects an appropriate dwell time. No fluid should enter the syringe. If the nodule is a cyst or partly cystic, the aspiration should be followed by FNAB of any residual solid component. Investigation of the cyst sediment rarely gives useful information.

Diagnostically useful FNAB specimens are obtained in about 80% of cases (Box 3.5.3.1). The number of insufficient samples depends on operator experience, number of aspirations, the character of the nodule (cystic/solid), the experience of the cytopathologist, and especially the criteria used for adequacy of a sample. The number of sufficient samples increases if FNAB is guided by ultrasound. Rebiopsy will typically halve the number of insufficient biopsies. Needle-steering devices and pistol-grip equipment are used by some. The specimens should be smeared immediately (pull-apart technique) and most are air dried. Staining is with May-Giemsa-Grünwald stain, which is good for cytoplasmic details, or alternatively Papanicolaou's stain, which is good for nuclear details.

Diagnostic accuracy of FNAB depends upon the handling of suspicious lesions. If considered negative, sensitivity will decrease and specificity will increase. If suspicious results are regarded as positive, the converse is true. In our opinion, patients with suspicious, malignant, and nondiagnostic cytology (after reaspiration) should be operated on (Table 3.5.3.1). The relevant question is what the false-negative rate is in the remaining 70–80% of cases in which nonsurgical treatment is an option. This has generally been estimated at 1% (2). Repeat FNAB during follow-up, to decrease the false-negative rate, will virtually eliminate the risk of overlooking thyroid malignancy.

Large-core needle biopsies can be considered when cytopathology expertise is not available. Its limitations include the need for local anaesthesia, local discomfort, and decreasing patient acceptance of repeat biopsies (11).

(a)

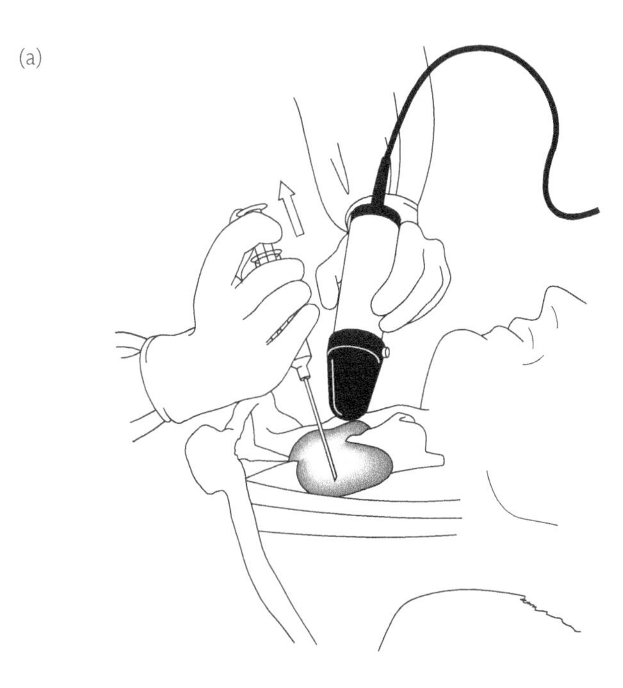

(b)

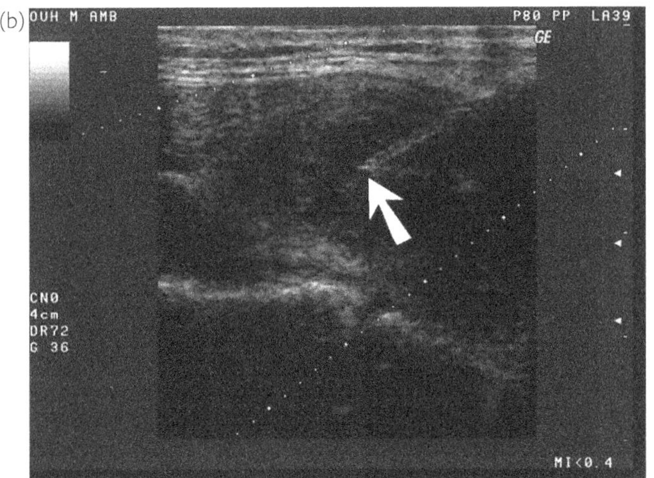

Fig. 3.5.3.1 (a) Ultrasound-guided fine-needle aspiration biopsy of a thyroid nodule. The needle is inserted into the nodule. Some use a free-hand technique, others use needle-steering devices. (b) Longitudinal ultrasound scan of the neck showing the needle tract and needle tip (arrow) inside a solid hypoechoic thyroid nodule.

Approach to the patient with a single thyroid nodule

- Initial evaluation of all patients with thyroid nodules using ultrasound-guided FNAB and a serum TSH assay is a cost-effective approach (Fig. 3.5.3.2) (2, 12).
- With the discovery of a thyroid nodule, a complete history and physical examination focusing on the thyroid gland and adjacent cervical lymph nodes should be performed.
- If the serum TSH is subnormal, a thyroid scintigraphy should be obtained to confirm tracer uptake in the nodule. Functioning nodules rarely harbour malignancy.
- Diagnostic ultrasonography should be performed unless the serum TSH is suppressed. FNAB guided by ultrasonography is recommended.
- Most impalpable thyroid nodules (incidentalomas) require observation alone, but ultrasound-guided FNAB is recommended for nodules larger than 10 mm, or for those exhibiting suspicious features.

Table 3.5.3.1 Treatment of the single thyroid nodule: comparison of various methods of treatment

Treatment type	Advantages	Disadvantages
Surgery	Nodule ablation, complete relief of symptoms, definite histological diagnosis	Inpatient, high cost, risks associated with surgery, vocal cord paralysis (approximately 1% of patients), hypoparathyroidism (<1%), hypothyroidism (1% in case of lobectomy)
L-thyroxine	Outpatient, low cost, may slow nodule growth, may prevent new nodule formation	Low efficacy, need for lifelong treatment, regrowth after cessation of treatment, cardiac tachyarrhythmias, reduced bone density, not feasible when thyrotropin level is suppressed
Radio-iodine[a]	Outpatient, low cost, high success rate (normalization of thyrotropin in >95% and nodule reduced by 40% in 1 year)	Hypothyroidism (10% in 5 years), risk of radiation thyroiditis and thyrotoxicosis, only gradual reduction of the nodule, use of contraceptives in fertile women
Ethanol injection	Outpatient, relatively low cost, no hypothyroidism, nodule reduced by >40% in 6 months	Limited experience with treatment, decreasing efficacy with increasing nodule size, operator dependency, painful (reducing compliance), risk of thyrotoxicosis and vocal cord paralysis (1–2%), seepage of ethanol[b], cytological/histological interpretation impeded in treated nodules, repeat injections often needed
Laser treatment[c]	Outpatient, relatively low cost, no hypothyroidism, nodule reduced by >40% in 6 months	Limited experience with treatment, operator dependency, cytological/histological interpretation impeded in treated nodules

[a] Treatment of the autonomous thyroid nodule.

[b] Side effects due to ethanol escaping outside the nodule or drainage of ethanol are rare (<1%) and comprise nerve damage, perinodular/periglandular fibrosis jeopardizing subsequent surgery, thrombosis of the jugular vein, and neck haematomas.

[c] Laser treatment is still experimental. The advantages are similar to those of ethanol injection, but side effects are fewer due to the higher degree of control with laser therapy which limits the risk of extranodular damage.

- Patients with benign nodules should be examined periodically (6-month to 1-year intervals). During follow-up any changes in the consistency or size of the nodules require another FNAB or surgery.
- Patients with malignant or suspicious lesions are referred for surgery.

Treatment

The optimal therapy for patients with thyroid nodules varies with the lesion and whether or not it is functioning (Table 3.5.3.1).

Surgery

The main indications for surgery are malignant or suspicious cytological features and symptoms due to the nodule itself. Certain clinical features raising the suspicion of thyroid malignancy (Box 3.5.3.2) are an indication for surgery despite a benign cytology as recommended by most European thyroidologists (1). The frequency of complications due to surgery decreases with increasing experience and specialized training. Results from a specialist department for thyroid surgery indicate very low rates of complications: temporary and permanent unilateral vocal cord paralysis (2% and 0.7%, respectively), temporary and permanent hypocalcaemia (0.6% and 0.7%, respectively), and wound haematomas and infections (0.5% and 0.3%, respectively) (13). The likelihood of surgical complications increases proportionally with the extent of operation. Patients with benign cytology, in whom clinical suspicion results in referral for surgery, may generally be managed with lobectomy (hemithyroidectomy). Endoscopic surgery has the advantage of improved cosmetic results but is limited due to decreased ability to control bleeding and evaluate nodal status and to perform definitive procedures when a frozen section is reported malignant. L-thyroxine postoperatively to prevent regenerative hyperplasia is not recommended routinely (1, 2, 14).

Thyroid hormone suppressive therapy

Thyroid suppression is intended to shrink or slow the growth of thyroid nodules, and also to prevent the occurrence of new nodules. However, most evidence suggests that changes in nodule size are similar in TSH suppressed and control groups and treatment seems at best beneficial in a subgroup of patients with smaller solid nodules (15). Twenty per cent or less of solitary nodules will actually regress as a result of L-thyroxine treatment, and regrowth is seen after cessation of therapy (8, 15). Long-term results confirm that the nodule-reducing effect of L-thyroxine is insignificant (16). Growth can be suppressed or slowed and the formation of new nodules may be prevented. Nodules grow less if serum TSH is suppressed to less than 0.1 mU/l, than if TSH is more than 0.1 mU/l (16). This degree of TSH suppression may, however, have adverse effects. Because suppressive treatment (by definition) produces subclinical hyperthyroidism, treated patients are at increased risk of atrial fibrillation, other cardiac abnormalities, and reduced bone density. These side effects, combined with the questionable efficacy, have led to recommendations that vary depending upon the age, sex, and menopausal status of the patient. L-thyroxine suppressive therapy is least tempting in elderly patients and in postmenopausal women. It should be reserved for small nodules—where treatment is least necessary—in younger patients living in borderline iodine-deficient areas. Based on management guidelines and meta-analyses, routine suppression therapy of benign thyroid nodules is discarded (2, 7, 12, 17).

Percutaneous tissue ablation with ethanol

Absolute ethanol (70–100%) can cause permanent tissue ablation due to coagulative necrosis and local small vessel thrombosis. It has proved useful in the treatment of autonomously functioning thyroid nodules, cystic thyroid nodules, and solid cold thyroid nodules (8). Using multiple ethanol injections, complete cure (normalization of scintigraphy and serum TSH) can be achieved in two-thirds of patients with toxic nodules and three-quarters of patients with pretoxic nodules. A single ethanol instillation in thyroid cysts prevents recurrence in 80% of patients (18). A single small dose of ethanol injected into benign cold solitary solid thyroid nodules results in relief of clinical symptoms in 50% of patients based on a nodule volume reduction of about one-half (2, 8).

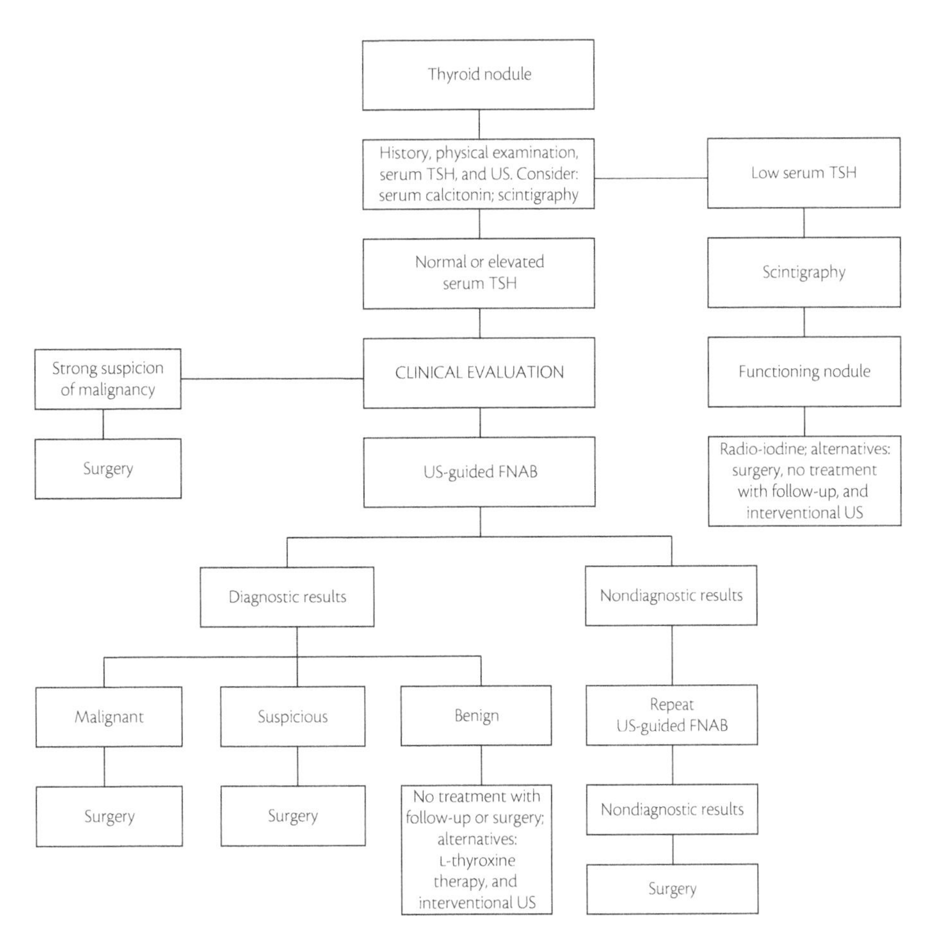

Fig. 3.5.3.2 Algorithm outlining a cost-effective strategy for evaluation and treatment of the palpable thyroid nodule. In case of strong suspicion of malignancy, surgery is advised irrespective of fine-needle aspiration biopsy (FNAB) results. In case of a nondiagnostic result, repeat FNAB yields a satisfactory aspirate in 50%. Ultrasound (US)-guided FNAB allows sampling from the periphery of a solid nodule or solid part of a mixed solid–cystic nodule, increasing the satisfactory rate. The options in case of a diagnostic FNAB covers both solid and cystic nodules. In case of recurrent cysts the possibilities are reaspiration, surgery, or interventional ultrasonography (ethanol injection or laser treatment).

Limitations are the need to repeat ethanol injections to achieve complete cure in toxic and pretoxic nodules and to prevent renewed growth in solid cold nodules. Furthermore, the procedure is often painful despite local anaesthesia. To minimize the risk of complications, each dose should be no more than 20% of the pretreatment nodule volume. The special technical skill obtained at a centre familiar with interventional ultrasonography reduces the risk of complications.

Percutaneous tissue ablation with laser treatment

Following an approximately 10-min session of ultrasound-guided laser thermal ablation, a 50% reduction (very similar to that of ethanol injection) in nodule volume can be achieved (10, 19). This effect seems independent of whether the nodule is hot or cold. One or two additional sessions augment this effect by up to 30% (10). Side effects are mainly related to various degrees of local and irradiating pain, which is much milder than with ethanol injection. Laser treatment has only been introduced in a few centres and, while awaiting long-term follow-up data, it should be considered experimental (10, 19).

Radioactive iodine (hot nodule)

In the clinically euthyroid patient, autonomous thyroid nodules may present as a hot lesion on scintigraphy with varying degrees of extranodular suppression. Most of these patients have suppressed serum TSH (see also Chapters 3.3.4 and 3.3.11). Treatment may be dictated either by the nodule size, causing compression of the adjacent structures, or cosmetic disturbances. Additionally, treatment is given to prevent thyrotoxicosis (annual risk about 5%), particularly in patients with heart disease or older patients (8, 20). A cure rate (normalization of scintigraphy and serum TSH) of 75% and volume reduction of 40% following a single dose of radio-iodine can be anticipated (8, 20). Side effects are few and consist of hypothyroidism in about 10% after 5 years and seem unrelated to any type of dose planning (20). Treatment must be individualized based on the patient's preference and risk factors for adverse effects. Table 3.5.3.1 summarizes the advantages and drawbacks of the treatment options.

Future

Recommendations on management of the single thyroid nodule are based on fair evidence and FNAB has been as the cornerstone for almost 30 years, despite significant shortcomings in sensitivity and specificity. The recent application of microarray analysis to tumour biology has provided a novel opportunity for classifying tumours based on gene expression profiles (21). This might provide a foundation for the future addition of gene profiling to thyroid FNAB and ultimately improve the distinction between follicular carcinomas and adenomas.

References

1. Bennedbæk FN, Perrild H, Hegedüs L. Diagnosis and treatment of the solitary thyroid nodule. Results of a European survey. *Clin Endocrinol*, 1999; **50**: 357–63.
2. Hegedüs L. The thyroid nodule. *N Engl J Med*, 2004; **351**: 1764–71.
3. Kaplan MM. Clinical evaluation and management of solitary thyroid nodules. In: Braverman LE, Utiger RD, eds. *Werner and Ingbar's The Thyroid: a fundamental and clinical text*. Philadelphia: Lippincott, Williams & Wilkins, 2005: 996–1010.
4. Frates MC, Benson CB, Doubilet PM, Kunreuther E, Contreras M, Cibas ES, *et al*. Prevalence and distribution of carcinoma in patients with solitary and multiple thyroid nodules on sonography. *J Clin Endocrinol Metab*, 2006; **91**: 3411–17.

5. Jarløv AE, Nygaard B, Hegedüs L, Hartling SG, Hansen JM. Observer variation in the clinical evaluation of patients with suspected thyroid disease. *Thyroid*, 1998; **8**: 393–8.
6. Boelaert K, Horacek j, Holder RL, Watkinson JC, Sheppard MC, Franklyn JA. Serum thyrotropin concentration as a novel predictor of malignancy in thyroid nodules investigated by fine-needle aspiration. *J Clin Endocrinol Metab*, 2006; **91**: 4295–301.
7. Pacini F, Schlumberger M, Dralle H, Elisei R, Smit JW, Wiersinga W, *et al.* European consensus for the management of patients with differentiated thyroid carcinoma of the follicular epithelium. *Eur J Endocrinol*, 2006; **154**: 787–803.
8. Hegedüs L, Bonnema SJ, Bennedæk FN. Management of simple and nodular goiter: current status and future perspectives. *Endocr Rev*, 2003; **24**: 102–32.
9. Bennedbæk FN, Nielsen LK, Hegedüs L. Effect of percutaneous ethanol injection therapy versus suppressive doses of L-thyroxine on benign solitary solid cold thyroid nodules. A randomized trial. *J Clin Endocrinol Metab*, 1998; **83**: 830–5.
10. Døssing H, Bennedbæk FN Hegedüs L. Effect of ultrasound-guided interstitial laser photocoagulation on benign solitary solid cold thyroid nodules: one versus three treatments. *Thyroid*, 2006; **16**: 763–8.
11. Pitman MB, Abele J, Ali SZ, Duick D, Elsheikh TM, Jeffrey RB. Techniques for thyroid FNA: a synopsis of the national cancer institute thyroid fine-needle aspiration state of the science conference. *Diagn Cytopathol*, 2008; **36**: 407–24.
12. Cooper DS, Doherty GM, Haugen BR, Kloos RT, Lee SL, Mandel SJ. Management guidelines for patients with thyroid nodules and differentiated thyroid cancer. *Thyroid*, 2006; **16**: 109–42.
13. Al Suliman NN, Ryttov NF, Qvist N, Blichert-Toft M, Graversen HP. Experience in a specialist thyroid surgery unit: a demographic study, surgical complications, and outcome. *Eur J Surg*, 1997; **163**: 13–20.
14. Hegedüs L, Nygaard B, Hansen JM. Is routine thyroxine treatment to hinder postoperative recurrence of nontoxic goitre justified?. *J Clin Endocrinol Metab*, 1999; **84**: 756–60.
15. Zelmanovitz F, Genro S, Gross JL. Suppressive therapy with levothyroxine for solitary thyroid nodules: a double-blind controlled clinical study and cumulative meta-analyses. *J Clin Endocrinol Metab*, 1998; **83**: 3881–5.
16. Papini E, Petrucci L, Guglielmi R, Panunzi C, Rinaldi R, Bacci V, *et al.* Long-term changes in nodular goitre: a 5-year prospective randomized trial of levothyroxine suppressive therapy for benign cold nodules. *J Clin Endocrinol Metab*, 1998; **83**: 780–3.
17. Sdano MT, Falciglia M, Welge JA, Steward DL. Efficacy of thyroid hormone suppression for benign thyroid nodules: meta-analysis of randomized trials. *Otolaryngol Head Neck Surg*, 2005; **133**: 391–6.
18. Bennedbæk FN, Hegedüs L. Treatment of recurrent thyroid cysts with ethanol: a randomized double-blind controlled trial. *J Clin Endocrinol Metab*, 2003; **88**: 5773–7.
19. Papini E, Guglielmi R, Bizzarri G, Graziano F, Bianchini A, Brufani C. Treatment of benign cold thyroid nodules: a randomized clinical trial of percutaneous laser ablation versus levothyroxine therapy or follow-up. *Thyroid*, 2007; **17**: 229–35.
20. Ferrari C, Reschini E, Paracchi A. Treatment of the autonomous thyroid nodule: a review. *Eur J Endocrinol*, 1996; **135**: 383–90.
21. Finley DJ, Zhu B, Barden CB, Fahey TJ. Discrimination of benign and malignant thyroid nodules by molecular profiling. *Ann Surg*, 2004; **240**: 425–36.

3.5.4 Pathogenesis of thyroid cancer

Dan Mihailescu, Arthur B Schneider, Leon Fogelfeld

Introduction

Both epidemiological and molecular biological studies have been used to understand the origins of thyroid cancer. Epidemiological studies have been used to identify factors that predispose to thyroid cancer. That is principally how we know that exposure to radiation leads to thyroid cancer (see Chapter 3.2.5). In fact, radiation is the only environmental factor for which the proof is incontrovertible. Molecular biological studies, reviewed in the second part of this chapter, have been used to investigate the events within thyroid cells that are initiated by predisposing factors, e.g. radiation, and lead, by one or multiple steps, to transformation and cancer. These studies have focused on cancer-related genes, particularly proto-oncogenes and tumour suppressor genes, and have led to the identification of potential therapeutic agents. They have also focused on the cellular pathways and processes, including epigenetic changes and microRNA expression, which accompany transformation of the thyroid cell. Epidemiology and molecular biology have interacted productively in the studies that have followed the Chernobyl accident. This interaction is described in the third part of this chapter in which the mutations found in radiation-related thyroid cancers are reviewed.

Factors predisposing to thyroid cancer

Trends in the prevalence of thyroid cancer

Throughout the world the incidence of thyroid cancer has been increasing and this increase may shed light on potential environmental risk factors (1). However, the analysis has been complicated as the methods used to diagnose thyroid cancer have changed markedly over time. The increase is largely as a result of relatively small papillary thyroid cancers; 50% of the increase between 1992–1995 and 2003–2005 in the USA was due to cancers no more than 1.0 cm diameter and 30% to cancers 1.1–2.0 cm diameter (2). This is consistent with the possibility that incidentally found lesions, principally by ultrasonography or other diagnostic images obtained for nonthyroid-related indications, play a dominant role in the increase. However, it may not be the only explanation, as large cancers have also increased; there was a 222% increase for those more than 5.0 cm diameter among white women (2). Also, the effects of radiation exposure continue for decades and exposure still occurs, especially from the increasing use of CT imaging. Even though the incidence has been increasing, there has been no corresponding increase in mortality due to thyroid cancer.

The incidence of thyroid cancer varies widely from country to country. The reasons for this variability are not known. Based on the observation that there is an approximately fivefold range in thyroid cancer incidence in the five Nordic countries, ascertainment is unlikely to be the explanation.

Radiation exposure

The thyroid is one of the most sensitive organs in the body to the cancer-producing effects of radiation (3). The relationship between radiation and thyroid cancer has been shown at doses as low as about 10 cGy and the slope of the dose–response curve for thyroid cancer is as steep or steeper than for any other neoplasm. Chapter 3.2.5 summarizes the neoplastic effects on the thyroid of external radiation, used to treat benign and malignant conditions, and Chapter 3.3.5 that of internal radiation (^{131}I), used for the diagnosis and treatment of thyroid diseases and the principal source of thyroid exposure after the Chernobyl accident (4).

Given the thyroid's sensitivity, it is reasonable to be concerned about possible effects from occupational exposure and exposure from geological sources. A comparison of about 25 000 physicians in China occupationally exposed to radiation and a similar number of unexposed physicians found an excess of thyroid cancer, especially if the exposure occurred before 1960, when the doses were higher (5). Radiology technicians surveyed in the USA had a higher incidence of thyroid cancer than the general population, especially if they were employed in that profession before 1950 (6). So far, natural background radiation has not been associated with thyroid cancer. Some areas in southern China have a relatively high level of background radiation whereas nearby areas, similar in other respects, do not. A comparison of about 1000 older women from each of these areas did not reveal a difference in palpable thyroid nodularity (7). With respect to exposure from diagnostic radiographic examinations, a large case–control study in Sweden found no relationship (8). This study largely avoided the problem of recall bias (i.e. if a person had thyroid cancer they are more likely to remember diagnostic radiographs) by using comprehensive regional medical records rather than questionnaires. However, this and other studies were performed before the dramatic increase in the use of CT scans, including among children, which result in much more radiation exposure than conventional diagnostic radiographs.

Familial factors

Nonmedullary thyroid cancer has a strong familial component (9). In the minority of familial cases a specific genetic syndrome can be identified, while for most instances of where multiple cases occur within a family the cause or causes remain unknown.

Familial adenomatous polyposis, including its variant Gardner's syndrome, predisposes to papillary thyroid cancer. In fact, thyroid cancer is the most frequent, nonintestinal neoplasm associated with the syndrome, reported in up to 12% of cases. Thyroid cancer in this syndrome is characterized by an early age of onset and a cribriform–morular histological pattern. In some cases the syndrome presents with thyroid cancer, before intestinal lesions are found, and is diagnosed by the pathological findings. Depending on the evaluation of the intestines, studies of the family may be necessary. The syndrome is caused by mutations in the *APC* (adenomatous polyposis coli) gene on chromosome 5q21.

Mutations in the *PTEN* gene at 10q23.3 cause Cowden's (hamartoma tumour) syndrome and related syndromes. Cowden's disease is most often associated with multiple adenomatous goitre. Follicular adenomas and follicular cancers also occur, the latter in 5–10% of cases. Carney's complex, Werner syndrome's, and multiple endocrine neoplasia syndrome type 2A are also associated with thyroid cancer.

Although it is now well accepted that there are familial factors in some cases of nonmedullary thyroid cancer, originally this was difficult to establish, partly because many families with two cases may arise by chance. Two large studies from Japan made the nearly identical observations that 5% of surgically confirmed cases were in families with multiple cases. A more precise estimate was made using the comprehensive Swedish cancer registry data from 1958 to 2002 (10). The standard incidence ratio for a child of a parent with thyroid cancer was 3.21 and was 6.24 for a sibling of a thyroid cancer case. However, given the nature of thyroid cancer, such findings could be influenced by ascertainment bias, in other words, the occurrence of thyroid cancer in one relative could lead to closer scrutiny for thyroid cancer in the relatives. In a few families with multiple cases, distinctive pathological features are present. For example, an autosomal dominant form of thyroid cancer with oxyphilia has been located at chromosomal location 19p13.2, but the gene has not been identified.

There is some evidence that familial thyroid cancers are more frequently multifocal and, in most reports, recur more often. This has led to the suggestion that near-total thyroidectomy is the preferred treatment. A large study from Japan noted that in 273 cases of familial papillary cancer, the prognosis was no different than for sporadic cases, but when the thyroidectomy was incomplete, recurrences were more common (11). Screening asymptomatic family members with ultrasonography is supported by a Japanese study; in 157 mostly first-degree relatives of familial cases (thyroid cancer in two or more first-degree relatives) there was a prevalence of 52% for nodules and 7% for cancer (12).

Pre-existing thyroid disease

Many studies have tried to determine whether people with a history of a benign thyroid disease are at increased risk for developing thyroid cancer. In addition to its clinical importance, this question has relevance to understanding the pathogenesis of thyroid cancer. Several studies have found such a relationship. For the most part, these are case–control studies where patients who have developed thyroid cancer are matched to controls and then compared for the frequency of prior thyroid disease. An international pooled analysis of 14 case–control studies provides the best evaluation of the potential risk factors analysed in these studies (1, 13). Perhaps surprisingly, after radiation exposure, goitre and benign nodules were the largest risk factor for developing thyroid cancer. However, these case–control studies are subject to at least two problems. The first is recall bias where a subject with thyroid cancer may have a stronger recollection, or even a false recollection, of being told that they had a thyroid problem. The second is the possibility that, given the long course of thyroid cancer, the original diagnosis was in error and that the cancer was already present.

These problems were, for the most part, obviated in prospective studies carried out in Denmark. In this study a roster of 57 326 hospitalized patients who were discharged with diagnoses of benign thyroid disease were matched to the Danish Cancer Registry (14). Thyroid cancers subsequently occurred more frequently in these patients than in the general population, especially in those for whom the original diagnosis was goitre. It is possible, however, that the original thyroid diagnosis led to more frequent or more thorough examinations of the thyroid gland.

In summary, the weight of evidence favours a relationship between pre-existing benign thyroid disease and thyroid cancer, but the evidence is subject to alternative explanations and the clinical significance is not yet clear. In part, the association must reflect the fact that many multinodular goitres harbour thyroid cancers. Most studies indicate that benign nodules seldom, if ever, progress to become thyroid cancers.

Iodine and other dietary factors

Many studies have addressed the question of how the levels of iodine in the diet affect the incidence and types of thyroid cancer. One approach has been to compare iodine-sufficient with iodine-deficient geographical areas. Another has been to look for time trends during the institution of iodine supplementation programmes. These studies have been complicated by other factors, particularly the advances in diagnosing thyroid cancer.

The clearest effect of iodine is that, compared to iodine-sufficient areas, follicular cancer is more prevalent in areas of iodine deficiency (15) (see also Chapter 3.2.3). Whether iodine affects the overall incidence of thyroid cancer is less clear. In Denmark, e.g., thyroid cancer incidence has been increasing, but at the same rates and at the same levels in areas with different iodine intake levels (16).

The relationship between dietary iodine and thyroid cancer also has been examined by determining the composition of individual diets in case–control studies. The amount of fish and shellfish in the diet is generally used as a marker of iodine intake. Unfortunately, the results have not been consistent (1). The international pooled analysis of 14 case–control studies did not find an association between fish consumption and thyroid cancer (13).

With respect to other constituents of the diet, data from the international pooled case–control study indicate that consumption of cruciferous vegetables was associated with a small, but non-significant protective effect for thyroid cancer. This was observed, despite the fact they contain thioglycosides that are metabolized into goitrogens. A high consumption of vegetables other than Cruciferae was associated with a significant protective effect.

Reproductive and hormonal factors

The reason for the striking female-to-male ratio of about 3:1 for papillary and follicular thyroid cancer remains an enigma. Exposure to oestrogens and/or other hormonal factors have long been suspected, but whether this is the case and, if so, by what mechanisms, is not known. Many studies have focused on the relationship between thyroid cancer and: (1) age at menarche, (2) parity and reproductive history, and (3) exposure to exogenous oestrogens. In general, the studies have been inconsistent and have shown, at most, small effects. The international pooled analysis provides the best estimates (1, 13). The analysis found a weak association between later age at menarche and later age at first birth and thyroid cancer. Parity was associated with a small increase in thyroid cancer risk (odds ratio = 1.2), but the risk did not change with the number of births. Similarly, use of birth control pills at any time was associated with a small risk (odds ratio = 1.2), but no increased risk was found for hormone replacement therapy.

Molecular and cellular pathogenesis

General principles

Neoplasms, including those of thyroid follicular cell origin, develop when the control of cell division and programmed cell death is disrupted by mutations at critical genomic sites. The general principles of molecular tumorigenesis, as they apply to thyroid tumours, are outlined here (17–19).

For a tumour to develop, the control of the cell cycle in dividing cells, at critical checkpoints, must be disrupted. In addition, resting cells may undergo an unplanned transition from the quiescent G_0 phase into the $G_1 \rightarrow S$ phase, as a prelude to unregulated cell division. Other perturbations of the cell cycle may result in the inability of dividing cells to arrest properly when they are subjected to genetic damage. Normally, cell cycle arrest allows for DNA repair mechanisms to be activated. Then, following successful repair, progression through the cell cycle resumes.

The arrest of the cell cycle, either at the $G_1 \rightarrow S$ or $G_2 \rightarrow M$ transition is necessary to repair DNA damage produced by genotoxic endogenous or exogenous agents. Cells that do not repair damaged DNA sufficiently may be eliminated by activation of programmed cell death (apoptosis). In instances where the complex apoptotic process is disrupted, some cells that survive may acquire genetic instability and pass this characteristic on to progeny cells, leading to the progressive accumulation of mutations. Some of these mutations may confer a clonal proliferative advantage, leading to the acquisition of neoplastic characteristics. This route conforms to the 'multistage hypothesis' of cancer development, the sequential accumulation of genetic mutations giving rise to clonal expansion and, eventually, the development of clinically overt cancers.

Different types of genetic mutations contribute to the development of cancer. Changes in one or more bases may cause missense mutations that give rise to altered proteins by amino acid substitutions or nonsense mutations that give rise to truncated proteins. Some gene products—tumour suppressor genes—have functions that help prevent cancers from developing and when they are inactivated, cancer may ensue. Their inactivation results in escape from control, leading to tumour progression. These genes are recessive because, in most cases, inactivation of both alleles is required to promote tumorigenesis. In other genes, point mutations lead to tumours by a dominant effect. The *RAS* genes, coding for specific guanosine triphosphate (GTP)-binding proteins involved in signal transduction are examples. Mutations in specific codons result in constitutive activation by inactivating the GTPase activity of the RAS protein. The GTPase activity is required for normal control by catalysing the transition from active GTP-RAS to inactive GDP-RAS. Activated RAS promotes downstream signalling that leads to tumorigenesis. *RAS* mutations are important in thyroid tumorigenesis. Point mutations in the *BRAF* gene, whose product is located downstream to *RAS*, are the most common genetic alterations in the papillary thyroid cancers. Genes such as *RAS* and *BRAF* are referred to as oncogenes. The more inclusive term 'cancer gene' is used to include all genes whose altered products play a role in carcinogenesis.

Mutations involving larger segments of DNA can lead to allelic loss. The loss of genetic material from one chromosome with additional loss or mutations on the other can inactivate tumour suppressor genes. The loss of a tumour suppressor gene on one of the two paired chromosomes is detected by loss of heterozygosity. When chromosomal sites near or in the tumour suppressor genes derived from paternal and maternal origins have different sequences (allelic heterozygosity), loss of heterozygosity is detected by finding both alleles in normal tissue and only one allele in cancer tissue. Usually, restriction enzyme analysis or microsatellite (areas of DNA with nucleotide repeats) analysis is used for this purpose. In thyroid cancer, loss of heterozygosity has been detected in specific regions of the genome and may be associated with a propensity for more aggressive behaviour.

The translocation of genetic material within or between chromosomes can result in activated cancer genes (oncogenes). When a promoter from an expressed gene is translocated and replaces the promoter of a silent gene, the silent gene becomes constitutively activated. When the translocation includes an active promoter and the first part of its adjacent gene, the rearrangement results in a constitutively activated gene that codes for a fusion protein. The classic example occurs in the formation of the Philadelphia chromosome where the tyrosine kinase gene, *ABL1*, is translocated to the breakpoint cluster region. The resulting protein is highly expressed and has increased kinase activity. In papillary thyroid cancer, the *RET* oncogene is created by such an activation mechanism. Another type of genetic mutation is gene amplification in which a cancer gene is present in multiple copies, either on one chromosome or as 'minute' chromosomes containing highly duplicated genetic material.

Many genes are involved in the control and progression of the cell cycle, but several emerge as key cell cycle checkpoint control genes with roles in the pathogenesis of cancer. The *TP53* gene is an important checkpoint gene causing the arrest of cells at the $G_1 \rightarrow S$ transition in response to DNA damage. Since cell cycle arrest allows for the activation of repair genes or activation of cell elimination by apoptosis, the inactivation of *TP53* plays a decisive role in the development of many cancers. The inactivation of *TP53* occurs through point mutations in single bases or through a dominant negative effect of increased expression of inactivating isoforms of the other TP53 family proteins and other modulators that interfere with *TP53* gene regulation. In thyroid cancer, *TP53* involvement mainly through point mutations has been found to occur in the more advanced and aggressive cancers and is thought to be associated with dedifferentiation and progression and not with initiation.

The improper activation of intracellular transduction pathways that regulate cell proliferation contributes to tumorigenesis. Normally, transduction pathways are activated and controlled by the interactions of extracellular ligands, typically hormones or growth factors, with their membrane bound receptors. Mutations in genes coding for key signalling proteins can result in constitutive and unregulated activation of specific transduction pathways, leading to improper cell proliferation. Mutated RAS proteins, mentioned above, activate a sequence of kinases which, in turn, activate the early proliferation-inducing genes *JUN*, *FOS*, and *MYC*. BRAF is downstream of RAS and mutations in its gene activate the same pathway. The *RET* gene product is a membrane-bound tyrosine kinase which is normally activated by glial-derived nerve factor. It is not normally expressed in thyroid follicular cells. In papillary thyroid cancers the *RET* oncogene is activated through intrachromosomal or interchromosomal translocation of strong promoters and the expression of a chimeric tyrosine kinase. Having lost its transmembrane domain, the chimeric protein is no longer bound to the membrane and it produces unregulated activation of its downstream signalling intermediates. The activation of another tyrosine kinase gene, *TRK1*, by rearrangement, is also involved in some papillary thyroid cancers. In thyroid follicular cancers the *PPAR-γ* gene, which promotes cellular differentiation and inhibits proliferation, can be inactivated by fusion with the DNA binding domain of the *PAX8* gene, which codes for a thyroid a transcription factor (20). Finally, point mutations in the transmembrane domain of the TSH receptor and mutations in G-stimulating protein (GSP) can lead to unregulated signal transduction pathway activation as found in toxic adenomas and rarely in thyroid cancers.

An additional intracellular signal transduction cascade, initiated by phosphatidylinositol 3-kinase (PI3K) has been shown to be activated in thyroid cancer (21). This pathway is activated when PI3K generates the active phosphatidylinositol triphosphate. A series of downstream activation events follow, among them the activation of AKTs, which promote additional phosphorylation events in the cytoplasm and in the nucleus of the cells. The increased expression of AKTs induces cell proliferation, invasion, enhanced cellular migration, and inhibition of apoptosis in thyroid cancer cells. The activation of the PI3K/AKT pathway may be induced by activated *RAS* and *RET* oncogenes. The PI3K/AKT pathway is also activated by reduced expression of its inhibitor PTEN, a tumour suppressor whose gene may be mutated or hypermethylated. Constitutive activation of PI3K/AKT pathway can occur through mutation or amplification of the *PIK3CA* gene, which codes for a catalytic subunit of the PI3K complex. Activated PI3K/AKT is thought to contribute to thyroid cancer progression and aggressiveness, including the transformation into anaplastic thyroid cancer.

Other types of molecular mechanisms that contribute to the development of cancer include mutations in DNA repair genes (e.g. in hereditary nonpolyposis colon cancers), mutations in cell cycle-controlling genes (such as the retinoblastoma gene and cyclin genes), alterations of angiogenesis, and dysregulation of cell spindle checkpoints. To what extent, if any, these play a role in thyroid cancer is under investigation.

New evidence is emerging regarding the importance of epigenetic changes in tumorigenesis, i.e. changes in the state of DNA methylation or histone conformation. Thus hypermethylation or hypomethylation of certain regulatory promoter regions of tumour suppressor genes or oncogenes result in their suppressed or enhanced expression, respectively. In thyroid cancers, cyclins and cyclin-dependent kinases (CKDs), which regulate and activate the cell cycle, may be up-regulated when the genes that code for the CKD inhibitors are hypermethylated and down-regulated (22). Hypermethylation of thyroid specific genes, including the sodium-iodide symporter, reduces their expression and partly explains the reduced iodine uptake capacity of thyroid cancers and may become a therapy target to enhance the iodine uptake. Changes in histone structure are induced mainly by acetylation and lead to altered expression of genes that may have oncogene or tumour suppressor gene activities in specific cancers. The importance of cancer epigenetics is now well recognized, not only in pathogenesis, but also in the diagnosis and as a potential target of cancer therapies, including thyroid cancers.

An additional type of molecular alteration has recently been found to be associated with thyroid cancer. MicroRNAs are small RNA segments that regulate gene expression by binding to the 3′ untranslated part of the mRNA, thus inhibiting their translation or enhancing their degradation. Increased expression of microRNAs miR-221, miR-222, and miR-181 has been found in some thyroid cancers. *In vitro* and animal studies suggest that they down-regulate the expression of the c-*KIT* gene (23).

Genetic alterations in papillary thyroid cancers

Papillary thyroid cancers frequently have genetic modifications that abnormally activate the mitogen-activated protein kinase (MAPK) signalling pathway (Fig. 3.5.4.1), leading to tumorigenic effects. Transmembrane tyrosine kinase receptors have extracellular domains which are physiologically activated by various growth factors. The activation of these receptors is followed by phosphorylation of RAS which subsequently activates BRAF. Activated BRAF induces phosphorylation of MEK which subsequently enables MAPK (also known as ERK) to translocate to the cell nucleus and activate various transcription factors and genes responsible for cellular proliferation and survival (24). The MAPK pathway can be abnormally activated by various mutations or gene rearrangements at different levels starting with tyrosine kinase receptor molecules (*RET*, *NTRK1*) or at the intracellular effectors level (*RAS*, *BRAF*). These molecular alterations can result in uncontrollable cellular proliferation and are found in about two-thirds of all papillary thyroid cancers (25).

Tyrosine kinase receptor gene alterations

Rearrangements of the genes coding for two tyrosine kinase receptors, *RET* and *NTRK1*, can generate activated chimeric proteins which induce downstream effectors leading to the malignant phenotype. In normal thyroid tissue RET is only expressed in parafollicular C cells, not in follicular cells. The *RET* gene is located at chromosomal locus 10q11.2 and several different alterations (translocations, inversions, etc.) producing the fusion of its 3′ portion to the 5′ portion of various other genes can result in activation and expression of the *RET* gene in thyroid follicular cells. These are known as *RET/PTC* rearrangements and, so far, at least 11 different types have been described (26).

RET/PTC1, the most common form, derives from an intrachromosomal inversion of a portion of the *RET* gene (its tyrosine kinase domain) and the *H4* gene (its promoter and N-terminal region), both situated on the long arm of chromosome 10 (Fig. 3.5.4.2). *RET/PTC3*, the next most common form, results from fusion with the *NCOA4* (also called *ELE1* or *RFG*) gene which is also on chromosome 10. *RET/PTC2* results from translocation of *RET* with the gene for the RIα regulatory subunit of protein kinase A located on a different chromosome, chromosome 17.

The pathogenetic role of *RET/PTC1* in papillary thyroid cancers has been confirmed by experiments *in vitro* and *in vivo*. Introducing the *RET/PTC1* gene into rat thyroid epithelial cells growing in culture resulted in independent growth and loss of differentiation. Transgenic mice created to express *RET/PTC1* or *RET/PTC3* in the thyroid, by placing these genes on thyroglobulin promoters, develop thyroid neoplasms with papillary cancer characteristics. *RET/PTC* rearrangements are found in 20–40% of sporadic papillary cancer in adults (Table 3.5.4.1) (27). This proportion is higher in children (about 60%) and in radiation-induced thyroid cancer (about 80%) (28, 29).

Rearrangements of the *NTRK1* gene are found in a small percentage of papillary thyroid cancers. The gene encodes for a transmembrane tyrosine kinase receptor that is activated by nerve growth factor in neuroectodermal tissues. The *NTRK1* gene is activated by translocation, in the same way as *RET*, by fusion of strong promoters of ubiquitously expressed genes to the intracellular tyrosine kinase domain of NTRK1. The rearranged forms lose their membrane links, resulting in intracellular constitutive activation by autophosphorylation and activation of downstream signalling proteins. Several rearranged *NTRK1* isoforms have been identified. One isoform (*TRK*) results from an intrachromosomal inversion that creates a fusion with the promoter of nonmuscle tropomyosin on the short arm of chromosome 1. Two other isoforms (*TRK-T1* and *TRK-T2*) result from intrachromosomal translocations to one of two breakpoints in the *TPR* (tumour-potentiating region) gene, also located on chromosome 1q. Another isoform (*TRK-T3*) involves an interchromosomal translocation with *TFG* (*TRK*-fused gene).

BRAF gene mutations

Point mutations of the *BRAF* gene are the most common genetic alteration in sporadic papillary thyroid cancer, accounting for approximately 45% of all these cancers (Table 3.5.4.1) (30). BRAF protein is a serine-threonine kinase which is normally activated by *RAS*. Activated BRAF triggers MAPK/ERK kinase (MEK) activation and subsequently the other downstream effectors of the MAPK cascade (Fig. 3.5.4.1). It belongs to the family of RAF proteins which also includes two other isoforms, ARAF and CRAF. BRAF is the predominant form in follicular cells and the vast majority of its mutations result from a T to A transversion at nucleotide 1799 producing a valine-to-glutamate substitution at residue 600 (V600E) (31, 32). This mutation results in constitutively activated BRAF kinase, resulting in MEK phosphorylation and activation of the MAPK cascade (33). *BRAF* gene mutations are usually found in papillary carcinomas with classic features or in the tall cell variant, but not in the follicular variant of papillary cancer (34). A significant association between *BRAF* gene mutations and more aggressive

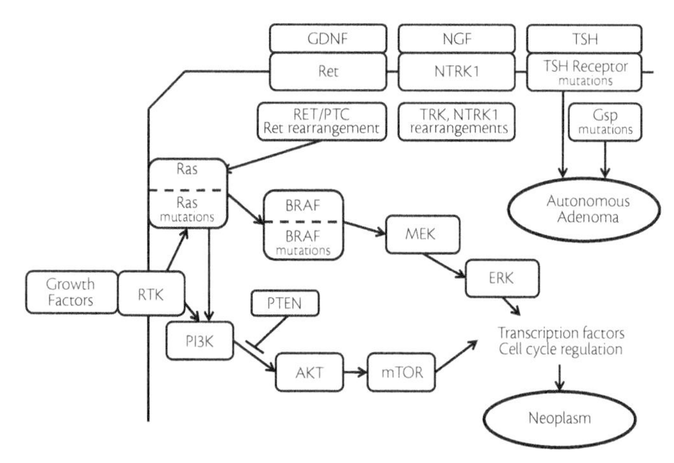

Fig. 3.5.4.1 Molecular pathogenesis of thyroid neoplasms. Rearrangements of the genes coding for the tyrosine kinase receptors RET or TRK can initiate the mitogen-activated protein kinase (MAPK) pathway by activating RAS proteins. Several mutations of the *RAS* genes can also produce molecules with intrinsic catalytic activity. Similarly, BRAF can be activated by either RAS or point mutations and induce the downstream effectors MEK and ERK which translocate to the nucleus and affect transcription factors that trigger neoplasia. The phosphatidylinositol 3-kinase (PI3K) pathway is activated when PI3K generates the active phosphatidylinositol triphosphate. This eventually results in activation of AKTs, which induces cell proliferation, invasion, enhanced cellular migration, and inhibition of apoptosis in thyroid cancer cells. The activation of the PI3K/AKT pathway may be induced by activated RAS or *RET/PTC* oncogenes. The PI3K/AKT pathway is also activated by reduced expression of its inhibitor *PTEN*, a tumour suppressor whose gene may be mutated or hypermethylated. Mutations in *p53*, normally involved in the cell response to DNA damage, lead to neoplasms by loss of its regulatory functions in cell cycle arrest and apoptosis. Point mutations in the transmembrane domain of the TSH receptor and mutations in its G-stimulating protein (Gsp) can lead to neoplastic transformation and autonomous function.

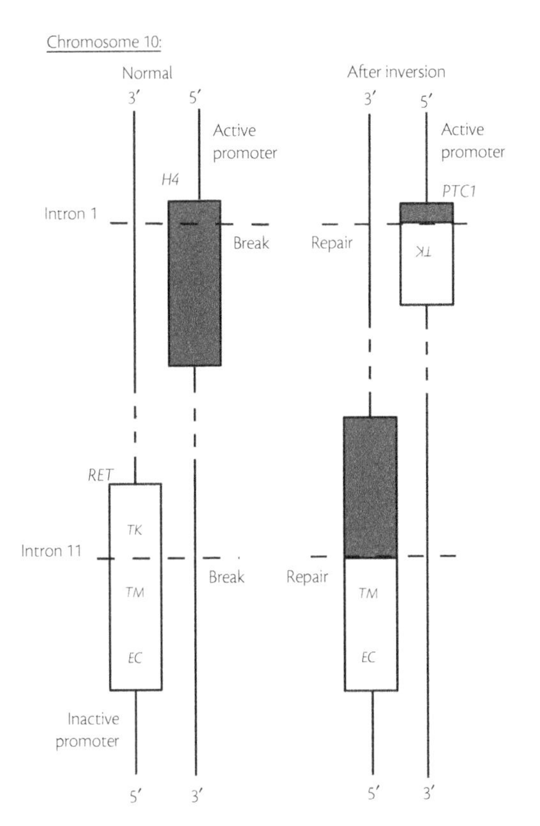

Fig. 3.5.4.2 Translocation of *RET* with *H4* to form *RET/PTC1*. The section of the normal gene (left) shown between the dashed lines is inverted to form *RET/PTC1* (right). The tyrosine kinase (TK) domain is transferred to the active promoter of *H4*. The extracellular domain (EC) and the transmembrane (TM) portion of *RET* remain on the inactive promoter. The other papillary thyroid cancer genes are formed by the translocation of *RET*'s tyrosine kinase to other genes.

features, such as extrathyroidal invasion, lymph node metastasis, and a higher risk of recurrence, has been reported and these tumours have a lower expression of both thyroperoxidase and the sodium-iodide symporter (35, 36). The latter finding could potentially explain why *BRAF*-positive tumours loose their ^{131}I avidity and are more refractory to treatment. Elisei *et al.*, using 15-year follow-up data, confirmed that papillary cancers that were positive for the *BRAF*-V600E mutation had a poorer prognosis in terms of having a higher risk of persistent disease and death (37). Besides the classic V600E mutation, the *BRAF* gene can also be activated by an inversion of chromosome 7q that leads to a fusion between *BRAF* and *AKAP9* genes (38). This alteration produces a fusion protein which includes the BRAF kinase domain but lacks the autoinhibitory N-terminal portion, resulting in constitutive activation of the MAPK cascade via ERK phosphorylation. The *AKAP9-BRAF* fusion is predominantly found in radiation-induced thyroid cancer and is very rare in sporadic papillary carcinoma (38).

BRAF gene mutations can also be found in anaplastic and poorly differentiated papillary carcinomas. They are considered to be an early event in malignancy because of their presence in both well-differentiated and poorly differentiated areas (33).

Mutations of *RAS* genes

Rarely, genetic alterations in papillary thyroid cancers involve mutations of one of the *RAS* genes, resulting in activated G-proteins that induce downstream signalling pathways. At present, it is estimated that *RAS* mutations have a prevalence of about 10% of papillary thyroid cancer and that they almost always occur in the follicular variant of the tumour (39). These mutations are more common in follicular adenomas and carcinomas, as discussed below.

Mutations in follicular adenomas and carcinomas

The most common genetic alterations seen in follicular carcinomas are *RAS* gene mutations and *PAX8-PPAR*γ rearrangements. These alterations are mutually exclusive pointing to a separate pathogenetic mechanism in the development of follicular thyroid cancer (34).

Mutations of *RAS* genes

There are four isoforms of *RAS* (*HRAS*, *KRAS A*, *KRAS B*, and *NRAS*) that encode for membrane-bound small G-proteins. These proteins play an important role in the intracellular signalling of the MAPK cascade pathway. In their inactive states, they bind to guanine diphosphate (GDP), but when activated they release GDP and bind guanine triphosphate (GTP) instead, which then activates BRAF (Fig. 3.5.4.1). Under normal conditions, RAS proteins have intrinsic phosphatase activity rapidly converting them back to the inactive RAS-GDP form. Point mutations in *RAS* genes (in codons 12 and 13) can result either in an increased affinity for GTP or in inactivation of the autocatalytic GTPase function (codon 61) (33).

RAS mutations are the most common somatic genetic alterations found in follicular adenomas and carcinomas. They are not specific for thyroid follicular cancer, also being seen in papillary, poorly differentiated, and anaplastic carcinomas and in many other cancers (pancreas, colon, lung, etc.). The frequency of these mutations is high in follicular adenomas and even higher in follicular cancers, representing about 45% of genetic alterations seen in these tumours (Table 3.5.4.1) (33). The presence of these mutations in follicular adenomas points to early involvement of RAS in the formation of follicular neoplasms. It supports the concept that follicular cancers arise from follicular adenomas. *RAS* mutations in follicular thyroid cancer appear to be associated with more aggressive clinical behaviour (40).

*PAX8-PPAR*γ rearrangements

Approximately one-third of all follicular thyroid cancers demonstrate an interchromosomal translocation t(2;3)(q13;p25) that produces a fusion between the paired box 8 gene (*PAX8*) and the peroxisome activator receptor γ gene (*PPAR*γ) (41). This rearrangement produces a paired box 8 / peroxisome proliferator activated receptor γ fusion protein (PPFP) which has been identified both in follicular thyroid cancers and, to a smaller extent, in follicular adenomas. The oncogenic mechanisms are not yet completely understood, but may involve the loss of function of the wild-type PPARγ nuclear receptor or modification of normal transcription of various genes controlled by PAX8 and PPARγ (41, 42).

Hürthle cell carcinomas

Hürthle cell cancers are usually classified as variants of follicular thyroid cancer, but some have histological features and mutations related to papillary carcinoma. Hürthle cell cancers have a more aggressive behaviour, being refractory to radioactive iodine treatment and showing more local and lymph node recurrences (43). The molecular genetics of Hürtle cell cancer appear to differ from follicular cancer, with some evidence pointing towards mutations in the mitochondrial DNA (mtDNA). Gasparre *et al.* sequenced the entire mitochondrial genome and showed a high prevalence

Table 3.5.4.1 Genetic and molecular changes in follicular cell derived thyroid tumours and their estimated prevalence

	Molecular alteration	Tumour	Prevalence
Oncogenes			
RAS	Point mutations inactivate GTPases and activate MAPK signalling cascade	Adenomas	May be present
		Papillary carcinoma	10%, associated with follicular variants
		Follicular carcinoma	40–50%, predisposes to tumour dedifferentiation
		Poorly differentiated/anaplastic	55%
TSHR and *GSP*	Point mutations in the transmembrane domain of TSHR and GSP lead to unregulated signal transduction pathway	Adenomas	Present in toxic thyroid adenomas
BRAF	Point mutations cause constitutive activation of MAPK signalling cascade	Papillary carcinoma	45%, associated with extrathyroidal extension and tumour recurrence
		Poorly differentiated/anaplastic	20%
RET/PTC	Rearrangement and fusion causes constitutive activation of tyrosine kinase	Papillary carcinoma	20%, prevalence higher in radiation-induced tumours (up to 60%)
TRK	Rearrangement and fusion causes constitutive activation of tyrosine kinase receptor	Papillary carcinoma	Uncommon, found in up 12% of tumours
PIK3CA	Point mutations and amplifications cause activations of the PI3K\AKT pathway	Papillary carcinoma	6–13% point mutations; 24–28% gene amplification
		Follicular carcinoma	<10%, mainly gene amplification
		Poorly differentiated/anaplastic	16–23% point mutations; 42% gene amplification
B-catenin	Point mutations in the CTNNB1 gene	Poorly differentiated	20%
		Anaplastic	65%
Tumour suppressor genes			
PTEN	Mutations in PTEN inactivate its inhibitory activity of PI3K\AKT pathway	Papillary carcinoma	<5%
		Follicular carcinoma	<10% in sporadic tumours. The prevalent mutation in Cowden's syndrome
		Poorly differentiated/anaplastic	About 14%
PAX8/PPARγ	Rearrangement and fusion inhibits PPARγ action on cell differentiation	Follicular carcinoma	35%, associated with vascular invasion
p53	Point mutations and deletions impair cell cycle arrest, damage repair, and apoptosis	Poorly differentiated/anaplastic	70%, late event in tumorigenesis
Extragenetic changes			
Hypermethylation of CKD inhibitors p27Kip1 and p16INK4a	Down-regulation of CKD inhibitors result in activation of cell cycle from G1 to S phase and overexpression of cyclin D1	Papillary carcinoma	60%, associated with lymph node metastasis
Overexpression of miR-221, miR-222, and miR-181b	Down-regulation of c-KIT protein	Papillary carcinoma	Common, prevalence not established

MAPK, mitogen-activated protein kinase.

of disruptive mutations in the complex I subunit genes of mtDNA (44). The authors caution that tumorigenesis probably does not arise from a single mitochondrial mutation and that a 'more-than-one hit hypothesis is more plausible'.

Poorly differentiated and anaplastic thyroid cancers

Anaplastic thyroid cancer can occur in the setting of pre-existent thyroid disease, including well-differentiated carcinomas, or *de novo*. Poorly differentiated thyroid cancers have a severity intermediate between that of differentiated and anaplastic cancer. Poorly differentiated and anaplastic types both show a high prevalence of mutations characteristically found in differentiated papillary and follicular carcinomas, predominantly mutations of the genes encoding for effectors of the MAPK pathway, suggesting that they are early events. It has been estimated that RAS mutations occur in 55%, and *BRAF* mutations in 20% of anaplastic thyroid cancers, with corresponding percentages of 35% and 15% for poorly differentiated cancers (33). It is generally believed that the progression from differentiated to anaplastic thyroid carcinoma is due to subsequent mutations of several genes including *TP53*, *CTNNB1* (β-catenin), and others encoding effectors of the PI3K pathway.

TP53 gene mutations in anaplastic and poorly differentiated thyroid carcinoma

The role of the *TP53* gene is to produce p53, a cyclin kinase inhibitor (p21), one of whose functions is to promote cell arrest in the $G_1 \rightarrow S$ phase in response to DNA damage. Since this process allows for the activation of repair genes or, alternatively, activation of apoptosis, the inactivation of p53 plays a decisive role in the development of many cancers. Mutations of the *TP53* gene are rare events in well-differentiated thyroid cancer but it can be seen in up to 20% of poorly differentiated and in about 70% of anaplastic carcinomas (33). In one series of anaplastic carcinoma cases, multiple genetic alterations involving *p53* in association with *BRAF* and *RAS* gene mutations were found. In contrast, none of the cases had *RET/PTC* gene mutations (45). This is consistent with *TP53* mutations as late events associated with dedifferentiation and tumour progression.

β-catenin pathway in anaplastic carcinoma

The β-catenin protein, encoded by *CTNNB1* gene, is a subunit of the transmembrane cadherin complex that has an important role in cell adhesion and in the Wnt signalling pathway. In the absence of WNT signals it is present in the cytoplasm at low concentrations. Normally the APC protein binds to cytosolic β-catenin and induces its degradation by phosphorylation. The Wnt pathway stabilizes β-catenin by inhibiting its phosphorylation and allows its transfer into the nucleus where it can function as a transcription factor (32, 46). Garcia-Rostan *et al.* found a high rate of various activating point mutations in the *CTNNB1* region coding for β-catenin in patients with anaplastic thyroid cancer (47). It is estimated that approximately 20% of poorly differentiated and 65% of anaplastic carcinomas have mutations of the β-catenin gene (33).

Molecular changes in radiation-related thyroid cancers

Ionizing radiation has sufficient energy to displace electrons from atoms to produce charged particles that cause damage to cells. Although ionizing radiation can affect several components of a cell, DNA damage is thought to be the primary event leading to transformation and cancer (48). Among the various forms of DNA damage, double-strand breaks are most important for tumour formation. These manifest themselves as losses of, or rearrangements of, large segments of chromosomes. Since cells have multiple mechanisms to maintain genomic integrity (see above), to induce cancer, radiation must produce damage that escapes these protective mechanisms. Thus, radiation could affect a key gene, a proto-oncogene, or tumour suppressor gene that leads, through multiple steps, to cancer. Alternatively, radiation could affect the mechanisms that maintain genomic integrity, allowing the cell to accumulate mutations that lead to cancer. These two possibilities are not mutually exclusive, since either one could lead to the other.

Radiation-related thyroid cancers are virtually always of the papillary form. Several studies have addressed the molecular pathogenesis of cancers occurring after childhood external radiation exposure. RET/PTC translocations are common in the thyroid cancers of patients exposed to external radiation, with the *RET/PTC1* form being the most prevalent. There have been many studies on somatic mutations in post-Chernobyl thyroid cancer cases. Genes already suspected to be involved with the pathogenesis of thyroid cancer have been studied. Although there are variations in the reports, so far only rearrangements, particularly of the *RET* gene, are clearly related to radiation-related cases (49). Rearrangements of the *RET* gene are frequent in papillary thyroid cancers, but more so in radiation-related cases. Since the post-Chernobyl cases are in children, the appropriate comparison is to nonirradiated children with thyroid cancer, a relatively rare condition. Nevertheless, there are two distinctive features of *RET* rearrangements in radiation-related cases (50). First, the frequency is very high, higher than in age-matched cases, and second, the pattern of *RET* mutations, specifically the selection of translocation partners, is distinctive. However, additional factors in the Chernobyl area, such as iodine deficiency, may play a role in these observations.

The findings from the Chernobyl cases show that radiation increases both the frequency and the types of *RET* rearrangements. The increased frequency of rearrangements involving *RET* is in accordance with a direct effect of radiation on DNA causing double-strand breaks and 'illegitimate' recombination. The rearrangements occurring after radiation may be facilitated by the chromosomal structure of normal thyroid cells where the *RET* gene and at least one of its translocation partners, *H4*, are in proximity (51). Presumably, cells with recombination events that give a growth advantage, such as the activation of the ret tyrosine kinase activity, undergo clonal expansion. There are two distinctive features to the pattern of ret rearrangements. The first is the increased proportion of cases with *RET/PTC3* compared to *RET/PTC1*, especially in the earliest cases after the accident. The frequency of *RET/PTC3* appears to be decreasing in the more recent cases. The second is the identification of unusual *RET* rearrangements that have not been seen in nonradiation-related cases of papillary thyroid cancer.

What is the relationship between radiation and translocations of ret gene? The simplest hypothesis is that radiation causes them directly. Two observations support this possibility. Transgenic animals made to express either *RET/PTC1* or *RET/PTC3* in the thyroid develop cancers with characteristics suggesting the papillary type. This indicates that *RET* activation alone is sufficient to cause thyroid cancer. Also, *RET* activation is very common in radiation-related cases, clearly more common than in other cases of thyroid cancer. However, radiation could initiate a series of events with the involvement of *RET* occurring later.

For other genes implicated in thyroid neoplasia in general, *RAS*, *TP53*, and *GSP*, some cases of mutations in radiation-related cases have been described, but the observed frequency and types are similar to cases not related to radiation. This is not entirely surprising; mutations in these genes are usually found in nonpapillary thyroid cancers, while papillary thyroid cancer is the most common after radiation exposure, and the alterations in these genes are usually point mutations, whereas radiation more commonly causes double-strand breaks.

Future directions

Impact of molecular pathogenesis on epidemiology

When a factor related to thyroid cancer, such as radiation exposure, is identified, the magnitude of the effect is determined by analysis of the dose–response relationship. However, it is not possible to distinguish which cases are due to radiation and which are sporadic cases. If it were possible to identify radiation-related cases, by some distinctive genetic changes, then a more specific dose–response relationship could be derived. This would improve the ability to make recommendations of public health relevance about medical and occupational radiation exposure. Some headway in this direction, but not complete success, has been made studying radiation-related cases occurring in the vicinity of Chernobyl.

Clinical importance of molecular pathogenesis

Some of the shortcomings of fine-needle aspiration of the thyroid may be overcome by the application of molecular techniques. The feasibility of detecting mutations by isolating DNA and RNA from aspiration samples has been demonstrated (52). The differentiation of benign and malignant follicular neoplasms, not possible using morphological criteria, could be approached by looking for specific mutations or for signs of increased genetic instability. The diagnosis of papillary cancer could be confirmed, e.g. by analysing the *RET* gene, and the prognosis predicted more accurately by analysing *TP53*, with a view to surgery and subsequent treatment planning. Finally, some cases with insufficient cellular yield to perform a morphological diagnosis may be susceptible to a molecular diagnosis, given the sensitivity of amplification by the polymerase chain reaction.

The prognosis of papillary thyroid cancer is very good and many factors related to long-term outcome are known with confidence. It is not clear how these factors are best combined to predict the behaviour of thyroid cancer in specific patients. There are cases where the course is more or less aggressive than predicted. It is likely that characterizing genetic changes will improve the ability to predict the behaviour of individual thyroid cancers. For example, with respect to BRAF, reports indicate that mutations are associated with a more aggressive course.

Molecular studies may lead to the identification of individuals with an increased susceptibility to thyroid cancer. The discovery of specific genes in families with thyroid cancer would make this possible, at least within the affected families. In the general population there are likely to be variations in susceptibility to factors such as radiation. Epidemiological and molecular studies will be necessary to discover the genetic factors underlying susceptibility. Finally, understanding the molecular pathogenesis of thyroid cancer has led, and will continue to lead to advances in treatment. Kinase inhibitors, as discussed elsewhere in this text, are currently the best examples of this.

References

1. Ron E, Schneider AB. Thyroid cancer. In: Schottenfeld D, Fraumeni Jr JF, eds. *Cancer Epidemiology and Prevention*. 3rd edn. Oxford: Oxford University Press, 2006: 975–94.
2. Enewold L, Zhu K, Ron E, Marrogi AJ, Stojadinovic A, Peoples GE, *et al.* Rising thyroid cancer incidence in the United States by demographic and tumor characteristics, 1980–2005. *Cancer Epidemiol Biomarkers Prev*, 2009; **18**: 784–91.
3. Ron E, Lubin JH, Shore RE, Mabuchi K, Modan B, Pottern LM, *et al.* Thyroid cancer after exposure to external radiation: a pooled analysis of seven studies. *Radiat Res*, 1995; **141**: 259–77.
4. Hatch M, Ron E, Bouville A, Zablotska L, Howe G. The Chernobyl disaster: cancer following the accident at the Chernobyl nuclear power plant. *Epidemiol Rev*, 2005; **27**: 56–66.
5. Wang JX, Inskip PD, Boice JD Jr, Li BX, Zhang JY, Fraumeni JF, Jr. Cancer incidence among medical diagnostic X-ray workers in China, 1950 to 1985. *Int J Cancer*, 1990; **45**: 889–95.
6. Zabel EW, Alexander BH, Mongin SJ, Doody MM, Sigurdson AJ, Linet MS, *et al.* Thyroid cancer and employment as a radiologic technologist. *Int J Cancer*, 2006; **119**: 1940–5.
7. Wang Z, Boice JD Jr, Wei L, Beebe GW, Zha YR, Kaplan MM, *et al.* Thyroid nodularity and chromosome aberrations among women in areas of high background radiation in China. *J Natl Cancer Inst*, 1990; **82**: 478–85.
8. Inskip PD, Ekbom A, Galanti MR, Grimelius L, Boice JD Jr. Medical diagnostic X-rays and thyroid cancer. *J Natl Cancer Inst*, 1995; **87**: 1613–21.
9. Nose V. Familial non-medullary thyroid carcinoma: an update. *Endocr Pathol*, 2008; **19**: 226–40.
10. Hemminki K, Eng C, Chen BW. Familial risks for nonmedullary thyroid cancer. *J Clin Endocrinol Metab*, 2005; **90**: 5747–53.
11. Ito Y, Kakudo K, Hirokawa M, Fukushima M, Yabuta T, Tomoda C, *et al.* Biological behavior and prognosis of familial papillary thyroid carcinoma. *Surgery*, 2009; **145**: 100–5.
12. Uchino S, Noguchi S, Yamashita H, Murakami T, Watanabe S, Ogawa T, *et al.* Detection of asymptomatic differentiated thyroid carcinoma by neck ultrasonographic screening for familial nonmedullary thyroid carcinoma. *World J Surg*, 2004; **28**: 1099–102.
13. Preston-Martin S, Franceschi S, Ron E, Negri E. Thyroid cancer pooled analysis from 14 case-control studies: what have we learned?. *Cancer Cause Control*, 2003; **14**: 787–9.
14. From G, Mellemgaard A, Knudsen N, Jorgensen T, Perrild H. Review of thyroid cancer cases among patients with previous benign thyroid disorders. *Thyroid*, 2000; **10**: 697–700.
15. Harach HR, Ceballos GA. Thyroid cancer, thyroiditis and dietary iodine: a review based on the Salta, Argentina model. *Endocr Pathol*, 2008; **19**: 209–20.
16. Sehestedt T, Knudsen N, Perrild H, Johansen C. Iodine intake and incidence of thyroid cancer in Denmark. *Clin Endocrinol (Oxf)*, 2006; **65**: 229–33.
17. Fagin JA. Molecular pathogenesis of tumors of thyroid follicular cells. In: Fagin J, ed. *Thyroid Cancer*. Boston: Kluwer Academic, 1998: 59–83.
18. Suarez HG. Genetic alterations in human epithelial thyroid tumours. *Clin Endocrinol (Oxf)*, 1998; **48**: 531–46.
19. Patel KN, Singh B. Genetic considerations in thyroid cancer. *Cancer Control*, 2006; **13**: 111–18.
20. Dwight T, Thoppe SR, Foukakis T, Lui WO, Wallin G, Höög A, *et al.* Involvement of the PAX8/peroxisome proliferator-activated receptor gamma rearrangement in follicular thyroid tumors. *J Clin Endocrinol Metab*, 2003; **88**: 4440–5.
21. Paes JE, Ringel MD. Dysregulation of the phosphatidylinositol 3-kinase pathway in thyroid neoplasia. *Endocrinol Metab Clin North Am*, 2008; **37**: 375–87.
22. Elisei R, Shiohara M, Koeffler HP, Fagin JA. Genetic and epigenetic alterations of the cyclin-dependent kinase inhibitors p15^{INK4b} and p16^{INK4a} in human thyroid carcinoma cell lines and primary thyroid carcinomas. *Cancer*, 1998; **83**: 2185–93.
23. Pallante P, Visone R, Ferracin M, Feraro A, Berlingieri MT, Troncone G, *et al.* MicroRNA deregulation in human thyroid papillary carcinomas. *Endocr Relat Cancer*, 2006; **13**: 497–508.
24. Ciampi R, Nikiforov YE. RET/PTC rearrangements and *BRAF* mutations in thyroid tumorigenesis. *Endocrinology*, 2007; **148**: 936–41.
25. Kimura ET, Nikiforova MN, Zhu Z, Knauf JA, Nikiforov YE, Fagin JA. High prevalence of *BRAF* mutations in thyroid cancer: genetic evidence for constitutive activation of the RET/PTC-RAS-BRAF signaling pathway in papillary thyroid carcinoma. *Cancer Res*, 2003; **63**: 1454–7.
26. Jhiang SM. The *RET* proto-oncogene in human cancers. *Oncogene*, 2000; **19**: 5590–7.
27. Nikiforov YE. *RET*/PTC rearrangement in thyroid tumors. *Endocr Pathol*, 2002; **13**: 3–16.

28. Smida J, Salassidis K, Hieber L, Zitzelsberger H, Kellerer AM, Demidchik EP, *et al.* Distinct frequency of *ret* rearrangements in papillary thyroid carcinomas of children and adults from Belarus. *Int J Cancer*, 1999; **80**: 32–8.
29. Fenton CL, Lukes Y, Nicholson D, Dinauer CA, Francis GL, Tuttle RM. The *ret*/PTC mutations are common in sporadic papillary thyroid carcinoma of children and young adults. *J Clin Endocrinol Metab*, 2000; **85**: 1170–5.
30. Ciampi R, Nikiforov YE. Alterations of the *BRAF* gene in thyroid tumors. *Endocr Pathol*, 2005; **16**: 163–71.
31. Davies H, Bignell GR, Cox C, Stephens P, Edkins S, Clegg S, *et al.* Mutations of the *BRAF* gene in human cancer. *Nature*, 2002; **417**: 949–54.
32. Fagin JA, Mitsiades N. Molecular pathology of thyroid cancer: diagnostic and clinical implications. *Best Pract Res Clin Endocrinol Metab*, 2008; **22**: 955–69.
33. Nikiforov YE. Thyroid carcinoma: molecular pathways and therapeutic targets. *Mod Pathol*, 2008; **21** (Suppl 2): S37–43.
34. Nikiforova MN, Kimura ET, Gandhi M, Biddinger PW, Knauf JA, Basolo F, *et al. BRAF* mutations in thyroid tumors are restricted to papillary carcinomas and anaplastic or poorly differentiated carcinomas arising from papillary carcinomas. *J Clin Endocrinol Metab*, 2003; **88**: 5399–404.
35. Xing M, Westra WH, Tufano RP, Cohen Y, Rosenbaum E, Rhoden KJ, *et al. BRAF* mutation predicts a poorer clinical prognosis for papillary thyroid cancer. *J Clin Endocrinol Metab*, 2005; **90**: 6373–9.
36. Romei C, Ciampi R, Faviana P, Agate L, Molinaro E, Bottici V, *et al.* $BRAF^{V600E}$ mutation, but not RET/PTC rearrangements, is correlated with a lower expression of both thyroperoxidase and sodium iodide symporter genes in papillary thyroid cancer. *Endocr Relat Cancer*, 2008; **15**: 511–20.
37. Elisei R, Ugolini C, Viola D, Lupi C, Biagini A, Giannini R, *et al.* $BRAF^{V600E}$ mutation and outcome of patients with papillary thyroid carcinoma: a 15-year median follow-up study. *J Clin Endocrinol Metab*, 2008; **93**: 3943–9.
38. Ciampi R, Knauf JA, Kerler R, Gandhi M, Zhu Z, Nikiforova MN, *et al.* Oncogenic *AKAP9-BRAF* fusion is a novel mechanism of MAPK pathway activation in thyroid cancer. *J Clin Invest*, 2005; **115**: 94–101.
39. Namba H, Rubin SA, Fagin JA. Point mutations of Ras oncogenes are an early event in thyroid tumorigenesis. *Mol Endocrinol*, 1990; **4**: 1474–9.
40. Garcia-Rostan G, Zhao H, Camp RL, Pollan M, Herrero A, Pardo J, *et al. ras* mutations are associated with aggressive tumor phenotypes and poor prognosis in thyroid cancer. *J Clin Oncol*, 2003; **21**: 3226–35.
41. Kroll TG, Sarraf P, Pecciarini L, Chen CJ, Mueller E, Spiegelman BM, *et al. PAX8-PPARγ1* fusion in oncogene human thyroid carcinoma. *Science*, 2000; **289**: 1357–60.
42. Au AYM, McBride C, Wilhelm KG Jr, Koenig RJ, Speller B, Cheung L, *et al.* PAX8-peroxisome proliferator-activated receptor γ (PPARγ) disrupts normal PAX8 or PPARγ transcriptional function and stimulates follicular thyroid cell growth. *Endocrinology*, 2006; **147**: 367–76.
43. Kushchayeva Y, Duh QY, Kebebew E, D'Avanzo A, Clark OH. Comparison of clinical characteristics at diagnosis and during follow-up in 118 patients with Hürthle cell or follicular thyroid cancer. *Am J Surg*, 2008; **195**: 457–62.
44. Gasparre G, Porcelli AM, Bonora E, Pennisi LF, Toller M, Iommarini L, *et al.* Disruptive mitochondrial DNA mutations in complex I subunits are markers of oncocytic phenotype in thyroid tumors. *Proc Natl Acad Sci U S A*, 2007; **104**: 9001–6.
45. Quiros RM, Ding HG, Gattuso P, Prinz RA, Xu XL. Evidence that one subset of anaplastic thyroid carcinomas are derived from papillary carcinomas due to *BRAF* and *p53* mutations. *Cancer*, 2005; **103**: 2261–8.
46. Gavert N, Ben Ze'ev A. β-catenin signaling in biological control and cancer. *J Cell Biochem*, 2007; **102**: 820–8.
47. Garcia-Rostan G, Tallini G, Herrero A, D'Aquila TG, Carcangiu ML, Rimm DL. Frequent mutation and nuclear localization of β-catenin in anaplastic thyroid carcinoma. *Cancer Res*, 1999; **59**: 1811–15.
48. Schneider AB, Robbins J. Ionizing radiation and thyroid cancer. In: Fagin J, ed. *Thyroid Cancer*. Boston: Kluwer Academic, 1998: 27–57.
49. Nikiforov YE, Fagin JA. Radiation-induced thyroid cancer in children after the Chernobyl accident. *Thyroid Today*, 1998; **21**: 1–11.
50. Rabes HM, Klugbauer S. Molecular genetics of childhood papillary thyroid carcinomas after irradiation: high prevalence of RET rearrangement. *Rec Results Cancer Res*, 1998; **154**: 248–64.
51. Nikiforova MN, Stringer JB, Blough R, Medvedec M, Fagin JA, Nikiforov YE. Proximity of chromosomal loci that participate in radiation-induced rearrangements in human cells. *Science*, 2000; **290**: 138–41.
52. Nikiforov YE, Steward DL, Robinson-Smith TM, Haugen BR, Klopper JP, Zhu Z, *et al.* Molecular testing for mutations in improving the fine needle aspiration diagnosis of thyroid nodules. *J Clin Endocrinol Metab*, 2009; **94**: 2092–8.

3.5.5 Pathology of thyroid cancer

Yolanda C. Oertel

Introduction

The majority of thyroid cancers arise from the follicular epithelium, are usually well differentiated, and thus many have a follicular architecture with varying amounts of colloid present. Medullary carcinoma constitutes a minority of thyroid cancers and arises from the C cells.

Fine-needle aspiration (FNA) biopsy is the accepted diagnostic test to determine whether a thyroid nodule is benign or malignant (1, 2). The role of the cytopathologist in the interpretation of smears has been considered crucial, and I believe this is partially valid. Based upon 30 years of experience as an 'interventional pathologist' who performs and interprets many aspirates, I emphasize that the quality of the sample is the crucial factor. The pathologist's interpretation is only as good as the sample he/she obtains or receives, and not enough attention has been paid to the technique of aspiration. I have trained numerous physicians to perform FNAs in a skilful fashion in a short period of time, and I refer the reader to my previous publications (3–5). The high rate of 'unsatisfactory specimens' reported in the literature is concerning. This was discussed at the National Cancer Institute Thyroid Fine-Needle Aspiration State of the Science Conference in October 2007 (6) and it was recommended that 'at the end of training and for re-credentialing 90% diagnostic samples should be documented'. Please note that FNA biopsy should not be confused with needle biopsies (e.g. Tru-cut, Vim-Silverman, etc.) that yield tissue fragments that are processed for histological diagnosis.

The usual classification of thyroid cancers is founded on their histological and cytological features, many of which have been correlated with the clinical behaviour of the tumours. In addition, the age of the patients and the extent of the tumours are particularly important to determine the prognosis. The classification I follow is that of the WHO (7) with some of the modifications by the Armed Forces Institute of Pathology (AFIP) (8). My discussion will be focused largely on the most common types (see Box 3.5.5.1). Prolonged follow-up of the patients and extensive modern studies

Box 3.5.5.1 Classification of thyroid cancer

- Papillary carcinoma
  - Microcarcinoma
  - Clinically apparent carcinoma: the most common is the classic pattern, but variants have been described (follicular variant, cystic, encapsulated, diffuse sclerosing, oxyphilic cell type, solid/trabecular, tall cell, columnar cell)
- Follicular carcinoma
  - Minimally invasive
  - Widely invasive
- Poorly differentiated carcinoma (rare)
- Anaplastic carcinoma (undifferentiated carcinoma) (rare): some of these tumours have features of squamous cell carcinoma
- Medullary carcinoma (C-cell carcinoma) (uncommon)
- Miscellaneous rare neoplasms (mucoepidermoid carcinoma, mucinous carcinoma, mixed medullary–follicular cell carcinoma)
- Secondary or metastatic tumours
- Malignant nonepithelial neoplasms: lymphoma, sarcoma

of the tumours indicate that papillary carcinomas and follicular carcinomas have histological similarities and are usually of a low grade of malignancy, but they also have a variety of inherent differences.

Papillary carcinoma

This is now the most common thyroid cancer that is clinically apparent, as well as constituting most of the microcarcinomas discovered incidental to excision of the gland for other thyroidal disorders or found at autopsy. The cancer cells have receptor tyrosine kinases in the proto-oncogenes *ret* (9) and *ntrk1*, which are activated by fusion with other genes (usually because of intrachromosomal inversions). The resulting chimeric proteins are expressed in the cytoplasm and are apparently mitogenic (10).

Over 80% of papillary cancers are invasive, with this characteristic evident either on gross examination or during histological study. Thus the border of the cancer is quite irregular. Fibrosis is common and it is irregularly distributed in and around the mass, frequently causing the tumour to be hard on palpation. An irregular pseudocapsule sometimes surrounds part of the mass, but typically this is uneven and incomplete, in contrast to the relatively uniform better-defined capsules nearly always present around follicular adenomas and follicular carcinomas. About 10–20% of papillary cancers do have well-developed capsules; often these tumours are cystic to a considerable extent.

Papillary cancers spread mostly through lymphatic vessels within and outside the thyroid gland. Invasion of blood vessels is much less common. They tend to be multifocal. Of course, when one or several small papillary cancers are found accompanying a larger one, the pathologist may not be able to determine if these are separate primary tumours or intraglandular spread from the principal cancer. Lymph nodes of the neck are frequently the sites of metastatic foci. When more than one focus of papillary cancer is present in the thyroid, determining which one has produced the metastases may not be possible. Calcification is common and occurs in two forms, as irregular masses in the stroma and as laminated calcospherites. The calcified material may cause the cut surfaces to be gritty on palpation. Ossification occurs occasionally in the calcific masses. Lymphoplasmacytic infiltrates are common around and within the cancers. In some instances the presence of this inflammation may have favourable prognostic implications (11), but that may not be true in all instances (12).

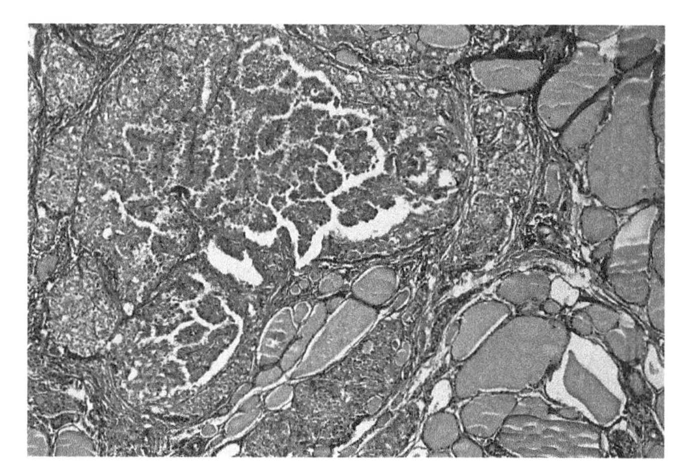

Fig. 3.5.5.1 Papillary carcinoma. Papillary structures are surrounded by solid foci of neoplastic cells. The tumour has infiltrated the normal parenchyma, which lies to the right. Haematoxylin and eosin, low magnification.

These neoplasms usually are composed of a mixture of papillae (Fig. 3.5.5.1) and abnormal follicles (Fig. 3.5.5.2). Great variations in the proportions of these structures are possible. Papillae vary from tiny buds protruding into follicular spaces to large complex structures which occasionally are large enough to be seen by the naked eye. Regardless of their sizes, they often cause the cut surfaces to have a granular appearance on gross examination. Large papillae have stroma which varies from myxoid to densely collagenous.

The neoplastic follicles may vary in size and shape (Fig. 3.5.5.2). A few are elongated and sinuous, appearing as tubules in the microscopic sections. A predominance of follicles (especially when

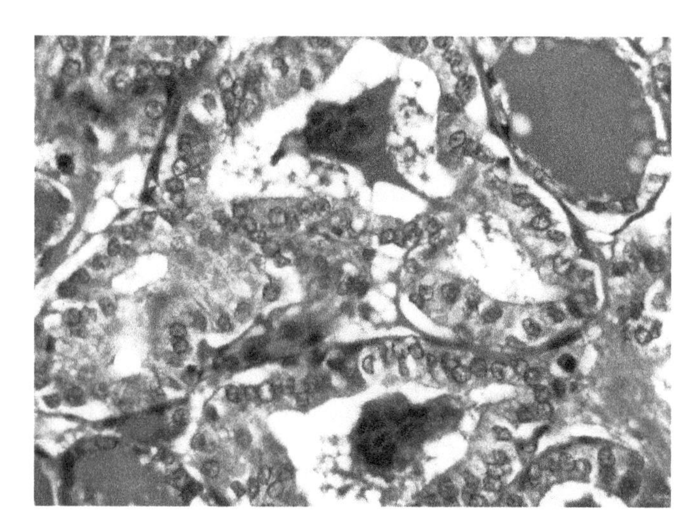

Fig. 3.5.5.2 Papillary carcinoma. The pattern is follicular with colloid apparent in a few follicles. Multinucleated histiocytes (giant cells) are conspicuous. Haematoxylin and eosin, high magnification.

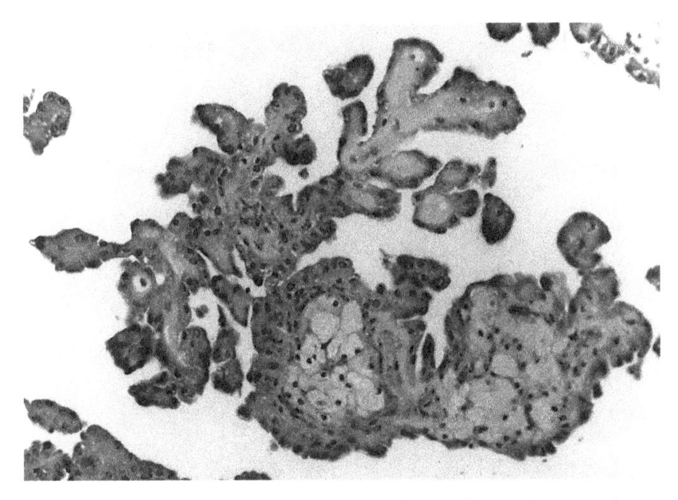

Fig. 3.5.5.3 Papillary carcinoma, cystic variant. The papillae vary in size, and their surfaces are covered by irregular neoplastic cells. Note the clusters of foamy histiocytes within the papillae. Haematoxylin and eosin, medium magnification.

the cancer is encapsulated) may lead to a misinterpretation of the tumour as follicular adenoma or follicular carcinoma. If the follicles are medium-sized and filled with colloid, the lesion may be mistaken for an adenomatoid nodule on both gross and microscopic examination (especially if the pathologist does not examine the lesion carefully).

Cystic change is fairly common in papillary carcinoma and occasionally it is so extensive that the neoplasm appears as a fluid-filled sac with only rare papillae visible (Fig. 3.5.5.3). Small solid foci are common in papillary cancers. Extensive solid regions are probably most common in papillary carcinomas of children and young adults. Occasionally a cancer appears solid, very rarely because of a true solid pattern, but more often because its follicles are closed and lack colloid or because papillae are crowded tightly together.

Although the name suggests otherwise, some of these cancers lack papillae. Instead, they are usually defined by the characteristic neoplastic cells which are two to four times the size of normal follicular cells with relatively large ovoid nuclei. Many of these nuclei are irregular in shape (Fig. 3.5.5.2) with grooves or folding. Variations in nuclear size may be notable. Rather frequently, cytoplasm extends into the nucleus, producing a pseudoinclusion. Nuclei frequently have a pale or clear (ground glass) appearance because the heterochromatin tends to lie next to the nuclear membrane and the nucleoli tend to be in the peripheral parts also. Not all nuclei are so distinctive; a considerable number may be generally regular in shape and sometimes may stain quite darkly.

On aspiration there is a gritty sensation as the needle is inserted (as if one would be piercing an apple). The smears show many neoplastic cells arranged in clusters and sheets with crowded and overlapping nuclei, papillary fragments (with or without vascular cores), and single cells. These cells are enlarged and their cytoplasm is often dense with well-demarcated borders (Fig. 3.5.5.4). Many nuclei are three times the size of the erythrocytes, but considerable variations in size and shape are evident. The chromatin is dense, the nuclear outline is sharp, and nucleoli are inconspicuous. Intranuclear cytoplasmic pseudoinclusions are seen frequently. Nuclear grooves are more readily seen in Papanicolaou-stained smears, multinucleated histiocytes are common, psammoma bodies occur in 30–40% of these cancers, and colloid is usually scant. In my experience, the presence of characteristic dense pink colloid

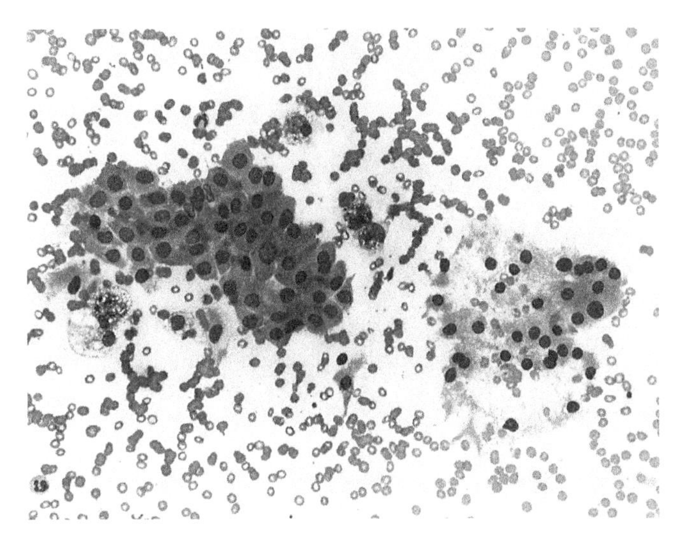

Fig. 3.5.5.4 Papillary carcinoma. The cluster of neoplastic cells to the left (with dense cytoplasm, sharply demarcated borders, and enlarged nuclei) contrast with the non-neoplastic follicular cells to the right. FNA smear, Diff-Quik, medium magnification.

(ropy colloid, bubble-gum colloid) is more important than the amount present. For more detailed descriptions of the cytological diagnostic criteria in the fine-needle aspirates, I refer the readers to previous publications (4, 13–15).

The follicular variant usually yields very cellular smears with empty follicles that are readily visible (Fig. 3.5.5.5). The cystic variant is one of the leading sources of false-negative diagnosis. The smears show evidence of old haemorrhage (cholesterol crystals, haemosiderin-laden macrophages), and some clusters of neoplastic cells with scalloped borders, enlarged nuclei, and cytoplasm that varies from clear to dense (Fig. 3.5.5.6). A small percentage of papillary carcinomas are more aggressive: some of the trabecular/solid variants (which merge with the poorly differentiated carcinomas), the tall cell variant, and the columnar cell type.

Follicular carcinoma

This tumour is uncommon in the industrialized nations where iodides are readily available. Unlike papillary thyroid cancer, it is

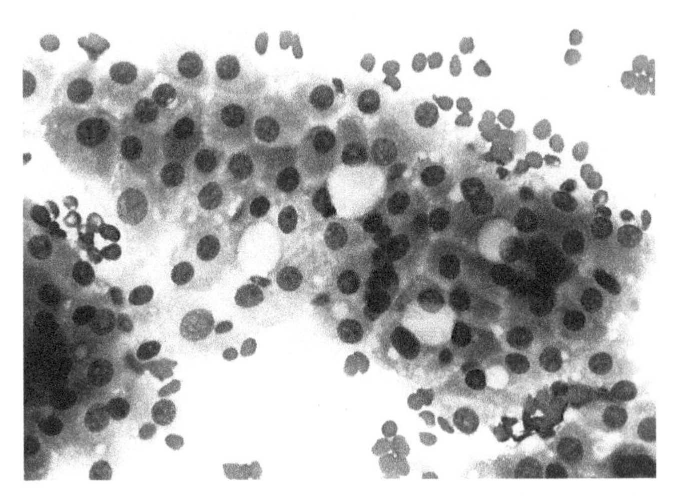

Fig. 3.5.5.5 Papillary carcinoma, follicular variant. The cluster of neoplastic cells has nuclei of various sizes and shapes. Empty follicles are evident. FNA smear, Diff-Quik, high magnification.

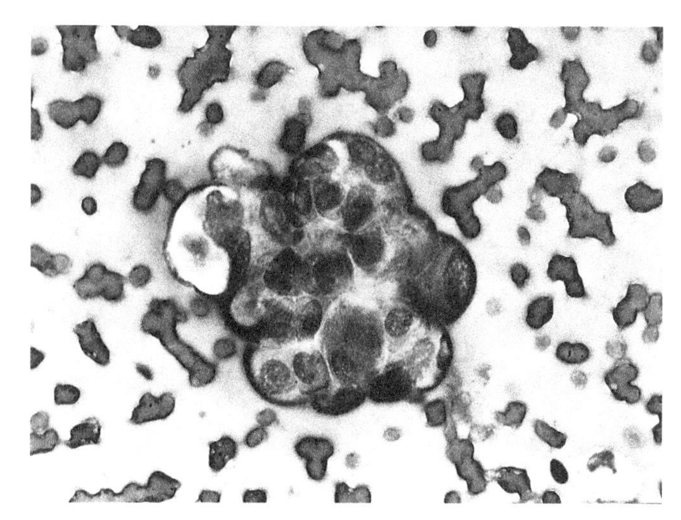

Fig. 3.5.5.6 Papillary carcinoma, cystic variant. The cluster of neoplastic cells has a scalloped outline. Note the variation in nuclear size and shape, and also the differences in the density of the cytoplasm. FNA smear, Diff-Quik, high magnification.

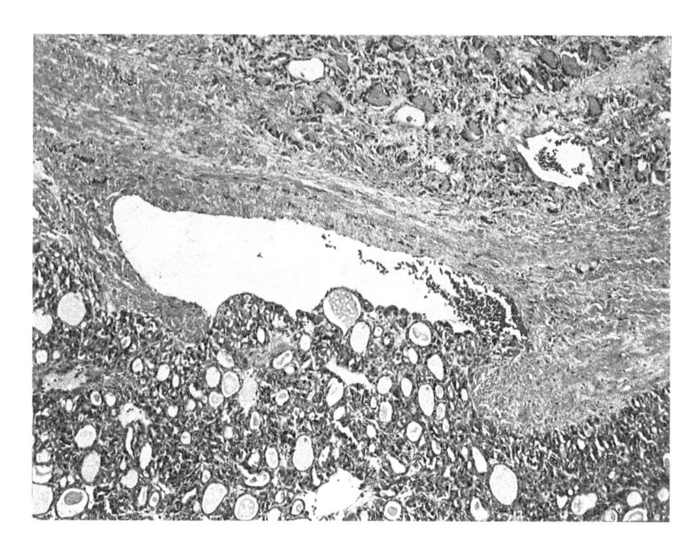

Fig. 3.5.5.7 Follicular carcinoma. Note the thick capsule and the presence of tumour in a capsular vessel. Haematoxylin and eosin, low magnification.

rare in young persons, and fairly often is present in a gland containing adenomatoid nodules. Loss of heterozygosity is common (much more than in papillary carcinoma), especially the result of fractional allelic loss (16, 17). The *ras* mutations have been detected frequently, which is different from their rarity in papillary carcinoma (18).

On gross examination the tumour is a firm fleshy mass, typically well encapsulated and solid, in contrast to any benign nodules also present. The cut surfaces generally are uniform, but while foci of haemorrhage, cystic change, necrosis, and fibrosis can occur, they are rare. In particular, cystic change and fibrosis are rather common in papillary carcinoma and in adenomatoid nodules (the nodules of a benign nodular goitre), but these alterations are uncommon in follicular cancers. Most follicular carcinomas have well-developed capsules, and the smaller ones often have capsules that appear relatively thick. This contrasts with most adenomatoid nodules and follicular adenomas, which have thin or incomplete capsules or none at all. Because these cancers usually do not contain much colloid, they lack the translucent, jelly-like appearance of many adenomatoid nodules.

The microscopic appearance is often monotonous: uniform, medium-sized cells with rounded nuclei, and forming microfollicular, trabecular, and solid patterns. Nuclei may have subtle irregularities of shape and size, but these are considerably less than those evident in papillary carcinoma. Sometimes nucleoli are conspicuous, often in contrast to follicular adenomas. Unfortunately, careful comparisons of nucleoli in the malignant cells with those of adenomas do not yield sufficient differences to permit their usefulness as reliable diagnostic tools. Mitotic figures may be evident, but they may be visible in adenomas also.

Invasion of neoplastic cells into blood vessels at the periphery of the tumour or invasion through the tumour's capsule are the criteria required for the definite diagnosis of malignancy (Fig. 3.5.5.7). Most follicular carcinomas are minimally invasive when diagnosed, which means they are difficult to differentiate from adenomas, but this feature also indicates a small chance of metastatic foci and a good prognosis. The widely invasive follicular carcinomas are uncommon and often have sufficient disruption of their capsules to be suspected on careful gross inspection. Also, these tumours are usually larger and occur in older patients. Follicular adenoma and follicular carcinoma cannot be differentiated cytologically; on aspirates, only the diagnosis of 'follicular neoplasm' can be made. Separating these two entities requires histological examination of the surgically excised specimen for capsular and vascular invasion, as previously stated.

These neoplasms bleed easily when aspirated, and many samples are diluted by blood and appear hypocellular. A more experienced aspirator may obtain hypercellular smears ('tumour cellularity'). The most characteristic cytological pattern consists of enlarged follicular cells arranged in rosettes, tubules, and microfollicles containing dark blue inspissated colloid (Diff-Quik stained smears) (Figs. 3.5.5.8 and 3.5.5.9). These neoplastic follicles have enlarged cells with delicate cytoplasm of pale pink or bluish tint. The rounded nuclei have chromatin of variable density which gives them a mottled appearance. The nuclear borders are slightly irregular, and the nucleoli are usually visible. There is no colloid in the background, but red blood cells are numerous.

It has been suggested that the follicular carcinomas that are better differentiated (forming follicles rather than composed mostly

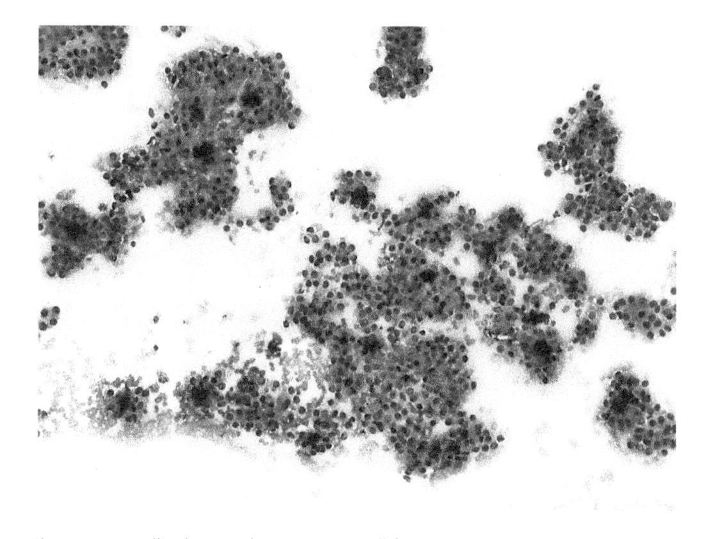

Fig. 3.5.5.8 Follicular neoplasm. Many small follicles are evident and have dense inspissated colloid. FNA smear, Diff-Quik, low magnification.

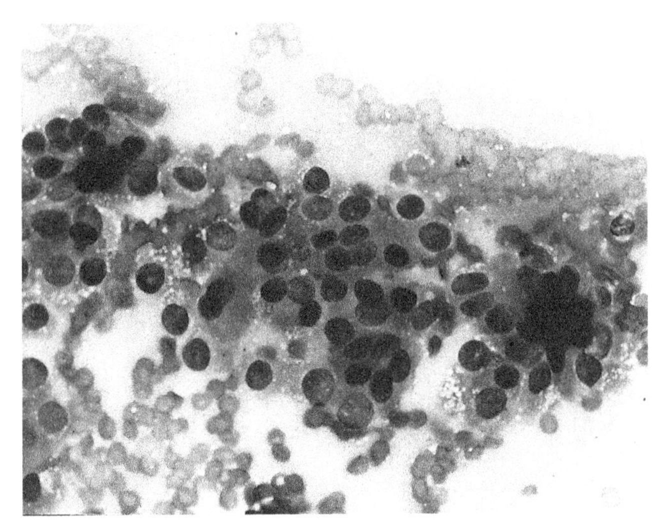

Fig. 3.5.5.9 Follicular neoplasm. To the left and right of the field there are two follicles with dense colloid filling their lumina. FNA smear, Diff-Quik, high magnification.

of trabeculae and solid regions) may have a better prognosis. This is difficult to evaluate because of the scarcity of the tumours and the difficulty of separating this factor from the size of the tumour, its extent, and the age and sex of the patient.

Follicular carcinoma of oxyphilic cells

Oxyphilic cells also are called oncocytes, Askanazy cells, Hürthle cells, and mitochondrion-rich cells. The tumours composed of these cells are probably of a higher grade of malignancy than those composed of nonoxyphilic cells. They tend to have trabecular and solid patterns, usually without much colloid, and often have large uniform cells. Binucleation is common and so too are conspicuous nucleoli; these cellular characteristics are evident in the cytological smears (14). Aspirates are cell-rich and have numerous tissue fragments. Neoplastic follicles with empty lumina are seen more frequently than those with inspissated colloid. Spontaneous infarction of the neoplasms as well as following aspiration is relatively common.

Poorly differentiated carcinoma

This is rare, occurs mostly in middle-aged and elderly patients, and seems to have a rather poor prognosis. The number of cases published is small, and a considerable number of the patients probably did not have the benefit of total thyroidectomy followed by prompt radioactive iodine therapy. An exact definition has not been developed. Sakamoto *et al.* (19) emphasized the presence of extensive trabecular and solid regions in neoplasms that could be recognized as papillary or follicular in type. Also, they believed that elongated strands of neoplastic cells embedded in dense fibrosis were indicative of an aggressive tumour. Carcangiu *et al.* (20) followed Langhans in emphasizing the presence of solid islands of relatively uniform small- to medium-sized cells (thus the term 'insular' carcinoma). Tiny follicles in the solid regions and immunoreactive thyroglobulin in many neoplastic cells have been described. Aspirates are markedly cellular and the neoplastic cells are arranged predominantly in rosettes and clusters with crowded nuclei. Some atypical cells with pleomorphic nuclei are seen, and occasionally cells with 'intranuclear cytoplasmic pseudoinclusions' (21).

Anaplastic carcinoma (undifferentiated carcinoma)

This is rare and is unlikely to occur in any patient before middle age and lacking a long history of a thyroid tumour or multinodular goitre. Very rapid growth is usually noted. Substantial evidence exists that these neoplasms arise from well-differentiated carcinomas, very rarely from poorly differentiated carcinoma, and perhaps from an adenomatoid nodule or adenoma that has been present for many years. Usually a careful search of an anaplastic carcinoma that has undergone extensive resection will demonstrate one or more small regions of well-differentiated carcinoma. Immunoreactive keratin is sometimes found in a putative anaplastic thyroid carcinoma, providing some evidence of epithelial differentiation, but detection of thyroglobulin in a convincing fashion rarely occurs. Consequently the diagnosis of an anaplastic carcinoma requires consideration of all aspects of the patient's history, clinical findings, and pathological data.

Multiple aspirates are required to obtain representative cellular material. Also, extensive necrosis and haemorrhage may be present, and therefore some smears may be hypocellular; the few cells that are observed may be bizarre. In other cases the smears are hypercellular and composed of spindled cells and/or pleomorphic cells. Multinucleated cells may be frequent; they are either histiocytic (osteoclast-like) or pleomorphic neoplastic cells (13, 14, 22).

Certain aspects of this neoplasm deserve comment. If the entire clinical and pathological findings are not characteristic of an anaplastic thyroid carcinoma, then the possibility of a sarcoma of the neck deserves consideration. These are rare, of course, and may be difficult to separate from the carcinoma. Very rarely, the anaplastic carcinoma is composed mostly of fibroblasts and inflammatory cells, with few neoplastic cells visible. This 'paucicellular' variant might be difficult to recognize by the pathologist, who could mistakenly suggest the fibrosing variant of Hashimoto's thyroiditis or fibrosclerosis (Riedel's struma). Because extensive fibrosis and inflammation can accompany an anaplastic carcinoma, a small biopsy or limited sampling by FNA could be misleading.

Squamous characteristics may occur in anaplastic thyroid cancer and anaplastic foci can occur in squamous thyroid cancers. Also, the squamous neoplasms are very aggressive. Consequently, some pathologists consider squamous thyroid carcinoma as a part of anaplastic thyroid carcinomas.

Medullary carcinoma

It apparently originates from C cells and usually has a distinctive appearance. Most of these cancers are solid and have an insular pattern (Fig. 3.5.5.10); they lack thyroglobulin and nearly always have demonstrable calcitonin. The cells are rounded, polygonal, or spindled. A common characteristic is the deposition of amyloid, which varies greatly in amount from one tumour to another and has to be differentiated from dense collagen (Fig. 3.5.5.11). Occasional examples have gland-like structures (simulating follicles), trabecular patterns can occur, and sometimes the neoplastic cells are quite small (simulating those of poorly differentiated carcinoma), so the pathologist must study these tumours carefully (23). All solid thyroid tumours should be evaluated with antibodies for calcitonin. Usually the tumours are invasive, and they spread through lymphatics and blood vessels.

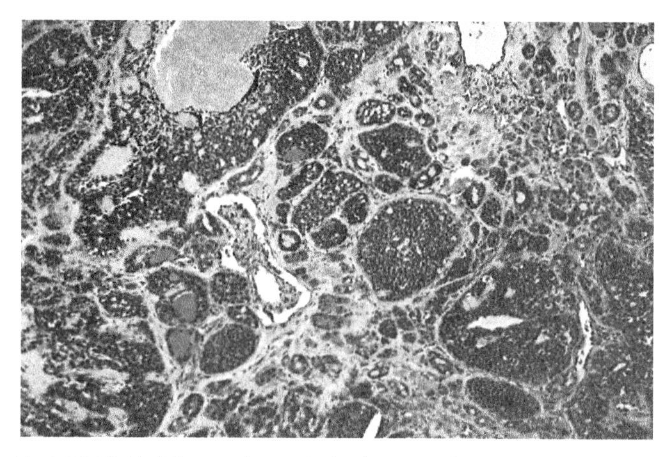

Fig. 3.5.5.10 Medullary carcinoma. An insular pattern is apparent. Haematoxylin and eosin, low magnification.

Germline mutations of the *ret* proto-oncogene are associated with multiple endocrine neoplasia types 2A and 2B, and familial medullary carcinoma. Some patients with sporadic medullary carcinoma have somatic mutations of *ret* (9). The familial type is typically bilateral.

Smears are markedly cellular. Loosely cohesive clusters of rounded polygonal or spindled cells (Fig. 3.5.5.12) are observed in a haemorrhagic background with many single neoplastic cells. In some cases the neoplastic cells have round nuclei, eccentrically located, which produces a plasmacytoid appearance (24, 25). In other cases the spindled cells predominate (Fig. 3.5.5.12). Frequently, large neoplastic cells with enlarged single or multiple nuclei are present (Fig. 3.5.5.13). Intranuclear cytoplasmic inclusions are observed in some cases (26), but nucleoli are rarely visible. The cytoplasm has variable tinctorial characteristics, from dense and bluish-pink in the plasmacytoid cells to attenuated and pale blue in the bizarre neoplastic cells. The presence of calcitonin cytoplasmic granules that stain bright pink with haematological stains has been overemphasized in the literature (27, 28). In my experience they are found in about one-third of the cases and only after a tedious search.

The features I find most helpful in making the cytological diagnosis are tumour cellularity, lack of cellular cohesiveness, plasmacytoid appearance of many cells (in some cases), scattered very large tumour cells with bizarre single or multiple nuclei

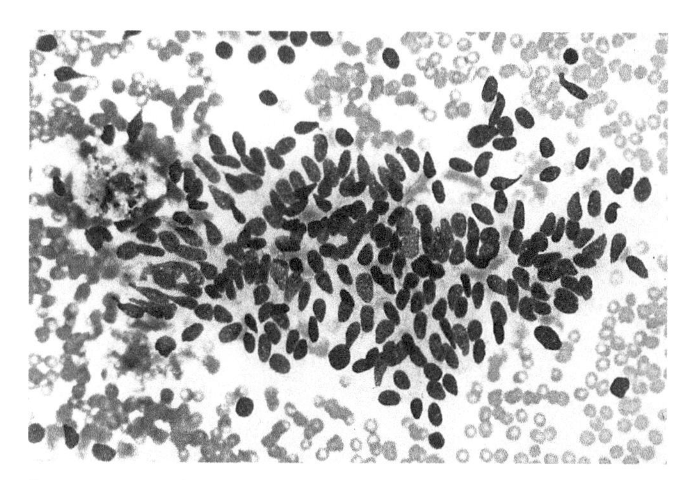

Fig. 3.5.5.12 Medullary carcinoma. The cluster of neoplastic cells has spindled nuclei and pale delicate cytoplasm. FNA smear, Diff-Quik, high magnification.

(Fig. 3.5.5.13), and the general absence of visible nucleoli. This is largely a diagnosis of exclusion because the smears are not typical of the most common thyroidal neoplasms.

Malignant lymphoma

Malignant lymphoma nearly always arises in a thyroid affected by diffuse or focal lymphocytic thyroiditis (autoimmune thyroiditis, Hashimoto's thyroiditis). The patients are usually middle-aged to elderly women. Rather often there is rapid enlargement of part of the gland. Unless multiple aspirations are performed, the varied infiltrate of autoimmune thyroiditis may be seen and the complete diagnosis is not made. Many lymphomas are B-cell types, often rather low grade, and are confined to the thyroid. Unfortunately, the patient with a long history of goitre (which suddenly has enlarged) may have a high-grade lymphoma which has originated in a low-grade lymphoma.

Microscopic examination of a thyroidal lymphoma reveals extensive effacement of the architecture of the gland by a monotonous infiltrate of abnormal lymphoid cells. Evidence of Hashimoto's thyroiditis usually can be found (e.g. lymphoid follicular centres, oxyphilic metaplasia of the thyroid epithelium). Some thyroid vessels may have their walls infiltrated by lymphoma cells.

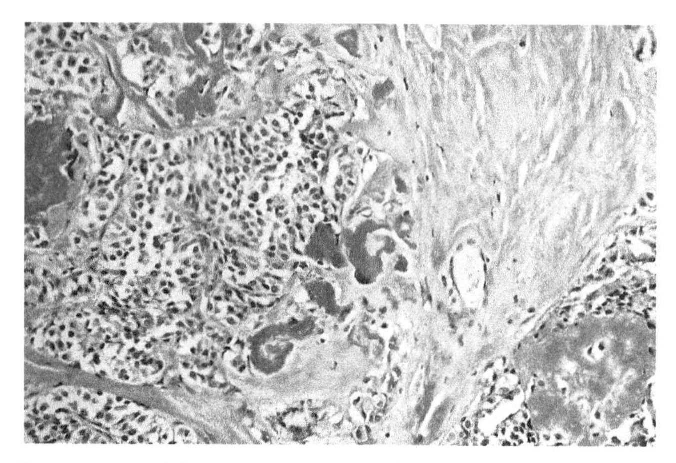

Fig. 3.5.5.11 Medullary carcinoma. Deposits of darker staining amyloid contrast with the considerable amount of collagenous tissue present. Haematoxylin and eosin, medium magnification.

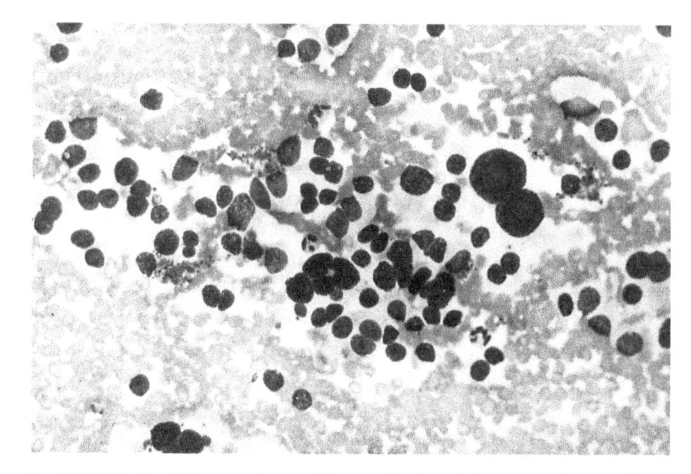

Fig. 3.5.5.13 Medullary carcinoma. The neoplastic cells have round to ovoid nuclei which vary markedly in size. Note bizarre binucleated cell. FNA smear, Diff-Quik, high magnification.

Many thyroid follicles have lost their colloid and are distended by lymphoma cells. Smears from FNAs contain a monotonous lymphoid population, fairly numerous mitotic figures, and general absence of follicular epithelial cells (22, 29).

Secondary or metastatic tumours

The neoplasms that most frequently spread to the thyroid gland are carcinomas of the lung, kidney, and breast. The metastasis may present as a dominant nodule. Malignant melanoma is also a frequent source of metastases. The histological and cytological appearance will depend on the site of the primary neoplasm. A feature that I find helpful in the cytological diagnosis of the smears is the presence of sheets of benign follicular epithelial cells (with their characteristic 'paravacuolar cytoplasmic granules') mixed with the neoplastic cells.

References

1. Gharib H, Papini E, Valcavi R. American Association of Clinical Endocrinologists and Associazione Medici Endocrinologi Medical Guidelines for clinical practice for the diagnosis and management of thyroid nodules. *Endocr Pract*, 2006; **12**: 63–102.
2. Cooper DS, Doherty GM, Haugen BR, Kloos RT, Lee S, Mandel S, *et al.* Management guidelines for patients with thyroid nodules and differentiated thyroid cancer. The American Thyroid Association Guidelines Taskforce. *Thyroid*, 2006; **16**: 1–33.
3. Oertel YC. Fine-needle aspiration: a personal view. *Lab Med*, 1982; **13**: 343–7.
4. Oertel YC. Fine-needle aspiration of the thyroid. In: Moore WT, Eastman RC, eds. *Diagnostic Endocrinology*. 2nd edn. St. Louis: Mosby, 1996: 211–28.
5. Oertel YC. Fine-needle aspiration of the thyroid: technique and terminology. *Endocrinol Metab Clin North Am*, 2007; **36**: 737–51.
6. Ljung B-M, Langer J, Mazzaferri EL, Oertel YC, Wells SA, Waisman J. Training, credentialing and re-credentialing for the performance of a thyroid FNA: a synopsis of the National Cancer Institute thyroid fine-needle aspiration state of the science conference. *Diagn Cytopathol*, 2008; **36**: 400–6.
7. Hedinger CE, Williams ED, Sobin LH. *Histological Typing of Thyroid Tumors*. 2nd edn. Berlin: Springer, 1988: 66.
8. Rosai J, Carcangiu ML, DeLellis RA. *Tumors of the Thyroid Gland*. 3rd series edn. Washington, DC: Armed Forces Institute of Pathology, 1993: 343.
9. Komminoth P. *RET* proto-oncogene and thyroid cancer. *Endocr Pathol*, 1997; **8**: 235–39.
10. Jossart GH, Grossman RF. Thyroid oncogenesis. In: Clark OH, Duh Q-Y, eds. *Textbook of Endocrine Surgery*. 3rd edn. Philadelphia: Saunders, 1997: 237–42.
11. Matsubayashi S, Kawai K, Matsumoto Y, Mukuta T, Morita T, Hirai K, *et al.* The correlation between papillary thyroid carcinoma and lymphocytic infiltration in the thyroid gland. *J Clin Endocrinol Metab*, 1995; **80**: 3421–4.
12. Takahashi MH, Thomas GA, Williams ED. Evidence for mutual interdependence of epithelium and stromal lymphoid cells in a subset of papillary carcinoma. *Br J Cancer*, 1995; **72**: 813–17.
13. Oertel YC. Fine-needle aspiration and the diagnosis of thyroid cancer. *Endocrinol Metab Clin North Am*, 1996; **25**: 69–91.
14. Oertel YC. Fine-needle aspiration in the evaluation of thyroid neoplasms. *Endocr Pathol*, 1997; **8**: 215–24.
15. Gallagher J, Oertel YC, Oertel JE. Follicular variant of papillary carcinoma of the thyroid: fine-needle aspirates with histologic correlation. *Diagn Cytopathol*, 1997; **16**: 207–13.
16. Tung WS, Shevlin DW, Kaleem Z, Tribune DJ, Wells Jr SA, Goodfellow PJ. Allelotype of follicular thyroid carcinomas reveals genetic instability consistent with frequent nondisjunctional chromosomal loss. *Genes Chromosomes Cancer*, 1997; **19**: 43–51.
17. Ward LS, Brenta G, Medvedovic M, Fagin JA. Studies of allelic loss in thyroid tumors reveal major differences in chromosomal instability between papillary and follicular carcinomas. *J Clin Endocrinol Metab*, 1998; **83**: 525–30.
18. Manenti G, Pilotti S, Re FC, Della Porta G, Pierotti MA. Selective activation of *ras* oncogenes in follicular and undifferentiated thyroid carcinomas. *Eur J Cancer*, 1994; **30A**: 987–93.
19. Sakamoto A, Kasai N, Suganu H. Poorly differentiated carcinoma of the thyroid. A clinicopathologic entity for a high-risk group of papillary and follicular carcinomas. *Cancer*, 1983; **52**: 1849–55.
20. Carcangiu ML, Zampi G, Rosai J. Poorly differentiated ('insular') thyroid carcinoma. A reinterpretation of Langhans' 'wuchernde Struma'. *Am J Surg Pathol*, 1984; **8**: 655–68.
21. Oertel YC, Miyahara-Felipe L. Cytologic features of insular carcinoma of the thyroid: a case report. *Diagn Cytopathol*, 2006; **34**: 572–5.
22. Kini SR. *Thyroid*. 2nd edn. New York: Igaku-Shoin, 1996: 521.
23. Bussolati G, Papotti M, Pagani A. Diagnostic problems in medullary carcinoma of the thyroid. *Pathol Res Pract*, 1995; **191**: 332–44.
24. Kini SR, Miller JM, Hamburger JI, Smith MJ. Cytopathologic features of medullary carcinoma of the thyroid. *Arch Pathol Lab Med*, 1984; **108**: 156–9.
25. Collins BT, Cramer HM, Tabatowski K, Hearn S, Raminhos A, Lampe H. Fine needle aspiration of medullary carcinoma of the thyroid. Cytomorphology, immunocytochemistry and electron microscopy. *Acta Cytol*, 1995; **39**: 920–30.
26. Schaffer R, Muller H-A, Pfeifer U, Ormanns W. Cytological findings in medullary carcinoma of the thyroid. *Pathol Res Pract*, 1984; **178**: 461–6.
27. Mendonca ME, Ramos S, Soares J. Medullary carcinoma of thyroid: a re-evaluation of the cytological criteria of diagnosis. *Cytopathology*, 1991; **2**: 93–102.
28. Bose S, Kapila K, Verma K. Medullary carcinoma of the thyroid: a cytological, immunocytochemical, and ultrastructural study. *Diagn Cytopathol*, 1992; **8**: 28–32.
29. Mazzaferri EL, Oertel YC. Thyroid lymphoma. In: Mazzaferri EL, Samaan NA, eds. *Endocrine Tumors*. 1st edn. Boston: Blackwell Scientific Publications, 1993.

Further reading

Hedinger C, Williams ED, Sobin LH. *Histological Typing of Thyroid Tumours. World Health Organization International Histological Classification of Tumours*. 2nd edn. Berlin: Springer, 1988. (This represents a widely utilized classification of thyroidal neoplasms.)

Rosai J, Carcangiu ML, DeLellis RA. Tumors of the thyroid gland. In: Rosai J, Sobin LH, eds. *Atlas of Tumor Pathology*. 3rd series. Fascicle 5. Washington, DC: Armed Forces Institute of Pathology, 1992. (This provides a useful survey of the pathological features of benign and malignant thyroid neoplasms.)

3.5.6 Papillary, follicular, and anaplastic thyroid carcinoma and lymphoma

Sophie Leboulleux, Martin Jean Schlumberger

Introduction

Papillary and follicular thyroid carcinomas are the most frequent forms of thyroid cancers and are among the most curable cancers. However, some patients are at high risk of recurrence or even death from their cancer, and can be identified at the time of diagnosis using well-established prognostic indicators (1–3). The apparent increase in the incidence of thyroid carcinomas observed in recent years is mainly related to an increased detection of low risk small carcinomas in adults, which is attributed to an improvement in diagnostic techniques (4, 5). This leads to the treatment of an increasing number of low-risk patients for whom an optimal quality of life should be maintained. However, the number of high-risk patients remains unchanged and these patients require aggressive treatment and follow-up. The extent of initial treatment and follow-up should therefore be individualized according to recent guidelines and consensus (6, 7).

Diagnosis

Most differentiated thyroid carcinomas present as asymptomatic thyroid nodules, but occasionally the first signs of the disease are lymph node metastases and rarely lung or bone metastases. Hoarseness, dysphagia, cough, and dyspnoea are suggestive of advanced stages of the disease. At physical examination, the carcinoma, usually single, is firm, freely moveable during swallowing, and not easily distinguishable from a benign nodule. A thyroid nodule should be suspected of being a carcinoma when it is found in children or adolescents or in men above 60 years of age, when it is hard and irregular, when ipsilateral lymph nodes are enlarged or compressive symptoms are present, and when there is a history of progressive increase in size. Virtually all patients are clinically euthyroid and have normal serum thyrotropin concentrations.

Thyroid ultrasonography is useful for assessing the characteristics of the nodule and detecting other nodules and lymph node enlargement, and to guide the fine-needle biopsy. Suspicious ultrasonographic findings are taller than wide shape, marked hypoechogenicity, spiculated margins, microcalcifications and macrocalcifications, and hypervascularization; isoechogenicity of the nodule in conjunction with a spongiform appearance are reliable criteria for benign nodules (8). Whatever the presentation, fine-needle aspiration cytology is the best test for diagnosing a papillary thyroid carcinoma. Provided an adequate specimen is obtained (6, 7, 9), three cytological results are possible: benign, malignant, and indeterminate (or suspicious). Among indeterminate results, only 20% are from malignant nodules, reflecting the difficulty of differentiating benign follicular or oncocytic adenomas from their malignant counterparts.

Prognostic indicators

The overall 10-year survival rates for middle-aged adults with thyroid carcinomas are about 80–95% (Table 3.5.6.1). Five to 15% of patients have local or regional recurrences and 5–10% have distant metastases. Prognostic indicators of recurrence and of death are age at diagnosis, histological type, and extent of the tumour (1–3, 10).

There are many scoring systems for thyroid carcinoma, among which the pTNM staging system is the most widely accepted (Table 3.5.6.2) (11). Based on this system, 80–85% of patients are classified as being at low risk of cancer-specific mortality. Some patients have a higher risk of recurrences. They include young (<16 years) and older (>45 years) patients, and those with large tumours, extension of the tumour beyond the thyroid capsule, or lymph node metastases. Finally, patients with certain histological subtypes (tall cell, columnar cell, and diffuse-sclerosing variants), and those with poorly differentiated carcinoma (12, 13) may have a higher risk of both recurrence and tumour-related death.

Table 3.5.6.1 Proportion of various histotypes among malignant thyroid tumours, and overall 10-year survival rates for each histotype in the absence of distant metastases

	Proportion (%)	Overall 10-year survival rates (%)
Differentiated thyroid cancer	85	
Papillary	65	95
Follicular	20	90
Poorly differentiated	<10	50
Other thyroid tumours	15	
Anaplastic	<5	<20
Medullary	5–10	65
Rare tumours	<5	

Initial treatment

Surgery

The goal of surgery is to remove all neoplastic neck tissue. A neck ultrasonography is performed preoperatively, but can detect only one-half of metastatic lymph nodes. Total thyroidectomy is advocated for all patients with thyroid cancer (6, 7). It reduces the recurrence rate as compared with more limited surgery because many papillary carcinomas are multifocal and bilateral. Removal of most if not all of the thyroid gland facilitates total ablation with ^{131}I. However, total thyroidectomy may increase the risk of recurrent laryngeal nerve injury and hypoparathyroidism, but morbidity remains low when performed by an experienced surgeon. A lobectomy may be appropriate only in patients with papillary carcinomas less than 1 cm in diameter, if unifocal and intralobar (6, 7, 14).

Table 3.5.6.2 TNM staging system for papillary and follicular thyroid carcinoma

Stage	Age <45 years	Age >45 years
I	Any T, Any N, M0	T1, N0, M0
II	Any T, Any N, M1	T2, N0, M0
III		T3, N0, M0 or any T1–3, N1a, M0
IVA		T1–3, N1b, M0 or T4a, Any N, M0 N, M0
IVB		T4b, Any N, M0
IVC		Any T, Any N, M1

Primary tumour (T): T1, tumour ≤2 cm limited to the thyroid; T2, tumour >2 to ≤4 cm limited to the thyroid; T3, tumour >4 cm limited to the thyroid or any tumour with minimal extrathyroidal extension (e.g. extension to sternothyroid muscle or perithyroidal soft tissues); T4a, tumour of any size with extension beyond the thyroid capsule and invading any of the following: subcutaneous soft tissues, larynx, trachea, oesophagus, recurrent laryngeal nerve; T4b, tumour invading prevertebral fascia, mediastinal vessels, or encases carotid artery.

Lymph nodes (N): To classify as N0 or N1, at least six lymph nodes should be examined at histology. Otherwise, the tumour is classified as Nx. N0, no regional lymph node metastasis; N1a, metastases in pretracheal and paratracheal, including prelaryngeal and Delphian lymph nodes; N1b, metastases in other unilateral, bilateral, or contralateral cervical or upper mediastinal lymph nodes.

Distant metastases (M): M0, no distant metastasis; M1, distant metastasis.

In patients who underwent a lobectomy for a supposedly benign tumour that proves to be a follicular carcinoma, a completion thyroidectomy should be offered to those patients for whom a near-total or total thyroidectomy would have been recommended had the diagnosis been available before the initial surgery.

Lymph node dissection is routinely performed in patients with known lymph node involvement, as demonstrated pre- or peroperatively. It includes a dissection of the central compartment (level VI), defined as the removal of lymph nodes and soft tissue from the hyoid bone superiorly, to the great vessels inferiorly and to the jugular veins laterally and may also include a dissection of the supraclavicular area and the lower one-third of the jugulo-carotid chain (levels III and IV). In the absence of demonstrated lymph node metastases, several arguments support its routine use in patients with large papillary carcinomas: (1) about two-thirds of patients have lymph node metastases, more than 80% of whom have involvement of the central compartment (15); (2) metastases are difficult to detect in lymph nodes located behind the vessels or in the paratracheal groove; and (3) it has improved the recurrence and survival rates in several series. In patients with small (T1–T2) papillary carcinomas, the indication for prophylactic lymph node dissection is controversial, but the knowledge of lymph node status will help to better define the indication for postoperative ^{131}I therapy (16).

Iodine-131 therapy

Iodine-131 therapy is given postoperatively for three reasons: (1) it destroys normal thyroid remnants, thereby increasing the sensitivity and the specificity of serum thyroglobulin measurement for the detection of persistent or recurrent disease; (2) it may destroy occult microscopic carcinoma, thereby decreasing the long-term recurrence rate; and (3) it permits a postablative total body scan, a sensitive tool for the detection of persistent carcinoma (6, 7).

Iodine-131 therapy is administered 4–6 weeks after surgery, during which no thyroid hormone treatment is given to achieve a serum thyroid-stimulating hormone (TSH) level above 30 mU/l. As an alternative, thyroxine treatment may be given after surgery and recombinant human TSH (rhTSH) injected (0.9 mg intramuscularly on two consecutive days) and ^{131}I given on the day after the second injection (17); this method avoids hypothyroidism, maintains the quality of life, reduces the body radiation exposure, and shortens the length of hospitalization (18–20). Patients should be instructed to avoid iodine-containing medications and iodine-rich foods, and urinary iodine should be measured in doubtful cases. Pregnancy must be excluded in women of childbearing age. Education of the patient with written documents is mandatory before any administration of radio-iodine. Total ablation (undetectable stimulated serum thyroglobulin with normal neck ultrasonography) is achieved 6–12 months later, after the administration of either 100 mCi (3700 MBq) or 30 mCi (1100 MBq) in almost all patients who had a total thyroidectomy (17, 21). Total ablation requires a dose of at least 300 Gy delivered to thyroid remnants, and a dosimetric study allows to estimate more precisely the activity of ^{131}I to be administered (22).

A total body scan is carried out 3–7 days later, and thyroxine therapy is maintained or is initiated in case of withdrawal. This total body scan is informative for the detection of neoplastic uptake foci outside the thyroid bed when uptake in thyroid remnants is less than 1%. The fusion of scintigraphy images with anatomical CT images on a dedicated gamma camera improves both the sensitivity and the specificity of the technique (23).

Simple methods are used for minimizing body irradiation, improving the quality of scanning images, and reducing the risk of false-positive images: lemon juice decreases uptake in salivary glands, ingestion of large quantities of liquid decreases bladder and gonad irradiation, and laxative treatment decreases colon contamination. Furthermore, patients are invited to take a shower and to wear clean clothes before scanning. False-positive results are rare and are usually easily recognized. They may be related to skin contamination, axillary perspiration, to salivary glands, to the presence of radioactive saliva in the mouth and oesophagus, to thymus hypertrophy, or to various conditions such as pleuropericardial cyst or inflammatory processes.

A diagnostic total body scan with 2 mCi (74 MBq) ^{131}I may be performed before ^{131}I therapy only when less than a total thyroidectomy has been performed, in order to assess the size of thyroid remnants; however, it may induce stunning (24). A low or undetectable serum thyroglobulin level obtained on the day of ^{131}I administration is predictive of a favourable outcome (25).

Postoperative ^{131}I therapy should be used selectively (Table 3.5.6.3) (6, 7). In very low-risk patients, the long-term prognosis after surgery alone is so favourable that ^{131}I ablation is usually not recommended. Patients who are at high risk of recurrence or in whom resection of the neoplastic tissue was incomplete, or who have known distant metastases are routinely treated with a high activity of ^{131}I (100 mCi or more) following thyroid hormone treatment withdrawal, because ^{131}I treatment improves the outcome. Finally, for the other patients, there is no firm evidence that ^{131}I treatment may improve the outcome, and a high (100 mCi or more) or a low (30 mCi) ^{131}I activity may be administered following either thyroid hormone treatment withdrawal or rhTSH.

External radiotherapy

External radiotherapy to the neck and mediastinum is indicated only in patients older than 45 years in whom surgical excision has been incomplete or impossible, and in whom the tumour tissue does not take up ^{131}I (26).

Follow-up

The goals of follow-up after initial therapy are to maintain adequate thyroxine therapy and to detect persistent or recurrent thyroid

Table 3.5.6.3 Indications for ^{131}I ablative treatment in patients with thyroid carcinoma after initial surgery

Patient group	Tumour staging	Comments
Very low risk patients	T <1 cm, unifocal, intrathyroidal, and N0	No benefits, no indication
High risk patients	T2–4, large or multiple N1, M1, persistent disease	Treatment with a high activity (100 mCi or more) following thyroid hormone withdrawal
Low risk patients	All others	Controversial benefits. Ablation may be performed with either a low (30 mCi) or high (100 mCi) activity and following either thyroid hormone withdrawal or rhTSH

carcinoma. Most recurrences occur during the first years of follow-up, but some occur late. Therefore, follow-up is necessary throughout the patient's life.

Thyroxine treatment

Thyroxine is given to all patients with thyroid carcinoma to restore euthyroidism. Also, the growth of thyroid tumour cells is stimulated by thyrotropin (TSH) and inhibition of thyrotropin secretion with thyroxine improves the recurrence and survival rates, but only in high-risk patients. TSH suppression is achieved in such patients and in those with any evidence of disease; in low-risk patients with no evidence of disease, the risk of recurrence is so low that total suppression is not justified and serum TSH is maintained within the normal range (27). The initial daily dose is 2.2 μg/kg body weight in adults; children require higher doses. The adequacy of therapy is monitored by measuring serum TSH 3 months after it is begun, the initial goal being a serum TSH concentration of not more than 0.1 μU/ml and a serum free triiodothyronine concentration within the normal range to avoid overdosing.

Early detection of recurrent disease

Clinical and ultrasonographic examinations

Palpation and ultrasonography of the thyroid bed and lymph node areas are routinely performed. Lymph nodes that are small, thin, or oval, in the posterior neck chains, and decrease in size after an interval of 3 months are considered benign; suspicious findings are short axis more than 0.5 cm, round shape, loss of fatty hyperechoic hilum, hypoechogenicity, cystic appearance, hyperechoic punctuations, and peripheral vascularization (Table 3.5.6.4) (28). Serum thyroglobulin is undetectable in 20% of patients receiving thyroxine treatment who have isolated lymph node metastases, and undetectable serum thyroglobulin values do not exclude metastatic lymph node disease (29). Suspicious cases should be submitted to an ultrasound-guided node biopsy for cytology and thyroglobulin measurement in the fluid aspirate (30, 31).

Serum thyroglobulin determinations

Thyroglobulin is a glycoprotein that is produced only by normal or neoplastic thyroid follicular cells. It should not be detectable in patients who have had total thyroid ablation, and its detection in them indicates persistent or recurrent disease. The production of thyroglobulin by both normal and neoplastic thyroid tissue is in part TSH dependent.

The functional sensitivity of first-generation thyroglobulin immunometric assays was 1 ng/ml. Because results of serum thyroglobulin determination may be different with various assays, the same assay should be used for the follow-up of a given patient. Serum antithyroglobulin antibodies that are found in about 15–25% of patients with thyroid carcinoma are always sought by a radioimmunoassay because they may induce falsely reduced or falsely negative serum thyroglobulin measurements (32, 33). In patients in complete remission after total thyroid ablation, serum antithyroglobulin antibodies decline with a median time of 3 years to low or undetectable values; their persistence or their reappearance during follow-up should be considered as suspicious for persistent or recurrent disease.

After total ablation in patients on thyroxine treatment, serum thyroglobulin is undetectable in 98% of individuals considered in complete remission. It is detectable in practically all patients with large metastases and often at high levels; however, in this context, about 20% of patients with isolated lymph node metastases and 5% of patients with small lung metastases have an undetectable serum thyroglobulin level. Following withdrawal of thyroid hormone treatment, thyroglobulin concentration will increase in most patients with neoplastic disease and will frequently reach high levels. In this situation, serum thyroglobulin will remain undetectable in less than 5% of patients with isolated lymph node metastases and in less than 1% of patients with small lung metastases. In contrast, serum thyroglobulin will remain undetectable in more than 90% of patients with no other evidence of disease (32, 34, 35). Intramuscular injection of rhTSH is an alternative to withdrawal (0.9 mg intramuscularly for two consecutive days and serum thyroglobulin determination 3 days after the second injection), because thyroxine treatment need not be discontinued and side effects are minimal. The efficacy of rhTSH for the detection of persistent and recurrent disease is similar to that of thyroid hormone withdrawal, and a major advantage of the use of rhTSH is that it avoids hypothyroidism and maintains the quality of life (19, 20, 36, 37). The serum thyroglobulin concentration is an excellent prognostic indicator, and recurrence rate after 12 years is 0.5% in patients with undetectable thyroglobulin following withdrawal or rhTSH stimulation (40, 41) (Box 3.5.6.1).

Table 3.5.6.4 Ultrasound criteria of malignancy for cervical lymph nodes. These criteria may be difficult to interpret in small lymph nodes

	Sensitivity (%)	Specificity (%)
Long axis (>1 cm)	68	75
Short axis (>0.5 cm)	61	96
Round shape	46	64
Loss of fatty hyperechoic hilum	c.100	29
Hypoechogenicity	32	21
Cystic appearance	11	100
Hyperechoic punctuations	46	100
Peripheral vascularization	86	82

From Leboulleux S, Girard E, Rose M, Travagli JP, Sabbah N, Caillou B, *et al.* Ultrasound criteria of malignancy for cervical lymph nodes in patients followed for differentiated thyroid cancer. *J Clin Endocrinol Metab*, 2007; **92**: 3590–4.

Box 3.5.6.1 Advantages of combining neck ultrasonography and serum thyroglobulin determination following recombinant human TSH stimulation at 9–12 months

- In >95% of patients: assessment of cure
  - Reassurance of patients and reassessment of prognosis
  - Decrease L-thyroxine dose to obtain a serum TSH level at 0.5–1 mU/l
  - Avoid any other test
  - Yearly follow-up with clinical examination and determination of serum TSH and thyroglobulin levels during thyroxine treatment
- In <5% of patients: detection of disease that indicates specific treatments

The availability of second-generation thyroglobulin assays with a functional sensitivity of 0.1 ng/ml or even less may reduce the need for routine rhTSH stimulation in low-risk patients with undetectable serum thyroglobulin on thyroxine treatment (38, 39). However, the significance of the frequently observed low but detectable serum thyroglobulin levels is currently unknown. Also, an undetectable serum thyroglobulin following rhTSH stimulation or thyroid hormone withdrawal allows to reassure the patient, to decrease the thyroxine dosage, and to avoid any other testing (Box 3.5.6.1), but whether this can also be done with an undetectable serum thyroglobulin obtained during thyroxine treatment with a second-generation assay has not yet been established.

Imaging modalities

Imaging modalities for the detection of persistent and recurrent disease are indicated only in selected patients. Control ^{131}I total body scan with a diagnostic activity (2–5 mCi) may be performed in patients who had large thyroid remnants at the time of ablation and in whom the post-therapy total body scan was not informative. In patients with an informative post-therapy total body scan that is normal, a control total body scan is not beneficial and for this reason is not recommended on a routine basis (40, 41).

Iodine-131 total body scan is more sensitive for detecting neoplastic foci when it is performed with a high activity (100 mCi or more) than with a low activity (42, 43). It is performed after thyroid hormone withdrawal in patients with high and increasing serum thyroglobulin levels. The discovery of lesions with ^{131}I uptake may indicate further ^{131}I treatments. However, in the absence of such lesions no further ^{131}I treatment should be given.

[^{18}F]2-fluoro-2-deoxy-D-glucose positron emission tomography (FDG-PET)/CT has a sensitivity of 50–100% for the localization of recurrent disease depending on tumour burden and histology subtype (44) (Box 3.5.6.2). Furthermore, treatment changes due to FDG-PET results occur in 20–38% of the cases. FDG-PET is particularly informative in patients with aggressive thyroid cancer such as tall cell, Hürthle cell, or poorly differentiated cancer. FDG-PET and neck–chest CT with contrast-medium injection are complementary, with FDG-PET being more sensitive for the detection of neck and mediastinum lymph nodes and bone metastases and chest CT being more sensitive for the detection of micronodular lung metastases. PET/CT with high-quality CT being performed with contrast-medium injection and respiratory gating will combine the advantages of the two methods. The drawback of FDG-PET is the risk of false-positive lesions that can occur in up to 17% of patients; neck inflammatory lymph nodes with low FDG uptake are frequently seen. FDG uptake increases following rhTSH stimulation, with rhTSH-stimulated FDG-PET showing more lesions than FDG-PET performed during thyroxine treatment (45). Whether rhTSH administration should be performed systematically before FDG-PET has, however, not yet been demonstrated.

Bone involvement is well visualized by MRI or CT and by FDG-PET in cases with FDG uptake. Because bone metastases are osteolytic, bone scintigraphy is usually poorly informative showing a decrease or a moderately increased uptake.

Box 3.5.6.2 Indications for FDG-PET scan in patients with thyroid cancer

- Localization of tumour foci in patients with elevated thyroglobulin/TSH level (>10 ng/ml) and negative imaging (CT scan, neck ultrasonography, ^{131}I total body scan)
- Initial staging and follow-up of patients with Hürthle cell carcinoma or poorly differentiated thyroid cancers unlikely to concentrate ^{131}I, in order to identify sites of disease that may be missed with ^{131}I scanning
- Identification among patients with known distant metastases those who are at highest risk for disease-specific mortality and those who are unlikely to respond to ^{131}I therapy
- Detection of progressive foci in patients with metastatic disease that may need local treatment
- Evaluation of response to external beam irradiation, surgical resection, embolization, radiotherapy, cement injection, or systemic therapy
- Low-risk patients are very unlikely to require FDG-PET scanning as part of initial staging or follow-up. The sensitivity of FDG-PET scanning may be marginally improved with rhTSH stimulation

Follow-up strategy

If the total body scan performed after the administration of ^{131}I to destroy the thyroid remnant does not show any uptake outside the thyroid bed, physical examination is performed and serum TSH, free triiodothyronine, and thyroglobulin are measured during thyroxine treatment 3 months later. Nine to 12 months after initial treatment, a determination of serum thyroglobulin following rhTSH stimulation and a neck ultrasonography are obtained (Fig. 3.5.6.1) (6, 7). The results of these two tests will guide the subsequent follow-up, and may allow to revise the initial prognostic assessment. If serum thyroglobulin following TSH stimulation is undetectable and neck ultrasonography is normal, the risk of recurrence is less than 0.5% at 12 years (40, 41). These low-risk patients are considered cured, and can be reassured; the dose of thyroxine is decreased to maintain serum TSH concentration around 0.5 mU/l. In higher risk patients, higher doses of thyroxine are given for 5 years, the goal being a low serum TSH concentration (around 0.1 mU/l). Clinical and biochemical evaluation is then performed annually; any other testing is unnecessary as long as the serum thyroglobulin concentration is undetectable, and repeating rhTSH stimulation is usually not necessary (46). In these patients, control ^{131}I total body scan does not provide any benefits and is usually not performed (47–49).

If serum thyroglobulin is detectable following TSH stimulation at 9–12 months, another determination following rhTSH is obtained 6–18 months later, because with longer follow-up serum thyroglobulin became undetectable following rhTSH stimulation in two-thirds of these patients (50). In those with high and increasing serum thyroglobulin levels, imaging tests should be performed, including a CT of the neck and chest, the administration of a large activity of ^{131}I (100 mCi (3700 MBq) or more) with a total body scan 3–5 days later, and an FDG-PET scan (42, 44). These imaging modalities are also performed during long-term follow-up in patients receiving thyroxine in whom serum thyroglobulin becomes detectable, and increases above 10 ng/ml after TSH stimulation.

In low-risk patients who have had a total thyroidectomy but who were not given ^{131}I postoperatively, and in those who have had less than a total thyroidectomy, the follow-up protocol is based on

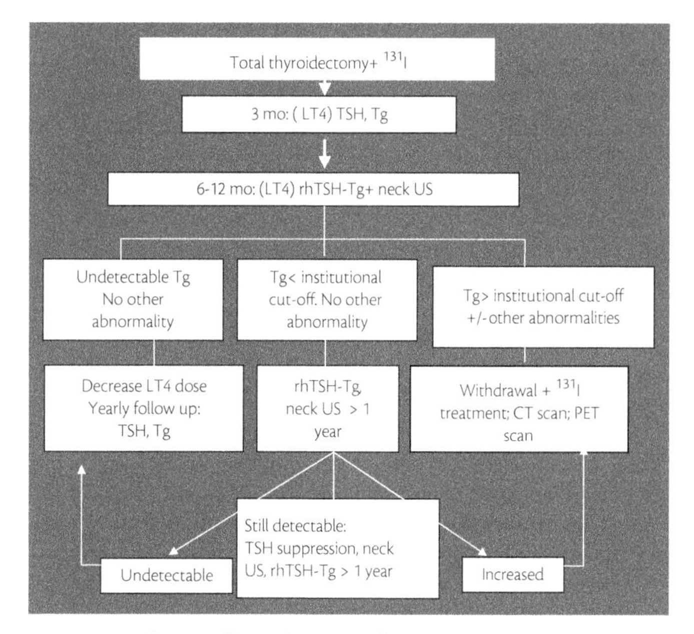

Fig. 3.5.6.1 Follow-up of low-risk patients after total thyroid ablation, based on serum thyroglobulin determinations and neck ultrasonography. The decision level of serum thyroglobulin depends upon the assay used to measure serum thyroglobulin. LT4, L-thyroxine; rhTSH, recombinant human TSH; Tg, thyroglobulin; TSH, thyrotropin; US, ultrasonography. (Adapted from Pacini F, Schlumberger M, Dralle H, Elisei R, Smit JW, Wiersinga W, *et al.* European consensus for the management of patients with differentiated thyroid cancer of the follicular epithelium. *Eur J Endocrinol*, 2006; **154**: 787–803.)

thyroglobulin determinations and neck ultrasonography. Further treatment may be given for increasing serum thyroglobulin level with time or for any imaging abnormality.

Local and regional recurrences

Local or regional recurrences occur in 5–20% of patients with differentiated thyroid carcinomas. Some are related to incomplete initial treatment (in a thyroid remnant or in lymph nodes), and others indicate tumour aggressiveness (in the thyroid bed after total thyroidectomy or in soft tissues) and are often associated with distant metastases (51, 52).

A local or regional recurrence that is palpable or easily visualized with ultrasonography or CT scan should be resected. Total excision may be facilitated by total body scanning 4 days after administration of 100 mCi (3700 MBq) ^{131}I, because additional tissue that should be excised may be identified. Surgery is performed 1 day later, preferably using an intraoperative probe. The completeness of resection is verified 1–2 days after surgery by another total body scan and was achieved in 92% of patients who underwent this protocol (53). Involvement of the trachea or oesophagus may indicate extensive surgery (54)

A local or regional recurrence that is small, less than 1 cm in diameter, may be treated with ^{131}I alone. Indeed, ^{131}I uptake will still be detectable in only 24% of patients after three ^{131}I treatments, and depending on disease location these patients may then undergo surgery (55). Preoperative charcoal tattooing under ultrasonographic guidance may facilitate the peroperative detection of small lymph node metastases.

From a practical point of view, there is no evidence that treatment of small lymph nodes (<5 mm in diameter) may provide a better outcome than treatment of lymph nodes that are more than 7–10 mm in diameter; for this reason, there is no usually need to explore small abnormalities found at neck ultrasonography. External radiotherapy is indicated in patients with soft tissue recurrences that cannot be completely excised and that do not take up ^{131}I.

Distant metastases

Distant metastases, mostly in the lungs and bones, occur in 5–10% of patients with differentiated thyroid carcinomas. Lung metastases are most frequent in young patients with papillary carcinoma. Bone metastases are more common in older patients and in those with follicular carcinoma. Other less common sites are the brain, liver, and skin (56–59).

Diagnosis

Clinical symptoms of lung involvement are uncommon. The pattern of lung involvement may vary from macronodular to diffuse infiltrates. The latter is usually diagnosed with ^{131}I total body scan and may be confirmed by CT; enlarged mediastinal lymph nodes are often present in children with papillary carcinomas. Pain, swelling, or fractures occur in more than 80% of patients with bone metastases. Nearly all patients with distant metastases have a high serum thyroglobulin concentration and two-thirds of patients have ^{131}I uptake in the metastases. ^{131}I uptake is more frequently found in younger patients, in those with small metastases, and in those with a well-differentiated thyroid carcinoma. FDG uptake on PET scan is more frequently seen in older patients with poorly differentiated thyroid carcinoma and large metastases. High FDG uptake is an adverse prognostic indicator for survival and for response to ^{131}I therapy (60, 61).

Treatment

Palliative surgery is required for bone metastases when there are neurological or orthopaedic complications or there is a high risk of such complications. Surgery may also be useful to debulk large tumour masses, and may be curative in patients with a single bone metastasis (62). Other local treatment modalities may include cement injection, radiofrequency, and external radiotherapy.

Patients with metastases that take up ^{131}I are treated with 100–150 mCi (3700–5550 MBq) following thyroid hormone withdrawal every 4–6 months. The effective radiation dose, which depends on the effective half-life of ^{131}I in the metastasis and on the ratio between total uptake and the mass of thyroid tissue, is correlated with the outcome of ^{131}I therapy (63–65). This was the rationale to administer higher activities (200 mCi or more, or based on dosimetry), but no clinical benefits have been demonstrated over standard treatment. Lower activities (1 mCi/kg (37 MBq) body weight) are given to children. There is no limit to the cumulative activity of ^{131}I that can be given to patients with distant metastases, although above a cumulative activity of 600 mCi (22 000 MBq) further ^{131}I therapy usually has little benefit but the risk of leukaemia increases significantly (56).

Cytotoxic chemotherapy with an anthracycline or taxane regimen is poorly effective in patients with advanced or metastatic disease that is refractory to ^{131}I treatment and is progressive (66). In these patients, treatment with drugs that are antiangiogenic and that interfere with the MAP kinase pathway provided significant benefits and are used as first-line treatment (67–70).

Box 3.5.6.3 Outcome of patients with distant metastases

- ^{131}I treatment may eradicate neoplastic foci (one-third of patients)
  - High radiation doses (high uptake, radiation doses >8000 cGy)
  - And radiosensitive: younger age, well-differentiated tumour, small tumour foci, absent or low FDG uptake
- ^{131}I treatment: pitfalls (two-thirds of patients)
  - Low radiation doses (no uptake or radiation doses <3500 cGy) or heterogeneous dose distribution (between lesions or inside a given lesion)
  - Or radioresistant: older age, poorly differentiated tumour, large tumour foci, high FDG uptake

Treatment results

Complete responses have been obtained in 45% of patients with distant metastases with initial ^{131}I uptake, more frequently in younger patients with well-differentiated tumours, and with metastases that are small when discovered and with no significant FDG uptake on PET (Box 3.5.6.3). Nearly all complete responses have been obtained with a cumulative activity of 600 mCi or less and nearly half with a cumulative activity of 200 mCi. Few relapses occurred after complete response, despite detectable serum thyroglobulin concentration in some patients (56).

Overall survival after the discovery of distant metastases is about 40% at 10 years. Young patients with well-differentiated tumours who have metastases that are small when discovered and that take up ^{131}I and have no FDG uptake on PET scan have a more favourable outcome: the large majority of these patients are cured and their overall survival is excellent. In the other groups of patients with distant metastases, median survival after the discovery of the metastases is about 3 years in those with no initial ^{131}I uptake, and about 5 years in those with initial ^{131}I uptake but who are not cured with ^{131}I treatment. When the tumour mass is considered, the location of the metastases, be it the lungs or bone, has no independent prognostic influence. The poor prognosis of bone metastases is linked to the bulkiness of their lesions and their clinical morbidity. Local treatment of bone lesions should be performed, even in the presence of ^{131}I uptake, including surgery, radiofrequency, cement injection, or external radiation therapy.

Complications of treatment with ^{131}I

Acute side effects

Acute side effects (nausea, sialadenitis, lost of taste) after treatment with ^{131}I are common but are usually mild and resolve rapidly. Radiation thyroiditis is usually trivial, but, if the thyroid remnant is large, the patient may have enough pain to warrant corticosteroid therapy for a few days. Tumour in certain locations, brain, spinal cord, and paratracheal, may swell in response to TSH stimulation or after ^{131}I therapy, causing compressive symptoms and may warrant corticosteroid therapy. Radiation fibrosis may develop in patients with diffuse lung metastases who have high ^{131}I uptake, if high activities (>150 mCi (5550 MBq)) are administered at short intervals (<3 months). Xerostomia (71) and obstruction of the lachrymal duct (72) may occur after ^{131}I treatment.

Genetic defects and infertility

Particular attention must be paid to avoid administration of ^{131}I in pregnant women. After ^{131}I treatment, in men spermatogenesis may be transiently depressed (73), and women may have transient ovarian failure (74). Pregnancy outcome is not affected by previous radio-iodine exposure (75, 76). Therefore, it is only recommended that conception be postponed for 6 months after treatment with ^{131}I. There is no evidence that pregnancy affects tumour growth in women receiving adequate thyroxine therapy, which should be monitored carefully before conception and during pregnancy.

Carcinogenesis and leukaemogenesis

Mild pancytopenia may occur after repeated ^{131}I therapy, especially in patients with bone metastases also treated with external radiotherapy. The overall relative risk of secondary carcinoma and of leukaemia was found to be increased in patients treated with a high cumulative activity of ^{131}I (>500 mCi (18 500 MBq)) or in association with external radiotherapy (77).

Anaplastic thyroid carcinoma

Anaplastic carcinoma of the thyroid is one of the most aggressive cancers encountered in humans. In most cases, it represents the ultimate stage in the dedifferentiation of a follicular or papillary carcinoma. In fact, anaplastic cells do not produce thyroglobulin, they are not able to concentrate iodine, and thyrotropin receptors are not found in their plasma cell membranes. Anaplastic carcinomas represent less than 5% of all thyroid cancers. Nearly all patients affected are older people. The peak incidence is in the seventh decade of life and the male to female ratio is 1:3 (78).

Diagnosis

More than one-third of the patients with anaplastic carcinoma have a long-standing goitre. The most common mode of presentation is a rapidly enlarging fixed neck mass, with palpable lymph nodes. Invasion of adjacent organs and compressive symptoms are frequent. Twenty to 50% of patients have distant metastases, most commonly in lungs, bones, brain, and liver. Anaplastic carcinomas are solid masses. Fine-needle aspiration biopsy is an effective diagnostic method but the diagnosis should be established by biopsy or at surgery. Neck ultrasonography, CT scan or MRI, FDG-PET scan, and endoscopy will assess the local extent of the tumour and will search for distant metastases (79).

Pathology

The tumour is typically composed of varying proportions of spindle, polygonal, and giant cells, often harbouring squamous cells and sarcomatoid foci. Keratin is the most useful epithelial marker and is present in 40–100% of the tumours. Many anaplastic carcinomas have a well-differentiated component. Conversely, differentiated carcinomas with small undifferentiated foci should be considered as anaplastic.

Immunohistochemical studies indicate that most tumours previously classified as small cell undifferentiated carcinomas were in fact primary malignant lymphomas (positive for leucocyte common antigen) or less often medullary carcinomas (positive for calcitonin and carcinoembryonic antigen), poorly differentiated thyroid carcinomas, or a thyroid metastasis from another primary tumour. Some tumours do not react with any antibody; they are considered as anaplastic carcinomas and carry the same prognosis.

Treatment

Survival is not altered by treatment with surgery, radiotherapy, or chemotherapy alone. In most patients, death is caused by local tumour invasion. The median survival is 2–6 months, and few patients have survived more than 12 months.

Only combined multimodality treatment improved the local control rate, thus avoiding death from suffocation. This includes surgical resection of all tumour masses present in the neck, followed by a combination of systemic chemotherapy and external radiotherapy to the neck and mediastinum. Chemotherapy consists of either fractionated doses of doxorubicin, 10 mg/m^2 per week, or a combination of doxorubicin, 60 mg/m^2, and cisplatin, 90 mg/m^2, every 3–4 weeks; a taxane regimen may also be used as first- or second-line treatment (80, 81).

External radiotherapy may be hyperfractionated and accelerated. This comprises fractions of 1.25 Gy given twice a day for 5 days a week to a total dose of 40–45 Gy. It is given either in combination with fractionated doxorubicin or between the second and third courses of the combination doxorubicin–cisplatin. Severe toxicity occurs in one-third of the patients. All protocols of combined multimodality treatment provide similar rates of local control and long-term survival: complete local control is obtained in 60–80% of patients, thus avoiding death from local invasion and suffocation; long-term survival is obtained in 20–30% of patients with most deaths being due to distant metastases.

Benefits are observed mostly in patients who had apparently complete surgery and in whom the anaplastic cancer component represented a small fraction of the thyroid tumour mass. No response was observed in patients with distant metastases. This underlines the need for treating these patients as soon as possible, before distant metastases appear.

Thyroid lymphoma

Primary non-Hodgkin's lymphomas of the thyroid are rare tumours accounting for 2.5% of all non-Hodgkin's lymphomas and less than 5% of all malignant thyroid tumours (82). Older people are predominantly affected with the peak incidence during the seventh decade of life and the male to female ratio is 1:3.

Pathology

Primary thyroid lymphoma almost always has a B-cell lineage. The majority are 'mucosa-associated lymphoid tissue' (MALT) lymphomas, and arise in patients with chronic autoimmune thyroiditis. These small cell lymphomas are characterized by a low grade of malignancy, a slow growth rate, and a tendency for recurrence at other MALT sites such as the gastrointestinal or respiratory tract, the thymus, or the salivary glands.

At diagnosis, diffuse large cell lymphomas account for about 70–80% of tumours, and a significant proportion of clinical cases arise from the transformation of low-grade MALT lymphoma to high-grade B-cell lymphoma.

Diagnosis

Thyroid lymphomas almost invariably present as a rapidly enlarging painless fixed neck mass with palpable lymph nodes. One-third of the patients have compressive symptoms. Clinically evident distant disease is uncommon. In patients with chronic autoimmune thyroiditis, the diagnosis of small cell lymphoma may be difficult and a lymphoma should be sought when the goitre increases in size, or when patients complain of neck discomfort, pain, or compressive symptoms.

The palpated mass is solid and hypoechoic on ultrasonography. A biopsy is needed for immunohistochemical staining to diagnose small cell lymphomas and the frequently associated chronic autoimmune thyroiditis. It is also needed to exclude an anaplastic carcinoma. Lymphocyte monoclonality for light chain immunoglobulin may be necessary to confirm malignant lymphoma.

Accurate staging is critical for treatment planning. Staging includes a physical examination, complete blood count, serum lactate dehydrogenase, liver function tests, bone marrow biopsy, CT scan or MRI of the neck, thorax, abdomen, and pelvis, FDG-PET scan, and appropriate biopsies at sites where tumour is suspected. Involvement of Waldeyer's ring and of the gastrointestinal tract have been associated with thyroid lymphomas and therefore upper gastrointestinal tract endoscopy should be performed.

Treatment

Treatment is guided by the histological subtype, the extent of the disease, and in case of diffuse large B-cell lymphoma by the age-adjusted international prognostic index. Small tumours are often treated initially as primary thyroid carcinomas with surgery, and additional radiotherapy may be necessary in case of indolent lymphoma. Surgical debulking of thyroid lymphomas is neither feasible nor necessary.

For diffuse large B-cell lymphoma, or transformation of MALT lymphoma to high-grade B-cell lymphoma, chemotherapy combined with rituximab (chimeric human-mouse anti-CD20 monoclonal antibody) has become the standard treatment (83). The chemotherapy usually consists of 4–6 cycles of the CHOP regimen (cyclophosphamide, 750 mg/m^2 on day 1, doxorubicin, 50 mg/m^2 on day 1, vincristine, 1.4 mg/m^2 on day 1 and prednisone, 40 mg/m^2 per day on days 1–5) every 3 weeks. Radiotherapy alone for aggressive lymphoma should be used only for elderly patients who cannot receive medical treatment. In fact, about one-third of the patients with disease apparently confined to the neck and treated with external radiotherapy alone, develop a recurrence at distant sites.

For localized MALT lymphomas, total thyroidectomy (predicted overall survival and freedom-from-progression survival, 100% at 5 years) or involved-field radiation therapy alone, 2 Gy/fraction for 5 days a week up to a total dose of 30–40 Gy, (5-year overall survival 90%) may be adequate if disease is localized after accurate staging (84, 85). For disseminated MALT lymphoma, chemotherapy alone with a single agent such as chlorambucil or combined with local radiation therapy can be used.

Other unusual tumours of the thyroid

Histiocytosis X

Isolated cases of thyroid involvement have been reported in patients with the malignant form of histiocytosis X. Chemotherapy with an anthracycline-based regimen induces long-term remission in most of these patients.

Sinus histiocytosis with massive lymphadenopathy (Rosai–Dorfman disease)

S100 protein-positive histiocytes with strong plasma cell reactions are the main histological features. Most affected patients have irregular goitre and enlarged cervical lymph nodes that simulate chronic autoimmune thyroiditis or a malignant process. The majority of the cases resolve spontaneously, but the disease may progress and is potentially lethal. In these cases, chemotherapy with an anthracycline-based regimen can be effective.

Mesenchymal tumours of the thyroid

Benign mesenchymal tumours of the thyroid such as lipoma and haemangioma are extremely rare and are usually treated with surgery alone. Primary fibrosarcomas and angiosarcomas of the thyroid are also rare and the differential diagnosis with anaplastic carcinoma may be difficult. They should be treated in the same manner as patients with anaplastic thyroid carcinoma.

Teratoma of the thyroid gland

There are two different types of thyroid teratomas. In infants, teratomas are often congenital and are composed of mature cystic tissue; these benign lesions are treated by total thyroidectomy. Teratomas in children and adults are composed of neuroepithelial tissue and are highly malignant, metastasizing early to lymph nodes and lungs. They require combined treatment with surgery, external radiotherapy, and chemotherapy.

Other primary tumours

Ectopic parathyroid or thymic tissue and primary paraganglioma may be found inside the thyroid gland.

Thyroid metastases

Microscopic metastases to the thyroid are a regular feature of necroptic findings in patients with malignant tumours. A thyroid nodule is rarely the initial sign of a tumour arising in a contiguous structure. Such cases ordinarily do not complicate the diagnosis. However, the discovery of a squamous or a neuroendocrine tumour should dictate a complete work-up including neck CT scan and endoscopies. Frequently, a thyroid mass is discovered in a patient who has been treated for another neoplasm such as cancer of the kidney, breast, lung, colon, or a malignant melanoma. This is a frequent finding on FDG-PET scan. Many years may elapse between the diagnosis of the primary lesion and the appearance of the thyroid mass. Furthermore, the thyroid mass may be the only known metastatic site. In such cases, fine-needle aspiration biopsy may be a useful diagnostic tool, but surgery is usually performed. Diagnosis may be difficult and immunohistochemical studies are warranted. Negative immunostaining with antithyroglobulin and anticalcitonin antibodies is firm evidence for the metastatic origin of the thyroid tumour. Although detection of metastasis to the thyroid gland often signifies a poor prognosis, aggressive surgical and medical therapy may be effective in a small percentage of patients.

References

1. Schlumberger M. Papillary and follicular thyroid carcinoma. *N Engl J Med*, 1998; **338**: 297–306.
2. Schlumberger MJ, Filetti S, Hay ID. Nontoxic diffuse and nodular goiter and thyroid neoplasia, In: Kronenberg HM, Melmed S, Polonsky KS, Larsen RP, eds. *Williams' Textbook of Endocrinology*. 11th edn. Philadelphia: Saunders Elsevier, 2007: 411–4.
3. Sherman SI. Thyroid carcinoma. *Lancet*, 2003; **361**: 501–11.
4. Davies L, Welch HG. Increasing incidence of thyroid cancer in the United States, 1973–2002. *JAMA*, 2006; **295**: 2164–7.
5. Leenhardt L, Bernier MO, Boin-Pineau MH, Conte Devolx B, Maréchaud R, Niccoli-Sire P, *et al.* Advances in diagnostic practices affect thyroid cancer incidence in France. *Eur J Endocrinol*, 2004; **150**: 133–9.
6. Cooper DS, Doherty GM, Haugen BR, Kloos RT, Lee SL, Mandel SJ, *et al.* Management guidelines for patients with thyroid nodules and differentiated thyroid cancer. *Thyroid*, 2006; **16**: 109–42.
7. Pacini F, Schlumberger M, Dralle H, Elisei R, Smit JW, Wiersinga W, *et al.* European consensus for the management of patients with differentiated thyroid cancer of the follicular epithelium. *Eur J Endocrinol*, 2006; **154**: 787–803.
8. Moon WJ, Jung SL, Lee JH, Na DG, Baek JH, Lee YH, *et al.* Benign and malignant thyroid nodules: US differentiation—multicenter retrospective study. *Radiology*, 2008; **247**: 762–70.
9. Hegedus L. Clinical practice. The thyroid nodule. *N Engl J Med*, 2004; **351**: 1764–71.
10. Hay ID, Thompson GB, Grant CS, Bergstralh EJ, Dvorak CE, Gorman CA, *et al.* Papillary thyroid carcinoma managed at the Mayo Clinic during six decades (1940–1999): temporal trends in initial therapy and long-term outcome in 2444 consecutively treated patients. *World J Surg*, 2002; **26**: 879–85.
11. American Joint Committee Thyroid Cancer. In: *AJCC Cancer Staging Handbook*. 6th edn. New York: Springer, 2002: 89–98.
12. Rosai J. *Ackerman's Surgical Pathology*. 8th edn. Saint Louis: Mosby, 1996: 1318.
13. Volante M, Rapa I, Papotti M. Poorly differentiated thyroid carcinoma: diagnostic features and controversial issues. *Endocr Pathol*, 2008; **19**: 150–5.
14. Hay ID, Grant CS, van Heerden JA, Goellner JR, Ebersold JR, Bergstralh EJ. Papillary thyroid microcarcinoma: a study of 535 cases observed in a 50-year period. *Surgery*, 1992; **112**: 1139–47.
15. Machens A, Hinze R, Thomusch O, Dralle H. Pattern of nodal metastasis for primary and reoperative thyroid cancer. *World J Surg*, 2002; **26**: 22–8.
16. Bonnet S, Hartl D, Leboulleux S, Baudin E, Lumbroso JD, Al Ghuzlan A, *et al.* Prophylactic lymph node dissection for papillary thyroid cancer less than 2 cm: implications for radioiodine treatment. *J Clin Endocrinol Metab*, 2008; **94**: 1162–7.
17. Pacini F, Ladenson PW, Schlumberger M, Driedger A, Luster M, Kloos RT, *et al.* Radioiodine ablation of thyroid remnants after preparation with recombinant human thyrotropin in differentiated thyroid carcinoma: results of an international, randomized, controlled study. *J Clin Endocrinol Metab*, 2006; **91**: 926–32.
18. Rémy H, Borget I, Leboulleux S, Guilabert N, Lavielle F, Garsi J, *et al.* ^{131}I effective half-life and dosimetry in thyroid cancer patients. *J Nucl Med*, 2008; **49**: 1445–50.
19. Schroeder PR, Haugen BR, Pacini F, Reiners C, Schlumberger M, Sherman SI, *et al.* A comparison of short-term changes in health-related quality of life in thyroid carcinoma patients undergoing diagnostic evaluation with recombinant human thyrotropin compared with thyroid hormone withdrawal. *J Clin Endocrinol Metab*, 2006; **91**: 878–84.
20. Schlumberger M, Ricard M, De Pouvourville G, Pacini F. How the availability of recombinant human TSH has changed the management of patients who have thyroid cancer. *Nat Clin Pract Endocrinol Metab*, 2007; **3**: 641–50.
21. Hackshaw A, Harmer C, Mallick U, Haq M, Franklyn JA. ^{131}I activity for remnant ablation in patients with differentiated thyroid cancer: a systematic review. *J Clin Endocrinol Metab*, 2007; **92**: 28–38.
22. Maxon HR, Thomas SR, Hertzberg VS, Kereiakes JG, Chen IW, Sperling MI, *et al.* Relation between effective radiation dose and outcome of radioiodine therapy for thyroid cancer. *N Engl J Med*, 1983; **309**: 937–41.

23. Aide N, Heutte N, Rame JP, Henry-Amar M, Bardet S. Clinical relevance of SPECT/CT of the neck and thorax in post-ablation ^{131}I scintigraphy. *J Clin Endocrinol Metab*, 2009; **94**: 2075–84.
24. Lassmann M, Luster M, Hanscheid H, Reiners C. Impact of $^{(131)}$I diagnostic activities on the biokinetics of thyroid remnants. *J Nucl Med*, 2004; **45**: 619–25.
25. Toubeau M, Touzery C, Arveux P, Chaplain G, Vaillant G, Berriolo A, *et al.* Predictive value for disease progression of serum thyroglobulin levels measured in the postoperative period and after (131)I ablation therapy in patients with differentiated thyroid cancer. *J Nucl Med*, 2004; **45**: 988–94.
26. Brierley JD, Tsang RW. External-beam radiation therapy in the treatment of differentiated thyroid cancer. *Semin Surg Oncol*, 1999; **16**: 42–9.
27. Biondi B, Filetti S, Schlumberger M. Thyroid-hormone therapy and thyroid cancer: a reassessment. *Nat Clin Pract Endocrinol Metab*, 2005; **1**: 32–40.
28. Leboulleux S, Girard E, Rose M, Travagli JP, Sabbah N, Caillou B, *et al.* Ultrasound criteria of malignancy for cervical lymph nodes in patients followed for differentiated thyroid cancer. *J Clin Endocrinol Metab*, 2007; **92**: 3590–4.
29. Bachelot A, Cailleux AF, Klain M, Baudin E, Ricard M, Bellon N, *et al.* Relationship between tumor burden and serum thyroglobulin level in patients with papillary and follicular thyroid carcinoma. *Thyroid*, 2002; **12**: 707–11.
30. Pacini F, Fugazzola L, Lippi F, Ceccarelli C, Centoni R, Miccoli P, *et al.* Detection of thyroglobulin in fine needle aspirates of nonthyroidal neck masses: a clue to the diagnosis of metastatic differentiated thyroid cancer. *J Clin Endocrinol Metab*, 1992; **74**: 1401–4.
31. Snozek CL, Chambers EP, Reading CC, Sebo TJ, Sistrunk JW, Singh RJ, *et al.* Serum thyroglobulin, high-resolution ultrasound, and lymph node thyroglobulin in diagnosis of differentiated thyroid carcinoma nodal metastases. *J Clin Endocrinol Metab*, 2007; **92**: 4278–81.
32. Spencer CA, Bergoglio LM, Kazarosyan M, Fatemi S, LoPresti JS. Clinical impact of thyroglobulin (Tg) and Tg autoantibody method differences on the management of patients with differentiated thyroid carcinomas. *J Clin Endocrinol Metab*, 2005; **90**: 5566–75.
33. Chiovato L, Latrofa F, Braverman LE, Pacini F, Capezzone M, Masserini L, *et al.* Disappearance of humoral thyroid autoimmunity after complete removal of thyroid antigens. *Ann Intern Med*, 2003; **139**: 346–51.
34. Francis Z, Schlumberger MJ. Serum thyroglobulin determination in thyroid cancer patients. *Best Pract Res Clin Endocrinol Metab*, 2008; **22**: 1039–46.
35. Eustatia-Rutten CF, Smit JW, Romijn JA, van der Kleij-Corssmit EP, Pereira AM, Stokkel MP, *et al.* Diagnostic value of serum thyroglobulin measurements in the follow-up of differentiated thyroid carcinoma, a structured meta-analysis. *Clin Endocrinol (Oxf)*, 2004; **61**: 61–74.
36. Haugen BR, Pacini F, Reiners C, Schlumberger M, Ladenson PW, Sherman SI, *et al.* A comparison of recombinant human thyrotropin and thyroid hormone withdrawal for the detection of thyroid remnant or cancer. *J Clin Endocrinol Metab*, 1999; **84**: 3877–85.
37. Borget I, Corone C, Nocaudie M, Allyn M, Iacobelli S, Schlumberger M, *et al.* Sick leave for follow-up control in thyroid cancer patients: comparison between stimulation with Thyrogen and thyroid hormone withdrawal. *Eur J Endocrinol*, 2007; **156**: 531–8.
38. Smallridge RC, Meek SE, Morgan MA, Gates GS, Fox TP, Grebe S, *et al.* Monitoring thyroglobulin in a sensitive immunoassay has comparable sensitivity to recombinant human TSH-stimulated thyroglobulin in follow-up of thyroid cancer patients. *J Clin Endocrinol Metab*, 2007; **92**: 82–7.
39. Schlumberger M, Hitzel A, Toubert ME, Corone C, Troalen F, Schlageter MH, *et al.* Comparison of seven serum thyroglobulin assays in the follow-up of papillary and follicular thyroid cancer patients. *J Clin Endocrinol Metab*, 2007; **92**: 2487–96.
40. Cailleux AF, Baudin E, Travagli JP, Ricard M, Schlumberger M. Is diagnostic iodine-131 scanning useful after total thyroid ablation for differentiated thyroid cancer? *J Clin Endocrinol Metab*, 2000; **85**: 175–8.
41. Pacini F, Capezzone M, Elisei R, Ceccarelli C, Taddei D, Pinchera A. Diagnostic 131-iodine whole-body scan may be avoided in thyroid cancer patients who have undetectable stimulated serum thyroglobulin levels after initial treatment. *J Clin Endocrinol Metab*, 2002; **87**: 1499–1501.
42. Schlumberger M, Mancusi F, Baudin E, Pacini F. 131-I Therapy for elevated thyroglobulin levels. *Thyroid*, 1997; **7**: 273–6.
43. Pacini F, Agate L, Elisei R, Capezzone M, Ceccarelli C, Lippi F, *et al.* Outcome of differentiated thyroid cancer with detectable serum thyroglobulin and negative diagnostic (131) I whole body scan: comparison of patients treated with high (131) I activities versus untreated patients. *J Clin Endocrinol Metab*, 2001; **86**: 4092–7.
44. Leboulleux S, Schroeder PR, Schlumberger M, Ladenson PW. The role of PET in follow-up of patients treated for differentiated epithelial thyroid cancers. *Nat Clin Pract Endocrinol Metab*, 2007; **3**: 112–21.
45. Leboulleux S, Schroeder PR, Busaidy NL, Auperin A, Corone C, Jacene HA, *et al.* Assessment of the incremental value of recombinant thyrotropin stimulation before 2-[18F]-fluoro-2-deoxy-D-glucose positron emission tomography/computed tomography imaging to localize residual differentiated thyroid cancer. *J Clin Endocrinol Metab*, 2009; **94**: 1310–16.
46. Castagna MG, Brilli L, Pilli T, Montanaro A, Cipri C, Fioravanti C, *et al.* Limited value of repeat recombinant thyrotropin (rhTSH)-stimulated thyroglobulin testing in differentiated thyroid carcinoma patients with previous negative rhTSH-stimulated thyroglobulin and undetectable basal serum thyroglobulin levels. *J Clin Endocrinol Metab*, 2008; **93**: 76–81.
47. Torlontano M, Attard M, Crocetti U, Tumino S, Bruno R, Costante G, *et al.* Follow-up of low risk patients with papillary thyroid cancer: role of neck ultrasonography in detecting lymph node metastases. *J Clin Endocrinol Metab*, 2004; **89**: 3402–7.
48. Pacini F, Molinaro E, Castagna MG, Agate L, Elisei R, Ceccarelli C, *et al.* Recombinant human thyrotropin-stimulated serum thyroglobulin combined with neck ultrasonography has the highest sensitivity in monitoring differentiated thyroid carcinoma. *J Clin Endocrinol Metab*, 2003; **88**: 3668–73.
49. Frasoldati A, Pesenti M, Gallo M, Caroggio A, Salvo D, Valcavi R. Diagnosis of neck recurrences in patients with differentiated thyroid carcinoma. *Cancer*, 2003; **97**: 90–6.
50. Baudin E, Do Cao C, Cailleux AF, Leboulleux S, Travagli JP, Schlumberger M. Positive predictive value of serum thyroglobulin levels, measured during the first year of follow-up after thyroid hormone withdrawal, in thyroid cancer patients. *J Clin Endocrinol Metab*, 2003; **88**: 1107–11.
51. Leboulleux S, Rubino C, Baudin E, Caillou B, Hartl DM, Bidart JM, *et al.* Prognostic factors for persistent or recurrent disease of papillary thyroid carcinoma with neck lymph node metastases and/or tumor extension beyond the thyroid capsule at initial diagnosis. *J Clin Endocrinol Metab*, 2005; **90**: 5723–9.
52. Kouvaraki MA, Lee JE, Shapiro SE, Sherman SI, Evans DB. Preventable reoperations for persistent and recurrent papillary thyroid carcinoma. *Surgery*, 2004; **136**: 1183–91.
53. Travagli JP, Cailleux AF, Ricard M, Baudin E, Caillou B, Parmentier C, *et al.* Combination of radioiodine (131I) and probe-guided surgery for persistent or recurrent thyroid carcinoma. *J Clin Endocrinol Metab*, 1998; **83**: 2675–80.
54. McCaffrey JC. Evaluation and treatment of aerodigestive tract invasion by well-differentiated thyroid carcinoma. *Cancer Control*, 2000; **7**: 246–52.
55. Pacini F, Cetani F, Miccoli P, Mancusi F, Ceccarelli C, Lippi F, *et al.* Outcome of 309 patients with metastatic differentiated thyroid carcinoma treated with radioiodine. *World J Surg*, 1994; **18**: 600–4.
56. Durante C, Haddy N, Baudin E, Leboulleux S, Hartl D, Travagli JP, *et al.* Long term outcome of 444 patients with distant metastases from papillary and follicular thyroid carcinoma: benefits and limits of radioiodine therapy. *J Clin Endocrinol Metab*, 2006; **91**: 2892–9.
57. Dinneen SF, Valimaki MJ, Bergstralh EJ, Goellner JR, Gorman CA, Hay ID. Distant metastases in papillary thyroid carcinoma: 100 cases observed at one institution during 5 decades. *J Clin Endocrinol Metab*, 1995; **80**: 2041–5.
58. Casara D, Rubello D, Saladini G, Masarotto G, Favero A, Girelli ME, *et al.* Different features of pulmonary metastases in differentiated thyroid cancer: natural history and multivariate statistical analysis of prognostic variables. *J Nucl Med*, 1993; **34**: 1626–31.
59. Chiu AC, Delpassand ES, Sherman SI. Prognosis and treatment of brain metastases in thyroid carcinoma. *J Clin Endocrinol Metab*, 1997; **82**: 3637–42.

60. Wang W, Larson SM, Tuttle RM, Kalaigian H, Kolbert K, Sonenberg M, *et al.* Resistance of [18f]-fluorodeoxyglucose-avid metastatic thyroid cancer lesions to treatment with high-dose radioactive iodine. *Thyroid*, 2001; **11**: 1169–75.
61. Robbins RJ, Wan Q, Grewal RK, Reibke R, Gonen M, Strauss HW, *et al.* Real-time prognosis for metastatic thyroid carcinoma based on 2-[18F] fluoro-2-deoxy-D-glucose-positron emission tomography scanning. *J Clin Endocrinol Metab*, 2006; **91**: 498–505.
62. Bernier MO, Leenhardt L, Hoang C, Aurengo A, Mary JY, Menegaux F, *et al.* Survival and therapeutic modalities in patients with bone metastases of differentiated thyroid carcinomas. *J Clin Endocrinol Metab*, 2001; **86**: 1568–73.
63. Schlumberger M, Lacroix L, Russo D, Filetti S, Bidart JM. Defects in iodide metabolism in thyroid cancer and implications for the follow-up and treatment of patients. *Nat Clin Pract Endocrinol Metab*, 2007; **3**: 260–9.
64. Kolbert KS, Pentlow KS, Pearson JR, Sheikh A, Finn RD, Humm JL, *et al.* Prediction of absorbed dose to normal organs in thyroid cancer patients treated with ^{131}I by use of ^{124}I PET and 3-dimensional internal dosimetry software. *J Nucl Med*, 2007; **48**: 143–9.
65. Kitamura Y, Shimizu K, Nagahama M, Sugino K, Ozaki O, Mimura T, *et al.* Immediate causes of death in thyroid carcinoma: clinicopathological analysis of 161 fatal cases. *J Clin Endocrinol Metab*, 1999; **84**: 4043–9.
66. Baudin E, Schlumberger M. New therapeutic approaches for metastatic thyroid carcinoma. *Lancet Oncol*, 2007; **8**: 148–56.
67. Sherman SI, Wirth LJ, Droz JP, Hofmann M, Bastholt L, Martins RG, *et al.* Motesanib diphosphate in progressive, differentiated thyroid cancer. *N Engl J Med*, 2008; **359**: 31–42.
68. Cohen EE, Rosen LS, Vokes EE, Kies MS, Forastiere AA, Worden FP, *et al.* Axitinib is an active treatment for all histologic subtypes of advanced thyroid cancer: results from a phase II study. *J Clin Oncol*, 2008; **26**: 4708–13.
69. Gupta-Abramson V, Troxel AB, Nellore A, Puttaswamy K, Redlinger M, Ransone K, *et al.* Phase II trial of Sorafenib in advanced thyroid cancer. *J Clin Oncol*, 2008; **26**: 4714–9.
70. Kloos RT, Ringel MD, Knopp MV, Hall NC, King M, Stevens R, *et al.* Phase II trial of sorafenib in metastatic thyroid cancer. *J Clin Oncol*, 2009; **27**: 1675–84.
71. Kloos RT, Duvuuri V, Jhiang SM, Cahill KV, Foster JA, Burns JA. Nasolacrimal drainage system obstruction from radioactive iodine therapy for thyroid carcinoma. *J Clin Endocrinol Metab*, 2002; **87**: 5817–20.
72. Mandel SJ, Mandel L. Radioactive iodine and the salivary glands. *Thyroid*, 2003; **13**: 265–71.
73. Ceccarelli C, Benicivelli W, Morciano D, Pinchera A, Pacini F. I-131 therapy for differentiated thyroid cancer leads to an earlier onset of menopause: results of a retrospective study. *J Clin Endocrinol Metab*, 2001; **86**: 3512–15.
74. Sawka AM, Lea J, Alshehri B, Tsang RW, Brierley JD, Thabane L, *et al.* A systematic review of the gonadal effects of therapeutic radioactive iodine in male thyroid cancer survivors. *Clin Endocrinol (Oxf)*, 2007; **68**: 610–17.
75. Garsi JP, Schlumberger M, Rubino C, Ricard M, Labbé M, Ceccarelli C, *et al.* Therapeutic administration of ^{131}I for differentiated thyroid cancer, radiation dose to ovaries and outcome of pregnancies. *J Nucl Med*, 2008; **49**: 845–52.
76. Garsi JP, Schlumberger M, Ricard M, Labbé M, Ceccarelli C, Schvartz C, *et al.* Health outcomes of children fathered by patients treated with radioiodine for thyroid cancer. *Clin Endocrinol (Oxf)*, 2009; [Epub ahead of print].
77. Rubino C, de Vathaire F, Dottorini ME, Hall P, Schvartz C, Couette JE, *et al.* Second primary malignancies in thyroid cancer patients. *Br J Cancer*, 2003; **89**: 1638–44.
78. Kebebew E, Greenspan FS, Clark OH, Woeber KA, McMillan A. Anaplastic thyroid carcinoma. Treatment outcome and prognostic factors. *Cancer*, 2005; **103**: 1330–5.
79. Bogsrud TV, Karantanis D, Nathan MA, Mullan BP, Wiseman GA, Kasperbauer JL, *et al.* 18F-FDG PET in the management of patients with anaplastic thyroid carcinoma. *Thyroid*, 2008; **18**: 713–19.
80. Ain KB, Egorin MJ, DeSimone PA. Treatment of anaplastic thyroid carcinoma with paclitaxel: phase 2 trial using ninety-six-hour infusion. Collaborative Anaplastic Thyroid Cancer Health Intervention Trials (CATCHIT) Group. *Thyroid*, 2000; **10**: 587–94.
81. De Crevoisier R, Baudin E, Bachelot A, Leboulleux S, Travagli JP, Caillou B, *et al.* Combined treatment of anaplastic thyroid carcinoma with surgery, chemotherapy, and hyperfractionated accelerated external radiotherapy. *Int J Radiation Oncology Biol Phys*, 2004; **60**: 1137–43.
82. Belal AA, Allam A, Kandil A, El Husseiny G, Khafaga Y, Al Rajhi N, *et al.* Primary thyroid lymphoma: a retrospective analysis of prognostic factors and treatment outcome for localized intermediate and high-grade lymphoma. *Am J Clin Oncol*, 2001; **24**: 299–305.
83. Coiffier B, Lepage E, Briere J, Herbrecht R, Tilly H, Bouabdallah R, *et al.* CHOP chemotherapy plus rituximab compared with CHOP alone in elderly patients with diffuse large-B-cell lymphoma. *N Eng J Med*, 2002; **346**: 235–42.
84. Mack LA, Pasieka JL. An evidence-based approach to the treatment of thyroid lymphoma. *World J Surg*, 2007; **5**: 978–86.
85. Tsang RW, Gosodarowicz MK, Pintilie M, Wells W, Hodgson DC, Sun A, *et al.* Localized mucosa-associated lymphoid tissue lymphoma treated with radiation therapy has excellent clinical outcome. *J Clin Oncol*, 2003; **21**: 4157–64.

3.5.7 Medullary thyroid carcinoma

Friedhelm Raue, Karin Frank-Raue

Classification and epidemiology

Medullary thyroid carcinoma (MTC) is a rare calcitonin-secreting tumour of the parafollicular or C cells of the thyroid. As the C cells originate from the embryonic neural crest, MTC often have the clinical and histological features of neuroendocrine tumours. They account for 8–12% of all thyroid carcinomas and occur in both sporadic and hereditary forms (1). The majority of patients have sporadic MTC (70%), while 30% have hereditary MTC. The sex ratio in sporadic MTC is 1:1.3 (male to female), while both sexes are nearly equally affected in the familial variety (2). The highest incidence of sporadic disease occurs in the fifth decade of life, while hereditary disease can be diagnosed earlier, depending on the possibility of genetic and biochemical screening.

The familial variety of MTC is inherited as an autosomal dominant trait with a high degree of penetrance and is associated with multiple endocrine neoplasia type 2 (MEN 2) syndrome (3). It is caused by germline-activating mutations of the *RET* proto-oncogene. Three distinct hereditary varieties of MTC are known, and each variant of MEN 2 results from a different *RET* gene mutation, with a good genotype–phenotype correlation:

1. The MEN 2A syndrome (OMIM 171400), characterized by MTC in combination with phaeochromocytoma and tumours of the parathyroids, is the most common form of all MEN 2 syndromes (55% of all cases) (4).
2. The MEN 2B syndrome (OMIM 162300), consisting of MTC, phaeochromocytoma, ganglioneuromatosis, and marfanoid habitus; it is the most aggressive form (5–10% of all cases).
3. Familial MTC (FMTC) (OMIM 155240), with a low incidence of any other endocrinopathies, is the mildest variant and has

been diagnosed more frequently in recent years (35–40% of all cases).

These four varieties of MTC, three hereditary and one nonhereditary, are clinically distinct with respect to incidence, genetics, age of onset, association with other diseases, histopathology of the tumour, and prognosis (Table 3.5.7.1). Many patients with MEN 2B have an earlier onset in the first year of life and more aggressive MTC with a higher morbidity and mortality than in patients with MEN 2A. They often do not have a family history of the disease. Their tumours and characteristic appearance are therefore due to *de novo* mutations that present as sporadic cases of potentially hereditary disease. In contrast, the clinical course of MTC in FMTC is more benign than in MEN 2A and MEN 2B with a late onset or no clinically manifest disease, and the prognosis is relatively good. Therefore a family history is often inadequate in establishing familial disease and more thorough evaluation by genetic and biochemical screening often reveals a family history of MTC in a patient originally thought to have the sporadic form of the disease.

Detection of MTC in patients has changed in recent years with the introduction of specific strategies: calcitonin screening in patients with thyroid nodules and screening with molecular methods for *RET* proto-oncogene mutations in patients with apparently sporadic MTC and in family members at risk for MTC. By earlier identification of patients with MTC, the presentation has changed from clinical tumours to preclinical disease, resulting in a high cure rate of affected patients with much better prognosis.

Pathology and biochemical markers

The histological appearance of MTC is enormously variable with regard to cytoarchitecture (solid, trabecular, or insular) and cell shape (spindle, polyhedral, angular, or round). The presence of stromal amyloid is characteristic in about 50–80% of MTC patients. This feature had been an auxiliary diagnostic criterion for MTC before the use of calcitonin immunocytochemistry.

Hereditary MTC characteristically presents as a multifocal process with C-cell hyperplasia in areas distinct from the primary tumour. Bilateral C-cell hyperplasia is a precursor lesion to hereditary MTC with a penetrance approaching nearly 100% in gene carriers (5). The time frame of the progression from C-cell hyperplasia to microscopic carcinoma remains unclear but may take years (6).

Table 3.5.7.1 Classification of medullary thyroid carcinoma

Variety of MTC	Incidence (%)	Age at onset	Associated endocrinopathies
Sporadic MTC	70	Fifth decade	None
Hereditary MTC	30		
FMTC	12	Fourth decade	Rare
MEN 2A	15	Third decade	Phaeochromocytoma, parathyroid adenoma/ hyperplasia
MEN 2B	3	First decade	Phaeochromocytoma, mucosal neuromas

FMTC, familial medullary thyroid carcinoma; MEN 2A, multiple endocrine neoplasia type 2A; MTC, medullary thyroid carcinoma.

The earliest reported finding of C-cell hyperplasia in MEN 2A is at 20 months of age, and children with MEN 2B may have this lesion at birth. Metastasis may be found first in central and lateral cervical and mediastinal lymph nodes of the neck in 10% of patients with a micro MTC operated on after discovery at familial screening, and in up to 90% of patients operated on for clinical MTC. Metastases outside the neck and mediastinum may occur during the course of the disease in the lung, liver, and bone.

The primary secretory product of MTC is calcitonin, which serves as a highly sensitive tumour marker. Measurement of monomeric calcitonin with two-site assays remains the definitive test for prospective diagnosis of MTC (7). The test is widely available, accurate, reproducible, and cost-effective. Normal calcitonin levels are below 3.6 pmol/l. Basal calcitonin concentrations usually correlate with tumour mass and are almost always high in patients with palpable tumours (8). Similarly, elevated plasma calcitonin levels following surgery to remove the tumour are indicative of persistent or recurrent disease. In patients with postoperative normal or slightly elevated basal calcitonin, provocative stimulation of calcitonin release using pentagastrin or calcium is done to confirm the absence or presence of residual tumour. The test is administered by giving pentagastrin 0.5 μg/kg body weight as an intravenous bolus over 5–10 s or calcium gluconate 2.5 mg/kg body weight as an intravenous infusion over 30 s; calcitonin measurements are made 2 and 5 min after initiation of the infusion. For patients with recurrence or persistence of MTC the peak observed after pentagastrin stimulation is usually 5–10 times higher than basal levels, while patients with normal basal and stimulated postoperative calcitonin levels are probably disease free.

Measurement of plasma calcitonin has been part of the routine evaluation of patients with thyroid nodules; up to 3% of patients with thyroid nodules have pathological calcitonin concentrations and about 0.6% have an MTC (9). The prevalence of MTC was nearly 100% when basal calcitonin levels were more than 36 pmol/l and pentagastrin-stimulated levels more than 360 pmol/l measured with specific and sensitive two-site assays. It is well known that basal calcitonin can also be elevated up to 36 pmol/l during normal childhood and pregnancy, as well as in different malignant tumours, Hashimoto's thyroiditis, and chronic renal failure. Many increases of calcitonin are unrelated to MTC and are commonly caused by C-cell hyperplasia not related to MTC. Patients with these conditions, however, usually have blunted or absent stimulatory responses to calcitonin secretagogues and should not be operated on. After careful evaluation, calcitonin measurement in nodular thyroid disease allows early diagnosis and early surgery of MTC, reducing the significant mortality associated with this malignant tumour. There are a number of other substances, including carcinoembryonic antigen (CEA), PDN-21 (katacalcin), chromogranin A, neuron-specific enolase, somatostatin, and ACTH, that are produced by MTC and which may help to differentiate it from other tumours.

Genetic abnormalities

The responsible gene for MEN 2 (OMIM 171400, 162300, 155240) was localized to centromeric chromosome 10 by genetic linkage analysis in 1987. Activating germline point mutations of the *RET* proto-oncogene were identified in 1993 (10). Analysis of *RET* in families with MEN 2 revealed that only affected family members had germline missense mutations in eight closely located exons (Fig. 3.5.7.1).

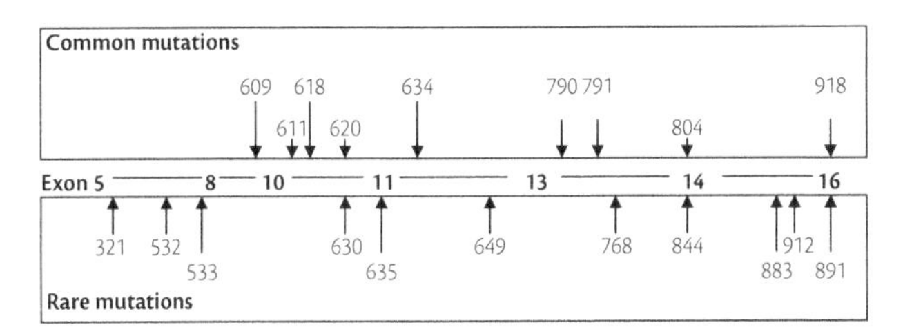

Fig. 3.5.7.1 Germline mutations of the *RET* proto-oncogene associated with MEN 2 and FMTC. Numbers indicated mutated codons of the *RET* gene.

The *RET* gene has 21 exons and encodes a receptor tyrosine kinase that appears to transduce growth and differentiation signals in several developing tissues including those derived from the neural crest. It is expressed in cells such as C cells, the precursors of MTC, and in phaeochromocytomas. The *RET* gene codes for a receptor that has a large extracellular cysteine-rich domain which is thought to be involved in ligand binding, a short transmembrane domain, and a cytoplasmic tyrosine kinase domain which is activated upon ligand-induced dimerization. Hereditary MTC is caused by autosomal dominant gain-of-function mutations in the *RET* proto-oncogene. Mutation of the extracellular cysteine at exon 11 codon 634 causes ligand-independent dimerization of receptor molecules, enhanced phosphorylation of intracellular substrates, and cell transformation. Mutation of the intracellular tyrosine kinase (codon 918) has no effect on receptor dimerization but causes constitutive activation of intracellular signalling pathways and also results in cellular transformation (11). There is a significant age-related progression from C-cell hyperplasia to MTC, which correlates with the transforming capacity of the respective *RET* mutations.

At present, mutation analysis has identified over 50 different missense mutations associated with the development of MEN 2. Although some overlap exists between *RET* mutations and the resulting clinical subtype of MEN 2, 85% of patients with MEN 2A have a mutation of codon 634 (exon 11); mutations of codons 609, 611, 618, and 620 account for an additional 10–15% of cases. Phaeochromocytomas are associated with codon 634 and 918 mutations in approximately 50% of patients, and are ssociated with mutations in exon 10 (codon 609, 611, 618, 620) in adout 20% of patients and rarely in exon 15 (codon 791, 804) (12). Hyperparathyroidism in MEN 2A is most commonly associated with codon 634 mutations, and in particular with the C634R mutation. In FMTC, germline mutations are distributed throughout the *RET* gene with an accumulation in exon 13 (codons 768, 790, and 791), exon 14 (codons 804 and 844), and rarely exon 10 (codons 618 and 620); some of these mutations have also been identified in families with MEN 2A. More than 95% of MEN 2B patients have mutations in codon 918 (exon 16), but mutations are rarely identified at codon 883 exon 15.

The association between disease phenotype and *RET* mutation genotype has important implications for the clinical management of MEN 2 patients and their families. There is a correlation between the specific germline *RET* mutation and the age of onset and aggressiveness of MTC development and the presence of nodal metastases. This information is used to stratify *RET* mutations into four risk levels: patients with ATA(American Thyroid Association)-A mutations (codons 609, 768, 790, 791, 804, and 891) have a high risk for MTC development and growth, patients with ATA-B mutations (codons 609, 611, 618, 620, and ATA-C (codon 634) are at a higher risk, and patients with ATA-D mutations (codons 883 and 918) are at the highest risk for early development and growth of MTC (13, 13a).

Approximately 23–60% of sporadic MTC have a codon 918 somatic (present in tumour only) mutation identical to the germline mutation found in MEN 2B. Some reports suggest that patients with sporadic MTC with codon 918 somatic mutations have more aggressive tumour growth and a poorer prognosis (14).

Clinical syndrome and diagnostic procedure

Sporadic medullary thyroid carcinoma

The most common clinical presentation of sporadic MTC is a single nodule or thyroid mass found incidentally during routine examination (1). The presentation does not differ from that observed in papillary or follicular thyroid carcinoma. A thyroid nodule identified by physical examination is generally evaluated by ultrasonography and radioisotopic scanning (Fig. 3.5.7.2). MTC shows hypoechogenic regions, sometimes with calcifications, and a thyroid scan almost always shows no trapping of radioactive iodine or technetium. Cytological examination of the cold hypoechogenic nodule will lead to a strong suspicion, or a correct diagnosis in most cases, of sporadic MTC. A plain radiograph of the neck sometimes reveals a characteristic dense coarse calcification pattern.

A plasma calcitonin measurement can clarify the diagnosis, since preoperative calcitonin levels correlate significantly with tumour size (8) and, in the presence of a palpable MTC, the plasma calcitonin concentration will usually be greater than 36 pmol/l. The CEA level will be elevated in most cases with clinically evident tumours. Therefore measurement of plasma calcitonin in patients with thyroid nodules has been advocated as a routine procedure by some European consensus groups (15).

Genetic testing for *RET* mutations in patients with elevated calcitonin levels may also be helpful in apparently sporadic cases of MTC, since, if a mutation is found, it will imply that the disease is hereditary and that the family should be screened. The frequency of germline mutations, either inherited or *de novo*, in a larger series of apparently sporadic MTC patients varied between 1% and 7% (16).

Metastases to cervical and mediastinal lymph nodes are found in two-third of patients at the time of initial presentation. Distant metastases to lung, liver, and bone occur late in the course of the disease. Diarrhoea is the most prominent of the hormone-mediated clinical features of MTC and is often seen in patients with

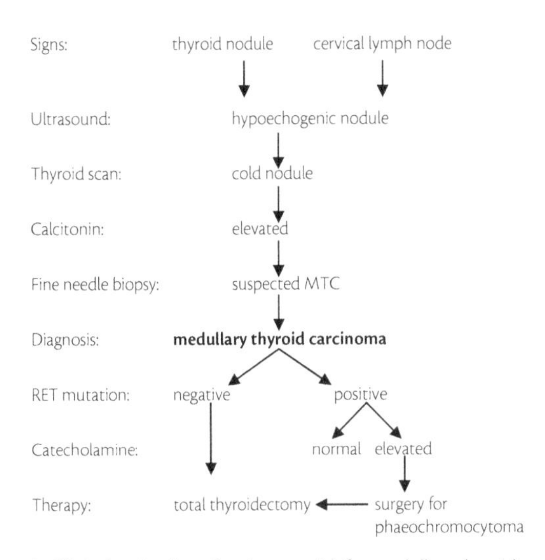

Fig. 3.5.7.2 Clinical evaluation of patients at risk for medullary thyroid carcinoma.

advanced disease. In addition, occasional tumours secrete ACTH causing Cushing's syndrome. Given the possibility that any patient with MTC may have MEN 2, preoperative testing must also include a 24-h urinary excretion of catecholamines (to rule out phaeochromocytoma) and measurement of calcium (to rule out hyperparathyroidism).

Hereditary medullary thyroid carcinoma

The clinical presentation and manifestation of familial MTC in index cases does not appear to differ from that in patients with sporadic MTC. MTC is often the initial manifestation of MEN 2 syndrome, as the other manifestations, phaeochromocytoma and hyperparathyroidism, develop later in the course of the disease (3). Less common presentations of MTC include recognition during search initiated after an associated disease such as bilateral phaeochromocytoma or multiglandular hyperparathyroidism becomes apparent. The diagnosis of familial MTC in index cases is often made postoperatively when pathohistological examination may show multifocal bilateral MTC accompanied by diffuse C-cell hyperplasia. Rare variants of MEN 2A exist, including MEN 2A with cutaneous lichen amyloidosis and FMTC (or MEN 2A) with Hirschsprung's disease.

MEN 2B has a typical phenotype with visible physical stigmata such as raised bumps on the lips and tongue (due to cutaneous neuromas), ganglioneuromas throughout the gastrointestinal tract, and a marfanoid habitus (long thin extremities, an altered upper–lower body ratio, slipped femoral epiphysis, pectus excavatum) with skeletal deformations and joint laxity. These patients have disease onset in the first year of life with the most aggressive form of MTC.

The diagnosis of FMTC can only be considered when four or more family members across a wide range of ages have isolated MTC. In general, the clinical course of MTC in familial MTC is more benign and typically has a late onset or is not a clinically manifest disease.

DNA testing becomes the optimal test for early detection of MEN 2 especially in 'at risk' families. At present, genetic testing is performed before the age of 5 years in all first-degree relatives of an index case (in MEN 2B patients directly after birth). Mutations in the *RET* proto-oncogene can be used to confirm the clinical diagnosis and identify asymptomatic family members with the syndrome (Fig. 3.5.7.3). Those who have a negative test can be reassured and require no further biochemical screening.

The age of onset of MTC and tumour aggressiveness in MEN 2 depends on the codon mutated. This genotype–phenotype correlation is the basis for stratifying mutations into four risk levels concerning the risk for MTC development and growth. Decision making in the clinical management of MEN 2 patients depends on the risk level classification, especially the timing of prophylactic thyroidectomy and the extent of surgical resection in presymptomatic *RET* mutation carriers (13, 13a).

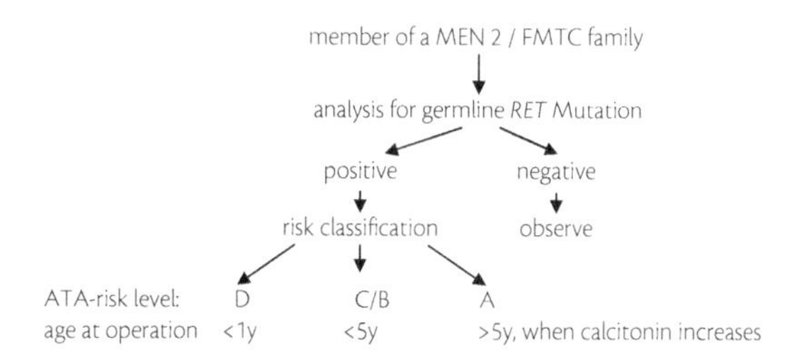

Fig. 3.5.7.3 Work-up of family members at risk for medullary thyroid carcinoma/multiple endocrine neoplasia type 2. Age at operation is age at recommended prophylactic thyroidectomy.

Phaeochromocytoma

Phaeochromocytomas occur in approximately 20–50% of MEN 2A patients depending on the mutation. Phaeochromocytomas are associated with codon 634 and 918 mutations in approximately 50% of patients, and are associated with mutations in exon 10 (codons 609, 611, 618, and 620) in about 20% of patients and rarely in exon 15 (codons 791 and 804) (13, 14). As with MTC, the phaeochromocytomas of MEN 2 are also multicentric with diffuse adrenomedullary hyperplasia developing bilateral phaeochromocytomas in one-half of the cases, but often after an interval of several years (12). Almost all phaeochromocytomas are located in an adrenal gland, and malignant phaeochromocytomas are rare. In index cases, the clinical manifestation of phaeochromocytoma associated with MEN 2 is similar to that in sporadic cases with signs and symptoms such as headache, palpitations, nervousness, tachycardia, and hypertension. However, phaeochromocytomas are usually identified early as a result of regular biochemical screening in gene carriers, and clinical manifestations are thus subtle or absent. It is unusual for phaeochromocytoma to precede the development of MTC and be the initial manifestation of MEN 2. Annual biochemical screening by measuring plasma and/or 24-h urinary excretion of catecholamines and metanephrines should be performed. Once the biochemical diagnosis is made, imaging studies such as MRI or *m*-iodobenzylguanidine (MIBG) scanning are appropriate. The presence of phaeochromocytoma must be ruled out before any surgical procedure. Patients with MTC should be evaluated for possible phaeochromocytoma. A coexisting phaeochromocytoma should be removed before thyroidectomy.

Primary hyperparathyroidism

Primary hyperparathyroidism, with hypercalcaemia and an elevated serum parathyroid hormone level occurs in 10–25% of MEN 2 gene carriers (especially codon 634). Hyperparathyroidism develops slowly, is usually mild, and clinical features do not differ from those seen in mild sporadic hyperparathyroidism. The diagnosis is established by finding high parathyroid hormone concentrations in the presence of hypercalcaemia. Pathological findings show chief cell hyperplasia involving multiple glands. Annual measurement of serum calcium concentration in gene carriers is probably adequate for screening purposes.

Treatment and prognosis

Surgery

The definitive treatment for MTC is surgery no matter whether MTC is sporadic or familial, primary or recurrent, or restricted to the thyroid gland or extending beyond it. Several studies have shown that survival in patients with MTC is dependent upon the adequacy of the initial surgical procedure. The appropriate surgery for MTC is total thyroidectomy and careful lymph node dissection of the central and if necessary lateral compartment of the neck. The latter is necessary for tumour staging and prevention of later midline complications related to local metastatic disease. If there is no evidence of local lymph node metastases during the primary surgical procedure, a surgical cure is likely and further neck dissection is probably unnecessary. Total thyroidectomy is absolutely necessary in hereditary cases because of the bilateral and multifocal nature of MTC. If the initial surgical procedure was inadequate, then reoperation with an appropriate surgical procedure is indicated. In contrast, unilateral lobectomy is sufficient in a patient with sporadic MTC showing a single unilateral tumour focus and normal plasma calcitonin levels after provocative testing. All patients should receive adequate L-thyroxine replacement therapy after total thyroidectomy (17).

Perhaps the most difficult problem associated with the management of MTC is what to do with the patient who has persistently elevated plasma calcitonin levels after an adequate surgical procedure. In almost all cases, persistent elevation of plasma calcitonin implies the presence of tumour. A thorough evaluation should be undertaken to define the extent of local and distant metastatic disease. Localization of metastases or recurrence can be done by different imaging methods such as ultrasonography of neck and abdomen, CT of neck, mediastinum, lung, and liver, or an MRI technique. Selective venous catheterization with blood sampling for calcitonin determination is helpful in detecting liver metastases at a very early stage and identifying a particular region of the neck or mediastinum that the surgeon should focus upon. Octreotide or [^{18}F]2-fluoro-2-deoxy-glucose positron emission tomography (FDG-PET) scanning may also be helpful, especially in identifying lung metastases at a very early stage of MTC. At the conclusion of these diagnostic procedures, a decision regarding reoperation must be made. If the primary operation was inadequate, if there is no evidence of distant metastases, and if local disease is found in the neck or/and mediastinum, reoperation is advocated. A successful cure, even long after the primary operation, is possible in a small number of patients by meticulous lymph node dissection of all compartments of the neck and mediastinum, with the complete removal of the lymphatic and fatty tissue between important anatomical structures. This surgical technique has produced a cure rate of 25% in such patients. If distant metastases are found, there is no indication for surgical intervention unless the patient develops diarrhoea or local complications, for which tumour debulking may be beneficial.

Recommendations for the timing of prophylactic thyroidectomy in MEN 2 patients are based upon a model that utilizes genotype–phenotype correlations to stratify mutations into four risk levels (13). In the cases of higher risk mutations, a thyroidectomy is recommended at the age of 5 years with ATA-C and B mutations (codons 609, 611, 618, 620, and 634), and as early as possible, preferably in the first year after birth, for patients with ATA-D mutations (codons 883 and 918) (6). For patients with ATA-A mutations (codons 768, 790, 791, 804, and 891) there are three alternatives concerning recommended age at prophylactic surgery: some authors suggest thyroidectomy at age 5, others at age 10, while others suggest that surgery may be postponed until an abnormal C-cell stimulation test result is observed (i.e. an abnormal calcitonin response to pentagastrin or calcium stimulation) (18). Further studies, particularly regarding rare mutations, are necessary before common recommendations can be made (19).

Surgery for phaeochromocytoma in MEN 2 should precede surgery for MTC. Before adrenalectomy all patients should receive appropriate pharmacotherapy (α- with/or without β-adrenergic antagonist). Approximately one-third of patients who undergo a unilateral adrenalectomy will eventually require a second operation for contralateral phaeochromocytoma, but this may not occur for many years, during which time the patient will not be steroid dependent. Adrenal cortical-sparing adrenalectomy is a promising technique for preventing adrenal insufficiency.

The parathyroid glands in MEN 2 patients are frequently found to be enlarged at thyroidectomy for MTC and should therefore be carefully evaluated. The goal in MEN 2 patients with primary hyperparathyroidism is to excise the enlarged glands and to leave at least one normal parathyroid gland intact. If they are all enlarged, a subtotal parathyroidectomy or total parathyroidectomy with autotransplantation should be performed.

Postsurgical follow-up and management

All patients with MTC should undergo calcitonin and CEA determination at regular intervals after total thyroidectomy. Normal basal and pentagastrin-stimulated calcitonin levels suggest a tumour-free state and thus patients require no further treatment. They can be followed-up at yearly intervals with physical examination and calcitonin determination (Fig. 3.5.7.4).

Patients with persistent elevation of plasma calcitonin after total thyroidectomy should be thoroughly evaluated to define the extent of local and distant disease (see above). If there is no evidence of distant metastases and if local disease is found in the neck, reoperation is advocated using meticulous dissection and microsurgical techniques.

In patients remaining calcitonin-positive with evidence of noncurable and nonoperable disease (diffuse distant metastases) or occult disease (no local recurrence is found and adequate operation has been done), close observation of changes in serum calcitonin and CEA concentration is required. Many patients may exhibit a remarkably stable course and no further treatment is recommended; a 'wait and see' approach is advocated, as experience with nonsurgical therapy in the management of slowly growing metastatic MTC has been disappointing (20, 21). In those patients whose disease shows rapid and steady progress, e.g. doubling of tumour marker in less than 1 year, intervention with chemotherapy, radiotherapy, or tyrosine kinase inhibitors can be considered as a palliative therapeutic modality.

The role of regional external radiotherapy in the treatment of MTC continues to be controversial. In patients with inoperable tumour, radiotherapy can offer prolonged palliation and achieve

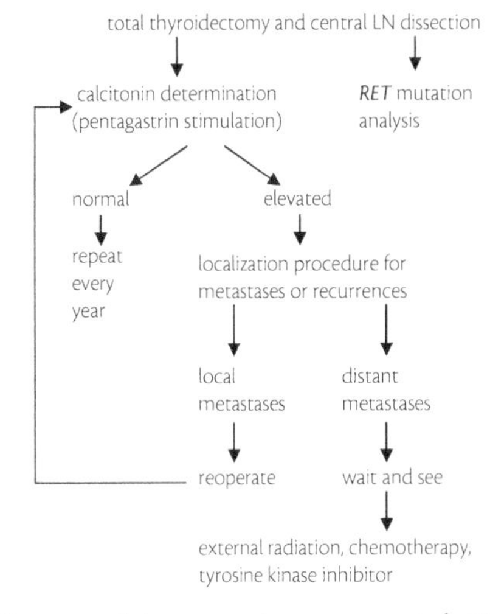

Fig. 3.5.7.4 Recommended postoperative management of patients with medullary thyroid carcinoma. LN, lymph node.

local tumour control. Radiotherapy may be helpful for patients with expanding final stage lesions or painful osseous metastases, but the response is poor.

As MTC is relatively insensitive to chemotherapy and the results are correspondingly poor, such treatment might be indicated when the tumour mass seems to have escaped local control and entered a more aggressive growth phase. Monotherapy with adriamycin (60 mg/m^2 every 3 weeks) or a combination of adriamycin and cisplatin has been used in some trials but with a response rate below 30%. Life quality, toxic side effects, and survival have to be taken into account when chemotherapy is recommended. Therefore chemotherapy in advanced MTC must be individualized based on clinical grounds.

Prognostic factors

The natural history of sporadic MTC is variable. The spectrum ranges from years of dormant residual disease after surgery to rapidly progressive disseminated disease and death related to either metastatic thyroid tumour or complications of phaeochromocytoma in MEN 2. The 10-year survival rates for all MTC patients ranges from approximately 61% to 76% (2, 22, 23). The overall prognosis is comparable to differentiated papillary and follicular carcinoma of the thyroid and much better than the more aggressive anaplastic thyroid cancer. There is general agreement that tumour stage and surgical management have a favourable influence on the clinical course of the disease. Early detection and surgical treatment of MTC is likely to be curative; more than 95% of patients detected at an early stage of disease remain disease-free (normal or undetectable calcitonin values). The main factors that influence survival are the stage of disease at the time of diagnosis, size of the tumour, and lymph node involvement. The excellent prognosis associated with identification of MTC at its earliest stage underscores the importance of prospective screening (calcitonin screening) and early diagnosis (*RET* mutation analysis) which must be followed by adequate therapy.

Future

Advances in our understanding of the molecular pathways underlying the different MEN 2 phenotypes may aid in the development of individualized therapeutic modalities based on codon-specific inhibition of tumour growth. RET seems to be a promising target for molecular therapy of patients with MTC. Different strategies that might obstruct the kinase function of RET are on the way (20). Some competitive inhibitors of ATP binding have been tested and are now in clinical trials. Vandetanib (ZD6474, AstraZeneca), a multikinase inhibitor, inhibits the wild-type enzyme and most of the activated forms of RET.

References

1. Leboulleux S, Baudin E, Travagli JP, Schlumberger M. Medullary thyroid carcinoma. *Clin Endocrinol (Oxf)*, 2004; **61**: 299–310.
2. Raue F. German medullary thyroid carcinoma/multiple endocrine neoplasia registry. *Langenbecks Arch Chir*, 1998; **383**: 334–6.
3. Raue F, Frank-Raue K. Multiple endocrine neoplasia type 2. 2007 Update. *Horm Res*, 2007; **68** (Suppl 5): 101–4.
4. Kouvaraki MA, Shapiro SE, Perrier ND, Cote GJ, Gagel RF, Hoff AO, *et al.* RET proto-oncogene: a review and update of genotype-phenotype correlations in hereditary medullary thyroid cancer and associated endocrine tumors. *Thyroid*, 2005; **15**: 531–44.
5. Etit D, Faquin WC, Gaz R, Randolph G, DeLellis RA, Pilch BZ. Histopathologic and clinical features of medullary microcarcinoma and C-cell hyperplasia in prophylactic thyroidectomies for medullary carcinoma a study of 42 cases. *Arch Pathol Lab Med*, 2008; **132**: 1767–73.
6. Machens A, Niccoli-Sire P, Hoegel J, Frank-Raue K, van Vroonhoven TJ, Roeher HD, *et al.* Early malignant progression of hereditary medullary thyroid cancer. *N Engl J Med*, 2003; **349**, 1517–25.
7. d'Herbomez M, Caron P, Bauters C, Cao CD, Schlienger JL, Sapin R, *et al.* Reference range of serum calcitonin levels in humans: influence of calcitonin assays, sex, age, and cigarette smoking. *Eur J Endocrinol*, 2007; **157**: 749–55.
8. Cohen R, Campos JM, Salaün C, Heshmati M, Kraimps JL, Proye C, *et al.* Preoperative calcitonin levels are predictive of tumor size and postoperative calcitonin normalization in medullary thyroid carcinoma. *J Clin Endocrinol Metab*, 2000; **85**: 905–18.
9. Costante G, Meringolo D, Durante C, Bianchi D, Nocera M, Tumino S, *et al.* Predictive value of serum calcitonin levels for preoperative diagnosis of medullary thyroid carcinoma in a cohort of 5817 consecutive patients with thyroid nodules. *J Clin Endocrinol Metab*, 2007; **92**: 450–5.
10. Donis-Keller H, Dou S, Chi D, Carlson KM, Toshima K, Lairmore TC, *et al.* Mutations in the RET proto-oncogene are associated with MEN 2A and FMTC. *Hum Mol Genet*, 1993; **2**: 851–6.
11. de Groot JW, Links TP, Plukker JTM, Lips C, Hofstra MW. RET as a diagnostic and therapeutic target in sporadic and hereditary endocrine tumours. *Endocr Rev*, 2006; **27**: 535–60.
12. Quayle FJ, Fialkowski EA, Benveniste R, Moley JF. Pheochromocytoma penetrance varies by RET mutation in MEN 2A. *Surgery*, 2007; **142**: 800–5.
13. Brandi ML, Gagel RF, Angeli A, Bilezikian JP, Beck-Peccoz P, Bordi C, *et al.* Guidelines for diagnosis and therapy of MEN type 1 and type 2. *J Clin Endocrinol Metab*, 2001; **86**: 5658–71.

13a. Kloos RT, Eng C, Evans DB, Francis GL, Gagel RF, Gharib H, *et al.* Medullary thyroid cancer: management guidelines of the American Thyroid Association. *Thyroid*, 2009; **19**(6): 565–612.

14. Schilling T, Bürck J, Sinn HP, Clemens A, Otto HF, Höppner W, *et al.* Prognostic value of codon 918 (ATG→ACG) RET proto-oncogene mutations in sporadic medullary thyroid carcinoma. *Int J Cancer*, 2001; **95**: 62–6.
15. Pacini F, Schlumberger M, Dralle H, Elisei R, Smit JW, Wiersinga W. European consensus for the management of patients with differentiated thyroid carcinoma of the follicular epithelium. *Eur J Endocrinol*, 2006; **154**, 787–803.
16. Elisei R, Romei C, Cosci B, Agate L, Bottici V, Molinaro E, *et al.* RET genetic screening in patients with medullary thyroid cancer and their relatives: experience with 807 individuals at one center. *J Clin Endocrinol Metab*, 2007; **92**: 4725–9.
17. Moley JF, Fialkowski EA. Evidence-based approach to the management of sporadic medullary thyroid carcinoma. *World J Surg*, 2007; **31**: 946–56.
18. Frank-Raue K, Buhr H, Dralle H, Klar E, Senninger N, Weber S, *et al.* Long-term outcome in 46 gene carriers of hereditary medullary thyroid carcinoma after prophylactic thyroidectomy: impact of individual *RET* genotype. *Eur J Endocrinol*, 2006; **155**: 229–36.
19. Frank-Raue K, Machens A, Scheuba, C, Niederle B, Dralle H, Raue F, *et al.* Difference in the development of medullary thyroid carcinoma among carriers of RET mutations in codon 790 and 791. *Clin Endocrinol*, 2008; **69**: 259–63.
20. Ball DW. Medullary thyroid cancer: monitoring and therapy. *Endocrinol Metab Clin North Am*, 2007; **36**: 823–37.
21. Vitale G, Canaglia M, Ciccarelli A, Lupoli G, Abruzzese A, Tagliaferri P, *et al.* Current approaches and perspectives in the therapy of medullary thyroid carcinoma. *Cancer*, 2001; **91**: 1797–808.
22. Kebebew E, Ituarte PHG, Siperstein AE, Duh QY, Clark OH. Medullary thyroid carcinoma, clinical characteristics, treatment, prognostic factors and a comparison of staging systems. *Cancer*, 2000; **88**: 1139–48.
23. Roman S, Lin R, Sosa J. Prognosis of medullary thyroid carcinoma: demographic, clinical, pathologic predictors of survival in 1252 cases. *Cancer*, 2006; **107**: 2134–42.

PART 4

Parathyroid, calcium, and bone metabolism

4.1

Parathyroid anatomy, hormone synthesis, secretion, action, and receptors

Geoffrey N. Hendy, David Goltzman

Parathyroid embryology, anatomy, and morphology

Humans have two pairs of parathyroid glands lying in the anterior cervical region. The fetal parathyroid glands begin developing at 5 weeks from the third and fourth pharyngeal pouches. The third pharyngeal pouch, which contains tissue that will become the thymus and parathyroid, migrates downward and gives rise to the two inferior parathyroid glands normally located at the lower poles of the thyroid. The fourth pharyngeal pouch does not migrate and gives rise to the two upper parathyroid glands, which normally are attached to the upper poles of the thyroid (1).

Eighty-five per cent of normal adults have four parathyroid glands, but the number can vary markedly in some individuals. The location of the glands is also variable with the upper glands sometimes located behind the pharynx or the oesophagus. The lower glands may be found close to or within the thymus in the superior mediastinum. Because of the variability in location surgical exploration of the neck can be problematic, especially in hyperparathyroidism of chronic kidney disease (2). Thus referral to an experienced parathyroid surgeon is essential to maximize localization of affected glands and minimize complications. Conversely, hypoparathyroidism most commonly occurs as a result of surgical excision of, or damage to, the parathyroid glands during non-parathyroid surgery, e.g. total thyroidectomy for thyroid cancer and radical neck dissection for laryngeal or oesophageal carcinoma, as well as repeated surgery for hyperparathyroidism.

Most patients with primary hyperparathyroidism, about 80%, have a single benign adenoma (3). Multiple (so-called) adenomas are rarely found and probably represent asynchronous parathyroid hyperplasia. Hyperplasia accounts for 15–20% of cases, and malignant parathyroid carcinoma is extremely rare, less than 1% of cases. In secondary hyperparathyroidism, all four glands are enlarged.

The chief cell is the predominant cell type in humans, with some oxyphil cells, which have an acidophilic cytoplasm and mitochondria are also present. Parathyroid cells have limited numbers of secretory granules containing parathyroid hormone (PTH), indicating that relatively little hormone is stored in the gland. Parathyroid cells normally divide at an extremely slow rate—mitoses are rarely observed.

Knowledge of the embryological formation of the parathyroids has been gained by study of mouse models in which deletion of specific genes has led to lack of parathyroid gland development (4), on the one hand, and of human familial hypoparathyroidism, in which the defective formation of the parathyroid glands is inherited in an autosomal-dominant, autosomal-recessive, or X-linked manner, on the other (1).

The mouse has a single pair of parathyroid glands, and at day e10 both the precursor thymus and parathyroid cells in the third pharyngeal pouch endoderm, express the four transcription factors, Hoxa3, Pax1, Eya1, and Pax9. The conjoined thymus and parathyroid rudiment develops at day e11 and the primordium also expresses transcription factors Six1 and Pbx1. At day e12, separate pathways distinct for the different parts of the rudiment that will develop into the thymus and parathyroid become apparent. Signalling molecules, including sonic hedgehog, bone morphogenetic protein-4, noggin, and fibroblast growth factor-8, act in a complex fashion to affect the outgrowth of the parathyroid precursor. By day e13.5, the parathyroid cell mass and thymus cell mass are separate. The thymic cells express *Foxn1* that is not present in the parathyroid cells that in turn specifically express glial cells missing-2 (Gcm2). *Gcm2* expression continues into adulthood; it transactivates the calcium-sensing receptor (*Casr*) gene and thereby influences the expression of the parathyroid calciostat (5).

In humans, hypoparathyroidism is part of the DiGeorge's syndrome, which occurs because of a 22q11 microdeletion. Congenital defects arise as a result of the failure to develop the derivatives of the third and fourth pharyngeal pouches, leading to agenesis or hypoplasia of the parathyroid glands and thymus (6). Haploinsufficiency of the *TBX1* transcription factor gene appears to play an important role although loss of other contiguous genes such as *CRKL*, encoding a tyrosine kinase signalling adaptor protein, probably contributes to the full expression of the syndrome. Hypoparathyroidism is a part of the Barakat's or HDR (hypoparathyroidism, nerve deafness, and renal dysplasia) syndrome, which maps to 10p14–10pter. HDR is due to haploinsufficiency and loss-of-function mutations in the *GATA3* gene, which encodes a zinc finger transcription factor (7). *GATA3* is essential for normal embryonic development of the parathyroids, auditory system, and kidney in humans. Hypoparathyroidism together with growth and mental retardation, and characteristic dysmorphism (HRD) occur in autosomal recessive Kenny–Caffey and Sanjad–Sakati syndromes. The HRD syndrome is due to mutations in the tubulin chaperone E (*TBCE*) gene, which maps to 1q42–43 (8). In an X-linked recessive form of hypoparathyroidism there is an interstitial deletion–insertion involving chromosomes 2p25.3 and Xq27.1 near the *SOX3* gene, which encodes a high mobility group box transcription factor. It is proposed that the hypoparathyroidism is caused by disruption of regulatory elements of the *SOX3* gene (1). Rare cases of primary hypoparathyroidism inherited in either an autosomal recessive or dominant manner due to mutations in the *GCM2* gene on chromosome 6p24 have been identified. In the latter case the mutated *GCM2* acts in a dominant-negative fashion (5).

Parathyroid hormone synthesis

PTH is the product of a single-copy gene and, in mammals, has 84 amino acids (9, 10) (Fig. 4.1.1). The gene, which encodes a larger precursor molecule of 115 amino acids, preproPTH, is organized into three exons. Exon I encodes the 5′ untranslated region of the messenger RNA, exon II encodes the NH_2-terminal pre- or signal peptide and a part of the short propeptide, and exon III encodes the Lys^{-2}–Arg^{-1} of the prohormone cleavage site, the 84 amino acids of the mature hormone, and the 3′ untranslated region of the mRNA (Fig. 4.1.2). The importance of correct splicing of the primary *PTH* gene transcript, or premessenger RNA, was emphasized by the identification of a donor splice mutation in the *PTH* gene in affected members of a family with autosomal recessive isolated hypoparathyroidism, resulting in the loss of exon II, which encodes the initiation codon and signal peptide (1).

The second member of the *PTH* gene family encodes the parathyroid hormone-related peptide (PTHrP), which is the causal factor responsible in the majority of cases of hypercalcaemia associated with malignancies. PTHrP plays a critical role in fetal development, especially skeletogenesis (11, 12), but is not involved in normal calcium homoeostatic control in the adult. In postnatal life, PTHrP regulates the epithelial mesenchymal interactions that are critical for development of the mammary gland, skin, and hair follicle. The *PTH* and *PTHrP* genes map to chromosome 11p15 and chromosome 12p12.1–11.2, respectively. These two human chromosomes are thought to have arisen by an ancient duplication of a single chromosome, and their respective gene clusters have been maintained as syntenic groups across the genomes of several species. Because of the similarity in NH_2-terminal sequence of their mature peptides, their gene organization, and chromosomal locations, it is likely that the *PTH* and *PTHrP* genes evolved from a single ancestral gene, with *PTHrP* being the more ancient gene.

The gene for tuberoinfundibular peptide of 39 residues (*TIP39*), a more distantly related member of the gene family, resides on chromosome 19q13.33. TIP39 is a neuropeptide (13). The *TIP39* gene shares organizational features with the *PTH* and *PTHrP* genes, having one exon encoding the 5′ untranslated region, one encoding the precursor leader sequence, and one encoding the prohormone cleavage site and the mature peptide (Fig. 4.1.2).

Transcription of the *PTH* gene occurs almost exclusively in the endocrine cells of the parathyroid gland, and is subject to strong repressor activity in all other cells. Ectopic PTH synthesis (i.e. synthesis outside parathyroid tissue) has been documented in only a very few cases of malignancies associated with hypercalcaemia. Activation of genes in a particular tissue is often related to demethylation of cytosine residues, and the *PTH* gene in parathyroid cells is hypomethylated at CpG residues relative to other tissues. In one of the few cases of true ectopic PTH production, involving a pancreatic tumour, the upstream regions of the *PTH* gene were abnormally hypomethylated (14). The human *PTH* gene has two functional TATA box-controlled transcription start sites, a cyclic AMP response element (CRE), and a negative vitamin D response element (VDRE) in its proximal promoter. While *PTH* gene transcription is negatively regulated by the hormonally active metabolite of vitamin D, 1,25-dihydroxvitamin D (1,25(OH)$_2$D), any regulation by extracellular calcium remains to be established. Also located distally are sequences that function to silence transcription in nonparathyroid cells. In a further case of ectopic PTH production, an ovarian carcinoma, this repressor regulatory region was replaced by a foreign sequence, which allowed inappropriate transcription of the *PTH* gene to take place (3).

The human PTH produced by patients with hyperparathyroidism is structurally normal (9, 10). In a small number of parathyroid tumours examined, the *PTH* gene sequence is rearranged, and the 5′ flanking region of the *PTH* gene is placed upstream of the cyclin D1 (*CCND1*) gene located on the long arm of chromosome 11.

Parathyroid hormone

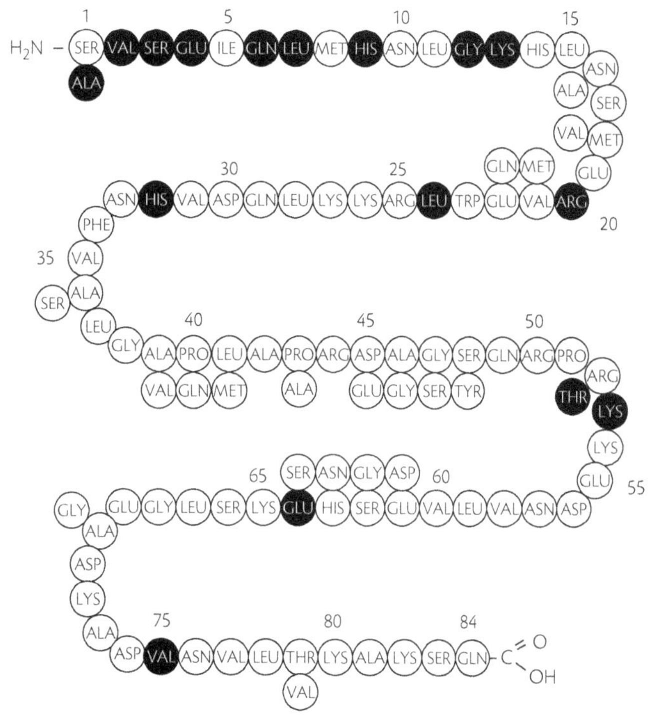

Fig. 4.1.1 Amino acid sequence of mammalian PTH. The backbone sequence is that of the human with substitutions in the rat hormone shown at specific sites. Biological activity is a property of the N-terminal one-third of the molecule (PTH(1–34)). The solid circles show those amino acids that are identical in the human and rat PTH and PTH-related peptide (PTHrP) molecules.

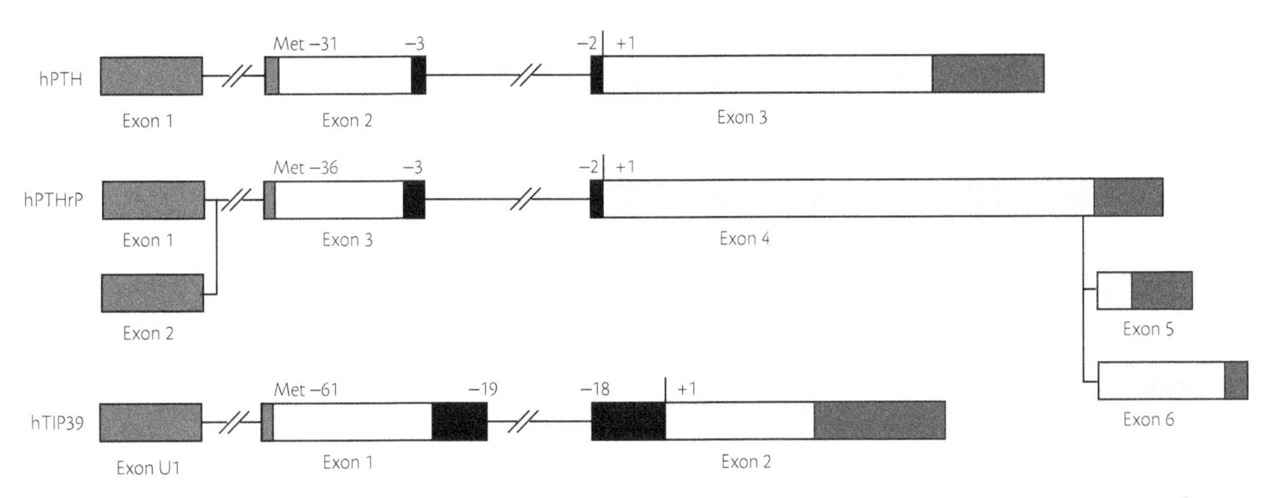

Fig. 4.1.2 Comparison of structural organization of the human *PTH, PTHrP*, and *TIP39* genes. Exons are boxed: from left to right, dark grey boxes denote 5′ untranslated regions, white boxes denote presequences, black boxes denote prosequences, light grey boxes denote mature polypeptide sequences, and dark grey boxes denote 3′ untranslated regions.

This is thought to lead to deregulated expression of the *CCND1* gene, which contributes to tumour development (3). However, this type of gene arrangement occurs very infrequently in parathyroid tumours. A more common event involves the loss or inactivation of the multiple endocrine neoplasia type 1 (*MEN1*) gene, also on the long arm of chromosome 11. The protein encoded by the *MEN1* gene (15, 16) called menin, is a 610-amino acid nuclear protein (17). Germ-line mutations in the *MEN1* gene cause familial and sporadic MEN 1 and are found in 20% of non-MEN 1 parathyroid adenomas. Loss of heterozygosity at 11q13 is found in MEN 1 tumours and sporadic parathyroid adenomas, consistent with *MEN1* being a tumour suppressor gene.

A target of the Wnt pathway, β-catenin, encoded by the *CTNNB1* gene, is a candidate for involvement in parathyroid neoplasia. Very few of the parathyroid adenomas examined so far have stabilizing missense *CTNNB1* mutations, suggesting that mutation of the β-catenin gene itself is unlikely to be involved in the initiation or early progression of parathyroid adenomatosis. However, other components of the Wnt signalling pathway, e.g. a constitutively active LRP5 receptor derived from an alternatively spliced mRNA, may be implicated in parathyroid tumorigenesis (18).

Early onset recurrent parathyroid tumours occur as part of the uncommon autosomal dominant hyperparathyroidism and jaw tumour syndrome, in which parathyroid carcinoma is frequent. The responsible gene, *HRPT2*, at 1q31.2, encodes a novel transcription factor, parafibromin, of 531 amino acids (19). Sporadic parathyroid carcinomas very commonly contain somatic mutations of the *HRPT2* gene and some of these patients harbour germline mutations. In these cases, genetic testing in family members provides for early diagnosis (6). Loss of heterozygosity at chromosome 1q occurs in carcinomas of the familial and sporadic disorder, usually by intragenic mutations.

PTH follows a pattern of biosynthesis and of vectorial transport through organelles of the cell similar to that of many other peptide hormones. It is biosynthesized on the polyribosomes of the rough endoplasmic reticulum of the parathyroid endocrine cell. The gene for PTH encodes a precursor, preproPTH, which is extended at the N-terminus of PTH 1–84 by 31 residues. The NH_2-terminal 25-residue portion, characterized by its hydrophobicity, is called the signal, leader, or pre sequence, and it facilitates entry of the nascent hormone into the cisternae of the endoplasmic reticulum. One patient with autosomal dominant hypoparathyroidism had a mutation within the protein coding region of the *PTH* gene in which there was a single base substitution (T→C) in exon II, resulting in the replacement of arginine (CGT) for cysteine (TGT) in the signal peptide. This places a charged amino acid in the hydrophobic core of the signal peptide, leading to inefficient processing of the mutant preproPTH to PTH (6). Further studies have suggested that the mutant polypeptide acts in a dominant-negative fashion by promoting endoplasmic reticulum stress leading to apoptosis (20).

Normally, as the signal sequence of the synthesized hormone emerges from the ribosome, it binds to a signal recognition particle, which stops further synthesis of the nascent protein. The signal recognition particle carrying the ribosome then binds to an integral membrane protein of the endoplasmic reticulum, called the docking protein or signal recognition particle receptor. This protein releases the block in protein synthesis, and the nascent peptide is transported across the membrane into the cisternae of the endoplasmic reticulum. The signal sequence is simultaneously removed at the inner surface of the endoplasmic reticulum, at a glycyl–lysyl bond, by a signalase enzyme. The resultant precursor molecule, proPTH, is extended at the NH_2-terminus of PTH 1–84 by only six amino acids. The pro sequence is necessary for efficient translocation and cleavage of the signal peptide. Once formed, proPTH is transported to the Golgi apparatus.

The prohormone hexapeptide has several basic residues, which serve as a recognition sequence to yield the mature hormone. Unlike many other prohormones, proPTH does not contain another sequence at the COOH-terminus and has not been detected within the circulation even in states of parathyroid gland hyperfunction. ProPTH has little biological activity until cleaved to create the hormonal form (21). The conversion of proPTH to PTH takes place within the *trans*-Golgi network rather than the secretory granules as occurs with other prohormones such as proinsulin. The enzymes involved include furin and PC7, mammalian proprotein convertases, which are related to bacterial subtilisins (22). Little proPTH is stored within the gland.

The resultant mature 84-amino acid form of the hormone is packaged in secretory granules and transported to the region of the plasma membrane. The hormone is released by exocytosis in response to the principal stimulus to secretion hypocalcaemia. The calcium ion does not influence the enzymatic cleavages involved in the processing of preproPTH or proPTH.

Parathyroid hormone secretion

Relatively little PTH is stored in secretory granules within the parathyroid glands. In the absence of a stimulus for release, intraglandular metabolism occurs, causing complete degradation to its constituent amino acids or partial degradation to fragments (Fig. 4.1.3). This has been postulated to occur through a specific calcium-regulated enzymatic mechanism. In the case of hypercalcaemia, the predominant hormonal entities released from the gland are fragments comprising midregion or COOH-terminal sequences. In response to hypocalcaemia, degradation of PTH within the parathyroid cell is minimized, and the major hormonal entity released is the bioactive PTH 1–84 molecule. Thus, in the presence of hypocalcaemia, increased amounts of bioactive PTH are secreted, even in the absence of additional synthesis of hormone. Hormone stores are insufficient, however, to maintain secretion for more than a few hours in the presence of a sustained, severe hypocalcaemic stimulus, and other mechanisms—transcriptional and post-transcriptional—come into play to increase hormone production. For example, hypocalcaemia promotes stabilization of the preproPTH mRNA, leading to increased PTH synthesis. In the presence of a sustained, severe hypocalcaemic stimulus, additional PTH secretion depends on an increase in the number of parathyroid cells. Such an increase may also be stimulated by the reduction in circulating 1,25-dihydroxvitamin D (1,25$(OH)_2$D) that often accompanies hypocalcaemia. Normally, the sterol inhibits parathyroid cell proliferation by inhibiting expression of early immediate response genes, such as the *MYC* proto-oncogene.

A circadian rhythm has been reported for PTH secretion, with increased blood levels occurring at night and small-amplitude pulses of PTH secretion occurring at much shorter intervals. This suggests neural or central nervous system influences on PTH secretion, or reflects circadian alterations in the levels of extracellular calcium.

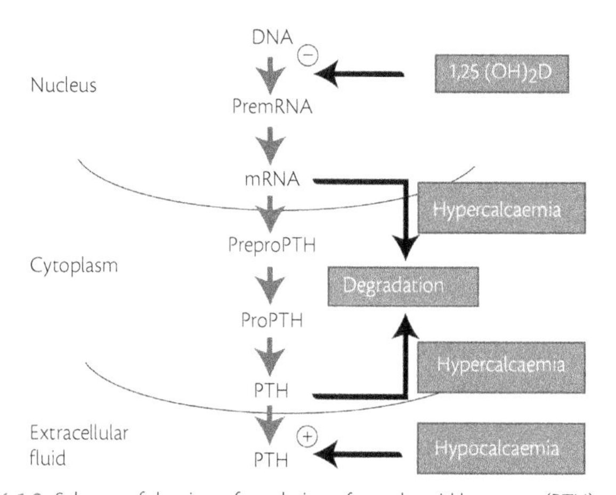

Fig. 4.1.3 Schema of the sites of regulation of parathyroid hormone (PTH) biosynthesis, intraglandular degradation, and secretion. Both extracellular fluid calcium and 1,25-dihydroxyvitamin D levels negatively regulate transcription of the PreproPTH gene. Hypercalcaemia increases PreproPTH mRNA turnover and PTH degradation while hypocalcaemia stabilizes PreproPTH mRNA and promotes the production and synthesis of mature PTH.

Calcium

There is an inverse relationship between ambient calcium levels and PTH release that is curvilinear rather than proportional (23). This relationship between PTH and extracellular calcium contrasts with the influence of the calcium ion as a secretagogue in most other secretory systems in which elevations in this ion enhance release of the secretory product. This distinction between the parathyroid cell and other secretory cells is maintained intracellularly, where elevations rather than decreases in cytosolic calcium correlate with decreased PTH release. Alterations in extracellular fluid calcium levels are transmitted through a parathyroid plasma membrane calcium-sensing receptor (CaSR) that couples through a Gq/11-protein complex to phospholipase C. Increases in extracellular calcium lead to increases in inositol 1,4,5-trisphosphate (IP_3) and mobilization of intracellular calcium stores. The CaSR also couples to a Gi-protein complex thereby inhibiting cyclic AMP production. The precise mechanisms whereby activation of the CaSR inhibits PTH secretion and synthesis and parathyroid cell proliferation are not known.

The human CaSR has 1078 amino acids with a large extracellular domain (ECD) (*c.* 600 amino acids) and a seven transmembrane-spanning domain and cytoplasmic tail (24). The CaSR is a member of group C of the G protein-coupled receptor (GPCR) superfamily that includes the metabotropic glutamate, γ-aminobutyric acid-B, and vomeronasal odorant receptors. These receptors function as dimers with the ECDs of each monomer having a so-called Venus flytrap domain consisting of two lobes, which close upon the ligand leading to conformation changes in the transmembrane domain of the receptor, allowing coupling of G proteins to the intracellular loops and the cytoplasmic tail. The CaSR has a low affinity for Ca^2+ appropriate for it monitoring the relatively high levels of the mineral ion in the blood. Besides the parathyroid, the CaSR is also expressed in other cells having Ca^2+-sensing functions, such as those of the kidney tubule, the calcitonin-secreting thyroid C-cells, and in diverse other organs and tissues such as brain, bone and cartilage, haematopoietic stem cells, keratinocytes, gastrointestinal tract, mammary gland, placenta, and vascular smooth muscle. Neomycin binds the receptor, which may account for the toxic renal effects of aminoglycoside antibiotics.

Inherited abnormalities of the *CASR* gene located on chromosome 3q13.3–21 can lead to either hypercalcaemia or hypocalcaemia depending upon whether they are inactivating or activating, respectively (25). Heterozygous loss-of-function mutations give rise to familial (benign) hypocalciuric hypercalcaemia (FHH) in which the lifelong hypercalcaemia is asymptomatic. The homozygous condition manifests itself as neonatal severe hyperparathyroidism (NSHPT), a rare disorder characterized by extreme hypercalcaemia and the bony changes of hyperparathyroidism. Several cases of NSHPT have normocalcaemic parents and seem to be sporadic. The disorder autosomal dominant hypocalcaemia (ADH) is due to gain-of-function mutations in the *CASR* gene. ADH may be asymptomatic or present with neonatal or childhood seizures. Because of the overactive CaSR in the nephron, these patients are at a greater risk of developing renal complications during vitamin D therapy than patients with idiopathic hypoparathyroidism. A common polymorphism in the intracellular tail of the CaSR, Ala to Ser at position 986, has a modest effect on the serum calcium concentrations in healthy individuals (26). *CASR* polymorphisms might also affect urinary calcium excretion and therefore *CASR* is a candidate gene for involvement in disorders such as idiopathic hypercalciuria and primary hyperparathyroidism.

The CaSR is a target for phenylalkylamine compounds—so-called calcimimetics—which are allosteric stimulators of the CaSR's affinity for cations. These orally active compounds have been approved for use in patients with uraemic secondary hyperparathyroidism and parathyroid cancer and by their direct action on the parathyroid gland CaSR they provide an effective medical means of lowering PTH secretion (27). Cinacalcet HCl is marketed as Sensipar in North America and Australia and Mimpara in the European Union. Ongoing clinical trials in patients with mild primary hyperparathyroidism (PHPT) have shown that calcimimetics reduce serum calcium and PTH levels and increase serum phosphate levels but do not significantly affect bone turnover or bone mineral density (BMD). While calcimimetics provide an important addition to the armamentarium of drugs to treat the secondary hyperparathyroidism of chronic kidney disease, their more widespread use in the medical management of PHPT is uncertain at present.

CaSR allosteric antagonists, calcilytics, are also being evaluated in clinical trials as a treatment of osteoporosis (27). As intermittent administration of exogenous PTH produces increases in BMD, it is proposed that once-daily administration of a short-acting calcilytic could achieve a similar result by producing a pulse of endogenous PTH secretion.

The CaSR expressed in the developing parathyroid glands—and in the placenta—plays an important role in regulating fetal calcium concentrations. Normally, the fetal blood calcium level is elevated above the maternal level. This depends upon the action of PTHrP released from the fetal parathyroids and placenta on placental calcium transport. Disruption of the CaSR, as shown by studies in CaSR-deficient mice, causes fetal hyperparathyroidism and hypercalcaemia due to fetal bone resorption. The transfer of calcium across the placenta is reduced and renal calcium excretion is increased.

Some patients with anti-CaSR autoantibodies (of the inactivating type) associated with autoimmune disorders such as sprue or autoimmune thyroid disease present as an FHH phenocopy, termed acquired hypocalciuric hypercalcaemia (AHH). The anti-CaSR antibodies are directed against the ECD and interfere with elevated extracellular Ca^{2}+-mediated suppression of PTH release and perturb Ca^{2}+ sensing in the kidney, thereby closely mimicking FHH (25). Autoantibodies from a subset of patients with autoimmune hypoparathyroidism that inhibited PTH secretion were identified several years ago. More recently, the CaSR has been identified as a self-antigen in patients with autoimmune polyendocrine syndrome type 1 (APS 1) or acquired hypoparathyroidism associated with autoimmune hypothyroidism or idiopathic hypoparathyroidism. The activating antibodies are directed against epitopes in the ECD of the receptor and inhibit PTH secretion from parathyroid cells.

In vivo, PTH mRNA levels are markedly stimulated by decreased circulating calcium concentrations. This occurs, in part, by a post-transcriptional mechanism whereby hypocalcaemia stabilizes and hypercalcaemia destabilizes the PTH mRNA. Prolonged hypocalcaemia *in vivo* may stimulate DNA replication, cell division, and the production of increased numbers of parathyroid cells or parathyroid hyperplasia. This would increase the synthesis of proteins, including PTH, within the hypercellular parathyroid gland and ultimately would increase PTH release. In primary parathyroid gland hyperfunction resulting in hyperparathyroidism, alterations in the calcium-sensing mechanism may manifest as a set-point error, producing a shift to the right of the curve relating PTH secretion to extracellular calcium levels. Consequently, elevated concentrations of extracellular fluid calcium may be required to reduce PTH secretion, resulting in an adenomatous or hyperplastic parathyroid gland that is incompletely suppressed by calcium. Such a mechanism may underlie the observation that an increase in the mass of parathyroid tissue like that produced by transplantation, can be associated with hypercalcaemia. The parathyroid glands of patients with primary and severe uraemic secondary hyperparathyroidism have reduced CaSR expression as assessed by immunostaining. Loss of a functional CaSR, as in humans with NSHPT or in mice in which the *Casr* gene has been ablated, leads to severe parathyroid hyperplasia. If basal secretion per cell produces a significant amount of bioactive PTH, the cumulative increase in this basal or non-calcium-suppressible secretion arising from an increase in parathyroid cells could also be responsible for the hypercalcaemia. The precise mechanistic relationship of extracellular calcium to parathyroid cell growth remains to be determined.

1,25-dihydroxyvitamin D

Vitamin D metabolites modulate PTH release. There is a feedback loop between PTH-induced increase in $1,25(OH)_2D$ and vitamin D metabolite-induced decrease of PTH levels (28). This latter effect is achieved by a direct action on *PTH* gene transcription, thus altering the quantities of hormone available for immediate release by secretagogues. 'Low calcaemic analogues' of vitamin D have been developed that appear to diminish PTH secretion *in vitro* and *in vivo* and that serve as therapeutics for hyperparathyroidism in chronic kidney disease.

Other factors

In addition to calcium and vitamin D metabolites, several other factors influence the release of PTH from parathyroid glands. The cation magnesium affects PTH release like calcium, although with reduced efficacy. (The CaSR is also a magnesium sensor.) High concentrations of aluminium also suppress PTH release. Hyperphosphataemia is associated with increased levels of PTH, an effect that is most often indirect and a result of the hypocalcaemia and/or the decreased $1,25(OH)_2D$ production that accompanies the rise in serum phosphate. However, the anion can exert a more direct effect on PTH synthesis with hyperphosphataemia stabilizing and hypophosphataemia destabilizing PTH mRNA levels. Glucocorticoids (in some studies) increase PTH secretion. Agents such as biogenic amines, which increase parathyroid gland cAMP levels, induce PTH secretion, and those that lower cAMP levels within the parathyroid gland decrease PTH secretion.

PTH measurement

Circulating PTH is heterogeneous. The major circulating bioactive moiety is similar or identical to intact PTH(1–84). This is metabolized by the liver, which releases midregion and COOH-terminal fragments into the circulation for subsequent clearance by the kidney. These biologically inert moieties generated by metabolism and secretion from the parathyroid gland are cleared more slowly than intact PTH. Circulating bioactive PTH is best measured by sensitive immunometric assays that simultaneously recognize NH_2 and COOH epitopes on the PTH molecule, and detect intact PTH(1–84). This is the method of choice for the accurate diagnosis of patients with hypercalcaemia, especially in distinguishing patients with primary hyperparathyroidism from those with hypercalcaemia of malignancy and in assessing hyperparathyroidism in chronic kidney disease.

Actions of PTH

The major function of PTH is the maintenance of a normal level of extracellular fluid calcium (23, 28) (Fig. 4.1.4). The hormone exerts important effects on bone and kidney and indirectly influences the gastrointestinal tract. In response to a fall in the extracellular fluid ionized calcium concentration, PTH is released from the parathyroid cell and acts directly on the kidney to enhance renal calcium reabsorption and promote the conversion of 25-hydroxyvitamin D to $1,25(OH)_2D$. The latter metabolite increases gastrointestinal absorption of calcium and, with PTH, induces skeletal resorption, causing the restoration of extracellular fluid calcium and the neutralization of the signal initiating PTH release. The opposite series of homoeostatic events occur in response to a rise in extracellular fluid calcium levels.

Although this scheme outlines the overall events that occur after a fall in calcium, aspects of the response may vary. Certain actions of PTH, such as renal calcium retention, may predominate at relatively low circulating concentrations of PTH. Furthermore, PTH appears to be essential as a bone anabolic factor in the fetus (29) and neonate (30) but may be predominantly resorptive in older animals (31) when the source of external calcium changes. PTH and PTHrP regulate osseous cellular differentiation, proliferation, and development, and are now considered to be anabolic skeletal agents when administered periodically rather than continuously *in vivo*. Thus, intermittent doses of PTH(1–34)—and PTHrP(1–34) and related analogues—promote bone formation. Daily injections of PTH(1–34) increase hip and spine bone mineral density, and prevent vertebral and non-vertebral fractures in osteoporosis, and human PTH is now used clinically as a bone anabolic agent.

Besides regulating calcium homoeostasis, PTH elicits various other responses. Among these responses are perturbations of other ions, the most marked of which are those involving phosphate. As a consequence of PTH-enhanced $1,25(OH)_2D$ production, the gastrointestinal absorption of phosphate is facilitated to some extent, and with PTH-induced skeletal lysis, phosphate and calcium are released. These effects increase the extracellular fluid phosphate levels, but the predominant effect of PTH on phosphate homeostasis is to inhibit renal phosphate reabsorption and produce phosphaturia. Consequently, a net decrease in extracellular fluid phosphate concentration occurs, which is adjunctive to the role of PTH in raising calcium levels.

PTH receptors

Like other peptide hormones, PTH interacts through a receptor on the plasma membrane of target cells. This same receptor binds PTHrP (32). The PTH/PTHrP receptor (PTHR1) is a seven-transmembrane G-protein linked receptor that has the 'signature' GPCR topology, a seven-membrane-spanning, 'serpentine' domain, as well as an extracellular ligand-binding domain and an intracellular COOH-terminal domain (33). It is a member of group B of the GPCR superfamily. The receptor can couple to the stimulatory G

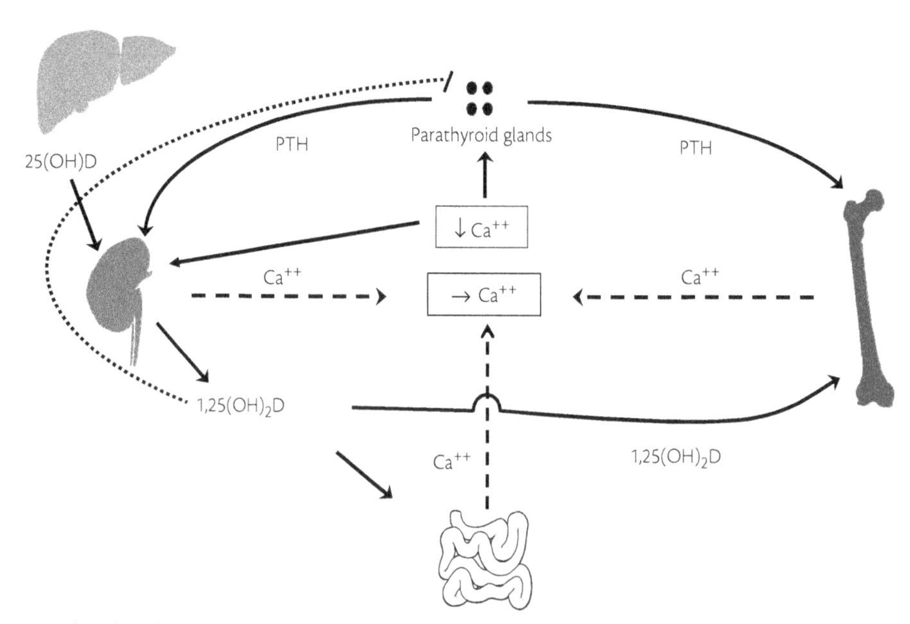

Fig. 4.1.4 Parathyroid hormone (PTH) and vitamin D control calcium (as shown) and phosphate homoeostasis. A fall in extracellular calcium concentration triggers PTH secretion. PTH directly acts on the kidney to promote renal calcium reabsorption and conversion of 25-hydroxyvitamin D (25(OH)D) to 1,25-dihydroxyvitamin D ($1,25(OH)_2D$). $1,25(OH)_2D$ increases intestinal absorption of calcium (and phosphate) and, with PTH, mobilizes calcium (and phosphate) from bone. Thus extracellular fluid (ECF) calcium is restored to normal, neutralizing the signal initiating PTH release. PTH inhibits renal phosphate reabsorption, promoting phosphaturia.

protein, G_s, leading to increased adenylate cyclase activity, the generation of cAMP, and activation of the protein kinase A (PKA) pathway, and can couple to G_q, leading to an increase in the protein kinase C (PKC) pathway and to an increase in IP_3, diacylglycerol, and intracellular Ca^{2+} (33). As with other GPCRs, PTHR1 undergoes cyclical receptor activation, desensitization, and internalization (34). After ligand binding and endocytosis, the PTHR1 is either recycled to the cell membrane or targeted for degradation. High circulating levels of PTH in hyperparathyroid states have been associated with hormonal desensitization in target tissues. Arrestins contribute to the desensitization of both G_s and G_q mediated PTHR1 signalling. PTHR1 activation and internalization can be selectively dissociated (35). PTHR1 signalling can be modified by scaffolding proteins such as the Na^+/H^+ exchanger regulatory factor (NHERF) 1 and 2 through PDZ1 and PDZ2 domains (36). PTHR1 signalling via the cAMP pathway, leading to PKA activation, results in phosphorylation of the cyclic AMP response element binding protein (CREB). CREB binds to the cyclic AMP response element (CRE) in the promoter region of many genes and transcriptionally modulates their expression.

The PTHR1 is highly expressed in kidney and bone, the primary target tissues of PTH, but is also expressed in a wide variety of embryonic and adult tissues, including cartilage, liver, brain, smooth muscle, spleen, testis, and skin. In most of these tissues, the receptor appears to mediate the autocrine/paracrine actions of locally produced and secreted PTHrP. Nevertheless, PTHrP may also exert some of its bioactivity through domains of the molecule that do not interact with PTHR1 (37).

The human PTH/PTHrP receptor gene *(PTHR1)* localizes to chromosome 3p21.1–22. A second related receptor, which is the product of a distinct gene (*PTHR2* on chromosome 2q33), and which binds PTH, TIP39, but not PTHrP, has been identified (38). It is expressed in brain, pancreas, testis and placenta and its endogenous ligand is TIP39.

Direct evidence that the PTHR1 mediates the calcium homoeostatic actions of PTH and the skeletal growth plate actions of PTHrP in humans has come from the study of rare genetic disorders. Jansen's metaphyseal chondrodysplasia (JMC) is inherited in an autosomal dominant fashion although most reported cases are sporadic (6). The disorder comprises short-limbed dwarfism secondary to severe growth plate abnormalities, asymptomatic hypercalcaemia, and hypophosphataemia. There is increased bone resorption similar to that in primary hyperparathyroidism and urinary cAMP levels are elevated, but circulating PTH and PTHrP levels are low or undetectable. Although PTHR1 is found widely in fetal and adult tissues, it is most abundant in three major organs, the kidney, bone, and metaphyseal growth plate. The changes in mineral ion homoeostasis and the growth plate in JMC are caused by heterozygous gain-of-function mutations (Fig. 4.1.5) in the *PTHR1* giving rise to constitutively active receptors.

Inactivating or loss-of-function mutations in the *PTHR1* have been implicated in the molecular pathogenesis of Blomstrand's lethal chondrodysplasia (BLC) (6). This rare disease is characterized by advanced endochondral bone maturation, short-limbed dwarfism, abnormal breast and tooth morphogenesis, and fetal death, thus mimicking the phenotype of *Pthr1*-less mice (39). The majority of BLC cases were born to phenotypically normal, consanguineous parents, suggesting an autosomal recessive mode of inheritance. Mutant PTHR1s (Fig. 4.1.5) identified in BLC fetuses

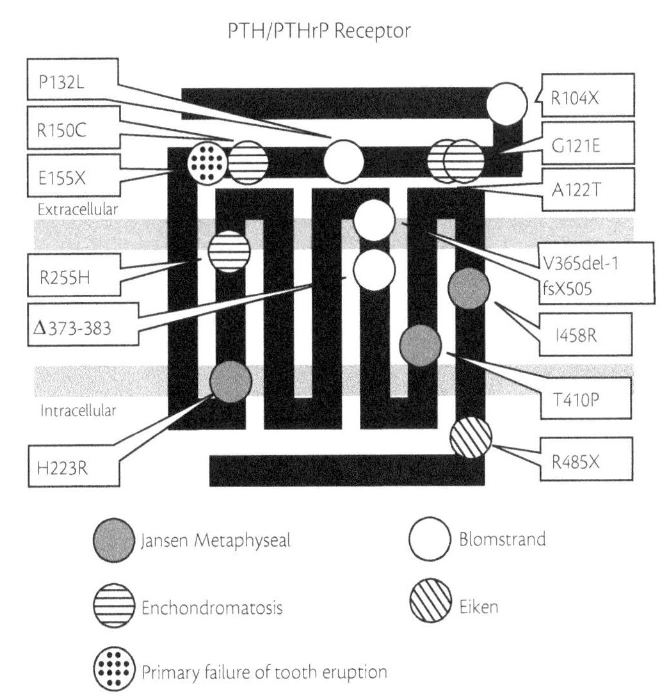

Fig. 4.1.5 Schematic representation of the human PTH/PTHrP receptor. The locations of the H223R, T410P, and I458R activating mutations identified in patients with Jansen's metaphyseal chondrodysplasia, the R104X, P132L, V365del-1fsX505, and Δ373–383 inactivating mutations found in patients with Blomstrand's chondrodysplasia, the R485X Eiken's syndrome mutation, the G121E, A122T, R150C, and R255H endochondromatosis mutations, and the E155X primary failure of tooth eruption (PFE) mutation are indicated. Splice-site mutations that would result in predicted mutant C351fsX485 and E182fsX203 proteins have been identified in additional PFE cases.

fail to bind ligand or stimulate cAMP or inositol phosphate production. A milder form of recessively inherited skeletal dysplasia, known as Eiken's syndrome, has been linked to mutations of *PTHR1*, suggesting a wider range of skeletal phenotypes to this gene. Dominantly acting heterozygous *PTHR1* mutations have been identified in familial, nonsyndromic primary failure of tooth eruption (40). Heterozygous *PTHR1* mutations have been identified in endochondromas of patients with endochondromatosis (Ollier's disease), a familial disorder with evidence of autosomal dominance characterized by multiple benign cartilage tumours, and a predisposition to malignant osteocarcinoma (41). As many patients with Ollier's disease do not apparently have *PTHR1* mutations, the condition may be genetically heterogeneous.

Heterozygous inactivating mutations in the *GNAS1* gene encoding Gαs cause an approximately 50% reduction in amount/ activity of the protein leading to resistance to PTH and other hormones in the disorder, pseudohypoparathyroidism (PHP) type 1a (42). In contrast, patients with PHP type 1b have end-organ resistance to PTH without the typical physical stigmata—termed Albright's hereditary osteodystrophy—of PHP type 1a. Linkage to chromosome 20q13.3, which includes the *GNAS1* locus, was established in kindreds with PHP type 1b (43). In addition, the genetic defect is imprinted paternally and is inherited in the same fashion as the PTH resistance in kindreds with PHP type 1a, and in a mouse model heterozygous for ablation of the *Gnas* gene (44). In PHP type 1b patients, mutations some distance upstream of the *GNAS1* coding regions affect the normal differential methylation of maternal and paternal alleles leading to silencing of the *GNAS* gene specifically in the renal proximal tubules (45).

PTH controls renal phosphate reabsorption. Mutations in the genes encoding the two renal sodium phosphate co-transporters, NPT2a and NPT2c, have been identified in a few patients with hyperphosphaturia. The NHERF1 interacts with the PTHR1 and NPT2a. Study of hyperphosphaturic patients referred initially for nephrolithiasis or osteopenia identified a few cases having NHERF1 mutations that could contribute to the renal phosphate loss (46).

Summary

PTH is responsible for the minute-to-minute maintenance of calcium homoeostasis. PTH secretion is controlled via the parathyroid CaSR, and inactivating or activating mutations in this receptor lead to inherited hypercalcaemic and hypocalcaemic disorders, respectively. Both PTH (and the related gene family member, PTHrP) act through the PTHR1 that is widely expressed and signals through multiple second messenger pathways. Inactivating mutations in the PTHR1 cause Blomstrand's lethal chondrodysplasia, whereas activating mutations are found in Jansen's metaphyseal chondrodysplasia.

References

1. Thakker RV. Genetic regulation of parathyroid gland development. In: Bilezikian JP, Martin TJ, Raisz LG, eds. *Principles of Bone Biology*. 3rd edn. San Diego: Academic Press, 2008: 1415–29.
2. Meakins JL, Milne CA, Hollomby DJ, Goltzman D. Total parathyroidectomy: parathyroid hormone levels and supernumerary glands in hemodialysis patients. *Clin Invest Med*, 1984; **7**: 21–5.
3. Hendy GN, Arnold A. Molecular basis of PTH overexpression. In: Bilezikian JP, Martin TJ, Raisz LG, eds. *Principles of Bone Biology*. 3rd edn. San Diego: Academic Press, 2008: 1311–26.
4. Miao D, He B, Karaplis AC, Goltzman D. Parathyroid hormone is essential for normal fetal bone formation. *J Clin Invest*, 2002; **109**: 1173–82.
5. Canaff L, Zhou X, Mosesova I, Cole DEC, Hendy GN. Glial cells missing-2 transactivates the calcium-sensing receptor gene: effect of a dominant-negative GCM2 mutant associated with autosomal dominant hypoparathyroidism. *Hum Mutat*, 2009; **30**: 85–92.
6. Hendy GN, Cole DEC. Parathyroid disorders. In: Rimoin DL, Connor JM, Pyeritz RE, Korf BE, eds. *Emery and Rimoin's Principles and Practice of Medical Genetics*. Vol. 2. 5th edn. Edinburgh: Churchill Livingstone, 2007: 1951–79.
7. Ali A, Christie PT, Grigorieva IV, Harding B, Van Esch H, Ahmed SF, *et al*. Functional characterization of GATA3 mutations causing the hypoparathyroidism-deafness-renal (HDR) dysplasia syndrome: insight into the mechanisms of DNA binding by the GATA3 transcription factor. *Hum Mol Genet*, 2007; **16**: 265–75.
8. Parvari R, Diaz GA, Hershkovitz E. Parathyroid development and the role of tubulin chaperone E. *Horm Res*, 2007; **67**: 12–21.
9. Keutmann HT, Sauer MM, Hendy GN, O'Riordan JLH, Potts JT Jr. Complete amino acid sequence of human parathyroid hormone. *Biochemistry*, 1978; **17**: 243–4.
10. Hendy GN, Kronenberg HM, Potts JT Jr, Rich A. Nucleotide sequence of cloned DNAs encoding human preproparathyroid hormone. *Proc Natl Acad Sci U S A*, 1981; **78**: 7365–9.
11. Karaplis AC, Luz A, Glowacki J, *et al*. Lethal skeletal dysplasia from targeted disruption of the parathyroid hormone-related peptide gene. *Gene Develop*, 1994; **8**: 277–89.
12. Amizuka N, Warshawsky H, Henderson JE, Goltzman D, Karaplis AC. Parathyroid hormone-related peptide-depleted mice show abnormal epiphyseal cartilage development and altered endochondral bone formation. *J Cell Biol*, 1994; **126**: 1611–23.
13. Fegley DB, Holmes A, Riordan T, Faber CA, Weiss JR, Ma S, *et al*. Increased fear- and stress-related anxiety-like behavior in mice lacking tuberoinfundibular peptide of 39 residues. *Genes Brain Behav*, 2008; **7**: 933–42.
14. VanHouten JN, Yu N, Rimm D, Dotto J, Arnold A, Wysolmerski JJ, Udelsman R, *et al*. Hypercalcemia of malignancy due to ectopic transactivation of the parathyroid hormone gene. *J Clin Endocrinol Metab*, 2006; **91**: 580–3.
15. Chandrasekharappa SC, Guru SC, Manickam P, Olufemi SE, Collins FS, Emmert-Buck MR, *et al*. Positional cloning of the gene for multiple endocrine neoplasia-type 1. *Science*, 1997; **276**: 404–7.
16. Lemmens I, Van der Ven WJ, Kas K, Zhang CX, Giraud S, Wautot V, *et al*. Identification of the multiple endocrine neoplasia type 1 (MEN1) gene. European Consortium on MEN1. *Hum Mol Genet*, 1997; **6**: 1177–83.
17. Hendy GN, Kaji H, Canaff L. Cellular functions of menin. *Adv Exp Med Biol*, 2009; **668**: 37–50.
18. Bjorklund P, Akerstrom G, Westin G. An LRP5 receptor with internal deletion in hyperparathyroid tumors with implications for deregulated WNT/β-catenin signalling. *PLoS Medicine*, 2007; **4**: e328.
19. Carpten JD, Robbins CM, Villablanca A, Forsberg L, Presciuttini S, Bailey-Wilson J, *et al*. HRPT2, encoding parafibromin, is mutated in hyperparathyroidism-jaw tumor syndrome. *Nat Genet*, 2002; **32**: 676–80.
20. Datta R, Waheed A, Shah GN, Sly WS. Signal sequence mutation in autosomal dominant form of hypoparathyroidism induces apoptosis that is corrected by a chemical chaperone. *Proc Natl Acad Sci USA*, 2007; **104**: 19989–94.
21. Rabbani SA, Kaiser SM, Henderson JE, *et al*. Synthesis and characterization of extended and deleted recombinant analogues of parathyroid hormone-(1–84): correlation of peptide structure with function. *Biochemistry*, 1990; **29**: 10080–9.
22. Hendy GN, Bennett HPJ, Gibbs BF, Lazure C, Day R, Seidah NG. Proparathyroid hormone (ProPTH) is preferentially cleaved to parathyroid hormone (PTH) by the prohormone convertase furin: a mass spectrometric analysis. *J Biol Chem*, 1995; **270**: 9517–25.
23. Brown EM. Physiology of calcium metabolism. In: Becker KL, Bilezikian JP, eds. *Principles and Practice of Endocrinology and Metabolism*. 3rd edn. Philadelphia: JB Lippincott, 2000: 478–89.
24. Brown EM. Biology of the extracellular Ca2+-sensing receptor. In: Bilezikian JP, Martin TJ, Raisz LG, eds. *Principles of Bone Biology*. 3rd edn. San Diego: Academic Press, 2008: 533–53.
25. Hendy GN, Guarnieri V, Canaff L. Calcium-sensing receptor and associated diseases. *Prog Mol Biol Transl Sci*, 2009; **89**: 31–95.
26. Cole DEC, Peltekova VD, Rubin LA, *et al*. A986S polymorphism of the calcium-sensing receptor and circulating calcium concentrations. *Lancet*, 1999; **353**: 112–5.
27. Nemeth EF. Drugs acting on the calcium receptor. Calcimimetics and calcilytics. In: Bilezikian JP, Martin TJ, Raisz LG, eds. *Principles of Bone Biology*. 3rd edn. San Diego: Academic Press, 2008: 1711–35.
28. Hendy GN. Calcium regulating hormones. Vitamin D and parathyroid hormone. In: Melmed S, Conn PM, eds. *Endocrinology. Basic and Clinical Principles*. Totowa, NJ: Humana Press Inc, 2005: 283–99.
29. Miao D, He B, Karaplis AC, Goltzman D. Parathyroid hormone is essential for normal fetal bone formation. *J Clin Invest*, 2002; **109**: 1173–82.
30. Miao D, He B, Lanske B, *et al*. Skeletal abnormalities in Pth-null mice are influenced by dietary calcium. *Endocrinology*, 2004; **145**: 2046–53.

31. Xue Y, Karaplis AC, Hendy GN, Goltzman D, Miao D. Genetic models show that parathyroid hormone and 1,25-dihydroxyvitamin D3 play distinct and synergistic roles in postnatal mineral ion homeostasis and skeletal development. *Hum Mol Genet*, 2005; **14**: 1515–28.
32. Goltzman D. Interactions of PTH and PTHrP with the PTH/PTHrP receptor and with downstream signaling pathways: exceptions that provide the rules. *J Bone Miner Res*, 1999; **14**: 173–7.
33. Mannstadt M, Jüppner H, Gardella TJ. Receptors for PTH and PTHrP: their biological importance and functional properties. *Am J Physiol*, 1999; **277**: F665–75.
34. Weinman EJ, Hall RA, Friedman PA, Liu-Chen LY, Shenolikar S. The association of NHERF adaptor proteins with G protein-coupled receptors and receptor tyrosine kinases. *Ann Rev Physiol*, 2006; **68**: 491–505.
35. Sneddon WB, Syme CA, Bisello A, Magyar CE, Rochdi MD, Parent JL, *et al.* Activation independent parathyroid hormone receptor internalization is regulated by NHERF1 (EBP50). *J Biol Chem*, 2003; **278**: 43787–96.
36. Mahon MJ, Donowitz M, Yun CC, Segre GV. Na^+/H^+ exchanger regulatory factor 2 directs parathyroid hormone 1 receptor signalling. *Nature*, 2002; **417**: 858–61.
37. Miao D, Su H, He B, Gao J, Xia Q, Zhu M, *et al.* Severe growth retardation and early lethality in mice lacking the nuclear localization sequence and C-terminus of PTH-related protein. *Proc Natl Acad Sci U S A*, 2008; **105**: 20309–14.
38. Usdin TB, Gruber C, Bonner TI. Identification and functional expression of a receptor selectively recognizing parathyroid hormone, the PTH2 receptor. *J Biol Chem*, 1995; **270**: 15455–8.
39. Lanske B, Karaplis AC, Lee K, Luz A, Vortkamp A, Pirro A, *et al.* PTH/PTHrP receptor in early development and Indian Hedgehog-regulated bone growth. *Science*, 1996; **273**: 663–6.
40. Decker E, Stellzig-Eisenhauer A, Fiebig BS, Rau C, Kress W, Saar K, *et al.* PTHR1 loss-of-function mutations in familial, nonsyndromic primary failure of tooth eruption. *Am J Hum Genet*, 2008; **83**: 781–6.
41. Couvineau A, Wouters V, Bertrand G, Rouyer C, Gérard B, Boon LM, *et al.* PTHR1 mutations associated with Ollier diseases result in receptor loss of function. *Hum Mol Genet*, 2008; **17**: 2766–75.
42. Bastepe M. The GNAS locus and pseudohypoparathyroidism. *Adv Exp Med Biol*, 2008; **626**: 27–40.
43. Juppner H, Schipani E, Bastepe M, Cole DE, Lawson ML, Mannstadt M, *et al.* The gene responsible for pseudohypoparathyroidism type 1b is paternally imprinted and maps in four unrelated kindreds to chromosome 20q13.3. *Proc Natl Acad Sci U S A*, 1998; **95**: 11798–803.
44. Yu S, Yu D, Lee E, Eckhaus M, Lee R, Corria Z, *et al.* Variable and tissue-specific hormone resistance in heterotrimeric Gs protein α-subunit (Gsα) knockout mice is due to tissue-specific imprinting of the Gsα gene. *Proc Natl Acad Sci U S A*, 1998; **95**: 8715–20.
45. Bastepe M, Frolich LF, Hendy GN, Indridason OS, Josse RG, Koshiyama H, *et al.* Autosomal pseudohypoparathyroidism type 1b is associated with a heterozygous microdeletion that likely disrupts a putative imprinting control element of GNAS. *J Clin Invest*, 2003; **112**: 1255–63.
46. Karim Z, Gérard B, Bakouh N, Alili R, Leroy C, Beck L, *et al.* NHERF1 mutations and responsiveness of renal parathyroid hormone. *N Engl J Med*, 2008; **359**: 1128–35.

4.2

Hypercalcaemia

Ronen Levi, Justin Silver

Introduction

Ionized calcium is essential for several physiological functions, including neuromuscular activation, endocrine and exocrine secretions, integrity of cellular bilayers, plasma coagulation, immune functions and bone metabolism. Extracellular fluid (ECF) calcium is uniquely controlled by its own calcium-sensing receptor, regulating the secretion of parathyroid hormone (PTH), synthesis of 1,25-dihydroxyvitamin D, and the renal reabsorption of filtered calcium (see Chapter 4.1). With the advent of the autoanalyser and routine determination of serum calcium levels, recognition of hypercalcaemia has become common. However, the clinical spectrum of hypercalcaemia varies from a laboratory-detected, asymptomatic mineral disorder to a life-threatening state.

Hypercalcaemia may be regarded as a pathological excessive manifestation of normal calcium recruitment. Since serum calcium level depends on intestinal absorption, bone resorption, and renal tubular reabsorption, hypercalcaemia is necessarily derived from an abnormal regulation of these processes. The bone serves as the major reservoir of calcium. Therefore, any disruption of the equilibrium between bone formation and resorption may have profound effects on serum calcium. When bone resorption is uncoupled with equivalent bone formation and calcium–phosphate complex skeletal deposition, hypercalcaemia may result. Calcium, unlike phosphate, is inefficiently absorbed from the gut. 1,25-dihydroxyvitamin D_3, stimulated by PTH, enhances both calcium and phosphate absorption. 1,25-dihydroxyvitamin D_3 binds to a nuclear vitamin D receptor and promotes, in the intestine, the transcription of a calcium binding protein, thereby increasing net influx of calcium from the intestine to the circulation (1).

Daily urinary calcium excretion is efficiently kept below 5% of daily calcium glomerular filtration (100–300 mg/day versus 6–10 g/day, respectively). Tubular calcium reabsorption is also dependent on PTH and takes place mainly in the proximal tubule (60%) and the loop of Henle (30%). However, the actions of PTH and calcium-sensing receptor (CaSR) in the distal tubule determine the fine tuning and the extent of calcium eventually excreted in the urine.

In the average adult human body, the total calcium content varies between 1 and 2 kg, of which nearly 99% is deposited in the bone. The remainder of the calcium serves for vital intracellular and extracellular functions. Twelve millimoles of calcium are exchanged daily between the bone and ECF. In practically every cell, calcium mediates essential steps in signal transduction. Intracellular calcium concentration is kept extremely low through a constantly active transport across the cell membrane and sequestration of ionized calcium in mitochondria and endoplasmic reticulum. Intracellular free calcium concentration is 2.5^{10-5}(10^{-4}mg/dl), while extracellular calcium concentration is 8–10 mg/dl. Hence, minute intracellular fluid (ICF) calcium changes have profound effects, while a gradient in the order of 10^4 higher is required for ECF effects.

To maintain homoeostasis both ICF and ECF calcium are tightly regulated. ECF calcium concentration is regulated by PTH, vitamin D, calcitonin, intake of calcium, urinary calcium excretion, ECF phosphate concentration, and bone mineral resorption and deposition. ECF calcium exists in three forms: 50% bound to plasma proteins, mainly albumin; 45% as free ionized calcium; and 5% as a diffusible complex with citrate, sulfate, bicarbonate, phosphate, or lactate anions (2).

Ionized calcium is biologically active and subject to the control mechanisms stated above. Acid–base balance affects the relative ratio of ionized calcium to the total calcium, but not the total calcium concentration. Acidosis inhibits calcium ion complex with albumin, thereby increasing ionized calcium concentration. Hence, chronic renal failure patients, despite being hypocalcaemic, are usually protected from manifestations of hypocalcaemia. Vice versa, alkalosis promotes binding of calcium ions to albumin, thereby reducing ionized calcium concentration. Acute hyperventilation may be associated with respiratory alkalosis and manifestations of hypocalcaemic tetany despite normal total calcium serum concentration. While 40–50% of calcium is bound to plasma proteins, 50–60% is ultrafilterable, or diffusible. Non-diffusible calcium is mainly bound to plasma albumin and to a much lesser extent to globulins. Hence, alterations in albumin concentration result in changes in total calcium concentration in the same direction. The diffusible calcium exists as free ionized calcium (45%), or as a diffusible complex (5–15%). Acidosis effect on calcium ion complex with albumin is evident by a non-diffusible calcium concentration elevation of 0.12 mg% for a pH decrease of 0.1 (3).

Definition

Hypercalcaemia is defined as a serum total calcium concentration above 2.62 mmol/l (10.5 mg/dl). Serum calcium is ordinarily measured as the sum of ionized and bound calcium. Since most calcium is bound to albumin, total serum calcium levels vary with the concentration of serum albumin. As a rule of thumb, serum total calcium levels rise or fall 0.2 mmol/l (0.8 mg/dl) per 1 g/l of albumin, and should therefore be corrected for serum albumin concentration. The upper limit of serum calcium may vary in different laboratories in accordance with the reference population and analytic method. Serum ionized calcium measures the physiologically active form of calcium, and is highly correlated with the total calcium concentration. Ionized calcium assays may detect subtle abnormalities in calcium homoeostasis, but are inversely affected by serum pH. Once hypercalcaemia is detected in an asymptomatic individual, the calcium level should be redetermined because of the broad overlap between the normal population and that of documented disease-associated hypercalcaemia. Even when hypercalcaemia is recurrent and its cause is determined, the increment in serum calcium is usually mild, often less than 1 mg/dl. Moreover, in a significant proportion of documented disorders leading to hypercalcaemia, for example, hyperparathyroidism, the serum calcium may even be below the upper limit of normal, that is 10.5 mg/dl.

Prevalence

The prevalence of persistent hypercalcaemia in the asymptomatic adult population varies from 1/100 to 1/1000, depending on the definition of the normal range and the study population. However, the prevalence of hypercalcaemia rises universally with age in postmenopausal women because of oestrogen deficiency. In fact two-thirds of newly diagnosed asymptomatic individuals are postmenopausal women.

Symptoms

Serum calcium levels below 2.7 mmol/l (11 mg/dl) are generally asymptomatic. However, a rapid rise in serum calcium correlates with a more symptomatic patient. Manifestations may also alter with the specific aetiology for hypercalcaemia. As symptoms are not pathognomonic, they are often overlooked and regarded as nonspecific. Signs and symptoms include, in descending order of frequency, fatigue, polydipsia, confusion, anorexia, depression, polyuria caused by reversible nephrogenic diabetes insipidus, nausea, proximal myopathy, constipation, nephrolithiasis, pancreatitis, and peptic ulcer disease (4). Neurological manifestations are especially conspicuous because the nervous system function is dependent on a narrow range of extracellular calcium concentration. In severe cases, unless treated, coma and death may supervene. Persistent hypercalcaemia, especially when phosphate levels are not decreased, may result in ectopic calcification in blood vessels, joints, cornea, and renal parenchyma. Additionally, hypertension may be aggravated with hypercalcaemia. Shortened Q–T interval in the electrocardiogram may be associated in some patients with arrhythmias. Bradycardia and first-degree atrioventricular block may also be observed. ST segment elevation mimicking acuter myocardial infarction has been reported (5–7). Mild metabolic alkalosis may follow bone dissolution and alkali release, and increased bicarbonate reclamation. Hyperparathyroidism overshadows the alkalosis by prompting chloride reabsorption for bicarbonate. Interestingly, symptoms are not universally correlated with serum calcium levels. Thus, although most patients become symptomatic when serum calcium is above 2.9 mmol/l (11.5 mg/dl), occasional patients may still be asymptomatic with calcium levels reach 3.0 mmol/l (12 mg/dl). Calcifications usually occur when serum calcium is above 3.2 mmol/l (13 mg/dl), or when hyperphosphataemia is also evident, as in renal failure, or with vitamin D overdose or tumoral calcinosis. Serum calcium levels above 13–15 mg% may represent a medical emergency because of the risk of a rapid deterioration to coma, cardiac arrest, and death. However, severe asymptomatic hypercalcaemia may be buffered by excessive calcium binding to albumin, resulting in near-normal ionized calcium concentration (8).

Pathophysiology

Since extracellular calcium, reflected by serum calcium levels, is the net result of intestinal calcium absorption, calcium efflux from bone, and renal excretion, any up-regulation of the former two and down-regulation of the latter, will result in hypercalcaemia. Of these, increased calcium efflux from bone, mediated by osteoclastic bone resorption, is the single most important factor. Less often, excessive intestinal calcium absorption, as in excess circulating 1,25-dihydroxyvitamin D from various causes, coupled with absence of skeletal capacity for calcium reclamation, may result in increased ECF total calcium content and hypercalcaemia. In general, the kidney does not contribute to hypercalcaemia. Rather it protects against the development of hypercalcaemia. Therefore hypercalciuria usually precedes hypercalcaemia unless renal calcium excretory capacity has been overwhelmed, as in familial hypercalcaemic hypocalciuria (FHH). FHH is therefore a unique predisposing factor for hypercalcaemia because the latter develops in subjects with normal skeletal calcium efflux and intestinal calcium absorption (9) (see Chapter 4.4).

As most cases of hypercalcaemia are associated with increased bone resorption, osteoclasts play a major role in the pathogenesis of the disorder. Both under normal and pathologic conditions, osteoclasts are stimulated by PTH or PTH-related protein (PTHrP) to degrade bone surface (10). However, osteoclasts do not have receptors for PTH and probably receive the signal via the osteoblast. Osteoclast progenitors are stimulated to differentiate and enhance bone resorption by osteoclast differentiation factor (ODF). ODF, identical to the T-cell growth factor TRANCE/RANKL, mediates the signal for differentiation of osteoclast progenitors into osteoclasts and thus regulates osteoclastogenesis and bone resorption (11).

Malignancy-induced hypercalcaemia is to a large extent the result of PTHrP production by the tumour (Fig. 4.2.1). This hormone is immunologically distinct but shares biological activity with PTH (12). These hormones have amino acid sequence homology in the N-terminal region. However, unlike the PTH gene, the gene encoding PTHrP is normally expressed in various tissues, such as epithelial, endocrine, breast, and other tissues. Moreover, the non-PTH-homologous part is highly conserved in evolution, indicating an important role in normal physiology, yet to be elucidated.

Malfunction of the recently discovered calcium-sensing receptor may lead to hypercalcaemia (see Chapter 4.4). The gene encoding this divalent-cation receptor is located on chromosome 3. In this disorder, effective regulation of serum calcium is lost and PTH secretion occurs at higher calcium levels. Additionally, renal tubular calcium reabsorption is enhanced for the same reason, leading to a very low fractional excretion of calcium, and hypocalciuric

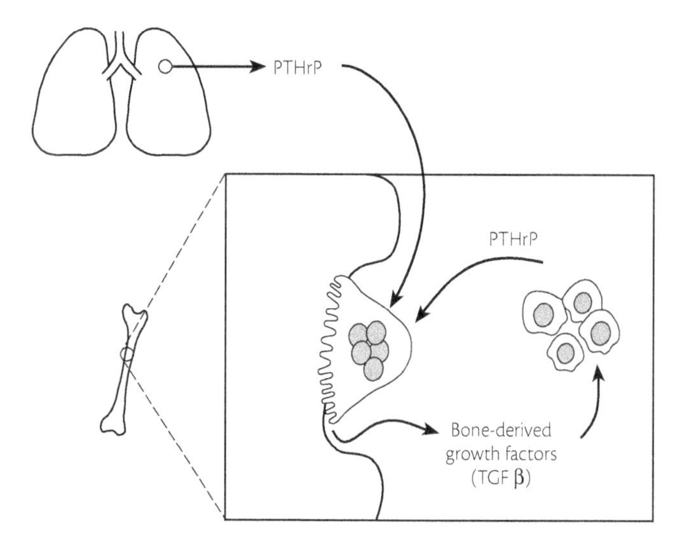

Fig. 4.2.1 PTHrP is the chief mechanism accounting for hypercalcaemia associated with malignancy. Local factors often also play a major role. (Adapted with permission from the New England journal of Medicine.)

hypercalcaemia ensues. The CaSR is in fact a divalent sensor, mediating magnesium metabolism as well. One abnormal allele results in FHH while homozygous individuals are affected early in life and develop severe hypercalcaemia and hyperparathyroidism, necessitating urgent parathyroidectomy (9, 13, 14).

Diagnostic work-up

Hyperparathyroidism and malignancy associated hypercalcaemia account for more than 90% of cases, contributing about an equal proportion each (Box 4.2.1). Therefore, one's approach to the problem will differ and depend upon whether the hypercalcaemia has a mild protracted course or an accelerating course. Clinical features of weight loss, low-grade fever, bone pain, night sweats, anaemia, or lumps detected on physical examination are suggestive of malignancy. Hyperparathyroidism is often asymptomatic, or limited to subtle neurologic symptoms, renal colic, or peptic complaints. Persistent and mild hypercalcaemia is most frequently caused by hyperparathyroidism, where calcium concentration is most commonly below 11.5–12 mg%. These patients may be free from complications or may have chronic complications, such as nephrolithiasis. Malignancy-related hypercalcaemia, however, is progressive and symptomatic, and may lead to severe hypercalcaemia. Rarely, hyperparathyroidism crisis may produce the 'malignant' presentation of hypercalcaemia, and an occult tumour may be associated with the 'hyperparathyroid' presentation. Taken together, the vast majority of hypercalcaemic episodes can be attributed to either of these two conditions, while granulomatous disorders, such as sarcoidosis, tuberculosis, and berylliosis, represent a small minority. Other aetiologies for hypercalcaemia are less commonly encountered, with serum calcium levels usually not sufficiently severe or protracted to account for severe complications.

The diagnostic work-up includes complete history, including drugs (especially calcium, lithium, and aluminium intake, vitamin D and A derivatives, thiazides, and those used for oestrogen replacement and in chronic renal failure). Family history, risk factors for malignancy, and its manifestations should be evaluated, as should be complications of hypercalcaemia, especially mental

Box 4.2.1 Aetiologies of hypercalcaemia

- Primary hyperparathyroidism
  - Adenoma
  - Hyperplasia
  - Carcinoma
  - Multiple endocrine neoplasias
- Malignancy
  - PTHrP secretion by solid tumours
  - Metastatic bone destruction
  - Osteoclast activating factors
  - Prostaglandins
  - 1,25-dihydroxyvitamin D_3
- Granulomatous disorders
  - Sarcoidosis
  - Tuberculosis
  - Berylliosis
  - Histoplasmosis
  - Coccidiodomycosis
  - Wegener's granulomatosis
- Drugs
  - Thiazides
  - Vitamin D
  - Vitamin A
- Renal failure associated
  - Tertiary hyperparathyroidism
  - Aluminium toxicity
  - Adynamic bone disease
  - Therapy with calcium and vitamin D
- High bone turnover
  - Paget's disease
  - Hyperthyroidism
  - Immobilization
- Recovery from pancreatitis
- CaSR mutation
  - FHH
  - Severe congenital hypercalcaemia
- Miscellaneous
  - Addison's disease
  - Milk alkali syndrome
  - Hypophosphatasia

The differential diagnosis of hypercalcaemia. Major aetiologies include parathyroid adenoma, malignancy, granulomatous disorders, drugs, endocrine disorders, high bone turnover, and FHH.

status changes, nephrolithiasis, and polyuria. Excruciating bone pain should direct a search for malignancy. Physical examination should be oriented to neurologic functions, lumps, and bone pain. Laboratory investigations should include a complete blood count and erythrocyte sedimentation rate (ESR). Anaemia and ESR above 100 mm/1st h should prompt a comprehensive evaluation for malignancy, such as multiple myeloma or lymphoma. Biochemistry profile should include total protein (may suggest hyperglobulinaemia), albumin, ionized calcium, alkaline phosphatase (marker of bone formation and turnover), and renal function tests. Hyperphosphataemia suggests granulomatous disorders or excessive vitamin D ingestion. Hypophosphataemia suggests primary hyperparathyroidism, after a malignancy has been ruled out. Hypermagnesaemia is a unique feature of familial hypocalciuric hypercalcaemia. Daily urine calcium excretion above 8 mmol (300 mg) is a definite risk factor for nephrolithiasis and may mandate therapy, at times before the development of frank hypercalcaemia. Excessive hypercalciuria is suggestive of malignant humoral-mediated hypercalcaemia due to PTHrP, which is associated with only a mild reabsorptive effect on calcium reabsorption in the proximal tubule. While a fractional calcium excretion above 0.01 is usually seen in most of the disorders, a fractional calcium excretion below 0.01 is suggestive of FHH. An abnormal chest radiograph may be the first clue for malignancy, sarcoidosis, or tuberculosis. The serum PTH level is an essential component of the work-up and may increase the diagnostic accuracy from 95% based on the above clinical and laboratory findings, to 99%. Elevated PTH accompanied by hypercalcaemia is almost diagnostic of primary hyperparathyroidism, since normal parathyroid tissue is effectively depressed by hypercalcaemia. Rare exceptions may be lithium therapy, FHH, or a tumour secreting intact PTH (and not the more common PTHrP), or primary hyperparathyroidism existing simultaneously with malignancy in a single patient (occurrence with a higher frequency than in the general population). Vitamin D metabolite levels are only rarely helpful for the diagnosis. In the occasional patient who denies ingestion of vitamin D, 25-hydroxyvitamin D_3 levels may be high, while an occult granulomatous disease or lymphoma may escape previous extensive evaluation and manifest as hypercalcaemia and increased 1,25-dihydroxyvitamin D_3 levels. 1,25-dihydroxyvitamin D_3 levels may be elevated in primary hyperparathyroidism and reduced in tumours secreting PTHrP, and should therefore not be used as a first step in the work-up.

Aetiology

The causes of hypercalcaemia are detailed in Box 4.2.1 and an approach to establishing a diagnosis in a hypercalcaemic patient is illustrated in Fig. 4.2.2. The two most common causes are primary hyperparathyroidism and malignancy.

Hyperparathyroidism

Primary hyperparathyroidism is often suspected when mild hypercalcaemia is detected in the course of routine biochemical screening profiles. Eighty-five percent are due to parathyroid adenoma and 15% are accounted for by gland hyperplasia and multiple endocrine neoplasia type 1 (pituitary and pancreatic tumours) or 2A (phaeochromocytoma and medullary carcinoma of the thyroid). In less than 1% of cases parathyroid carcinoma is responsible. Most of the individuals with primary hyperparathyroidism (often postmenopausal women) remain asymptomatic for a long period following the diagnosis. However, complications may include bone pain, nephrolithiasis, peptic ulcer disease, or manifestations of hypercalcaemia *per se*, as described above. When normal PTH secretion fails to establish a normal calcium homoeostasis, or when vitamin D and calcium absorption are deficient, the result may be hypocalcaemia, with the development of second-

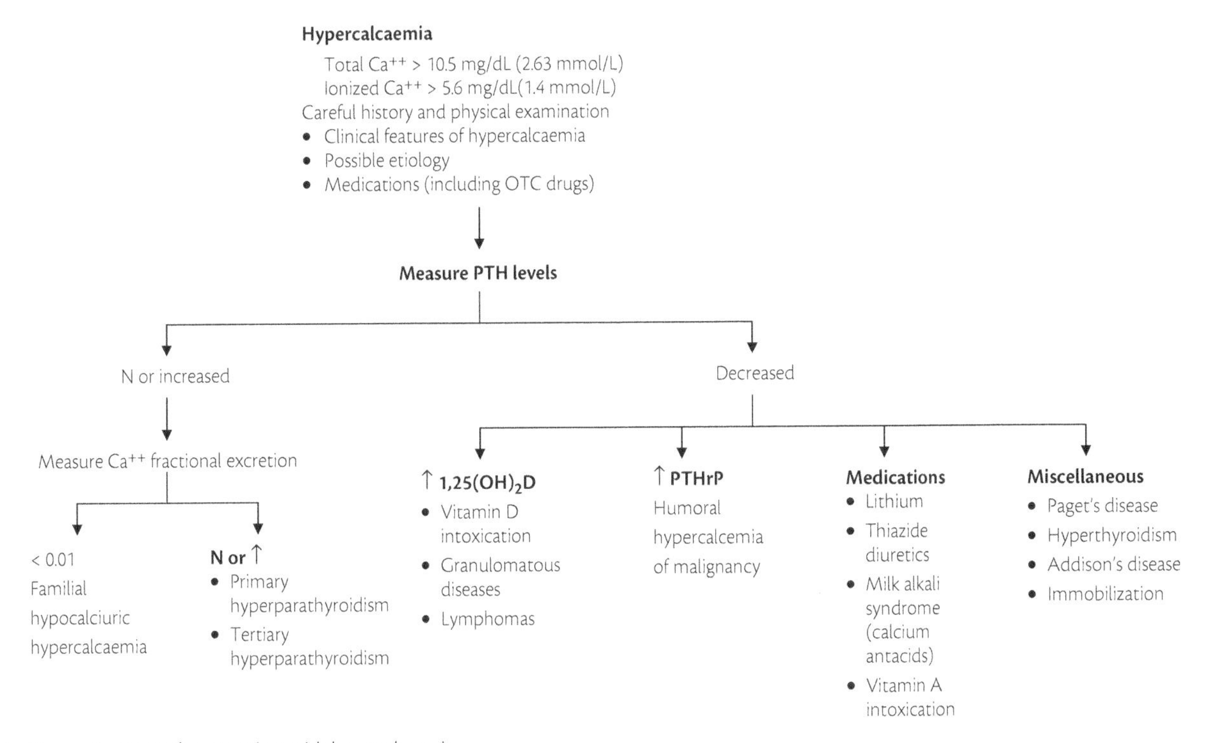

Fig. 4.2.2 Diagnostic approach to a patient with hypercalcaemia.

ary hyperparathyroidism (see Chapters 4.5 and 4.10). This is most often the case in chronic renal failure, where PTH resistance, hyperphosphataemia, and 1,25-dihydroxyvitamin D_3 deficiency result in protracted hypocalcaemia. Such patients with chronic renal failure may eventually develop hypercalcaemia associated with raised PTH levels, and this has been referred to as tertiary hyperparathyroidism (Box 4.2.1).

Malignancies

Severe symptomatic hypercalcaemia often results from malignancy, although most tumour-associated hypercalcaemia is mild. Unless the tumour is of an endocrine type, the prognosis is often poor once hypercalcaemia is detected, and mean survival may be a few weeks to a few months. Multiple metastases resulting in bone lytic lesions often cause symptomatic hypercalcaemia, at times uncontrollable and implying end-stage disease. Various types of malignancies are associated with hypercalcaemia. The leading aetiologies in men and women, respectively, are carcinomas of the lung and breast. Another common aetiology is multiple myeloma, but many other types could lead to symptomatic hypercalcaemia (15).

Once hypercalcaemia appears in the course of malignancy, the disease is often overt. Hypercalcaemia associated with malignancy can be classified into four types (Table 4.2.1):

Local osteolytic hypercalcaemia Hypercalcaemia results from marked increased in bone resorption due to release of cytokines, chemokines, and PTHrP by the tumour cells invading bone marrow. This is the case in breast cancer, multiple myeloma (see below) and lymphomas.

Humoral hypercalcaemia of malignancy (HMM) This occurs in about 80% of cases, and is caused by systemic release of PTHrP by malignant tumours. This peptide has an autocrine or paracrine effect and is a normal fetal constituent, playing a role in skeletal development. It is produced by mammary glands (and found in human milk), placenta, heart and lungs, pancreas, endothelium, and smooth muscle tissue. PTHrP effect differs from PTH by less renal tubular calcium reabsorption, less bone turnover effect, less 1,25-dihydroxyvitamin D_3 stimulation, and a more prominent effect on bone reabsorption in hypercalcaemia production. The typical net effect for PTHrP-induced hypercalcaemia is markedly increased hypercalciuria (16).The receptor binding and activating domains of PTH and PTHrP are contained within the first 34 amino acids, interacting with the same receptor. The chief role of PTHrP in humoral hypercalcaemia of malignancy was shown by resolution of hypercalcaemia in rodents with PTHrP-producing tumours that were passively immunized with antibodies against N-terminal PTHrP, followed by inhibition of bone resorption and calcium reabsorption.

Despite sequence and functional homology, PTH and PTHrP are products of different genes. Normal paracrine activity may be associated with undetectable plasma levels of PTHrP. However, squamous cell carcinomas may significantly overproduce PTHrP, leading to binding and activation of the PTH receptor at the intestinal, bone and renal target sites, and resulting in hypercalcaemia. PTHrP mRNA and protein are expressed in many tumour types. At least in human T-cell leukaemia virus type 1 (HTLV1) associated T-cell lymphoma leukaemia, PTHrP gene transcription is promoted by the transcription factors *tax* and *ets1*. PTHrP may also contribute to bone metastases, as it is observed more often in patients with breast carcinoma metastatic to bone than with metastases to other organs. In mice injected with breast carcinoma cell line producing PTHrP, PTHrP antibody can inhibit bone metastases. Moreover, despite the prior common belief that in patients with multiple bone metastases, the mechanism of hypercalcaemia involves mainly local bone destruction, increased cAMP and phosphate clearance, suggest a role for PTHrP. Indeed, up to 65% of hypercalcaemic patients with breast carcinoma may have detectable levels of PTHrP. PTHrP may also account for hypercalcaemia in rare cases where it is associated with phaeochromocytoma, prostatic cancer, pituitary, thyroid, parathyroid, testicular and ovarian adenomas (17).

PTHrP is normally produced locally and has a paracrine effect in several tissues. In fact, it may be the mediator of some of the extrarenal and extraskeletal effects of PTH, as well as a paracrine or autocrine factor in cell growth and differentiation.

Squamous cell carcinomas (most likely to be derive from lung, female genital tract, head and neck, or midoesophagus), renal cancer, ovarian cancer, endometrial cancer, HTLV1-associated lymphoma, and breast cancer are most commonly associated with humoral malignant hypercalcaemia.

1,25-dihydroxyvitamin D-secreting lymphomas 1,25-dihydroxyvitamin D is secreted by all lymphomas.

Ectopic hyperparathyroidism This is rare and accounts for less than 1% of malignancy-associated hypercalcaemia.

Discrete local bone lesions or diffuse bone destruction may cause hypercalcaemia in 30% of patients with multiple myeloma

Table 4.2.1 Types of hypercalcaemia associated with cancer

Type	Frequency (%)	Bone metastases	Causal agent	Typical tumours
Local osteolytic hypercalcaemia	20	Common, extensive	Cytokines, chemokines, PTHrP	Breast cancer, multiple myeloma, lymphoma
Humoral hypercalcaemia of malignancy	80	Minimal or absent	PTHrP	Squamous cell cancer (e.g. of head and neck, oesophagus, cervix or lung), renal cancer, ovarian cancer, endometrial cancer, HTLV-associated lymphoma, breast cancer
$1,25(OH)_2D$-secreting lymphomas	1<	Variable	$1,25(OH)_2D$	Lymphoma (all types)
Ectopic hyperparathyroidism	1<	Variable	PTH	Variable

PTHrP, parathyroid hormone-related peptide; HTLV, human T-cell leukaemia virus; $1,25(OH)_2D$, 1,25-dihydroxyvitamin D.

sometime in the course of their disease. Osteoclasts are activated by various cytokines secreted by monoclonal plasma cells. Tumour necrosis factor-α, known also as lymphotoxin, is considered one of these mediators. It is normally secreted by the macrophage lineage and prompts the replication of osteoclast precursors, their differentiation into mature osteoclasts, and the formation of ruffled border in multinucleated osteoclasts, where bone resorption occurs. Additional macrophage-derived cytokines, such as IL-1α and β, IL-6, transforming growth factor-α and β, and tumour necrosis factor may also be involved in the locally mediated bone destruction and resultant hypercalcaemia in myeloma. Moreover, Wnt signalling inhibitor, Dickhopf-1 has recently been identified as an important factor that inhibits osteoblast by myeloma cells (18, 19). Osteoblast proliferation is also inhibited by IL-3 and hepatocyte growth factor. Thus the mechanism of lytic bone destruction in multiple myeloma involves uncoupling of bone remodelling caused by osteoclast activation and inhibition of osteoblast precursors. Transforming growth factor-α and IL-6 may potentiate the hypercalcaemic effect of PTHrP. Despite the extensive bone destruction that occurs in most myeloma patients, only 30% become hypercalcaemic. The reason is probably the contribution of a reduced glomerular filtration rate in these myeloma patients. Lymphomas result in hypercalcaemia via several mechanisms. Locally secreted bone resorbing factors, pathologically high 1,25-dihydroxyvitamin D_3 levels and PTHrP secretion may all play a role in maintaining the elevated calcium levels.

Drugs

Thiazides

Thiazides are frequently associated with hypercalcaemia. Thiazide diuretics cause hypercalcaemia in 2% of patients taking the drug. The mechanism involves reduction of urinary calcium excretion. However, most of these patients continue to be hypercalcaemic even when the drug is stopped, thereby prompting the unravelling of occult hyperparathyroidism (usually parathyroid adenoma) by the drug. In the normal subject, the calcium-elevating properties of thiazides are offset by counteraction of homoeostatic controls. However, when administered in a state of a high-turnover bone disorder, hypercalcaemia ensues. The hypocalciuric effect of thiazides is mediated mainly by enhanced proximal tubular reabsorption triggered by mild sodium depletion. Additionally, increased renal tubular response to PTH and potentiation of an already existing bone resorption state may also play a role. More recently, the molecular pathways controlling distal calcium reabsorption and their regulation have been elucidated. Active calcium reabsorption fine-tunes the final amount of calcium excreted into the urine. One of the key regulators of active calcium reabsorption in the distal tubule is the epithelial calcium channel TRPV5 (transient receptor potential, vanilloid subfamily, member 5) the expression of which is affected by various calciotropic hormones and other factors. These include PTH vitamin D, klotho, and WNK4 (20). The mechanism whereby WNK4 affects renal calcium handling and hence changes in calcium excretion is intriguing. WNK4 has been shown to be a multifunctional protein regulating renal ion transport. It does so by affecting surface abundance of several ion transporters including the thiazide-sensitive Na^+–Cl^- cotransporter (NCCT) and TRPV5. Specifically, WNK4 decreases membrane expression of NCCT, while increasing activity of TRPV5 by upregulating its surface abundance (21). Moreover, the positive effect of WNK4 on TRPV5 is greatly reduced when NCCT is upregulated. Thus blocking the NCCT by thiazide diuretics may serve to enhance the effect of WNK4 on TRPV5 with consequent increase in active calcium reabsorption. Other than chlorthalidone, all other diuretics do not reduce urinary calcium excretion, and loop diuretics enhance calciuresis.

Vitamin D

1,25-dihydroxyvitamin D_3 increases intestinal calcium (and phosphate) absorption, and bone resorption, leading to hypercalciuria and hypercalcaemia. The vitamin and its derivatives may be taken enterally as food supplementation, capsules, or parenterally, mainly in the therapy of secondary hyperparathyroidism, hypoparathyroidism, rickets or osteomalacia, and osteoporosis. Calcium is often prescribed along with vitamin D and increases the risk for hypercalcaemia. Unlike derivatives of vitamin D, the hormone itself may exert a prolonged effect on calcium absorption resulting in hypercalcaemia because of its long half-life. Although the daily recommended vitamin D intake is 400 IU, as much as 10 000 IU may be needed to be taken per day for prolonged periods, in order to result in hypercalcaemia. In patients with reduced renal function, however, the dose may be much lower. Glucocorticoids are helpful in restoring calcium levels to normal, especially if calcium excretion is not feasible. Vitamin D increases intestinal calcium (and phosphate) absorption and bone resorption leading to hypercalciuria and hypercalcaemia. The appearance of hypercalcaemia in patients taking vitamin D is unpredictable because the therapeutic range between normocalcaemia and hypercalcaemia is narrow. Also, this hormone is lipid soluble and may be stored in adipose tissues, thereby it may be responsible for hypercalcaemia even weeks after it was stopped. 1,25-dihydroxyvitamin D_3 administration, however, may result in shorter-lived period, of only several days after its withdrawal. Menopause and thiazides increase the risk for hypercalcaemia in patients taking vitamin D derivatives.

Vitamin A

The daily recommended vitamin A intake is limited to 5000 IU; however, chronic daily ingestion of 50 000 IU may already result in vitamin A intoxication associated with increased bone resorption and hypercalcaemia, sometimes severe. Metastatic calcification may accompany the intoxication. Vitamin A toxicity is usually observed in suicide attempts, in patients with acute myeloid leukaemia treated with all-*trans* retinoic acid, and in patients with dermatological disorders for which vitamin A analogues are applied topically. A major symptom of vitamin A toxicity may be painful swellings along the limbs accompanied by periosteal bone deposition visible on radiographs, but the diagnosis is based on elevated serum vitamin A levels. Therapy consists mainly of drug cessation. In severe cases, intravenous hydrocortisone prompts the return of serum calcium levels to normal.

Lithium carbonate

Lithium-induced hypercalcaemia was first described in 1973, and was initially attributed to hyperparathyroidism (22). Up to 25–30% of lithium-treated patients develop mildly elevated serum calcium concentrations. In these patients, false hypercalcaemia resulting from plasma volume depletion due to lithium-induced nephrogenic diabetes insipidus should be excluded. The prevalence of hyperparathyroidism in chronic lithium users (above 10 years) was estimated at about 10–15% (23). The prevalence is highest in patients with renal failure in whom calciuria is reduced. Hypercalcaemia may be seen even in the presence of therapeutic drug levels. Nephrolithiasis and nephrocalcinosis can occur. Lithium-induced hyperparathyroidism is caused by parathyroid adenomas in two-thirds of cases, and multiglandular hyperplasia in one-third but the mechanism is not yet clear. One possibility is that lithium directly stimulates PTH production. Alternatively, lithium may reduce the set point for PTH secretion by interacting with the calcium-sensing receptor in the parathyroid gland. Hypocalciuria due to mild renal insufficiency is another possibility.

Oestrogens

Oestrogens and partial oestrogen agonists may be associated with hypercalcaemia in patients with bone metastases from breast carcinoma. Local skeletal destruction is not responsible for the hypercalcaemia in these patients because the mineral disorder develops along with regression of these lesions. Potentiation of humoral factors may be the mechanism responsible for the increased bone resorption.

Granulomatous disorders

Granulomatous disorders, such as sarcoidosis, Wegener's granulomatosis, tuberculosis, and berylliosis may be associated with hypercalcaemia. The mechanism seems to involve autonomous overproduction of 1,25-dihydroxyvitamin D_3 in macrophages, uninfluenced by serum calcium or PTH levels, but related to sun exposure. This supports the theory of vitamin D as a substrate for the macrophage 1 α-hydroxylase. Thus, hypercalcaemia in these disorders is directly associated with increased intestinal calcium absorption. Hypercalciuria ensues and may often result in nephrolithiasis. PTH levels are characteristically low because the parathyroids are amenable to inhibition by stimulation of the CaSR by the high extracellular calcium levels, and transcriptional inhibition by the high circulating 1,25-dihydroxyvitamin D_3 levels. Relative hyperphosphataemia is characteristic and suggests a diagnosis other than hyperparathyroidism. The incidence of hypercalcaemia in sarcoidosis approximates to 10–17%, but hypercalciuria may be detected in 50% of patients at some time during the course of their disease. However, despite the unequivocal role of 1,25-dihydroxyvitamin D_3 in the pathogenesis of hypercalcaemia in granulomatous disorders, low calcium diet often fails to correct the hypercalcaemia. Additionally, urinary calcium excretion usually exceeds the intestinal calcium absorption in sarcoid patients. Therefore, increased bone resorption is probably also a major factor in the development of the abnormal calcium homoeostasis in granulomatous diseases. The production of 1,25-dihydroxyvitamin D_3 is extrarenal and not subjected to the normal physiological regulatory mechanisms. This is manifested by the rapid conversion of 25-hydroxyvitamin D_3 to 1,25-dihydroxyvitamin D_3, insensitivity to PTH stimulation and 1,25-dihydroxyvitamin D_3 inhibition of 1-hydroxylase, by control of hypercalcaemia with agents such as glucocorticoids, that inhibit mononuclear cell proliferation, and by insensitivity of 1,25-dihydroxyvitamin D_3 synthesis to calcium levels. Rather than stimulated by PTH, macrophage 1 α-hydroxylase is positively controlled by β-interferon, secreted chiefly by activated inflammatory (formerly TH1) CD4T lymphocytes, and by nitric oxide. Consequently, glucocorticoids may be used to inhibit mononuclear proliferation and to control hypercalcaemia caused by granulomatous processes (24).

High bone turnover

Immobilization prompts a higher rate of bone resorption than bone formation, as evidenced by mobilization of skeletal calcium, resulting in osteopenia and hypercalciuria. Occasionally, especially in younger people, or in the elderly with previously unrecognized high bone turnover, such as Paget's disease, this mobilization may overwhelm the renal excretory capacity, resulting in hypercalcaemia. Prolonged bed rest may also expose a previously unsuspected, subclinical, mildly hypercalcaemic state, such as hyperparathyroidism or occult malignancy. However, hypercalcaemia related solely to immobilization is promptly reversible upon resumption of normal weight bearing. In patients that are developing severe skeletal calcium loss due to prolonged immobilization, the use of bisphosphonates may be of help (25). Thyroid hormone also directly increases bone resorption. Hyperthyroidism is often associated with hypercalciuria. As in immobilization, this high calcium load derived from bone may eventually result in hypercalcaemia in 10–20% of patients. However, when accompanied by partial inhibition of intestinal calcium absorption, hypercalciuria and hypercalcaemia in hyperthyroidism may be associated with a negative calcium balance, correctable by antithyroid therapy. Additionally, hyperthyroid patients are probably more susceptible to the effect of PTH, even at normal physiological levels, and hyperparathyroidism and hyperthyroidism may coincide.

Paget's disease may be associated infrequently with hypercalcaemia. In this disease, localized bone remodelling is abnormal, because of increased bone resorption by osteoclasts, and subsequent reactive bone formation. When immobilized, patients with Paget's disease develop uncoupled bone resorption and formation because of a decrease in the gravitational stimulus for bone formation, and this results in hypercalciuria, and less often hypercalcaemia. Additionally, primary hyperparathyroidism may coexist with Paget's disease.

Low bone turnover

Aluminium toxicity in dialysis patients is associated with a dynamic bone disease. These patients typically have osteomalacia, not responding to vitamin D. In the hypocalcaemic dialysis patient, low serum alkaline phosphatase activity should direct the astute physician to divert from the diagnosis and therapy of secondary hyperparathyroidism to establish the diagnosis of osteomalacia, possibly induced by aluminium intoxication. In this case, improper therapy with vitamin D derivatives will inadvertently lead to hypercalcaemia and will not heal the bone disease. Hypercalcaemia results when increased intestinal calcium absorption, induced by vitamin D derivatives, is coupled with aluminium inhibition of osteoblast activity, thereby blocking calcium incorporation into the bone. Once established, aluminium toxicity may respond to administration of chelating agent deferoxamine and removal of the complex by high-flux dialysis.

Milk alkali syndrome

This syndrome is now only rarely observed. Combined hypercalcaemia and alkalosis may be observed in a small minority of patients treated for peptic ulcer disease with calcium carbonate. The hypercalcaemia occurs only if the intestinal calcium absorption rate exceeds the renal excretory mechanism. In some patients decreased renal calcium excretion and hypocalciuria is mediated by concomitant thiazide administration or occult hyperparathyroidism. Once hypercalcaemia develops, several factors contribute to its maintenance; these are: (1) volume depletion from natriuresis and diuresis caused by activation of the CaSR by hypercalcaemia; (2) reduced GFR which reduces calcium filtration; and (3) metabolic alkalosis and volume depletion that increase renal reabsorption of calcium. In addition, PTH suppression by high serum calcium probably contributes to low bone turnover, which in turn reduces calcium buffering capacity of bone. Acute and chronic forms may exist, whereas renal failure may complicate the latter (26).

Addison's disease

The mechanism of hypercalcaemia in Addison's disease is obscure. Volume depletion with avid sodium retention may be coupled with proximal tubular calcium reabsorption. Additionally, potentiation of intestinal calcium absorption by 1,25-dihydroxyvitamin D_3 in a state of glucocorticoid deficiency prompts the development of hypercalcaemia. Increased concentration of albumin-bound calcium may also cause an artefactual hypercalcaemia without a clinical effect.

Total parenteral nutrition

Hypercalcaemia caused by excessive content of calcium or vitamin D in the solution is observed following the short-term administration of total parenteral nutrition, and is easily correctable. However, in some patients on chronic total parenteral nutrition for short bowel syndrome, skeletal calcium mobilization may result in osteomalacia and hypercalciuria. Since hyperoxaluria is also a common feature in these patients, renal calcium excretory function is often reduced, leading to hypercalcaemia. Until recently, total parenteral nutrition aluminium content was not negligible and was associated with reduced bone turnover and hypercalcaemia.

Familial hypocalciuric hypercalcaemia

FHH (also called familial benign hypercalcaemia) is characterized by hypercalcaemia, hypocalciuria (fractional excretion of calcium below 1%) and familial involvement (see Chapter 4.4). Other than occasional fatigue, this hypercalcaemic disorder is often asymptomatic. Serum calcium levels are only mildly to moderately elevated, and serum PTH levels are inappropriately normal in the presence of hypercalcaemia or mildly elevated. The disease results from inactivating mutation of the CaSR and has an autosomal dominant inheritance. The inactivating mutations make the parathyroid gland less sensitive to calcium so that higher than normal levels of calcium are necessary to suppress PTH release. More than 100 mutations, most of them missense mutations, have been described.

A clue to the diagnosis is the extremely low fractional calcium excretion in the face of hypercalcaemia, and the normal serum levels of phosphate, 1,25-dihydroxyvitamin D_3, PTH, and bone mineral density. As a rule, hypercalcaemic states, excluding those attributed to prolonged renal failure, are necessarily accompanied by significant calcium excretion secondary to increased ECF calcium load on the kidneys. FHH is an exception because it is characterized by uncoupling of ECF calcium level and urinary calcium excretion. The CaSR, located on the basolateral membrane of the distal renal tubular site, fails to sense the true ionized calcium concentration and triggers directly or indirectly the continued tubular calcium and magnesium reabsorption. One abnormal allele of the gene of the CaSR is associated with FHH, while two mutated alleles are manifested as neonatal hypercalcaemia, necessitating early parathyroidectomy. FHH is usually detectable in the first decade, but may be diagnosed only at a later stage.

Hypercalcaemia in infants

Hypercalcaemia in infants, in addition to the above conditions, may be associated with several other unique conditions. Williams' syndrome is characterized by supravalvular aortic stenosis, elfin-face, and hypercalcaemia. The latter usually disappears spontaneously within the first year of life, but hypercalciuria may persist. The pathogenesis is unknown, but vitamin D metabolites have been implicated in this disorder, and a minority may involve maternal hypervitaminosis D. Rarely, hypercalcaemia in infants may be associated with postnatal subcutaneous fat necrosis, where granulomatous changes have been implicated in the autonomous production of 1,25-dihydroxyvitamin D_3 (27). Hypophosphatasia, resulting from alkaline phosphatase deficiency and expressed as deficient bone mineralization, may also be evident by hypercalcaemia and very low serum levels of alkaline phosphatase.

Management

When considering therapy for hypercalcaemia, target organ damage should be evaluated. On the one hand, severe, symptomatic hypercalcaemia is life threatening and necessitates urgent therapy, while mild, chronic, asymptomatic hypercalcaemia does not always require therapy. Diagnosis of the underlying disease is mandatory, in order to address the primary disorder and to reverse the mechanism of the impaired calcium balance. The definitive treatment depends on the primary disorder and on an understanding of the pathophysiology of the hypercalcaemia in the individual patient. Thus, in cases of hyperparathyroidism, surgical parathyroidectomy may be indicated (discussed in Chapter 4.3). Specific therapy for the other causes of hypercalcaemia is aimed at decreasing intestinal absorption, reducing bone resorption, and increasing urinary calcium excretion. Specific options include saline diuresis and loop diuretics, cellulose phosphate, sodium phytate, bisphosphonates, calcitonin, glucocorticoids, mithramycin, and gallium nitrate, and renal dialysis, all of which are reviewed below. The nonspecific measures include avoiding excessive exposure to sun, limiting calcium, vitamin D, vitamin A, and polyvitamin preparation intake, eliminating offending drugs and antacids, mobilization when possible, and hydration. An approach to the management of acute hypercalcaemia is illustrated in Fig. 4.2.3. Patients with chronic hypercalcaemia and hypercalciuria may need to be evaluated for daily urinary oxalate, uric acid, and citrate excretion, and should be treated to prevent future nephrolithiasis. However, in patients with FHH, all therapy, including parathyroidectomy, should be avoided.

Volume expansion with *saline* enhances urinary calcium excretion because calcium handling by the kidney is coupled to sodium. Additionally, hypercalcaemia is often associated with dehydration induced by the reduced concentrating renal capacity and reduced fluid intake. Therefore, unless the patient has end-stage renal failure, the initial consideration for hypercalcaemic patient should be volume expansion with saline. Sodium sulfate may have an additional advantage in the patient with normal renal function, as it forms nonreabsorbable urinary calcium sulfate complexes. Loop diuretics, such as *furosemide*, have calciuretic effect, but are efficient only after initial volume expansion. Thiazides should not be

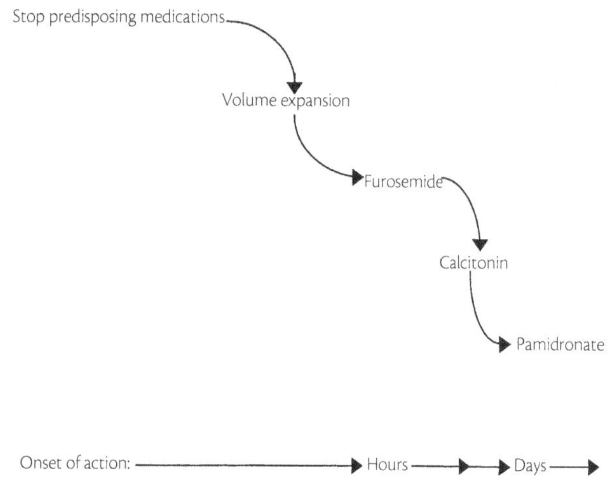

Fig. 4.2.3 The recommended general management of acute hypercalcaemia. Offending drugs should always be stopped. In patients with intact kidneys rehydration is essential. In granulomato us disorders and vitamin A and D intoxication, corticosteroids may be the drug of choice. When all measures fail to control hypercalcameia, dialysis against a low calcium dialysate may be indicated.

administered for diuresis. In the chronic hypercalcaemic patient, intestinal calcium reabsorption can be reduced by ingesting *cellulose phosphate* or *sodium phytate* that bind calcium and form complexes secreted in the faeces. However, extreme care should be undertaken in the follow-up of these patients, because hyperphosphataemia and hyperoxaluria may result, causing metastatic calcification and nephrolithiasis respectively (28).

Bisphosphonates (see Chapter 4.9) have emerged as the first-line measure to inhibit bone resorption in chronic hypercalcaemia. These compounds are effective in conditions of enhanced bone resorption such as bone metastases, humoral hypercalcaemia, multiple myeloma, and Paget's disease, as well as in osteoporosis.

Structurally, bisphosphonates are chemically stable derivatives of naturally occurring inorganic pyrophosphate (PPi), in which two phosphates are linked by esterification. Like their natural analogue they have a very high affinity for bone mineral because they bind to hydroxyapatite crystals. Bisphosphonates are preferentially incorporated into sites of active bone remodelling. In addition to their ability to inhibit calcification, bisphophonates inhibit hydroxyapatite breakdown, and thus effectively suppressing bone resorption. Moreover, modification of the chemical structure of bisphosphonates led to the development of new compounds with higher antiresorptive potency relative to their ability to decrease bone mineralization. This was accomplished by the introduction of nitrogen or amino group to the molecule. These drugs also contain central nonhydrolysable carbon, and thus have a prolonged half-life of weeks in some cases, for example, pamidronate. Moreover, the local effect on bone destruction may be therapeutic against the primary disease, especially in multiple myeloma. Bisphosphonates exert their negative effect on osteoclasts by inhibiting several processes:

- Direct effect on bone resorption. Bisphosphonates bind to and directly decrease hydroxyapatite crystals degradation rate.
- Effect on osteoclast and osteoblast function. These drugs inhibit monocyte–macrophage differentiation into osteoclast, osteoclast proton pump activity, osteoclast secretion of acid hydrolase from lysozomes in the ruffled border, integrin secretion, and osteoblast and osteoclast cytokine release.
- Induction of osteoclast apoptosis. First-generation bisphosphonates, because of their close similarity to PPi, become incorporated into newly formed molecules of adenosine triphosphate (ATP). Intracellular accumulation of these nonhydrolysable ATP analogues inhibit multiple ATP-dependent cellular processes, thus leading to osteoclast apoptosis (29). Unlike early bisphosphonates, second- and third-generation bisphosphonates (alendronate, risedronate, rbandronate, pamidronate, and zoledronic acid) have nitrogen-containing side chains. The mechanism by which they promote osteoclast apoptosis is distinct from that of the nonnitrogen containing bisphosphonates. As illustrated in recent studies, nitrogen-containing bisphosphonates bind to and inhibit the activity of farnesyl pyrophosphate synthase, a key regulatory enzyme in the mevalonic acid pathway critical to the production of cholesterol, other sterols, and isoprenoid lipids (30, 31). As such, post-translational modification of proteins, which plays a central role in the regulation of osteoclast cellular activities, is inhibited, ultimately leading to osteoclast apoptosis (32).

Since second- and third- generation bisphosphonates are 100–10 000 times more efficient in inhibiting osteoclast activity and do not adversely affect bone mineralization; these drugs are now considered as the bisphosphonate of choice for severe hypercalcaemia (33, 34). Pamidronate is administered in a dose of 30–90 mg (alternatively, zoledronic acid 4 mg intravenously), exerts its effect within 2–3 days for a mean period of 2–3 weeks. It is the drug of choice for severe hypercalcaemia associated with multiple myeloma, malignancy, and Paget's disease, and may have a potent analgesic effect. Bisphosphonates may also reduce the number of osteolytic lesions and pathologic fractures caused by metastatic carcinomas or myeloma lesions. The first response to bisphosphonates is often rapid, manifested by increased urinary excretion of hydroxyproline within days. Reduction of bone formation rate follows, expressed by a decline in levels of alkaline phosphatase. However, side-effects include flu-like symptoms, which may be mediated by cytokine secretion by macrophage lineage. Alendronate is a potent inhibitor of bone resorption and has been approved for oral therapy of chronic hypercalcaemia in Europe and for osteoporosis in the USA. Third generation bisphosphonates may improve the ratio of bone resorption to demineralization even more (32).

The chief effect of *calcitonin* is the inhibition of osteoclast bone resorption, while it also enhances calcium and phosphate urinary excretion. Therefore, in addition to its hypocalcaemic effect, it also prompts reduction of serum phosphate levels, resulting in a reduced risk for metastatic calcification. Calcitonin may exert its effect within hours, has virtually no side-effects, and is recommended in the management of both acute and chronic hypercalcaemia. It may also have an independent analgesic effect. However, its half-life is shorter and its potency is less than pamidronate.

Glucocorticoids may be used for treatment of hypercalcaemia in granulomatous disorders, vitamin D intoxication, and malignancy, especially multiple myeloma, lymphoma, leukaemia, and breast carcinoma. Glucocorticoids generally have a negative effect on both intestinal absorption and bone resorption, and in malignant disease they may inhibit the osteoclast activating factors.

Table 4.2.2 Pharmacological management of hypercalcaemia

Intervention	Dose	Averse effect
Hydration or calciuresis		
Intravenous saline	200–500 ml/h, depending on the cardiovascular and renal status of the patient	Congestive heart failure
Furosemide	20–40 mg intravenously, after rehydration has been achieved	Dehydration, hypokalaemia
Phosphate repletion		
Oral phosphorus (if serum phosphorus ≤3.0 mg/dl)	For example, 250 mg Neutraphos orally, four times daily until serum phosphorus >1.0 mmol/l (3.0 mg/dl) or until serum creatinine level increases	Renal failure, hypocalcaemia, seizures, abnormalities of cardiac conduction, diarrhoea
First-line medications		
Intravenous bisphosphonates		
Pamidronate	60–90 mg intravenously over a 2-h period in a solution of 50–200 saline or 5% dextrose in water	Renal failure, transient flu-like syndrome
Zoledronate	4 mg intravenously over a 15-min period in a solution of 50 ml of saline or 5% dextrose in water	Renal failure, transient flu-like syndrome
Second-line medications		
Glucocorticoids	e.g. prednisone, 60 mg orally daily for 10 days	Potential interference with chemotherapy, hypokalaemia, hyperglycaemia, hypertension, Cushing's syndrome, immunosuppression
Mithramycin	A single dose of 25 μg/kg of body weight over a 4–6-h period in saline	Thrombocytopenia, platelet-aggregation defect, anaemia, leucopenia, hepatitis renal failure
Calcitonin	4–8 IU/km subcutaneously or intramuscularly every 12 h	Flushing, nausea
Gallium nitrate	100–200 mg/m^2 of body-surface area intravenously given continuously over a 24-h period for 5 days	Renal failure

The hypocalcaemic effect of glucocorticoids is not evident before 24–48 h after its administration.

Mithramycin/plicamycin, is a cytotoxic antibiotic agent that suppresses bone resorption by blocking osteoclast RNA transcription. It is indicated mainly in acute hypercalcaemia associated with malignancy. Its main advantage is the rapid correction of serum calcium (levels may decline within 12 h and may be effective for several days). However, because of possible renal, hepatic, and bone marrow toxicity, and because of the availability of bisphosphonates, it is not considered a first-line drug in the management of chronic hypercalcaemia.

Gallium nitrate probably exerts its hypocalcaemic effect by reducing hydroxyapatite solubility and bone resorption. However, the effect of gallium is only observed after several days of administration and it is contraindicated in renal failure. Therefore, gallium has been replaced by safer and more potent hypocalcaemic agents. The pharmacologic management of hypercalcaemia is summarized in Table 4.2.2.

Dialysis is a very effective mode of reversing hypercalcaemia. In the chronic dialysis patient, dialysis is the treatment of choice using low calcium, very low, or calcium-free solutions. In the haemodialysis patient with severe hypercalcaemia, regional citrate infusion removes excess calcium, without being infused into the patient. However, severe hypocalcaemia and alkalosis may result. Additionally, these patients are often receiving oral calcium carbonate for phosphate binding, and oral or intravenous 1 α hydroxyvitamin D_3 ($1\alpha\ (OH)_2\ D_3$). These agents should be withheld until calcium levels are normal. Dialysis against very low calcium, in the form of haemodialysis or acute peritoneal dialysis, may be used as the definitive treatment for hypercalcaemia, when all other means fail. However, it is only rarely necessary with the current availability of effective drugs, and more importantly, with the regular monitoring of serum calcium in patients at risk.

Acknowledgements

The authors are indebted to Drs G. W. Mundy and T. A. Guise for approving the use of their figure.

References

1. Bushinsky DA, Monk RD. Calcium. *Lancet*, 1998; **352**: 306–11.
2. Popovtzer MM, Knochel JP. Disorders of calcium, phosphate, vitamin D, and parathyroid hormone activity. In: Scrier RW, ed. *Renal and Electrolyte Disorders*. 4th edn. Boston: Little, Brown, 1992.
3. Slatopolsky E, Klahr S. Disorders of calcium, magnesium and phosphate metabolism. In: Schrier RW, Gottschalk CW, eds. *Diseases of the Kidney*. 5th edn. Boston: Little, Brown, 1993.
4. Shane E. Hypercalcaemia: pathogenesis, clinical manifestations, differential diagnosis, and management. In: Flavus MJ, ed. *Primer on the Metabolic Bone Diseases and Disorders of Mineral Metabolism*. Philadelphia: Lippincott-raven, 1996: 177–81.
5. Nishi SP, Barbagelata NA, Atar S, Birnbaum Y, Tuero EJ. Hypercalcemia-induced ST-segment elevation mimicking acute myocardial infarction. *Electrocardiology*, 2006; **39**: 298–300.
6. Turhan S, Kilickap M, Kilinc S. ST segment elevation mimicking acute myocardial infarction in hypercalcaemia. *Heart*, 2005; **91**: 999.
7. Ashizawa N, Arakawa S, Koide Y, Toda G, Seto S, Yano K. Hypercalcemia due to vitamin D intoxication with clinical features mimicking acute myocardial infarction. *Intern Med*, 2003; **42**: 340–4.
8. Nussbaum SR. Pathophysiology and management of severe hypercalcemia. *Endocrinol Metab Clin North Am*, 1993; **22**: 343–62.

9. Mancilla EE, De-Luca E, Baron J. Activating mutations of the Ca^{2+}-sensing receptor. *Mol Genet Metab*, 1998; **64**: 198–204.
10. Wysolomerski JJ, Stewart FF. The physiology of PTH-related protein: an emerging role as a developmental factor. *Ann Rev Physiol*, 1998; **60**: 431–60.
11. Yasuda H, Shima N, Nakagawa N Yamaguchi K, Kinosaki M, Mochizuki S, *et al.* Osteoclast differentiation factor is a ligand for osteoprotegerin/osteoclastogenesis-inhibitory factor and is identical to TRANCE/RANKL. *Proc Natl Acad Sci U S A*, 1998; **95**: 3597–602.
12. Rankin W, Grill V, Martin TJ. Parathyroid-related protein and hypercalcaemia. *Cancer*, 1997; **80** (Suppl. 8): 1564–71.
13. Brown EM, Pollak M, Seidman CE *et al.* Calcium-ion-sensing cell surface receptors. *N Engl J Med*, 1995; **333**: 234–40.
14. Brown EM, Gamba G, Riccardi D, Lombardi M, Butters R, Kifor O, *et al.* Cloning and characterization of an extracellular calcium-sensing receptor from bovine parathyroid. *Nature*, 1993; **366**: 575–80.
15. Stewart AF, Insogna KL, Broadus AE. Malignancy-associated hypercalcemia. In: DeGroot L, ed. *Endocrinology*. 3rd edn. Philadelphia: WB Saunders, 1995: 1061–74.
16. Ratcliffe WA. PTH-related protein and hypercalcemia of malignancy (editorial). *J Pathol*, 1994; **173**: 79–80.
17. Grill V, Rankin W, Martin TJ. Parathyroid hormone-related protein (PTHrP) and hypercalcaemia. *Eur J Cancer*, 1998; **34**: 222–9.
18. Tian E, Zhan F, Walker R, Rasmussen E, Ma Y, Barlogie B, Shaughnessy JD Jr. The role of the Wnt-signaling antagonist DKK1 in the development of osteolytic lesions in multiple myeloma. *N Eng J Med*, 2003; **349**: 2483–94.
19. Qiang YW, Barlogie B, Rudikoff S, Shaughnessy JD Jr. Dkk1-induced inhibition of Wnt signaling in osteoblast differentiation is an underlying mechanism of bone loss in multiple myeloma. *Bone*, 2008; **42**: 669–80.
20. De Groot T, Bindels RJ, Hoenderop JG. TRPV5: an ingeniously controlled calcium channel. *Kidney Int*, 2008; **74**: 1241–6.
21. Jiang Y, Ferguson WB, Peng JB. WNK4 enhances TRPV5-mediated calcium transport: potential role in hypercalciuria of familial hyperkalemic hypertension cuased by gene mutation in WNK4. *Am J Physiol Renal Physiol*, 2007; **292**: F545–54.
22. Christiansen C, Baastrup PC, Lindgreen P, Transbol I. Endocrine effects of lithium: II. 'Primary hyperparathyroidism'. *Acta Endocrinol (Copenh.)*, 1978; **88**: 528–34.
23. Hundly JC, Woodrum DT, Saunders BD, Doherty GM, Gauger PG. Revisiting lithium-associated hyperparathyroidism in the era of intraoperative parathyroid hormone monitoring. *Surgery*, 2005; **138**: 1027–31.
24. Rizzato G. Clinical impact of bone and calcium metabolism changes in sarcoidosis. *Thorax*, 1998; **53**: 425–9.
25. Singer FR, Minoofar PN. Bisphosphonates in the treatment of disorders of mineral metabolism. *Adv Endocrinol Metab*, 1995; **6**: 259–88.
26. Felsenfeld AJ, Levine BS. Milk alkali syndrome and the dynamics of calcium homeostasis. *Clin J Am Soc Nephrol*, 2006; **1**: 641–54.
27. Kruse K, Irle U, Uhlig R. Elevated 1,25-dihydroxyvitamin D serum concentrations in infants with subcutaneous fat necrosis. *J Pediatrics*, 1993; **122**: 460–3.
28. Bilezikian JP. The management of acute hypercalcemia. *N Engl J Med*, 1992; **326**: 1196.
29. Russell RG. Bisphosphonates: from bench to bedside. *Ann N Y Acad Sci*, 2006; **1068**: 367–401.
30. Dunford JE, Thompson K, Coxon FP, Luckman SP, Hahn FH, Poulter CD, *et al.* Structure-activity relationships for inhibition of farnesyl diphosphate synthase in vitro and inhibition of bone resorption in vivo by nitrogen-containing bisphosphonates. *J Pharmacol Exp Therap*, 2001; **296**: 235–42.
31. Kavanagh KL, Guo K, Dunford JE, Wu X, Knapp S, Ebetino FH, *et al.* The molecular mechanism of nitrogen-containing bisphosphonates as antiosteoporosis drugs. *Proc Natl Acad Sci U S A*, 2006; **103**: 7829–34.
32. Luckman SP, Hughes DE, Coxon FP, Graham R, Russell G, Rogers MJ. Nitrogen-containing bisphosphonates ingibit the mevalonate pathway and prevent post-translational prenylation of GTP-binding proteins, including Ras. *J Bone Min Res*, 1998; **13**: 581–9.
33. Rogers MJ, Watts DJ, Russle RG. Overview of bisphosphonates. *Cancer*, 1997; **80** (Suppl. 8): 1652–60.
34. Geddes AD, D'Souza SM, Ebetino FH. Bisphosphonates structure–activity relationship and therapeutic implications. *J Bone Miner Res*, 1994; **8**: 265–306.

4.3

Primary hyperparathyroidism

Shonni J. Silverberg, John P. Bilezikian

Introduction

Primary hyperparathyroidism is no longer the severe disorder of 'stones, bones, and groans' described by Fuller Albright and others in the 1930s (1,2). Osteitis fibrosa cystica, with its brown tumours of the long bones, subperiosteal bone resorption, distal tapering of the clavicles and phalanges, and 'salt-and-pepper' appearance of erosions of the skull on radiograph is rare, and kidney stones are seen in only 20% of patients. Asymptomatic disease is the rule in the vast majority of patients, with the diagnosis commonly following the finding of hypercalcaemia on routine serum chemistry analysis (Table 4.3.1) (3–5). Primary hyperparathyroidism is due to a solitary parathyroid adenoma in 80% of patients (5). Most cases are sporadic, although some are associated with a history of neck irradiation, or prolonged use of lithium therapy for bipolar disease (6, 7). Multiple parathyroid adenomas have been reported in 2 to 4% of cases (8). Parathyroid adenomas can be discovered in many unexpected anatomic locations, including within the thyroid gland, the superior mediastinum, and within the thymus. Occasionally, the adenoma may ultimately be identified in the retroesophageal space, the pharynx, the lateral neck, and even the alimentary submucosa of the oesophagus (9). In approximately 15% of patients with primary hyperparathyroidism, all four parathyroid glands are involved. There are no clinical features that differentiate single versus multiglandular disease. In nearly one-half of cases, four-gland disease is associated with a familial hereditary syndrome, such as multiple endocrine neoplasia 1 (MEN 1) or MEN 2a.

Clinical presentation

Primary hyperparathyroidism affects individuals of all ages, although incidence peaks between the ages of 50 and 60 years. Women are affected approximately three times more commonly than men. At the time of diagnosis, most patients are asymptomatic (5). Hypertension, peptic ulcer disease, gout, or pseudogout have been described in association with the disease, but are not causally linked (except in cases of MEN). Patients often complain of weakness. Easy fatigability, depression, and intellectual weariness are seen with some regularity (see below). Despite these complaints, the physical examination is generally unremarkable, including a normal neuromuscular and neck examination in those with benign disease.

Diagnosis and biochemical features

The biochemical hallmark of primary hyperparathyroidism is hypercalcaemia with elevated or inappropriately normal levels of parathyroid hormone (PTH). The disease is readily distinguished from malignancy, the other main cause of hypercalcaemia, in which PTH levels are suppressed. Rarely, a patient with malignancy will be shown to have elevated PTH levels due to ectopic secretion of PTH (10). Malignancy can also present in association with primary hyperparathyroidism. Ninety percent of patients with hypercalcaemia have primary hyperparathyroidism or malignancy. The broader differential diagnosis of hypercalcaemia is discussed in Chapter 4.2 (10).

Improved PTH assay methodology for PTH measurement, especially the immunoradiometric (IRMA) and immunochemiluminometric assays, has facilitated the diagnosis, although the 'intact' IRMA measures a large non-(1–84) PTH fragment in addition to biologically active PTH (11). A more specific assay detects only the full-length parathyroid hormone molecule, PTH (1–84) (12). While this assay has clear utility in uraemic patients, in whom the 'intact'-IRMA has been shown to considerably overestimate elevations in biologically active hormone concentration (13), it is not clear whether this assay will aid in the routine diagnosis of primary hyperparathyroidism.

A small percentage of patients with primary hyperparathyroidism have PTH levels that are within the normal reference range as measured by either assay. In these patients, levels tend to be in the upper range of normal. In primary hyperparathyroidism, such values, although within the normal range, are clearly abnormal in a hypercalcaemic setting. This is even more evident in those under the age of 45 years. Because PTH levels normally rise with age, in an individual who is under 45 years old, one expects a more narrow, lower normal range (10–45 pg/ml). Thus, a PTH level of 50 pg/ml is distinctly abnormal in an individual under 45 who has hypercalcaemia. Occasionally, in either a younger or older patient, the PTH level as measured by the established IRMA, will be rather low, although not suppressed (i.e. in the 30 pg/ml range). Although these individuals require a more careful consideration of other causes of hypercalcaemia, in the end, they are also likely to have primary hyperparathyroidism because non-PTH-dependent hypercalcaemia should suppress the PTH concentration to levels that are either undetectable or at the lower limits of the reference range. Souberbielle *et al.* (14) have illustrated that the normal range

Table 4.3.1 Changing profile of primary hyperparathyroidism

	Cope (1930–1965)	Heath *et al.* (1965–1974)	Mallette *et al.* (1965–1972)	Silverberg *et al.* (1984–2009)
Nephrolithiasis (%)	57	51	37	17
Skeletal disease (%)	23	10	14	1.4
Hypercalciuria (%)	NR	36	40	39
Asymptomatic (%)	0.6	18	22	80

NR, not reported.

is very much a function of whether or not the reference population is, or is not, vitamin D deficient. When vitamin D deficient individuals are excluded, the upper limit of the PTH reference interval decreases from 65 to 46 pg/ml. When vitamin D deficient individuals were excluded from the subjects used to establish a reference interval for 'whole PTH', the upper limit decreased from 44 to 34 ng/l.

There are a few exceptions to the rule that PTH is suppressed in all hypercalcaemic individuals who do not have primary hyperparathyroidism. These involve individuals who have a history of prolonged use of lithium or thiazide diuretics, and those with familial hypocalciuric hypercalcaemia (FHH). If the patient can be safely withdrawn from lithium or thiazide, this should be attempted. Serum calcium and PTH levels are then reassessed 3 months later. If the serum calcium and PTH levels continue to be elevated, the diagnosis of primary hyperparathyroidism is made. FHH is differentiated from primary hyperparathyroidism by: (1) family history, (2) markedly low urinary calcium excretion, and (3) the specific gene abnormality. In addition, subjects with FHH often demonstrate hypercalcaemia much earlier than patients with primary hyperparathyroidism, typically before 40 years of age.

Normocalcaemic primary hyperparathyroidism There has been considerable controversy concerning the accuracy of this diagnosis. In many cases, the increases in PTH levels were due to measurement of inactive fragments by earlier generation PTH assays. Many other patients were vitamin D deficient, which can give the semblance of normal calcium levels when there is concomitant primary hyperparathyroidism (15). Furthermore, it is now accepted that the normal range of 25-hydroxyvitamin D is higher than previous designations. A diagnosis of normocalcaemic primary hyperparathyroidism requires that the patient has levels of 25-hydroxyvitamin D within the normal physiological range, namely above 30 ng/ml. Patients who have normal calcium levels, elevated PTH, and no causes for secondary hyperparathyroidism may represent the earliest manifestations of primary hyperparathyroidism. Several reports describing these individuals have recently been published, demonstrating that some, but not all, patients progress to overt hypercalcaemia while under observation (16, 17). Some even undergo successful parathyroid surgery with removal of a single or multiple adenomas, or hyperplastic glands. However, little is known about the natural history of patients with this variant of the disorder. The 2008 International Workshop on the Management of Asymptomatic Primary Hyperparathyroidism designated normocalcaemic primary hyperparathyroidism, for the first time, as a recognized phenotype of the disease (18). In order to make this diagnosis, all causes of secondary hyperparathyroidism (including vitamin D deficiency, hypercalciuria, malabsorption, liver disease, renal disease, etc.) must first be eliminated.

In addition to abnormalities in serum calcium and PTH levels, there are other biochemical features typical of primary hyperparathyroidism. The serum phosphorus tends to be in the lower range of normal but frank hypophosphataemia is present in less than one-fourth of patients. Average total urinary calcium excretion is at the upper end of the normal range, with about 40% of all patients having frank hypercalciuria. Serum 25-hydroxyvitamin D levels tend to be low, as now defined by 25-hydroxyvitamin D levels below 30 ng/ml. The average serum calcium in our series is approximately 20 ng/ml. While mean values of 1,25-dihydroxyvitamin D_3 are in the high-normal range, approximately one-third of patients have frankly elevated levels of 1,25-dihydroxyvitamin D_3. This is due to parathyroid hormone-mediated conversion of 25-hydroxyvitamin D to 1,25-dihydroxyvitamin D. A mild hyperchloraemia is seen occasionally, due to the effect of PTH on renal acid–base balance. A typical biochemical profile is shown in Table 4.3.2.

The skeleton

Although osteitis fibrosa cystica is rarely seen today, over the past several decades we have come to understand that there is a typical picture of skeletal involvement in modern-day primary hyperparathyroidism.

Table 4.3.2 Biochemical profile in primary hyperparathyroidism

	Patients (mean ± SEM)	Normal range
Serum calcium	10.7 ± 0.1 mg/dl	8.2–10.2 mg/dl
Serum phosphorus	2.8 ± 0.1 mg/dl	2.5–4.5 mg/dl
Total alkaline phosphatase	114 ± 5 IU/l	<100 IU/l
Serum magnesium	2.0 ± 0.1 mg/dl	1.8–2.4 mg/dl
PTH (IRMA)	119 ± 7 pg/ml	10–65 pg/ml
25 (OH) vitamin D	19 ± 1 ng/ml	30-100 ng/ml
$1,25(OH)_2$ vitamin D	54 ± 2 pg/ml	15–60 pg/ml
Urinary calcium	240 ± 11 mg/g creatinine	
Urine DPD	17.6 ± 1.3 nmol/mmol creatinine	<14.6 nmol/mmol creatinine
Urine PYD	46.8 ± 2.7 nmol/mmol creatinine	<51.8 nmol/mmol creatinine

N = 137.

DPD, deoxypyridinoline; PTH (IRMA), parathyroid hormone (immunoradiometric assay); PYD, pyridinoline.

Bone densitometry Bone mineral densitometry can provide important information about the hyperparathyroid state, because the technique measures bone mass at sites containing differing amounts of cortical and cancellous bone. The known physiologic proclivity of parathyroid hormone to be catabolic at sites of cortical bone establishes the distal third of the radius, a readily accessible cortical site, as the key measurement site in this disease. Early densitometric studies in primary hyperparathyroidism revealed another physiological property of parathyroid hormone, namely to be anabolic at cancellous sites. In this regard, the lumbar spine, a predominantly cancellous bone, best demonstrates this proclivity. In primary hyperparathyroidism, bone density at the distal third of the radius is decreased, while bone density of the lumbar spine tends to be only minimally involved or even spared (19). The hip, which contains a relatively equal mixture of cortical and cancellous elements, shows bone density values intermediate between the cortical and cancellous sites (Fig. 4.3.1). In postmenopausal women, this pattern is opposite to what one typically experiences in the context of oestrogen deficiency, namely preferential loss of cancellous bone. Bone mineral density testing is important in the evaluation of all patients with primary hyperparathyroidism, because it is a key factor in clinical decision making regarding management and monitoring.

While this densitometric pattern is seen in the vast majority of patients with primary hyperparathyroidism, a small group of patients with mild disease have evidence of vertebral osteopenia at the time of presentation. In our natural history study, approximately 15% of patients had a lumbar spine Z-score of less than −1.5 at the time of diagnosis (20). Not all vertebral bone loss could be attributed to the effects of antecedent oestrogen deficiency, as half of these individuals were not postmenopausal women.

Finally, when primary hyperparathyroidism is more advanced, there will be more generalized involvement, and the lumbar spine will not appear to be protected. In this setting, when primary hyperparathyroidism is severe or more symptomatic, all bones can be extensively involved.

Bone markers Both bone resorption and bone formation are increased in primary hyperparathyroidism (21). These skeletal dynamics can be measured by circulating markers of bone formation, such as bone-specific alkaline phosphatase activity, osteocalcin, and type 1 procollagen peptide. Levels are typically mildly elevated, but in many patients the more general marker, total alkaline

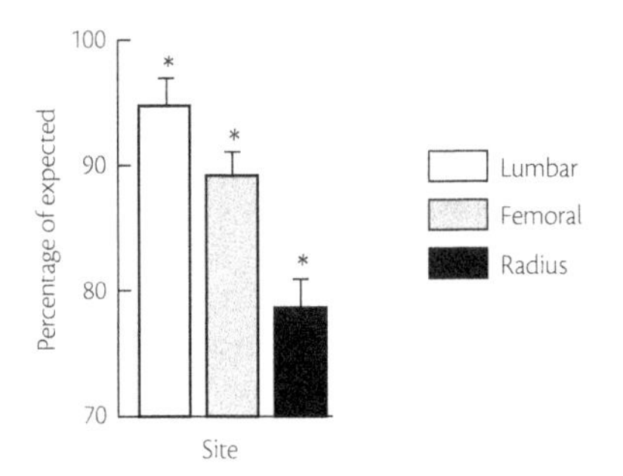

Fig. 4.3.1 Bone densitometry in primary hyperparathyroidism. Data are shown in comparison to age- and sex-matched normal subjects. Divergence from expected values is different at each site (p = 0.0001). (From Silverberg SJ, Shane E, DeLaCruz L, Dempster DW, Feldman F, Seldin D, *et al*. Skeletal disease in primary hyperparathyroidism. *J Bone Miner Res*, 1989; **4**: 283–91 (19).)

phosphatase activity, is often within normal limits. In a small pilot study from our group, bone-specific alkaline phosphatase activity correlated with PTH levels and with bone mineral density (BMD) at the lumbar spine and femoral neck. Osteocalcin is also often increased in patients with primary hyperparathyroidism while procollagen extension peptides have not been shown to have significant predictive or clinical utility in the disease. Bone resorption markers also have potential clinical utility. Urinary hydroxyproline, once the resorption marker of choice, was frankly elevated in patients with osteitis fibrosa cystica, but is generally normal in mild, asymptomatic, primary hyperparathyroidism. The test is not used anymore as a marker of bone resorption in primary hyperparathyroidism. Hydroxypyridinium cross-links of collagen, pyridinoline, and deoxypyridinoline, on the other hand, are often elevated in primary hyperparathyroidism, and return to normal after parathyroidectomy. N- and C-terminal peptides of type I collagen are likely to have utility but they have not been studied extensively in primary hyperparathyroidism. Other markers of bone resorption have been limited also in their application to bone turnover in primary hyperparathyroidism. Studies of bone markers in the longitudinal follow-up of patients with primary hyperparathyroidism are limited, but indicate a reduction in these turnover markers following parathyroidectomy (21–23).

Bone histomorphometry Analyses of percutaneous bone biopsies from patients with primary hyperparathyroidism have provided additional insight into the skeleton. (Fig. 4.3.2). Using the percutaneous bone biopsy of the iliac crest, cortical thinning is clearly seen and quantitated (24), consistent with the known effect of PTH to be catabolic at endocortical surfaces of bone. Osteoclasts are thought to erode more widely along the corticomedullary junction under the influence of PTH. Also as suggested by bone densitometry, cancellous bone volume is clearly well preserved in primary hyperparathyroidism. Cancellous bone is actually increased in primary hyperparathyroidism as compared to normal subjects (25, 26). When cancellous bone volume is compared among age- and sex-matched subjects with primary hyperparathyroidism or postmenopausal osteoporosis, cancellous bone volume is lowest in those with osteoporosis and highest in women with primary hyperparathyroidism. Preservation of cancellous bone volume even extends to comparisons with the expected losses associated with the effects of ageing on cancellous bone physiology. In primary hyperparathyroidism, there is no relationship between trabecular number or separation and age, suggesting that the actual plates and their connections were being maintained over time more effectively than one would have expected through the ageing process. Thus, primary hyperparathyroidism seems to retard the normal age-related processes leading to trabecular loss. In primary hyperparathyroidism, indices of trabecular connectivity are greater than expected, while indices of disconnectivity are decreased (26). Thus cancellous bone is preserved in primary hyperparathyroidism through the maintenance of well-connected trabecular plates.

Recent analyses of trabecular microarchitecture using newer technologies have largely been confirmatory. Using three-dimensional microCT technology, higher bone volume, higher bone surface area, higher connectivity density, and lower trabecular separation are seen in primary hyperparathyroidism (27, 28). There were also less marked age-related declines in bone volume and connectivity

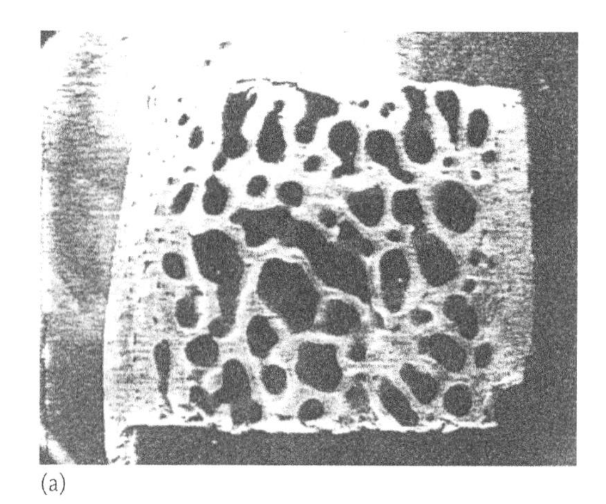

(a)

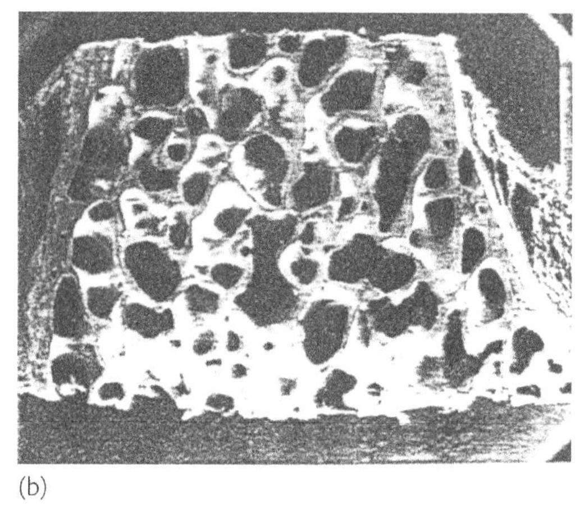

(b)

Fig. 4.3.2 Scanning electron micrograph of bone biopsy specimens in a normal subject (a) and age- and sex-matched patient with primary hyperparathyroidism (b). The cortices of the hyperparathyroid sample are markedly thinned, but cancellous bone and trabecular connectivity appear to be well preserved. (Magnification × 31.25.) (From Parisien MV, Silverberg SJ, Shane E, *et al.* Bone disease in primary hyperparathyroidism. *Endocrinol Metab Clin North Am*, 1990; **19**: 19–34.)

density as compared to controls, with no decline in bone surface area. Using the technique of backscattered electron imaging to evaluate trabecular BMD distribution in iliac crest bone biopsies (29), Roschger *et al.* showed reduced average mineralization density and increase in the heterogeneity of the degree of mineralization, consistent with reduced mean age of bone tissue. Studies of collagen maturity using Fourier transform infrared spectroscopy provide further support for these observations (30). Thus characteristics other than bone density are important determinants of bone strength in primary hyperparathyroidism. Together they suggest a mixed picture with regard to fracture risk. While reduced cortical bone density might argue for increased fracture risk, improved microarchitectural parameters would argue for reduced fracture risk.

Fractures Reports on fracture incidence in the milder presentation of primary hyperparathyroidism seen today have been conflicting (28, 31). A definitive, prospective study is unfortunately lacking. Of the larger studies that are available, one population-based prospective analysis (17 years' duration; 23 341 person-years) showed no increase in hip fractures in women with primary hyperparathyroidism in Sweden (32). On the other hand, the Mayo Clinic retrospective review of 407 cases of primary hyperparathyroidism over a 28-year period, 1965 to 1992, suggested an increase in fracture incidence at the vertebral spine, the distal forearm, ribs, and the pelvis (33). There was no increase in hip fractures. After multivariate analysis, age and female sex remained significant independent predictors of fracture risk. These data, however, are subject to potential ascertainment bias. Patients with primary hyperparathyroidism are typically followed more conscientiously and thus fractures at some of these sites may have been recognized by greater surveillance. Recently, Vignali, Marcocci, and their associates studied the incidence of vertebral fractures in primary hyperparathyroidism as determined by dual-energy X-ray absorptiometry-based vertebral fracture assessment (34) in 150 consecutive patients and 300 healthy women matched for age and menopausal age. Vertebral fractures were detected in more subjects with primary hyperparathyroidism (24.6%) than the control subjects (4.0%; $p < 0.001$). Among asymptomatic primary hyperparathyroidism patients, only those who met surgical guidelines showed a higher incidence of vertebral fractures compared with controls. Thus, the matter of fracture risk in primary hyperparathyroidism remains unclear.

Nephrolithiasis

Although the incidence of nephrolithiasis has decreased, kidney stones remain the most common manifestation of symptomatic primary hyperparathyroidism (see Table 4.3.1), affecting 15% to 20% of all patients (35). Other renal manifestations of primary hyperparathyroidism include hypercalciuria, which is seen in approximately 40% of patients, and nephrocalcinosis, the frequency of which is unknown. It is important to note that in patients with primary hyperparathyroidism who do not have renal stone disease, there is no relationship between extent of hypercalciuria and the development of kidney stones (36).

While in the 1930s it was generally accepted that bone and stone disease did not coexist in the same patient with classic primary hyperparathyroidism (1), today there is no clear evidence for two distinct subtypes of primary hyperparathyroidism. There is no distinctive set of biochemical data for patients with stone disease (37). Urinary calcium excretion per gram of creatinine, levels of 1,25-dihydroxyvitamin D, and BMD at all sites were indistinguishable among patients with and without nephrolithiasis. Furthermore, cortical bone demineralization is as common and as extensive in those with and without nephrolithiasis (37, 38).

Other organ involvement

Neurocognitive and neuropsychological features Over the years, primary hyperparathyroidism has been associated with complaints referable to many different organ systems. Perhaps the most common complaints have been those of weakness and easy fatigability (18). Classical primary hyperparathyroidism used to be associated with a neuromuscular syndrome, characterized by easy fatigability, symmetrical proximal muscle weakness, and type II muscle cell atrophy (39). These findings were reversible after parathyroid surgery. This disorder is rarely seen today (18).

The neuropsychiatric features of primary hyperparathyroidism remain a source of controversy today. While complaints are common, association of specific symptomatology with primary hyperparathyroidism is unclear, as are expectations for postoperative improvement (18). Although much of the available literature has been limited by design issues (lack of controls, etc.) three randomized, prospective trials have been conducted recently (41–43). Unfortunately, data from these studies do not offer clarity on specific symptoms or improvement following successful parathyroid surgery. Recent data from Walker *et al.* suggest that there are cognitive features of primary hyperparathyroidism, some of which do improve after parathyroidectomy (44).

Cardiovascular system Both calcium and parathyroid hormone are well known to have significant cardiovascular effects. Hypercalcaemia has been associated with increases in blood pressure, left ventricular hypertrophy, heart muscle contractility, and arrhythmias, as well as calcification of the myocardium, heart valves, and coronary arteries. However, the association of overt cardiovascular symptomatology with modern-day primary hyperparathyroidism is unclear. Inconsistencies in the literature on the cardiovascular manifestations of primary hyperparathyroidism relate to the fact that the clinical profile of the disease has changed. Data from cohorts with marked hypercalcaemia and hyperparathyroidism show most cardiovascular involvement

Cardiovascular mortality While cardiovascular mortality is increased in patients with moderate to severe primary hyperparathyroidism (45–47), the limited data on mild disease have not shown any increase in mortality (48, 49). In the Mayo Clinic study, patients whose serum calcium was in the highest quartile, and thus had levels that could not have been considered mild, had increased cardiovascular mortality (48).

Hypertension Hypertension, a common feature of primary hyperparathyroidism when it is part of a MEN with phaeochromocytoma or hyperaldosteronism, has also been reported to be more prevalent in sporadic asymptomatic primary hyperparathyroidism than in appropriately matched control groups. The mechanism of this association is unknown, and the condition does not clearly remit following cure of the hyperparathyroid state (50).

Coronary artery disease Coronary atherosclerosis was seen in autopsy studies such as those of Roberts and Waller (51) but these individuals had very marked hypercalcaemia (16.8–27.4 mg/dl). The incidence of coronary artery disease in primary hyperparathyroidism is more likely to be present as a function of the serum calcium level. (52) The same is true of valvular and myocardial calcification (53, 54).

Left ventricular hypertrophy Left ventricular hypertrophy (LVH) is considered separately because it is itself a strong predictor of cardiovascular events and mortality. Moreover, as opposed to the indices described above, in which involvement seems to be a function of the serum calcium level, LVH has been seen across a wide range of calcium levels (55, 56). The idea has been advanced that LVH is more a function of the parathyroid hormone level than it is the serum calcium. Some studies suggest that LVH is reversible after parathyroidectomy, a finding that could have important management implications (54–57).

Electrocardiographic manifestations While marked hypercalcaemia is associated with a reduced Q–T interval, most patients with mild hypercalcaemia do not demonstrate such electrocardiographic abnormalities. Moreover, no other conduction abnormalities or arrhythmogenic potential are observed(58, 59).

Vascular function The evidence implicating vascular dysfunction in primary hyperparathyroidism has out focused upon those with severe disease (60–62). However, in those with lower calcium levels, Baykan *et al.* also found impaired flow-mediated (endothelial) dilation that negatively correlated with calcium levels.[168] There is a preliminary report on endothelial dysfunction in primary hyperparathyroidism (63) and two studies that have reported increased vascular stiffness (64, 65).

Gastrointestinal system Once thought to be associated with an increased incidence of peptic ulcer disease, recent studies suggest that the incidence in primary hyperparathyroidism, approximately 10%, is similar to the general population. The exception is in patients with primary hyperparathyroidism due to MEN 1, in which approximately 40% of patients have clinically apparent gastrinomas (Zollinger–Ellison syndrome). In these patients, primary hyperparathyroidism is associated with increased clinical severity of gastrinoma, and treatment of the associated primary hyperparathyroidism has been reported to ameliorate the Zollinger–Ellison syndrome (66). Despite this, current recommendations (Consensus Conference Guidelines for Therapy of MEN 1) state that the co-existence of Zollinger–Ellison syndrome does not represent sufficient indication for parathyroidectomy, since medical therapy is so successful (67).

Although hypercalcaemia can be associated with pancreatitis, the incidence of pancreatitis in patients with primary hyperparathyroidism with serum calcium levels under 12 mg/dl is not increased. The Mayo Clinic experience from 1950 to 1975 found that only 1.5% of those with primary hyperparathyroidism had coexisting pancreatitis, and alternative explanations for pancreatitis were found for several patients (68). Similarly, although pancreatitis and pregnancy may coexist in patients with primary hyperparathyroidism, there is no evidence for a causal relationship between the disorders.

Other organ involvement Many organ systems were affected by the hyperparathyroid state in the past. Anaemia, band keratopathy, and loose teeth are no longer seen, while gout and pseudogout are rare and the nature of the association with primary hyperparathyroidism is not clear.

Natural history

The availability of data on the longitudinal course of primary hyperparathyroidism with or without surgery has led to a reconsideration of the need for surgery in all patients with asymptomatic primary hyperparathyroidism. The 15-year data from the longest prospective observational trial have recently been reported by Silverberg, Bilezikian and their colleagues (69, 70).

Natural history with surgery Parathyroidectomy resulted in normalization of the serum calcium and PTH levels permanently. Postoperatively, there was a marked improvement in BMD at all sites (lumbar spine, femoral neck, and distal third radius) amounting to gains above 10%. The improvement was most rapid at the lumbar spine but all sites showed persistent gains at all sites for the 15 years of follow-up (Fig. 4.3.3). The improvements were seen in those who met and did not meet surgical criteria at study entry, confirming the salutary effect of parathyroidectomy in this regard on all patients.

Natural history without surgery In subjects who did not undergo parathyroid surgery, serum calcium remained stable for about 12 years with a tendency for the serum calcium level to rise in

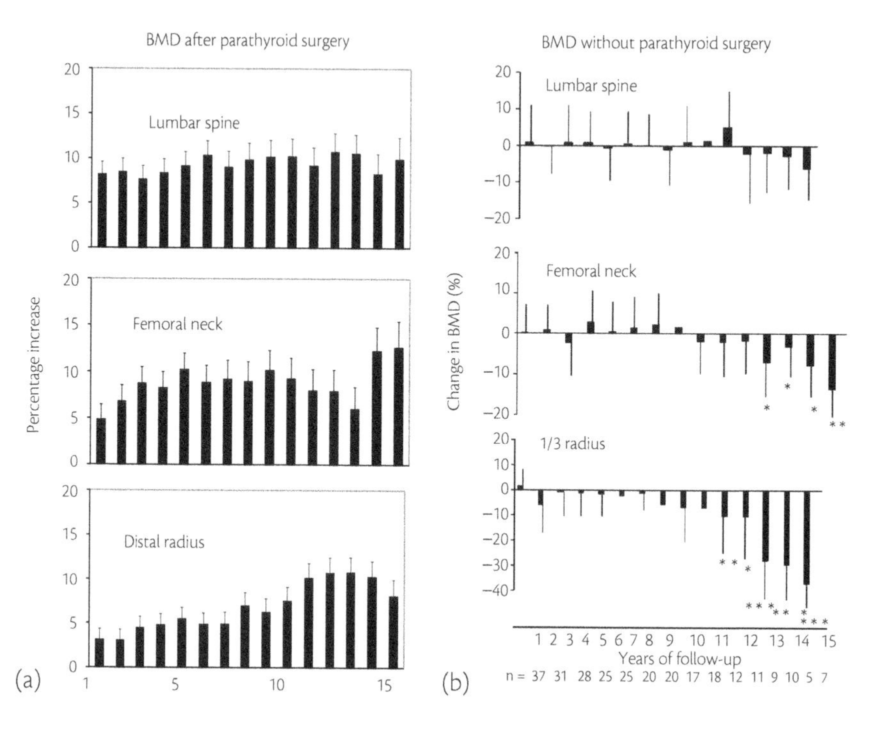

Fig. 4.3.3 Longitudinal course of bone density in primary hyperparathyroidism. Data are presented as percentage change from preoperative baseline bone density measurement by site following parathyroidectomy (a) or in patients followed with no intervention (b). (Adapted from Rubin MR, Bilezikian JP, McMahon DJ, Jacobs T, Shane, E, Siris E, *et al.* The natural history of primary hyperparathyroidism with or without parathyroid surgery after 15-years. *J Clin Endocrinol Metab*, 2008; **93**: 3462–70.)

years 13 to 15. Other biochemical indices, such as the PTH, vitamin D metabolites, and urinary calcium, did not change for the entire 15 years of follow-up in the group as a whole. Bone density at all three sites remained stable for the first 8–10 years. However, after this period of stability, declining cortical BMD was seen at the hip and the distal third site.

Randomized clinical trial data Data from three randomized trials of surgery in mild primary hyperparathyroidism, were remarkably consistent with those from the longer observational study (41–43). The three trials are limited by their short duration. In 2004, Rao *et al.* reported on 53 subjects, assigned either to parathyroid surgery (n = 25) or to no surgery (n = 28) followed for at least 2 years. BMD significantly increased at the femoral neck and total hip along with normalization of the serum calcium and PTH. In those who did not undergo parathyroid surgery, there were no changes in the lumbar spine or femoral neck bone density but total hip significantly declined. Forearm BMD increased, an oddity considering the vulnerability of this site to the catabolic actions of PTH. Biochemical indices were all stable. In 2007, Bollerslev *et al.* reported interim results of their randomized trail of parathyroidectomy versus no surgery. In this larger study (191 patients), after surgery, biochemical indices normalized and BMD increased. In the group that did not undergo parathyroid surgery, bone mineral density did not change. Also in 2007, Ambrogini *et al.* reported that surgery was associated with a significant increase in bone mineral density of the lumbar spine and hip after 1 year.

Surgical guidelines

Parathyroidectomy remains the only currently available option for cure of primary hyperparathyroidism. In an effort to address the need for surgery in all patients with asymptomatic primary hyperparathyroidism, there have been two conferences on the management of asymptomatic primary hyperparathyroidism and recently by a third international conference to review the most up to date information (71–73). The guidelines that emerged from the 2008 conference should be helpful to the clinician faced with the asymptomatic hyperparathyroid patient. All symptomatic patients are advised to undergo parathyroidectomy. Surgery is advised in asymptomatic patients who meet any one of the following criteria: (1) serum calcium greater than 1 mg/dl above the upper limits of normal; (2) reduction in creatinine clearance to less than 60 cc/min; (3) reduced bone density (T-score less than −2.5 at any site or the presence of a fragility fracture); (4) age less than 50 years. The updated guidelines are shown in Table 4.3.3. It is important to note that urinary calcium excretion is no longer regarded to be a guideline for surgery, because this measurement is not predictive of the risk for subsequent nephrolithiasis in subjects with primary hyperparathyroidism who have not had a kidney stone.

Table 4.3.3 A comparison of new and old guidelines for surgery in asymptomatic primary hyperparathyroidism

Measurement	Guidelines 1990	Guidelines 2002	Guidelines 2008
Serum calcium (above normal)	1–1.6 mg/dl	1.0 mg/dl	1.0 mg/dl
24-h urinary calcium	>400 mg	>400 mg	
Creatinine clearance	Reduced by 30%	Reduced by 30%	< 60 cc/min
Bone mineral density	Z-score < −2.0 (forearm)	T-score < −2.5 (any site)	T-score < −2.5/ fragility fracture
Age	50	50	50

Surgery

Preoperative localization of hyperfunctioning parathyroid tissue

In the hands of an expert parathyroid surgeon, 95% of abnormal parathyroid glands will be discovered and removed at the time of initial surgery (74). However, in the patient with previous neck surgery, such high success rates are not generally achieved. Preoperative localization is extremely helpful in these cases. In addition, preoperative localization is important if a minimally invasive approach (see below) is contemplated.

Noninvasive parathyroid imaging studies include technetium Tc-99m Sestamibi, ultrasound, CT scanning, MRI, and PET scanning. Tc-99m Sestamibi is generally regarded to be the most sensitive and specific imaging modality, especially when it is combined with single photon emission computed tomography. In disease caused by a single parathyroid adenoma, sensitivity has ranged from 80 to 100% with a 5 to 10% false-positive rate. However, sestamibi scintigraphy has a poor record in the context of multiglandular disease (75). Ultrasonography is highly operator dependent (76) with experience needed to differentiate a possible parathyroid adenoma from a thyroid nodule or lymph node. Rapid spiral thin slice CT scanning of the neck and mediastinum with evaluation of axial, coronal, and sagittal views can add much to the search for elusive parathyroid tissue (77). MRI can also identify abnormal parathyroid tissue, but it is expensive and less sensitive than the other noninvasive modalities. PET with or without simultaneous CT scan is also costly and of unclear utility.

Invasive localization techniques include parathyroid aspiration and arteriography. Fine needle aspiration of a parathyroid gland, identified by any of the aforementioned modalities, can be performed and the aspirate can be analysed for PTH. This technique is not recommended for routine *de novo* cases, and could lead to seeding of the area with parathyroid cells (78). Arteriography and selective venous sampling for PTH may be done when the gland has not been identified by any of the techniques described. The combination of arteriography and selective venous sampling can provide both anatomical and functional localization of abnormal parathyroid tissue. This approach, however, is costly and requires an experienced interventional radiologist. It is also performed in only a few centres in the USA (79).

Surgical procedures

The four-gland parathyroid gland exploration under general or local anaesthesia, with or without preoperative localization, has long been considered the gold standard surgical approach, and led to cure in over 95% of cases. However, unilateral approaches are appealing in a disease in which only a single gland is involved (in approximately 85% of cases). The procedure of choice in many centres today is the minimally invasive parathyroidectomy (MIP) (74). Preoperative parathyroid imaging is necessary, and the procedure is directed only to the site where the abnormal parathyroid gland has been visualized. Preoperative blood is obtained for comparison of the PTH concentration with an intraoperative sample obtained after removal of the 'abnormal' parathyroid gland. The availability of a rapid parathyroid hormone assay in or near the operating room is necessary for this procedure. If the level falls by more than 50% following resection, into the normal range, the gland that has been removed is considered to be the sole source of overactive parathyroid tissue and the operation is terminated. If the parathyroid hormone level does not fall by more than 50%, into the normal range, the operation is extended to permit a search for other overactive parathyroid tissue. There is a small risk that a minimally invasive procedure may miss another overactive gland(s) that are suppressed in the presence of a dominant gland. In Europe, MIP is being performed with an endoscopic camera (80). Yet another variation on this theme is the use of preoperative sestamibi scanning with an intraoperative gamma probe to help locate enlarged parathyroid glands. The MIP procedure seems to be as successful as more standard approaches, in the range of 95–98%.

Postoperative course

After surgery, serum calcium and PTH levels normalize and urinary calcium excretion falls by as much as 50%. Postoperative hypocalcaemia ('hungry bone syndrome') is now rare. Occasionally, postoperative hypocalcaemia still occurs, especially if preoperative bone turnover markers are elevated. Although typically the early postoperative course is not complicated by symptomatic hypocalcaemia, it is important that patients be instructed to take calcium supplementation following parathyroidectomy.

Nonsurgical management

There are new guidelines for monitoring those patients who are not going to have parathyroid surgery (Table 4.3.4). This includes annual measurements of the serum calcium concentration, a calculated creatinine clearance, and regular monitoring of bone mineral density. In addition, patients should be instructed to remain well hydrated and to avoid thiazide diuretics and prolonged immobilization. Dietary calcium intake in patients can safely be liberalized to 1000 mg/day if 1,25-dihydroxyvitamin D_3 levels are not increased, but should be more tightly controlled if 1,25-dihydroxyvitamin D levels are elevated.

Drug therapy

The 2008 Workshop on Primary Hyperparathyroidism concluded that there is no drug for which there are sufficient data to recommend its use in patients with this disorder (81). Drugs that are sometimes used in patients with primary hyperparathyroidism are reviewed in this section.

Phosphate While oral phosphate can lower the serum calcium by up to 1 mg/dl this drug is no longer used in primary hyperparathyroidism due to its limited gastrointestinal tolerance, possible

Table 4.3.4 A comparison of new and old management guidelines for patients with asymptomatic primary hyperparathyroidism who do not undergo parathyroid surgery

Measurement	Older guidelines	Newer guidelines
Serum calcium	Semiannually	Annually
24-h urinary calcium	Annually	Not recommended
Creatinine clearance	Annually	Not recommended
Serum creatinine	Annually	Annually
Bone density	Annually	Annually or biannually
Abdominal radiograph	Annually	Not recommended

(From reference #183).

further increase in PTH levels, and the possibility of soft tissue calcifications after long-term use.

Oestrogens and SERM's Serum calcium reductions of 0.5 to 1.0 mg/dl in postmenopausal women with primary hyperparathyroidism who receive oestrogen replacement therapy is generally seen, while PTH is unchanged (82–84). Studies of BMD in oestrogen-treated patients with primary hyperparathyroidism have documented an increase in BMD at the femoral neck and lumbar spine (85). Data on raloxifene, a selective oestrogen receptor modulator, in primary hyperparathyroidism are limited. In a short-term (8-week) trial of 18 postmenopausal women, raloxifene (60 mg/day) was associated with a statistically significant although small (0.5 mg/dl) reduction in the serum calcium concentration and in markers of bone turnover (86). No long-term data or data on bone density are available.

Bisphosphonates By reducing bone turnover, bisphosphonates could be beneficial in primary hyperparathyroidism. The most extensive data are available with alendronate. With alendronate (87–89) bone mineral density of the lumbar spine and hip regions increases and bone turnover markers decline. A bisphosphonate such as alendronate could be useful in patients with low bone density in whom parathyroid surgery is not an option.

Inhibition of parathyroid hormone Targeted medical therapy for primary hyperparathyroidism is inhibition of the synthesis and secretion of PTH from the parathyroid glands. Calcimimetics that bind to the parathyroid cell calcium-sensing receptor and inhibit PTH secretion would be an example of targeted therapy. The calcimimetic, phenylalkylamine (*R*)-*N*(3-methoxy-α-phenylethyl)-3-(2-chlorophenyl)-1-propylamine (R-568), has been shown to inhibit PTH secretion in postmenopausal women with primary hyperparathyroidism (90). A second-generation calcimimetic, cinacalcet, has been the subject of recent more extensive investigation in primary hyperparathyroidism. The studies, conducted by Peacock, Shoback, Bilezikian, and their colleagues indicate that this drug can reduce the serum calcium concentration to normal in primary hyperparathyroidism (Fig. 4.3.4) (91,92). Despite normalization of the serum calcium concentration, PTH levels fell but did not return to normal, and BMD did not change, even after 3 years of cinacalcet. Marcocci *et al.* have recently shown that cinacalcet is effective in subjects with intractable primary hyperparathyroidism (93). Silverberg *et al.* have shown that cinacalcet reduces calcium levels effectively in inoperable parathyroid carcinoma (94).

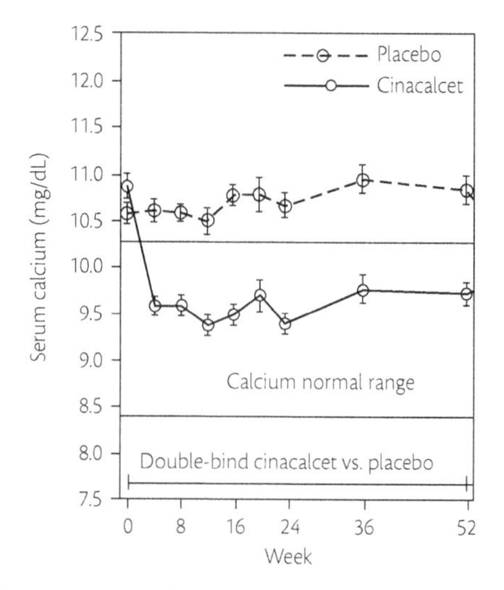

Fig. 4.3.4 Changes in serum calcium concentrations with administration of the calcimimetic cinacalcet (*solid line*) or placebo (*broken line*) in patients with primary hyperparathyroidism. (Modified with permission from Shoback DM, Bilezikian JP, Turner SA, McCary LC, Guo MD, Peacock M. The calcimimetic AMG 073 normalizes serum calcium in patients with primary hyperparathyroidism. *J Clin Endocrinol Metab*, 2003; **88**: 5644–9 (91). All rights reserved.)

Unusual presentations

Neonatal primary hyperparathyroidism

Neonatal primary hyperparathyroidism is a rare form of primary hyperparathyroidism caused by homozygous inactivation of the calcium-sensing receptor (95). When present in a heterozygous form, it is a benign hypercalcaemic state, known as familial hypocalciuric hypercalcaemia (FHH). However, in the homozygous, neonatal form, hypercalcaemia is severe and the outcome is fatal unless it is recognized early. The treatment of choice is early subtotal parathyroidectomy to remove the majority of hyperplastic parathyroid tissue.

Primary hyperparathyroidism in pregnancy

Complications of primary hyperparathyroidism in pregnancy impact on the fetus and neonate, and include spontaneous abortion, low birth weight, supravalvular aortic stenosis, and neonatal tetany (96). Tetany occurs due to fetal parathyroid gland suppression by high levels of maternal calcium, which readily crosses the placenta during pregnancy. These infants have functional hypoparathyroidism after birth, and can develop hypocalcaemia and tetany in the first few days of life. Today, with most pregnant patients presenting with only mild hypercalcaemia, an individualized approach to the management is advised. Many of those with very mild disease can be followed safely, with successful neonatal outcomes without surgery. However, parathyroidectomy during the second trimester remains the traditional recommendation for this condition.

Acute primary hyperparathyroidism

Known variously as parathyroid crisis, parathyroid poisoning, parathyroid intoxication, and parathyroid storm, acute primary hyperparathyroidism describes an episode of life-threatening hypercalcaemia in a patient with primary hyperparathyroidism (97). Clinical manifestations are associated with severe hypercalcaemia, and may include nephrocalcinosis or nephrolithiasis, subperiosteal bone resorption, and altered mental state. Laboratory evaluation is remarkable for very high serum calcium levels and PTH elevations to approximately 20 times normal. A history of persistent mild hypercalcaemia has been reported in 25% of patients. Intercurrent severe medical illness with immobilization may precipitate acute primary hyperparathyroidism (i.e. stroke, myocardial infarction, etc.). Early diagnosis, with aggressive medical management followed by surgical cure, is essential for a successful outcome.

Parathyroid cancer

Parathyroid carcinoma accounts for less than 0.5% of cases of primary hyperparathyroidism (98, 99) and is not associated with a malignant degeneration of previously benign parathyroid adenomas. The disease does not tend to have a bulk tumour effect, spreading slowly in the neck and causing symptoms related to hypercalcaemia. Metastatic disease is a late finding, with lung (40%), liver (10%), and lymph node (30%) involvement seen most commonly. There is no female predominance and serum calcium and PTH are far higher than are seen in benign disease. Nephrolithiasis or nephrocalcinosis is seen in up to 60% of patients, while overt radiological evidence of skeletal involvement is seen in 35 to 90% of patients. A palpable neck mass is reported in 30 to 76% of patients with parathyroid cancer.

Parathyroid carcinoma has also been reported in hereditary syndromes of hyperparathyroidism, (100–102) particularly in hyperparathyroidism-jaw tumour syndrome, a rare autosomal disorder, in which as many as 15% of patients will have malignant parathyroid disease. Parathyroid carcinoma has also been reported in familial isolated hyperparathyroidism. Recently, parathyroid carcinoma, as defined pathologically, has been reported in MEN 1 syndrome and with somatic *MEN1* mutations (103, 104). Only one case of parathyroid carcinoma has been reported in the MEN 2A syndrome (105).

Parathyroid carcinomas from 10 of 15 (66%) patients with sporadic parathyroid cancer carried a mutation in the *HRPT2* gene. The *HRPT2* gene that encodes for the parafibromin protein has been shown to be mutated in a substantial number of patients with parathyroid cancer, as reviewed by Marcoccci *et al.* (98).

Surgery is the only effective therapy currently available for this disease. The greatest chance for cure occurs with the first operation. Once the disease recurs, cure is unlikely, although the disease may smoulder for many years thereafter. The tumour is not radiosensitive, although there are isolated reports of tumour regression with localized radiation therapy. Traditional chemotherapeutic agents have not been useful. When metastasis occurs, isolated removal is an option, although never curative. Chemotherapy has had a very limited role in this disease. Bradwell and Harvey have attempted an immunotherapeutic approach by injecting a patient who had severe hypercalcaemia due to parathyroid cancer with immunogenic PTH. Coincident with a rise in antibody titre to PTH, previous refractory hypercalcaemia fell impressively (106). A more recent report provided evidence of antitumour effect in a single case of PTH immunization in metastatic parathyroid cancer (107). Recent attention has been focused instead on control of hypercalcaemia. Intravenous bisphosphonates treat severe hypercalcaemia, but do not have a lasting effect. The calcimimetic agents hold promise for offering calcium-lowering effects on an outpatient basis (108). Cinacalcet has been shown to have utility in the management of parathyroid cancer (94) and has been approved by the US Food and Drug Administration for the treatment of hypercalcaemia in patients with parathyroid cancer.

References

1. Albright F, Reifenstein EC. *The Parathyroid Glands, Metabolic Bone Disease*. Baltimore: Williams, Wilkins, 1948.
2. Albright F, Aub JC, Bauer W. Hyperparathyroidism: A common and polymorphic condition as illustrated by seventeen proven cases from one clinic. *JAMA*, 1934; **102**: 1276–87.
3. Silverberg SJ, Bilezikian, JP. Clinical presentation of primary hyperparathyroidism in the United States. Marcus R, Levine MA, eds. *The Parathyroids*. New York: Academic Press, 2001: 349–60.
4. Heath H, Hodgson SF, Kennedy MA. Primary hyperparathyroidism: Incidence, morbidity, and economic impact in a community. *N Engl J Med*, 1980; **302**: 189–93.
5. Bilezikian JP, Silverberg SJ. Primary hyperparathyroidism. In: Rosen C, ed. *Primer on the Metabolic Bone Diseases and Disorders of Calcium Metabolism*. 7th edn. American Society for Bone and Mineral Research, 2008: 302–6.
6. Rao SD, Frame B, Miller MJ, Kleerekoper M, Block MA, Parfitt AM. Hyperparathyroidism following head and neck irradiation. *Arch Intern Med*, 1980; **140**: 205–7.
7. Nordenström J, Strigård K, Perbeck L, Willems J, Bågedahl-Strindlund M, Linder J. Hyperparathyroidism associated with treatment of manic-depressive disorders by lithium. *Eur J Surg*, 1992; **158**: 207–11.
8. Attie JN, Bock G, Auguste L. Multiple parathyroid adenomas: Report of 33 cases. *Surgery*, 1990; **108**: 1014–19.
9. Gilmour JR. Some developmental abnormalities of the thymus and parathyroids. *J Pathol Bacteriol*, 1941; **52**: 213–18.
10. Jacobs TP, Bilezikian JP. Rare causes of hypercalcemia. *J Clin Endo Metab*, 2005; **90**: 6316–22.
11. Lepage R, Roy L, Brossard JH, Rousseau L, Dorais C, Lazure C, D'Amour P: A non (1-84) circulating parathyroid hormone (PTH) fragment interferes significantly with intact PTH commercial assay measurements in uremic samples. *Clin Chem*, 1998; **44**: 805–9.
12. Gao, P, Scheibel S, D'Amour P, John MR, Rao SD, Schmidt-Gayk H, Cantor TL. Development of a novel immunoradiometric assay exclusively for biologically active whole parathyroid hormone 1-84. *J Bone Miner Res*, 2001; **16**: 605–14.
13. Silverberg SJ, Brown I, LoGerfo P, Gao P, Cantor T, Bilezikian JP. Clinical utility of an immunoradiometric assay for whole PTH (1-84) in primary hyperparathyroidism. *J Clin Endocrinol Metab*, 2003; **88**: 4725–30.
14. Souberbielle JC, Cormier C, Kindermans C, Gao P, Cantor T, Forette F, Baulieu EE. Vitamin D status and redefining serum parathyroid hormone reference range in the elderly. *J Clin Endocrinol Metab*, 2001; **86**: 3086–90.
15. Silverberg SJ, Shane E, Dempster DW, Bilezikian JP. Vitamin D deficiency in primary hyperparathyroidism. *Am J Med*, 1999; **107**: 561–7.
16. Silverberg SJ, Bilezikian JP. "Incipient" primary hyperparathyroidism: a "forme fruste" of an old disease. *J Clin Endocrinol Metab*, 2003; **88**: 5348–52.
17. Lowe H, McMahon DJ, Rubin MR, Bilezikian JP, Silverberg SJ. Normocalcemic primary hyperparathyroidism: further characterization of a new clinical phenotype. *J Clin Endocrinol Metab*, 2007; **92**: 3001–5.
18. Silverberg SJ, Lewiecki EM, Mosekilde L, Peacock M, Rubin MR. Presentation of asymptomatic primary hyperparathyroidism: Proceedings of the Third International Workshop. *J Clin Endocrinol Metab*, 2009; **94**: 351–65.
19. Silverberg SJ, Shane E, DeLaCruz L, Dempster DW, Feldman F, Seldin D, *et al.* Skeletal disease in primary hyperparathyroidism. *J Bone Miner Res*, 1989; **4**: 283–91.
20. Silverberg SJ, Locker FG, Bilezikian JP. Vertebral osteopenia: A new indication for surgery in primary hyperparathyroidism. *J Clin Endocrinol Metab*, 1996; **81**: 4007–12.
21. Seibel MJ. Molecular markers of bone metabolism in primary hyperparathyroidism. In: Bilezikian JP, ed. *The Parathyroids: Basic and Clinical Concepts*. New York: Academic Press, 2001: 399–410.
22. Guo CY, Thomas WER, Al-Dehaimi AW, Assiri AM, Eastell R. Longitudinal changes in bone mineral density and bone turnover in women with primary hyperparathyroidism. *J Clin Endocrinol Metab*, 1996; **81**: 3487–91.
23. Tanaka Y, Funahashi H, Imai T, Tominaga Y, Takagi H. Parathyroid function and bone metabolic markers in primary and secondary hyperparathyroidism. *Semin Surg Oncol*, 1997; **13**: 125–33.
24. Parfitt AM. Surface specific bone remodeling in health and disease. In: Kleerekoper M, ed. *Clinical Disorders of Bone and Mineral Metabolism*. New York: Mary Ann Liebert, 1989: 7–14.

25. Parisien M, Cosman F, Mellish RWE, Schnitzer M, Nieves J, Silverberg SJ, *et al.* Bone structure in postmenopausal hyperparathyroid, osteoporotic and normal women. *J Bone Miner Res*, 1995; **10**: 1393–9.
26. Dempster DW, Parisien M, Silverberg SJ, Liang XG, Schnitzer M, Shen V, *et al.* On the mechanism of cancellous bone preservation in postmenopausal women with mild primary hyperparathyroidism. *J Clin Endocrinol Metab*, 1999; **84**: 1562–6.
27. Dempster DW, Müller R, Zhou H, Kohler T, Shane E, Parisien M, *et al.* Preserved three-dimensional cancellous bone structure in mild primary hyperparathyroidism. *Bone*, 2007; **41**: 19–24.
28. Dauphine RT, Riggs BL, Scholz DA. Back pain and vertebral crush fractures: An unemphasized mode of presentation for primary hyperparathyroidism. *Ann Intern Med*, 1975; **83**: 365–7.
29. Roschger P, Dempster DW, Zhou H, Paschalis EP, Silverberg SJ, Shane E, *et al.* New observations on bone quality in mild primary hyperparathyroidism as determined by quantitative backscattered electron imaging. *J Bone Min Res*, 2007; **22**: 717–23.
30. Zoehrer R, Dempster DW, Bilezikian JP, Zhou H, Silverberg SJ, Shane E, *et al.* Bone quality determined by Fourier transform infrared imaging analysis in mild primary hyperparathyroidism. *J Clin Endocrinol Metab*, 2008; **93**: 3484–9.
31. Wilson RJ, Rao S, Ellis B, Kleerekoper M, Parfitt AM. Mild asymptomatic primary hyperparathyroidism is not a risk factor for vertebral fractures. *Ann Intern Med*, 1988; **109**: 959–62.
32. Larsson K, Ljunghall S, Krusemo UB, Naessén T, Lindh E, Persson I. The risk of hip fractures in patients with primary hyperparathyroidism: A population-based cohort study with a follow-up of 19 years. *J Intern Med*, 1993; **234**: 585–93.
33. Khosla S, Melton LJ, Wermers RA, Crowson CS, O'Fallon W, Riggs B. Primary hyperparathyroidism and the risk of fracture: A population-based study. *J Bone Miner Res*, 1999; **14**: 1700–7.
34. Vignali E, Viccica C, Diacinti D, Cetani F, Cianferotti L, Ambrogini E, *et al.* Morphometric vertebral fractures in postmenopausal women with primary hyperparathyroidism. *J Clin Endocrinol Metab*, 2009; **94**: 2306–12.
35. Klugman VA, Favus M, Pak CYC. Nephrolithiasis in primary hyperparathyroidism. In: Bilezikian JP, ed. *The Parathyroids: Basic and Clinical Concepts.* New York: Academic Press, 2001: 437–50.
36. Peacock M. Primary hyperparathyroidism and the kidney: biochemical and clinical spectrum. *J Bone Miner Res*, 2002; **17** (Suppl 2): N87–N94.
37. Silverberg SJ, Shane E, Jacobs TP, Siris ES, Gartenberg F, Seldin D, *et al.* Nephrolithiasis and bone involvement in primary hyperparathyroidism, 1985–1990. *Am J Med*, 1990; **89**: 327–34.
38. Pak CY, Nicar MJ, Peterson R, Zerwekh JE, Snyder W. Lack of unique pathophysiologic background for nephrolithiaisis in primary hyperparathyroidism. *J Clin Endocrinol Metab*, 1981; **53**: 536–42.
39. Patten BM, Bilezikian JP, Mallette LE, Prince A, Engel WK, Aurbach GD. Neuromuscular disease in hyperparathyroidism. *Ann Intern Med*, 1974; **80**: 182–93.
40. Turken SA, Cafferty M, Silverberg SJ, De La Cruz L, Cimino C, Lange DJ, *et al.* Neuromuscular involvement in mild, asymptomatic primary hyperparathyroidism. *Am J Med*, 1989; **87**: 553–7.
41. Rao DS, Phillips ER, Divine GW, Talpos GB. Randomized, controlled clinical trial of surgery vs no surgery in mild asymptomatic primary hyperparathyroidism. *J Clin Endocrinol Metab*, 2004; **89**: 5415–22.
42. Bollerslev J, Jansson S, Mollerup CL, Nordenström J, Lundgren E, Tørring O, *et al.* Medical observation compared with parathyroidectomy, for asymptomatic primary hyperparathyroidism: a prospective, randomized trial. *J Clin Endocrinol Metab*, 2007; **92**: 1687–92.
43. Ambrogini E, Cetani F, Cianferotti L, Vignali E, Banti C, Viccica G, *et al.* Surgery or no surgery for mild asymptomatic primary hyperparathyroidism: a prospective, randomized clinical trial. *J Clin Endocrinol Metab*, 2007; **92**: 3114–21.
44. Walker MD, McMahon DJ, Inabnet WB, Lazar RM, Brown I, Vardy S, *et al.* Neuropsychological features of primary hyperparathyroidism: a prospective study. *J Clin Endocrinol Metab*, 2009; **94**: 1951–9.
45. Palmer M, Adami HO, Bergstrom R, Akerstrom G, Ljunghall S. Mortality after surgery for primary hyperparathyroidism: a follow-up of 441 patients operated on from 1956 to 1979. *Surgery*, 1987; **102**: 1–7.
46. Hedback G, Tisell LE, Bengtsson BA, Hedman I, Oden A. Premature death in patients operated on for primary hyperparathyroidism. *World J Surg*, 1990; **14**: 829–35; discussion 36.
47. Ljunghall S, Jakobsson S, Joborn C, Palmer M, Rastad J, Akerstrom G. Longitudinal studies of mild primary hyperparathyroidism. *J Bone Miner Res*, 1991; **6** (Suppl 2): S111–6.
48. Wermers RA, Khosla S, Atkinson EJ, Grant CS, Hodgson SF, O'Fallon M, Melton LJ III. Survival after the diagnosis of hyperparathyroidism: a population-based study. *Am J Med*, 1998; **104**: 115–22.
49. Soreide JA, van Heerden JA, Grant CS, Yau Lo C, Schleck C, Ilstrup DM. Survival after surgical treatment for primary hyperparathyroidism. *Surgery*, 1997; **122**: 1117–23.
50. Bradley EL III, Wells JO. Primary hyperparathyroidism and hypertension. *Am Surg*, 1983; **49**: 569–70.
51. Roberts WC, Waller BF. Effect of chronic hypercalcemia on the heart. An analysis of 18 necropsy patients. *Am J Med*, 1981; **71**: 371–84.
52. Vestergaard P, Mollerup CL, Frokjaer VG, Christiansen P, Blichert-Toft M, Mosekilde L. Cardiovascular events before and after surgery for primary hyperparathyroidism. *World J Surg*, 2003; **27**: 216–22.
53. Stefenelli T, Mayr H, Bergler-Klein J, Globits S, Woloszczuk W, Niederle B. Primary hyperparathyroidism: incidence of cardiac abnormalities and partial reversibility after successful parathyroidectomy. *Am J Med*, 1993; **95**: 197–202.
54. Dalberg K, Brodin LA, Juhlin-Dannfelt A, Farnebo LO. Cardiac function in primary hyperparathyroidism before and after operation. *An echocardiographic study. Eur J Surg*, 1996; **162**: 171–6.
55. Nuzzo V, Tauchmanova L, Fonderico F, Trotta R, Fittipaldi MR, Fontanta D, *et al.* Increased intima-media thickness of the carotid artery wall, normal blood pressure profile and normal left ventricular mass in subjects with primary hyperparathyroidism. *Eur J Endocrinol*, 2002; **147**: 453–9.
56. Nilsson IL, Aberg J, Rastad J, Lind L. Left ventricular systolic and diastolic function and exercise testing in primary hyperparathyroidism-effects of parathyroidectomy. *Surgery*, 2000; **128**: 895–902.
57. Piovesan A, Molineri N, Casasso F, Emmolo I, Ugliengo G, Cesario F, Borretta G. Left ventricular hypertrophy in primary hyperparathyroidism. Effects of successful parathyroidectomy. *Clin Endocrinol (Oxf)*, 1999; **50**: 321–8.
58. Rosenqvist M, Nordenstrom J, Andersson M, Edhag OK. Cardiac conduction in patients with hypercalcaemia due to primary hyperparathyroidism. *Clin Endocrinol (Oxf)*, 1992; **37**: 29–33.
59. Barletta G, De Feo ML, Del Bene R, Lazzeri C, Vecchiarino S, La Villa G, *et al.* Cardiovascular effects of parathyroid hormone: a study in healthy subjects and normotensive patients with mild primary hyperparathyroidism. *J Clin Endocrinol Metab*, 2000; **85**: 1815–21.
60. Nilsson IL, Aberg J, Rastad J, Lind L. Endothelial vasodilatory dysfunction in primary hyperparathyroidism is reversed after parathyroidectomy. *Surgery*, 1999; **126**: 1049–55.
61. Neunteufl T, Katzenschlager R, Abela C, Kostner K, Niederie B, Weidinger F, Stefenelli T. Impairment of endothelium-independent vasodilation in patients with hypercalcemia. *Cardiovasc Res*, 1998; **40**: 396–401.
62. Kosch M, Hausberg M, Vormbrock K, Kisters K, Gabriels G, Rahn KH, Barencrobk M. Impaired flow-mediated vasodilation of the brachial artery in patients with primary hyperparathyroidism improves after parathyroidectomy. *Cardiovasc Res*, 2000; **47**: 813–18.

63. Baykan M, Erem C, Erdogan T, Hacihasanoglu A, Gedikli O, Kiris A, *et al.* Impairment of flow mediated vasodilatation of brachial artery in patients with primary hyperparathyroidism. *Int J Cardiovasc Imaging*, 2007; **23**: 323–8.
64. Smith JC, Page MD, John R, Wheeler MH, Cockcroft JR, Scanlon MF, Davies JS. Augmentation of central arterial pressure in mild primary hyperparathyroidism. *J Clin Endocrinol Metab*, 2000; **85**: 3515–19.
65. Rubin MR, Maurer MS, McMahon DJ, Bilezikian JP, Silverberg SJ. Arterial stiffness in mild primary hyperparathyroidism. *J Clin Endocrinol Metab*, 2005; **90**: 3326–30.
66. Marx S. Multiple endocrine neoplasia type 1. In: Bilezikian JP, ed. *The Parathyroids*. New York: Academic Press, 2001: 535–84.
67. Brandi ML, Gagel RF, Angeli A. Consensus guidelines for diagnosis and therapy of MEN type 1 and type 2. *J Clin Endocrinol Metab*, 2001; **86**: 5658–71.
68. Khoo TK, Vege SS, Abu-Lebdeh HS, Ryu E, Nadeem S, Werners RA. Acute pancreatitis in primary hyperparathyroidism, a population-based study. *J Clin Endocrinol Metab*, 2009; **94**: 2115–18.
69. Silverberg SJ, Shane E, Jacobs TP, Siris E, Bilezikian JP. A 10-year prospective study of primary hyperparathyroidism with or without parathyroid surgery. *New Eng J Med*, 1999; **341**: 1249–55.
70. Rubin MR, Bilezikian JP, McMahon DJ, Jacobs T, Shane, E, Siris E, *et al.* The natural history of primary hyperparathyroidism with or without parathyroid surgery after 15-years. *J Clin Endocrinol Metab*, 2008; **93**: 3462–70.
71. National Institutes of Health. Consensus development conference statement on primary hyperparathyroidism. *J Bone Miner Res*, 1991; **6**: s9–s13.
72. Bilezikian JP, Potts JT Jr, El-Hajj Fuleihan G, Kleerekoper M, Neer R, Peacock M, *et al.* Summary statement from a workshop on asymptomatic primary hyperparathyroidism: a perspective for the 21st century. *J Clin Endocrinol Metab*, 2002; **87**: 5353–61.
73. Bilezikian JP, Khan AA, Potts JT Jr. on behalf of the Third International Workshop on the Management of Asymptomatic Primary Hyperthyroidism. Summary statement: Guidelines for the management of asymptomatic primary hyperparathyroidism: Summary statement from the Third International Workshop. *J Clin Endocrinol Metab*, 2009; **94**: 335–9.
74. Udelsman R, Pasieka JL, Sturgeon C, Young JEM, Clark OH. Surgery for asymptomatic primary hyperparathyroidism: Proceedings of the Third International Workshop. *J Clin Endocrinol Metab*, 2009; **94**: 366–72.
75. Civelek A, Ozalp E, Donovan P, Udelsman R. Prospective evaluation of delayed technetium-99M sestamibi SPECT scintigraphy for preoperative localization of primary hyperparathyroidism. *Surgery*, 2002; **131**: 149–57.
76. Van Husen R, Kim LT. Accuracy of surgeon-performed ultrasound in parathyroid localization. *World J Surg*, 2004; **28**: 1122–6.
77. Mortenson ME, Evans DB, Hunter GJ, Shellingerhout D, Vu T, Edeiken BS, *et al.* Parathyroid exploration in the reoperative neck improved preoperative localization with 4D-computer tomography. *J Am Coll Surg*, 2008; **206**: 888–95.
78. Maser C, Donovan P, Satos F, Donabedian R, Rinder C, Scoutt L, Udelsman R. Sonographically guided fine needle aspiration with rapid parathyroid hormone assay. *Ann Surg Oncol*, 2006; **13**: 1690–5.
79. Udelsman R, Donovan PI. Remedial parathyroid surgery: changing trends in 130 consecutive cases. *Ann Surg*, 2006; **244**: 471–9.
80. Miccoli P, Berti P, Materazzi G, Ambrosini CE, Fregoli L, Donatini G. Endoscopic bilateral neck exploration versus quick intraoperative parathormone assay (qPTHa) during endoscopic parathyroidectomy: A prospective randomized trial. *Surg Endosc*, 2008; **22**: 398–400.
81. Khan AA, Bilezikian JP, Potts JT Jr. Guest editors for the Third International Workshop on Asymptomatic Primary Hyperparathyroidism. The diagnosis and management of asymptomatic primary hyperparathyroidism revisited. *J Clin Endocrinol Metab*, 2009; **94**: 333–4.
82. Gallagher JC, Nordin BEC. Treatment with oestrogens of primary hyperparathyroidism in post-menopausal women. *Lancet*, 1972; **1**: 503–7.
83. Marcus R, Madvig P, Crim M, Pont A, Kosek J. Conjugated estrogens in the treatment of postmenopausal women with hyperparathyroidism. *Ann Intern Med*, 1984; **100**: 633–40.
84. Selby PL, Peacock M. Ethinyl estradiol and norethinedrone in the treatment of primary hyperparathyroidism in postmenopausal women. *N Engl J Med*, 1986; **314**: 1481–5.
85. Grey AB, Stapleton JP, Evans MC, Tatnell MA, Reid IR. Effect of hormone replacement therapy on BMD in post-menopausal women with primary hyperparathyroidism. *Ann Intern Med*, 1996; **125**: 360–8.
86. Rubin MA, Lee KH, McMahon DJ, Silverberg SJ. Raloxifene lowers serum calcium and markers of bone turnover in postmenopausal women with primary hyperparathyroidism. *J Clin Endocrinol Metab*, 2003; **88**: 1174–8.
87. Rossini M, Gatti D, Isaia G, Sartori L, Braga V, Adami S. Effects of oral alendronate in elderly patients with osteoporosis and mild primary hyperparathyroidism. *J Bone Miner Res*, 2001; **16**: 113–19.
88. Chow CC, Chan WB, Li JKY, Chan NN, Chan MHM, Ko GTC, *et al.* Oral alendronate increases bone mineral density in postmenopausal women with primary hyperparathyroidism. *J Clin Endocrinol Metab*, 2003; **88**: 581–7.
89. Kahn AA, Bilezikian JP, Kung AWC, Ahmed MM, Dubois SJ, Ho AYY, *et al.* Alendronate in primary hyperparathyroidism: a double-blind, randomized, placebo-controlled trial. *J Clin Endocrinol Metab*, 2004; **89**: 3319–25.
90. Silverberg SJ, Marriott TB, Bone HG III, Locker FG, Thys-Jacobs S, Dziem G, *et al.* Short term inhibition of parathyroid hormone secretion by a calcium receptor agonist in primary hyperparathyroidism. *N Engl J Med*, 1997; **307**: 1506–10.
91. Shoback DM, Bilezikian JP, Turner SA, McCary LC, Guo MD, Peacock M. The calcimimetic AMG 073 normalizes serum calcium in patients with primary hyperparathyroidism. *J Clin Endocrinol Metab*, 2003; **88**: 5644–9.
92. Peacock M, Bilezikian JP, Klassen PS, Guo MD, Turner SA, Shoback DM. Cinacalcet hydrochloride maintains long-term normocalcemia in patients with primary hyperparathyroidism. *J Clin Endocrinol Metab*, 2005; **90**: 135–41.
93. Marcocci C, Chanson P, Shoback D, Bilezikian JP, Fernandez-Cruz L, Orgiazzi J, *et al.* Cinacalcet reduces serum calcium concentrations in patients with intractable primary hyperparathyroidism. *J Clin Endocrinol Metab*, 2009; **94**: 2766–72.
94. Silverberg SJ, Rubin MR, Faiman C, Peacock M, Shoback DM, Smallridge R, *et al.* Cinacalcet HCI reduces the serum calcium concentration in inoperable parathyroid carcinoma. *J Clin Endocrinol Metab*, 2007; **92**: 3803–8.
95. Marx SJ, Fraser D, Rapoport A. Familial hypocalciuric hypercalcemia: Mild expression of the gene in heterozygotes and severe expression in homozygotes. *Am J Med*, 1985; **78**: 15–22.
96. Lowe DK, Orwoll ES, McClung MR, Cawthon ML, Peterson CG. Hyperparathyroidism and pregnancy. *Am J Surg*, 1983; **145**: 611–19.
97. Fitzpatrick LA. Acute primary hyperparathyroidism. In: Bilezikian JP, ed. *The Parathyroids: Basic and Clinical Concepts*. New York: Academic Press, 2001: 527–34.
98. Marcocci C, Cetani F, Rubin MR, Silverberg SJ, Pinchera A, Bilezikian JP. Parathyroid carcinoma. *J Bone Min Res*, 2008; **23**: 1869–80.
99. Shane E. Parathyroid carcinoma. *J Clin Endocrinol Metab*, 2001; **86**: 485–93.
100. Marx SJ, Simonds WF, Agarwal SK, Burns AL, Weinstein LS, Cochran C, *et al.* Hyperparathyroidism in hereditary syndromes: special expressions and special managements. *J Bone Miner Res*, 2002; **17** (Suppl 2): N37–43.

101. Chen JD, Morrison C, Zhang C, Kahnoski K, Carpten JD, Teh BT. Hyperparathyroidism-jaw tumour syndrome. *J Intern Med*, 2003; **253**: 634–42.
102. Simonds WF, James-Newton LA, Agarwal SK, Yang B, Skarulis MC, Hendy GN, Marx SJ. Familial isolated hyperparathyroidism: clinical and genetic characteristics of 36 kindreds. *Medicine (Baltimore)*; 2002: **81**: 1–26.
103. Dionisi S, Minisola S, Pepe J, De Geronimo S, Paglia F, Memeo L, Fitzpatrick LA. Concurrent parathyroid adenomas and carcinoma in the setting of multiple endocrine neoplasia type 1: presentation as hypercalcemic crisis. *Mayo Clin Proc*, 2002; **77**: 866–9.
104. Haven CJ, van Puijenbroek M, Tan MH, Teh BT, Fleuren GJ, van Wezel T, Morreau H. Identification of MEN1 and HRPT2 somatic mutations in paraffin-embedded (sporadic) parathyroid carcinomas. *Clin Endocrinol (Oxf)*, 2007; **67**: 370–6.
105. Jenkins PJ, Satta MA, Simmgen M, Drake WM, Williamson C, Lowe DG, *et al.* Metastatic parathyroid carcinoma in the MEN2A syndrome. *Clin Endocrinol (Oxf)*, 1997; **47**: 747–51.
106. Bradwell AR, Harvey TC. Control of hypercalcemia of parathyroid carcinoma by immunisation. *Lancet*, 1999; **353**: 370–3.
107. Betea D, Bradwell AR, Harvey TC, Mead GP, Schmidt-Gayk H, Ghaye B, *et al.* Hormonal and biochemical normalization and tumor shrinkage induced by anti-parathyroid hormone immunotherapy in a patient with metastatic parathyroid carcinoma. *J Clin Endocrinol Metab*, 2004; **89**: 3413–20.
108. Collins MT, Skarulis MC, Bilezikian JP, Silverberg SJ, Spiegel AM, Marx SJ. 1998 Treatment of hypercalcemia secondary to parathyroid carcinoma with a novel calcimimetic agent. *J Clin Endocrinol Metab*, 1998; **83**: 1083–8.

4.4

Familial hypocalciuric hypercalcaemia

Edward M. Brown

Introduction

Familial hypocalciuric hypercalcaemia (FHH) is a generally asymptomatic form of mild to moderate, parathyroid hormone (PTH)-dependent hypercalcaemia, which was initially confused with the more common hypercalcaemic disorder, primary hyperparathyroidism (PHPT) (1–3). Subsequent studies showed that FHH differs from PHPT in several important respects, although distinguishing between these two conditions can still be difficult on a clinical basis alone (4). Urinary calcium excretion is lower in the former than in the latter, and in FHH, unlike PHPT, hypercalcaemia recurs rapidly following surgical treatment with anything less than total parathyroidectomy. Indeed, given FHH's generally benign natural history, surgery is usually ill advised (3).

The phenotype of FHH implicated some abnormality in the sensing and/or handling of calcium by parathyroid and kidney (3, 5). For more than two decades after its initial description, however, the genetic defect in FHH was unknown. In 1992, the major genetic locus for this condition was identified on the long arm of chromosome 3 (6). The following year saw the cloning of a G protein-coupled extracellular calcium (Ca^{2+}_{o})-sensing receptor (CaSR) mediating direct regulation of PTH secretion by Ca^{2+}_{o} (7). The CaSR's function and its location of its gene on the same region chromosome 3 in humans made it an obvious candidate gene for FHH. Shortly thereafter, heterozygous inactivating mutations in the *CaSR* were identified in several FHH families (8). Moreover, patients with a related condition, neonatal severe hyperparathyroidism (NSHPT), also turned out to harbour inactivating *CaSR* mutations in the homozygous, compound heterozygous, and in a milder disorder, neonatal hyperparathyroidism (NHPT), in the heterozygous state (8). This chapter reviews the clinical and biochemical features of FHH, its genetics, pathophysiology, and pathogenesis, and its relationship to NSHPT.

Familial hypocalciuric hypercalcaemia

Clinical and biochemical features of FHH

In 1972, Foley, *et al.* described a family with an asymptomatic, unexpectedly benign form of hypercalcaemia that they called familial benign hypercalcaemia (9). Their report first detailed the distinctive clinical features of this syndrome, although in retrospect a family described in 1966 (10) proved to have the same condition when re-evaluated later. Subsequent work confirmed and refined these initial observations. Marx *et al.* studied families with the same syndrome and renamed it FHH to emphasize its characteristic alteration in renal Ca^{2+} handling (e.g. absolute or relative hypocalciuria, the latter being an inappropriately low urinary Ca^{2+} excretion in the face of hypercalcaemia) (3). The terms FHH and familial benign hypercalcaemia are both employed to describe this condition (or the hybrid term, familial benign hypocalciuric hypercalcaemia), but we shall use the first of these here.

FHH is an uncommon condition; its prevalence is thought to be 1% or less of that of PHPT. It exhibits an autosomal dominant inheritance of lifelong, generally asymptomatic hypercalcaemia of mild to moderate severity. FHH's penetrance approaches 100% (3) and its biochemical abnormalities appear immediately postnatally. The degree of hypercalcaemia varies, but the serum calcium concentrations within a given family tend to be clustered within a relatively narrow range. Occasional families have serum calcium concentrations that are consistently within the upper part of the normal range or only intermittently elevated. Most families have serum total calcium concentrations of 2.6–2.9 mmol/l, while rare kindreds have values as high as 3–3.3 mmol/l or even higher (3, 11). Affected individuals do not, in general, exhibit the symptoms and complications of other hypercalcaemic disorders (1–3). These typical manifestations of hypercalcaemia include gastrointestinal (nausea, anorexia, and constipation), mental, and renal disturbances (nephrolithiasis, nephrocalcinosis, impaired renal function, and defective urinary concentrating capacity) (12). Even in FHH kindreds with unusually high serum calcium concentrations, affected individuals are remarkably asymptomatic. Nonspecific symptoms encountered in other hypercalcaemic disorders, such as fatigue, were initially reported in patients with FHH (3), but were not confirmed subsequently to be related to this condition and are thought to be the result of ascertainment bias (13).

Some persons with FHH have experienced pancreatitis or chondrocalcinosis, raising the possibility of a causal relationship between FHH and these complications (3). Some studies have found pancreatitis to be no more common in affected than in unaffected members of families with FHH or in the population as a whole (13).

More recent studies, however, have suggested that the presence of FHH may increase the risk of pancreatitis in individuals with mutations in other genes, such as *SPINK1*, which by themselves confer increased risk of pancreatitis (14). In the case of chondrocalcinosis, follow-up studies failed to confirm that chondrocalcinosis occurs with increased frequency in FHH (13).

The degree of hypercalcaemia in FHH is comparable to that in mild to moderate PHPT, and both conditions exhibit equivalent increases in serum total and ionized calcium concentrations (3, 13). The serum phosphate concentration tends to be somewhat reduced in FHH but usually remains within the normal range. Serum magnesium is high-normal or mildly elevated. There is a positive relationship between the serum calcium and magnesium concentrations in FHH; PHPT, in contrast, exhibits an inverse relationship between these parameters (3).

A common abnormality in FHH is an inappropriately normal (i.e. nonsuppressed) PTH level or, less commonly, a mildly elevated level of this hormone (13), especially when measured with an intact PTH assay (6, 15). Thus Ca^{2+}_o-regulated PTH release must be abnormal, since hypercalcaemia would otherwise suppress PTH secretion. One factor that can cause an unusually high level of PTH in FHH is coexistent vitamin D deficiency (16). It is in patients with FHH who have PTH levels that are in the upper part of the normal range or are frankly elevated that differentiating this condition from mild PHPT on the basis of serum calcium and PTH alone may be difficult (4), since 10–15% of hyperparathyroid patients exhibit intact PTH levels in the upper normal range and many have levels that are only mildly to moderately elevated.

Studies modulating serum calcium concentration in FHH by infusing calcium to raise it and citrate (or ethylenediamine tetraacetic acid (EDTA)) to lower it have revealed an increase in parathyroid 'set-point' (the level of Ca^{2+}_o half-maximally suppressing PTH levels) (17). Thus FHH exhibits mild to moderate 'resistance' to the normal inhibitory effect of Ca^{2+}_o on PTH release. PHPT exhibits an analogous, but somewhat greater, increase in set-point (17). PHPT also commonly exhibits additional defects in secretory control, including elevated maximal and minimal secretory rates at low and high Ca^{2+}_o, respectively. The parathyroid glands in FHH appear normal or mildly hyperplastic (18), although occasional families have overt parathyroid enlargement and hyperplasia (19).

A number of individuals with FHH have undergone partial or total parathyroidectomy in an attempt to cure their hypercalcaemia, usually following an erroneous diagnosis of PHPT. Their unusual postoperative course has provided further evidence that FHH differs fundamentally from PHPT. Among 27 individuals with FHH who underwent from one to four neck explorations, hypercalcaemia recurred within days to weeks in most (21 patients), and only two remained normocalcaemic indefinitely without additional treatment (1). Cure of hypercalcaemia in FHH usually occurred only after total parathyroidectomy (5 of 27 persons). Recurrent hypercalcaemia after resecting a parathyroid adenoma, in contrast, occurs in less than 5–10% of cases, usually several years postoperatively. Recurrent hypercalcaemia is more common in primary parathyroid hyperplasia, particularly in familial disorders, such as multiple endocrine neoplasia type 1 (MEN 1). The incidence of recurrence in the latter condition increases progressively to approximately 50% at 10 years after subtotal parathyroidectomy (20).

Serum 25-hydroxyvitamin D (25(OH)D) and 1,25-dihydroxyvitamin D ($1,25(OH)_2D$) levels are generally normal in FHH (15), and intestinal Ca^{2+} absorption is normal or modestly reduced (13). Some persons with FHH show a blunted rise in $1,25(OH)_2D$ and gastrointestinal Ca^{2+} absorption when dietary calcium intake is reduced (13). Patients with PHPT exhibit higher levels of $1,25(OH)_2D$ than those in patients with FHH (15), accompanied by increased calcium absorption. Markers of bone turnover (i.e. urinary deoxypyridinoline excretion) can be mildly elevated in FHH, but bone mineral density is generally normal (21) and is higher in the hip and forearm—areas relatively rich in cortical bone—than in patients with PHPT, who typically exhibit loss of cortical bone. As might be expected from their bone mineral density, fracture risk is not increased in FHH patients (13). Several affected persons in an FHH kindred in Oklahoma, USA exhibited osteomalacia (22). However, osteomalacia is not a feature of other FHH kindreds, and this Oklahoma kindred has a form of FHH that is genetically distinct from that in most kindreds (see below).

Another characteristic finding in FHH is excessively avid renal tubular reabsorption of Ca^{2+} and Mg^{2+} (Fig. 4.4.1a) (3, 9, 13), particularly given the concomitant hypercalcaemia, which normally increases urinary Ca^{2+} excretion (12). The parameter of renal Ca^{2+} handling utilized most frequently to document this abnormality is the ratio of the clearance of calcium to that of creatinine, calculated as (urinary calcium/ serum total calcium)×(serum creatinine/ urinary creatinine). This clearance ratio is lower than 0.01 in approximately 80% of individuals with FHH but in only about 20% of patients with PHPT (23). Persons with other, non-PTH-dependent forms of hypercalcaemia generally exhibit markedly greater rates of calcium excretion. In a recent study, a calcium to creatinine clearance ratio of 0.0115 provided 80% sensitivity and 88% specificity in distinguishing FHH from PHPT (24). Thus the clinical constellation of autosomal dominant inheritance of mild, asymptomatic hypercalcaemia in two or more first-degree family members, a low urinary calcium to creatinine clearance ratio, and a normal PTH level usually makes the diagnosis of FHH straightforward. The excessive renal tubular reabsorption of Ca^{2+} in FHH patients exhibiting the usual hypocalciuric phenotype persists even after total parathyroidectomy (5), showing that it is not dependent upon PTH but is an intrinsic defect in renal sensing/ handling of Ca^{2+} (Fig. 4.4.1b).

Confusion can arise in distinguishing patients with FHH from those with mild PHPT in the setting of conditions that would be expected to lower urinary calcium excretion in PHPT, such as vitamin D deficiency, very low calcium intake, concomitant use of thiazide diuretics, coexistent hypothyroidism, or during treatment with lithium for psychiatric disorders (lithium can also predispose to and/ or unmask PTH-dependent hypercalcaemia) (2, 12). Moreover, in persons with PHPT and greater than a 50% reduction in glomerular filtration rate owing to chronic renal dysfunction, urinary calcium excretion decreases due to the renal insufficiency *per se*. Use of the calcium to creatinine clearance ratio to distinguish between FHH and PHPT may be of limited utility in the circumstances just noted, although correction of coexistent medical conditions, e.g. vitamin D or calcium deficiency, and studies of additional family members may clarify the diagnosis. Moreover, as discussed later, genetic testing is appropriate in some settings for unequivocal diagnosis of FHH. An additional parameters of renal function that is altered in FHH is urinary concentrating ability. While hypercalcaemia of other causes can produce defective urinary concentrating ability (25), individuals with FHH concentrate their urine to a greater extent than do patients with PHPT who have a comparable degree of hypercalcaemia (26).

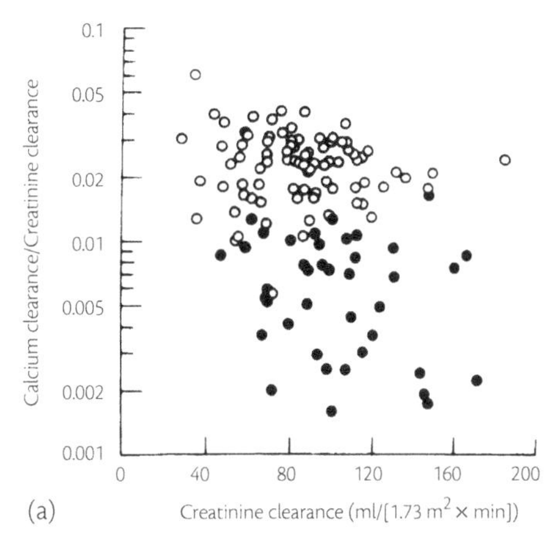

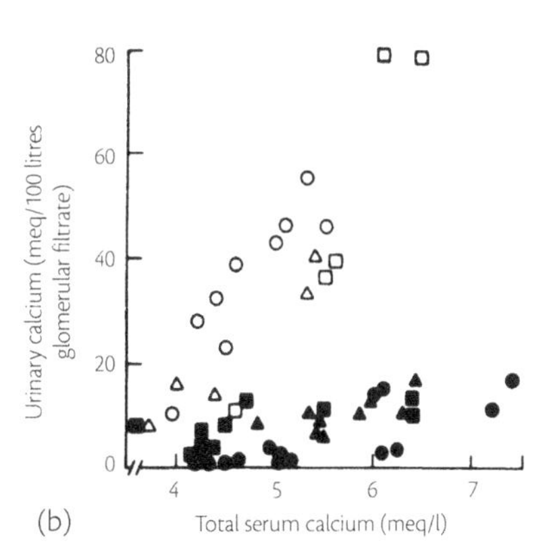

Fig. 4.4.1 Comparison of the renal handling of calcium in FHH compared to other conditions. (a) The calcium to creatinine clearance ratio in FHH (closed circles) expressed as a function of creatinine clearance and compared to that seen in typical PHPT (open circles). Note that about 80% of persons with FHH exhibit a clearance ratio less than 0.01, while a single patient with PHPT falls below this value. (From Marx SJ, Attie, MF, Levine MA, Spiegel AM, Downs Jr RW, Lasker RD. The hypocalciuric or benign variant of familial hypercalcaemia: Clinical and biochemical features in fifteen kindreds. *Medicine* (Baltimore), 1981; **60**: 397–412 (3).)
(b) The relationship between the level of serum calcium concentration and excretion of calcium in the urine in FHH patients rendered surgically hypoparathyroid (closed symbols) compared to those with hypoparathyroidism alone (open symbols). (From Attie M, Gill J, Stock J, Spiegel AM, Downs RW Jr, Levine MA, Marx SJ. Urinary calcium excretion in familial hypocalciuric hypercalcaemia. *J Clin Invest* 1983; **72**: 667–76 (5).)

In occasional FHH kindreds, hypercalcaemia has accompanied by hypercalciuria and even overt renal stone disease (27, 28). In one such kindred, in which FHH was caused by the most common genetic form of FHH linked to chromosome 3 (see Genotype–phenotype relationships, below), hypercalciuria and/or nephrolithiasis were present in several affected family members and were corrected in most cases by subtotal parathyroidectomy (27). The parathyroid glands in this family differed from the norm in FHH in that many revealed nodular hyperplasia.

Thus both the clinical and biochemical manifestations of FHH suggested that it was an inherited abnormality in the responsiveness of parathyroid, kidney, and perhaps other tissues to $Ca^{2+}{}_{o}$. In the latter regard, there is a notable lack, for instance, of the usual gastrointestinal or mental symptoms of hypercalcaemia in FHH, even in kindreds with higher than average serum calcium concentrations (3, 9, 13). Given the benign natural history of FHH and the difficulty in achieving a biochemical 'cure', a consensus has emerged that surgical intervention is unwise in this condition except in unusual circumstances detailed below. Therefore, differentiating FHH from PHPT is very important to avoid unnecessary neck exploration in the former.

Physiological roles of the $Ca^{2+}{}_{o}$-sensing receptor in $Ca^{2+}{}_{o}$ homoeostasis

Studies converging from two different directions established, on the one hand, that the extracellular CaSR is a key player in the maintenance of extracellular Ca^{2+} homoeostasis while, on the other hand, also representing the disease gene for the most common form of FHH. By briefly describing the biochemistry and biology of the CaSR and how it maintains $Ca^{2+}{}_{o}$ homoeostasis, this section provides a foundation for the ones that follow detailing the molecular genetics and pathophysiology of FHH.

Expression cloning in *Xenopus laevis* oocytes enabled isolation of the CaSR from bovine parathyroid (7). The bovine CaSR and the same receptor in other mammalian species, including humans, have three key structural domains: The first is a large N-terminal extracellular domain (ECD) comprising over 600 amino acids. The second comprises an approximately 250 amino acid transmembrane domain (TMD) that includes seven transmembrane helices, and three extracellular and three intracellular loops. These structural features of the TMD are characteristic of the large superfamily of G protein-coupled receptors (GPCR). The last domain is the CaSR's approximately 200 amino acid cytoplasmic, carboxyl (C)-terminal tail. The CaSR resides on the cell surface as a disulfide-linked dimer (29). Sensing of $Ca^{2+}{}_{o}$ occurs largely within its ECD (30), although elements within the TMD probably also participate in $Ca^{2+}{}_{o}$-sensing, as a 'headless' CaSR, totally lacking its ECD, retains some responsiveness to $Ca^{2+}{}_{o}$. Changes in the conformations of the ECD, transmembrane helices and extra- and/or intracellular loops occurring following binding of extracellular $Ca^{2+}{}_{o}$ to the CaSR are thought to activate G proteins (especially $G_{q/11}$ and G_i) and enable the receptor to couple its intracellular effector systems. These comprise numerous signalling cascades, including activation of phospholipases C, A_2, and D and mitogen-activated kinases (MAPK) and inhibition of adenylate cyclase (31). The relative contributions of these signalling pathways to the CaSR's biological actions in its various target tissues remain to be fully elucidated in most cases.

CaSR-expressing tissues with clear homoeostatic roles include the parathyroid chief cells, thyroidal C-cells, and kidney (32). The *CaSR* is also expressed in bone cells, including osteoblasts, osteoclasts, and osteocytes, but its physiological roles in these cell types remain somewhat controversial and are the subject of active investigation. Available data, however, support physiologically relevant roles of the CaSR in promoting osteoblastic bone formation and in inhibiting osteoclastogenesis and osteoclastic bone resorption, physiological functions that have been recently reviewed in detail elsewhere (33).

In the parathyroid, activating the CaSR inhibits PTH secretion, parathyroid cellular proliferation, and PTH gene expression (34). In C-cells, in contrast, the CaSR stimulates, rather than inhibiting, hormonal secretion (e.g. of calcitonin) (34). Since PTH is a $Ca^{2+}{}_{o}$-elevating hormone and calcitonin a $Ca^{2+}{}_{o}$-lowering hormone, the CaSR-mediated inhibition of PTH secretion and stimulation of calcitonin secretion are homoeostatically essential for defending against hypercalcaemia. Conversely, stimulation of PTH secretion is a key defence against hypocalcaemia.

The CaSR is present along most of the renal tubule, including proximal convoluted and straight tubules, medullary and cortical thick ascending limbs (MTAL and CTAL, respectively), distal convoluted tubule, and cortical, outer medullary, and inner medullary collecting ducts (35). In CTAL, which synthesizes the highest level of the CaSR in the kidney, the receptor resides principally on the basolateral cell surface, where it senses systemic (i.e. blood) levels of Ca^{2+}_o. The CaSR in CTAL, and perhaps also in the distal convoluted tubule, directly regulates tubular Ca^{2+} and Mg^{2+} handling, increasing their reabsorption when Ca^{2+}_o is low and diminishing it if Ca^{2+}_o is high (36). The CaSR and the PTH receptor are both expressed in CTAL, where they antagonize one another's actions on Ca^{2+} reabsorption—the CaSR inhibiting and the PTH receptor enhancing it. In the inner medullary collecting ducts, the CaSR is on the apical (e.g. luminal) plasma membrane and monitors Ca^{2+}_o within the urine (37). This apical CaSR probably mediates the high Ca^{2+}_o-evoked decrease in vasopressin-stimulated water reabsorption noted above (36). This action could potentially reduce the risk of forming renal stones when urinary Ca^{2+} is high. The CaSR probably also diminish maximal urinary concentration by inhibiting NaCl reabsorption in the MTAL, thereby reducing the medullary hypertonicity needed to drive vasopressin-stimulated water reabsorption in the collecting duct (36).

To summarize, the CaSR's roles in defending against hypercalcaemia include the following: High Ca^{2+}_o inhibits PTH secretion, which reduces net release of Ca^{2+} from bone owing to the fact that PTH is a stimulator of bone resorption. Decreased PTH release also has two key effects on the kidney, enhancing renal Ca^{2+} excretion and reducing proximal tubular synthesis of $1,25(OH)_2D_3$, both of which are normally enhanced by PTH. The reduced synthesis of $1,25(OH)_2D$ decreases gastrointestinal absorption of Ca^{2+}. As a result, there is decreased influx of Ca^{2+} into the extracellular fluid from intestine and bone and increased excretion of Ca^{2+} via the kidneys, thereby normalizing Ca^{2+}_o. Additional consequences of high Ca^{2+}_o-elicited activation of the CaSR that contribute to the defence against hypercalcaemia include stimulation of calcitonin, direct inhibition of distal renal tubular Ca^{2+} reabsorption in the CTAL, direct inhibition of 1-hydroxylation of 25(OH)D in the proximal tubule, and, perhaps, CaSR-mediated stimulation of osteoblastic activity and inhibition of osteoclastic function (33). Hypocalcaemia elicits reciprocal changes in these various parameters, permitting an effective defence against hypocalcaemic challenges.

While the preceding is a well-accepted description of the body's homoeostatic responses to hyper- and hypocalcaemia, recent studies utilizing mice with knockout of the CaSR suggest that low Ca^{2+}_o-evoked, CaSR-mediated enhancement of PTH secretion may serve primarily to defend against hypocalcaemia, in effect acting as a homoeostatic 'floor', and play a less essential role in defending against hypercalcaemia. CaSR-mediated inhibition of renal Ca^{2+} reabsorption and stimulation of calcitonin secretion (although the latter may be less important in humans than in calcitonin-responsive species such as rodents), in contrast, may be key elements of the homoeostatic 'ceiling' defending against hypercalcaemia (Kantham, *et al.*, in press).

Molecular genetics of FHH

Chou *et al.* first mapped the FHH disease gene in four families to the long arm of chromosome 3 (q21–24) (6), although this locus has subsequently been refined to 3q13.3-q21 (see http://www.casrdb.mcgill.ca). Identification of this genetic locus made it possible to show, using closely linked genetic markers, that persons with FHH are heterozygous for the disease gene (38). Subsequent studies demonstrated that most (*c.* 90% or more) FHH kindreds sufficiently large for genetic analysis exhibit linkage to chromosome 3. This genetic form of FHH is called hypocalciuric hypercalcaemia, type 1 (HHC 1, OMIM 145980) in the Online Mendelian Inheritance in Man (OMIM) database. In one family, however, a disorder clinically indistinguishable from FHH was linked to the short arm of chromosome 19, band 19p13.3 (39), and this variant of FHH is termed HHC 2 (OMIM 145981). Moreover, the Oklahoma kindred mentioned earlier with unusual clinical features (e.g. osteomalacia and rising PTH levels with age) was shown to be linked to chromosome 19, band q13 (22), and this variant of FHH is called HHC 3 (OMIM 600740). Therefore, FHH is genetically heterogeneous, but only the disease gene causing HHC 1 has been identified (see next section). A severe neonatal form of hyperparathyroidism (neonatal severe hyperparathyroidism (NSHPT)) is sometimes encountered in FHH kindreds (38). It represents the homozygous form of FHH linked to chromosome 3 in most cases. The clinical, biochemical, and genetic features of NSHPT are described below.

Identification of *CaSR* mutations in FHH

Because of the abnormal Ca^{2+}_o-sensing by kidney and parathyroid in FHH, the *CaSR* was a good candidate for the disease gene. Pollak *et al.* showed that point mutations (i.e. a change in a single nucleotide base producing a nonconservative change in the receptor's coding sequence) were present in the *CaSR* gene in three FHH families that were linked to chromosome 3 (Fig. 4.4.2) (8). Subsequent studies have identified nearly 200 *CaSR* mutations in kindreds with FHH, many of which can be accessed at http://www.casrdb.mcgill.ca/. Generally, each family harbours its own unique mutation, although several mutations have recurred in apparently unrelated kindreds (e.g. p.R185Q, p.P55L, p.T138M, and p.T151M—in current terminology p.R185Q designates mutation of the arginine at amino acid 185 in the CaSR protein sequence to glutamine) (http://www.casrdb.mcgill.ca/). Most mutations are missense mutations (a new amino acid is substituted for the one normally coded for) (21, 30–33, 35), but additional types of mutations that have been identified include: (1) nonsense mutations (e.g. point mutations introducing a stop codon), (2) frame shift mutations (loss or gain of one or more nucleotides, thereby modifying the downstream coding sequence), (3) insertion of a substantial segment of unrelated nucleotide sequence (e.g. an Alu repetitive element), and (4) a mutation of a splice site at the *CaSR* gene's intron–exon boundaries (for summary, see http://www.casrdb.mcgill.ca/). These mutations reside throughout most of the receptor's amino acid sequence.

Mutations within the *CaSR* coding region have only been identified, however, in about two-thirds of FHH families linked to the locus on chromosome 3 (although linkage analysis has been carried out in only a minority of FHH families). The remaining families presumably have mutations in other areas of the gene,

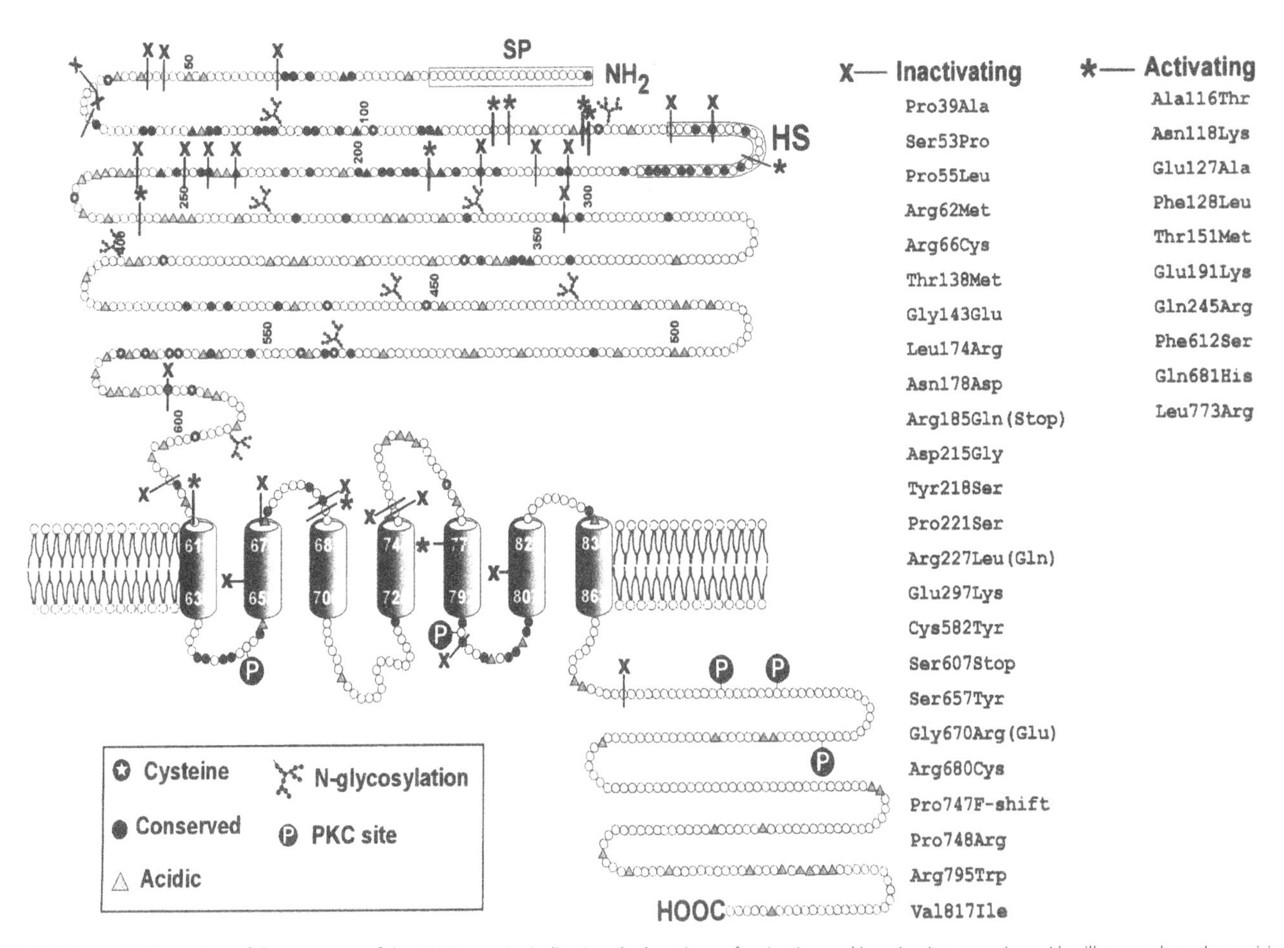

Fig. 4.4.2 Schematic illustration of the structure of the CaSR protein, indicating the locations of activating and inactivating mutations. Also illustrated are the positions of missense and nonsense mutations causing either familial hypocalciuric hypercalcaemia (FHH) or autosomal dominant hypocalcaemia; mutations are denoted with the three letter amino acid code. The normal amino acid is given prior to and the mutant amino acid after the number of the relevant codon. HS, hydrophobic segment; SP, predicted signal peptide. (From Brown EM, Bai M, Pollak M. Familial benign hypocalciuric hypercalcaemia and other syndromes of altered responsiveness to extracellular calcium. In: *Metabolic Bone Diseases*. Krane SM, Avioli LV, eds. 3rd edn. San Diego, CA; Academic Press, 1997: 479–99.)

such as regulatory regions, which impact its level of expression, but further studies are needed. Several polymorphisms reside within the *CaSR* coding region or within the intervening sequences between coding exons (http://www.casrdb.mcgill.ca). Some studies have shown subtle effects of polymorphisms within the *CaSR* C-tail on parameters such as serum calcium concentration (40), urinary calcium excretion (41), or the severity of hyperparathyroidism, but these observations have not always been reproducible.

The expanding clinical presentation of FHH

The ability to identify FHH by genotype, rather than just by phenotype, has considerably expanded the spectrum of clinical presentations resulting from inactivating mutations of the *CaSR*. About 15–20% of kindreds thought to have familial isolated PHPT have been shown to harbour inactivating mutations of the *CaSR* gene (28). Members of these kindreds present with a clinical picture typical of PHPT, without the characteristic relative or absolute hypocalciuria of FHH. It remains to be determined whether specific functional properties of the *CaSR* mutations in these kindreds can explain their clinical presentation and whether their clinical management should differ from that of typical FHH. The family described earlier with hypercalciuria and kidney stones (27) was shown to have a mutation within the *CaSR* C-tail and represents an example of an FHH kindred with features of familial isolated hyperparathyroidism.

Several cases of FHH have presented with coexistent parathyroid adenomas and more marked hypercalcaemia than is the norm in FHH (42). Removal of the adenoma produced a return of serum calcium concentration to a level more characteristic of FHH. It is not currently known whether the presence of FHH caused a predisposition to the development of an adenoma in these cases or the latter was coincidental. Some infants with heterozygous inactivating mutations of the *CaSR* present with hyperparathyroid bone disease, high PTH levels and moderate hypercalcaemia that is more severe than in typical FHH but less severe than is usually encountered in NSHPT (43). Such cases have been termed neonatal primary hyperparathyroidism (NHPT) and not infrequently revert to a picture compatible with FHH following conservative medical management or occasionally after partial parathyroidectomy (32). The clinical features of NSHPT and NHPT are discussed in more detail below. Finally, cases have been described of individuals homozygous for inactivating mutations of the *CaSR* that were only identified serendipitously in adulthood (44). Despite serum calcium concentrations, presumably lifelong, in the range of 3.75 mmol/l, these individuals were remarkably asymptomatic. They appear to harbour *CaSR* mutations sufficiently mild in their functional impairment to permit the affected individuals to survive undetected throughout childhood. This broader spectrum of clinical manifestations of inactivating *CaSR* mutations makes it important for the clinician to remain vigilant in order to correctly diagnose such patients.

Functional impact of FHH mutations

Transient transfection in human embryonic kidney (HEK293) cells has been utilized to express *CaSRs* harbouring a number of the mutations identified in FHH kindreds (11). These studies have suggested several mechanisms through which these mutations alter not only the function of the mutated receptor but also that of the normal CaSR, which coexists in the cells of persons with FHH since it is a heterozygous condition.

Figure 4.4.3 illustrates the impact of several missense mutations on high Ca^{2+}_{o}-evoked increases in the cytosolic calcium concentration. Mutations within the CaSR ligand-binding ECD probably interfere with its activity via two mechanisms: (1) by reducing the mutant receptors' affinity for calcium (10) and/or (2) by decreasing its cell surface expression. The mutation, p.R185W, for example, markedly reduces both maximal response and apparent affinity of the CaSR (11) without substantially lowering its cell surface expression. However, as discussed in more detail later, this mutation's negative impact extends beyond its effect on the mutant receptor, because it also exerts a dominant negative action on the coexpressed normal receptor (11).

Some mutant CaSRs exhibit almost complete loss of biological activity owing to a markedly reduced level of cell surface expression. For instance, the mutation, p.R66C, creates an unpaired cysteine within the ECD that probably forms mispaired intra- and/or intermolecular disulfide bonds, thereby producing a structurally distorted receptor protein(s) that fails to reach the cell surface (11).

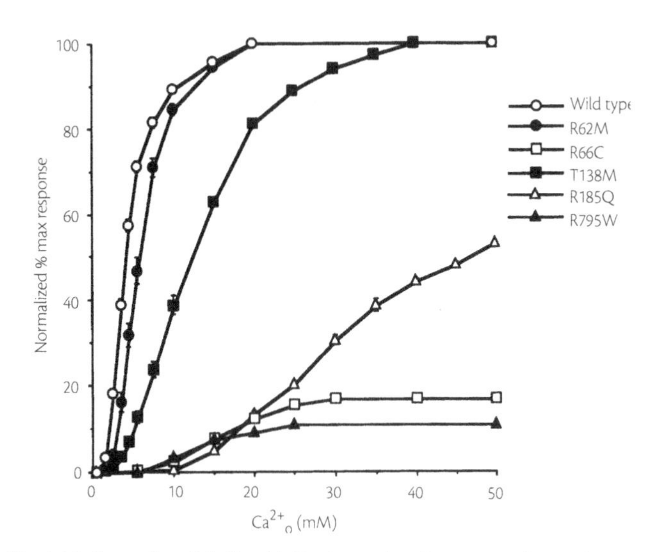

Fig. 4.4.3 Expression of *CaSRs* with FHH mutations in HEK293 cells. Results indicate the effects of varying levels of Ca^{2+}_{o} on the cytosolic calcium concentration normalized to per cent of the normal CaSR maximal response in HEK293 cells transiently transfected with the wild type *CaSR* or the mutant *CaSRs* that are indicated. (From Bai M, Quinn S, Trivedi S, Kifor O, Pearce S, Pollak M, *et al*. Expression and characterization of inactivating and activating mutations of the human Ca^{2+}_{o}-sensing receptor. *J Biol Chem*, 1996; **271**: 19537–45 (11), with permission.)

Mutant CaSRs may also: (1) fail to enter the endoplasmic reticulum from their ribosomal site of synthesis because of missense mutations within the CaSR signal peptide—the latter is needed for translocation of the nascent receptor protein into the endoplasmic reticulum (45); (2) fail to exit the endoplasmic reticulum and are degraded (46); or (3) leave the endoplasmic reticulum but encounter a biosynthetic block at the level of the Golgi apparatus (46). Another class of mutations severely reducing biological activity is nonsense mutation, because the resultant truncated receptor protein lacks structural determinants needed for biological activity.

Mutations within the CaSR transmembrane domains, extracellular loops, intracellular loops, or C-terminal tail probably also impact negatively on the receptors' function through several mechanisms: (1) Mutations producing truncated CaSRs, such as a frame shift mutation at codon 747, produce receptors with gross structural alterations that both abolish biological activity and severely diminish cell surface expression; and (2) missense mutations may interfere with steps involved in receptor signalling, e.g. the mutation, p.R795W, within the CaSR third intracellular loop, probably interferes directly with G protein binding and/or activation (11).

Genotype–phenotype relationships

Of interest, the degree of elevation in serum calcium concentration in families with *CaSR* mutations greatly reducing its cell surface expression (i.e. p.R66C) and/or producing nonfunctional receptors (e.g. p.S607X—where X refers to a stop codon) (43) can be relatively mild (e.g. ≤0.25 mmol/l) above that of unaffected family members. Conversely, mutant receptors exhibiting robust cell surface expression, such as p.R185Q and p.R795W, can cause more severe hypercalcaemia (11). How can these observations be explained? Several developments have provided significant insights into the factors contributing to the severity of hypercalcaemia in FHH. First, the cell surface form of the receptor is known to be a disulfide-linked dimer (29) and, second, the development of mice with targeted disruption (e.g. 'knockout') of one allele of the *CaSR* gene has provided a useful animal model of FHH (47).

In contrast to null mutations, the p.R795W or p.R185Q mutations produce serum calcium concentrations in affected family members that are 0.5 mmol/l and 0.75 mmol/l higher, respectively, than in unaffected family members (11). These mutations exert a so-called dominant negative effect on the wild type receptor when the two *CaSRs* are cotransfected. That is, coexpression of receptors bearing the p.R795W or p.R185Q mutation with the wild type *CaSR* (to mimic the heterozygous state in FHH) causes a rightward shift in the EC_{50} relative to that of the normal receptor (the concentration of agonist evoking half of the maximal response) (Fig. 4.4.4) (11). In contrast, cotransfection of the normal *CaSR* with mutant receptors whose cell surface expression is greatly reduced often has much less or no effect on the normal receptor's function. This dominant negative action results from the formation of heterodimers of the wild type and mutant receptors. Since the CaSR normally functions as a dimer, if these heterodimers are less active than wild type homodimers, then the number of normally functioning CaSRs on the cell surface (e.g. homodimers of the normal receptor) will be less than when the normal CaSR is cotransfected with mutant *CaSRs* functioning as null mutants. In other words, on a purely statistical basis, the proportion of wild type homodimers, heterodimers, and mutant homodimers in the former situation will be 1:2:1 (i.e. 25% wild type homodimers, 50% wild type-mutant heterodimers, and

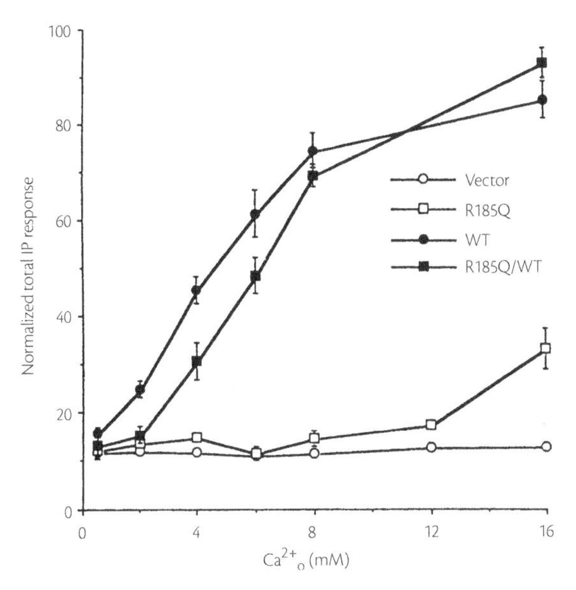

Fig. 4.4.4 Co-expression of a mutant *CaSR* bearing an inactivating *CaSR* mutation (Arg185Gln) and the normal human *CaSR* in HEK293 cells. The results show the high Ca^{2+}_{o}-elicited increases in total cellular inositol phosphates (IP; an index of CaSR-mediated activation of phospholipase C) in HEK293 cells transiently transfected with empty vector (i.e. not containing the cDNA for the *CaSR*), wild type *CaSR*, a mutant *CaSR* bearing the inactivating *CaSR* mutation, Arg185Gln, or both the mutant and wild type *CaSRs*. Note the 'dominant negative' effect of the *CaSR* containing the mutation, Arg185Gln, when cotransfected with the wild type *CaSR*, thereby shifting the EC_{50} of the wild type receptor rightward. (From Bai M, Pearce S, Kifor O, Trivedi S, Stauffer U, Thakker R, *et al.* In vivo and in vitro characterization of neonatal hyperparathyroidism resulting from a de novo, heterozygous mutation in the $Ca2^{+}$-sensing receptor gene—normal maternal calcium homoeostasis as a cause of secondary hyperparathyroidism in familial benign hypocalciuric hypercalcaemia. *J Clin Invest*, 1997; **99**: 88–96 (48).)

25% mutant homodimers), and the 25% wild type homodimers will be the only normally functioning form of the CaSR present on the cell surface. In contrast, with true null mutations, the mutant receptor is not present and will not interfere with the function of the wild type receptor homodimers arising from the remaining normal *CaSR*-encoding allele.

In heterozygous *CaSR* knockout mice, the levels of *CaSR* expression in parathyroid and kidney are about 50% of those in wild type (i.e. normal) mice (47). Thus loss of one *CaSR* allele does not produce any substantial increase in the expression of the remaining normal allele, and the 50% reduction in *CaSR* expression is associated with mild PTH-dependent hypercalcaemia and relative hypocalciuria. The pathophysiology of the heterozygous mice appears to be similar to that in FHH families with 'null' mutations. Presumably in these patients, as in the heterozygous mice, the reduced complement of normal *CaSRs* resulting from loss of one *CaSR* allele causes a mild increase in parathyroid set-point and increased renal tubular reabsorption of calcium with resultant mild hypercalcaemia.

In the family described earlier with a mutation in the *CaSR* C-terminal tail, it is possible that this particular mutation more substantially reduces the mutant receptor's function and/or cell surface expression in parathyroid than in kidney (27). That is, the kidney might respond more normally to Ca^{2+}_{o} than the parathyroid in affected family members, producing PTH-dependent hypercalcaemia in association with hyper- rather than hypocalciuria. Thus, while we remain at a relatively early stage in our ability to predict phenotype from genotype, specific examples now exist of individual mutations that modify the degree of elevation in the serum calcium concentration and/or urinary calcium excretion. It should be pointed out, however, that among the nearly 200 FHH mutations that have been described to date, there is a large degree of overlap in serum and urine parameters, and, in the majority of these mutations, studies of the respective receptors' functional properties *in vitro*, including the use of cotransfection with the mild type receptor, have not yet been performed.

Issues in diagnosis and management of FHH

With the identification of the *CaSR* gene as the disease gene in the most common form of FHH came the ability to perform genetic testing to confirm the diagnosis in probands and other affected family members. When should genetic testing be carried out? As noted above, the constellation of asymptomatic, mild hypercalcaemia with an autosomal dominant pattern of inheritance, a normal serum PTH level, and a urinary calcium to creatinine clearance ratio of 0.01 or less is essentially diagnostic of FHH. No further evaluation is warranted in such cases. There are several instances, however, in which genetic testing is appropriate. These include: (1) apparently sporadic or *de novo* cases of FHH or those who do not have any other family members available for testing, (2) affected members of kindreds with familial isolated hyperparathyroidism, as approximately 15–20% of such kindreds have mutations in the *CaSR*, and (3) as described in more detail in the next section, in children shown to have PTH-dependent hypercalcaemia prior to the age of 10 years.

Experience with a large number of FHH kindreds indicates that conservative medical follow-up, similar to that used to follow patients with asymptomatic PHPT, is an appropriate course of action (1, 3, 13). The rare instances in which parathyroid surgery might be contemplated are: (1) in cases in which hypercalcaemia and the degree of elevation in PTH are unusually severe, particularly if accompanied by hypercalcaemic symptoms and/or complications of hyperparathyroidism (e.g. bone disease, kidney stones), including patients with *CaSR* mutations presenting as FIH; and (2) perhaps in patients with recurrent pancreatitis who have mutations in other genes predisposing to pancreatitis (i.e. the *SPINK1* gene). The calcimimetic, cincalcet, is an allosteric activator of the CaSR, which is approved as a medical therapy for severe hyperparathyroidism in patients receiving dialysis treatment for kidney failure (49) or for parathyroid cancer (in the USA) as well as for PHPT in Europe. It provides a novel medical therapy of potential utility in patients with FHH being considered for parathyroid surgery.

Neonatal severe primary hyperparathyroidism (NSHPT)

Clinical and biochemical features of NSHPT

NSHPT presents at birth or shortly thereafter, often during the first week of life (1, 32, 50), with varying combinations of anorexia, constipation, failure to thrive, hypotonia, and respiratory distress. Respiratory compromise can be due to thoracic deformity, sometimes owing to a flail chest syndrome resulting from multiple fractures of severely demineralized ribs (1, 50). Hypercalcaemia in NSHPT can be severe, on the order of 3.5 to 5 mmol/l, and levels as high as 8 mmol/l have been recorded. Serum magnesium concentrations, when available, have sometimes been well above the normal range (1, 32). Serum PTH is often 5–10-fold elevated, although the increase can be more modest (1, 32, 50). Despite marked hypercalcaemia, affected infants can exhibit relative hypocalciuria. Skeletal radiographs frequently show profound demineralization, fractures of long bones and ribs, metaphyseal widening, subperiosteal erosion, and occasionally rickets (50). Skeletal histology reveals typical osteitis fibrosa cystica of severe hyperparathyroidism. All four parathyroid glands are enlarged and exhibit chief cell or water-clear cell hyperplasia (1, 50).

Before 1982 (1), NSHPT often had a fatal outcome without a prompt and aggressive combination of medical and surgical treatment. More recent series have described infants with neonatal hyperparathyroidism and hyperparathyroid bone disease but less severe hypercalcaemia (2.75–3 mmol/l) (43). Moreover, these cases can run a self-limited course with medical therapy alone, exhibiting healing of bone disease and reversion to a milder form of hypercalcaemia resembling FHH after several months (43). The genetic basis for this less severe form of neonatal hyperparathyroidism (NHPT) is described below. In symptomatic cases of NSHPT, initial management should include vigorous hydration, inhibitors of bone resorption such as the bisphosphonate, pamidronate, and respiratory support. It should be emphasized that each patient must be treated individually, as even several patients homozygous for FHH mutations within the same family may have varying degrees of clinical severity. If the infant's condition is very severe or deteriorates during medical therapy, total parathyroidectomy within the first month of life with autotransplantation of a portion of one gland is usually recommended (1). Some authors recommend total parathyroidectomy followed by management of the resultant hypoparathyroidism using calcium and vitamin D supplementation to prevent symptomatic hypocalcaemia (50). The activity of many mutant *CaSR*s is enhanced by calcimimetics. Accordingly, a potential addition to the other modalities of the therapy for NSHPT is the use of cinacalcet to determine whether it is capable of lowering the serum calcium concentration.

NSHPT caused by homozygous or compound heterozygous *CaSR* mutations

Infants with NSHPT were described in FHH kindreds, suggesting that the former could be the homozygous form of the latter (50). Pollak *et al.* (38) utilized genetic markers to show that NSHPT was the homozygous form of FHH in three families with consanguineous marriages. Since homozygous infants have no normal *CaSR* genes, they manifest much more severe clinical and biochemical manifestations as a result of marked 'resistance' to $Ca^{2+}{}_{o}$ than in FHH. NSHPT can also be caused by compound heterozygous *CaSR* mutations, i.e. the inheritance two different *CaSR* mutations from two unrelated parents (51). Not surprisingly, having no normal *CaSRs*, this infant, similar to those with homozygous FHH, exhibited severe hypercalcaemia (6.6 mmol/l). Mutational analysis of the *CaSR* gene in NSHPT is important to document the presence of *CaSR* mutations. The parents should also be tested and receive appropriate genetic counselling regarding the risk that future offspring will be affected with FHH or NSHPT.

Neonatal hyperparathyroidism caused by heterozygous inactivating *CaSR* mutations

As noted above, a clinical picture has been described in the neonatal period and during early childhood that is intermediate in severity between the usual asymptomatic presentation of FHH and the marked hypercalcaemia, hyperparathyroidism and bone disease of NSHPT. Such infants have proven in some cases to be heterozygous for inactivating *CaSR* mutations. Why do infants with NHPT present with a more severe phenotype than those with typical FHH? A factor potentially contributing to NHPT in a heterozygous child with an affected father and an unaffected mother is the impact of normal maternal calcium homoeostasis on the fetus' abnormal $Ca^{2+}{}_{o}$-sensing *in utero*. Calcium is transported actively across the placenta from mother to fetus, producing a higher fetal than maternal calcium concentration. Therefore, a normal mother would expose her affected fetus' parathyroid glands to a level of $Ca^{2+}{}_{o}$ that would be sensed as 'hypocalcaemic' by the latter. 'Overstimulation' of the fetal parathyroids would then ensue, causing superimposition of secondary fetal/ neonatal hyperparathyroidism on top of the abnormal $Ca^{2+}{}_{o}$-sensing already present. Support for this hypothesis has been provided by the occurrence NSHPT in cases where the father had FHH and the mother appeared normal (1). Postnatally, the 'secondary' hyperparathyroidism would gradually resolve over several months, eventually reverting to typical features of FHH. Most children with FHH born to normal mothers, however, do not manifest more severe hypercalcaemia than those born to affected mothers. Some FHH families may be more susceptible to the development of NHPT in heterozygous infants because their mutant *CaSRs* exert a dominant negative effect (48). A third contributory factor might be the presence of vitamin D deficiency in the mother and/or her infant.

FHH and NSHPT represent a form of generalized $Ca^{2+}{}_{o}$-resistance, analogous to other forms of hormonal resistance

The discovery of the CaSR proved that extracellular calcium ions can act in a hormone-like fashion via their own cell surface, G protein-coupled receptor. In other words, the cells and tissues expressing the *CaSR* can communicate with one another using $Ca^{2+}{}_{o}$ as an extracellular first messenger. A corollary is that FHH and NSHPT are disorders of reduced hormone action, analogous to better recognized hormone resistance syndromes, such as androgen or insulin resistance (52). FHH is a condition in which the target tissues expressing the *CaSR* are mildly to moderately 'resistant' to the actions of $Ca^{2+}{}_{o}$, while the $Ca^{2+}{}_{o}$-resistance in NSHPT is moderate to severe. Both are examples of generalized $Ca^{2+}{}_{o}$-resistance, while PHPT exhibits 'tissue-selective' $Ca^{2+}{}_{o}$-resistance (i.e. only the pathological parathyroid gland(s) show reduced responsiveness to the $Ca^{2+}{}_{o}$). Furthermore, although not discussed here (see Chapter 4.6), activating mutations in the *CaSR* have been identified as a cause of sporadic and, in some cases, an autosomal dominant form of hypocalcaemia associated with relative hypercalciuria (53). In contrast to FHH and NSHPT, these hypocalcaemic syndromes represent generalized 'over responsiveness' or 'oversensitivity' to $Ca^{2+}{}_{o}$. They are analogous to the rapidly expanding group of disorders caused by activating mutations in various other types of receptors (54).

References

1. Heath DA. Familial hypocalciuric hypercalcemia. In: Bilezikian JP, Marcus R, Levine MA, eds. *Familial Hypocalciuric Hypercalcemia.* New York, NY: Raven Press, 1994: 699–710.
2. Egbuna OI, Brown EM. Hypercalcaemic and hypocalcaemic conditions due to calcium-sensing receptor mutations. *Best Pract Res Clin Rheumatol*, 2008; **22**: 129–48.
3. Marx SJ, Attie MF, Levine MA, Spiegel AM, Downs Jr RW, Lasker RD. The hypocalciuric or benign variant of familial hypercalcemia: clinical and biochemical features in fifteen kindreds. *Medicine (Baltimore)*, 1981; **60**: 397–412.
4. Heath HD. Familial benign (hypocalciuric) hypercalcemia. A troublesome mimic of mild primary hyperparathyroidism. *Endocrinol Metab Clin North Am*, 1989; **18**: 723–40.
5. Attie MF, Gill JR Jr, Stock JL, Spiegel AM, Downs RW Jr, Levine MA, *et al.* Urinary calcium excretion in familial hypocalciuric hypercalcemia. Persistence of relative hypocalciuria after induction of hypoparathyroidism. *J Clin Invest*, 1983; **72**: 667–76.
6. Chou YH, Brown EM, Levi T, Crowe G, Atkinson AB, Arnqvist HJ, *et al.* The gene responsible for familial hypocalciuric hypercalcemia maps to chromosome 3q in four unrelated families. *Nat Genet*, 1992; **1**: 295–300.
7. Brown EM, Gamba G, Riccardi D, Lombardi M, Butters R, Kifor O, *et al.* Cloning and characterization of an extracellular Ca(2^+)-sensing receptor from bovine parathyroid. *Nature*, 1993; **366**: 575–80.
8. Pollak MR, Brown EM, Chou YH, Hebert SC, Marx SJ, Steinmann B, *et al.* Mutations in the human Ca(2^+)-sensing receptor gene cause familial hypocalciuric hypercalcemia and neonatal severe hyperparathyroidism. *Cell*, 1993; **75**: 1297–303.
9. Foley Jr T, Harrison H, Arnaud C, Harrison H. Familial benign hypercalcemia. *J Pediatr*, 1972; **81**: 1060–7.
10. Jackson CE, Boonstra CE. Hereditary hypercalcemia and parathyroid hyperplasia without definite hyperparathyroidism. *J Lab Clin Med*, 1966; **68**: 883–90.
11. Bai M, Quinn S, Trivedi S, Kifor O, Pearce SH, Pollak MR, *et al.* Expression and characterization of inactivating and activating mutations in the human $Ca2^+o$-sensing receptor. *J Biol Chem*, 1996; **271**: 19537–45.
12. Bringhurst FR, Demay MB, Kronenberg HM. Hormones and disorders of mineral metabolism. In: Wilson JD, Foster DW, Kronenberg HM, Larsen PR, eds. *Hormones and Disorders of Mineral Metabolism.* 9th edn. Philadelphia: W.B. Saunders, 1998: 1155–209.
13. Law Jr WM, Heath III H. Familial benign hypercalcemia (hypocalciuric hypercalcemia). Clinical and pathogenetic studies in 21 families. *Ann Int Med*, 1985; **105**: 511–19.
14. Felderbauer P, Klein W, Bulut K, Ansorge N, Dekomien G, Werner I, *et al.* Mutations in the calcium-sensing receptor: a new genetic risk factor for chronic pancreatitis?. *Scand J Gastroenterol*, 2006; **41**: 343–8.
15. Christensen SE, Nissen PH, Vestergaard P, Heickendorff L, Rejnmark L, Brixen K, *et al.* Plasma 25-hydroxyvitamin D, 1,25-dihydroxyvitamin D, and parathyroid hormone in familial hypocalciuric hypercalcemia and primary hyperparathyroidism. *Eur J Endocrinol*, 2008; **159**: 719–27.
16. Zajickova K, Vrbikova J, Canaff L, Pawelek PD, Goltzman D, Hendy GN. Identification and functional characterization of a novel mutation in the calcium-sensing receptor gene in familial hypocalciuric hypercalcemia: modulation of clinical severity by vitamin D status. *J Clin Endocrinol Metab*, 2007; **92**: 2616–23.
17. Auwerx J, Demedts M, Bouillon R. Altered parathyroid set point to calcium in familial hypocalciuric hypercalcaemia. *Acta Endocrinologica (Copenh)*, 1984; **106**: 215–18.
18. Law Jr WM, Carney JA, Heath III H. Parathyroid glands in familial benign hypercalcemia (familial hypocalciuric hypercalcemia). *Am J Med*, 1984; **76**: 1021–6.
19. Thogeirsson U, Costa J, Marx SJ. The parathyroid glands in familial hypocalciuric hypercalcemia. *Hum Pathol*, 1981; **12**: 229–37.
20. Norton JA, Venzon DJ, Berna MJ, Alexander HR, Fraker DL,Libuttie SK, *et al.* Prospective study of surgery for primary hyperparathyroidism (HPT) in multiple endocrine neoplasia-type 1 and Zollinger-Ellison syndrome: long-term outcome of a more virulent form of HPT. *Ann Surg*, 2008; **247**: 501–10.
21. Christensen SE, Nissen PH, Vestergaard P, Heickendorff L, Rejnmark L, Brixen K, *et al.* Skeletal consequences of familial hypocalciuric hypercalcaemia versus primary hyperparathyroidism, *Clin Endocrinol (Oxf)*, 2009; Nov 11 [Epub ahead of print].
22. Trump D, Whyte MP, Wooding C, Pang JT, Pearce SH, Kocher DB, *et al.* Linkage studies in a kindred from Oklahoma. with familial benign (hypocalciuric) hypercalcaemia (FBH) and developmental elevations in serum parathyroid hormone levels, indicate a third locus for FBH, *Hum Genet*, 1995; **96**: 183–7.
23. Marx S, Spiegel AM, Brown EM, Koehler JO, Gardner DG, Brennan MF, *et al.* Divalent cation metabolism. Familial hypocalciuric hypercalcemia versus typical primary hyperparathyroidism. *Am J Med*, 1978; **65**: 235–42.
24. Christensen SE, Nissen PH, Vestergaard P, Heickendorff L, Brixen K, Mosekilde L. Discriminative power of three indices of renal calcium excretion for the distinction between familial hypocalciuric hypercalcaemia and primary hyperparathyroidism: a follow-up study on methods. *Clin Endocrinol (Oxf)*, 2008; **69**: 713–20.
25. Gill JJ, Bartter F. On the impairment of renal concentrating ability in prolonged hypercalcemia and hypercalciuria in man. *J Clin Invest*, 1961; **40**: 716–22.
26. Marx SJ, Attie MF, Stock JL, Spiegel AM, Levine MA. Maximal urine-concentrating ability: familial hypocalciuric hypercalcemia versus typical primary hyperparathyroidism. *J Clin Endocrinol Metab*, 1981; **52**: 736–40.
27. Carling T, Szabo E, Bai M, Westin G, Gustavsson P, Trivedi S, *et al.* Autosomal dominant mild hyperparathyroidism. A novel hypercalcemic disorder caused by a mutation in the cytoplasmic tail of the calcium receptor. *J Clin Endocrinol Metab*, in press.
28. Simonds WF, James-Newton LA, Agarwal SK, Yang B, Skarulis MC, Hendy GN, *et al.* Familial isolated hyperparathyroidism: clinical and genetic characteristics of 36 kindreds. *Medicine (Baltimore)*, 2002; **81**: 1–26.
29. Bai M, Trivedi S, Brown EM. Dimerization of the extracellular calcium-sensing receptor (CaR) on the cell surface of CaR-transfected HEK293 cells. *J Biol Chem*, 1998; **273**: 23605–10.
30. Brauner-Osborne H, Jensen AA, Sheppard PO, O'Hara P, Krogsgaard-Larsen P. The agonist-binding domain of the calcium-sensing receptor is located at the amino-terminal domain. *J Biol Chem*, 1999; **274**: 18382–6.
31. Brown EM, MacLeod RJ. Extracellular calcium sensing and extracellular calcium signaling. *Physiol Rev*, 2001; **81**: 239–97.
32. Brown EM. Clinical lessons from the calcium-sensing receptor. *Nat Clin Pract Endocrinol Metab*, 2007; **3**: 122–33.
33. Theman TA, Collins MT. The role of the calcium-sensing receptor in bone biology and pathophysiology. *Curr Pharm Biotechnol*, 2009; **10**: 289–301.
34. Brown EM. Is the calcium receptor a molecular target for the actions of strontium on bone. *Osteoporos Int*, 2003; **14** (Suppl 3): S25–34.
35. Riccardi D, Hall AE, Chattopadhyay N, Xu JZ, Brown EM, Hebert SC. Localization of the extracellular $Ca2^+$/polyvalent cation-sensing protein in rat kidney. *Am J Physiol*, 1998; **274**: F611–622.
36. Hebert SC, Brown EM, Harris HW. Role of the Ca(2^+)-sensing receptor in divalent mineral ion homeostasis. *J Exp Biol*, 1997; **200**: 295–302.
37. Sands JM, Naruse M, Baum M, Jo I, Hebert SC, Brown EM, *et al.* Apical extracellular calcium/polyvalent cation-sensing receptor regulates vasopressin-elicited water permeability in rat kidney inner medullary collecting duct. *J Clin Invest*, 1997; **99**: 1399–405.

38. Pollak MR, Chou YH, Marx SJ, Steinmann B, Cole DE, Brandi ML, *et al.* Familial hypocalciuric hypercalcemia and neonatal severe hyperparathyroidism. Effects of mutant gene dosage on phenotype. *J Clin Invest*, 1994; **93**: 1108–12.
39. Heath HD, Jackson CE, Otterud B, Leppert MF. Genetic linkage analysis in familial benign (hypocalciuric) hypercalcemia: evidence for locus heterogeneity. *Am J Hum Genet*, 1993; **53**: 193–200.
40. Scillitani A, Guarnieri V, De Geronimo S, Muscarella LA, Battista C, D'Agruma L, *et al.* Blood ionized calcium is associated with clustered polymorphisms in the carboxyl-terminal tail of the calcium-sensing receptor. *J Clin Endocrinol Metab*, 2004; **89**: 5634–8.
41. Corbetta S, Eller-Vainicher C, Filopanti M, Saeli P, Vezzoli G, Arcidiacono T, *et al.* R990G polymorphism of the calcium-sensing receptor and renal calcium excretion in patients with primary hyperparathyroidism. *Eur J Endocrinol*, 2006; **155**: 687–92.
42. Brachet C, Boros E, Tenoutasse S, Lissens W, Andry G, Martin P, *et al.* Association of parathyroid adenoma and familial hypocalciuric hypercalcaemia in a teenager. *Eur J Endocrinol*, 2009; **161**: 207–10.
43. Pearce SH, Trump D, Wooding C, Besser GM, Chew SL, Grant DB, *et al.* Calcium-sensing receptor mutations in familial benign hypercalcemia and neonatal hyperparathyroidism. *J Clin Invest*, 1995; **96**: 2683–92.
44. Chikatsu N, Fukumoto S, Suzawa M, Tanaka Y, Takeuchi Y, Takeda S, *et al.* An adult patient with severe hypercalcaemia and hypocalciuria due to a novel homozygous inactivating mutation of calcium-sensing receptor. *Clin Endocrinol (Oxf)*, 1999; **50**: 537–43.
45. Pidasheva S, Canaff L, Simonds WF, Marx SJ, Hendy GN. Impaired cotranslational processing of the calcium-sensing receptor due to signal peptide missense mutations in familial hypocalciuric hypercalcemia. *Hum Mol Genet*, 2005; **14**: 1679–90.
46. White E, McKenna J, Cavanaugh A, Breitwieser GE. Pharmacochaperone-mediated rescue of calcium-sensing receptor loss-of-function mutants. *Mol Endocrinol*, 2009; **23**: 1115–23.
47. Ho C, Conner DA, Pollak MR, Ladd DJ, Kifor O, Warren HB, *et al.* A mouse model of human familial hypocalciuric hypercalcemia and neonatal severe hyperparathyroidism (see comments). *Nat Genet*, 1995; **11**: 389–94.
48. Bai M, Pearce SH, Kifor O, Trivedi S, Stauffer UG, Thakker RV, *et al.* In vivo and in vitro characterization of neonatal hyperparathyroidism resulting from a de novo. heterozygous mutation in the $Ca2^{+}$-sensing receptor gene: normal maternal calcium homeostasis as a cause of secondary hyperparathyroidism in familial benign hypocalciuric hypercalcemia, *J Clin Invest*, 1997; **99**: 88–96.
49. Block GA, Martin KJ, de Francisco AL, Turner SA, Avram MM, Suranyi MG, *et al.* Cinacalcet for secondary hyperparathyroidism in patients receiving hemodialysis. *N Engl J Med*, 2004; **350**: 1516–25.
50. Marx SJ, Fraser D, Rapoport A. Familial hypocalciuric hypercalcemia. Mild expression of the gene in heterozygotes and severe expression in homozygotes. *Am J Med*, 1985; **78**: 15–22.
51. Kobayashi M, Tanaka H, Tsuzuki K, Tsuyuki M, Igaki H, Ichinose Y, *et al.* Two novel missense mutations in calcium-sensing receptor gene associated with neonatal severe hyperparathyroidism. *J Clin Endocrinol Metab*, 1997; **82**: 2716–19.
52. Jameson L, ed *Hormone Resistance Syndromes*. Towata, NJ; Humana Press, 1999.
53. Pollak MR, Brown EM, Estep HL, McLaine PN, Kifor O, Park J, *et al.* Autosomal dominant hypocalcaemia caused by a $Ca(2^{+})$-sensing receptor gene mutation. *Nat Genet*, 1994; **8**: 303–7.
54. Spiegel AM. Mutations in G protein and G protein-coupled receptors in endocrine disease. *J. Clin Endocrinol Metab*, 1996; **81**: 2434–42.

4.5

Hypocalcaemic disorders, hypoparathyroidism, and pseudohypoparathyroidism

Rajesh V. Thakker

Introduction

Extracellular calcium ion concentration is tightly regulated through the actions of parathyroid hormone (PTH) on kidney and bone (Fig. 4.5.1). The intact peptide is secreted by the parathyroid glands at a rate that is appropriate to and dependent upon the prevailing extracellular calcium ion concentration. The causes of hypocalcaemia (Box 4.5.1) can be classified according to whether serum PTH concentrations are low (that is hypoparathyroid disorders) or high (that is disorders associated with secondary hyperparathyroidism) (1–6). The most common causes of hypocalcaemia are hypoparathyroidism, a deficiency or abnormal metabolism of vitamin D, acute or chronic renal failure, and hypomagnesaemia. This chapter will initially review the clinical features and management of hypocalcaemia, and then discuss the specific hypocalcaemic disorders.

Hypocalcaemia

Clinical features and investigations

The clinical presentation of hypocalcaemia ranges from an asymptomatic biochemical abnormality to a severe, life-threatening condition. Normal total serum calcium is 2.15–2.65 mmol/l and in mild hypocalcaemia (serum calcium 2.00–2.15 mmol/l) patients may be asymptomatic. Those with more severe (serum calcium less than 1.9 mmol/l) and long-term hypocalcaemia may develop: acute symptoms of neuromuscular irritability (Box 4.5.2); ectopic calcification (e.g. in the basal ganglia, which may be associated with extrapyramidal neurological symptoms); subcapsular cataract; papilloedema; and abnormal dentition. Investigations should be directed at confirming the presence of hypocalcaemia and establishing the cause, e.g. in hypoparathyroidism, serum calcium is low, phosphate is high, and PTH is undetectable; renal function and concentrations of the 25-hydroxy and 1,25-dihydroxy metabolites of vitamin D are normal (2, 3, 5). The features of *pseudohypoparathyroidism* (PHP) are similar to those of hypoparathyroidism except for PTH, which is markedly increased (3, 5). In *chronic renal failure*, which is the commonest cause of hypocalcaemia, serum phosphate is high and alkaline phosphatase activity, creatinine, and PTH are elevated; 25-hydroxyvitamin D3 is normal and 1,25-dihydroxyvitamin D3 is low. In *vitamin D deficiency osteomalacia*, serum calcium and phosphate are low, alkaline phosphatase activity and PTH are elevated, renal function is normal, and 25-hydroxyvitamin D3 is low. The commonest artefactual cause of hypocalcaemia is hypoalbuminaemia, such as occurs in liver disease or the nephrotic syndrome.

Management of acute hypocalcaemia

The management of acute hypocalcaemia depends on the severity of the hypocalcaemia, the rapidity with which it developed, and the degree of neuromuscular irritability (Box 4.5.2). Treatment should be given to: symptomatic patients (for example, with tetany); and asymptomatic patients with a serum calcium of less than 1.90 mmol/l who may be at high risk of developing complications. The preferred treatment for acute symptomatic hypocalcaemia is calcium gluconate, 10 ml 10% w/v (2.20 mmol of calcium) intravenous, diluted in 50 ml of 5% dextrose or 0.9% sodium chloride and given by slow injection (more than 5 min); this can be repeated as required to control symptoms. Serum calcium should be assessed regularly (4, 5). Continuing hypocalcaemia may be managed acutely by administration of a calcium gluconate infusion; for example, dilute 10 ampoules of calcium gluconate, 10 ml 10% w/v (22.0 mmol of calcium), in 1 litre of 5% dextrose or 0.9% sodium chloride, start infusion at 50 ml/h and titrate to maintain serum calcium in the low normal range. Generally, 0.30–0.40 mmol/kg of elemental calcium infused over 4–6 h increases serum calcium by 0.5–0.75 mmol/l. If hypocalcaemia is likely to persist, oral vitamin D therapy should also be commenced. It is important to note that, in hypocalcaemic patients who are also hypomagnesaemic, the hypomagnesaemia must be corrected before the hypocalcaemia will resolve. This may occur in the postparathyroidectomy period or in those with severe intestinal malabsorption, e.g. as in coeliac disease.

Management of persistent hypocalcaemia

The two major groups of drugs available for the treatment of hypocalcaemia are supplemental calcium, about 10–20 mmol calcium 6–12 hourly, and vitamin D preparations (5). Patients with

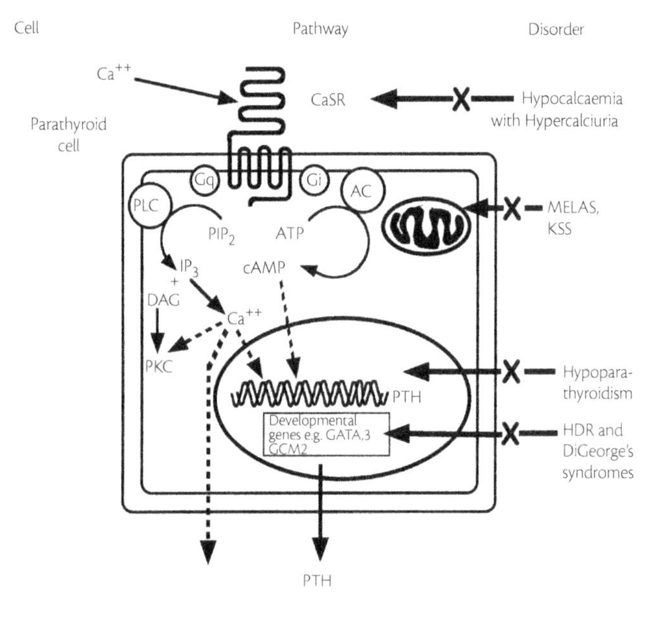

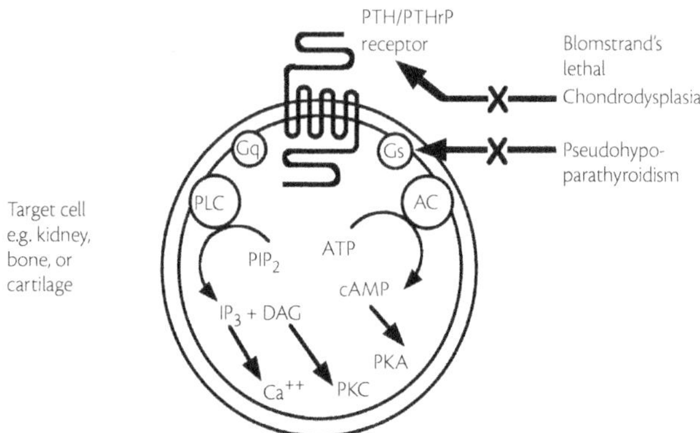

Fig. 4.5.1 Schematic representation of some of the components involved in calcium homoeostasis. Alterations in extracellular calcium are detected by the calcium-sensing receptor (CaSR), which is a 1078 amino acid G-protein coupled receptor. The PTH/PTHrP-receptor is also a G-protein coupled receptor. Thus, Ca^2+, parathyroid hormone (PTH), and parathyroid hormone-related protein (PTHrP) involve G-protein coupled signalling pathways, and interaction with their specific receptors can lead to activation of Gs, Gi and Gq. Gs stimulates adenylate cyclase (AC), which catalyses the formation of cAMP from ATP. Gi inhibits AC activity. cAMP stimulates protein kinase A (PKA), which phosphorylates cell-specific substrates. Activation of Gq stimulates PLC, which catalyses the hydrolysis of phosphoinositide (PIP_2) to inositol triphosphate (IP_3), which increases intracellular calcium, and diacylglycerol (DAG), which activates protein kinase C (PKC). These proximal signals modulate downstream pathways, which result in specific physiological effects. Abnormalities in several genes and encoded proteins in these pathways have been identified in patients with hypoparathyroid disorders (Table 4.5.1). KSS, Kearns–Sayre syndrome; MELAS, mitochondrial encephalopathy, lactic acidosis, and stroke-like episodes. (Adapted from Thakker RV. Parathyroid disorders: molecular genetics and physiology. In: Morris PJ, Wood WC, eds. *Oxford Textbook of Surgery*. Oxford University Press, 2000: 1121–9 (1).)

hypoparathyroidism seldom require calcium supplements after the early stages of stabilization on vitamin D. A variety of vitamin D preparations have been used (Table 4.5.1). These include: vitamin D_3 (cholecalciferol) or vitamin D_2 (ergocalciferol), 25 000–100 000 units (1.25–5 mg/day); dihydrotachysterol (now seldom used), 0.25–1.25 mg/day; alfacalcidol (1α-hydroxycholecalciferol), 0.25–1.0 µg/day; and calcitriol (1,25-dihydroxycholecalciferol), 0.25–2.0 µg/day. In children, these preparations are prescribed in

Box 4.5.1 Causes of hypocalcaemia

- Low serum parathyroid hormone levels (hypoparathyroidism)
  - Parathyroid agensis
    - Isolated or part of complex developmental anomaly (e.g. DiGeorge's syndrome)
  - Parathyroid destruction
    - Surgery[a]
    - Radiation
    - Infiltration by metastases or systemic disease(e.g. haemochromatosis, amyloidosis, sarcoidosis, Wilson's disease, thalassaemia)
  - Autoimmune
    - Isolated
    - Polyglandular (type 1)[a]
  - Reduced parathyroid function (i.e. parathyroid hormone secretion)
    - Parathyroid hormone gene defects
    - Hypomagnesaemia[a]
    - Neonatal hypocalcaemia (may be associated with maternal hypercalcaemia)
    - Hungry bone disease (postparathyroidectomy)
    - Calcium-sensing receptor mutations
- High serum parathyroid hormone levels (secondary hyper-parathyroidism)
  - Vitamin D deficiency[a]
    - As a result of nutritional lack,[a] malabsorption,[a] liver disease, or acute or chronic renal failure[a]
  - Vitamin D resistance (rickets)
    - As a result of renal tubular dysfunction (Fanconi's syndrome), or vitamin D receptor defects
  - Parathyroid hormone resistance (e.g. pseudohypoparathyroidism, hypomagnesaemia)
  - Drugs
    - Calcium chelators (e.g. cirated blood transfusions, phosphate)
    - Inhibitors of bone resorption (e.g. bisphosphonate, calcitonin, plicamycin)
    - Altered vitamin D metabolism (e.g. phenytoin, ketaconazole)
  - Miscellaneous
    - Acute pancreatitis
    - Acute rhabdomyolysis
    - Massive tumour lysis
  - Osteoblastic metastases (e.g. from prostate or breast carcinoma)
  - Toxic shock syndrome
  - Hyperventilation

[a] Most common causes.

Box 4.5.2 Hypocalcaemic clinical features of neuromuscular irritability

- Paraesthesia, usually of fingers, toes and circumoral regions
- Tetany, carpopedal spasm, muscle cramps
- Chvostek's sign[a]
- Trousseau's sign[b]
- Seizures of all types (that is, focal or petit mal, grand mal or syncope)
- Prolonged QT interval on ECG
- Laryngospasm
- Bronchospasm

[a] Chvostek's sign is twitching of the circumoral muscles in response to gentle tapping of the facial nerve just anterior to the ear; it may be present in 10 per cent of normal individuals.

[b] Trousseau's sign is carpal spasm elicited by inflation of a blood pressure cuff to 20 mm Hg above the patient's systolic blood pressure for 3 min.

doses based on body weight. Cholecalciferol and ergocalciferol are the least expensive preparations, but have the longest durations of action and may result in prolonged toxicity. The other preparations, which do not require renal 1α-hydroxylation, have the advantage of shorter half-lives and thereby minimize the risk of prolonged toxicity. Calcitriol is probably the drug of choice because it is the active metabolite and, unlike alfacalcidol, does not require hepatic 25-hydroxylation. Close monitoring (at about 1–2 week intervals) of the patient's serum and urine calcium are required initially, and at 3–6 monthly intervals once stabilization is achieved. The aim is to avoid hypercalcaemia, hypercalciuria, nephrolithiasis, and renal failure. It should be noted that hypercalciuria may occur in the absence of hypercalcaemia.

Hypocalcaemic disorders

The application of the recent developments in molecular biology to the study of hypocalcaemic disorders (Table 4.5.2) has enabled the characterization of some of the mechanisms involved in the regulation of parathyroid gland development, of PTH secretion, and of PTH-mediated actions in target tissues (6). Thus, mutations in the *TBX1* gene have been identified in patients with the DiGeorge's syndrome and mutations in the *CaSR* gene have been reported in patients with autosomal dominant hypocalcaemia with hypercalciuria. In addition, mutations in the *PTH* gene, the transcriptional factor *GATA3*, and the mitochondrial genome have been demonstrated to be associated with some forms of hypoparathyroidism; defects in the *PTH/PTHrP* receptor gene have been identified in patients with Blomstrand's chondrodysplasia; and inactivating mutations in the stimulatory G protein have been found in individuals with PHP type Ia, PHP type Ib, and pseudopseudohypoparathyroidism (PPHP). Furthermore, the gene causing the polyglandular autoimmune syndrome (*APECED*) has been characterized. These molecular genetic studies have provided unique opportunities to elucidate the pathogenesis of some hypocalcaemic disorders such that these may be classified according to whether they arise from a deficiency of PTH, a defect in the PTH-receptor (that is the parathyroid hormone/ parathyroid hormone-related protein (PTH/PTHrP) receptor), or an insensitivity to PTH caused by defects down-stream of the PTH/PTHrP receptor (Fig. 4.5.1). These advances together with the clinical features of these disorders will be reviewed in this chapter.

Hypoparathyroidism

Hypoparathyroidism is characterized by hypocalcaemia and hyperphosphataemia, which are the result of a deficiency in PTH secretion or action (Table 4.5.3) (2, 5). Hypoparathyroidism may result from agenesis (e.g. the DiGeorge syndrome) or destruction of the parathyroid glands (e.g. following neck surgery, in autoimmune diseases), from reduced secretion of PTH (e.g. neonatal hypocalcaemia or hypomagnesaemia), or resistance to PTH (which may occur as a primary disorder (e.g. pseudohypoparathyroidism) or secondary to hypomagnesaemia). In addition, hypoparathyroidism may occur as an inherited disorder (Table 4.5.2) which may either be part of a complex congenital defect (e.g. the DiGeorge syndrome), or as part of a pluriglandular autoimmune disorder, or as a solitary endocrinopathy, which has been referred to as *isolated or idiopathic* hypoparathyroidism.

Isolated hypoparathyroidism

Isolated hypoparathyroidism may either be *inherited* as an autosomal or X-linked disorder (7–11), or it may be *acquired* by damage to the parathyroids at surgery, or by infiltrating metastases, or systemic disease (Box 4.5.1).

Table 4.5.1 Pharmaceutical preparations of vitamin D and active metabolites

	Drug				
	Calciferol[a]	**Dihydrotachysterol**	**Calcifediol**	**Calcitriol**	**Alfacalcidiol**
	Vitamin D_3 or D_2	DHT	25(OH) D_3	1,25$(OH)_2D_3$	1α$(OH)D_3$
Preparation	Capsules, 0.25 mg and 1.25 mg	Liquid, 0.25 mg/ml	Capsules, 20 and 50 μg	Capsules, 0.25 and 0.5 μg	Capsules, 0.25, 0.50 and 1 μg
				Injection, 1 μg/ml	Liquid, 2 μg/ml Injection, 2 μg/ml in propylene glycol
Time to maximum effect	4–10 weeks	2–4 weeks	4–20 weeks	0.5–1 week	0.5–1 week
Persistence of effect after cessation	6–30 weeks	2–8 weeks	4–12 weeks	0.5–1 week	0.5–1 week

[a] Calciferol may contain cholecalciferol or ergocalciferol.

Table 4.5.2 Inherited forms of hypoparathyroidism and their chromosomal locations

Disease	Inheritance	Gene product	Chromosomal location
Isolated hypoparathyroidism	Autosomal dominant	PTH[a]	11p15
	Autosomal recessive	PTH[a], GCMB	11p15, 6p24.2
	X-linked recessive	SOX3	Xq27
Hypocalcaemic hypercalciuria	Autosomal dominant	CaSR	3q21.1
Hypoparathyroidism associated with complex congenital syndromes			
DiGeorge type 1 (DGS 1)	Autosomal dominant	TBX1	22q11.2
DiGeorge type 2 (DGS 2)	Autosomal dominant		10p13–14
HDR	Autosomal dominant	GATA3	10p15
Hypoparathyroidism associated with Kearns–Sayre and MELAS	Maternal	Mitochondrial genome	
Blomstrand lethal chondrodysplasia	Autosomal recessive	PTH/PTHrPR	3p21.3
Kenney–Caffey, Sanjad–Sakati	Autosomal dominant[b]	TBCE	1q42.3
Barakat	Autosomal recessive[b]	Unknown	?
Lymphoedema	Autosomal recessive	Unknown	?
Nephropathy, nerve deafness	Autosomal dominant[b]	Unknown	?
Nerve deafness without renal dysplasia	Autosomal dominant	Unknown	?
Hypoparathyroidism associated with APECED	Autosomal recessive	AIRE	21q22.3
PHP Ia	Autosomal dominant parentally imprinted	GNAS1	20q13.3
PHP Ib	Autosomal dominant parentally imprinted	GNAS1	20q13.3

[a] Mutations of PTH gene identified only in some families.
[b] Most likely inheritance shown.
APECED, polyglandular autoimmune syndrome; HDR, hypoparathyroidism, deafness, and renal anomalies; MELAS, mitochondrial encephalopathy, stroke-like episodes and lactic acidosis; PHP, pseudohypoparathyroidism;?, location not known.

Autosomal hypoparathyroidism

Patients with autosomal forms of hypoparathyroidism may develop hypocalcaemic seizures in the neonatal or infantile periods and require lifelong treatment with oral vitamin D preparations, e.g. calcitriol. These patients have been investigated for mutations in the *PTH* gene, which consists of three exons and is located on chromosome 11p15 (2, 6, 7). Exon 1 of the *PTH* gene is untranslated, whereas exons 2 and 3 encode the 115-amino acid pre-pro-PTH peptide. Exon 2 encodes the initiation (ATG) codon, the prehormone sequence, and part of the prohormone sequence, whilst exon 3 encodes the remainder of the prohormone sequence, the mature 84-amino acid PTH peptide, and the 3′ untranslated region. DNA sequence analysis of the *PTH* gene from one patient with *autosomal dominant isolated hypoparathyroidism* has revealed a single base substitution (T→C) in exon 2 (11), which resulted in the substitution of arginine (CGT) for cysteine (TGT) in the signal peptide. The presence of this charged amino acid in the midst of the hydrophobic core of the signal peptide was shown, by *in vitro* studies, to impede the processing of the mutant preproPTH. This revealed that the mutation impaired the interaction between the nascent protein and the translocation machinery and cleavage of the mutant signal sequence by solubilized signal peptidase was ineffective (11, 12). In another family with *autosomal recessive hypoparathyroidism* a single base substitution (T→C) involving codon 23 of exon 2 was detected. This resulted in the substitution of proline (CCG) for the normal serine (TCG) in the signal peptide (13). This mutation alters the −3 position of the pre-pro-PTH protein cleavage site. Indeed, amino acid residues at the −3 and −1 positions of the signal peptidase recognition site have to conform to certain criteria for correct processing through the rough endoplasmic reticulum, and one of these is an absence of proline in the region −3 and +1 of the site. Thus, the presence of a proline, which is a strong helix-breaking residue, at the −3 position is likely to disrupt cleavage of the mutant pre-pro-PTH, which would be subsequently degraded in the rough endoplasmic reticulum, and PTH would not be available (13). Another abnormality of the *PTH* gene, involving a donor splice site at the exon 2–intron 2 boundary, has been identified in one family with autosomal recessive isolated hypoparathyroidism (14). This mutation involved a single base transition (G→C) at position 1 of intron 2 and an assessment of the effects of this alteration in the invariant GT dinucleotide of the 5′ donor splice site consensus on mRNA processing revealed that the mutation resulted in exon skipping, in which exon 2 of the *PTH* gene was lost and exon 1 was spliced to exon 3. The lack of exon 2 would lead to a loss of the initiation codon (ATG) and the signal peptide sequence, which are required, respectively, for the commencement of PTH mRNA translation and for the translocation of the PTH peptide.

Mutations of the *PTH* gene have been detected in only a minority of autosomal forms of hypoparathyroidism (9–14) and this indicates that other genes are likely to be involved (Table 4.5.2). Two of these are the *CASR* gene (see below), and the *GCM2* (*glial cells missing 2*) (8, 15–17). *GCMB* (glial cells missing B), which is the human homologue of the *Drosophila* gene *Gcm* and of the mouse *Gcm2* gene, is expressed exclusively in the parathyroid glands, suggesting that it may be a specific regulator of parathyroid gland development (18). Mice that were homozygous (−/−) for deletion of *Gcm2* lacked parathyroid glands and developed the hypocalcaemia and hyperphosphataemia as observed in hypoparathyroidism (18). However, despite their lack of parathyroid glands, Gcm2 deficient (−/−) mice did not have undetectable serum PTH levels, but instead had levels indistinguishable from those of normal (+/+, wild type) and heterozygous (+/−) mice. This endogenous level of PTH in the Gcm2 deficient (−/−) mice was too low to correct the hypocalcaemia, but exogenous continuous PTH infusion could correct the hypocalcaemia (18). Interestingly, there were no compensatory increases in PTHrP or $1,25(OH)_2$ vitamin D_3. These findings indicate that Gcm2 mice have a normal response (and not resistance) to PTH, and that the PTH in the serum of Gcm2-deficient mice was active. The auxiliary source of PTH was identified to be a cluster of PTH-expressing cells under the thymic capsule. These thymic PTH-producing cells also expressed the *CaSR*, and long-term treatment of the Gcm2-deficient mice with $1,25(OH)_2$ vitamin D_3 restored the serum calcium concentrations to normal and reduced the serum PTH levels, thereby indicating that the thymic production of PTH can be downregulated (18). However, it appears that this thymic production of PTH cannot be upregulated as serum PTH levels are not high despite the hypocalcaemia in the Gcm2-deficient mice. This absence of up-regulation would be consistent with the very small size of the thymic PTH-producing cell cluster when compared to the size of normal parathyroid glands.

Studies of patients with isolated hypoparathyroidism have shown that *GCMB* mutations are associated with autosomal recessive and dominant forms of hypoparathyroidism (15–17). Thus, a homozygous intragenic deletion of *GCMB* has been identified in a patient with autosomal recessive hypoparathyroidism (16), whilst in another family a homozygous missense mutation (Arg47Leu) of the DNA binding domain has been reported (15). Functional analysis, using electrophoretic mobility shift assays, of this Arg47Leu GCMB mutation revealed that is resulted in a loss of DNA binding to the GCM DNA binding site (15). More recently, heterozygous *GCMB* mutations, which consist of single nucleotide deletions (c1389deT and c1399delC) that introduce frame shifts and premature truncations, have been identified in two unrelated families with autosomal dominant hypoparathyroidism (17). Both of these mutations were shown, by using a GCMB-associated luciferase reporter, to inhibit the action of the wild-type transcription factor, thereby indicating that these GCMB mutants have dominant-negative properties (17).

X-linked recessive hypoparathyroidism

X-linked recessive hypoparathyroidism has been reported in two multigenerational kindreds from Missouri, USA (19). In this disorder only males are affected and they suffer from infantile onset of epilepsy and hypocalcaemia, which is due to an isolated defect in parathyroid gland development (20). Relatedness of the two kindreds has been established by demonstrating an identical mitochondrial DNA sequence, which is inherited via the maternal lineage, in affected males from the two families (21). Studies utilizing X-linked polymorphic markers in these families localized the mutant gene to chromosome Xq26-q27 (22), and a molecular deletion–insertion that involves chromosome 2p25 and Xq27 has been identified (23). This deletion–insertion is located approximately 67 kb downstream of *SOX3*, and hence it is likely to exert a position effect on *SOX3* expression. Moreover, *SOX3* was shown to be expressed in the developing parathyroids of mouse embryos, and this indicates a likely role for *SOX3* in the embryonic development of the parathyroid glands (23). *SOX3* belongs to a family of genes encoding high-mobility group box transcription factors and is related to *SRY*, the sex determining gene on the Y chromosome. The mouse homologue is expressed in the prestreak embryo and subsequently in the developing central nervous system, that includes the region of the ventral diencephalon which induces development of the anterior pituitary and gives rise to the hypothalamus, olfactory placodes, and parathyroids (23). The location of the deletion–insertion ~67 kb downstream of *SOX3* in X-linked recessive hypoparathyroid patients is likely to result in altered *SOX3* expression, as *SOX3* expression has been reported to be sensitive to position-effects caused by X-chromosome abnormalities (24). Indeed, reporter-construct studies of the mouse *Sox3* gene have demonstrated the presence of both 5′ and 3′ regulatory elements (25), and thus it is possible that the deletion–insertion in the X-linked recessive hypoparathyroid patients may have a position effect on *SOX3* expression, and parathyroid development from the pharyngeal pouches. Indeed such position effects on *SOX* genes, which may be exerted over large distances, have been reported; e.g. the very closely related *SOX2* gene has been shown to have regulatory regions spread over a long distance, both 5′ and 3′ to the coding region and disruption of sequences at some distance 3′ have been reported to lead to loss of expression in the developing inner ear, and absence of sensory cells, whereas expression in other sites is unaffected (26). Similarly for the *SRY* gene, which probably originated from *SOX3*, both 5′ and 3′ deletions result in abnormalities of sexual development, and translocation breakpoints over 1 Mb upstream of the *SOX9* gene have been reported to result in campomelic dysplasia due to removal of elements that regulate *SOX9* expression (24). The molecular deletion–insertion identified in X-linked recessive hypoparathyroidism may similarly cause position effects on *SOX3* expression, and this points to a potential role for the *SOX3* gene in the embryological development of the parathyroid glands from the pharyngeal pouches.

Acquired forms of hypoparathyroidism

Hypoparathyroidism may occur after neck *surgery*, *irradiation*, or because of *infiltration by metastases or systemic disease*, e.g. haemochromatosis, amyloidosis, sarcoidosis, Wilson's disease, or thalassaemia (2, 4, 5) (Box 4.5.1). Surgical damage to the parathyroids occurs most commonly after a radical neck dissection, e.g. for laryngeal or oesophageal carcinoma, or a total thyroid resection, or after repeated parathyroidectomies for multigland disease, e.g. in multiple endocrine neoplasia type 1 or type 2. Hypocalcaemic symptoms begin 12–24 h postoperatively and may need treatment with oral or intravenous calcium. Parathyroid function often returns, but persistent hypocalcaemia requires treatment with vitamin D preparations (2, 4, 5).

Neonatal hypoparathyroidism resulting in hypocalcaemia may occur in the baby of a mother with hypercalcaemia caused by primary hyperparathyroidism (2, 4, 5). Maternal hypercalcaemia results in increased calcium delivery to the fetus, and this fetal hypercalcaemia suppresses fetal PTH secretion. Postpartum, the infant's suppressed parathyroids are unable to maintain normocalcaemia. The disorder is usually self-limiting, but occasionally therapy may be required.

Hypoparathyroidism may occur secondary to *severe hypomagnesaemia* (less than 0.40 mmol/l), which may be due to a severe intestinal malabsorption disorder (e.g. Crohn's disease) or a renal tubular disorder (2, 4, 5). It is associated with hypoparathyroidism because magnesium is required for the release of PTH from the parathyroid gland and also for PTH action via adenyl cyclase. Magnesium chloride, 35–50 mmol intravenous in 1 l of 5% glucose or other isotonic solution given over 12–24 h may be repeatedly required to restore normomagnesaemia.

Complex syndromes associated with hypoparathyroidism

Hypoparathyroidism may occur as part of a complex syndrome which may either be associated with a congenital development anomaly or with an autoimmune syndrome (2). The congenital developmental anomalies associated with hypoparathyroidism include the DiGeorge, the hypoparathyroidism, deafness, and renal anomalies (HDR), the Kenney–Caffey and the Barakat syndromes, and also syndromes associated with either lymphoedema or dysmorphic features and growth failure (Table 4.5.2).

DiGeorge syndrome

Patients with the DiGeorge syndrome (DGS) typically suffer from hypoparathyroidism, immunodeficiency, congenital heart defects, and deformities of the ear, nose, and mouth (2). The disorder arises from a congenital failure in the development of the derivatives of the third and fourth pharyngeal pouches with resulting absence or hypoplasia of the parathyroids and thymus. Most cases of DGS are sporadic but an autosomal dominant inheritance of DGS has been observed and an association between the syndrome and an unbalanced translocation and deletions involving 22q11.2 have also been reported (27), and this is referred to as DGS type 1 (DGS 1). In some patients, deletions of another locus on chromosome 10p have been observed in association with DGS (28) and this is referred to as DGS type 2 (DGS 2). Mapping studies of the *DGS1* deleted region on chromosome 22q11.2 have defined a 250 kb to 3000 kb critical region (29), which contained approximately 30 genes. Studies of DGS 1 patients have reported deletions of several of the genes (e.g. *RNEX40, NEX2.2–NEX3, UDFIL*, and *TBX1*) from the critical region and studies of transgenic mice deleted for such genes (e.g. *Udf1l, Hira*, and *Tbx1*) have revealed developmental abnormalities of the pharyngeal arches (29, 30). However, point mutations in DGS 1 patients have only been detected in the *TBX1* gene (31), and *TBX1* is now considered to be the gene causing DGS 1 (32). *TBX1* is a DNA binding transcriptional factor, of the T-box family, which is known to have an important role in vertebrate and invertebrate organogenesis and pattern formation. The *TBX1* gene is deleted in approximately 96% of all DGS 1 patients. Moreover, DNA sequence analysis of unrelated DGS 1 patients who did not have deletions of chromosome 22q11.2, revealed the occurrence of three heterozygous point mutations (31). One of these mutations resulted in a frameshift with a premature truncation, whilst the other two were missense mutations (Phe148Tyr and Gly310Ser). All of these patients had the complete pharyngeal phenotype but did not have mental retardation or learning difficulties. Interestingly, transgenic mice with deletion of *Tbx1* have a phenotype that is similar to that of DGS 1 patients (30). Thus, *Tbx1* null mutant mice (−/−) had all the developmental anomalies of DGS 1 (i.e. thymic and parathyroid hypoplasia, abnormal facial structures and cleft palate, skeletal defects, and cardiac outflow tract abnormalities), whilst *Tbx1* haploinsufficiency in mutant mice (+/−) was associated only with defects of the fourth branchial pouch (i.e. cardiac outflow tract abnormalities). The basis of the phenotypic differences between DGS 1 patients, who are heterozygous, and the transgenic +/− mice remain to be elucidated. It is plausible that *Tbx1* dosage, together with the downstream genes that are regulated by *Tbx1* could provide an explanation, but the roles of these putative genes in DGS 1 remains to be elucidated.

Some patients may have a late-onset DGS 1 and these develop symptomatic hypocalcaemia in childhood or during adolescence with only subtle phenotypic abnormalities (33). These late-onset DGS 1 patients have similar microdeletions in the 22q11 region. It is of interest to note that the age of diagnosis in the families of the three DGS 1 patients with inactivating *TBX1* mutations ranged from 7 to 46 years, which is in keeping with late-onset DGS 1 (31).

Hypoparathyroidism, deafness, and renal anomalies syndrome

The combined inheritance of hypoparathyroidism, deafness, and renal dysplasia (HDR) as an autosomal dominant trait was reported in one family in 1992 (34). Patients had asymptomatic hypocalcaemia with undetectable or inappropriately normal serum concentrations of PTH, and normal brisk increases in plasma cAMP in response to the infusion of PTH. The patients also had bilateral, symmetrical, sensorineural deafness involving all frequencies. The renal abnormalities consisted mainly of bilateral cysts which compressed the glomeruli and tubules, and lead to renal impairment in some patients. Cytogenetic abnormalities were not detected and abnormalities of the *PTH* gene were excluded (34). However, cytogenetic abnormalities involving chromosome 10p14–10pter were identified in two unrelated patients with features that were consistent with HDR. These two patients suffered from hypoparathyroidism, deafness, and growth and mental retardation; one patient also had a solitary dysplastic kidney with vesicoureteric reflux and a uterus bicornis unicollis and the other patient, who had a complex reciprocal, insertional translocation of chromosomes 10p and 8q, had cartilaginous exostoses (35). Neither of these patients had immunodeficiency or heart defects, which are key features of DGS 2 (see above), and further studies defined two nonoverlapping regions; thus, the *DGS2* region was located on 10p13–14 and *HDR* on 10p14–10pter. Deletion mapping studies in two other HDR patients further defined a critical 200 kb region that contained *GATA3* (35), which belongs to a family of zinc finger transcription factors involved in vertebrae embryonic development. DNA sequence analysis in other HDR patients identified mutations that resulted in a haploinsufficiency and loss of GATA3 function (35, 36). GATA3 has two zinc fingers, and the C-terminal finger (ZnF2) binds DNA, whilst the N-terminal finger (ZnF1) stabilizes this DNA binding and interacts with other zinc finger proteins, such as the friends of GATA (FOG) (36). HDR-associated mutations involving GATA3 ZnF2 or the adjacent basic amino acids were found to result in a loss of DNA binding, whilst those involving ZnF1 either lead to a loss of interaction with FOG2 ZnFs or altered DNA binding affinity (36). These findings are consistent with the proposed three-dimensional model of GATA3 ZnF1, which has separate DNA and protein binding surfaces (36). Thus, the HDR-associated GATA3 mutations can be subdivided into two broad classes, depending upon whether they disrupt ZnF1 or ZnF2, and their subsequent effects on interactions with FOG2 and altered DNA binding, respectively. The majority (>75%) of these HDR-associated mutations are predicted to result in truncated forms of the GATA3 protein. Each proband and family will generally have its own unique mutation and there appears to be no correlation with the underlying genetic defect and the phenotypic variation, e.g. the presence or absence of renal dysplasia. Over 90% of patients with two or three of the major clinical features of the HDR syndrome, i.e. hypoparathyroidisim, deafness, or renal abnormalities, have a *GATA3* mutation (36). The remaining 10% of HDR of patients who do not have a *GATA3* mutation of the coding region, may harbour mutations in the regulatory sequences flanking the *GATA3* gene, or else they may represent heterogeneity. The phenotypes of HDR patients with *GATA3* mutations appear to be similar to those without *GATA3* mutations (36). The HDR phenotype is consistent with the expression pattern of *GATA3* during human and mouse embryogenesis in the developing kidney, otic vesicle, and parathyroids. However, *GATA3* is also expressed in developing central nervous system and the haematopoietic organs in man and mice, and this suggests that GATA3 may have a more complex role. Indeed, homozygous *Gata3* knockout mice have defects of the central nervous system and a lack of T-cell development. The heterozygous *Gata3* knockout mice appear to have no abnormalities other than deafness (37, 38). It is important to note that HDR patients with *GATA3* haploinsufficiency do not have immune deficiency, and this suggests that the immune abnormalities observed in some patients with 10p deletions are most likely to be caused by other genes on 10p. Similarly, the facial dysmorphism, growth, and development delay, commonly seen in patients with larger 10p deletions, were absent in the HDR patients with *GATA3* mutations, further indicating that these features were probably due to other genes on 10p (35). These studies of HDR patients indicate an important role for GATA3 in parathyroid development and in the aetiology of hypoparathyroidism.

Mitochondrial disorders associated with hypoparathyroidism

Hypoparathyroidism has been reported to occur in three disorders associated with mitochondrial dysfunction: the Kearns–Sayre syndrome, the MELAS syndrome, and a mitochondrial trifunctional protein deficiency syndrome. Kearns–Sayre syndrome is characterized by progressive external ophthalmoplegia and pigmentary retinopathy before the age of 20 years, and is often associated with heart block or cardiomyopathy. The MELAS syndrome consists of a childhood onset of *m*itochondrial *e*ncephalopathy, Lactic Acidosis, and Stroke-like episodes. In addition, varying degrees of proximal myopathy can be seen in both conditions. Both the Kearns–Sayre syndrome and MELAS syndromes have been reported to occur with insulin-dependent diabetes mellitus and hypoparathyroidism (39, 40). A point mutation in the mitochondrial gene tRNA leucine (UUR) has been reported in one patient with the MELAS syndrome who also suffered from hypoparathyroidism and diabetes mellitus (40). Large deletions, consisting of 6741 and 6903 base pairs and involving more than 38% of the mitochondrial genome, have been reported in other patients who suffered from Kearns–Sayre syndrome, hypoparathyroidism, and sensorineural deafness (41). Rearrangements and duplication of mitochondrial DNA have also been reported in Kearns–Sayre syndrome (2). Mitochondrial trifunctional protein deficiency is a disorder of fatty-acid oxidation that is associated with peripheral neuropathy, pigmentary retinopathy, and acute fatty liver degeneration in pregnant women who carry an affected fetus. Hypoparathyroidism has been observed in one patient with trifunctional protein deficiency (42). The role of these mitochondrial mutations in the aetiology of hypoparathyroidism remains to be further elucidated.

Kenney–Caffey, Sanjad–Sakati, and Kirk–Richardson syndromes

Hypoparathyroidism has been reported to occur in over 50% of patients with the Kenney–Caffey syndrome, which is associated with short stature, osteosclerosis and cortical thickening of the long bones, delayed closure of the anterior fontanel, basal ganglia calcification, nanophthalmos, and hyperopia (43). Parathyroid tissue could not be found in a detailed post mortem examination of one patient (44) and this suggests that hypoparathyroidism may be due to an embryological defect of parathyroid development. In the Kirk–Richardson and Sanjad–Sakati syndromes, which are similar, hypoparathyroidism is associated with severe growth failure and dysmorphic features (45, 46). This has been reported in patients of Middle Eastern origin. Consanguinity was noted in the majority of the families, indicating that this syndrome is inherited as an autosomal recessive disorder. Homozygosity and linkage disequilibrium studies located this gene to chromosome 1q42-q43 and molecular genetic investigations have identified that mutations of the tubulin-specific chaperone (TBCE) are associated with the Kenney–Caffey and Sanjad–Sakati syndromes (47). *TBCE* encodes one of several chaperone proteins required for the proper folding of α-tubulin subunits and the formation of α–β tubulin heterodimers (Fig. 4.5.1) (47).

Additional familial syndromes

Single familial syndromes in which hypoparathyroidism is a component have been reported (Table 4.5.2). The inheritance of the disorder in some instances has been established and molecular genetic analysis of the *PTH* gene has revealed no abnormalities. Thus, an association of hypoparathyroidism, renal insufficiency, and developmental delay has been reported in one Asian family in whom autosomal recessive inheritance of the disorder was established. An analysis of the *PTH* gene in this family revealed no abnormalities. The occurrence of hypoparathyroidism, nerve deafness, and a steroid-resistant nephrosis leading to renal failure, which has been referred to as the *Barakat's syndrome*, has been reported in four brothers from one family, and an association of hypoparathyroidism with congenital lymphoedema, nephropathy, mitral valve prolapse, and brachytelephalangy has been observed in two brothers from another family. Molecular genetic studies have not been reported from these two families.

Blomstrand disease

Blomstrand chondrodysplasia is an autosomal recessive disorder characterized by early lethality, dramatically advanced bone maturation, and accelerated chondrocyte differentiation. Affected infants, who usually have consanguineous unaffected parents, develop pronounced hyperdensity of the entire skeleton with markedly advanced ossification, which results in extremely short and poorly modelled long bones. Mutations of the PTH/PTHrP receptor that impair its function are associated with Blomstrand disease (48). Thus, it seems likely that affected infants will, in addition to the skeletal defects, also have abnormalities in other organs, including secondary hyperplasia of the parathyroid glands, presumably due to hypocalcaemia.

Pluriglandular autoimmune hypoparathyroidism

This syndrome (Fig. 4.5.2) comprises of hypoparathyroidism, Addison disease, candidiasis, and two or three of the following: insulin-dependent diabetes mellitus, primary hypogonadism, autoimmune thyroid disease, pernicious anaemia, chronic active hepatitis, steatorrhoea (malabsorption), alopecia (totalis or areata), and vitiligo. The disorder has also been referred to as either the autoimmune polyendocrinopathy–candidiasis–ectodermal dystrophy (APECED) syndrome or the polyglandular autoimmune type 1 syndrome (49).

This disorder has a high incidence in Finland, and a genetic analysis of Finnish families indicated autosomal recessive inheritance of the disorder. In addition, the disorder has been reported to have a high incidence among Iranian Jews, although the occurrence of candidiasis was less common in this population. Linkage studies of Finnish families mapped the *APECED* gene to chromosome 21q22.3 (50). Further positional cloning approaches led to the isolation of a novel gene from chromosome 21q22.3. This gene, referred to as *AIRE* (autoimmune regulator), encodes a 545 amino acid protein, which contains motifs suggestive of a transcriptional factor and includes two zinc finger motifs, a proline-rich region, and three LXXLL motifs (51, 52). Four *AIRE1* mutations are commonly found in APECED families and these are: Arg257stop in Finnish, German, Swiss, British, and Northern Italian families; Arg139stop in Sardinian families; Tyr85Cys in Iranian Jewish families; and a 13 bp deletion in exon 8 in British, Dutch, German, and Finnish families (51, 53). AIRE1 has been shown to regulate the elimination of organ-specific T cells in the thymus, and thus APECED is likely to be caused by a failure of this specialized mechanism for deleting forbidden T cells, and establishing immunological tolerance (54). Patients with autoimmune polyglandular syndrome type 1 (APS 1) may also develop other autoimmune disorders in association with organ-specific autoantibodies, which are similar to those in patients with non-APS 1 forms of the disease. Examples of such autoantibodies and related diseases are GAD6S autoantibodies in diabetes mellitus type 1A and 21-dydroxylase autoantibodies in Addison disease. Patients with APS 1 may also develop autoantibodies that react with specific autoantigens that are not found in non-APS 1 patients, and examples of this are autoantibodies to type 1 interferon, which are present in all APS 1 patients (55), and to NACHT leucine-rich-repeat-protein 5 (NALP5), which is a parathyroid-specific autoantibody present in 49% of patients with APS 1-associated hypoparathyroidism (56). NALP proteins are essential components of the inflammasone and activate the innate immune system in different inflammatory and autoimmune disorders, such as vitiligo, which involves NALP1, and gout, which involves NALP3 (57). The precise role of NALP5 in APS 1-associated hypoparathyroidism remains to be elucidated.

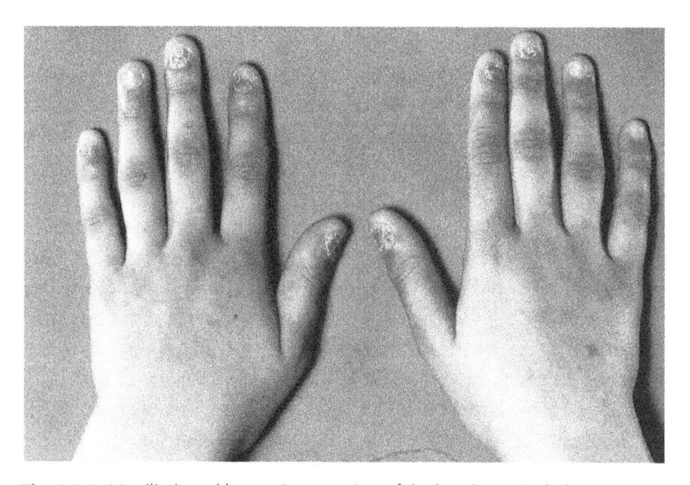

Fig. 4.5.2 Moniliasis and hyperpigmentation of the hands, particularly over the knuckles, is seen in this 8-year-old patient with hypoparathyroidism and Addison disease. The patient also had vitiligo, and thus had some of the features of the polyglandular autoimmune syndrome type 1. (Reproduced with permission from Thakker RV. Hypocalcaemic disorders. In: Thakker RV, Wass JAH, ed. *Medicine. Vol 25.* Abingdon, Oxon, UK: The Medicine Group (Journals), 1997; 68–70.) (See also Plate 19)

Calcium-sensing receptor abnormalities

The CaSR, which is located in the plasma membrane of the cell (Fig. 4.5.1), is at a critical site to enable the cell to recognize changes in extracellular calcium concentration. Thus, an increase in extracellular calcium leads to CaSR activation of the G-protein signalling pathway, which in turn increases the free intracellular calcium concentration and leads to a reduction in transcription of the *PTH* gene. *CaSR* mutations that result in a loss of function are associated with familial benign (hypocalciuric) hypercalcaemia (58). CaSR abnormalities are associated with three hypocalcaemic disorders, which are autosomal dominant hypocalcaemic hypercalciuria (ADHH), Bartter syndrome type V (i.e. ADHH with a Bartter-like syndrome), and a form of autoimmune hypoparathyroidism due to CaSR autoantibodies (Table 4.5.2). *CaSR* missense mutations that result in a gain of function (or added sensitivity to extracellular calcium) lead to ADHH (59). These hypocalcaemic individuals are generally asymptomatic and have serum PTH concentrations that are in the low-normal range, and because of the insensitivities of previous PTH assays in this range, such patients have often been diagnosed to be hypoparathyroid. In addition, such patients may have hypomagnesaemia. Treatment with Vitamin D or its active metabolites to correct the hypocalcaemia in these patients results in marked hypercalciuria, nephrocalcinosis, nephrolithiasis, and renal impairment. Thus, these patients need to be distinguished from those with hypoparathyroidism. Patients with Bartter syndrome type V have the classical features of the syndrome, i.e. hypokalaemic metabolic alkalosis, hyperreninaemia, and hyperaldosteronism (60, 61). In addition, they develop hypocalcaemia, which may be symptomatic and lead to carpopedal spasm, and an elevated fractional excretion of calcium that may be associated with nephrocalcinosis (60, 61). Such patients have been reported to have heterozygous gain-of-function *CaSR* mutations, and *in vitro* functional expression of these mutations has revealed a more severe set-point abnormality for the receptor than that found in patients with ADHH (60, 61). This suggests that the additional features occurring in Bartter's syndrome type V, but not in ADHH, are due to severe gain-of-function mutations of the *CaSR*.

Autoimmune acquired hypoparathyroidism

Twenty per cent of patients who had acquired hypoparathyroidism in association with autoimmune hypothyroidism, were found to have autoantibodies to the extracellular domain of the CaSR (62, 63). The CaSR autoantibodies did not persist for long; 72% of patients who had acquired hypoparathyroidism for less than 5 years had detectable CaSR autoantibodies, whereas only 14% of patients with acquired hypoparathyroidism for more than 5 years had such autoantibodies (62). The majority of the patients who had CaSR autoantibodies were females, a finding that is similar to that found in other autoantibody-mediated diseases. Indeed, a few acquired hypoparathyroidism patients have also had features of autoimmune polyglandular syndrome type 1 (APS 1). These findings establish that the CaSR is an autoantigen in acquired hypoparathyroidism (62, 63).

Pseudohypoparathyroidism

Patients with pseudohypoparathyroidism (PHP), which may be inherited as an autosomal dominant disorder, are characterized by hypocalcaemia and hyperphosphataemia due to PTH resistance rather than PTH deficiency (2, 3, 6). Five variants are recognized on the basis of biochemical and somatic features (Table 4.5.3) and three of these—PHP type Ia (PHP Ia), PHP type 1b (PHP Ib), and pseudopseudohypoparathyroidism (PPHP)—will be reviewed in further detail. Patients with PHP Ia exhibit PTH resistance (hypocalcaemia, hyperphosphataemia, elevated serum PTH, and an absence of an increase in serum and urinary cyclic AMP and urinary phosphate following intravenous human PTH infusion), together with the features of Albright's hereditary osteodystrophy, which includes short stature, obesity, subcutaneous calcification, mental retardation, round facies, dental hypoplasia, and brachydactyly (i.e. shortening of the metacarpals, particularly the third, fourth, and fifth) (3). In addition to brachydactyly, other skeletal abnormalities of the long bones and shortening of the metatarsals may also occur. Patients with PHP Ib exhibit PTH resistance only and do not have the somatic features of Albright's hereditary osteodystrophy, whilst patients with PPHP exhibit the somatic features of Albright's hereditary osteodystrophy in the absence of PTH resistance (3). The absence of a normal rise in urinary excretion of cyclic AMP excretion after an infusion of PTH in PHP Ia indicated a defect at some site of the PTH receptor–adenyl cyclase system. This receptor system is regulated by at least two G proteins, one of which stimulates (Gsα) and another which inhibits (Giα) the activity of the membrane-bound enzyme that catalyses the formation of the intracellular second messenger cyclic AMP. Interestingly, patients with PHP Ia may also show resistance to other hormones, for example thyroid-stimulating hormone, follicle-stimulating hormone, and luteinizing hormone, which act via G-protein coupled receptors (3). Inactivating mutations of the Gsα gene (referred to as *GNAS1*), which is located on chromosome 20q13.2, have been identified in PHP Ia and PPHP patients (64, 65). However, *GNAS1* mutations do not fully explain the PHP Ia or PPHP phenotypes, and studies of PHP Ia and PPHP that occurred within the same kindred revealed that the hormonal resistance is parentally imprinted (66). Thus, PHP Ia occurs in a child only when the mutation is inherited from a mother affected with either PHP Ia or PPHP; and PPHP occurs in a child only when the mutation is inherited from a father affected with either PHP Ia or PPHP. *GNAS1* mutations have not been detected in PHP Ib, which has been considered to be due to a defect of the PTH/PTHrP receptor. However, studies of the *PTH/PTHrP* receptor gene and mRNA in PHP Ib patients have not identified mutations (67), and linkage

Table 4.5.3 Clinical, biochemical, and genetic features of hypoparathyroid and pseudohypoparathyroid disorders

	Hypoparathyroidism	Pseudohypoparathyroidism (PHP)				
		PHP Ia	PPHP	PHP Ib	PHP Ic	PHP II
AHO manifestations	No	Yes	Yes	No	Yes	No
Serum calcium	↓	↓	N	↓	↓	↓
Serum PO_4	↑	↑	N	↑	↑	↑
Serum PTH	↓	↑	N	↑	↑	↑
Response to PTH:						
Urinary cAMP[a] (Chase–Aurbach test)	↑	↓	↑	↓	↓	↑
Urinary PO_4 (Ellsworth–Howard test)	↑	↓	↑	↓	↓	↓
Gsα activity	N	↓	↓	N	N	N
Inheritance	AD/AR/X	AD	AD	AD	AD	Sporadic
Molecular defect	PTH/CaSR/ GATA3/ Gcm2/ others	GNAS1	GNAS1	GNAS1	?adenyl cyclase	?cAMP targets
Other hormonal resistance	No	Yes	No	No	Yes	No

↓ = decreased, ↑ = increased, N = normal,? = presumed, but not proven.
[a] Plasma cAMP responses are similar to those of urinary cAMP.
AD, autosomal dominant; AHO, Albright's hereditary osteodystrophy; AR, autosomal recessive; X, X-linked.

studies in four unrelated kindreds have mapped the PHP Ib locus to chromosome 20q13.3, a location that also contains the *GNAS1* gene. In addition, parental imprinting of the genetic defect was observed and this is similar to the findings in kindreds with PHP Ia and/or PPHP. Detailed analyses of the *GNAS1* gene in PHP Ib families have revealed a large 3 kb deletion involving upstream exon(s) referred to as A/B (68). In affected individuals, the deletion involved the maternal allele, whereas its occurrence on the paternal allele resulted in unaffected healthy carriers (68). This is consistent with parental imprinting of the *GNAS1* abnormality causing PHP Ib.

Acknowledgements

I am grateful: to the Medical Research Council (UK) for support; and to Mrs Tracey Walker for typing the manuscript and expert secretarial assistance.

References

1. Thakker RV. Parathyroid disorders: molecular genetics and physiology. In: Morris PJ, Wood WC, eds. *Oxford Textbook of Surgery*. Oxford University Press, 2000: 1121–9.
2. Thakker RV. Molecular basis of PTH under expression. In: Bilezikian JP, Raisz LG, Rodan GA, eds. *Principles of Bone Biology*. 2nd edn. San Diego: Academic Press, 2002: 1105–16.
3. Rubin MR, Levine MA. Hypoparathyroidism and pseudohypoparathyroidism. In: Rosen CJ, ed. *Primer on the Metabolic Bone Diseases and Disorders of Mineral Metabolism*. 7th edn. Washington DC: American Society of Bone and Mineral Research, 2008: 354–61.
4. Shoback D. Hypocalcaemia: definition, etiology, pathogenesis, diagnosis and management. In: Rosen CJ, ed. *Primer on the Metabolic Bone Diseases and Disorders of Mineral Metabolism*. 7th edn. Washington DC: American Society of Bone and Mineral Research, 2008: 313–17.
5. Thakker RV. Hypocalcaemic disorders. In: Thakker RV, Wass JAH, ed. *Medicine*. Vol. 25. Abingdon, Oxon, UK: The Medicine Group (Journals) Limited, 1997: 68–70.
6. Thakker RV, Juppner H. Genetic disorders of calcium homeostasis caused by abnormal regulation of parathyroid hormone secretion or responsiveness. In: DeGroot LJ, Jameson JL, eds. *Endocrinology*, 5th edn. Philadelphia. Elsevier Saunders, 2006: 1511–31.
7. Marx SJ. Hyperparathyroid and hypoparathyroid disorders. *N Engl J Med*, 2000; **343**: 1803–75.
8. Thakker RV. Diseases associated with the extracellular calcium-sensing receptor. *Cell Calcium*, 2004; **35**: 275–82.
9. Ahn TG, Antonarakis SE, Kronenberg HM, Igarashi T, Levine MA. Familial isolated hypoparathyroidism: a molecular genetic analysis of 8 families with 23 affected persons. *Medicine*, 1986; **65**: 73–81.
10. Parkinson DB, Shaw NJ, Himsworth RL, Thakker RV. Parathyroid hormone gene analysis in autosomal hypoparathyroidism using an intragenic tetranucleotide $(AAAT)_n$ polymorphism. *Hum Genet*, 1993; **91**: 281–4.
11. Arnold A, Horst SA, Gardella TJ, Baba H, Levine MA, Kronenberg HM. Mutations of the signal peptide encoding region of preproparathyroid hormone gene in isolated hypoparathyroidism. *J Clin Invest*, 1990; **86**: 1084–7.
12. Karaplis AC, Lim SC, Baba H, Arnold A, Kronenberg HM. Inefficient membrane targeting, translocation, and proteolytic processing by signal peptidase of a mutant preproparathyroid hormone protein. *J Biol Chem*, 1995; **27**: 1629–35.
13. Sunthornthepvarakul T, Churesigaew S, Ngowngarmratana S. A novel mutation of the signal peptide of the pre-pro-parathyroid horome gene associated with autosomal recessive familial isolated hypoparathyroidism. *J Clin Endocrinol Metab*, 1999; **84**: 3792–6.
14. Parkinson DB, Thakker RV. A donor splice site mutation in the parathyroid hormone gene is associated with autosomal recessive hypoparathyroidism. *Nat Genet*, 1992; **1**: 149–52.
15. Baumber L, Tufarelli C, Patel S, King P, Johnson CA, Maher ER, Trembath RC. Identification of a novel mutation disrupting the DNA binding activity of GCM2 in autosomal recessive familial isolated hypoparathyroidism. *J Med Genet 2005*, 2005; **42**: 443–8.
16. Ding C, Buckingham B, Levine M. Familial isolated hypoparathyroidism caused by a mutation in the gene for the transcription factor GCMB. *J Clin Invest*, 2001; **108**: 1215–20.
17. Mannstadt M, Bertrand G, Grandechamp B, Jueppner H, Silve C. Dominant-negative GCMB mutations cause hypoparathyroidism. *JBMR*, 2007; **22**: S9.
18. Günther T, Chen ZF, Kim J, Priemel M, Rueger JM, Amling M, *et al.* Genetic ablation of parathyroid glands reveals another source of parathyroid hormone. *Nature*, 2000; **406**: 199–203.
19. Whyte MP, Weldon VV. Idiopathic hypoparathyroidism presenting with seizures during infancy: X-linked recessive inheritance in a large Missouri kindred. *J Pediatr*, 1981; **99**: 608–11.
20. Whyte MP, Kim GS, Kosanovich M. Absence of parathyroid tissue in sex-linked recessive hypoparathyroidism (letter). *J Pediatr*, 1986; **109**: 915.
21. Mumm S, Whyte MP, Thakker RV, Buetowk H, Schlessinger D. mtDNA analysis shows common ancestry in two kindreds with X-linked recessive hypoparathyroidism and reveals a heteroplasmic silent mutation. *Am J Hum Genet*, 1997; **1**: 153–9.
22. Thakker RV, Davies KE, Whyte MP, Wooding C, O'Riordan JLH. Mapping the gene causing X-linked recessive idiopathic hypoparathyroidism to Xq26–Xq27 by linkage studies. *J Clin Invest*, 1990; **6**: 40–5.
23. Bowl MR, Nesbit MA, Harding B, Levy E, Jefferson A, Volpi E, *et al.* An interstitial deletion-insertion involving chromosomes 2p25.3 and Xq27.1, near SOX3, causes X-linked recessive hypoparathyroidism. *J Clin Invest*, 2005; **115**: 2822–31.
24. Kleinjan DA, van Heyningen V. Long-range control of gene expression: emerging mechanisms and disruption in disease. *Am J Hum Genet*, 2005; **76**: 8–32.
25. Brunelli S, Silva Casey E, Bell D, Harland R, Lovell-Badge R. Expression of SOX3 throughout the developing central nervous system is dependent on the combined action of discrete, evolutionarily conserved regulatory elements. *Genesis*, 2003; **36**: 12–24.
26. Kiernan AE, Pelling AL, Leung KK Tang AS, Bell DM, Tease C, *et al.* Sox2 is required for sensory organ development in the mammalian inner ear. *Nature*, 2005; **434**: 1031–5.
27. Scambler PJ, Carey AH, Wyse RKH, Roach S, Dumanski JP, Nordenskjold M, Williamson R. Microdeletions within 22q11 associated with sporadic and familial DiGeorge syndrome. *Genomics*, 1991; **10**: 201–6.
28. Monaco G, Pignata C, Rossi E, Mascellaro O, Cocozza S, Ciccimarra F. DiGeorge anomaly associated with 10p deletion. *Am J Med Genet*, 1991; **39**: 215–6.
29. Scambler PJ. The 22q11 deletion syndromes. *Hum Mol Genet*, 2000; **9**: 2421–6.
30. Jerome LA, Papaioannou VE. DiGeorge syndrome phenotype in mice mutant for the T-box gene, Tbx1. *Nat Genet*, 2001; **27**: 286–91.
31. Yagi H, Furutani Y, Hamada H, Sasaki T, Asakawa S, Minoshima S, *et al.* Role of TBX1 in human del22q11.2 syndrome. *Lancet*, 2003; **362**: 1366–73.

32. Baldini A. DiGeorge's syndrome: a gene at last. *Lancet*, 2003; **362**: 1342–3.
33. Sykes K, Bachrach L, Siegel-Bartelt J, Ipp M, Kooh SW, Cytrynbaum C, *et al.* (1997). Velocardio-facial syndrome presenting as hypocalcemia in early adolescence. *Arch Pediatr Adolesc Med*, **151**: 745–7.
34. Bilous RW, Murty G, Parkinson DB, Thakker RV, Coulthard MG, Burn J, *et al.* Autosomal dominant familial hypoparathyroidism, sensorineural deafness and renal dysplasia. *N Engl J Med*, 1992; **327**: 1069–84.
35. Van Esch H, Groenen P, Nesbit MA, Schuffenhauer S, Lichtner P, Vanderlinden G, *et al.* GATA3 haploinsufficiency causes human HDR syndrome. *Nature*, 2000; **406**: 419–22.
36. Ali A, Christie PT, Grigorieva IV, Harding B, Van Esch H, Ahmed SF, *et al.* Functional characterisation of GATA3 mutations causing the hypoparathyroidism-deafness-renal (HDR) dysplasia syndrome: insight into mechanisms of DNA binding by the GATA3 transcription factor. *Hum Mol Genet*, 2007; **3**: 265–75.
37. Pandolfi PP, Roth ME, Karis A, Leonard MW, Dzierzak E, Grosveld FG, *et al.* Targeted disruption of the GATA3 gene causes severe abnormalities in the nervous system and in fetal liver haematopoiesis. *Nat Genet*, 1995; **11**: 40–4.
38. van Looij M, van der Burg H, van der Giessen R, de Tuiter M, van der Wees J, van Doorninck J, *et al.* GATA3 haploinsufficiency causes a rapid deterioration of distortion product otoacoustic emissions (DPOAEs) in mice. *Neurobiol Dis*, 2005; **20**: 890–7.
39. Moraes CT, DiMauro S, Zeviani M, Lombes A, Shanske S, Miranda AF, *et al.* Mitochondrial deletions in progressive external ophthalmoplegia and Kearns–Sayre syndrome. *N Engl J Med*, 1989; **320**: 1293–9.
40. Morten KJ, Cooper JM, Brown GK, Lake BD, Pike D, Poulton J. A new point mutation associated with mitochondrial encephalomyopathy. *Hum Mol Genet*, 1993; **2**: 2081–7.
41. Isotani H, Fukumoto Y, Kawamura H, Furukawa K, Ohsawa N, Goto Y, *et al.* Hypoparathyroidism and insulin-dependent diabetes mellitus in a patient with Kearns–Sayre syndrome harbouring a mitochondrial DNA deletion. *Clin Endocrinol*, 1996; **45**: 637–41.
42. Dionisi-Vici C, Garavaglia B, Burlina AB, Bertini E, Saponara I, Sabetta G, *et al.* Hypoparathyroidism in mitochondrial trifunctional protein deficiency. *J Pediatr*, 1996; **129**: 159–62.
43. Franceschini, P, Testa, A, Bogetti, G, Girardo, E, Guala, A, Lopez-Bell, G, *et al.* Kenny-Caffey syndrome in two sibs born to consanguineous parents: Evidence for an autosomal recessive variant. *Am J Med Genet*, 1992; **42**: 112–16.
44. Boynton JR, Pheasant TR, Johnson BL, Levin DB, Streeten BW. Ocular findings in Kenny's syndrome. *Arch Ophthalmol (Chicago)*, 1979; **97**, 896–900.
45. Richardson RJ, Kirk JM. Short stature, mental retardation, and hypoparathyroidism: a new syndrome. *Arch Dis Child*, 1990; **65**: 1113–17.
46. Sanjad SA, Sakati NA, Abu-Osba YK, Kaddoura R, Milner RD. A new syndrome of congenital hypoparathyroidism, severe growth failure, and dysmorphic features. *Arch Dis Child*, 1991; **66**: 193–6.
47. Parvari R, Hershkovitz E, Grossman N, Gorodischer R, Loeys B, Zecic A, *et al.* Mutation of TBCE causes hypoparathyroidism-retardation-dysmorphism and autosomal recessive Kenny-Caffey syndrome. *Nat Genet*, 2002; **32**: 448–52.
48. Jobert AS, Zhang P, Couvineau A, Bonaventure J, Roume J, Le Merrer M, Silve C . Absence of functional receptors parathyroid hormones and parathyroid hormone-related peptide in Blomstrand chondrodysplasia. *J Clin Invest*, 1998; **102**: 34–40.
49. Ahonen P, Myllarniemi S, Sipila I, Perheentupa J. Clinical variation of autoimmune polyendocrinopathy-candidiasis ectodermal dystrophy (APECED) in a series of 68 patients. *N Engl J Med*, 1990; **322**: 1829–36.
50. Aaltonen J, Bjorses P, Sandkuijl L, Perheentupa J, Peltonen L . An autosomal locus causing autoimmune disease: autoimmune polyglandular disease type 1 assigned to chromosome 21. *Nat Genet*, 1994; **8**: 83–7.
51. Nagamine K, Peterson P, Scott HS, Heino M, Minoshima S, Kudoh J, *et al.* Positional cloning of the APECED gene. *Nat Genet*, 1997; **17**: 393–8.
52 The Finnish-German APECED consortium. An autoimmune disease, APECED, caused by mutations in a novel gene featuring two PHD-type zinc finger domains. *Nat Genet*, 1997; **17**: 399–403.
53. Pearce SH, Cheetham T, Imrie H, Vaidya B, Barnes ND, Bilous RW, *et al.* A common and recurrent 13-bp deletion in the autoimmune regulator gene in British kindreds with autoimmune polyendocrinopathy type 1. *Am J Hum Genet*, 1998; **63**: 1675–84.
54. Liston A, Lesage S, Wilson J, Goodnow CC, Peltonen L. Aire regulates negative selection of organ-specific T cells. *Nat Immunol*, 2003; **4**: 350–4.
55. Meaager A, Visvalingam K, Peterson P, Moll K, Murumagi A, Krohn K, *et al.* Anti-interferon autoantibodies in autoimmune polyendocrinopathy syndrome type 1. *PLoS Med*, 2006; **3**: e289.
56. Alimohammadi M, Bjorklund P, Hallgren A, Pontynen N, Szinnai G, Shikama N, *et al.* Autoimmune polyendocrine syndrome type 1 and NALP5, a parathyroid autoantigen. *N Engl J Med*, 2008; **358**: 1018–28.
57. Eisenbarth SC, Colegio OR, O'Connor W, Sutterwala FS, Flavell RA. Crucial role for the Nalp3 inflammasome in the immunostimulatory properties of aluminium adjuvants. *Nature*, 2008; **453**: 1122–6.
58. Pollak MR, Brown EM, Chou YH, Hebert SC, Marx SJ, Steinmann B, *et al.* Mutations in the human Ca^{2}+-sensing receptor gene cause familial hypocalciuric hypercalcaemia and neonatal severe hyperparathyroidism. *Cell*, 1993; **75**: 1297–303.
59. Pearce SH, Williamson C, Kifor O, Bai M, Coulthard MG, Davies M, *et al.* A familial syndrome of hypocalcaemia with hypocalciuria due to mutations in the calcium-sensing receptor gene. *N Engl J Med*, 1996; **335**: 1115–22.
60. Watanabe S, Fukumoto S, Chang H, Takeuchi Y, Hasegawa Y, Okazaki R, *et al.* Association between activating mutations of calcium-sensing receptor and Bartter's syndrome. *Lancet*, 2002; **360**: 692–4.
61. Vargas-Poussou R, Huang C, Hulin P, Houillier P, Jeunemaitre X, Paillard M, *et al.* Functional characterization of a calcium-sensing receptor mutation in severe autosomal dominant hypocalcemia with a Bartter-like syndrome. *J Am Soc Nephrol*, 2002; **13**: 2259–66.
62. Li Y, Song YH, Rais N, Connor E, Schatz D, Muir A, Maclaren N. Autoantibodies to the extracellular domain of the calcium sensing receptor in patients with acquired hypoparathyroidism. *J Clin Invest*, 1996; **97**: 910–4.
63. Kifor O, Moore FD, Jr., Delaney M, Garber J, Hendy GN, Butters R, *et al.* A syndrome of hypocalciuric hypercalcemia caused by autoantibodies directed at the calcium-sensing receptor. *J Clin Endocrinol Metab*, 2003; **88**: 60–72.
64. Weinstein LS, Gejman PV, Friedman E, Kadowaki T, Collins RM, Gershon ES, *et al.* Mutations of the Gsα-subunit gene in Albright hereditary osteodystrophy detected by denaturing gradient gel electrophoresis. *Proc Natl Acad Sci USA*, 1990; **87**: 8287–90.
65. Yu S, Yu D, Hainline BE, Brener JL, Wilson KA, Wilson LC, *et al.* A deletion hot-spot in exon 7 of the $G_s\alpha$ gene (GNAS1) in patients with Albright hereditary osteodystrphy. *Hum Mol Genet*, 1995; **4**: 2001–2.
66. Wilson LC, Oude-Luttikhuis MEM, Clayton PT, Fraser WD, Trembath RC, *et al.* Parental origin of Gsα gene mutations in Albright's hereditary osteodystrophy. *J Med Genet*, 1994; **31**: 835–9.

67. Schipani E, Weinstein LS, Bergwitz C, Iida-Klein A, Kong XF, Stuhrmann M, *et al.* Pseudohypoparathyroidism type Ib is not caused by mutations in the coding exons of the human parathyroid hormone (PTH)/PTH-related peptide receptor gene. *J Clin Endocrinol Metab*, 1995; **80**: 1611–21.

68. Jüppner H, Schipani E, Bastepe M, Cole DE, Lawson ML, Mannstadt M, *et al.* The gene responsible for pseudohypoparathyroidism type Ib is paternally imprinted and maps in four unrelated kindreds to chromosome 20q13.3. *Proc Natl Acad Sci USA*, 1998; **95**: 11798–803.

4.6

Hypercalcaemic and hypocalcaemic syndromes in children

Laleh Ardeshirpour, Thomas O. Carpenter

Introduction

The calcium-regulating system employs an intricate network of homoeostatic signals and targets in order to meet the body's mineral demands. Mineral requirements vary considerably throughout progressive stages of development, in large part reflecting the changing mineral demands of skeletal growth, and representing characteristic features of the calcium homoeostatic system during childhood years. As a consequence, this system must be adaptable to the wide-ranging mineral demands occurring throughout the life cycle. Furthermore, the numerous factors involved in calcium homoeostasis allow for compensatory mechanisms to limit the severity of disease when an isolated insult occurs to the system. Indeed, many heritable disorders of mineral homoeostasis become evident in early childhood and are best recognized when viewed in the light of mineral requirements during infancy and childhood. As understanding of the relevant physiology is central to formulating approaches to management of such problems, we review these disorders in the context of physiology specific to childhood to provide the basis for understanding hypocalcaemia and hypercalcaemia in this age group.

Features of calcium homoeostasis specific to children

Perinatal calcium metabolism

Skeletal development and mineral requirements of the fetus

The growing fetus must be supplied with sufficient calcium for the formation and growth of a mineralizing skeleton. In addition, the physiological milieu of the fetus must be maintained in an environment appropriate for normal cellular function. Thus adequate extracellular calcium must be provided for normal function of the clotting factors, and avoidance of neuromuscular hyperexcitation. Yet, at the same time, the supply must be appropriately limited to prevent damaging soft tissue calcification or other toxicity to the developing fetus. A critical calcium-dependent process in fetal life is skeletal development. Most of the skeleton is formed by the complex process referred to as endochondral ossification (1). Cartilage templates are organized in concert with the transition of undifferentiated mesenchymal cells to differentiated chondrocytes. The cartilage templates serve as a nidus for eventual development into the skeleton. A system of chondrocyte maturation and proliferation occurs at what will become the ends of long bones, allowing for the continued linear growth of the skeleton. Regulation of this early formative process is dependent upon a variety of local and systemic factors, such as insulin-like growth factors, fibroblast growth factors, parathyroid hormone-related protein (PTHrP), and Indian hedgehog protein (2). Once mature cartilage forms, chondrocytes hypertrophy, and blood vessels penetrate the region, with the appearance of marrow stroma and osteoblasts soon to follow. Mineralization of the newly established skeleton begins, and growth results in a continuing mineral demand in order to effectively mineralize the newly formed tissue. Indeed, the fetus has substantial mineral demands: approximately 21 g of calcium accumulate in the human through a term gestation, and accretion of more than three-quarters of this amount occurs in the third trimester (3). Calcium supply from the maternal circulation must be regulated by specific mechanisms in order to meet these demands throughout the later weeks of gestation.

The fetal calcium-regulating system

The maternal circulation is the source of calcium provided to the fetus. An abundance of calcium occurs in the mother primarily as a result of a pregnancy-induced doubling of maternal circulating 1,25-dihydroxyvitamin D (1,25 $(OH)_2D$) levels, which in turn increases fractional absorption of calcium at the intestine (4). This occurs with no significant increases in circulating levels of parathyroid hormone (PTH) in the mother.

The placenta is the site of transfer of nutrients from the maternal circulation to the fetus. Calcium may be transported by several mechanisms across the placenta; the dominant direction of flow is from maternal to the fetal circulation, requiring active transport. A Ca^{2+}-ATPase located in the fetus-directed basement membrane of the syncytial trophoblast cells appears to mediate this important function (5). Although it is not clear exactly when in gestation active calcium transport begins, it is present by the beginning of the third trimester. The fetal circulating calcium level is maintained at a slightly higher concentration than the maternal circulation. Active placental calcium transfer plays an important role in determining fetal circulating calcium level, but other factors may play a role, including PTH and PTHrP. The relative hypercalcaemia in the fetus is ample for normal skeletal growth and development. Placental calcium transfer seems to be mainly regulated by PTHrP, and to a lesser extent PTH (5–7). The mid- and C-terminal portions of the PTHrP molecule are required, whereas the N-terminus (most related to PTH in sequence) does not have activity in this regard (3, 5). PTHrP plays an important role in embryonic growth and development of many tissues, and is produced by multiple tissues. Major sources of PTHrP production are the placenta, and to a lesser extent, the parathyroid glands. In a fetal mouse model, disruption of PTHrP results in hypocalcaemia and severe chondrodysplasia (7, 8). Fetal circulating PTH levels are low, probably due to Ca-sensing receptor (CaSR) mediated suppression of PTH secretion by fetal parathyroid glands (5). Nevertheless, aparathyroid fetal mice develop hypocalcaemia and defective bone mineralization, pointing towards a role for PTH in maintaining normal serum calcium, and thereby perhaps supporting normal bone mineralization (9). PTH may also exert its effect on bone formation, to some extent, via direct interaction with osteoblasts.

Fetal circulating 1,25 $(OH)_2D$ levels are low. This may be related to low PTH and high serum phosphorus levels. 1,25 $(OH)_2D$ does not play a major role in placental calcium transfer or maintenance of serum calcium level as evidenced by the fully mineralized skeleton and normal fetal serum calcium levels at term in vitamin D receptor-null (*Vdr*-null) mice. In human cases of maternal vitamin D deficiency, skeletal mineralization seems to be unaffected but the newborn will be at risk of developing hypocalcaemia (5) The presence of CaSR in both human and murine placenta suggests a possible role for this membrane receptor in fetal calcium homoeostasis. Some insight has been provided by CaSR knockout mice: fetuses of this strain demonstrate increased PTH levels, reduced placental calcium transport, increased amniotic fluid calcium, and increased markers of bone resorption. This constellation of findings suggests that an increase in resorption of the skeleton can occur, when inadequate calcium levels are sensed by the fetus (9, 10). The fetal kidneys and skeleton may be involved in regulation of fetal calcium levels as well, but their roles are less defined. Excreted calcium is not lost from the fetal unit as it remains in the amniotic fluid.

Transition from fetal life to infancy

With birth the supply of maternal calcium is abruptly withdrawn from the fetus, as well as any placental sources of PTHrP and 1,25 $(OH)_2D$. A resultant acute decrease in serum calcium of approximately 1 mg/dl occurs in term infants, and slightly more in preterm infants. One study indicates that the decrement in serum calcium and rise in PTH is greater in babies born by caesarean section than in babies born spontaneously by the vaginal route. This decrease in calcium then stimulates secretion of PTH, suppressed during fetal life, which in turn, stimulates the kidney to generate adult normal levels of 1,25 $(OH)_2D$ within the next several days. Levels of PTHrP are reduced; this hormone probably plays a lesser role in postnatal calcium homoeostasis than *in utero*. The serum calcium gradually increases to normal childhood levels within a few days of the acute postnatal decrement.

The intestine and kidney assume major roles in mineral homoeostasis with this transition. The neonatal skeleton continues to accrue calcium at rates close to that attained in late gestation (averaging 100–150 mg/kg per day). Thus the newborn infant becomes critically dependent upon its nutritional environment for nonmaternal sources of calcium. Renal excretion of calcium increases over the first few weeks of life, as glomerular filtration rate (GFR) increases. As the kidney matures, it begins to play a minor role in regulation of calcium. The newborn infant, however, becomes primarily dependent upon the intestine to maintain its calcium supply. In the first few days to weeks of neonatal life, passive or facilitated calcium transport (not vitamin D-mediated mechanisms) are the dominant means by which calcium is brought into the body. After several weeks, vitamin D appears to be useful in enhancing calcium absorption in term infants. Fractional calcium absorption can be relatively high in infancy, particularly in very low birthweight children, who may develop hypercalcaemia during high calcium intake, as may occur with the administration of breast-milk fortifiers. This phenomenon may occur independently of vitamin D status (with normal circulating levels of 25 (OH)D, and appropriately low circulating PTH and 1,25 $(OH)_2D$), implying that passive or facilitated, nonvitamin D mediated calcium transport in the immature intestine can be remarkably efficient.

Childhood growth: a period of intensive mineral accretion

Growth and accrual of bone density

Skeletal growth and mineralization continue at a very rapid pace throughout the first 2 years of life. The growth velocity on average during the first 4 months of life can be annualized to approximately 28 cm/year. From that time on, a child's growth rate asymptotically decreases from a rate of 1 cm/month (approximately 12.5 cm/year) to about 5–6 cm/year at the time of the pubertal growth spurt, when a rate of about 10 cm/year is transiently achieved prior to the cessation of growth. This linear growth represents the growth of the appendicular skeleton, which must be adequately mineralized; thus rapid growth in infancy places considerable mineral demands on the skeleton. Bone mineral content and areal bone mineral density, as assessed by standard two-dimensional techniques, such as dual energy X-ray absorptiometry proceeds at a steady pace until approximately age 11 in girls and slightly later in boys (11). Specific guidelines for the use and interpretation of bone densitometry in children have recently been published by the International Society of Clinical Densitometry (12).

Although the focus on bone activity during these years is primarily on formation and mineralization, there must also be extremely active turnover in general. The growing bone must be constantly modelled in order to maintain an appropriate structure. Weight-bearing forces begin to correct the physiological bow of childhood, as lower extremity alignment becomes more linear. As metaphyseal long bone segments accrue mineral at growth plate cartilage, extending the length of the long bone calls for an eventual narrowing of the former metaphyseal segment as it assumes a diaphyseal position. These processes require extensive bone resorptive activity. Thus, when investigating disorders of the bone and mineral system, one must recognize this relatively hyperdynamic state of bone turnover. None of the established normal ranges of bone activity apply, and the remarkably high numbers (by adult standards) can be the norm (13). In fact, the normal range of values for such markers as serum osteocalcin, alkaline phosphatase activity, or urinary excretion of deoxypyridinoline cross-links of collagen, or the N-telopeptide of type I collagen are quite wide (Table 4.6.1). Several investigators have compiled normative data on these and other biomarkers of bone turnover throughout childhood and/or adolescent age groups (14). There is a consistent peak in the concentrations of most serum markers of bone formation and resorption in adolescence, and this rise occurs approximately 2.5 years earlier in girls than in boys (14). Values in adolescence for the more widely used markers are shown in Table 4.6.1. Although studies are limited, there appears to be less variation by age with serum tartrate-resistant acid phosphatase (17).

Puberty

In addition to the rapid growth spurt beginning in early puberty in girls, and later stages of puberty in boys, bone mineral density accrues at an accelerated pace. The rate of increase in bone mineral density in girls between the ages of 11 and 16 years is more rapid than at any time in late childhood or during adult life. The National Academy of Sciences, USA, has set 'adequate intake' levels for calcium by age ranges. These levels are 210 mg/day through the first 6 months of life, 270 mg/day for months 6–12, 500 mg/day from years 1–3, and 800 mg/day for ages 4–8. In keeping with the rapid rate of bone accretion in adolescence, calcium 'adequate intake' has been set at 1300 mg/day for the 9–18 year-old group (18). Some have thought this number underestimates calcium requirements

Table 4.6.1 Normal values of biochemical markers of bone turnover in childhood

Marker	Age (years)	Value	
		Male	Female
Formative markers			
Serum osteocalcin (ng/ml)[a]	<10	6–35	6–40
	10–18	9–84	7–50
Serum alkaline phosphatase activity (IU/l)[b]	<10	100–300	100–300
	10–18	50–400	50–375
Serum PINP (N-terminal propeptide of type 1 procollagen) (ng/ml)[c]	6–12		250–1500
	6–14		250–1800
	12–16		80–1000
	14–18		80–1500
	16–26		20–200
	18–26		40–300
Resorptive markers			
Serum N-Tx (cross-linked N-terminal-telopeptide of type I collagen) (pmol/ml)[d]	6–12		25–120
	6–14	20–200	
	12–18		8–120
	14–16	14–180	
	18–26		5–25
	16–26		7–50
Urinary N-Tx (pmol equivalent of bone collagen/ μmol creatinine)[e]	<1	500–5000	870–5700
	1	120–2800	475–2750
	2–4	320–2100	155–2010
	5–10	110–1275	115–1620
	11–12	210–2600	235–2430
	13–14	105–1900	45–1335
	15–18	34–1146	45–400
Serum C-Tx (cross-linked C terminal-telopeptide of type I collagen) (pmol/ml)[f]	10–17	3–20	2–12

[a] Extrapolated from Figs 5 and 8, Calvo, *et al.* (13). Note that values will vary with respect to the assay employed and to the laboratory performing the test.
[b] Extrapolated from Figs 5 and 8, Calvo, *et al.* (13). Note that values will vary with respect to the assay employed and to the laboratory performing the test.
[c] Extrapolated from Fig. 2, van der Sluis, *et al.* (14).
[d] Extrapolated from Fig. 3, van der Sluis, *et al.* (14).
[e] Values rounded from Bollen and Eyre (15).
[f] Extrapolated from Fig. 3, Fares, *et al.* (16).

and have suggested that teenage girls consume 1500 mg of calcium daily.

Commensurate with the pubertal growth spurt are transient rises in the markers of bone formative activity, serum osteocalcin and alkaline phosphatase activity. The bone resorptive markers, which decrease somewhat throughout later childhood, decrease substantially in late puberty (Tanner stages IV and V), reflecting more quiescent bone turnover than in earlier childhood, as described above and in Table 4.6.1. The postpubertal period of elevation in turnover markers persists in males longer than in females, suggesting a longer period in young men of active mineral accrual than in young women.

In addition to the changes in bone markers, geometric properties of long bones change during puberty, and appear to differ between boys and girls. These changes may be reflected in the differential changes in biomarker levels described above. However, the finding of wider long bones of males remains largely unexplained. Male long bones progressively grow in circumferential diameter beyond female growth in this regard, in part due to a prolonged period of generalized prepubertal growth (19). Furthermore, recent data suggests that such sex differences in geometry are evident in prepubertal years, determined by complex genetic traits and environmental stimuli (19).

Age-dependent changes in serum minerals and calciotropic hormones

Appropriate diagnosis of disease or monitoring of therapy require an understanding of changes in the biochemical parameters used to facilitate an evaluation of mineral metabolism in children. Figure 4.6.1 illustrates the changes in circulating minerals and related hormones during early infancy. The serum levels of calcium and magnesium do not change significantly after the first few days of life until adulthood. On the other hand urinary excretion of calcium is much greater in infancy than in later childhood and adulthood. A convenient measure for urinary excretion of calcium is the ratio of calcium to creatinine (Ca/Cr) in a random urine sample. Urinary calcium excretion varies with type of feedings, vitamin D nutrition, and gestational age (20). In the older child a fasting urine sample should have a Ca/Cr less than 0.21 (mg/mg). A 24-h urine collection should be confirmed by measurement of total creatinine (which should be 10–20 mg/kg per 24 h in most children), and the calcium should be less than 4 mg/kg per 24 h. Circulating phosphate concentrations decrease considerably throughout the first year of life, and even further throughout later childhood. The normal ranges are substantially greater than that seen in older adults. This change is primarily due to increased reclamation of filtered phosphate in the proximal renal tubule early in life. The confusion in interpretation of age-related normal ranges has continued to result in missed diagnoses and inappropriate interpretation of mineral status. The assessment of urinary phosphate excretion should be performed on a 2-h fasting urine specimen, with a blood sample obtained at the midpoint of the urine collection. The tubular reabsorption of phosphate (TRP) is calculated as:

$$\%TRP = 1- \varphi\, U_P \times P_{Cr}\, \kappa \times 100$$

$$\lambda\, P_p \times U_{Cr}\, \mu$$

The %TRP can be plotted on the nomogram of Walton and Bijvoet (21) to obtain the TMP/GFR, or tubular maximum for phosphate expressed per GFR. This value reflects the value of serum phosphate above which one will tend to stop reclaiming phosphate in the tubule. The normal ranges vary with age and approximate the normal phosphate concentrations for age.

Finally, values for circulating PTH do not change after early infancy throughout childhood. Circulating 1,25 $(OH)_2D$ levels tend to be slightly higher in childhood than in later life. This is particularly true during the first 2 years of life. The authors generally have observed values up to 30% in excess of the adult normal range in normal children at his institution. Furthermore, there appears to be

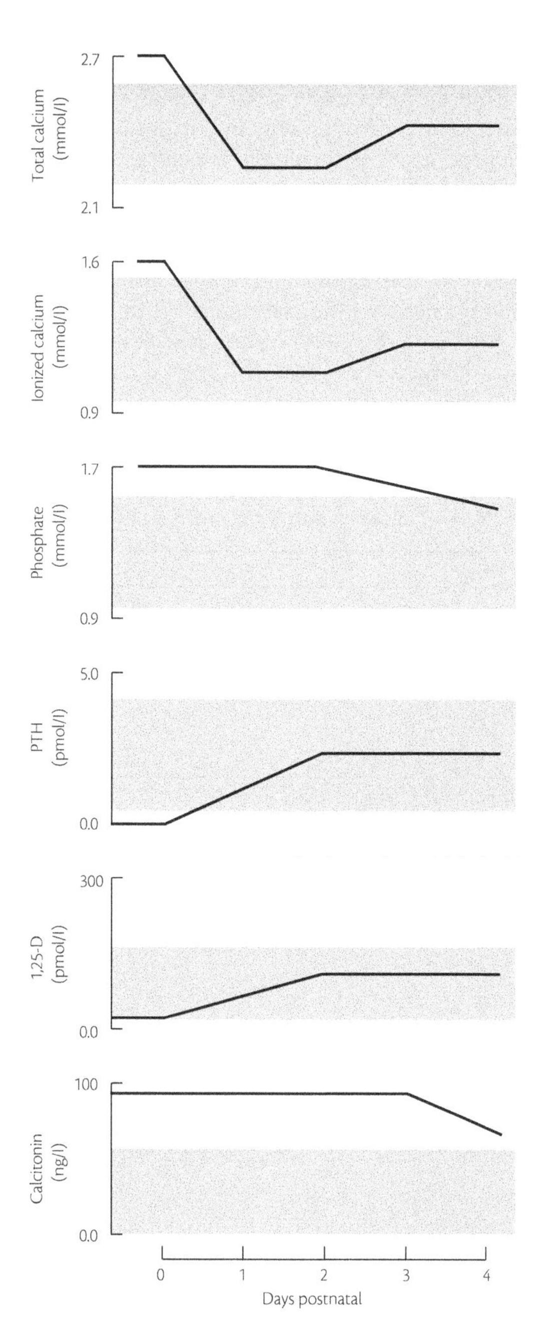

Fig. 4.6.1 Longitudinal change in circulating concentrations of minerals, parathyroid hormone (PTH), calcitonin, and 1,25-dihydroxyvitamin D (1,25 D) during the first few days of life. Shaded areas represent the adult normal range for the parameter. (From Kovacs CS, Kronenberg HM, Maternal-fetal calcium and bone metabolism during pregnancy, puerpium, and lactation. *Endocr Rev*, 1997; 18: 832–72, with permission (3).)

less stringent regulation of conversion of 25 (OH)D to 1,25 $(OH)_2D$ in early life.

Disorders of hypocalcaemia

Serum calcium

Total serum calcium is comprised of a free or ionized calcium component, a protein (primarily albumin) bound component, and a small component of filterable calcium that is complexed to other ions such as sulfate, citrate, or phosphate. The ionized and protein-bound components each represent approximately 45–50% of the total calcium. The ionized fraction is the active component, and derangements in this fraction result in symptoms. As discussed elsewhere, serum calcium can be low with a simultaneously normal ionized fraction. This finding is typical of hypoalbuminaemia or acidosis. Various correction factors have been proposed, and are applicable to children as well as adults, however accurate measures of ionized calcium are preferable to calculated corrections.

Hypocalcaemia in childhood

This section discusses disorders of calcium homoeostasis in childhood, with a primary focus on abnormalities in the maintenance of serum calcium. Several of these disorders, however, primarily affect the skeletal calcium compartment, and bone disease may be a more significant abnormality than perturbations in the serum concentrations. Thus certain disorders are described in which serum calcium levels are often normal in the clinical setting, but at the expense of osteopenic or rachitic abnormalities.

The presentation of hypocalcaemia in the newborn period typically includes facial twitching, limb jitteriness, or other features of neuromuscular irritability, occasionally progressing to focal or generalized convulsions. Poor feeding, hyperacusis, and laryngospasm have been described. On the other hand, nonspecific findings such as apnoea, tachypnoea, tachycardia, cyanosis, or vomiting may be the only features evident. In older children tetany or perioral tingling, presentations more characteristically seen in adults, are more likely to be encountered. As with infants, focal seizures and generalized convulsions may occur. Carpopedal spasm in school-age children has often been attributed to a writer's cramp. This phenomenon may be exacerbated by the hypomagnesaemia and alkalosis frequently encountered in states of parathyroid insufficiency. Lethargy, vomiting, and other nonspecific signs have also been reported. The electrocardiogram may reveal a prolonged corrected Q–T interval, $Q–T_c$, which is determined by dividing the Q–T interval by the square root of the EKG cycle. The upper limit of normal in children is 0.44. The musculature may be affected by chronic hypocalcaemia. Serum creatine kinase activity may be elevated in chronic hypocalcaemia; over time actual myopathic changes may occur.

Neonatal hypocalcaemia

Neonatal hypocalcaemia seen transiently in the first few days of life is commonly referred to as early neonatal hypocalcaemia. This is often seen in preterm infants and has been explained as an exaggeration of the normal postnatal decrease in serum calcium levels. Early neonatal hypocalcaemia appears to occur with greater frequency in asphyxiated babies and in infants of diabetic mothers than otherwise. The hypocalcaemia seen in infants of diabetic mothers is probably multifactorial. Magnesium deficiency has been implicated, as well as alterations in maternal metabolism secondary to poor glucose control throughout gestation. Whether the normal postnatal increase in PTH secretion is blunted is not entirely clear.

Late neonatal hypocalcaemia occurs after 5–7 days of life and is a syndrome more characteristic of the term infant. Late neonatal hypocalcaemia often presents with seizures and is less likely to be transient in nature. Hypoparathyroidism and magnesium deficiency often present in this time frame. Hypocalcaemia in babies with congenital heart disease of many types has been reported as a relatively common finding. Hypocalcaemia related to vitamin D deficiency may present at several weeks of age, however radiographic evidence of rickets is usually not observed until the child is over 2 months old.

One classic situation in which prolonged neonatal hypocalcaemia occurs is in the infant of the hyperparathyroid mother. Presumably the maternal hypercalcaemia results in increased transport of calcium from the maternal to fetal circulation. The resultant excess calcium supply to the fetus is thought to suppress parathyroid responsivity, and prolonged hypoparathyroidism results. Symptomatic hypocalcaemia and hyperphosphataemia are typical biochemical features; hypomagnesaemia may occur as well. The disorder is usually transient, but some cases have been prolonged for months. Unrecognized maternal hyperparathyroidism should be carefully investigated in children that present with the characteristic features of the disorder. Maternal familial hypocalciuric hypercalcaemia (FHH) can result in this syndrome; it is presumed that any cause of chronic maternal hypercalcaemia can result in a similar clinical picture.

Hypocalcaemia in the newborn setting may also occur during blood transfusions using citrated blood products. Citrate complexes with ionized calcium, reducing its circulating concentration to a level where neuromuscular hyperexcitability may occur. Total serum calcium is usually not decreased. Hypocalcaemia can occur in the congenital nephrotic syndrome. Persistent hypocalcaemia may present in this time frame as well. Congenital hypoparathyroidism may be present, as in the DiGeorge syndrome. The classic triad of this chromosome 22 deletion syndrome (hypoparathyroidism, athymia, and conotruncal defects of the heart) typically results in long-standing hypoparathyroidism, although 'partial' hypoparathyroidism has been described. Mitochondrial diseases also may present as congenital hypoparathyroidism. Severe osteopetrosis may present with hypocalcaemia secondary to impaired mobilization of calcium from bone. Typically PTH levels are elevated in this situation. Severe vitamin D deficiency is generally an acquired condition manifest as hypocalcaemia as early as 2–3 months, but low maternal stores have rarely contributed to its development in an even younger age range.

Osteopenia of prematurity is commonly encountered in premature infants. Poor bone mineralization is evident on radiographs or other measures of bone mineral density. In general, the problem is more severe in children of lower birthweight. With increasing survival of children with birthweights less than 1000 g the severity of this problem is increasing. Classical rachitic changes of flared and frayed epiphyses, craniotabes, and a rachitic rosary may develop over the first months of life. The histological pattern of bone is thought to be a combined lesion with components of osteomalacia and osteoporosis. This disorder is a consequence of premature withdrawal of the maternal mineral supply. The enteral route, even with maximum feeding delivery, cannot provide for the mineral demands of the skeleton as it rapidly grows and mineralizes throughout the latter weeks of gestation. The problem often occurs in the setting of normocalcaemia. In preterm infants fed solely with breast milk, a phosphate deficiency syndrome may occur, as the phosphate content of breast milk is considerably less than that of commonly used cow's milk formulas. Although breast milk phosphate is adequate for the growth of the term infant's skeleton, human breast milk fortifiers are routinely used to increase the mineral intake of the preterm infant. One caveat regarding the use of such fortifiers: calcium intake, if excessive, can result in hypercalcaemia, as its absorption is not tightly regulated in early infancy, and the fractional absorption of calcium can be very high in a low birthweight premature infant.

Treatment of neonatal hypocalcaemia

Symptomatic infants are replaced with calcium, but there is controversy regarding treatment of hypocalcaemic infants who are asymptomatic. The emergency treatment of neonatal hypocalcaemia consists of the intravenous administration of 1 ml/min of 10% calcium gluconate, which should not exceed 2.0 ml/kg. This may be repeated three to four times in 24 h. After acute symptoms have been managed, 5.0 ml/kg of 10% calcium gluconate may be given with intravenous fluids over 24 h. Calcium supplements may be introduced orally if tolerated. In persistent cases, the load of dietary phosphate should be lessened with a formula such as Similac PM 60/40. When hypomagnesaemia is identified, it can be treated with 0.1–0.2 ml/kg of a 50% solution of magnesium sulfate ($MgSO_4 \cdot 7H_2O$).

Hypocalcaemia of later onset

Disorders of parathyroid insufficiency

Congenital hypoparathyroidism A wide variety of hypocalcaemic syndromes occur in children due to abnormalities in parathyroid synthesis or secretion. These syndromes provide classic examples of the critical role PTH plays in protecting the organism from acute decreases in the serum calcium level. The clinical manifestations of hypocalcaemia described above are the typical presenting features of hypoparathyroidism. Biochemical features usually include low blood total and ionized calcium levels, and an elevated blood phosphate level. The serum magnesium level may be low, and alkalosis may be present.

Hypoparathyroidism may result from a variety of causes (Box 4.6.1). A number of genetic disorders may cause agenesis of parathyroid glands, disrupt PTH synthesis, processing, and secretion, and/or result in autoimmune destruction of parathyroid glands. As noted above, agenesis of the parathyroid glands occurs in the classic DiGeorge (OMIM 530000) triad of hypoparathyroidism, athymia, and conotruncal heart defects. This syndrome is now known to be part of the larger spectrum of disease referred to as CATCH 22, a sequence of contiguous microdeletion syndromes localized to chromosome 22q11.2. These mutations are most notable in the *TBX1* gene, a transcription factor which plays an important role in development of thymus and parathyroid glands (22, 23). Hypoparathyroidism usually occurs in those disorders most related to the classic DiGeorge's syndrome, but has also been described in the velocardiofacial syndrome, another CATCH-22 pattern of anomalies. Fluorescent *in situ* hybridization using DNA probes that hybridize to the 22q11.2 locus are helpful in establishing the diagnosis.

Box 4.6.1 Aetiology of hypoparathyroidism

- Congenital
  - Processing defects in parathyroid hormone synthesis
  - Aplasia (DiGeorge/velocardiofacial syndromes)
  - Mitochondrial disease
  - Ca-sensing receptor (autosomal dominant hypocalcaemia)
  - Familial hypomagnesaemia
- Acquired
  - Autoimmune
  - Surgical
  - Magnesium deficiency
  - Thalassaemia, Wilson's disease
  - Burns

Mutations of the preproPTH gene, resulting in disruption of PTH secretion (24), or processing and translocation of PTH (OMIM 146200) from the endoplasmic reticulum, (25) can cause familial isolated hypoparathyroidism (24). Likewise, mutations of the transcription factor glial cells missing 2 (*GCM2*; also referred to as glial cell missing B (*GCMB*)), resulting in loss of activity, will result in familial isolated hypoparathyroidism (26–29). A form of X-linked hypoparathyroidism has been reported in patients with mutation in the gene for the transcription factor Syr box 3 (*SOX3*) (30).

A number of other patients with congenital hypoparathyroidism have concomitant involvement of other organ systems. The syndrome of hypoparathyroidism, sensorineural deafness, and renal anomalies (HDR syndrome) (OMIM 146255) is an autosomal dominant disorder due to mutations or deletions of the gene for the transcription factor GATA3 on chromosome 10 (31–34). Loss-of-function mutations in tubulin chaperone E (*TBCE*) gene cause the autosomal recessive syndrome of hypoparathyroidism, mental retardation, and dysmorphism (Sanjad–Sakati syndrome) (OMIM 241410) (35–37) and Kenny–Caffey syndrome (hypoparathyroidism, dwarfism, medullary stenosis of the long bones, and eye abnormalities) (OMIM 244460). Mitochondrial gene defects, ranging from deletions to mutations and rearrangement, have been associated with hypoparathyroidism in patients with Kearns–Sayre syndrome (OMIM 53000) (external ophthalmoplegia, pigmentary retinopathy, cardiomyopathy, diabetes, and hypoparathyroidism), MELAS (OMIM 540000) syndrome (diabetes and hypoparathyroidism), and MTPDS syndrome (peripheral neuropathy, retinopathy, hypoparathyroidism) (24, 38, 39). Other mitochondrial disorders associated with hypoparathyroidism include mitochondrial trifunctional protein deficiency (OMIM 609015), long-chain 3-hydroxyacyl-coenzyme A dehydrogenase deficiency (LCHAD) (OMIM 609016), and propionic acidaemia (OMIM 606054). We have recently observed hypoparathyroidism in a mitochondrial DNA deletion syndrome initially diagnosed as Pearson's syndrome (OMIM 557000).

Gain-of-function mutations of the recently discovered calcium-sensing receptor (*CaSR*) on parathyroid cells have been found to cause an autosomal dominant variety of hypocalcaemia. The CaSR has increased affinity for ionized calcium, such that relatively low concentrations of this ion effectively suppress PTH secretion, and a steady state serum calcium level in the hypocalcaemic range is established. One family with previously diagnosed autosomal dominant hypoparathyroidism has been shown to actually have this disorder. It may be possible to distinguish autosomal dominant hypocalcaemia from other forms of parathyroid insufficiency because of the relative hypercalciuria that occurs. Circulating PTH levels may not be undetectable in the untreated state (40). This distinction from hypoparathyroidism has important consequences regarding long-term management. That is, the standard treatments for hypoparathyroidism, vitamin D or its metabolites, and calcium, can further exaggerate this hypercalciuria such that nephrocalcinosis, nephrolithiasis, and renal impairment may result, particularly when serum calcium levels are kept in the usual normal range. The CaSR and associated disorders are discussed in Chapter 4.4.

Acquired hypoparathyroidism A major cause of acquired hypoparathyroidism is due to the autoimmune polyglandular syndrome (APS) type I. The disorder is also referred to by other names such as autoimmune polyendocrinopathy, candidiasis, and ectodermal dystrophy (APECED) (41). The primary manifestations of this disorder include hypoparathyroidism, primary adrenal insufficiency, and mucocutaneous candidiasis. A variety of other autoimmune phenomena may occur, often grouped with the endocrine, gastrointestinal, or dermatological systems (Box 4.6.2). Defects in cellular or humoral immunity may occur. The presentation typically begins in early childhood with candidiasis. In later childhood the onset of hypocalcaemic symptoms related to hypoparathyroidism occurs, and Addison disease often presents during adolescence. There is considerable variability, however, and often patients do not develop the classic triad. The elevation in serum calcium that may occur during an acute adrenal crisis in an undiagnosed individual may result in an increase of the serum calcium from a hypocalcaemic to a normocalcaemic value, thus masking a coexistent presentation of hypoparathyroidism. Serum calcium should be determined during the initial presentation of suspected Addison's disease, but also shortly after recovery from the acute crisis.

APS 1 syndrome is due to mutations in the gene encoding the autoimmune regulator protein AIRE (42–44). Mutations resulting in a single amino acid substitution at position 257 (arginine→glutamic acid) were present in more than three-quarters of the affected Finnish cases. The same mutation has been identified in the majority of cases in another series from Italy and Switzerland. Autoantibodies directed to parathyroid cells have been described in patients with APS 1, but the frequency of these findings vary greatly dependent upon the series studied (45). In one recent series, antibodies to the parathyroid CaSR were detected in the sera of approximately half the affected individuals.

In addition to the usual measures taken in the management of hypoparathyroidism, treatment of this disorder may require aggressive mineral replacement, due to the often complicating issue of malabsorption. Acute illness can be associated with such severe impairment of gastrointestinal absorption of calcium and magnesium that parenteral replacement of these minerals may be required. Continuous nocturnal nasogastric calcium supplementation may be a useful temporary measure in the affected child unable to tolerate standard bolus feeding, and where prolonged parenteral infusions are not practical.

Box 4.6.2 Clinical features of autoimmune polyendocrinopathy syndrome type I

- Major manifestations
  - Chronic hypoparathyroidism
  - Chronic candidiasis
  - Autoimmune Addison disease
- Other manifestations
  - Autoimmune hypogonadotropic hypogonadism
  - Alopecia
  - Chronic hepatitis
  - Chronic atrophic gastritis
  - Pernicious anaemia
  - Vitiligo
  - Malabsorption
  - Sjögren's syndrome
  - Autoimmune thyroid disease
  - Keratoconjunctivitis
  - Hypophysitis
  - Insulin-dependent diabetes mellitus
  - Vasculitis
  - Haemolytic anaemia
  - Turner syndrome

In decreasing order of incidence. (Adapted from Betterle C, Greggio NA, Volpato M. Autoimmune polyglandular syndrome type 1. *J Clin Endocrinol Metab*, 1998; 83: 1049–55 (41)).

The long-term prognosis of this condition has improved greatly over the past generation. Early cases succumbed to such problems as unrecognized adrenal crises or diabetic ketoacidosis. Although numerous complications of this disorder are recorded, including overwhelming *Candida* sepsis, oesophageal carcinoma, and chronic active hepatitis, these severe features are rare. One review records a 50-year survival of greater than 75%.

Surgical hypoparathyroidism is rarely encountered in childhood. Standard guidelines for thyroid surgery include identification and preservation of parathyroid tissue. The use of radioactive iodine to ablate any thyroid remnants following surgery for cancer has resulted in a less aggressive approach to thyroid surgery. Transient hypocalcaemia in the 36 hours acutely following thyroid surgery is common, although no mechanism has been clearly established which accounts for this finding. Early (1 hour) postoperative intact PTH measurement has been proposed as a sensitive way of identifying patients who are at risk of becoming hypocalcaemic (46, 47).

Hypoparathyroidism may occur as a complication in disorders related to metal toxicity. Thalassaemia has been shown to result in a variety of endocrinopathies related to iron deposition. Although hypoparathyroidism was recognized as an occasional complication in most clinics managing such patients, the incidence of this complication has decreased over the past 20 years with increasing use of chelating therapies such as desferoxamine (48). Hypoparathyroidism has been reported to occur in Wilson's disease presumably related to copper deposition in the parathyroid glands (49).

Functional hypoparathyroidism occurs in severe magnesium deficiency. Both impairment of parathyroid secretion and resistance to PTH activity at the renal tubule have been described in the setting of chronic magnesium deficiency. In classic studies by Anast *et al.* (50), the dependence of the parathyroid glands on magnesium for secretion of PTH was described in a girl with a congenital magnesium wasting syndrome. It appears that more subtle defects in PTH secretion may occur with less severe magnesium depletion. The serum magnesium level may not reflect total body magnesium status, as magnesium is predominantly an intracellular ion. However, magnesium deficiency associated with a serum level of greater than 1.3 mg/dl is unlikely to result in clinically significant changes in parathyroid secretion. In children, chronic magnesium deficiency occurs in familial hypomagnesaemia (51). Familial hypomagnesaemia (OMIM 602014) with secondary hypocalcaemia is an autosomal recessive disease due to mutations in the TRPM6 ion channel, resulting in electrolyte abnormalities in the newborn period (52). This disorder may present with hypocalcaemic/ hypomagnesaemic seizures in the first 2 months of life. If diagnosed early, severe neurologic impairment may be prevented. Mutations in paracellin (encoded by *CLDN16*), a renal tubular paracellular transport protein of the claudin family, may also cause hypomagnesaemia, hypocalcaemia, and hypercalciuria (53) (OMIM 248250). Another member of this family, *CLDN19*, may also cause a similar syndrome (54) (OMIM 248190). Gitelman's syndrome (OMIM 263800) is an autosomal recessive disorder of magnesium and potassium wasting with metabolic alkalosis and hypocalciuria, due to mutations in *SLC12A3*, which encodes a thiazide-sensitive Na–Cl cotransporter (55).

Hypomagnesaemia in children occurs more frequently in children with the use of chemotherapeutic agents such as cisplatin, and with aminoglycoside diuretics such as tobramycin. Hypomagnesaemia has been reported with ibuprofen overdosage in a 21-month old child simultaneously treated with furosemide (56), and following ingestion of ammonium bifluoride-containing automobile wheel cleaner (57). Recent data have suggested that moderate decreases in serum magnesium levels accompany the hypocalcaemia encountered during rehabilitation from burn injuries in children (58).

Treatment of chronic hypoparathyroidism The mainstay of the management of chronic hypoparathyroidism is replacement with oral calcium supplements and an active metabolite of vitamin D, such as 1,25 $(OH)_2D_3$ (calcitriol) or 1α $(OH)D_3$. Various liquid forms of calcium carbonate (often sold as antacids for children) are useful for the small child unable to take tablets. The doses are titrated to maintain the serum calcium in the slightly low to low-normal range, with care not to render the child hypercalciuric. This is especially a concern in patients with autosomal dominant hypocalcaemia due to activating mutations in the CaSR. Teraparatide (parathyroid hormone (1–34)) and calcilytic agents (antagonists of CaSR) are currently being studied as potential therapeutics for these disorders.

PTH resistance and pseudohypoparathyroidism

Resistance to parathyroid hormone has been termed pseudohypoparathyroidism (PHP). The classical form of the disease, PHP type 1A is due to mutations in the alpha subunit of the heterotrimeric guanine nucleotide binding protein, G_s. The change in conformation of this protein, induced by interaction of PTH with its receptor, activates membrane adenylate cyclase, thus initiating the protein kinase C signal transduction pathway. Patients with PHP 1a fail to transduce PTH (and various other peptide hormone) signals in target tissues. The syndrome represents a fascinating aspect of hormone receptor biology, and is discussed in detail in Chapter 4.5. For our purposes here, we will describe only a few of the clinical features pertinent to children with the disorder.

The major clinical features of PHP 1a (OMIM 103580) are: (1) resistance to PTH, manifest by hypocalcaemia and hyperphosphataemia; (2) a specific phenotype of short stature, round facies, and other skeletal features such as the presence of shortened fourth metacarpal bones, collectively referred to as Albright's hereditary osteodystrophy; and (3) generalized resistance to peptide hormones that require intact $G_s\alpha$ for signal transduction. PHP may be suspected in child within a family because of other affected members or individuals that manifest the PHP 1a phenotype, but have no biochemical abnormalities or other endocrine deficiencies. Presentations in infancy may include short stature and congenital hypothyroidism, but manifestations of hypocalcaemia usually appear in later in childhood.

PHP 1b (OMIM 603233) is also linked to the $G_s\alpha$ gene on chromosome 21, but isolated PTH resistance occurs with none of skeletal features manifest in type 1a Associated endocrine abnormalities are usually mild or absent. PHP 1c (OMIM 612462) refers to syndromes of PTH resistance, with other associated endocrine abnormalities, but without Albright's hereditary osteodystrophy. Evidence as been presented indicating that PHP types 1a and 1b are subject to expression by genomic imprinting (59–62).

Type II PHP (OMIM 203330) refers to PTH resistance mediated by a pathway not resulting from interference with the generation of cAMP by adenylate cyclase. No specific phenotype, or associated hormone resistance, occurs.

Treatment of PHP is similar to that for primary hypoparathyroidism, although there is usually little risk of hypercalciuria in the classic (1a) form of the disease. Other features of the disease may require therapy, such as hypothyroidism, and monitoring of subcutaneous ectopic ossification, which if severe may require surgical removal.

Disorders related to vitamin D

Hypocalcaemia may result from a deficiency of vitamin D, usually related to limited dietary content of vitamin D or limited exposure to ultraviolet light, critical in the early steps of endogenous vitamin D production in skin. Sufficient UV light is necessary for the production of previtamin D in the stratum spinosum of the dermis. UVB light of wavelength 290–315 nm provides the energy to disrupt the 9–10 C–C bond in the B ring of the steroid nucleus of 7-dehydrocholesterol (Fig. 4.6.2). Previtamin D is then rapidly isomerized in the skin to vitamin D. Thus vitamin D deficiency is most frequent in parts of the world where sunlight exposure is limited or exposure to sunlight is prevented. In North America, there have been numerous recent reports of vitamin D deficiency rickets in breast-fed children not supplemented with vitamin D. Breast milk contains little vitamin D, unless the mother is taking pharmacological doses of the vitamin. Pigmented individuals are at higher risk for this problem, as melanin absorbs UV light external to the layer of skin where vitamin D synthesis occurs. There is a greater

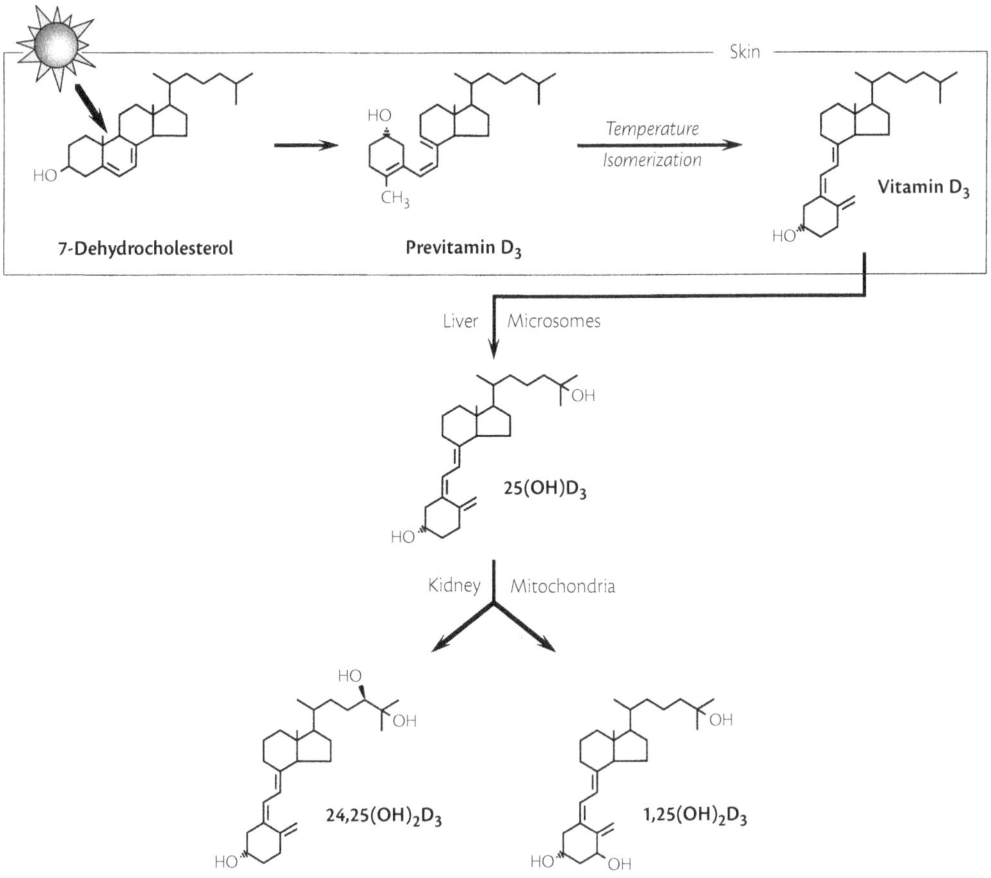

Fig. 4.6.2 The vitamin D biosynthetic pathway. The steroid nucleus of 7-dehydrocholesterol is converted in skin to previtamin D_3 with exposure to UVB light and rapidly isomerized to vitamin D_3, which is found in nmol/L concentrations in the circulation. This metabolite is converted to 25 $(OH)D_3$ in hepatic microsomes, and is also found in nmol/L amounts in the circulation. Measurement of circulating 25 $(OH)D_3$ is a biomarker of total body vitamin D stores. 25 $(OH)D_3$ is converted in renal mitochondria to the best-known active metabolite, 1,25 $(OH)_2D_3$ which circulates in pg/ml concentrations in serum. Conversion of 25 $(OH)D_3$ to 24,25 $(OH)_2D_3$ also occurs in renal mitochondria.

incidence of the problem in the late winter as compared to other times of the year. In some children, vitamin D deficiency is compounded by the coincident problem of calcium deficiency. This problem may occur in lactose intolerant children avoiding dairy products, or when the diet has a very high phytate content (as with certain grains and cereals) which can limit the bioavailability of ingested calcium.

Vitamin D deficiency may often present with rachitic bone disease. Symptomatic hypocalcaemia generally occurs late in the course of development of vitamin D deficiency. The initial decreases in intestinal calcium absorption which result from vitamin D deficiency are readily compensated for by the resultant secondary elevations in PTH. When frank hypocalcaemia with tetany or seizures occurs due to vitamin D deficiency, substantial chronicity of vitamin D deficiency has usually been present.

Vitamin D is further metabolized to its most abundant circulating metabolite, 25 (OH)D, and its best-known active metabolite, 1,25 $(OH)_2D$. The critical mechanism of action for this involves binding to its receptor, a DNA binding protein which is part of the large superfamily of steroid/ thyroid/ retinoid receptors. Pathophysiology similar to vitamin D deficiency may result from defects in the 1α hydroxylase enzyme instrumental in the synthesis of 1,25 $(OH)_2D$, or in mutations in the vitamin D receptor.

Clinical features of rickets in children include bowing of the lower extremities, craniotabes, and rachitic rosary (hypertrophy of the costochondral junctions). These syndromes are discussed in detail in Chapter 4.10. The laboratory findings of vitamin D-related hypocalcaemic disorders are compared in Table 4.6.2.

Establishment of an appropriate biochemical threshold for the definition of vitamin D deficiency has received considerable attention recently. In the adult population the circulating 25(OH)D level of 32 ng/ml (80 nmol/l) has been suggested as an appropriate target threshold for the definition of vitamin D deficiency (63). Recent reports of various health benefits have been associated with vitamin D status, mostly related to a variety of associations of 25 (OH)D level and prevalence of certain disorders, including diabetes, multiple sclerosis, cancers (particularly colorectal), and obesity (64). These data are epidemiological in nature, and the possibility that vitamin D status serves as a marker for other unidentified contributors to disease remains. Perhaps the most convincing direct evidence of 'nonclassical' vitamin D effects (i.e. effects apart from those influencing systemic calcium homoeostasis) comes from immunological studies demonstrating important effects of vitamin D on macrophages (65). In the presence of activated toll-like receptors 1/2, macrophages are able to express their own 1α hydroxlase and its own vitamin D receptor. Thus the macrophage has the capacity to metabolize 25 (OH)D and to use the activated product, 1,25 $(OH)_2D$, in autocrine fashion, as it can produce this molecule's receptor. The stimulation of the macrophage in this way leads to the production of a unique antimicrobial peptide, cathelicidin, which is inhibitory to the growth of *Mycobacterium tuberculosis*. Thus a clear mechanism exists by which vitamin D may play a role in fighting infection. In other studies based on linear regression analysis of small population data, elevations in circulating PTH occur as levels of circulating 25 (OH)D decrease. However the threshold values of 25 (OH)D at which an increase

Table 4.6.2 Laboratory findings in childhood syndromes presenting with hypocalcaemia

Syndrome	Serum biochemical measures					
	Ca	P	Alkaline phosphatase	PTH	25D	1,25D
Vitamin D deficiency	N,9	N,9	8	8	9	9,N,8
Calcium deficiency	N,9	N,9	8	8	N	8
Vitamin D 1-α hydroxylase defect	9,N	9,N	8	8	N	9,N
Hereditary resistance to vitamin D	9,N	9,N	8	8	N	8
Hypoparathyroidism	9	8	N	9	N	9,N,8
Pseudohypoparathyroidism	9	8	N	9	N	9,N

PTH, parathyroid hormone; 25D, 25-hydroxyvitamin D; 1,25D 1,25 dihydroxyvitamin D; N, normal level; 9, decreased level; 8, increased level.

in PTH levels occurs is quite variable (67), suggesting caution in using this measure as a generalizable means of establishing vitamin D deficiency. Nevertheless, these findings, in sum, raise the issue of revising the threshold for 25 (OH)D level as a measure of optimal vitamin D status, and toxicity information in adults appear to indicate that modest increases in supplementation is safe. Data are not yet available to establish a clear benefit to this approach, and the application of such measures to infants and children needs to be carefully examined. Indeed, the administration of vitamin D to infants and children at the increased levels recently suggested for supplementation in adults could be risky. The authors have recently observed hypercalcaemia in an infant given 1400 units of supplemental vitamin D daily, with concomitant circulating 25 (OH)D levels over 225 nmol/l (90 ng/ml). Thus we have continued to support a conservative definition of vitamin D deficiency, using threshold values for 25 (OH)D of 37.5–50 nmol/l (15–20 ng/ml). Likewise, in the normal healthy term infant we advise adherence to current recommendations of a daily vitamin D intake of 400 IU.

Treatment Vitamin D in dosages of 1000–2000 IU/day is a standard approach to the initial treatment of vitamin D deficiency. As rachitic lesions heal, the dosage is decreased to 400 IU/day, the generally recognized recommended daily allowance. A single intramuscular dose of 6 00 000 units of vitamin D, or in two oral doses of 3 00 000 units each can be given in the outpatient clinic if the clinical situation would indicate that limited follow-up will occur.

The specialty clinician may happen to evaluate such a patient after a change in season, and sunlight exposure has concomitantly increased since the onset of the disease, or after vitamin supplementation has begun. This situation should be recognized clinically, as low-normal values of the 25 (OH)D level may confuse the diagnosis. Radiographs may demonstrate a thin, dense line of opacity at the metaphyses of long bones, which indicates that recent rapid mineralization has occurred at the edge of the growth plate.

As mentioned above, children with vitamin D deficiency often require supplemental calcium. Some children may manifest hungry bone syndrome, in which mineralization is rapid and serum calcium levels may decrease as the bone mineralizes. Thus supplemental calcium is given in many cases to provide a total daily intake of 30–50 mg/kg of elemental calcium. Vitamin D stores may be depleted rapidly during calcium insufficiency (68), suggesting that dietary calcium deficiency itself may be yet another risk factor for the development of vitamin D deficiency.

Deficiency of 1α hydroxylase is best treated with physiological doses of 1,25 $(OH)_2D_3$. Hereditary resistance to vitamin D may respond to high dosages of 1,25 $(OH)_2D_3$, but some patients require parenteral calcium infusions (69).

Other causes of hypocalcaemia

Hypocalcaemia may also result from rapid loading of phosphate into the circulation. This phenomenon occurs in settings of tissue destruction, such as in tumour lysis syndrome observed during early phases of chemotherapy of large solid tumours. Rhabdomyolysis may decrease serum calcium levels for similar reasons. Several cases of hypocalcaemia and seizures have occurred following high-dose administration of phosphate either by enema or by the oral route. The use of phosphate-based cathartics in infants and small children is contraindicated. We are aware of one case in which severe hyperphosphataemia and hypocalcaemia occurred repetitively in a small child surreptitiously administered oral phosphate by her mother. Hypocalcaemia may also occurs in the setting of pancreatitis due to precipitation of calcium-containing salts in the inflamed pancreatic tissue and it often correlates with the severity of the episode. Children with acute or chronic renal failure will also develop mild hypocalcaemia which is due to a multitude of precipitating factors, such as hyperphosphataemia, and decreased 1α hydroxylation of 25-hydroxyvitamin D. Hypocalcaemia has recently been associated with high volume (1.5 litres or more per week) of soft drinks containing phosphoric acid (70). Hypocalcaemia solely due to low dietary calcium intake has been reported (71). This syndrome has occurred in areas of South Africa in areas where food content is relatively low in calcium, and rickets is the usual presenting feature. The combination of dietary vitamin D and calcium deficiency is more commonly seen in North American children (see above).

Disorders of hypercalcaemia

Persistent hypercalcaemia is usually attributed to some combination of the following mechanisms: (1) excessive intestinal absorption of calcium; (2) excessive bone resorption of mineral; and (3) abnormal renal retention of calcium. Infants are usually asymptomatic with mild to moderate hypercalcaemia (11.0–13.0 mg/dl). More severe hypercalcaemia may lead to failure to thrive, poor feeding, hypotonia, vomiting, seizures, lethargy, polyuria, and hypertension. Hypercalcaemia is discussed in detail in Chapter 4.2. Several syndromes with specific childhood features are described below.

Severe neonatal hyperparathyroidism (OMIM 239200) is a rare condition presenting with hypercalcaemic symptoms in the first few days of life. Serum calcium levels may range as high as 15 to 30 mg/dl. The serum phosphate level is usually low, and serum PTH is elevated. The hypercalcaemia is predominantly due to increased bone resorption, but elevated intestinal absorption of calcium, as well as increased renal calcium retention, probably occur. Radiographs of the clavicles typically reveal features of primary hyperparathyroidism. Nephrocalcinosis may be present on ultrasonographic examination. Severe neonatal hyperparathyroidism may occur in families with familial hypocalciuric hypercalcemia (FHH) (OMIM 145980). This autosomal dominant trait is manifest by modest asymptomatic hypercalcaemia with relative hypocalciuria and normal or slightly increased serum PTH levels. A loss-of-function mutation in the *CaSR* gene on parathyroid cells, acts in a dominant negative manner in FHH; severe neonatal hyperparathyroidism has been shown to result in individuals homozygous for such a mutation (72). Severe neonatal hyperparathyroidism usually requires emergency extirpation of the parathyroid glands. Hypercalcaemia of sufficient severity to warrant surgery has also been described in infants in FHH families that have only one mutant copy of the *CaSR* gene (73).

In severe Williams syndrome (OMIM 194050), symptoms may be present from the neonatal period, but more frequently recognized later in the first few years of life. Infantile hypercalcaemia may be a presenting feature, in addition to pre- and postnatal growth failure. A characteristic, unusual facies (Fig. 4.6.3) is often present, as well as cardiovascular abnormalities (usually supravalvular aortic stenosis or peripheral pulmonic stenosis), delayed psychomotor development, and selective mental deficiency. A deletion of the elastin gene is found in many cases of Williams' syndrome. The serum calcium levels may range as high as 12–19 mg/dl. The hypercalcaemia usually subsides spontaneously by the age of 4 years.

The pathogenesis of hypercalcaemia (OMIM 143880) is uncertain, although various disturbances in vitamin D metabolism have been described. Treatment has traditionally consisted of placing the child on a low calcium diet, free of vitamin D. Short-term therapy with corticosteroids may also be necessary. More recently we have found that intravenous bisphosphonate therapy is quite effective in controlling hypercalcaemia in Williams' syndrome patients. We usually use pamidronate at a dose of 0.25–0.5 mg/kg per dose, and have found that one to three doses have been sufficient to manage this problem permanently.

Milder forms of idiopathic infantile hypercalcaemia have been described with less severe hypercalcaemia and less overt clinical features, however the degree of hypercalcaemia can be quite variable among children with a classic phenotype. Elevations in PTHrP have been reported in some of these individuals.

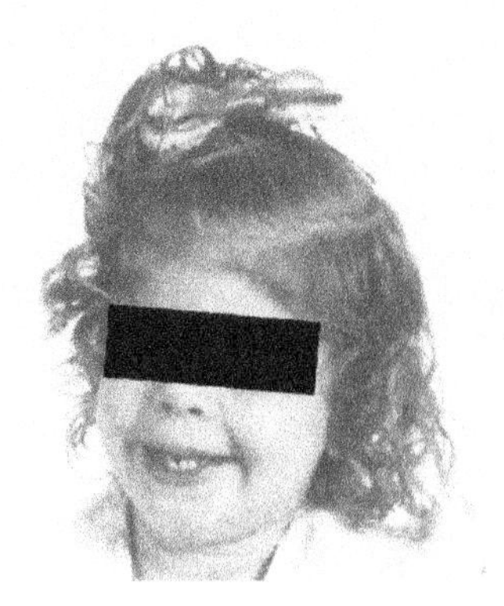

Fig. 4.6.3 The characteristic facies of a child affected with Williams' syndrome.

Subcutaneous fat necrosis is a self-limited disorder which presents in infancy with symptoms of hypercalcaemia and violacious discoloration of the skin. These areas of discoloration consist of a mononuclear cell infiltrate, sometimes coexistent with small calcification. Increased production of 1,25 $(OH)_2D$ has been described. Thus a vitamin D-free, low calcium diet and glucocorticoids have traditionally been used to treat the disorder. More recently, we have employed pamidronate (0.25 mg/kg body weight) to successfully control hypercalcaemia in this condition. Often a single dose is sufficient.

Intoxication with vitamin D or vitamin A should be excluded in the older infant with hypercalcaemia. In vitamin D intoxication, it is important to measure the circulating level of 25 (OH)D, the most abundant circulating vitamin D metabolite. Levels of 1,25 $(OH)_2D$ are usually low. Toxicity may be mediated by the overwhelming large dosages of 25 (OH)D interacting with the vitamin D receptor. Alternatively because 25 (OH)D has a far greater affinity than 1,25 $(OH)_2D$ for the circulating vitamin D binding protein, it has been proposed that the latter, more active metabolite is displaced from vitamin D binding protein, with toxicity resulting from the increase in free levels of 1,25 $(OH)_2D$. Excess intestinal absorption of calcium is present, and in some cases there is evidence for increased bone resorption.

Vitamin A intoxication results in bone pain, hypercalcaemia, headache, pseudotumour cerebri, and a characteristic erythematous skin rash with exfoliation. Alopecia and profuse ear discharge may be present. The hypercalcaemia is thought to be mediated by bone resorption. Although toxicity is not thought to occur when less than 50 000 units of vitamin A or equivalent is ingested on a daily basis, reports of toxicity with less ingestion have been recorded in children (74). Unrecognized liver disease may decrease the tolerance of vitamin A. In order to establish the diagnosis of vitamin A intoxication, serum retinyl ester levels should be determined in addition to the more common test for serum retinol.

Other conditions in which hypercalcaemia may be manifest in children include Down's syndrome, skeletal dysplasias (such as Jansen's), and in osteogenesis imperfecta. Indeed we have observed mild elevations in serum calcium during infancy in association with a variety of skeletal dysplasias. This appears to be a transient phenomenon. Endogenous overproduction of 1,25 $(OH)_2D$ has been described in twins with cat-scratch disease induced granulomata (75). Other major causes of hypercalcaemia include those commonly encountered in adults: immobilization, malignancy, and acquired hyperparathyroidism, including parathyroid adenomas. It may be useful to measure PTHrP levels in the setting of undiagnosed hypercalcaemia. Elevated circulating levels of PTHrP would prompt a careful search for neoplastic disease.

Treatment of hypercalcaemia

The medical management of acute symptomatic hypercalcaemia consists of the administration of intravenous saline. Additionally, furosemide, in a dose of 1 mg/kg, is frequently given intravenously at 6- to 8-h intervals. Intravenous infusion of pamidronate has also been useful in this setting. Specific long-term therapy depends on the specific hypercalcaemic disorder.

The use of bisphosphonate therapy in children has increased in recent years. Pamidronate has been highly successful in the management of hypercalcaemia associated with childhood cancers (76). We have successfully used this medication for the treatment of hypercalcaemia in Williams' syndrome and subcutaneous fat necrosis as noted above. Short-term data would suggest that side effects are minimal and that the therapy is safe. One should be aware of the potential complications of electrolyte disturbances, particularly hypocalcaemia, hypophosphataemia, and hypomagnesaemia.

References

1. Marks SC, Hermey DC. The structure and development of bone. In: Bilezikian JP, Raisz LG, Rodan GA, eds. *Priniciples of Bone Biology*. San Diego: Academic Press, 1996: 3–14.
2. Vortkamp A, Lee K, Lanske B, Segre GV, Kronenberg HM, Tabin CJ. Regulation of rate of cartilage differentiation by Indian hedgehog and PTH-related protein. *Science*, 1996; **273**: 613–22.
3. Kovacs CS, Kronenberg HM. Maternal-fetal calcium and bone metabolism during pregnancy, puerpium, and lactation. *Endocr Rev*, 1997; **18**: 832–72.
4. Gertner JM, Coustan DR, Liger AS, Mallette LE, Ravin N, Broadus AE. Pregnancy as a state of physiologic absorptive hypercalciuria. *Am J Med*, 1986; **81**: 451–6.
5. Care AD. The placental transfer of calcium. *J Dev Physiol*, 1991; **15**: 253–7.
6. Kovacs CS. F *etal* calcium metabolism. In: Rosen CJ, Compston JE, Lian JB, eds. *Primer on the Metabolic Bone Diseases and Disorders of Mineral Metabolism*. Washington, DC: American Society for Bone and Mineral Research, 2008: 108–12.
7. Kovacs CS, Lanske B, Hunzelman JL, Guo J, Karaplis AC, Kronenberg HM. Parathyroid hormone-related peptide (PTHrP) regulates fetal-placental calcium transport through a receptor distinct from the PTH/PTHrP receptor. *Proc Natl Acad Sci U S A*, 1996; **93**: 15233–8.
8. Karaplis AC, Luz A, Glowacki J, Bronson RT, Tybulewicz VL, Kronenberg HM, *et al.* Lethal skeletal dysplasia from targeted disruption of the parathyroid hormone-related peptide gene. *Genes Dev*, 1994; **8**: 277–89.
9. Kovacs CS, Chafe LL, Fudge NJ, Friel JK, Manley NR. PTH regulates fetal blood calcium and skeletal mineralization independently of PTHrP. *Endocrinol*, 2001; **142**: 4983–93.
10. Kovacs CS, Ho-Pao CL, Hunzelman JL, Lanske B, Fox J, Seidman JG, *et al.* Regulation of murine fetal-placental calcium metabolism by the calcium-sensing receptor. *J Clin Invest*, 1998; **101**: 2812–20.
11. Zanchetta JR, Plotkin H, Alvarez Filgueira ML. Bone mass in children: normative values for the 2–20-year-old population. *Bone*, 1995; **16** (Suppl.): 393S–9S.
12. Gordon CM, Bachrach LK, Carpenter TO, Crabtree N, El-Hajj Fuleihan G, Kutilek S, *et al.* Dual energy X-ray absorptiometry interpretation and reporting in children and adolescents: the 2007 ISCD pediatric official positions. *J Clin Densitom*, 2008; **11**: 43–58.
13. Calvo MS, Eyre DR, Gundberg CM. Molecular basis and clinical application of biological markers of bone turnover. *Endocr Rev*, 1996; **17**: 333–68.
14. Van der Sluis IM, Hop WC, Van Leeuwen JPTM, Pols HAP, De Muinck Keizer-Schrama SMPF. A cross-sectional study on biochemical parameters of bone turnover and vitamin D metabolites in healthy Dutch children and young adults. *Horm Res*, 2002; **57**: 170–9.
15. Bollen AM, Eyre DR. Bone resorption rates in children monitored by the urinary assay of collagen type I cross-linked peptides. *Bone*, 1994; **15**: 31–4.
16. Fares JE, Choucair M, Nabulsi M, Salamoun M, Shahine CH, Fuleihan Gel-H, *et al.* Effect of gender, puberty and vitamin D status on biochemical markers of bone remodeling. *Bone*, 2003; **33**: 242–7.
17. Szulc P, Seeman E, Delmas PD. Biochemical measurements of bone turnover in children and adolescents. *Osteoporos Int*, 2000; **11**: 281–94.
18. Institute of Medicine Standing Committee on the Scientific Evaluation of Dietary Reference Intakes. *Dietary Reference Intakes for Calcium, Phosphorus, Magnesium, Vitamin D, and Fluoride*. Washington, USA: National Academy Press, 1997.
19. Iuliano-Burns S, Hopper J, Seeman E. The age of puberty determines sexual dimorphism in bone structure: a male/female co-twin control study. *J Clin Endocrinol Metab*, 2009; **94**: 1638–43.
20. Hillman LS, Chow W, Salmons SS, Weaver E, Erickson M, Hansen J. Vitamin D metabolism mineral homeostasis, and bone mineralization in term infants fed human milk, cows milk-based formula, or soy-based formula. *J Pediatr*, 1988; **112**: 864–74.
21. Walton RJ, Bijvoet OLM. Nomogram for derivation of renal threshold phosphate concentration. *Lancet*, 1975; **ii(7929)**: 309–10.
22. Zweier, C, Sticht H, Aydin-Yaylagul I, Campbell CE, Rauch A. Human TBX1 missense mutations cause gain of function resulting in the same phenotype as 22q11.2 deletions. *Am J Hum Genet*, 2007; **80**: 510–17.
23. Kobrynski, LJ, Sullivan KE. Velocardiofacial syndrome, DiGeorge syndrome: the chromosome 22q11.2 deletion syndromes. *Lancet*, 2007; **370**: 1443–52.
24. Craigen WJ, Lindsay EA, Bricker JT, Hawkins EP, Baldini A. Deletion of chromosome 22q11 and pseudohypoparathyroidism. *Am J Med Genet*, 1997; **72**: 63–5.
25. Thakker, RV. Genetics of endocrine and metabolic disorders: parathyroid. *Rev Endocr Metab Disord*, 2004; **5**: 37–51.
26. Arnold A, Horst SA, Gardella TJ, Baba H, Levine MA, Kronenberg HM. Mutation of the signal peptide-encoding region of the preproparathyroid hormone gene in familial isolated hypoparathyroidism. *J Clin Invest*, 1990; **86**: 1084–7.
27. Baumber L, Tufarelli C, Patel S, King P, Johnson CA, Maher ER, Trembath RC. Identification of a novel mutation disrupting the DNA binding activity of GCM2 in autosomal recessive familial isolated hypoparathyroidism. *J Med Genet*, 2005; **42**: 443–8.
28. Ding C, Buckingham B, Levine MA. Familial isolated hypoparathyroidism caused by a mutation in the gene for the transcription factor GCMB. *J Clin Invest*, 2001; **108**: 1215–20.
29. Thomee C, Schubert SW, Parma J, Lê PQ, Hashemolhosseini S, Wegner M, Abramowicz MJ. GCMB mutation in familial isolated hypoparathyroidism with residual secretion of parathyroid hormone. *J Clin Endocrinol Metab*, 2005; **90**: 2487–92.
30. Canaff L, Zhou X, Mosesova I, Cole DE, Hendy GN. Glial cells missing-2 (GCM2) transactivates the calcium-sensing receptor gene: effect of a dominant-negative GCM2 mutant associated with autosomal dominant hypoparathyroidism. *Hum Mutat*, 2009; **30**: 85–92.
31. Bowl MR, Nesbit MA, Harding B, Levy E, Jefferson A, Volpi E, *et al.* An interstitial deletion-insertion involving chromosomes 2p25.3 and Xq27.1, near SOX3, causes X-linked recessive hypoparathyroidism. *J Clin Invest*, 2005; **115**: 2822–31.
32. Ali A, Christie PT, Grigorieva IV, Harding B, Van Esch H, Ahmed SF, *et al.* Functional characterization of GATA3 mutations causing the hypoparathyroidism-deafness-renal (HDR) dysplasia syndrome: insight into mechanisms of DNA binding by the GATA3 transcription factor. *Hum Mol Genet*, 2007; **16**: 265–75.
33. Ferraris S, Del Monaco AG, Garelli E, Carando A, De Vito B, Pappi P, *et al.* HDR syndrome: a novel "de novo" mutation in GATA3 gene. *Am J Med Genet A*, 2009; **149A**: 770–5.
34. Saito T, Fukumoto S, Ito N, Suzuki H, Igarashi T, Fujita T. A novel mutation in the GATA3 gene of a Japanese patient with PTH-deficient hypoparathyroidism. *J Bone Miner Metab*, 2009; **27**: 386–9.
35. Van Esch H, Groenen P, Nesbit MA, Schuffenhauer S, Lichtner P, Vanderlinden G, *et al.* GATA3 haplo-insufficiency causes human HDR syndrome. *Nature*, 2000; **406**: 419–22.

36. Padidela R, Kelberman D, Press M, Al-Khawari M, Hindmarsh PC, Dattani MT. Mutation in the TBCE gene is associated with Hypoparathyroidism-Retardation-Dysmorphism syndrome featuring pituitary hormone deficiencies and hypoplasia of the anterior pituitary and the corpus callosum. *J Clin Endocrinol Metab*, 2009; **94**: 2686–91.
37. Parvari R, Diaz GA, Hershkovitz E. Parathyroid development and the role of tubulin chaperone E. *Horm Res*, 2007; **67**: 12–21.
38. Parvari R, Hershkovitz E, Grossman N, Gorodischer R, Loeys B, Zecic A, *et al.* Mutation of TBCE causes hypoparathyroidism-retardation-dysmorphism and autosomal recessive Kenny-Caffey syndrome. *Nat Genet*, 2002; **32**: 448–52.
39. Shoback D. Clinical practice. Hypoparathyroidism. *N Engl J Med*, 2008; **359**: 391–403.
40. Labarthe F, Benoist JF, Brivet M, Vianey-Saban C, Despert F, de Baulny HO. Partial hypoparathyroidism associated with mitochondrial trifunctional protein deficiency. *Eur J Pediatr*, 2006; **165**: 389–91.
41. Pearce SH, Williamson C, Kifor O, Bai M, Coulthard MG, Davies M, *et al.* A familial syndrome of hypocalcaemia with hypercalciuria due to mutations in the calcium-sensing receptor. *N Eng J Med*, 1996; **335**: 1115–22.
42. Betterle C, Greggio NA, Volpato M. Autoimmune polyglandular syndrome type 1. *J Clin Endocrinol Metab*, 1998; **83**: 1049–55.
43. Alimohammadi M, Bjorklund P, Hallgren A, Pöntynen N, Szinnai G, Shikama N, *et al.* Autoimmune polyendocrine syndrome type 1 and NALP5, a parathyroid autoantigen. *N Engl J Med*, 2008; **358**: 1018–28.
44. Perheentupa J. Autoimmune polyendocrinopathy-candidiasis-ectodermal dystrophy. *J Clin Endocrinol Metab*, 2006; **91**: 2843–50.
45. Shikama N, Nusspaumer G, Hollander GA. Clearing the AIRE: on the pathophysiological basis of the autoimmune polyendocrinopathy syndrome type-1. *Endocrinol Metab Clin North Am*, 2009; **38**: 273–88.
46. Brown, EM. Anti-parathyroid and anti-calcium sensing receptor antibodies in autoimmune hypoparathyroidism. *Endocrinol Metab Clin North Am*, 2009; **38**: 437–45.
47. Gentileschi P, Gacek IA, Manzelli A, Coscarella G, Sileri P, Lirosi F, *et al.* Early (1 hour) post-operative parathyroid hormone (PTH) measurement predicts hypocalcaemia after thyroidectomy: a prospective case-control single-institution study. *Chir Ital*, 2008; **60**: 519–28.
48. Lim JP, Irvine R, Bugis S, Holmes D, Wiseman SM. Intact parathyroid hormone measurement 1 hour after thyroid surgery identifies individuals at high risk for the development of symptomatic hypocalcemia. *Am J Surg*, 2009; **197**: 648–53.
49. Gamberini MR, De Sanctis V, Gilli G. Hypogonadism, diabetes mellitus, hypothyroidism, hypoparathyroidism: incidence and prevalence related to iron overload and chelation therapy in patients with thalassaemia major followed from 1980 to 2007 in the Ferrara Centre. *Pediatr Endocrinol Rev*, 2008; **6** (Suppl. 1): 158–69.
50. Carpenter TO, Carnes Jr DL, Anast CS. Hypoparathyroidism in Wilson's disease. *N Engl J Med*, 1983; **309**: 873–7.
51. Anast CS, Mohs JM, Kaplan SL, Burns TW. Evidence for parathyroid failure in magnesium deficiency. *Science*, 1972; **177**: 606–8.
52. Shalev H, Phillip M, Galil A, Carmi R, Landau D. Clinical presentation and outcome in primary familial hypomagnesaemia. *Arch Dis Child*, 1998; **78**: 127–30.
53. Schlingmann KP, Weber S, Peters M, Niemann Nejsum L, Vitzthum H, Klingel K, *et al.* Hypomagnesaemia with secondary hypocalcaemia is caused by mutations in TRPM6, a new member of the TRPM gene family. *Nat Genet*, 2002; **31**: 166–70.
54. Simon DB, Lu Y, Choate KA, Velazquez H, Al-Sabban E, Praga M, *et al.* Paracellin-1, a renal tight junction protein required for paracellular Mg2- resorption. *Science*, 1999; **285**: 103–6.
55. Konrad M, Schaller A, Seelow D, Pandey AV, Waldegger S, Lesslauer A, *et al.* Mutations in the tight-junction gene claudin 19 (CLDN19) are associated with renal magnesium wasting, renal failure, and severe ocular involvement. *Am J Hum Genet*, 2006; **79**: 949–57.
56. Schlingmann KP, Konrad M, Seyberth HW. Genetics of hereditary disorders of magnesium homeostasis. *Pediatr Nephrol*, 2004; **19**: 13–25.
57. al-Harbi NN, Domrongkitchaiporn S, Lirenman DS. Hypocalcemia and hypomagnesemia after ibuprofen overdose. *Ann Pharmacother*, 1997; **31**: 432–4.
58. Klasaer AE, Sealzo AJ, Blume C, Johnson P, Thompson MW. Marked hypocalcemia and ventricular fibrillation in two pediatric patients exposed to a fluoride-containing wheel cleaner. *Ann Emerg Med*, 1998; **28**: 713–18.
59. Klein GL, Nicolai M, Langman CB, Cuneo BF, Sailer DE, Herndon DN. Dysregulation of calcium homeostasis after severe burn injury in children: possible role of magnesium depletion. *J Pediatr*, 1997; **131**: 246–51.
60. Bastepe M. The GNAS locus and pseudohypoparathyroidism. *Adv Exp Med Biol*, 2008; **626**: 27–40.
61. Bastepe M. The GNAS locus: quintessential complex gene encoding GSALPHA, XLALPHAS, and other imprinted transcripts. *Curr Genomics*, 2007; **8**: 398–414.
62. Juppner H, Schipani E, Bastepe M, Cole DE, Lawson ML, Mannstadt M, *et al.* The gene responsible for pseudohypoparathyroidism type Ib is paternally imprinted and maps in four unrelated kindreds to chromosome 20q13.3. *Proc Natl Acad Sci U S A*, 1998; **95**: 798–803.
63. Wilson LC, Oude Luttikhuis ME, Clayton PT, Fraser WD, Trembath RC. Parental origin of Gsα gene mutations in Albright's hereditary osteodystrophy. *J Med Genet*, 1994; **31**: 835–9.
64. Hollis BW. Circulating 25-hydroxyvitamin D levels indicative of vitamin D sufficiency: Implications for establishing a new effective dietary intake recommendation for vitamin D. *J Nutr*, 2005; **135**: 317–22.
65. Maalouf NM. The noncalciotropic actions of vitamin D: recent clinical developments. *Curr Opin Nephrol Hypertens*, 2008; **17**: 408–15.
66. Adams JS, Ren S, Liu PT, Chun RF, Lagishetty V, Gombart AF, *et al.* Vitamin d-directed rheostatic regulation of monocyte antibacterial responses. *J Immunol*, 2009; **182**: 4289–95.
67. Lips P. Which circulating level of 25-hydroxyvitamin D is appropriate? *J Steroid Biochem Mol Biol*, 2004; **89–90**: 611–14.
68. Clements MR, Johnson L, Fraser DR. A new mechanism for induced vitamin D deficiency in calcium deprivation. *Nature*, 1987; **325**: 62–5.
69. Balsan S, Garabedian M, Larchet M, Gorski AM, Cournot G, Tau C, *et al.* Long-term nocturnal calcium infusions can cure rickets and promote normal mineralization in hereditary resistance to 1,25-dihydroxyvitamin D. *J Clin Invest*, 1986; **77**: 1661–7.
70. Mazariegos-Ramos E, Guerrero-Romero E, Rodriguez-Moran M, Lazcano-Burciaga G, Paniagua R, Amato D. Consumption of soft drinks with phosphoric acid as a risk factor for the development of hypocalcemia in children: a case-control study. *J Pediatr*, 1995; **126**: 940–2.
71. Marie PJ, Pettifor JM, Ross FP, Glorieux FH. Histological osteomalacia due to dietary calcium deficiency in children. *N Eng J Med*, 1982; **307**: 584–8.
72. Pollack MR, Chou Y-HW, Marx SJ, Steinmann B, Cole DE, Brandi ML, *et al.* Familial hypocalciuric hypocalcemia and neonatal severe hyperparathyroidism: effects of mutant gene dosage on phenotype. *J Clin Invest*, 1994; **93**: 1108–12.
73. Schwarz P, Larsen NE, Lonborg Friis IM, Lillquist K, Brown EM, Gammeltoft S. Familial hypocalciuric hypercalcemia and neonatal

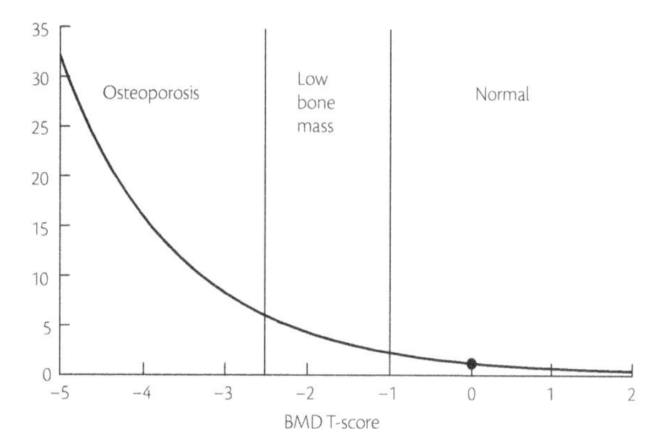

Fig. 4.7.1 The risk of fracture increases by a factor of 2 for every 1–SD decrease in bone mineral density (BMD). The WHO definition of osteoporosis is based on the BMD in relation to SDs from the young normal mean (the T score). Osteoporosis is defined as a BMD that is equal to or less than 2.5 SD below the young normal mean.

skeletal site. It is likely that several genes regulate bone mass, each with a modest effect, and likely candidates include the genes for type I collagen (*COL1A1*) and for the lipoprotein related protein (*LRP5*). The nongenetic factors include low calcium intake during childhood, low body weight at maturity and at 1 year of life, sedentary lifestyle, and delayed puberty. Each of these results in decreased bone mass.

Bone loss

Mechanisms of bone loss

Bone loss occurs in the postmenopausal woman as a result of an increase in the rate of bone remodelling and an imbalance between the activity of osteoclasts and osteoblasts. Bone remodelling occurs at discrete sites within the skeleton and proceeds in an orderly fashion with bone resorption always being followed by bone formation, a phenomenon referred to as 'coupling'. In cortical and cancellous bone the sequence of bone remodelling is similar (8). The quiescent bone surface is converted to activity (origination) and the osteoclasts resorb bone (progression) forming a cutting cone (cortical bone) or a trench (cancellous bone). The osteoblasts synthesize bone matrix which subsequently mineralizes. The sequence takes up to 8 months. If the processes of bone resorption and bone formation are not matched then there is 'remodelling imbalance'. In postmenopausal women, this imbalance is magnified by the increase in the rate of initiation of new bone remodelling cycles (activation frequency).

Remodelling imbalance results in irreversible bone loss. There are two other causes of irreversible bone loss, referred to as 'remodelling errors'. First is excavation of overlarge haversian spaces in cortical bone (9). Radial infilling is regulated by signals from the outermost osteocytes and is generally no more than 90 μm. Hence, large external diameters, which may simply occur randomly, lead to large central haversian canals, which then accumulate with age, leading to increased cortical porosity. In a similar way, osteoclast penetration of trabecular plates, or severing of trabecular beams, removes the scaffolding needed for osteoblastic replacement of resorbed bone. In both ways random remodelling errors tend to reduce both cancellous and cortical bone density and structural integrity.

Causes of bone loss

Oestrogen deficiency

Bone loss in the postmenopausal woman occurs in two phases (10). There is a phase of rapid bone loss that lasts for 5 years (about 3% per year in the spine). Subsequently, there is lower bone loss that is more generalized (about 0.5% per year at many sites). This slower phase of bone loss affects men, starting at about age 55 years. The rapid phase of bone loss in women is caused by oestrogen deficiency. The circulating level of oestradiol decreases by 90% at the time of the menopause. This bone loss can be prevented by the administration of oestrogen and progestins to the postmenopausal woman. It has been estimated that this rapid phase of bone loss contributes 50% to the spinal bone loss across life in women. The main effect of oestrogen deficiency is on bone, where it increases activation frequency, and may contribute to the remodelling imbalance. Oestrogen deficiency may increase bone resorption by stimulating the synthesis of RANKL by osteoblasts (or their precursors). RANKL binds to its receptor RANK on the osteoclast and promotes differentiation to osteoclasts, increases osteoclast activity and inhibits osteoclast apoptosis. Oestrogen deficiency also increases the apoptosis of osteoblasts and osteocytes.

Oestrogen deficiency may be a determinant of bone loss in men (11). Decreased BMD has been reported in men with an inactivating mutation of the genes for the oestrogen receptor or for aromatase (the enzyme that converts androgens to oestrogens). In older men, oestrogen levels correlate more closely with BMD than testosterone levels. In men with osteoporosis, oestradiol (but not testosterone) levels have been reported to be decreased.

Ageing

The slow phase of bone loss is attributed to age-related factors such as an increase in parathyroid hormone (PTH) levels (Fig. 4.7.2) and to osteoblast senescence. An increase in PTH levels (and action) occurs in both men and women with ageing. PTH levels correlate with those of biochemical markers of bone turnover and both may be returned to those found in young adults by the intravenous infusion of calcium. The increase in PTH results from decreased renal calcium reabsorption and decreased intestinal

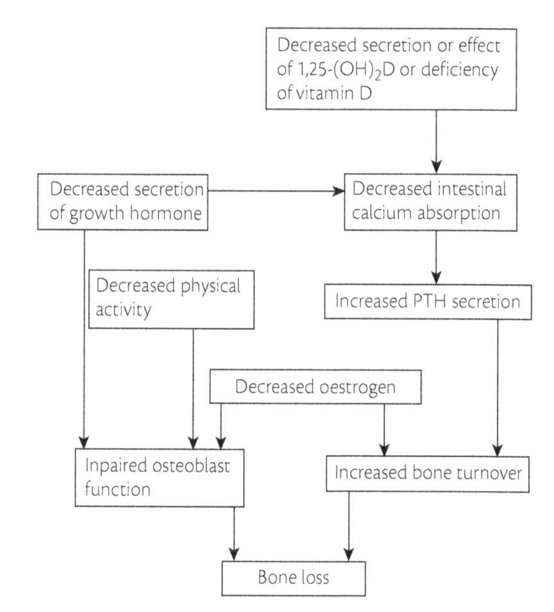

Fig. 4.7.2 The causes of bone loss with ageing.

calcium absorption. The latter may result from vitamin D deficiency (e.g. in the housebound elderly), decreased 1α-hydroxylase activity in the kidney resulting in decreased synthesis of 1,25-dihydroxyvitamin D, or resistance to vitamin D. Whatever the cause, a diet high in calcium returns both PTH and bone turnover markers to levels found in healthy young adults. It has been proposed that the age-related increase in PTH could result from indirect effects of oestrogen deficiency (10). This proposal is based on the following evidence. In older women treated with oestrogen, (1) there is a decrease in bone turnover markers and PTH levels; (2) there is an increase in calcium absorption, possibly mediated by an increase in 1,25-dihydroxyvitamin D; (3) there is an increase in the PTH-independent calcium reabsorption in the kidney; and (4) there is a decrease in the parathyroid secretory reserve.

Accelerating factors

A number of diseases and drugs are clearly related to accelerated bone loss (Box 4.7.1). Their effects are superimposed on those described above. Thus, a patient starting on corticosteroid therapy is more likely to have an osteoporosis-related fracture if she has low BMD resulting from low peak bone mass and the accelerated bone loss of the menopause.

Identification of mechanism of bone loss in an individual

In a woman presenting with osteoporosis at age 70 years it is often possible to identify several reasons for the low BMD (Fig. 4.7.3). Some of these may be identified from history taking (early menopause, drugs that accelerate bone loss), but some cannot be identified in retrospect (low peak bone mass and rapid losers).

Other determinants of bone strength (3)

Bone geometry

Bone geometry has a major effect on fracture risk. One example is hip axis length, the distance from the lateral surface of the trochanter to the inner surface of the acetabulum, along the axis of the femoral neck. Short hip axis length results in an architecturally stronger structure for any given bone density. This is probably the reason why Japanese and other Orientals have about half the hip fracture rate of Caucasians, despite similar bone density values.

Fatigue damage

Fatigue damage consists of ultramicroscopic rents in the basic bony material, resulting from the inevitable bending that occurs when a structural member is loaded. Fatigue damage is the principal cause of failure in mechanical engineering structures; its prevention is the responsibility of the remodelling apparatus which detects and removes fatigue-damaged bone. Fractures related to fatigue damage occur whenever the damage occurs faster than remodelling can repair it or whenever the remodelling apparatus is defective. March fractures and the fractures of radiation necrosis are well-recognized examples of fractures due to these two mechanisms.

Loss of trabecular connectivity

Bone structures loaded vertically, such as the vertebral bodies and femoral and tibial metaphyses, derive a substantial portion of their structural strength from a system of horizontal, cross-bracing trabeculae which support the vertical elements and limit lateral bowing and consequent snapping under vertical loading. Severance of such

Box 4.7.1 Risk factors for osteoporosis in postmenopausal women

- Genetic factors
  - First-degree relative with low-trauma fracture, e.g. mother with hip fracture
- Environmental factors
  - Cigarette smoking
  - Alcohol abuse
  - Physical inactivity or prolonged immobilization
  - Thin habitus, e.g. less than 57 kg
  - Diet low in calcium, e.g. less than 500 mg/day
  - Little exposure to sunlight, e.g. housebound elderly
- Menstrual status
  - Early menopause, that is, before age 45 years
  - Previous amenorrhoea, e.g. anorexia nervosa, hyperprolactinaemia
- Drug therapy
  - Glucocorticoids, e.g. 7.5 mg/day of prednisolone or more, for 6 months or more
  - Antirejection therapy after organ transplantation, e.g. ciclosporin
  - Antiepileptic drugs, e.g. phenytoin
  - Excessive substitution therapy, e.g. thyroxine, hydrocortisone
  - Anticoagulant therapy, e.g. heparin, warfarin
  - Aromatase inhibitors and gonadotropin-releasing hormone agonist therapy for breast (and prostate) cancer
- Endocrine diseases
  - Primary hyperparathyroidism
  - Thyrotoxicosis
  - Cushing's syndrome
  - Addison's disease
- Haematological diseases
  - Multiple myeloma
  - Systemic mastocytosis
  - Lymphoma, leukaemia
  - Pernicious anaemia
- Rheumatological diseases
  - Rheumatoid arthritis
  - Ankylosing spondylitis
- Gastrointestinal diseases
  - Malabsorption states, e.g. coeliac disease, Crohn's disease, surgery for peptic ulcer
  - Chronic liver disease, e.g. primary biliary cirrhosis

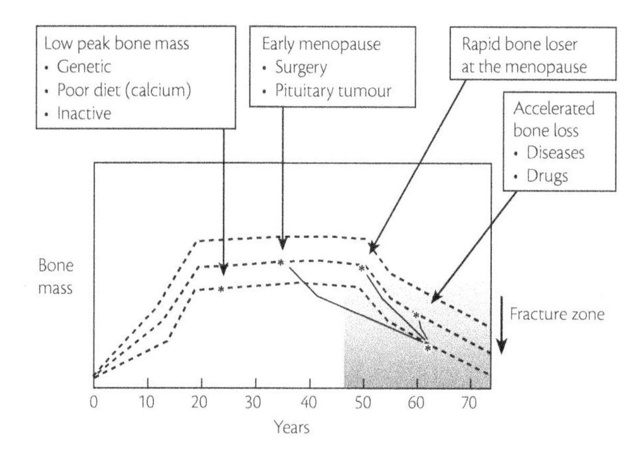

Fig. 4.7.3 The possible causes of low bone mass in a 70-year-old woman. Note how peak bone mass is attained about the age of 30 years and the phase of accelerated bone loss begins at the menopause. The lower the bone density falls, the greater the risk of fracture.

trabecular connections is known to occur preferentially in postmenopausal women and is considered to be an important reason for the large female/male preponderance of low-trauma vertebral fractures.

Risk factors for osteoporosis

A number of risk factors have been identified for osteoporosis (Box 4.7.1). Bone loss can be stopped, or reversed, if risk factors such as primary hyperparathyroidism (see Chapter 4.3) are identified and treated. The patient who presents with a vertebral fracture and low BMD is likely to have had one of four causes (Fig. 4.7.3). It is impossible to know the importance of peak bone mass and the rate of bone loss in retrospect. Questions can be asked about early menopause and about the drugs and diseases known to accelerate bone loss. We usually assess risk factors by administering a questionnaire before first attendance at the clinic, by carrying out a limited biochemical work-up before the clinic visit (Box 4.7.2), and, after the clinical, evaluation exploring alternative diagnoses.

Genetic factors

Family history

A maternal history of hip fracture increases the risk of hip fracture in an individual.

Osteogenesis imperfecta

Late-onset forms (e.g. Sillence type I) may present with vertebral fracture. The clinical clues are the blue sclerae, hypermobile joints, lax skin, cardiac murmurs, and deafness (see Chapter 4.11).

Environmental factors

Cigarette smoking and chronic obstructive pulmonary disease

Smoking results in lower oestrogen levels and early menopause, and smokers often have a slender stature (see below). Chronic lung disease is associated with chronic respiratory acidosis and decreased physical activity.

Alcohol abuse

The relationship between alcohol and bone loss is complex (and there may even be a protective effect at a low level of intake) (12). Alcoholism results in low BMD because of poor nutrition and pseudo-Cushing's syndrome, and a direct suppressive effect of alcohol on osteoblasts. Fractures result from the increased propensity to fall.

Physical inactivity and immobilization (neurological)

Athletes have high BMD. However, bone loss only results from complete immobilization (or space flight). The bone loss after paralysis (e.g. stroke) is regional.

Thin habitus

This is a risk factor for fracture through decreased oestrogen production from adrenal androgens (in adipose tissue) and through decreased padding (to cushion a fall). Women with hip fracture weigh about 8 kg less than the average woman.

Diet—low dietary calcium

Low dietary calcium and high dietary sodium are considered risk factors for osteoporosis. Calcium requirement increases during growth and in the postmenopausal period. A postmenopausal woman should take 1500 mg/day of calcium.

Little exposure to ultraviolet light

Ultraviolet light (UVB) acts on the skin as the main source of vitamin D (see Chapter 4.10). The housebound are liable to vitamin D insufficiency. This does not result in clinical osteomalacia, but the decreased calcium absorption (see above) results in secondary hyperparathyroidism.

Menstrual status

Early menopause

A menopause before the age of 45 years is associated with increased risk of fracture. A menopause before the age of 40 years is often associated with some endocrine cause and should be investigated further.

Box 4.7.2 Diagnostic evaluation of osteoporosis

- Establish presence of low-trauma fracture (fall from standing height or less)
  - Spine radiographs
- Evaluate degree of bone loss
  - Bone densitometry (see Box 4.7.3)
- Laboratory tests to exclude secondary osteoporosis
  - Primary hyperparathyroidism (serum calcium)
  - Thyrotoxicosis (thyroid-stimulating hormone)
  - Multiple myeloma (erythrocyte sedimentation rate, protein electrophoresis, and urinary Bence Jones protein)
  - Osteomalacia (serum calcium, phosphate (fasting, morning), alkaline phosphatase, 24-h urinary calcium and creatinine)
  - Malabsorption syndrome (full blood count and, if necessary, red cell folate, serum vitamin B_{12}, antiendomysial antibodies, magnesium)
  - Hypogonadism in men (testosterone and, if necessary, sex hormone binding globulin, luteinizing hormone, follicle-stimulating hormone, prolactin)

Amenorrhoea

A late onset of the menarche and periods of amenorrhoea of any cause, e.g. exercise related, are associated with decreased bone mass later in life.

Anorexia nervosa

This is associated with bone loss and increased risk of fracture. The bone loss is probably irreversible after 4 years of amenorrhoea. The mechanism of the bone loss is not just oestrogen deficiency. The diet is low in calcium and serum IGF-1 levels are low, and cortisol secretion may be increased.

Hyperprolactinaemia

This results in oestrogen deficiency. Not all studies have reported bone loss, and it may be that prolactin has some beneficial effects on calcium homoeostasis, such as an increase in calcium absorption.

Drug therapy

Corticosteroids

In the UK, over 250 000 patients take continuous oral glucocorticoids, yet no more than 14% receive any therapy to prevent bone loss, a serious complication of glucocorticoid treatment. Bone loss is rapid, particularly in the first year, and fracture risk may double (13). The mechanism of the bone loss is mainly a suppression of osteoblast activity. This differs from oestrogen deficiency, in which the mechanism is mainly increased activation frequency. A treatment algorithm has been presented for adults receiving glucocorticoid doses for 6 months or more (14). General measures, e.g. alternative glucocorticoids and routes of administration, and therapeutic interventions such as bisphosphonates, are recommended. Glucocorticoid-induced osteoporosis is discussed in greater detail in Chapter 4.11.

Antiepileptic drugs

Phenobarbitone and phenytoin are known to affect vitamin D metabolism and result in osteomalacia. More commonly, they may cause secondary hyperparathyroidism and osteoporosis.

Excessive substitution therapy

Thyroxine doses sufficient to suppress thyroid-stimulating hormone, and hydrocortisone doses that result in 24-h urinary free cortisol above the reference range, have adverse effects on bone turnover and bone density (see Chapter 4.8).

Anticoagulant drugs

Heparin stimulates bone resorption by a direct effect on osteoclasts. Its long-term use (e.g. in pregnancy) results in bone loss at the spine and hip of 8–10% over 6 months. Warfarin may interfere with the γ-carboxylation of bone proteins, and its use is associated with an increased risk of fracture.

Endocrine diseases

Primary hyperparathyroidism

This is associated with an increase in bone turnover and a decrease in bone mass, particularly at sites rich in cortical bone. It is likely that there is an increase in fracture rates. These changes are reversible with surgical removal of the tumour (see Chapter 4.3).

Thyrotoxicosis

This topic is discussed in Chapter 4.8.

Cushing's syndrome

Cushing's disease may present with vertebral fracture. The bone loss in the first few years after pituitary surgery is between 10 and 20% at the spine.

Addison's disease

This is associated with decreased bone mass, resulting from excess substitution therapy and deficiency of adrenal androgens (precursors for oestrogen synthesis in men and postmenopausal women).

Haematological diseases

Multiple myeloma

This may present with vertebral fracture. It is usually identified with serum protein electrophoresis, and urinary Bence Jones testing, but occasionally the myeloma may be nonsecretory and can usually be diagnosed by bone marrow examination.

Systemic mastocytosis

This may cause decreased or increased bone density. It can be identified by urticaria pigmentosa, and mast cells are identified in the bone biopsy (see Chapter 6.17).

Pernicious anaemia

This has been associated with low bone density and increased risk of fractures. The mechanism is unclear, as the absorption of calcium from food is normal despite the absence of gastric acid.

Rheumatological diseases

Rheumatoid arthritis and ankylosing spondylitis

The immobility may be an important cause, as may be the local (and circulating) cytokines, which promote bone resorption. The corticosteroid therapy for rheumatoid arthritis may also contribute.

Gastrointestinal diseases

Malabsorption syndrome

Diseases such as coeliac disease may present with osteoporosis. Other inflammatory bowel diseases, such as Crohn's disease, may require treatment with corticosteroids. Patients who have had peptic ulcer surgery have low bone density and increased risk of fracture. This may also be due to their habits—such patients are usually thin, and commonly smoke and may take excess alcohol.

Chronic liver disease

Chronic obstructive liver diseases, such as primary biliary cirrhosis, are associated with osteoporosis. Bilirubin has been associated with osteoblast suppression *in vitro*. Liver transplantation results in further bone loss and about one-third of patients suffer fractures (15). This bone loss is likely to be related to the immunosuppression (corticosteroids and ciclosporine).

Clinical presentation of vertebral fracture

Osteoporosis does not cause pain or deformity in the absence of fractures. Its importance lies in the fact that it greatly increases the risk of fracture, notably forearm (Colles') fracture, hip fracture, and vertebral fracture. The commonest presentation in clinical practice is vertebral fracture and so this will be described in more detail.

History of back pain

The back pain of vertebral fracture has some characteristic features. The pain often comes on within a day of some strain on the back, such as lifting a suitcase or a grandchild, a jolt on a bus or working in the garden. The pain soon becomes very severe and the patient may need to stay in bed for several days. The pain is usually localized to the back and it is uncommon for pain to radiate into the legs, and symptoms of cord compression such as bladder dysfunction are rare. The pain is present throughout the day and night. The pain gradually eases and goes by 4 to 6 months. If pain persists longer, or if there is a second peak of pain during the first 6 months, this usually indicates a second vertebral fracture. This is not an uncommon occurrence. Patients commonly do not complain of back pain. Indeed, it has been estimated that at least half of vertebral fractures are asymptomatic. These asymptomatic fractures appear to be particularly common in patients taking corticosteroids. Episodes of back pain may have been forgotten. The patient commonly recalls a painful episode when confronted with the appearance of a fracture on the spinal radiograph. This incontrovertible evidence prompts the recall of a painful event occurring many decades previously, often in relation to heavy manual work in a man or after pregnancy in a woman.

Loss of height

Loss of height is an effect of ageing, resulting from the change of posture caused by degenerative changes in the intervertebral discs. Patients do not report this symptom often and it needs to be sought by asking the patient's height in early adult life. The patient may have noticed that it is more difficult to reach high shelves. It is unusual to have sudden height loss as the presenting complaint for vertebral fracture.

Kyphosis

This may have been noticed by a relative or the patient may report being 'round-shouldered'. Clothes may no longer fit. These symptoms are not specific to vertebral fracture and are more commonly caused by disc degeneration. In a young person, kyphosis may be caused by Scheuermann's disease (see below).

Other symptoms of vertebral fracture

Vertebral fractures in the lumbar region result in decreased abdominal volume. This causes the abdomen to protrude. Patients with osteoporosis are commonly slender, so this appearance is new. They may also result in impingement of the costal margin on the iliac crest. This 'iliocostal friction syndrome' causes pain and a grating sensation. This pain is postural, occurring on sitting. Vertebral fractures in the thoracic spine result in reduced lung volume. This may result in respiratory symptoms, such as dyspnoea, or in delayed recovery from chest infections.

Clinical examination

Two aspects of the clinical examination are useful in the patient with suspected vertebral fracture. The first relates to the location of the pain. It is often assumed that the deformity on the radiograph and the patient's back pain are associated. However, a careful palpation of the spinal processes counting down from vertebra prominens (seventh cervical vertebra) often reveals that the site of the pain does not correspond with the level of the deformity on the radiograph. It is helpful to evaluate the size of the gap between the costal margin and the iliac crest. This is normally three finger's breadths (as measured by the patient's fingers).

Diagnostic evaluation (Box 4.7.2)

Spinal radiographs

Plain radiographs are required of the thoracic and lumbar spine in the anteroposterior and lateral position. It is a common mistake to take the radiograph only of the painful area. This would miss asymptomatic fractures in other parts of the spine. It is common only to take lateral radiographs. The anteroposterior radiograph is useful to identify the vertebral level of the fracture and to exclude other causes of deformity, such a malignancy (associated with absent pedicles).

Types of deformity

Vertebral deformities may be wedge, endplate ('biconcave', when both endplates are affected), and compression (also called 'crush') (16). Wedge deformities are particularly common in the thoracic spine, because the normal kyphosis in this region results in the main force running anteriorly. Biconcavity deformities are particularly common in the lumbar spine, because the normal lordosis results in the main force running through the middle of the vertebra. There appears to be no association between the type of deformity and the severity of pain or with the level of BMD. The level of the deformities should be recorded to allow comparison at follow-up visits.

Deformities that mimic fractures

The most common deformity to mimic fracture is Scheuermann's disease. This is a form of epiphysitis that occurs during adolescence ('juvenile epiphysitis') and gives the appearance of wedging and elongation of the vertebral bodies. The characteristic feature is the wavy appearance of the superior and inferior borders.

Malignancy may cause vertebral deformity. The isotope bone scan is particularly useful in this situation as it is unusual to have a single bone lesion. Increased uptake in multiple sites in the skeleton is typical of malignancy. This may occur in prostate cancer, which affects the sacrum, lumbar spine, and ribs (via Batson's venous plexus). Malignancy may cause erosion of the pedicle, a typical appearance not found with osteoporotic vertebral fractures.

Paget's disease of bone commonly affects the spine (see Chapter 4.9). The bone may appear sclerotic, but it is weak and can fracture. The bone texture has a disorganized appearance and the vertebra may be enlarged.

Osteomalacia may result in vertebral deformities (see Chapter 4.10). Often adjacent vertebrae are affected and the endplates are deformed. This gives rise to a 'cod-fish' appearance. There may be other radiological clues, such as the ground-glass appearance of the vertebral body bone and the presence of pseudofractures (Looser's zones) in the pelvis, long bones, or ribs.

Use of vertebral morphometry in the clinic

Dual-energy X-ray absorptiometry (DXA) can be used to image the spine as well as to obtain a measurement of bone density (see below). Vertebral fractures may be identified by careful focus on the appearance of the vertebral endplate (16). Fracture is likely if the endplate is deformed and should be confirmed with a radiograph.

Isotope bone scan

This can be a useful diagnostic tool in certain cases. There is increased isotope uptake in a vertebra for at least 6 months after it has fractured and typically has a uniform distribution in the vertebral body. This can be useful if the radiological appearances are borderline and yet the symptoms are characteristic. In patients with a suspicion of malignancy (previous breast cancer and history of weight loss) the scan is helpful in that metastases often affect many bones. The scan is helpful in a patient with corticosteroid-induced osteoporosis with pelvic pain. These patients commonly develop insufficiency fractures and these show up as symmetrical appearance affecting the sacral alae and the pubic rami. Single photon emission computed tomography is a variant of the isotope bone scan and is particularly useful in identifying the cause of back pain. If the facet joints show increased uptake then the patient may benefit from an injection of local anaesthetic into the facet joint.

Magnetic resonance imaging

This approach can be useful in identifying a recent deformity and distinguishing a fracture from a malignant deposit. It is very useful in identifying cord compression. It is an essential test before kyphoplasty or vertebroplasty are considered (see below); only recent fractures clearly benefit from these procedures.

Bone density measurement (Table 4.7.1)

DXA is precise, accurate, involves exposure to only low doses of X-rays, and allows measurement of sites of clinical interest (that is, lumbar spine and proximal femur). In DXA, two energy peaks of X-rays are absorbed to different extents by bone and soft tissue, and the density of bone is calculated, in g/cm^2, using simultaneous equations. The measurement is compared with two reference ranges—one for young adults (age 30 years) to give T scores and one for age-matched adults to give Z scores. This has become the standard technique for bone density assessment and guidelines have been proposed (Box 4.7.3). The two sites most commonly used in practice are lumbar spine and total hip. Low BMD at the total hip is a strong predictor of hip fracture (17).

Single energy X-ray (or photon) absorptiometry has similar advantages to DXA, and the equipment is less expensive. However, the sites in which bone density can be measured (distal forearm and calcaneum) may not be of clinical interest.

Box 4.7.3 Clinical indications for bone densitometry

- Presence of strong risk factors (see Box 4.7.1)
- Radiological evidence of vertebral fracture or osteopenia
- Previous fragility fracture of the spine, hip, or wrist (after age 40 years)
- Monitoring of therapy

Quantitative CT allows three-dimensional measurements of the bone density of the lumbar spine. This technique also allows measurement of trabecular bone alone (i.e. the type of bone usually lost first in the development of osteoporosis). In the research setting, finite element modelling can be applied to the information provided by this technique to estimate bone strength. However, quantitative CT is more expensive, less precise, and involves a higher radiation dose then DXA.

Quantitative ultrasound measurements are usually made on the calcaneum. The ultrasound signal has a lower frequency (200–600 kHz) than that used in obstetrics (more than 1 MHz). The attenuation of the signal (broad-band ultrasound attenuation) may reflect both the density and the architecture of bone, and the velocity of the signal reflects the density and biomechanical properties (elasticity). Quantitative ultrasonometry is currently used only in research but, if recent studies of its predictive ability in osteoporosis are confirmed, it could become an established technique.

Investigating secondary osteoporosis

A secondary cause is present in approximately 40% of women and 60% of men with osteoporosis. The most commonly found abnormalities are those of low vitamin D and either high or low urinary calcium (18). Investigations to identify a secondary cause are recommended if the BMD is more than 2 SD below the age-matched mean or if the patient has low-trauma vertebral fractures (Box 4.7.2).

Bone biopsy This may be useful in unusual forms of osteoporosis (e.g. idiopathic osteoporosis in young adults). It provides information

Table 4.7.1 Techniques for the noninvasive measurement of bone mass

Technique	Site	Comments
Single (or dual) energy X-ray absorptiometry	Forearm and heel	Inexpensive, precise, uses low doses of radiation, measures sites unresponsive to therapy
Dual-energy X-ray absorptiometry	Lumbar spine	Fairly expensive, precise, uses low doses of radiation, measures site responsive to therapy, needs skilled operator, subject to artefacts (spondylosis)
	Proximal femur	Fairly expensive, less precise, uses low doses of radiation, measures site best for fracture prediction, needs skilled operator
	Total body	Expensive, precise, uses low doses of radiation, measures sites unresponsive to therapy, needs skilled operator, allows assessment of body composition
Quantitative computed tomography	Spine	Expensive, less precise, uses high doses of radiation, measures sites responsive to therapy, needs skilled operator, allows assessment of trabecular bone alone
	Forearm and ankle	Inexpensive, precise, uses low doses of radiation, measures sites unresponsive to therapy, does not need skilled operator
Ultrasonometry	Heel, fingers, etc.	Inexpensive, less precise, uses no radiation, measures sites unresponsive to therapy, does not need skilled operator, fairly portable

Box 4.7.4 Biochemical markers of bone turnover

- Bone formation markers (products of the osteoblast)
  - Serum alkaline phosphatase (bone isoform)
  - Serum osteocalcin
  - Serum C- and N-propeptides of type I collagen
- Bone resorption markers (degradation products of type I collagen or enzymes)
  - Urinary excretion of pyridinium cross-links of collagen, e.g. deoxypyridinoline
  - Serum or urinary excretion of C- and N-telopeptides of type I collagen
  - Serum or urinary excretion of galactosyl hydroxylysine
  - Urinary excretion of hydroxyproline
  - Serum tartrate-resistant acid phosphatase

about the rate of bone turnover and the presence of secondary forms of osteoporosis (e.g. systemic mastocytosis). Patients with high bone turnover usually respond better to antiresorptive drugs.

Biochemical markers of bone turnover These reflect the processes of bone resorption and bone formation (Box 4.7.4). Markers that are specific to bone (e.g. osteocalcin and deoxypyridinoline) may be useful for monitoring the effect of drugs used in the treatment of osteoporosis (19). Biochemical markers of bone resorption may be particularly useful because they are maximally suppressed by 3 months' treatment with oestrogens or bisphosphonates (see below and Chapter 4.9). They could be more useful than bone density for monitoring treatment because changes in bone density may not be detected for 2 years and not all patients have access to bone densitometry.

Treatment

General measures

The treatment of acute back pain due to a recent vertebral fracture includes:

- bed rest (as short as possible), back support
- analgesics/nonsteroidal anti-inflammatory drugs (NSAIDs)
- heat and gentle massage
- insertion of cement into the vertebral body (balloon kyphoplasty (http://www.nice.org.uk/Guidance/IPG166) or percutaneous vertebroplasty (http://www.nice.org.uk/Guidance/IPG12)).

The treatment of chronic back pain due to vertebral fractures is difficult but includes:

- analgesics/NSAIDs
- physiotherapy
- intermittent use of spinal support for some activities
- exercise programme to maintain muscle strength and flexibility of the spine
- injection of local anaesthetic into the facet joints of the spine.

In all patients (with or without fractures), it is important to treat diseases that can increase bone loss and contribute to osteoporosis (Box 4.7.1). An important part of the management of patients with osteoporosis, especially those following hip fracture or other frail patients, consists of attention to their general health status, such as ensuring adequate dietary protein intake, and measures to decrease the risk of falls or the degree of trauma that results from falling. These included better lighting, provision of hand rails, removal of obstacles, attention to drugs such as sedatives and antihypertensives that may predispose to falls, or carpeted surfaces rather than hard floors. Regular exercise may be of value in maintaining mobility and improving muscle mass, thus reducing the risk of falling. Heavy weight-bearing and vigorous exercise programmes should be avoided by patients with osteoporosis as they may trigger the occurrence of a new fracture.

Calcium and vitamin D

Low calcium intake and vitamin D deficiency should be prevented or effectively treated in all patients. As many hip fractures occur in patients over age 80 years and this population is particularly prone to low calcium intake and vitamin D deficiency (see Chapter 4.10), it is particularly important to ensure that these patients receive adequate calcium and vitamin D as part of their management. Ambulatory patients who receive periodic sunlight exposure generally produce sufficient vitamin D through skin photoconversion, but others should receive a supplement containing at least 800 IU of vitamin D daily. Total intake of calcium, including supplements if necessary, should be at least 1000 mg. Despite the necessity of adequate calcium and vitamin D for bone health, it should be appreciated that treatment with calcium and vitamin D alone is insufficient to prevent postmenopausal bone loss or to markedly reduce fracture risk in patients with osteoporosis.

Pharmacological intervention (20)

Drugs to increase bone mass inhibit bone resorption or stimulate bone formation. Most drugs approved for use in osteoporosis inhibit bone resorption, but some of these (e.g. hormone replacement therapy (HRT), bisphosphonates) increase BMD by 5–10% over the first 2 years of treatment.

Antiresorptive drugs—bisphosphonates—are considered the treatment of choice (Table 4.7.2). Their strict dosing instructions may reduce compliance in the elderly. In the UK, five agents are currently approved for use in osteoporosis: etidronate, alendronate, risedronate, ibandronate, zoledronic acid, and raloxifene. The most effective alternative treatments are raloxifene and HRT.

- Calcium, 1000 mg/day, and vitamin D, 500 IU/day, have been shown to prevent hip fracture in housebound, elderly patients. This treatment is safe and inexpensive, and does not require monitoring. It is commonly given with other treatments for osteoporosis.
- Etidronate is given in a cyclical regimen in a dose of 400 mg/day for 2 weeks, followed by elemental calcium, 500 mg/day for 11 weeks. The effects on spine BMD are similar to those of HRT; etidronate is licensed for 'spinal osteoporosis'. Side-effects are uncommon. Etidronate must be taken on an empty stomach (2 h after the last meal and 2 h before the next meal).
- Alendronate is given in a dose of 10 mg/day continuously or 70 mg once weekly. Alendronate must be taken at least 30 min

Table 4.7.2 Evidence for fracture prevention from randomized clinical trials

	Spine	Nonvertebral	Hip
Alendronate	A	A	A
Calcitonin	A	B	B
Calcitriol	A	A	ND
Calcium	A	B	B
Calcium/vit D	ND	A	A
Cyclic etidronate	A	B	B
Denosumab	A	A	A
Hip protectors	–	–	A
HRT	A	A	A
Ibandronate	A	ND	ND
Physical exercise	ND	B	B
Raloxifene	A	ND	ND
Resedronate	A	A	A
Strontium	A	A	A
Tibolone	A	A	ND
Vitamin D	ND	B	B
Zoledronic acid	A	A	A

Level of evidence: Grade A, meta-analysis of randomized controlled trials or from at least one randomized controlled trial; Grade B, from at least one well-designed, quasiexperimental study, or from well-designed nonexperimental descriptive studies such as comparative, correlation, or case–control studies; Grade C, from expert committee reports/opinions and/or clinical experience of authorities.

In most studies, the control group received calcium supplements and adequate vitamin D so these effects are in excess of this supplementation.

ND, not determined.

(Updated from Compston J. Prevention and treatment of osteoporosis. Clinical guidelines and new evidence. *Journal of the Royal College of Physicians, London*, 2000; **34**: 518–21.)

before breakfast (to help absorption) with a full glass of water, and the patient must not lie down after taking the tablet (to avoid oesophagitis). Alendronate is equally effective on the hip, forearm, and spine and has been shown to prevent fracture at all of these sites.

- Risedronate is given in a dose of 5 mg/day continuously or 35 mg once weekly. Risedronate can be taken at least 30 min before breakfast or 2 h after a meal. It has been shown to prevent spine, hip, and other fractures.
- Ibandronate is given in a dose of 150 mg once monthly; calcium recommendations and instructions for use are as for risedronate. Ibandronate reduces the risk of vertebral fracture (and other fractures, if the BMD T score is ≤ 3). This treatment can also be given by intravenous injection (3 mg) given every 3 months.
- Zoledronic acid is given by intravenous infusion (5 mg over 15 min) given every 12 months. It reduces fractures at the spine and hip and all other fracture sites; it has been shown to reduce further fractures in patients presenting with hip fractures.
- Raloxifene is given in a dose of 60 mg/day continuously. Raloxifene has been shown to reduce the risk of spine (but not other) fracture, and may reduce the risk of breast cancer. It may increase the risk of deep vein thrombosis and does not prevent hot flushes.
- HRT is no longer recommended for the first-line prevention of osteoporosis because the risks outweighs the benefits. Risks with HRT include breast cancer (50% increase in risk after 10 years' treatment) and deep vein thrombosis (threefold increase in risk, particularly in patients with previous deep vein thrombosis); it is associated with increased risk of stroke and ischaemic heart disease. The benefits of HRT include relief of hot flushes and vaginal dryness. Tibolone (21) has the advantage that it reduces fractures (spine and nonvertebral) and the risk of breast cancer, but it does increase the risk of stroke.
- Testosterone therapy is effective in men with hypogonadism. It is not currently used in eugonadal men, because of concerns about the increased risk of prostate cancer and ischaemic heart disease (via lowering of high-density lipoprotein).

Three other agents can be useful in special circumstances.

- Strontium ranelate works by mechanisms that are not yet fully elucidated. It reduces the risk of spine and non-spine fracture and is given in a dose of 2 g/day in water, preferably at bedtime.
- Calcitonin (salmon calcitonin, 50 IU SC on alternate days) is not as effective as HRT and bisphosphonates, and has several side effects (e.g. nausea, diarrhoea, flushing). It has an analgesic effect and can be useful in patients with acute vertebral fracture. A nasal preparation is now available (200 μg/day).
- Calcitriol stimulates calcium absorption and may stimulate osteoblasts directly. It appears to be effective in corticosteroid-induced osteoporosis, in which it can be considered an alternative to HRT or bisphosphonates, particularly in younger patients. Regular monitoring of serum calcium is required because hypercalcaemia is a common adverse effect.

Formation-stimulating drugs have been licensed for osteoporosis.

- Use of a recombinant fragment of parathyroid hormone (teriparatide) may be advised by specialists in osteoporosis for patients who have failed to respond to antiresorptive therapy or are intolerant of it and have severe osteoporosis. Teriparatide treatment increases the thickness of cortical bone and the connectivity of trabecular bone. These improvements in bone quality (and in quantity—spine BMD is increased by about 9% on average at 1 year) are associated with reductions in fractures of the spine and elsewhere. The treatment is given by daily subcutaneous injection (20 μg/day), with calcium supplementation for a period of 2 years. Parathyroid hormone (1–84) is now available for the treatment of severe osteoporosis and it reduces the risk of vertebral fractures. It is administered at a dose of 100 μg daily given subcutaneously.

Follow-up

Once patients have been identified and treatment initiated, it is important to ensure adequate follow-up to reinforce the importance of compliance to treatment and evaluate response. At a minimum, all treated patients should be seen initially after 3 to 6 months and thereafter at least annually. The importance of adherence to treatment should be stressed.

Monitoring of response to therapy can be achieved with the use of biochemical markers or repeated BMD measurements, and may be of value in assessing compliance and providing feedback to patients. Although not required, treatment response to oral

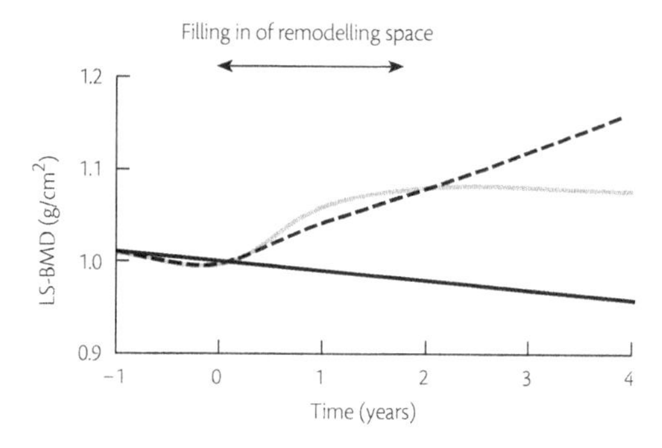

Fig. 4.7.4 Changes in bone mineral density (BMD) with treatment. If no treatment is given (solid line) to someone with osteoporosis there is progressive bone loss. Antiresorptive treatments (stippled line) prevent this bone loss and result in bone gain because of filling in of the remodelling space (over a period of about 2 years). Formation-simulating treatments result in a year-on-year increase in BMD (broken line).

antiresorptive treatments, such as bisphosphonates, can be evaluated after 3 to 6 months by assessing the change in biochemical markers of bone turnover, such as N-terminal or C-terminal cross-links of type I collagen, serum osteocalcin or serum procollagen I N-propeptide (Box 4.7.4). In most patients these markers decrease by more than 30% relative to pretreatment baseline measurements, and/or are reduced to within the premenopausal reference range, providing evidence that the treatment is having its desired effect to decrease bone turnover. Changes in BMD occur over a longer time frame, and it is generally not useful to repeat the BMD measurement before the end of 1 to 2 years of therapy, and every 2 years thereafter (Fig. 4.7.4). Most patients receiving efficacious therapy can be expected to have a measurable increase in BMD at the spine and hip (especially the trochanter subregion) after 2 years of treatment. The increases in BMD are small at the peripheral sites of measurement, such as the heel or forearm, in relation to the precision of these measurements. Therefore, peripheral sites are unreliable for assessing response in individual patients.

Other forms of primary osteoporosis—male osteoporosis

Although osteoporosis is generally regarded as a disease of women, up to 30% of hip fractures and 20% of vertebral fractures occur in men (11). The risk factors for osteoporotic fractures in men include low body mass index, smoking, high alcohol consumption, corticosteroid therapy, physical inactivity, diseases that predispose to low bone mass, and conditions increasing the risk of falls. The key drugs and diseases that definitely produce a decrease in BMD and/or an increase in fracture rate in men are long-term corticosteroid use, hypogonadism, alcoholism, and transplantation. Age-related bone loss may be a result of declining renal function, vitamin D deficiency, increased PTH levels, low serum testosterone levels, low calcium intake, and absorption. Osteoporosis can be diagnosed on the basis of radiological assessments of bone mass or clinically when it becomes symptomatic. Various biochemical markers have been related to bone loss in healthy and osteoporotic men. Their use as diagnostic tools, however, needs further investigation. A practical approach would be to consider a bone density more than 2.5 SD below the young normal mean value ($T \leq -2.5$) as an indication for therapy (17). The treatment options for men with osteoporosis include agents to influence bone resorption or formation and specific therapy for any underlying pathological condition. Testosterone treatment increases BMD in hypogonadal men and is most effective in those whose epiphyses have not closed completely. Bisphosphonates (such as alendronate and risedronate) are the treatment of choice in idiopathic osteoporosis (22, 23), with teriparatide in more severe cases (24).

References

1. NIH Consensus Development Panel on Osteoporosis Prevention, Diagnosis, and Therapy, March 7-29, 2000: highlights of the conference. *South Med J*, 2001; **94**: 569–73.
2. Kanis JA, Melton LJIII, Christiansen C, Johnston CC, Khaltaev N. The diagnosis of osteoporosis. *J Bone Miner Res*, 1994; **9**: 1137–41.
3. Seeman E, Delmas PD. Bone quality—the material and structural basis of bone strength and fragility. *N Engl J Med*, 2006; **354**: 2250–61.
4. Kanis JA, McCloskey EV, Johansson H, Strom O, Borgstrom F, Oden A. Case finding for the management of osteoporosis with FRAX—assessment and intervention thresholds for the UK. *Osteoporos Int*, 2008; **19**: 1395–408.
5. Eastell R. Role of oestrogen in the regulation of bone turnover at the menarche. *J Endocrinol*, 2005; **185**: 223–34.
6. Walsh JS, Henry YM, Fatayerji D, Eastell R. Lumbar spine peak bone mass and bone turnover in men and women: a longitudinal study. *Osteoporos Int*, 2008; **16**: 355–62.
7. Liu YJ, Shen H, Xiao P, Xiong DH, Li LH, Recker RR, *et al.* Molecular genetic studies of gene identification for osteoporosis: a 2004 update. *J Bone Miner Res*, 2006; **21**: 1511–35.
8. Eastell R. Treatment of postmenopausal osteoporosis. *N Engl J Med*, 1998; **338**: 736–46.
9. Seeman E, Delmas PD. Bone quality—the material and structural basis of bone strength and fragility. *N Engl J Med*, 2006; **354**: 2250–61.
10. Riggs BL, Khosla S, Melton LJ, III. Sex steroids and the construction and conservation of the adult skeleton. *Endocr Rev*, 2002; **23**: 279–302.
11. Ebeling PR. Clinical practice. Osteoporosis in men. *N Engl J Med*, 2008; **358**: 1474–82.
12. Kanis JA, Johansson H, Johnell O, Oden A, De Laet C, Eisman JA, *et al.* Alcohol intake as a risk factor for fracture. *Osteoporos Int*, 2005; **16**: 737–42.
13. van Staa TP. The pathogenesis, epidemiology and management of glucocorticoid-induced osteoporosis. *Calcif Tissue Int*, 2006; **79**: 129–37.
14. Compston J. Glucocorticoid-induced osteoporosis. *Horm Res*, 2003; **60** (Suppl 3): 77–9.
15. Maalouf NM, Shane E. Osteoporosis after solid organ transplantation. *J Clin Endocrinol Metab*, 2005; **90**: 2456–65.
16. Jiang G, Eastell R, Barrington NA, Ferrar L. Comparison of methods for the visual identification of prevalent vertebral fracture in osteoporosis. *Osteoporos Int*, 2004; **15**: 887–96.
17. Cummings SR, Bates D, Black DM. Clinical use of bone densitometry: scientific review. *JAMA*, 2002; **288**: 1889–97.
18. Tannenbaum C, Clark J, Schwartzman K, Wallenstein S, Lapinski R, Meier D, *et al.* Yield of laboratory testing to identify secondary contributors to osteoporosis in otherwise healthy women. *J Clin Endocrinol Metab*, 2002; **87**: 4431–7.
19. Eastell R, Hannon RA. Biomarkers of bone health and osteoporosis risk. *Proc Nutr Soc*, 2008; **67**: 157–62.
20. Sambrook P, Cooper C. Osteoporosis. *Lancet*, 2006; **367**: 2010–8.
21. Cummings SR, Ettinger B, Delmas PD, Kenemans P, Stathopoulos V, Verweij P, *et al.* The effects of tibolone in older postmenopausal women. *N Engl J Med*, 2008; **359**: 697–708.

22. Orwoll E, Ettinger M, Weiss S, Miller P, Kendler D, Graham J, *et al.* Alendronate for the treatment of osteoporosis in men. *N Engl J Med*, 2000; **343**: 604–10.
23. Boonen S, Orwoll ES, Wenderoth D, Stoner KJ, Eusebio R, Delmas PD. Once-weekly risedronate in men with osteoporosis: results of a 2-year, placebo-controlled, double-blind, multicenter study. *J Bone Miner Res*, 2009; **24**: 719–25.
24. Orwoll ES, Scheele WH, Paul S, Adami S, Syversen U, Perez A, *et al.* The effect of teriparatide [human parathyroid hormone (1–34)] therapy on bone density in men with osteoporosis. *J Bone Miner Res*, 2003; **18**: 9–17.

4.8

Thyroid disorders and bone disease

Moira S. Cheung, Apostolos I. Gogakos, J.H. Duncan Bassett, Graham R. Williams

Introduction

Osteoporosis is defined as a bone mineral density (BMD) of 2.5 or more standard deviations below that of a young adult (T score ≤ −2.5). It is characterized by reduced bone mass, low BMD, deterioration of bone microarchitecture, and an increased susceptibility to fragility fracture. The prevalence of postmenopausal osteoporosis increases with age from 6% at 50 years of age to over 50% at age 80 and the lifetime incidence of fracture for a 50 year old in the UK is 40% for women and 13% for men. Osteoporosis is a worldwide public health burden that costs an estimated £1.7 billion in the UK, $15 billion in the USA, and £32 billion in Europe per annum (see Chapter 4.7).

Low BMD, a prior or parental history of fracture, low body mass index, use of glucocorticoids, smoking, excessive alcohol consumption, untreated thyrotoxicosis, and other risk factors increase susceptibility to osteoporosis and fracture. Even subclinical hyperthyroidism, defined by a suppressed thyroid stimulating hormone (TSH) level in the presence of normal thyroid hormone concentrations, is associated with fracture while treatment with thyroxine (T_4) at doses that suppress TSH is associated with increased bone turnover and low BMD in postmenopausal women (1).

Thyroid disease occurs 10-fold more frequently in women and its prevalence increases with age. Hypothyroidism is a common disorder with a prevalence of 0.5% in women between the ages of 40 and 60 and greater than 2% over the age of 70. Thyrotoxicosis has a prevalence of 0.45% in women between the ages of 40 and 60 and 1.4% over the age of 60. As a result, 3% of women over 50 receive T_4 replacement for either primary hypothyroidism or the consequences of surgical or radio-iodine treatment for thyrotoxicosis, and at least 20% of them are overtreated (2). Moreover, subclinical hyperthyroidism affects an additional 1.5% of women over 60 and its prevalence also increases with age. Nevertheless, the role of thyroid hormone in the pathogenesis of osteoporosis has been under-recognized and the extent of its contribution remains uncertain.

Bone strength and fracture susceptibility are determined by the acquisition of peak bone mass and the rate of bone loss in adulthood (3). In children, congenital hypothyroidism is the most common congenital endocrine disorder with an incidence of 1 in 1800. Hypothyroidism in children results in delayed bone age and growth arrest and treatment with T_4 reverses these changes by inducing rapid 'catch-up' growth. Although juvenile Graves' disease is rare, it remains the commonest cause of thyrotoxicosis in children, being characterized by advanced bone age and accelerated growth that results in short stature due to premature fusion of the growth plates (4). In adults, histomorphometry studies reveal that hypothyroidism results in reduced bone turnover but a net gain in bone mass per remodelling cycle, whereas thyrotoxicosis increases bone resorption and bone formation but induces a net 10% loss of bone per remodelling cycle (5, 6). Taken together, these studies indicate the juvenile and adult skeleton is exquisitely sensitive to thyroid hormones. Thus, euthyroid status is essential for skeletal development, bone mineralization, and acquisition of peak bone mass, and the regulation of bone maintenance in adults. Importantly, recent large population studies have shown that both hypothyroidism and thyrotoxicosis are associated with an increased risk of fracture, demonstrating the physiological importance of euthyroid status for optimization of skeletal integrity and bone strength (7–11).

In this chapter we provide an up to date analysis of the role of thyroid hormone in skeletal development and adult bone maintenance by discussing evidence from animal models and basic science in relation to a detailed review of the current clinical literature.

Thyroid hormone action

Circulating thyroid hormone levels are maintained in the euthyroid range by a classical endocrine negative feedback loop. Thyrotropin-releasing hormone is synthesized in the paraventricular nucleus of the hypothalamus and stimulates synthesis and secretion of TSH from thyrotrophs in the anterior pituitary gland. TSH, acting via the G-protein coupled TSH receptor (TSHR), stimulates growth of thyroid follicular cells and the synthesis and release of thyroid hormones. Thyroid hormones act via thyroid hormone receptors in the hypothalamus and pituitary to inhibit thyrotropin-releasing hormone and TSH synthesis and secretion. This negative feedback loop maintains circulating thyroid hormones and TSH in a physiological inverse relationship, which defines the hypothalamic–pituitary–thyroid (HPT) axis set point (4).

The thyroid gland secretes the prohormone T_4 and a small amount of the physiologically active hormone 3,5,3′-L-triiodothyronine (T_3). The majority of circulating T_3, however, is thought to be generated via 5′-deiodination of T_4 by the type 1 iodothyronine deiodinase enzyme (DIO1) in liver and kidney. Circulating free T_4 levels are maintained at approximately three to fourfold higher concentrations than free T_3. Intracellular availability of T_3 is determined by active uptake of the free hormones by specific cell membrane transporters, including monocarboxylate transporter-8 and -10, and organic acid transporter protein-1c1, and by the activities of the type 2 and 3 deiodinase enzymes (DIO2 and DIO3). DIO2 converts T_4 to the active hormone T_3 by catalysing removal of a 5′-iodine atom. By contrast, DIO3 prevents activation of T_4 and inactivates T_3 by removal of a 5-iodine atom to generate the metabolites 3,3′,5′-L-triiodothyronine (reverse T_3) and 3,3′-diiodothyronine (T_2), respectively. Thus, the relative levels of DIO2 and DIO3 ultimately determine the concentration of intracellular T_3 available to the nuclear T_3 receptors (TRs) (12).

TRs act as hormone-inducible transcription factors that regulate expression of T_3-responsive target genes. The *THRA* and *THRB* genes encode three functional TRs: TRα1, TRβ1, and TRβ2. TRα1 and TRβ1 are expressed widely but their relative levels differ during development and in adulthood due to tissue-specific and temporospatial regulation. Expression of TRβ2, however, is restricted. In the hypothalamus and pituitary it mediates inhibition of thyrotropin-releasing hormone and TSH expression whilst in the cochlea and retina it has a key role to control the timing of sensory organ development (13).

Skeletal development and bone maintenance

The skeleton develops via two distinct processes. Endochondral ossification is the process by which long bones form and linear growth occurs. A cartilage anlage forms from mesenchyme condensations to form a scaffold for subsequent bone formation. Mesenchyme progenitor cells differentiate into chondrocyte precursors, which undergo a tightly regulated sequence of clonal expansion, proliferation, hypertrophic differentiation, and apoptosis. Chondrocytes secrete a cartilage matrix that mineralizes and is subsequently remodelled by the activities of bone resorbing osteoclasts and bone forming osteoblasts, resulting in formation of the diaphysis. Linear growth continues throughout development by a similar process within the epiphyseal growth plates, which are located at the proximal and distal ends of long bones. By contrast, the skull vertex forms by intramembranous ossification, in which mesenchymal cells differentiate directly into osteoblasts, resulting in bone formation in the absence of a cartilage scaffold. Linear growth continues until fusion of the growth plates during puberty but bone mineralization and consolidation of bone mass accrual continues into early adulthood so that peak bone mass is achieved during the third to fourth decade (14, 15).

Functional integrity and strength of the skeleton is maintained by the process of bone remodelling, which is achieved by the integrated and coupled activities of osteocytes, osteoclasts, and osteoblasts. Osteocytes comprise 90–95% of all adult bone cells. They derive from osteoblasts that have become embedded in bone matrix. The osteocyte network is thought to sense changes in mechanical load and regulate local initiation of bone remodelling by the release of cytokines and chemotactic signals or by osteocyte apoptosis. Bone remodelling begins with the recruitment of mature osteoclasts and their precursors to sites of altered mechanical load or micro-damage. Osteoclasts excavate a resorption cavity over a period of 3–5 weeks until this process is terminated by apoptosis and followed by recruitment of osteoblast precursors. Subsequently, osteoblasts undergo a programme of maturation during which they secrete and mineralize osteoid to replace the resorbed bone over a period of approximately 3 months. Coupling of osteoclast and osteoblast activities via signalling between the two cell lineages regulates the bone remodelling cycle and results in skeletal homoeostasis with preservation of bone strength. In summary, the bone remodelling cycle is initiated and orchestrated by osteocytes, and regulated by coupled crosstalk between osteoblasts and osteoclasts.

Thyroid hormone action in bone

TRα1 and TRβ1 are expressed in growth plate chondrocytes, bone marrow stromal cells, and osteoblasts but it is uncertain whether they are present in osteoclasts (4, 16).

In vivo and *in vitro* studies have shown that T_3 acts via the Indian hedgehog/ parathyroid hormone-related peptide feedback loop, growth hormone/ insulin-like growth factor-1, and fibroblast growth factor receptor-3 (FGFR3) signalling pathways to inhibit growth plate chondrocyte proliferation and stimulate hypertrophic chondrocyte differentiation. In childhood hypothyroidism, growth arrest and delayed bone formation are consequences of gross disruption of growth plate architecture (epiphyseal dysgenesis), which results from disorganization of the growth plates and a failure of hypertrophic chondrocyte differentiation. By contrast, thyroid hormone excess accelerates hypertrophic chondrocyte differentiation resulting in advanced bone formation (4, 16).

Studies of bone marrow stromal cells suggest that many of the actions of T_3 involve complex cytokine and growth factor signalling pathways that regulate communication between osteoblast and osteoclast cell lineages within the bone marrow microenvironment. *In vivo* and *in vitro* studies have further shown that T_3 regulates osteoblast differentiation and activity at least in part via the FGFR1 signalling pathway. Activating mutations of *FGFR1* cause Pfeiffer's craniosynostosis syndrome and, consistent with this, craniosynostosis is a recognized manifestation of severe juvenile thyrotoxicosis in which FGFR1 activity is increased in osteoblasts.

The regulation of adult bone turnover by thyroid hormones has been investigated by bone histomorphometry (5, 6). The skeletal manifestations of hypothyroidism include reduced osteoblast activity, impaired osteoid apposition, and a prolonged period of secondary bone mineralization. Consistent with a state of low bone turnover, osteoclast activity and bone resorption are also reduced. The effect of the low bone turnover state in hypothyroidism is a net increase in mineralization without a change in bone volume. By contrast, thyrotoxicosis results in a state of high bone turnover. The frequency of initiation of bone remodelling is markedly increased and the duration of the bone remodelling cycle is reduced. The net result is that the duration of bone formation and mineralization is reduced to a greater extent than the reduction in duration of bone resorption. This leads to a net 10% loss of bone per remodelling cycle, resulting in high bone turnover osteoporosis.

Studies in genetically modified mice

In vivo studies in mutant mice have demonstrated that TRα1 mediates T_3 action in bone (17). Mutation or deletion of TRα results in transient growth retardation, impaired ossification, and reduced bone mineralization during growth (Table 4.8.1). In adults, there is a defect in bone remodelling, a marked increase in bone mass, and increased bone mineralization. By contrast, mutation or deletion of TRβ results in an opposite phenotype of accelerated growth, advanced ossification with increased mineralization during growth but short stature, which results from premature quiescence of the growth plates (Table 4.8.1). In adults, increased bone remodelling results in osteoporosis and reduced bone mineralization. Taken together, these features indicate that thyroid hormones exert anabolic actions during skeletal growth but catabolic responses in adult bone (17). Mutation of TRα disrupts T_3 action in bone cells resulting in skeletal hypothyroidism, whereas mutation of TRβ disrupts the HPT axis, leading to elevated levels of circulating thyroid hormones which activate TRα in bone cells, resulting in skeletal hyperthyroidism. Consistent with these phenotypes, levels of TRα mRNA expression are 10- to 100-fold greater than TRβ in adult bone.

Recently, a direct role for TSH as a negative regulator of bone turnover has also been proposed (4). Osteoblasts and osteoclasts were shown to express the TSHR, and congenitally hypothyroid TSHR knockout mice treated with thyroid hormone displayed a phenotype of high bone turnover osteoporosis. As a result of these findings, it was suggested that bone loss was a consequence of TSH deficiency. However, the susceptibility of patients with Graves' disease to osteoporosis and fracture is inconsistent with the hypothesis that TSH negatively regulates bone turnover because the presence of TSHR-stimulating antibodies would be predicted to protect patients from osteoporosis. Thus, the skeletal consequences of thyrotoxicosis are most likely to result primarily from thyroid hormone excess although TSH deficiency cannot be excluded as a contributing factor (4).

These two possibilities cannot be differentiated readily because the HPT axis maintains thyroid hormones and TSH in a physiological reciprocal relationship. Nevertheless, studies in mutant mice have enabled the issue to be addressed *in vivo*. Thus, the skeletal phenotypes of two different mouse models of congenital hypothyroidism were compared. Pax8 knockout mice lack a transcription factor that is essential for thyroid follicular cell development and have undetectable thyroid hormone levels, a 2000-fold elevation of TSH, and a fully functional TSHR. By contrast, hyt/hyt mice have gross congenital hypothyroidism also accompanied by a 2000-fold increase in TSH but they harbour a point mutation in the *Tshr* gene, leading to complete loss of TSHR protein function. Both mutants exhibited a similar phenotype of growth retardation and delayed ossification typical of hypothyroidism despite the divergence in TSH signalling (4).

In summary, the skeleton is exquisitely sensitive to thyroid status during growth and in adulthood. T_3 exerts important anabolic responses during skeletal growth and has significant catabolic effects on adult bone. Both of these actions are mediated by TRα1.

Skeletal consequences of altered thyroid status in humans

Studies in children

Childhood hypothyroidism

Congenital hypothyroidism results in growth arrest, epiphyseal dysgenesis, delayed bone age, and short stature. Thyroxine replacement therapy induces rapid catch-up growth and as a result children that are treated early ultimately reach their predicted adult height and achieve normal BMD after 8.5 years' follow-up. Nevertheless, a single study has suggested that adult BMD may be reduced despite treatment from the neonatal period. Children with juvenile acquired hypothyroidism also display growth arrest, delayed bone maturation, and short stature. T_4 replacement again induces rapid catch-up growth, but these individuals may fail to achieve final predicted height and the resulting permanent height deficit is related to the duration of thyroid hormone deficiency prior to replacement (18).

Childhood hyperthyroidism

Juvenile thyrotoxicosis results in accelerated growth, advanced bone age, and short stature, which is a consequence of the premature fusion of the epiphyseal growth plates due to accelerated skeletal maturation. In severe cases in young children, early closure of the cranial sutures may result in craniosynostosis (19). To date, there

Table 4.8.1 Skeletal phenotypes of thyroid hormone receptor mutant mice

	TRα mutant mice	TRβ mutant mice
Systemic thyroid status	Euthyroid	Elevated T_4, T_3 and TSH
Skeletal thyroid status	Hypothyroid	Thyrotoxic
Juvenile skeleton	Transient growth delay Delayed endochondral and intramembranous ossification Impaired chondrocyte differentiation Reduced calcified bone	Persistent short stature Advanced endochondral and intramembranous ossification Enhanced chondrocyte differentiation Increased calcified bone
Adult skeleton	Osteosclerosis Increased bone volume Increased mineralization Reduced osteoclastic bone resorption	Osteoporosis Reduced bone volume Reduced mineralization Increased osteoclastic bone resorption

See review (17).
TR, 3,5,3′-L-triiodothyronine receptor.

are no data relating to the effects of childhood thyrotoxicosis on BMD.

Resistance to thyroid hormone

Resistance to thyroid hormone is an autosomal dominant condition resulting from a dominant negative mutation of TRβ (20). The mutant TRβ protein disrupts negative feedback in the HPT axis, leading to increased circulating thyroid hormone concentrations in the presence of inappropriately normal or elevated TSH levels. The syndrome results in a complex mixed phenotype of hyperthyroidism and hypothyroidism depending on the target tissue studied and the specific mutation present in TRβ. Thus, an individual patient can have symptoms of both thyroid hormone deficiency and excess. A broad range of skeletal abnormalities have been described in association with resistance to thyroid hormone. These include craniofacial abnormalities, craniosynostosis, delayed or advanced bone age, short stature, increased bone turnover, osteoporosis, and fracture, although only a few patients have been studied in detail.

Studies in adults

A large number of studies have attempted to characterize the skeletal consequences of altered thyroid function in adults. Unfortunately, many of these studies have been confounded by inclusion of patients with a variety of thyroid diseases and by comparison of mixed cohorts of patients, which have included pre- and postmenopausal women or men. Furthermore, many studies have lacked sufficient statistical power because of the inclusion of small numbers of patients and the absence of long-term follow-up. In addition, in many studies there has been inadequate control for other confounding factors that influence bone mass and fracture susceptibility, including: age, prior or family history of fracture, body mass index, physical activity, use of oestrogens, glucocorticoids, bisphosphonates, and vitamin D, prior history of thyroid disease or use of thyroxine, and smoking or alcohol intake. For these reasons, the literature in this field has been difficult to investigate by meta-analysis and conclusions can only be uncertain (1).

Studies of normal individuals

Bone turnover markers

Few studies have determined bone turnover markers in euthyroid populations. Zofkova *et al.* in a study of bone turnover markers in a population of 60 healthy postmenopausal women reported that high circulating TSH levels correlated with low urinary deoxypyridinoline concentrations but not with serum procollagen type I C propeptide levels (21). This study illustrates difficulties with interpretation of thyroid hormone effects on bone turnover as only a small number of subjects were investigated and individuals with treated hypothyroidism, subclinical hyperthyroidism, and secondary hyperparathyroidism were not excluded.

Bone mineral density and fracture

Four large population studies have investigated the relationship between thyroid status and BMD (Table 4.8.2). van der Deure *et al.* studied a population of 1151 euthyroid men and women over 55 from Rotterdam (22). BMD at the femoral neck was positively correlated with TSH levels and inversely correlated with free T_4, and the association with free T_4 was much stronger than the association with TSH. No relationships between free T_4 or TSH and fracture were identified in this study. Kim *et al.* studied 959 Korean postmenopausal women and showed that individuals with low-normal TSH levels between 0.5 and1.1 mU/l had lower lumbar spine and femoral neck BMD than women with high-normal TSH between 2.8 and 5.0 mU/l, although no fracture data were reported (23). Morris studied 581 postmenopausal American women and showed that subjects with a low-normal TSH were nearly five times more likely to have osteoporosis than women with a high-normal TSH (24). Grimnes *et al.* studied a population of 993 postmenopausal women and 968 men from Tromso. This study revealed that individuals with TSH below the 2.5th percentile had a low forearm BMD whereas those with TSH above the 97.5th percentile had a high femoral neck BMD compared with the rest of the population (25). Neither of these studies investigated the incidence of fracture. Finally, the incidence of fracture in 367 UK women over 50 was prospectively studied for 10 years by Finigan *et al.* and no associations between free T_3, free T_4, or TSH and incident vertebral fracture were identified (26).

In summary, these studies suggest the hypothesis that thyroid status in the upper normal range is associated with reduced BMD whereas thyroid status in the lower normal range is associated with increased BMD. A definitive conclusion, however, is not possible as these studies unfortunately did not account for a number of confounding variables. Prospective population studies of sufficient size and duration will be required to determine the relationship between thyroid status and fracture risk.

Studies of patients with hypothyroidism

Bone turnover markers and BMD

Histomorphometric analyses have demonstrated that bone turnover is decreased in hypothyroidism (5, 6) but studies of the effect of

Table 4.8.2 Large studies of thyroid status and BMD

First author (reference)	Study design	Subjects (n)	Patient group	Fracture risk
Van der Deure (22)	Prospective cohort	479 men 672 women	Men and women >55 years of age	Free T_4 negatively associated with spine and hip BMD
Grimnes (25)	Cross-sectional	968 men 993 women	Men and women >55 years of age	Decreased forearm BMD associated with low-normal TSH
Morris (24)	Cross-sectional	581 women	Postmenopausal women	Decreased spine BMD associated with low-normal TSH
Kim (23)	Cross-sectional	959 women	Postmenopausal women	Decreased spine and hip BMD associated with low-normal TSH
Jamal (9)	Cross-sectional	15 316 women	Postmenopausal women	Decreased hip BMD associated with abnormally low TSH

Abbreviations: BMD, bone mineral density; TSH, thyroid stimulating hormone.

hypothyroidism on bone turnover markers have included only very small numbers of patients and were inconclusive. Consistent with histomorphometric data showing normal bone volume in hypothyroid patients, Vestergaard and Mosekilde, and Stamato *et al.* have reported that BMD is normal in patients newly diagnosed with hypothyroidism (10, 27).

Fracture

Large population studies, however, have demonstrated an association between hypothyroidism and fracture. Patients with a prior history of hypothyroidism had a two to three-fold increased relative risk of fracture, which persisted for up to 10 years following initial diagnosis (7, 10, 11, 28) (Table 4.8.3).

In summary, hypothyroidism results in low bone turnover and an increased risk of fracture.

Studies of patients with thyrotoxicosis

The severe bone disease associated with overt uncontrolled thyrotoxicosis in now rare because of early diagnosis and treatment, although several studies have investigated the skeleton in thyrotoxic patients prior to treatment.

Bone turnover markers and BMD

The effect of thyrotoxicosis on bone turnover markers is consistent with histomorphometric data reported by Eriksen *et al.* (5). Thus, levels of bone resorption markers such as urinary pyridinoline and deoxypyridinoline are increased. Bone formation markers, including bone-specific alkaline phosphatase and osteocalcin, are also elevated. A meta-analysis of 20 eligible studies by Vestergaard and Mosekilde (37) calculated that BMD at the time of diagnosis of thyrotoxicosis was reduced compared to age-matched controls (Table 4.8.4).

Fracture

Two cross-sectional case–controlled (11, 43) and four population studies (7, 8, 29, 30) have identified an association between fracture and a prior history of thyrotoxicosis (Table 4.8.3). Similarly, a meta-analysis of patients with thyrotoxicosis revealed an increased relative risk of hip fracture (37). The majority of these studies did not determine whether the increased fracture risk could be accounted for by reduced BMD, although one prospective study (29) showed that a prior history of thyroid disease is associated with hip fracture even after adjustment for BMD. Furthermore, Bauer *et al.* (8, 44)

Table 4.8.3 Large studies of thyroid status and fracture risk

Reference	Study design	Subjects (n)	Patient group	Fracture risk
Positive studies				
Ahmed (7)	Cross-sectional	27 159 men and women	Nonvertebral fractures	Increased risk of fractures with both thyrotoxicosis and hypothyroidism
Vestergaard (11)	Cross-sectional case–control	124 655 men and women 373 962 controls	All fractures	Fracture risk increased for 5 years after thyrotoxicosis and 10 years after hypothyroidism
Jamal (9)	Cross-sectional	15 316 women	Postmenopausal women	Increased risk of vertebral fracture with low TSH
Vestergaard (10)	Cross-sectional	11 776 thyrotoxic 4473 hypothyroid 48 710 controls	National register	Increased risk of femur fracture with thyrotoxicosis and hypothyroidism
Sheppard (35)	Cross-sectional	23 183 men and women	T_4 replacement	Increase risk of femur fracture in males
Bauer (8)	Prospective longitudinal	686 women	Women >65 years of age	Increased risk of hip and vertebral fracture with suppressed TSH
Lau (36)	Cross-sectional	1176 Asian men and women 1162 controls	>50 years with hip fracture	Increase risk of hip fracture with T_4 treatment
Franklyn (31)	Retrospective cohort	1226 men 5983 women	Radio-iodine treated thyrotoxicosis	Increase risk of death from hip fracture
Seeley (30)	Longitudinal	9704 women	Women >65 years of age	Increased risk of foot fractures if prior thyrotoxicosis
Cummings (29)	Longitudinal	9516 women	Women >65 years of age	Increased fracture risk with prior thyrotoxicosis
Negative studies				
Van der Deure (22)	Prospective cohort	479 men 672 women	>55 years of age	Free T_4 and TSH not associated with fracture
Van den Eeden (34)	Cross-sectional case–controlled	501 women 533 controls	Hip fracture	No association with T_4 replacement
Melton (33)	Retrospective cohort	630 men and women	Thyroidectomy	No association with fracture
Leese (32)	Cross-sectional	1180 men and women	Thyroid register	No association between fracture risk and TSH

TSH, thyroid stimulating hormone.

Table 4.8.4 Meta-analyses and literature reviews

First author (reference)	Population	Studies (n)	Type	Conclusions
Heemstra (39)	Suppressive T_4	21 BMD	Literature review	Postmenopausal women at risk of reduced BMD; no effect in premenopausal women or men
Murphy (1)	Suppressive T_4 T_4 replacement Thyroid disease	19 BMD 9 BMD 15 Fracture	Literature review	Prior history of thyrotoxicosis is associated with increased fracture risk Subclinical hyperthyroidism is associated with reduced BMD in postmenopausal women A suppressed TSH from any cause is associated with an increased fracture risk in postmenopausal women Appropriate T_4 replacement does not affected BMD or fracture risk Suppressive T_4 treatment does not affect BMD in premenopausal women or men; the situation is less clear in postmenopausal women
Vestergaard (37)	Thyrotoxicosis	20 BMD 5 Fracture	Meta-analysis	Spine and hip BMD reduced in untreated thyrotoxicosis Fractures risk increases with age at diagnosis
Schneider (42)	T_4 replacement	63 BMD	Literature review	Insufficient evidence to draw formal conclusion
Quan (40)	Suppressive T_4	11 BMD	Literature review	Effect in postmenopausal women unclear No effect in premenopausal women or men
Uzzan (41)	T_4 replacement Suppressive T_4	13 BMD 27 BMD	Meta-analysis	Suppressive doses of T_4 associated with reduced BMD at radius, spine, and hip in postmenopausal women but not in premenopausal women or men
Faber (38)	Suppressive T_4	13 BMD	Meta-analysis	Suppressive T_4 associated with reduced BMD in postmenopausal women and an excess annual bone loss of 1% per year No effect in premenopausal women

BMD, bone mineral density; T_4, thyroid hormone; TSH, thyroid stimulating hormone.

demonstrated that low TSH was associated with a three to fourfold increased risk of fracture even though a relationship between TSH and BMD was not identified. In agreement with these observations, Franklyn *et al.* showed an increased standardized mortality ratio due to fractured femur in a follow-up register of thyrotoxic patients treated with radio-iodine (31). Nevertheless, several studies have failed to demonstrate an association between thyrotoxicosis and fracture (32–34).

In summary, a prior history of thyrotoxicosis may be associated with reduced bone density and a long-term increased risk of fracture, although data are conflicting and limited by confounding factors.

Studies of individuals with subclinical hyperthyroidism

Bone turnover markers and BMD

Either elevated or normal levels of the bone resorption markers urinary deoxypyridinoline and hydroxyproline have been reported in patients with subclinical hyperthyroidism. Similarly, levels of the bone formation markers osteocalcin, alkaline phosphatase, and procollagen I C-terminal extension propeptide have been reported to be elevated or normal. Subclinical hyperthyroidism has also been associated with reduced BMD at the femoral neck and other sites, although other studies have not found such a relationship. Accordingly, a meta-analysis was inconclusive (38) (Table 4.8.4).

Fracture

Although no prospective studies of fracture risk in subclinical hyperthyroidism have been published, data from Bauer *et al.* suggest that suppressed TSH levels may be associated with an increased risk of fracture (8). Additionally, Jamal *et al.* reported a subanalysis of the Fracture Intervention Trial and demonstrated that a TSH level suppressed below 0.5 mIU/l was associated with an increased risk of vertebral fracture (9). Unfortunately, there was insufficient information provided to determine whether patients in this study had subclinical hyperthyroidism or untreated thyrotoxicosis.

In summary, subclinical hyperthyroidism may be associated with increased bone turnover, reduced BMD, and increased fracture risk although again insufficient data are currently available to draw definitive conclusions.

Studies in patients treated with suppressive doses of thyroxine

The long-term management of patients with differentiated thyroid cancer frequently involves treatment with doses of thyroxine that suppress circulating TSH concentrations and which may have detrimental effects on the skeleton.

Bone turnover markers

A number of small studies have investigated the effect of suppressive doses of T_4 on bone turnover markers. Three studies reported increased levels of bone resorption markers in patients receiving T_4 and two of these also demonstrated an increase in bone formation markers (45). Nevertheless, other studies reported no effect on markers of bone resorption or formation (46).

Bone mineral density

A large number of studies have investigated the effects of suppressive doses of T_4 on BMD in pre- and postmenopausal women and in men at various anatomical locations.

Most studies showed no effect of TSH suppression therapy on BMD at the lumber spine, femur, or radius in premenopausal women. By contrast, three studies have reported reduced BMD at the femur in premenopausal women receiving suppressive doses of T_4. Heemstra *et al.* analysed 12 cross-sectional and four prospective studies of premenopausal women receiving suppressive doses of T_4, but a meta-analysis could not be performed due to heterogeneity of the cohorts (39). The authors concluded that treatment with suppressive doses of T_4 did not affect BMD in premenopausal women (Table 4.8.4). This finding supported results of an earlier review of eight studies by Quan *et al.* (40).

The effects of suppressive doses of T_4 on BMD in postmenopausal women are less clear as the two most rigorous cross-sectional studies reported conflicting results (47, 48). Franklyn *et al.* investigated 26 UK postmenopausal women treated for 8 years and demonstrated no effect of TSH suppression on BMD (47), whereas Kung and Yeung studied 34 postmenopausal Asian women and found a decrease in total body, lumbar spine, and femoral BMD in patients treated with suppressive doses of T_4 (48). However, direct comparison between the two studies is difficult because in the study by Franklyn *et al.* TSH was fully suppressed in only 80% of patients, whilst mean calcium intake was low in the study by Kung *et al.* Similar conflicting results have been reported at various anatomical sites in less well-controlled cross-sectional and longitudinal studies. Eight cross-sectional studies also included investigation of male patients, but only Jodar *et al.* reported a reduction in lumber spine and femur BMD in men receiving suppressive doses of T_4 (49).

A meta-analysis of 27 studies investigating the effect of suppressive doses of T_4 on BMD (41) concluded there were no effects on BMD in premenopausal women or men, although such treatment in postmenopausal women for up to 10 years led to reductions in BMD at the distal radius, lumbar spine, and femoral neck of between 5 and 7% (Table 4.8.4). Although the long-term effects of suppressive doses of T_4 on BMD in postmenopausal women remain uncertain, further reviews of this topic support the findings of Uzzan *et al.* and recommend monitoring of BMD in such patients (1, 39, 40).

Fracture

No studies with sufficient statistical power to determine the effect of treatment with suppressive dose of T_4 on fracture risk have been reported.

In summary, treatment with suppressive dose of T_4 does not affect BMD in premenopausal women or men but may lead to reduced BMD in postmenopausal women. Effects on bone turnover are inconclusive and there are no data regarding fracture risk.

Studies of patients treated for hypothyroidism

Bone turnover markers, BMD, and fracture

Histomorphometric studies have suggested an increase in bone turnover in response to T_4 replacement in hypothyroidism (5) but the effect on bone markers has not been reported. The majority of cross-sectional studies of pre- and postmenopausal women receiving long-term T_4 replacement for hypothyroidism have not identified any significant effect on BMD. However, in premenopausal women Paul *et al.* (50) reported a 10% reduction BMD in the femur but no change at the lumbar spine following T_4 replacement, whilst Kung and Pun (51) reported reduced BMD at both lumbar spine and hip. There are no prospective studies investigating the effects of T_4 replacement in hypothyroid patients on fracture risk, although population studies have not identified an association between T_4 replacement therapy and fracture (29, 33, 34).

Studies of patients treated for thyrotoxicosis

Bone turnover markers, BMD, and fracture

Two prospective studies of patients with thyrotoxicosis have shown that elevated levels of bone resorption and bone formation markers return to normal levels within 1 month of initiation of treatment. A meta-analysis of 20 studies investigating the effect of treatment for thyrotoxicosis on BMD (37) demonstrated that the low BMD at diagnosis returned to normal after 5 years (Table 4.8.4). In a subsequent study, treatment for thyrotoxicosis was shown to result in a 4% increase in BMD within 1 year (52). Nevertheless, in a large population study Vestergaard *et al.* (11) reported that an increased relative risk of fracture risk persisted for 5 years following a diagnosis of thyrotoxicosis (Table 4.8.3).

In summary, treatment of patients with thyrotoxicosis results in normalization of bone turnover and BMD by 5 years, although the increased risk of fracture may persist for longer.

Human genetics

In healthy individuals free T_3, free T_4, and TSH levels fluctuate over a range that is less than 50% of the normal reference range. Thus, variation in thyroid status within an individual is narrower than the broad interindividual variation seen in the population. Each person has a unique HPT axis set point that lies within the population reference range, indicating there is variation in tissue sensitivity to thyroid hormones between normal individuals (53). Data from the UK Adult Twin Registry estimate heritability for free T_3 concentration at 23%, free T_4 at 39%, and TSH at 65%, whilst estimates from a Danish twin study were 64%, 65%, and 64%, respectively (54, 55). A genome-wide screen identified eight quantitative trait loci linked to circulating free T_3, free T_4, and TSH levels, indicating that thyroid status is inherited as a complex genetic trait (56). Similarly, unbiased genome-wide association studies and candidate gene approaches have shown that osteoporosis is a polygenic disorder in which many genes and signalling pathways exert small contributions that influence bone size, BMD, and fracture susceptibility (57).

These observations raise the possibility that variations in bone turnover, BMD, and fracture susceptibility in normal individuals may be associated with differences in their HPT axis set points. Furthermore, genes that establish the HPT axis set point and thus regulate thyroid status may also influence the acquisition of peak bone mass, skeletal growth, and bone turnover and thereby contribute to the genetic determination of fracture risk. This hypothesis is consistent with observations in other physiological complex traits including body mass index, blood pressure, heart rate, atherosclerosis, serum cholesterol, and psychological well-being, in which variations have been associated with small alterations in thyroid function and with polymorphisms in thyroid pathway genes that are themselves associated with altered serum thyroid hormone and TSH concentrations (58). These new developments in our understanding the physiological regulation of the HPT axis and thyroid hormone action in target tissues have been extended recently to investigation of the skeleton and these studies suggest common genetic factors may be involved in the determination of thyroid status, bone turnover, and BMD (22, 59).

Future prospective studies investigating the relationships between variations in the HPT axis set point and genes regulating thyroid hormone transport, metabolism, and action with bone mass and fracture risk will need to be well designed and adequately powered. Stringent exclusion criteria will be required to define large populations of individuals which can be followed up prospectively for prolonged periods. Nevertheless, such studies have the potential to individualize fracture risk prediction and inform the choice of preventative therapy (58).

Conclusions

- Bone strength and fracture susceptibility are determined by peak bone mass acquisition during growth and the rate of bone loss in adulthood.
- Large population studies indicate that both hypothyroidism and thyrotoxicosis are associated with increased fracture susceptibility, demonstrating the importance of euthyroid status for optimal bone strength.
- A negative feedback loop maintains circulating thyroid hormones and TSH in an inverse relationship which defines the HPT axis set point.
- The skeleton is exquisitely sensitive to thyroid status during growth and in adulthood. T_3 exerts anabolic responses during skeletal growth and has catabolic effects on adult bone.
- Many studies have investigated the consequences of altered thyroid function on bone. Unfortunately, many of these have been confounded by poor study design, lack of statistical power, and an absence of long-term follow-up analysis. Thus, definitive conclusions cannot be obtained from the current literature.
- Population studies suggest that reduced BMD is associated with thyroid status in the upper normal range whereas increased BMD is associated with thyroid status in the lower normal range.
- Hypothyroidism results in low bone turnover and may be associated with an increased risk of fracture.
- Untreated hyperthyroidism results in increased bone turnover, reduced BMD, and an increased risk of fracture. A prior history of thyrotoxicosis may be associated with reduced BMD and a long-term increased risk of fracture. Subclinical hyperthyroidism may be associated with increased bone turnover, reduced BMD, and increased risk of fracture. Treatment with suppressive dose of T_4 may lead to reduced BMD in postmenopausal women.
- Treatment of patients with thyrotoxicosis results in normalization of bone turnover and BMD within 5 years, although the increased risk of fracture may persist for much longer.

References

1. Murphy E, Williams GR. The thyroid, the skeleton. *Clin Endocrinol*, 2004; **61**: 285–98.
2. Parle JV, Franklyn JA, Cross KW, Jones SR, Sheppard MC. Thyroxine prescription in the community: serum thyroid stimulating hormone level assays as an indicator of undertreatment or overtreatment. *Br J Gen Pract Mar*, 1993; **43**: 107–9.
3. Ralston SH, de Crombrugghe B. Genetic regulation of bone mass and susceptibility to osteoporosis. *Genes Dev*, 2006; **20**: 2492–506.
4. Bassett JH, Williams GR. Critical role of the hypothalamic-pituitary-thyroid axis in bone. *Bone*, 2008; **43**: 418–26.
5. Eriksen EF, Mosekilde L, Melsen F. Kinetics of trabecular bone resorption and formation in hypothyroidism: evidence for a positive balance per remodeling cycle. *Bone*, 1986; **7**: 101–8.
6. Mosekilde L, Eriksen EF, Charles P. Effects of thyroid hormones on bone and mineral metabolism. *Endocrinol Metab Clin North Am*, 1990; **19**: 35–63.
7. Ahmed LA, Schirmer H, Berntsen GK, Fonnebo V, Joakimsen RM. Self-reported diseases and the risk of non-vertebral fractures: the Tromso study. *Osteoporos Int*, 2006; **17**: 46–53.
8. Bauer DC, Ettinger B, Nevitt MC, Stone KL. Risk for fracture in women with low serum levels of thyroid-stimulating hormone. *Ann Intern Med*, 2001; **134**: 561–8.
9. Jamal SA, Leiter RE, Bayoumi AM, Bauer DC, Cummings SR. Clinical utility of laboratory testing in women with osteoporosis. *Osteoporos Int*, 2005; **16**: 534–40.
10. Vestergaard P, Mosekilde L. Fractures in patients with hyperthyroidism and hypothyroidism: a nationwide follow-up study in 16,249 patients. *Thyroid*, 2002; **12**: 411–9.
11. Vestergaard P, Rejnmark L, Mosekilde L. Influence of hyper- and hypothyroidism, and the effects of treatment with antithyroid drugs and levothyroxine on fracture risk. *Calcif Tissue Int*, 2005; **77**: 139–44.
12. St Germain DL, Galton VA, Hernandez A. Minireview: Defining the roles of the iodothyronine deiodinases: current concepts and challenges. *Endocrinology*, 2009; **150**: 1097–107.
13. Yen PM. Physiological and molecular basis of thyroid hormone action. *Physiol Rev*, 2001; **81**: 1097–142.
14. Karsenty G, Wagner EF. Reaching a genetic and molecular understanding of skeletal development. *Dev Cell*, 2002; **2**: 389–406.
15. Kronenberg HM. Developmental regulation of the growth plate. *Nature*, 2003; **423**: 332–6.
16. Bassett JH, Williams GR. The molecular actions of thyroid hormone i n bone. *Trends Endocrinol Metab*, 2003; **14**: 356–64.
17. Bassett JH, Williams GR. The skeletal phenotypes of TRalpha and TRbeta mutant mice. *J Mol Endocrinol*, 2009; **42**: 269–82.
18. Rivkees SA, Bode HH, Crawford JD. Long-term growth in juvenile acquired hypothyroidism: the failure to achieve normal adult stature. *N Engl J Med*, 1988; **318**: 599–602.
19. Segni M, Leonardi E, Mazzoncini B, Pucarelli I, Pasquino AM. Special features of Graves' disease in early childhood. *Thyroid*, 1999; **9**: 871–7.
20. Weiss RE, Refetoff S. Resistance to thyroid hormone. *Rev Endocr Metab Disord*, 2000; **1**: 97–108.
21. Zofkova I, Hill M. Biochemical markers of bone remodeling correlate negatively with circulating TSH in postmenopausal women. *Endocr Regul*, 2008; **42**: 121–7.
22. van der Deure WM, Uitterlinden AG, Hofman A, Rivadeneira F, Pols HA, Peeters RP, *et al.* Effects of serum TSH and FT4 levels and the TSHR-Asp727Glu polymorphism on bone: the Rotterdam Study. *Clin Endocrinol*, 2008; **68**: 175–81.
23. Kim DJ, Khang YH, Koh JM, Shong YK, Kim GS. Low normal TSH levels are associated with low bone mineral density in healthy postmenopausal women. *Clin Endocrinol*, 2006; **64**: 86–90.
24. Morris MS. The association between serum thyroid-stimulating hormone in its reference range and bone status in postmenopausal American women. *Bone*, 2007; **40**: 1128–34.
25. Grimnes G, Emaus N, Joakimsen RM, Figenschau Y, Jorde R. The relationship between serum TSH and bone mineral density in men and postmenopausal women: the Tromso study. *Thyroid*, 2008; **18**: 1147–55.
26. Finigan J, Greenfield DM, Blumsohn A, Hannon RA, Peel NF, Jiang G, *et al.* Risk factors for vertebral and nonvertebral fracture over 10 years: a population-based study in women. *J Bone Miner Res*, 2008; **23**: 75–85.
27. Stamato FJ, Amarante EC, Furlanetto RP. Effect of combined treatment with calcitonin on bone densitometry of patients with treated hypothyroidism. *Rev Assoc Med Bras*, 2000; **46**: 177–81.
28. Vestergaard P, Rejnmark L, Weeke J, Mosekilde L. Fracture risk in patients treated for hyperthyroidism. *Thyroid*, 2000; **10**: 341–8.
29. Cummings SR, Nevitt MC, Browner WS, Stone K, Fox KM, Ensrud KE, *et al.* Risk factors for hip fracture in white women, Study of Osteoporotic Fractures Research Group. *N Engl J Med*, 1995; **332**: 767–73.
30. Seeley DG, Kelsey J, Jergas M, Nevitt MC. Predictors of ankle and foot fractures in older women. The Study of Osteoporotic Fractures Research Group. *J Bone Miner Res*, 1996; **11**: 1347–55.
31. Franklyn JA, Maisonneuve P, Sheppard MC, Betteridge J, Boyle P. Mortality after the treatment of hyperthyroidism with radioactive iodine. *N Engl J Med*, 1998; **338**: 712–8.

32. Leese GP, Jung RT, Guthrie C, Waugh N, Browning MC. Morbidity in patients on L-thyroxine: a comparison of those with a normal TSH to those with a suppressed TSH. *Clin Endocrinol*, 1992; **37**: 500–3.
33. Melton LJ, 3rd, Ardila E, Crowson CS, O'Fallon WM, Khosla S. Fractures following thyroidectomy in women: a population-based cohort study. *Bone*, 2000; **27**: 695–700.
34. Van Den Eeden SK, Barzilay JI, Ettinger B, Minkoff J. Thyroid hormone use and the risk of hip fracture in women > or = 65 years: a case-control study. *J Womens Health*, 2003; **12**: 27–31.
35. Sheppard MC, Holder R, Franklyn JA. Levothyroxine treatment and occurrence of fracture of the hip. *Arch Intern Med*, 2002; **162**: 338–43.
36. Lau EM, Suriwongpaisal P, Lee JK, Das De S, Festin MR, Saw SM, *et al.* Risk factors for hip fracture in Asian men and women: the Asian osteoporosis study. *J Bone Miner Res*, 2001; **16**: 572–80.
37. Vestergaard P, Mosekilde L. Hyperthyroidism, bone mineral, and fracture risk—a meta-analysis. *Thyroid*, 2003; **13**: 585–93.
38. Faber J, Galloe AM. Changes in bone mass during prolonged subclinical hyperthyroidism due to L-thyroxine treatment: a meta-analysis. *Eur J Endocrinol*, 1994; **130**: 350–6.
39. Heemstra KA, Hamdy NA, Romijn JA, Smit JW. The effects of thyrotropin-suppressive therapy on bone metabolism in patients with well-differentiated thyroid carcinoma. *Thyroid*, 2006; **16**: 583–91.
40. Quan ML, Pasieka JL, Rorstad O. Bone mineral density in well-differentiated thyroid cancer patients treated with suppressive thyroxine: a systematic overview of the literature. *J Surg Oncol*, 2002; **79**: 62–9.
41. Uzzan B, Campos J, Cucherat M, Nony P, Boissel JP, Perret GY. Effects on bone mass of long term treatment with thyroid hormones: a meta-analysis. *J Clin Endocrinol Metab*, 1996; **81**: 4278–89.
42. Schneider R, Reiners C. The effect of levothyroxine therapy on bone mineral density: a systematic review of the literature. *Exp Clin Endocrinol Diabetes*, 2003; **111**: 455–70.
43. Wejda B, Hintze G, Katschinski B, Olbricht T, Benker G. Hip fractures and the thyroid: a case-control study. *J Intern Med*, 1995; **237**: 241–7.
44. Bauer DC, Nevitt MC, Ettinger B, Stone K. Low thyrotropin levels are not associated with bone loss in older women: a prospective study. *J Clin Endocrinol Metab*, 1997; **82**: 2931–6.
45. Karner I, Hrgovic Z, Sijanovic S, Bukovic D, Klobucar A, Usadel KH, *et al.* Bone mineral density changes and bone turnover in thyroid carcinoma patients treated with supraphysiologic doses of thyroxine. *Eur J Med Res*, 2005; **10**: 480–8.
46. Reverter JL, Holgado S, Alonso N, Salinas I, Granada ML, Sanmarti A. Lack of deleterious effect on bone mineral density of long-term thyroxine suppressive therapy for differentiated thyroid carcinoma. *Endocr Relat Cancer*, 2005; **12**: 973–81.
47. Franklyn JA, Betteridge J, Daykin J, Holder R, Oates GD, Parle JV, *et al.* Long-term thyroxine treatment and bone mineral density. *Lancet*, 1992; **340**: 9–13.
48. Kung AW, Yeung SS. Prevention of bone loss induced by thyroxine suppressive therapy in postmenopausal women: the effect of calcium and calcitonin. *J Clin Endocrinol Metab*, 1996; **81**: 1232–6.
49. Jodar E, Begona Lopez M, Garcia L, Rigopoulou D, Martinez G, Hawkins F. Bone changes in pre- and postmenopausal women with thyroid cancer on levothyroxine therapy: evolution of axial and appendicular bone mass. *Osteoporos Int*, 1998; **8**: 311–6.
50. Paul TL, Kerrigan J, Kelly AM, Braverman LE, Baran DT. Long-term L-thyroxine therapy is associated with decreased hip bone density in premenopausal women. *JAMA*, 1988; **259**: 3137–41.
51. Kung AW, Pun KK. Bone mineral density in premenopausal women receiving long-term physiological doses of levothyroxine. *JAMA*, 1991; **265**: 2688–91.
52. Udayakumar N, Chandrasekaran M, Rasheed MH, Suresh RV, Sivaprakash S. Evaluation of bone mineral density in thyrotoxicosis. *Singapore Med J*, 2006; **47**: 947–50.
53. Andersen S, Bruun NH, Pedersen KM, Laurberg P. Biologic variation is important for interpretation of thyroid function tests. *Thyroid*, 2003; **13**: 1069–78.
54. Hansen PS, Brix TH, Sorensen TI, Kyvik KO, Hegedus L. Major genetic influence on the regulation of the pituitary-thyroid axis: a study of healthy Danish twins. *J Clin Endocrinol Metab*, 2004; **89**: 1181–7.
55. Panicker V, Wilson SG, Spector TD, Brown SJ, Falchi M, Richards JB, *et al.* Heritability of serum TSH, free T4 and free T3 concentrations: a study of a large UK twin cohort. *Clin Endocrinol*, 2008; **68**: 652–9.
56. Panicker V, Wilson SG, Spector TD, Brown SJ, Kato BS, Reed PW, *et al.* Genetic loci linked to pituitary-thyroid axis set points: a genome-wide scan of a large twin cohort. *J Clin Endocrinol Metab*, 2008; **93**: 3519–23.
57. Zmuda JM, Kammerer CM. Snipping away at osteoporosis susceptibility. *Lancet*, 2008; **371**: 1479–80.
58. Peeters RP, van der Deure WM, Visser TJ. Genetic variation in thyroid hormone pathway genes; polymorphisms in the TSH receptor and the iodothyronine deiodinases. *Eur J Endocrinol*, 2006; **155**: 655–62.
59. Heemstra KA, van der Deure WM, Peeters RP, Hamdy NA, Stokkel MP, Corssmit EP, *et al.* Thyroid hormone independent associations between serum TSH levels and indicators of bone turnover in cured patients with differentiated thyroid carcinoma. *Eur J Endocrinol*, 2008; **159**: 69–76.

4.9

Paget's disease of bone

Socrates E. Papapoulos

Introduction

In 1876, Sir James Paget presented to the Royal Medical and Chirurgical Society of London an account of his experience with a previously unrecognized disease of the skeleton, which he termed osteitis deformans and has since born his name. Paget's disease of bone is a focal skeletal disorder which progresses slowly and leads to changes in the shape and size of affected bones and to skeletal, articular, and vascular complications. In some parts of the world it is the second most common bone disorder after osteoporosis. The disease is easily diagnosed and effectively treated but its pathogenesis is largely unknown (1–3).

Epidemiology

Paget's disease affects typically the elderly, slightly more men than women, and seldom presents before the age of 35 years. Its prevalence increases with age and it affects 1 to 5% of those above 50 years of age. There is a distinct geographical distribution; the disease is common in central, western, and parts of southern Europe, the USA, Australia, New Zealand, and some countries of South America, while it is uncommon in Scandinavia, Asia, and Africa. There may also be variations within the same country, as shown in studies in the USA, UK, Italy, and Spain. For example, in northeast USA the prevalence is about fivefold higher than in south USA (4) and in parts of northwest England in 1974 the age- and gender-standardized prevalence rate was 8.3% compared to 4.6% in southern towns and cities (5). Interestingly, a more recent radiographic survey in the same centres with identical methodology (6) reported a decline in the overall prevalence of the disease, as has also been observed in other, but not all, regions where comparative studies were performed. In addition, reports from New Zealand, UK, and Spain suggested that the clinical severity of the disease has attenuated in recent years (3). These changes in prevalence and severity of the disease strongly suggest that environmental factors are involved in its pathogenesis.

Pathogenesis

Normal bone metabolism

The adult skeleton is continuously renewed throughout life by the process of bone remodelling. Old bone is removed by the osteoclasts whereas new bone is formed in the same location by the osteoblasts. This occurs in an orderly fashion through temporary anatomic structures called basic multicellular units (BMUs). A basic multicellular unit comprises a team of osteoclasts at the front and a team of osteoblasts at the back supported by blood vessels, nerves, and loose connective tissue. Osteoclasts and osteoblasts are derived from different precursors in the bone marrow. Osteoclasts originate from haematopoietic precursors of the monocyte/ macrophage lineage while osteoblasts originate from multipotent mesenchymal stem cells, which give also rise to bone marrow stromal cells, chondrocytes, adipocytes, and muscle cells. The formation and lifespan of bone cells are controlled by mechanical, systemic, and local factors through mediator molecules in the bone marrow. Important regulators of osteoclast formation and activity belong to a ligand/ receptor/ soluble (decoy) receptor system involving proteins of the TNF receptor superfamily (7, 8). These are RANK-ligand, RANK, and OPG. RANKL is produced by osteoblastic/ stromal cells, reacts with RANK, which is localized in haematopoietic osteoclast precursors, stimulates the formation and activity of osteoclasts, and prolongs their life span. RANKL is essential and sufficient for osteoclastogenesis. Bone resorbing factors up-regulate the expression of RANKL and thereby of osteoclastogenesis. On the other hand, OPG is a soluble receptor which counteracts the biological effects of RANKL preventing its binding to RANK and thereby suppressing bone resorption.

Pathology

Paget's disease of bone is a focal disorder of bone remodelling characterized by an increase in the number and size of osteoclasts in affected sites while the rest of the skeleton remains normal. The typically large osteoclasts, which may contain up to 100 nuclei per cell, induce excessive bone resorption associated with an increased recruitment of osteoblasts to the remodelling sites, resulting in increased bone formation and, hence, an overall increase in the rate of bone turnover. The increase in bone formation is thought to be secondary to the increased rate of bone resorption due to the coupling of the two processes. Some evidence, however, suggests that osteoblastic/ stromal cells may also be primarily affected in Paget's disease and contribute to the increased rate of bone formation (9, 10). The accelerated rate of bone turnover is responsible for the deposition of bone with disorganized architecture and structural weakness. The bone packets lose their lamellar structure and are replaced by woven bone with a characteristic mosaic pattern while bone marrow is infiltrated by fibrous tissue and blood vessels.

Cell biology

In clinical studies the likelihood of a bone being affected by Paget's disease was related to the amount of bone marrow present in that bone, leading to the postulation that the development of bone lesions may be related to specific properties of pagetic bone marrow (11). In bone marrow cultures from patients with Paget's disease the rate of formation of osteoclasts and their number is markedly increased, suggesting that intrinsic abnormalities of the bone marrow microenvironment and/or of osteoclast precursors may contribute to the up-regulation of osteoclastogenesis. A number of studies supported these notions and documented two major abnormalities. First, pagetic osteoclasts and their precursors express high levels of osteotropic factors, e.g. IL-6, a bone resorbing cytokine which has been proposed as a possible paracrine/autocrine factor contributing to the pathogenesis of the disease (10, 12, 13). In addition, enhanced expression of RANKL was detected in bone marrow stromal cells from patients with Paget's disease and may contribute to the increased number of osteoclasts (14). Second, compared to controls, bone marrow and peripheral cells from patients are hypersensitive to the action of RANKL and calcitriol (15, 16) and there is evidence suggesting that TAFII-17, a component of the transcription complex that binds vitamin D receptor, may be responsible for the hypersensitivity to calcitriol (17). Thus, while the molecular characteristics of the cellular abnormalities of the disease are currently understood, the precise mechanism(s) that trigger these changes remain to be elucidated.

Aetiology

Several, not mutually exclusive, hypotheses have been proposed to explain the pathology of the disease, the most relevant being the viral and the genetic hypotheses. Studies of the distribution of bone lesions in patients with Paget's disease showed that the probability of a bone being affected is very similar to the probability of a bone being affected with haematogenous osteomyelitis, suggesting that the disease may be caused by a circulating infectious agent. An infection by a slow virus of the paramyxovirus family (measles virus, respiratory syncytial virus, canine distemper virus) was supported by the detection of nuclear and cytoplasmic inclusions resembling paramyxoviral nucleocapsids in osteoclasts and of measles virus nucleocapsid transcripts in bone marrow and peripheral blood monocytes from patients with the disease (18). However, paramyxoviral-like structures have also been found in specimens from patients with other bone diseases, questioning the specificity of this finding. In addition, further search for viral presence in the osteoclasts provided conflicting results (19). However, although the presence or not of paramyxoviruses in pagetic bone is currently debated, there is good evidence that paramyxoviruses and viral proteins can promote the formation of osteoclasts with features similar to those of pagetic osteoclasts (20).

In familial aggregation studies the risk of first-degree relatives of patients with Paget's disease to develop the disorder was seven to 10 times greater than the risk of individuals without such relatives (21, 22). Furthermore, a positive family history has been reported in up to 25% of patients and a small but detailed study from Spain showed that 40% of 35 patients with Paget's disease had at least one affected first-degree relative (23). Familial Paget's disease is inherited as an autosomal dominant trait and initial genetic analyses showed evidence of linkage to chromosome 18q21–22 in some families (24, 25). This chromosome also contains the locus of the rare disease familial expansile osteolysis, which resembles Paget's disease and was found to be associated with activating mutations in the gene *TNFRSF11A*, which encodes RANK (26), while abnormalities of the same gene are responsible for another rare skeletal disease, expansile skeletal hyperphosphatasia (27). Subsequent studies, however, failed to detect such mutations in patients with familial or sporadic Paget's disease. Other abnormal genes that have been identified in diseases with bone phenotypes similar to that of Paget's disease include *TNFRSF11B*, which encodes OPG in juvenile Paget's disease (28), and *VCP*, which encodes p97 in the syndrome of inclusion body myopathy associated with Paget's disease of bone and frontotemporal dementia (29). All these genetic defects have in common the up-regulation of the NF-kB-signal transduction, an essential process in the differentiation and activation of osteoclasts. These genes have also been investigated in patients with familial or sporadic Paget's disease but no mutations were identified. Analysis of families with Paget's disease identified further possible loci in other chromosomes indicating genetic heterogeneity. However, studies in different parts of the world have now identified mutations in the *SQSTM1* gene, located on chromosome 5q35, in up to 50% of patients with familial Paget's disease and up to 10% of those with sporadic disease (3, 19, 22, 30). Moreover, the most common mutation associated with Paget's disease (P329L) has been detected in patients from different European countries suggesting a founder gene defect. In addition, animals overexpressing this mutation in cells of the osteoclast lineage formed more osteoclasts, which were hypersensitive to RANKL but did not develop bone lesions resembling those of Paget's disease in one study while in another they did (19). Whether mutations of genes associated with Paget's disease are the cause of the disease or whether individuals with a mutation have an increased susceptibility to the disease when exposed to environmental factors, such as paramyxoviruses, is currently unclear. The current view is, therefore, that the disease is caused by interactions between environmental and genetic factors, the nature of which remains to be determined.

Clinical manifestations

The most commonly affected bones are the pelvis (in about two-thirds of patients), the spine, the femora, and the skull but practically any bone of the skeleton may be affected and there is remarkable similarity in the frequency of affected bones in large series of patients from different countries (1, 31, 32). About one-third of patients have only one lesion (Fig. 4.9.1) but the frequency of single lesions varies among series, probably reflecting referral patterns, and is higher in asymptomatic patients. The anatomical spread of the disease is not related to age or gender, shows no particular symmetry in the body, and remains largely unchanged throughout life. The disease progresses slowly within the affected bone but does not generally appear in other bones. Patients with limited bone involvement should, therefore, be reassured that the disease will not progress to other bones with time.

The majority of patients are asymptomatic and the disease may be diagnosed incidentally during investigation of an unrelated

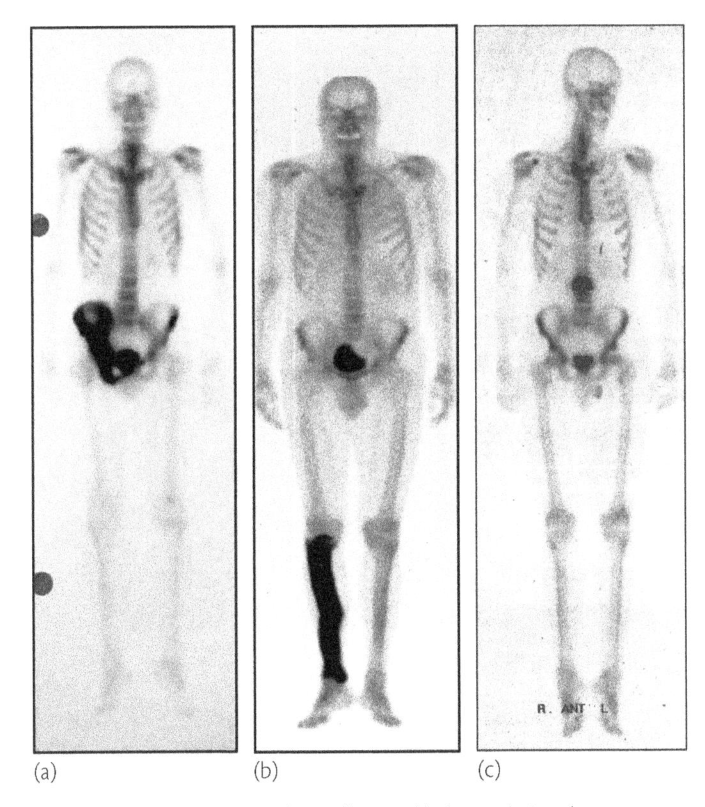

(a) (b) (c)

Fig. 4.9.1 Monostotic Paget's disease illustrated by bone scintigraphy: (a) left pelvis; (b) right tibia (with deformity and fracture); (c) vertebra.

complaint by skeletal radiographs or by the finding of an unexplained elevation of serum alkaline phosphatase activity (33). About 5 to 10% of affected patients have symptoms. Skeletal morbidity in Paget's disease is determined by the damage caused and the progression of the disease in affected sites as well as by the number and the localization of the lesions. Extensive disease, as originally described by Sir James Paget, occurs in about 5% of symptomatic patients. This is in agreement with the limited chance of an individual to develop extensive disease, as predicted by the distribution of lesions, but changing patterns of the disease to milder forms may also contribute to that.

The symptoms and complications of Paget's disease, summarized in Table 4.9.1, can have a great impact on the quality of life of affected individuals (34, 35). In the majority of patients the presenting complaint is pain. This is related to the extent and site of the disease, it is usually persistent and present at rest, but is not specific. Pain due to secondary osteoarthritis is common and may hamper assessment of the relative contribution of bone and joint pains to the patient's disability. The origin of such pain can be assessed only retrospectively after treatment which reduces mainly the disease-related pain, having a rather limited effect on the arthritic pain. Deformities are present in about 15% of patients at the time of diagnosis and affect mainly weight bearing bones, the most common deformity being bowing of the lower limbs. About 9% of patients present with fractures, which can be complete or fissure (incomplete) fractures. The latter occur more frequently, can be multiple, can cause pain, and may develop to complete fractures. Fractures heal generally well although in an older, large series of 182 fractures of the femur the incidence of nonunion was 40% (36). The skin overlying an affected bone may be warm as a result of increased blood flow and bone turnover locally and hypervascularity of affected bones may cause ischaemia of adjacent structures (steal syndrome). Irreversible hearing loss is the most common neurological complication occurring in about one-third of patients with skull involvement. This is thought to be related to structural and/or density changes in the cochlear capsule bone (37). Malignant transformation of pagetic bone and development of osteosarcoma is a rare (less than 1%) but extremely serious complication.

Table 4.9.1 Symptoms and complications of Paget's disease of bone

System	Complication
Musculoskeletal	Bone pain Bone deformity Osteoarthritis of adjacent joints Acetabular protrusion Fractures Spinal stenosis
Neurological	Hearing loss Cranial nerve deficits (rare) Basilar impression Increased cerebrospinal fluid pressure Spinal stenosis Vascular steal syndrome
Cardiovascular	Congestive heart failure and angina Increased cardiac output Aortic stenosis Generalized atherosclerosis Endocardial calcification
Metabolic	Immobilization hypercalcaemia Hypercalciuria Hyperuricaemia Nephrolithiasis
Neoplasia	Sarcoma (osteosarcoma, chondrosarcoma, and fibrosarcoma) Giant cell tumour

From Lyles KW, Siris ES, Singer FR, Meunier PJ. A clinical approach to diagnosis and management of Paget's disease of bone. *J Bone Miner Res* 2001; **16**: 1379–87 (34).

Investigations

Radiographic changes are characteristic of the disease (Fig. 4.9.2). Increased bone resorption may be detected as a decrease in the density of affected bones; sometimes a wedge- or flame-segment of bone resorption may be seen in long bones and extensive osteolytic areas in the skull (osteoporosis circumscripta). The osteolytic changes in long bones progress at a rate of about 1 cm/year. Older lesions usually have a mixed sclerotic and lytic appearance and in the last stage of the disease sclerotic lesions predominate. The involved parts of the skeleton are enlarged and deformed and the cortex can be thickened and dense. The radiological changes can be considered pathognomonic but in some cases differential diagnosis may include fibrous dysplasia and bone metastases, particularly from prostate cancer. Bone scintigraphy is used to assess the extent of the disease. It is not specific but it is more sensitive than plain radiographs; up to 15% of lesions detected by bone scintigraphy may have normal radiographic appearance. Bone scintigraphy

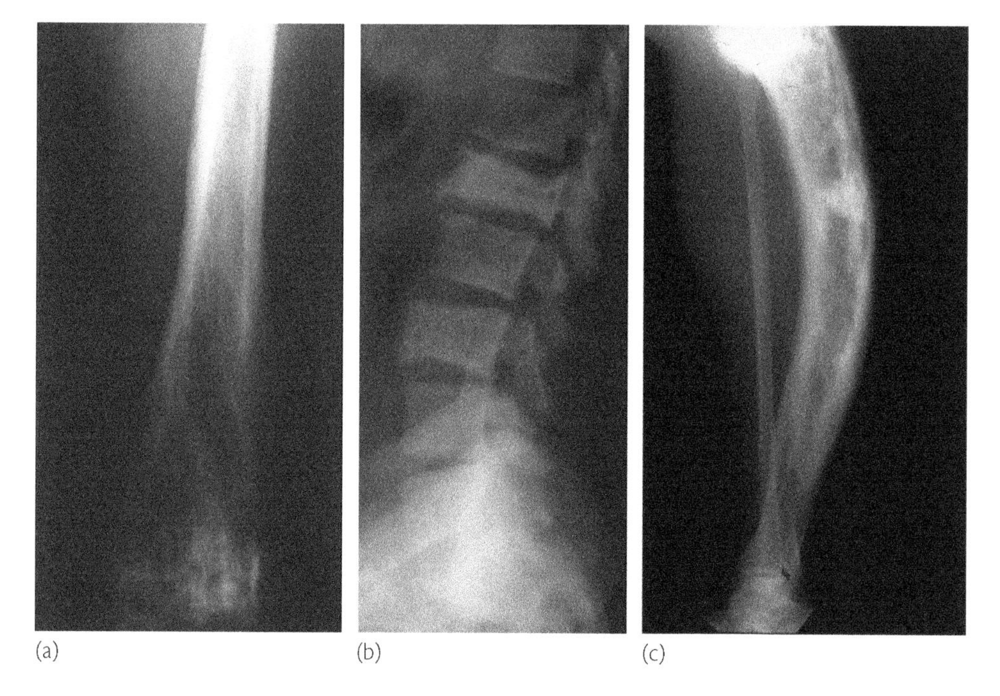

Fig. 4.9.2 Radiographs of patients with Paget's disease: (a) distal femur showing extensive and flame-shaped osteolysis; (b) lumbar spine; (c) tibia with characteristic deformity.

should always be included in the investigation of patients with Paget's disease and plain radiographs of the areas of increased radioisotope uptake should be subsequently made to confirm the diagnosis (Fig. 4.9.3).

The pathology of Paget's disease is reflected in the proportional increase in biochemical indices of bone turnover (38). Classically, urinary hydroxyproline excretion was used as an index of bone resorption and serum total alkaline phosphatase activity as an index of bone formation. These can be markedly increased in patients with extensive disease but can be also found within the reference range in patients with limited bone involvement. Patients with skull disease tend to have the highest values of serum alkaline phosphatase activity. More specific and sensitive biochemical indices of bone formation include the bone-specific isoenzyme of alkaline phosphatase and the N-terminal extension peptide of collagen type I (procollagen I N-terminal peptide). Serum osteocalcin concentrations are within the normal range in about half of the patients with elevated serum alkaline phosphatase values and should not be used in the management of patients with Paget's disease. Urinary hydroxyproline is neither specific nor sensitive enough and its determination depends on specific dietary advice. Deoxypyridinoline and peptides of the cross-linking domains of collagen type I, such as the N-telopeptide or the C-telopeptide, measured in urine or serum are the most sensitive biochemical markers of bone resorption. Impaired isomerization of C-telopeptide has been reported in patients with Paget's disease but not in patients with increased bone turnover from other causes, leading to the postulation that this abnormality may reflect the defect in bone structure (39). Degradation products of collagen type II are not increased in urines of patients (40).

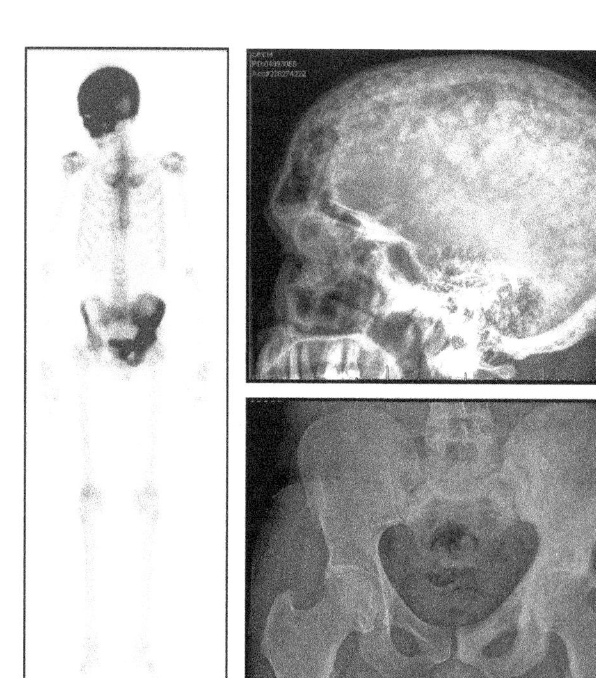

Fig. 4.9.3 Bone scintigram of a patient with Paget's disease showing two areas of increased uptake of the isotope. Radiographs of these areas were diagnostic.

In Paget's disease, despite the marked changes in the rate of bone and calcium turnover, extracellular calcium homoeostasis is generally maintained but some disturbances may occur. Hypercalcaemia may develop in immobilized patients with active, extensive disease or may be due to concurrent primary hyperparathyroidism, the incidence of which is thought to be higher in Paget's disease compared to the general population. Secondary hyperparathyroidism is present in about 20% of patients while serum concentrations of calcitriol are generally normal. Hypercalciuria and renal stone disease occur also more frequently in patients with Paget's disease.

Management

During the past 30 years, the management of patients with Paget's disease has changed dramatically due to the discovery of the therapeutic potential of the calcitonins and later of the bisphosphonates. Other, less frequently used treatments were plicamycin (mithramycin) and gallium nitrate. Bisphosphonates are currently the preferred treatment of Paget's disease.

Aims and indications of treatment

Classically treatment is given to patients with Paget's disease to relieve symptoms and improve their quality of life. The disease, however, is progressive and patients with symptoms were previously asymptomatic (Fig. 4.9.4). It is currently impossible to identify patients who will develop symptoms and complications and no way to quantify the risk of complications in an individual. Treatment with potent bisphosphonates does not only relieve symptoms due to the disease but restores bone quality and improves or even normalizes radiological appearances. Moreover, the bulk of evidence obtained with bisphosphonates strongly suggests that complications can be prevented if bone turnover is adequately suppressed, whereas there are indications that the contrary is true if bone turnover does not normalize (41). Firm evidence, however, from prospective randomized controlled trials is lacking. Recently, in an attempt to answer this question Langston *et al.* (42) compared intensive bisphosphonate treatment and symptomatic management in a large cohort of patients with Paget's disease followed for 3 years and found no differences in clinical outcomes between the two groups. Limitations of the study were the already advanced disease in most of the patients, use of bisphosphonates by the majority of patients before trial entry, and the fact that the disease was in biochemical remission in about half of the patients.

Currently, the following treatment indications are recommended: (1) symptomatic disease; (2) preoperative treatment in preparation for an orthopaedic procedure on pagetic bone to reduce the increased blood flow and excessive bleeding; (3) treatment of asymptomatic patients with skeletal localizations at higher risk of future complications, such as those adjacent to large joints, in the skull, the spine, and the weight-bearing bones; and (4) young patients. The goal of treatment should be to normalize

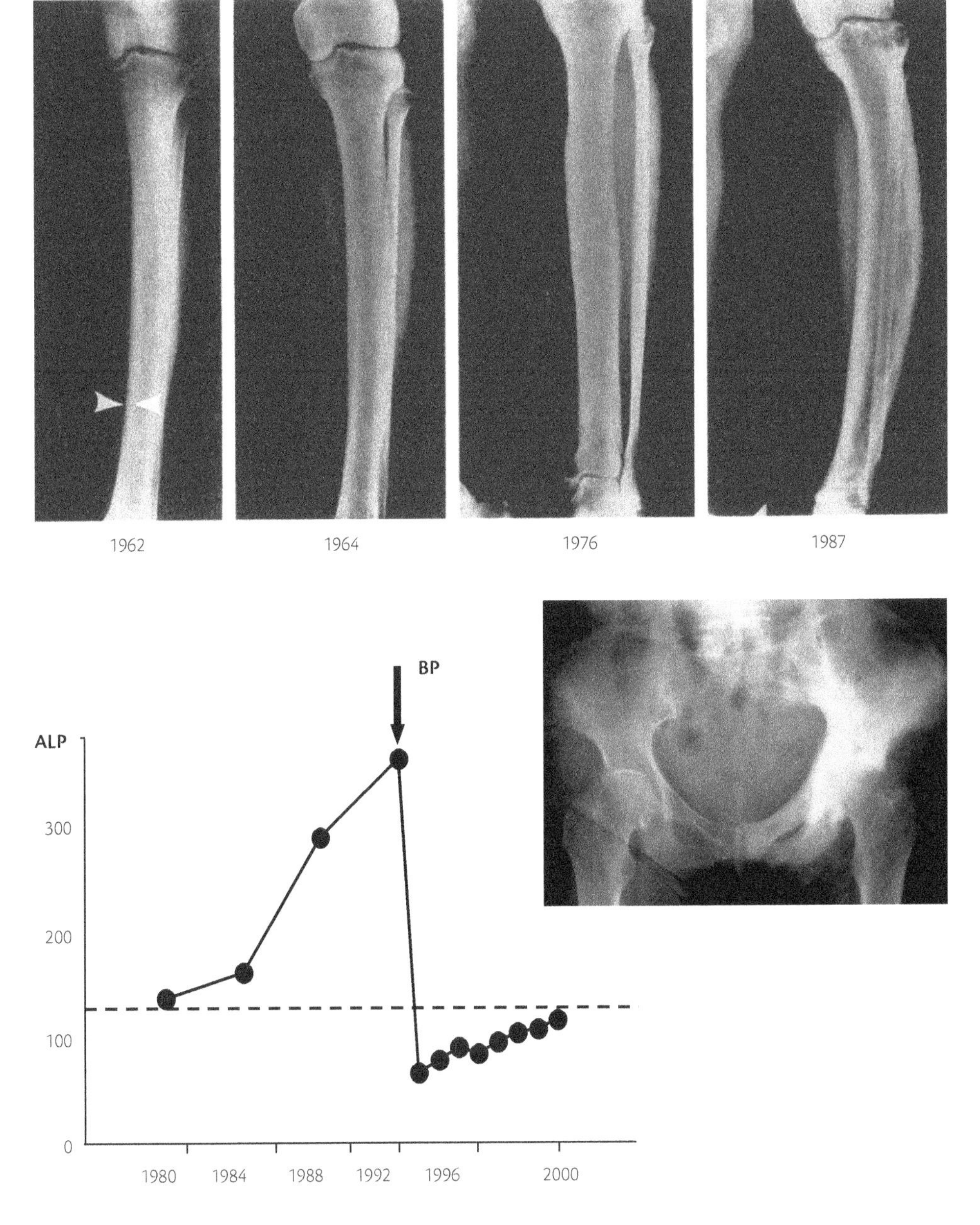

Fig. 4.9.4 (upper panel) Serial radiographs (anteroposterior view) of the tibia of an untreated 68-year-old man with Paget's disease illustrating the progression of the disease. (From Siris ES, Feldman F. Natural history of untreated Paget's disease of the tibia. *J Bone Miner Res* 1997; **12**: 691–2.) (lower panel) Sequential measurements of serum alkaline phosphatase (ALP) activity (U/l) over 20 years in a 51-year-old woman with Paget's disease of the pelvis. Note the progressive threefold increase in serum ALP activity on no treatment. Arrow indicates treatment with oral olpadronate 200 mg/day for 1 month inducing complete, long-lasting remission. Horizontal line represents the upper limit of the normal range. At the time of intervention, the patient had already developed osteoarthritis and required total hip arthroplasty despite successful treatment. BP, bisphosphonate.

bone turnover, suppress serum alkaline phosphatase activity well within the normal range, and keep it adequately suppressed, if necessary with additional courses of treatment. Retreatment is generally advocated when a previously normal value of serum alkaline phosphatase activity exceeds the upper limit of normal or when it increases by 20 to 25% above its nadir value.

Bisphosphonates

The following properties render bisphosphonates as ideal agents for the treatment of Paget's disease: selective uptake at active skeletal sites; specific inhibition of bone resorption; short plasma half-life and lack of circulating metabolites; and persistence of the effect after stopping treatment. The general structure of the molecule of germinal bisphosphonates allows numerous substitutions, which has led to the synthesis of a variety of compounds with considerable differences in potency, activity to toxicity ratio, and mechanism of action (43). Bisphosphonates are divided into two groups according to the presence or absence of a nitrogen atom in the molecule. The nitrogen increases the potency of the bisphosphonates and determines their mechanism of action. Compounds without a nitrogen atom in the side chain are etidronate, clodronate, and tiludronate. Nitrogen-containing bisphosphonates include alendronate, ibandronate, incandronate, neridronate, olpadronate, pamidronate, risedronate, and zolendronate. Practically all bisphosphonate, either approved or in clinical development, have been used in the treatment of Paget's disease, which in turn has served as a human model for investigating the pharmacological properties of these agents. The bisphosphonates approved around the world for the treatment of Paget's disease are listed in Table 4.9.2.

Pharmacodynamics

For the design of optimal therapeutic strategies of Paget's disease with bisphosphonates their pharmacodynamic properties need to be taken into consideration (44). When a potent bisphosphonate is given to a patient with Paget's disease, the first measurable effect is the suppression of bone resorption. This occurs within a few days of starting treatment. During this initial period, bone formation does not change. This will decrease secondarily, at a slower rate, due to the coupling of bone resorption to bone formation, so that a new equilibrium will be reached after 3–6 months (Fig. 4.9.5). Thus, adequate suppression of bone resorption will be predictably followed by an adequate suppression of bone formation. Suppression of biochemical indices of bone resorption early during the course of treatment provides, therefore, an indication of the pharmacological efficacy of the bisphosphonate and can subsequently determine the length of treatment (45). Because of the predictable changes in bone remodelling that follow bisphosphonate therapy in Paget's disease, it is not necessary to prolong treatment until the lowest level of serum alkaline phosphatase is reached and short courses are usually sufficient to achieve remissions. Moreover, the retention of bisphosphonate in the skeleton is proportional to disease activity and inversely proportional to renal function (46). Therefore, dose adjustments may be required in patients with impaired renal function but no specific studies have addressed this issue. These pharmacodynamic principles indicate that bisphosphonate treatment regimens of Paget's disease should be different from those used in osteoporosis. In addition, the wide variability of disease activity of affected patients strongly suggest that treatment needs to be individualized.

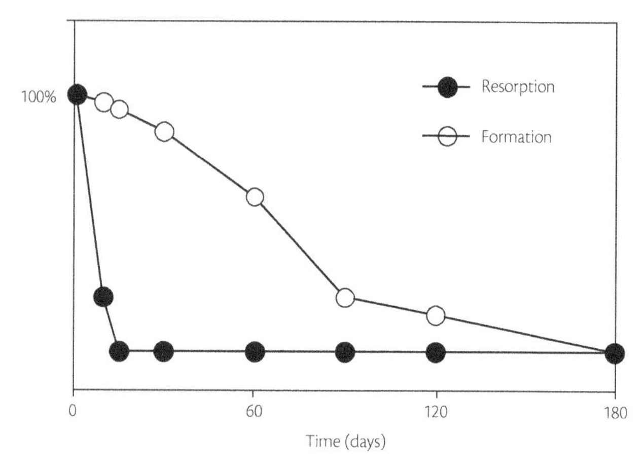

Fig. 4.9.5 Schematic presentation of the changes in biochemical indices of bone resorption and bone formation following bisphosphonate treatment of Paget's disease.

Table 4.9.2 Bisphosphonates approved for the treatment of Paget's disease

Generic name	Dose
Alendronate	Oral, 40 mg daily for 6 months
Clodronate	Oral, 1600 mg daily for 3 to 6 months
Etidronate	Oral, 400 mg daily for 6 months
Pamidronate	Intravenous, 30 to 60 mg daily for 3 days[a]
Risedronate	Oral, 30 mg daily for 2 months
Tiludronate	Oral, 400 mg daily for 3 months
Zoledronate	Intravenous, 5 mg (one 15 min infusion)

[a] Lower dose recommended by the pharmaceutical industry, higher dose recommended by investigators.

The long-term efficacy of treatment is best assessed by measuring biochemical indices of bone formation, serum alkaline phosphatase activity being still the most commonly used. In the past, the efficacy of treatment was evaluated by its ability to decrease serum alkaline phosphatase activity by more than 50% of its initial value. With the available potent bisphosphonates, this is no longer appropriate and treatment efficacy should be assessed only by its ability to decrease serum alkaline phosphatase values to the normal range (remission). In clinical practice there is no need to measure serum alkaline phosphatase activity earlier than 3 months after the start of treatment, 6 months being the optimal time.

During the initial phase of bisphosphonate treatment, when bone resorption and bone formation are still dissociated, the increased retention of calcium in the skeleton leads to changes in calcium metabolism. There is a fall in serum calcium concentration, which stimulates the secretion of parathyroid hormone secretion and consequently the renal production of calcitriol. These hormones, in turn, increase the renal tubular reabsorption of calcium (parathyroid hormone) and its intestinal absorption (calcitriol). The result is a marked, but transient, increase in calcium balance. The concomitant decrease in serum phosphate concentrations is due to the renal action of parathyroid hormone. Such responses are not observed during etidronate treatment, which has a weak action on bone metabolism. With the attainment of the new equilibrium of bone remodelling, calcium balance returns towards pretreatment levels and the values of the biochemical indices of calcium metabolism normalize. The adaptive changes of calcium metabolism to the marked alterations in bone remodelling prevent the development of symptomatic hypocalcaemia in calcium-replete patients. However, elderly patients frequently have calcium-deficient diets and some investigators advocate the use of calcium supplements during treatment of Paget's disease with potent bisphosphonates, especially if these are given intravenously or the disease is very active. Support for this logical assumption by clinical trials is, however, limited.

Treatment responses

Clinical responses to treatment include the disappearance or clear improvement of pain in more than 80% of treated patients, when this is due to the activity of the disease. A decrease of bone pain is generally observed 1 to 3 months after the start of treatment and the effect is maximal after 6 months and is maintained for as long as biochemical indices of bone turnover remain within the normal range. Soon after the start of therapy with a potent bisphosphonate, particularly if given intravenously, there may be a transient increase in pain at affected sites and patients should be reassured. Pain due to osteoarthritis is unresponsive to treatment in about 75% of patients; nonsteriodal anti-inflammatory drugs can then be used. If the hip joint is affected, hip arthroplasty may be required to control the symptoms. Back pain resulting from involvement of lumbar vertebrae is frequently not relieved by treatment. About half of the patients with pain associated with deformity of the femur or the tibia will respond favourably to bisphosphonate therapy but pain may persist and a corrective osteotomy may be necessary. Deafness is usually not affected but its progression appears to be arrested. There have been also reports of improvement of spinal cord compression with bisphosphonate therapy and fracture frequency of pagetic bones appears to decrease with treatment.

Improvement in bone histology and formation of bone with normal lamellar structure and no evidence of a mineralization defect has been reported with currently used bisphosphonates. Radiologically, an arrest of the progression of the disease is usually seen. Radiological improvement can be dramatic, however, if lesions are lytic and are localized in long bones or in the skull. In other areas, improvement is slow and sometimes difficult to demonstrate by nonexperienced radiologists. Treatment induces an exponential decrease in isotope uptake on bone scintigrams. However, even with normalization of disease activity, only about 10 to 30% of lesions normalize completely and residual uptake (up to 20% of the original) is detected (47). The possible relation of these scintigraphic changes to future recurrences has not been adequately studied but some investigators advocate normalization of bone scintigrams as one of the aims of treatment.

These clinical, histological, and radiological responses emphasize the need for an intervention with a bisphosphonate early in the course of the disease and before the development of complications.

All bisphosphonates given to patients with Paget's disease significantly decrease biochemical indices of bone turnover (48–55). Considerable differences exist, however, in their ability to induce remissions. Generally, potent bisphosphonates induce better responses. Head to head clinical trials have been performed with etidronate 400 mg daily for 6 months as comparator. In all these clinical trials, etidronate was less effective. The limited efficacy, relative to other bisphosphonates, together with the increased risk of osteomalacia, have made etidronate a treatment of the past. Normalization of serum alkaline phosphatase activity has been reported with tiludronate 400 mg daily for 3 months (35%), clodronate 1600 mg daily for 6 months (up to 70%), alendronate 40 mg daily for 6 months (63%), risedronate 30 mg daily for 2 months (up to 70%), and pamidronate, intravenously or orally in variable regimens (up to 90%). It should be noted that comparison of results obtained in different studies is not appropriate due to different selection criteria and disease activity of treated patients. The results of these studies show, in addition, that despite the availability of effective and convenient treatment regimens with bisphosphonates, there is still need for further improvement. More recently, the efficacy and tolerability of a single 15-min intravenous infusion of zolendronate was compared to oral risedronate 30 mg per day for 2 months in patients with Paget's disease of moderate activity (56). Results showed that zoledronate was significantly more efficacious than risedronate in inducing biochemical remission associated with improvements in some aspects of the quality of life of the patients. Zoledronate should be currently considered the treatment of choice of Paget's disease.

Follow-up of patients in remission is indicated every 6–12 months. Remissions, estimated from the time of normalization of serum alkaline phosphatase activity, can be long and can last even longer than 10 years in some patients. We have observed, however, recurrences 12 or 13 years after induction of complete biochemical remission which illustrates the need for continuous follow-up. The duration of remission is determined by the degree of suppression of serum alkaline phosphatase activity and the number of affected bones but is not related to the length or to the mode of treatment (oral or intravenous) as long as a potent, efficacious bisphosphonate is given (57–59). The lower the serum alkaline phosphatase activity reached with treatment, the longer the period of remission. Suppression of serum alkaline phosphatase activity well within the normal range is a prerequisite for long-term remissions and should be part of treatment strategies.

Resistance to bisphosphonate treatment

Impaired response to repeated treatment courses with bisphosphonates is usually referred to as acquired resistance and should be distinguished from an intrinsic resistance to a particular compound. Acquired resistance has been reported for etidronate and pamidronate (60, 61) but the underlying mechanism is not known and it is important to differentiate between real and apparent resistance. Some patients may not respond to oral bisphosphonate but may show a prompt response to the same compound given intravenously. In such cases, factors interfering with the already low intestinal absorption of the drug are most likely responsible for the impaired response to oral treatment. Patients retreated with the same bisphosphonate during a recurrence of their disease may show a reduced fractional decrease in biochemical indices of bone turnover compared to earlier treatments. Some consider this response compatible with development of resistance to therapy. However, it has been shown in studies with clodronate and pamidronate that the actual level, rather than the fractional decrease of biochemical indices of bone turnover following every treatment, should be compared to those obtained after the initial therapy (Fig. 4.9.6). This is because patients who are offered a new treatment course have generally a lower rate of bone turnover compared to

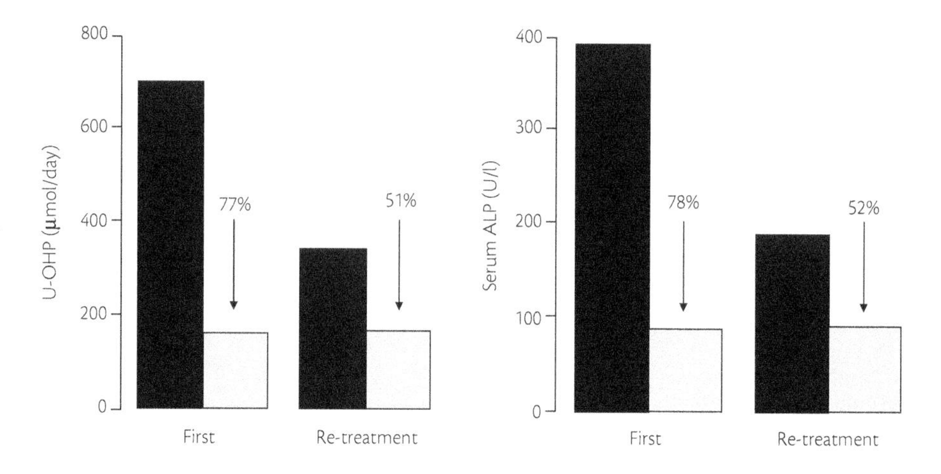

Fig. 4.9.6 Apparent resistance to bisphosphonate therapy in Paget's disease. Absolute and percent changes of urinary hydroxyproline excretion (U-OHP) and serum alkaline phosphatase (ALP) activity after first treatment with pamidronate or retreatment with the same bisphosphonate for a recurrence of the disease. (Modified from Harinck HI, Bijvoet OL, Blanksma HJ, Dahlinghaus-Nienhuys PJ. *Clin Orthop Relat Res*, 1987; **217**: 79–98.)

that before the first treatment. Finally, in patients with Paget's disease and concurrent hyperparathyroidism, completeness of response is generally less and recurrences occur quicker which might be considered reduced responsiveness. For optimal responses of patients with Paget's disease and autonomous hyperparathyroidism to be bisphosphonates, parathyroidectomy should be considered. However, real resistance to pamidronate can develop. We showed, for example, progressive reduction in responsiveness to this bisphosphonate, which was mainly related to the extent of skeletal involvement but not to the dose of pamidronate or to the biochemical activity of the disease. Patients with three or more affected bones were most likely to develop resistance to pamidronate, a finding consistent with other reports. These patients respond readily to other bisphosphonates. There are scarce data of resistance to other nitrogen-containing bisphosphonates. Using the same approach as in the pamidronate studies, we found no resistance to consecutive treatments of patients with Paget's disease with olpadronate. Thus, within the limitations of existing studies, it appears that acquired resistance is specific for pamidronate and is limited to patients with extensive disease. Such resistance does not seem to occur with other nitrogen-containing bisphosphonates but the evidence for that is still weak. Finally, primary resistance to a specific bisphosphonate, if it exists, is rare.

Adverse effects

All bisphosphonates given at very high doses can impair the mineralization of newly formed bone and induce osteomalacia. In clinical practice this is, however, relevant only for etidronate. Doses of potent nitrogen-containing bisphosphonates that induce osteomalacia exceed, by many orders of magnitude, those required for effective suppression of bone turnover. Consequently, in all reported controlled studies no adverse effects on bone mineralization have been observed. In only a few patients treated with intravenous pamidronate, at doses higher than those recommended, has impaired bone mineralization been reported. Histological osteomalacia induced by either etidronate or pamidronate is reversible.

In some patients treated for the first time with nitrogen-containing bisphosphonates there is a rise in body temperature and flu-like symptoms during the first 3 days of treatment. These symptoms are transient and subside with no specific measures even when treatment is continued (62, 63). This response is dose-dependent and is associated more frequently with intravenous than oral treatment. Moreover, it does not generally recur upon retreatment, and, if it does, it is of lower intensity. Previous exposure to another nitrogen-containing bisphosphonate, but not to etidronate, precludes the development of this response. Laboratory findings are consistent with an acute phase reaction (63). There is a transient decrease in blood lymphocytes and a transient increase in serum C-reactive protein, possibly due to increases in proinflammatory cytokines, such as IL-6 and TNF-α produced by γ,δ T-lymphocytes in response to a metabolite of the mevalonate pathway, upstream farnesyl pyrophosphate synthase, which is inhibited by nitrogen-containing bisphosphonates (63, 64). Rarely, high doses of nitrogen-containing bisphosphonates may induce ophthalmic reactions such as conjunctivitis, iritis, or uveitis. There are case reports of ototoxicity and central nervous toxicity after intravenous pamidronate. Allergic skin reactions have been occasionally observed with most of the bisphosphonates.

Mild gastrointestinal complaints occur with low frequency with the use of all bisphosphonates. Some nitrogen-containing bisphosphonates can induce more severe symptoms such as heartburn, nausea, and vomiting in a few patients, associated with oesophagitis or gastritis. The use of oral alendonate 40 mg daily was associated with higher frequency of epigastric complaints in an open, but not in a controlled, study and the latter was also the case with oral risedronate 30 mg daily. In a comparative study of alendronate 40 mg/day and risedronate 30 mg/day gastric ulcers and/or large numbers of gastric erosions were detected endoscopically in approximately 3% of patients, and their occurrence was comparable with both bisphosphonates. Nitrogen-containing bisphosphonates should be administered orally with one full glass of water and the patient should remain in an upright position for one half hour to allow quick passage through the oesophagus and to avoid oesophageal irritation. Rapid intravenous injection of bisphosphonates may chelate calcium in the circulation and form complexes, which can be nephrotoxic or can damage directly the renal tubule. Bisphosphonates should, therefore, be given by slow infusion. Zoledronate is administered by short intravenous infusion (15 min) because of the low effective dose. Aminobisphosphonates should not be injected intramuscularly because they can cause severe local irritation and necrosis but clodronate has been given intramuscularly. Osteonecrosis of the jaw is extremely rare in patients with Paget's disease treated either with oral or intravenous bisphosphonates.

References

1. Kanis JA. *Pathophysiology and Treatment of Paget's Disease of Bone*. 2nd edn. London: Dunitz, 1998.
2. Siris ES, Roodman GD. Paget's disease of bone. In: Rosen CJ, ed. *Primer on the Metabolic Bone Diseases and Disorders of Mineral Metabolism*. 7th edn. Washington DC: American Society for Bone and Mineral Research, 2008: 335–43.
3. Cundy T, Bolland M. Paget disease of bone. *Trends Endocrinol Metab*, 2008; **19**: 246–53.
4. Altman RD, Bloch DA, Hochberg MC, Murphy WA. Prevalence of pelvic Paget's disease of bone in the United States. *J Bone Miner Res*, 2000; **15**: 461–5.
5. Barker DJP, Clough PWL, Guyer PB, Gardner MJ. Paget's disease of bone in 14 British towns. *BMJ*, 1977; **1**: 1181–3.
6. Cooper C, Schafheutle K, Dennison E, Kellingray S, Guyer P, Barker D. The epidemiology of Paget's disease in Britain: is the prevalence decreasing? *J Bone Miner Res*, 1999; **14**: 192–7.
7. Suda T, Takahashi N, Udagawa N, Jimi E, Gillespie MT, Martin TJ. Modulation of osteoclast differentiation and function by the new members of the tumor necrosis factor receptor and ligand families. *Endocr Rev*, 1999; **20**: 345–57.
8. Kearns AE, Khosla S, Kostenuik PJ. Receptor activator of nuclear factor κB ligand and osteoprotegerin regulation of bone remodeling in health and disease. *Endocr Rev*, 2008; **29**: 155–92.
9. Gehron-Robey P, Bianco P. The role of osteogenic cells in the pathophysiology of Paget's disease. *J Bone Miner Res*, 1999; **14** (Suppl 2): 9–16.
10. Naot D, Bava U, Mattews B, Callon KE, Gamble GD, Black M, *et al.* Differential gene expression in cultured osteoblasts and bone marrow stromal cells from patients with Paget's disease of bone. *J Bone Miner Res*, 2007; **22**: 298–309.
11. Reddy SV, Menaa S, Singer FR, Demulder A, Roodman GD. Cell biology of Paget's disease. *J Bone Miner Res*, 1999; **14** (Suppl 2): 3–8.
12. Hoyland JA, Freemond AJ, Sharpe PT. Interleukin-6, IL-6 receptor, and IL-6 nuclear factor gene expression in Paget's disease. *J Bone Miner Res*, 1994; **9**: 75–80.
13. Roodman GD, Kurihara N, Ohsaki Y, Kukita A, Hosking D, Demulder A, *et al.* Interleukin-6: a potential autocrine/paracrine factor in Paget's disease of bone. *J Clin Invest*, 1992; **89**: 46–52.
14. Menaa C, Reddy SV, Kurihara N, Anderson D, Roodman GD. Enhanced RANK ligand expression and responsivity of bone marrow cells in Paget's disease of bone. *J Clin Invest*, 2000; **105**: 1833–8.
15. Neale SD, Smith R, Wass JA, Athanasou NA. Osteoclast differentiation from circulating mononuclear precursors in Paget's disease is hypersensitive to 1,25-dihydroxyvitamin D3 and RANKL. *Bone*, 2000; **27**: 409–16.
16. Menaa C, Barsony J, Reddy SV, Cornish J, Cundy T, Roodman D, *et al.* 1,25-dihydroxyvitamin D3 hypersensitivity of osteoclast precursors from patients with Paget's disease. *J Bone Miner Res*, 2000; **15**: 228–34.
17. Kurihara N, Reddy SV, Araki N, Ishizuka S, Ozono K, Cornish J, *et al.* Role of TAFII-17, a VDR binding protein, in the increased osteoclast formation in Paget's disease. *J Bone Miner Res*, 2004; **19**: 1154–64.
18. Singer FR. Update on the viral etiology of Paget's disease of bone. *J Bone Miner Res*, 1999; **14** (Suppl 2): 29–33.
19. Ralston SH. Pathogenesis of Paget's disease of bone. *Bone*, 2008; **43**: 819–25.
20. Reddy SV, Kurihara N, Menaa C, Landucci G, Forthal D, Koop BA, *et al.* Osteoclasts formed by measles virus-infected osteoclast precursors from hCD46 transgenic mice express characteristics of Pagetic osteoclasts. *Endocrinology*, 2001; **142**: 2898–905.
21. Siris ES, Ottman R, Flaster E, Kelsey JL. Familial aggregation of Paget's disease of bone. *J Bone Miner Res*, 1991; **6**: 495–500.
22. Eekhoff EWM, Karperien M, Houtsma D, Zwinderman AH, Dragoiescu C, Kneppers ALT, Papapoulos SE. Familial Paget's disease in the Netherlands. *Arthritis Rheum*, 2004; **50**: 1650–4.
23. Morales-Piga AA, Rey-Rey JS, Corres-Gonzales J, Garcia-Sagredo JM, Lopez-Abente G. Frequency and characteristics of familial aggregation of Paget's disease of bone. *J Bone Miner Res*, 1995; **10**: 663–70.
24. Haslam SI, van Hul W, Morales-Piga A, Balemans W, San-Millan JL, Nakatsuka K, *et al.* Paget's disease of bone: evidence for a susceptibility locus on chromosome 18q and for genetic heterogeneity. *J Bone Miner Res*, 1998; **13**: 911–17.
25. Hocking L, Slee F, Haslam SI, Cundy T, Nicholson G, van Hul W, Ralston SH. Familial Paget's disease of bone: Patterns of inheritance and frequency of linkage to chromosome 18q. *Bone*, 2000; **26**: 1095–103.
26. Hughes AE, Ralston SH, Marken J, Bell C, MacPherson H, Wallace RG, *et al.* Mutations in TNFRSF11A, affecting the signal peptide of RANK, cause familial expansile osteolysis. *Nat Genet*, 2000; **24**: 45–8.
27. Whyte MP, Hughes AE. Expansile skeletal hyperphosphatasia is caused by a 15-base pair tendem dublication in TNFRSF11A encoding RANK and is allelic to familial expansile osteolysis. *J Bone Miner Res*, 2002; **17**: 26–9.
28. Whyte MP, Obrecht SE, Finnegan PM, Jones JL, Podgornik MN, McAlister WH, *et al.* Osteoprotegerin deficiency and juvenile Paget's disease. *N Engl J Med*, 2002; **347**: 175–84.
29. Watts GD, Wymer J, Kovach MJ, Mehta SG, Mumm S, Darvush D, *et al.* Inclusion body myopathy associated with Paget's disease of bone and frontotemporal dementia is caused by mutant valosin-containing protein. *Nat Genet*, 2004; **36**: 377–81.
30. Laurin N, Brown JP, Lemainque A, Duchesne A, Huot D, Lacourcière Y, *et al.* Paget's disease of bone: mapping of two loci at 5q35-qter and 5q31. *Am J Hum Genet*, 2001; **69**: 528–43.
31. Harinck HIJ, Bijvoet OLM, Vellenga CJLR, Blanksma HJ, Frijlink WB. Relation between signs and symptoms in Paget's disease of bone. *Q J Med*, 1986; **58**: 133–51.
32. Meunier PJ, Salson C, Mathieu L, Chapuy MC, Delmas P, Alexandre C, *et al.* Skeletal distribution and biochemical parameters of Paget's disease. *Clin Orthop Rel Res*, 1987; **217**: 37–44.
33. Eekhoff EWM, van der Klift M, Kroon HM, Cooper C, Hofman A, Pols HAP, Papapoulos SE. Paget's disease of bone in the Netherlands: a population-based radiological and biochemical survey; the Rotterdam study. *J Bone Miner Res*, 2004; **19**: 566–70.
34. Lyles KW, Siris ES, Singer FR, Meunier PJ. A clinical approach to diagnosis and management of Paget's disease of bone. *J Bone Miner Res*, 2001; **16**: 1379–87.
35. Gold DT, Boisture J, Shipp KM, Pieper CF, Lyles KW. Paget's disease of bone and quality of life. *J Bone Miner Res*, 1996; **11**: 1897–904.
36. Dove J. Complete fractures of the femur in Paget's disease of bone. *J Bone Joint Surg Br*, 1980; **62-B**: 12–17.
37. Monsell EM, Cody DD, Bone HG, Divine GW. Hearing loss as a complication of Paget's disease of bone. *J Bone Miner Res*, 1999; **14** (Suppl 2): 92–5.
38. Alvarez L, Peris P, Pons F, Guañabens N, Herranz R, Monegal A, *et al.* Relationship between biochemical markers of bone turnover and bone scintigraphy indices in assessment of Paget's disease activity. *Arthritis Rheum*, 1997; **40**: 461–8.
39. Garnero P, Fledelius C, Gineyts E, Serre CM, Vignot E, Delmas PD. Decreased ß-isomerization of C-telopeptides of α1 chain of type I collagen in Paget's disease of bone. *J Bone Miner Res*, 1997; **12**: 1407–15.
40. Christgau S, Garnero P, Fledelius C, Moniz C, Ensig M, Gineyts E, *et al.* Collagen type II C-telopeptide fragments as an index of cartilage degradation. *Bone*, 2001; **29**: 209–15.
41. Meunier PJ, Vignot E. Therapeutic strategies in Paget's disease of bone. *Bone*, 1995; **17** (Suppl 5): 489S–91S.

42. Langston AL, Cambell MK, Fraser WD, MacLennan GS, Selby PL, Ralston SH. Randomised trial of intensive bisphosphonate treatment versus symptomatic management in Paget's disease of bone. *J Bone Miner Res*,2010; **25**: 20–31.
43. Papapoulos SE. Bisphosphonates: How do they work? *Best Pract Res Clin Endocrinol Metab*, 2008; **22**: 831–47.
44. Papapoulos SE. Pharmacodynamics of bisphosphonates in man; implications for treatment. In: Bijvoet OLM, Fleisch HA, Canfield RE, Russell RGG, eds. *Bisphosphonates on Bones*. Amsterdam: Elsevier, 1995: 231–63.
45. Papapoulos SE, Frölich M. Prediction of the outcome of treatment of Paget's disease of bone with bisphosphonates from short-term changes in the rate of bone resorption. *J Clin Endocrinol Metab*, 1996; **81**: 3993–7.
46. Cremers SCLM, Eekhoff MEMW, den Hartigh J, Vermeij P, Papapoulos SE. Relationships between pharmacokinetics and rate of bone turnover after intravenous bisphosphonate (olpadronate) in patients with Paget's disease of bone. *J Bone Miner Res*, 2003; **18**: 868–75.
47. Vellenga CJLR. Quantitative bone scintigraphy in the evaluation of Paget's disease of bone. In: Bijvoet OLM, Fleisch HA, Canfield RE, Russell RGG, eds. *Bisphosphonates on Bones*. Amsterdam: Elsevier, 1995: 279–91.
48. Delmas PD, Meunier PJ. The management of Paget's disease of bone. *N Engl J Med*, 1997; **336**: 558–66.
49. Miller PD, Brown JP, Siris ES, Hoseyni MS, Axelrod DW, Bekker PJ. A randomized, double-blind comparison of risedronate and etidronate in the management of Paget's disease of bone. *Am J Med*, 1999; **106**: 513–20.
50. Reid IR, Nicholson GC, Weinstein RS, Hosking DJ, Cundy T, Kotowicz MA, *et al.* Biochemical and radiological improvement in Paget's disease of bone treated with alendronate: a randomized, placebo-controlled trial. *Am J Med,* 1996; **101**: 341–8.
51. Roux C, Gennari C, Farrerons J, Devogelaer JP, Mulder H, Kruse HP, *et al.* Comparative prospective, double-blind, multicenter study of the efficacy of tiludronate and etidronate in the treatment of Paget's disease of bone. *Arthritis Rheumat*, 1995; **38**: 851–8.
52. Schweitzer DH, Zwinderman AH, Vermeij P, Bijvoet OLM, Papapoulos SE. Improved treatment of Paget's disease with dimethylaminohydroxypropylidene bisphosphonate. *J Bone Miner Res*, 1993; **8**: 175–82.
53. Siris E, Weinstein RS, Altman R, Conte JM, Favus M, Lombardi A, *et al.* Comparative study of alendronate versus etidronate for the treatment of Paget's disease of bone. *J Clin Endocrinol Metab*, 1996; **81**: 961–7.
54. Siris ES, Chines AA, Altman RD, Brown JP, Johnston CC Jr, Lang R, *et al.* Risedronate on the treatment of Paget's disease of bone; an open label, multicenter study. *J Bone Miner Res*, 1998; **13**: 1032–8.
55. Brown JP, Chines AA, Myers WR, Eusebio RA, Ritter-Hrncirik C, Hays CW. Improvement of pagetic bone lesions with risedronate treatment: a radiologic study. *Bone*, 2000; **26**: 263–7.
56. Reid IR, Miller P, Lyles K, Fraser W, Brown JP, Saidi Y, *et al.* Comparison of a single infusion of zoledronic acid and risedronate for Paget's disease. *N Engl J Med*, 2005; **353**: 898–908.
57. Harinck HIJ, Papapoulos SE, Blanksma HJ, Moolenaar AJ, Vermeij P, Bijvoet OLM. Paget's disease of bone; early and late responses to three different modes of treatment with aminohydroxypropylidene bisphosphonate. *BMJ*, 1987; **295**: 1301–5.
58. Schweitzer DH, Zwinderman AH, Bijvoet OLM, Vermey P, Papapoulos SE. Improved treatment of Paget's disease with dimethyl-aminohydroxypropylidene bisphosphonate (dimethyl-APD). *J Bone Miner Res*, 1993; **8**: 175–82.
59. Eekhoff EMW, Zwinderman AH, Haverkort DMAD, Cremers SCLM, Hamdy NAT, Papapoulos SE. Determinants of induction and duration of remission of Paget's disease of bone after bisphosphonate (olpadronate) therapy. *Bone*, 2003; **33**: 831–8.
60. Cutteridge DH, Ward LC, Stewart GO, Retallack RW, Will RK, Prince RE, *et al.* Paget's disease: acquired resistance to one aminobisphosphonate with retained response to another. *J Bone Miner Res*, 1999; **14** (Suppl 2): 79–84.
61. Papapoulos SE, Eekhoff EMW, Zwinderman AH. Acquired resistance to bisphosphonates in Paget's disease of bone. *J Bone Miner Res*, 2006; **21** (Suppl 2): 88–91.
62. Adami S, Zamberlan N. Adverse effects of bisphosphonates. *Drug Safety*, 1996; **14**: 158–70.
63. Schweitzer DH, Oostendorp-van de Ruit M, van der Pluijm G, Löwik CWGM, Papapoulos S. Interleukin-6 and the acute phase reaction during treatment of patients with Paget's disease with the nitrogen-containing bisphosphonate dimethylaminohydroxypropylidene bisphosphonate. *J Bone Miner Res*, 1995; **10**: 956–62.
64. Coxon FP, Thompson K, Rogers MJ. Recent advances in understanding the mechanism of action of bisphosphonates. *Curr Opin Pharmacol*, 2006; **6**: 307–12.

4.10

Rickets and osteomalacia (acquired and heritable forms) and skeletal dysplasias

Michael P. Whyte, Uri A. Liberman

Introduction

Background

Mineralization of newly formed organic matrix of bone is a complex and highly ordered process. The requirements include adequate extracellular concentrations of calcium (Ca^{2+}) and phosphorous, as inorganic phosphate (Pi), and normal function of bone-forming cells. Disturbances in either requirement can lead to a stereotypic response of impaired skeletal mineralization (1).

Rickets describes the clinical consequences of diminished mineralization of matrix throughout a growing skeleton. Infants, children, and adolescents can be affected. Osteomalacia results from the same disturbance after growth plates fuse. However, neither term denotes a specific disease. Each is a generic label for the signs and symptoms that follow perturbations that disrupt the orderly deposition of hydroxyapatite crystals into skeletal tissue. Nevertheless, in nearly all patients, there are low extracellular levels of Ca^{2+} and/or Pi. Often, diminished stores or impaired bioactivation of vitamin D are involved and cause hypocalcaemia, secondary hyperparathyroidism, and hypophosphataemia (1). Occasionally, it is kidney tubule dysfunction that results directly in urinary Pi wasting and leads to hypophosphataemia, sometimes associated with impaired bioactivation of vitamin D. Rarely, disturbances involving chondrocytes and osteoblasts, defective bone matrix, or other disruptions interfere with Ca^{2+} and Pi deposition into the skeleton. The number of conditions that cause rickets and osteomalacia is considerable—some are acquired and some are inherited (Box 4.10.1).

Successful medical therapy for rickets or osteomalacia must address the specific disturbance(s) leading to aberrant mineral homoeostasis. It may be possible to correct the fundamental disorder, or it may be necessary to circumvent it. Except for dosage, pharmacological regimens for specific conditions will generally be the same regardless of patient age. However, distinctive disease manifestations trouble paediatric compared to adult patients, and the goals for treatment and follow-up differ.

In rickets, all three processes of skeletal formation are adversely affected (1):

- Growth: for long bones to lengthen, chondrocytes in columnar arrangement within growth plates (physes) must proliferate, hypertrophy, and then degenerate, allowing the matrix they produce to mineralize (endochondral bone formation).
- Modelling: correct shaping of growing bones requires simultaneous deposition and removal of osseous tissue at the outer and inner surfaces (subperiosteum and endosteum, respectively) of cortical bone.
- Remodelling: cortical (compact) and trabecular (spongy) bone are resorbed and then reformed throughout life in numerous and changing microscopic areas to fulfil the metabolic, structural, and repair requirements of the skeleton.

Rickets features short stature (physeal disturbances), skeletal distortions (modelling defects), as well as fractures (impaired remodelling). Osteomalacia is usually not deforming (unless there are fractures) because growth plates are fused and modelling has essentially ceased; only remodelling is deranged. Accordingly, impaired mineralization of skeletal matrix is less apparent clinically and less distinctive radiographically in osteomalacia. In both conditions, however, defective bone remodelling (turnover) can appear on radiographs as generalized osteopenia or, occasionally, as osteosclerosis (coarse trabecular bone).

Alternatively, some refer to rickets as the disturbance in endochondral bone growth and modelling, and to osteomalacia as the disturbance in bone remodelling. In this context, osteomalacia is also present in paediatric patients.

Most of the clinical, radiological, and histological features of rickets and/or osteomalacia are the same and independent of the primary disorder. Thus, bone matrix mineralization can be impaired from: (1) primary Ca^{2+} deficiency (i.e. nutritional deficiency of the element, or more commonly from disruption of vitamin D metabolism) and called hypocalcaemic rickets and/or osteomalacia;

Box 4.10.1 Causes of rickets or osteomalacia

Vitamin D deficiency

- Deficient endogenous synthesis
  - Inadequate sunshine
  - Other factors, e.g. ageing, pigmentation, sunscreens, clothing
- Dietary
  - Classic 'nutritional'
  - Fat-phobic

Malabsorption

- Gastric
  - Partial gastrectomy
- Intestinal
  - Small bowel disorders, e.g. coeliac disease (gluten-sensitive enteropathy)
- Hepatobiliary
  - Cirrhosis
  - Biliary fistula
  - Biliary atresia
- Pancreatic
  - Chronic pancreatic insufficiency

Calciopenic

Disorders of vitamin D bioactivation

- Hereditary
  - Vitamin D dependency, type I (1α-hydroxylase deficiency)
  - Vitamin D dependency, type II (hereditary vitamin D-resistant rickets)
- Acquired
  - Anticonvulsant therapy
  - Renal insufficiency
- Acidosis
- Distal renal tubular acidosis (classic, type I)
  - Primary (specific aetiology not determined)
    - Sporadic
    - Familial
  - Secondary
    - Galactosaemia
    - Hereditary fructose intolerance with nephrocalcinosis
    - Fabry's disease
  - Hypergammaglobulinaemic states
  - Medullary sponge kidney
  - Post renal transplantation
- Acquired
  - Ureterosigmoidostomy

Box 4.10.1 *(Contd.)* Causes of rickets or osteomalacia

  - Ileal conduit
  - Obstructive uropathies
  - Drug-induced
  - Acetazolamide
  - Ammonium chloride

Chronic renal failure

Phosphate depletion

- Dietary
  - Low phosphate intake
  - Aluminium hydroxide antacid abuse (or other nonabsorbable hydroxides)
- Impaired renal tubular phosphate reabsorption ('phosphate diabetes')
  - Hereditary
    - X-linked hypophosphataemia
    - Adult-onset vitamin D-resistant hypophosphataemia
    - Syndrome of lipoatrophic diabetes, vitamin D resistant rickets, persistent Müllenian ducts
    - Dent's disease
  - Acquired
    - Sporadic hypophosphataemic osteomalacia
    - Oncogenic (tumour-associated)
    - Neurofibromatosis
    - McCune–Albright syndrome
    - Ifosfamide treatment
    - Epidermal nevus syndrome

General renal tubular disorders (Fanconi's syndrome)

- Primary renal
  - Idiopathic
    - Sporadic
    - Familial
  - Associated with a systemic metabolic disease
    - Cystinosis
    - Glycogenosis
    - Lowe's syndrome
- Systemic disorder with associated renal disease
  - Hereditary
    - Inborn errors
      - Wilson's disease
      - Tyrosinaemia
  - Acquired
    - Multiple myeloma

Box 4.10.1 *(Contd.)* Causes of rickets or osteomalacia

- Nephrotic syndrome
- Transplanted kidney
- Toxins
  - Cadmium
  - Lead
  - Outdated tetracycline

Primary mineralization defects

- Hereditary
  - Hypophosphatasia
- Acquired
  - Bisphosphonate intoxication
  - Fluorosis
  - Aluminium intoxication
  - Gallium intoxication

States of rapid bone formation

- Postoperative hypoparathyroidism with osteitis fibrosa cystica

Defective matrix synthesis

- Fibrogenesis imperfecta ossium

Miscellaneous

- Mg^{2+}-dependent
- Steroid-sensitive
- Axial osteomalacia
- Osteopetrosis ('osteopetrorickets')

(2) primary phosphorous deficiency (e.g. increased renal Pi clearance as in X-linked hypophosphataemia) and called hypophosphataemic rickets and/or osteomalacia; and (3) primary defects in local bone processes (e.g. hypophosphatasia due to alkaline phosphatase (ALP) deficiency) causing rickets and/or osteomalacia with normal or increased extracellular levels of mineral (1).

Vitamin D and mineral metabolism

Vitamin D

Much is now known about the biosynthesis, bioactivation, and physiological actions of vitamin D (2, 3) and the control of mineral homoeostasis (4). Despite fortification of foods with vitamin D in several countries (e.g. 400 IU per quart of milk or infant formula in the USA) or use of vitamin supplements, most antirachitic activity in healthy people comes from cutaneous synthesis of vitamin D (5). In the skin, 7-dehydrocholesterol is converted by 290–310 nm ultraviolet (UV) light to cholecalciferol (vitamin D_3). Age, skin pigmentation, and clothing as well as duration, angle, and intensity of UV light exposure all condition how much vitamin D_3 is made (5). Ergocalciferol (vitamin D_2) is the product of UV irradiation of ergosterol extracted from animal or plant tissues, and is used as a supplement or as a drug (2, 3).

Both vitamin D_2 and D_3 are prohormones, which are transported in the circulation by a high-affinity binding protein to muscle or fat for storage, or to the liver and subsequently to the kidney for bioactivation (2, 3). First, with little regulation, vitamin D is hydroxylated in hepatocyte mitochondria by the enzyme P450c25 to form the 25-hydroxyvitamin D metabolite called calcidiol. Then, with precise control mediated by Ca^{2+}, Pi, and parathyroid hormone (PTH), 25-hydroxyvitamin D is further hydroxylated in kidney proximal convoluted tubule cells by mitochondrial P450c1α, more commonly referred to as 25-hydroxyvitamin D,1α–hydroxylase (or 1α–hydroxylase) to 1,25-dihydroxyvitamin D, also called calcitriol (6, 7, 8). Other cells can have 1α-hydroxylase activity: placental decidual cells, keratinocytes, macrophages from various origins, and some tumour cells (7, 8). However, the role of extrarenal production of 1,25-dihydroxyvitamin D is unknown, and under physiological conditions does not significantly add to circulating levels of this hormone. Hydroxylation at carbon 24 to produce 24,25-dihydroxyvitamin D, or 1,24,25-trihydroxyvitamin D, occurs in a wide range of normal tissues and is considered important for deactivation and removal of vitamin D metabolites. All of these enzymes are mitochondrial mixed function oxidases containing cytochrome P450 with ferredoxin and haem-binding domains. Vitamin D_2 and D_3 seem equally susceptible to these hydroxylations, and their bioactivated forms are essentially equipotent in influencing mineral homoeostasis (2, 3). However, there is some evidence that suggests vitamin D_2 is less effective than vitamin D_3 in humans. Rightfully, vitamin D is regarded as a steroid hormone, not as a nutrient, because cholecalciferol undergoes this series of bioactivation steps, and then circulates as 1,25-dihydroxyvitamin D to target organs where it binds to the vitamin D receptor (VDR) (6, 7, 8).

In target tissues, there are genomic and nongenomic actions of 1,25-dihydroxyvitamin D (9). 1,25-dihydroxyvitamin D couples to the VDR encoded by a gene of the nuclear hormone receptor superfamily. The VDR has both 1,25-dihydroxyvitamin D-binding and DNA-binding domains. After also combining with a retinoid X receptor heterodimeric partner, this VDR complex activates transcription of genes in bone, kidney, and enterocytes to assure adequate extracellular concentrations of minerals (9). 1,25-dihydroxyvitamin D is the active metabolite of vitamin D assessed by its potency and rapidity of action to augment gut absorption of Ca^{2+}. Urinary Ca^{2+} reclamation by the kidneys and bone resorption are also increased. Furthermore, 1,25-dihydroxyvitamin D suppresses PTH synthesis (2, 3). The nomenclature of vitamin D and its activated forms emphasizes the hormonal nature of these secosterols (Table 4.10.1).

Minerals

Extracellular concentrations of Ca^{2+} and Pi are maintained by three organs: intestine (mainly by absorption), bone (principally by in and out fluxes, as well as by resorption and formation), and kidney (by ultrafiltration and tubular reabsorption) (4). At least three hormones interact and control this homoeostatic mechanism. PTH activates bone cells, increases renal tubular reabsorption of Ca^{2+} while causing phosphaturia, and promotes 1,25-dihydroxyvitamin D production in the proximal renal tubule. Vitamin D (1,25-dihydroxyvitamin D) promotes Ca^{2+} absorption from the gut, probably affects osteoblasts, and controls the synthesis of PTH and a phosphatonin, fibroblast growth factor-23 (FGF-23) (10). FGF-23, produced by cells of the osteoblast lineage, diminishes renal tubular

Table 4.10.1 Nomenclature of vitamin D (calciferol) and its metabolites

Chemical	Vitamin	Abbreviation
Ergocalciferol	Vitamin D_2	D_2
Cholecalciferol	Vitamin D_3	D_3
25-Hydroxyergocalciferol	25-hydroxyvitamin D_2	25(OH) D_2
25-Hydroxycholecalciferol	25-hydroxyvitamin D_3	25(OH) D_3
1α-Hydroxyergocalciferol	1α-hydroxyvitamin D_2	1α(OH) D_2
1,25-Dihydroxyergocalciferol	1,25-dihydroxyvitamin D_2	1,25$(OH)_2D_2$
1,25-Dihydroxycholecalciferol	1,25-dihydroxyvitamin D_3	1,25$(OH)_2D_3$

Throughout the text, the abbreviations D, 25-hydroxyvitamin D, and 1,25-dihydroxyvitamin D are used to indicate either the D_2 or D_3 compound, or a mixture of both.

reabsorption of Pi and production of 1,25-dihydroxyvitamin D (7). The interplay of these hormones on net fluxes and each other creates a precise mechanism for controlling mineral homoeostasis; circulating levels of Ca^{2+} being more tightly controlled than Pi concentrations (4). Increments in extracellular Ca^{2+} reflect direct actions of PTH on the skeleton and kidneys to augment bone turnover and reclaim filtered Ca^{2+}, respectively, but an indirect action on the gut mediated by the enhanced 1,25-dihydroxyvitamin D production (2, 3). Extracellular Pi levels are regulated primarily by the kidney (11). Although PTH is known to cause phosphaturia, how other factors control Pi homoeostasis remains incompletely understood, but now importantly includes the action of a variety of phosphatonins, such as FGF-23 (10).

Diagnosis

Medical history

Depending on the patient's age, disturbances in vitamin D and mineral homoeostasis can engender a considerable variety of signs and symptoms. They can be metabolic or skeletal in origin (Box 4.10.2), and are likely to be severe when extracellular Ca^{2+} levels are low (Box 4.10.3). Furthermore, many somatic changes may manifest (Boxes 4.10.2 and 4.10.3). Reduced levels or ineffective action of vitamin D can be particularly harmful for infants and children. In osteomalacia in adults, there may be axial skeleton pain with focal areas of discomfort due to fractures or pseudofractures, but other symptoms can be vague. The importance of the medical history to capture this information for diagnosing and treating metabolic bone disease has been emphasized and reviewed (12).

Physical examination

Rickets affects especially the most rapidly growing bones (13, 14). Thus, the location and severity of the clinical features will depend on the age of onset. Children with hereditary disorders will usually appear normal at birth because Ca^{2+} and Pi levels in fetal plasma are unregulated and sustained by placental transport from maternal plasma. These patients usually develop the characteristic features of rickets within the first 2 years of life. During infancy, this includes the cranium, wrist, and ribs. Rickets at this time will lead to widened cranial sutures, frontal bossing, posterior flattening of the skull (craniotabes), widening of the wrists, bulging of costochondral junction (rachitic rosary), and indentation of the ribs at the diaphragmatic insertion (Harrison's groove). The rib cage may be so deformed that it contributes to recurrent pneumonia and respiratory failure. Dental eruption is delayed, and teeth can show enamel hypoplasia. After infancy, with standing and rapid linear growth, deformities are most severe in the legs. Bow legs (genu varum) or knock-knee (genu valgum) deformities of variable severity develop as well as widening of the ends of long bones from metaphyseal expansion. If, however, soft bones develop later in childhood or during the adolescent growth spurt, knock-knee

Box 4.10.2 Vitamin D deficiency: age-dependent signs and symptoms

- Metabolic
  - Hypocalcaemia
  - (See also Box 4.10.3)
- Muscle
  - Asthenia
  - Pot belly with lumbar lordosis
  - Proximal myopathy
  - Waddling gait
- Dental
  - Caries
  - Delayed eruption
  - Enamel defects
- Skeletal and other features
  - Bone tenderness
  - Cranial sutures widened
  - Craniotabes (skull asymmetry)
  - Dystocia
  - Flared wrists and ankles
  - Fracture
  - Frontal bossing
  - Harrison's groove
  - Hypotonia
  - Kyphosis
  - Lax ligaments
  - Limb deformity
  - Listlessness
  - Low back pain
  - Pneumonia
  - Rachitic rosary
  - Rib deformity → respiratory compromise
  - Short stature
  - Sternal indention or protrusion
  - 'String-of-pearls' deformity in hands

Box 4.10.3 Signs and symptoms of hypocalcaemia

- Nervous system
  - Increased irritability with latent or overt tetany
  - Seizures
  - Mental status change, retardation
  - Basal ganglia calcification
- Cardiovascular
  - Prolonged ST interval with arrhythmia
  - Cardiomyopathy with congestive heart failure
  - Hypotension
- Other
  - Papilloedema
  - Lenticular cataracts
  - Intestinal malabsorption
  - Dysplastic teeth
  - Rickets/osteomalacia
  - Integument changes
  - Joint contractures
  - Vertebral ligament calcification

Reproduced with permission from Whyte MP. Hypocalcemia. In: *Metabolic Bone and Stone Disease*, 3rd edn. Nordin BEC, Need AG, Morris HA, eds. Edinburgh: Churchill Livingstone, 1993: 147–62.

deformity can occur. Occasionally, the lower limbs curve in the same direction ('windswept' legs) (13). However, deformity may not manifest if the child cannot bear weight or is not growing. If not treated, rickets may cause severe lasting deformities, compromise adult height, and increase susceptibility to pathological fractures. Bone pain and tenderness can reflect fracture or deformity. In osteomalacia, compression of the ribs or sternum, percussion of the vertebrae, and squeezing of long bones may elicit tenderness.

In infants with deranged vitamin D homoeostasis and hypocalcaemia, floppiness and hypotonia are common. They are often listless and irritable (13). Symptoms of latent or overt tetany may be elicited during the medical history, but signs appear during the physical examination (Box 4.10.3). Such abnormalities are particularly striking with severe and/or rapid reductions in circulating Ca^{2+} levels. Hypocalcaemia enhances neuromuscular excitability (4). Depending on the severity, patients can experience paresthesias of the lips and fingertips and spontaneous muscle contractions in the limbs, face, or elsewhere. Carpopedal spasm manifests with thumb adduction, metacarpophalangeal joint flexion, and interphalangeal joint extension. Latent tetany is unmasked by Chvostek's or Trousseau's sign, yet both signs can be negative despite severe hypocalcaemia. Profound hypocalcaemia can also cause mental status changes, epileptic seizures, lethal stridor from laryngeal muscle spasm, and cardiomyopathy (Box 4.10.3) (4).

Additional problems include a 'metabolic myopathy' with reduced muscle tone and strength as well as a waddling gait, but no (or nonspecific) changes on electromyography (13). Myopathy is a prominent feature of vitamin D deficiency and tumour-induced rickets or osteomalacia. Proximal muscle weakness is suspected because of difficulty negotiating stairs, combing hair, or rising from a sitting position. Gower's sign detects this problem when patients must push with their hands on their thighs to stand. Routine assessments of muscle strength should be performed, before and after treatment.

Skull shape and size can be distorted. Premature fusion of the sagittal suture often causes dolichocephaly in X-linked hypophosphataemia, but usually this is only a cosmetic difficulty. In hypophosphatasia, functional or true premature fusion of cranial sutures can lead to a scafalocephalic skull, sometimes with raised intracranial pressure (15).

Total alopecia is a distinctive finding in some patients with hereditary resistance to 1,25-dihydroxyvitamin D (6, 7). There can also be lax ligaments, pectus excavatum from diaphragmatic and intercostal muscle traction, delayed eruption of permanent teeth, and obvious enamel defects (13, 14).

Dystocia (narrowed birth canal) resulting from childhood vitamin D deficiency was a major cause of puerperal mortality at the turn of the past century (14). This deformity should be considered for women with a history of rickets.

In oncogenic (tumour-induced) rickets or osteomalacia, the causal neoplasm may be visible, if not palpable, although some lesions are no more than pea-size. Typically, they are found subcutaneously, but can be anywhere. Some have occurred intravaginally or in the nasopharynx, and some are discovered in the skeleton. Because extirpation of these tumours is curative, thorough physical examination is essential. If the neoplasm is also elusive on radiological studies, patients should conduct self-examination periodically for subcutaneous masses. Lesions grow slowly and may gradually manifest.

Radiological studies

For rickets, an anteroposterior radiograph of a knee and a posteroanterior radiograph of a wrist best document the severity of physeal and metaphyseal distortion, and are used for diagnosis and to judge response to therapy (16). Rickets initially widens growth plates uniformly (Fig. 4.10.1a and b). However, chronic disease with skeletal deformity alters mechanical forces acting on lower limb physes, which can become asymmetrically broad in the knees (Fig. 4.10.1c). Typically, metaphyses are splayed and appear ragged and concave with epiphyses seemingly held within a cup (Fig. 4.10.1b). For a few years after the major growth plates fuse, indistinct apophyses can still be seen in the ischium and ilium (16). Long cassette films of the lower limbs, taken while the patient stands, help to explain and to quantify bowing or knock-knee deformity.

Radiographs can also provide clues to the aetiology or pathogenesis of rickets (12, 16). Disturbances in vitamin D homoeostasis, which result in secondary hyperparathyroidism, often lead to osteopenia and sometimes subperiosteal bone resorption. Conversely, X-linked hypophosphataemia features normal or sometimes increased radiodensity, and changes of hyperparathyroidism are generally absent. In hypophosphatasia, peculiar 'tongues' of radiolucency project from physes into metaphyses where there can be

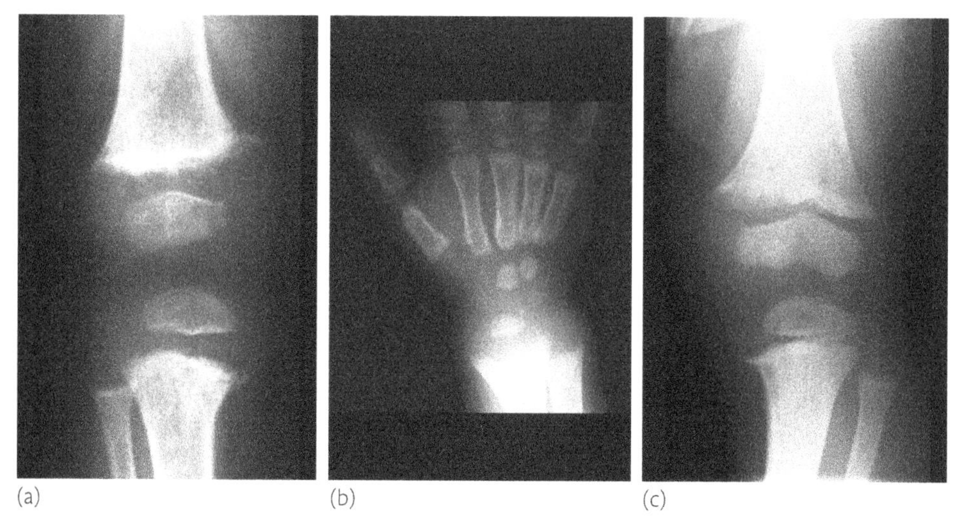

Fig. 4.10.1 Rickets: (a) Before treatment, uniform physeal widening and metaphyseal irregularity and flaring affect the knee of this 2-year-old black child with vitamin D deficiency, poor dietary $Ca^{2}+$ intake, and seizures treated with phenobarbital. (b) Physes are widened and metaphyses are irregular and flared in the right wrist of this 2-year-old girl with untreated X-linked hypophosphataemia. A 'ball-in-cup' deformity is developing at the distal radius. (c) Physeal widening is less apparent in the left knee of this 2-year-old girl beginning treatment for X-linked hypophosphataemia. Asymmetrical physeal widening is due to the bowing deformity of the lower limbs. Also, there is beaking of the medial tibial metaphysis.

paradoxical areas of osteosclerosis (Fig. 4.10.2) (15). However, not all disorders that cause growth plate distortions and limb bowing are forms of rickets (16). Epiphyseal and metaphyseal dysplasias or Blount's disease may mimic rickets, but they do not alter vitamin D homoeostasis and rarely produce overt abnormalities in mineral metabolism (4).

Radiographic signs of secondary hyperparathyroidism are seen best as subperiosteal erosions involving the radial border of the middle phalanx of the index finger, and erosion of the distal ends of the clavicles and symphysis pubis (16). The vertebrae may develop a 'rugger-jersey' appearance. In osteomalacia, pseudofractures (Looser's zones) can occur anywhere except in the skull, and most often affect the pubic and ischial rami, ribs, scapulae, and the medial cortex of the proximal femora (Fig. 4.10.3). Intervertebral discs may compress softened endplates causing biconcave ('cod fish') vertebrae (16).

In addition, the rapidity of response to therapy may be of diagnostic significance for rickets. In primary vitamin D deficiency, radiographic improvement occurs just several weeks after a single large oral dose of vitamin D and correction of circulating 25-hydroxyvitamin D levels (13). Other forms of rickets, especially those due to renal Pi wasting, often take months to improve with current medical treatments (11).

Bone scintigraphy is useful for uncovering abnormalities in the skeleton, but does not provide a diagnosis. Enhanced radioisotope uptake in bone occurs where there is osteoidosis; hence, rickets or

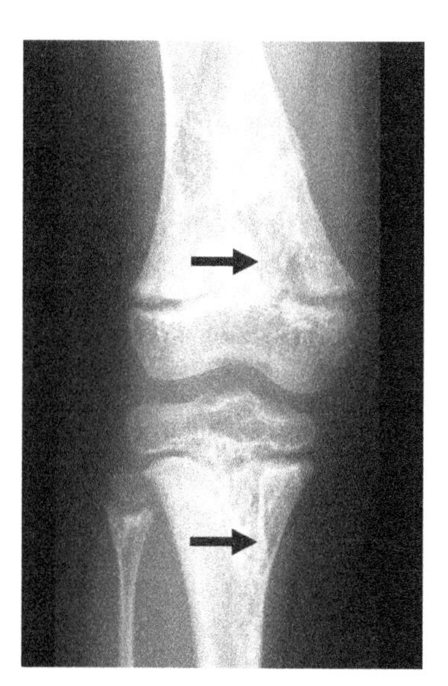

Fig. 4.10.2 Hypophosphatasia: Characteristic tongues of radiolucency project from the physes (arrows) into the metaphyses of this 5-year-old girl who survived infantile hypophosphatasia.

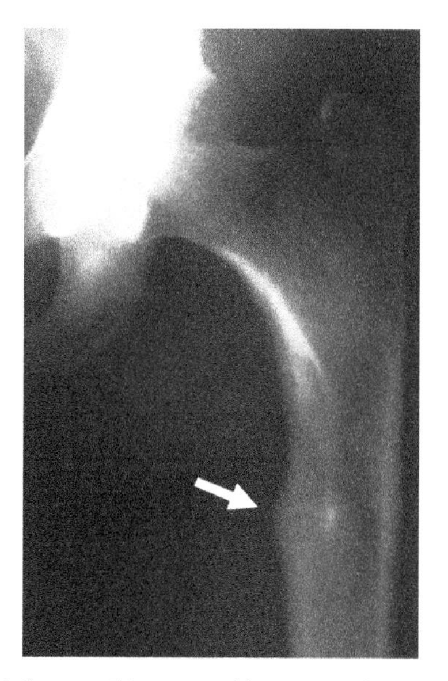

Fig. 4.10.3 Pseudofracture: This 20-year-old woman with X-linked hypophosphataemia has a 'Looser zone' (arrow), characteristic of an osteomalacia, in her proximal femur.

osteomalacia can produce a 'superscan' featuring also no apparent renal uptake of radioisotope. This procedure is usually unnecessary in children with rickets. However, when physical examination fails to disclose the cause of tumoral rickets or osteomalacia, bone scanning helps detect skeletal sources. In adults, this procedure also discloses complications of osteomalacia, such as fractures and pseudofractures.

Bone densitometry, especially by dual-energy X-ray absorptiometry, can be imprecise in rickets or osteomalacia because of short stature, bone deformities, and osteoid accumulation.

Biochemical investigation

Measurements of serum Ca^{2+}, Pi, PTH, and bone-specific ALP are essential to differentiate among the three principal aetiologies of rickets and/or osteomalacia; 24-hour urinary Ca^{2+} excretion and serum 1,25-dihydroxyvitamin D levels help differentiate among aetiological groups of primary hypophosphataemic rickets and/or osteomalacia due to defects in renal tubular Pi reabsorption.

Hypocalcaemia is usually more severe in vitamin D-deficiency rickets versus osteomalacia, and sometimes paradoxically results in hyperphosphataemia due to a direct disturbance in the kidney tubule (13). Secondary hyperparathyroidism causes a mild hyperchloraemic metabolic acidosis, reflecting enhanced renal excretion of bicarbonate. Significant acidosis, however, suggests Fanconi's syndrome (11).

Although quantitation of circulating vitamin D_2 and D_3 levels directly assesses vitamin D status, assays for these prohormones are not readily available (2, 3). Fortunately, measuring serum 25-hydroxyvitamin D is an excellent surrogate. 25-hydroxyvitamin D assays are generally offered by reference laboratories and detect both 25-hydroxyvitamin D_2 and 25-hydroxyvitamin D_3 together. Assays for serum 1,25-dihydroxyvitamin D are also obtained commercially, but their utility is limited because levels can be high, normal, or low in vitamin D deficiency, depending upon the degree of secondary hyperparathyroidism and how much 25-hydroxyvitamin D substrate remains for 1,25-dihydroxyvitamin D production (13, 14). Quantitation of these two vitamin D compounds is, however, essential to differentiate among the various disturbances in vitamin D action: vitamin D deficiency, 1,25-dihydroxyvitamin D deficiency, and resistance to 1,25-dihydroxyvitamin D (Table 4.10.2).

Serum ALP activity (bone isoform) from osteoblasts is elevated in nearly all patients with rickets or osteomalacia. The exception is hypophosphatasia, which features hypophosphatasaemia (15). Levels of other markers of skeletal turnover can be altered, but are sometimes confusing in rickets or osteomalacia and need not be measured routinely.

Histopathological findings

Although the patient's medical history, physical findings, and routine biochemical and radiographic abnormalities usually suffice to diagnose and to treat rickets or osteomalacia, histopathological studies showing defective mineralization of bone tissue provide the definitive evidence for these disturbances (1).

Because in clinical practice bone biopsy specimens are routinely acquired only from the iliac crest, the histological picture obtained is osteomalacia, not rickets. Osteomalacia is defined as excess osteoid (hyperosteoidosis) together with quantitative and dynamic proof of defective bone matrix mineralization using time-spaced tetracycline labelling (17).

Transiliac bone biopsy is taken at a standard location: 2 cm behind the anterosuperior iliac spine and just below the crest, using a trephine of 5.0 or 7.5 mm inner diameter for adults, or 5 mm diameter for children. The specimen should contain the inner and outer cortex and intervening trabeculae. Two 3-day courses of oxytetracycline or demeclocycline hydrochloride (20 mg/kg body weight per day in divided doses) are given (separated by a 2-week interval) for *in vivo* tetracycline labelling of mineralizing bone surfaces. The final dose is swallowed several days before the biopsy. The core is sectioned undecalcified and used unstained, or with different stains and techniques to assess qualitative and quantitative histomorphometric parameters (Fig. 4.10.4).

In rickets or osteomalacia, properly stained, nondecalcified sections will reveal increased quantities of unmineralized osteoid (width and extent) covering bone surfaces (Fig. 4.10.4a), and fluorescence microscopy will fail to show two discrete tetracycline 'labels' produced by ongoing mineralization (Fig. 4.10.4b). Instead, absent or smeared fluorescence is noted. Commonly used histomorphometric parameters (17) include trabecular bone volume, osteoid volume, osteoid surface, osteoid thickness, osteoblast surface, osteoclast surface, osteoclast number, double labelled surface, mineral appositional rate, bone formation rate, and mineralization lag time. Although bone biopsy is not required routinely for rickets, which is defined radiographically, bone histology in osteomalacia is useful because radiographic studies are less helpful (16).

Guidelines for therapy and follow-up

Most forms of rickets or osteomalacia can be treated with considerable success. However, an accurate diagnosis and appropriate follow-up are essential for a favourable clinical outcome, while

Table 4.10.2 Biochemical parameters of mineral and bone metabolism in rickets and/or osteomalacia, by aetiology

Aetiology	Biochemical properties				
	Serum concentrations				
	Calcium	Phosphorous	PTH	Bone-specific ALP	24th urinary Ca^{2}+ excretion
Hypocalcaemic e.g. vitamin D deficiency	Low to low normal	Low	Elevated	Elevated	Low
Hypophosphataemic e.g. X-linked hypophosphataemia	Normal	Low	Normal to elevated	Elevated	Low to elevated
Tissue defects e.g. hypophosphatasia	Normal or elevated	Normal or elevated	Low to normal	Low	Normal to elevated

PTH, parathyroid hormone; ALP, alkaline phosphatase.

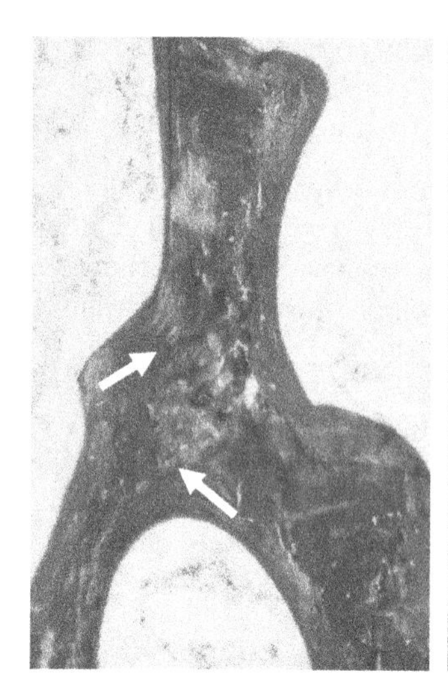

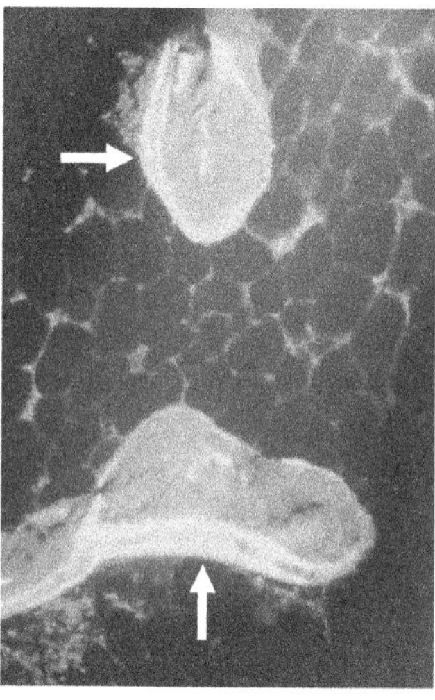

Fig. 4.10.4 (a) Osteomalacia: Undecalcified bone shows excessive red-staining osteoid covering all surfaces of blue-staining, mineralized trabeculae. Osteoid also forms 'halos' (arrows) surrounding osteocytes indicative of X-linked hypophosphataemia (Masson stain; × 250). (b) Normal bone formation: Two discrete yellow bands at the surface of trabeculae (arrows) indicate that bone mineralization is ongoing. In osteomalacia, such fluorescent 'labels' are absent or smeared (x 250). (See also Plate 20)

avoiding intoxication with vitamin D or mineral supplements. Ideally, the primary pathological process is corrected (Box 4.10.1). However, this may not be possible, and pharmacological doses of vitamin D (or an active metabolite), sometimes with mineral supplementation, will be necessary. Currently, five sterols with vitamin D activity are available as pharmaceuticals: vitamin D_2 or D_3, 25-hydroxyvitamin D_3, 1,25-dihydroxyvitamin D_3, alfacalcidiol (1α-hydroxyvitamin D_3), and dihydrotachysterol. They differ importantly in potency and biological half-life (Table 4.10.3).

Wisely chosen, medical therapy for rickets or osteomalacia can be rewarding for patient and physician. Given sufficient time before growth plate closure, the three disturbances of skeletal development can be corrected (1). Reversal of short stature and deformity are major goals of treatment of rickets. Relief from bone pain and fracture prevention also follow effective management of osteomalacia.

Physical examination provides critical information. Linear growth rates are important parameters to monitor in infants, children, and especially adolescents. Height is determined best with a wall-mounted stadiometer. Rapid increases in body size during the pubertal growth spurt can significantly augment dose requirements for chronic forms of rickets. Furthermore, inordinate weight gain in girls can accelerate puberty and the growth spurt can increase limb deformity and compromise final height. When growth is complete, dosage requirements may unexpectedly diminish.

Measurements of arm span and height as well as upper and lower segment lengths will help to quantify skeletal distortion. With chronic forms of rickets, treatment may be necessary throughout growth, and some time can pass before control is achieved. It may be the individual who sees the patient only every 6 months who best appreciates changes in deformities. Accordingly, clinical photography, gait analysis, and even videotaping can help to document gradual alterations. Radiographic changes, such as widening of the growth plates and metaphyseal irregularity, are essential not only for diagnosis but also to assess for follow-up. Pseudofractures can heal with treatment. Osteopenia and coarsening of trabecular bone are observed in only some patients (16). Other radiographic findings are less helpful.

The most useful biochemical parameters are serum Ca^{2+} and Pi concentrations, ALP, and PTH levels. Depending on the aetiology and pathogenesis of the rickets or osteomalacia, serum 25-hydroxyvitamin D and 1,25-dihydroxyvitamin D concentrations may be helpful. Ca^{2+} excretion in 24-h urine collections (corrected for creatinine content) guides therapy, and helps monitor for drug toxicity. Maintenance of normal urinary levels of Ca^{2+} often indicates that treatment is effective. If, however, incomplete healing of rickets or osteomalacia is suspected, nondecalcified iliac crest histomorphometry is definitive (1).

The causes of rickets and osteomalacia are numerous (Box 4.10.1). Successful treatment will depend upon a correct diagnosis and understanding of the mechanism for the aberration in vitamin D stores or bioactivation and/or the changes in mineral homoeostasis. The optimum regimen will correct or circumvent the defect, but a range of effective doses should be anticipated among patients. Significant adverse consequences (failed treatment, hypercalcaemia, kidney stones, secondary or tertiary hyperparathyroidism, or renal damage) may result from an incorrect diagnosis or excessive therapy.

Treatment with active metabolites of vitamin D can circumvent defective bioactivation of vitamin D (7), and also be useful

Table 4.10.3 Pharmaceutical preparations of vitamin D and active metabolites

	Ergocalciferol	**Dihydrotachysterol**[a]	**Calcifediol**[a]	**Calcitriol**	**Alfacalcidol**
Abbreviation	D_2	DHT	25(OH) D_3	$1,25(OH)_2D_3$	1α(OH)D
Dosage form	Capsules: 1.25 mg Liquid: 200 μg/ml Intramuscular injection: 12.5 mg/ml in sesame oil	Tablets: 0.125, 0.200, and 0.400 mg Liquid: 0.250 mg/ml	Capsules: 20 and 50 μg	Capsules: 0.25 and 0.50 μg Injection: 1.0 μg/ml Liquid: 1.0 μ/ml	Capsules: 0.25 and 1.0 μg Liquid: 0.20 μg/ml Injection: 2.0 μg/ml in propylene glycol
Time to reach maximum biological effects	4–10 weeks	2–4 weeks	4–20 weeks	0.5–1 week	0.5–1 week
Persistence of biological effect after cessation	6–30 weeks	2–8 weeks	4–12 weeks	0.5–1 week	0.5–1 week

[a] These forms of vitamin D are no longer generally available, but are listed for historical interest and for reference.

for hereditary defects in the VDR (see below) (7). These drugs are more potent than vitamin D_2 or D_3, have more rapid onset of action, and have shorter biological half-lives (Table 4.10.3). Thus, toxicity can be corrected rapidly (7). Unfortunately, they do not replete deficient stores of vitamin D, if present. Many preparations are available for Ca^{2+} and Pi supplementation (17). Ca^{2+} dose will be dependent on the primary disturbance, and Ca^{2+} salt on the individual patient. $CaCO_3$ given orally is least expensive, but Ca^{2+} citrate is better absorbed under certain conditions. Ca^{2+} gluconate is especially costly. Tablets rather than liquid preparations for Pi supplementation are more convenient, taste better, and seem less prone to cause diarrhoea. Those with high amounts of sodium should be avoided.

Follow-up clinic visits are essential for all types of rickets and osteomalacia, but the interval should reflect the specific diagnosis as well as the formulation and track record of therapy. Because rickets and osteomalacia reflect correctable deficiencies in skeletal mineral content, decreases in dose might be necessary when healing is complete. Satiation of 'hungry bones' may abruptly increase urinary Ca^{2+} excretion because the skeleton no longer acts avidly as a sump for mineral deposition. Correction of previously abnormal biochemical findings should herald hypercalciuria. Lower doses or cessation of vitamin D and mineral supplements may then be needed. Unless there is renal failure or fixed elevation in circulating PTH levels (reclaiming Ca^{2+} from the glomerular filtrate), hypercalciuria generally precedes hypercalcaemia. Thus, 24-h urine collections, not random specimens, assayed for Ca^{2+} and creatinine are especially important for follow-up. Because hypocalciuria characterizes most forms of rickets or osteomalacia, rising urinary Ca^{2+} levels will also indicate effective therapy.

Consultation and follow-up with the orthopaedic surgeon is often important for treating rickets. Leg bracing, physeal stapling (epiphysiodesis), or osteotomy may be helpful. Straight lower limbs when growth ceases, with alignment of physes parallel to the ground, helps prevent osteoarthritis. Intramedullary rodding may be necessary to heal pseudofractures or to prevent fractures for some patients with osteomalacia (18).

Pharmacological regimens for specific types of rickets or osteomalacia are outlined in the following sections, representing the different aetiologies; i.e. hypocalcaemic, hypophosphataemic, and with no abnormalities in mineral homoeostasis.

Acquired rickets and osteomalacia

Primary vitamin D deficiency

Pathogenesis

Vitamin D deficiency can be caused by decreased acquisition and/or increased clearance. Primary ('nutritional') rickets or osteomalacia is a man-made disorder involving social, economic, and/or cultural factors that prevent sufficient exposure to sunlight and insufficient photosynthesis of vitamin D_3 in the skin. Decreased input may be exacerbated by diminished intake from dietary (nutritional) deficiency or intestinal malabsorption. Increased vitamin D clearance could result from accelerated catabolism, mainly in the liver, or increased loss via the kidneys or intestine.

Vitamin D content of various unfortified food substances is very low, with the exception of fatty fish such as herring and mackerel, or cod liver oil. It is estimated that during unfortified food consumption less than 20% of total circulating 25-hydroxyvitamin D is contributed by nutritional vitamin D. However, in some countries, dietary vitamin D is enhanced by supplementation of certain food products. In the USA, milk is fortified with 400 IU per quart. Greater vitamin D intake could also result from habitual use of multivitamins, which usually contain 400 IU per tablet, or some Ca^{2+} salt preparations that also contain vitamin D. These supplements will increase the relative contribution of dietary vitamin D to the total body pool, and be beneficial especially when cutaneous production is limited. Now in the USA, substantially higher doses of vitamin D can be purchased over-the-counter.

Vitamin D synthesis in the skin requires UV light with a maximal effective wave length between 290 and 310 nm, and is affected by the intensity, surface area of the skin exposed, and intrinsic properties of the epidermis (5). In northern latitudes during winter, almost no UV light reaches the ground. In the north of the USA, Canada, and North-western Europe very little or practically no vitamin D is produced in exposed skin between October and March. Clothing, glass, plastic, and sunscreens effectively block UV radiation and prevent cutaneous vitamin D synthesis. Furthermore, vitamin D production is lower in dark skin (because melanin absorbs UV radiation), and in the elderly. Even in the elderly, however, dermal vitamin D production persists (5). It has been estimated that, in summer, a 20-min exposure three times weekly of the skin of the head and arms prevents vitamin D deficiency in the elderly.

Diagnosis

Vitamin D deficiency is diagnosed by a low serum concentration of 25-hydroxyvitamin D, which is a reliable measure of vitamin D status in almost all clinically relevant situations. All additional biochemical parameters, as well as clinical signs and symptoms, reflect the subsequent perturbations in bone and mineral metabolism, and are shared by all disorders in vitamin D action and Ca^{2+} deficiency (Tables 4.10.2 and 4.10.4). Included are low to low-normal serum Ca^{2+} levels, hypocalciuria, secondary hyperparathyroidism, hypophosphataemia, increased levels of biochemical markers of bone turnover (e.g. bone-specific ALP and osteocalcin). Therefore, these parameters can support (but not establish) the diagnosis of rickets and/or osteomalacia, and help assess the relative severity of the vitamin D deficiency and the response to treatment. Importantly, circulating levels of 1,25-dihydroxyvitamin D can vary from low to elevated (Table 4.10.4), and thus are unhelpful for this diagnosis.

Population-based reference values for serum 25-hydroxyvitamin D levels were, for a considerable time, debatable and uncertain.

Table 4.10.4 Serum levels of vitamin D metabolites in disorders of vitamin D action, by aetiology

Aetiology	Serum levels	
	25-hydroxyvitamin D	**1,25-dihydroxyvitamin D**
Vitamin D deficiency	Low	Low to elevated
25-hydroxyvitamin D, 1α-hydroxylase deficiency	Normal to elevated	Very low
Resistance to 1,25-dihydroxyvitamin D	Normal to elevated	Markedly elevated

They differ according to age, geography, season, dress habits, confinement to bed or home (affecting sunshine exposure and thus vitamin D synthesis) as well as eating habits, local regulation on food fortification, and customs of vitamin supplementation (affecting vitamin D intake). A better alternative, however, is to define health-based parameters, i.e. serum 25-hydroxyvitamin D levels below which adverse health outcomes may occur. Actually, this represents an intervention threshold below which therapy may prevent detrimental effects on the skeleton, including milder vitamin D deficiency states which may not compromise matrix mineralization but, via disruption of mineral homoeostasis, cause secondary hyperparathyroidism, increased bone turnover, and bone loss (19). The relationship between serum 25-hydroxyvitamin D and PTH levels has been analysed in multiple studies to define serum 25-hydroxyvitamin D concentrations below which serum PTH levels increase, or baseline 25-hydroxyvitamin D levels above which vitamin D supplementation significantly decreased serum PTH concentrations (19). Both approaches yielded similar functional thresholds. Accordingly, diagnostic staging of vitamin D states, based on serum 25-hydroxyvitamin D levels and secondary perturbations in mineral and bone metabolism, has been proposed. Vitamin D 'adequacy' is serum 25-hydroxyvitamin D at or above 30 ng/ml (75 nmol/l). This is accepted by most clinicians, though not by all, and some argue that the threshold level is instead somewhere between 50–75 nmol/l (20 and 30 ng/ml). However, there is no debate that serum 25-hydroxyvitamin D below 50 nmol/l (20 ng/ml) is inadequate. Vitamin D 'inadequacy' is subdivided into vitamin D 'insufficiency' levels between 25 nmol/l (10 ng/ml) and the threshold value, and vitamin D 'deficiency' below 25 nmol/l (10 ng/ml). Vitamin D deficiency represents a state in which Ca^{2+} homoeostasis begins to fail, i.e. a decrease in serum Ca^{2+} (up to overt hypocalcaemia) despite markedly increased serum PTH concentrations, with the high risk of developing rickets and/or osteomalacia. The same threshold of approximately 75 nmol/l (30 ng/ml) was observed in studies that correlated serum 25-hydroxyvitamin D levels to additional physiological variables, such as intestinal Ca^{2+} absorption, changes in bone mineral density, and lower extremity physical performance (20). Further support for this threshold was obtained by a meta-analysis of intervention studies with vitamin D. Reduction of falls and fractures was positively correlated to the doses of vitamin D and serum 25-hydroxyvitamin D levels (up to a certain threshold) (21).

Prevalence of vitamin D insufficiency and deficiency

Although we understand the biosynthetic and bioactivation pathways for vitamin D, primary deficiency is still common worldwide (14, 22). In the UK, the condition resurged in the 1970s within the immigrant Asian community (13). Because vitamin D status depends upon both cutaneous photosynthesis and dietary intake, serum 25-hydroxyvitamin D levels vary widely depending on latitude, season, urban living, clothing, skin pigmentation, use of sunscreens, age, gender, etc., and local rules and customs concerning vitamin D supplementation. The most vulnerable are those who cannot move freely, and therefore are at the beginning or end of life. However, any age can be affected, especially those with physical or mental handicaps. Limited sunshine exposure due to cultural practices and prolonged breastfeeding without vitamin D supplementation contributes considerably to vitamin D deficiency in some regions worldwide (5). Now, use of sunscreens may also block skin access to UV light (5). Additionally, a 'safety-net' created by fortifying certain foods with vitamin D may not be provided (13, 22). Among adults, institutionalized or housebound individuals, the poor, the elderly, food faddists, and some religious groups (because of diet and dress) are at greater risk. Infants who breast feed beyond 6 months of age or drink nonfortified milk or formula are also susceptible (13). In some populations, low dietary Ca^{2+} intake can be an important exacerbating factor (22).

In 1998, investigation of patients on a general medicine ward in Boston, Massachusetts revealed that secondary hyperparathyroidism was common when serum 25-hydroxyvitamin D levels were at or below 15 ng/ml (23), and led to subsequent studies which have redefined vitamin D insufficiency and deficiency.

In postmenopausal women treated for osteoporosis in various parts of the world, vitamin D inadequacy, serum 25-hydroxyvitamin levels below 75 nmol/l (30 ng/ml), was observed in 52% of those in North America, 58% in Europe, 53% in Latin America, 71% in Asia, and 82% in the Middle East (24). Pronounced variability was observed among countries, ranging from 30% in Sweden in the summer to approximately 90% in Japan and South Korea in the winter and summer. Deficiency, however, was much less common; approximately 1% in North America, and approximately 6% and 8% in Latin America and the Middle East, respectively.

Furthermore, serum levels below 50 nmol/l (20 ng/ml) were observed in 78% of healthy hospital staff in India, and 90% of young women in Beijing and Hong Kong. Values below 25 nmol/l (10 ng/ml) were reported in about 40% of those tested in Sri Lanka and Beijing, and 18% in Hong Kong (25).

An additional concern is the high prevalence, in some regions, of vitamin D deficiency in pregnant women, their children, adolescent girls, and the elderly. Maternal serum 25-hydroxyvitamin D levels correlate negatively with PTH, and positively with 25-hydroxyvitamin D levels in cord blood. Of pregnant women in India, 84% had serum 25-hydroxyvitamin D levels less than 20 ng/ml. In Saudi Arabia, Israel, Kuwait, the United Arab Emirates, and Iran 10–60% of mothers and 40–80% of their neonates had levels at or below 25 nmol/l (10 ng/ml) at delivery (25).

In adolescent girls, 70% in Iran, 80% in Saudi Arabia, and 32% in Lebanon had serum 25-hydroxyvitamin D levels below 25 nmol/l (10 ng/ml); 91% of healthy school girls from Northern India and 89% of adolescent girls from North China had levels below 20 ng/ml (50 nmol/l).

In multiple studies worldwide, vitamin D deficiency was detected in 35 to 65% of the elderly; more so in institutionalized individuals (26). In patients hospitalized for an osteoporotic fracture, deficiency was recorded in 20–68%; only 1–3% had levels above 75 nmol/l (30 ng/ml).

Fortunately, the prevalence of osteomalacia is lower, but depends on the criteria for diagnosis, i.e. clinical, biochemical, or bone histology or histomorphometry. In a review of multiple publications describing histomorphometry of the femoral head or iliac crest in approximately 1400 patients with hip facture, osteomalacia ranged from none to over 30% of patients. Perhaps this reflects separate populations and different magnitudes and durations of vitamin D deficiency, but also the histological criteria used to define osteomalacia. Nevertheless, the high prevalence of vitamin D deficiency in patients with hip fractures supports the hypothesis that this event is a complication of frank osteomalacia as well as secondary hyperparathyroidism and the consequent acceleration in bone turnover. In fact, there is a positive relationship between serum 25-hydroxyvitamin D levels (below a certain threshold) and hip bone mineral density, and a negative correlation between hip density and serum PTH. Moreover, vitamin D plus Ca^{2+} supplementation reduced the incidence of hip and other nonvertebral fractures in several studies of vitamin D deficiency.

Treatment

Although patient or parent education and correction of adverse socioeconomic factors would be optimal for preventing and treating primary vitamin D deficiency, this is often difficult to achieve. Fortunately, pharmacological or supplementation therapy is inexpensive, effective, and works rapidly. Vitamin D deficiency should be treated using vitamin D_2 or D_3. Although 25-hydroxyvitamin D_3, 1α-hydroxyvitamin D_3, and 1,25-dihydroxyvitamin D_3 may be more potent and act more rapidly, none corrects depleted stores of vitamin D, and the therapeutic window is narrow.

Adequate vitamin D intake was recommended recently by the National Osteoporosis Foundation of the USA to be 800–1000 IU/day in adults age 50 years or older (27). Also, the recommendation for infants was increased to 400 IU/day of vitamin D_3. It will probably become routine to recommend the adult dose for adolescents and older children. However, these intakes are usually unachievable unless additional foods are fortified with vitamin D. Thus, the population at large, and the elderly in particular, are dependent upon both cutaneous vitamin D synthesis and vitamin D supplementation.

Treatment must be targeted to those at greatest risk. Vitamin D supplementation for infants up to 1 year of age is mandatory in many, but not all, countries. Unfortunately, this is not routine for the elderly. Nursing home residents, institutionalized and hospitalized elderly, patients with hip fractures, and those with neurological disorders are among those most in jeopardy (26). Thus, it may be necessary to treat with recommended doses of vitamin D and Ca^{2+} (see below) even before biochemical confirmation because of the high incidence of deficiency in this population, and the fact that tight physiological control of serum 1,25-dihydroxyvitamin D production makes toxicity unlikely.

It is important to remember that, together with vitamin D treatment, the recommended daily Ca^{2+} allowance must be achieved, often by Ca^{2+} salt supplementation. Low Ca^{2+} intake, common in some regions of Africa and North China, may also cause or exacerbate rickets.

The typical oral maintenance dose of vitamin D is 800 to 1000 IU daily. In severe vitamin D deficiency, 4000–8000 IU daily could be given for the first 4–6 weeks. Alternatively, 50 000 IU of vitamin D could be given two or three times a week for the first 2 weeks, followed by lower doses. Because vitamin D is stored in fat and released slowly, and the serum half-life of 25-hydroxyvitamin D is 2–3 weeks, dosing can be once weekly, monthly, or every 3–6 months. An oral dose of 100 000 IU every 4 months for 5 years increased serum 25-hydroxyvitamin D to adequate levels. This approach can improve compliance, both in independent elderly and especially in dependent, institutionalized patients, but experience with this mode of vitamin D administration is relatively limited.

The response to vitamin D supplementation will depend on the degree and severity of deficiency and the secondary changes in mineral and bone metabolism. In severe cases with rickets or osteomalacia, dramatic responses in the signs, symptoms, and laboratory parameters will occur. Bone pain and muscle weakness will improve quickly, pseudofractures can heal, and serum Ca^{2+}, PTH, and biochemical markers of bone turnover will return towards normal. In moderate or mild vitamin D deficiency or insufficiency, the response is more subtle. Muscle weakness and bone pain may improve as serum 25-hydroxyvitamin D and PTH return to normal (this will reflect the severity of the initial vitamin D deficiency). Bone mineral density can increase somewhat, and the incidence of fractures may decrease in adults with osteomalacia.

For infants and young children with vitamin D-deficiency rickets, liquid preparations of vitamin D_2 are available (Table 4.10.3). They can be given 4000 IU of vitamin D_2 (100 μg) orally each day for several months to heal their rickets and replenish vitamin D stores (13, 14). If capsules can be swallowed, one 50 000 IU (1.25 mg) dose of vitamin D_2 orally each week for three or four doses is also an inexpensive and straight-forward treatment. It is prudent for the physician to see that at least the first capsule is swallowed. Biochemical and radiographic improvement then typically occurs within just a few weeks (13, 14).

After healing, children who persist without adequate sunlight exposure should receive 400 IU vitamin D_2 or D_3 per day, either by consuming fortified foods or using over-the-counter multivitamin or vitamin D supplements (2, 3).

For patients with severe vitamin D deficiency causing symptomatic hypocalcaemia, it is helpful to administer a 'loading dose' of vitamin D_2 to replete body stores rapidly. Ca^{2+} intake must also be supplemented. Insufficient Ca^{2+} for the suddenly mineralizing skeleton could exacerbate the hypocalcaemia. A single oral dose of 5000 IU of vitamin D per kg body weight can be given. For a 70 kg adult, this is 350 000 IU of vitamin D. Although this quantity of vitamin D seems great, it illustrates the storage capacity for vitamin D (2, 3). With symptomatic hypocalcaemia, Ca^{2+} can be given intravenously over 24 hours (as much as 20 mg of elemental Ca^{2+} per kg of body weight per day). Ca^{2+} infusions should be given continuously, or slowly in portions, and always regulated by serum Ca^{2+} levels determined several times daily. Oral Ca^{2+} supplementation (1–2 g of elemental Ca^{2+} each day) can be initiated at this time. For patients who are not lactose intolerant and no longer hypocalcaemic, three to four glasses of milk each day will provide both Ca^{2+} and Pi to help remineralize the skeleton.

Failure to show biochemical and radiographic improvement with persistently low serum 25-hydroxyvitamin D levels could reflect failed compliance or malabsorption. Use of inexpensive vitamin D capsules may help to assure that the medication is taken. Alternatively, and if available, intramuscular injection of vitamin D in sesame oil will assure long-term access to antirachitic activity if patient compliance for oral treatment is poor, or if there is malabsorption (Table 4.10.3). Visits to a 'tanning salon' have also proved effective. If skeletal disease persists despite sustained correction of circulating 25-hydroxyvitamin D levels, calciopenia or one of the vitamin D-dependent or resistant syndromes (Box 4.10.1) must be considered (see below) (7, 9, 13, 22).

Prophylaxis against vitamin D-deficiency rickets could involve outdoor activity, occasional exposure to UV light using protective goggles, consumption of vitamin D-fortified foods, or vitamin D supplements (2, 3). 'Stoss therapy', used in Europe, consists of one depot intramuscular injection of 600 000 IU of vitamin D_2 during the autumn. However, this dose given orally has caused hypercalcaemia and renal damage (28).

Secondary vitamin D deficiency

Vitamin D deficiency due to enhanced clearance is relatively uncommon and usually accompanies systemic disorders (e.g. protein losing nephropathy, intestinal malabsorption) or increased liver catabolism sometimes caused by certain drugs (e.g. barbiturates, other antiepileptics, etc.). Gastrointestinal malabsorption interferes with vitamin D input from the gut, but sometimes also with the enterohepatic recirculation of vitamin D metabolites. Thus, intestinal malabsorption may contribute to vitamin D deficiency by both decreasing input and increasing excretion. Vitamin D deficiency caused by decreased input is discussed below.

Vitamin D deficiency can be caused by malabsorption, perhaps despite normal amounts of sunlight exposure (5). Gastrointestinal, pancreatic, or hepatobiliary disease may be the explanation (Box 4.10.1) (2, 3). The mechanism for the vitamin D deficiency and associated derangements in mineral metabolism is often complex. Gut malabsorption may also interfere with influx of minerals.

Vitamin D is a fat-soluble secosterol, and bile salts are necessary for its absorption (2, 3). Additionally, there is enterohepatic circulation of vitamin D and its derivatives (2, 3). Hence, hepatobiliary or pancreatic disease or short bowel syndrome can cause deficiency of bile salts, steatorrhoea, and malabsorption leading to depletion of vitamin D. Furthermore, the small bowel mediates dietary Ca^{2+} uptake, and malabsorption of Ca^{2+} can exacerbate vitamin D deficiency. With secondary hyperparathyroidism, conversion of 25-hydroxyvitamin D to both 1,25- and 24,25-dihydroxyvitamin D is enhanced, and 25-hydroxyvitamin D is depleted also by this mechanism. Nevertheless, in some conditions where osteomalacia might be anticipated (for example, primary biliary cirrhosis) the associated osteopathy is often osteoporosis. Iliac crest biopsy is especially useful in such patients. Vitamin D deficiency and its clinical and biochemical consequences may be the first sign of occult malabsorption due, for example, to coeliac disease (nontropical sprue).

Although the pathogenesis of secondary vitamin D-deficiency rickets or osteomalacia is complicated, pharmacological therapy should produce gratifying results. These patients reflect heterogeneous disturbances, and there must be individualized therapy and follow-up. Assay of serum 25-hydroxyvitamin D documents vitamin D deficiency and is essential for monitoring progress (23). Sufficient doses of vitamin D_2 or D_3 given orally should prove effective, and are relatively inexpensive. Vitamin D repletes exhausted stores, and is readily converted to 25-hydroxyvitamin D by hepatocytes despite parenchymal liver disease (2, 3).

Here too, a single oral 'loading' dose of about 125 μg (5000 IU) of vitamin D per kg of body weight can expedite treatment prior to maintenance dosing. Intravenous Ca^{2+} (as much as 20 mg of elemental Ca^{2+} per kg of body weight daily) over 24 hours by continuous infusion, or slowly in divided doses, is regulated by frequent measurements of serum Ca^{2+} and is helpful for symptomatic hypocalcaemia and 'hungry bones'. Serum Mg^{2+} should be assayed for newly diagnosed hypocalcaemia, and treated if levels are low (17).

After the loading dose of vitamin D, patients with secondary vitamin D deficiency will require supplemental vitamin D unless the primary disorder is also corrected. It is impossible to predict the maintenance dose. Hence, clinical and biochemical follow-up is mandatory. Initially, patients should be seen every few weeks. Adjustments in dosing will be needed when the rickets or osteomalacia heals, or the gastrointestinal, hepatobiliary, or pancreatic disturbance evolves or responds to treatment.

For milder disease, a reasonable starting dose of vitamin D_2 or D_3 is 50 000 IU (1.25 mg) orally twice weekly. Assay of the circulating 25-hydroxyvitamin D level about 1 month later, and about every 4 months thereafter, will determine what dose of vitamin D is effective. Serum 25-hydroxyvitamin D levels should be maintained above the threshold value of 30 ng/ml (75 nmol/l). Ca^{2+} supplements can be added. Then, assay of the Ca^{2+} and creatinine content 24-h urine collections periodically can be used to monitor therapy. This should show correction of any hypocalciuria unless circulating levels of PTH (which reclaims urinary Ca^{2+}) are persistently elevated and do not suppress with treatment. In this situation, assay of serum Ca^{2+} levels becomes especially important. Attention to urinary Ca^{2+} levels will help to guard against vitamin D toxicity manifesting as hypercalciuria.

Although oral vitamin D therapy is nearly always successful (unless there has been almost complete resection of the small intestine requiring total parenteral nutrition), intramuscular injection (if available) of depot vitamin D_2 in oil can be an alternative. Here, 12.5 mg of vitamin D_2 (500 000 IU) is dissolved in 1 ml of sesame oil (Table 4.10.3), providing prolonged bioavailability of vitamin D_2 (29). An increment in the circulating 25-hydroxyvitamin D level may not appear for several weeks, but vitamin D_2 release will persist for months. Injections of 500 000 IU of vitamin D_2 every few months should provide effective and continuous supplementation for an adult, but biochemical monitoring is important.

Calciopenic

Hypophosphataemia due to secondary hyperparathyroidism or primary renal Pi wasting contributes importantly to the pathogenesis of defective mineralization of skeletal matrix in most patients. However, some individuals with hypocalcaemia alone from hypoparathyroidism or pseudohypoparathyroidism develop rickets or osteomalacia despite elevated serum Pi levels.

Severe deficiency of dietary Ca^{2+} despite intact stores of vitamin D can also lead to defective skeletal mineralization (13, 22). So-called calciopenic rickets has been described in children fed a cereal-based diet (13), and in premature infants (14). Poor dietary Ca^{2+} intake can also exacerbate vitamin D-deficiency rickets (22). Several religious, ethnic, and other groups have vegetarian members who are at risk because they do not consume dairy products. Altering the diet, or using Ca^{2+} supplements, should readily reverse this disorder.

Drug-induced

Anticonvulsant-induced

Rickets and osteomalacia have been reported in institutionalized people receiving anticonvulsants, especially multiple pharmaceuticals (2, 3, 14). Phenobarbital can alter hepatic vitamin D metabolism predisposing to vitamin D depletion (2, 3). However, primary deficiency of vitamin D also afflicts many such individuals.

If serum 25-hydroxyvitamin D levels are low, epileptics who take phenobarbital and other anticonvulsants can receive a 50 000 IU dose of vitamin D orally once weekly, thereafter adjusted by following serum 25-hydroxyvitamin D concentrations.

Phosphate binders

Osteomalacia can result from excessive use of Pi-binders (e.g. magnesium and aluminium hydroxide antacids) (17). Rickets complicated by craniosynostosis has occurred when such preparations were added to infant formula to treat colic (30). Significant hypophosphataemia can occur. Assay of urinary phosphorous will reveal low levels. Conversely, patients may hyperabsorb dietary Ca^{2+} and become hypercalciuric because hypophosphataemia stimulates renal 25-hydroxyvitamin D, 1α-hydroxylase activity and augments the biosynthesis of 1,25-dihydroxyvitamin D. Rarely, kidney stones develop. Despite the increased Ca^{2+} levels, hypophosphataemia impairs skeletal mineralization, but elimination of the Pi-binder will rapidly correct the hypophosphataemia and skeletal defect. Pi supplementation or vitamin D therapy will not be necessary. However, it may take several months for serum ALP activity to correct.

Ifosfamide

This chemotherapeutic drug can cause transient or permanent kidney tubule damage leading to urinary Pi wasting and hypophosphataemic skeletal disease (31).

Etidronate

This first-generation bisphosphonate used for Paget's bone disease and hypercalcaemia of malignancy can, with excessive or prolonged exposure, cause rickets or osteomalacia. Etidronate retains sufficient similarity to inorganic pyrophosphate to act as an inhibitor of mineralization (4).

Toxin-induced

Rickets or osteomalacia follow long-term exposure to several other inhibitors of skeletal mineralization.

Aluminium

Patients with uraemia who were exposed to aluminium-containing antacids or contaminated dialysis fluid or parenteral feedings have developed osteomalacia (17). Treatment with desferoxamine has been helpful (17). Unusual case reports suggest that bone mineralization can be impaired in healthy individuals if sufficient aluminium is leached from cookware. With use of newer agents for Pi-binding, this disorder is now rare.

Fluoride

Excessive fluoride from well water, industrial exposure, inordinate tea drinking, or sodium fluoride given for osteoporosis can cause osteomalacia (17). Defective bone mineralization will respond gradually to cessation of fluoride poisoning and Ca^{2+} supplementation.

Oncogenic

Oncogenic rickets or osteomalacia is a rare, sporadic disorder that is often caused by a benign 'mixed mesenchymal' tumour in soft tissues (Fig. 4.10.5) (11, 17). However, a considerable variety of other indolent neoplasms, nonossifying fibroma, and (rarely) malignant bone tumours or other cancers can cause this condition (17). Patients are often profoundly weak. These tumours secrete FGF-23 and sometimes other phosphatonins that cause phosphaturia and profoundly inhibit renal 25-hydroxyvitamin D, 1α-hydroxylase activity (10). Low circulating 1,25-dihydroxyvitamin D levels can cause malabsorption of dietary Ca^{2+} and mild hypocalcaemia,

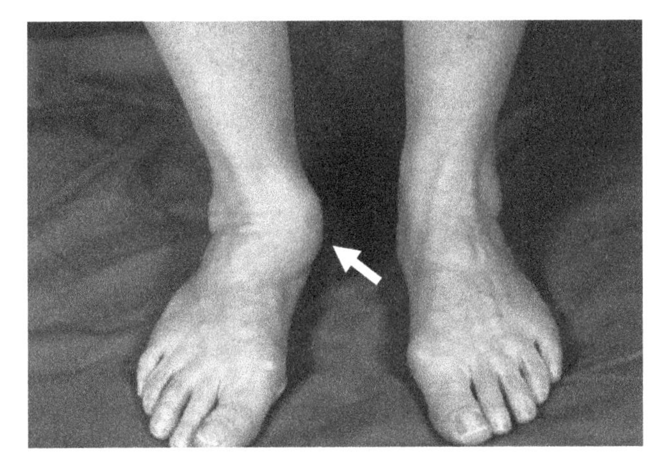

Fig. 4.10.5 Oncogenic osteomalacia: A mass over the medial malleolus (arrow) had been present for 7 years in this 57-year-old woman. She was cured by resection of this mixed mesenchymal tumour. (See also Plate 21)

secondary hyperparathyroidism, and hypocalciuria. Hypophosphataemia is, however, the major biochemical abnormality, and sufficiently lowers the blood $Ca^{2+} \times$ Pi product to impair skeletal mineralization.

Definitive diagnosis and treatment of oncogenic rickets or osteomalacia is achieved by resection of the neoplasm. Therefore, thorough diagnostic evaluation is especially important in sporadic, acquired hypophosphataemic skeletal disease. If a soft tissue tumour is not apparent, bone scintigraphy and/or octreotide scanning is performed. If these studies are not revealing, the nasopharynx should be examined, sometimes by computed tomography. Whole body magnetic resonance imaging and positron emission tomography scanning have proven useful (17).

When removal of the causal neoplasm is not possible, Pi supplementation with 1,25-dihydroxyvitamin D_3 or 1α-hydroxyvitamin D_3 treatment will reverse patient weakness and heal the osteomalacia.

Metabolic acidosis

Metabolic acidosis can cause rickets or osteomalacia (Box 4.10.1). The pathogenesis is not well understood, and seems complex. Nevertheless, the skeletal disease responds well to vitamin D and alkali therapy. Ca^{2+} and potassium supplementation may be necessary at the onset of alkali therapy to prevent hypocalcaemia and hypokalaemia. Vitamin D (50 000 IU orally thrice weekly) can be used for adults, with careful follow-up until healing occurs. Alkali therapy should be continued after the mineralization defect is corrected. Urinary Ca^{2+} and creatinine levels must be monitored frequently because metabolic acidosis *per se* causes hypercalciuria.

Renal failure

In uraemia, skeletal disease usually reflects secondary or tertiary hyperparathyroidism leading to rapid bone remodelling (osteitis fibrosa cystica) (4). However, some patients manifest defective mineralization of skeletal matrix that is caused mainly by calcitriol deficiency. Additional causes have been proposed as well.

Aluminium intoxication

Aluminium is toxic to osteoblasts and inhibits skeletal mineralization (4). Contamination of dialysate caused 'Newcastle bone disease'. Uraemic patients who used aluminium-containing antacids to bind dietary Pi also deposited this metal in skeletal tissue. Serum assays and bone histochemistry for aluminium support the diagnosis (4). Therapy includes substituting new Pi-binders. Desferoxamine has been a useful chelating agent (17).

Hypophosphataemia

Excessive use of Pi-binders in uraemic patients can cause hypophosphataemia leading to rickets or osteomalacia.

Parathyroid insufficiency

Severe osteomalacia has occurred in renal failure after excessive parathyroidectomy for secondary or tertiary hyperparathyroidism (4). PTH is necessary for bone turnover in uraemia. Pharmacological doses of calcitriol and Ca^{2+} supplementation have had some therapeutic success.

Epidermal nevus syndrome

Infants and children with epidermal nevus syndrome can develop rickets due to renal Pi wasting (32). 1,25-dihydroxyvitamin D_3 and Pi supplementation therapy is effective.

Miscellaneous disorders

A few rare, sporadic conditions manifest with osteomalacia despite normal circulating concentrations of Ca^{2+} and Pi (17). There is no established therapy. A correct diagnosis is important in part because massive doses vitamin D, either as the calciferol or active metabolite form, and Ca^{2+} supplementation could lead to hypercalcaemia and hypercalciuria.

Fibrogenesis imperfecta ossium, reported in about a dozen patients, is an acquired abnormality within skeletal matrix. Axial osteomalacia is characterized radiographically by coarsening of trabecular bone in the axial skeleton, seemingly from a primary defect in osteoblasts, and perhaps is a heritable disorder (33).

Heritable rickets and osteomalacia

Heritable disorders that cause rickets or osteomalacia are included in Box 4.10.1. Some feature renal Pi wasting; some reflect disturbances in the bioactivation or action of vitamin D. Several have proven to be inborn errors of metabolism due to enzyme deficiencies (throughout this section, heritable disorders are referred to by their McKusick symbol and number provided in Online Mendelian Inheritance In Man) (33).

Hypophosphataemic bone disease

Most forms of rickets or osteomalacia reflect aberrations in vitamin D homoeostasis leading to reduced levels of Ca^{2+} in extracellular fluid (14). However, these disorders also diminish extracellular Pi concentrations partly from phosphaturia due to secondary hyperparathyroidism. Hypocalcaemia and hypophosphataemia then act in concert to impair mineralization of newly synthesized osteoid, and are reflected by a decreased blood $Ca^{2+} \times$ Pi product (1).

The importance of Pi for skeletal mineralization is especially well illustrated by types of rickets or osteomalacia due to renal phosphate leak causing osteopathy without significantly diminishing circulating Ca^{2+} levels (11). 'Hypophosphataemic bone disease' is a generic term which emphasizes the critical nature of this biochemical disturbance. Although pharmacological treatment for these disorders has certain themes, each entity is unique and optimal regimens can differ.

X-linked hypophosphataemia

X-linked hypophosphataemia (XLH) is the most common heritable form of rickets or osteomalacia (OMIM #307800) (11). The prevalence in North America is approximately 1:20 000 live births. All races seem to have affected individuals.

XLH was first described in 1937 after vitamin D-deficiency rickets, a plague of Northern industrialized cities at the turn of the last century, had waned (34). Discovery of vitamin D in 1919, and then successful treatment and preventive measures for 'nutritional' rickets, represented a major triumph of medical science (2, 3). Nevertheless, some cases of rickets were puzzling because they were not cured even by massive doses of vitamin D_2 (34). XLH became the prototypic 'vitamin D-resistant rickets'. In 1958, the disorder was recognized to manifest X-linked dominant inheritance (35). Girls and boys (2:1) are affected. Hypophosphataemia from renal Pi wasting was appreciated as a key pathogenetic factor in 1969 (36). Inappropriately normal circulating levels of 1,25-dihydroxyvitamin D despite hypophosphataemia were documented in 1982. In 1995, an international consortium identified the gene they called *PHEX* (phosphate-regulating gene with homology to endopeptidases on the X-chromosome) that was altered in most patients with XLH (37).

XLH causes short stature and bowing of the lower limbs after toddlers begin to bear weight (Fig. 4.10.6). They are clumsy, but otherwise strong and well. The skull is often dolichocephalic and Chiari 1 malformation can occur. The chest and upper extremities are not deformed. There is no muscle weakness in contrast to nearly all other forms of rickets. Fractures are uncommon. Skeletal disease occasionally presents with knock-knees. Without treatment, height Z scores will be minus 2–3 standard deviations (38, 39).

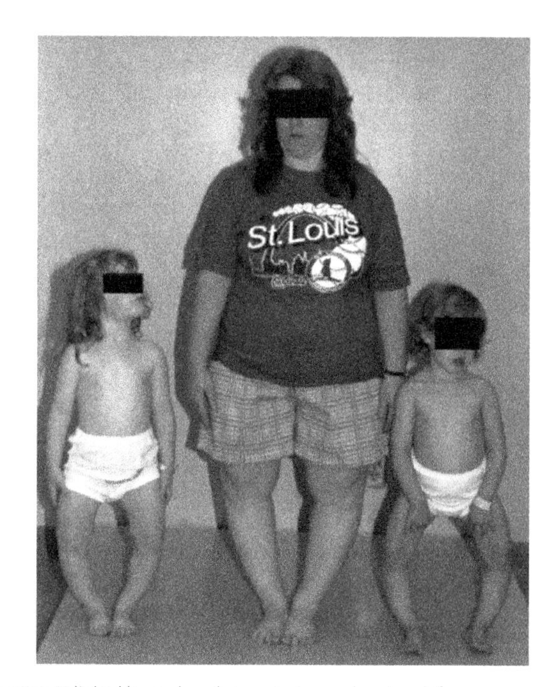

Fig. 4.10.6 X-linked hypophosphataemia: Severe bowing deforms an untreated mother and her daughters. However, there is no muscle weakness.

Adults with XLH can suffer five principal complications (38). Arthralgias, primarily involving the lower limbs and especially the knees, are due to osteoarthritis. The degree of lower extremity rachitic deformity predicts the likelihood of knee joint deterioration (38). Bone pain in the thighs is often explained by femoral pseudofractures (Fig. 4.10.3). Dental abscesses develop because brittle 'shell' teeth form early in life due to defective mineralization of dentin. Enthesopathy (calcification of tendons, ligaments, joint capsules, etc.) is common, but it is unclear the degree to which symptoms develop. Sensorineural hearing loss and spinal stenosis may also occur. Obstetrical histories seem benign (38). The impact of XLH during old age has not been studied, but life expectancy is probably not compromised.

Radiographs of children with XLH and bowing deformity of the lower limbs show physeal widening in the knees, which becomes especially pronounced medially (Fig. 4.10.1c). Osteopenia and evidence of secondary hyperparathyroidism is generally absent unless dietary Ca^{2+} intake is poor. In fact, the skeleton in XLH often appears dense, contrasting with other forms of rickets which characteristically increase circulating PTH levels. In adults, axial skeletal mass is typically normal, although sometimes bones appear sclerotic (40).

The biochemical hallmark of XLH is hypophosphataemia (11). Serum Ca^{2+} levels are low-normal, but usually not distinctly reduced (38, 39). Hypophosphataemia is documented if age-related changes in the normal range for serum Pi are appreciated. Healthy children have considerably higher serum Pi concentrations (and ALP activity) compared with adults. Because serum Pi levels may increase or decrease depending upon what is eaten, fasting blood specimens are necessary for diagnosis (39). In XLH, quantitation of renal Pi reclamation by calculating the transport maximum for phosphorous per glomerular filtration rate (TmP/GFR) shows that hypophosphataemia is due to decreased renal tubular reabsorption of phosphate (phosphate diabetes) (38, 39). Occasionally, trace glucosuria is detected, however, other parameters of renal proximal tubular function (e.g. serum potassium, bicarbonate, or uric acid levels) are normal; that is, Fanconi's syndrome (see later) is absent. Serum 1,25-dihydroxyvitamin D levels in XLH are generally normal or low-normal despite hypophosphataemia, which typically increases renal 25-hydroxyvitamin D, 1α-hydroxylase activity (11). Unless patients receive Pi supplements that are insufficiently matched by doses of 1,25-dihydroxyvitamin D_3 (see below), circulating PTH levels are usually normal (38, 39). Without treatment, serum ALP is always increased in children, but not always in adults. Serum FGF-23 levels are elevated in most XLH patients (10).

Histopathological examination of the skeleton shows rickets or osteomalacia in untreated patients with XLH (Fig. 4.10.4a) (38). Elevated circulating PTH levels predict features of hyperparathyroidism, including abundant osteoclasts and peritrabecular fibrosis. Additionally, in appropriately stained, nondecalcified sections (1), there are halos of hypomineralized bone surrounding osteocytes (Fig. 4.10.4a) (38). This peculiarity is considered diagnostic of XLH, reflecting an osteoblast defect persisting when these cells become osteocytes and despite successful 1,25-dihydroxyvitamin D_3 and Pi therapy.

The pathogenesis of XLH is incompletely understood (10, 11). Transport of Pi is defective across renal proximal tubule cells, where PTH and somehow dietary phosphorous control urinary Pi reclamation (11). Here, Pi movement across brush border membranes is the rate-limiting step. The murine (*Hyp*) model for XLH implicates a decrease in a high-affinity, low-capacity, Na^+-dependent Pi transport system (11). However, there is also a blunted response to activators of 1,25-dihydroxyvitamin D biosynthesis in kidney mitochondria (11). Pi deprivation and supplementation accelerate and suppress, respectively, 1,25-dihydroxyvitamin D catabolism. Nevertheless, the precise intracellular disturbances that diminish Pi transport and alter vitamin D bioactivation are not known (10, 11). Parabiosis and renal transplantation studies using the *Hyp* mouse implicated a phosphaturic factor(s) (41), now appreciated to be principally FGF-23 (10). Tissue culture studies of *Hyp* mouse and XLH patient bone indicate that osteoblast function is also directly impaired (11). Malabsorption of dietary Ca^{2+} is poorly understood, but considered a manifestation of the vitamin D resistance.

In XLH, no gene dosage effect emerges from a study of prepubertal heterozygous girls and hemizygous boys (Fig. 4.10.6) (42). Nevertheless, complications such as pseudofractures and enthesopathy seem more severe in men compared to women (38). Accordingly, gender (sex steroids and/or physical labour, etc.) does appear to affect the long-term outcome (38).

XLH maps to chromosome Xp22.31–21.3 (33). More than 150 different mutations involving the splice sites or coding sequence of the *PHEX* gene have been discovered worldwide (33). They are expected to diminish PHEX protein function. However, such defects are detected in only approximately 50% of patients (43). Mutations involving the noncoding regions could be involved. A preliminary study indicates that defects compromising the structure of the PHEX protein *per se* cause severe XLH (44). Nevertheless, the putative substrate for PHEX remains uncertain (10, 11). PHEX could act at cell surfaces to inactivate a phosphaturic factor, or activate a suppressor of phosphatonins such as FGF-23 (10, 11, 45).

Renal Pi wasting is a major pathogenetic abnormality in XLH. TmP/GFR correlates positively with height Z score in paediatric patients (42), and decreases reflect the degree of bowing deformity in affected adults (38). Accordingly, this disturbance is targeted by medical therapy. Decreases in 1,25-dihydroxyvitamin D biosynthesis are also compensated.

The bioactivated forms of vitamin D are used to treat XLH. High doses of vitamin D_2 (e.g. 100 000 IU daily) can improve, but will not heal, the rickets (46). Large doses of vitamin D_2 are readily converted to 25-hydroxyvitamin D, however, the affinity of the VDR for 25-hydroxyvitamin D is two to three orders of magnitude lower than for 1,25-dihydroxyvitamin D (2, 3). Conversely, excessive vitamin D_2 therapy sometimes causes prolonged hypercalcaemia, hypercalciuria, nephrocalcinosis, and renal failure (47)reflecting the long biological half-life of vitamin D (Table 4.10.3). Hypercalcaemia can persist for months, requiring dietary Ca^{2+} restriction and glucocorticoid treatment. Additionally, high-dose vitamin D_2 therapy requires cessation months in advance of osteotomy to avoid hypercalciuria or hypercalcaemia if postoperative immobilization is prolonged.

When the pathogenetic renal Pi wasting of XLH was addressed, improved clinical, biochemical, and radiographic responses were noted (36, 39). Transient augmentation of circulating Pi levels is achieved using frequent oral Pi dosing to supply, depending on body size, about 1–2 g of phosphorous (as Pi) each day. Now, combined use of 1,25-dihydroxyvitamin D_3 and Pi supplementation currently seems to be the best regimen for XLH (39). 1,25-dihydroxyvitamin D_3 augments both Ca^{2+} and Pi uptake from the gut. Improved dietary Ca^{2+} absorption prevents secondary or tertiary hyperparathyroidism provoked by Pi lowering blood Ca^{2+} levels directly or binding Ca^{2+} in the gut. Recently, a monoclonal antibody to neutralize circulating FGF-23 has begun clinical trials.

Treatment of XLH requires a medical/ orthopaedic approach best provided by experienced centres. 1,25-dihydroxyvitamin D_3 and Pi supplementation can reverse defects in skeletal growth, modelling, and remodelling in compliant patients (39). There are two principal goals of therapy. Correction of limb deformity by the time growth plates fuse is paramount. Additionally, boys and girls both can achieve normal heights. Two potential complications of treatment are: (1) secondary or tertiary hyperparathyroidism compromising the clinical outcome and perhaps necessitating parathyroidectomy and osteotomies, and (2) renal damage.

Treatment should begin with toddlers to help promote growth and to avoid lower extremity distortions. However, dosing and monitoring will understandably be difficult at first. Control, but not complete correction, of the rickets is a reasonable objective early on. Both 0.25 and 0.50 μg capsules of 1,25-dihydroxyvitamin D_3 are commercially available. The contents can be put into applesauce, etc., but a liquid preparation is also now marketed (Table 4.10.3). Approximately 40 ng (i.e. 0.040 μg) per kg of body weight of 1,25-dihydroxyvitamin D_3 daily (divided doses is ideal) may be achieved safely over 2 to 3 months by gradually increasing the dose and monitoring its biochemical effects. In the UK and Europe, a solution of 1α-hydroxyvitamin D is available. Pi supplementation, given three to four times daily, is introduced simultaneously and also gradually increased. Tablets of neutral sodium/ potassium phosphate (e.g. K-Phos Neutral®; Beach Pharmaceuticals, Tampa, Florida) are most convenient and generally well tolerated. Occasionally, Pi causes diarrhoea. In some ways, 1,25-dihydroxyvitamin D_3 and Pi produce opposite effects on Ca^{2+} homoeostasis (39). Accordingly, if either Pi or 1,25-dihydroxyvitamin D_3 is stopped, both should stop. Sudden decreases or especially cessation in Pi supplementation alone should be avoided, because 1,25-dihydroxyvitamin D effects can persist and urinary and then blood Ca^{2+} levels may rapidly rise. Accordingly, patients should be cautioned not to run out of medications.

Careful biochemical surveillance is essential because 1,25-dihydroxyvitamin D_3 is especially potent in increasing gastrointestinal Ca^{2+} absorption. Ca^{2+} and creatinine should be assayed in 24-h urine collections (not random specimens) (39). Initially, monitoring should occur monthly, but then every 3 months. Urinary Ca^{2+} to creatinine ratios of about 150–180 mg/g reflect adequate gut effects of 1,25-dihydroxyvitamin D_3 helping to suppress circulating PTH levels. If hypocalciuria is a persisting problem, increased milk consumption or Ca^{2+} supplementation may be helpful. Unless PTH levels are elevated and nonsuppressable (predicting hypercalcaemia before hypercalciuria), hypercalciuria will herald excessive 1,25-dihydroxyvitamin D_3 dosing. Fortunately, 1,25-dihydroxyvitamin D_3 has a short biological half-life, permitting rapid corrections (Table 4.10.3). Urine levels of 3–3.5 g phosphorous per g creatinine are efficacious, and seem less likely than greater values to cause nephrocalcinosis. Renal ultrasonography, creatinine clearance, and serum PTH levels should be monitored at least yearly. Dosage increases will be necessary as the child grows. Nephrocalcinosis in XLH seems to represent Ca^{2+}–Pi deposits. Perhaps, subradiographic abnormalities will not compromise renal function (46). Partial parathyroidectomy may become necessary when elevated serum PTH levels are associated with hypercalcaemia and/or difficulty controlling the skeletal disease. Hypercalciuria (>4 mg Ca^{2+} per kg of body weight, or >220 mg Ca^{2+} per g creatinine) can occur when skeletal mineralization is fully restored or when growth plates fuse. Halving doses may provide maintenance therapy until skeletal 'consolidation' is complete and cessation of medical treatment can be considered.

Orthopaedic evaluation should occur at least yearly during childhood and twice yearly during the adolescent growth spurt, because limb bracing or epiphysiodesis may be necessary. Osteotomies are sometimes postponed until growth ceases to minimize the possibility of postoperative deformity. Unless patients are weight-bearing within 2 days of surgery (or fracture, etc.), 1,25-dihydroxyvitamin D_3 and then Pi therapy should be held to avoid immobilization hypercalciuria and hypercalcaemia.

Closure of physes after puberty does not mean that XLH is cured (38). The metabolic derangements persist life-long. Accordingly, affected adults should be followed perhaps yearly. Some may benefit from 1,25-dihydroxyvitamin D_3 and Pi therapy to prevent fractures or worsening deformity (38). The efficacy and benefits of medical therapy for adults with XLH are poorly understood.

Dent's disease

X-linked recessive hypophosphataemia (Dent's disease) maps to chromosome Xp11.22 and is due to deactivation of the *CLCN5* gene involved in chloride transport (48). Hypercalciuria nephrocalcinosis, β_2-microglobinuria, and progressive glomerular disease affect males. Renal Pi wasting sometimes causes mild rickets. Treatment consists of Pi supplementation with caution not to cause hyperparathyroidism, or to exacerbate nephrocalcinosis.

Autosomal dominant hypophosphataemic rickets

This rare form of renal Pi wasting (OMIM #193100) causes relatively mild rickets appearing during adolescence. The disorder has been mapped to chromosome 12p13 and involves activating mutations in the gene encoding FGF-23 (45). Treatment is similar to XLH, but lower doses of 1,25-dihydroxyvitamin D_3 and Pi are required.

Autosomal recessive hypophosphataemic rickets

Deactivating mutation in the gene that encodes dentin matrix protein 1 (*DMP1*) causes a very rare, autosomal recessive form of hypophosphataemic rickets (OMIM #241520).

Fanconi's syndrome

Fanconi's syndrome features renal Pi wasting together with other manifestations of proximal renal tubule dysfunction causing low serum levels of Pi, potassium, bicarbonate, and uric acid as well as aminoaciduria. There are many aetiologies including cystinosis, tyrosinaemia, and Lowe's syndrome (Table 4.10.1). Therapy with 1,25-dihydroxyvitamin D_3 and Pi supplementation (see XLH) seems helpful, but urinary Ca^{2+} levels must be monitored carefully because hypercalciuria can be present.

McCune–Albright syndrome

McCune–Albright syndrome (OMIM #174800) often causes acquired hypophosphataemic rickets (17). Treatment with 1,25-dihydroxyvitamin D_3 and Pi helps control the added skeletal disease, but therapy may be especially difficult to assess because of premature closure of growth plates and the underlying fibrodysplastic disease. In fact, even bone biopsy looking for osteomalacia may not be helpful because of the widespread fibrous dysplasia.

Vitamin D-dependent rickets

Vitamin D-dependent rickets (VDDR) types I and II (VDDR I and VDDR II) are rare, autosomal recessive disorders that mimic vitamin D-deficiency rickets (5–8, 49). However, there is no defect in cutaneous synthesis or accelerated loss of vitamin D. Patients are typically replete with vitamin D as shown by normal serum levels of 25-hydroxyvitamin D. In fact, heritable defects in hepatic vitamin D 25-hydroxylation have not been established (50).

VDDR I and II feature diminished biosynthesis of, and target tissue resistance to, 1,25-dihydroxyvitamin D, respectively. Because there is either disturbed conversion of 25-hydroxyvitamin D to 1,25-dihydroxyvitamin D (VDDR I) or peripheral resistance to 1,25-dihydroxyvitamin D (VDDR II), serum levels of 1,25-dihydroxyvitamin D are low and high, respectively (Table 4.10.4) (5–8, 49). Nevertheless, both types of VDDR alter mineral homoeostasis in a similar way. Dietary Ca^{2+} is malabsorbed, leading to hypocalcaemia, secondary hyperparathyroidism, and hypophosphataemia. Decreased extracellular fluid levels of Ca^{2+} and Pi together impair mineralization of skeletal matrix. Because the pathogenesis of VDDR I involves defective production of 1,25-dihydroxyvitamin D by the kidney, physiological doses of 1,25-dihydroxyvitamin D_3 control the disorder (49). However, in VDDR II even enormous doses of 1,25-dihydroxyvitamin D_3 may prove ineffective (5–8). Both VDDR I and II are now understood at the gene level and therefore have more informative names (17, 33).

25-Hydroxyvitamin D, 1α-hydroxylase deficiency (vitamin D-dependent rickets, type I)

1,25-dihydroxyvitamin D deficiency can be defined as low circulating levels of this hormone with normal or elevated (depending on preceding vitamin D therapy) concentrations of 25-hydroxyvitamin D. In theory, this situation could result from decreased production or increased clearance of 1,25-dihydroxyvitamin D. Decreased production can be hereditary or acquired. Acquired deficiency is usually explained by systemic disease, such as chronic renal failure or acquired Fanconi's syndrome, etc., which affect bone and mineral metabolism in multiple and complex ways (beyond the scope of this chapter). Increased clearance is uncommon, and typically accompanies loss of other vitamin D metabolites, such as 25-hydroxyvitamin D, and would therefore fit within the definition of vitamin D deficiency. The genetic entity discussed here (OMIM #264700) is now also called hereditary 1,25-dihydroxyvitamin D deficiency, and is an inborn error of metabolism featuring defective biosynthesis of 1,25-dihydroxyvitamin D.

Prader and colleagues were the first to characterize this disorder when they described two young children who showed all of the usual clinical features of vitamin D deficiency despite adequate input of the vitamin. Complete remission depended upon continuous therapy with high doses of vitamin D—thus, the term 'vitamin D-dependent rickets'. They coined the term 'pseudovitamin D deficiency'. Remission could, however, be achieved by physiological (microgram) doses of 1α-hydroxylated vitamin D metabolites (51, 52). VDDR I is now understood at the molecular level and is, therefore, best described as 25-hydroxyvitamin D, 1α-hydroxylase deficiency (49).

Patients with 1α-hydroxylase deficiency appear healthy at birth. Features consistent with nutritional rickets are usually noticed before 2 years of age, and often during the first 6 months of life. There is growth retardation and poor gross motor development. Muscle weakness, irritability, pneumonia, seizures, and failure to thrive are prominent findings.

Serum 1,25-dihydroxyvitamin D levels are low or undetectable despite normal levels of 25-hydroxyvitamin D. Malabsorption of dietary Ca^{2+} leads to hypocalcaemia, secondary hyperparathyroidism, and hypophosphataemia. Serum ALP activity is elevated.

Radiographic changes are in keeping with nutritional rickets. In addition to growth plate abnormalities and rachitic deformities, osteopenia and other features of secondary hyperparathyroidism are present. Undecalcified bone documents defective matrix mineralization and secondary hyperparathyroidism including osteoclastosis and peritrabecular fibrosis (49).

Early reports of affected siblings in inbred kindreds indicated that VDDR I is an autosomal recessive condition especially prevalent in French-Canadians (33). A founder effect seems to have occurred in this population and, in 1990, linkage studies mapped the disorder to chromosome l2q14 (49). The molecular defect involves the kidney mitochondrial cytochrome P450clα enzyme responsible for rate-limiting, hormonally regulated, 25-hydroxyvitamin D bioactivation to 1,25-dihydroxyvitamin D (i.e. 25-hydroxyvitamin D, lα-hydroxylase). Actually, this enzyme has several components, cytochrome P-450D10t, ferredoxin, and ferredoxin reductase (49). Several mutations have been found in the P450clα gene (*CYP27B1*: OMIM 609506) (51). French-Canadian patients are commonly homozygous for a 958ΔG defect in this single copy gene. None of these mutations engenders an enzyme with decreased (rather than absent) activity (51).

Serum concentrations of 25-hydroxyvitamin D are normal in VDDR I (elevated if pharmacological doses of vitamin D or 25-hydroxyvitamin D are given), yet 1,25-dihydroxyvitamin D levels are subnormal, or remain only partially corrected by vitamin D or 25-hydroxyvitamin D therapy (49). Because pharmacological doses of vitamin D_2 or D_3 or 25-hydroxyvitamin D_3 produce therapeutic responses in VDDR I similar to physiological (replacement) doses of 1,25-dihydroxyvitamin D_3, it is apparent that 25-hydroxyvitamin D (or some metabolite) at sufficient levels can activate the VDR. Alternatively, perhaps enhanced local 1,25-dihydroxyvitamin D biosynthesis occurs with pharmacological doses of the prohormones.

The 1α-hydroxylase gene from more than 25 families has been studied by site-directed mutagenesis and cDNA expression in transfected cells. All patients had homozygous mutations. Most French-Canadian patients had the same mutation causing a frame shift and a premature stop codon in the putative haem-binding domain. The same mutation was observed in additional families of diverse origin. All other patients had either a base-pair deletion causing premature termination codon upstream from the putative ferredoxin and haem-binding domains, or missense mutations. No 1α-hydroxylase activity was detected when the mutant enzyme was expressed in various cells. The sequence of the human 1α-hydroxylase gene from keratinocytes and peripheral blood mononuclear cells has been shown to be identical with the renal gene.

The differential diagnosis includes especially defects in the VDR-effector system, where serum concentrations of 1,25-dihydroxy-vitamin D and the response to treatment with 1-α hydroxylated vitamin D metabolites are greatly different (Table 4.10.2).

Clinical remission has followed daily, high-dose therapy with 1–3 mg of vitamin D_2, or with 0.2–0.9 mg of 25-hydroxyvitamin D. Because there is no defect in hepatic conversion of vitamin D to 25-hydroxyvitamin D, vitamin D rather than 25-hydroxyvitamin D is cheap yet effective. However, a physiological ('replacement') dose of 1,25-dihydroxyvitamin D, 0.25–1.0 μg daily, bypasses the lα-hydroxylase defect and provides effective treatment (49). Although 25-hydroxyvitamin D_3 or 1,25-dihydroxyvitamin D_3 therapy is expensive, it has advantages. The physiological half-lives of these metabolites are much shorter than vitamin D, and excessive dosing will respond more rapidly to temporary cessation of therapy. Most patients, however, can be managed with vitamin D, but follow-up is essential for any regimen.

Hereditary resistance to 1,25-dihydroxyvitamin D (vitamin D-dependent rickets, type II)

This disorder was characterized in 1978 when a patient with features of 'pseudovitamin D deficiency' (see above) was found to have high serum levels of 1,25-dihydroxyvitamin D (51). Thus, 'hereditary resistance to 1,25-dihydroxyvitamin D' or VDDR II refers to this condition (OMIM #277440) (5, 6). Autosomal recessive inheritance is well established, and parental consanguinity has been reported in approximately 50% of cases (33).

Most patients have been from the Mediterranean region. Obligate heterozygotes do not have clinical manifestations. Patients appear normal at birth, but then develop features of vitamin D deficiency during the first year in a few patients (5–8), similar to vitamin D deficiency or VDDR I within the first 2 years of life. Although several sporadic cases developed skeletal disease as late as their teenage years or middle age, these patients represent the mildest form of the disease and had complete remission when treated with vitamin D or its active metabolites. It is unclear if the adult-onset patients belong to this entity. In general, the earlier the presentation, the more severe the clinical and biochemical features (5–8).

Hypocalcaemia causes secondary hyperparathyroidism, hypophosphataemia, and elevated serum ALP activity. However, 1,25-dihydroxyvitamin D levels are elevated, sometimes as much as 10-fold (5–8). This abnormality reflects peripheral resistance to 1,25-dihydroxyvitamin D causing malabsorption of dietary Ca^{2+} and the combined effects of four subsequent activators of renal 25-hydroxy-vitamin D, lα-hydroxylase activity: hypocalcaemia, increased serum PTH, hypophosphataemia and also diminished feedback inhibition by 1,25-dihydroxyvitamin D on the kidney 1α-hydroxylase.

The radiographic and histological findings of VDDR II resemble those of nutritional rickets, as described before, including growth plate disturbances, rachitic deformities, osteopenia, and evidence of secondary hyperparathyroidism. In a patient with total alopecia, hair follicles were present.

A peculiar feature, appearing in more than half of the subjects, is total alopecia or sparse hair. Alopecia usually appears during the first year of life and in one patient, at least, has been associated with additional ectodermal anomalies as oligodentia, epidermal cysts, and cutaneous milia (5–8).

Alopecia seems to be a marker for a more severe form of the disease, as judged by earlier onset, severity of the clinical features, proportion of patients who do not respond to treatment with high doses of vitamin D or its active metabolites, and the extremely elevated serum levels of 1,25-dihydroxyvitamin D during therapy. Although some patients with alopecia achieve clinical and biochemical remission of their bone disease, none have shown hair growth. The notion that total alopecia reflects a defective VDR-effector system is supported by the fact that alopecia has only been associated with hereditary defects in the VDR system, i.e. with end-organ resistance to the action of the hormone. Hair follicles normally contain the VDR.

Patients with VDDR II with normal hair can respond fully to high doses of bioactive vitamin D metabolites. However, only some with total alopecia do so. Remarkably, however, some patients with VDDR II may no longer need 1,25-dihydroxyvitamin D_3 therapy, or require lower doses, later in life (5–8).

The nature of the resistance to 1,25-dihydroxyvitamin D and aberrations in the VDR/effector system have been elucidated (5–8, 9). A variety of VDR, or post-VDR, defects block the peripheral action of 1,25-dihydroxyvitamin D. There can be an absence of the VDR, diminished or absent 1,25-dihydroxyvitamin D-binding capacity or decreased binding affinity, and failure of the 1,25-dihydroxyvitamin D–VDR complex to localize to the nucleus or bind to DNA (8). A mouse model has been developed by targeted ablation of the *VDR* gene. Patients without VDR hormone or DNA binding are the most difficult to treat (5, 6).

A VDR-positive, mild variant has been reported in Columbia, South America (OMIM %600785) (33, 53).

If untreated, most patients with VDDR II die in early childhood (5–8). However, good control of the disorder is possible with therapy, especially in individuals without alopecia. Depending upon severity, VDDR II may require treatment with calciferols, which enhance endogenous production of 1,25-dihydroxyvitamin D, administration of high doses of both calciferols and Ca^{2+} to compensate for the target tissue resistance to 1,25-dihydroxyvitamin D, or the use of high doses of Ca^{2+} alone (given orally or intravenously) to circumvent the target cell 1,25-dihydroxyvitamin D resistance (8, 46). Whereas most patients may respond to very high oral doses of 1,25-dihydroxyvitamin D_3 (10–40 μg daily), some can have clinical, radiographic, and biochemical corrections with high doses of vitamin D_2 or 25-hydroxyvitamin D_3 (5–8). Some patients have unexplained disease fluctuation.

Before therapy, serum 1,25-dihydroxyvitamin D concentrations range from the upper normal limit to markedly elevated. With vitamin D treatment, they may reach the highest levels found in any living system (≥100 times the upper normal limit). Such values may reflect four different mechanisms acting synergistically to drive renal 25-hydroxyvitamin D, 1α-hydroxylase: hypocalcaemia, secondary hyperparathyroidism, hypophosphataemia, and perhaps failure of the negative feedback loop by which 1,25-dihydroxyvitamin D inhibits the renal enzyme activity (8).

In approximately half of the reported kindreds, parental consanguinity and multiple siblings with the same defect indicate autosomal recessive inheritance. Parents or siblings of patients who are obligate heterozygotes have been reported to be normal, i.e. no bone disease or alopecia, and have normal blood biochemistry findings. There is a striking clustering of patients around the Mediterranean, including patients reported form Europe and America who originated from the same area (7, 8). A notable exception is a cluster of kindreds from Japan (33).

The near ubiquity of a similar if not identical VDR-effector system among various cell types helped clarify the nature of the intracellular and molecular defects in these patients (7, 8).

Defects in the 1,25-dihydroxyvitamin D-binding region range from no hormone binding (the most common abnormality), to defective hormone binding capacity and defective hormone binding affinity. A defect that compromises RXR heterodimerization with the VDR (which is essential for nuclear localization and probably for recognition of the vitamin D responsive element in the DNA as well) was characterized in several kindreds with and without alopecia (7, 8). In one patient, the receptor exhibited a marked impairment in binding coactivators essential for transactivation of the hormone–VDR complex and initiation of the physiological response. In kindreds with defects in the VDR binding to DNA, different single nucleotide mutations in the DNA binding region were found (7, 8). All point mutations affected the region of the two zinc fingers of the VDR essential for functional interaction of the hormone–receptor complex with DNA. Interestingly, all altered amino acids are highly conserved in the steroid receptor superfamily. In all of those patients, no response followed very high doses of vitamin D or its active 1α-hydroxylated metabolites.

Normal hair is usually associated with milder and usually complete clinical and biochemical remission on high doses of vitamin D or its metabolites (7, 8). Only about half of the patients with alopecia have shown satisfactory clinical and biochemical remission to high doses of vitamin D or its active 1α-hydroxylated metabolites, but the dose requirement is about 10-fold higher than in patients with normal hair.

It seems that defects characterized as deficient hormone binding affinity and deficient heterodimerization with RXR achieve remission on high doses of vitamin D or its active 1α-hydroxylated metabolites. Most with other defects could not be cured. However, not all patients received prolonged treatment and with sufficiently high doses (see below).

Typical clinical and biochemical features (Table 4.10.4) support the diagnosis. The issue becomes more complicated when the clinical features are atypical, i.e. late onset, sporadic cases, and normal hair. Failure of a therapeutic trial with Ca^{2+} and/or physiological replacement doses of vitamin D or its active metabolites may support the diagnosis but direct proof requires demonstration of a cellular, molecular, and functional defect in the VDR–effector system.

Based on the clinical and biochemical features, the following additional disease states should be considered: (1) extreme Ca^{2+} deficiency: e.g. some children from South Africa who consume a very low calcium diet of about 125 mg/day with severe bone disease and histologically proven osteomalacia, biochemical features of hypocalcaemic rickets with elevated levels of serum 1,25-dihydroxyvitamin D, and sufficient vitamin D. Ca^{2+} repletion caused complete clinical and biochemical remission. Nutritional history and the response to Ca^{2+} supplementation support this diagnosis; and (2) severe vitamin D deficiency: during the initial stages of vitamin D therapy in children with severe vitamin D-deficient rickets, the biochemical picture may resemble 1,25-dihydroxyvitamin D resistance, i.e. hypocalcaemic rickets with elevated 1,25-dihydroxyvitamin D levels. This may represent a 'hungry bone syndrome', i.e. high Ca^{2+} demands of the abundant osteoid tissue becoming mineralized. However, this is a transient condition that may be differentiated from hereditary resistance to 1,25-dihydroxyvitamin D by a history of vitamin D deficiency and the final therapeutic response to vitamin D.

In about half of the kindreds, the bioeffects of 1,25-dihydroxyvitamin D_3 were measured *in vitro*. Nearly always, correlation was documented between the *in vitro* effect and the therapeutic response *in vivo*, i.e. patients with no calcaemic response to high levels of 1,25-dihydroxyvitamin D_3 showed no effects of 1,25-dihydroxyvitamin D_3 on their cells *in vitro* (either induction of 25-hydroxyvitamin D-24-hydroxylase or inhibition of lymphocyte proliferation) and *vice versa* (7, 8). If the predictive therapeutic value of the *in vitro* cellular response to 1,25-dihydroxyvitamin D_3 could be substantiated convincingly, it may eliminate the need for time consuming and expensive therapeutic trials with massive doses of vitamin D or its active metabolites. In the meantime, it is mandatory to treat every patient with this disease irrespective of the type of receptor defect.

An adequate therapeutic trial must include vitamin D at sufficient doses to maintain high serum concentrations of 1,25-dihydroxyvitamin D because patients can produce high serum 1,25-dihydroxyvitamin D levels if supplied with substrate. If high serum levels are not achieved, 1α-hydroxylated vitamin D metabolites should be given in daily doses up to 6 μg/kg weight or a total of 30–60 μg and up to 3 g of elemental Ca^{2+} orally daily; therapy must continue for a period sufficient to mineralize the abundant osteoid (usually 3–5 months). Therapy may be considered a failure if no change in the clinical, radiological, or biochemical parameters occurs while serum 1,25-dihydroxyvitamin D concentrations are maintained at approximately 100 times average normal values.

In some patients unresponsive to vitamin D or its metabolites, clinical and biochemical remission, including catch-up growth, accompanied large amounts of Ca^{2+} achieved by long-term (months) intracaval infusions of up to 1000 mg of Ca^{2+} daily. Alternatively, increasing oral Ca^{2+} intake was used successfully in only very few patients and this approach is limited by dose and patient tolerability.

Several patients have shown unexplained fluctuations in response to therapy or in presentation of the disease (7, 8). One patient, after a prolonged remission, became completely unresponsive to much higher doses of active 1α-hydroxylated vitamin D metabolites, and another patient seemed to show amelioration of resistance to serum 1,25-dihydroxyvitamin D_3 after a brief therapeutic trial with 24,25-dihydroxyvitamin D. In several patients, spontaneous healing occurred in their teens or rickets did not recur for 14 years after cessation of therapy.

VDRs are abundant and widely distributed among most tissues studied and multiple effects of 1,25-dihydroxyvitamin D are observed on various cell functions *in vitro*. Yet, the clinical and biochemical features in patients with hereditary 1,25-dihydroxyvitamin D deficiency and resistance seems to demonstrate that the only disturbances of clinical relevance are perturbations in mineral and bone metabolism. This emphasizes the pivotal role of 1,25-dihydroxyvitamin D in transepithelial net Ca^{2+} fluxes. Moreover, the fact that in patients with extreme end-organ resistance to 1,25-dihydroxyvitamin D, Ca^{2+} infusions correct the disturbances in mineral homoeostasis and cure the bone disease may support the notion that defective bone matrix mineralization is secondary to disturbances in mineral homoeostasis.

Hypophosphatasia

In 1948, hypophosphatasia (OMIM #241500, #146300, #241510) was coined to distinguish a rare form of heritable rickets characterized biochemically by hypophosphatasaemia and deficient activity of the tissue-nonspecific (liver/ bone/ kidney) isoenzyme of ALP (TNSALP) (15). At least 200 different mutations in the *TNSALP* gene (OMIM *171760) have been discovered in patients worldwide (55). Hence, hypophosphatasia is an instructive inborn error of metabolism which verifies the theory promulgated by Robert Robison, beginning in 1923, that ALP conditions mineralization of cartilage and bone matrix.

Approximately 300 cases of hypophosphatasia have been described. However, the severity of this disorder is remarkably variable and spans intrauterine death from profound skeletal hypomineralization to merely premature loss of teeth in adults (15). Traditionally, six clinical forms are reported depending on patient age when skeletal disease is documented. Although TNSALP is ubiquitous in tissues, and especially rich in liver and kidney as well as in cartilage and bone, hypophosphatasia seems to affect directly only hard tissues (55). Perinatal, infantile, childhood, and adult hypophosphatasia feature rickets and osteomalacia, respectively, and dental disease (15). Children and adults who manifest premature tooth loss without skeletal disease (radiographically or on bone biopsy) have odontohypophosphatasia. Although artificial and somewhat conflicting, this clinical classification has provided a sense of recurrence risk and prognosis.

Perinatal hypophosphatasia is diagnosed at birth and is almost invariably lethal (15, 55). Stillbirth is common. Profound skeletal hypomineralization with caput membranaceum and short and deformed limbs is obvious. Severe osteogenesis imperfecta or cleidocranial dysplasia may be suspected, but can be distinguished radiographically and by gene testing (16). Occasionally, bony spurs protrude from the shafts of major long bones. Failure to gain weight, irritability with a high-pitched cry, unexplained fever, anaemia, periodic apnoea with bradycardia, and intracranial haemorrhage can occur. Respiratory compromise from pulmonary hypoplasia and chest deformity proves fatal.

Infantile hypophosphatasia becomes clinically apparent before 6 months of age with failure to thrive, widened fontanelles, hypotonia, and sometimes vitamin B_6-responsive seizures (15). Poor feeding and rickets are noted. Hypercalcaemia and hypercalciuria may explain bouts of vomiting and nephrocalcinosis, sometimes with significant renal impairment. Rachitic deformity of the chest and rib fractures predispose to recurrent pneumonia. Seizures and spells of apnoea may occur. Despite the impression from palpation or radiographs that skull hypomineralization reflects widely open fontanelles, functional craniosynostosis is common. Infantile hypophosphatasia often features progressive clinical and radiographic deterioration, and about 50% of patients die within the first year of life. However, the prognosis seems better if there is survival past infancy, although persisting skeletal disease seems likely (15).

Childhood hypophosphatasia is especially variable (14). Premature loss of deciduous teeth (age <5 years) from hypoplasia of cementum may be the most remarkable manifestation. Cementum anchors dentition to the periodontal ligament, therefore, teeth are shed without root resorption. Incisors are usually lost first, but the entire dentition can be exfoliated. Enlarged pulp chambers and root canals result in 'shell' teeth. Skeletal deformity can include scaphalocephaly with frontal bossing, a rachitic rosary, bowed legs or knock-knees, short stature, and wrist, knee, or ankle enlargement. When radiographs disclose rickets, delayed walking and a characteristic waddling gait are common. Childhood hypophosphatasia may improve when growth plates fuse after puberty, but recurrence of symptoms seems likely during the adult years (15, 55).

Adult hypophosphatasia presents during middle age (15, 55). Approximately 50% of patients mention rickets and/or premature loss of teeth during childhood. Often, there are recurrent, poorly healing, metatarsal stress fractures. Subtrochanteric femoral pseudofractures may be found proximally in the lateral cortices (18). Chondrocalcinosis is common, but Ca^{2+} pyrophosphate dihydrate crystal deposition rarely causes arthritis or pseudogout.

Radiographic findings in hypophosphatasia are helpful for diagnosis, especially in paediatric patients. Perinatal hypophosphatasia features pathognomonic changes. The skeleton can be so hypomineralized that only the skull base is apparent. Individual vertebrae appear to be 'missing', and bony spurs may protrude from major long bones. Alternatively, severe rachitic changes are seen. Calvarial bones can be mineralized only centrally, giving the illusion that sutures are widely patent. Fractures are not uncommon. In infants, abrupt transition from well mineralized diaphyses to hypomineralized metaphyses suggests sudden metabolic deterioration. Relentless skeletal demineralization, worsening rachitic disease, and progressive deformity or vitamin B_6-responsive seizures predict a lethal outcome. Bone scintigraphy showing little tracer uptake in widely separated cranial 'sutures' suggests functional suture closure. Patients who survive infancy can have true premature cranial sutures fusion causing a 'beaten-copper' radiographic appearance and raised intracranial pressure (Fig. 4.10.7). In children, characteristic tongues of radiolucency extend from physes into metaphyses of major long bones (Fig. 4.10.2). Adult hypophosphatasia causes recurrent, poorly healing, metatarsal stress fractures and femoral pseudofractures occur laterally (rather than medially as in other forms of osteomalacia). There can also be

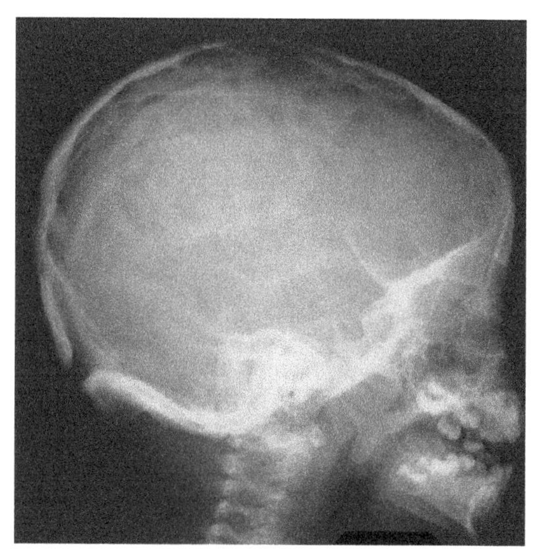

Fig. 4.10.7 Hypophosphatasia: The 'beaten copper' skull of this 2-year-old boy with the childhood form of hypophosphatasia results from premature closure of cranial sutures. Previously, he underwent craniotomy.

osteopenia and chondrocalcinosis with changes of pyrophosphate arthropathy.

Subnormal serum ALP activity for age and sex (hypophosphatasaemia) is the biochemical hallmark of hypophosphatasia. The levels reflect disease severity (15, 55). Patients with odontohypophosphatasia have mild but discernible decreases. In fact, this finding is especially impressive because rickets or osteomalacia typically cause hyperphosphatasaemia (14). Several other conditions, some with skeletal manifestations, lower blood ALP levels (15), but are readily distinguished from hypophosphatasia, partly because patients do not accumulate TNSALP substrates (see below). Serum levels of Ca^{2+} and Pi are not diminished. Hypercalciuria and hypercalcaemia often complicate the infantile form. The pathogenesis seems to involve a 'dyssynergy' between gut absorption of dietary Ca^{2+} and defective skeletal mineralization; however, skeletal demineralization may also be a factor. Serum levels of PTH, 25-hydroxyvitamin D, and 1,25-dihydroxyvitamin D are usually unremarkable unless there is hypercalcaemia or renal compromise. Serum Pi concentrations are above control mean levels, and mild hyperphosphataemia occurs in about one-half of children and adults. The pathogenesis involves enhanced renal reclamation of Pi only sometimes explained by suppressed serum PTH levels (55).

Three phosphocompounds, natural substrates for TNSALP, accumulate endogenously in hypophosphatasia: phosphoethanolamine, inorganic pyrophosphate (PPi), and pyridoxal 5′-phosphate (PLP) (15, 55). Assays are commercially available for urinary phosphoethanolamine and plasma PLP. Mild phosphoethanolaminuria occurs in several metabolic bone diseases (15), and fortunately increased plasma PLP concentration is a particularly sensitive and specific marker for hypophosphatasia. However, patients must not be taking vitamin B_6 when tested. Endogenous accumulation of PPi seems to be a key pathogenetic factor (see below), yet quantitation of PPi remains a research technique.

Defective skeletal mineralization occurs in all clinical forms of hypophosphatasia except odontohypophosphatasia (2). Unless evaluation of the ALP activity in bone is undertaken, the histopathological findings are those of other types of rickets or osteomalacia lacking secondary hyperparathyroidism.

Hypophosphatasia occurs in all races, but seems to be especially common among Mennonites and Hutterites in Canada, where the incidence of severe disease is approximately 1/100 000 live births (15). Perinatal and nearly all cases of infantile hypophosphatasia are transmitted as autosomal recessive traits. Obligate carriers can have diminished or low-normal levels of serum ALP activity, and sometimes demonstrate modest elevations in plasma PLP levels, especially after a vitamin B_6 challenge (15, 55). The inheritance pattern(s) for childhood, adult, and odonto forms of hypophosphatasia is autosomal recessive for some cases. In others, there is generation to generation transmission with mild clinical expression.

The gene for TNSALP has 12 exons and appears to exist as a single copy in the haploid genome on the tip of the short arm of chromosome 1 (lp36.1–lp34). In 1988, a missense mutation in the *TNSALP* gene was identified in a severely affected infant from an inbred Canadian kindred (55). Studies of patients with severe hypophosphatasia have disclosed approximately 200 different mutations in the *TNSALP* gene (55). Most are missense mutations. Perinatal and infantile hypophosphatasia reflect homozygosity or compound heterozygosity for these defects. The childhood and adult forms of hypophosphatasia can indeed be the 'same' disease (15). Mouse models that recapitulate the infantile form of hypophosphatasia have been developed by *TNSALP* gene knock-out (56).

ALP (orthophosphoric monoester phosphohydrolase (alkaline optimum), EC 3.1.3.1), found in nearly all organisms, is a glycosylated, plasma membrane-bound, ectoenzyme (55). Discovery of the accumulation of three phosphocompounds, phosphoethanolamine, PPi, and PLP, in hypophosphatasia revealed how TNSALP may function (15, 55). Accumulation of PLP, the principal cofactor form of vitamin B_6, indicates that TNSALP acts primarily as an ectoenzyme. Patients with hypophosphatasia do not have symptoms or signs of vitamin B_6, deficiency or toxicity despite their markedly increased plasma PLP levels.

In 1965, discovery of elevated urinary levels of PPi in hypophosphatasia disclosed the pathogenesis of the rickets and osteomalacia. Excess PPi was found to be a potent inhibitor of biomineralization. PPi levels are increased in plasma and urine in hypophosphatasia. Matrix vesicles are devoid of ALP activity but do contain hydroxyapatite crystals (4). However, only a few isolated crystals are observed outside these extracellular structures. Excess PPi blocks hydroxyapatite crystal formation in the extracellular matrix of bone.

Conventional treatments for rickets or osteomalacia are generally best avoided in hypophosphatasia because patients are usually vitamin D replete and serum levels of Ca^{2+} and Pi are not reduced (15). Indeed, such treatment could exacerbate or provoke hypercalcaemia and hypercalciuria. Hypercalcaemia in infantile hypophosphatasia generally responds to reduction in dietary Ca^{2+} intake, but may require glucocorticoid or calcitonin therapy. Enzyme replacement by intravenous infusion of various soluble forms of ALP has generally been disappointing (55), but administration of an investigational, bone-targeted, TNSALP fusion protein is showing considerable success (56). Additionally, two infants who seemed destined to die from infantile hypophosphatasia showed clinical and radiographic improvement following transplantation of marrow or bone-derived cells (57). Supportive therapy is important for hypophosphatasia. Fractures do mend, but delayed healing after casting or osteotomy has been observed. In affected adults, placement of intramedullary rods, rather than load-sparing devices (e.g. plates), seems to be preferable for the acute or prophylactic treatment of fractures and pseudofractures (18). Expert dental care is especially important for children, because their nutrition can be impaired by premature tooth loss. Craniotomy may be crucial in cases with craniosynostosis. Fetuses that are severely affected (perinatal form) can be detected reliably *in utero* by ultrasonography, but a relatively mild 'benign prenatal' form of hypophosphatasia must be considered. *TNSALP* gene mutation studies have improved prenatal diagnosis (15).

Acknowledgements

Supported in part by Shriners Hospitals for Children, The Clark and Mildred Cox Inherited Metabolic Bone Disease Research Fund, and The Barnes-Jewish Hospital Foundation.

References

1. Parfitt AM. Vitamin D and the pathogenesis of rickets and osteomalacia. In: Feldman D, Pike JW, Glorieux FH, eds. *Vitamin D*. 2nd edn. Amsterdam: Elsevier Academic Press, 2005: 1029–48.

2. Holick MF, ed. *Vitamin D: Physiology, Molecular Biology, and Clinical Applications*. Totawa, New Jersey: Humana Press, 1999.
3. Feldman D, Pike JW, Glorieux FH, eds. *Vitamin D*. 2nd edn. Amsterdam: Elsevier Academic Press, 2005.
4. Bilezikian JP, Raisz LG, Martin, TJ, eds. *Principles of Bone Biology*. 3rd edn. San Diego: Academic Press, 2008.
5. Holick MF. Photobiology of vitamin D. In: Feldman D, Pike JW, Glorieux FH, eds. *Vitamin D*. 2nd edn. Amsterdam: Elsevier Academic Press, 2005: 37–45.
6. Malloy PJ, Pike JW, Feldman D. Hereditary 1,25-dihydroxyvitamin D resistant rickets. In: Feldman D, Pike JW, Glorieux FH, eds. *Vitamin D*. 2nd edn. Amsterdam: Elsevier Academic Press, 2005: 1207–37.
7. Liberman UA, Marx SJ. Vitamin D and other calciferols. In: Scriver CR, Beaudet AL, Sly WS, Valle D, eds. *The Metabolic and Molecular Bases of Inherited Disease*. 8th edn. New York: McGraw-Hill, 2001: 4223–40.
8. Liberman UA. Hereditary deficiencies in vitamin D action. In: Bilizikian JP, Raisz LG, Rodan GA, eds. *Principles in Bone Biology*. 3rd edn. Academic Press, 2008: 1195–1208.
9. Haussler MR, Haussler CA, Jurutka PW, Thompson PD, Hsieh JC, Remus LS, *et al.* The vitamin D hormone and its nuclear receptor: molecular actions and disease states. *J Endocrinol*, 1997; **154**: S57–73.
10. White KE, Larsson TE, Econs MJ. The roles of specific genes implicated as circulating factors involved in normal and disordered phosphate homeostasis: frizzled related protein-4, matrix extracellular phosphoglycoprotein, and fibroblast growth factor 23. *Endocr Rev*, 2006; **27**: 221–41.
11. Tenenhouse HS, Econs MJ. Mendelian hypophosphatemias. In: Scriver CR, Beaudet AL, Sly WS, Valle D, eds. *The Metabolic and Molecular Bases of Inherited Disease*. 8th edn. New York: McGraw-Hill, 2001: 5039–67.
12. Whyte MP. Approach to the patient with metabolic bone disease. In: Feldman D, Pike JW, Glorieux FH, eds. *Vitamin D*. 2nd edn. Amsterdam: Elsevier Academic Press, 2005: 913–29.
13. Pettifor JM. Vitamin D deficiency and nutritional rickets in children. In: Feldman D, Pike JW, Glorieux FH, eds. *Vitamin D*. 2nd edn. Amsterdam: Elsevier Academic Press, 2005: 1065–83.
14. Glorieux FH, ed. *Rickets*. New York: Raven Press, 1991.
15. Whyte MP. Hypophosphatasia. In: Scriver CR, Beaudet AL, Sly WS, Valle D, eds. *The Metabolic and Molecular Bases of Inherited Disease*. 8th edn. New York: McGraw-Hill, 2001: 5313–29.
16. Resnick D, Niwayama G. *Diagnosis of Bone and Joint Disorders*. Vol. 3. Philadelphia: WB Saunders, 1981.
17. Rosen CF, ed. *Primer on the Metabolic Bone Diseases and Disorders of Mineral Metabolism*. 7th edn. Philadelphia: Lippincott Williams & Wilkins, 2008.
18. Coe JD, Murphy WA, Whyte MP. Management of femoral fractures and pseudofractures in adult hypophosphatasia. *J Bone Joint Surg Am*, 1986; **68**: 981–90.
19. Lips P, Duong D, Oleksik A, Black D, Cummings S, Cox D, Nickelsen T. A global study of vitamin D status and parathyroid function in postmenopausal with osteoporosis: baseline data from the Multiple Outcomes of Raloxifene Evaluation Clinical Trial. *J Clin Endocrinol Metab*, 2001; **86**: 1212–21.
20. Bischoff-Ferrari HA, Giovannucci E, Willett WC, Dietrich T, Dawson-Hughes B. Estimation of optimal serum concentrations of 25-hydroxyvitamin D for multiple health outcomes. *Am J Clin Nutr*, 2006; **84**: 18–28.
21. Bischoff-Ferrari HA, Willett WC, Wong JB, Giovanucci E, Dietrich T, Dawson-Hughes B. Fracture prevention with vitamin D supplementation: a meta-analysis of randomized control trials. *JAMA*, 2005; **293**: 2257–64.
22. Thacher TD, Fischer PR, Pettifor JM, Lawson JO, Isichei CO, Reading JC, Chan GM. A comparison of calcium, vitamin D, or both for nutritional rickets in Nigerian children. *N Engl J Med*, 1999; **341**: 563–8.
23. Thomas MK, Lloyd-Jones DM, Thadhani RI, Shaw AC, Deraska DJ, Kitch BT, Vamvakas EC, *et al.* Hypovitaminosis D in medical inpatients. *N Engl J Med*, 1998; **338**: 777–83.
24. Lips P, Hosking D, Lippunes K, Norquist JM, Wehren L, Maalouf G, *et al.* The prevalence of vitamin D inadequacy amongst women with osteoporosis: an international epidemiological investigation. *Journal of Internal Medicine*, 2006; **260**: 245–54.
25. Mithal A, Wahl DA, Bonjour JP, Burckhardt P, Dawson-Hughes B, Eisman JA, *et al.* Global vitamin D status and determinants of hypovitaminosis D. *Osteoporos Int*, 2009; **20**: 1807–20.
26. Bischoff-Ferrari HA. How to select the dose of vitamin D in the management of osteoporosis. *Osteoporos Int*, 2007; **18**: 401–7.
27. National Osteoporosis Foundation. Physician Guide to Prevention and Treatment of Osteoporosis. Updated recommendation for calcium and vitamin D intake. Available at: www.nof.org/prevention/calcium_and_vitamin D.htm
28. Hoppe B, Gnehm HE, Wopmann M, Neuhaus T, Willi U, Leumann E. Vitamin D poisoning in infants: a preventable cause of hypercalciuria and nephrocalcinosis. *Schweiz Med Wochenschr*, 1992; **122**: 257–62.
29. Whyte MP, Haddad JG Jr., Walters D, Stamp TCB. Vitamin D bioavailability: Serum 25-hydroxyvitamin D levels in man following oral, subcutaneous, intramuscular, and intravenous Vitamin D administration. *J Clin Endocrinol Metab*, 1979; **48**: 906–11.
30. Pivnick EK, Kerr NC, Kaufman RA, Jones DP, Chesney RW. Rickets secondary to phosphate depletion. A sequela of antacid use in infancy. *Clin Pediatr*, 1995; **34**: 73–78.
31. Skinner R, Pearson AD, English MW, Price L, Wyllie RA, Coulthard MG, *et al.* Risk factors for ifosfamide nephrotoxicity in children. *Lancet*, 1996; **348**: 578–80.
32. Ivker R, Resnick SD, Skidmore RA. Hypophosphatemic vitamin D-resistant rickets, precocious puberty, and the epidermal nevus syndrome. *Arch Dermatol*, 1997; **133**: 1557–61.
33. Online Mendelian Inheritance in Man, OMIM (TM). *McKusick-Nathans Institute of Genetic Medicine*, Johns Hopkins University (Baltimore, MD) and National Center for Biotechnology Information, National Library of Medicine (Bethesda, MD), 12–21-2009. World Wide Web URL: http://www.ncbi.nlm.nih.gov/omim/, accessed 4 June 2010.
34. Albright F, Butler AM, Bloomberg E. Rickets resistant to vitamin D therapy. *Am J Dis Child*, 1937; **54**: 529–47.
35. Winters RW, Graham JB, Williams TF, McFalls VW, Burnett CH. A genetic study of familial hypophosphatemia and vitamin D resistant rickets with a review of the literature. *Medicine (Baltimore)*, 1958; **37**: 97–142.
36. Menking M, Sotos JF. Effect of administration of oral neutral phosphate in hypophosphatemic rickets. *J Pediatr*, 1969; **75**: 1001–7.
37. The HYP Consortium. A gene (PEX) with homologies to endopeptidases is mutated in patients with X-linked hypophosphatemic rickets. *Nat Genet*, 1995; **11**: 130–6.
38. Reid IR, Hardy DC, Murphy WA, Teitelbaum SL, Bergfeld MA, Whyte MP. X-linked hypophosphatemia: a clinical, biochemical, and histopathologic assessment of morbidity in adults. *Medicine (Baltimore)*, 1989; **68**: 336–52.
39. Petersen DJ, Boniface AM, Schranck FW, Rupich RC, Whyte MP. X-linked hypophosphatemic rickets: a study (with literature review) of linear growth response to calcitriol and phosphate therapy. *J Bone Miner Res*, 1992; **7**: 583–97.
40. Reid IR, Hardy DC, Murphy WA, Teitelbaum SL, Bergfeld MA, Whyte MP. X-linked hypophosphatemia: skeletal mass in adults assessed by histomorphometry, computed tomography, and absorptiometry. *Am J Med*, 1991; **90**: 63–9.
41. Nesbitt T, Coffman TM, Griffiths R, Drezner MK. Cross-transplantation of kidneys in normal and Hyp mice: evidence that the Hyp mouse phenotype is unrelated to an intrinsic renal defect. *J Clin Invest*, 1992; **89**: 1453–9.

42. Whyte MP, Schranck FW, Armamento-Villareal R. X-linked hypophosphatemia: a search for gender, race, anticipation, or parent-of-origin effects on disease expression in children. *J Clin Endocrinol Metab*, 1996; **81**: 4075–80.
43. Dixon PH, Christie PT, Wooding C, Trump D, Grieff M, Holm I, Gertner JM, Schmidtke J, Shah B, Shaw N, Smith C, Tau C, Schlessinger D, Whyte MP, Thakker RV. Mutational analysis of PHEX gene in X-linked hypophosphatemia. *J Clin Endocrinol Metab*, 1998; **83**: 3615–23.
44. Whyte MP, Christie PT, Podgornik MN, Dixon PH, Eddy MC, Wooding C, *et al.* X-linked hypophosphatemia (XLH): mutations compromising PHEX structure reflect a severe phenotype (abstract). *Am J Hum Genet*, 1999; **65**: A114.
45. White KE, Evans WE, O'Riordan JLH, Speer MC, Econs MJ, Lorenz-Depiereux B, Grabowski M, Meitinger T, Strom TM. Autosomal dominant hypophosphataemic rickets is associated with mutations in FGF-23. *Nat Genet*, 2000; **26**: 345–8.
46. Glorieux FH, Marie PJ, Pettifor JM, Delvin EE. Bone response to phosphate salts, ergocalciferol, and calcitriol in hypophosphatemic vitamin D-resistant rickets. *N Engl J Med*, 1980; **303**: 1023-31.
47. Eddy MC, McAlister WH, Whyte MP. X-linked hypophosphatemia: normal renal function despite medullary nephrocalcinosis 25 years after vitamin D_2-induced azotemia. *Bone*, 1997; **21**: 515–20.
48. Scheinman SJ, Guay-Woodford LM, Thakker RJ, Warnock DG. Genetic disorders of renal electrolyte transport. *Mechanisms of Disease*, 1999; **340**: 1177–87.
49. Glorieux FH, St-Arnaud R. Vitamin D pseudodeficiency. In: Feldman D, Pike JW, Glorieux FH, eds. *Vitamin D*. 2nd edn. Amsterdam: Elsevier Academic Press, 2005; 1197–205.
50. Casella SJ, Reiner BJ, Chen TC, Holick MF, Harrison HE. A possible genetic defect in 25-hydroxylation as a cause of rickets. *J Pediatr*, 1994; **124**: 929–32.
51. Wang JT, Lin CJ, Burridge SM, Fu GK, Labuda M, Portale AA, *et al.* Genetics of vitamin D 1alpha-hydroxylase deficiency in 17 families. *Am J Hum Genet*, 1998; **63**: 1694–702.
52. Miller WL, Portale AA. Genetic causes of rickets. *Curr Opin Pediatr*, 1999; **11**: 333–9.
53. Giraldo A, Pino W, Garcia-Ramirez LF, Pineda M, Iglesias A. Vitamin D dependent rickets type II and normal vitamin D receptor cDNA sequence. A cluster in a rural area of Cauca, Colombia, with more than 200 affected children. *Clin Genet*, 1995; **48**: 57–65.
54. Wong GW, Leung SS, Law WY, Cheung NK, Oppenheimer SJ. Oral calcium treatment in vitamin D-dependent rickets type II. *J Paediatr Child Health*, 1994; **30**: 444–6.
55. Whyte MP. Hypophosphatasia: nature's window on alkaline phosphatase function in humans. In: Bilezikian JP, Raisz LG, Martin TJ, eds. *Principles of Bone Biology*. 3rd edn. San Diego: Academic Press, 2008: 1573–98.
56. Millán JL, Narisawa S, Lemire I, Loisel TP, Boileau G, Leonard P, *et al.* Enzyme replacement therapy for murine hypophosphatasia. *J Bone Miner Res*, 2008; **23**: 876–86.
57. Cahill RA, Wenkert D, Perlman SA, Steele A, Coburn SP, McAlister WH, *et al.* Infantile hypophosphatasia: Trial of transplantation therapy using bone fragments and cultured osteoblasts. *J Clin Endocrinol Metab*, 2007; **92**: 2923–30.

4.11

Glucocorticoid-induced osteoporosis

Gherardo Mazziotti, Andrea Giustina, Ernesto Canalis, John P. Bilezikian

Introduction

Synthetic glucocorticoids are used in a wide variety of disorders including autoimmune, pulmonary, and gastrointestinal diseases, as well as in patients following organ transplantation and with malignancies. Although the indications for glucocorticoids in these various conditions are clear, their use is fraught with a host of potential side effects. In particular, glucocorticoids are detrimental to bone and glucocorticoid-induced osteoporosis (GIO) is the most common form of secondary osteoporosis (1). Despite the fact that glucocorticoids can cause bone loss and fractures, many patients receiving or initiating long-term glucocorticoid therapy are not evaluated for their skeletal health. Furthermore, patients often do not receive specific preventive or therapeutic agents when indicated. New knowledge of the pathophysiological mechanisms underlying GIO has been accompanied by the availability of effective strategies to prevent and treat GIO (1).

Epidemiology

GIO is almost always caused by exogenous glucocorticoids, which are widely used in the treatment of several diseases. Approximately 1% of the population in the UK is receiving oral glucocorticoid therapy, and this prevalence may rise in the elderly (2). Up to 30–50% of chronic glucocorticoid users may develop fractures (3). Fracture risk increases rapidly after starting oral glucocorticoid treatment and is also related to the dose and duration of exposure. Published reports suggest that there is no dose of glucocorticoid therapy that is safe for the skeleton (3). Regimens of daily prednisolone at doses as low as 2.5 mg have been associated with an increased risk of hip and vertebral fractures. The risk increases by fivefold with prednisone doses above 7.5 mg daily. A dramatic 17-fold increase in vertebral fracture incidence was observed in subjects who used prednisone continuously more than 10 mg/day for longer than 3 months (3). Prolonged use at higher doses is accompanied by even greater fracture risk. As expected, the greatest increase in fracture incidence was seen in postmenopausal females and elderly males. The risk of osteoporotic fractures remains increased in patients undergoing cyclic corticosteroid treatment at high doses. It is noteworthy that fracture risk decreases after discontinuation of oral corticosteroids, although the time it takes to reduce the risk appears to be variable.

Inhaled glucocorticoids have minimal effects on bone metabolism since their systemic absorption is low (3). Endogenous hypercortisolism is a less frequent cause of GIO but up to 10% of subjects attending an outpatient clinic for osteoporosis were suspected of subclinical Cushing's syndrome (4). Either clinical or subclinical fragility fractures can be the presenting manifestation of Cushing's syndrome (5). Limited data from cross-sectional studies show that 30–50% of patients with overt Cushing's syndrome experience fractures, particularly at vertebral sites. Although remission of Cushing's syndrome may lead to improvement in osteoporosis, recovery of bone loss is gradual and often incomplete (5).

Pathophysiology

Glucocorticoids have both direct and indirect effects on bone metabolism (6). The central pathophysiological mechanism of bone loss during long-term use of glucocorticoids is reduced bone formation, due to actions on osteoblast differentiation and function. However, during the first phases of glucocorticoid excess, a significant increase in bone resorption (ultimately leading to the observed early increase in the risk of fractures) may occur.

Direct effects of glucocorticoids on bone cells

Glucocorticoids decrease the number and the function of osteoblasts. These effects lead to a suppression of bone formation, a central feature in the pathogenesis of GIO. Glucocorticoids decrease the replication of cells of the osteoblastic lineage, reducing the pool of cells that may differentiate into mature osteoblasts. In addition, glucocorticoids impair osteoblastic differentiation and maturation. Under certain experimental conditions, glucocorticoids have been reported to favour osteoblastic differentiation. In murine models, physiological levels of glucocorticoids seem to be required for cortical bone acquisition and osteoblast differentiation.

In the presence of glucocorticoids, bone marrow stromal cells are directed towards cells of the adipocytic lineage. Mechanisms involved in this redirection of stromal cells include induction of nuclear factors of the CCAAT/enhancer binding protein family and the induction of peroxisome proliferator-activated receptor γ 2, both of which play essential roles in adipogenesis (7).

An additional mechanism by which glucocorticoids inhibit osteoblast cell differentiation is by opposing Wnt/β-catenin signalling. Wnt signalling has emerged as a key regulator of osteoblastogenesis (7). In skeletal cells Wnt uses the canonical Wnt/β-catenin signalling pathway. In this pathway, when Wnt is absent, β-catenin is phosphorylated by glycogen synthase kinase-3β (GSK3β), and then degraded by ubiquitination. When Wnt is present, it binds to specific receptors, called Frizzled, and to coreceptors, low density lipoprotein receptor related proteins-5 and -6, leading to an inhibition of GSK3β activity. When GSK3β is not active, stabilized β-catenin translocates to the nucleus, where it associates with transcription factors to regulate gene expression. Deletions of either Wnt or β-catenin result in the absence of osteoblastogenesis, and increased osteoclastogenesis. The Wnt pathway can be inactivated by Dickkopf, an antagonist that prevents Wnt binding to its receptor complex. Glucocorticoids enhance Dickkopf expression, and maintain GSK3β in an active state, leading to the inactivation of β-catenin (6).

In addition to inhibiting the differentiation of osteoblasts, glucocorticoids inhibit the function of the differentiated mature cell. Glucocorticoids inhibit osteoblast-driven synthesis of type I collagen, the major component of the bone extracellular matrix, with a consequent decrease in bone matrix available for mineralization. The decrease in type I collagen synthesis occurs by transcriptional and post-transcriptional mechanisms.

Glucocorticoids have proapoptotic effects on osteoblasts and osteocytes due to activation of caspase 3, a common downstream effector of several apoptotic signalling pathways. Caspases are synthesized as proenzymes and are activated through autocatalysis or a caspase cascade. Active caspases contribute to apoptosis by cleaving target cellular proteins. Caspase 3 is a key mediator of apoptosis and is a common downstream effector of multiple apoptotic signalling pathways. The inhibitory effects of glucocorticoids on osteoblastic cell replication and differentiation and the increased apoptosis of mature osteoblasts, all contribute to the depletion of the osteoblastic cellular pool and decreased bone formation (6).

Osteocytes serve as mechanosensors, and play a role in the repair of bone microdamage (8). Loss of osteocytes disrupts the osteocyte–canalicular network, resulting in failure to detect signals that normally stimulate processes associated with the replacement of damaged bone. Disruption of the osteocyte–canalicular network can disrupt fluid flow within the network, adversely affecting the material properties of the surrounding bone independently of changes in bone remodelling or architecture. Glucocorticoids affect the function of osteocytes, by modifying the elastic modulus surrounding osteocytic lacunae. Glucocorticoids induce the apoptosis of osteocytes. As a result, the normal maintenance of bone through this mechanism is impaired and the biomechanical properties of bone are compromised (6).

The initial bone loss occurring in patients exposed to glucocorticoids may be secondary to increased bone resorption. Glucocorticoids increase the expression of receptor activator of NF-κB ligand (RANKL) and decrease the expression of its soluble decoy receptor, osteoprotegerin, in stromal and osteoblastic cells (6). The combination of an increase in RANK-L, a necessary signal for osteoclastogenesis, and a reduction in osteoprotegerin, an inhibitor of RANK-L action, can explain the initial phase of rapid bone loss after glucocorticoid exposure. Glucocorticoids also enhance the expression of colony-stimulating factor 1, which in the presence of RANK-L induces osteoclastogenesis. Glucocorticoids up-regulate receptor subunits for osteoclastogenic cytokines of the gp130 family. Furthermore, glucocorticoids may decrease apoptosis of mature osteoclasts. Consequently, there is increased formation of osteoclasts with a prolonged lifespan explaining, at the cellular level, the enhanced and prolonged bone resorption observed in the initial phases of GIO.

Effects of glucocorticoids on bone cells mediated by growth factors

In addition to the direct actions of glucocorticoids on bone target cells, other effects are mediated by changes in the synthesis, receptor binding, or binding proteins of growth factors present in the bone microenvironment. Glucocorticoids inhibit the expression of insulin-like growth factor (IGF) 1 (9). IGF-1 increases bone formation and the synthesis of type I collagen, and decreases bone collagen degradation and osteoblast apoptosis. Glucocorticoids suppress IGF-1 gene transcription, but increase IGF-1 receptor number in osteoblasts (10). The activity of IGFs is regulated by six classic IGF binding proteins, all of which are expressed by the osteoblast. The effects of glucocorticoids on IGF-1 expression by the osteoblast are reversed by parathyroid hormone (PTH), an observation that may help explain why PTH may be effective in the treatment of GIO (11).

Indirect effects of glucocorticoids on bone metabolism

Glucocorticoids inhibit calcium absorption from the gastrointestinal tract, by opposing vitamin D actions, and by decreasing the expression of specific calcium channels in the duodenum (1). Renal tubular calcium reabsorption also is inhibited by glucocorticoids. As a consequence of these effects, secondary hyperparathyroidism could exist in the context of glucocorticoid use, but a hyperparathyroid state does not explain the bone disorder observed in GIO. Most patients with GIO do not exhibit serum levels of PTH that are frankly elevated. Nevertheless, there may be subtle, but important, effects of glucocorticoids on the secretory dynamics of PTH. In healthy subjects, PTH is secreted by low amplitude and high frequency pulses superimposed upon tonic secretion. PTH bursts are thought to mediate the anabolic actions of the hormone on bone. In glucocorticoid-treated patients, a decrease in the tonic release of PTH and an increase in pulsatile bursts of the hormone may be observed (12). Abnormal PTH pulsatility is found not only following glucocorticoid exposure, but also in postmenopausal women and in acromegaly. Additionally, glucocorticoids may enhance the sensitivity of skeletal cells to PTH, by increasing the number and affinity of PTH receptors.

In addition to the direct effects of glucocorticoids on skeletal IGF-1, glucocorticoids decrease the secretion of growth hormone and may alter the systemic growth hormone/ IGF-1 axis (13). However, serum levels of IGF-1 are normal in GIO. Growth hormone secretion is blunted by glucocorticoids by an increase in hypothalamic somatostatin tone, and growth hormone administration could reverse some of the negative effects of chronic glucocorticoid treatment in bone. Secretion of growth hormone is blunted in asthmatic patients receiving inhaled corticosteroids, suggesting that inhaled steroids may alter the synthesis or release of growth hormone (6). However, the cause or consequence of this effect is not clear, since serum levels of cortisol and of IGF-1 are not suppressed. Glucocorticoids inhibit the release of gonadotropins, and as a result oestrogen and testosterone production. This effect of glucocorticoids on the gonadal axis may be an additional factor playing a role in the pathogenesis of GIO.

Effects on muscle

In addition to the direct effects of glucocorticoids on bone cells, the catabolic effects of glucocorticoids on muscle may contribute to fracture risk because of muscular weakness, which can increase the incidence of falls (6). Glucocorticoid-induced myopathy may occur following early exposure to glucocorticoids, may affect up to 60% of patients, and is generally manifested by proximal weakness, particularly of the pelvic girdle musculature. The muscle loss is due to glucocorticoid-induced proteolysis of myofibrils, which is mediated by activation of lysosomal and ubiquitin-proteasome enzymes. Glucocorticoids induce myostatin, a negative regulator of muscle mass. Deletion of the myostatin gene, prevents glucocorticoid-induced myofibril proteolysis and muscle loss in experimental murine models. This would suggest that myostatin plays a role in the mechanism of muscular atrophy in GIO.

Effects of the underlying chronic disease

An important point that should be considered is that many disorders for which the glucocorticoids are prescribed are themselves a cause of osteoporosis. One has to take into account the underlying disease itself along with the use of glucocorticoids, when considering the management of GIO. Inflammatory bowel disease, rheumatoid arthritis, and chronic obstructive pulmonary disease, for example, are associated with bone loss, independent of glucocorticoid treatment (6). The systemic release of inflammatory cytokines, which affect bone formation and bone resorption, seem to underlie the pathophysiology of the bone loss in these settings (6). However, there are additional factors that may play a role in the bone loss. In inflammatory bowel disease, bone loss may be, in part, secondary to malabsorption of vitamin D, calcium, and other nutrients (6). In chronic obstructive pulmonary disease, hypoxia, acidosis, reduced physical activity, and smoking may all contribute to bone loss, independent of the use of glucocorticoids (6).

Differential skeletal susceptibility to glucocorticoids

Individual susceptibility to glucocorticoids varies considerably, possibly because of differences in the absorption, distribution, or metabolism of the steroid, or because of differences in the number and affinity of glucocorticoid receptors. Polymorphisms of the glucocorticoid receptor gene, are associated with differences in bone mineral density (BMD) and body composition (1). An attractive explanation for the interindividual variability among those exposed to glucocorticoids is related to peripheral enzymes that interconvert active and inactive glucocorticoids (14). 11β-hydroxysteroid dehydrogenases regulate the interconversion of the inactive hormone cortisone and hormonally active cortisol, thereby playing a critical role in the regulation of glucocorticoid activity (14). Two distinct 11β-hydroxysteroid dehydrogenase enzymes have been described in humans. 11β-hydroxysteroid dehydrogenase type 2 is expressed in tissues, which express high levels of mineralocorticoid receptors, such as kidney and colon tissue, and acts as an inactivating enzyme by converting cortisol to cortisone. This enzyme was identified also in rat and human osteosarcoma cells where glucocorticoid inactivation by this mechanism was demonstrated. In contrast, 11β-hydroxysteroid dehydrogenase type 1 is primarily a glucocorticoid activator, converting cortisone to cortisol. This enzyme is widely expressed in target tissues of glucocorticoid action, including liver, fat, and bone. The activity of 11β-hydroxysteroid dehydrogenase type 1 and its potential to generate cortisol from cortisone in human osteoblasts is increased by proinflammatory cytokines and by glucocorticoids (14). These effects of glucocorticoids appear to be mediated by the C/EBP family of transcription factors (1). An inverse relationship between 11β-hydroxysteroid dehydrogenase type 1 activity and osteoblast differentiation appears to occur, although mice with a targeted deletion of the 11β-hydroxysteroid dehydrogenase type 1 gene do not develop a skeletal phenotype (1). An increase of 11β-hydroxysteroid dehydrogenase type 1 activity occurs with ageing, possibly providing an explanation for the enhanced glucocorticoid effects in the skeleton of elderly subjects (1).

Clinical manifestations

Despite the recognition that glucocorticoids can cause bone loss and fractures, many patients receiving, or being considered for, long-term glucocorticoid therapy are not evaluated for their skeletal health. Many patients do not receive specific prophylaxis or treatment when indicated. This observation is particularly evident in males taking glucocorticoids, in accordance with the general inadequate awareness of male osteoporosis (15).

Fractures occur more frequently at sites enriched in cancellous bone, such as the vertebrae and femoral neck. As with vertebral fractures occurring in postmenopausal osteoporosis, vertebral fractures associated with glucocorticoid therapy often are asymptomatic, in which case a radiological evaluation with morphometric analysis is often necessary (16). Vertebral fractures occur early after exposure to glucocorticoids, at a time when BMD declines rapidly. However, a direct relationship between BMD and fracture risk in GIO has not been established. It is likely to be different from that established in postmenopausal osteoporosis because fractures in GIO occur at higher BMD values (6). This point has to be considered when making treatment decisions in GIO. The Royal College of Physicians (RCP) recommends a vertebral T score of −1.5 or lower as the intervention threshold (17). The American College of Rheumatology (ACR) recommends a more stringent therapeutic intervention at a T score of −1 or lower (18). These scores are different from the treatment threshold T scores of below −2.5, used in the management of postmenopausal osteoporosis.

Although bone density is an important therapeutic benchmark, consensus is still lacking on when to perform BMD measurements in GIO. Some intervention guidelines recommend to obtain densitometries in individuals starting glucocorticoid therapy and before administering bisphosphonates (18). The RCP guidelines recommend evaluation of calcium metabolism in all subjects to select those individuals in need of vitamin D and calcium supplementation (17). ACR guidelines do not recommend a metabolic assessment and recommend vitamin D supplementation in all patients with GIO (18).

The role of biochemical markers of bone turnover in the diagnostic work-up of GIO has not been established, and their levels vary and are dependent on the different stages of the disease. Following the initial exposure to glucocorticoids, there is an increase in biochemical markers of bone resorption, which is followed by a prolonged suppression of markers of bone formation and bone resorption.

The assessment of gonadal function may be useful for the subsequent treatment of GIO. In men taking glucocorticoids, low total and free-testosterone concentrations are frequently found. Combined with low or normal serum gonadotropin levels, such low testosterone levels are likely to be as manifestation of secondary hypogonadism (1).

Therapy

The ACR and RCP advocate the following measures for the prevention and treatment of GIO: general health awareness, administration of sufficient calcium and vitamin D, use of the minimal effective dose of corticosteroids, and, when indicated, therapeutic intervention with bisphosphonates and other agents (17, 18). Prevention is considered in patients exposed to glucocorticoids for 3 months or less and therapy in individuals exposed to glucocorticoids for 6 months or longer.

The RCP guidelines suggest that treatment in GIO is indicated in: (1) patients who are at high risk of osteoporosis, such as those taking prednisone equivalents at or above 7.5 mg daily, or those with a personal history of fractures or with lifestyle risk factors for osteoporosis; (2) patients with low risk of osteoporosis, but with T scores at or below −1.5, as assessed by vertebral densitometry; and (3) patients with low risk of osteoporosis and T score at or above −1.5, but with a decline in vertebral BMD of at least 4.0% after 1 year on glucocorticoid treatment (17). The ACR recommends prevention in patients exposed to glucocorticoids for 3 months or less at doses at or below 5 mg prednisone equivalents daily. ACR recommends lifestyle changes, such as tobacco cessation and reduction of alcohol consumption, an exercise programme, restriction of sodium intake (in the presence of hypercalciuria), sufficient calcium intake, and adequate vitamin D supplementation (18). The ACR recommends the use of bisphosphonates for the prevention and treatment of GIO (18). Treatment should be initiated in all individuals who are on glucocorticoid treatment for periods 6 months or longer at doses at or above 5 mg prednisone equivalents and whose T score is at or below −1.0, as assessed by densitometry (18). Despite these clear and authoritative guidelines, their application is suboptimal. In clinical practice, treatment with bisphosphonates seems to be prevalently based on low BMD, whereas these drugs are rarely prescribed for the prevention of GIO. The designation and selection of patients for prevention and treatment measures is somewhat arbitrary and controversial. A recent cost-effectiveness analysis demonstrated that treatment of GIO is cost-effective in patients with a prior fracture, in individuals 75 years of age and older or in younger subjects with T scores at or below −2.0 (19).

Various pharmacological agents have been assessed for the prevention and treatment of GIO. In most studies, the primary endpoint was BMD; and fracture outcomes were measured in selected studies as secondary endpoints (20).

Calcium and vitamin D

Vitamin D and calcium supplementation are recommended in subjects exposed to glucocorticoids, and vitamin D and its analogues prevent bone loss during glucocorticoid therapy and restoration of serum calcium suppresses the synthesis and release of PTH (21). Vitamin D increases the intestinal absorption of calcium and its reabsorption in the distal renal tubule leading to higher serum calcium levels and decreased secretion of PTH. In addition to its role in calcium homoeostasis, vitamin D increases muscular strength. In a 2-year randomized trial, subjects with rheumatoid arthritis receiving prednisone therapy (mean dose 5.6 mg/day) exhibited a decline in BMD of 2.0% and 0.9% per year in the lumbar spine and trochanter, respectively. Patients randomized to calcium (1 g/day) and vitamin D (500 IU/day) gained BMD at an annual rate of 0.72% at the spine and 0.85% in the trochanter (22). It is important to note that subjects receiving glucocorticoids may display vitamin D resistance. Consequently, patients often require up to 1000–2000 IU of vitamin D_3 daily, in an effort to maintain supra optimal 25 hydroxyvitamin D_3 levels at or above 110 nmol/l (40 ng/ml) (23).

Hormonal replacement therapy

GIO can be associated with suppressed gonadal function in men and women since glucocorticoids inhibit gonadotropin release and, as a consequence, oestrogen and androgen synthesis. In men with GIO, testosterone administered intramuscularly induced a significant increase in lumbar BMD, without significant effects on BMD at the femoral neck. The studies had BMD as primary endpoint, and no information on bone fractures is available. Testosterone also was shown to improve muscular performance and quality of life in men with GIO (24). Therefore, substitution treatment of hypogonadal men may be useful in the management of GIO, although the potential benefits should be balanced against the risk of androgen therapy, such as prostate enlargement.

Antiresorptive therapy

Bisphosphonates are currently the drugs most commonly used for the treatment of osteoporosis, including GIO (20). Several bisphosphonates are effective and are approved for the treatment of GIO. These include alendronate, risedronate, and zoledronic acid. Bisphosphonates are stable analogues of naturally occurring inorganic pyrophosphate. Stability is conferred by a carbon atom replacing the oxygen atom that connects two phosphate groups. The R1 and R2 side chains attached to the carbon atom are responsible for the wide spectrum of activity observed among bisphosphonates. R1 substitutes, such as a hydroxyl or amino group, enhance the adsorption of the bisphosphonate to mineral, whereas the R2 substitutes determine the antiresorptive potency. The different antiresorptive potency observed with different R2 groups is linked to their ability to inhibit farnesyl pyrophosphate synthase and to bind to hydroxyapatite.

Currently, bisphosphonates are considered the gold standard for the prevention and treatment of GIO. The ACR and the RCP have recommended bisphosphonates as first-line of therapy (17, 18). Alendronate, risedronate, and zoledronic acid as well as other bisphosphonates prevent the loss and restore BMD in GIO. Oral alendronate at 10 mg/day for 48 weeks significantly increased BMD at the lumbar spine and femoral neck, when compared to untreated control subjects, and after 2 years alendronate decreased the incidence of vertebral fractures (25, 26). Oral risedronate, at 5 mg/day was tested in two placebo-controlled 12-month clinical trials in patients either on long-term glucocorticoid therapy (treatment) or in subjects initiating glucocorticoid treatment (prevention) (20). In the prevention trial, risedronate stabilized BMD, whereas in the treatment trial risedronate increased BMD. Pooled data from the two trials revealed a 70% reduction in the incidence of vertebral fractures compared to control subjects after 12 months (20). Recently, zoledronic acid was shown to have a greater effect on BMD than risedronate in both prevention and treatment trials (27). The benefits of bisphosphonates in GIO have been ascribed primarily to their antiresorptive activity, although an inhibition of glucocorticoid-induced apoptosis of osteoblasts and osteocytes may contribute to the therapeutic effectiveness of bisphosphonates. Bisphosphonates are more effective than vitamin D in the prevention of fractures in GIO, although bisphosphonates should be given with supplemental calcium and vitamin D. A meta-analysis revealed that among antiresorptive therapies, bisphosphonates are the most effective in the management of GIO (28). The use of bisphosphonates in eugonadal premenopausal women has to be considered carefully, since bisphosphonates cross the placenta and may affect embryonic skeletal development.

Unresolved issues with the use of bisphosphonates in GIO include the mechanism responsible for the increase in BMD, whether they are effective reducing nonvertebral fractures, the duration of therapy, and the incidence of side effects in the context of GIO. Patients with GIO may be more susceptible to osteonecrosis of the jaw, particularly with the use of intravenous bisphosphonates. However, this did not seem to be the case in a recent trial comparing zoledronic acid and risedonate in GIO.

Anabolic therapy

PTH is an attractive candidate for the treatment of GIO because it protects against osteoblast apoptosis and increases osteoblast cell number and activity. The use of PTH in GIO has been examined in postmenopausal women with rheumatoid arthritis receiving prednisone and oestrogens (11). In this population, daily treatment with teriparatide (PTH(1–34)) increased spinal BMD and, more modestly, hip BMD. PTH administration induces an initial uncoupling of bone remodelling with an early increase in bone formation followed by a more gradual increase of bone resorption (7). According to the concept of the 'anabolic window', PTH rapidly stimulates osteoblastic function, inducing an up-regulation of osteoblast derived cytokines such as sRANK-L, IL-6, and a suppression of osteoprotegerin. These actions eventually lead to osteoclast activation and gradual rebalancing of bone formation and resorption.

Recently, a multicenter, randomized, controlled study was performed to compare the effects of teriparatide with those of alendronate on lumbar spine BMD in patients undergoing long-term glucocorticoid therapy at high risk for osteoporotic fractures, i.e. with mean baseline lumbar T score of −2.5 or less and with high prevalence of fragility fractures (29). In this clinical setting, teriparatide was more effective than alendronate in increasing BMD at the lumbar spine and total hip during an 18-month period. Similar results were obtained after 36 months of therapy (30). A secondary endpoint of the study was the reduction of new vertebral fractures after 18 months, and 6.1% patients receiving alendronate suffered vertebral fractures, whereas the incidence was 0.6% in the teriparatide arm. Teriparatide treatment was associated with a higher frequency of undesired side effects, such as injection-site reactions, headache, and dizziness. Teriparatide was approved by the FDA in the USA for the treatment of glucocorticoid-induced osteoporosis in July, 2009.

Unresolved issues with the use of teriparatide and other forms of PTH in GIO are its use in the prevention of GIO, its use in patients who are resistant to bisphosphonate therapy, its use in younger populations, and whether teriparatide should be followed by antiresorptives in GIO, as it is recommended in postmenopausal osteoporosis (31).

Growth hormone or IGF-1 administration could reverse some of the negative effects of chronic glucocorticoids on the skeleton (9). However, glucocorticoids decrease the activity of growth hormone on skeletal cells and there are no controlled trials to determine the effectiveness of either growth hormone or IGF-1 as treatments for GIO. Increases in serum osteocalcin, C-terminal propeptide of type I procollagen, and C-terminal telopeptide of type I collagen are observed following short-term use of recombinant human growth hormone treatment in a selected population of patients receiving chronic corticosteroid treatment for nonendocrine diseases (32). Combined therapy of growth hormone and IGF-1 counteracts selected negative effects of glucocorticoids on bone in healthy volunteers receiving short-term glucocorticoid therapy (9). Observational and controlled studies in children receiving glucocorticoid therapy for juvenile idiopathic arthritis demonstrated that growth hormone restored normal height velocity with a concomitant enhancement of bone mineralization (9). However, the efficacy and safety of growth hormone and IGF-1 treatment in GIO is unknown and well designed prospective controlled studies are necessary before their use can be recommended.

References

1. Mazziotti G, Angeli A, Bilezikian JP, Canalis E, Giustina A. Glucocorticoid-induced osteoporosis: an update. *Trends Endocrinol Metab*, 2006; 7: 144–9.
2. van Staa TP, Leufkens HG, Abenhaim L, Begaud B, Zhang B, Cooper C. Use of oral corticosteroids in the United Kingdom. *QJM*, 2000; 93: 105–11.
3. Civitelli R, Ziambaras K. Epidemiology of glucocorticoid-induced osteoporosis. *J Endocrinol Invest*, 2008; 31 (7 Suppl): 2–6.
4. Chiodini I, Mascia ML, Muscarella S, Battista C, Minisola S, Arosio M, *et al*. Subclinical hypercortisolism among outpatients referred for osteoporosis. *Ann Intern Med*, 2007; 147: 541–8.
5. Mancini T, Doga M, Mazziotti G, Giustina A. Cushing's syndrome and bone. *Pituitary*, 2005; 7: 1–4.
6. Canalis E, Mazziotti G, Giustina A, Bilezikian JP. Glucocorticoid-induced osteoporosis: pathophysiology and therapy. *Osteoporos Int*, 2007; 18: 1319–28.
7. Canalis E, Giustina A, Bilezikian JP. Mechanisms of anabolic therapies for osteoporosis. *N Engl J Med*, 2007; 357: 905–16.
8. Verborgt O, Gibson GJ, Schaffler MB. Loss of osteocyte integrity in association with microdamage and bone remodeling after fatigue damage in vivo. *J Bone Miner Res*, 2000; 15: 60.
9. Giustina A, Mazziotti G, Canalis E. Growth hormone, insulin-like growth factors, and the skeleton. *Endocr Rev*, 2008; 29: 535–59.
10. Bennett A, Chen T, Feldman D, Hintz RL, Rosenfeld RG. Characterization of insulin-like growth factor I receptors on cultured rat bone cells: regulation of receptor concentration by glucocorticoids. *Endocrinology*, 1984; 115: 1577–83.

11. Lane NE, Sanchez S, Modin GW, Genant HK, Pierini E, Arnaud CD. Parathyroid hormone treatment can reverse corticosteroid-induced osteoporosis. Results of a randomized controlled clinical trial. *J Clin Invest*, 1998; 102: 1627–33.
12. Bonadonna S, Burattin A, Nuzzo M, Bugari G, Rosei EA, Valle D, *et al.* Chronic glucocorticoid treatment alters spontaneous pulsatile parathyroid hormone secretory dynamics in human subjects. *Eur J Endocrinol*, 2005; 152: 199–205.
13. Giustina A, Veldhuis JD. Pathophysiology of the neuroregulation of growth hormone secretion in experimental animals and the human. *Endocr Rev*, 1998; 19: 717–97.
14. Tomlinson JW, Walker EA, Bujalska IJ, Draper N, Lavery GG, Cooper MS, *et al.* 11beta-hydroxysteroid dehydrogenase type 1: a tissue-specific regulator of glucocorticoid response. *Endocr Rev*, 2004; 25: 31–66.
15. Guzman-Clark JR, Fang MA, Sehl ME, Traylor L, Hahn TJ. Barriers in the management of glucocorticoid-induced osteoporosis. *Arthritis Rheum*, 2007; 57: 140–6.
16. Angeli A, Guglielmi G, Dovio A, Capelli G, de Feo D, Giannini S, *et al.* High prevalence of asymptomatic vertebral fractures in post-menopausal women receiving chronic glucocorticoid therapy: a cross-sectional outpatient study. *Bone*, 2006; 39: 253–9.
17. Eastell R, Reid DM, Compston J, Cooper C, Fogelman I, Francis RM, *et al.* A UK Consensus Group on management of glucocorticoid-induced osteoporosis: an update. *J Intern Med*, 1998; 244: 271–92.
18 American College of Rheumatology. Ad Hoc Committee on Glucocorticoid-Induced Osteoporosis recommendations for the prevention and treatment of glucocorticoid- induced osteoporosis. *Arthritis Rheum*, 2001; 44: 1496–503.
19. Kanis JA, Stevenson M, McCloskey EV, Davis S, Lloyd-Jones M. Glucocorticoid-induced osteoporosis: a systematic review and cost-utility analysis. *Health Technol Assess*, 2007; 11: 1–231.
20. Doga M, Mazziotti G, Bonadonna S, Patelli I, Bilezikian JP, Canalis E, Giustina A. Prevention and treatment of glucocorticoid-induced osteoporosis. *J Endocrinol Invest*, 2008; 31 (7 Suppl): 53–8.
21. Boonen S, Vanderschueren D, Haentjens P, Lips P. Calcium and vitamin D in the prevention and treatment of osteoporosis–a clinical update. *J Intern Med*, 2006; 259: 539–52.
22. Buckley LM, Leib ES, Cartularo KS, Vacek PM, Cooper SM. Calcium and vitamin D3 supplementation prevents bone loss in the spine secondary to low-dose corticosteroids in patients with rheumatoid arthritis. A randomized, double-blind, placebo-controlled trial. *Ann Intern Med*, 1996; 125: 961–8.
23. Heaney RP. The Vitamin D requirement in health and disease. *J Steroid Biochem Mol Biol*, 2005; 97: 13–9.
24. Tracz MJ, Sideras K, Boloña ER, Haddad RM, Kennedy CC, Uraga MV, *et al.* Testosterone use in men and its effects on bone health. A systematic review and meta-analysis of randomized placebo-controlled trials. *J Clin Endocrinol Metab*, 2006; 91: 2011–6.
25. Saag KG, Emkey R, Schnitzer TJ, Brown JP, Hawkins F, Goemaere S, *et al.* Alendronate for the prevention and treatment of glucocorticoid-induced osteoporosis. Glucocorticoid-Induced Osteoporosis Intervention Study Group. *N Engl J Med*, 1998; 339: 292–9.
26. de Nijs RN, Jacobs JW, Lems WF, Laan RF, Algra A, Huisman AM, *et al.* Alendronate or alfacalcidol in glucocorticoid-induced osteoporosis. *N Engl J Med*, 2006; 355: 675–84.
27. Reid DM, Devogelaer JP, Saag K, Roux C, Lau CS, Reginster JY, *et al.* Zoledronic acid and risedronate in the prevention and treatment of glucocorticoid-induced osteoporosis (HORIZON): a multicentre, double-blind, double-dummy, randomised controlled trial. *Lancet*, 2009; 373 (9671): 1253–63.
28. Amin S, Lavalley MP, Simms RW, Felson DT. The comparative efficacy of drug therapies used for the management of corticosteroid-induced osteoporosis: a meta-regression. *J Bone Miner Res*, 2002; 17: 1512–26.
29. Saag KG, Shane E, Boonen S, Marín F, Donley DW, Taylor KA, *et al.* Teriparatide or alendronate in glucococorticoid-induced osteoporosis. *N Engl J Med*, 2007; 357: 2028–39.
30. Saag KG, Zanchetta JR, Devogelaer JP, *et al.* Effects of teriparatide versus alendronate for treating glucocorticoid-induced osteoporosis: thirty-six-month results of a randomized, double-blind, controlled trial. *Arthritis Rheum*, 2009; 60:3346–55.
31. Black DM, Bilezikian JP, Ensrud KE, Greenspan SL, Palermo L, T, *et al.* One year of alendronate after one year of parathyroid hormone (1–84) for osteoporosis. *N Engl J Med*, 2005; 353: 555–65.
32. Giustina A, Bussi AR, Jacobello C, Wehrenberg WB. Effects of recombinant human growth hormone (GH) on bone and intermediary metabolism in patients receiving chronic glucocorticoid treatment with suppressed endogenous GH response to GH-releasing hormone. *J Clin Endocrinol Metab*, 1995; 80: 122–9.

PART 5

The adrenal gland and endocrine hypertension

5.1

Adrenal imaging

Peter Guest

Introduction

Evaluating the adrenal gland with imaging can be challenging. The adrenal glands may be morphologically within normal limits even in the presence of clear hyperfunction. Hyperplasia and small nodules may coexist. Nonfunctioning nodules are frequent and need to be differentiated from culpable hyperfunctioning adenomas or carcinomas. However, the increasingly sophisticated anatomical imaging provided by CT and MRI, together with the functional characterization afforded by radionuclide imaging, allows good correlation with clinical and endocrine parameters.

Embryologically, the adrenal cortex derives from coelomic mesoderm and the medulla from neural crest cells. Development is independent of the kidney and adrenal glands will normally be present in the absence of a kidney. In the newborn the adrenal glands are large structures, being one-third of the size of the kidneys. They involute rapidly, however, and in the adult are small structures. They are situated immediately above and anteromedial to the upper pole of the kidneys, although the left is less suprarenal. The right lies immediately behind the cava, alongside the right diaphragmatic crus. The left lies behind the splenic vein, lateral to the left crus.

The normal adrenal has a characteristic inverted Y- or V-shape with the two limbs fusing anteromedially. The most cranial section has a triangular appearance. Cross-sectional appearance varies according to the exact level. Each limb measures 2.5–4 cm in length and 3–6 mm in thickness. Greater than 1 cm thickness is definitely abnormal. Accessory adrenal tissue (rests) may be found in the kidney, testis, or ovary, and elsewhere in the retroperitoneum.

Arterial supply is from three sources: superior–multiple arteries from the inferior phrenic; middle from the aorta; and inferior from the renal artery. A single vein drains each adrenal. The left is a tributary of the left renal vein, the right leads directly to the cava, although rarely may join a hepatic vein first. The right adrenal vein is shorter and narrower.

Imaging modalities

The diagnosis of hyperfunction is made clinically and endocrinologically, not radiologically. Imaging is reserved for localization and characterization of adrenal lesions (1, 2).

Radiography

The adrenals may be calcified as a result of previous haemorrhage infarction or granulomatous infection, e.g. due to tuberculosis. Adrenal cysts may be large and show calcification of the wall. Of adrenal tumours, 10–14% are calcified on CT, but this is rarely demonstrable on plain films. Large adrenal masses may be inferred from displacement or distortion of bowel gas or adjacent organs such as the kidney. Rarely, malignant adrenal lesions will invade the kidney and masquerade as a renal tumour on intravenous urography.

Ultrasonography

Ultrasonography is widely available and accessible, and does not involve exposure to radiation. It is, however, very poor at visualizing the normal adrenal or small masses, and a normal examination would therefore not exclude an adenoma, adrenal hyperplasia, or small malignant tumours. It could be expected to demonstrate tumours of 2 cm or more in size if the examination is technically complete (Fig. 5.1.1). It is more helpful in children where body fat is less of a problem, and when it is particularly desirable to avoid the radiation exposure of a CT examination.

Computed tomography

CT is the mainstay of modern adrenal imaging. The normal adrenal gland can almost always be visualized. The right may be more difficult to identify, being in close apposition to the back wall of the cava and being affected by partial volume effect from the overlying liver. If hyperplasia or a small tumour is suspected, definitive assessment of the adrenals requires thin (1–3 mm) contiguous sections. Modern multidetector CT scanners are currently capable of resolving tumours as small as 5 mm. The use of contrast media is not necessary for detection of adrenal masses, the anatomical demonstration being more important. In some instances however, the pattern of enhancement may help characterize the lesion.

Staging of malignant adrenal tumours requires scanning of the chest and abdomen for local organ invasion, lymphadenopathy, and metastases. Intravenous contrast medium is necessary for maximum sensitivity for hepatic metastases. Hypervascular metastases (e.g. phaeochromocytoma) may be more conspicuous with scans obtained in the arterial phase rather than the portal venous phase of enhancement.

Magnetic resonance imaging

As with CT, MRI allows visualization of the normal and abnormal adrenal gland in the majority of cases. It does not involve exposure to ionizing radiation and hence is preferred in children, the young adult, and the pregnant patient. It has a valuable role particularly in characterization of the indeterminate adrenal

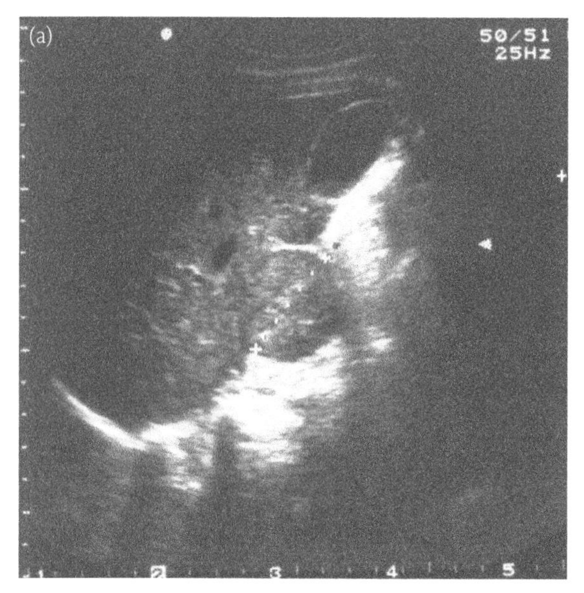

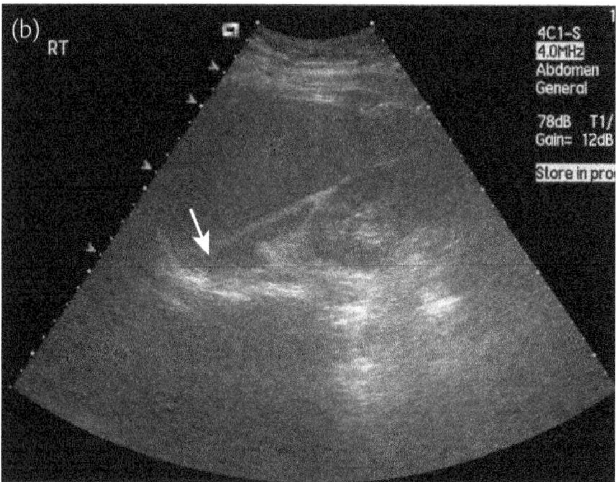

Fig. 5.1.1 (a) Ultrasonography demonstration of a 3 cm right adrenal mass and its relation to liver and right kidney. (b) Ultrasonographic demonstration of a v-shaped hyperplastic adrenal in a patient with congenital adrenal hyperplasia.

lesion using chemical shift imaging (in- and opposed-phase sequences). The ability to image in multiple planes allows improved recognition of adjacent organ involvement, and possibly determination of an adrenal origin of an upper-quadrant mass (Fig. 5.1.2). However, when staging malignancy, it is usually difficult to evaluate the whole body as the examination time would be prolonged, and it is as yet poorly sensitive to small metastases in the lung.

Radionuclide imaging

The functional information afforded by imaging with radioisotopes is unique and is complementary to the anatomical demonstrations of CT and MRI. Isotope imaging of the adrenal medulla uses the noradrenaline analogue meta-iodobenzylguanidine (MIBG) (3). The tracer is actively taken up in postsynaptic nerve terminals where it is resistant to degradation and can hence be used to demonstrate accumulations of such tissue as in phaeochromocytomas, paragangliomas, and neuroblastomas. Carcinoid tumours and medullary carcinomas of the thyroid also take up the radiopharmaceutical.

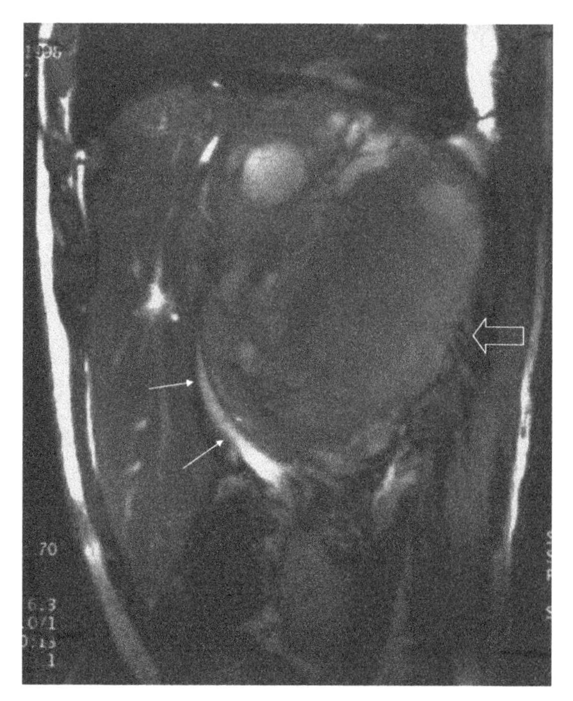

Fig. 5.1.2 Large phaeochromocytoma (open arrow). Sagittal T2-weighted magnetic resonance image with flowing blood and areas of fluid as white. Note anterior displacement of inferior vena cava (arrows) and heterogeneity of tumour.

The pharmaceutical is labelled with ^{123}I- or ^{131}I-iodine; ^{123}I-iodine gives a lower radiation dose and better quality images but is less readily available and more expensive. A number of drugs inhibit MIBG uptake: opioids, tricyclic antidepressants, sympathomimetics, antipsychotics, cocaine, and importantly antihypertensive agents including labetalol and calcium channel blockers, and such drugs need to be withdrawn if possible before this examination (3, 4).

Scans are usually performed at 24 and 48 h. Uptake is normal in liver, spleen, myocardium, and salivary glands. Urinary excretion may obscure primary or metastatic disease in the pelvis or bladder. Occasionally, bowel uptake is seen which may hinder interpretation. Normal adrenal glands are usually not well visualized although there may be faint uptake.

An alternative radiopharmaceutical is the somatostatin analogue octreotide acetate labelled with ^{123}I or ^{111}In (indium), which localizes to somatostatin receptor-bearing tumours including phaeochromocytomas and neuroblastomas (5).

Isotope imaging of the adrenal cortex uses labelled cholesterol analogues: 6-β-iodomethyl-19-norcholesterol labelled with ^{131}I (NP-59). Adrenocortical scintigraphy is not widely available or used. This may be due to the number of patient visits required, the lag time to final result, a relatively high radiation dose, limited availability, but perhaps most importantly the use of endocrine assessments in conjunction with high resolution anatomical imaging with CT.

Positron emission tomography (PET) has an increasingly recognized role in the assessment of adrenal masses (6, 7). The most commonly used radiopharmaceutical is [^{18}F]2-fluoro-2-deoxy-D-glucose (FDG), a glucose analogue that is actively taken up and trapped in hypermetabolic cells, usually reflecting malignancy. PET can thus be used to detect metastases to the adrenals, and to indicate that the likelihood that a mass is malignant. Although not yet widely available, other pharmaceuticals such as ^{18}F-fluorodopamine, ^{18}F-fluroDOPA and have been used for evaluation of adrenal and other neuroendocrine tumours (4).

Arteriography

The vascular supply and drainage have been described above. Arteriography is rarely indicated for diagnostic purposes. Occasionally it may help indicate an adrenal origin of an uncertain abdominal mass, or be used as a prelude to embolization of vascular tumours.

Venous sampling

Sampling of the adrenal effluent is used to determine whether hormone production originates from one or both adrenals, and to determine if nodules detected on CT are functional or not. The left adrenal vein is relatively easy to cannulate via the renal vein but the anatomy of the right is less favourable (direct drainage to the inferior vena cava) and high failure rates have been reported. Nevertheless, some investigators approach 100% success rates (8). Extravasation and venous infarction may complicate injection of the adrenal veins. However, adrenal venography is not necessary for diagnostic purposes, although it may help confirm correct catheter placement.

Biopsy

The indeterminate lesion that is discovered when imaging for other purposes may need histological evaluation. However, endocrine assessment and the newer CT and MR characterization techniques have significantly reduced the requirement for biopsy (9). Biopsy accuracy rates range between 80 and 100% (10, 11). Biopsy cannot differentiate between an adenoma and a carcinoma and thus should be avoided if an adrenocortical carcinoma is suspected; violation of the tumour capsule of an adrenocortical carcinoma significantly worsens the prognosis and metastases in the biopsy needle canal have been described. However, biopsy can be helpful to differentiate between a tumour of adrenal origin and an adrenal metastasis of a solid organ tumour distinct from the adrenal. An adrenal biopsy should only be carried out if the outcome would have a therapeutic consequence. Haemorrhage and pneumothorax are the most common complications of adrenal biopsy.

CT guidance is usual except where the tumour is relatively large when ultrasonography is a good alternative. A posterior approach with the patient prone is the least hazardous but the posterior costophrenic angles may be deep, and transgression of the lungs may be unavoidable with consequent risk of pneumothorax. A transhepatic approach is an alternative on the right, or on rare occasions a safe anterior approach may be identified (9).

Most operators remain reluctant to biopsy adrenal masses that may be phaeochromocytomas due to the risk of precipitating a hypertensive crisis (9). Prior blood or urine biochemistry for exclusion of catecholamine excess is therefore mandatory before any adrenal biopsy.

Cushing's syndrome

Cushing's syndrome is the result of overproduction of cortisol by the adrenal cortex. The distinction between pituitary or ectopic ACTH-driven cortisol production and primary adrenal disorders is made on a clinical and biochemical basis and imaging directed appropriately.

MRI is the best imaging modality for pituitary tumours, which account for about 80% of cases of Cushing's (Fig. 5.1.3a). The multiplanar presentation is ideal, and intravenous contrast medium administration mandatory, for the detection of small tumours. CT is a reasonable alternative. Thin-section coronal examinations with intravenous contrast are most sensitive for small tumours. There is no justification for imaging the adrenals in pituitary-driven or ectopic Cushing's, although bilateral adrenal hyperplasia can be expected (Fig. 5.1.3b). Adrenal hyperplasia is manifest as thickening and elongation of the limbs of the adrenal gland. The hyperplasia may be smooth or multinodular, but the glands may look normal.

Adrenal tumours are the cause of Cushing's syndrome in 15–25% of cases and are well shown with CT and MRI (12, 13). Adenomas are usually between 2 and 4 cm in size. They are uniform in attenuation, rounded, and well demarcated (Fig. 5.1.3c), identical to nonfunctioning tumours. They may be large enough to be seen on ultrasonography although increased body fat may hinder the examination. An active adrenal adenoma will be accompanied by atrophy of the rest of the gland and the contralateral adrenal. Carcinomas are usually larger (more than 4 cm) and may show necrosis, haemorrhage, or calcification (12, 13). Histology cannot indicate malignancy but large tumours are predictive of subsequent malignant behaviour, that is, metastasis or recurrence. Multiplanar imaging as with ultrasonography, MRI, and multidetector CT studies may clarify the organ of origin of large tumours more readily than axial CT. Growth over time (Fig. 5.1.4a) or local invasion of adjacent organs are features of malignancy (Fig. 5.1.4b). As with renal cell carcinoma, there may be invasion of the adrenal vein and extension into the cava (Fig. 5.1.4c).

Rarely Cushing's syndrome is the result of primary pigmented nodular hyperplasia when multiple small nodules are shown arising from an otherwise atrophic gland; or ACTH independent macronodular hyperplasia when the glands are markedly enlarged and nodular but maintain their shape (12).

There are other radiological features of Cushing's syndrome. Increased body fat may be radiologically evident, especially on CT and MRI. Chronic steroid overproduction results in skeletal osteoporosis. Diagnosis of osteoporosis is best done with bone mineral densitometry.

Primary hyperaldosteronism (Conn's syndrome)

Conn's syndrome results from overproduction of aldosterone either from an adrenal adenoma or bilateral hyperplasia (14). The distinction is crucial as it directly affects surgical management. A unilateral adrenalectomy is often curative for an aldosterone-secreting adenoma but has no role to play in bilateral hyperplasia. The pitfall is to remove a nonfunctional nodule or to fail to appreciate subtle hyperplasia in addition to a nodule. Conn's is very rarely (less than 1%) the result of an adrenocortical carcinoma.

Aldosterone-producing adenomas are often small (less than 2 cm), compared to cortisol-producing adenomas requiring thin-section (3 mm) CT for detection (Fig. 5.1.5a). The average diameter is between 12 and 18 mm and 20% are less than 10 mm

(a)

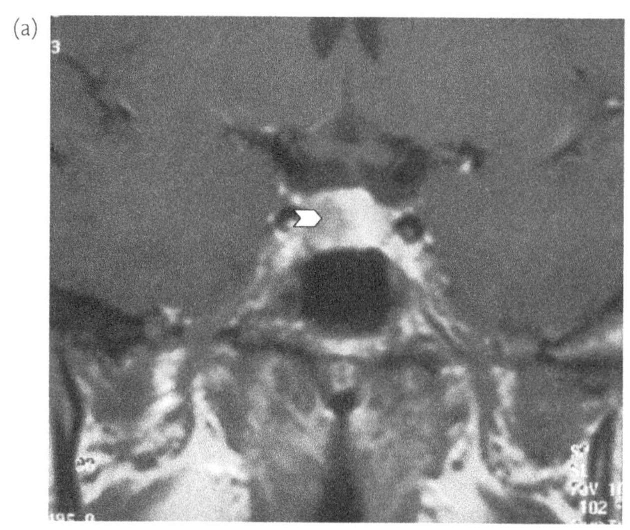

(b)

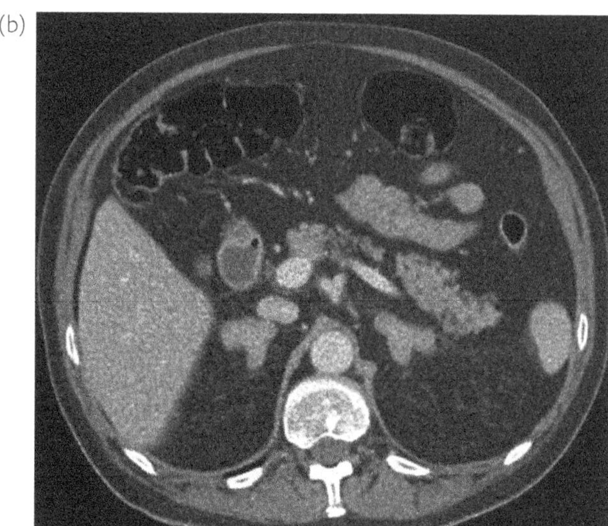

(c)

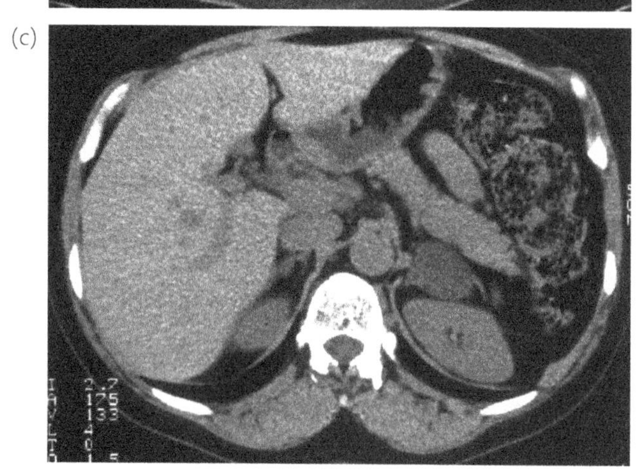

Fig. 5.1.3 (a) Cushing's disease: pituitary adenoma (arrowhead) on coronal gadolinium-enhanced MR image. (b) Cushing's syndrome due to ectopic ACTH production. Marked bilateral adrenal hyperplasia secondary to an unidentified source of ectopic ACTH. The patient was subjected to bilateral adrenalectomy for treatment. (c) Adrenal Cushing's syndrome: unenhanced CT. Low attenuation, 3 cm left adrenal mass.

(15). CT can detect 82–88% (16, 17). Tumours less than 1 cm can be difficult to identify. Conn's tumours usually have the lowest attenuation values of all hyperfunctioning adenomas (Fig. 5.1.5b) (18).

Hyperplastic glands may appear normal or show obvious symmetric enlargement. MRI has no real advantage over CT although high signal returned from the lesion on T2-weighted imaging may aid detection.

The definitive test is adrenal venous sampling with an accuracy rate of close to 100% (8, 14, 19). The ratio between aldosterone and cortisol in the venous blood from each adrenal is compared with peripheral samples. Baseline samples and samples following ACTH stimulation may be taken. A high ratio is present on the side with an adenoma, and a low ratio on the opposite side.

Androgen excess and oestrogen excess

Androgen excess may be of ovarian or adrenal origin. Tumorous adrenal causes are mostly malignant. Imaging choices are similar to the investigation of Conn's syndrome, that is, CT or MRI with venous sampling (with the addition of ovarian venous aspirates) or dexamethasone-suppressed adrenal scans in diagnostically difficult cases (10).

Feminization, for example gynaecomastia, due to adrenal oestrogen excess is rare. As with androgen excess of adrenal origin, the cause is most often an adrenocortical carcinoma of such a size that CT and ultrasonography are invariably helpful (Fig. 5.1.4c).

Adrenocortical carcinoma

This may be responsible for any of the above syndromes or be relatively nonfunctional. They are readily seen on ultrasonography, CT, or MRI, as tumours are usually large at presentation although hyperfunctioning tumours are usually smaller at presentation, as a result of the endocrine effects (Fig. 5.1.4a–d) (20). Heterogeneity of some degree is usual. Calcification occurs in 30%. An adrenal origin may be difficult to determine on standard axial CT imagng if the tumours are large and invasive but CT reconstructions or MRI is more informative, using multiple planes and different sequences. Vascular and adjacent organ invasion is diagnostic of malignancy. They rarely contain significant amounts of intracellular lipid, which can be exploited diagnostically as malignant tumours therefore rarely lose signal on opposed MRI and generally feature low attenuation density values (<10 Hounsfield units (HU)) on CT.

Addison's disease

This term refers to adrenal insufficiency. Autoimmune mechanisms are the commonest cause now that the incidence of tuberculosis has been reduced. CT may show atrophy or calcification. Tuberculous infection in the subacute stage produces enlarged adrenals, which may show peripheral enhancement around central necrosis. In the long term the glands calcify (Fig. 5.1.6a,b). Histoplasmosis produces similar appearances and half of patients with disseminated disease develop Addison's disease (10, 15).

Bilateral adrenal metastases, even when large, rarely result in adrenal insufficiency (less than 20%), but symptoms of Addison's disease may be confused for those of the malignancy (Fig. 5.1.7) (21).

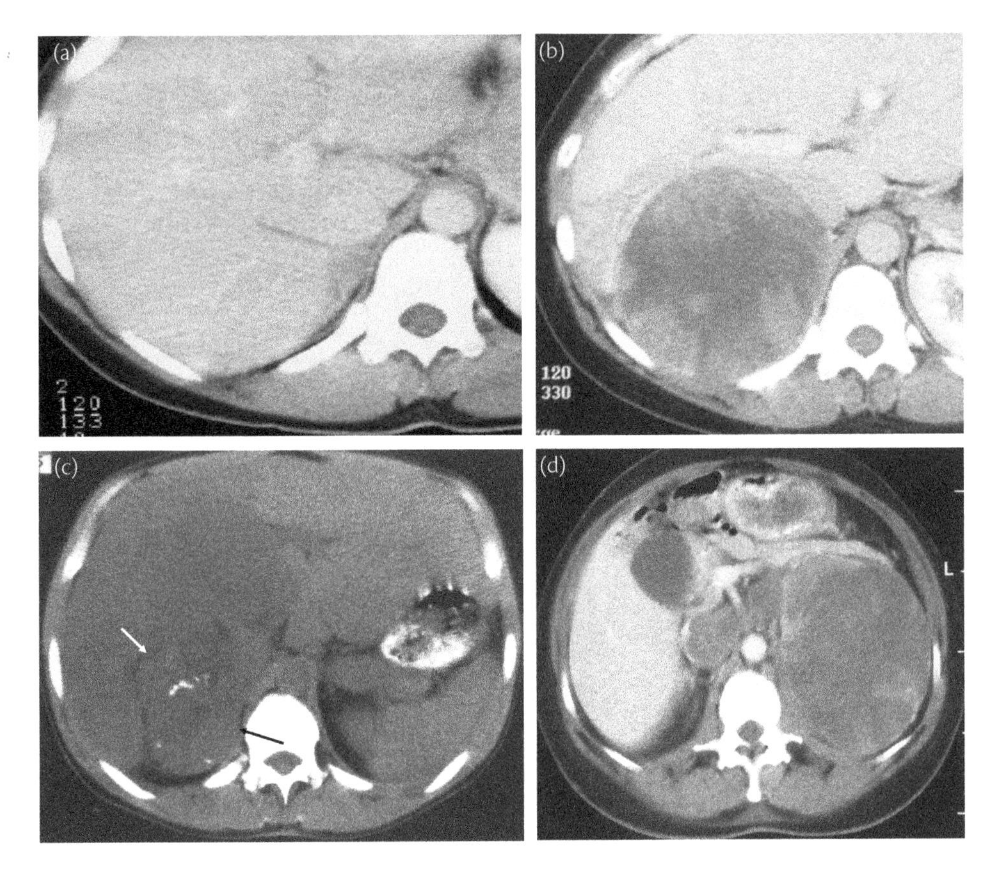

Fig. 5.1.4 (a and b) CT images demonstrating growth over time of an adrenocortical carcinoma. (c) Adrenocortical carcinoma: unenhanced CT showing a large, partly calcified mass (between arrows) in the suprarenal region, invading liver. There was a history of gynaecomastia. (d) Left-sided adrenocortical carcinoma invading left renal vein and inferior vena cava.

Acute adrenal insufficiency as the result of bilateral adrenal haemorrhage or hypotension may complicate shock, sepsis, or bleeding disorders. High-attenuation swelling of the adrenals is the finding on CT performed acutely.

Rare causes of hypoadrenalism include haemochromatosis, when CT may demonstrate increased attenuation of liver and pancreas as a result of iron deposition and Wolman's disease (lipid storage abnormality due to a deficiency of liposomal acid lipase) when the adrenals are enlarged and show diffuse punctate calcification.

Secondary hypoadrenalism is usually due to prolonged steroid therapy, but more rarely is a result of pituitary infarction or haemorrhage.

Phaeochromocytomas

These tumours arise from the chromaffin cells of the sympathetic nervous system. Thus they most commonly arise in the adrenal medulla but can also be found in the neck, the mediastinum (including intrapericardiac), in a para-aortic position, in an accumulation of sympathetic ganglia at the base of the inferior mesenteric artery known as the organ of Zuckerkandl, and in the pelvis and bladder (Fig. 5.1.2 and 5.1.8) (22).

About 25% of apparently sporadic tumours are associated with familial conditions such as neurofibromatosis, and von Hippel–Lindau and multiple endocrine neoplasia (MEN) syndromes. These patients are more likely to have bilateral or multiple lesions (Fig. 5.1.9) (23).

Phaeochromocytomas are usually but not always benign. As with other adrenal tumours, benign and malignant phaeochromocytomas are distinguished by behaviour (i.e. metastasis or local invasion) rather than histology. However, the results of genetic analysis are usually predictive of malignancy risk and determine screening and follow-up strategies.

Adrenomedullary tumours are usually sizeable (greater than 5 cm) except when associated with the MEN syndromes. Therefore they can often be shown with ultrasonography and appear either homogeneous or heterogeneous with cystic or necrotic elements. CT is preferred, however, and will demonstrate the majority of adrenal phaeochromocytomas (77–98%) (23). About 10% may show calcification. These lesions usually enhance strongly on CT and heterogeneity corresponding to haemorrhage or necrosis is better appreciated after contrast medium enhancement, or on T2-weighted MR images. They are characteristically of high signal on T2-weighted MR sequences (20).The older intravenous iodinated ionic contrast agents can precipitate hypertensive crisis in the absence of pharmacological alpha and beta blockade (24). The almost ubiquitous nonionic contrast media used now do not carry the same risk and blockade is not now regarded as necessary (25).

CT is generally used to evaluate the adrenals and to search for ectopic sources (4). MR does not usually have any additional benefit.

Surgical planning for large or locally invasive tumours is helped by the multiplanar capabilities of multidetector CT or MR (Fig. 5.1.2). The mediastinal tumours, and especially the intrapericardiac lesions, are well shown with electrocardiographically gated MRI. The tumour can be expected to be markedly hyperintense on T2-weighted imaging. These lesions are often heterogeneous and vascular. Haemorrhage may occur leading to fluid–fluid levels and

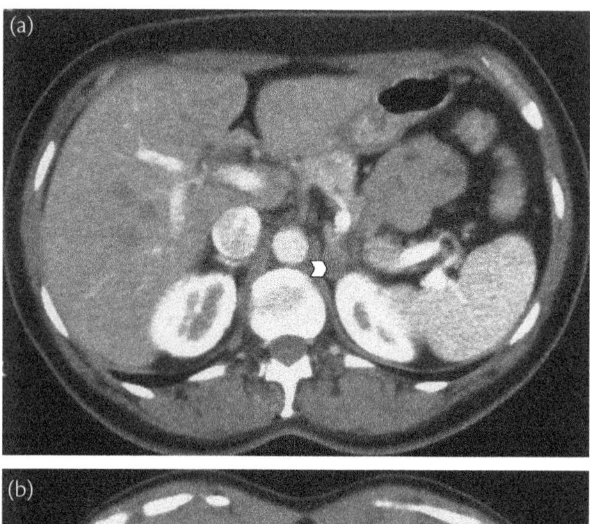

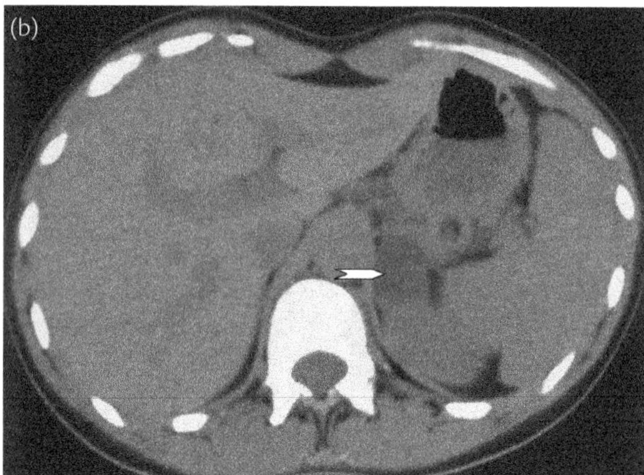

Fig. 5.1.5 (a) Small Conn's tumour: enhanced CT showing a small mass (arrowhead) arising from the medial limb of the left adrenal. (b) Large Conn's tumour: unenhanced CT showing a typically low attenuation left adrenal mass (arrowhead) causing Conn's syndrome.

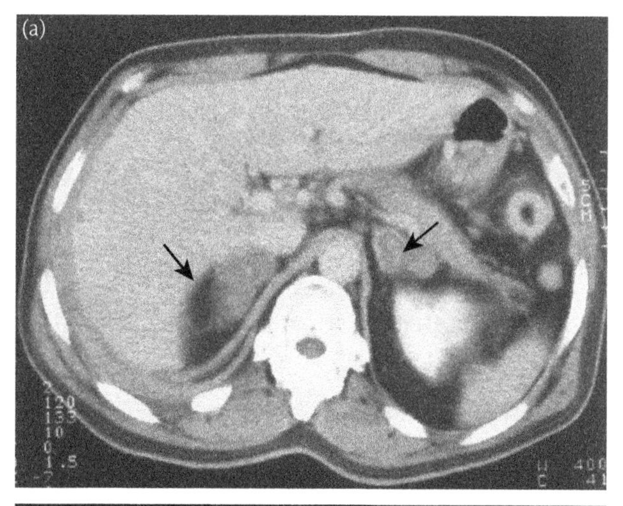

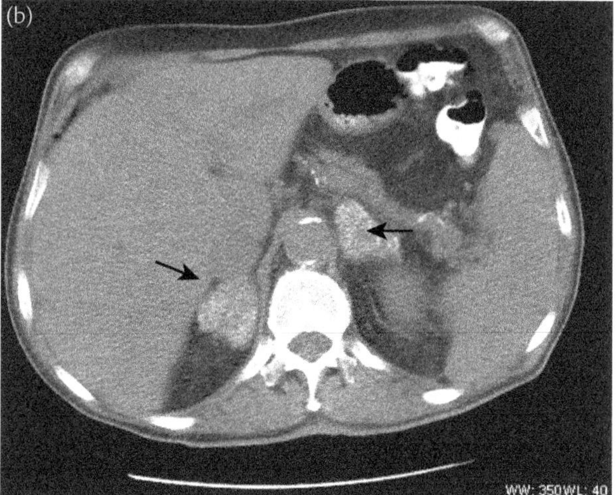

Fig. 5.1.6 (a) Active tuberculosis of adrenals. (b) Calcified enlarged adrenals following previous tuberculous infection.

areas of high signal on T1-weighted images. Extension into the inferior vena cava is shown with flow-sensitive sequences, or with intravenous contrast enhancement (22, 28).

MIBG scanning is of great value in the imaging of phaeochromocytomas (Fig. 5.1.8). It is especially useful for the detection of extra-abdominal tumours and for the staging of malignant lesions, as the metastases are active (Fig. 5.1.10). It is 87% sensitive, and 97% specific (2, 4, 10). Whole-body imaging is straightforward and may be used for the initial imaging test, or to search for an ectopic tumour following a negative adrenal CT. CT, MRI, and MIBG scanning are equally accurate for detection of primary adrenal tumours.

MIBG is not specific for phaeochromocytoma; other tumours of neural crest origin such as neuroblastoma, carcinoid tumours, medullary carcinoma of the thyroid, Merkel-cell skin tumours, and nonfunctioning paragangliomas also show uptake, but this is not usually a clinical problem.

Other radionuclide methods used to demonstrate phaeochromocytomas include ^{111}In-octreotide scanning (2) and positron emission tomography with FDG (Fig. 5.1.11) or other radiopharmaceuticals such as ^{18}F-fluoroDOPA, ^{18}F-fluorodopamine, or ^{11}C-hydroxyephedrine (4, 6, 22). ^{111}In octreotide is more useful for demonstration of metastatic disease than benign tumours (1). FDG and ^{18}F-fluorodopamine appear to be better than MIBG for metastatic disease and FDOPA is superior for extra-adrenal tumours and paragangliomas (23).

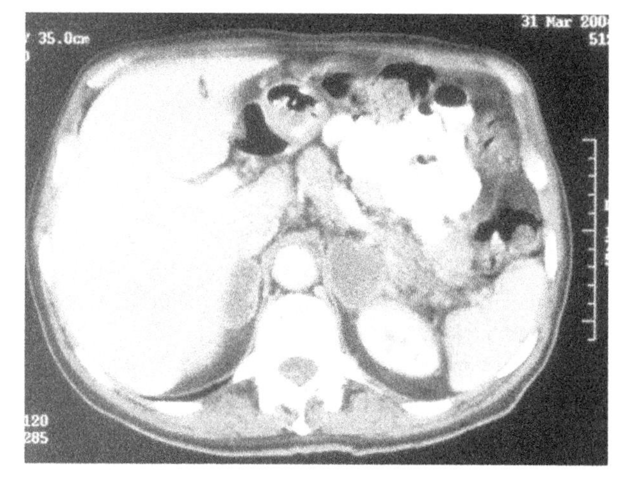

Fig. 5.1.7 Bilateral adrenal metastases that unusually resulted in adrenal failure.

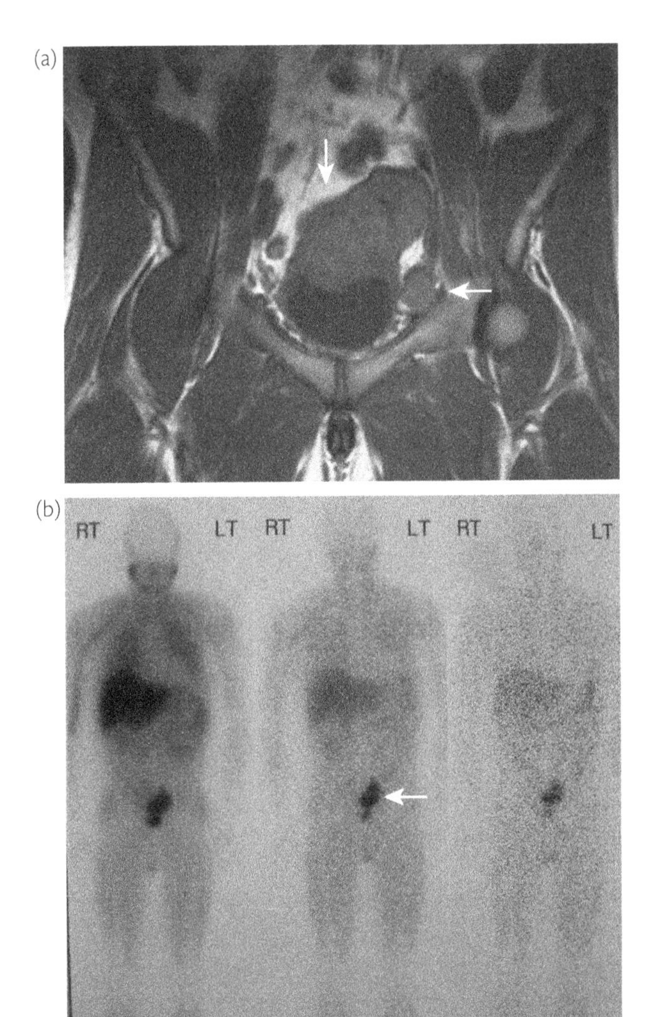

Fig. 5.1.8 Bladder phaeochromocytoma. (a) Coronal MR of bladder showing a polypoid tumour arising from the left side of the bladder dome (and an enlarged metastatic left pelvic node). (b) Corresponding anterior whole body MIBG images at 1, 2 and 3 days.

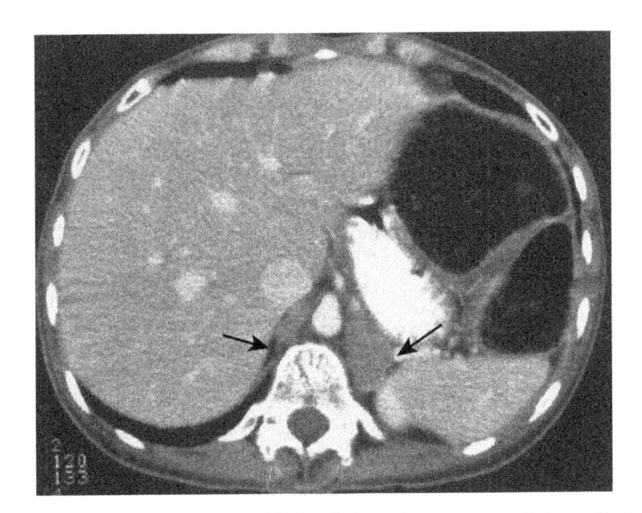

Fig. 5.1.9 MEN type 2 associated bilateral phaeochromocytoma. Enhanced CT showing moderate-sized left adrenal and small right adrenal masses in a patient with a positive family history and a previous medullary cell carcinoma of the thyroid.

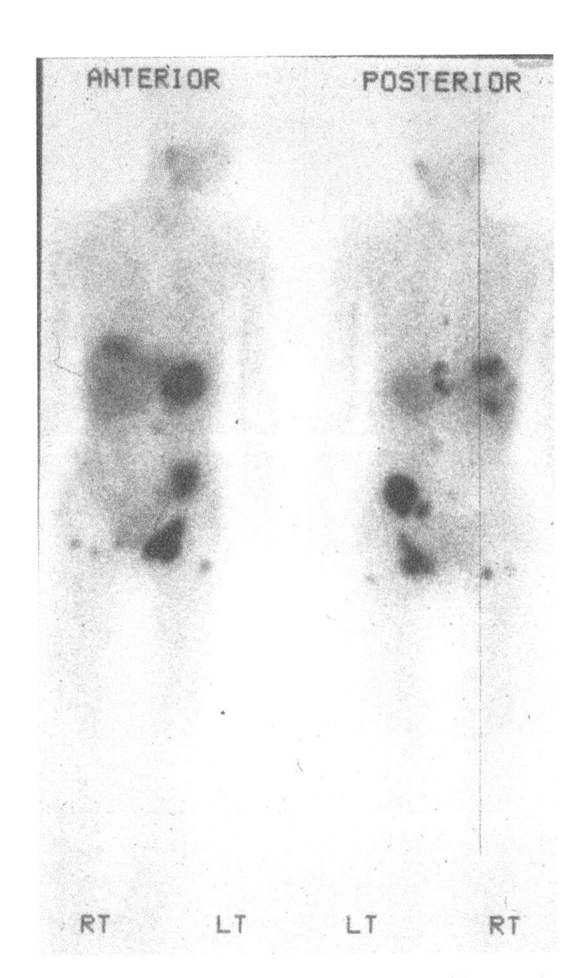

Fig. 5.1.10 Metastatic phaeochromocytoma. MIBG scan of thorax and abdomen showing multiple areas of abnormal uptake.

Neuroblastoma

This tumour of infancy and childhood can arise in the adrenals (50%), in the abdominal sympathetic chain, or in the mediastinum. MIBG uptake is a feature, and can therefore be used for assessment of metastatic disease, although CT or MRI is more appropriate for the assessment of the local disease. Tumours are often nonhomogeneous on CT and MRI, and calcification is characteristic (which helps differentiate it from Wilm's tumour of the kidney). Local invasion into the spine, and skeletal metastatic disease, can occur. The multiplanar capability of MRI allows demonstration of vascular and liver involvement, intraspinal spread, and marrow disease (29).

The incidental adrenal mass

With the exponential increase in the use of modern imaging techniques adrenal masses are often recognized as incidental findings (4–6%). These are almost invariably benign in patients with no history of malignancy. They may be functional in terms of hormone synthesis and this is determined endocrinologically. The vast majority are, however, endocrinologically irrelevant, and are likely, statistically, to be benign if small. They are much more likely to be malignant if there is known primary malignancy, although less than 50% are metastatic. The differentiation of metastasis

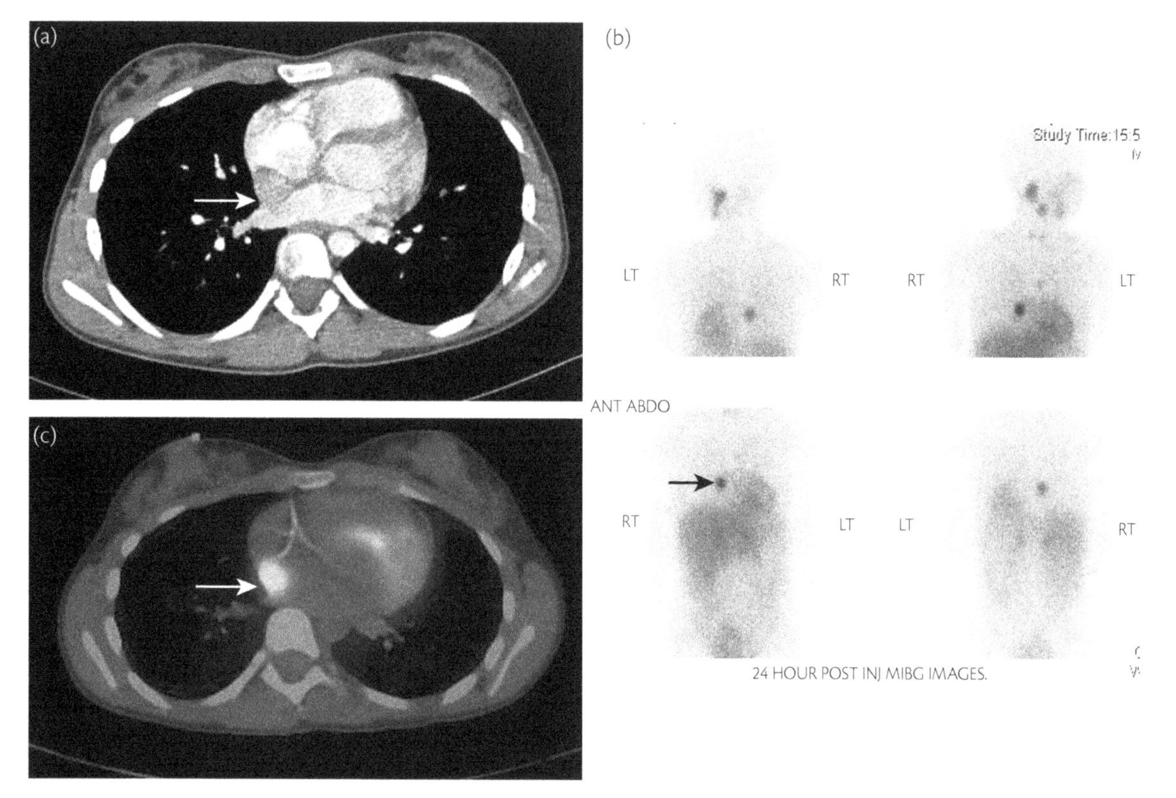

Fig. 5.1.11 Paracardiac paraganglioma demonstrated on (a) CT (not prospectively identified), (b) MIBG, and (c) 18-FDG scanning.

or malignancy from an incidental adenoma is therefore very important (30).

Comparison with old scans or follow-up examination is important—a lesion that changes in size over 6 months is highly likely to be malignant. A positive biopsy result might be regarded as the most definitive test short of surgery. However, these lesions may be small and difficult to sample without morbidity. A negative result is less reassuring because of concerns about sampling error. However, noninvasive techniques now often allow distinction of an adrenal adenoma from a metastasis.

The CT appearance may give some indication of the nature of an incidentally discovered adrenal mass. It may be evidently a cyst (i.e. thin-walled, well-defined, and of fluid density). If solid, benign lesions are usually homogeneous, although there may rarely be calcification. Frank areas of fat may indicate a myelolipoma. Malignant lesions may be irregular in outline, heterogeneous, perhaps with necrotic areas. The morphological appearance following contrast may be of value. Adjacent organ invasion or demonstration of metastasis is diagnostic.

The presence of a high proportion of intracellular fat in 70% of adenomas allows the use of CT density measurements and chemical shift MR imaging.

Adenomas are often readily apparent as hypoattenuating compared to kidney or liver on unenhanced CT (Fig. 5.1.3c and 5.1.5b). Mean attenuation values of adenomas are 2 HU,and of nonadenomas 30 HU (31). On thin-section unenhanced scans a density of 10 HU or less is indicative of a high proportion of intracellular fat, which suggests an adenoma with high specificity (98%) though poorer sensitivity (71%) (32–33).An upper threshold of 2 HU will be 100% specific for benign adrenal lesions at the cost of sensitivity. Quantitative enhancement and wash-out characteristics have been used effectively

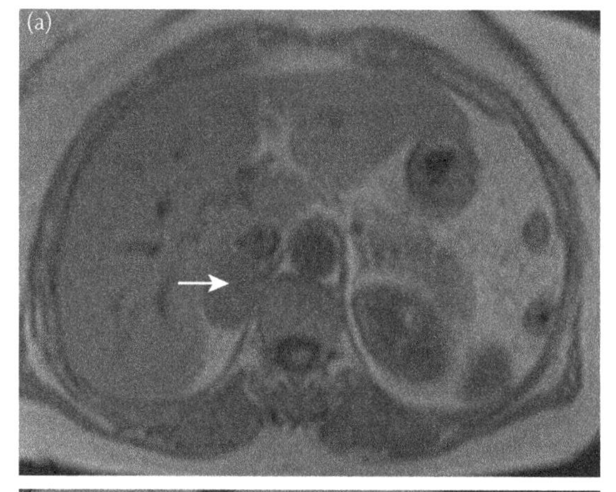

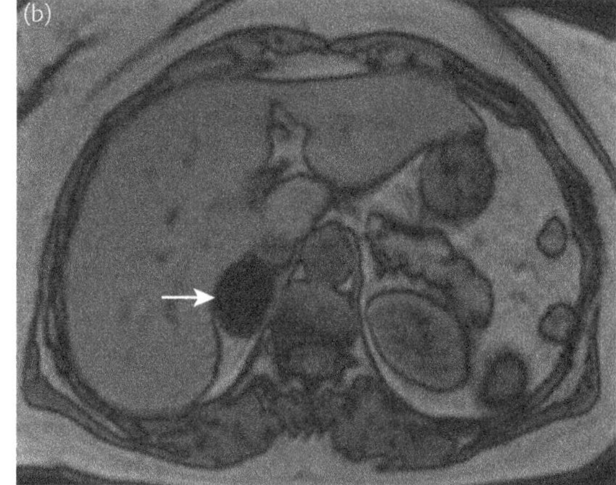

Fig. 5.1.12 (a) In-phase T1-weighted MR; (b) opposed-phase T1-weighted MR showing marked signal loss of a moderate-sized right adrenal adenoma.

by many authors and relates to the fact that benign lesions lose enhancement more rapidly than malignant. The most commonly used threshold is 40% relative wash-out on a 15 min delayed scan (30, 34). This technique is proven even for lipid-poor adenomas.

Early users of MRI suggested that high signal intensity on T2-weighted images indicated a malignant lesion, benign lesions generally having signal intensity similar to normal adrenal; however, it became apparent that there was too much overlap (20–30%) for this to be a useful feature. Gadolinium contrast medium enhancement was likewise unreliable, even with the use of dynamic acquisitions (34). The most robust technique appears to be the use of chemical-shift imaging (30, 35). This utilizes the fact that the presence of fat within benign adenomatous cells alters the local magnetic environment, and hence the resonant frequency of the precessing protons. This results in a reduction of signal intensity of benign lesions (whose cells contain both lipid and water) on out-of-phase imaging. This feature can be seen in 95% of adrenal adenomas (Fig. 5.1.12). Normal adrenals also display this phenomenon but nonadenomatous lesions do not.

There is recent work indicating that MR spectroscopy can characterize adrenal masses as adenomas, carcinomas, phaeochromocytomas, or metastases but at present this can only be used for masses larger than 2 cm (36).

FDG-PET relies on the altered metabolism of cancer cells trapping this radiopharmaceutical which enters the glycolytic pathway in the place of glucose. It has been shown to accurately differentiate benign and malignant adrenal masses in the cancer patient with specificities of 90–96%, and sensitivities of 93–100% (6, 7). It is the most accurate test therefore to confirm that an adrenal mass is metastatic in the cancer patient. It is expensive but availability has rapidly increased in recent years.

A reasonable approach to the incidentally discovered adrenal lesion, whether in the setting of a known malignancy or not, is to perform density measurement on thin-section unenhanced CT, or delayed wash-out if indeterminate. On unenhanced CT if the density is less than 0 HU, malignancy is excluded. If less than 10 HU, malignancy is almost certainly excluded. In the range 10–20 HU in- and out-of-phase MRI is helpful. If greater than 20 HU it is less likely to resolve the issue due to the lack of intracellular lipid, and FDG-PET may be helpful.

Nonadenomatous adrenal abnormalities

Myelolipomas are benign and contain elements of fat and bone marrow (30). The fat is diagnostic and can be demonstrated on ultrasonography (hyperechoic), CT (low attenuation), or MRI (high signal on T1-weighting, focal loss of signal on fat-suppressed images, but not on opposed-phase sequences) (Fig. 5.1.13). However, fat is not always a dominant feature and the appearance of the lesion is then nonspecific. Haemorrhage may complicate the imaging features.

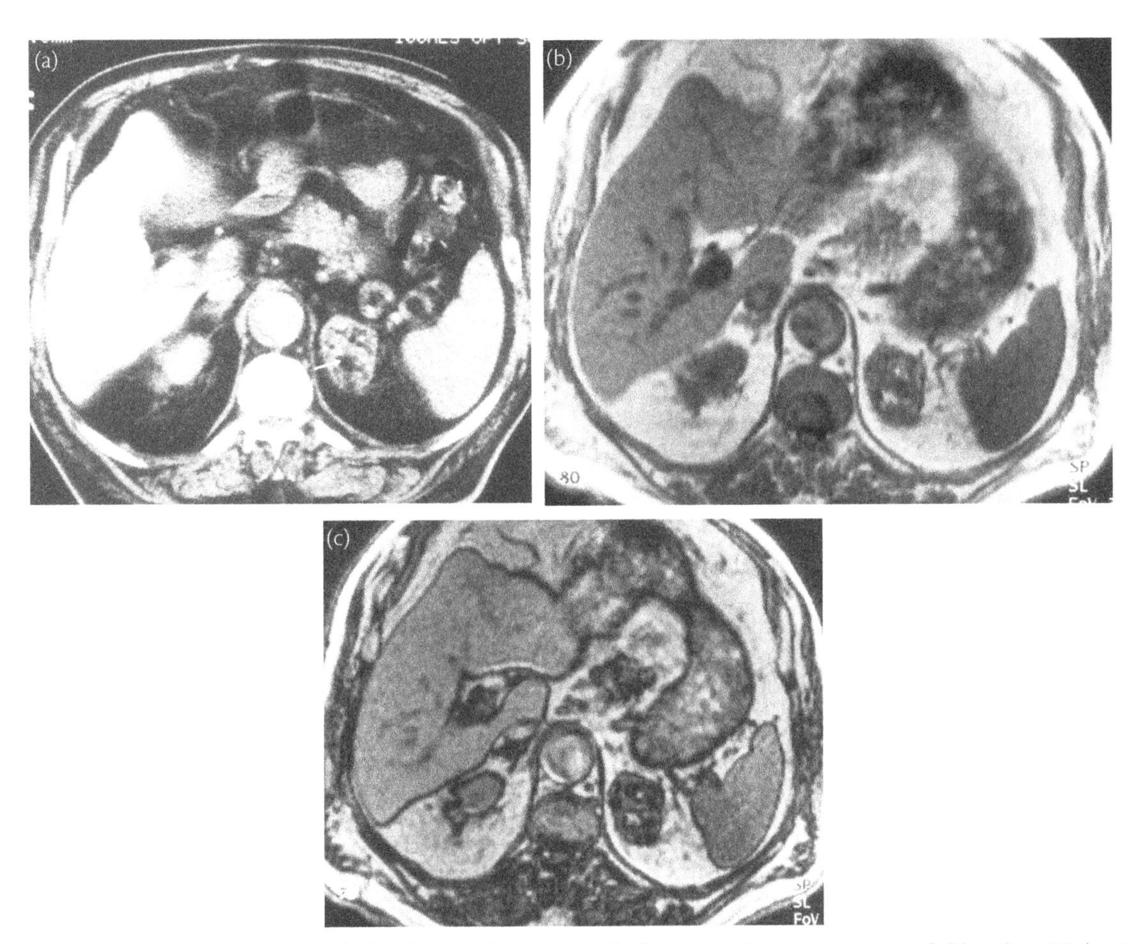

Fig. 5.1.13 Adrenal myelolipoma. (a) CT showing a left adrenal mass with macroscopic fat (low attenuation elements—arrowed); (b) in-phase MR showing the macroscopic fat to be of high intensity with no loss of intensity on (c) the opposed-phase image.

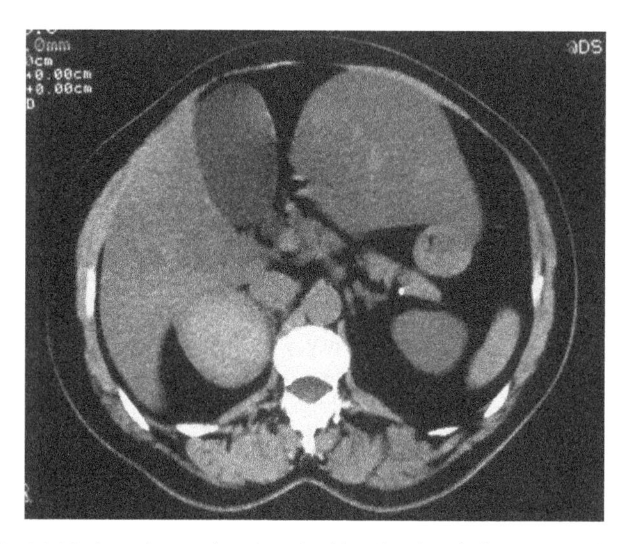

Fig. 5.1.14 Acute haemorrhage into the right adrenal. High-density material is expanding the right adrenal gland on unenhanced CT.

Adrenal cysts are endothelial (lymphangiomas and haemangiomas), epithelial (retention cysts, embryonal, or cystic adenomas), pseudocysts (resulting from previous haemorrhage), or echinococcal (hydatid). Of adrenal cysts, 15% show mural calcification, particularly in hydatid disease (37, 38).

The CT appearance of acute adrenal haemorrhage is of high-attenuation material expanding the adrenal gland or periadrenal haemorrhage leading to stranding, and an indistinct adrenal contour (Fig. 5.1.14). The high density may not be appreciated if only contrast-enhanced scans are available. Subacute haematomas are isodense with normal adrenal and indistinguishable from adenomas. Old adrenal haematomas may lead to calcification. Because of the paramagnetic effects of blood such as haemosiderin and methaemoglobin, MRI can be diagnostic of adrenal haematoma, although there will be a complex variation depending on the age of the lesion.

Adrenal rests

Adrenal tissue can be found in ectopic sites such as the coeliac plexus region, the broad ligaments, the testes, and the ovaries. These rests may then enlarge in pathological conditions such as congenital adrenal hyperplasia (Fig. 5.1.15) (39), or following ACTH stimulation such as occurs in Addison's or Cushing's diseases. This phenomenon may lead to the misdiagnosis of testicular or other tumours (40).

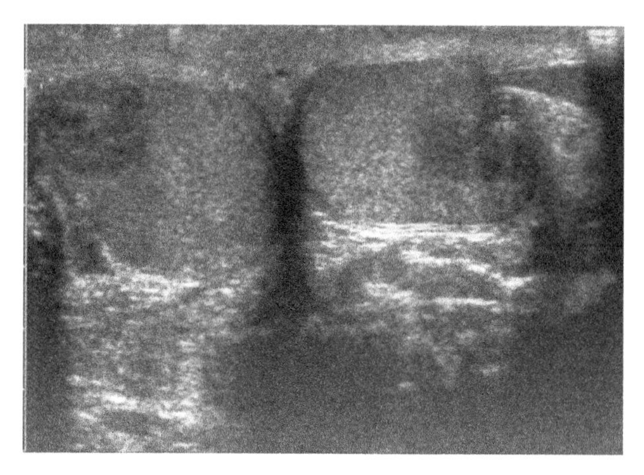

Fig. 5.1.15 Bilateral adrenal rest 'tumours' in congenital adrenal hyperplasia (same patient as Fig. 5.1.1b).

References

1. Ilias I, Sahdev A, Reznek R, Grossman A, Pacak K. The optimum imaging of adrenal tumours: a comparison of different methods. *Endocr Relat Cancer*, 2007; 14: 587–99.
2. Mayo-Smith WW, Boland GW, Noto RB, Lee M. State-of-the-art adrenal imaging. *Radiographics*, 2001; 21: 995–1012.
3. Bombardieri E, Aktolun C, Baum R, Bishof-Delaloye A, Buscombe J, Chatal JF, *et al.* $^{131}I/^{123}I$-Metaiodobenzylguanidine (MIBG) scintigraphy 2003. Available at: *http://www.eanm.org/scientific_info/guidelines/guidelines_intro.php* (accessed 7 May 2010).
4. Ilias J, Pacak K. Current approaches and recommended algorithm for the diagnostic localization of pheochromocytoma. *J Clin Endocrinol Metab*, 2004; 89: 479–91.
5. Bombardieri E, Aktolun C, Baum R, Baum RP, Bishof-Delaloye A, Buscombe J, *et al.* ^{111}In-pentetreotide scintigraphy—procedure guidelines for tumour imaging 2003. Available at: *http://www.eanm.org/scientific_info/guidelines/guidelines_intro.php* (accessed 7 May 2010).
6. Elaini AB, Shetty SK, Chapman VM, Sahani DV, Boland GW, Sweeney AT, *et al.* Improved detection and characterization of adrenal disease with PET-CT. *Radiographics*, 2007; 27: 755–67.
7. Chong S, Lee KS, Kim HY, Kim YK, Kim BT, Chung MJ, *et al.* Integrated PET-CT for the characterization of adrenal gland lesions in cancer patients: diagnostic efficacy and interpretation pitfalls. *Radiographics*, 2006; 26: 1811–26.
8. Daunt N. Adrenal vein sampling: how to make it quick, easy and successful. *Radiographics*, 2005: 25 (Suppl 1); S143–S158.
9. Paulsen S, Hghiem H, Korobkin M, Caoili E, Higgins E. Changing role of imaging-guided biopsy of adrenal masses: evaluation of 50 adrenal biopsies. *Am J Roentgenol*, 2004; 182: 1033–7.
10. Francis IR, Gross MD, Shapiro B, Korobkin M, Quint LE. Integrated imaging of adrenal disease. *Radiology*, 1992; 184: 1–13.
11. Mody MK, Kazeroooni EA, Korobkin M. Percutaneous CT-guided biopsy of adrenal masses: immediate and delayed complications. *J Comput Assist Tomogr*, 1985; 144: 67–9.
12. Rockall AG, Babar SA, Sohaib SA, Isidori AM, Diaz-Cano S, Monson JP, *et al.* CT and MR imaging of the adrenal glands in ACTH-independent Cushing syndrome. *Radiographics*, 2004; 24: 435–52.
13. Krebs TL, Wagner BJ. The adrenal gland. Radiologic-pathologic correlation. *Magn Reson Imaging Clin N Am*, 1997; 5: 127–46.
14. Patel SM, Lingam R, Beaconsfield TI, Tran TL, Brown B. Role of radiology in the management of primary aldosteronism. *Radiographics*, 2007; 27: 1145–57.
15. Korobkin M, Francis IR. Adrenal imaging. *Semin Ultrasound CT MRI*, 1995; 16: 317–30.
16. Dunnick NR, Leight GS, Jr, Roubidoux MA, Leder RA, Paulson E, Kurylo L. CT in the diagnosis of primary aldosteronism: sensitivity in 29 patients. *Am J Roentgenol*, 1993; 160: 321–4.
17. Ikeda D, Francis I, Glazer G, Amendola M, Gross M, Aisen A. The distinction of adrenal tumours and hyperplasia in patients with primary hyperaldosteronism: comparison of scintigraphy, CT and MR imaging. *Am J Roentgenol*, 1989; 153: 301–6.
18. Kawashima A, Sandler CM, Fishman EK, Charnsangavej C, Yasumori K, Honda H, *et al.* Spectrum of CT findings in nonmalignant disease of the adrenal gland. *Radiographics*, 1998; 18: 393–412.
19. Nwariaku FE, Miller BS, Auchus R, Holt S, Watumull L, Dolmatch B, *et al.* Primary hyperaldosteronism. Effect of adrenal vein sampling on surgical outcome. *Arch Surg*, 2009; 141: 497–503.

20. Elsayes KM, Mukundan G, Narra VR, Lewis JS Jr, Shirkhoda A, Farooki A, *et al.* Adrenal masses:MR imaging features with pathologic correlation. *Radiographics,* 2004; 24: S73-S86.
21. Seidenwurm DJ, Elmer EB, Kaplan LM, Williams EK, Morris DG, Hoffman AR, *et al.* Metastases to the adrenal gland and development of Addison's disease. *Cancer,* 1984; 54: 552–7.
22. Francis I, Korobkin M. Phaeochromocytoma. *Radiol Clin N Am,* 1996; 34: 1101–12.
23. Chrisoulidou A, Kaltsas G, Ilias I, Grossman A. The diagnosis and management of malignant phaeochromocytoma and paraganglioma. *Endocr Relat Cancer,* 2007; 14: 569–85.
24. Raisanen J, Shapiro B, Glazer GM, Desai S, Sisson JC. Plasma catecholamines in phaeochromocytoma: effect of urographic contrast media. *Am J Roentgenol,* 1984; 143: 43–6.
25. Mukherjee JJ, Peppercorn PD, Reznek RH, Patel V, Kaltsas G, Besser M, *et al.* Pheochromocytoma: effect of non-ionic contrast medium in CT on circulating catecholamine levels. *Radiology,* 1997; 202: 227–31.
26. Bessel-Browne R, Malley ME. CT of pheochromocytoma and paraganglioma: risk of adverse events with IV administration of nonionic contrast material. *Am J Roentgenol,* 2007; 188: 970–4.
27. Baid S, Lai E, Wesley, Ling A, Timmers HJ, Adams KT, *et al.* Brief communication: radiographic contrast infusion and catecholamine release in patients with pheochromocytoma. *Ann Intern Med,* 2009; 150: 27–32.
28. Gilfeather M, Woodward P. MR imaging of the adrenal glands and kidneys. *Semin Ultrasound CT MRI,* 1998; 19: 53–66.
29. Bilal MM, Brown JJ. MR imaging of renal and adrenal masses in children. *MRI Clin N Am,* 1997; 5: 179–97.
30. Boland G; Blake M, Hahn P, Mayo-Smith W. Incidental adrenal lesions: principles, techniques, and algorithms for imaging characterization. *Radiology,* 2008; 249: 756–75.
31. Boland GW, Lee ML, Gazelle GS, Halpern EF, McNicholas MJM, Mueller PR. Characterization of adrenal masses using unenhanced CT: an analysis of the CT literature. *Am J Roentgenol,* 1998; 171: 201–4.
32. Korobkin M, TJ Giordano, FJ Brodeur, Francis IR, Siegelman ES, Quint LE, *et al.* Adrenal adenomas: relationship between histological lipid and CT and MR findings. *Radiology,* 1996; 200: 743–7.
33. Francis IR, Korobkin M. Incidentally discovered adrenal masses. *MRI Clin N Am,* 1997; 5: 147–64.
34. Korobkin M, Brodeur FJ, Francis IR, Quint LE, Dunnick NR, Londy F. CT time-attenuation washout curves of adrenal adenomas and nonadenomas. *Am J Roentgenol,* 1998; 170: 747–52.
35. Israel G, Korobkin M, Wand C, Hecht E, Krinsky G. Comparison of unenhanced CT and chemical shift MRI in evaluating lipid-rich adrenal adenomas. *Am J Roentgenol,* 2004; 183: 215–19.
36. Faria J, Goldman S, Szejnfeld J, Melo H, Kater C, Kenney P, *et al.* Adrenal masses: characterization with in vivo proton MR spectroscopy–initial experience. *Radiology,* 2007; 245: 788–97.
37. Pender SM, Boland GW, Lee MJ. The incidental nonhyperfunctioning adrenal mass: an imaging algorithm for characterization. *Clin Radiol,* 1998; 53: 796–804.
38. Rozenblit A, Morehouse HT, Amis ES. Cystic adrenal lesions: CT features. *Radiology,* 1996; 201: 541–8.
39. Martinez-Aguayo A, Rocha A, Rojas N, García C, Parra R, Lagos M, *et al.* Testicular adrenal rest tumors and Leydic and Seroli cell function in boys with classical congenital adrenal hyperplasia. *J Clin Endocrinol Metab,* 2007; 92: 4583–9.
40. Avila NA, Premkumar A, Shawker TS, Jones JV, Laue L, Cutler GB. Testicular adrenal rest tissue in congenital adrenal hyperplasia: findings at gray-scale and color Doppler US. *Radiology,* 1996; 198: 99–104.

Further reading

Blake MA, Boland GWL, eds. *Adrenal Imaging.* Totowa, NJ: Springer, 2009.

5.2

Adrenal surgery

Sabapathy P. Balasubramanian,
Barney J. Harrison

Introduction

The indications for adrenal surgery and techniques employed have evolved significantly in the last 20 years. The need for adrenalectomy has increased due to:

- increased use of abdominal CT/MRI that identifies adrenal incidentalomas
- the more frequent biochemical diagnosis of subclinical hormonal syndromes.

The operative approach has changed with the availability of minimal access surgery; this has significant advantages for the patient in terms of reduced morbidity and faster recovery (1).

Despite these changes, the fundamental principles of adrenal surgery have remained unchanged:

- Biochemical investigations should be performed *before* localization studies and/or surgical intervention.
- Biopsy is rarely indicated in the investigation of adrenal lesions and is confined to confirmation of adrenal metastasis, suspected lymphoma, tuberculosis, or histoplasmosis. It should only be performed *after* biochemical assessment has excluded phaeochromocytoma.
- Close collaboration with colleagues in endocrinology, biochemistry, and radiology is essential for good outcomes.

This chapter will focus on the surgical aspects of treatment. The pathology of adrenal disease, details of biochemical and radiological investigations, and the nonsurgical modalities of treatment are covered elsewhere.

Historical perspective

The existence of the adrenal glands has been known for several centuries but its importance as an endocrine organ was only highlighted in the 19th century after the description by Thomas Addison of the clinical features of patients with adrenal insufficiency. The first reported adrenalectomy was performed by Knowsley-Thornton, in London in 1889, for a 9-kg tumour where the adrenal and the kidney were removed via an anterior transperitoneal operation. The patient survived the operation despite significant postoperative sepsis. The posterior approach was initially described by Hugh Young, a urologist from Baltimore, who attempted this approach when he was unable to access the adrenals at laparotomy. Surgery for phaeochromocytomas, first performed successfully in 1926 by Cesar Roux in Switzerland, was considered a formidable challenge and associated with a high mortality until the advent of adrenergic receptor blockers in the 1960s (2).

Adrenal surgery underwent a rapid transformation with the advent of laparoscopic adrenalectomy in the early 1990s. First described by surgeons in Japan and Canada, it was initially adopted for small tumours and soon became rapidly accepted as the gold standard of treatment for most adrenal tumours.

Applied anatomy

The adrenal glands are located in the retroperitoneum in relation to the upper poles of the kidneys at the levels of T11–T12 vertebrae (Fig. 5.2.1). The right adrenal is pyramidal in shape and located partly behind the inferior vena cava with the base of the pyramid abutting the upper pole of the right kidney. The left adrenal gland is semilunar in shape and situated anteromedial to the upper pole of the left kidney. The adrenal glands are enclosed in a layer of fat within Gerota's fascia. During adrenalectomy for Cushing's disease, the surgeon will remove the adrenal glands with their fatty envelope to ensure complete removal of hyperfunctioning adrenocortical tissue. The close relationship of the adrenal gland to the inferior vena cava and liver on the right side and the aorta, spleen, stomach, and tail of the pancreas on the left side requires special care during dissection. Clinicians should also be aware of ectopic adrenal tissue or adrenal rests which may exist along the path of testicular descent in males and near the broad ligament and uterus in females. This can be a source of continued cortisol production after bilateral adrenalectomy.

Superior, middle, and inferior adrenal arteries arise from the inferior phrenic, aorta, and renal arteries respectively. The middle adrenal artery is the most variable and not uncommonly absent. Venous drainage is usually via a single, large vein which drains into the inferior vena cava on the right, and the upper border of the renal vein on the left side. The vein on the right side is short and if torn or inadequately secured during surgery can cause profuse bleeding from the vena cava. Additional accessory veins are sometimes found draining into the inferior phrenic veins, renal, and portal veins. The lymphatic drainage of the adrenal glands is to adjacent para-aortic and paracaval lymph nodes.

The adrenal gland has an outer cortex derived from the embryonic mesoderm and an inner medulla derived from ectoderm.

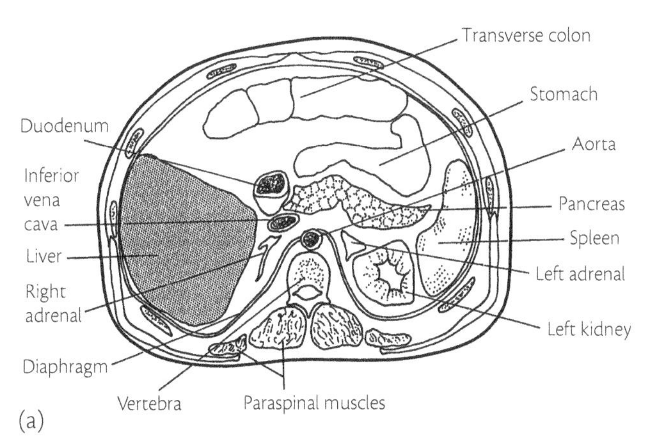

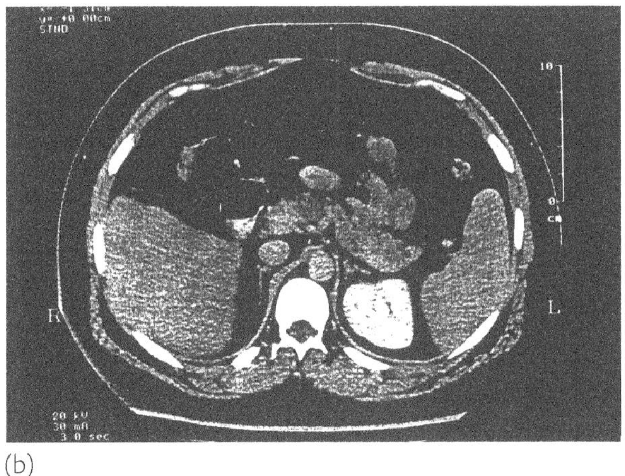

Fig. 5.2.1 (a,b) Normal-appearing right and left adrenal glands and their anatomical relationships on cross-sectional imaging at the level of T12–L1 vertebrae.

The cortex in turn is divided into three layers: the outer zona glomerulosa, the middle zona fasciculata, and the inner zona reticularis. These layers predominantly secrete aldosterone, cortisol, and sex steroids, respectively. The adrenal medulla is part of the sympathetic nervous system and functions as postganglionic neural tissue, secreting catecholamines and their metabolites.

Indications for surgery

ACTH-independent hypercortisolism The adrenal glands are the site of pathology in 15% of patients with hypercortisolism. Of these, adenoma (two-thirds) and carcinoma (one-thirds) are the usual causes. Rarely, other lesions such as bilateral nodular hyperplasia, primary pigmented nodular adrenal disease, and McCune–Albright syndrome are encountered (3). Surgery offers the potential for complete biochemical cure. Cushing's syndrome-related symptoms and signs can be expected to improve after surgery, although this can take from a few weeks to years (4). Surgery is also of benefit in patients with subclinical Cushing's syndrome. A recent randomized controlled trial of 45 patients compared surgery with nonintervention. Adrenalectomy resulted in significant 'improvement', not only of biochemical parameters, but also associated medical conditions such as diabetes, hypertension, hyperlipidaemia, and obesity (5).

ACTH-dependent hypercortisolism Pituitary tumours are the commonest (70%) cause of cortisol excess. The primary treatment of the pituitary lesion is trans-sphenoidal excision, associated with recurrence rates of up to 10% at 5 years and 20% at 10 years (6). Although persistent or recurrent Cushing's disease can be treated with reoperative pituitary surgery or pituitary radiotherapy, bilateral laparoscopic adrenalectomy is an alternative that provides rapid control of the hormonal syndrome with low morbidity (3, 6). In patients with ectopic ACTH secretion, the primary source of ACTH may not be identified. In such patients and in patients where the primary source is unresectable due to extensive or metastatic disease, bilateral adrenalectomy may be indicated to control symptoms of cortisol excess (7).

Primary hyperaldosteronism Adrenalectomy is indicated in unilateral disease (Conn's syndrome) and in some patients with bilateral disease when there is evidence of unilateral dominant secretion on selective venous sampling. Adrenal morphology on CT/MRI may be inconclusive or misleading as the adrenals are often nodular in hypertensive patients and 'obvious nodules' are not always the source of hormone hypersecretion. The key issues for the surgeon are that unilateral disease is distinguished from bilateral disease, and the laterality is clearly defined in all cases prior to operation. This is achieved in many centres by the performance of selective venous sampling before a decision is made to proceed with adrenalectomy (8). Laparoscopic adrenalectomy for unilateral disease results in significant long-term benefits. Hypertension is cured in one-third of patients and in the majority of the remainder there is a significant reduction in the dosage and number of antihypertensive medications (9, 10).

Phaeochromocytoma Surgery is indicated in patients with phaeochromocytoma/extra-adrenal chromaffin tumours (paraganglioma). Malignant phaeochromocytomas are very rare and account for less than 10% of all cases. Despite earlier concerns, the laparoscopic approach is now considered safe for patients with phaeochromocytoma (11). Recurrent phaeochromocytoma and extra adrenal phaeochromocytomas (paragangliomas) can also be effectively treated with surgery (Fig. 5.2.2).

Adrenocortical cancer (primary) Surgery is indicated in adrenal tumours that are potentially or overtly malignant. A 'curative resection' has a favourable impact on outcome in this uncommon disease, which has an overall 5-year survival of 38% (12). Clinical features that indicate an increased risk of malignancy include young age, rapid onset of hormonal symptoms/signs, pain, mixed hormonal secretion, virilizing or feminizing features, and other organ metastases. CT features of malignancy include large tumour size, heterogeneous tumour with bleeding or necrosis, rapidly enlarging tumour on serial scans, invasion into adjacent structures, and regional lymph node enlargement. An MRI scan can sometimes help in evaluating lesions that are indeterminate (lesions with a density of more than 10 Hounsfield units on unenhanced CT). Features of malignancy on MRI include reduced fat content, isointensity to liver on T1 images, intermediate to moderate intensity on T2 images, and enhancement after gadolinium contrast with slow washout. Surgery should be considered in patients with locally advanced or recurrent tumours as resection may improve survival and help in the control of hormonal symptoms (13).

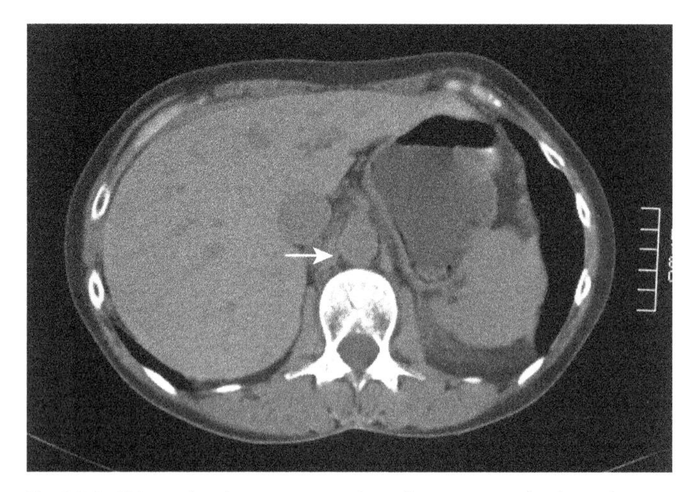

Fig. 5.2.2 CT scan showing a recurrent phaeochromocytoma (as shown by the tip of the arrow) in a patient with von-Hippel–Lindau syndrome who had a bilateral adrenalectomy 20 years prior to her current presentation.

Adrenal metastases Patients with recently diagnosed cancer or a past history of cancer have a 50% chance of an incidentally discovered adrenal lesion being a metastasis (14). Adrenal metastases most frequently arise from primary malignancy in the lung, kidneys, gastrointestinal tract, and melanoma (15). Adrenalectomy in selected patients with isolated adrenal metastasis may be associated with an improvement in survival (15, 16).

Incidentalomas An adrenal lesion detected on cross-sectional imaging performed for an unrelated indication requires thorough biochemical and radiological assessment. Surgery should be considered in all patients with functioning lesions (clinical and subclinical syndromes) and patients with malignant or potentially malignant tumours. The size of an incidentaloma correlates with the risk of malignancy— less than 2% in lesions smaller than 4 cm in size, compared with 25% in lesions larger than 6 cm in size (17). Surgery is indicated for all lesions larger than 6 cm in size, while nonfunctioning lesions smaller than 4 cm may be managed conservatively. For NIH guidelines from 2002 state that surgery or observation are reasonable options. However, in many centres, an incidentaloma larger than 4cm in size is an indication for surgery. Decision making in such cases is also based on considerations such as radiological features, increasing tumour size on sequential scans, and patient choice (17).

Rare lesions Adrenal cysts may be neoplastic (cystic degeneration of cortical or medullary neoplasms) or non-neoplastic, the latter being very rare. Non-neoplastic cysts may be lined by an endothelial or epithelial layer or simply fibrous tissue (as in pseudocysts). Large adrenal cysts, if symptomatic, can be successfully treated by image-guided aspiration alone. This is done after exclusion of a cystic phaeochromocytoma by biochemical tests. Recurrent cysts that are symptomatic may be considered for excision both to treat symptoms and to exclude cystic neoplasms.

Virilizing/feminizing syndromes result from adrenocortical tumours that secrete sex hormones. Cosecretion of androgens/androgen precursors in conjunction with corticosteroids indicates an increased risk of adrenocortical cancer. Surgery is curative in benign tumours.

Other rare lesions in adults that require surgery include adrenal sarcoma and medullary tumours such as ganglioneuroma, ganglioneuroblastoma, and neuroblastoma. Ganglioneuroma is a benign tumour that may present with symptoms of catecholamine excess. Ganglioneuroblastoma and neuroblastomas are malignant tumours which occur more frequently in children. These conditions are amenable to surgery, but patients with neuroblastoma often need chemotherapy and carry a poor prognosis.

Adrenalectomy—perioperative management

I would like to see the day when somebody would be appointed surgeon somewhere who had no hands, for the operative part is the least part of the work.

(Harvey Cushing)

General measures

All patients require a thorough preoperative clinical assessment to determine comorbidities that may need optimization prior to surgery. A full blood count, renal and liver function tests, clotting screen, and blood grouping are performed. Prophylaxis against venous thromboembolism with low molecular weight heparin (especially in patients with hypercortisolism) is given unless specifically contraindicated. For patients with large tumours/phaeochromocytoma, the availability of critical care facilities in the early postoperative period is recommended.

Specific measures

Patients with hypercortisolism Hypertension, diabetes, and ischaemic heart disease are commonly associated with cortisol excess; measures should be taken to reduce their adverse impact on surgical outcomes. A single dose of prophylactic antibiotics is given at induction because of the increased risk of wound infection. Patients with cortisol excess have fragile skin and special care is required to avoid soft tissue injury during patient movement, positioning on the operating table, and during surgery. Adhesive dressings and sticky tape are best avoided in this situation. All patients should receive perioperative hydrocortisone before surgery. Our practice is to give 100 mg intramuscular hydrocortisone 6-hourly starting on the morning of surgery, continuing with parenteral administration at a reducing dose until the patient can take steroids orally (tds). On the third postoperative day, the evening dose of hydrocortisone (20 mg) is omitted and basal cortisol levels measured the following morning prior to the first daytime dose. In patients who have undergone bilateral adrenalectomy, undetectable cortisol levels confirm cure. These patients require lifelong glucocorticoid and mineralocorticoid replacement therapy. In patients who have undergone adrenalectomy for unilateral disease, low levels of cortisol mandate that a short synacthen test is performed to identify contralateral adrenal hypofunction (observed in 75% of patients). These patients require glucocorticoid replacement for a variable period of time ranging from months to years until recovery of the HPA axis is confirmed on biochemistry. Post operative in hospital care is provided in conjunction with endocrinologists according to clearly defined local protocols, robust arrangements should be in place for subsequent follow-up. Patients on steroid replacement must be counselled on the need for compliance with steroid medication and the need for increased steroid requirements during acute illness. The patient should be given an emergency 'steroid' pack and a card detailing their steroid regimen.

Patients with primary hyperaldosteronism Hypokalaemia is corrected preoperatively. Aldosterone antagonists are stopped postoperatively followed by regular monitoring of blood pressure and appropriate modification of antihypertensive medications. Preoperative biochemical screening sometimes identifies concomitant cortisol secretion in patients with aldosteronomas. For these patients, appropriate perioperative steroid cover and postoperative testing for contralateral adrenal suppression is performed. Plasma aldosterone concentrations and renin activity are also measured in the follow up period to confirm biochemical cure.

Patients with phaeochromocytoma The principles of preoperative preparation of a patient with phaeochromocytoma include 'maximum tolerated' α-blockade and adequate hydration. In our practice, patients are started on phenoxybenzamine (10 or 20 mg twice daily) at diagnosis and the dose is increased until symptoms are controlled. Patients are admitted to the ward a week prior to surgery. Lying and standing blood pressure is monitored at 6-hourly intervals. Each dose of phenoxybenzamine is increased by 10 mg every 48 h until symptomatic postural hypotension and nasal stuffiness occurs. β-blockers are only used to limit tachycardia, and only when α-blockade has been achieved. An adequate oral fluid intake is encouraged and patients are prescribed 1–2 litres of intravenous fluids over 12 h prior to the operation. Intraoperative invasive monitoring of central venous pressure, arterial blood pressure and the judicious use of vasodilators and inotropes by an experienced anaesthetist minimizes the risk of cardiovascular instability during surgery. In the immediate postoperative period (up to several hours), patients should be monitored for hypoglycaemia and appropriately treated.

Consent for operation

As with any operative procedure, it is the duty of the surgeon to ensure that the patient scheduled to undergo adrenalectomy understands the indications, implications, and risks of surgery (see below). In primary hyperaldosteronism and subclinical Cushing's syndrome, the alternative (nonsurgical) options should be discussed so that a fully informed choice can be made by the patient with appropriate guidance from the surgeon. Patients should be made aware that some clinical features of their illness (e.g. hypertension in Conn's syndrome and features of Cushing's syndrome) may persist after surgery. Conversion to open surgery may be required with the laparoscopic approach in up to 10% of patients. This is a consequence of intraoperative complications or technical limitations of the laparoscopic approach, the most significant predictor of conversion being a large tumour size (18).

Surgery

Laparoscopy versus open surgery

Laparoscopic adrenalectomy should be the standard surgical approach to most adrenal lesions (Fig. 5.2.3). This is due to the distinct advantages seen with laparoscopy in large observational studies. The advantages include reduction in postoperative pain, blood loss, wound infection, hospital stay, and time to return to normal activity.

The choice of an open or laparoscopic surgical approach for the 'potentially' malignant adrenal mass is controversial (19). Proponents of the open approach quote the risk of peritoneal seeding and local recurrence after laparoscopic adrenalectomy (20).

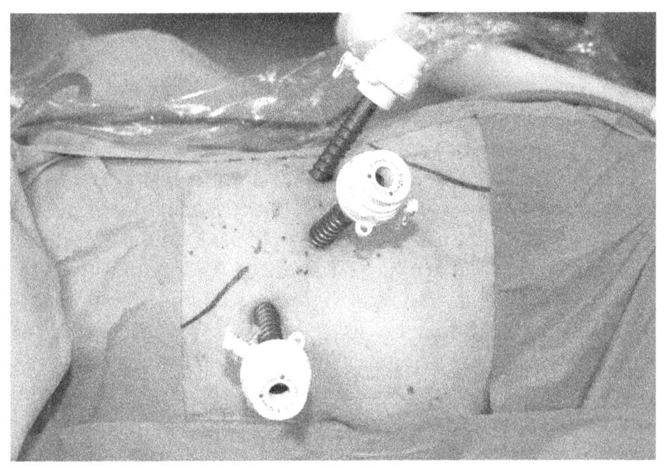

(a)

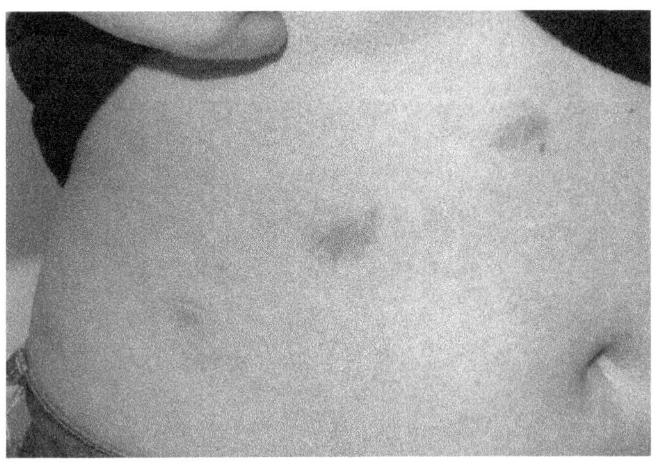

(b)

Fig. 5.2.3 Transperitoneal laparoscopic right adrenalectomy. (a) The position of laparoscopic ports and the surface marking of the costal margin as an interrupted line and the iliac crest as a solid line. (b) The postoperative photograph showing scars at port sites.

In contrast, laparoscopic surgery is associated with lower postoperative morbidity (21) and in selected patients has the same potential for complete resection as open surgery (22). Our practice is to use an open approach for patients with obvious radiological features of malignancy and lesions larger than 10 cm in size. The latter tumours have a significant risk of cancer and are often difficult to mobilize without capsular rupture at laparoscopy (23). Some surgeons who perform laparoscopic adrenalectomy for large tumours make use of a hand-assist device which enables direct handling and aids the dissection of large tumours (24).

Anterior, lateral, and posterior

Both open and laparoscopic procedures can be performed via the anterior, lateral, or posterior approach. In the 'open' era, the approach adopted was based on the underlying pathology, unilateral or bilateral disease, and the likelihood of ectopic or extra-adrenal lesions. The posterior approach was an option for small to medium sized tumours thought to be benign. The lateral approach was adopted in the case of large unilateral lesions as this approach is suited to a thoracic extension (thoracoabdominal approach) when a large malignant tumour infiltrates the diaphragm and/or vena cava.

The anterior transperitoneal approach was used most frequently, in patients with bilateral tumours, or in patients with malignancy when abdominal exploration for metastatic disease was required. Preoperative imaging with CT/MRI has changed the decision-making process in many of these cases.

The approach in the 'laparoscopic' era is principally determined more by the surgeon's experience and his/her familiarity with a specific procedure. The transperitoneal (Fig. 5.2.3) and the posterior retroperitoneal approach (Fig. 5.2.4) are most commonly used. No significant difference in clinical outcomes have been demonstrated in randomized controlled trials of these two approaches (25, 26); surgeons familiar with both techniques base their choice upon specific patient characteristics. In patients with bilateral tumours and/or previous intra-abdominal surgery, the posterior approach would be preferred and in patients with large tumours the anterior approach has the advantage of a larger working space. Table 5.2.1 gives a flavour of the approaches used in our practice in different clinical situations and their underlying rationale.

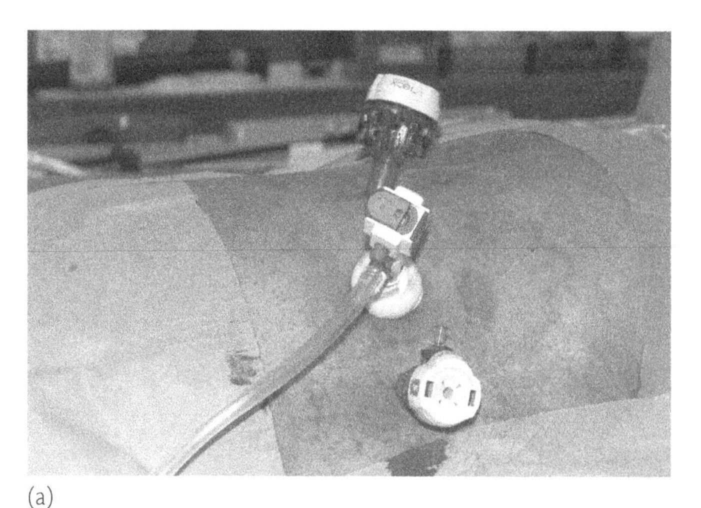

(a)

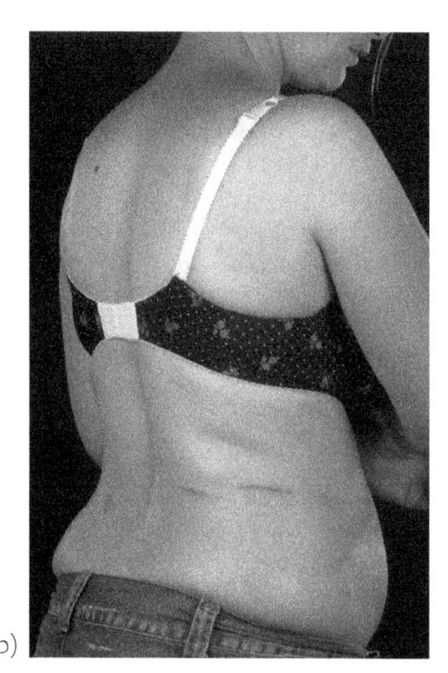

(b)

Fig. 5.2.4 Posterior retroperitoneoscopic right adrenalectomy. (a) The position of the laparoscopic ports for this procedure. The right side is the superior end of the patient. (b) The postoperative photograph showing scars at port sites.

General principles

The key steps to performing adrenalectomy are correct positioning of the patient, use of appropriate port sites or incisions, identification of the anatomical landmarks and careful dissection of the adrenal gland. The term 'radical adrenalectomy' is often used to describe the surgical approach in adrenal malignancy. The nature and extent of this procedure is poorly defined. An *en bloc* resection of the entire adrenal gland, periadrenal fat, and involved lymph nodes is usually performed. Occasionally, resection of involved adjacent organs such as the liver and kidney may be required for complete macroscopic clearance. Cortical-sparing adrenalectomy can be performed in patients with bilateral (i.e. genetically determined) phaeochromocytoma. These patients would otherwise undergo bilateral (total) adrenalectomy, which necessitates lifelong steroid replacement and places them at risk of adrenal insufficiency. Inadvertently retained adrenal medulla in patients treated by cortex-sparing surgery can however result in recurrent disease. Other proposed indications for subtotal adrenalectomy include patients who have previously undergone contralateral adrenalectomy and those with Conn's adenomas where tumours are small, benign, and eccentrically located (27). The tumour is excised with surrounding normal tissue aiming to preserve sufficient adrenal tissue to preserve cortical function.

Complications

General complications of adrenalectomy include venous thromboembolism, and respiratory and cardiac failure. The reported overall postoperative mortality of adrenalectomy is up to 2.8% (28). Specific risks of adrenalectomy are:

- Those related to surgical access and exposure—wound infection, delayed healing, wound dehiscence (increased risk in patients with hypercortisolism), hernia formation, and injury to adjacent viscera such as the bowel, kidneys, great vessels, diaphragm, and liver on the right side; spleen and pancreas on the left side.
- Those consequent to incomplete removal of tumour/ gland, and rupture of the tumour capsule. Incomplete removal of adrenal tissue during bilateral adrenalectomy for Cushing's disease can result in persistent or recurrent hypercortisolism (29). Rupture of the tumour capsule in phaeochromocytoma (30) and in adrenal cancers (20) can result in local tumour recurrence.
- Those secondary to perioperative hormonal dysfunction. Patients with phaeochromocytoma are at risk of potentially fatal intraoperative blood pressure fluctuations, and postoperative hypotension and hypoglycaemia. The risks of contralateral adrenal suppression in patients who have undergone unilateral adrenalectomy for Cushing's syndrome and the risks of acute steroid deficiency after unilateral/ bilateral adrenalectomy are outlined above.

Summary

Adrenal surgery is required for the treatment for syndromes of hormonal excess arising from the adrenal gland and adrenal neoplasms. A multidisciplinary approach, careful preoperative planning, and an experienced surgeon are essential for a good outcome.

Table 5.2.1 Surgical approaches in adrenalectomy

Surgical procedure/approach	Clinical situation	Rationale
Lateral transperitoneal laparoscopic approach	Unilateral lesions >5 cm in size	Large working space provided by the transperitoneal approach would be an advantage.
Lateral transperitoneal or posterior retroperitoneal approach	Bilateral adrenalectomy for Cushing's disease or familial phaeochromocytoma	Laparoscopy has distinct advantages. The trans or retroperitoneal approach would depend on surgeon's preference and familiarity. The retroperitoneal approach avoids need for repositioning the patient intraoperatively.
Posterior retroperitoneal approach	Tumours <5 cm, history of multiple previous upper abdominal operations	Smaller tumours are ideal for the posterior approach. Intraperitoneal adhesions from previous surgery can be avoided.
Anterior open/thoracoabdominal approach	Large (>10 cm) adrenal tumour	This facilitates *en bloc* resection of adjacent organs if necessary.

Several areas in the surgical treatment of adrenal disease are still in evolution. These include

- the appropriateness of laparoscopic surgery in suspected or proven adrenal malignancy
- the indications for specific surgical approaches—transperitoneal versus retroperitoneal versus open
- the use of cortical sparing/ subtotal adrenalectomy
- the role of adrenalectomy in patients with adrenal metastasis.

The rarity of adrenal disease, the heterogeneity of clinical conditions, and the multifactorial influences on outcome will make it difficult (if not impossible) for surgical strategies to be based on evidence from randomized trials. Good quality data from observational series and the insight and judgement of experienced endocrine surgeons should be considered an acceptable alternative.

References

1. Linos DA, Stylopoulos N, Boukis M, Souvatzoglou A, Raptis S. Anterior, posterior, or laparoscopic approach for the management of adrenal diseases? *Am J Surg*, 1997; **173**: 120–5.
2. Welbourn RB. *The History of Endocrine Surgery*. New York: Praeger Publishers, 1990: 385.
3. Newell-Price J, Bertagna X, Grossman AB, Nieman LK. Cushing's syndrome. *Lancet*, 2006; **367**: 1605–17.
4. Sippel RS, Elaraj DM, Kebebew E, Lindsay S, Tyrrell JB, Duh QY. Waiting for change: symptom resolution after adrenalectomy for Cushing's syndrome. *Surgery*, 2008; **144**: 1054–60; discussion 1060–1.
5. Toniato A, Merante-Boschin I, Opocher G, Pelizzo MR, Schiavi F, Ballotta E. Surgical versus conservative management for subclinical Cushing syndrome in adrenal incidentalomas: a prospective randomized study. *Ann Surg*, 2009; **249**: 388–91.
6. Biller BM, Grossman AB, Stewart PM, Melmed S, Bertagna X, Bertherat J, *et al.* Treatment of adrenocorticotropin-dependent Cushing's syndrome: a consensus statement. *J Clin Endocrinol Metab*, 2008; **93**: 2454–62.
7. Porterfield JR, Thompson GB, Young WF Jr, Chow JT, Fryrear RS, van Heerden JA, *et al.* Surgery for Cushing's syndrome: an historical review and recent ten-year experience. *World J Surg*, 2008; **32**: 659–77.
8. Rossi GP, Seccia TM, Pessina AC. Primary aldosteronism: part II: subtype differentiation and treatment. *J Nephrol*, 2008; **21**: 455–62.
9. Rossi GP, Bolognesi M, Rizzoni D, Seccia TM, Piva A, Porteri E, *et al.* Vascular remodeling and duration of hypertension predict outcome of adrenalectomy in primary aldosteronism patients. *Hypertension*, 2008; **51**: 1366–71.
10. Pang TC, Bambach C, Monaghan JC, Sidhu SB, Bune A, Delbridge LW, *et al.* Outcomes of laparoscopic adrenalectomy for hyperaldosteronism. *ANZ J Surg*, 2007; **77**: 768–73.
11. Toniato A, Boschin IM, Opocher G, Guolo A, Pelizzo M, Mantero F. Is the laparoscopic adrenalectomy for pheochromocytoma the best treatment? *Surgery*, 2007; **141**: 723–7.
12. Icard P, Goudet P, Charpenay C, Andreassian B, Carnaille B, Chapuis Y, *et al.* Adrenocortical carcinomas: surgical trends and results of a 253-patient series from the French Association of Endocrine Surgeons study group. *World J Surg*, 2001; **25**: 891–7.
13. Allolio B, Fassnacht M. Clinical review: Adrenocortical carcinoma: clinical update. *J Clin Endocrinol Metab*, 2006; **91**: 2027–37.
14. Lenert JT, Barnett CC Jr, Kudelka AP, Sellin RV, Gagel RF, Prieto VG, *et al.* Evaluation and surgical resection of adrenal masses in patients with a history of extra-adrenal malignancy. *Surgery*, 2001; **130**: 1060–7.
15. Kim SH, Brennan MF, Russo P, Burt ME, Coit DG. The role of surgery in the treatment of clinically isolated adrenal metastasis. *Cancer*, 1998; **82**: 389–94.
16. Gittens PR Jr, Solish AF, Trabulsi EJ. Surgical management of metastatic disease to the adrenal gland. *Semin Oncol*, 2008; **35**: 172–6.
17. NIH state-of-the-science statement on management of the clinically inapparent adrenal mass ('incidentaloma'). *NIH Consens State Sci Statements*, 2002; **19**: 1–25.
18. Shen ZJ, Chen SW, Wang S, Jin XD, Chen J, Zhu Y, *et al.* Predictive factors for open conversion of laparoscopic adrenalectomy: a 13-year review of 456 cases. *J Endourol*, 2007; **21**: 1333–7.
19. Harrison BJ. Surgery of adrenocortical cancer. *Ann Endocrinol (Paris)*, 2009; **70**: 195–6.
20. Gonzalez RJ, Shapiro S, Sarlis N, Vassilopoulou-Sellin R, Perrier ND, Evans DB, *et al.* Laparoscopic resection of adrenal cortical carcinoma: a cautionary note. *Surgery*, 2005; **138**: 1078–85; discussion 1085–6.
21. Lee J, El-Tamer M, Schifftner T, Turrentine FE, Henderson WG, Khuri S, *et al.* Open and laparoscopic adrenalectomy: analysis of the National Surgical Quality Improvement Program. *J Am Coll Surg*, 2008; **206**: 953–9; discussion 959–61.
22. McCauley LR, Nguyen MM. Laparoscopic radical adrenalectomy for cancer: long-term outcomes. *Curr Opin Urol*, 2008; **18**: 134–8.
23. Sturgeon C, Kebebew E. Laparoscopic adrenalectomy for malignancy. *Surg Clin North Am*, 2004; **84**: 755–74.
24. Liao CH, Chueh SC, Lai MK, Hsiao PJ, Chen J. Laparoscopic adrenalectomy for potentially malignant adrenal tumors greater than 5 centimeters. *J Clin Endocrinol Metab*, 2006; **91**: 3080–3.
25. Fernandez-Cruz L, Saenz A, Benarroch G, Astudillo E, Taura P, Sabater L. Laparoscopic unilateral and bilateral adrenalectomy for Cushing's syndrome. Transperitoneal and retroperitoneal approaches. *Ann Surg*, 1996; **224**: 727–34; discussion 734–6.
26. Rubinstein M, Gill IS, Aron M, Kilciler M, Meraney AM, Finelli A, *et al.* Prospective, randomized comparison of transperitoneal versus retroperitoneal laparoscopic adrenalectomy. *J Urol*, 2005; **174**: 442–5; discussion 445.
27. Walz MK. Extent of adrenalectomy for adrenal neoplasm: cortical sparing (subtotal) versus total adrenalectomy. *Surg Clin North Am*, 2004; **84**: 743–53.

28. Turrentine FE, Henderson WG, Khuri SF, Schifftner TL, Inabnet WB 3rd, El-Tamer M, *et al.* Adrenalectomy in veterans affairs and selected university medical centers: results of the patient safety in surgery study. *J Am Coll Surg*, 2007; **204**: 1273–83.
29. Kemink L, Hermus A, Pieters G, Benraad T, Smals A, Kloppenborg P. Residual adrenocortical function after bilateral adrenalectomy for pituitary-dependent Cushing's syndrome. *J Clin Endocrinol Metab*, 1992; **75**: 1211–4.
30. Li ML, Fitzgerald PA, Price DC, Norton JA. Iatrogenic pheochromocytomatosis: a previously unreported result of laparoscopic adrenalectomy. *Surgery*, 2001; **130**: 1072–7.

5.3

Adrenal incidentaloma

Massimo Terzolo

Introduction

Adrenal incidentaloma is an adrenal mass that is discovered serendipitously with a radiological examination performed for indications unrelated to adrenal disease (1). The incidental discovery of an adrenal mass has become an increasingly common problem, because of the widespread use of ultrasonography, CT, and MRI in clinical practice (2, 3). These techniques have greatly improved their power of resolution over recent years, thereby increasing the possibility of detection of tiny adrenal lumps.

Several factors hinder a clear characterization of the phenomenon 'adrenal incidentaloma', which may be considered as a byproduct of technology applied to medical practice. Adrenal incidentaloma is not a single pathological entity and the likelihood of any specific diagnosis depends both on the circumstances of discovery and the applied definition of incidentaloma. Unfortunately, published reports are inconsistent in applying inclusion and exclusion criteria for these various factors, making the results difficult to interpret. A further issue is the lack of specific clinical features of the patients carrying an adrenal incidentaloma.

Epidemiology

In autopsy series, the mean prevalence of clinically inapparent adrenal masses is about 2.0%, ranging from 1.0 to 8.7% (4). This variability reflects different definitions and also the difficulty in distinguishing larger nodules within adrenal hyperplasia from distinct adrenocortical adenomas. The mean prevalence of adrenal incidentalomas in CT scan series published from 1982 to 1994 was 0.64%, ranging from 0.35 to 1.9% (4). More recently, we have found a frequency of benign adrenal masses of 4.2% in middle-aged subjects who were enrolled in a screening programme of lung cancer (5). The frequency of incidental adrenal masses is up to 4.4% in patients with a clinical history of cancer and 50–75% of adrenal nodules diagnosed in such patients are metastases, since the adrenal gland is frequently involved by metastatic spread. Many malignancies can metastasize to the adrenals, most frequently lung cancer, breast cancer, kidney cancer, melanoma, and lymphoma (4).

Adrenal incidentalomas show different distribution in the population dependent on the patient's age and sex. In clinical reports, adrenal incidentalomas show a peak incidence between 50 and 60 years of age (4). This pattern could merely reflect a higher number of diagnostic procedures in these age decades or be the consequence of the ageing process of the adrenal glands, which may lead to increased formation of cortical nodules secondary to vascular changes (4). The frequency of adrenal incidentalomas is very low in childhood and adolescence (0.3–0.4% of all neoplasms in children). Unfortunately, the frequency of adrenocortical carcinoma within adrenal neoplasms in children is very high, about 80%. Adrenal cancer represents 1.3% of all malignancies in patients less than 20 years and frequency is higher in children under 6 years (4).

The sex distribution is characterized by a male to female ratio of 1:3 to 1:5. A higher prevalence of adrenal incidentalomas in women is likely to be partly explained by a referral bias (i.e. more imaging studies are done in women due to higher prevalence of biliary disease) as nonfunctioning adrenal adenomas occurred with comparable frequency in men and women in autopsy series (4).

Adrenal incidentalomas are more frequent in the Caucasian population and the right adrenal gland is affected in 50–60% of cases, the left one in 30–40%, while bilateral lesions are found in 10–15% (4). This right-side predominance reflects the fact that in most series adrenal masses were discovered by ultrasonography, which is less accurate in detecting masses on the left side (5). No side-related difference was reported in CT scan and autopsy series (4, 6).

Aetiology

Aetiology of adrenal incidentalomas includes either benign or malignant lesions. However, an adrenal incidentaloma is generally benign, being an adrenal adenoma in approximately 70% of cases (cortisol-secreting in 1–29%, aldosterone-secreting in 1.6–2.3%) (7). The frequency of phaeochromocytoma is estimated at 1.5–23% (7), that of adrenal cancer varies from 1.2% to 11% (7). The risk of an adrenal incidentaloma being an adrenal cancer is linearly related to the mass size, but this correlation is not apparent for metastases of extra-adrenal cancers (7). Other causes of adrenal incidentaloma are adrenal cysts, ganglioneuromas, myelolipomas, haematomas, and metastases of other malignancies. Moreover, adrenal lesions are found in inherited endocrine cancer syndromes (McCune–Albright syndrome, multiple endocrine neoplasia) and in insufficiently controlled congenital adrenal hyperplasia.

In a multi-institutional, retrospective survey performed in Italy including 1004 patients, of whom 380 underwent surgery, the most frequent pathological diagnoses were adrenocortical adenoma (52%), adrenocortical carcinoma (12%), phaeochromocytoma

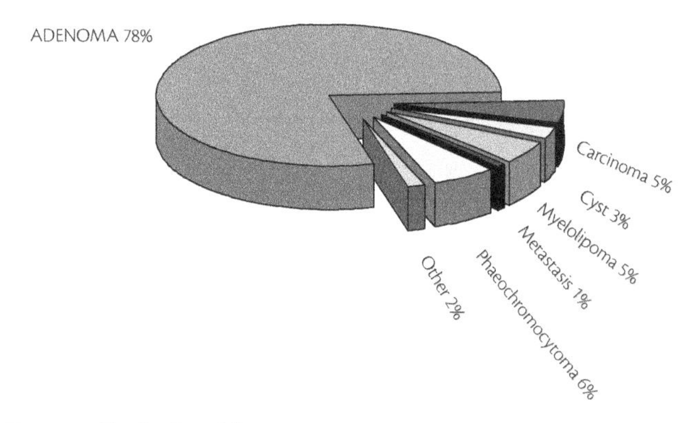

Fig. 5.3.1 Distribution of diagnoses among 181 patients with adrenal incidentaloma referred to San Luigi Hospital between 1991 and 2005.

(11%), and myelolipoma (8%) (6). Obviously, the frequency of adrenocortical carcinoma and phaeochromocytoma was likely to be overestimated in this surgical cohort. Between 1991 and 2005, we collected a series of 181 patients at our institution and found adrenal adenoma to be the by far most frequent tumour type (Fig. 5.3.1). Establishing the precise aetiology of adrenal incidentaloma is difficult because surgical series have usually a selection bias towards masses that have a higher probability of being malignant or functioning, while series collected in medical departments have the limitation that most diagnoses are ascertained only by imaging and clinical criteria.

Differential diagnosis

Adrenal incidentaloma is a growing public health challenge since the serendipitous detection of an adrenal mass increases with age and is expected to rise in populations that are getting older and have widespread access to ever improving radiological techniques (3). An impressive variety of tumoural and nontumoural lesions arising from the adrenal glands or extra-adrenal tissues may present as an adrenal mass detected serendipitously. Before embarking on a cumbersome diagnostic process, it is important to determine the most important questions the diagnostic work-up has to answer (Box 5.3.1). Following these concepts, it may be recommended to identify either primary adrenocortical carcinoma (ACC) or secondary adrenal malignancy (metastasis), and to rule out phaeochromocytoma (Fig. 5.3.2).

There is no doubt that ACC may significantly affect patients' health and there is sufficient evidence to recommend surgery whenever possible. MacFarlane has reported that patients with untreated ACC have a median survival of 3 months (8), while

Box 5.3.1 Key points on the differential diagnosis of adrenal incidentalomas

- Consider the potential of causing harm to the patient of a given tumour type
- Consider the prevalence in the general population of a given tumour type
- Consider the possibility of effective diagnosis and treatment of a given tumour type

(a)

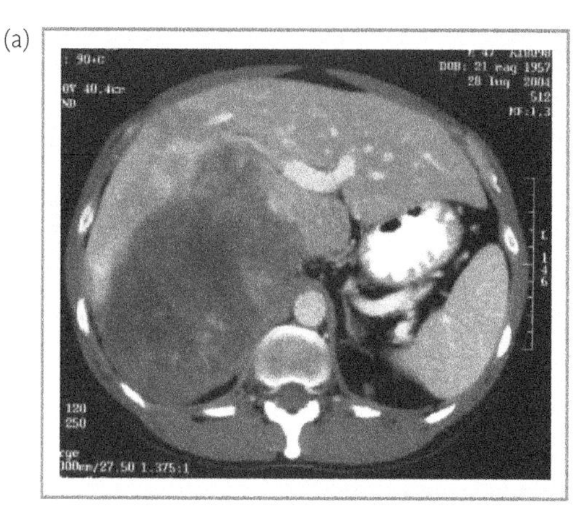

(b)

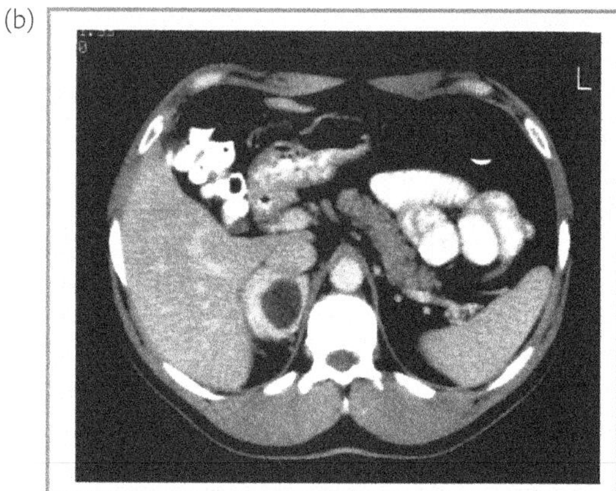

(c)

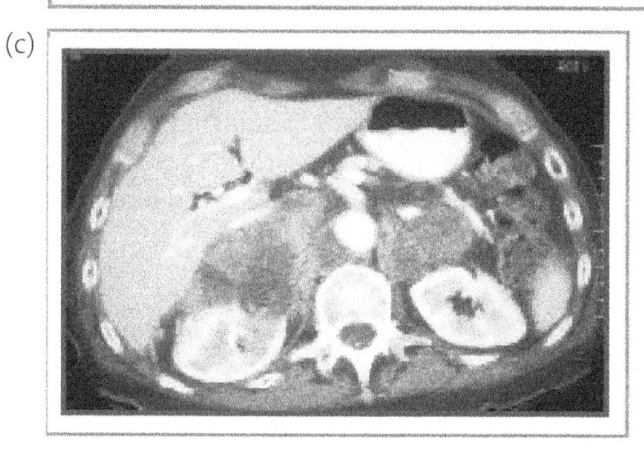

Fig. 5.3.2 CT images of (a) adrenocortical carcinoma, (b) phaeochromocytoma, and (c) metastases from extra-adrenal cancer.

complete surgical resection continues to be the treatment of choice for ACC and a margin-free resection is a strong predictor of long-term survival (7). The suspicion of ACC is raised by radiological criteria and finally verified by histopathology; fine-needle aspiration biopsy (FNAB) is currently not indicated for the diagnosis of primary ACC because of poor differentiation from adenoma and safety issues (9). The risk of ACC is related to the mass size, even if the correlation is far from perfect (Fig. 5.3.3). In the multicentre Italian experience, a cut-off at 4 cm had the highest sensitivity to differentiate ACC from benign lesions. The positive predictive value, however, was low because benign lesions greatly exceeded the incidence of ACC at any tumour size (6).

Despite that, only a limited number of patients with ACC have been included in imaging studies, current criteria suggestive of a benign adenoma include attenuation values less than 10 Hounsfield units (HU) on unenhanced CT scans and less than 30 HU on

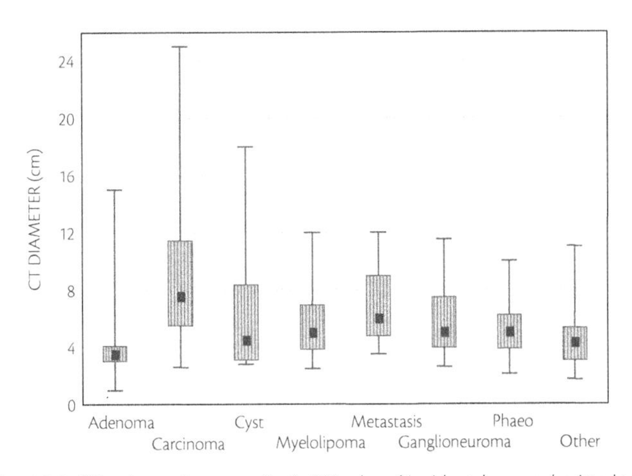

Fig. 5.3.3 CT-estimated tumour size in 380 adrenal incidentalomas submitted to surgery. Data are expressed as range (whisker), 25–75% centile (box), and median. Phaeo, phaeochromocytoma. Data from Mantero *et al*., 2000.

enhanced scans. Tumours with more than 10 HU include adrenal adenomas with a low lipid content, phaeochromocytoma, metastasis, and ACC (see Chapter 5.1).

Recently, the analysis of the SEER database, a comprehensive national cancer registry compiled by the NCI, confirmed that an increased tumour size correlates with a higher likelihood of malignancy (10). The subset of data on 192 ACCs presenting with localized disease showed that a tumour size of 4 cm had a sensitivity of 96% and specificity of 52% for ACC (10), a figure very close to that observed in the Italian survey on adrenal incidentaloma (6). However, since the prevalence of malignant neoplasms is low among adrenal incidentalomas, the post-test probability of malignancy associated with any tumour size remains low (10).

It is also important to rule out phaeochromocytoma because it can lead to significant morbidity and mortality, particularly if it remains undiagnosed. An increasingly higher number of patients harbouring a phaeochromocytoma are found to be normotensive or have stable, low-grade hypertension. In a large, multi-institutional series of adrenal incidentalomas collected in Italy and Sweden, approximately 50% of the patients bearing incidental phaeochromocytoma were normotensive or had stable, low-grade hypertension, which was indistinguishable from essential hypertension (6, 11). On the contrary, approximately 10% of the benign sporadic adrenal phaeochromocytomas diagnosed at the Mayo Clinic from 1978 to 1995 presented as incidentalomas. About 90% of these cases were hypertensive and had diagnostic values of urinary catecholamines or metanephrines (12). Furthermore, in a multi-institutional survey performed in France, the frequency of incidentally detected phaeochromocytomas was 15.9% in the whole series, while the proportion of clinically silent phaeochromocytomas was as high as 25% among patients operated in more recent times (13). These findings confirm that phaeochromocytomas may present with mild symptoms, if any (4). In fact, several series reported that in a relevant number of cases phaeochromocytoma may only be discovered by autopsy (4).

In general, incidental phaeochromocytomas are large masses, greater than 4 cm (14). Large phaeochromocytomas are able to extensively metabolize catecholamines prior to secretion; they may therefore exhibit fewer clinical symptoms than small tumours (15). Unenhanced CT is accurate in the detection of adrenal phaeochromocytoma with a sensitivity ranging from 93 to 100% (16). Intravenous contrast enhancement is not generally essential even if most tumours enhance markedly after intravenous contrast medium (14). MRI may have higher specificity than CT in diagnosing adrenal phaeochromocytoma and is also more accurate in detecting the infrequent extra-adrenal phaeochromocytoma (17). T2-weighted MRI may be particularly helpful, as this tumour usually shows a high signal intensity (higher than ACC or metastasis) (4). Adrenal scintigraphy with [^{131}I]metaiodobenzylguanidine (MIBG) provides anatomical localization and functional characterization of the tumour. This technique has lower sensitivity (78%) compared with CT or MRI but superior specificity (100%). MIBG scintigraphy may be useful in patients with equivocal imaging and biochemical data, or when a malignant or multifocal phaeochromocytoma is suspected (15).

Since nearly one-third of all phaeochromocytomas show a nonspecific appearance upon imaging, it is mandatory to perform an appropriate biochemical screening in every patient with an adrenal mass. Screening is of utmost importance whenever FNAB or surgical removal of the mass is scheduled (6). Prompt surgical resection remains the standard curative modality after specific preparation of the patient because up to 80% of patients with unsuspected phaeochromocytoma who underwent surgery or anaesthesia have died (8).

The adrenal glands are a common site of metastasis, with a reported rate in patients with an extra-adrenal malignancy ranging from 32 to 73% in different series (8). The morphological CT imaging features of metastases are nonspecific and in selected cases FNAB may be helpful in patients with a history of extra-adrenal cancer, no other metastatic sites, and a heterogeneous adrenal mass with more than 20 HU, after exclusion of phaeochromocytoma (8), but only if the FNA information is likely to change management. When an extra-adrenal malignancy is not obvious, search for the primary tumour should be undertaken and total body scan and adrenal FNB are reasonable in this context. In only a limited number of cases an effective treatment of adrenal metastasis is available; however, the diagnosis of adrenal metastasis may change the therapeutic approach and has important implications on the clinical history of a cancer patient.

Radiological assessment

When evaluating the literature on radiological assessment of adrenal incidentalomas, we have to consider that almost all studies lack a definitive ascertainment of outcome since a pathological diagnosis based on the tumour specimen was available in a minority of cases. Final diagnosis was mainly based on the change in size of the adrenal mass over variable periods of observation.

Only two retrospective studies have evaluated ultrasonography in patients with adrenal incidentalomas and their outcomes were contradictory . The first study proposed ultrasonography as a first-line test in the follow-up of patients with adrenal incidentaloma, reporting that mass size was well correlated between ultrasonography and CT measurements, although ultrasonography could not differentiate mass type (18). The second study found that ultrasonography may detect only 65% of masses less than 3 cm (19).

CT is an accurate tool for detecting the presence of adrenal masses and differentiating between benign and malignant lesions. Using a fast scanner and 1-cm scanning intervals, both adrenals can be identified in 97–99% of patients. In previous studies, size has been reported to be the most reliable way to distinguish benign adenomas from ACCs, but more recent studies found that attenuation value is a superior parameter. Noncontrast CT attenuation coefficient expressed in Hounsfield units has been increasingly used to differentiate adrenal adenomas from nonadenomas (20). This is based on the fact that intracytoplasmic fat is often abundant in adrenal adenoma but is scarce in metastasis, phaeochromocytoma, or ACC (20). Threshold values for noncontrast CT ranging from 0 to 20 HU have been suggested and a cut-off value of 10 HU was recommended by a consensus panel organized by the National Institutes of Health (21). A density of 10 HU had the best accuracy, with a sensitivity of 96–100% and still a broad variability in specificity ranging from 50 to 100%. Adrenal masses with a density more than 10 HU on unenhanced CT required other tests for characterization (30% of adrenal adenomas have a low lipid content and may show higher attenuation values). Some studies suggested that lesions with density more than 43 HU on unenhanced CT should be considered as malignant (21).

In addition to lipid content, there have been a variety of other CT characteristics that may differentiate adrenal adenomas from nonadenomas. Such characteristics include smooth border, round or oval shape, sharp margins, maintenance of adrenal configuration, lack of calcification within or on the edge of the tumour, homogeneity of the mass, and lack of enhancement after contrast (22). Although these features are helpful in the characterization of a mass, none of them individually rules out malignancy with great confidence. Adrenal adenomas are often small, well-defined, homogeneous lesions that do not enhance on CT, and are believed to remain constant in size on serial CT scans (21). ACCs are usually large, dense, irregular, heterogeneous, enhancing lesions that invade other structures (21). However, small masses, in the range of 1 to 6 cm, may be difficult to discriminate (21, 22).

Enhanced CT is indicated when the mass density is more than 10 HU on unenhanced CT. An absolute washout at or above 40–60% 10 min after the administration of the contrast medium has a sensitivity of 82–96% and a specificity of 81–100% to differentiate benign from malignant masses. A relative washout of 37.5–50% 10 min after the administration of the contrast medium has sensitivity of 100% and specificity of 95–100% to differentiate benign from malignant masses (22).

MRI has also been used to differentiate between adrenal adenoma, metastasis, and phaeochromocytoma. Chemical shift MRI, similar to CT densitometry, is dependent on the detection of intracellular lipid in adenomas, but chemical shift MRI does so by relying on the different resonant frequencies of fat and water protons in a given voxel rather than on attenuation differences. Both T_1 and T_2 relaxation times have been studied. Signal intensity ratios between the adrenal mass and various organs, including spleen, fat, liver, and muscle, have been tested to discriminate adrenal masses. In general, malignant masses are denser than benign masses, though various benign lesions can mimic malignancies (21). The loss of signal on out-of-phase images in relation to spleen (to avoid the confounding of liver steatosis) differentiated adenomas from nonadenomas with a sensitivity of 84–100% and a specificity of 92–100% (21, 22). Studies suggest that there is no significant difference between CT and MRI for characterizing lipid-rich adenomas, whereas MRI might be superior when evaluating adrenal adenomas with a low lipid content with an attenuation value of up to 30 HU (22).

Two radioisotopes, ^{131}I-iodomethyl-norcholesterol (NP-59) and 6-methyl-75-selenomethyl-19-norcholesterol have been used for imaging of adrenal masses of presumed adrenocortical origin. Various methods of analysing scintigraphy have been used to differentiate adrenal masses, including relative uptake of tracer, concordance with CT, and imaging patterns: adrenal nonadenomas have absent or significantly reduced uptake compared with adenomas (21). In addition to its potential role in diagnosing malignancy, scintigraphy may also be capable of differentiating autonomously secreting adenomas from nonfunctioning adenomas, adrenal hyperplasia, and other adrenal diseases (21). However, NP-59 adrenal scintigraphy is not reliable for lesions less than 2 cm in size. In recent years, the use of adrenal scintigraphy has declined because of the lack of widespread availability and parallel technical improvement of other radiological procedures (22).

[^{18}F]2-fluoro-2-deoxy-D-glucose positron emission tomography (FDG PET) or PET/CT has also been reported to have a high sensitivity and specificity in characterizing adrenal lesions, although not as a routine imaging technique (22, 23), with a reported sensitivity of 93–100% and specificity of 80–100%. Necrotic or haemorrhagic malignant adrenal lesions may cause false-negative results showing poor FDG uptake. Metomidate-PET had a sensitivity of 89% and a specificity of 96% to differentiate masses of adrenal origin from masses of extra-adrenal origin. PET imaging is not reliable for lesions less than 1 cm in size, as metastatic lesions of this size may demonstrate less radiotracer uptake than normal liver. The use of PET/CT offers advantages over PET alone, as the morphology of the lesion can be assessed by CT while its metabolic activity can be measured concomitantly by PET, allowing for accurate anatomical localization of any focal FDG uptake. CT densitometry and washout measurements (if a delayed contrast-enhanced CT is performed) can be incorporated into the analysis. PET or PET/CT should be used when CT densitometry or washout analysis are inconclusive (22, 23).

Transcutaneous needle biopsy or FNAB, of an adrenal mass has been advocated by some for the investigation of incidentally discovered adrenal masses (21). FNAB is indicated only in patients with known extra-adrenal cancer when an adrenal adenoma has been reasonably excluded by CT or MRI (after biochemical exclusion of phaeochromocytoma). FNAB may be also useful in selected cases with discordant results of imaging tests and/or when rare tumours are suspected. The biopsy is generally performed under either CT or ultrasonography guidance. While accuracy appears to be high, up to 15% of biopsies are inconclusive (21). Complications of adrenal mass needle biopsy include pneumothorax, bleeding, and bacteraemia (21). Rare instances of metastatic seeding of the cancer along the needle track have been reported (21). A summary of recommendations for radiological assessment is outlined in Box 5.3.2.

Hormonal assessment

With the exception of patients with imaging characteristics typical for myelolipoma or adrenal cyst, in all of the subjects with incidentally discovered adrenal mass either phaeochromocytoma or overt Cushing's syndrome should be excluded (Box 5.3.3). Including patients with signs and symptoms attributable to an adrenal tumour that were overlooked before detection of an adrenal mass, will increase the proportion of secretory tumours. Conversely, using the strictest inclusion criteria and the purest definition of incidentaloma eliminates the need for considering overt Cushing's syndrome.

Box 5.3.2 Take-home points on radiological assessment

- Mass density on unenhanced CT scan is superior to tumour size to predict malignancy.
- Lesions with density >10 HU on unenhanced CT are considered indeterminate and other tests are generally required for characterization (enhanced CT).
- A relative washout of about 50% 10 min after the administration of the contrast medium is the best parameter to differentiate the typical lipid-poor adrenal adenoma from nonadenomas.
- MRI is possibly as accurate as CT but there is less experience with this technique.
- PET or PET/CT may be useful when CT or MRI are inconclusive.
- FNAB may have a role in the diagnostic work-up of metastases or when rare adrenal neoplasms are suspected.

As for ACC, there is little doubt that an early diagnosis of phaeochromocytoma is beneficial for the patient. Early recognition of the tumour may prevent potentially lethal hypertensive crises or arrhythmias (24). In the Italian survey, the frequency of phaeochromocytoma among adrenal incidentalomas was roughly comparable to that of adrenal carcinoma (approximately 4%) (6). Since an increasingly higher number of patients bearing a phaeochromocytoma are normotensive or have stable, low-grade hypertension, and phaeochromocytoma may not be easily recognized by imaging studies, it is mandatory to perform an appropriate biochemical screening in every patient with an adrenal mass according to the current guidelines (24).

Following recent epidemiological evidence that shows primary aldosteronism is the most frequent cause of endocrine hypertension, it was recommended to obtain a paired upright plasma aldosterone concentration and plasma renin activity in hypertensive patients with clinically inapparent adrenal adenoma in patients who are hypertensive. This measurement should be carried out after correction of hypokalaemia, if present. Dietary salt intake should be unrestricted. Hypokalaemia is no longer a mandatory prerequisite for suspecting primary hyperaldosteronism since more than 50% of patients are normokalaemic. Screening for primary aldosteronism should be pursued according to current guidelines (25).

Box 5.3.3 Take-home points on hormonal assessment

- Phaeochromocytoma should be ruled out in all patients with adrenal incidentalomas; hypertension is no longer a prerequisite to suspect phaeochromocytoma.
- Primary aldosteronism should be ruled out in all hypertensive patients with adrenal incidentalomas. Hypokalaemia is no longer a prerequisite to suspect primary aldosteronism.
- The overnight 1 mg dexamethasone suppression test should be used to screen for subclinical Cushing's syndrome; however, there is no consensus on the cutpoint to consider the test as positive.
- The value of employing further tests (urinary free cortisol, plasma ACTH, cortisol rhythm, other dexamethasone tests) in addition to the 1 mg dexamethasone suppression test is uncertain.

In all patients with an incidentally discovered adrenal mass, the presence of overt cortisol excess must be suspected in the presence of one out the following four signs, which are relatively specific for Cushing's syndrome: (1) easy bruising, (2) facial plethora, (3) proximal myopathy or muscle weakness, and (4) reddish-purple striae (>1 cm wide) (26). However, most patients with adrenal incidentalomas do not present signs or symptoms suggestive of hypercortisolism. If overt Cushing's syndrome is not an issue, an endocrine work-up may frequently disclose subtle derangements of the hypothalamic–pituitary–adrenal axis (HPA) axis consistent with autonomous cortisol secretion by an incidental adrenal adenoma, the so-called subclinical Cushing's syndrome (Box 5.3.4).

Subclinical Cushing's syndrome

Subclinical Cushing's syndrome may be defined as an autonomous cortisol secretion not fully restrained by pituitary feedback and variably exceeding the physiological daily production rate in the absence of an overt cushingoid phenotype (12, 27). Although the term 'preclinical' Cushing's syndrome has been proposed previously, 'subclinical' Cushing's syndrome more accurately describes this condition, not implying any assumption on the further development of a clinically overt syndrome (2). Since the prevalence of overt Cushing's syndrome caused by adrenal adenoma in the general population is significantly lower than the prevalence of subclinical Cushing's syndrome in patients with clinically nonfunctioning adrenal adenoma, it is rather inappropriate to consider subclinical Cushing's syndrome as an early stage of development of overt hypercortisolism (27).

Although the pathophysiological concept of autonomous cortisol secretion sustained by an adrenal adenoma is straightforward, demonstration of subclinical Cushing's syndrome is extremely difficult in practice. In fact, the standard biochemical tests used to screen Cushing's syndrome are generally ill-suited to the assessment of patients who have no, or only mild, signs of cortisol excess. In this clinical setting, the *a priori* probability of subclinical Cushing's syndrome is roughly comparable with the false-positive rate of the tests used for screening (2, 3). In the absence of reliable clinical clues it is indeed challenging to distinguish between true-positive and false-positive test results. Moreover, many tests used to study the HPA axis do not have sufficient sensitivity to recognize a very mild degree of cortisol excess. This is the case for the determination of urinary free cortisol, which has also the drawback of a remarkable daily variation in either cortisol excretion in the urine or daily urine output (the latter problem is amplified by the difficulty in obtaining complete urine collections) (27).

Box 5.3.4 Diagnostic criteria for subclinical Cushing's syndrome

1. Adrenal adenoma of serendipitous discovery
2. Lack of apparent cushingoid phenotype
3. Biochemical evidence of functional autonomy/hypercortisolism

The reported prevalence of subclinical Cushing's syndrome among patients with adrenal incidentaloma ranges from 5 to 20% (4, 8, 12, 27). This heterogeneity is explained, at least in part, by the different work-up protocols and variable criteria used to define subclinical cortisol excess as well as in different inclusion criteria and size of the reported series. Methodological limits add to the intrinsic biological problems associated with identification of subclinical cortisol excess, thus explaining the great uncertainty surrounding this entity. A number of alterations of the HPA axis have been associated to clinically inapparent adrenal adenomas and various biochemical criteria, alone or in combination, have been employed to qualify subclinical Cushing's syndrome but the optimal diagnostic strategy remains to be defined (4, 8, 12, 27).

To provide a standard, in 2002, the National Institutes of Health state-of-the-science conference panel recommended the 1-mg dexamethasone suppression test as screening for subclinical Cushing's syndrome with the traditional threshold of 5 μg/dl (138 nmol/l) to define adequate suppression (21). However, some experts advocate lower cut-points to increase detection of subclinical Cushing's syndrome following the recommendations for screening of overt Cushing's syndrome (4, 8). The rationale for this choice is that in most healthy subjects cortisol is barely detectable following 1 mg dexamethasone. However, specificity decreases when lower post-dexamethasone cortisol thresholds are used, which are likely to result in more false-positive test results (26). Conversely, other authors have suggested employing high-dose (3 or even 8 mg) dexamethasone tests since the diagnosis of pituitary Cushing's syndrome is not a consideration (4, 8). At present, there is insufficient evidence to solve this controversy. However, the recommendation to use the overnight 1 mg suppression test seems sound since this test has been extensively employed for screening purposes, and the cut-off of 1.8 μg/dl (50 nmol/l) seems too low to assess individuals without specific features of hypercortisolism. The patients with an adrenal incidentaloma should be indistinguishable from the general population and in this setting the test specificity using this cut-off may be unacceptably low (12, 27).

Some experts require that two concomitant alterations in the tests aimed to study the HPA axis should be demonstrated to qualify a patient for subclinical Cushing's syndrome, in order to circumvent the problem of false positivity of biochemical testing, and a number of tests have been employed for this purpose, thus making the screening procedure complicate and expensive (6). Blunting of the circadian rhythm of cortisol seems more frequent than elevation of urinary free cortisol and this confirms the view that derangement of the daily secretory pattern of cortisol is an early marker of (subclinical) hypercortisolism (27). Also, low to undetectable ACTH levels have been frequently reported, even if technical problems associated with measurement of ACTH concentrations close to the detection limits of the assay affect the utility of ACTH determination to demonstrate functional autonomy of an adrenal adenoma. Use of the corticotropin-releasing hormone test does not seem to add significant information to baseline ACTH levels (27). Recently, it has been demonstrated that the efficacy of midnight salivary cortisol in diagnosing subclinical Cushing's syndrome is clearly lower than that found for overt Cushing's syndrome (28).

The current uncertainty on what strategy is best suited to detect adrenal cortical autonomy might be solved by finding at what point cortisol excess becomes clinically significant, causing clinical morbidity. We are at present unable to answer this question because we do not know to what extent subclinical Cushing's syndrome may affect patients' health and life expectancy (12, 27).

Since many patients with clinically nonfunctioning incidentalomas are exposed to a chronic, even if only minimal to mild, cortisol excess, it is biologically plausible to anticipate that they should suffer, at least to some extent, from the classic, long-term consequences of overt Cushing's syndrome, such as arterial hypertension, obesity, or diabetes (12, 21, 27). Several data from autopsy series, cross-sectional studies, and case–control studies (4, 8, 12, 17) consistently point to an association between clinically inapparent adrenal adenoma, subclinical Cushing's syndrome, and the metabolic syndrome. There are also data suggesting that subclinical Cushing's syndrome may predispose to osteoporosis, another well-established consequence of overt cortisol excess, and confers an increased risk of vertebral fractures (4, 12, 27). However, caution should be taken in generalizing results from series gathered in academic centres referral bias is an obvious issue since these studies are not population-based and there is the potential for confounding due to their case–control design. The complexity of an accurate matching between patients and controls for the many factors that may affect cardiovascular risk should also be disclosed. Moreover, the demonstration of an association should not imply a cause and effect relationship (27).

At present, subclinical Cushing's syndrome presents a vexing problem as to diagnosis and management. The major areas of uncertainty are summarized in Box 5.3.5.

Natural history and management

Management of adrenal incidentaloma is a complex decision-making process, which involves considering a range of possible diagnoses and their natural history, and weighing the risks and benefits of interventions in light of the patient's age and the tumour size. Surgery is the appropriate therapeutic measure for ACC, phaeochromocytoma, and others functional adrenal tumours causing overt glucocorticoid, mineralocorticoid, or adrenal sex hormone; treatment of metastasis depends on individual clinical circumstances. Treatment of adrenal adenomas is much more difficult to outline because the natural history of these tumours is not well known (Box 5.3.6).

The available follow-up data of patients with clinically inapparent adrenal mass suggests that the large majority of adrenal lesions classified as benign at diagnosis remain stable over time. The risk of malignant transformation at long-term follow-up is very low, and it is estimated to be about 1:1000 incidentalomas (4). In 5–20% of cases mass size increases over time; however, most growing adrenal masses are not malignant (4, 27). The presence of isolated

Box 5.3.5 Unsolved issues with subclinical Cushing's syndrome

- Which are the best diagnostic criteria and evaluation algorithms?
- At what point does cortisol autonomy lead to clinical morbidity?
- Does subclinical Cushing's syndrome predispose to the classic complications of full-blown cortisol excess?
- What is the natural history of subclinical Cushing's syndrome?

Box 5.3.6 Issues concerning the natural history of adrenal adenomas

- Increase in size
- Malignant transformation
- Development of overt endocrine syndromes
- Long-term consequences of subclinical hormone hypersecretion

endocrine abnormalities at diagnosis may be considered a risk factor for mass enlargement or development of bilateral masses during follow-up (4). Occasional reduction or even disappearance of adrenal masses have been also reported in about 4% of adrenal incidentalomas, most often when cystic lesions, haematomas, or adrenal pseudotumours were the underlying diagnosis (12, 27).

The risk of progression from subclinical to overt Cushing's syndrome is minimal (<1% of cases) (27). However, the occurrence of silent biochemical alterations during follow-up has been reported in a percentage ranging from 0 to 11% across different studies. The development of HPA axis abnormalities is unlikely in lesion smaller than 3 cm and appears to plateau after 3–4 years (4). A spontaneous regression of the alterations of the HPA axis may be observed, suggesting that cortisol output may have a cyclical or intermittent pattern (27).

The management of patients with subclinical Cushing's syndrome is a very controversial issue. It is tempting to speculate that this condition represents a very mild variant of the syndrome of endogenous glucocorticoid excess sharing similar target-organ damages and long-term complications with the full-blown variant (12, 27). Evidence of increased morbidity and mortality in patients with clinically inapparent adrenal adenoma, with or without subclinical Cushing's syndrome, is at present lacking and data are insufficient to indicate the superiority of a surgical or nonsurgical approach in the management of such patients (12, 27).

It is important to remember that patients with subclinical Cushing's syndrome should receive perioperative glucocorticoids after removal of the functioning mass because they are at risk for hypoadrenalism. Factors such as young patient age, coexistence of hypertension, or diabetes, or osteoporosis might influence the decision in favour of surgery (4). The significant decrease in surgical morbidity and economic costs using a laparoscopic approach to adrenalectomy is actually widening indications to surgery (4). While adrenalectomy has been demonstrated to correct the HPA axis abnormalities, its effect on long-term patient outcome and quality of life is unknown. Until the risks and benefits of surgical removal of silent hyperfunctioning adrenocortical adenomas has been elucidated, we should elect to surgery patients with silent hypercortisolism who display diseases potentially attributable to cortisol excess that are of recent onset, or are resistant to medical intervention, or are rapidly worsening (12, 27). This strategy is based purely on pragmatism and not evidence. Box 5.3.7 outlines key issues with surgery in subclinical Cushing's syndrome. Patients not submitted to surgery (possibly the majority) should undergo careful clinical monitoring and receive adequate treatment of the associated clinical conditions according to the specific guidelines (i.e. hypertension, diabetes) (27).

The limited and incomplete evidence available precludes making any stringent recommendation for periodic hormonal testing and repeat imaging evaluation for follow-up purposes. However, a repeat CT after 3 to 6 months from diagnosis should be recommended to recognize a rapidly growing mass whose malignant potential has escaped detection by the first imaging study, and then after 12 to 48 months (12). Hormonal testing (low-dose dexamethasone suppression test) is usually recommended in all patients with adrenal adenomas annually for 3–5 years. If no change in the functional state or imaging occurs further investigation may not be required (12, 27). However, it is important to stress the concept that little evidence is available to define the follow-up strategy, which should also consider the economic costs of follow-up investigations and the risk of cancer due to radiation exposure from multiple CT scans. Further research is urgently needed to inform a rational follow-up strategy, as outlined in Box 5.3.8.

Box 5.3.7 Key points on surgery in subclinical Cushing's syndrome

- There are no randomized trials or long-term follow-up studies supporting the benefits of adrenalectomy in all patients with subclinical Cushing's syndrome.
- Few small studies with methodological limits reported improvement in blood pressure, metabolic parameters, and osteoporosis after surgery.
- It is current practice to elect for surgery younger patients with subclinical Cushing's syndrome and manifestations potentially related to cortisol excess (hypertension, diabetes, abdominal obesity, and osteoporosis) that are difficult to manage.
- We suggest considering adrenalectomy in patients with subclinical Cushing's syndrome showing clinical deterioration despite optimal medical treatment.
- Laparoscopic adrenalectomy is the procedure of choice.
- Patients with subclinical Cushing's syndrome require postoperative glucocorticoid replacement to prevent the risk of adrenal insufficiency. Treatment may be required also in some patients with nonfunctioning adenomas.

Box 5.3.8 Research agenda

- Increase knowledge on the natural history of subclinical Cushing's syndrome
- Identify the level of cortisol excess that may have a negative impact on patients' health status
- Identify biochemical markers predictive of cortisol-induced target-organ damage
- Identify subsets of patients at increased risk of adverse outcome
- Compare the long-term outcome of surgery versus medical treatment in subclinical Cushing's syndrome
- Establish cost-effective follow-up schedules for imaging and biochemical work-up of patients managed conservatively

References

1. Young WF Jr. Management approaches to adrenal incidentalomas: a view from Rochester, Minnesota. *Endocrinol Metab Clin North Am*, 2000; **29**: 159–85.
2. Gross MD, Shapiro B. Clinical review 50. Clinically silent adrenal masses. *J Clin Endocrinol Metab*, 1993; **77**: 885–8 Review.
3. Chidiac RM, Aron DC. Incidentalomas. A disease of modern technology. *Endocrinol Metab Clin North Am*, 1997; **26**: 233–53 Review.
4. Barzon L, Sonino N, Fallo F, Palu G, Boscaro M. Prevalence and natural history of adrenal incidentalomas. *Eur J Endocrinol*, 2003; **149**: 273–85. Review.
5. Bovio S, Cataldi A, Reimondo G, Sperone P, Novello S, Berruti A, *et al.* Prevalence of adrenal incidentaloma in a contemporary computerized tomography series. *J Endocrinol Invest*, 2006; **29**: 298–302.
6. Mantero F, Terzolo M, Arnaldi G, Osella G, Masini AM, Alì A, *et al.* A survey on adrenal incidentaloma in Italy. *J Clin Endocrinol Metab*, 2000; **85**: 637–44.
7. Singh PK, Buch HN. Adrenal incidentaloma: evaluation and management. *J Clin Pathol*, 2008; **61**: 1168–73 Review.
8. Kloos RT, Gross MD, Francis IR, Korobkin M, Shapiro B. Incidentally discovered adrenal masses. *Endocr Rev*, 1995; **16**: 460–84.
9. Herrera MF, Grant CS, van Heerden JA, Sheedy PF, Ilstrup DM. Incidentally discovered adrenal tumours: an institutional perspective. *Surgery*, 1991; **110**: 1014–21.
10. Sturgeon C, Shen WT, Clark OH *et al.* Risk assessment in 457 adrenal cortical carcinomas: how much does tumour size predict the likelihood of malignancy? *J Am Coll Surg*, 2006; **202**: 423–430.
11. Bulow B, Ahren B & Swedish Research Council Study Group of Endocrine Abdominal Tumours. Adrenal incidentaloma-experience of a standardized diagnostic programme in the Swedish prospective study. *J Int Med*, 2002; **252**: 239–246.
12. Young WF Jr. Clinical practice. The incidentally discovered adrenal mass. *N Engl J Med*, 2007; **356**: 601–10. Review.
13. Amar L, Servais A, Gimenez-Roqueplo A-P, Zinzindohoue F, Chatellier G, Plouin P-F. Year of diagnosis, features at presentation, and risk of recurrence in patients with pheochromocytoma or secreting paraganglioma. *J Clin Endocrinol Metab*, 2005; **90**: 2110–2116.
14. Bravo EL, Tagle R. Pheochromocytoma: state-of-the-art and future prospects. *Endocr Rev*, 2003; **24**: 539–553. Review.
15. Lenders JW, Pacak K, Walther MM *et al.* Biochemical diagnosis of pheochromocytoma: which test is best? *JAMA*, 2002; **287**: 1427–1434.
16. Szolar DH, Korobkin M, Reittner P *et al.* Adrenocortical carcinomas and adrenal pheochromocytomas: mass and enhancement loss evaluation at delayed contrast-enhanced CT. *Radiology*, 2005; **234**: 479–485.
17. Kasperlik-Zaluska AA, Roslonowska E, Slowinska-Srzednicka J, Tolloczko T, Szamowska R, Leowska E *et al.* Incidentally discovered adrenal mass (incidentaloma): investigation and management of 208 patients. *Clin Endocrinol*, 1997; **46**: 29–37.
18. Fontana D, Porpiglia F, Destefanis P, Fiori C, Alì A, Terzolo M, *et al.* What is the role of ultrasonography in the follow-up of adrenal incidentalomas? The Gruppo Piemontese Incidentalomi Surrenalici. *Urology*, 1999; **54**: 612–6.
19. Suzuki Y, Sasagawa, Suzuki H, Izumi T, Kaneko H, Nakada T *et al.* The role of ultrasonography in the detection of adrenal masses: comparison with computed tomography and magnetic resonance imaging. *Int Urol Nephrol*, 2001; **32**: 303–6.
20. Hamrahian AH, Ioachimescu AG, Remer EM, Motta-Ramirez G, Bogabathina H, Levin HS, *et al.* Clinical utility of noncontrast computed tomography attenuation value (hounsfield units) to differentiate adrenal adenomas/hyperplasias from nonadenomas: Cleveland Clinic experience. *J Clin Endocrinol Metab*, 2005; **90**: 871–7.
21. NIH state-of-the-science statement on management of the clinically inapparent adrenal mass ("incidentaloma"). *NIH Consens State Sci Statements*, 2002; **19**: 1–25. Review.
22. Giles WL, Boland GWL, Blake MA, Hahn PF, Mayo-Smith WW. Incidental adrenal lesions: principles, techniques, and algorithms for imaging characterization. *Radiology*, 2008; **249**: 756–75.
23. Park BK, Kim CK, Kim B, Choi JY. Comparison of delayed enhanced CT and 18F-FDG PET/CT in the evaluation of adrenal masses in oncology patients. *J Comput Assist Tomogr*, 2007; **31**: 550–6.
24. Lenders JW, Eisenhofer G, Mannelli M, Pacak K. Phaeochromocytoma. *Lancet*, 2005; **366**(9486): 665–75. Review.
25. Funder JW, Carey RM, Fardella G, Gomez-Sanchez CE, Mantero F, Stowasser M, *et al.* Case detection, diagnosis, and treatment of patients with primary aldosteronism: an Endocrine Society Clinical Practice Guideline. *J Clin Endocrinol Metab*, 2008; **93**: 3266–81.
26. Nieman LK, Biller BM, Findling JW, Newell-Price J, Savage MO, Stewart PM, *et al.* The diagnosis of Cushing's syndrome: an Endocrine Society Clinical Practice Guideline. *J Clin Endocrinol Metab*, 2008; **93**: 1526–40.
27. Terzolo M, Bovio S, Reimondo G, Pia A, Osella G, Borretta G, *et al.* Subclinical Cushing's syndrome in adrenal incidentalomas. *Endocrinol Metab Clin North Am*, 2005; **34**: 423–39. Review.
28. Masserini B, Morelli V, Bergamaschi S, Ermetici F, Eller-Vainicher C, Barbieri AM, *et al.* The limited role of midnight salivary cortisol levels in the diagnosis of subclinical hypercortisolism in patients with adrenal incidentaloma. *Eur J Endocrinol*, 2009; **160**: 87–92.
29. Terzolo M, Reimondo G, Bovio S, Daffara F, Allasino B, Minetto M, *et al.* Management of adrenal incidentalomas. *Exp Clin Endocrinol Diabetes*, 2007; **115**(3):166–70. Review.

5.4

Adrenocortical cancer

Rossella Libè, Lionel Groussin, Xavier Bertagna, Jérôme Bertherat

Introduction

Adrenocortical cancer (ACC) is among the most aggressive endocrine tumours with an overall very poor prognosis. Morbidity and mortality can be secondary to steroid hormone excess and/or tumour growth and metastases. This potentially poor outcome justifies the importance of considering malignancy in the management of an adrenal mass. The diagnosis of malignancy in a patient with an adrenal tumour relies on careful investigations of clinical, biological, and imaging features before surgery and pathological examination after tumour removal. Appropriate management and follow-up by an expert multidisciplinary team is important to improve prognosis and to progress in these rare neoplasms.

Pathogenesis and genetics

ACC consists of monoclonal populations of cells, suggesting that tumour progression is the end result of an intrinsic genetic or epigenetic alteration. Monoclonal tumours result from alterations conferring a growth advantage to the cell initially affected.

These genetic events can be studied at the scale of the whole genome, as losses or gains of part or all of a chromosome. A large number of molecular techniques, such as comparative genomic hybridization and microsatellite analysis, have been used in genome-wide screens for such chromosomal alterations. It has been demonstrated by comparative genomic hybridization that chromosomal alterations are very frequent in ACC. Chromosomal losses were observed at 1p, 17p, 22p, 22q, 2q, and 11q in up to 62% of cases of ACC. Studies using microsatellite markers have demonstrated a high percentage of loss of heterozygosity or allelic imbalance at 11q13 (≥90%), 17p13 (≥85%), and 2p16 (92%) in ACC (1).

The genes involved in these molecular alterations could be classified as tumour suppressor genes on the one hand, and oncogenes on the other hand. Molecular alterations would lead to inactivation of the tumour suppressor genes and activation of the oncogenes. In various cancers the study of chromosomal rearrangement led to the identification of the oncogenes or tumour suppressor genes involved in their development. However, currently in ACC, such genes have been mostly identified by the study of familial diseases associated with adrenocortical tumours. Nevertheless, the loci of these genes are frequently altered in sporadic ACC, suggesting the importance of these loci and genes in the development of these tumours (Table 5.4.1; Fig. 5.4.1).

TP53 and the 17p13 locus

The tumour suppressor gene *TP53* is located at 17p13 and its product is involved in the control of cell proliferation. Germline mutations in *TP53* are responsible for the Li–Fraumeni syndrome. This syndrome displays dominant inheritance and confers susceptibility to breast cancer, soft tissue sarcoma, brain tumours, osteosarcoma, leukaemia, and ACC. Germline mutations in *TP53* have been observed in 50–80% of children with apparently sporadic ACC in North America and Europe. In Southern Brazil, a specific germline mutation has been identified in exon 10 of the *TP53* gene, R337H, which is observed in almost all paediatric cases (2). In sporadic ACC in adults, somatic mutations of *TP53* are found in only 25–35% of the cases. Interestingly, loss of heterozygosity at 17p13 occurs in 85% of sporadic ACC (1).

IGF2 (insulin-like growth factor 2) and the 11p15 locus

The *IGF2* gene, located at 11p15, encodes an important fetal growth factor which is maternally imprinted and expressed only from the paternal allele. Genetic or epigenetic changes in the imprinted 11p15 region, resulting in increased *IGF2* expression, and mutations of the *p57kip2* gene have been implicated in the Beckwith–Wiedemann syndrome. This overgrowth disorder is characterized by macrosomia, macroglossia, organomegaly, and developmental abnormalities (in particular abdominal wall defects with exomphalos), embryonal tumours (such as Wilms' tumour), and ACC, neuroblastoma, and hepatoblastoma. Several studies have demonstrated that *IGF2* is strongly overexpressed in approximately 90% of ACC (3).

The Wnt/β-catenin pathway

Genetic alterations of the Wnt signalling pathway were initially identified in familial adenomatous polyposis coli and have been extended to a variety of cancers. Furthermore, familial adenomatous polyposis coli patients with germline mutations of the *APC* (adenomatous polyposis coli) gene, which lead to an activation of the Wnt signalling pathway, may develop adrenocortical tumour. The Wnt signalling pathway is normally activated during

Table 5.4.1 The genetic predisposition to adrenocortical tumours and the molecular genetics of sporadic ACC

Genetic hereditary syndrome and OMIM reference number	Genes, chromosomal localization, and type of defect	Tumours and nontumoural manifestations observed in the hereditary syndrome	Somatic genetic defect observed in sporadic adrenocortical tumours
Li–Fraumeni syndrome (OMIM 151623)	*TP53* (17p13) Inactivation heterozygous mutations of the tumour suppressor gene *TP53*	Soft-tissue sarcoma, breast cancers, brain tumours, leukaemia, ACC	*TP53* somatic mutations in sporadic ACC (30%) 17p13 LOH in sporadic ACC (>80%)
Multiple endocrine neoplasia type 1 (OMIM 131100)	*Menin* (11q13) Inactivation heterozygous mutations of the tumour suppressor gene *Menin*	Parathyroid, pituitary, pancreas tumours, adrenal cortex (25–40%), among which are adrenocortical adenomas, adrenocortical hyperplasia, and rare ACC	Very rare somatic *menin* gene mutations in sporadic adrenocortical tumours Frequent 11q13 LOH in ACC (90%)
Beckwith–Wiedemann syndrome (OMIM 130650)	11p15 locus alterations *IGF2* overexpression *p57kip2* (*CDKN1C*) (genetic defect) *KCNQ10T* (epigenetic defect) *H19* (epigenetic defect)	Omphalocele, macroglossia, macrosomia, hemilhypertrophy, Wilms' tumour, ACC	ACC: 11p15 LOH (>80%) ACC: *IGF2* overexpression (>85%)
Familial adenomatous polyposis coli (OMIM 175100)	*APC* (5q12–22) Inactivation heterozygous mutations of the tumour suppressor gene *APC*	Multiple adenomatous polyps and cancer of the colon and rectum Possible extracolonic manifestations include periampullary cancer, thyroid tumours, hepatoblastoma Adrenocortical tumours can be diagnosed as adrenocortical adenomas, possibly multiples and/or bilateral, and ACC	Transcriptome analysis shows overexpression of targets of the Wnt-signalling pathway in ACC Immunohistochemistry shows abnormal localization of β-catenin in ACC, suggesting activation of the Wnt/b-catenin pathway β-catenin activating somatic mutations in ACC (20–30%)

The table describes the main hereditary syndromes associated with adrenocortical tumours for which the locus and/or genes have been identified at the germline level. The alterations of these genes and chromosomal regions as somatic defect observed on tumour DNA of sporadic tumours are listed.
LOH, loss of heterozygosity; ACC, adrenocortical cancer.

embryonic development. β-catenin is a key component of this signalling pathway. In ACC, β-catenin delocalization can be observed, consistent with an abnormal activation of the Wnt-signalling pathway. In a subset of adrenocortical tumours, this is explained by somatic activating mutations in the β-catenin gene (4).

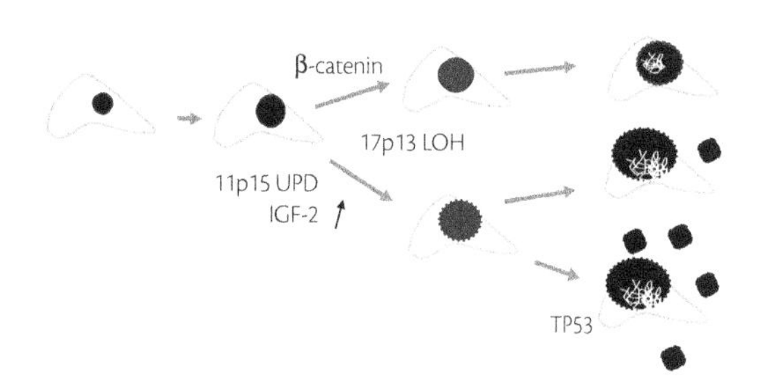

Fig. 5.4.1 Schematic view of adrenocortical cancer pathogenesis—summary of current knowledge on the molecular pathogenesis of ACC. Some chromosomal alterations as 17p13 loss of heterozygosity (LOH) or 11p15 unipaternal disomy (UPD) might occur early in tumour development. Insulin-like growth factor (IGF-2) overexpression is associated with 11p15 alterations. Somatic β-catenin mutations and/or abnormal β-catenin immunohistochemistry lead to activation of the Wnt signalling pathway. Some events, such as *TP53* somatic mutations, might be found in a subset of aggressive ACC. Tumour phenotype will be determined by a combination of the various molecular alterations and their timing of appearance. Accordingly, some ACC will have a very low growth potential and might not recur after complete tumour removal. Other ACC will have a very aggressive growth with a high potential to develop metastasis.

MEN1 gene and the 11q13 locus

The *MEN1* gene, located at the 11q13 locus, is a tumour suppressor gene. A heterozygous inactivating germline mutation of *MEN1* is found in about 90% of families affected by multiple endocrine neoplasia type 1 (MEN 1). The principal clinical features of this autosomal dominant syndrome include parathyroid (95%), endocrine pancreatic (45%), and pituitary (45%) tumours and thymic carcinoids. Adrenocortical tumours and/or hyperplasia are observed in 25–40% of MEN 1 patients. ACC has rarely been observed in MEN 1 patients. Somatic mutations in the *MEN 1* gene are very rare in sporadic adrenocortical tumours. By contrast, loss of heterozygosity at 11q13 is observed in more than 90% of informative ACC and only 20% of adrenocortical adenomas. However, loss of heterozygosity in ACC involves almost all the 11q domain, suggesting that an, as yet unidentified, tumour suppressor gene located on the long arm of the chromosome is involved in ACC formation (5).

Gene profiling in adrenocortical cancer

The use of large-scale analysis of gene expression, or transcriptome analysis, to study various cancers has been a source of important advances both in tumour classification and understanding of pathogenesis. This method has been applied recently to adrenocortical tumours and it appears that gene expression profiles of benign tumours differ markedly from that of ACC (6). A cluster of genes overexpressed in ACC are related to IGF-2 and other growth factors, and this has been termed the IGF-2 cluster. This cluster contains mainly growth factors and growth factor receptor genes.

By contrast, a steroidogenic cluster of genes (such as *CYP11A*, *CYP11B1*, *HSD3B*, encoding steroidogenic enzymes) is expressed only at low level in ACC as compared to adrenocortical adenomas. As most of these genes are related to steroidogenesis, a dedifferentiation process might occur during malignant transformation (1). The observed differences in gene expression profile between benign and malignant ACC suggest that transcriptome analysis could potentially offer new diagnostic tools for the discrimination of benign from malignant tumours (7).

Epidemiology

ACC is a rare tumour with an estimated incidence between 1 and 2 per million per year in adults, in North America and Europe. The prevalence has been estimated to be between 4 and 12 per million population (8). As observed in many rare tumours, the incidence is difficult to determine and the true numbers might be higher than the current estimations. For instance, the prevalence of adrenal incidentaloma range in the general population from 1% in subjects younger than 30 years to 7% in subjects older than 70 years. Among the group of adrenal incidentalomas selected for surgery, the frequency of ACC ranges between 3 and 10%.

In children, the incidence of ACC is considered as 10 times lower than in adults, except in South Brazil where there is a higher incidence of paediatric ACC due to the high prevalence of a specific germline *TP53* mutation, as discussed above.

In some series there is a slightly increased female to male ratio (9), although not always reported. Among female patients with Cushing's syndrome diagnosed during pregnancy, the frequency of ACC is higher than in nonpregnant female patients with Cushing's syndrome (10).

Clinical features and hormonal investigations

Circumstances leading to the initial diagnosis

Signs and symptoms leading to the diagnosis of ACC can be due to steroid excess, tumour mass, and effects of metastases (11). Although ACC is not the most frequent diagnosis in adrenal incidentalomas, nowadays the diagnosis of ACC is made with an increasing frequency during the diagnostic work-up of an incidentally discovered adrenal mass. This is important since it might be a way to diagnose an ACC at an earlier stage and to improve the prognosis by an early, complete surgical removal. This underlines the need for careful investigations of adrenal incidentalomas in order to decide whether to go for surgery if malignancy is suspected. Other specific features may be associated with rare genetic diseases such as the Li–Fraumeni and Beckwith–Wiedemann syndromes where ACC is part of a more complex syndrome, as discussed above.

Less than a third of ACCs are really 'nonhypersecretory' after careful hormonal investigations (11, 12). In these cases, one should be cautious not to overdiagnose a tumour of the adrenal area as an ACC. These nonhypersecretory ACCs can be diagnosed after investigation of adrenal incidentalomas or due to the consequences of local expansion of the tumour mass, e.g. local symptoms (pain, palpation of a tumour, venous thrombosis), or distant metastases (liver, lung, bones). Fever may occur, in some cases after tumour necrosis, but is a rather rare sign. Similarly, weight loss is rarely observed in ACC. Characteristically, the general health condition of patients affected by apparently endocrine inactive ACC is remarkably good, even during the early stages of metastasis. However, the general condition of the patient is most often preserved except at a very late stage when the tumour is nonsecreting. This explains why nonhypersecretory ACCs may be diagnosed only at a relatively late stage of the disease.

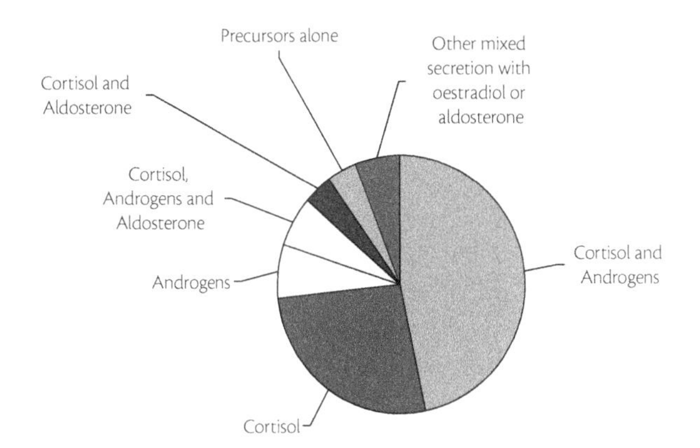

Fig. 5.4.2 Steroid secretion patterns in adrenocortical carcinoma. The frequency of each steroid secretion profile (expressed as a percentage) is shown according to hormonal investigations in secreting ACC (Cochin Endocrinology Department series, investigated as reported in Abiven, *et al.* 2006). Note that almost half of the secreting tumours will be responsible for a mixed secretion of cortisol and androgens.

Steroid excess

Most patients will present with signs of steroid excess. Cushing's syndrome associated with signs of androgens excess progressing for a few months is the most characteristic presentation (Fig. 5.4.2). Signs of mineralocorticoid or oestrogen excess are less frequent but highly suggestive of the diagnosis of ACC in a patient with an adrenal mass above 3 cm.

More than three-quarters of ACC patients suffer from steroid-secreting tumours when based on biochemical diagnosis following careful hormonal investigations of plasma and urine. In the near future, it is expected that mass spectrometry urine analysis will allow detection of alterations of adrenal steroid profile in all patient with ACC (12). In the absence of steroid excess, one should be cautious before diagnosing a mass of the adrenal area, which does not appear as a benign adrenal adenoma on imaging, as an adrenocortical tumour. Hormonal investigations are important for the diagnosis of the nature of an adrenal mass. Evidence of steroid excess can link an adrenal mass to its cortical origin. Some patterns of steroid oversecretion are very suggestive of malignancy. Hormonal investigations also give important information for patient management and may serve as a tumour marker during postoperative follow-up and treatment of the metastatic stage of the disease. In 2006, the ACC working group of the European Network for the Study of Adrenal Tumours (ENSAT) recommended a minimal hormonal work-up in patient with ACC (12, 13) (Box 5.4.1).

In contrast to benign adrenocortical tumours, which characteristically secrete a single class of steroid, usually either cortisol or

Box 5.4.1 Hormonal investigations in patients with ACC

These assays are adapted from the recommendation of the ACC working group of the European Network for the Study of Adrenal Tumours (ENSAT); the steroids in italics are not part of the minimal ENSAT work-up. This implies prior exclusion of a phaeochromocytoma by the urinary or plasma metanephrine and normetanephrine assay.

1 Glucocorticoid secretion (a minimum of three tests):
   - 24-h urinary free cortisol and urinary creatinine
   - Dexamethasone suppression test (1 mg)
   - Basal ACTH
   - Basal cortisol
2 Sex steroids:
   - Testosterone (in female)
   - Oestradiol (in male and postmenopausal women)
   - Androstenedione
   - DHEA-S (*or DHEA*)
3 Precursors:
   - 17-OH-progesterone
   - *S-compound*
   - *Deoxycorticosterone*
4 Mineralocorticoids:
   - Aldosterone/renin ratio (patients with hypertension or hypokalaemia)

aldosterone, ACC often secrete several types of steroids. Cosecretion of androgens and cortisol is the most frequent and is highly suggestive of a malignant adrenocortical tumour. Cortisol oversecretion will induce centripetal obesity, protein wasting with skin thinning, and striae, muscle atrophy (myopathy), and osteoporosis. Cortisol excess can also cause impaired defence against infection, diabetes, hypertension, psychiatric disturbances, and gonadal dysfunction in men and women. Androgen oversecretion may induce various manifestations in women: hirsutism, menstrual abnormalities, infertility, and eventually frank virilization (alopecia, deepening of the voice, clitoris hypertrophy). ACC can also secrete mineralocorticoids and steroids precursors. Oversecretion of oestrogens can be observed in rare cases and is very suggestive of ACC in a male patient with an adrenal tumour, where it often results in gynaecomastia.

ACTH-independent cortisol oversecretion is easily demonstrable by increased urinary cortisol excretion, cortisol secretion that is not suppressible with high doses of dexamethasone, and associated undetectable plasma ACTH levels. Plasma 17-hydroxyprogesterone is often elevated as well as the specific adrenal androgen DHEA-S, which leads to increased plasma testosterone in females. Other steroids, such as compound S, 11-deoxycorticosterone (DOC), δ4-androstenedione, and oestradiol, can be overproduced by the tumour. Secretion of aldosterone by ACC is not frequent and can be detected by plasma aldosterone and renin assays.

Imaging investigations

Computed tomography scan and magnetic resonance imaging

Imaging is an essential diagnostic step for ACC, especially in cases of adrenal incidentaloma. It is important both for the diagnosis of malignancy of an adrenal mass but also for the extension work-up. Adrenal CT scan is a very informative imaging procedure for adrenocortical tumours (14) (see also Chapter 5.1). In ACC, it shows a unilateral mass, which is most often large (above 5–6 cm, and typically 10 cm and above), lowering the kidney. Apart from the size of the tumour, the features suggestive of malignancy are: the lack of homogeneity with foci of necrosis and irregular margins; and a high spontaneous density observed before contrast media injection during CT scan (above 10 HU), indicating a low fat content in contrast to a usually characteristic high fat content observed in adrenocortical adenomas (Fig. 5.4.3). Dynamic measurement of contrast-enhanced densities may provide a more sensitive way to distinguish between benign and malignant lesions. A CT scan also contribute to the detection of local invasion, and distant metastases (liver, lung). This emphasizes the need to perform a CT scan of the abdomen and the chest prior to any surgery of a suspected ACC. Locoregional vessel invasion through the renal veins and the inferior vena cava can extend up to the right atrium and may result in metastatic lung embolism (15). MRI can be used, and might be as effective as CT scan when dynamic-gadolinium enhanced and chemical shift are used to characterize an adrenal mass. MRI can also participate to the detection of liver metastasis and venous invasions.

Nuclear imaging

More recently studies have demonstrated that ACCs almost always have a high uptake of [^{18}F]2-fluoro-2-deoxy-D-glucose (FDG).

(a)
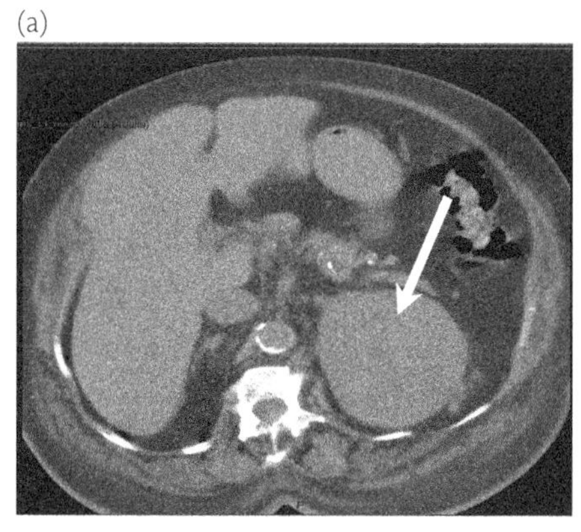
(b)
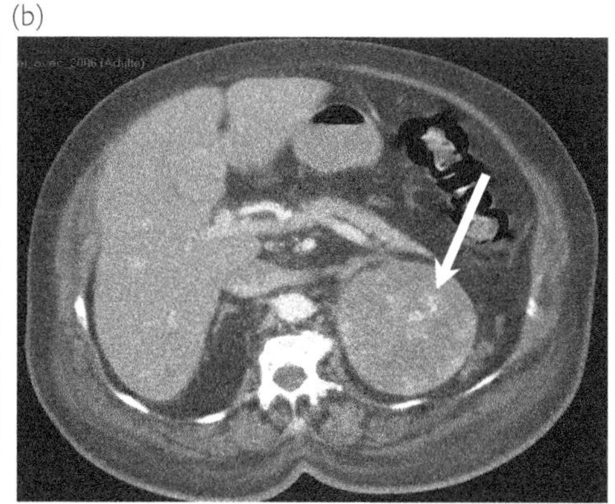

Fig. 5.4.3 Computed tomography scan of an adrenocortical cancer. The white arrow points to an ACC located in the left adrenal gland. The maximal diameter of the tumour on CT scan is 11 cm. The spontaneous density in the noninjected scan (a) is 38 HU (i.e. above the 20 HU cut-off suggestive of malignancy). After injection (b) the mass appear heterogeneous and the wash-out is below 50%.

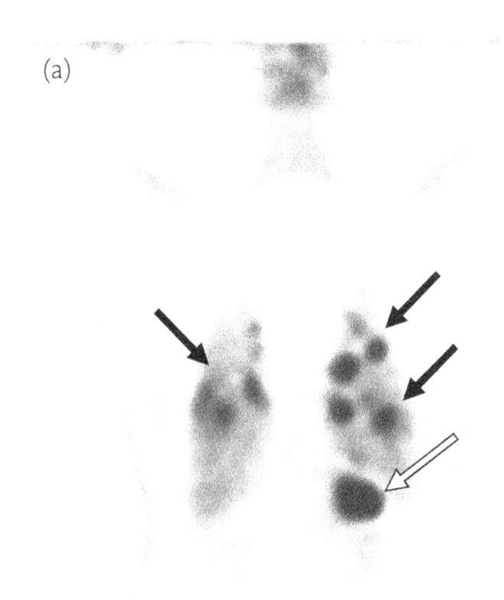

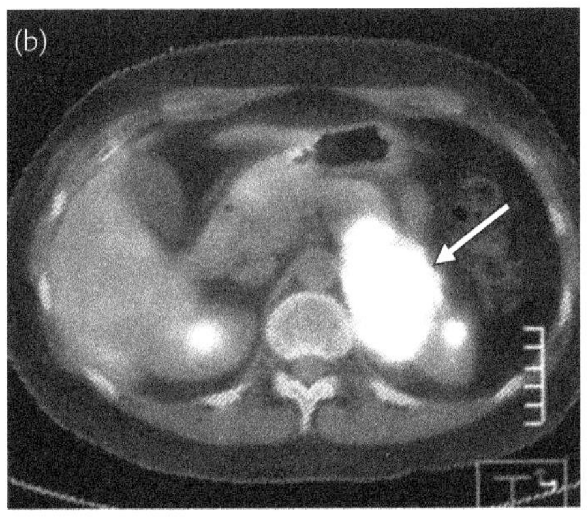

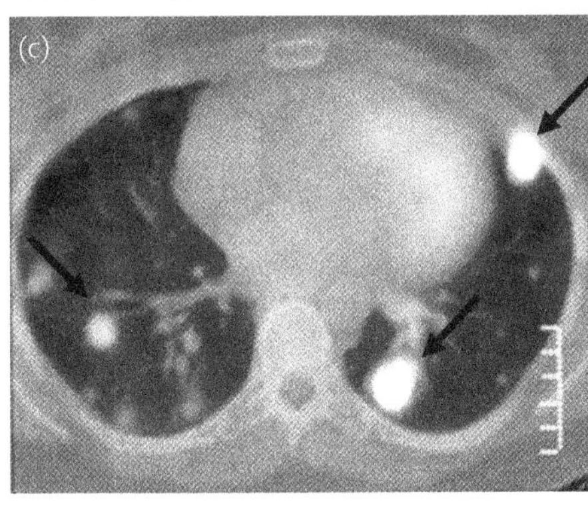

Fig. 5.4.4 ^{18}F-fluorodeoxyglucose positron emission tomography (FDG-PET) of a metastatic adrenocortical cancer. (a) The left adrenal tumour presents a high uptake on the FDG-PET scan (white arrow) and pulmonary metastasis are detected at diagnosis (black arrows) in this patient with a Stage 4 tumour. Combination of the PET imaging with a CT-scan (PET/CT) shows the adrenal primary tumour (b) and the pulmonary metastases (c). (See also Plate 22)

Thus FDG positron emission tomography (FDG-PET) appears to distinguish between benign and malignant adrenal tumours (16). This simple, noninvasive imaging procedure is part of the extended work-up in ACC (17) (Fig. 5.4.4). It is especially informative when it is combined with a CT scan (PET/CT). Currently FDG-PET is used as a very sensitive method prior to surgery of an adrenal tumour considered as an ACC; it is also used to exclude metastasis and during follow-up of ACC, in particular if recurrence is biochemically suspected but not visualized by CT.

Adrenal scintigraphy with iodocholesterol is not routinely needed but can help in some situations. Bone scintigraphy may help evaluate bone metastases. However, in patients with Cushing's syndrome bone remodelling and fractures can lead to false-positive results of bone scintigraphy and the wider use of FDG-PET might in the future replace it. New adrenal cortex specific scintigraphy imaging, using radiolabelled tracers such as metomidate, are under investigation and might be a promising tool in the not too distant future (18).

Diagnostic criteria and prognosis

Pathological diagnosis and the Weiss score

As discussed above, clinical, hormonal, and imaging investigations can be very suggestive of an ACC. Large adrenocortical tumours (>6 cm) are more likely to be malignant (Fig. 5.4.5), but tumour size is clearly not a valid criterion to diagnose or exclude malignancy. On the other hand, evidence of a metastatic adrenal mass with ACTH-independent steroid excess is almost diagnostic for ACC, with a few exception. However, histopathological diagnosis is always a very important step. In the case of nonhypersecreting and/or localized tumours, pathology is key to diagnose both the adrenocortical origin and the malignant nature of the mass. The adrenocortical origin of the tumour is based on the histological analysis, but also immunohistochemistry. Immunohistochemical markers are especially used to exclude other types of tumour, for instance a phaeochromocytoma will stained with a chromogranin A antibody but an ACC will not. The immunostains that can be positive in an adrenocortical tumour are either not specific (such as Melan A) or not used on a routine basis (such as SF-1 or steroidogenic enzyme).

As often is the case with endocrine tumours, the diagnosis of malignancy in adrenocortical lesions can be difficult for the pathologist. There is not a single pathological feature that allows the conclusive diagnosis of a malignant adrenal cortical tumour

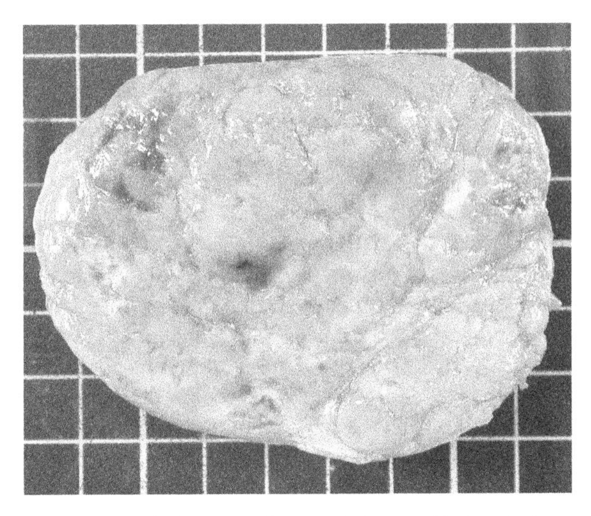

Fig. 5.4.5 Macroscopic view of an adrenocortical cancer. The length of each square is 1 cm. Note the characteristic large size and heterogeneous appearance of the tumour.

Box 5.4.2 The nine items of the Weiss score for the diagnosis of malignancy of an adrenocortical tumour

- The presence of three or more criteria classifies the tumour as a malignant one.
- High nuclear grade
- Mitotic rate above 5 per 50 high-power fields
- Atypical mitosis
- Less than 25% of clear cells
- Diffuse architecture
- Necrosis
- Venous invasion
- Sinusoidal structures invasion
- Tumour capsule invasion

based on the adrenal mass histology alone. Combinations of various histological parameters that allow establishment of a 'score' for a given tumour have been developed. The most widely used is the Weiss score, featuring nine different items (19) (Box 5.4.2). Each item is given a value of one when it is present and zero when it is absent. The total score is obtained by adding up the values of each individual item. It is assumed that a score of 3 or above is most probably associated with a malignant tumour. Other approaches based on microscopic feature analysis have been developed but have been less widely used and are therefore less validated than the Weiss score. However, all these approaches suffer limitations and are dependent on the experience of the pathologist. Therefore, efforts towards developing informative molecular markers of malignancy in ACC are under way. As described previously, IGF-2 overexpression and allelic losses at 17p13 have been suggested as potential molecular markers (3). Immunohistochemistry of cyclin E or Ki-67, which are higher in malignant adrenocortical tumours, has also been suggested as potentially useful diagnostic tools (12, 13). More recently, large-scale transcriptome analysis using DNA chips has been used to develop molecular markers based on the expression level of two genes for the diagnosis of malignancy (7). In the near future, such research efforts into translation are likely to have an important impact on our ability to accurately diagnose and classify adrenocortical tumours.

Tumour staging

Tumour staging is the most important prognostic factor in the diagnosis of ACC. The McFarlane staging, as modified by Sullivan, is the most commonly used and relies on surgical finding and extension work-up (20). It has been followed by the UICC/WHO TNM classification of ACC in 2004 (12). Four stages are differentiated with this score. Stage 1 and Stage 2 tumours are localized to the adrenal cortex and present a maximum diameter below or above 5 cm, respectively. Stage 3 tumours present with local infiltration reaching the surrounding adipose tissue or lymph node. Stage 4 tumours are associated with infiltration of the surrounding tissue and lymph nodes, invasion into adjacent organs, or distant metastases. The prognosis of Stage 1 and 2 tumours is better than that of Stage 3 or 4 tumours (11, 15) (Fig. 5.4.6). A score with slight

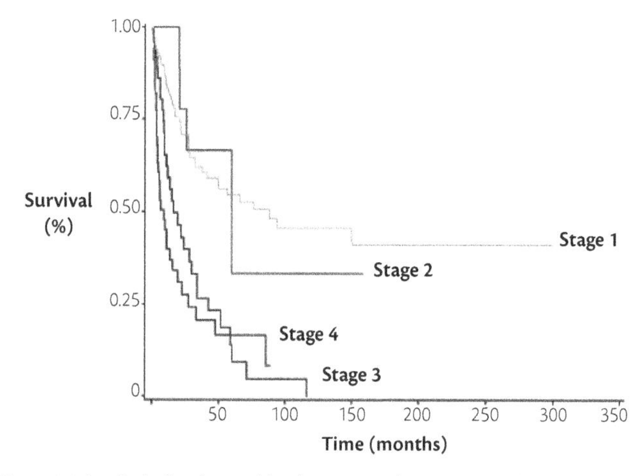

Fig. 5.4.6 Survival of patients with adrenocortical cancer according to initial staging. The survival time (expressed in months) according to Macfarlane stage is shown. (Cochin series, as described in Abiven G, Coste J, Groussin L, Anract P, Tissier F, Legmann P, *et al.* Clinical and biological features in the prognosis of adrenocortical cancer: poor outcome of cortisol-secreting tumors in a series of 202 consecutive patients. *J Clin Endocrinol Metab*, 2006; 91: 2650–5. (11)).

modification offering a better discrimination of the survival between the Stage 2 and 3 tumours has recently been defined by ENSAT (21).

Outcome and long-term survival

The metastatic spread of ACC involves mostly liver and lung, observed in about 35 to 50% of patients for each organ. Bone metastases are only diagnosed in 10 to 15% of cases. Metastatic spread to other organs is rare (11, 12).

The overall survival of patients with ACC is poor, with a 5-year survival rate below 35% in most series. However, this depends on tumour stage. It is likely that progress in medical management of adrenal incidentalomas and more sensitive investigations of modest signs of steroid excess will increase the detection of localized ACC (stages 1 or 2). This should improve the overall survival rate. A better survival has been reported in younger patients, but this is not a constant finding (11). Cortisol-secreting tumours might be associated with a worse prognosis (11, 22). This could be due to the morbidity associated with Cushing's syndrome or to differences in tumour progression. Some pathological features, such as a high mitotic rate or atypical mitotic figures as well as a high Ki-67 labelling, have been shown to be associated with a poor prognosis (12, 23, 24). This suggests that tumour biology plays a role in the prognosis. Here again, gene profiling has been used for tumour classification in research programmes to define molecular markers that might be useful in the near future for prognostication and therefore patient management (7).

Treatment

Treatment aims at correcting both steroid oversecretion and its clinical consequences in cases of secreting tumours and to eradicate the tumour in all cases. The best way to achieve both goals is the complete removal of the tumour whenever it is possible, depending on tumour stage and the patient's condition (Fig. 5.4.7).

Steroid oversecretion when clinically significant and not curable by tumour removal requires anticortisolic and/or symptomatic

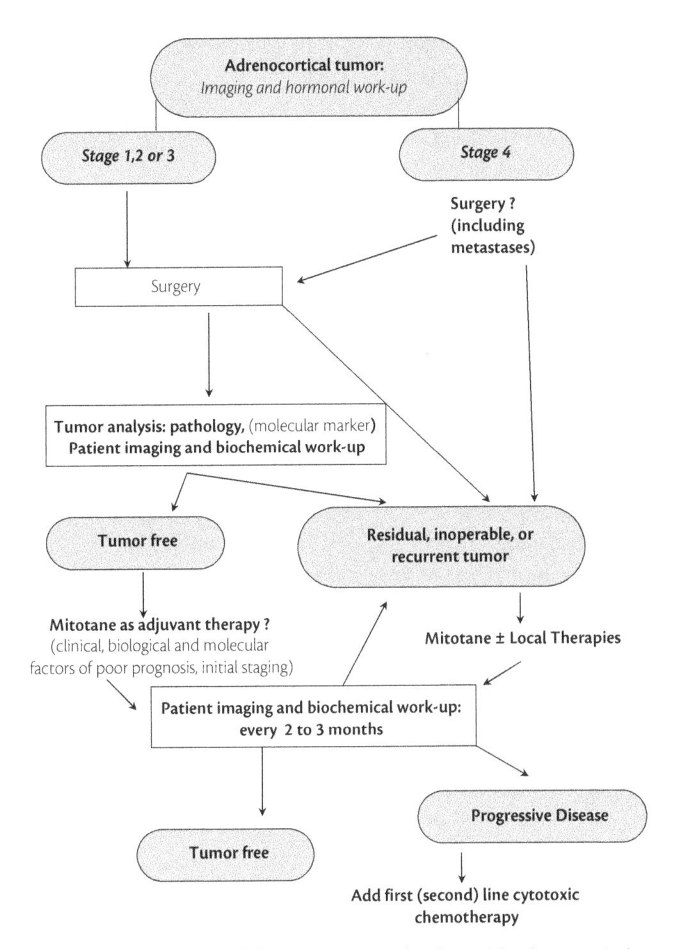

Fig. 5.4.7 Schematic view of the management of patient with adrenocortical cancer. Except in case of major contraindication to anaesthesia, surgery is indicated in patients with localized tumours (McFarlane Stage 1, 2 and 3). In patients with distant metastasis (Stage 4) surgery should be discussed to reduce tumour mass, particularly in patients with tumour-related hormone excess. Where possible, i.e. if all visible tumour mass can be removed, surgery of metastasis may be considered. Local recurrence without distant metastasis usually requires surgery. Other treatment options include radiotherapy (especially for bone metastasis), chemoembolization (mostly for liver metastasis), radiofrequency thermal ablation of lung or liver metastasis, as well as surgical removal of limited metastasis. The intervals between follow-up work-up, including imaging and biochemical work-up, can be extended to 3–4 months in patients presenting with complete remission and good prognostic factors, and might be extended to 6 months if there is still no recurrence after 2–3 years of continuous follow-up.

treatment. In this indication, mitotane is the drug most often used because it also has a cytotoxic effect on the adrenocortical cells, as discussed below. In some situation of severe Cushing's syndrome requiring rapid control of steroid excess, other drugs can also be used, eventually as combined therapy (e.g. ketoconazol, metyrapone, etomidate).

Surgery

Surgery of the adrenal tumour is the major treatment of stage 1–3 ACC. It can also be discussed in Stage 4 patients. The initial surgery is a crucial therapeutic step in the management of ACC. It should therefore be performed by trained surgeons, with experience of the management of adrenal tumours, to achieve complete tumour removal and avoid tumour spillage. Complete tumour removal and avoidance of violation of the tumour capsule is very important to increase the probability of long-term remission (15, 25). Open adrenalectomy is currently recommended as laparoscopic removal of malignant adrenocortical tumours could be associated with a high risk of peritoneal dissemination (26). Glucocorticoid replacement therapy should be started at the time of surgery of cortisol-secreting tumours to avoid adrenal deficiency resulting from long-term ACTH suppression by the ACC-associated cortisol oversecretion and thus functional suppression of the contralateral adrenal gland.

In Stage 4 patients with distant metastasis, tumour debulking with removal of the adrenal tumour can be discussed in order to reduce steroid excess and sometimes also tumour bulk, and requires multidisciplinary consideration. Surgery is discussed depending of the tumour bulk and spread as well as the growth velocity of the tumour. However, it is important to weigh the post-operative recovery period and the expected residual tumour mass and the systemic options for treatment in the discussion. When the number of metastasis is limited, their surgical removal can also be discussed.

In cases of local recurrence, surgery represents the preferred therapeutic option. If the patient had a long disease-free interval prior to development of the local recurrence, surgery can offer a good probability of long-lasting disease-free survival.

Local therapies and radiotherapy

Radiofrequency thermal ablation of liver and lung metastasis below 4 to 5 cm maximum diameter can be an alternative to surgical removal (13). Bone metastasis, e.g. in cases of spinal compression, can be operated to improve neurological impairment, but is also responsive in many cases to radiotherapy. Radiation therapy in ACC has often been considered as not very effective to control tumour growth. However, it has been recently suggested that it could help to prevent local recurrence, if not to prolong survival (12). Whether the tumour bed should be irradiated following initial, presumed curative surgery is widely debated and currently not established.

Medical therapy

When completed tumour removal is not possible or in cases of recurrence, medical treatment with o,p′DDD (*ortho, para′*, dichlorodiphenyldichloroethane, or mitotane) is recommended (21). Mitotane has a specific cytotoxic effect on adrenal cortical cells; it also inhibits steroid synthesis by an action on steroidogenic enzymes. Interestingly, mitotane is usually effective to control steroid excess in patients with secreting ACC. Most series reported in the literature on the efficacy of o,p′DDD in ACC are retrospective analyses with variable results regarding tumour progression. An objective tumour regression has been observed in about 25% of the cases (13). Patients with a cortisol-secreting ACC might have a better survival when treated with mitotane started in the 3 months following surgery of the adrenal tumour (11). A mitotane blood level of at least 14 mg/l seems to improve the tumour response (12, 13). However, side effects (mainly gastrointestinal and, at higher mitotane levels, neurological) often limit the ability to reach this suggested therapeutic plasma level. The daily mitotane dose required to achieve 14 mg/l varies from patients to patients. Therefore close monitoring of mitotane blood level is very helpful to remain in the narrow range between 14 and 20 mg/l, considered by most authors as the therapeutic range of mitotane in ACC. Since o,p′DDD invariably induces adrenal insufficiency, glucocorticoid replacement has to be initiated concurrently with mitotane and should be administered at increased doses (e.g. 40 to 80 mg per day) due to induction of Cortisol Binding Globulin (CBG) and cortisol metabolism by mitotane. The benefit of mitotane treatment as an adjuvant medical treatment after 'complete' surgical removal of a Stage 1 or 2 ACC remains to be conclusively demonstrated; however, at present, based on data from retrospective series, adjuvant mitotane is recommended for patients with a high risk of tumour recurrence (large tumour, potential capsule violation, high Ki-67) (27). Randomized international trials are expected to clarify whether mitotane should be recommended postoperatively in all patients with ACC.

Several cytotoxic chemotherapy regimens have been used in ACC. They are usually considered in patients with tumour progression under mitotane therapy. Various drugs have been used and the experience is still limited. It is currently accepted, since the Ann Arbor international conference on adrenocortical cancer (25), that combined treatment with cisplatin, etoposide, and doxorubicin together with mitotane or streptozotocin plus mitotane are the better regimens. The first phase III trial in ACC, the international FIRM-ACT trial, comparing these two regimens is currently in its final phase and will inform future management (12).

Conclusions

Considering the rarity of ACC, significant advances have been made in the last decade in the understanding of the pathophysiology. The advances have also been important for a better diagnosis and might ultimately lead to a better assessment of prognosis. However, much more progress needs to be achieved, especially to improve therapeutic efficiency. Due to the rarity of ACC, collaborative work performed in national and international networks dedicated to adrenocortical tumours will be key for ensuring the development of better diagnostic and therapeutic tools. In Europe this is the goal of ENSAT, which has been developed in the background of several national networks (in France, Italy, Germany, and UK) already working successfully in this field.

Areas of uncertainty or controversy

The pathological diagnosis of malignancy of an adrenocortical tumour can be difficult in some cases. Although careful analysis by an expert pathologist solves most cases, there are still some suspicious tumours with a borderline Weiss score (3) that are difficult to classify. The prognosis of a tumour diagnosed as malignant, especially after complete surgical resection of a Stage 1 or 2 ACC, is heterogeneous and still difficult to predict.

The surgical procedure has not been defined in a homogeneous way. The benefit of large *en bloc* aggressive surgical resection, which could lead to kidney ablation, and the strategy for lymph node removal need to be discussed. The possibility, by expert surgeons, to use laparoscopic resection of small ACC restricted to the adrenal without increasing the risk of local recurrence or peritoneal metastasis needs to be determined.

The benefit of radiotherapy has been suggested recently in retrospective studies, while ACC has usually been considered to be nonsensitive to radiotherapy. The place for radiotherapy as adjuvant or curative therapy will have to be established. The benefit of mitotane as adjuvant therapy is most often accepted but needs to be demonstrated in prospective trials.

Likely developments over the next 5–10 years

The development of new immunohistochemical markers should improve the pathological diagnosis and prognostication of ACC. Genomic studies will allow a better classification of adrenocortical tumours leading to the development of molecular markers for the classification and prognostication of adrenocortical tumours. These studies are also giving new insights on the pathophysiology of ACC and this should help to define new targeted therapies. The use of gas chromatography/mass spectrometry assays of urinary steroid currently investigated will help to define steroid profile for the diagnosis and follow-up of ACC. Similar proteomic approaches on urine and plasma are also expected. The development of new specific scintigraphies (such as ^{123}I-iodometomidate or ^{11}C-metomidate) is in progress and should improve tumour diagnosis and follow-up. Radiolabelled tracers could also be used for metabolic radiotherapy. The results of the FIRM-ACT study will determine the respective role of the two cytotoxic chemotherapies currently considered as the best options (cisplatin, etoposide, doxorubicin or streptozotocin). New targeted therapies are currently in preclinical and clinical studies. Among these, inhibitors of the IGF receptors are very attractive in view of the strong evidence for a major role of IGF-2 overexpression in the pathogenesis of ACC.

Acknowledgment

Dr Frédérique Tissier (Service d'Anatomopathologie, Hôpital Cochin) for help with the figures for this chapter.

References

1. Bertherat J, Bertagna X. Pathogenesis of adrenocortical cancer. *Best Pract Res Clin Endocrinol Metab*, 2009; **23**: 261–71.
2. Ribeiro RC, Sandrini F, Figueiredo B, Zambetti GP, Michalkiewicz E, Lafferty AR, *et al.* An inherited p53 mutation that contributes in a tissue-specific manner to pediatric adrenal cortical carcinoma. *Proc Natl Acad Sci U S A*, 2001; **98**: 9330–5.
3. Gicquel C, Bertagna X, Gaston V, Coste J, Louvel A, Baudin E, *et al.* Molecular markers and long-term recurrences in a large cohort of patients with sporadic adrenocortical tumors. *Cancer Res*, 2001; **61**: 6762–7.
4. Tissier F, Cavard C, Groussin L, Perlemoine K, Fumey G, Hagnere AM, *et al.*. Mutations of beta-catenin in adrenocortical tumors: activation of the Wnt signaling pathway is a frequent event in both benign and malignant adrenocortical tumors. *Cancer Res*, 2005; **65**: 7622–7.
5. Libe R, Bertherat J. Molecular genetics of adrenocortical tumours, from familial to sporadic diseases. *Eur J Endocrinol*, 2005; **153**: 477–87.
6. Giordano TJ, Thomas DG, Kuick R, Lizyness M, Misek DE, Smith AL, *et al.* Distinct transcriptional profiles of adrenocortical tumors uncovered by DNA microarray analysis. *Am J Pathol*, 2003; **162**: 521–31.
7. de Reynies A, Assie G, Rickman DS, Tissier F, Groussin L, Rene-Corail F, *et al.* Gene expression profiling reveals a new classification of adrenocortical tumors and identifies molecular predictors of malignancy and survival. *J Clin Oncol*, 2009; **27**: 1108–15.
8. Grumbach MM, Biller BM, Braunstein GD, Campbell KK, Carney JA, Godley PA, *et al.* Management of the clinically inapparent adrenal mass ("incidentaloma"). *Ann Intern Med*, 2003; **138**: 424–9.
9. Luton JP, Cerdas S, Billaud L, Thomas G, Guilhaume B, Bertagna X, *et al.* Clinical features of adrenocortical carcinoma, prognostic factors, and the effect of mitotane therapy. *N Engl J Med*, 1990; **322**: 1195–201.

10. Lindsay JR, Nieman LK. The hypothalamic-pituitary-adrenal axis in pregnancy: challenges in disease detection and treatment. *Endocr Rev*, 2005; **26**: 775–99.
11. Abiven G, Coste J, Groussin L, Anract P, Tissier F, Legmann P, *et al.* Clinical and biological features in the prognosis of adrenocortical cancer: poor outcome of cortisol-secreting tumors in a series of 202 consecutive patients. *J Clin Endocrinol Metab*, 2006; **91**: 2650–5.
12. Fassnacht M, Allolio B. Clinical management of adrenocortical carcinoma. *Best Pract Res Clin Endocrinol Metab*, 2009; **23**: 273–89.
13. Libe R, Fratticci A, Bertherat J. Adrenocortical cancer: pathophysiology and clinical management. *Endocr Relat Cancer*, 2007; **14**: 13–28.
14. Hamrahian AH, Ioachimescu AG, Remer EM, Motta-Ramirez G, Bogabathina H, Levin HS, *et al.* Clinical utility of noncontrast computed tomography attenuation value (hounsfield units) to differentiate adrenal adenomas/hyperplasias from nonadenomas: Cleveland Clinic experience. *J Clin Endocrinol Metab*, 2005; **90**: 871–7.
15. Icard P, Goudet P, Charpenay C, Andreassian B, Carnaille B, Chapuis Y, *et al.* Adrenocortical carcinomas: surgical trends and results of a 253-patient series from the French Association of Endocrine Surgeons study group. *World J Surg*, 2001; **25**: 891–7.
16. Groussin L, Bonardel G, Silvera S, Tissier F, Coste J, Abiven G, *et al.* 18F-Fluorodeoxyglucose positron emission tomography for the diagnosis of adrenocortical tumors: a prospective study in 77 operated patients. *J Clin Endocrinol Metab*, 2009; **94**: 1713–22.
17. Leboulleux S, Dromain C, Bonniaud G, Auperin A, Caillou B, Lumbroso J, *et al.* Diagnostic and prognostic value of 18-fluorodeoxyglucose positron emission tomography in adrenocortical carcinoma: a prospective comparison with computed tomography. *J Clin Endocrinol Metab*, 2006; **91**: 920–5.
18. Hahner S, Stuermer A, Kreissl M, Reiners C, Fassnacht M, Haenscheid H, *et al.* [^{123}I]Iodometomidate for molecular imaging of adrenocortical cytochrome. P450 family 11B enzymes. *J Clin Endocrinol Metab*, 2008; **93**: 2358–65.
19. Lau SK, Weiss LM. The Weiss system for evaluating adrenocortical neoplasms: 25 years later. *Hum Pathol*, 2009; **40**: 757–68.
20. Sullivan M, Boileau M, Hodges CV. Adrenal cortical carcinoma. *J Urol*, 1978; **120**: 660–5.
21. Fassnacht M, Johanssen S, Quinkler M, Bucsky P, Willenberg HS, Beuschlein F, *et al.* Limited prognostic value of the 2004 International Union Against Cancer staging classification for adrenocortical carcinoma: proposal for a Revised TNM Classification. *Cancer*, 2009; **115**: 243–50.
22. Berruti A, Terzolo M, Sperone P, Pia A, Casa SD, Gross DJ, *et al.* Etoposide, doxorubicin and cisplatin plus mitotane in the treatment of advanced adrenocortical carcinoma: a large prospective phase II trial. *Endocr Relat Cancer*, 2005; **12**: 657–66.
23. Stojadinovic A, Ghossein RA, Hoos A, Nissan A, Marshall D, Dudas M, *et al.* Adrenocortical carcinoma: clinical, morphologic, and molecular characterization. *J Clin Oncol*, 2002; **20**: 941–50.
24. Assie G, Antoni G, Tissier F, Caillou B, Abiven G, Gicquel C, *et al.* Prognostic parameters of metastatic adrenocortical carcinoma. *J Clin Endocrinol Metab*, 2007; **92**: 148–54.
25. Schteingart DE, Doherty GM, Gauger PG, Giordano TJ, Hammer GD, Korobkin M, *et al.* Management of patients with adrenal cancer: recommendations of an international consensus conference. *Endocr Relat Cancer*, 2005; **12**: 667–80.
26. Harrison BJ. Surgery of adrenocortical cancer. *Ann Endocrinol (Paris)*, 2009; **70**: 195–6.
27. Terzolo M, Angeli A, Fassnacht M, Daffara F, Tauchmanova L, Conton PA, *et al.* Adjuvant mitotane treatment for adrenocortical carcinoma. *N Engl J Med*, 2007; **356**: 2372–80.

5.5

Phaeochromocytomas, paragangliomas, and neuroblastoma

Isla S. Mackenzie, Morris J. Brown

Introduction

Phaeochromocytomas are rare neuroendocrine tumours of neural crest origin, which often produce excess catecholamines (1). Although usually arising from the chromaffin cells of the adrenal medulla, phaeochromocytomas may also arise at other sites of sympathetic or parasympathetic chromaffin tissue anywhere from the base of the skull to the pelvis. Extra-adrenal phaeochromocytomas are called paragangliomas. Some patients with phaeochromocytoma or paraganglioma present with the classical triad of symptoms of headaches, palpitations, and sweating but many others present with less specific features such as hypertension or with an unidentified mass lesion.

Owing to the rarity of the condition and the relatively nonspecific symptoms with which it often presents, it is not unusual for several years to pass from symptom onset until the diagnosis of phaeochromocytoma is made. However, the consequences of not finding a phaeochromocytoma can be severe and may even result in death. In fact, in one study, around 50% of cases of phaeochromocytoma found at post mortem were unsuspected during life. Interestingly, a former US President, Dwight Eisenhower, was found to have a 1.5 cm adrenal phaeochromocytoma at post mortem, which was undiagnosed during life despite a history of severe hypertension and headaches (2). Patients with untreated phaeochromocytoma are at risk of the cardiovascular consequences of catecholamine surges, including hypertensive emergencies, intracerebral haemorrhage, and acute heart failure. Approximately 10% of phaeochromocytomas are malignant and some represent part of familial syndromes. The genetic basis of many phaeochromocytomas is becoming increasingly apparent as more mutations are found.

Historical perspective

The first report in the literature of a likely case of phaeochromocytoma was made in 1886 by Frankel, who treated an 18-year-old patient with hypertension and bilateral adrenal tumours. The term 'paraganglioma' was introduced in 1908 by Alezais and Peyron, describing chromaffin tumours arising in paraganglia. The adrenal condition was named phaeochromocytoma in 1912 by a pathologist, Pick, who described the features of the tumour in more detail. The name is derived from the Greek terms *phaios* (dark, dusky), *chroma* (colour, referring to the chromium staining characteristics of phaeochromocytoma tissue), and *cytoma* (cell body). The first successful operative removal of a phaeochromocytoma took place in 1926.

Over the years, associations of phaeochromocytoma with other conditions now known to be of a genetic nature were described. Firstly, an association of phaeochromocytoma with neurofibromatosis (1910), then an association with retinal angioma (1953), which was later recognized to be part of von Hippel–Lindau disease. In the 1960s, the term multiple endocrine neoplasia (MEN) type 2 was introduced to describe the association of familial phaeochromocytoma with multiple endocrine tumours (3). Gradually, the genetic abnormalities responsible for these conditions have been elucidated. Recently, other genetic mutations contributing to phaeochromocytoma and paraganglioma syndromes have been described, most notably mutations in succinate dehydrogenase (SDH) subunits.

Aetiology, genetics, pathogenesis, and pathology

The majority of phaeochromocytomas and paragangliomas arise sporadically and the aetiology is not clearly understood. There are no definite known environmental triggers. However, up to 25% of apparently sporadic phaeochromocytomas and paragangliomas are due to germline mutations (4), a higher incidence than previously thought. There is a lack of clear pathological definition between benign and malignant tumours and it is not known whether apparently benign tumours would progress to malignant ones if left untreated for long enough.

Genetics

The genetic syndromes associated with phaeochromocytoma or paraganglioma include MEN type 2A and 2B, von Hippel–Lindau disease, neurofibromatosis, tuberous sclerosis, Carney's triad, Sturge–Weber syndrome, ataxia–telangectasia, and the familial paraganglioma syndromes. Identification of a phaeochromocytoma or paraganglioma, certainly in a younger patient, should precipitate consideration of whether it is an isolated lesion or is part of a genetic syndrome.

While some cases associated with a genetic syndrome may be strongly suspected due to family history or other clinical features, the decision whether patients presenting with sporadic phaeochromocytoma or paraganglioma should undergo genetic testing for the more commonly associated genetic mutations (*ret* proto-oncogene (*MEN2*), von Hippel–Lindau disease (*VHL*), and malignant phaeochromocytoma and paraganglioma (*SDHB*, *SDHC*, and *SDHD* mutations)) (Table 5.5.1) is somewhat controversial. A reasonable practice is to test all those presenting under the age of 50 years, those with multiple or malignant lesions, extra-adrenal lesions, positive family history, or features leading to clinical suspicion of one of the genetic syndromes. Some economies can be achieved by a focused staged approach, screening for the most likely affected genes first, based on the clinical features and history (5, 6, 7).

Pathogenesis and pathology

Around 90% of phaeochromocytomas arise in the adrenal gland. The remainder of phaeochromocytomas (extra-adrenal phaeochromocytomas or paragangliomas) mainly arise within the abdomen—the majority either occurring in the perirenal area or around the abdominal aorta (often in the organ of Zuckerkandl). They may, however, arise in any region from the base of the skull to the pelvis. Around 10% of the tumours are malignant and about 10% are bilateral. The traditional 'rule of 10s', often quoted with regard to phaeochromocytoma, stated that '10% are extra-adrenal, 10% bilateral, 10% malignant, and 10% genetic.' Although much of this rule has held true over the years, we now know that more than 10% of the tumours probably have a genetic basis (see above).

The pathology of phaeochromocytoma is complex (8, 9) (Fig. 5.5.1). Macroscopically, the tumours are often grey or haemorrhagic in appearance, with areas of necrosis and sometimes calcification. Sometimes the normal adrenal cortex is visible at the edge of the tumour. Benign phaeochromocytomas are often well encapsulated, although capsular invasion is not in itself evidence of malignancy. Most tumours have reached at least 2 cm in size by the time of clinical presentation and they can occasionally be

Table 5.5.1 Genetic syndromes associated with phaeochromocytoma

		Inheritance	Gene	Mutation(s)	Clinical features	Risk of phaeochromocytoma/ other features
MEN 2A 2B		Autosomal dominant	*RET* proto-oncogene; 10q11.2; 21 exons	Several described; 90% in tyrosine kinase domain	Medullary thyroid cancer, parathyroid hyperplasia, phaeochromocytoma Medullary thyroid cancer, mucosal neuromas, phaeochromocytoma	50% risk Mean age for phaeochromocytoma diagnosis 40 years. Rarely extra-adrenal. Usually benign
VHL	Types 2A 2B 2C	Autosomal dominant Renal cell carcinoma Phaeochromocytoma only	*VHL*; 3p25–26; 3 exons	Several described	Retinal angiomas, cerebellar haemangioblastomas, phaeochromocytoma, renal cell carcinoma. Renal, pancreatic and epididymal cysts. Pancreatic islet tumours	10–15% risk Mean age for phaeochromocytoma diagnosis 29 years. 10% extra-adrenal 5% malignant Most commonly noradrenaline excess.
NF1		Autosomal dominant	*NF1*; 17q11.2; 59 exons	Several Usually clinical diagnosis	*Café-au-lait* patches, cutaneous neurofibromas, axillary freckling, Lisch nodules, phaeochromocytoma	*c.* 2% risk Mean age at diagnosis of phaeochromocytoma 40 years.
SDH						
B			*SDHB* (*PGL4*); 1p36.13; 59 exons		Phaeochromocytoma adrenal and extra-adrenal, head + neck paraganglioma, renal cell carcinoma, GIST	Mean age at diagnosis of phaeochromocytoma ~28 years. 80% penetrance by 50yrs. High malignant potential.
C			*SDHC* (*PGL3*); 1q21		Head + neck paraganglioma GIST Rarely phaeochromocytoma	
D			*SDHD* (*PGL1*); 11q23; 4 exons	Maternal imprinting	Head + neck paraganglioma, phaeochromocytoma, often extra-adrenal. GIST	

MEN, multiple endocrine neoplasia; VHL, von Hippel–Lindau; NF, neurofibromatosis; PGL, paraganglioma; SDH, succinate dehydrogenase; GIST, gastrointestinal stromal tumours.

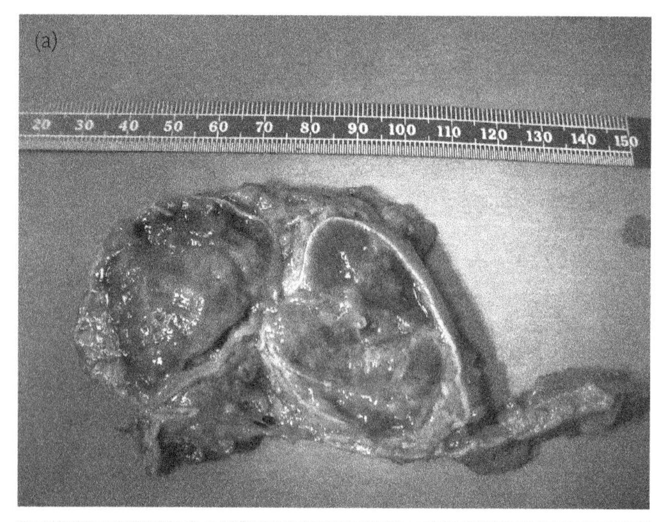

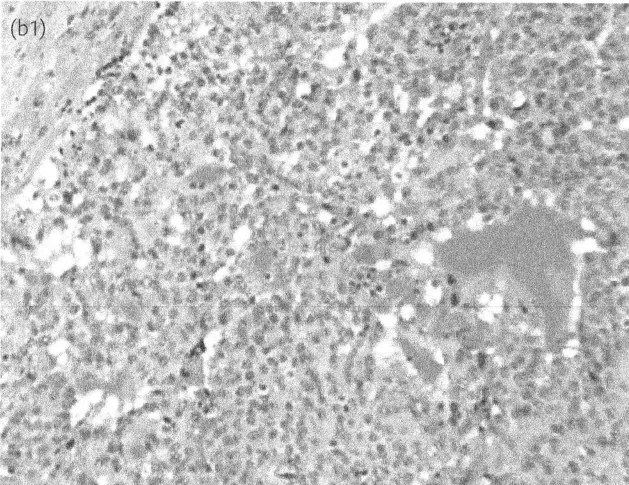

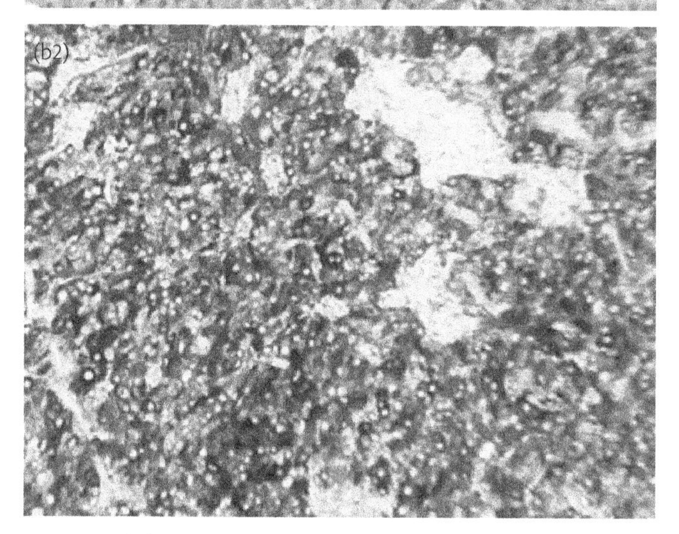

Fig. 5.5.1 Pathological appearances of phaeochromocytoma.
(a) Macroscopically, phaeochromocytomas are often greyish or haemorrhagic in appearance and there may be areas of necrosis. A capsule may be present around the tumour and a rim of normal adrenal cortex is sometimes seen.
(b) Microscopically, phaeochromocytomas consist of clusters of cells with variable degrees of mitotic figures and containing catecholamine secretory granules. (b1) The cells have amphophilic granular cytoplasm and eccentric nucleoli. (b2) Phaeochromocytomas usually stain positively for neuroendocrine and neural tissue markers including chromogranin, synaptophysin, neurospecific enolase, and S-100. (See also Plate 23)

very large, e.g. around 20 cm in size. Smaller tumours are occasionally detected in cases of familial screening such as MEN 2. Microscopically, the tumours consist of chromaffin tissue and usually contain secretory granules of catecholamines within the cells. Immunological staining can be used to identify the origin of the tissue. Phaeochromocytomas usually stain positively with neural tissue stains. It is generally not possible to differentiate between benign and malignant phaeochromocytomas based on histological appearance, but features that raise slightly the need to watch for malignant behaviour include large size, extra-adrenal location, and evidence of local vascular invasion. The finding of frequent mitoses in tumour sections or the presence of a germline *SDHB* mutation increase markedly the likelihood of malignancy—up to 60% in the case of *SDHB*-positive patients. However, the only definite diagnosis of malignancy comes from the finding of chromaffin tissue at a site where no chromaffin tissue should be present. Attempts have been made to develop pathological scoring systems to predict the likelihood of subsequent malignant disease, but the general consensus is that these are of limited utility. The most common sites of metastases from phaeochromocytoma include bones, lungs, liver, and lymph nodes. Following resection of adrenal phaeochromocytoma, local recurrence in the adrenal bed is also commonly described.

Epidemiology

Phaeochromocytomas and paragangliomas affect both genders equally, or with a slight male predominance, and no racial predilection has been described for sporadic tumours. There is no known geographical influence on the incidence of phaeochromocytoma or paraganglioma, except that clusters of familial cases have been described due to geographical isolation of populations carrying one of the genetic mutations, e.g. in remote mountainous village communities in Italy.

Phaeochromocytomas and paragangliomas affect all age groups. Those occurring in childhood are more commonly related to one of the genetic syndromes, especially von Hippel–Lindau disease or MEN 2. Phaeochromocytomas are rare in infancy and become more common in older children from 6–14 years of age (peak incidence in children is 11 years of age). Those presenting in early adulthood are again more likely to be associated with a genetic syndrome. Most phaeochromocytomas in adults present between the ages of 20 and 50 years but there is probably also a higher incidence than previously thought in the elderly, perhaps because elderly patients may not undergo such intensive investigation if they develop hypertension or perhaps because the elderly may develop less clinically obvious phaeochromocytomas. Certainly, post mortem studies in the elderly have confirmed that phaeochromocytomas are a more common finding than might be expected.

The true incidence of phaeochromocytoma is difficult to ascertain as many cases are probably never detected during life. Around 0.1–0.6% of patients attending hypertension clinics are found to have phaeochromocytomas and around 4% of patients presenting with an incidental adrenal mass found on abdominal imaging have a phaeochromocytoma. Most cases of phaeochromocytoma or paraganglioma are detected following investigation for symptoms or signs, but some are detected earlier as part of screening programmes in individuals with known familial syndromes such as MEN 2 or von Hippel–Lindau disease. For more common conditions such as hypertension, it is more difficult to decide who to screen for phaeochromocytoma. Some clinicians favour screening all hypertensive patients at least once, since phaeochromocytoma can be asymptomatic, but overall this results in a very low rate of detection and is probably not cost-effective. An alternative approach is to only screen younger patients and those with any suggestive symptoms. Other patients who should be considered for screening for phaeochromocytoma include those with unexplained heart failure or ischaemic heart disease, for example in young patients with no other risk factors.

Clinical features and differential diagnosis

The clinical features of phaeochromocytoma vary widely in different patients but are largely due to the effects of catecholamine excess and local effects of the tumour (Box 5.5.1). The most common presentation is with headache, sweating, and palpitations—usually associated with hypertension. Classically, these symptoms are paroxysmal in nature, although in some patients they are present most of the time. Some patients notice certain triggers for their symptoms, such as lying on one side in a case of a patient with adrenal phaeochromocytoma and passing urine in the case of a patient with a bladder phaeochromocytoma. Other common presenting features include anxiety, nausea, vomiting, weight loss, abdominal or chest pain, fatigue, tremor, blurred vision, and episodes of flushing or grey pallor. Orthostatic hypotension is a feature in some patients and hyperglycaemia is present in around 40% of patients at presentation.

Box 5.5.1 Clinical features of phaeochromocytoma

- Headache
- Palpitations
- Sweating
- Hypertension
- Grey pallor
- Flushing
- Abdominal pain
- Chest pain
- Nausea
- Vomiting
- Weight loss
- Blurred vision
- Anxiety
- Tremor
- Paraesthesiae
- Feelings of 'impending doom'
- Fatigue
- Postural hypotension
- Hyperglycaemia
- Constipation

Box 5.5.2 Substances secreted by phaeochromocytomas

- Noradrenaline[a]
- Adrenaline[a]
- Dopamine[a]
- Adrenocorticotrophic hormone
- Vasoactive intestinal peptide
- Neuropeptide Y
- Atrial natriuretic factor
- Growth hormone releasing factor
- Somatostatin
- Parathyroid hormone
- Calcitonin
- Serotonin
- Insulin-like growth factor-2
- Endothelin
- Calcitonin gene-related peptide
- Histamine

[a] Most commonly.

More rarely, other features are seen, sometimes in relation to the cosecretion of other substances in addition to catecholamines, for example hypoglycaemia in a patient cosecreting insulin-like growth factor-2 and Cushingoid features in patients cosecreting ACTH. Many other substances may also be cosecreted from phaeochromocytomas. Predominantly, the symptoms and signs in any one patient depend upon the location of the tumour and the relative amounts of secretion of the different catecholamines (noradrenaline, adrenaline, and dopamine) but also on any other substances secreted by that particular tumour (Box 5.5.2). For example, patients with pure dopamine-secreting phaeochromocytomas (extremely rare) classically present with hypotension rather than hypertension.

Tumours located outwith the adrenal gland rarely secrete adrenaline because the conversion of noradrenaline to adrenaline depends on the presence of the enzyme phenylethanolamine *N*-methyltransferase (PNMT), which is restricted to the adrenal medulla and certain regions of the brain (Fig. 5.5.2). Interestingly, very large or necrotic adrenal phaeochromocytomas may lose the ability to secrete adrenaline. This is because PNMT requires the presence of cortisol for enzyme induction. If the architecture of the adrenal gland is sufficiently disrupted by the presence of a large tumour, this impairs the delivery of cortisol from the adrenal cortex to the site of PNMT location in the medulla, preventing the conversion of noradrenaline to adrenaline by the tumour. Patients with von Hippel–Lindau disease often have normal adrenaline secretion, despite the usual adrenal site of the tumours.

Occasionally, patients with phaeochromocytoma present acutely with hypertensive crisis or shock. Such crises may be induced by sudden surges of catecholamine release, e.g. following tumour palpation or following haemorrhage or infarction of the tumour.

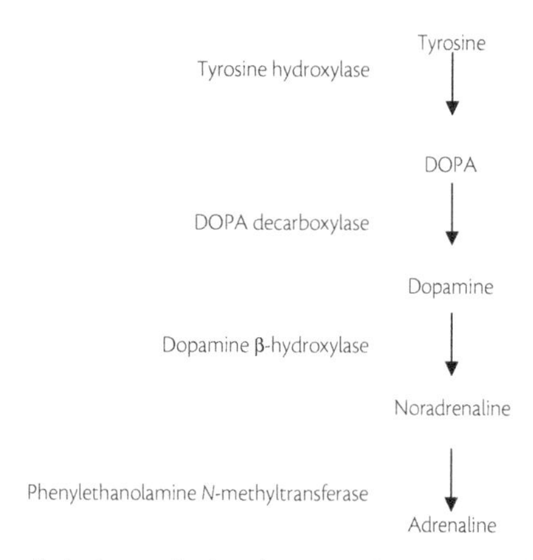

Fig. 5.5.2 Catecholamine synthesis pathway. Tyrosine is converted to dihydroxyphenylalanine (DOPA) then to dopamine, noradrenaline, and adrenaline. The conversion of noradrenaline to adrenaline is catalysed by the enzyme phenoxyethanolamine *N*-methyltransferase (PNMT) in the adrenal medulla, which is dependent on cortisol as a cofactor.

Administration of certain medications or chemical agents may also induce phaeochromocytoma crisis, e.g. dopamine antagonists (antiemetics or neurotropic drugs), some anaesthetic agents, tricyclic antidepressants, steroids (10) or synthetic ACTH, and radiographic contrast media. Phaeochromocytoma may also present acutely with accelerated hypertension (Fig. 5.5.3), hypertensive encephalopathy, acute myocardial infarction, acute heart failure, aortic dissection, arrhythmias, or sudden death.

The presenting features of paragangliomas vary depending on whether they are secretory. Those that secrete excess levels of catecholamines (usually abdominal paragangliomas) tend to present in a similar way to phaeochromocytomas. The majority of head and neck paragangliomas present initially as lumps, which on later investigation are found to be chromaffin tumours, or with other local features such as pain or mass effect.

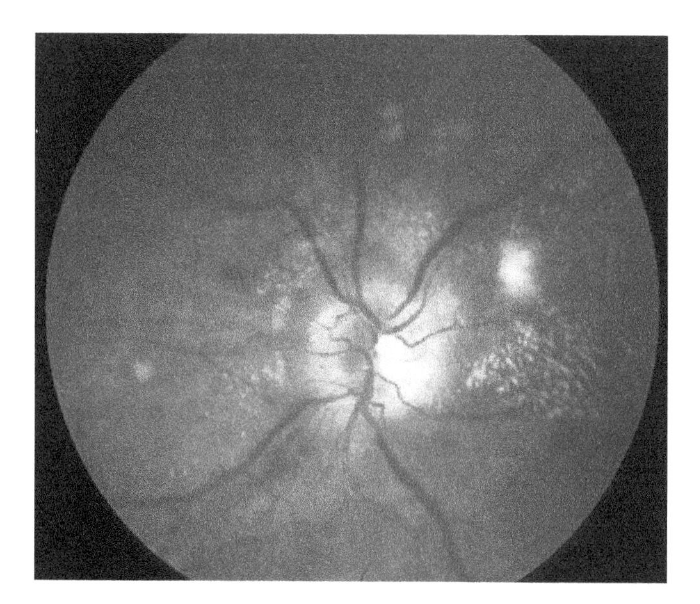

Fig. 5.5.3 Accelerated hypertension—retinal changes. This 23-year-old woman presented with accelerated hypertension. She had a history of several years of treated hypertension, headaches, and sweating. Retinal changes seen in accelerated hypertension include flame-shaped haemorrhages, papilloedema, and macular exudates (macular star). She was found to have an adrenal phaeochromocytoma. (See also Plate 24)

Differential diagnosis

The differential diagnosis of phaeochromocytoma is wide and patients may present to many different health professionals before the condition is finally recognized. Conditions causing sympathetic overactivity present with very similar features to phaeochromocytoma. These include anxiety or panic disorder, drug use (e.g. sympathomimetics, cocaine, monoamine oxidase inhibitors), baroreflex failure, and heart failure. Similar sweating may be seen in other endocrine conditions such as hyperthyroidism, hypoglycaemia, or even as part of the menopause. Other causes of headache (e.g. migraine) and palpitations (e.g. ischaemic heart disease) must also be considered. Pseudophaeochromocytoma shares many features with phaeochromocytoma and is often associated with mild catecholamine excess, but no anatomical lesion can be found. It is a diagnosis of exclusion and is thought to be associated with childhood traumatic experiences (11).

Clinical investigation and diagnostic criteria

Most phaeochromocytomas secrete excess catecholamines, therefore initial investigation is biochemical with the aim of establishing whether catecholamine excess is present (either continually or intermittently). Once catecholamine excess has been confirmed, attention then turns to localizing the tumour—with the most likely location being the adrenal gland. Both anatomical and functional imaging techniques are useful in establishing the location of the phaeochromocytoma.

Biochemical investigation

Catecholamines or their metabolic products can be measured in blood or urine (12, 13) (Table 5.5.2). Plasma or urine levels of noradrenaline, adrenaline, and dopamine can be measured directly. One or more of these are often elevated in cases of phaeochromocytoma, particularly if the patient is symptomatic (or hypertensive) at the time of measurement. However, if secretion is intermittent, as can sometimes be the case in phaeochromocytoma, the diagnosis may be missed. Collecting 24-h urine samples increases the sensitivity further, but, even then, false-negative results can occur. In order to confidently exclude phaeochromocytoma in a patient with suggestive symptoms, more than one negative collection is required. Measurement of plasma or urine total metadrenalines (normetadrenalines and metadrenalines) is a more sensitive test for phaeochromocytoma. Vanillyl mandelic acid measurement in the urine is highly specific but not very sensitive for the detection of phaeochromocytoma and in current practice its use has been replaced by the measurement of catecholamines and metadrenalines. Urine homovanillic acid is commonly used in the detection and monitoring of childhood neuroblastoma. Measurement of chromogranin A in plasma may also be useful in the detection of some phaeochromocytomas and other neuroendocrine tumours. However, the best test currently available is probably plasma metadrenalines measurement, with a close second best being urine metadrenalines. Limited availability of these methods results in the most commonly used test being measurement of urinary catecholamines.

A common problem in the biochemical diagnostic process for phaeochromocytoma is the finding of falsely positive borderline

Table 5.5.2 Biochemical tests for phaeochromocytoma

	Sensitivity (%)	Specificity (%)
Plasma metadrenalines	96–98	87–90
Urinary metadrenalines	93–99	45–80
Plasma catecholamines	70–92	69–72
Urinary catecholamines	83–93	59–80
Urinary vanillyl mandelic acid	63–76	86–94
Chromogranin A	83	96

elevated levels of catecholamines. Often this is caused by interference by concomitant medications, e.g. tricyclic antidepressants, paracetamol, labetalol, L-dihydroxyphenylalanine (L-DOPA), methyldopa, so the first step is to repeat the measurements without the influence of any potentially interfering medications. However, in other cases, it can be difficult to establish whether there is a true excess of catecholamines due to a phaeochromocytoma or whether the borderline excess catecholamine level is due to sympathetic overactivity of another cause such as anxiety. In such cases where the diagnosis is doubted, one way to differentiate between truly autonomous secretion from a tumour and general sympathetic overactivity is to perform a suppression test.

Suppression testing—pentolinium or clonidine

Suppression testing in the investigation of phaeochromocytoma may be performed using either pentolinium (ganglion blocker) or clonidine (central α_2-agonist and imidazoline (I_1) agonist). Both of these tests are useful for excluding phaeochromocytoma in patients with baseline elevated levels of noradrenaline. In the pentolinium suppression test (14), after a period of supine rest, baseline blood samples are collected for catecholamine or metadrenaline measurement. Then 2.5 mg intravenous pentolinium is administered. Further blood samples are taken at 10 and 20 min. In a patient without a phaeochromocytoma, over 40% suppression of baseline noradrenaline or normetadrenaline levels would be expected. In a patient with an autonomously secreting phaeochromocytoma, no significant suppression should occur. Similarly, in the clonidine suppression test (15), 300 μg of clonidine is administered orally after baseline blood samples have been collected. Further blood samples are collected hourly for 3 h. Again, suppression of baseline noradrenaline or normetadrenaline levels is expected in patients without phaeochromocytoma but no significant suppression in patients with a phaeochromocytoma. Both pentolinium and clonidine can cause marked hypotension and these tests should be performed under specialist supervision only. After pentolinium, hypotension is usually postural and transient, providing renal function is normal. Other antihypertensive medications are usually withheld, if possible, for 24 h prior to the tests.

Stimulation tests to diagnose phaeochromocytoma are dangerous and are no longer performed.

Anatomical imaging of phaeochromocytoma

CT and MRI are the mainstay of anatomical imaging techniques to localize phaeochromocytoma. As the majority of phaeochromocytomas are located in the adrenal glands, imaging focuses on this region. Both techniques have a high sensitivity but lower specificity for locating phaeochromocytomas. Lesions greater than around 0.5 cm are usually easily detected on either technique, although in our experience, on two occasions, smaller phaeochromocytomas have been mistaken for the inferior vena cava during initial CT investigations for adrenal phaeochromocytoma (Fig. 5.5.4). On CT, phaeochromocytomas typically have a heterogeneous appearance with Hounsfield units above 20 and may contain flecks of calcification (Fig. 5.5.5). On T_2-weighted MRI, phaeochromocytomas have a typically bright appearance, again with features of heterogeneity (Fig. 5.5.6). With the increasing use of abdominal CT and MRI, more phaeochromocytomas are being detected as incidental findings than ever before.

(a)

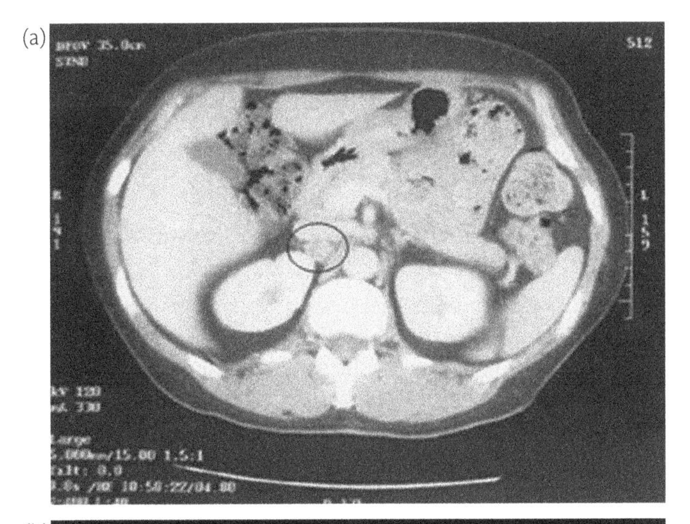

(b)

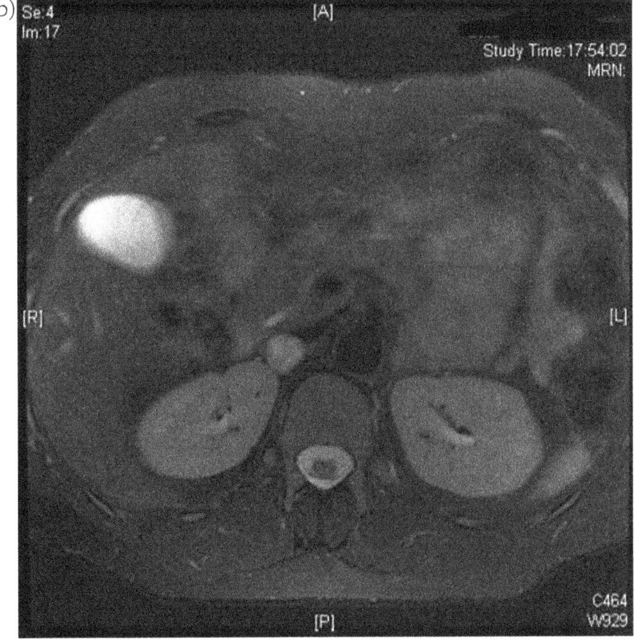

Fig. 5.5.4 Small adrenal phaeochromocytomas may be mistaken for the inferior vena cava on CT imaging. (a) This 48-year-old woman presented with hypertension and symptoms suggestive of phaeochromocytoma. Catecholamine measurements were borderline. The initial abdominal CT scan was reported as normal; the small right adrenal lesion (circled) was mistaken for the inferior vena cava. (b) Subsequent MR scanning clearly showed a right adrenal lesion consistent with phaeochromocytoma.

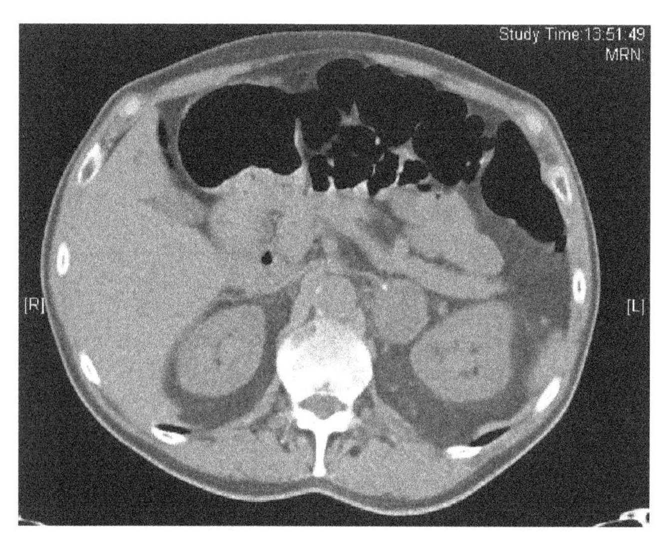

Fig. 5.5.5 CT image of an adrenal phaeochromocytoma. This lesion is located in the left adrenal gland and displays the typical heterogeneous appearance of a phaeochromocytoma, with areas of necrosis and flecks of calcification.

Functional imaging of phaeochromocytoma

Phaeochromocytoma provides an ideal opportunity to use functional imaging techniques because the cells contain specialized uptake mechanisms for catecholamines and their precursors. These can be exploited to create specific scanning techniques which will differentiate phaeochromocytomas and other neuroendocrine tumours from other causes of mass.

^{123}I-Metaiodobenzylguanidine (MIBG) scanning

MIBG is a structural analogue of noradrenaline which is taken up by most phaeochromocytoma cells and stored in catecholamine storage vesicles. Both ^{131}I- and ^{123}I-MIBG scanning have been used in phaeochromocytoma imaging but the ^{123}I-isotope gives better image quality and is generally preferred (Fig. 5.5.7). Around 85% of adrenal phaeochromocytomas are positive on MIBG imaging, but a lower proportion of extra-adrenal, malignant and familial tumours are positive. ^{123}I-MIBG uptake can be inhibited by medications such as reserpine, tricyclic antidepressants, labetalol, and calcium channel blockers; although high concentrations of phenoxybenzamine inhibit catecholamine uptake *in vitro*, it is probably not a problem in patients, and should not routinely be discontinued in order to undertake scanning. Iodine therapy is given for 3 days prior to the scan to block thyroid uptake of ^{123}I-MIBG. MIBG scanning is useful to confirm whether an adrenal lesion is likely to be a phaeochromocytoma and is also used to look for any other unsuspected extra-adrenal lesions, and in some cases as an initial attempt to localize an extra-adrenal phaeochromocytoma where anatomical imaging of the adrenal gland has been negative. MIBG is the most widely available and commonly used functional imaging technique at present for phaeochromocytoma. It can also be used to determine whether uptake is present with a view to evaluating a patient with malignant phaeochromocytoma for the possibility of therapeutic high-dose ^{131}I-MIBG therapy.

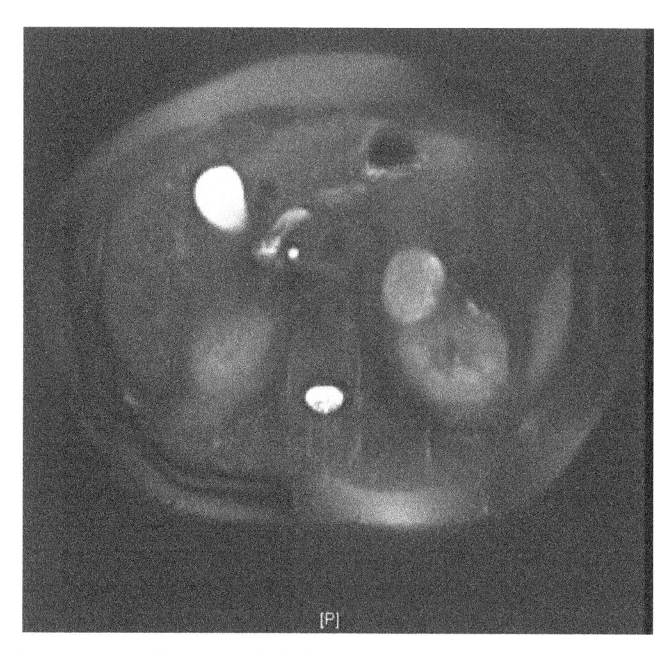

Fig. 5.5.6 T2-weighted MRI of left adrenal phaeochromocytoma. The phaeochromocytoma has a bright appearance on T2-weighted MR.

^{111}In-Octreotide scanning

^{111}In-octreotide scanning is useful in the imaging of head and neck paragangliomas, around 75% of which are positive. However, only around 25% of adrenal phaeochromocytomas will take up significant amounts of ^{111}In-octreotide (16). Again this scan is widely available and is often used as a second-line approach to imaging phaeochromocytomas if MIBG scanning is negative.

Positron emission tomography (PET) scanning

Several different tracers have been developed that may be used in imaging phaeochromocytoma (Table 5.5.3). Accounts of the use of some of these tracers are so far largely anecdotal. At present, the most useful ^{18}F-PET tracers targeting primary phaeochromocytoma tissue appear to be ^{18}F-DOPA (17) and ^{18}F-dopamine (18). ^{18}F-DOPA and ^{18}F-dopamine PET have sensitivities for phaeochromocytoma of 80–100% in studies to date but are currently only available in a few specialist centres. The more widely available [^{18}F]2-fluoro-2-deoxy-D-glucose (FDG)-PET scan is less specific for phaeochromocytoma (any highly metabolically active tissue will take up FDG), and probably less sensitive than the other ^{18}F-tracers for primary phaeochromocytoma, but it may be more useful for detecting metastatic phaeochromocytoma (Fig. 5.5.8). In some patients, the primary tumour and different metastatic deposits image differently with the more-specific and less-specific PET tracers, suggesting that dedifferentiation of the tumour has occurred in some of the metastatic deposits, causing them to lose their uptake mechanisms for the more specific tracers but still allowing the uptake of FDG. Newer PET tracers, such as ^{68}Ga-DOTATATE, ^{68}Ga-DOTATOC, and ^{68}Ga-DOTANOC, are still under evaluation in phaeochromocytoma but have shown some promise (19, 20).

Treatment and prognosis

Medical management

When the diagnosis of phaeochromocytoma has been made, medical treatment is commenced in the first instance to control symptoms, blood pressure, and to prepare the patient for surgery. α-blockade is the mainstay of treatment, and should be started

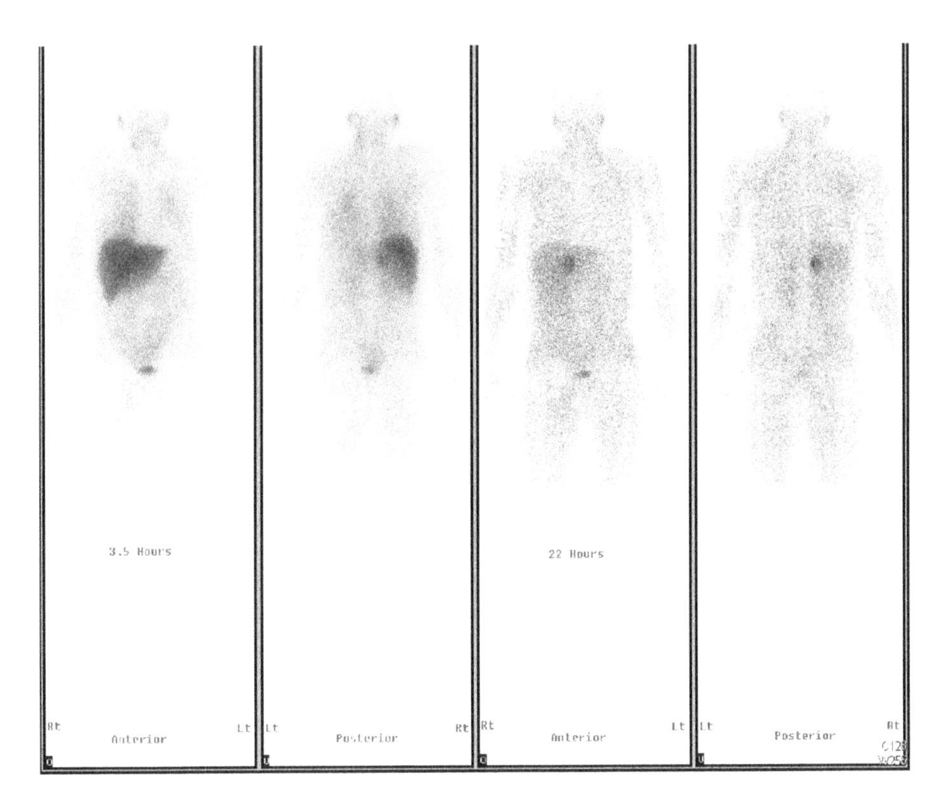

Fig. 5.5.7 ^{123}I-MIBG radioisotope scan showing a right adrenal phaeochromocytoma. Normal uptake is also seen in the liver, spleen, salivary glands, and excretion via the kidneys and bladder. Some adrenal uptake of ^{123}I-MIBG may be seen in normal adrenal glands, but strongly lateralized uptake into one adrenal gland, as in this image, suggests the presence of an adrenal phaeochromocytoma.

first, with the addition of low-dose selective β_1-blockade if necessary to counteract excessive tachycardia on α-blockade. Purely noradrenaline-secreting tumours are less likely to require adjuvant β_1-blockade, while tumours secreting large amounts of adrenaline are likely to require significant β_1-blockade to control symptoms adequately. Nonselective β-adrenoceptor antagonists are usually avoided due to the risk of blocking peripheral vasodilatation via a β_2-mediated effect, which can lead to hypertensive crisis. Once α-blockade has been initiated, β_2-blockade ceases to be dangerous, but can still make blood pressure control more difficult. In the exceptional patient where adrenaline secretion is similar in quantity to noradrenaline, the β-blocker may need to be changed to a nonselective β-blocker such as timolol. The α-blocker of choice is phenoxybenzamine. This irreversibly antagonizes the α-adrenoceptors by alkylating the receptors, so that the blockade cannot be overcome even by large surges of catecholamine release from the tumour, such as may occur during handling of the tumour during surgery. Alternatives include the reversible α-blocker doxazosin or the intravenous preparation phentolamine, which is also used to treat hypertensive crisis in phaeochromocytoma. Our usual practice is to titrate the dose of phenoxybenzamine upwards over a period of 4–6 weeks prior to surgery, increasing the dose more rapidly in the few days prior to surgery under close medical supervision and with intravenous fluid support if necessary. Careful, unrushed preoperative preparation of patients with phaeochromocytoma is essential to avoid perioperative catastrophes. Most cases of perioperative morbidity in phaeochromocytoma occur where the tumour was removed in haste without preoperative diagnosis or without preoperative α-blockade. The role of α-blockade is to permit expansion of the intravascular volume, which is nearly always low in phaeochromocytoma as a consequence of the purely vasoconstrictor hypertension and chronic compensatory pressure natriuresis. Indeed, normotension at presentation is a reason for, not against, instituting α-blockade since these are often the patients where pressure natriuresis has been most 'effective'. Careful, and regular, examination of the neck veins is part of the clinical skill in titrating the dose of α-blockade and deciding when postural hypotension is due to too little rather than too much treatment. If the venous pressure is low after prolonged α-blockade, intravenous saline should be administered during the 48 h prior to surgery.

Table 5.5.3 Radiotracers commonly used in PET scanning for phaeochromocytoma

Radiotracer	Comments
^{11}C-hydroxyephedrine	Catecholamine analogue. Good sensitivity and specificity for phaeochromocytoma but short half-life of ^{11}C necessitates on-site production of radiotracer.
^{18}F-fluoroDOPA	Amino acid uptake mechanism. Good sensitivity and specificity for phaeochromocytoma. Longer half-life of ^{18}F allows off-site production of radiotracer.
^{18}F-fluorodopamine	Dopamine analogue. Good sensitivity and specificity for phaeochromocytoma.
^{18}F-fluorodeoxyglucose	Nonspecific uptake into highly metabolically active tissues. Particularly useful in imaging malignant phaeochromocytoma. Advantage of being more widely available than the other PET tracers.

Surgical management

Most adrenal phaeochromocytomas are now removed by laparoscopic adrenalectomy. This procedure has very low perioperative morbidity and mortality in experienced hands. Occasionally—about

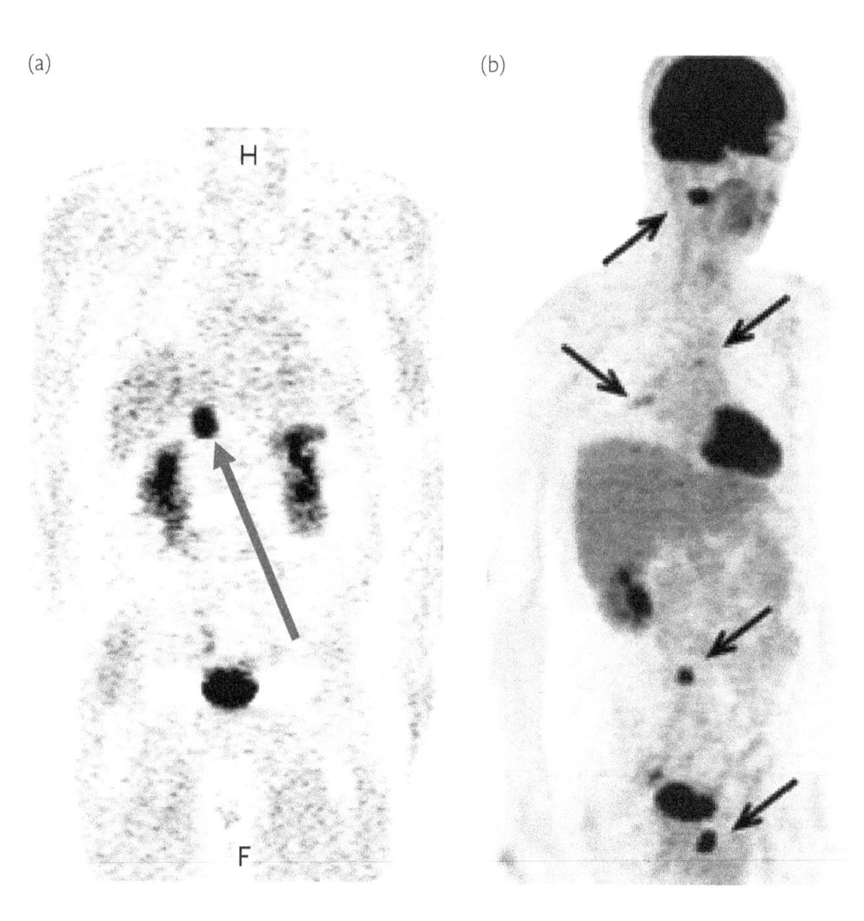

Fig. 5.5.8 PET imaging of phaeochromocytoma. (a) ^{18}F-DOPA PET scan in a patient with a right adrenal phaeochromocytoma. An abnormal focus of uptake is seen in the region of the right adrenal gland. Normal excretion of radiotracer occurs via the kidneys. Uptake of ^{18}F-DOPA is dependent on the expression of the neutral amine precursor uptake and decarboxylation system in tumour cells. (b) ^{18}F-FDG PET scan in a patient with malignant phaeochromocytoma. Uptake of ^{18}F-FDG is related to the metabolic activity of the tumour tissue and foci of abnormal uptake are seen at the sites of multiple metastases from the phaeochromocytoma (arrows).

1 in 20 operations—conversion to an open procedure is necessary where anatomy is difficult or unexpected haemorrhage occurs. More recently, cortical-sparing adrenalectomy has been tried in selected cases, mainly patients with MEN 2 in whom 95% of adrenal phaeochromocytomas are benign and in whom contralateral metachronous adrenal lesions requiring further surgery are more likely. Sparing the adrenal cortex may avoid the need for physiological glucocorticoid replacement if bilateral phaeochromocytomas develop (traditionally requiring bilateral adrenalectomy) but some clinicians have expressed concern about the risk of local recurrence of phaeochromocytoma if this technique is used. Prophylactic bilateral adrenalectomy is not currently recommended in MEN 2 as the lifetime risk of developing phaeochromocytoma is only around 50%, the lesions are usually benign and detected early through screening programmes, and the risks of being dependent on glucocorticoid replacement therapy are probably greater than the risks associated with an early phaeochromocytoma developing.

Good preoperative preparation usually leads to a smooth intraoperative course without dramatic fluctuations in blood pressure. However, hypertensive surges may be controlled with intravenous phentolamine. Hypotension following removal of the tumour is more difficult to treat, especially if irreversible α-blockade has been used, as the patient will be relatively unresponsive to noradrenaline and other pressor agents. However, where available, angiotensin II infusion may be used to support the circulation.

Surgical treatment of phaeochromocytoma is curative in most cases. Exceptions include when the tumour is unresectable due to involvement of other local organs or structures or when metastasis has already occurred. Even in metastatic cases, it is worth considering debulking surgery to reduce tumour load and hence catecholamine secretion, reducing symptoms, and the risk of catecholamine-induced cardiomyopathy (Takotsubo's cardiomyopathy), which may occur with high circulating levels of catecholamines.

Follow-up after surgical excision

Following excision of phaeochromocytoma, it is usually possible to stop most or all antihypertensive therapy and most patients have an excellent prognosis. Postoperative catecholamines should be checked within a few weeks of surgery once any acute effects of the surgery have passed. Patients should be kept under at least annual lifelong follow-up monitoring for recurrence of hypertension, symptoms, or excess catecholamine secretion. Patients who have had a phaeochromocytoma are at increased risk of a second metachronous lesion, and of recurrence at the site of the first lesion or of unexpected metastasis, which may sometimes appear years after the first presentation. Any familial screening considered necessary should be completed with appropriate genetic counselling.

Malignant phaeochromocytoma

Around 10% of cases of phaeochromocytoma are malignant. The rate of progression of malignant phaeochromocytoma is highly variable in different individuals and the prognosis may range from rapidly progressive disease causing death within days to disease which progresses very slowly over 20 years or more. Further research is ongoing into the optimal treatment of malignant phaeochromocytoma (21, 22). There are currently no curative treatments for malignant phaeochromocytoma. Surgical debulking is recommended, if feasible, to reduce catecholamine secretion. If the

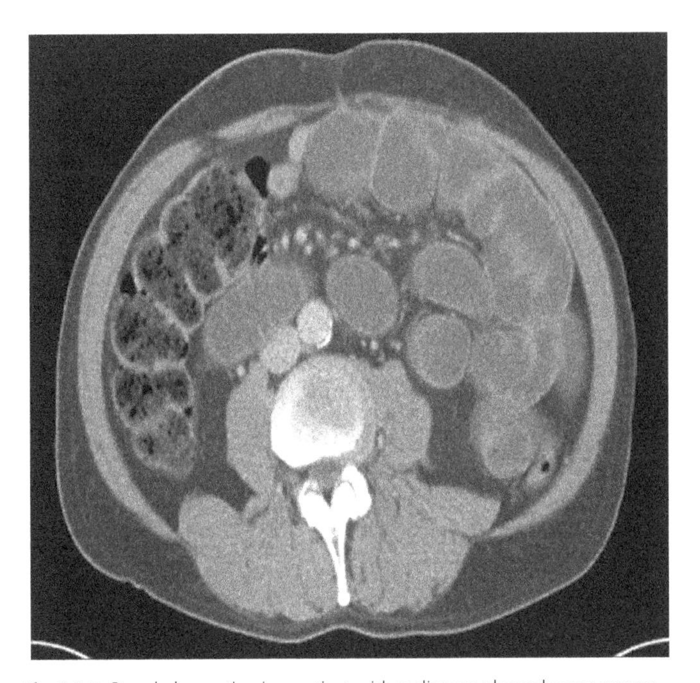

Fig. 5.5.9 Bowel obstruction in a patient with malignant phaeochromocytoma. This patient with inoperable malignant phaeochromocytoma presented with a 10-day history of absolute constipation. The large bowel obstruction was thought to be caused by a combination of mechanical effects of the tumour and inhibition of bowel function due to very high circulating noradrenaline levels. A life-saving emergency colostomy was performed using intravenous phentolamine treatment to control the blood pressure and the patient made a good recovery. Bowel obstruction and chronic constipation are common in malignant phaeochromocytoma.

disease is slowly progressive, many clinicians and patients would choose to manage symptoms medically using α-blockade, adding β_1-blockade as necessary. Regular laxative therapy may be necessary to reduce the risk of bowel obstruction secondary to noradrenaline effects on the gastrointestinal tract smooth muscle, a common cause of death in malignant phaeochromocytoma (Fig. 5.5.9). If the disease is more progressive or if symptoms are difficult to control, other treatment options may be considered. If the tumour takes up ^{123}I-MIBG on a diagnostic scan, radiotherapy with higher therapeutic doses of ^{131}I-MIBG may be beneficial. Only around 30–70% of suitable patients respond to therapy, and usually the treatment improves symptoms but only prolongs survival by a few months. Similarly, chemotherapy regimens based on cyclophosphamide, vincristine, and dacarbazine may improve symptoms and extend survival by a mean of 21 months, but again, only around 50% of patients will respond to treatment. Therapeutic ^{111}In-octreotide therapy may be used if the phaeochromocytoma tissue expresses somatostatin receptors and takes up octreotide, but there has been limited success with this therapy and problems include deterioration in renal function. Painful bone metastases may be treated by radiotherapy, radiofrequency ablation, or embolization. If there are very high levels of circulating catecholamines, α-methylparatyrosine therapy can be used to decrease the production of noradrenaline, which may be particularly helpful in cases of catecholamine-induced cardiomyopathy. However, side effects of α-methylparatyrosine include severe depression.

There are some early data suggesting the possibility that some phaeochromocytomas may respond to treatment with sunitinib (23) but clinical trials are necessary to investigate this further. Other possible future treatments include heat shock protein 90 inhibitors, other antiangiogenic agents and substances used to sensitize tumour tissue to improve uptake of therapeutic ^{131}I-MIBG. There is a theoretical possibility, and some anecdotal evidence, that angiotensin receptor antagonists may promote apoptosis and hence delay the growth of phaeochromocytoma by stimulation of the AT2 subtype of angiotensin receptor (24). Collaborative clinical trials would be needed to support this strategy. The rarity of malignant phaeochromocytoma has made proper scientific assessment of new treatment strategies difficult and there is a move to set up global collaborations to recruit adequate numbers of patients to treatment studies to draw meaningful conclusions. Improvements in the availability of the newer PET imaging techniques may improve the ability to accurately measure tumour response in treatment studies in malignant phaeochromocytoma.

Phaeochromocytoma in pregnancy

It is not uncommon for phaeochromocytoma to present during pregnancy, either with elevated blood pressure during routine antenatal screening, or later in pregnancy with complications of pre-eclampsia, severe hypertension, or hypertensive crisis during labour. Maternal and fetal mortality is significant if phaeochromocytoma is present and undiagnosed during pregnancy. However, if correctly diagnosed, maternal mortality is less than 1% and fetal mortality up to 15%. Adrenal phaeochromocytomas have been surgically removed laparoscopically during pregnancy, with the usual preoperative preparation using α-blockade (with or without β-blockade) and the safest time for surgery is probably the middle trimester, when the risk of miscarriage is lower, but the mass effects caused by the developing fetus are not yet too great.

Treatment of paraganglioma

Treatment of secretory paragangliomas is medical and surgical, similarly to adrenal phaeochromocytomas. Head and neck paragangliomas, derived from parasympathetic tissue, are often nonsecretory and are managed by surgical excision where possible, radioisotope therapy, or radiotherapy. The prognosis of patients with paraganglioma is highly variable, as for phaeochromocytoma, and depends on the rate of tumour growth, the ability to achieve complete surgical resection, and on any local effects caused by the tumour.

Neuroblastoma

Neuroblastoma is a tumour of infancy and childhood arising from sympathetic tissue of neural crest origin in the adrenal medulla or sympathetic chain (25). It may occur as early as prenatally and the majority of cases occur in the first year of life. Very occasionally, it occurs in adults. Neuroblastoma typically presents as a large abdominal mass but can also affect the posterior mediastinum, pelvis, or neck. Other presenting symptoms include fatigue, apathy, loss of appetite, and bone pain or limping. Neuroblastoma accounts for up to 10% of childhood malignancies and is the most common solid cancer after brain tumours in childhood. Up to 50% of cases are metastatic at the time of presentation, usually involving the vertebral bones, but haematogenous metastatic spread also commonly involves liver, brain, and the skull, particularly the orbits. Local spread to intra-abdominal organs, especially the kidneys, also occurs. The differential diagnosis includes Wilm's tumour, lymphoma, rhabdomyosarcoma, and Ewing's sarcoma.

Around 80–90% of neuroblastomas secrete excess catecholamines, therefore symptoms of catecholamine excess may be present, but many neuroblastomas are relatively asymptomatic considering the large size they may reach. Dopamine, homovanillic acid, and vanillyl mandelic acid levels are typically raised. It should be noted that dopamine levels are best estimated in plasma if not measured as one of its metabolites. Most dopamine in urine is derived from DOPA rather than plasma dopamine. Complications include spinal cord compression, due to infiltration of tumour along the sympathetic nerve fibres through the intervertebral foramina, and myoclonic encephalopathy secondary to an immunological response to the tumour.

Elevated catecholamine levels may be present and radiological imaging shows a large solid or necrotic lesion with flecks of calcification. Diagnosis is confirmed histologically. Tumours are often very large and necrotic. Tumour cells are small, round, and blue and are typically arranged in Homer–Wright pseudorosette formations. Areas of well-differentiated, relatively benign tissue and very poorly differentiated, highly malignant tissue may be found in different parts of the same tumour.

Overall genomic pattern within the tumour predicts clinical outcome. A recent study suggests that tumours presenting with whole chromosome copy number changes only are associated with excellent survival, while those presenting with segmental chromosome copy number changes are associated with a high risk of relapse. Within tumours with segmental changes, reduced survival is associated with deletions of 1p and 11q, gain of 1q, and N-*myc* amplification (26).

Full staging of the tumour is performed at time of presentation, including genetic analysis, imaging, iliac crest bone marrow biopsy, and technetium bone scanning. The International Neuroblastoma Staging System has traditionally been used and classification is based on anatomical involvement at presentation—ranging from Stage 1 disease (localized) to Stage 4 disease (disseminated). The International Neuroblastoma Risk Group Staging System was introduced more recently to allow prediction of risk and to facilitate the comparison of results of clinical trials in neuroblastoma.

Curiously, spontaneous regression of neuroblastomas (Stage 4) has been reported in infants, often despite multiple metastases at presentation. Treatment options for neuroblastoma depend on the stage and likely risk of the disease at presentation. Observation alone may be appropriate in some cases expected to resolve spontaneously. Other treatment options include surgery for localized disease and chemotherapy, sometimes followed by surgery. Most neuroblastomas are ^{123}I-MIBG avid and high-dose 131I-MIBG may be used therapeutically. Advanced cases of neuroblastoma are often treated with combinations of intensive chemotherapy, surgery, ^{131} I-MIBG therapy, and isotretinoin therapy. Stem cell or bone marrow transplantation is used in some cases. In recent years, attempts have been made to reduce the intensity of treatment given to patients with favourable initial prognosis to reduce the long-term sequelae of treatment, while increasing the intensity of treatment given to those with initial poor prognosis. Clinical trials assessing various chemotherapy regimes, biological therapies, and transplant regimens are ongoing. Patients with advanced disease at presentation (except those infants in whom disease spontaneously regresses) have a poor prognosis with 5-year survival around 20%. Older children with advanced disease have a worse prognosis than infants with advanced disease.

References

1. Lenders JW, Eisenhofer G, Mannelli M, Pacak K. Phaeochromocytoma. *Lancet*, 2005; **366**: 665–75.
2. Messerli FH, Loughlin KR, Messerli AW, Welch WR. The president and the pheochromocytoma. *Am J Cardiol*, 2007; **99**: 1325–9.
3. Manger WM. An overview of pheochromocytoma: history, current concepts, vagaries, and diagnostic challenges. *Ann N Y Acad Sci*, 2006; **1073**: 1–20.
4. Neumann HP, Bausch B, McWhinney SR, Bender BU, Gimm O, Franke G, *et al*. Germ-line mutations in nonsyndromic pheochromocytoma. *N Engl J Med*, 2002; **346**: 1459–66.
5. Erlic Z, Neumann HP. When should genetic testing be obtained in a patient with phaeochromocytoma or paraganglioma?. *Clin Endocrinol (Oxf)*, 2009; **70**: 354–7.
6. Timmers H, Gimenez-Roqueplo AP, Mannelli M, Pacak K: Clinical aspects of SDHx-related pheochromocytoma and paraganglioma. *Endocr Relat Cancer* 2009;**16**: 391–400.
7. Cascón A, López-Jiménez E, Landa I, Leskelä S, Leandro-García LJ, Maliszewska A, *et al*.: Rationalization of genetic testing in patients with apparently sporadic pheochromocytoma/ paraganglioma. *Horm Metab Res* 2009; **41**: 672–5.
8. McNicol AM. Histopathology and immunohistochemistry of adrenal medullary tumors and paragangliomas. *Endocr Pathol*, 2006; **17**: 329–36.
9. Tischler AS, Kimura N, McNicol AM. Pathology of pheochromocytoma and extra-adrenal paraganglioma. *Ann N Y Acad Sci*, 2006; **1073**: 557–70.
10. Takahashi N, Shimada T, Tanabe K, Yoshitomi H, Murakami Y, Ishibashi Y, *et al*.: Steroid-induced crisis and rhabdomyolysis in a patient with pheochromocytoma: A case report and review. *Int J Cardiol* 2009, in press.
11. Mann SJ. Severe paroxysmal hypertension (pseudopheochromocytoma). *Curr Hypertens Rep*, 2008; **10**: 12–18.
12. Pacak K, Eisenhofer G, Ahlman H, Bornstein SR, Gimenez-Roqueplo AP, Grossman AB, *et al*. Pheochromocytoma: recommendations for clinical practice from the First International Symposium. October 2005. *Nat Clin Pract Endocrinol Metab*, 2007; **3**: 92–102.
13. Grossman A, Pacak K, Sawka A, Lenders JW, Harlander D, Peaston RT, *et al*. Biochemical diagnosis and localization of pheochromocytoma: can we reach a consensus?. *Ann N Y Acad Sci*, 2006; **1073**: 332–47.
14. Brown MJ, Allison DJ, Jenner DA, Lewis PJ, Dollery CT. Increased sensitivity and accuracy of phaeochromocytoma diagnosis achieved by use of plasma-adrenaline estimations and a pentolinium-suppression test. *Lancet*, 1981; **1** (8213): 174–7.
15. Bravo EL, Tarazi RC, Fouad FM, Vidt DG, Gifford RW, Jr. Clonidine-suppression test: a useful aid in the diagnosis of pheochromocytoma. *N Engl J Med*, 1981; **305**: 623–6.
16. van der Harst E, de Herder WW, Bruining HA, Bonjer HJ, de Krijger RR, Lamberts SW, *et al*. [(^{123})I]metaiodobenzylguanidine and [(^{111})In] octreotide uptake in benign and malignant pheochromocytomas. *J Clin Endocrinol Metab*, 2001; **86**: 685–93.
17. Hoegerle S, Nitzsche E, Altehoefer C, Ghanem N, Manz T, Brink I, *et al*. Pheochromocytomas: detection with ^{18}F DOPA whole body PET—initial results. *Radiology*, 2002; **222**: 507–12.
18. Ilias I, Yu J, Carrasquillo JA, Chen CC, Eisenhofer G, Whatley M, *et al*. Superiority of 6-[^{18}F]-fluorodopamine positron emission tomography versus [^{131}I]-metaiodobenzylguanidine scintigraphy in the localization of metastatic pheochromocytoma. *J Clin Endocrinol Metab*, 2003; **88**: 4083–7.
19. Khan MU, Khan S, El-Refaie S, Win Z, Rubello D, Al-Nahhas A. Clinical indications for Gallium-68 positron emission tomography imaging. *Eur J Surg Oncol*, 2009; **35**: 561–7.
20. Forrer F, Riedweg I, Maecke HR, Mueller-Brand J. Radiolabeled DOTATOC in patients with advanced paraganglioma and pheochromocytoma. *Q J Nucl Med Mol Imaging*, 2008; **52**: 334–40.

21. Scholz T, Eisenhofer G, Pacak K, Dralle H, Lehnert H: Current treatment of malignant pheochromocytoma. *J Clin Endocrinol Metab* 2007; **92**: 1217–25.
22. Eisenhofer G, Bornstein SR, Brouwers FM, Cheung NK, Dahia PL, de Krijger RR, *et al.* Malignant pheochromocytoma: current status and initiatives for future progress. *Endocr Relat Cancer*, 2004; **11**: 423–36.
23. Joshua AM, Ezzat S, Asa SL, Evans A, Broom R, Freeman M, *et al.* Rationale and evidence for sunitinib in the treatment of malignant paraganglioma/ pheochromocytoma. *J Clin Endocrinol Metab*, 2009; **94**: 5–9.
24. Brown MJ, Mackenzie IS, Ashby MJ, Balan KK, Appleton DS. AT2 receptor stimulation may halt progression of pheochromocytoma. *Ann N Y Acad Sci*, 2006; **1073**: 436–43.
25. Park JR, Eggert A, Caron H. Neuroblastoma: biology, prognosis, and treatment. *Pediatr Clin North Am*, 2008; **55**: 97–120.
26. Janoueix-Lerosey I, Schleiermacher G, Michels E, Mosseri V, Ribeiro A, Lequin D, *et al.* Overall genomic pattern is a predictor of outcome in neuroblastoma. *J Clin Oncol*, 2009; **27**: 1026–33.

5.6

Primary aldosteronism and other steroid-related causes of endocrine hypertension

John M.C. Connell, E. Marie Freel

Introduction

Mineralocorticoid hypertension is characterized by increased distal renal tubular sodium reabsorption, raised body sodium content, plasma volume expansion, markedly reduced body potassium content, with a metabolic alkalosis and suppression of renin production by the juxtaglomerular cells of the kidney (and correspondingly low levels of angiotensin II). Primary aldosteronism is the most common cause of mineralocorticoid hypertension (1); less frequent causes include the rare inborn errors of adrenal steroid synthesis (11β-hydroxylase and 17α-hydroxylase deficiency), alterations in corticosteroid metabolism (syndrome of apparent mineralocorticoid excess), and constitutive activation of the epithelial sodium channel (Liddle's syndrome).

Mineralocorticoid synthesis

Aldosterone is produced from cholesterol in a series of biochemical reactions which involve sequential hydroxylation and dehydrogenation reactions (Fig. 5.6.1). These reactions are performed in cells of the zona glomerulosa of the adrenal cortex. The unique steps in the formation of aldosterone are an 18-hydroxylation of corticosterone to form 18-hydroxycorticosterone which, following a second hydroxylation reaction, is spontaneously dehydrated to form aldosterone. Both of these steps are carried out by a single enzyme, aldosterone synthase, encoded by the gene *CYP11B2* (2). This enzyme also converts 11-deoxycorticosterone, the preferred substrate, to corticosterone in zona glomerulosa cells.

CYP11B2 is highly homologous to the gene that encodes 11β-hydroxylase (*CYP11B1*) (3); in the zona fasciculata, this enzyme converts 11-deoxycortisol to cortisol and 11-deoxycorticosterone to corticosterone. It can also catalyse 18-hydroxylation, thus forming 18-hydroxy-deoxycorticosterone and 18-hydroxycorticosterone in this zone. In normal circumstances, zonation of the adrenal cortex results in distinct separation of functions, so that 17α-hydroxysteroids such as 11-deoxycortisol and cortisol are not available to act as substrates for aldosterone synthase. However, in some circumstances, loss of strict zonation does occur, in which case cortisol becomes available as a substrate, resulting in the production of large quantities of steroids such as 18-hydroxycortisol and 18-oxocortisol, which are normally minor products of 11β-hydroxylase (4). The clearest example of this occurs in glucocorticoid-remediable aldosteronism, where aldosterone synthase is expressed at a high level throughout the zona fasciculata (see Chapter 5.1) (5). In Conn's adenomas, there is also loss of strict zonal separation of hydroxylase activity, so that aldosterone synthase can convert cortisol to 18-hydroxy- and 18-oxocortisol, which can be detected in both urine and plasma (6). It is unlikely that either of these steroids has a significant effect on the clinical presentation of Conn's syndrome.

Regulation of aldosterone secretion

Normally, aldosterone secretion is regulated by changes in body sodium status, through the renin/ angiotensin system (7). Loss of sodium stimulates this system, whereas high intake suppresses it. Potassium is also a powerful direct stimulus to aldosterone secretion; very small increments, which do not alter plasma levels perceptibly, raise aldosterone secretion rate. In normal subjects, ACTH can acutely stimulate aldosterone release, but chronic pharmacological doses of ACTH given over several days results in suppression of aldosterone synthesis by mechanisms that remain incompletely understood. Importantly, electrolyte status affects the sensitivity of the zona glomerulosa to all agonists. Thus, sodium depletion enhances sensitivity to angiotensin II, potassium, and ACTH, while sodium loading has the opposite effect. The converse is true for potassium status, so that the sensitivity of aldosterone to angiotensin II stimulation is set by the prevailing potassium levels.

In primary aldosteronism, aldosterone levels are, by definition, inappropriate for the prevailing angiotensin II and potassium levels. The volume expansion and high extracellular sodium concentration caused by aldosterone suppress release of renin from the juxtaglomerular cells of the kidney; as renin activity determines angiotensin II production, levels of the peptide are low. Furthermore, the aldosterone excess leads to increased potassium loss in the urine, resulting in hypokalaemia. Despite this, aldosterone secretion remains higher than normal. However, but for the hypokalaemia, aldosterone levels would be higher still (8, 9).

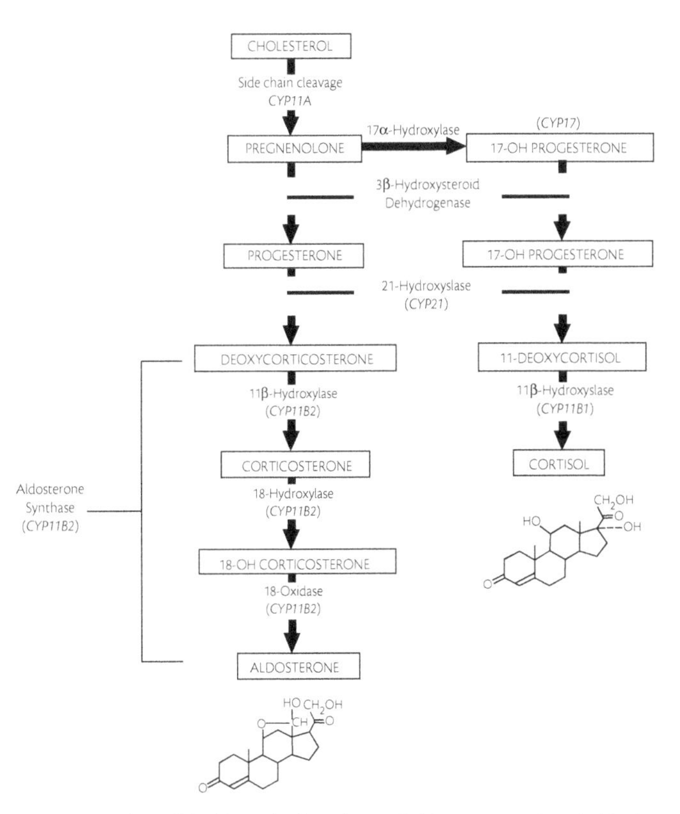

Fig. 5.6.1 Outline of the biosynthetic pathway of aldosterone and cortisol in the human adrenal cortex.

In normal subjects, aldosterone levels show diurnal variation, upon which are superimposed fluctuations entrained by acute posture-induced changes in renin release. Levels of the steroid are highest in the morning and have a nadir, which mirrors the pattern of plasma cortisol. In the majority of patients with primary aldosteronism, suppression of renin leads to loss of posture-induced changes. Indeed, paradoxically, concentrations may fall on assuming an upright posture, while the diurnal variation in aldosterone concentration is blunted but not completely absent (10). Thus, aldosterone levels tend to be highest after overnight recumbency and are lower in the later part of the day. In patients with an aldosterone-producing adenoma, aldosterone will respond acutely to administration of ACTH (indeed, the aldosterone response to ACTH may be greater than in normal subjects) but usually shows no response to administration of angiotensin II, which is, at least in part, due to the increased total body sodium content. However, in patients with bilateral adrenal hyperplasia and in a subgroup of subjects with aldosterone-producing adenomas, aldosterone does respond acutely to administration of angiotensin II (11). These patients may also show a small aldosterone rise after ambulation (reflecting their angiotensin II responsiveness). However, apart from the fact that patients with typical solitary Conn's adenomas are less likely to show responsiveness to angiotensin II than those with bilateral adrenal hyperplasia, there are no real practical advantages arising from this observation.

In normal subjects, a variety of other amines and peptides are reported to influence aldosterone secretion (12). These are summarized in Table 5.6.1. Of these, atrial natriuretic peptide may be one of the more important mechanisms that inhibits aldosterone production by the adrenal cortex. In patients with primary

Table 5.6.1 Factors other than angiotensin II, potassium, and ACTH involved in regulation of aldosterone secretion

Control factors	Effect	Receptor/mechanism
Atrial natriuretic peptide	Inhibitory ↓ Aldosterone	Atrial natriuretic peptide receptor ↓ Pregnenolone
Adrenaline, noradrenaline	Stimulatory ↑ Aldosterone	β-adrenergic receptors
Acetylcholine	Stimulatory ↑ Aldosterone	Muscarinic receptors
Vasoactive intestinal peptide	Stimulatory ↑Aldosterone	Synergizes with ACTH
Dopamine	Inhibitory ↓ Aldosterone	Tonic inhibition via dopamine receptor

aldosteronism, volume expansion results in increased secretion of atrial natriuretic peptide from the heart. However, despite this, aldosterone secretion remains elevated and patients with primary aldosteronism are reported not to respond to infusion of exogenous atrial natriuretic peptide (13). In some subjects with aldosterone-producing adenomas, other hormones, including gonadotrophins and gastrointestinal-derived peptides such as GIP-1, have, rarely, been reported to regulate aldosterone production (14). In these cases, expression of receptors for the peptides has been demonstrated in the tumour material. However, this appears to be a relatively unusual circumstance.

Production of 18-hydroxy- and 18-oxocortisol is modestly increased in patients with Conn's adenomas (in contrast with patients with glucocorticoid-remediable aldosteronism, where levels are considerably higher). In addition to excessive aldosterone production, patients with primary aldosteronism often have increased plasma levels of the immediate precursor, 18-hydroxycorticosterone (15). It is possible that hypokalaemia reduces the efficiency of its conversion to aldosterone. Levels of this hormone are greater in patients with Conn's adenomas than those with bilateral adrenal hyperplasia, but the observation, in itself, is of little practical importance in patient investigation or management. Furthermore, there is no good evidence that steroids other than aldosterone contribute in a major way to the clinical and pathophysiological features of primary aldosteronism.

Some patients with adrenocortical carcinomas produce excessive 11-deoxycorticosterone (16), which, in marked excess, can also cause mineralocorticoid hypertension. In these subjects, a range of other steroids is often present and diagnosis is usually obvious by imaging and measurement of plasma and urinary steroid concentrations.

The mineralocorticoid receptor and epithelial actions of aldosterone

The mineralocorticoid receptor mediates the classical effects of aldosterone, acting as a ligand-activated transcription factor (17). The receptor is found in the cytosol of epithelial cells, particularly in the renal collecting duct; other major target sites include the colon and the salivary gland. However, mineralocorticoid receptors have also been identified in nonepithelial sites such as heart, brain, vascular smooth muscle, liver, and peripheral blood leucocytes (18). The mineralocorticoid receptor belongs to the nuclear receptor superfamily of proteins and consists of an N-terminal domain, a DNA-binding domain, and a C-terminal ligand-binding domain (19). Aldosterone binds to this latter domain and causes a conformational change to the mineralocorticoid receptor, whereupon it dissociates from various heat-shock proteins and immunophilins, and translocates to the cell nucleus where it binds as a homodimer to the hormone response element of aldosterone-responsive genes in order to activate or repress gene transcription (the classical genomic effect of aldosterone).

The most important physiological action of aldosterone is to increase the reabsorption of sodium in the kidney and other epithelial sites at the expense of potassium and hydrogen ions (20). The cortical collecting tubules and the distal convoluted tubule are the principal sites of aldosterone-mediated sodium and potassium transport. The major determinant of renal sodium reabsorption is the epithelial sodium channel (ENaC) located on the apical membrane of the distal convoluted tubule (21). Its availability in open conformation at the apical membrane of the cell is increased by aldosterone, vasopressin, glucocorticoids, and insulin whilst elevated intracellular levels of calcium and sodium lead to its down-regulation (22).

Aldosterone induces the expression of the ENaC's α-, β-, and γ-subunits although its major effect appears to be achieved either by increasing the number of channels in the plasma membrane or by increasing the probability that the channels are open to allow the passage of Na+. This regulation of ENaC is achieved via the expression of a wide range of aldosterone-induced proteins, some of which appear to act by preventing tonic inhibition of ENaC activity. The best-characterized of these proteins is the serine–threonine kinase, SGK1 (23). Aldosterone causes phosphorylation and activation of SGK1, which in turn increases ENaC activity by an increase in the number of channels at the cell surface (Fig. 5.6.2). The principal ENaC inhibitory accessory protein is Nedd4 (neuronal precursor cells expressed developmentally down-regulated). This ubiquitin protein ligase binds to the C-terminal regions of β- and γ-subunits of ENaC, leading to channel internalization and degradation. It has been demonstrated that the stimulatory action of SGK on ENaC is mediated through phosphorylation of serine residues on Nedd4. Such phosphorylation reduces the interaction between Nedd4 and ENaC, leading to elevated ENaC cell surface expression (24, 25).

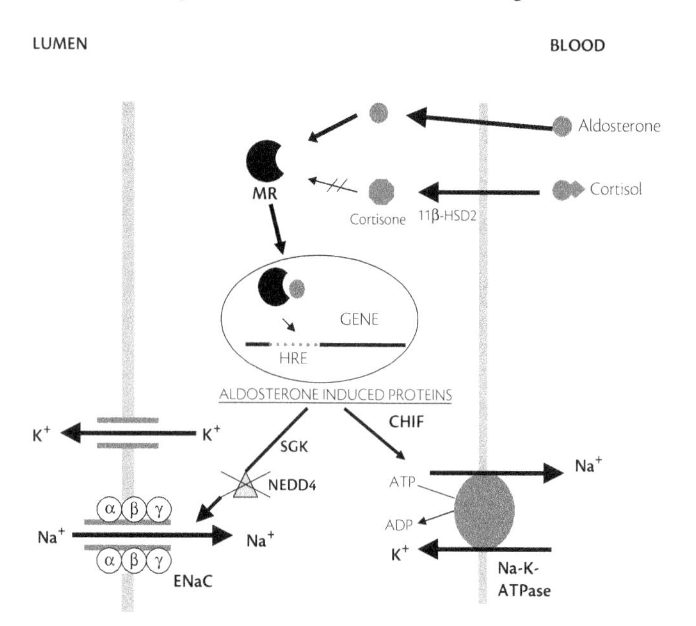

Fig. 5.6.2 Mechanism of action of aldosterone in epithelial cells. Aldosterone binds to mineralocorticoid receptor (MR) and leads to alteration in gene transcription by binding to hormone responsive elements (HRE) in relevant genes. ENaC, epithelial sodium channel; SKG, serine–threonine kinase; CHIF, ; 11β-HSD2, 11β-hydroxysteroid dehydrogenase.

Hydrogen ion excretion by the kidney in the distal nephron is also regulated by aldosterone. Hydrogen ion secretion is through a sodium-insensitive route, since it occurs principally in the intercalated cells of the collecting tubule. This segment of the nephron exhibits little or no aldosterone-induced sodium transport, and so aldosterone-induced natriuresis and hydrogen ion secretion appear to be independent events. This effect is mediated via an effect of aldosterone on the activity of the ATP-dependent apical hydrogen ion pump and parallel regulation of the basolateral membrane Cl–/ HCO_3– exchanger (26).

The net effect of aldosterone on the renal tubule is therefore to promote sodium retention at the expense of potassium and also to promote hydrogen ion excretion by the kidney. This explains the clinical features observed in cases of primary aldosterone excess, i.e. plasma hypokalaemia, alkalosis, a raised exchangeable sodium content, and low total body potassium.

The 11β-hydroxysteroid dehydrogenase system

Aldosterone and cortisol have equal affinities for the mineralocorticoid receptor; given that cortisol is found at much higher levels in plasma (up to 1000-fold in comparison to aldosterone levels) the vast majority of these receptors would be expected to be transactivated by glucocorticoid, particularly at times when cortisol levels are highest. This is clearly not the case *in vivo*, due in part, at least, to the activity of the enzyme 11β-hydroxysteroid dehydrogenase (11β-HSD), which acts as a gatekeeper to prevent activation of the mineralocorticoid receptor by much higher available levels of cortisol (Fig. 5.6.3) (27). The type 2 isoform of this enzyme is found in the renal distal nephron as well as other aldosterone-sensitive target tissues (colon, salivary glands, and placenta) and converts cortisol to its inactive metabolite, cortisone, which has does not transactivate the mineralocorticoid receptor (28). Whenever 11β-HSD2 activity is absent, inhibited, or overwhelmed, this 'protective' mechanism is lost and cortisol gains access to the mineralocorticoid receptor to act as a potent mineralocorticoid. However, this may be an oversimplification, as it has been pointed out that the capacity of the enzyme is insufficient to lead complete conversion of cortisol to cortisone, and it appears that cortisol may still be able to bind the mineralocorticoid receptor but fail to transactivate it; the ability of cortisol to act as an agonist may depend on other factors, including availability of NADH, generated as a consequence of the activity of 11β-HSD2, and local (intracellular) redox state (29). In particular, it has been proposed that NADH acts as a

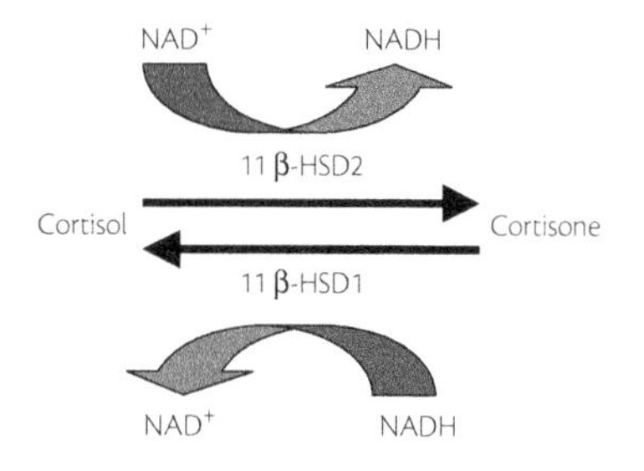

Fig. 5.6.3 The 11β-hydroxysteroid dehydrogenase (HSD) system.

corepressor of mineralocorticoid receptor activation when cortisol is a ligand, and may provide an alternate (or additional) way in which reduced 11β-HSD2 activity permits cortisol to transactivate the receptor. The clinical consequences of this are described later in this chapter.

Nongenomic and nonepithelial effects of aldosterone

It is now accepted that, as well as classical genomic effects through ligand–receptor binding of DNA regulatory elements, aldosterone also exerts rapid, nongenomic, effects (30). Nongenomic effects are associated with rapid activation (occurring within minutes), in the absence of a need for transcription or protein synthesis (31). Because of the brief response time, it is presumed that nongenomic actions are initiated at the membrane level, and membrane signalling transduction pathways have been intensively studied. These suggest the existence of novel steroid hormone receptors or possibly classical receptors embedded in the membrane that initiate the nongenomic signal cascade, although none have yet been found. However, two recent studies have demonstrated a role for intracellular calcium as well as protein kinase C activity as a potential mechanism of action of the nongenomic receptor (31, 32). In addition, several of these rapid responses can be blocked by the mineralocorticoid receptor antagonist spironolactone, suggesting that at least some nongenomic effects may be mediated via the classic mineralocorticoid receptor. Reports of rapid, nongenomic effects of aldosterone have been described in smooth muscle, cardiac muscle, skeletal muscle, colonic epithelial cells, and myocardial cells (33). These effects have been linked to the development of increased systemic vascular resistance and so could, theoretically, contribute to hypertension and cardiovascular disease.

Classical mineralocorticoid receptors have been localized in a number of nonepithelial tissues, particularly in the cardiovascular system and central nervous system. While the functional properties of the receptors in these tissues are largely similar (in terms of transactivation and downstream signalling), the effects they mediate are extremely diverse. In contrast to its established effects on electrolyte balance in epithelial tissue, aldosterone in the cardiovascular system promotes cardiac hypertrophy, fibrosis, and abnormal vascular endothelial function. In the central nervous system, mineralocorticoid receptor activation appears to regulate blood pressure, salt appetite, and sympathetic tone. In contrast to epithelial tissues, mineralocorticoid receptors in the central nervous system do not appear to colocalize with 11β-HSD2 (34). The lack of 11β-HSD2 in mineralocorticoid receptor-rich areas suggests that the majority of brain receptors are likely to be occupied by glucocorticoid although infusion of aldosterone intracerebroventricularly raises blood pressure in experimental circumstances, suggesting that the hormone may have central actions to influence cardiovascular function (35, 36).

Causes of mineralocorticoid hypertension

Primary aldosteronism is the most common cause of secondary hypertension (1, 37). By definition, the syndrome is a consequence of excessive autonomous aldosterone production. Solitary benign adenomas of the adrenal cortex (Conn's adenomas; APA) account for approximately 40% of presentations with primary aldosteronism; bilateral adrenal hyperplasia, in which several autonomous nodules are present throughout the adrenal cortex, is the most common cause, accounting for around 60%. A very small number of patients with primary aldosteronism have an inherited form (glucocorticoid-remediable aldosteronism) due to the presence of a chimeric gene, expression of which in the adrenal cortex is regulated by ACTH but which encodes aldosterone synthase (5); this is discussed in Chapter 5.7. Very rarely, primary aldosteronism can be due to carcinoma of the adrenal cortex and this is discussed below.

Epidemiology

In the years following the first description by Conn in 1955, the frequency of primary aldosteronism was thought to be low. This probably reflected the reliance on hypokalaemia as a diagnostic pointer in hypertensive patients. More recently, however, sensitive screening tests have been used to detect primary aldosteronism, principally based on the ratio of aldosterone to renin (ARR) (37–39). The widespread introduction of these tests has undoubtedly led to a rise in the detection rate for primary aldosteronism, worldwide. Interestingly, this has resulted in a change in the pattern of disease seen; in the Mayo clinic, earlier experience was that the majority of patients with primary aldosteronism had an APA, while more recent series have clearly shown that the majority of patients with primary aldosteronism have bilateral adrenal hyperplasia (40). Despite this, the true prevalence of primary aldosteronism remains unclear, probably due to differences in definition and source population. A range of prevalence figures for primary aldosteronism has been reported, with some groups suggesting figures as high as 12% (41). Even higher rates (up to 20%) have been reported in populations of patients with resistant hypertension (42), although such studies rarely categorize the type of primary aldosteronism being found. However, in one large series of patients with hypertension (3900 patients), who were very thoroughly screened for the condition with a series of measurements, including urinary corticosteroid levels as well as plasma measurements of aldosterone and renin, a prevalence of 6.5% was reported, with only half these subjects (3.7%) harbouring adrenal adenomas (43). Another study in Italy, using careful confirmatory tests for the disorder, reported a prevalence of 11% for primary aldosteronism in an unselected hypertensive cohort, with 4.8% of subjects harbouring an aldosterone-producing adenoma (44), while a comprehensive study in Greece of patients with resistant hypertension reported a figure of 11.3% (45). This figure is in keeping with other series and is probably a realistic estimate of the frequency of primary aldosteronism in a hypertensive population.

The frequency of Conn's adenomas is slightly greater in female patients; the age at diagnosis of patients with adenomas is less than that for patients with bilateral adrenal hyperplasia. For patients with adenomas, most series report that tumours occur more commonly on the left-hand side.

Bilateral adrenal hyperplasia more frequently affects older patients. It has been suggested that this syndrome is part of the spectrum of low renin essential hypertension and does not, in itself, constitute a distinct diagnostic entity (46). Thus, post mortem series of patients with essential hypertension report increased adrenal nodularity and hyperplasia (discussed above), and it is unclear whether patients with low renin essential hypertension differ in any substantial way from those diagnosed as having bilateral

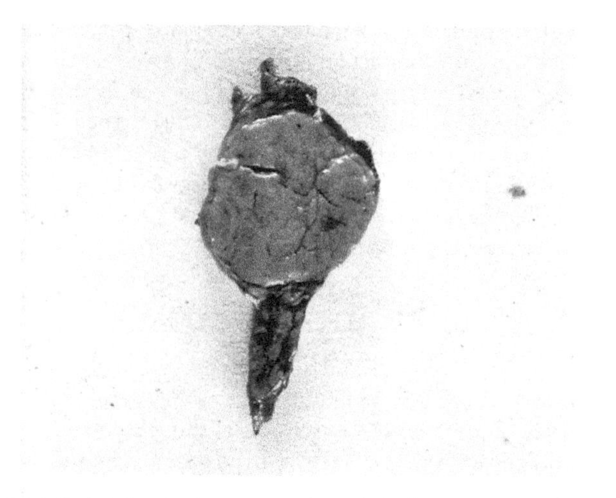

Fig. 5.6.4 Typical Conn's adenoma: note the typical yellow appearance of the cut surface. (See also Plate 25)

adrenal hyperplasia. Indeed, the distinction may be artificial and a consequence of rather arbitrary diagnostic criteria.

Pathology

Aldosterone-producing adenomas

The majority of Conn's tumours are benign. Grossly, they are characteristically around 1 cm in diameter or less and the cut surface has a bright yellow appearance (Fig. 5.6.4), which reflects the lipid-laden nature of the cells (47). On histological examination, the tumour contains cells which are typical of adrenal cortex. In the normal adrenal, it is possible to distinguish zona glomerulosa type cells, which have a high nuclear/cytoplasmic ratio and moderate amounts of lipid. Zona fasciculata type cells have a lower nuclear/cytoplasmic ratio and greater amount of lipid, and cells of the zona reticularis are lipid-depleted and appear eosinophilic. Furthermore, there are distinct differences in the morphological appearance of the mitochondria of these cell types on electron microscopy (48). Conn's adenomas are often composed of relatively uniform zona fasciculata type cells (Fig. 5.6.5) but may contain a mixture of fasciculata, glomerulosa, and reticularis cell types. Some cells may display features of both fasciculata and glomerulosa, so-called hybrid cells. It has been proposed that these histological differences reflect contrasting responsiveness to angiotensin II (tumours which contain predominantly zona glomerulosa type cells are responsive, whereas those with mainly zona fasciculata type cells are unresponsive (49)). Again, the practical value of this differentiation is limited.

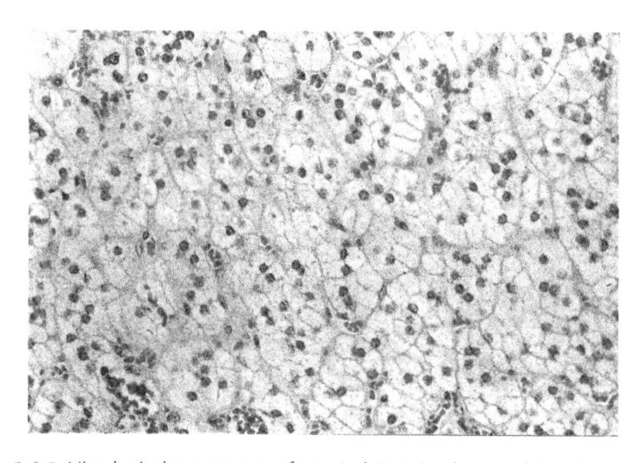

Fig. 5.6.5 Histological appearance of a typical Conn's adenoma (H and E: ×200). Typical lipid-laden cells with zona fasciculata type morphology are seen. (See also Plate 26)

Bilateral adrenal hyperplasia

In some cases there may be evidence of diffuse hyperplasia of the zona glomerulosa. The mechanisms underlying this are unknown. Alternatively, the adrenal cortex may be enlarged because it contains multiple nodules, which are histologically typical of zona fasciculata (50). Routine post mortem examinations in patients with essential hypertension and, indeed, in older normotensive subjects, show a high frequency of nodular change in the adrenal cortex (51). Thus, there may be no clear demarcation between essential hypertension and adrenal hyperplasia, either pathologically or clinically (see below).

Adrenocortical carcinoma

Aldosterone-producing adrenal carcinomas are rare. In any individual tumour it may be difficult to define malignant potential, and multifactorial analysis of histological features is usually required. In general, malignant tumours tend to be larger (over 100 g) and show a very abnormal pattern of corticosteroids in plasma and urine. Rarely, some tumours will secrete both aldosterone and cortisol.

Molecular pathology of Conn's adenomas

The molecular basis for development of Conn's adenomas, adrenal carcinomas, and hyperplasia remains uncertain. In carcinomas, there is evidence that tumours are monoclonal and there may be an association with abnormal expression of p53 protein (52). Furthermore, increased levels of insulin-like growth factor-II have been reported in these tumours. In contrast, aldosterone-producing Conn's adenomas may be polyclonal, and no single molecular pathology has been identified to account for their development. Increased expression of *CYP11B2*, leading to increased aldosterone synthase activity, has been reported, but the reason for this is uncertain. There are also reports of increased expression of renin in Conn's adenomas and it may be that in some the primary fault relates to overactivity of a local intra-adrenal renin/angiotensin system, leading to overexpression of aldosterone synthase. Gross chromosomal rearrangements have been sought in typical Conn's adenomas and have not been consistently found. Other studies have included screens for mutations in the subunits of the stimulatory G protein, G_s, and in the angiotensin II receptor (53). There is one report of increased *RAS* oncogene expression in Conn's adenomas, a report that remains unconfirmed (54). Other reports have demonstrated that a minority of Conn's adenomas display aberrant expression of G-protein-coupled receptors, including those that act as ligands for gut hormones and other peptides (14). However, these appear to be relatively rare. Finally, overexpression of a potassium channel (TASK) in the mouse leads to development of a syndrome that recapitulates features of primary aldosteronism (55); however, is not clear whether TASK channel abnormalities play any role in the genesis of this syndrome in humans.

Rarely, aldosterone-producing adenomas are associated with other genetic mutations. For example, Conn's adenomas have been reported in association with multiple endocrine neoplasia type I and also with the Beckwith–Wiedemann syndrome. However, these inherited conditions are extremely rare. Familial aldosterone-producing adenomas, designated FH II (to distinguish them from GRA (FH I)) are described, where an autosomal dominant pattern of inheritance is found (56). These are relatively rare, although detection of kindreds requires assiduous case detection. Family studies have suggested that a locus on chromosome 7 is associated with FH II, but the precise gene responsible has not been identified. None the less, it is prudent to enquire about the family history of hypertension and consider inherited conditions in any apparent sporadic cases of primary aldosteronism.

Genesis of hypertension in primary aldosteronism

Aldosterone binds to mineralocorticoid receptors in the distal renal tubule to increase sodium reabsorption (by activating the epithelial sodium–hydrogen exchanger). Activation of mineralocorticoid receptors also results in activation of sodium–potassium pump activity. The precise molecular events that link mineralocorticoid receptor activation to sodium reabsorption and potassium loss are discussed above. Mineralocorticoid receptor activation actions lead to expansion of body sodium and depletion of body potassium content; the excess body sodium results in expansion of both extracellular fluid volume and plasma volume. Although there is a reasonable correlation between body sodium and blood pressure in primary aldosteronism (57), it is likely that the rise in blood pressure reflects mechanisms other than, or in addition to, simple plasma volume expansion with the associated rise in cardiac output. For example, mineralocorticoid receptors are present in vascular smooth muscle and their activation leads to alteration in pressor responsiveness to adrenergic stimulation. Furthermore, there is good evidence that mineralocorticoid receptors in cardiac tissue regulate collagen formation (58, 59), and a similar action in the peripheral vasculature might be expected to result in remodelling which would help sustain blood pressure. Thus, there is good evidence that aldosterone levels are inversely related to arterial compliance in essential hypertension, while therapy with a mineralocorticoid receptor antagonist (eplerenone) in patients with essential hypertension leads to a reduction in arteriolar media thickness, in comparison with treatment using a β-blocker (60). Patients with primary aldosteronism would, by analogy, be expected to have vascular remodelling, reduced vascular compliance, effects which will increase systolic hypertension. This concept is supported by a study which shows that the outcome of surgical removal of an aldosterone-producing adenoma is directly related to the degree of vascular remodelling in resistance arterioles removed preoperatively (61).

Finally, receptors for aldosterone are present in the central nervous system and may regulate central sympathetic outflow as well as thirst and sodium appetite (62). It is known that central administration of aldosterone raises blood pressure without altering circulating concentrations of the hormone and that the rise in blood pressure is not associated with sodium retention. Thus, sustained excessive aldosterone is likely to raise blood pressure through a variety of different mechanisms, all of which are dependent on activation of mineralocorticoid receptors. The fact that blood pressure can be lowered effectively and specifically by a mineralocorticoid receptor antagonist, such as spironolactone, confirms this notion without giving any major insight into the relative importance of the pressor mechanisms involved.

Consequences of aldosterone excess

Biochemical consequences

Increased aldosterone secretion causes expansion of body sodium content, with a consequent rise in both extracellular fluid volume and plasma volume. However, unless water is restricted, plasma sodium is generally within the normal range. The increased distal sodium reabsorption and potassium loss are associated with hydrogen ion depletion, resulting in a systemic metabolic alkalosis.

The excess sodium reabsorption is invariably associated with total body potassium depletion, although this need not result in hypokalaemia. Potassium levels are generally at the lower end of the normal range or frankly subnormal; in only 50% of patients is plasma potassium distinctly low (40). Several factors may account for the relative normality of plasma potassium in this syndrome. First, relatively mild aldosterone excess may be less likely to lead to profound hypokalaemia. Secondly, other factors, including intercurrent drug therapy, may determine the prevailing potassium level in this syndrome. Thus, calcium-channel antagonist treatment can reduce aldosterone secretion in Conn's syndrome, leading to normalization of serum potassium levels. Conversely, drugs that increase sodium delivery to the distal renal tubule (for example, thiazide diuretics) will increase the tendency to hypokalaemia. Thirdly, hypokalaemia is more likely to be observed in circumstances of increased sodium intake. Thus, relative restriction of dietary sodium may result in a reduced tendency to develop hypokalaemia.

There is a tendency for magnesium concentrations to be reduced in primary aldosteronism, although this is generally not a major therapeutic issue. It is important to bear in mind that profound hypokalaemia may be associated with magnesium deficiency and that both ions should be replaced in such circumstances. A proportion of patients with primary aldosteronism have impaired glucose tolerance: in a small minority, frank diabetes mellitus may develop. This may be a consequence of potassium deficiency.

A few of the above changes give rise to characteristic physical findings. Occasionally, when hypokalaemia is severe, patients may develop muscular weakness or a frank proximal myopathy. In a small number of patients, the alkalosis which accompanies the other electrolyte abnormalities can become sufficiently severe to result in tetany.

Haemodynamic consequences

The rise in blood pressure in primary aldosteronism is generally mild or moderate, but rare patients have been described with malignant-phase hypertension. Under this unusual circumstance plasma renin concentrations will not be suppressed, due to the severe renal ischaemia present in the malignant phase. The blood pressure in patients with primary aldosteronism is often resistant to conventional antihypertensive drug treatment (63). This gives a clue to the need to investigate patients further. As noted above, there is a reported increase in frequency of primary aldosteronism in patients with resistant hypertension, suggesting that the degree of blood pressure elevation in patients with aldosterone excess is particularly severe.

There are no clear distinguishing features of cardiovascular function in primary aldosteronism to differentiate patients with essential hypertension. For example, baroreflex activity is normal, although recent studies have suggested that aldosterone may alter function of the autonomic nervous system (64). Studies of blood pressure variability in primary aldosteronism have been performed and show no distinct pattern on ambulatory recording over a 24-h period (65).

Vascular consequences

As mentioned above, aldosterone has effects on both vascular contractility and vascular structure. For example, administration of aldosterone to animals increases cardiac collagen content and there is a good correlation between aldosterone levels and cardiac collagen content in humans. Furthermore, there are changes in left ventricular mass and left ventricular function in patients with primary aldosteronism. Such analyses have been difficult to perform, as it is important to ensure that patients and controls are carefully matched for age, gender, body mass index, and other factors that can affect left ventricular hypertrophy. Nonetheless, several studies have shown that primary aldosterone excess leads to more severe left ventricular hypertrophy than is seen in patients with similar levels of blood pressure due to essential hypertension (66, 67). Moreover, abnormalities of left ventricular function, including abnormal diastolic relaxation, have been described. Whether these changes regress with effective aldosterone receptor antagonism or with removal of the source of aldosterone has not been thoroughly evaluated in humans. However, in animal studies, aldosterone-related cardiac hypertrophy can be blocked effectively by spironolactone, while experiments in hypertensive rats show that aldosterone is responsible for severe vascular damage and that this can be prevented by mineralocorticoid receptor antagonism (68). In these animal models the damage caused by mineralocorticoid excess is dependent on concomitant sodium loading and, often, partial nephrectomy; there is not only structural change but development of marked inflammatory change including infiltrate with lymphocytes and evidence of local synthesis of proinflammatory cytokines (69). It is not clear whether similar changes are seen in humans with primary aldosteronism, although a careful comparison of cardiovascular outcomes in patients with aldosterone excess with essential hypertension shows that primary aldosteronism is associated with a substantial excess of risk of left ventricular hypertrophy, atrial fibrillation, myocardial infarction, and stroke (70).

Renal consequences

There are no detailed studies of the effect of primary aldosteronism renal structure. Severe hypokalaemia, which can occur in primary aldosteronism, results in vacuolation within the kidney. However, such severe potassium depletion in primary aldosteronism is very uncommon. In animal models of hypertension, aldosterone excess causes significant renal damage due to deoxycorticosterone, while mineralocorticoid excess is associated with substantial histological evidence of inflammation and glomerular damage (71). Although primary renal impairment is not commonly reported in patients with aldosterone excess, there is evidence that aldosterone can determine the rate of progression of other forms of renal disease. For example, in patients with essential hypertension, aldosterone appears to interact with sodium intake to determine the excretion of protein loss in the urine (42), while analysis of renal function in the large Italian study of prevalence of primary aldosteronism (the PAPY study) showed that patients with primary aldosteronism had higher urinary albumen excretion subjects with essential hypertension (72). Thus, aldosterone excess appears to cause significant increased renal damage beyond that anticipated for the level of blood pressure.

Diagnosis

The diagnosis of primary aldosteronism falls into two distinct parts. First, aldosterone excess needs to be suspected and the primary nature of the disorder established. Secondly, the cause must be identified. If one accepts that primary aldosteronism may affect around 11% of the hypertensive population and that just less than half of those subjects may harbour a Conn's adenoma, it is reasonable to consider which screening procedures are appropriate in patients with hypertension. A comprehensive guideline on the detection and classification of primary aldosteronism is of particular value in this regard (73).

Screening for primary aldosteronism

Some authors have advocated very widespread screening for primary aldosteronism (74). However, it is difficult to justify screening of all hypertensive patients for a condition that may affect only around 10%; in this circumstance, it would be more appropriate to screen selected subgroups at high risk. Clearly, hypokalaemia (either spontaneous or provoked by diuretic therapy) is an important diagnostic clue. Patients who are resistant to conventional antihypertensive therapy (generally defined as not achieving target blood pressure despite use of three appropriate agents) are another group in whom screening is justified. Furthermore, although the true frequency of familial primary aldosteronism (either due to glucocorticoid-remediable aldosteronism or other less well-defined entities) remains uncertain, patients with hypertension who have a positive family history of primary aldosteronism should be screened for the condition. Finally, screening is reasonable in subjects developing hypertension at a young age (<40 years).

Simultaneous measurement of aldosterone and renin (either renin activity or active renin concentration) provides the most reliable single screening test for primary aldosteronism. Either measure on its own is prone to the influence of drug therapy, posture, or other confounding factors. The ARR circumvents many of these problems, as both measurements change in a parallel manner in response to most manoeuvres and is therefore of value as an initial screen (38). Additionally, there is no need to control dietary sodium intake.

The cut-off value for an abnormal ratio that merits further investigation must be determined using local assay conditions. A figure of 750 has been suggested as sufficiently sensitive and specific when plasma aldosterone is expressed in pmol/l and renin activity in ng/ml per h. Some screening algorithms demand not only a raised ARR but a cut-off of a minimal level of aldosterone (e.g. greater than 300 pmol/l) as this substantially increases the positive predictive value of the ARR in detecting the syndrome, a practice that we endorse (73). Finally, the performance of many assays (particularly those for renin) varies and it is necessary to establish a ratio for the normal population locally. It should be noted that in the ARR, renin, as the denominator, has an undue weight on the derived value (75). For this reason, care must be taken in the interpretation using new assays; the great majority of studies defining the prevalence of primary aldosteronism have used renin activity assays, and it is not safe to assume that similar data would be achieved using high throughput renin concentration assays. Factors that affect renin, including gender, age, and body mass index, must also be taken into account.

Drug therapy also has a substantial influence on the ARR, mainly through effects on renin (76). For example, β-blockers depress renin in plasma leading to raised (and therefore false-positive) levels of the ARR. Angiotensin-converting enzyme inhibitors will raise renin and lower aldosterone and, for that reason, reduce the ARR. Diuretics will raise renin and aldosterone and tend to reduce the ARR or have no significant effect. For these reasons, confirmation of the abnormal screening measurement should be made under more stringent conditions, where drug treatment has been either discontinued or altered to avoid confounding agents—α-blockers are unlikely to influence the ratio and can be safely used in this circumstance. Once a positive screening test using reliable methodology, and where it is clear that this is not an artefact caused by interfering antihypertensive agents, confirmation of the diagnosis is then required using a range of possible methods outlined below.

Confirmatory tests for primary aldosteronism

It is important to demonstrate that aldosterone secretion is autonomous to confirm the diagnosis of primary aldosteronism. It should be noted, of course, that all of the tests described show that aldosterone is independent of control of the renin/angiotensin system and do not provide information about other regulatory mechanisms (such as ACTH in GRA). Four main tests are described; the most appropriate needs to be selected to suit local circumstances and investigation facilities. In all of the sodium-loading tests (including the fludrocortisone test) it is important to maintain plasma potassium levels as near normal as possible, both for safety reasons and as hypokalaemia itself will reduce aldosterone secretion and affect the performance of the test being used. Oral potassium supplements are likely to be required in each instance (e.g. Slow K 600 mmol three times per day).

Oral sodium loading

This test can be simply performed in an outpatient setting (40). Patients need to be given low sodium tablets to raise intake to 200 mmol/day for a 4-day period; for the final 24 h a 24-h urine collection should be made to measure aldosterone excretion, and blood taken for measurement of renin and aldosterone. In normal subjects, aldosterone excretion should be suppressed to less than 5 μg/24 h. As described above, potassium supplements should be used to maintain plasma potassium levels within the normal reference range if possible during the period of sodium loading.

Saline infusion

The simplest test to confirm the presence of primary aldosteronism is infusion of normal saline (2 L over a 4-h period) (77). If plasma aldosterone levels remain elevated (in practice above 140 pmol/l) at the end of this manoeuvre, the diagnosis is confirmed. However, there is a small risk of provoking cardiac failure, particularly in elderly patients, and the test should be performed with caution.

Fludrocortisone suppression test

A more elaborate version of the sodium-loading test is the administration of the synthetic mineralocorticoid fludrocortisone (0.5 mg four times daily for 2 days), with measurements of aldosterone at the beginning and end of this manoeuvre. Some authorities regard this as a definitive test in primary aldosteronism. Although doubtless reliable, it does necessitate admission of patients to hospital, which may not be cost-effective. In the test described by Gordon, fludrocortisone is given in a dose of 400 mg/day in association with additional sodium chloride tablets (90 mmol daily) (78). In normal subjects, aldosterone should be fully suppressed, and failure to suppress is diagnostic of primary aldosteronism. However, the test carries with it a substantial risk of significant potassium depletion and profound hypokalaemia, with the attendant dangers of cardiac dysrythmia.

Captopril test

Administration of captopril (25 mg), with measurement of renin and aldosterone before and 2 h after drug therapy, is described as a diagnostic manoeuvre for primary aldosteronism (79). In normal subjects, aldosterone levels will be suppressed by a single dose of captopril (as a consequence of inhibition of angiotensin II formation), while this is not the case in patients with Conn's adenomas.

In summary, confirmation of primary aldosteronism can often be had simply by careful measurements of aldosterone and renin in patients in whom dietary sodium intake is not restricted and in whom confounding drug therapy (principally calcium-channel blockers, which can lower aldosterone levels in Conn's adenoma patients) has been eliminated. In such circumstances, it may be justifiable to proceed to definitive tests for the differential diagnosis of primary aldosteronism.

Differential diagnosis of primary aldosterone excess

When primary aldosteronism is confirmed, the principal problem is to distinguish between a Conn's adenoma and bilateral adrenal hyperplasia. The distinction is important since subsequent treatment of the two variants is different. A small number of patients will have glucocorticoid-remediable aldosteronism (see Chapter 000); this can be readily diagnosed on the basis of a simple genetic test (80). The distinction is important since subsequent treatment of the two variants is different.

Aldosterone levels are generally higher in patients with Conn's adenomas than in those with bilateral adrenal hyperplasia, but this is not, in itself, a reliable discriminant. Similarly, concentrations of other corticosteroids, including 18-hydroxycorticosterone, 18-hydroxycortisol, and 18-oxocortisol, are higher in patients with adenomas but are not routinely measured in the diagnostic workup of patients with primary aldosteronism and, in any case, do not reliably improve discrimination.

Dynamic tests of aldosterone responsiveness do not help discriminate accurately between Conn's adenomas and bilateral adrenal hyperplasia. Although aldosterone does not respond to the administration of angiotensin II, in the majority of patients with adenomas (in contrast to patients with bilateral hyperplasia, where a very brisk response may be seen), a positive response is reported in a substantial minority of patients with adenomas. For this reason, reliance on aldosterone response to upright posture or angiotensin II is not a secure means of discriminating between the two main causes of primary aldosteronism.

Imaging

Imaging of the adrenal glands is a key step in differential diagnosis. Ultrasonography is of no value, although large adrenal carcinomas

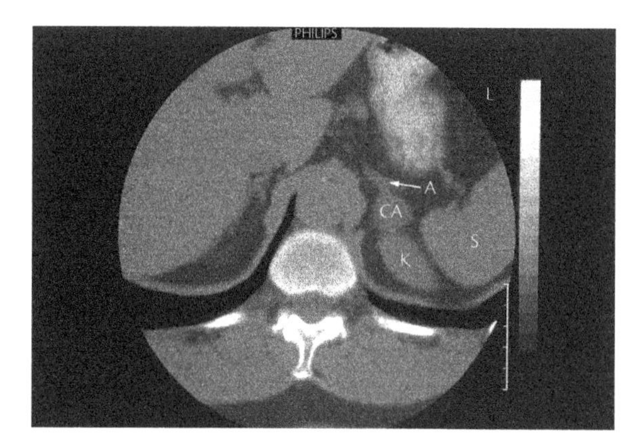

Fig. 5.6.6 CT scan in a patient with a left-sided Conn's adenoma (CA). Adjacent limb of adrenal (A), upper pole of left kidney (K), and spleen (S) are identified.

will be readily identified. In all patients with confirmed primary aldosteronism, careful imaging of the adrenal glands with either CT or MRI is necessary. CT scans of the abdomen with 3 to 5 mm slices of the adrenal regions will provide accurate identification of the adrenal glands and should demonstrate the majority of adenomas, although very small lesions (in practice, those less than 5 mm) may be missed by this technique. A typical lesion identified by CT scanning is shown in Fig. 5.6.6. MRI scanning of the abdomen also gives good resolution of the adrenal glands but offers no advantage over carefully performed CT imaging. Radiolabelled cholesterol scanning (generally carried out after dexamethasone suppression to reduce normal adrenal gland uptake of cholesterol) has been used to identify adrenal adenomas in patients with primary aldosteronism. However, this is not a sensitive technique. In some patients with bilateral adrenal hyperplasia, CT scanning may show enlargement of the glands; small nodules can be visualized. Due to the heterogeneity in nodule size, the CT scan appearance in these patients may be confused with that of a single adenoma, and the definitive diagnosis of a solitary aldosterone-producing adenoma requires selective adrenal vein sampling.

Selective adrenal vein sampling

This technique is indicated in any patient in whom surgical adrenalectomy is contemplated and in whom the presence of a unilateral adenoma is not clear cut. As small adrenal incidentalomas are commonly seen in normal subjects, particularly with advancing years, it is therefore not safe to assume that a lesion on CT scanning is responsible for the syndrome of primary aldosteronism. A reasonable approach is to consider sampling in any patient over the age of 40 in whom surgery is indicated (there is clearly no need to perform sampling if the patient or clinician does not feel that surgery, regardless of the diagnosis, is appropriate). Furthermore, the procedure is absolutely necessary when radiology is uncertain and when adrenal gland surgery is being considered in patients with no definite radiological abnormality.

In performing the technique, simultaneous measurement of both aldosterone and cortisol in the adrenal effluent is required (81). It is necessary to measure cortisol in order to confirm the technical success of the procedure by demonstrating a concentration gradient between adrenal vein and low inferior vena cava. Unfortunately, it is not always possible to achieve bilateral adrenal vein catheterization (the failure rate may be up to 25%, with greatest difficulty occurring in cannulation of the right adrenal vein) and this limits the value of the procedure. The confirmation of lateralization is achieved by demonstrating a ratio of aldosterone:cortisol that is at least twofold when comparing right with left (or vice versa). Some authors recommend use of ACTH during the procedure to stimulate secretion of aldosterone from an adenoma, and improve the sensitivity of the test; we suggest that this adds to the complexity of what is already a technically demanding test (82). Finally, real-time measurement of cortisol during the test has been advocated as a means of improving technical success rates for cannulation of the adrenal veins; this is not a widely available assay.

Although it has been suggested that adrenal vein sampling is not necessary in patients with a clear adenoma visualized on CT scanning, there are reports of removal of nonfunctional adrenal 'incidentalomas' which were not responsible for aldosterone excess. Thus, where there is any doubt, adrenal vein sampling should be performed.

Summary of investigation of suspected primary aldosteronism

The diagnosis of primary aldosteronism can be problematic but has been assisted by the recent publication of a clear investigative strategy by the Endocrine Society (73). Figure 5.6.7 summarizes a coherent diagnostic approach to investigate the patient with

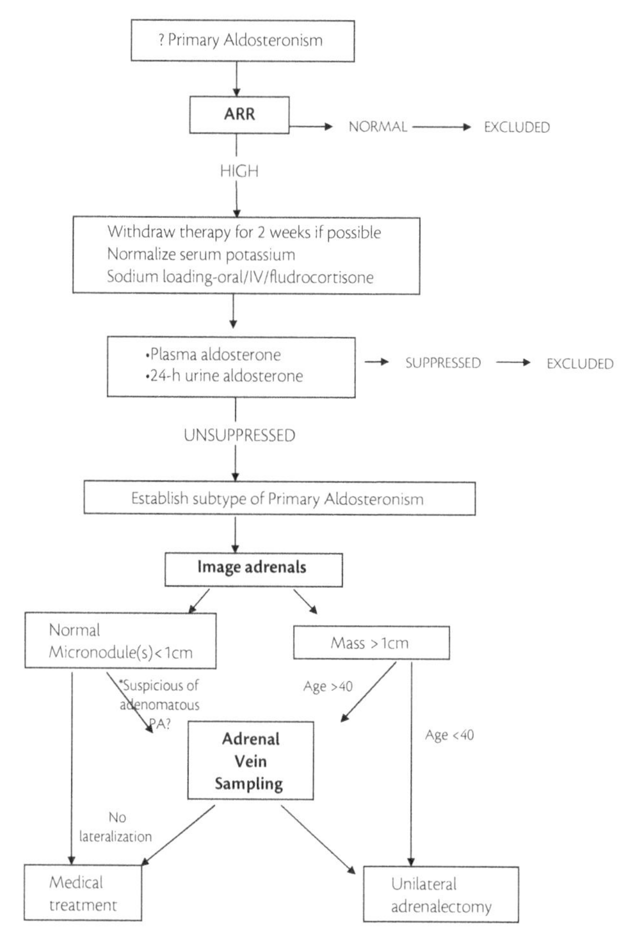

Fig. 5.6.7 Proposed algorithm for the screening, diagnostic confirmation, and management of primary aldosteronism. *Clinical features that make adenomatous primary aldosteronism more likely include: hypokalaemia, severe hypertension, younger age, higher levels of aldosterone. ARR, aldosterone to renin ratio.

suspected primary aldosteronism, which is based upon both Endocrine Society and Mayo Clinic guidelines (40). It should always be noted that, before performing specific diagnostic tests, serum potassium should be normalized, if necessary by oral supplementation, and patients should be encouraged to maintain a liberal dietary salt intake prior to ARR testing and throughout subsequent investigations for primary aldosteronism.

Medical therapy

The mineralocorticoid receptor antagonist, spironolactone, is effective as an antihypertensive agent in primary aldosteronism. Fairly high dosage may be required (historically use of up to 400 mg/day was reported), although it is appropriate to start with low doses (25 mg/day) and increase gradually until blood pressure control is achieved. The high dose necessary to cure hypertension may, however, limit use of spironolactone, particularly in male patients. Principal side effects of spironolactone include gynaecomastia, diminished libido, and impotence, and reflect transactivation of the androgen receptor. The alternative mineralocorticoid receptor antagonist, eplerenone, does not have significant affinity for the androgen receptor and is free of these unwanted effects. It can be used in primary aldosteronism, although it appears less effective as a mineralocorticoid antagonist compared with spironolactone; high doses (up to 150 mg twice daily) may be required.

Amiloride, which blocks the epithelial sodium channel in the distal renal tubule, is also effective in lowering blood pressure in primary aldosteronism. Indeed, earlier studies which compared amiloride with spironolactone show that the drugs were equally effective in lowering body sodium content and reducing blood pressure in this condition. As with spironolactone, amiloride must be given in relatively high dosage (up to 40 mg/day).

In treating patients with either drug, it is important to monitor plasma potassium concentrations. In patients with renal impairment, there is a risk of hyperkalaemia and dosage of both drugs should be kept to the minimum under these circumstances. Plasma renin concentrations give some guide to the effectiveness of drug therapy in patients with primary aldosteronism. Thus, persistent suppression of renin levels suggests that the drug is not being given at an effective aldosterone-antagonist dosage.

Patients with primary aldosteronism are often resistant to other antihypertensive drug therapy. Clearly, angiotensin-converting enzyme inhibitor treatment is illogical in patients in whom renin and angiotensin II levels are suppressed. Calcium-channel blockers, particularly of the dihydropyridine class, are reported to reduce aldosterone secretion in patients with Conn's adenomas. They can be combined safely with spironolactone or amiloride and may provide effective blood pressure control in patients resistant to single-drug therapy.

Surgical management

Surgical removal of an aldosterone-producing adenoma is normally the most appropriate treatment for patients with a unilateral lesion. However, before surgery is performed it is necessary to optimize blood pressure control and to correct any significant electrolyte disturbance. Previous studies have shown that the blood pressure response to either spironolactone or amiloride can predict the blood pressure outcome following surgical adrenalectomy. One practical consequence of this may be to help predict those patients in whom surgical treatment may not be curative; in these circumstances or where surgery is contraindicated, combination therapy with aldosterone antagonist drugs, with or without other antihypertensive treatments, may be appropriate.

Treatment with either spironolactone (or amiloride) will normally fully correct potassium depletion in primary aldosteronism before surgery. Effective therapy with either drug will also minimize the risk of postoperative hypoaldosteronism, which can occur due to atrophy of the normal zona glomerulosa caused by the excessive autonomous aldosterone secretion. Potassium supplementation may also be given, although administration of adequate doses of either spironolactone or amiloride is normally sufficient over a longer period of time to maintain a normal body potassium content.

The surgical approach to the adrenal gland in patients with unilateral adenomas was previously either by an anterior or a lateral open operation but laparoscopic adrenalectomy is the now the surgical approach of choice. In experienced hands the operation has a relatively low morbidity and a high success rate (83). It is important to inform patients about the likely success rates of adrenal surgery; this is often poorly documented in series of surgical adrenalectomy, and some do not fully differentiate between 'cure' of hypertension (where patients require no antihypertensive therapy) and 'improvement', where patients may need less medication than before the procedure. It is likely that surgery will cure the tendency to hypokalaemia if the adenoma is correctly removed; however, absolute cure rates of blood pressure elevation may be less than 30%, with improvement in blood pressure in a further 30% (84). It is possible that the duration of the syndrome before diagnosis influences the ultimate outcome following surgery; there is evidence that vascular structural changes predict the achieved blood pressure level after successful adrenalectomy.

Bilateral adrenal hyperplasia should be treated medically using either spironolactone or amiloride in conjunction with other antihypertensive drugs, as necessary. Although it has been suggested that partial adrenalectomy can improve blood pressure control, it is difficult to justify this when effective drug therapy is available.

Suspected adrenal carcinomas should be surgically resected at the earliest opportunity. It may not be possible to diagnose, with certainty, the malignant nature of a lesion on histological grounds alone, and the presence of recurrent or metastatic disease is the only certain way of doing so. Malignant adrenal lesions do not respond to external radiotherapy and are generally resistant to combination chemotherapy. Some patients with adrenocortical malignancy may show a response to the use of mitotane (*ortho, para'*, dichlorodiphenyldichloroethane (o,p'DDD)), but consistent good responses are unusual.

Rare causes of mineralocorticoid hypertension

Other causes of mineralocorticoid hypertension, listed in Table 5.6.2, are uncommon and are discussed briefly below.

Liddle's syndrome

This syndrome was first described by Grant Liddle, in 1963, in a family in which the siblings appeared to have features of aldosterone excess (early onset hypertension and hypokalaemia) but with suppressed plasma renin and aldosterone levels (85). It is now known that this syndrome is inherited as an autosomal dominant

Table 5.6.2 Classification of mineralocorticoid excess syndromes

Mechanism	Classification	Ligand
Post receptor	Liddle's syndrome	
Adrenal receptor	Progesterone-induced hypertension (MR) Glucocorticoid resistance (GR)[a]	Progesterone Cortisol
Abnormal ligand	Syndrome of apparent mineralocorticoid excess Congenital adrenal hyperplasia[a] DOC-producing tumours Ectopic ACTH syndrome	Cortisol DOC DOC Cortisol
Normal ligand	Primary aldosteronism Glucocorticoid remediable[a] Aldosteronism	Aldosterone

[a] Discussed elsewhere in Part 5.

DOC, deoxycorticosterone; GR, glucocorticoid receptor; MR, mineralocorticoid receptor.

trait and occurs due to mutations in the genes encoding the β or γ subunits of the ENaC. (Fig. 5.6.2). Thirteen mutations in the β ENaC and four in γ ENaC subunits have been identified in patients with Liddle's syndrome so far (86, 87). Most either alter or delete a highly conserved PY-motif at the C-terminal end of the channel that is involved in its normal regulation by virtue of its interaction with Nedd4 (see above). The effect of the mutations is to alter the interaction so that trafficking of ENaC to the proteosome is disrupted, and the likelihood of the channel being in open conformation in the apical membrane is greatly increased. The exception to this is one isolated mutation in γ ENaC (Asn530Ser) which is located in the extracellular loop of the gamma subunit and does not affect the PY-motif (88). These various mutations all lead to constitutive activation of the sodium channel, resulting in excessive sodium reabsorption in the distal nephron irrespective of circulating mineralocorticoid levels, which are suppressed. The laboratory findings include increased urinary potassium excretion, hypokalaemia, and suppression of plasma renin activity and of circulating levels of angiotensin II and aldosterone.

Interestingly, in the proband of one of Liddle's original cases, renal transplantation resulted in normalization of blood pressure and electrolyte abnormalities. In practice, however, blockers of the sodium channel, such as amiloride or triamterene, effectively treat the electrolyte abnormalities and hypertension. Mineralocorticoid antagonists such as spironolactone are ineffective, as this disorder is not a consequence of activation of the mineralocorticoid receptor.

Progesterone-induced hypertension

This rare disorder was first described in 2000 and is characterized by constitutive activation of the mineralocorticoid receptor as well as an alteration in receptor sensitivity (89). A missense mutation in the hormone binding domain of the mineralocorticoid receptor has been identified as the cause, leading to the substitution of leucine for serine at codon 810 (S810L). The S810L mutation alters mineralocorticoid receptor sensitivity; most significantly, both progesterone and spironolactone, which usually act as antagonists at the mineralocorticoid receptor, become potent agonists. Subjects with this mutation are characterized by early onset of severe hypertension with suppression of aldosterone and plasma renin. This mutation and the resulting phenotype were described in eight out of 23 of the index patient's family, suggesting an autosomal dominant mode of transmission. Progesterone levels increase by up to 100-fold in pregnancy, and carriers of the S810L tend to develop severe pregnancy-associated hypertension.

Syndrome of apparent mineralocorticoid excess

Apparent mineralocorticoid excess (AME) is a rare syndrome of hypertension and hypokalaemia associated with suppression of plasma renin activity and low plasma concentrations of aldosterone and other known mineralocorticoids (90). As described above, 11β-HSD2 normally oxidizes cortisol to cortisone, which does not transactivate the mineralocorticoid receptor. In this manner, 11β-HSD2 acts as a 'gatekeeper' to prevent the mineralocorticoid receptor becoming saturated with cortisol which is present at a much higher level than aldosterone. The molecular basis of this syndrome was described in 1995; 11β-HSD2 activity is reduced or absent such that cortisol overwhelms the mineralocorticoid receptor causing cortisol-mediated mineralocorticoid hypertension.

Classically, this syndrome, inherited in an autosomal recessive manner, usually presents in childhood with failure to thrive, short stature, significant hypertension, and hypokalaemia. The potassium depletion may be severe, leading to nephrogenic diabetes insipidus and rhabdomyolysis. Biochemical diagnosis of AME can be made by measuring the ratio of cortisol (compound F) to cortisone (compound E) as indicated by the ratios of their tetrahydro (allo)-urinary metabolites (THF + alloTHF:THE) (91). Normal subjects excrete two- to threefold more urinary free cortisone than urinary free cortisol, reflecting the significant activity of renal 11β-HSD2. In AME, however, urinary free cortisone excretion is extremely low, leading to an increased THF + alloTHF:THE ratio in urine. Despite a marked increase in the half life of plasma cortisol, AME patients are not cushingoid since the normal negative feedback system remains intact, leading to a marked reduction in cortisol secretion rates.

The gene encoding 11β-HSD2 is 6.2 kb long, comprises five exons, and is located on chromosome 16q22 (Fig. 5.6.8) (92).

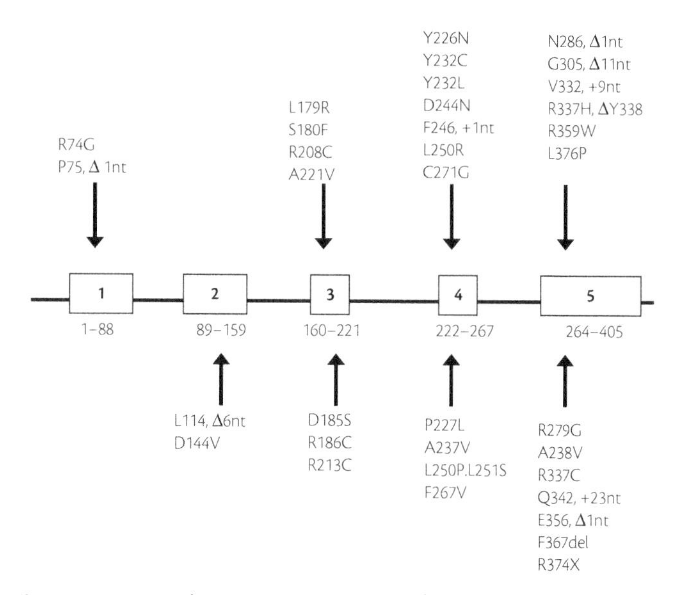

Fig. 5.6.8 Location of *HSD11B2* mutations. The 11β-hydroxysteroid dehydrogenase gene is located on chromosome 16 and has five exons. The numbers below the exons indicate the amino acid number.

Less than 100 cases of AME have been reported, with more than 35 different nonsilent mutations identified clustered in exons 1–5 (Fig. 5.6.8). Complete abolition of enzymatic activity results in the classical and severe AME phenotype described above. Milder cases of AME, so-called 'type II apparent mineralocorticoid excess' with isolated hypertension and normal or low-normal potassium have been described in Italian patients (93). In this kindred, a homozygous mutation in the 11β-HSD2 gene (R279C) has been identified which causes a reduction but not complete abolition of 11β-HSD2 activity. It can be seen, therefore, that AME comprises a spectrum of mineralocorticoid hypertension with a good correlation between genotype and phenotype.

AME can be effectively treated with amiloride, although high doses (up to 40 mg daily) can be required for therapeutic benefit. Mineralocorticoid receptor antagonism with spironolactone offers an alternative therapy, but its use may be limited by the relatively high doses required to competitively antagonize the agonist effects of cortisol in this circumstance; this consideration is particularly important in young male patients where unwanted androgen effects can limit use of this drug. Dexamethasone has also been used therapeutically but its use is limited by the need to employ a dose sufficiently high to inhibit endogenous cortisol production, exposing patients to unwanted glucocorticoid side effects. As well as improving blood pressure, a major aim of treatment is correction of hypokalaemia, which contributes to the poor growth rate seen in children with this disorder. As is common in secondary hypertension, definitive therapy may not always normalize blood pressure (or potassium levels) and additional antihypertensive agents may be required. Deficiency of 11β-HSD and consequent mineralocorticoid hypertension can also occur as a result of ingestion of liquorice or carbenoxolone (previously used for the treatment of peptic ulcer disease). The active component of liquorice is glycyrrhizic acid and its hydrolytic product glycyrrhetinic acid, which have been shown to inhibit the activity of 11β-HSD2 in the renal tubule allowing cortisol-driven mineralocorticoid hypertension (94). Carbenoxolone is a semisynthetic hemisuccinate derivative of glycyrrhetinic acid and has its effect through a mechanism analogous to that of liquorice.

Subjects consuming excessive quantities of liquorice may present with hypertension and hypokalaemia associated with suppression of plasma renin activity and aldosterone as well as an increase in exchangeable sodium levels. This condition responds to treatment with spironolactone or amiloride, but is best dealt with by cessation of liquorice ingestion.

Deoxycorticosterone hypertension

Other mineralocorticoids rarely circulate in sufficient levels to cause hypertension. The aldosterone precursor deoxycorticosterone, which binds and activates the mineralocorticoid receptor, circulates at concentrations around 2% of those of aldosterone and so, under normal circumstances, does not contribute to electrolyte and blood pressure regulation. However, excessive plasma levels of deoxycorticosterone can be found, rarely, in patients with adrenal carcinomas (16). The result is hypertension similar to that caused by excess aldosterone, and is associated with sodium retention and potassium loss leading to hypokalaemia. Less commonly, raised deoxycorticosterone levels are found in adult patients with the rare inborn errors of adrenal steroid synthesis due to defective 17α-hydroxylase or 11β-hydroxylase activity. In both of these circumstances, increased ACTH drive to the adrenal causes chronic excess deoxycorticosterone secretion (95). The resultant sodium retention causes suppression of renin release and, as a consequence, aldosterone levels are generally low. Most presentations occur shortly after birth or in early childhood. Adrenal androgens are produced in excessive amounts in patients with 11β-hydroxylase deficiency, leading to virilization of female subjects. In 17-hydroxylase deficiency, there is inability to synthesize sex hormones, with the result that affected males fail to develop normal masculine external genitalia, while females fail to progress through adrenarche or puberty. Diagnosis is confirmed by measurement of corticosteroid metabolite excretion in the urine. A more complete description of these autosomal recessive disorders and their management is given in Chapter 000.

Ectopic ACTH syndrome

Approximately 80% of patients with Cushing's syndrome have hypertension, increasing to 95% in subjects with Cushing's syndrome due to ectopic ACTH production. Ectopic ACTH syndrome is generally associated with hypokalaemic alkalosis (in 95–100%) consistent with mineralocorticoid hypertension. Several studies have demonstrated that the mineralocorticoid excess state is explained by saturation of 11β-HSD2 by the very high cortisol concentrations seen in the ectopic ACTH syndrome. Both the urinary ratios of tetrahydrocortsol and allotetrahydrocortisol/ tetrahydrocortisone and free cortisol/ cortisone are elevated, not because of impaired 11β-HSD2 function but due to saturation of the enzyme by high levels of cortisol (96). Thus, the enzyme is overwhelmed by substrate and cortisol cannot be inactivated to cortisone in the renal tubule leading to activation of the mineralocorticoid receptor by cortisol.

Gordon's syndrome; pseudohypoaldosteronism type II

Gordon's syndrome (also known as pseudohypoaldosteronism type II), is a rare autosomal dominant disorder characterized by hypertension, hyperkalaemia, hyperchloraemia, acidosis, and sodium retention leading to suppression of plasma renin and aldosterone (97). The molecular basis of this disorder has been found to be explained by mutations in the WNK (with no K (lysine)) kinases. These are a family of protein kinases with unusual protein kinase domains due to the unusual placement of the catalytic lysine when compared to all other protein kinases (98). Pseudohypoaldosteronism type II develops due to mutations in either WNK1 or WNK4 (99)

WNK4 normally inhibits the thiazide sensitive Na–Cl cotransporter of the distal nephron; thus missense mutations increase the activity of the Na–Cl cotransporter, leading to thiazide-sensitive hypertension; systolic and diastolic blood pressure fall by approximately 45 mm Hg and 25 mm Hg respectively after treatment with 25 mg of hydrochlorothiazide per day (100). The mechanism of hypertension in subjects with WNK1 mutations is less clear. It has been demonstrated that WNK1 mutations abolishes the WNK4-mediated inhibition of the Na–Cl cotransporter in the distal convoluted tubule. However, WNK1-mediated Gordon's syndrome is less sensitive to thiazide diuretic treatment, suggesting that other mechanisms may be involved (101). There are reports that WNK1-mediated hypertension may also occur through activation of ENaC and inhibition of ROMK (inwardly rectifying K) channel, which controls potassium secretion in the renal distal nephron.

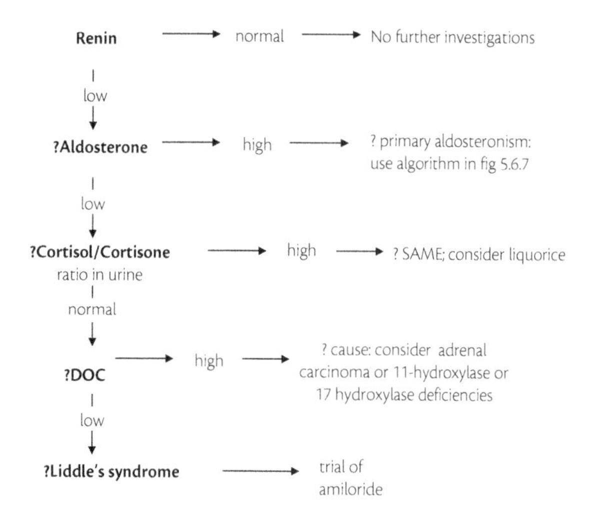

Fig. 5.6.9 Approach to initial investigation of mineralocorticoid excess. SAME, syndrome of apparent mineralocorticoid excess; DOC, deoxycorticosterone.

Summary

Primary aldosteronism is the commonest cause of mineralocorticoid hypertension, although other rare causes should be considered as discussed above and an algorithm outlining a potential approach to the investigation of mineralocorticoid excess is illustrated in Fig. 5.6.9. Importantly, primary aldosteronism is now considered to be the commonest cause of secondary hypertension; reported prevalence in the hypertensive population ranges from 6–12%. Much of this increase in detection of primary aldosteronism is due to more widespread screening of hypertensive populations using the ARR (which is driven by the level of renin) as a first step. The subsequent investigation of suspected mineralocorticoid hypertension can follow a logical pattern thereafter, and the algorithm shown in Fig. 5.6.9 offers one such simple approach, although it should be stressed that it relies on availability of reliable endocrine biochemical and imaging services. The publication of the recent consensus clinical guideline for the investigation of primary aldosteronism by the Endocrine Society (summarized in Fig. 5.6.7) provides a clear approach, thereafter, to the investigation and management of the patient suspected of having primary aldosteronism.

References

1. Young WF. Primary aldosteronism: renaissance of a syndrome. *Clin Endocrinol*, 2007; **66**: 607–18.
2. Rainey WE. Adrenal zonation: clues from 11beta-hydroxylase and aldosterone synthase. *Mol Cell Endocrinol*, 1999; **151**: 151–60.
3. Mornet E, Dupont J, Vitek A, White PC. Characterization of two genes encoding human steroid 11 beta- hydroxylase (P-450(11) beta). *J Biol Chem*, 1989; **264**: 20961–7.
4. Freel EM, Shakerdi LA, Friel EC, Wallace AM, Davies E, Fraser R, *et al.* Studies on the origin of circulating 18-hydroxycortisol and 18-oxocortisol in normal human subjects. *J Clin Endocrinol Metab*, 2004; **89**: 4628–33.
5. Lifton RP, Dluhy RG, Powers M, Rich GM, Cook S, Ulick S, *et al.* A chimaeric 11β-hydroxylase/aldosterone synthase gene causes glucocorticoid-remediable aldosteronism and human hypertension. *Nature*, 1992; **355**: 262–5.
6. Stowasser M, Bachmann AW, Tunny TJ, Gordon RD. Production of 18-oxo-cortisol in subtypes of primary aldosteronism. *Clin Exp Pharmacol Physiol*, 1996; **23**: 591–3.
7. Connell JM, Davies E. The new biology of aldosterone. *J Endocrinol*, 2005; **186**: 1–20.
8. Ganguly A. Potassium and aldosterone secretion in glucocorticoid-remediable aldosteronism. *J Clin Endocrinol Metab*, 1997; **82**: 4276–7.
9. Ganguly A. Current concepts—primary aldosteronism. *N Engl J Med*, 1998; **339**: 1828–34.
10. Vallotton MB. Primary aldosteronism.1. Diagnosis of primary hyperaldosteronism. *Clin Endocrinol*, 1996; **45**: 47–52.
11. Wisgerhof M, Brown RD, Hogan MJ, Carpenter PC, Edis AJ. The plasma-aldosterone response to angiotensin-II infusion in aldosterone-producing adenoma and idiopathic hyper-aldosteronism. *J Clin Endocrinol Metab*, 1981; **52**: 195–8.
12. Quinn SJ, Williams GH. Regulation of aldosterone secretion. *Annu Rev Physiol*, 1988; **50**: 409–26.
13. Rocco S, Opocher G, Carpene G, Mantero F. Atrial-natriuretic-peptide infusion in primary aldosteronism—renal, hemodynamic and hormonal effects. *Am J Hypertens*, 1990; **3**: 668–73.
14. Lampron A, Bourdeau I, Oble S, Godbout A, Schurch W, Arjane P, *et al.* Regulation of aldosterone secretion by several aberrant receptors including for glucose-dependent peptide in a patient with an aldosteronoma. *J Clin Endocrinol Metab* 2009; **94**: 750–6.
15. Biglieri EG, Schambelan M. Significance of elevated levels of plasma 18-hydroxycorticosterone in patients with primary aldosteronism. *J Clini Endocrinol Metab*, 1979; **49**: 87–91.
16. Stone NN, Janoski A, Muakkassa W, Shpritz L. Mineralocorticoid excess secondary to adrenal-cortical carcinoma. *J Urol*, 1984; **132**: 962–5.
17. Funder JW. Aldosterone action. *Annu Rev Physiol*, 1993; **55**: 115–30.
18. Connell JMC, MacKenzie SM, Freel EM, Fraser R, Davies E. A lifetime of aldosterone excess: Long-term consequences of altered regulation of aldosterone production for cardiovascular function. *Endocr Rev*, 2008; **29**: 133–54.
19. Arriza JL, Weinberger C, Cerelli G, Glaser TM, Handelin BL, Housman DE, *et al.* Cloning of human mineralocorticoid receptor complementary DNA: structural and functional kinship with the glucocorticoid receptor. *Science*, 1987; **237**: 268–75.
20. Horisberger JD, Diezi J. Effects of mineralocorticoids on Na+ and K+ excretion in the adrenalectomised rat. *Am J Physiol*, 1983; **245**: F89–F99.
21. Rossier BC, Canessa CM, Schild L, Horisberger JD. Epithelial sodium channels. *Curr Opin Nephrol Hypertens*, 1994; **437**: 487–96.
22. Garty H, Palmer LG. Epithelial sodium channels: Function, structure, and regulation. *Physiol Rev*, 1997; **77**: 359–96.
23. Naray-Fejes-Toth A, Canessa C, Cleaveland ES, Aldrich G, Fejes-Toth G. Sgk is an aldosterone-induced kinase in the renal collecting duct—effects on epithelial Na+ channels. *J Biol Chem*, 1999; **274**: 16973–8.
24. Staub O, Abriel H, Plant P, Ishikawa T, Kanelis V, Saleki R, *et al.* Regulation of the epithelial Na+ channel by Nedd4 and ubiquitination. *Kidney Int*, 2000; **57**: 809–15.
25. Rotin D. Regulation of the epithelial sodium channel (ENaC) by accessory proteins. *Curr Opin Nephrol Hypertens*, 2000; **9**: 529–34.
26. Hays S. Mineralocorticoid modulation of apical and basolateral membrane $H^+/OH^-/HCO^{3-}$ transport processes in the rabbit inner stripe of outer medullary collecting duct. *J Clin Invest*, 1992; **90**: 180–7.
27. Funder JW, Pearce PT, Smith R, Smith IA. Mineralocorticoid action: target tissue specificity is enzyme, not receptor, mediated. *Science*, 1988; **242**: 583–5.
28. Edwards CR, Stewart PM, Burt D, Brett L, McIntyre MA, Sutanto WS, *et al.* Localisation of 11 beta-hydroxysteroid dehydrogenase—tissue specific protector of the mineralocorticoid receptor. *Lancet*, 1988; **2** (8618): 986–9.
29. Funder JW. Reconsidering the roles of the mineralocorticoid receptor. *Hypertension*, 2009; **53**: 286–90.
30. Funder JW. Non-genomic actions of aldosterone: role in hypertension. *Curr Opin Nephrol Hypertens*, 2001; **10**: 227–30.

31. Winter C, Schulz N, Giebisch G, Geibel JP, Wagner CA. Nongenomic stimulation of vacuolar H+-ATPases in intercalated renal tubule cells by aldosterone. *Proc Natl Acad Sci USA*, 2004; **101**: 2636–41.
32. Mihailidou AS, Mardini M, Funder JW. Rapid, nongenomic effects of aldosterone in the heart mediated by epsilon protein kinase C. *Endocrinology*, 2004; **145**: 773–80.
33. Maguire D, MacNamara B, Cuffe JE, Winter D, Doolan CM, Urbach V, *et al.* Rapid responses to aldosterone in human distal colon. *Steroids*, 1999; **64**: 51–63.
34. Diaz R, Brown RW, Seckl JR. Distinct ontogeny of glucocorticoid and mineralocorticoid receptor and 11beta-hydroxysteroid dehydrogenase types I and II mRNAs in the fetal rat brain suggest a complex control of glucocorticoid actions. *J Neurosci*, 1998; **18**: 2570–80.
35. Gomez-Sanchez EP. Intracerebroventricular infusion of aldosterone induces hypertension in rats. *Endocrinology*, 1986; **118**: 819–23.
36. Gomez-Sanchez EP, Fort CM, Gomez-Sanchez CE. Intracerebroventricular infusion of RU28318 blocks aldosterone-salt hypertension. *Am J Physiol*, 1990; **258**: 482–4.
37. Mulatero P, Stowasser M, Loh KC, Fardella CE, Gordon RD, Mosso L, *et al.* Increased diagnosis of primary aldosteronism, including surgically correctable forms, in centers from five continents. *J Clin Endocrinol Metabol*, 2004; **89**: 1045–50.
38. Hiramatsu K, Yamada T, Yukimura Y, Komiya I, Ichikawa K, Ishihara M, *et al.* A screening test to identify aldosterone-producing adenoma by measuring plasma renin activity. Results in hypertensive patients. *Arch Intern Med*, 1981; **141**: 1589–93.
39. Gordon RD, Stowasser M, Tunny TJ, Klemm SA, Rutherford JC. High incidence of primary aldosteronism in 199 patients referred with hypertension. *Clin Exp Pharmacol Physiol*, 1994; **21**: 315–8.
40. Young WF, Jr. Minireview: primary aldosteronism—changing concepts in diagnosis and treatment. *Endocrinology*, 2003; **144**: 2208–13.
41. Gordon RD, Ziesak MD, Tunny TJ, Stowasser M, Klemm SA. Evidence that primary aldosteronism may not be uncommon: 12% incidence among hypertensive drug trial volunteers. *Clin Exp Pharmacol Physiol*, 1993; **20**: 296–8.
42. Calhoun DA, Nishizaka MK, Zaman MA, Thakkar RB, Weissmann P. Hyperaldosteronism among black and white subjects with resistant hypertension. *Hypertension*, 2002; **40**: 892–6.
43. Abdelhamid S, MullerLobeck H, Pahl S, Remberger K, Bonhof JA, Walb D, *et al.* Prevalence of adrenal and extra-adrenal Conn syndrome in hypertensive patients. *Arch Intern Med*, 1996; **156**: 1190–5.
44. Rossi GP, Bernini G, Caliumi C, Desideri G, Fabris B, Ferri C, *et al.* A prospective study of the prevalence of primary aldosteronism in 1,125 hypertensive patients. *J Am Coll Cardiol*, 2006; **48**: 2293–300.
45. Douma S, Petidis K, Doumas M, Papaefthimiou P, Triantafyllou A, Kartali N, *et al.* Prevalence of primary hyperaldosteronism in resistant hypertension: a retrospective observational study. *Lancet*, 2008; **371**: 1921–6.
46. Padfield PL, Brown JJ, Davies D, Fraser R, Lever AF, Morton JJ, *et al.* The myth of idiopathic hyperaldosteronism. *Lancet*, 1981; **2** (8237): 83–4.
47. Neville AM, MacKay AM. The structure of the human adrenal cortex in health and disease. *Clin Endocrinol Metab*, 1972; **1**: 361–95.
48. Neville AM, Ohare MJ. Histopathology of the human adrenal-cortex. *Clin Endocrinol Metab*, 1985; **14**: 791–820.
49. Fallo F, Barzon L, Biasi F, Altavilla G, Boscaro M, Sonino N. Zone fasciculata-like histotype and aldosterone response to upright posture are not related in aldosterone-producing adenomas. *Exp Clin Endocrinol Diabetes*, 1998; **106**: 74–8.
50. Davis WW, Newsome HH, Wright LD, Hammond WG, Easton J, Bartter FC Bilateral adrenal hyperplasia as a cause of primary aldosteronism with hypertension hypokalemia and suppressed renin activity. *Am J Med*, 1967; **42**: 642–7.
51. Russell RP, Masi AT. Prevalence of adrenal cortical hyperplasia at autopsy and its association with hypertension. *Ann Intern Med*, 1970; **73**: 195–205.
52. Reincke M. Mutations in adrenocortical tumors. *Horm Metab Res*, 1998; **30**: 447–55.
53. Davies E, Bonnardeaux A, Plouin PF, Corvol P, Clauser E. Somatic mutations of the angiotensin II (AT(1)) receptor gene are not present in aldosterone-producing adenoma. *J Clin Endocrinol Metab*, 1997; **82**: 611–15.
54. Higaki J, Miya A, Miki T, Morishita R, Mikami H, Takai S, *et al.* Contribution of the activation of the Ras oncogene to the evolution of aldosterone-secreting and renin-secreting tumors. *J Hypertens*, 1991; **9**: 135–7.
55. Davies LA, Hu C, Guagliardo NA, Sen N, Chen X, Talley EM, *et al.* TASK channel deletion in mice causes primary hyperaldosteronism. *Proc Natl Acad Sci U S A*, 2008; **105**: 2203–8.
56. Stowasser M, Gordon RD, Tunny TJ, Klemm SA, Finn WL, Krek AL. Familial hyperaldosteronism type II: Five families with a new variety of primary aldosteronism. *Clin Exp Pharmacol Physiol*, 1992; **19**: 319–22.
57. Davies DL, Berettapiccoli C, Brown JJ, Cumming AMM, Fraser R, Lasaridis A, *et al.* Body sodium and blood-pressure - abnormal and different correlations in Conns-syndrome, renal-artery stenosis and essential-hypertension. *Proc Eur Dial Transplant Assoc*, 1983; **20**: 483–8.
58. Funder JW. Steroids, hypertension and cardiac fibrosis. *Blood Press*, 1995; **4**: 39–42.
59. Young M, Funder JW. Aldosterone and the heart. *Trends Endocrinol Metab*, 2000; **11**: 224–6.
60. Savoia C, Touyz RM, Amiri F, Schiffrin EL. Selective mineralocorticoid receptor blocker eplerenone reduces resistance artery stiffness in hypertensive patients. *Hypertension*, 2008; **51**: 432–9.
61. Rossi GP, Bolognesi M, Rizzoni D, Seccia TM, Piva A, Porteri E, *et al.* Vascular remodeling and duration of hypertension predict outcome of adrenalectomy in primary aldosteronism patients. *Hypertension*, 2008; **51**: 1366–71.
62. Funder JW. Corticosteroid receptors and the central nervous system. *J Steroid Biochem Mol Biol*, 1994; **49**: 381–4.
63. Gonzaga CC, Calhoun DA. Resistant hypertension and hyperaldosteronism. *Curr Hypertens Rep*, 2008; **10**: 496–503.
64. Yee KM, Struthers AD. Aldosterone blunts the baroreflex response in man. *Clin Sci*, 1998; **95**: 687–92.
65. Mansoor GA, White WB. Circadian blood pressure variation in hypertensive patients with primary hyperaldosteronism. *Hypertension*, 1998; **31**: 843–7.
66. Shigematsu Y, Hamada M, Okayama H, Hara Y, Hayashi Y, Kodama K, *et al.* Left ventricular hypertrophy precedes other target-organ damage in primary aldosteronism. *Hypertension*, 1997; **29**: 723–7.
67. Muiesan ML, Salvetti M, Paini A, Agabiti-Rosei C, Monteduro C, Galbassini G, *et al.* Inappropriate left ventricular mass in patients with primary aldosteronism. *Hypertension*, 2008; **52**: 529–34.
68. Rocha R, Chander PN, Khanna K, Zuckerman A, Stier CT, Jr. Mineralocorticoid blockade reduces vascular injury in stroke-prone hypertensive rats. *Hypertension*, 1998; **31**: 451–8.
69. Rocha R, Stier CT, Jr., Kifor I, Ochoa-Maya MR, Rennke HG, Williams GH, *et al.* Aldosterone: a mediator of myocardial necrosis and renal arteriopathy. *Endocrinology*, 2000; **141**: 3871–8.
70. Milliez P, Girerd X, Plouin PF, Blacher J, Safar ME, Mourad JJ. Evidence for an increased rate of cardiovascular events in patients with primary aldosteronism. *J Am Coll Cardiol*, 2005; **45**: 1243–8.
71. Blasi ER, Rocha R, Rudolph AE, Blomme EA, Polly ML, McMahon EG. Aldosterone/salt induces renal inflammation and fibrosis in hypertensive rats. *Kidney Int*, 2003; **63**: 1791–800.
72. Rossi GP, Bernini G, Desideri G, Fabris B, Ferri C, Giacchetti G, *et al.* Renal damage in primary aldosteronism—Results of the PAPY study. *Hypertension*, 2006; **48**: 232–8.
73. Funder JW, Carey RM, Fardella C, Gomez-Sanchez CE, Mantero F, Stowasser M, *et al.* Case detection, diagnosis, and treatment of patients

with primary aldosteronism: an endocrine society clinical practice guideline. *J Clin Endocrinol Metab*, 2008; **93**: 3266–81.

74. Stowasser M, Gordon RD. Primary aldosteronism—careful investigation is essential and rewarding. *Mol Cell Endocrinol*, 2004; **217**: 33–9.
75. Montori VM, Young WF, Jr. Use of plasma aldosterone concentration-to-plasma renin activity ratio as a screening test for primary aldosteronism. A systematic review of the literature. *Endocrinol Metab Clin North Am* 2002; **31**: 619–32, xi.
76. Mulatero P, Rabbia F, Milan A, Paglieri C, Morello F, Chiandussi L, *et al.* Drug effects on aldosterone/plasma renin activity ratio in primary aldosteronism. *Hypertension*, 2002; **40**: 897–902.
77. Holland OB, Brown H, Kuhnert L, Fairchild C, Risk M, GomezSanchez CE. Further evaluation of saline infusion for the diagnosis of primary aldosteronism. *Hypertension*, 1984; **6**: 717–23.
78. Gordon RD, Jackson RV, Strakosch CR, Tunny TJ, Rutherford JC, Mccosker J, *et al.* Aldosterone producing adenoma—fludrocortisone suppression and left adrenal vein catheterization in definitive diagnosis and management. *Aust N Z J Med*, 1979; **9**: 676–82.
79. Lyons DF, Kem DC, Brown RD, Hanson CS, Carollo ML. Single dose captopril as a diagnostic-test for primary aldosteronism. *J Clin Endocrinol Metab*, 1983; **57**: 892–6.
80. MacConnachie AA, Kelly KF, McNamara A, Loughlin S, Gates LJ, Inglis GC, *et al.* Rapid diagnosis and identification of cross-over sites in patients with glucocorticoid remediable aldosteronism. *J Clin Endocrinol Metab*, 1998; **83**: 4328–31.
81. Young WF, Stanson AW. What are the keys to successful adrenal venous sampling (AVS) in patients with primary aldosteronism? *Clin Endocrinol (Oxf)* 2009; **70**:14–17.
82. Rossi GP, Pitter G, Bernante P, Motta R, Feltrin G, Miotto D. Adrenal vein sampling for primary aldosteronism: the assessment of selectivity and lateralization of aldosterone excess baseline and after adrenocorticotropic hormone (ACTH) stimulation. *J Hypertens*, 2008; **26**: 989–97.
83. McCallum RW, Connell JMC. Laparoscopic adrenalectomy. *Clin Endocrinol*, 2001; **55**: 435–6.
84. Pang TC, Bambach C, Monaghan JC, Sidhu SB, Bune A, Delbridge LW, *et al.* Outcomes of laparoscopic adrenalectomy for hyperladosteronism. *ANZ J Surg*, 2007; **77**: 768–73.
85. Liddle GW, Bledsoe T, Coppage WS. A familial renal disorder simulating primary aldosteronism but with negligible aldosterone secretion. *Trans Assoc Am Physicians*, 1963; **76**: 199–213.
86. Shimkets RA, Warnock DG, Bositis CM, Nelsonwilliams C, Hansson JH, Schambelan M, *et al.* Liddles syndrome—heritable human hypertension caused by mutations in the beta-subunit of the epithelial sodium-channel. *Cell*, 1994; **79**: 407–14.
87. Rossi E, Farnetti E, Debonneville A, Nicoli D, Grasselli C, Regolisti G, *et al.* Liddle's syndrome caused by a novel missense mutation (P617L) of the epithelial sodium channel beta subunit. *J Hypertens*, 2008; **26**: 921–7.
88. Hiltunen TP, Hannila-Handelberg T, Petajaniemi N, Kantola I, Tikkanen I, Virtamo J, *et al.* Liddle's syndrome associated with a point mutation in the extracellular domain of the epithelial sodium channel gamma subunit. *J Hypertens*, 2002; **20**: 2383–90.
89. Geller DS, Farhi A, Pinkerton N, Fradley M, Moritz M, Spitzer A, *et al.* Activating mineralocorticoid receptor mutation in hypertension exacerbated by pregnancy. *Science*, 2000; **289**: 119–23.
90. Stewart PM, Corrie JE, Shackleton CH, Edwards CR. Syndrome of apparent mineralocorticoid excess. A defect in the cortisol-cortisone shuttle. *J Clin Invest*, 1988; **82**: 340–9.
91. Palermo M, Shackleton CHL, Mantero F, Stewart PM. Urinary free cortisone and the assessment of 11β-hydroxysteroid dehydrogenase activity in man. *Clin Endocrinol*, 1996; **45**: 605–11.
92. White PC, Mune T, Agarwal AK. 11 beta-Hydroxysteroid dehydrogenase and the syndrome of apparent mineralocorticoid excess. *Endocr Rev*, 1997; **18**: 135–56.
93. Li A, Tedde R, Krozowski ZS, Pala A, Li KXZ, Shackleton CHL, *et al.* Molecular basis for hypertension in the "type II variant" of apparent mineralocorticoid excess. *Am J Hum Genet*, 1998; **63**: 370–79.
94. Stewart PM, Wallace AM, Valentino R, Burt D, Shackleton CHL, Edwards CRW. Mineralocorticoid activity of licorice - 11-beta-hydroxysteroid dehydrogenase-deficiency comes of age. *Lancet*, 1987; **2** (8563): 821–4.
95. White PC. Inherited forms of mineralocorticoid hypertension. *Hypertension*, 1996; **28**: 927–36.
96. Stewart PM, Walker BR, Holder G, O'Halloran D, Shackleton CHL. 11beta-Hydroxysteroid dehydrogenase activity in Cushing's syndrome: explaining the mineralocorticoid excess state of the ectopic adrenocorticotropin syndrome. *J Clin Endocrinol Metab*, 1995; **80**: 3617–20.
97. Gordon RD. The syndrome of hypertension and hyperkalemia with normal glomerular-filtration rate—Gordons syndrome. *Aust N Z J Med*, 1986; **16**: 183–4.
98. Xu BE, English JM, Wilsbacher JL, Stippec S, Goldsmith EJ, Cobb MH. WNK1, a novel mammalian serine/threonine protein kinase lacking the catalytic lysine in subdomain II. *J Biol Chem*, 2000; **275**: 16795–801.
99. Wilson FH, Disse-Nicodeme S, Choate KA, Ishikawa K, Nelson-Williams C, Desitter I, *et al.* Human hypertension caused by mutations in WNK kinases.. *Science*, 2001; **293**: 1107–12.
100. Mayan H, Vered I, Mouallem M, Tzadok-Witkon M, Pauzner R, Farfel Z. Pseudohypoaldosteronism type II: marked sensitivity to thiazides, hypercalciuria, normomagnesemia, and low bone mineral density. *J Clin Endocrinol Metab*, 2002; **87**: 3248–54.
101. Disse-Nicodeme S, Achard JM, Desitter I, Houot AM, Fournier A, Corvol P, *et al.* A new locus on chromosome 12p13.3 for pseudohypoaldosteronism type II, autosomal dominant form of hypertension. *Am J Hum Genet*, 2000; **67**: 302–10.

5.7

Cushing's syndrome

John Newell-Price

I would like to see the day when somebody would be appointed surgeon somewhere who had no hands, for the operative part is the least part of the work

Harvey Cushing: Letter to Dr Henry Christian, 20 November 1911

Introduction and historical perspective

Harvey Cushing described the first case of Cushing's syndrome with a severe phenotype in 1912. Since that time, investigation and management of Cushing's syndrome has remained a significant clinical challenge (1, 2) and patients suspected of this diagnosis warrant referral to major centres.

Endogenous Cushing's syndrome is due the chronic, excessive, and inappropriate secretion of cortisol. When presentation is florid diagnosis is usually straightforward, but in modern practice Cushing's syndrome is frequently and increasingly considered in mild cases in the absence of the classical signs in the context of osteoporosis, diabetes, hypertension, gynaecology, and psychiatric clinics, and achieving a diagnosis can be difficult. Appropriate management of Cushing's syndrome is dependent on correctly identifying the cause of excess cortisol. Separating non-ACTH-dependent causes (adrenal tumours) from ACTH-dependent causes (pituitary or ectopic secretion of ACTH) is usually simple. However, many ectopic sources are occult and the differentiation of the source of ACTH secretion may require meticulous and repeated investigation to enable the appropriate surgery to be undertaken.

In most circumstances the mainstay of therapy remains surgery to either an ACTH-secreting tumour or directly to the adrenal glands, but additional treatment with cortisol-lowering drugs and tumour-directed radiotherapy is often needed.

Aetiology, genetics, pathogenesis, and pathology

Endogenous Cushing's syndrome is usually sporadic and divided into ACTH-dependent, and ACTH-independent causes (Table 5.7.1). Overall, ACTH-dependent causes account for approximately 80% of cases, and of these 80% are due to corticotroph pituitary adenomas (Cushing's disease) with an excess female predominance, and the remaining 20% due to the ectopic ACTH syndrome (2). Cushing's disease, the ectopic ACTH syndrome, and adrenal adenomas may also be found in the context of multiple endocrine neoplasia 1 (MEN 1).

Most cases of Cushing's disease are due to corticotroph microadenomas, a few millimetres in diameter, only being larger than 1 cm (macroadenoma) in 6% of cases (1, 3). These tumours express the proopiomelanocortin gene (*POMC* 176830), the peptide product of which is subsequently cleaved to ACTH. POMC-processing is usually efficient in corticotroph microadenomas, but less so in macroadenomas, which may secrete relatively large amounts of unprocessed POMC. Some pituitary macroadenomas are 'silent corticotroph adenomas', and may present with tumour mass effects (e.g. optic chiasm compression) alone; on follow-up, initial absence of cushingoid features may progress to overt clinical Cushing's syndrome. Approximately 90% of tumours express the corticotropin-releasing hormone (CRH)-1 receptor, as evidenced by the release of ACTH in response to exogenously administered CRH. Tumours also express the vasopressin-3 receptor, and respond to vasopressin and desmopressin.

Tumours causing Cushing's disease are relatively resistant to the effects of glucocorticoids, but *POMC* expression and ACTH secretion are reduced by higher doses of dexamethasone in 80% of cases (2, 4). This may be caused by 'miss-expression' of the 'bridging protein' Brg1 (which is important for glucocorticoid inhibitory feedback on *POMC* expression) found in corticotroph tumours, and may be one event determining tumourogensis (5). Corticotroph tumours also show overexpression of cyclin E, low expression of the cyclin-dependent inhibitor, p27, and a high Ki-67 expression, all indicative of a relatively high proliferative activity (4). The excess number of reproductive-aged women with Cushing's disease, and the fact that there is a male preponderance in prepubertal cases (6) suggest a potential aetiological role for oestrogens.

Carcinoid tumours causing the ectopic ACTH syndrome, most frequently bronchial, show a molecular phenotype close to that of pituitary corticotroph tumours. In contrast, data in small cell lung cancer cells have shown that *POMC* is activated by transcription factors distinct from those in the pituitary, including E2F factors (7), which are able to bind the promoter when it is in an unmethylated state (8), suggesting a different pathogenesis.

In ACTH-independent macronodular hyperplasia excess cortisol secretion may be associated with either ectopically-expressed receptors or increased eutopic receptor expression (9), and activation by ligands not usually associated with adrenal steroidogenesis: gastric inhibitory peptide (food-dependent Cushing's); vasopressin; interleukin-1; lutenizing hormone; and serotonin. Activation of receptors increasing intracellular cAMP is thought to cause hyperplasia over many years, and hence Cushing's syndrome.

Table 5.7.1 Aetiology of Cushing's syndrome

Cause of Cushing's syndrome	F:M	%
ACTH-dependent[a]	3.5:1[b]	70%
Cushing's disease	1:1	10%
Ectopic ACTH syndrome	5:1	5%
Unknown source of ACTH[c]		
ACTH-independent	4:1	10%
Adrenal adenoma	1:1	5%
Adrenal carcinoma		<2%
Other causes (PPNAD; AIMAH; McCune–Albright)		

[a] In women 9:1 ratio of Cushing's disease to ectopic ACTH.
[b] Male preponderance in children.
[c] Patients may ultimately prove to have Cushing's disease.
PPNAD, primary pigmented nodular adrenal disease; AIMAH, ACTH-independent massive adrenal hyperplasia.

Primary pigmented nodular adrenal disease (PPNAD) causes small ACTH-secreting nodules on the adrenal, often not visualized on imaging. PPNAD can be sporadic or part of the Carney's complex and most cases occur in late childhood or in young adults, often with a mild or cyclical presentation (10, 11). Germ line mutations of the regulatory subunit R1A of PKA (*PRKAR1A*) are present in approximately 45% of patients with Carney's complex (12, 13) and as well as in sporadic PPNAD. Interestingly, these patients show a paradoxical increase in cortisol secretion in response to dexamethasone.

McCune–Albright syndrome is due to a postzygotic activating mutation in the *GNAS1* gene. The resulting tissue mosaicism results in a varied phenotype, and the disease may present in the first few weeks of life. These mutations lead to constitutive steroidogenesis in the affected adrenal nodules (14). Mutations of *GNAS1* have also been found in ACTH-independent macronodular hyperplasia.

Epidemiology

The true prevalence of Cushing's syndrome is difficult to quantify. Earlier data suggest an incidence from 0.7 to 2.4/million population per year depending on the population studied (1). More recently, biochemical Cushing's syndrome with no clear clinical features has been shown to be common. Incidental adrenal lesions found on CT scans are now a very common clinical problem and approximately 1% of the population aged 70 or more will have evidence of low-grade hypercortisolaemia from such a lesion. In addition, Cushing's syndrome is found in 1–5% of obese patients with type 2 diabetes, and up to 10.8% of older patients with osteoporosis and vertebral fracture (15). The difficulty here, however, is whether detection of mild Cushing's syndrome in these populations is of clinical value as the outcomes of small and uncontrolled intervention studies are mixed. These data indicate that formal intervention trials are needed before widespread screening in these populations can be recommended, and there is a need for clinical decision-making tools to allow stratification for intervention on an individualized basis.

Clinical features of Cushing's syndrome

Glucocorticoid receptors are present in virtually all cells, reflecting the diverse actions of cortisol, and hence the symptoms and signs of hypercortisolaemia encompass all organ systems. Many of the symptoms associated with hypercortisolaemia are common and of little specificity, such as weight gain, lethargy, weakness, menstrual irregularities, loss of libido, hirsutism, acne, depression, and psychosis (Table 5.7.2). Whilst each symptom itself may be mild, the presence of a greater number of features in any given patient increases the likelihood of Cushing's syndrome. The signs most useful in differentiating Cushing's syndrome include the presence of proximal myopathy, and easy bruising, purplish striae, thinness, and fragility of the skin (2). The sign of proximal weakness is most easily demonstrated by asking the patient to stand from sitting position without the use hands; an initial backwards movement of the buttocks is present in early myopathy, whilst in more severe cases rising from a chair may not be possible.

Table 5.7.2 Clinical features of Cushing's syndrome

Feature	%
Obesity or weight gain	95
Facial plethora	90
Rounded face	90
Decreased libido	90
Thin skin	85
Decrease linear growth in children	70–80
Menstrual irregularity	80
Hypertension	75
Hirsutism	75
Depression/emotional lability	70
Easy bruising	65
Glucose intolerance	60
Weakness	60
Acne	50
Osteopenia or fracture	50
Nephrolithiasis	50

Presentation differs between genders, with purple striae, muscle atrophy, osteoporosis, and kidney stones being more common in men (16). Gonadal dysfunction is common in both sexes. The adverse effects of glucocorticoids on bone metabolism are evidenced by decreased bone mineral density. Over 70% of patients with Cushing's syndrome may present with psychiatric symptoms ranging from anxiety to frank psychosis; if present, depression is often agitated in nature, and some degree of psychiatric disturbance often persists following remission of Cushing's syndrome (17). Impairment in short-term memory and cognition is common and can persist for at least a year following treatment. Cortisol excess predisposes to hypertension and glucose intolerance.

Classically, the ectopic ACTH syndrome due to small cell lung cancer may have a rapid onset with severe features: profound weakness, myopathy, hyperpigmentation, diabetes mellitus, and hypokalaemic alkalosis, while there is often neither weight gain nor the classical cushingoid appearance. In contrast, the clinical phenotype and biochemical features of carcinoid and other neuroendocrine tumours (of any tissue origin) may be indistinguishable from that of Cushing's disease, causing diagnostic difficulty.

Clinical and biochemical features may commonly vary in a 'cyclical fashion', causing diagnostic difficulty. Signs and symptoms fluctuate with the cortisol, such as facial plethora, myopathy, mood, blood pressure, and blood glucose, and all investigations may be normal when hypercortisolaemia is absent. Great care is needed to seek for evidence of 'cyclicity' in the clinical history.

Clinical investigation and diagnostic criteria

Who to test

Most patients initially suspected of possibly having Cushing's syndrome will not have this condition. The complete assessment of a patient known to have some form of Cushing's syndrome is complex, expensive, and often stressful for the patient, who is usually already significantly ill emotionally, psychologically, and physically. Thus efficient screening procedures are needed to identify the minority who will need intensive and expensive investigation leading to an accurate and precise differential diagnosis (1, 17).

It is recommended that clinical judgement is used to select patients for testing, which should be considered in: (1) patients with features that are unusual for age, such as hypertension and osteoporosis; (2) those with multiple and progressive features, especially if these include the signs that most reliably distinguish Cushing's syndrome: the presence of thin skin in the young, easy bruising, proximal myopathy, and purple striae; (3) in children with increasing weight percentile and decreased linear growth; and (4) patients with adrenocortical lesions consistent with an adenoma found on CT scans performed for other reasons, so-called adrenal 'incidentaloma' (15).

It is essential that a careful drug history is taken prior to any biochemical testing seeking to exclude exogenous sources of glucocorticoids that may be present in prescribed oral, rectal, inhaled, topical, or parenteral medication as well as in many 'over the counter' preparations, including skin creams, 'skin-whitening' agents, and various 'tonics' and herbal preparations.

Biochemical assessment

The biochemical hallmark of the condition is inappropriate cortisol secretion not subject to the normal negative feedback effects of circulating glucocorticoids. The tests are based on demonstration of excessive cortisol secretion, loss of its circadian rhythm, and the abnormal feedback regulation of the hypothalamic–pituitary– adrenal axis (Fig. 5.7.1).

In florid cases of Cushing's syndrome the diagnosis may be obvious, but biochemical confirmation is still needed. Investigation of Cushing's syndrome is a two-step process. Hypercortisolaemia *must* be confirmed and *then* the cause identified. Failure to follow this approach will result in inappropriate treatment and management.

Step 1: diagnosis of hypercortisolaemia

Several tests are usually needed. Investigation should be performed when there is no acute concurrent illness, such as infection or heart failure, as these may cause false-positive results. The three main tests in use are: 24-h urinary free cortisol; 'low-dose' dexamethasone-suppression tests; and assessment of midnight plasma or late-night salivary cortisol. The best approach is to perform at least two different tests; if concordantly positive or negative, Cushing's syndrome is either likely or unlikely, respectively (2, 15). When there are discrepancies between tests further evaluation and repeated testing is often required. Hypercortisolaemia is also found in some patients with depression, alcohol dependence, anorexia nervosa, and late pregnancy. However, in contrast to true endogenous Cushing's syndrome, the biochemistry improves when the underlying condition has resolved.

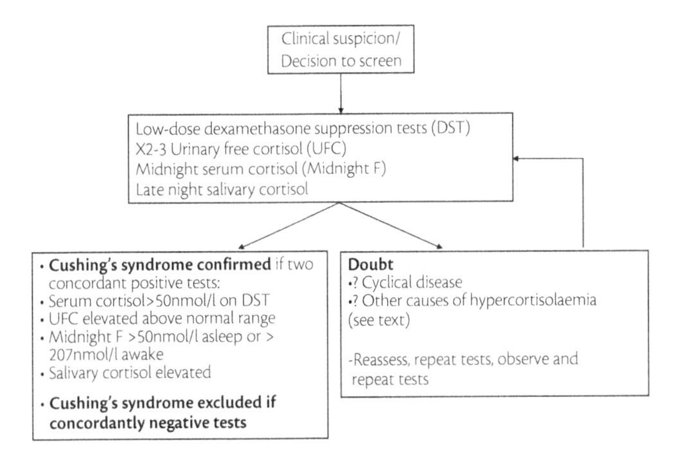

Fig. 5.7.1 Biochemical diagnosis of Cushing's syndrome.

Urinary free cortisol

Urinary cortisol is a direct assessment of circulating free (biologically active) cortisol. Excess circulating cortisol saturates the binding proteins (cortisol binding globulin) and is excreted in urine as free cortisol, and when collected for 24 h gives an integrated estimation of the level of hypercortisolaemia. A single measurement has low sensitivity, and three 24-h collections should be performed (2, 17). Values fourfold greater than the upper limit of normal are rare except in Cushing's syndrome. In contrast, if values are normal on repeated occasions Cushing's syndrome is unlikely. Specificity is a common problem with antibody-based assays, but (2, 17) high performance liquid chromatography (HPLC) and tandem mass spectrometry improves diagnostic accuracy, although substances such as digoxin and carbamazepine may produce peaks in the HPLC assay that give falsely high values (17). Moreover, if there is renal impairment with a GFR of less than 30.0 ml/min, or an incomplete collection, the urinary free cortisol may be falsely low (15, 17). Review of the collection volume and correction for creatinine concentration may be helpful in assessing whether the collection is complete. Use of urinary free cortisol is advised in the very rare situation of Cushing's syndrome being considered during pregnancy.

Low-dose dexamethasone-suppression tests

Two tests are in common use. In the overnight dexamethasone-suppression test, 1 mg of dexamethasone is administered at 23.00 hours and serum cortisol measured the next day at 08.00–09.00 hours. In the 48-h dexamethasone-suppression test, dexamethasone is administered at the dose of 0.5 mg every 6 h for 2 days at 09.00, 15.00, 21.00, and 03.00 hours with measurements of serum cortisol at 09.00 hours at the start and end of the test. To exclude Cushing's syndrome the serum cortisol value should be less than 50 nmol/l following either test (1, 2, 15, 17). The 48-h test, though more cumbersome, is more specific and with adequate regular instructions can easily be performed by outpatients. In both tests, caution needs to be exercised if there is potential malabsorption of dexamethasone or if patients are on drugs that increase hepatic clearance of dexamethasone, including carbamazepine, phenytoin, phenobarbital, or rifampicin. Patients taking oestrogen therapy, or who are pregnant, may have an increase in the cortisol binding globulin. As commercial cortisol assays measure total cortisol, this may give a false-positive result on dexamethasone-suppression testing. Oral oestrogens need to be stopped for a period of 4–6 weeks so that cortisol binding globulin may return to basal values. Even transdermal oestrogens may cause false-positive results, and tests should be repeated off transdermal oestrogens if positive results are obtained. In renal failure, suppression on dexamethasone testing is likely to exclude Cushing's syndrome.

It is important to note that 3–8% of patients with proven Cushing's disease show suppression of serum cortisol to less than 50 nmol/l on either test. Thus, if clinical suspicion remains high, repeated tests and other investigations are indicated.

Midnight plasma cortisol or late-night salivary cortisol

The normal circadian rhythm of cortisol secretion is lost in patients with Cushing's syndrome. A single sleeping midnight plasma cortisol of less than 50 nmol/l effectively excludes Cushing's syndrome at the time of the test. This is one of the harder tests to perform as it requires hospitalization for at least 48 h, and lack of intercurrent illness, but it can be of great utility to exclude Cushing's syndrome, especially when the patient is on drugs known to enhance metabolism of dexamethasone causing a false positive on dexamethasone testing. Values above 50 nmol/l when asleep or above 207 nmol/l when awake are found in Cushing's syndrome, even in those who suppress on dexamethasone (18, 19). An elevated midnight plasma cortisol does not provide additional information if clinical signs are florid and there is clear lack of suppression on dexamethasone testing.

Late-night salivary cortisol

Salivary cortisol reflects free circulating cortisol and its ease of collection and stability at room temperature make it a highly suitable screening tool for outpatient assessment. The diagnostic ranges vary between reports due to the different assays and the comparison groups used to set cut-off points. The test has a sensitivity and specificity of between 95% and 98% (15, 17). As the values of salivary cortisol are an order of magnitude lower than serum cortisol, it is essential that the performance of the local assay be known and that the appropriate cut-off point is utilized. The test is of particular use in the assessment of cyclical Cushing's syndrome, and in children. Despite these advantages, salivary cortisol is not yet used widely in the UK.

Diagnostic doubt

In cases of doubt the best option is to repeat the tests at a later date, or seek further opinion. The dexamethasone-suppressed CRH test, and the desmopressin test have been proposed as useful diagnostic tools but more recent data confirm that the dexamethasone-suppressed CRH test is not more accurate than the 48-h low-dose dexamethasone-suppression test (20).

Step 2: establishing the aetiology of Cushing's syndrome: differential diagnosis

Once a diagnosis of Cushing's syndrome is established the next step is establish the cause. Investigation will vary depending upon the availability of the biochemical tests and imaging and expertise detailed below.

The first key procedure is to measure plasma ACTH. The plasma should be separated rapidly and stored at −40 °C to avoid degradation and a falsely low result. Levels consistently below 5 ng/l indicate ACTH-independent Cushing's syndrome and attention can be turned to imaging the adrenal with CT. Levels of ACTH persistently above 15 ng/l almost always reflect ACTH-dependent pathologies and require investigation, as detailed below. The values between these two need cautious interpretation as patients with Cushing's disease and adrenal pathologies may have intermediate values (2, 17, 21). A positive CRH test (see below) can identify an occasional patient with Cushing's disease with low baseline ACTH plasma levels.

Non-ACTH-dependent Cushing's syndrome

In established Cushing's syndrome, when plasma ACTH has been sampled and handled carefully, and levels are persistently undetectable, the cause is of adrenal origin. The next diagnostic procedure is to proceed to imaging with CT or MRI, which will most likely show an adrenocortical adenoma or carcinoma. If imaging is negative the diagnosis may either be PPNAD, or due surreptitious hydrocortisone absorption.

ACTH-dependent Cushing's syndrome

Localization of the source of ACTH secretion in ACTH-dependent Cushing's syndrome can constitute one of the most formidable challenges of clinical endocrinology. Carcinoid tumours may be clinically indistinguishable from Cushing's disease, and are frequently difficult to identify with imaging, especially if radiological (pituitary, thoracic, pancreatic) 'incidentalomas' complicate interpretation. As a result, biochemical evaluation rather than imaging is used to differentiate between pituitary and nonpituitary causes. In women with ACTH-dependent Cushing's syndrome, 9 out of 10 cases will be due to Cushing's disease. It is against this pretest likelihood that the performance of any test needs to be judged. On occasion, despite all investigation, in some patients it may not be possible to locate the source of ACTH with confidence, and management of hypercortisolaemia may be needed without a precise diagnosis being reached.

Basal testing: plasma ACTH and potassium

Whilst very high levels of plasma ACTH may be seen in ectopic ACTH, the values frequently overlap those seen in Cushing's disease. High levels of cortisol of any aetiology may overwhelm the 11β-hydroxysteroid dehydrogenase type II enzyme in the kidney, allowing cortisol to act as a mineralocorticoid; approximately 70% of patients with ectopic ACTH syndrome due to carcinoid tumours have hypokalaemia, but it is also present in approximately 10% of patients with Cushing's disease with extremely high cortisol production (2).

Dynamic testing

The relative merits of each investigation will be discussed, but ultimately local experience of a given investigation, dependent on assays and radiological skill, will be an important determinant of the overall diagnostic success.

Dynamic noninvasive tests

High-dose dexamethasone-suppression test The high-dose dexamethasone-suppression tests (2 mg given every 6 h for 48 h and serum cortisol measure at 09.00 h at the beginning and end, or a single 8 mg dose given at 23.00 h and serum cortisol measured the next day at 09.00 h) have been in widespread use for many years. The test relies upon the relative sensitivity of pituitary corticotroph adenomas to the effects of glucocorticoids, compared to the resistance exhibited by nonpituitary tumours. Approximately 80% of patients with Cushing's disease will demonstrate suppression of the serum cortisol to a value of less than 50% of the basal level (2). This is less than the pretest likelihood of Cushing's disease and, thus, by itself the high-dose dexamethasone-suppression test has little diagnostic utility. Moreover, when utilizing the 48-h low-dose dexamethasone-suppression test, if there has already been the demonstration of suppression of serum cortisol by more than 30%, there is no further advantage to utilizing the high-dose dexamethasone-suppression test. Therefore, continued routine use of the high-dose dexamethasone-suppression test can no longer be recommended except when bilateral inferior petrosal sinus sampling (BIPSS) is not available. The positive predictive value for Cushing's disease is, however, high if there is a positive response (suppression of serum cortisol <50%) *and* a positive response on CRH testing (see below and Fig. 5.7.2), but the negative predictive value for exclusion of Cushing's disease when both tests are negative, is low.

The corticotropin-releasing hormone test CRH was identified and sequenced in 1981, and is available for clinical practice as either the ovine (oCRH) or human sequence (hCRH) which differ by seven amino acid residues. oCRH has a longer duration of action and is the form available in North America, while the experience of hCRH dominates in Europe. In practice, the value of the test is the same (22, 23). CRH is well tolerated, with side effects from systemic administration consisting of mild, short-lived facial flushing, a sensation of a metallic taste, and a transient sinus tachycardia. A single intravenous bolus of CRH (100 μg or 1 μg/kg) administered at 09.00 hours stimulates pituitary ACTH and cortisol release in healthy individuals, excessively in patients with pituitary-dependent Cushing's syndrome, but generally not in patients with ectopic ACTH secretion or adrenal tumours. The very variable baseline cortisol and ACTH levels in patients with Cushing's syndrome means that a response to corticotropin-releasing hormone is defined in terms of the increment rather than the peak values.

Desmopressin testing Since the vasopressin-3 receptor is expressed in pituitary and many ectopic tumours secreting ACTH, the desmopressin test is of limited utility in the differential diagnosis of ACTH-dependent Cushing's syndrome.

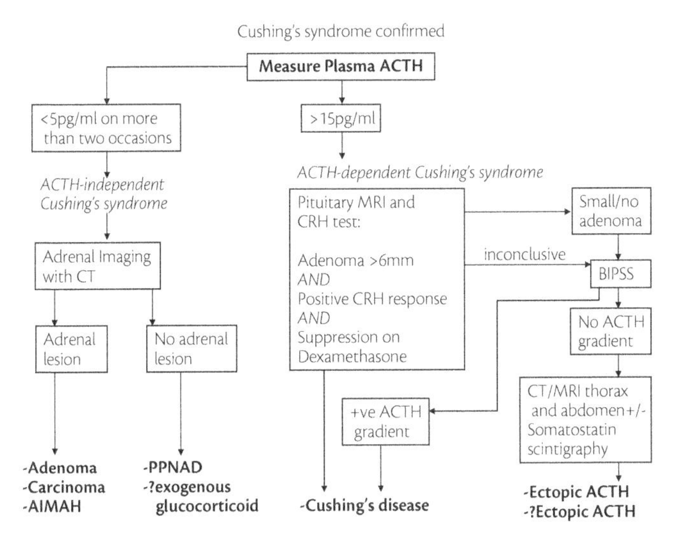

Fig. 5.7.2 Diagnosis of cause of Cushing's syndrome. BIPSS, bilateral inferior petrosal sinus sampling; PPNAD, primary pigmented nodular adrenal disease; AIMAH, ACTH-independent macronodular hyperplasia.

Dynamic invasive testing

Bilateral inferior petrosal sinus sampling If a patient has ACTH-dependent Cushing's syndrome, with responses *both* on dexamethasone-suppression *and* CRH testing suggesting pituitary disease, and the pituitary MRI scan shows an isolated lesion of 6 mm or more, most will regard the diagnosis of Cushing's disease to have been made. A major problem is that up to 40% of patients with proven Cushing's disease have normal pituitary MRI scans (21). In these cases, sampling of the gradient of ACTH from the pituitary to the periphery is the most reliable means for discriminating between pituitary and nonpituitary sources of ACTH, and is strongly recommended for most cases of ACTH-dependent Cushing's syndrome. Since the pituitary effluent drains via the cavernous sinuses to the petrosal sinuses and then jugular bulb, there is a gradient of the value of plasma ACTH compared to the simultaneous peripheral sample when there is a central source of ACTH. BIPSS is a highly skilled and invasive technique, requiring placement of catheters in both inferior petrosal sinuses. Plasma ACTH levels in peripheral blood fluctuate spontaneously by up to a factor of two, and hence a central to peripheral ratio greater than 2 is required to have confidence that ACTH secretion is pituitary and not the result of random variation from either a pituitary or ectopic source. Via a needle in a femoral vein, two catheters are passed up the inferior and superior vena cavae into the neck. One each is then placed in a jugular vein and advanced into the inferior petrosal sinus. Catheter position and venous anatomy require confirmation by venography, as nonuniform drainage is not uncommon. The diagnostic accuracy of the test is improved with the administration of CRH. A basal central: peripheral ratio of more than 2:1 or a CRH-stimulated ratio of more than 3:1 is consistent with Cushing's disease. The combined data for many series indicate a sensitivity and a specificity of 94% (24). Where CRH is unobtainable or too costly, desmopressin offers a reasonable alternative, but few patients with ectopic ACTH secretion have been studied in this way.

False-positive results may be caused by inadequate suppression of the normal corticotrophs; the duration and amount of hypercortisolism should be assessed prior to the test. For this reason pretreatment with cortisol-lowering agents prior to BIPSS is to be strongly discouraged as this increases the likelihood of a false-positive response in a patient with ectopic disease. ACTH secretion will always be localized to the pituitary in normal individuals and hence it is crucial to establish that all patients truly have ACTH-dependent Cushing's syndrome before undertaking this procedure. A false-negative result may be found in patients with cyclical Cushing's disease if the procedure is undertaken when the disease is inactive, and thus it is imperative to measure serum cortisol in the 24 h prior to sampling to establish activity.

In adults, BIPSS is only 70% accurate for lateralization of the source of ACTH within the pituitary gland (2, 17), but in children it may have greater accuracy for this purpose than MRI. False negatives may also occur if there is atrophic or plexiform venous drainage of the petrosal sinuses and this possibility should be checked for by venography at the time of BIPSS.

Imaging

Adrenal (Fig. 5.7.3)

Multidetector CT gives the best resolution of adrenal anatomy, whilst MRI and sequence manipulation can give information on the probability of malignancy. Cortisol-secreting adenomas are typically less than 4 cm in diameter and associated with atrophy of

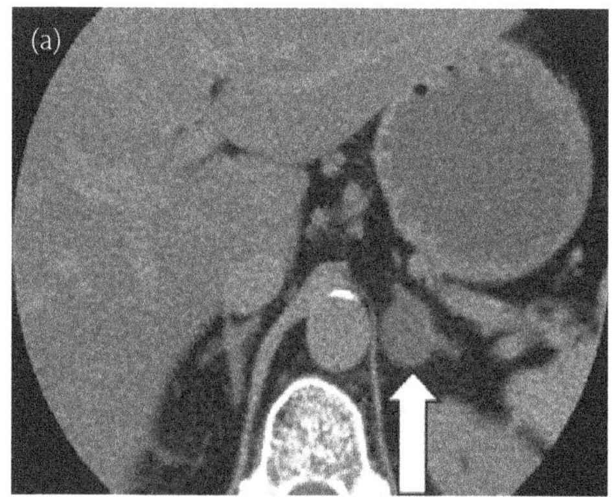

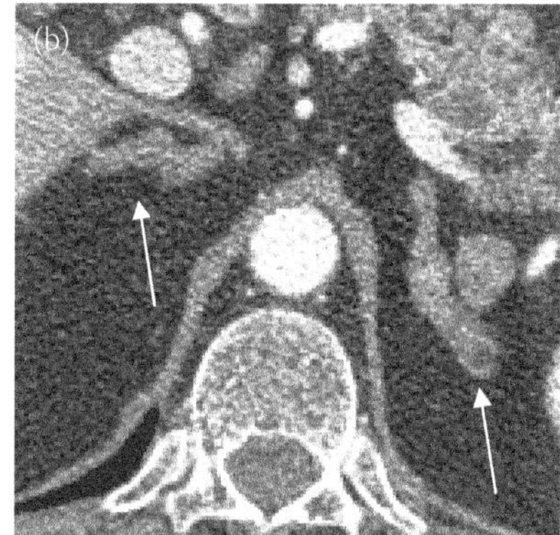

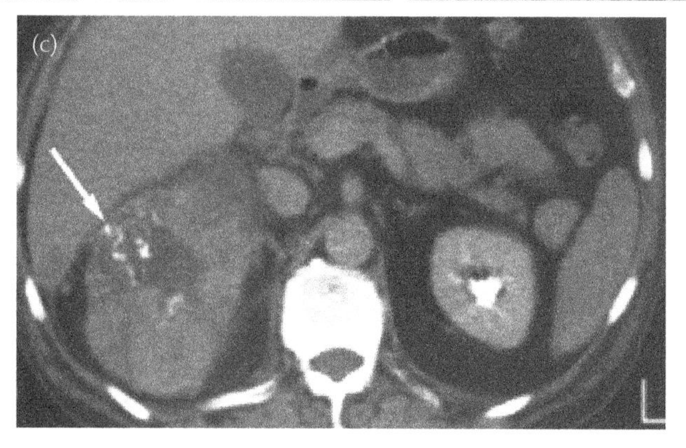

Fig. 5.7.3 Adrenal imaging in Cushing's syndrome. (a) Noncontrast CT scan of left adrenal adenoma with low Hounsfield unit density; (b) bilateral adrenal hyperplasia in ACTH-dependent Cushing's syndrome; (c) right-sided adrenocortical carcinoma.

the unaffected adrenal tissue, and the contralateral adrenal gland. Malignancy is more common with increasing tumour size and radiological evidence of vascular invasion, or cosecretion of sex steroids. In ACTH-dependent Cushing's syndrome nodules may occur and adrenal hyperplasia is not always symmetrical, causing diagnostic confusion with a unilateral primary adrenal cause if the biochemistry is not strictly assessed; in 30% of Cushing's disease the adrenal glands appear normal, whilst in ectopic ACTH the adrenals are virtually always homogeneously enlarged (25).

Pituitary

Up to 40% of corticotroph adenomas causing Cushing's disease in adults are not visible on MRI scanning (21). Those that are visible usually fail to enhance following gadolinium on T1-weighted imaging. The use of dynamic MRI, with the administration of intravenous contrast media and rapid sequence acquisition following this, does not improve the overall diagnostic rate. There is also a 10% rate of pituitary incidentalomas in the normal population (26), emphasizing the need for careful biochemical discrimination of pituitary from nonpituitary sources of ACTH. In the absence of a pituitary macroadenoma, an abnormal MRI alone is *not* conclusive evidence in favour of Cushing's disease.

Imaging in the ectopic ACTH syndrome

Small cell lung cancer may be obvious, but in most cases thoracic and abdominal imaging by fine-cut CT is needed to identify small neuroendocrine tumours, which may be extremely hard to localize, as a source of ACTH (27, 28). Other than small cell lung cancer, bronchial carcinoid tumours are the most common sources of ectopic ACTH secretion, and are usually less than 1 cm in diameter. High-resolution dynamic CT scanning is need with 1 mm cuts and studies early after intravenous contrast administration. However, small, typically enhancing carcinoid tumours may be confused with pulmonary vascular shadows, but bronchial carcinoid tumours usually have high signal intensity on T2-weighted and short-inversion-time inversion recovery on MRI. ACTH-secreting thymic carcinoid tumours are generally larger than 2 cm and readily visualized by CT. Although ectopic ACTH-secreting tumours often express somatostatin receptors and can be seen on radiolabelled octreotide scintigraphy, they are also almost always identified by CT.

Treatment and prognosis

To deliver high-quality treatment to patients with Cushing's syndrome requires a team that includes specialized surgeons and physicians, radiologists, cytologists, histopathologists, and radiotherapists. The sustained hypercortisolaemia of Cushing's syndrome, of any aetiology, suppresses ACTH secretion from healthy corticotrophs and hence hypoadrenalism will be the consequence of complete excision of any tumour causing Cushing's syndrome, be it adrenal, pituitary, or an ectopic source of ACTH secretion, and this may be prolonged.

Management is aimed at lowering cortisol levels, removing tumour tissue, and, in the case of Cushing's disease, causing the least harm to remaining pituitary function. Some centres use medical therapy to control hypercortisolaemia prior to surgery, and this makes intuitive sense, but there are no published data that this affects overall outcome. Hypertension and diabetes require treatment on their own merits, but both tend to improve, often dramatically, with control of hypercortisolaemia. Severe hypokalaemia secondary to Cushing's syndrome is extremely difficult to treat unless hypercortisolaemia is corrected. If it persists, or while cortisol control is being effected, trimaterone or high-dose amiloride is helpful.

Medical therapies to lower cortisol

The only consistently effective drugs for controlling hypercortisolaemia are those that act on the adrenal glands to inhibit cortisol secretion: metyrapone and ketoconazole. These are not curative, and cortisol oversecretion will recur when they are discontinued. Drugs are used to regulate cortisol secretion in very specific circumstances, namely: in preparation for surgery, in patients not cured by surgery, while waiting for radiotherapy to be effective, after chemotherapy, and to correct acute severe physical or psychiatric consequences of hypercortisolaemia. Cortisol-induced psychosis usually responds rapidly to lowering of circulating cortisol levels.

A potential side effect of all drugs used to control cortisol secretion is hypoadrenalism, particularly in patients with cyclical Cushing's syndrome, and hence all patients require close monitoring. Although urinary free cortisol is easy to use for monitoring therapy, it has major limitations in that hypoadrenalism may be difficult to establish accurately, and failure to ensure a complete 24-h collection will result in spuriously low results. Calculation of the mean of five serum cortisol measurements obtained via a cannula between 09.00 h and 21.00 h in a single day offers both the ability to identify transient hypoadrenalism and allows accurate monitoring, since a mean serum cortisol between 150 and 300 nmol/l has been demonstrated to equate to a normal cortisol production rate (29).

Metyrapone is effective in controlling hypercortisolaemia in 80% of patients with Cushing's disease and adrenal tumours, and in 70% of cases with the ectopic ACTH syndrome. It inhibits cortisol secretion by blocking the final step in cortisol synthesis, namely conversion from 11-deoxycortisol by the cytochrome P450 enzyme 11-hydroxylase. Serum cortisol levels fall within 2 h of instigating therapy, but the effect is short lived and metyrapone requires to be taken three times daily. Treatment is initiated at 500 mg thrice daily and the dose titrated against mean serum cortisol, with dose increments being every 72 h to a maximum dose of 6 g/day. The average daily dose in patients with Cushing's disease is approximately 2 g/day, while in the ectopic ACTH the average dose required to control cortisol secretion is 4 g/day. Hypoadrenalism is the major unwanted effect of metyrapone and can occur for several reasons: overtreatment, inability to mount a cortisol response to intercurrent infection, cyclical Cushing's syndrome (see above), and problems with cortisol assays. Metyrapone therapy results in gross elevation of circulating levels of the cortisol precursor 11-deoxycortisol. A small amount of cross-reactivity of 11-deoxycortisol in some cortisol assays will produce artificially elevated apparent serum cortisol, potentially masking hypoadrenalism. Hirsutism and acne, if present in women patients before treatment, may worsen due to the accumulation of androgenic precursors secondary to the blockade of cortisol synthesis. Gastrointestinal upset is frequently attributed to metyrapone but is rare in the absence of hypoadrenalism. Mean serum cortisol levels through the day of between 150 and 300 nmol/l should be the aim, but cross-reactivity with 11-deoxycortisol must be excluded (29).

Ketoconazole is an orally active antimycotic but in larger doses is an inhibitor of cortisol synthesis. It is important to note that achlorhydria and antacid therapy interfere with ketoconazole absorption. Ketoconazole acts at several points in adrenal steroidogenesis to inhibit cortisol synthesis; however, its principal site of action is early in corticosteroidogenesis. In contrast to metyrapone, adrenal androgen concentrations fall with treatment. An additional desirable characteristic is that ketoconazole lowers serum cholesterol concentrations, which are characteristically raised in Cushing's syndrome. Treatment is initiated with 200 mg three times per day and adjusted depending on serum cortisol concentrations; with between 200 and 1200 mg/day required to normalize cortisol secretion rates in patients with Cushing's disease. Ketoconazole is of slower onset of action than metyrapone, and dose adjustments should only be made every 2 to 3 weeks, although in patients with adrenal adenomas responsiveness is more rapid and hypoadrenalism has occurred within 24 h. Ketoconazole consistently induces a reversible rise in liver transaminase and γ-glutamyltransferase levels, and rarely fulminant hepatic failure has been seen. Liver function must be monitored on initiation of treatment and closely thereafter. Hypoadrenalism can occur, but is less common than with metyrapone. Ketoconazole is teratogenic to male fetuses and is contraindicated in pregnancy. Ketoconazole and metyrapone may be given in combination, allowing doses to be used that are lower than required as monotherapy, with ketoconazole lowering androgen levels and thereby greatly increases the acceptability of metyrapone in women.

Etomidate, is an imidazole, and its principal clinical use is as an anaesthetic agent. At low, subhypnotic doses intravenous etomidate is a potent inhibitor of cortisol secretion. The use of intravenous etomidate in an intensive care situation is reported when oral adrenolytic therapy is not possible. Doses between 1.2 and 2.5 mg/h lower serum cortisol, sometimes to undetectable levels, when the patient needs to be maintained on a 'block and replace' regimen with the concomitant use of intravenous hydrocortisone (1–2 mg/h) (30).

High-dose *o,p'*DDD (*ortho,para'*dichlorodiphenyl dichloroethane, mitotane) has been used widely in the treatment of inoperable adrenocortical carcinoma, but when given at a lower dose is effective in controlling cortisol secretion in Cushing's syndrome. It has a direct adrenolytic action, destroying adrenocortical cells, but also blocks cortisol synthesis by inhibiting 11-βhydroxylation and cholesterol side-chain cleavage. It is of slow onset of action, with changes in dose requiring 6 weeks to be fully effective. Use of mitotane in adrenocortical cancer is addressed in Chapter 5.4.

Low-dose treatment with mitotane for benign Cushing's syndrome, with a starting dose of 0.5 to 1 g/day, with gradual dose titration is well tolerated, with rare gastrointestinal upset and few neurological side effects, and is used more frequently in mainland Europe. Currently, it is mainly used for Cushing's disease only when metyrapone and ketoconazole cannot be used effectively. The major limitation of treatment is that it consistently causes hypercholesterolaemia, but if mitotane therapy is necessary, then the hypercholesterolaemia can be reversed by the use of a statin or ketoconazole.

RU 486 (mifepristone) is a potent glucocorticoid receptor antagonist that blocks cortisol action and reverses the consequences of hypercortisolaemia. A trial of its use in ectopic ACTH syndrome is in progress. It is reported to have reversed cortisol-induced psychosis in a patient with Cushing's syndrome. Its use, however, depends on clinical assessment only, as cortisol levels remain high in the blood, and this has limited its widespread use.

New therapies to lower ACTH

Over the past 30 years many agents have been used in an attempt to inhibit the secretion of ACTH by corticotroph tumours, including sodium valproate and cyproheptadine, but to date none has been shown to consistently lower plasma ACTH. If a compound were to be developed for the treatment Cushing's disease with the equivalent efficacy that dopamine agonists have for prolactinomas, this would be a huge step forwards.

Recently, the PPAR-γ agonist rosiglitazone has been tried in mouse models of Cushing's disease, but data in humans is disappointing. Corticotroph tumours may also express the dopamine-2 receptor and short-term administration of cabergoline at a dose of 1–3 mg/week may reduce hypercortisolism in up to 40% of case (31), but often with escape after this and larger studies are needed. The newer multiligand somatostatin analogue, pasireotide, appears to lower cortisol levels in some patients with Cushing's disease (32), but larger studies are awaited.

Surgery

Transsphenoidal surgery

Transsphenoidal selective microadenectomy, by an experienced pituitary surgeon, is the treatment of choice for Cushing's disease, as it offers the prospect of a dramatic, rapid, and longlasting cure without other hormonal deficiency (31) (Fig. 5.7.4a,b).

In most cases, control of tumour volume is not a priority as the majority have either microadenomas (Fig. 5.7.4c) or no visible tumour on MRI. Numerous series have reported the results and long-term follow-up following trans-sphenoidal surgery for Cushing's disease. Taking all series in the world literature together, the initial remission rate is between 60 and 80%, but with a relapse rate of up to 20% when followed for many years, emphasizing the need for lifelong follow-up (Fig. 5.7.5) (31). It is likely that these variations reflect surgical skill as well as the controversy regarding the characterization of remission or continuing disease in the postoperative period. Overall, with careful and prolonged follow-up (10 years) the long-term remission rate is approximately 60%; series suggesting rates higher than this either have shorter follow-up or less stringent criteria for remission. Patients who are hypocortisolaemic (low 09.00 h serum cortisol) in the immediate postoperative period require glucocorticoid therapy until the hypothalamic–pituitary–adrenal axis recovers, usually 6–18 months postoperatively. While long-term remission is most likely when postoperative serum cortisol is low (<50 nmol/l), there is no threshold value that fully excludes possible recurrence (31). Care needs to be taken in the interpretation of postoperative serum cortisol in those patients who have received high-dose perioperative glucocorticoids, as these may suppress the level of cortisol in any remaining corticotroph tumour cells, with the patient appearing to be in remission, but then for the tumour cells to grow slowly and relapse appear years

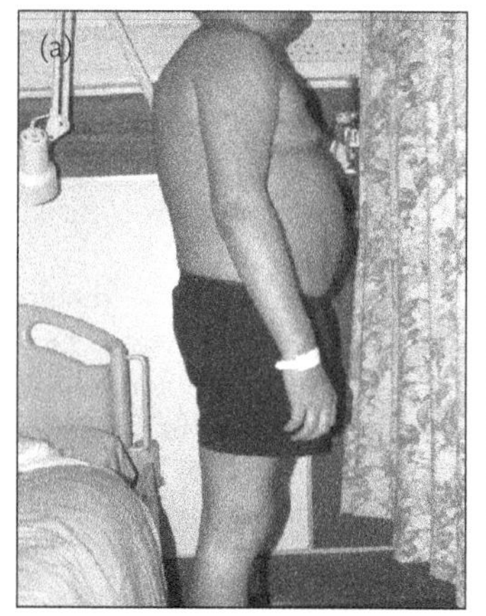

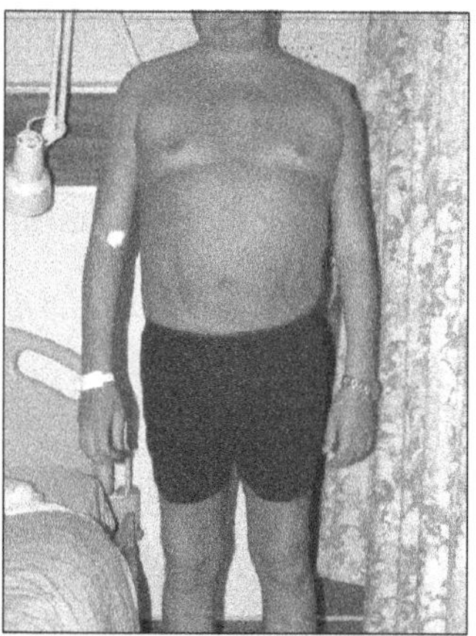

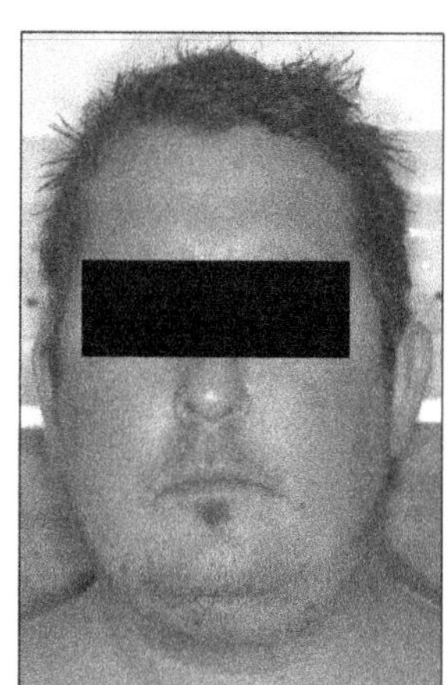

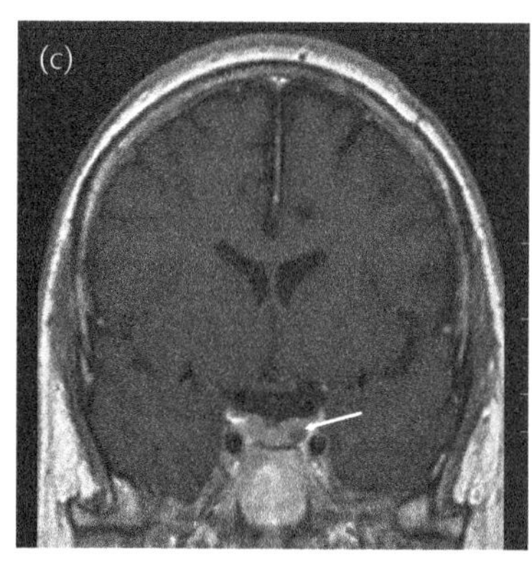

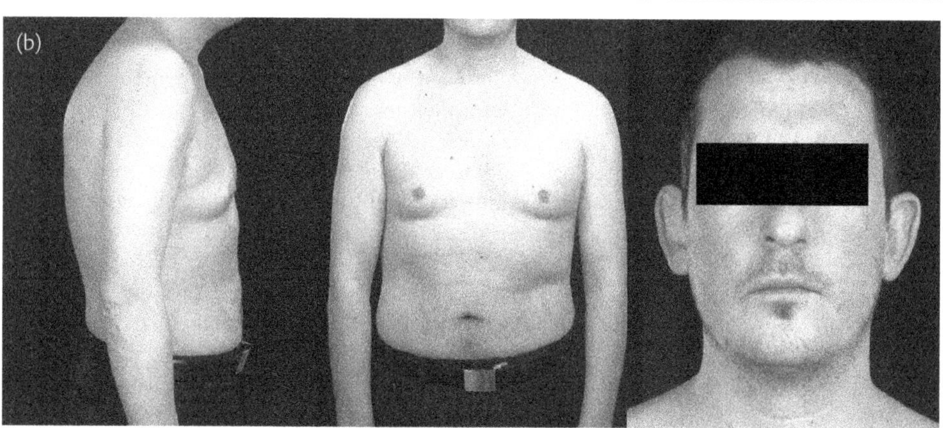

Fig. 5.7.4 Resolution of clinical features following selective trans-sphenoidal microadenomectomy. (a) 33-year-old man with florid Cushing's syndrome; note truncal obesity, striae, proximal muscle wasting, and facial plethora. (b) Dramatic resolution of clinical features 4 months after selective removal of ACTH-secreting microadenoma. (c) T1-weighted gadolinium-enhanced MRI scan from the same patient showing 2 × 3 mm pituitary microadenoma causing Cushing's disease. Note nonenhancement (arrow). Patient underwent bilateral inferior petrosal sinus sampling to confirm pituitary source of ACTH. (See also Plate 27)

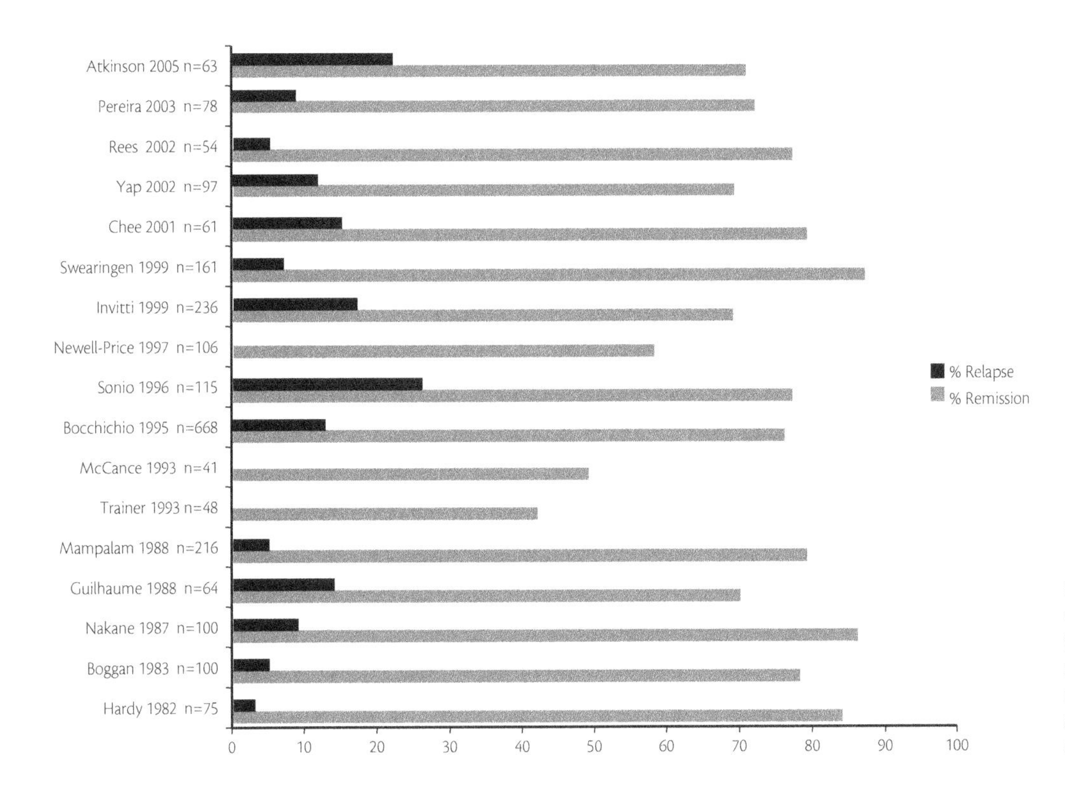

Fig. 5.7.5 Modified from long-term out come of trans-sphenoidal surgery for Cushing's disease. Initial remission rates in grey, relapse in black. Note that the lower initial remission rates are frequently associated with less relapse on follow-up.

later. Similarly, suppression of serum cortisol on dexamethasone testing in the postoperative period is a poor indicator of long-term remission. Levels of postoperative serum cortisol of 100–200 nmol/l do not necessarily indicate failure of surgery, as some patients may remain in long-term remission. On the other hand levels above 200 nmol/l will almost always indicate failure of surgery. Prompt postoperative assessment of the hypothalamic–pituitary–adrenal axis is important, as in patients in whom hypercortisolaemia persists after an initial operation, repeat surgery, within 10 days, will allow remission in a further 50% of patients having a second operation. There is no agreement as to whether the presence or absence of a microadenoma on MRI makes remission more likely, but remission for macroadenomas is less than 15%.

Complications of pituitary surgery include cerebrospinal fluid leakage (less than 5%) or meningitis (under 2%), but are unusual in experienced hands. Hypopituitarism may occur, but successful microadenectomy will leave pituitary function intact in more than 50%. Pituitary function needs to be tested in full, pre- and postoperatively. The importance of preserving pituitary function has to be balanced against fitness for surgery and the consequences of deficiency, such as future fertility plans. It is important to note that functional deficiencies of growth hormone secondary to hypercortisolaemia may remain for 2 years after achieving remission by surgery. Thus the frail elderly patient, in whom a second operation would not be possible, might need an attempted total hypophysectomy at first operation, whereas in a fit young patient the tumour may be treated by a more limited procedure to attempt selective removal of the apparent local microadenoma, on the understanding that a second operation may be necessary if cure does not follow the first attempt, with almost inevitable hypopituitarism afterwards.

Adrenal surgery

For patients with an adrenocortical adenoma causing Cushing's syndrome the treatment of choice is a laparoscopic adrenalectomy by an experienced surgeon, as this is a safe and well-tolerated procedure. The adrenal contralateral to a cortisol-secreting adrenal tumour will be atrophic, and glucocorticoid, but not mineralocorticoid, replacement therapy may be required for months or sometimes years. In any cause of ACTH-dependent Cushing's syndrome, total bilateral adrenalectomy induces a rapid resolution of the clinical features. Following bilateral surgery, patients require lifelong treatment with glucocorticoid and mineralocorticoid. With the low morbidity associated with laparoscopic adrenal surgery, this approach is being considered more frequently, and possibly even as primary therapy in some patients with Cushing's disease, especially when disease is severe or because of patient preference. A major concern following bilateral adrenalectomy in patients with Cushing's disease is the development of Nelson's syndrome—a locally aggressive pituitary tumour that secretes high levels of ACTH, resulting in pigmentation. It remains controversial as to whether the tumour progression is a result of the lack of cortisol feedback following adrenalectomy, or whether the progression reflects corticotroph tumours that were always programmed to behave in an aggressive manner (33). If no tumour is visible on pituitary MRI at the time of adrenalectomy the likelihood of Nelson's syndrome is much less. Monitoring is by MRI and measurement of plasma ACTH. The tumour itself may be treated with further surgery or radiotherapy. Some advocate pituitary radiotherapy at the time of adrenalectomy to reduce the risk of this syndrome (34), but others have not confirmed this (33).

Fractionated external pituitary radiotherapy

Conventional external-beam radiotherapy has been available for 40 years, with large amounts of data demonstrating it to be safe and effective at controlling tumour growth and hormone secretion (31). In Cushing's disease, its use is reserved for patients not cured by surgery, those in whom surgery is deemed inappropriate, and in the treatment of Nelson's syndrome. While waiting for the effect of radiotherapy to happen, which appears to be quicker in children, patients will usually require continued treatment with cortisol-lowering drugs, and regular biochemical assessment. Long-term hypopituitarism is likely in most cases.

Stereotactic radiosurgery

Stereotactic radiotherapy, the most widely used variety being the 'gamma knife', is a means of delivering a high dose of radiation to a small volume in a single session without surrounding tissues being exposed to significant radiation. The main advantages of stereotactic over conventional radiotherapy are the convenience of a single session, more rapid correction of hypersecretion, and preservation of the function of surrounding healthy pituitary tissue. Rare, larger tumours are less easily treated, and the dose to the optic chiasm limited to less than 6–8 Gy. Despite enthusiasm for the 'gamma knife', there appears to be a relapse rate of up to 20% following treatment (31), which does not compare favourably to conventional radiotherapy. It is likely that this poorer outcome reflects case selection. In some circumstances gamma knife radiotherapy can be extremely effective, even as primary therapy, and may be more rapid in onset and in efficacy. This depends on absolute confidence in diagnosis, and an anatomically favourable lesion, especially if not approachable by surgery (Fig. 5.7.6). Except in highly selected cases such as this, gamma knife radiosurgery is not yet recommended.

Prognosis

Uncontrolled and severe Cushing's syndrome has a 5-year survival of just 50%, with death due mainly to vascular and infective complications. With modern management control of hypercortisolaemia is associated with a normalization of the standard mortality ratio (15). Patients are, however, still left with features of cardiovascular risk for years after remission, and quality of life is frequently significantly impaired (17, 35).

Childhood Cushing's syndrome

Cushing's syndrome should be considered in any child with obesity in combination with short stature, as children with simple obesity tend to be tall whereas hypercortisolaemia stunts growth. The elevated circulating androgens seen in Cushing's syndrome, particularly in adrenal adenomas, can result in apparent puberty and virilization without gonadal enlargement (pseudoprecocious puberty). Contrary to earlier reports, bone age is normal in 80% of children with Cushing's syndrome as although androgens accelerate bone maturation, with a consequent loss of linear growth potential, hypercortisolaemia appears to delay maturation.

The specific features that may be present on examination include: inappropriate axillary or pubic hair, penile enlargement, scrotal pigmentation, and clitoral hypertrophy. Acne vulgaris can develop in children of any age. These features of hyperandrogenism are likely to be more pronounced with androgen-secreting adrenal tumours, but also occur with ACTH-dependent Cushing's syndrome. Primary or secondary amenorrhoea may be a feature in girls. Blood pressure is often mildly or moderately elevated, but diabetes mellitus is very unusual. School performance can suffer and psychiatric and emotional symptoms may occur.

Aetiology

The distribution of causes in childhood is different from that encountered in adults; there is a male predominance in Cushing's disease (6). Fetal- and neonatal-onset Cushing's syndrome have been described, but the diagnosis remains exceptionally rare until approximately 8 years of age (36, 37). Under 2 years of age, adrenal carcinoma accounts for 80% of cases of Cushing's syndrome, of which 80% occur in females.

Investigation in childhood

Cushing's syndrome presenting in childhood is rare but, if considered, the diagnosis should be relatively straightforward to confirm. Any child with weight gain and growth failure should be investigated but, as described above, the presenting symptoms may vary. The investigative algorithm is as described for adults, and experience shows that it is not necessary to alter the dose of dexamethasone or corticotropin-releasing hormone used in adults. Although more technically challenging in children, inferior petrosal sinus sampling is, as in adults, vital for localizing the source of ACTH secretion. (37)

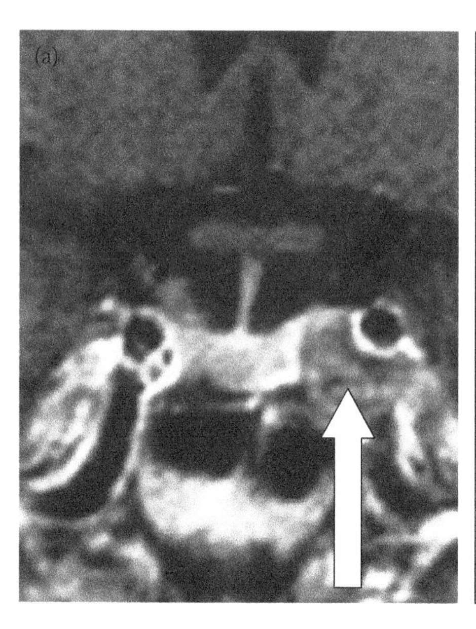

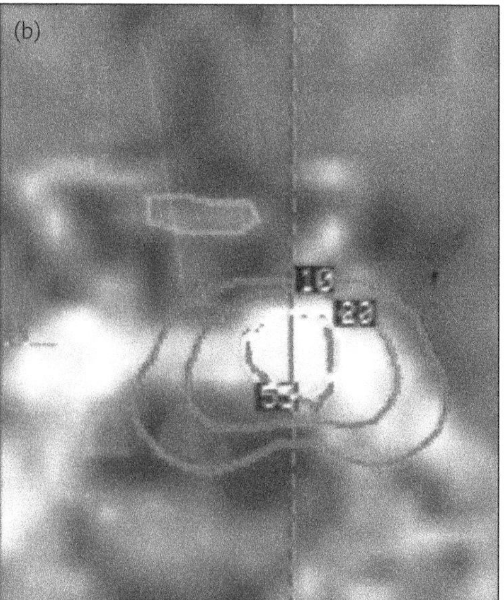

Fig. 5.7.6 Gamma knife stereotactic radiosurgery for Cushing's disease. Figure shows diagnostic and planning MRI images of a patient with severe Cushing's disease treated by gamma knife radiosurgery as the primary and only definitive therapy at the author's institution, and who remains in remission with no pituitary deficit 10 years later.
(a) Pretreatment the laterally placed tumour (arrow) was inaccessible to surgical approaches. (b) Tumour targeting with gammaknife—50% isodose to the tumour margin is shown; note the margin of safety from the 10% isodose to optic chiasm (outlined). (See also Plate 28)

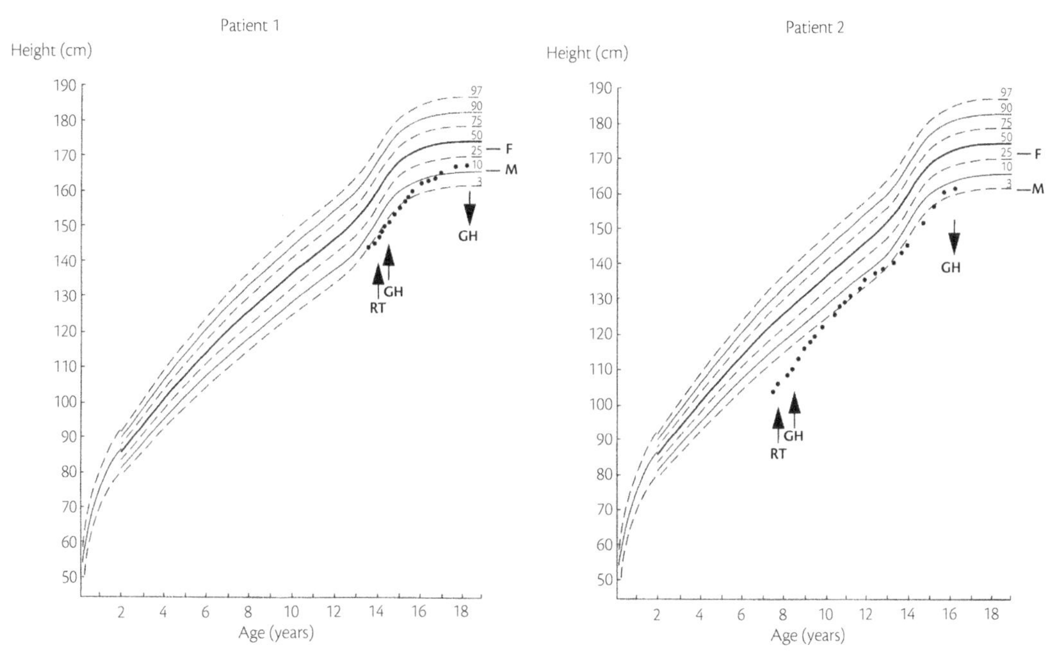

Fig. 5.7.7 Growth charts of two children with Cushing's disease treated with pituitary irradiation. GHT, growth hormone therapy; RT, radiotherapy; M, mother's height; F, father's height. (Reproduced with permission from Johnston L Grossmann AB, Plowman PN, Besser GM, Savage MO. *Clinical Endocrinology*, 1998; **48**: 663–7.)

Treatment

The principles of treatment of hypercortisolaemia are the same in children as adults. Ketoconazole is preferable to metyrapone in children, as the former lowers, rather than increases, circulating androgen levels, but both are safe. Trans-sphenoidal surgery achieves remission in the majority of children with Cushing's disease. Pituitary radiotherapy is reserved for surgical failures, or those whose surgery is impossible because of the small size of the pituitary fossa; however, when required it controls ACTH secretion more promptly in children than in adults with Cushing's disease, but residual pituitary function requires close monitoring to ensure normal pubertal development and growth. Growth hormone deficiency occurs early after radiotherapy in children, but may recover in some (38).

Once hypercortisolaemia has been controlled, the management of growth and puberty is a major challenge. Glucocorticoids both inhibit growth hormone secretion and induce epiphyseal insensitivity to growth hormone action, and correction of hypercortisolaemia is a prerequisite to re-establishing linear growth. Adrenal androgen-induced pseudoprecocious puberty causes premature true gonadotropin-dependent puberty, and hence, even once adrenal androgen secretion has been controlled, bone age will continue to advance and potential for linear growth diminish. These factors can be regulated by the combined use of gonadotropin-releasing hormone analogues to inhibit gonadotropin secretion and control puberty, and growth hormone treatment to induce linear growth. With effective treatment of hypercortisolaemia and careful management of puberty and growth, children with Cushing's syndrome will achieve a normal final height (39) (Fig. 5.7.7).

Likely developments over the next 5–10 years

There is a clear need for multinational databases to better establish the prevalence and complications Cushing's syndrome, especially in at risk populations, and these are being established. Formal intervention studies are needed in mild Cushing's syndrome in the context of hypercortisolaemia in adrenal incidentaloma and osteoporosis. The outcome of treatment for Cushing's disease remains disappointing in many patients, and further developments are needed in this area, especially novel approaches to medical therapy to lower ACTH.

References

1. Newell-Price J, Bertagna X, Grossman AB, Nieman LK. Cushing's syndrome. *Lancet*, 2006; **367**: 1605–17.
2. Newell-Price J, Trainer P, Besser M, Grossman A. The diagnosis and differential diagnosis of Cushing's syndrome and pseudo-Cushing's states. *Endocr Rev*, 1998; **19**: 647–72.
3. Woo YS, Isidori AM, Wat WZ, Kaltsas GA, Afshar F, Sabin I, *et al.* Clinical and biochemical characteristics of adrenocorticotropin-secreting macroadenomas. *J Clin Endocrinol Metab*, 2005; **90**: 4963–9.
4. Dahia PL, Grossman AB. The molecular pathogenesis of corticotroph tumors. *Endocr Rev*, 1999; **20**: 136–55.
5. Bilodeau S, Vallette-Kasic S, Gauthier Y, Figarella-Branger D, Brue T, Berthelet F, *et al.* Role of Brg1 and HDAC2 in GR trans-repression of the pituitary POMC gene and misexpression in Cushing disease. *Genes Dev*, 2006; **20**: 2871–86.
6. Storr HL, Isidori AM, Monson JP, Besser GM, Grossman AB, Savage MO. Prepubertal Cushing's disease is more common in males, but there is no increase in severity at diagnosis. *J Clin Endocrinol Metab*, 2004; **89**: 3818–20.
7. Picon A, Bertagna X, de Keyzer Y. Analysis of the human proopiomelanocortin gene promoter in a small cell lung carcinoma cell line reveals an unusual role for E2F transcription factors. *Oncogene*, 1999; **18**: 2627–33.
8. Newell-Price J, King P, Clark AJ. The CpG island promoter of the human proopiomelanocortin gene is methylated in nonexpressing normal tissue and tumors and represses expression. *Mol Endocrinol*, 2001; **15**: 338–48.
9. Lacroix A, Ndiaye N, Tremblay J, Hamet P. Ectopic and abnormal hormone receptors in adrenal Cushing's syndrome. *Endocr Rev*, 2001; **22**: 75–110.

10. Storr HL, Mitchell H, Swords FM, Main KM, Hindmarsh PC, Betts PR, *et al.* Clinical features, diagnosis, treatment and molecular studies in paediatric Cushing's syndrome due to primary nodular adrenocortical hyperplasia. *Clin Endocrinol (Oxf)*, 2004; **61**: 553–9.
11. Stratakis CA, Kirschner LS, Carney JA. Clinical and molecular features of the Carney complex: diagnostic criteria and recommendations for patient evaluation. *J Clin Endocrinol Metab*, 2001; **86**: 4041–6.
12. Kirschner LS, Carney JA, Pack SD, Taymans SE, Giatzakis C, Cho YS, *et al.* Mutations of the gene encoding the protein kinase A type I-alpha regulatory subunit in patients with the Carney complex. *Nat Genet*, 2000; **26**: 89–92.
13. Casey M, Vaughan CJ, He J, Hatcher CJ, Winter JM, Weremowicz S, *et al.* Mutations in the protein kinase A R1alpha regulatory subunit cause familial cardiac myxomas and Carney complex. *J Clin Invest*, 2000; **106**: R31–8.
14. Weinstein LS, Shenker A, Gejman PV, Merino MJ, Friedman E, Spiegel AM. Activating mutations of the stimulatory G protein in the McCune-Albright syndrome. *N Engl J Med*, 1991; **325**: 1688–95.
15. Nieman LK, Biller BM, Findling JW, Newell-Price J, Savage MO, Stewart PM, *et al.* The diagnosis of Cushing's syndrome: an Endocrine Society Clinical Practice Guideline. *J Clin Endocrinol Metab*, 2008; **93**: 1526–40.
16. Pecori Giraldi F, Moro M, Cavagnini F. Gender-related differences in the presentation and course of Cushing's disease. *J Clin Endocrinol Metab*, 2003; **88**: 1554–8.
17. Arnaldi G, Angeli A, Atkinson AB, Bertagna X, Cavagnini F, Chrousos GP, *et al.* Diagnosis and complications of Cushing's syndrome: a consensus statement. *J Clin Endocrinol Metab*, 2003; **88**: 5593–602.
18. Newell-Price J, Trainer P, Perry L, Wass J, Grossman A, Besser M. A single sleeping midnight cortisol has 100% sensitivity for the diagnosis of Cushing's syndrome. *Clin Endocrinol (Oxf)*, 1995; **43**: 545–50.
19. Papanicolaou DA, Yanovski JA, Cutler GB, Jr, Chrousos GP, Nieman LK. A single midnight serum cortisol measurement distinguishes Cushing's syndrome from pseudo-Cushing states. *J Clin Endocrinol Metab*, 1998; **83**: 1163–7.
20. Martin NM, Dhillo WS, Banerjee A, Abdulali A, Jayasena CN, Donaldson M, *et al.* Comparison of the dexamethasone-suppressed corticotropin-releasing hormone test and low-dose dexamethasone suppression test in the diagnosis of Cushing's syndrome. *J Clin Endocrinol Metab*, 2006; **91**: 2582–6.
21. Invitti C, Pecori Giraldi F, de Martin M, Cavagnini F. Diagnosis and management of Cushing's syndrome: results of an Italian multicentre study. Study Group of the Italian Society of Endocrinology on the Pathophysiology of the Hypothalamic-Pituitary-Adrenal Axis. *J Clin Endocrinol Metab*, 1999; **84**: 440–8.
22. Newell-Price J, Morris DG, Drake WM, Korbonits M, Monson JP, Besser GM, *et al.* Optimal response criteria for the human CRH test in the differential diagnosis of ACTH-dependent Cushing's syndrome. *J Clin Endocrinol Metab*, 2002; **87**: 1640–5.
23. Nieman LK, Oldfield EH, Wesley R, Chrousos GP, Loriaux DL, Cutler GB, Jr. A simplified morning ovine corticotropin-releasing hormone stimulation test for the differential diagnosis of adrenocorticotropin-dependent Cushing's syndrome. *J Clin Endocrinol Metab*, 1993; 77: 1308–12.
24. Lindsay JR, Nieman LK. Differential diagnosis and imaging in Cushing's syndrome. *Endocrinol Metab Clin North Am*, 2005; **34**: 403–21.
25. Sohaib SA, Hanson JA, Newell-Price JD, Trainer PJ, Monson JP, Grossman AB, *et al.* CT appearance of the adrenal glands in adrenocorticotrophic hormone-dependent Cushing's syndrome. *AJR Am J Roentgenol*, 1999; **172**: 997–1002.
26. Hall WA, Luciano MG, Doppman JL, Patronas NJ, Oldfield EH. Pituitary magnetic resonance imaging in normal human volunteers: occult adenomas in the general population. *Ann Intern Med*, 1994; **120**: 817–20.
27. Ilias I, Torpy DJ, Pacak K, Mullen N, Wesley RA, Nieman LK. Cushing's syndrome due to ectopic corticotropin secretion: twenty years' experience at the National Institutes of Health. *J Clin Endocrinol Metab*, 2005; **90**: 4955–62.
28. Isidori AM, Kaltsas GA, Pozza C, Frajese V, Newell-Price J, Reznek RH, *et al.* The ectopic adrenocorticotropin syndrome: clinical features, diagnosis, management, and long-term follow-up. *J Clin Endocrinol Metab*, 2006; **91**: 371–7.
29. Trainer PJ, Besser M. Cushing's syndrome. Therapy directed at the adrenal glands. *Endocrinol Metab Clin North Am*, 1994; **23**: 571–84.
30. Drake WM, Perry LA, Hinds CJ, Lowe DG, Reznek RH, Besser GM. Emergency and prolonged use of intravenous etomidate to control hypercortisolemia in a patient with Cushing's syndrome and peritonitis. *J Clin Endocrinol Metab*, 1998; **83**: 3542–4.
31. Biller BM, Grossman AB, Stewart PM, Melmed S, Bertagna X, Bertherat J, *et al.* Treatment of adrenocorticotropin-dependent Cushing's syndrome: a consensus statement. *J Clin Endocrinol Metab*, 2008; **93**: 2454–62.
32. Boscaro M, Ludlam WH, Atkinson B, Glusman JE, Petersenn S, Reincke M, *et al.* Treatment of pituitary-dependent Cushing's disease with the multireceptor ligand somatostatin analog pasireotide (SOM230): a multicenter, phase II trial. *J Clin Endocrinol Metab*, 2009; **94**: 115–22.
33. Assie G, Bahurel H, Bertherat J, Kujas M, Legmann P, Bertagna X. The Nelson's syndrome. *revisited. Pituitary*, 2004; **7**: 209–15.
34. Jenkins PJ, Trainer PJ, Plowman PN, Shand WS, Grossman AB, Wass JA, *et al.* The long-term outcome after adrenalectomy and prophylactic pituitary radiotherapy in adrenocorticotropin-dependent Cushing's syndrome. *J Clin Endocrinol Metab*, 1995; **80**: 165–71.
35. Lindsay JR, Nansel T, Baid S, Gumowski J, Nieman LK. Long-term impaired quality of life in Cushing's syndrome despite initial improvement after surgical remission. *J Clin Endocrinol Metab*, 2006; **91**: 447–53.
36. Magiakou MA, Mastorakos G, Oldfield EH, Gomez MT, Doppman JL, Cutler GB Jr, *et al.* Cushing's syndrome in children and adolescents. Presentation, diagnosis, and therapy. *N Engl J Med*, 1994; **331**: 629–36.
37. Weber A, Trainer PJ, Grossman AB, Afshar F, Medbak S, Perry LA, *et al.* Investigation, management and therapeutic outcome in 12 cases of childhood and adolescent Cushing's syndrome. *Clin Endocrinol (Oxf)*, 1995; **43**: 19–28.
38. Storr HL, Plowman PN, Carroll PV, François I, Krassas GE, Afshar F, *et al.* Clinical and endocrine responses to pituitary radiotherapy in pediatric Cushing's disease: an effective second-line treatment. *J Clin Endocrinol Metab*, 2003; **88**: 34–7.
39. Davies JH, Storr HL, Davies K, Monson JP, Besser GM, Afshar F, *et al.* Final adult height and body mass index after cure of paediatric Cushing's disease. *Clin Endocrinol (Oxf)*, 2005; **62**: 466–72.

5.8

Glucocorticoid resistance—a defect of the glucocorticoid receptor

Elisabeth F.C. van Rossum, Steven W.J. Lamberts

Introduction

The first case of glucocorticoid resistance was reported in 1976 by Vingerhoeds *et al.* (1). The patient was suffering from hypercortisolism with none of the tissue effects of Cushing's disease. Further evaluation revealed that the ligand-binding affinity of the glucocorticoid receptor (GR) was diminished. His son and nephew were mildly affected and their GR also showed a reduced hormone affinity, although this was to a lesser extent. Later, the *GR* gene of the index patient was sequenced and showed a homozygous mutation at position 2054, yielding a valine for aspartic acid substitution at amino acid residue 641 (2). The other two family members appeared to be heterozygous carriers of the same mutation, which can explain their milder clinical picture. Since then, other patients with mutations in the *GR* gene leading to the syndrome of generalized glucocorticoid resistance have been described (Table 5.8.1) (18).

Familial glucocorticoid resistance is a rare disease, characterized by reduced cortisol action at the tissue level, which is compensated for by elevation of ACTH levels, resulting in an increase of adrenal steroids (glucocorticoids, androgens, mineralocorticoids) (18). It is rather unfamiliar and may confuse clinicians, since the signs and symptoms can be nonspecific. This syndrome has an autosomal recessive or dominant mode of inheritance.

The hypothalamic–pituitary–adrenal axis and the glucocorticoid receptor

As shown in Fig. 5.8.1a, the production of glucocorticoids is regulated by the hypothalamus. In response to signals from the central nervous system, the secretion of corticotropin-releasing hormone (CRH) and vasopressin is stimulated (19). These hormones stimulate the pituitary to secrete proopiomelanocortin (POMC). After splitting POMC into several proteins, ACTH is released to the circulation, stimulating the adrenal glands to secrete glucocorticoids. To control the activity of the hypothalamic–pituitary–adrenal (HPA) axis, negative feedback action by glucocorticoids is crucial.

If this feedback regulation, mediated by the GR, is disturbed, ACTH levels increase, and the adrenals are stimulated to produce supraphysiological levels of cortisol (Fig. 5.8.1b). However, due to the GR defects, the effects of cortisol on target genes in the nucleus are impaired. The elevated glucocorticoid levels also exert a mineralocorticoid effect, since the capacity of the enzyme 11β-hydroxysteroid dehydrogenase type II, which normally protects the kidneys from an excessive cortisol effect by rapid inactivation, is overridden. In addition, since ACTH levels are increased the adrenal production of androgens (dehydroepiandrosterone (DHEA), DHEA-sulphate, and δ-4-androstenedione) and adrenal corticosteroids with mineralocorticoid activity (corticosterone and deoxycorticosterone) is elevated (3).

The effects of cortisol on target genes are the result of a cascade of events. First, the ligand passively diffuses through the cell membrane and binds to the GR. This receptor is present in the cytoplasm of virtually all human cells. In its unbound form the GR is surrounded by chaperone proteins, which keep it inactivated. When the ligand binds to the receptor, its conformation changes, the heat shock proteins dissociate from the receptor, and the GR translocates to the nucleus (3, 20). Within the nucleus there are two major modes of GR action. The 'classical' pathway comprises transcription initiation through binding to positive or negative glucocorticoid responsive elements of the target gene, resulting in, respectively, stimulation or inhibition of transcription. The GR can also act as a transcription factor and indirectly, through interacting with other proteins, stimulate or repress transcription (20).

Pathogenesis

Glucocorticoid receptor gene mutations

Several *GR* gene mutations have been reported as the cause of the syndrome of generalized glucocorticoid resistance. These are predominantly located in the ligand-binding domain, but some have been identified in the DNA-binding domain (3). These mutations lead to a variety of alterations in the GR signalling pathway, e.g. decreased transactivating or transrepressional capacity (11), disturbances in ligand binding (2), decreased GR expression (9), a delay in translocation to the nucleus, changes in interaction with coactivators, alternative splicing, or a combination of these changes in GR function (4, 6–9, 11 ,12, 15, 16).

Interestingly, one mutation, close to the boundary of exon 9 in the *GR* gene, resulted in an increased expression of the GR-β splice variant. In the literature, GR-β is suggested to function as a dominant negative inhibitor of the active GR-α. Therefore

Table 5.8.1 Mutations leading to the syndrome of generalized glucocorticoid resistance (a nonsuppressable hypercortisolaemia was present in all patients)

Year	Domain	(non) coding region	Mutation	Ligand affinity	Transactivating capacity	Other *in vitro* observations	Clinical features	References
1982	LB	Exon 7	Asp641Val	↓ (3-fold)	↓↓	Transrespressional capacity = Delayed nuclear translocation Abnormal interaction with the GR-interacting protein 1 coactivator mRNA GR copy number after EBV transformation ↓	Hypertension, hypokalaemia	(2, 3, 4, 5)
1990	LB	Exon 9α	Val729Ile	↓	↓ (4-fold)	Delayed nuclear translocation Abnormal interaction with the GR-interacting protein 1 coactivator	Isosexual precocious pseudopuberty in a boy, hyperandrogenism	(3, 6, 7)
1993	LB	Exon 6/ intron 6	4-base deletion (2013delGAGT)	Not tested	↓	Removal of a donor splice site, expression of only one allele and a 50% decrease of GR protein on PBMLs and EBV transformed lymphoblasts	Hirsutism, menstrual irregularities, male-pattern baldness	(4, 8)
1996	DB	Exon 5	Ile559Asn	= binding sites by 50% ↓	Dominant-negative effect on transactivation of the wild-type GR	Transrespressional capacity↓ mRNA GR copy number after EBV transformation ↓ Delayed nuclear translocation Abnormal interaction with the GR-interacting protein 1 coactivator	Hypertension, infertility, oligospermia, and secondary pituitary Cushing's disease	(3, 4, 9 10)
2001	DB	Exon 4	Arg477His	=	↓↓	In a structural model the mutant GR seems to have no contact with the GRE of the target gene	Hypertension, hirsutism, fatigue, obesity	(11, 12)
2001	LB	Exon 8	Gly679Ser	↓(2-fold)	↓	In heterozygous carriers the effect of the mutation was abolished when also the ER22/23EK polymorphism was present	Asymptomatic, hypertension, hypokalaemia hirsutism, fatigue, hyperandrogenism A dosage–allele effect was observed	(11, 12, 13)
2002	DB	Exon 5	Val571Ala	↓ (6-fold)	↓ (10- to 50-fold)	Delayed nuclear translocation	Hypertension, hypokalaemia, hyperandrogenism, female pseudohermaphroditism	(3, 14)
2002	LB	Exon 9α	Ile747Met	↓ (2-fold)	↓↓ (20- to 30-fold) Dominant negative effect on the wild-type GR	Abnormal interaction with p160 coactivators due to an ineffective AF-2 domain	Asymptomatic, cystic acne, hirsutism, oligoamenorrhoea	(3, 15)
2005	LB	Exon 9α	Leu773Pro	↓ (2.6-fold)	↓(2-fold)	Delayed nuclear translocation Abnormal interaction with the GR-interacting protein 1 coactivator Dominant negative effect on the wild-type GR	Hypertension, chronic fatigue, anxiety, hyperandrogenism,	(16)
2006	LB	Intron 8	G→A, +81 bp exon 8 and C→G -9 bp exon 9	Not tested	↓	Transrespressional capacity = Expression of the GR-β splice variant ↑ (4-fold)	Despite low dose immunosuppressive medication 33 years after post mortem renal transplantation still uneventful	(4)
2007	LB	Exon 9α	Phe737Leu	↓ (1.5-fold)	↓	Delayed nuclear translocation	Hypertension, hypokalaemia	(17)

↓, reduced; ↓↓, severely reduced; =, unaltered.

DB, DNA binding domain; EBV, Epstein–Barr virus; GR, glucocorticoid receptor; GRE, glucocorticoid responsive element; LB, ligand-binding domain; PBML, peripheral blood mononuclear leucocytes .

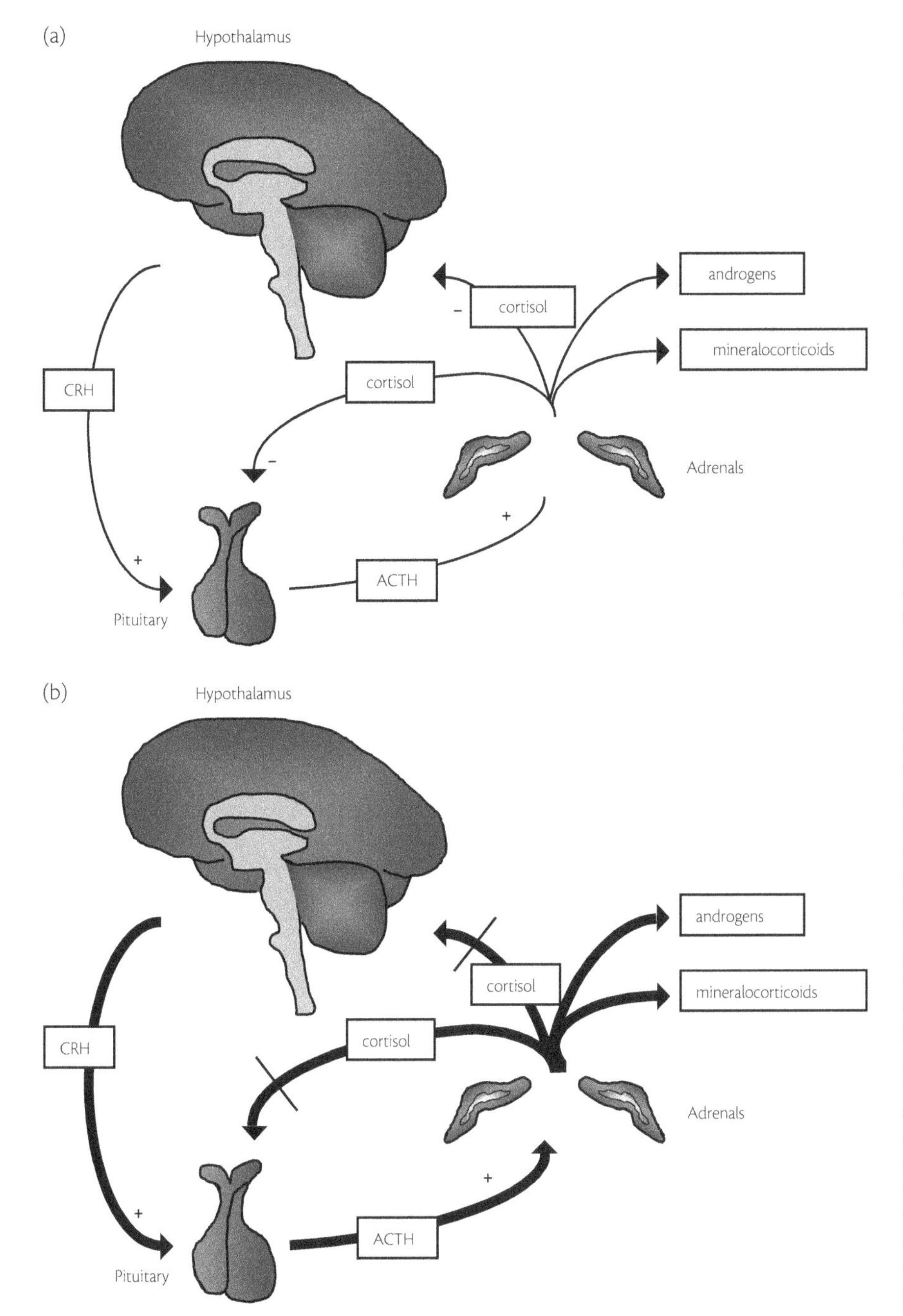

Fig. 5.8.1 (a) A simplified schematic overview showing the regulation of the hypothalamic–pituitary–adrenal (HPA) axis in a healthy situation. Corticotrophin releasing hormone (CRH), secreted by the hypothalamus, stimulates the production of adrenocorticotropin (ACTH) by the pituitary, resulting in increased secretion of cortisol, mineralocorticoids, and androgens by the adrenal glands. Cortisol controls its own production through a feedback loop to the pituitary, hippocampus (not shown), and hypothalamus. (b) In the syndrome of glucocorticoid resistance this negative feedback mechanism, mediated by the glucocorticoid receptor (GR), is impaired. As a consequence, the HPA axis becomes hyperactivated, resulting in an increased production of the adrenal steroid hormones. Patients suffer from signs and symptoms of overproduction of mineralocorticoids and, of particular importantance in women, androgens. However, no classical signs of glucocorticoid excess are present due to the impaired glucocorticoid signalling.

increased intracellular presence of the GR-β could lead to either an acquired or an inherited form of glucocorticoid resistance (4).

In some cases, no mutations in the *GR* gene were found and the mechanism leading to the glucocorticoid resistance is unknown (21). Several mechanisms leading to glucocorticoid resistance, have been suggested in the literature: altered phosphorylation status; hormone-induced conformation changes of the GR and nuclear transformation; thermolability of the GR; and enhanced expression of 90-kDa heat shock protein (hsp90), a chaperone protein (21, 22).

Acquired glucocorticoid resistance

Besides hereditary forms of systemic glucocorticoid resistance acquired forms also occur, in particular in some types of neoplasms. Examples are pituitary tumours (Nelson's syndrome/Cushing's disease), ectopic ACTH-producing tumours, as well as haematological malignancies (23). In a wide variety of other diseases, local or systemic, and temporary or chronic forms of glucocorticoid resistance have also been shown, e.g. major depression, AIDS, and several autoimmune diseases (24).

In asthma also, glucocorticoid resistance is a well-known clinical problem (25). Potential mechanisms involved in steroid-resistant asthma are increased expression of the dominant negative GR-β splice variant and local glucocorticoid resistance by diminished binding affinity in inflammatory cells induced by certain cytokines (e.g. interleukin (IL)-2, IL-4, IL-13). Also impaired nuclear localization, and leukaemia inhibitory factor, a cytokine decreasing GR expression in animal studies, may both be contributing factors in the development of glucocorticoid resistance (25).

Mild forms of glucocorticoid resistance

Within the normal population, variation in glucocorticoid sensitivity has been demonstrated, for which several single-nucleotide polymorphisms in the *GR* gene seem to be at least partially responsible (26). About 6–9% of the Caucasian population are carriers of the ER22/23EK polymorphism, which is associated with a mild glucocorticoid resistance and results in beneficial effects with respect to insulin sensitivity, lipid profile, body composition, cognition, and longevity (26). Russcher *et al.* showed that this *GR* gene variant causes an increased amount of the GR-α translational isoform, which has a lower transcriptional activity compared to the GR-β isoform (27). A polymorphism in the 3′ untranslated region of exon 9β of the *GR* gene has been associated with mild glucocorticoid resistance with respect to transrepressional effects, which is important for the immune system. *In vitro* this variant yielded more stable GR-β mRNA, possibly leading to a dominant negative effect on GR-α functioning, and showed diminished transrepressional activity (28, 29). Jiang *et al.* showed another exon 9 polymorphism in eight out of 39 lupus nephritis patients, resulting in addition of 20 amino acids to the GR protein, potentially affecting GR functioning and thereby increasing the risk of developing autoimmune diseases (30).

Hypersensitivity to glucocorticoids

In contrast to glucocorticoid resistance, hyperreactivity to endogenous cortisol has also been reported, resulting in clinical features consistent with Cushing's syndrome despite normal or decreased cortisol levels (22). In the healthy population two polymorphisms of the GR (Asn363Ser and *Bcl*I) have been demonstrated to be associated with mild hypersensitivity to glucocorticoids. Several studies have shown evidence for tissue-specific increased cortisol effects (26).

Clinical features

Glucocorticoid-resistant patients do not suffer from the classical cushingoid effects, such as a moon face, abdominal obesity with red striae, hyperglycaemia, myopathy, etc., despite their elevated cortisol levels. The symptoms in patients with cortisol resistance result from the compensatory increased activation of the HPA axis. Due to these elevated ACTH levels, patients experience symptoms related to an increased production of mineralocorticoids, leading to hypertension, hypokalaemic alkalosis, and fatigue. Female patients also suffer from symptoms of hyperandrogenism, such as hirsutism, male pattern of baldness, and menstrual disturbances, due to increased production of androgens by the adrenals. In male patients, the testicular production of androgens is much higher and outweighs the increased adrenal androgen production. However, some patients with glucocorticoid resistance are asymptomatic or complain only about chronic fatigue. The fatigue could also be attributed to a relative glucocorticoid deficiency in some tissue levels due to insufficient compensatory elevation of cortisol levels (21).

Clinical investigations and diagnostic criteria of glucocorticoid resistance

Figure 5.8.2 shows a practical scheme of clinical and biochemical tests for the diagnosis of glucocorticoid resistance. Plasma ACTH and serum cortisol concentrations are increased but, in contrast to Cushing's syndrome, the diurnal rhythm is maintained, although cortisol levels are on average higher (2, 5). Important for the diagnosis is nonsuppression after a 1 mg overnight dexamethasone suppression test with cortisol levels above 70 nmol/l or even higher—above 140 nmol/l being indicative for glucocorticoid resistance. Urinary cortisol excretion is increased. Serum concentrations of adrenal androgens (DHEA, DHEA-S, and androstenedione) and of ACTH-dependent mineralocorticoids (deoxycorticosterone and corticosterone) are also increased. Imaging may show slightly enlarged adrenal glands.

As shown in Fig. 5.8.2, the standard tests to evaluate hypercortisolism are not sufficient to differentiate between glucocorticoid resistance and Cushing's syndrome. Some clinical investigations, however, can be used to discriminate between these syndromes. A simple test is measurement of bone mineral density (BMD), which is normal or even increased in patients with glucocorticoid resistance. In contrast, in patients with Cushing's disease BMD is usually decreased. The increased BMD in glucocorticoid resistance may be explained by a combination of diminished cortisol effects on bone due to the defective GR, and increased adrenal androgen production as a result of elevated ACTH levels. If persistent doubt exists concerning the correct diagnosis, additional endocrine tests can be helpful, e.g. demonstration of a normal response of serum thyroid-stimulating hormone (TSH) to thyrotropin releasing hormone (TRH) administration and/or a normal response of growth hormone to an insulin-induced hypoglycaemia, which would be the case in conditions of glucocorticoid resistance. These responses are invariably reduced in patients with Cushing's disease. Recently, tests to confirm the diagnosis of glucocorticoid resistance have been developed (Fig. 5.8.2). Disadvantages are that, at present, these tests are labour-intensive and are performed only in research laboratories (4). A fast, alternative way to confirm the diagnosis of hereditary glucocorticoid resistance is to perform a dexamethasone-suppression tests in family members of the patient (22).

Treatment of glucocorticoid resistance

Morning ACTH levels can be suppressed by a low dose of dexamethasone taken around midnight. This leads to a reduction in adrenal overproduction of mineralocorticoids and androgens. It is essential that the treatment should be adjusted to the individual signs and symptoms of the patient. Titration to a dose of dexamethasone that normalizes androgens, blood pressure, and serum potassium seems the optimal therapy. After normalization of mineralocorticoids and androgens, the dexamethasone dose to maintain this suppression can be carefully titrated down. To minimize the risks of an effect of dexamethasone in addition to the remaining endogenous cortisol, it is important to slowly decrease the dose of dexamethasone as low as possible. A yearly measurement of BMD is recommended to monitor effects of too high doses of dexamethasone in combination with the endogenous cortisol production. In general, treatment can be started with a dose of about 1 mg dexamethasone at night. This dose can be slowly reduced to 0.5 mg/day or even 0.25 mg/day. To treat hypertension aldosterone antagonists are recommended, since these have additional effects. In particular, their potassium-sparing and antiandrogenic effects are beneficial for glucocorticoid-resistant patients. Thiazide or loop diuretics should not be used to control blood pressure because of their potassium-losing effects.

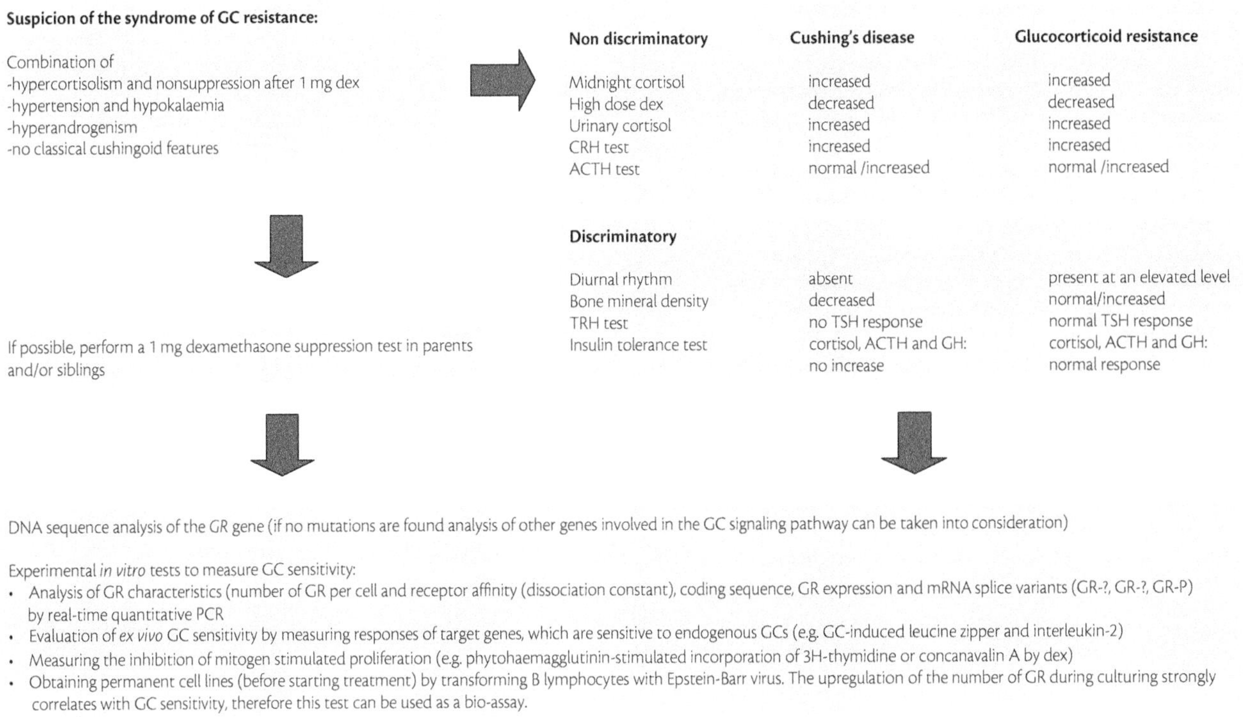

Suspicion of the syndrome of GC resistance:

Combination of
-hypercortisolism and nonsuppression after 1 mg dex
-hypertension and hypokalaemia
-hyperandrogenism
-no classical cushingoid features

Non discriminatory	**Cushing's disease**	**Glucocorticoid resistance**
Midnight cortisol	increased	increased
High dose dex	decreased	decreased
Urinary cortisol	increased	increased
CRH test	increased	increased
ACTH test	normal /increased	normal /increased

Discriminatory		
Diurnal rhythm	absent	present at an elevated level
Bone mineral density	decreased	normal/increased
TRH test	no TSH response	normal TSH response
Insulin tolerance test	cortisol, ACTH and GH: no increase	cortisol, ACTH and GH: normal response

If possible, perform a 1 mg dexamethasone suppression test in parents and/or siblings

DNA sequence analysis of the *GR* gene (if no mutations are found analysis of other genes involved in the GC signaling pathway can be taken into consideration)

Experimental *in vitro* tests to measure GC sensitivity:

- Analysis of GR characteristics (number of GR per cell and receptor affinity (dissociation constant), coding sequence, GR expression and mRNA splice variants (GR-?, GR-?, GR-P) by real-time quantitative PCR
- Evaluation of *ex vivo* GC sensitivity by measuring responses of target genes, which are sensitive to endogenous GCs (e.g. GC-induced leucine zipper and interleukin-2)
- Measuring the inhibition of mitogen stimulated proliferation (e.g. phytohaemagglutinin-stimulated incorporation of 3H-thymidine or concanavalin A by dex)
- Obtaining permanent cell lines (before starting treatment) by transforming B lymphocytes with Epstein-Barr virus. The upregulation of the number of GR during culturing strongly correlates with GC sensitivity, therefore this test can be used as a bio-assay.

Fig. 5.8.2 Clinical and biochemical evaluation of suspected generalized glucocorticoid resistance. dex, dexamethasone; GC, glucocorticoid; GR, glucocorticoid receptor.

References

1. Vingerhoeds AC, Thijssen JH, Schwarz F. Spontaneous hypercortisolism without Cushing's syndrome. *J Clin Endocrinol Metab*, 1976; **43**: 1128–33.
2. Hurley DM, Accili D, Stratakis CA, Karl M, Vamvakopoulos N, Rorer E, *et al.* Point mutation causing a single amino acid substitution in the hormone binding domain of the glucocorticoid receptor in familial glucocorticoid resistance. *J Clin Invest*, 1991; **87**: 680–6.
3. Charmandari E, Kino T, Souvatzoglou E, Vottero A, Bhattacharyya N, Chrousos GP. Natural glucocorticoid receptor mutants causing generalized glucocorticoid resistance: molecular genotype, genetic transmission, and clinical phenotype. *J Clin Endocrinol Metab*, 2004; **89**: 1939–49.
4. Russcher H, Smit P, van Rossum EF, van den Akker EL, Brinkmann AO, de Heide LJ, *et al.* Strategies for the characterization of disorders in cortisol sensitivity. *J Clin Endocrinol Metab*, 2006; **91**: 694–701.
5. Chrousos GP, Vingerhoeds A, Brandon D, Eil C, Pugeat M, DeVroede M, *et al.* Primary cortisol resistance in man. A glucocorticoid receptor-mediated disease. *J Clin Invest*, 1982; **69**: 1261–9.
6. Brufsky AM, Malchoff DM, Javier EC, Reardon G, Rowe D, Malchoff CD. A glucocorticoid receptor mutation in a subject with primary cortisol resistance. *Trans Assoc Am Physicians*, 1990; **103**: 53–63.
7. Malchoff DM, Brufsky A, Reardon G, McDermott P, Javier EC, Bergh CH, *et al.* A mutation of the glucocorticoid receptor in primary cortisol resistance. *J Clin Invest*, 1993; **91**: 1918–25.
8. Karl M, Lamberts SW, Detera-Wadleigh SD, Encio IJ, Stratakis CA, Hurley DM, *et al.* Familial glucocorticoid resistance caused by a splice site deletion in the human glucocorticoid receptor gene. *J Clin Endocrinol Metab*, 1993; **76**: 683–9.
9. Karl M, Lamberts SW, Koper JW, Katz DA, Huizenga NE, Kino T, *et al.* Cushing's disease preceded by generalized glucocorticoid resistance: clinical consequences of a novel, dominant-negative glucocorticoid receptor mutation. *Proc Assoc Am Physicians*, 1996; **108**: 296–307.
10. Kino T, Stauber RH, Resau JH, Pavlakis GN, Chrousos GP. Pathologic human GR mutant has a transdominant negative effect on the wild-type GR by inhibiting its translocation into the nucleus: importance of the ligand-binding domain for intracellular GR trafficking. *J Clin Endocrinol Metab*, 2001; **86**: 5600–8.
11. Charmandari E, Kino T, Ichijo T, Zachman K, Alatsatianos A, Chrousos GP. Functional characterization of the natural human glucocorticoid receptor (hGR) mutants hGRalphaR477H and hGRalphaG679S associated with generalized glucocorticoid resistance. *J Clin Endocrinol Metab*, 2006; **91**: 1535–43.
12. Ruiz M, Lind U, Gafvels M, Eggertsen G, Carlstedt-Duke J, Nilsson L, *et al.* Characterization of two novel mutations in the glucocorticoid receptor gene in patients with primary cortisol resistance. *Clin Endocrinol*, 2001; **55**: 363–71.
13. Raef H, Baitei EY, Zou M, Shi Y. Genotype-phenotype correlation in a family with primary cortisol resistance: possible modulating effect of the ER22/23EK polymorphism. *Eur J Endocrinol*, 2008; **158**: 577–82.
14. Mendonca BB, Leite MV, de Castro M, Kino T, Elias LL, Bachega TA, *et al.* Female pseudohermaphroditism caused by a novel homozygous missense mutation of the GR gene. *J Clin Endocrinol Metab*, 2002; **87**: 1805–9.
15. Vottero A, Kino T, Combe H, Lecomte P, Chrousos GP. A novel, C-terminal dominant negative mutation of the GR causes familial glucocorticoid resistance through abnormal interactions with p160 steroid receptor coactivators. *J Clin Endocrinol Metab*, 2002; **87**: 2658–67.
16. Charmandari E, Raji A, Kino T, Ichijo T, Tiulpakov A, Zachman K, *et al.* A novel point mutation in the ligand-binding domain (LBD) of the human glucocorticoid receptor (hGR) causing generalized glucocorticoid resistance: the importance of the C terminus of hGR LBD in conferring transactivational activity. *J Clin Endocrinol Metab*, 2005; **90**: 3696–705.
17. Charmandari E, Kino T, Ichijo T, Jubiz W, Mejia L, Zachman K, *et al.* A novel point mutation in helix 11 of the ligand-binding domain of the human glucocorticoid receptor gene causing generalized glucocorticoid resistance. *J Clin Endocrinol Metab* 2007; **92**: 3986–90.

18. Charmandari E, Kino T, Chrousos GP. Familial/sporadic glucocorticoid resistance: clinical phenotype and molecular mechanisms. *Ann N Y Acad Sci*, 2004; **1024**: 168–81.
19. Chrousos GP, Gold PW. The concepts of stress and stress system disorders. Overview of physical and behavioral homeostasis. *JAMA*, 1992; **267**: 1244–52.
20. Yudt MR, Cidlowski JA. The glucocorticoid receptor: coding a diversity of proteins and responses through a single gene. *Mol Endocrinol*, 2002; **16**: 1719–26.
21. Bronnegard M, Werner S, Gustafsson JA. Primary cortisol resistance associated with a thermolabile glucocorticoid receptor in a patient with fatigue as the only symptom. *J Clin Invest*, 1986; **78**: 1270–8.
22. van Rossum EF, Lamberts SW. Glucocorticoid resistance syndrome: A diagnostic and therapeutic approach. *Best Pract Res Clin Endocrinol Metab*, 2006; **20**: 611–26.
23. Lamberts SW. Glucocorticoid receptors and Cushing's disease. *Mol Cell Endocrinol*, 2002; **197**: 69–72.
24. Pariante CM. Glucocorticoid receptor function in vitro in patients with major depression. *Stress*, 2004; **7**: 209–19.
25. Adcock IM, Barnes PJ. Molecular mechanisms of corticosteroid resistance. *Chest*, 2008; **134**: 394–401.
26. van Rossum EFC, Lamberts SWJ. Polymorphisms in the glucocorticoid receptor gene and their associations with metabolic parameters and body composition. *Recent Prog Horm Res*, 2004; **59**: 333–57.
27. Russcher H, van Rossum EF, de Jong FH, Brinkmann AO, Lamberts SW, Koper JW. Increased expression of the glucocorticoid receptor-A translational isoform as a result of the ER22/23EK polymorphism. *Mol Endocrinol*, 2005; **19**: 1687–96.
28. Derijk RH, Schaaf MJ, Turner G, Datson NA, Vreugdenhil E, Cidlowski J, *et al.* A human glucocorticoid receptor gene variant that increases the stability of the glucocorticoid receptor beta-isoform mRNA is associated with rheumatoid arthritis. *J Rheumatol*, 2001; **28**: 2383–8.
29. van den Akker EL, Russcher H, van Rossum EF, Brinkmann AO, de Jong FH, Hokken A, *et al.* Glucocorticoid receptor polymorphism affects transrepression but not transactivation. *J Clin Endocrinol Metab*, 2006; **91**: 2800–3.
30. Jiang T, Liu S, Tan M, Huang F, Sun Y, Dong X, *et al.* The phase-shift mutation in the glucocorticoid receptor gene: potential etiologic significance of neuroendocrine mechanisms in lupus nephritis. *Clin Chim Acta*, 2001; **313**: 113–7.

5.9

Adrenal insufficiency

Wiebke Arlt

Introduction

In 1855, Thomas Addison identified a clinical syndrome characterized by wasting and hyperpigmentation as the result of adrenal gland destruction (1). This landmark observation paved the way for progress in understanding and treating adrenal insufficiency, with the introduction of adrenal extracts for treatment of Addison's disease by the groups of Hartman and Pfiffner in 1929. However, long-term survival of patients with adrenal insufficiency only became possible after the seminal work of Edward Kendall, Philip Hench, and Tadeus Reichstein on the characterization and therapeutic use of cortisone. In 1946, Lewis Sarrett, a Merck scientist, achieved a partial synthesis of cortisone, which marked the beginning of industrial-scale production of cortisone. In 1948, in a fundamental clinical experiment at the Mayo Clinic, the first patient with Addison's received intravenous injections of Kendall's Compound E, cortisone, resulting in 'notable improvement of his condition'. This was followed by the groundbreaking trials on the use of cortisone in rheumatoid arthritis yielding unanticipated clinical improvements, which quickly led to the labelling of cortisone as 'the wonder drug'. In November 1950, cortisone was made available to all physicians in the USA, a rapid translational development process, which culminated in the award of the 1950 Nobel Prize in Medicine to Kendall, Hench, and Reichstein. This progress reached other countries with variable delay and widespread availability of cortisone in the UK was achieved by joint efforts of Glaxo and the Medical Research Council. Though almost 150 years have passed since Addison's landmark observations and 60 years since the introduction of life-saving cortisone, there are still advances and challenges in the management of adrenal insufficiency, summarized in this chapter.

Physiology of adrenal steroid synthesis

Adrenal steroids and steroidogenesis

When extracting steroids from the adrenal Kendall and Reichstein identified 28 separate steroids and today we classify the steroids produced by the adrenal glands, the corticosteroids, in three major classes—glucocorticoids (cortisol, corticosterone), mineralocorticoids (aldosterone, deoxycorticosterone), and adrenal sex steroid precursors (dehydroepiandrosterone (DHEA), androstenedione).

Cholesterol is the precursor for all adrenal steroidogenesis. The principal source of cholesterol is provided from the circulation in the form of low-density lipoprotein (LDL) cholesterol. Uptake is by specific cell-surface LDL receptors present on adrenal tissue; LDL is then internalized via receptor-mediated endocytosis, the resulting vesicles fuse with lysozymes, and free cholesterol is produced following hydrolysis. However, it is clear that this cannot be the sole source of adrenal cholesterol as patients with abetalipoproteinaemia, who have undetectable circulating LDL, and patients with defective LDL receptors in the setting of familial hypercholesterolaemia still have normal basal adrenal steroidogenesis. Cholesterol can be generated *de novo* within the adrenal cortex from acetyl coenzyme A. In addition, there is evidence that the adrenal can utilize high-density lipoprotein (HDL) cholesterol following uptake through the HDL receptor, scavenger receptor.

The biochemical pathways involved in adrenal steroidogenesis start with the rate-limiting step of the transport of intracellular cholesterol from the outer to the inner mitochondrial membrane. Within the mitochondrion cholesterol is then converted to pregnenolone by the cholesterol side chain cleavage enzyme, cytochrome P450scc (CYP11A1). The rapid transport of cholesterol into the mitochondria is importantly facilitated by steroidogenic acute regulatory protein, which is induced by an increase in intracellular cAMP following binding of ACTH to its receptor.

Steroidogenesis involves the concerted action of several enzymes, including a series of cytochrome P450 (CYP) enzymes (for schematic overview, see Chapter 5.11). CYP11A1 and the CYP11B1 and CYP11B2 enzymes are localized to the mitochondria and require an electron shuttle system—provided through adrenodoxin/adrenodoxin reductase—for functional activity. Other CYP enzymes involved in steroidogenesis, namely 17α-hydroxylase (CYP17A1) and 21-hydroxylase (CYP21A2), are localized to the microsomal/endoplasmic reticulum fraction and depend on electron transfer from NADPH via the electron donor enzyme P450 oxidoreductase (POR).

After the uptake of cholesterol to the mitochondrion cleavage of cholesterol forms pregnenolone, which is converted in the cytoplasm to progesterone by the type II isoenzyme of 3β-hydroxysteroid dehydrogenase. Progesterone is hydroxylated to 17OH-progesterone through the activity of 17α-hydroxylase. 17-hydroxylation is an essential prerequisite for glucocorticoid synthesis CYP17 also possesses 17,20 lyase activity, which crucially facilitates the synthesis of the sex steroid precursor DHEA, a reaction that also requires allosteric interaction of the flavoprotein cytochrome b5 with both CYP17A1 and POR. In humans, 17-OH progesterone is not an efficient substrate for CYP17, and there is negligible conversion of 17-OH progesterone to androstenedione. Adrenal androstenedione secretion is dependent upon the conversion of dehydroepiandrosterone to androstenedione by 3β-hydroxysteroid dehydrogenase (3β-HSD). 21-hydroxylation of either progesterone (zona glomerulosa) or 17-OH-progesterone (zona fasciculata) is carried out by 21-hydroxylase (CYP21A2) to yield deoxycorticosterone or 11-deoxycortisol, respectively The final step in cortisol biosynthesis takes place in the mitochondria and involves the conversion of 11-deoxycortisol to cortisol by the enzyme CYP11B1, 11β-hydroxylase. In the zona glomerulosa, 11β-hydroxylase may also convert deoxycorticosterone to corticosterone. However, the enzyme CYP11B2, or aldosterone synthase, may also carry out this reaction and, in addition, is required for the conversion of corticosterone to aldosterone via the intermediate 18-OH corticosterone. Thus CYP11B2 can carry out 11β-hydroxylation, 18-hydroxylation, and 18-methyl oxidation to yield the characteristic C11–18 hemiacetyl structure of aldosterone.

Cortisol is inactivated to cortisone by action of the enzyme 11β-hydroxysteroid dehydrogenase type 2 (11β-HSD2) mainly in the kidney, while the opposite reaction, activation of cortisone to cortisol, is carried out by 11β-HSD1 mainly in the liver (Fig. 5.9.1). However, both enzymes are expressed in many tissues and recent years have highlighted the important role of this system in the tissue-specific activation and inactivation of glucocorticoids. Without the action of hepatic 11β-HSD1 Kendall would have observed no activity of his 'Compound E', as cortisone does not bind the glucocorticoid receptor and conversion to cortisol is a mandatory requirement for biological activity.

Glucocorticoids are secreted in relatively high amounts (cortisol 10–20 mg/day) from the zona fasciculata, whilst mineralocorticoids are secreted in low amounts (aldosterone 100–150 μg/day) from the zona glomerulosa. The adrenal androgen precursors DHEA, its sulphate ester DHEAS, and androstenedione are produced in the adrenal zona reticularis and represent the most abundant steroids secreted by the adult adrenal gland (>20 mg/day). In each case this is facilitated through the expression of steroidogenic enzymes in a specific 'zonal' manner. The zona glomerulosa cannot synthesize cortisol because it does not express 17α-hydroxylase. In contrast, aldosterone secretion is confined to the outer zona glomerulosa through the restricted expression of CYP11B2. Although CYP11B1 and CYP11B2 share 95% homology, the 5′ promoter sequences differ and permit regulation of the final steps in glucocorticoid and mineralocorticoid biosynthesis by ACTH and angiotensin II, respectively. DHEA is sulphated in the zona reticularis by the DHEA sulphotransferase (SULT2A1) to form DHEAS.

Regulation of adrenal corticosteroid synthesis

Classical endocrine feedback loops are in place to control the secretion of both hormones—cortisol inhibits the secretion of both corticotrophin releasing factor and ACTH from the hypothalamus and pituitary, respectively, and the aldosterone-induced sodium retention inhibits renal renin secretion (Fig. 5.9.2).

Glucocorticoid synthesis is under negative feedback control of the hypothalamic–pituitary–adrenal (HPA) axis (Fig. 5.9.2a). Adrenocorticotropic hormone (ACTH) secretion from the anterior pituitary is stimulated by hypothalamic corticotrophin-releasing

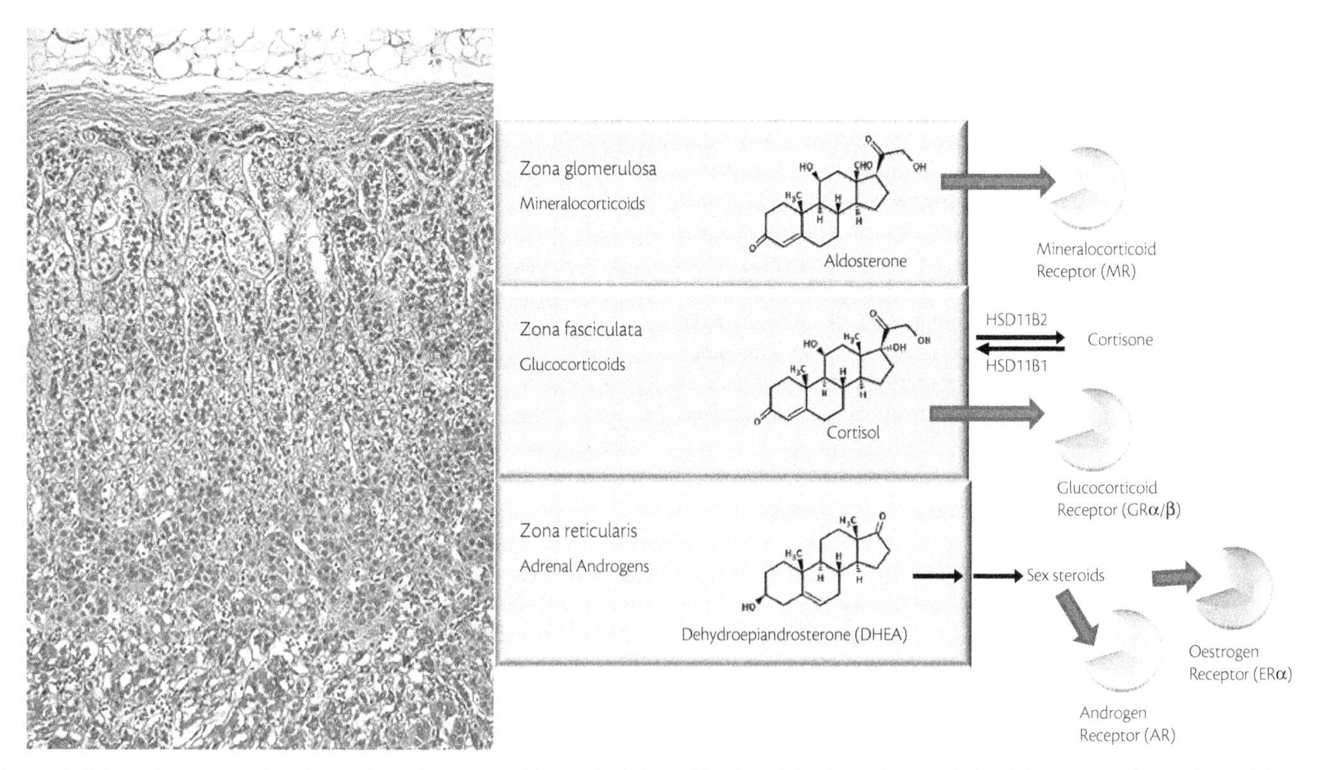

Fig. 5.9.1 Schematic representation of adrenal zonation and steroidogenesis, depicting histology of the three adrenocortical and the major corticosteroids and the receptors mediating their action. While cortisol and aldosterone can bind and activate the glucocorticoid and mineralocorticoid receptor, respectively, DHEA requires conversion to active androgens and further aromatization to oestrogens prior to exerting sex steroid action. (See also Plate 29)

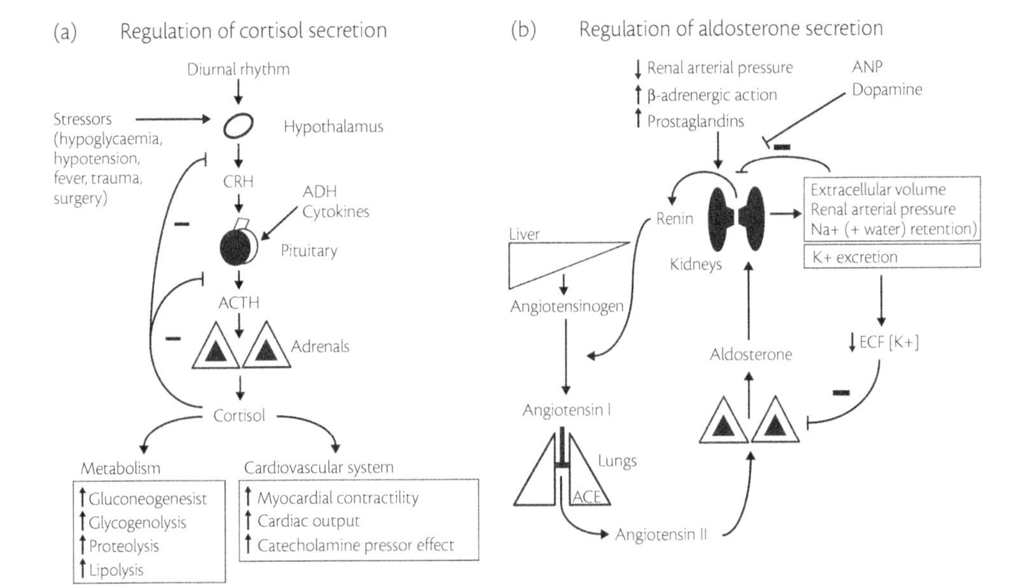

Fig. 5.9.2 Negative feedback regulation of cortisol and aldosterone secretion. (a) Glucocorticoid feedback regulation by the hypothalamic–pituitary–adrenal (HPA) axis. CRH, corticotropin-releasing hormone; ACTH, adrenocorticotropic hormone; ADH, antidiuretic hormone. (b) Mineralocorticoid regulation by the renin–angiotensin–aldosterone system (RAAS). The extracellular fraction (ECF) of potassium has an important direct influence on aldosterone secretion. ACE, angiotensin converting enzyme; ANP, atrial natriuretic peptide. Schematic graph: Dr Nils Krone, Birmingham.

hormone (CRH) following a circadian rhythm with a peak around 3.00 to 4.00 hours. Other major effectors on CRH secretions are various forms of stress, including hypoglycaemia, hypotension, fever, trauma, and surgery. ACTH binds to its receptor (melanocortin receptor 2, MC2R) on the adrenal cell and stimulates import of cholesterol into the mitochondrion by steroidogenic acute regulatory protein. In parallel, transcription of genes encoding steroidogenic enzymes and proteins of the electron transfer shuttle is increased.

Mineralocorticoid synthesis is mainly under the control of the renin–angiotensin–aldosterone system (RAAS) and a potassium feedback loop (Fig. 5.9.2b). A variety of factors stimulate renin secretion from renal juxtaglomerula cells, with renal perfusion being the most important regulator. Several other stimulators (β-adrenergic stimulation, prostaglandins) and inhibitors (α-adrenergic stimulation, dopamine, atrial natriuretic peptides, angiotensin II) are known. Angiotensinogen is an α_2-globulin synthesized within the liver which is cleaved by renin to form angiotensin I. Angiotensin I is converted to angiotensin II by angiotensin-converting enzyme in the lung and many other peripheral tissues. Angiotensin I has no apparent biological activity but angiotensin II is a potent stimulator of aldosterone secretion. In addition, angiotensin II acts is a potent vasconstrictor. The rate-limiting step in the RAAS is the secretion of renin, which is also controlled through a negative feedback loop. Renin is secreted from juxtaglomerular epithelial cells within the macula densa of the renal tubule in response to underlying renal arteriolar pressure, oncotic pressure, and sympathetic drive. Thus low perfusion pressure and/or low tubular fluid sodium content, as seen in haemorrhage, renal artery stenosis, dehydration, or salt loss, increase renin secretion. Conversely, secretion is suppressed following a high salt diet and by factors that increase blood pressure. Hypokalaemia increases and hyperkalaemia decreases renin secretion; in addition, potassium exerts a direct effect upon the adrenal cortex to increase aldosterone secretion. Angiotensin II and potassium stimulate aldosterone secretion principally by increasing the transcription of *CYP11B2* through common intracellular signalling pathways. The potassium effect is mediated through membrane depolarization and opening of calcium channels, and the angiotensin II effect following binding of angiotensin II to the surface AT_1 receptor and activation of phospholipase C.

The separate control of glucocorticoid biosynthesis through the HPA axis and mineralocorticoid synthesis via the renin–angiotensin system has important clinical consequences. Patients with primary adrenal failure invariably have both cortisol and aldosterone deficiency, whereas patients with ACTH deficiency due to pituitary disease have glucocorticoid deficiency, but aldosterone concentrations are normal because the renin–angiotensin system is intact.

Corticosteroid hormone action

Both cortisol and aldosterone exert their effects following uptake of free hormone from the circulation and binding to intracellular receptors, termed the glucocorticoid and mineralocorticoid receptors (GR, MR). These are both members of the thyroid/steroid hormone receptor superfamily of transcription factors, comprising a C-terminal ligand binding domain, a central DNA binding domain, interacting with specific DNA sequences on target genes, and an N-terminal hypervariable region. In both cases, although there is only a single gene encoding the GR and MR, splice variants have been described resulting in α and β variants.

The binding of glucocorticoid to the GR-α in the cytosol results in activation of the steroid–receptor complex through a process which involves the dissociation of heat-shock proteins HSP 90 and HSP 70. Following translocation to the nucleus, gene transcription is stimulated or repressed following binding of dimerized GR–ligand complexes to specific DNA sequences (glucocorticoid-response element) in the promoter regions of target genes. The GR-β variant may act as a dominant negative regulator of GR-α transactivation.

In contrast to the diverse actions of glucocorticoids, mineralocorticoids have a more restricted role, principally to stimulate epithelial sodium transport in the distal nephron, distal colon, and salivary glands. This is mediated through the induction of the apical sodium channel (comprising three subunits α, β, and γ) and the α_1 and β_1 subunits of the basolateral Na^+K^+ATPase through transcriptional regulation of a specific aldosterone-induced gene that encodes serum and glucocorticoid-induced kinase. Aldosterone binds to the MR, principally in the cytosol (though there is evidence for expression of the unoccupied MR in the nucleus) followed by translocation of the hormone–receptor complex to the nucleus.

The MR and GR share considerable homology—57% in the steroid binding domain and 94% in the DNA binding domain. It is perhaps not surprising therefore that there is promiscuity of ligand binding with aldosterone binding to the GR and cortisol binding to the MR. For the MR this is particularly impressive—*in vitro* the MR has the same inherent affinity for aldosterone, corticosterone, and cortisol. Specificity upon the MR is conferred through the 'prereceptor' metabolism of cortisol via the enzyme 11β-HSD2, which inactivates cortisol and corticosterone to inactive 11-keto metabolites, enabling aldosterone to bind to the MR.

For both glucocorticoids and mineralocorticoids there is accumulating evidence for so-called 'nongenomic' effects involving hormone response obviating the genomic GR or MR effects. A series of responses have been reported within seconds/minutes of exposure to corticosteroids and are thought to be mediated by, as yet uncharacterized, membrane coupled receptors.

Cortisol-binding globulin and corticosteroid hormone metabolism

Over 90% of circulating cortisol is bound, predominantly to the α_2-globulin cortisol-binding globulin (CBG). This 383-amino acid protein is synthesized in the liver and binds cortisol with high affinity. Affinity for synthetic corticosteroids (except prednisolone, which has an affinity for CBG of approximately 50% of that of cortisol) is negligible. Circulating CBG concentrations are approximately 700 nmol/l; levels are increased by oestrogens and in some patients with chronic active hepatitis but reduced in patients with cirrhosis, nephrosis, and hyperthyroidism. The oestrogen effect can be marked, with levels increasing two- to threefold across pregnancy, and this should also be taken into account when measuring plasma 'total' cortisol in pregnancy and in women taking oestrogens. Inherited abnormalities in CBG synthesis are much rarer than those described for thyroid-binding globulin but include patients with elevated CBG, partial and complete deficiency of CBG, or CBG variants with reduced affinity for cortisol. In each case, alterations in CBG concentrations change total circulating cortisol concentrations accordingly but 'free' cortisol concentrations are normal. Only this free circulating fraction is available for transport into tissues for biological activity. The excretion of 'free' cortisol through the kidneys is termed urinary free cortisol and represents only 1% of the total cortisol secretion rate. Approximately 50% of secreted cortisol appears in the urine as Tetrahydrocortisol (THF), 5alpha-tetrahydrocortisol (allo-THF), and tetrahydrocortisone (THE), 25% as cortols/cortolones, 10% as C19 steroids, and 10% as cortolic/cortolonic acids.

Aldosterone is also metabolized in the liver and kidneys. In the liver it undergoes tetrahydro reduction and is excreted in the urine as a 3-glucuronide tetrahydroaldosterone derivative. However, glucuronide conjugation at the 18 position occurs directly in the kidney, as does 3α and 5α/5β metabolism of the free steroid. Because of the aldehyde group at the C18 position, aldosterone is not metabolized by 11β-HSD2. Hepatic aldosterone clearance is reduced in patients with cirrhosis, ascites, and severe congestive heart failure.

Epidemiology of adrenal insufficiency

The prevalence of Addison's disease, mostly due to autoimmune adrenalitis, is 93–140 per million while secondary insufficiency, mostly due to hypothalamic–pituitary tumours, has a prevalence of 125–280 per million (2). The overall prevalence of adrenal insufficiency is 5 in 10 000 population, with three patients suffering from secondary adrenal insufficiency, one from primary adrenal insufficiency due to autoimmune adrenalitis, and one from congenital adrenal hyperplasia.

Primary adrenal insufficiency

According to recent studies, chronic primary adrenal insufficiency has a prevalence of 93 to 140 per million and an incidence of 4.7 to 6.2 per million in Caucasian populations (2, 3). These numbers are considerably higher than reported earlier, despite a continuous decline in tuberculous adrenalitis in the developed world, and suggest an increasing incidence of autoimmune adrenalitis. The age at diagnosis peaks in the fourth decade of life, with women more frequently affected.

Secondary adrenal insufficiency

Secondary adrenal insufficiency has an estimated prevalence of 150 to 280 per million (2, 3). Again, women are more frequently affected and age at diagnosis peaks in the sixth decade.

It has been suggested that therapeutic glucocorticoid administration is the most common cause of adrenal insufficiency, as exogenous glucocorticoids induce atrophy of both pituitary corticotroph and adrenocortical cells. However, iatrogenic adrenal insufficiency only becomes potentially relevant during or after glucocorticoid withdrawal. As iatrogenic adrenal insufficiency is transient in the majority of cases it can be suspected that the prevalence of permanent iatrogenic adrenal insufficiency is clearly lower than that of endogenous adrenal insufficiency.

Causes of adrenal insufficiency

A large number of frequent and rare causes of adrenal insufficiency are summarized in Tables 5.9.1 and 5.9.2, and in the following sections more detailed information on some of the more frequent causes is provided. Two reviews have given an excellent overview of causes of adrenal insufficiency including citation of all original literature which cannot be provided here because of space constraints (2, 3).

Causes of primary adrenal insufficiency

During the times of Thomas Addison, tuberculous adrenalitis was by far the most prevalent cause of adrenal insufficiency. In the developing world, tuberculosis still remains a major cause of adrenal insufficiency. In active tuberculosis, the incidence of adrenal involvement is 5%.

In North American and European countries, autoimmune adrenalitis accounts for more than 90% of cases with primary adrenal insufficiency; in 40% adrenal insufficiency is isolated while in 60% it arises as part of an autoimmune polyglandular syndrome

Table 5.9.1 Causes of primary adrenal insufficiency

Diagnosis	Clinical features	Pathogenesis/genetics
Autoimmune adrenalitis (AA)		
Isolated AA	AI	Associations with HLA-DR3, CTLA-4
AA as part of autoimmune polyendocrine syndromes (APS)		
APS 1 (= APECED) APS 2	AI + hypoparathyroidism + chronic mucocutaneous candidiasis ± other autoimmune disorders AI + thyroid disease (= Schmidt's syndrome) + type 1 diabetes mellitus (= Carpenter's syndrome) ± other autoimmune diseases	*AIRE* gene mutations (21q22.3) Associations with HLA-DR3, CTLA-4
Infectious adrenalitis		
Tuberculous adrenalitis	AI + other organ manifestations of tuberculosis	Tuberculosis
AIDS	AI +other AIDS-associated diseases	HIV, CMV
Fungal adrenalitis	AI + mostly immunosupppressed patients	Cryptococcosis, histoplasmosis, coccidioidomycosis
Genetic disorders leading to AI		
Adrenoleucodystrophy (ALD) Adrenomeyloneuropathy (AMN)	AI + demyelination of CNS (cerebral ALD) or spinal cord/peripheral nerves (AMN)	Mutation of the *X-ALD* gene encoding for the peroxisomal adrenoleucodystrophy protein (ALDP)
Congenital adrenal hyperplasia (CAH)		
21-hydroxylase deficiency 11β-hydroxylase deficiency 3β-HSD type 2 deficiency 17α-hydroxylase deficiency P450 oxidoreductase deficiency	AI + ambiguous genitalia in females AI + ambiguous genitalia in females + hypertension AI + ambiguous genitalia in males + postnatal virilization in females AI + ambiguous genitalia in males + lack of puberty in both sexes + hypertension AI + ambiguous genitalia in both sexes + skeletal malformations	*CYP21A2* mutation *CYP11B1* mutation *HSD3B2* mutation *CYP17A1* mutation *POR* mutation
Congenital lipoid adrenal hypoplasia (lipoid CAH)	AI + XY sex reversal	Mutations in the steroidogenic acute regulatory protein (*STAR*) gene Mutations in *CYP11A1* (encoding P450scc)
Smith–Lemli–Opitz syndrome (SLOS)	AI, mental retardation, craniofacial malformations, growth failure	Sterol delta-7-reductase gene (*DHCR7*) mutations
Adrenal hypoplasia congenita (AHC)		
X-linked AHC Xp21 contiguous gene syndrome SF-1 linked AHC	AI + hypogonadotropic hypogonadism AI + Duchenne muscular dystrophy + glycerol kinase deficiency (psychomotor retardation) AI + XY sex reversal	Mutation in *NROB1* (encoding DAX1) Deletion of the Duchenne muscular dystrophy, glycerol kinase, and *DAX1* genes Mutation in *NR5A1* (encoding SF-1)
IMAGe syndrome	Intrauterine growth retardation + metaphyseal dysplasia + AI + genital anomalies	?
Kearns–Sayre syndrome	Progressive external ophthalmoplegia, pigmentary retinal degeneration and cardiac conduction defects; endocrinopathies include gonadal failure, hypoparathyroidism, type 1 diabetes, only rarely AI	Mitochondrial DNA deletions
ACTH insensitivity syndromes = familial glucocorticoid deficiency (FGD)	Glucocorticoid deficiency, excess plasma ACTH; no (or only very mild) impairment of mineralocorticoid synthesis; lack of adrenarche	
FGD 1 FGD 2 FGD 3 Triple A syndrome (= Allgrove's syndrome)	AI, tall stature AI AI AI + alacrimia + achalasia; additional symptoms (neurological impairment, deafness, mental retardation, hyperkeratosis)	Mutations in melanocortin-2-receptor (*MC2R*) encoding the ACTH receptor Mutations in MC2R accessory protein (*MRAP*) ? Mutations in the triple A gene (*AAAS*) encoding a WD repeat protein
Bilateral adrenal haemorrhage	AI + symptoms of underlying disease	Septic shock, specifically meningococcal sepsis (Waterhouse–Friderichsen syndrome) Primary antiphospholipid syndrome

(Contd.)

Table 5.9.1 *(Contd.)* Causes of primary adrenal insufficiency

Diagnosis	Clinical features	Pathogenesis/genetics
Adrenal infiltration	AI + symptoms of underlying disease	Adrenal metastases primary adrenal lymphoma sarcoidosis, amyloidosis, haemochromatosis
Bilateral adrenalectomy	AI + symptoms of underlying disease	e.g. in the management of Cushing's due to ectopic ACTH secretion of unknown source or following tumour nephrectomy
Drug-induced AI	AI	Treatment with mitotane, aminoglutethimide, arbiraterone, trilostane, etomidate, ketoconazole, suramin, RU486

AI, adrenal insufficiency; APECED, autoimmune polyendocrinopathy–candidiasis–ectodermal dystrophy.

Table 5.9.2 Causes of secondary adrenal insufficiency

Diagnosis	Comment
AI as the consequence of growth or therapeutic management of hypothalamic–pituitary mass lesions	
Pituitary tumours	Generally adenomas, carcinomas very rare Additional signs and symptoms consequent to impairment of other pituitary axes (thyroid, gonads, PRL, GH), visual field impairment due to compression of the optic chiasm
Other tumours of the hypothalamic–pituitary region	Craniopharyngioma, meningioma, ependymoma, intra-/suprasellar metastases
Pituitary irradiation	Radiation therapy for pituitary tumours, brain tumours outside the HPA axis and craniospinal irradiation in leukaemia and other cancers
Nontumoural causes	
Lymphocytic hypophysitis isolated	Autoimmune hypophysitis; most frequently in relation to pregnancy; commonly associated with panhypopituitarism, but also presenting with isolated ACTH deficiency only
as part of autoimmune polyglandular syndromes (APS)	associated with autoimmune thyroid disease, less frequently also with vitiligo, primary gonadal failure, type 1 diabetes, and pernicious anaemia
Genetic disorders leading to secondary AI	
Congenital isolated ACTH deficiency	Tpit or T-box 19 (*TBX19*) mutations; neonatal presentation; autosomal recessive
Combined pituitary hormone deficiency (CPHD)	Prophet of Pit-1 (*PROP1*) mutations: progressive development of CPHD in the order GH, PRL, TSH, LH/FSH, (ACTH— late onset); anterior pituitary may be hypoplastic, normal or enlarged; autosomal recessive Homeobox gene 1 (*HESX1*) mutations: CPHD + optic nerve hypoplasia and midline brain defects/agenesis of corpus callosum (= septo-optic dysplasia); anterior pituitary hypoplastic or ectopic; autosomal recessive, autosomal dominant Lim homeobox 3 (*LHX3*) mutations: CPHD with involvement of GH, TSH, gonadotrophins, PRLs; ACTH may be deficient; limited neck rotation, short cervical spine, sensorineural deafness; anterior pituitary hypoplastic, normal or enlarged; autosomal recessive LIM homeobox 4 (*LHX4*) mutations: CPHD with involvement of GH, thyrotropin, and ACTH secretion, cerebellar abnormalities; anterior pituitary hypoplastic or ectopic; autosomal dominant SRY-box 3 (*SOX3*) mutations: infundibular hypoplasia, CPHD, variable: mental retardation
Proopiomelanocortin (POMC) deficiency syndrome	*POMC* gene mutations; clinical triad AI + early-onset obesity + red hair pigmentation
Prader–Willi syndrome	Imprinting disorder, manifests with AI, obesity, hypogonadism, variable learning difficulties, and hypotonia
Pituitary apoplexy—Sheehan's syndrome	Onset mainly with abrupt severe headache, visual disturbance, nausea/vomiting Pituitary apoplexy/necrosis with peripartal onset (e.g. due to high blood loss and/or hypotension)
Pituitary infiltration/granuloma	Tuberculosis, actinomycosis, sarcoidosis, histiocytosis X, Wegener's granulomatosis
Trauma	Pituitary stalk lesions, traumatic brain injury
Drugs	Chronic glucocorticoid excess: exogenous glucocorticoid administration for more than 4 weeks endogenous glucocorticoid hypersecretion due to Cushing's syndrome

GH, growth hormone; LH/FSH, luteinizing hormone/follicle-stimulating hormone; PRL, prolactin; TSH, thyroid-stimulating hormone.

(APS) (2, 4). APS type 1, also termed autoimmune polyendocrinopathy–candidiasis–ectodermal dystrophy, accounts for 15% of cases and is characterized by adrenal insufficiency, hypoparathyroidism, and chronic mucocutaneous candidiasis, the latter being the primary manifestation in most cases and already apparent in childhood (5). APS 1 is caused by mutations in the autoimmune regulator gene (*AIRE*) (6–8) while APS 2 is thought to be inherited as a complex trait, associated with loci within the major histocompatibility complex (4) and distinct susceptibility genes (9–11). APS 2 is much more common than APS 1 and in addition to adrenal insufficiency most frequently comprises autoimmune thyroid disease, albeit more often autoimmune hypothyroidism than Graves' disease.

X-linked adrenoleucodystrophy (ALD) is caused by a mutation in the *X-ALD* gene, which encodes a peroxisomal membrane protein (adrenoleucodystrophy protein), leading to accumulation of very long chain fatty acids (>24 carbon atoms). The clinical picture comprises adrenal insufficiency and neurological impairment due to white matter demyelination. The two major forms are cerebral ALD (50% of cases; early childhood manifestation, rapid progression) and adrenomyeloneuropathy (35% of cases; onset in early adulthood, slow progression) with restriction of demyelination to spinal cord and peripheral nerves. Adrenal insufficiency may precede the onset of neurological symptoms and is the sole manifestation of disease in 15% of cases.

Other causes of primary adrenal insufficiency (Table 5.9.1), e.g. adrenal infiltration or haemorrhage, are rare. Congenital or neonatal primary adrenal insufficiency accounts for only 1% of all cases. However, the recent elucidation of the genetic basis of underlying diseases has highlighted the importance of specific genes for adrenal development and steroidogenesis.

Causes of secondary adrenal insufficiency

The most common cause of secondary adrenal insufficiency is a tumour of the hypothalamic–pituitary region, usually associated with panhypopituitarism as a result of tumour growth or treatment with surgery and/or irradiation (Table 5.9.2). Autoimmune lymphocytic hypophysitis is less frequent, mostly affecting women during or shortly after pregnancy. Isolated ACTH deficiency may also be of autoimmune origin as some patients concurrently suffer from other autoimmune disorders, most frequently thyroid disease. The differential diagnosis of postpartal autoimmune hypophysitis includes Sheehan's syndrome, which results from pituitary apoplexy, mostly due to pronounced blood loss during delivery. Very rarely mutations of genes important for pituitary development or for synthesis and processing of the corticotropin precursor proopiomelanocortin cause secondary adrenal insufficiency (Table 5.9.2).

Clinical presentation of adrenal insufficiency

The clinical signs and symptoms of both acute and chronic adrenal insufficiency are a logical consequence of the underlying pathology, i.e. mostly the deficiency of adrenal corticosteroid production arising from primary or secondary adrenal failure (Table 5.9.3).

Acute adrenal insufficiency, i.e. life-threatening adrenal crisis, typically presents with severe hypotension or hypovolaemic shock, acute abdominal pain, vomiting, and often with fever, and, therefore, is sometimes mistaken for acute abdomen. In a series of 91 patients with Addison's disease, adrenal crisis led to the initial diagnosis of adrenal insufficiency in half of the patients. In children, acute adrenal insufficiency often presents as hypoglycaemic seizures. Deterioration of glycaemic control with recurrent hypoglycaemia may be the presenting sign of adrenal insufficiency in patients with pre-existing type 1 diabetes. In APS 2, onset of autoimmune hyperthyroidism (or thyroxine replacement for newly diagnosed hypothyroidism) may precipitate adrenal crisis due to enhanced cortisol clearance.

The leading symptom of chronic adrenal insufficiency is fatigue, accompanied by lack of stamina, loss of energy, reduced muscle strength, and increased irritability. In addition, chronic glucocorticoid deficiency leads to weight loss, nausea, and anorexia (in children, failure to thrive) and may account for muscle and joint pain. Unfortunately, most of these symptoms are nonspecific. Thus, every second patient suffers from signs and symptoms of Addison's disease for more than 1 year before diagnosis is established. In secondary adrenal insufficiency, diagnosis is mostly prompted by a history of pituitary disease, but may also be delayed, e.g. in isolated ACTH deficiency. A more specific sign for primary adrenal failure is hyperpigmentation (Fig. 5.9.3), which is most pronounced in areas of the skin exposed to increased friction (e.g. hand lines, knuckles, scars, oral mucosa). Hyperpigmentation is due to enhanced stimulation of skin MC1-receptor by ACTH and other pro-opiomelanocortin-related peptides. Accordingly, patients with secondary adrenal insufficiency often present with pale, alabaster-coloured skin. Laboratory findings in glucocorticoid deficiency may include mild anaemia, lymphocytosis, and eosinophilia. Cortisol physiologically inhibits thyrotropin release. Thus, thyrotropin is often increased at initial diagnosis of primary adrenal insufficiency, but returns to normal during glucocorticoid replacement unless there is coincident autoimmune thyroid failure. In rare cases, glucocorticoid deficiency may result in hypercalcaemia, which is due to increased intestinal absorption and decreased renal excretion of calcium and usually coincides with autoimmune hyperthyroidism, facilitating calcium release from bone.

Mineralocorticoid deficiency, which is only present in primary adrenal insufficiency, leads to dehydration and hypovolaemia, resulting in low blood pressure, postural hypotension, and sometimes even in prerenal failure. Deterioration may be sudden and is often due to exogenous stress such as infection or trauma. Combined mineralocorticoid and glucocorticoid replacement in primary adrenal insufficiency reconstitutes the diurnal rhythm of blood pressure and reverses cardiac dysfunction. Glucocorticoids contribute to this amelioration not only by mineralocorticoid receptor binding, but also by permissive effects on catecholamine action. The latter may account for the relative unresponsiveness to catecholamines in patients with unrecognized adrenal crisis. Mineralocorticoid deficiency accounts for hyponatraemia (90%), hyperkalaemia (65%), and salt craving (15%). Low serum sodium may also be present in secondary adrenal insufficiency due to the syndrome of inappropriate antidiuretic hormone secretion, which results from the loss of physiological inhibition of pituitary vasopressin release by glucocorticoids.

Adrenal insufficiency inevitably leads to DHEA deficiency. DHEA is the major precursor of sex steroid synthesis and loss of its synthesis results in pronounced androgen deficiency in women. As a consequence, women with adrenal insufficiency frequently show loss of axillary and pubic hair (absence of pubarche in children),

Table 5.9.3 Clinical manifestations of adrenal insufficiency

Manifestations	Explained by deficiency of
Symptoms	
Fatigue, lack of energy/stamina, reduced strength	Glucocorticoids (adrenal androgens)
Anorexia, weight loss (in children: failure to thrive)	Glucocorticoids
Abdominal pain, nausea, vomiting (more frequent in primary AI)	Mineralocorticoids, glucocorticoids
Myalgia, joint pain	Glucocorticoids
Dizziness, postural hypotension	Mineralocorticoids
Salt craving (primary AI only)	Mineralocorticoids
Dry and itchy skin (in women)	Adrenal androgens
Loss/impairment of libido (in women)	Adrenal androgens
Signs	
Skin hyperpigmentation (primary AI only)	*Excess*-of pro-opiomelanocortin (POMC) derived peptides (primary AI)
Alabaster-coloured pale skin (secondary AI only)	Deficiency of POMC derived peptides (secondary AI)
Loss of axillary/pubic hair (in women)	Adrenal androgens
Fever	Glucocorticoids
Low blood pressure (systolic RR <100 mm Hg), postural hypotension (pronounced in primary AI)	Mineralocorticoids, glucocorticoids
Anaemia, lymphocytosis, eosinophilia	Glucocorticoids
Serum creatinine ↑ (primary AI only)	Mineralocorticoids
Hyponatraemia	Mineralocorticoids, (glucocorticoids = SIADH)
hyperkalaemia (primary AI only)	mineralocorticoids
TSH ↑ (primary AI only)	Glucocorticoids (or autoimmune hypothyroidism)
Hypercalcaemia (primary AI only)	Glucocorticoids (rare, mostly observed if concurrent hyperthyroidism)
Hypoglycaemia	Glucocorticoids, (epinephrine deficiency?) (more frequent in children)

SIADH, syndrome of inappropriate antidiuretic hormone secretion; TSH, thyroid-stimulating hormone..

dry skin, and reduced libido. DHEA also exerts direct action as a neurosteroid with potential antidepressant properties. Thus DHEA deficiency may contribute to the impairment of well-being that is observed in patients with adrenal insufficiency despite adequate glucocorticoid and mineralocorticoid replacement.

Diagnostic laboratory evaluation of adrenal insufficiency

Presentation with acute adrenal insufficiency, i.e. life-threatening adrenal crisis, requires an immediate, combined diagnostic and therapeutic approach (Fig. 5.9.4). Haemodynamically stable patients may undergo a cosyntropin stimulation test; if in doubt, baseline bloods for serum cortisol and plasma ACTH will suffice and if cortisol is less than 100 nmol while ACTH is considerably elevated, there is no doubt about the diagnosis. Formal confirmation of diagnosis can be performed following clinical improvement. Diagnostic measures must never delay treatment, which should be initiated upon strong clinical suspicion of adrenal insufficiency. It is of negligible risk to start hydrocortisone and stop it after adrenal insufficiency has been safely excluded; withholding potentially life-saving treatment, however, could have fatal consequences.

Adrenal insufficiency is readily diagnosed by the cosyntropin test, a safe and reliable diagnostic tool with excellent long-term predictive value (12, 13); it is important to be aware of the considerable variability between results of different cortisol assays (14) and when defining the cut-off for failure, commonly set at 500 nmol/l, one should ideally refer to results from a local reference cohort obtained with the same assay. The diagnostic value of the cosyntropin test is only compromised within the first 4 weeks following a pituitary insult (13, 15), as during this period the adrenals will still respond to exogenous ACTH stimulation despite the loss of endogenous ACTH drive. When suspecting secondary adrenal insufficiency, the insulin tolerance test is an alternative choice for diagnostic confirmation, considered by many as the gold standard, however it is associated with side effects and requires exclusion of cardiovascular disease and history of seizures. Formal confirmation of diagnosis by the cosyntropin stimulation test should include blood samples for plasma ACTH, which will guide the way for further diagnostic assessment, by reliably differentiating primary from secondary adrenal insufficiency, i.e. adrenal from hypothalamic–pituitary disease (Fig. 5.9.4).

Possible glucocorticoid deficiency is also indicated by normocytic anaemia as sufficient levels of cortisol are required for maturation of blood progenitor cells; other blood count changes may include lymphocytosis and eosinophilia. Sometimes also, mild metabolic acidosis or hypercalcaemia can be observed in affected patients, the latter mostly in the context of coincident hyperthyroidism. Serum glucose may be low; however, significant hypoglycaemia as a presenting sign plays a more important role in childhood adrenal insufficiency where it can result in significant brain damage. However, in a patient with pre-existing type 1 diabetes onset of recurrent hypoglycaemic episodes despite unchanged insulin regimen should raise the suspicion of adrenal insufficiency.

Mineralocorticoid deficiency is present in primary adrenal insufficiency only; the renin–angiotensin–aldosterone system in patients with hypothalamic–pituitary disease and intact adrenals is usually preserved. Mineralocorticoid deficiency is not only reflected by the arterial hypotension and deranged potassium and sodium but intravascular volume depletion is also indicated by the slightly raised creatinine, a common finding in Addison patients. Hyponatraemia is observed in about 80% of acute cases while less than half present with hyperkalaemia. In the first instance, baseline levels of serum aldosterone and plasma renin should be taken.

Diagnosis of primary adrenal insufficiency

The combined measurement of early morning serum cortisol and plasma ACTH separates patients with primary adrenal insufficiency from normal subjects and patients with secondary adrenal insufficiency. Plasma ACTH is usually grossly elevated and

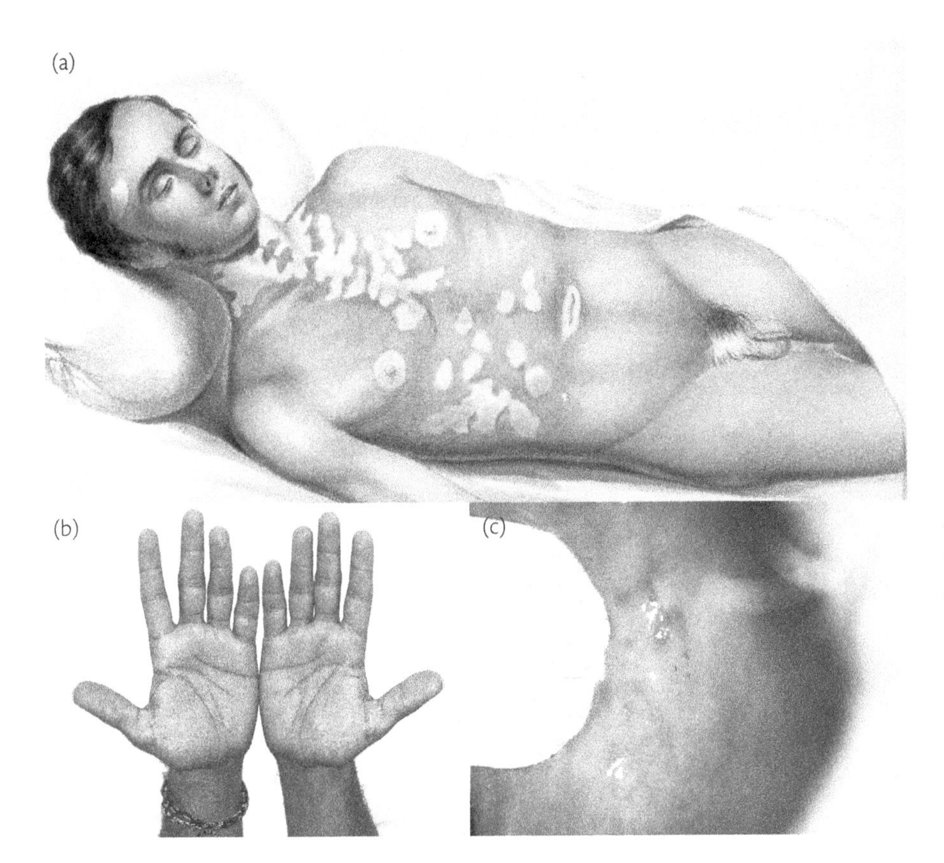

Fig. 5.9.3 Skin changes observed in primary adrenal insufficiency (Addison's disease). (a) Panel drawn by Thomas Addison (1855) of a patient with Addison's disease, depicting generalized hyperpigmentation, in particular in areas of increased friction, and patchy vitiligo, indicative of autoimmune polyglandular syndrome. (b) Hyperpigmentation of the palmar creases in a patient with acute primary adrenal insufficiency. (c) Patchy hyperpigmentation of the oral mucosa in a patient with acute primary adrenal insufficiency. (See also Plate 30)

invariably higher than 22 pmol/l with serum cortisol usually below the normal range (<165 nmol/l), sometimes also in the lower normal range. Establishment of the diagnosis of primary adrenal insufficiency always depends on the *combined* measurement of ACTH and cortisol. Serum aldosterone concentrations are subnormal or within the lower normal range with plasma renin activity concurrently increased above the normal range. In patients with adrenal insufficiency, serum DHEAS is invariably low, in women often below the limit of detection.

The impaired ability of the adrenal cortex to respond to ACTH is readily demonstrated by the short synacthen test (SST), employing serum cortisol measurements before and 30 (or 60) min after IV (or IM) injection of 250 μg 1–24 ACTH. In normal subjects, this leads to a physiological increase in serum cortisol to peak concentrations above 500 nmol/l. In primary adrenal insufficiency, the adrenal cortex is already maximally stimulated by endogenous ACTH, exogenous ACTH administration therefore usually does not evoke any further increase in serum cortisol.

Adrenal cortex autoantibodies and/or antibodies against 21-hydroxylase are found in more than 80% of patients with recent-onset autoimmune adrenalitis. While 21-hydroxylase has been identified as the major autoantigen in autoimmune adrenalitis, autoantibodies against other steroidogenic enzymes (P450scc, P450c17) and steroid-producing cell antibodies are present in a lower percentage of patients. Measurement of autoantibodies is particularly helpful in patients with isolated primary adrenal insufficiency and no family history of autoimmune disease. In APS 2, autoimmune adrenalitis may be associated with autoimmune thyroid disease or type 1 diabetes and screening for concomitant disease should involve measurements of thyrotropin and fasting glucose but not of other organ-related antibodies.

In male patients with isolated primary adrenal insufficiency without unequivocal evidence of autoimmune adrenalitis, serum very long chain fatty acids (chain length of 24 carbons and more; C26, C26/C22, and C24/C22 ratios) should be measured to exclude adrenoleucodystrophy/adrenomyeloneuropathy.

Diagnosis secondary adrenal insufficiency

Baseline hormone measurements only poorly separate patients with secondary adrenal insufficiency from normal subjects. However, a morning cortisol below 100 nmol/l indicates adrenal insufficiency whereas a serum cortisol greater than 500 mmol/l is consistent with an intact HPA axis. Thus in most cases dynamic tests of the HPA axis are required to establish the diagnosis of secondary adrenal insufficiency.

The insulin tolerance test (ITT) is still regarded as the 'gold standard' in the evaluation of suspected secondary adrenal insufficiency, as hypoglycaemia (blood glucose <2.2 mmol/l) is a powerful stressor resulting in rapid activation of the HPA axis. An intact HPA axis is demonstrated by a peak cortisol above 500 nmol/l at any time during the test. The occasional patient will pass the ITT while exhibiting clinical evidence for adrenal insufficiency responding to hydrocortisone substitution and a higher cut-off value (550 nmol/l) may help to reduce misclassification. During ITT close supervision is mandatory and cardiovascular disease and history of seizures represent contraindications.

Another test for the diagnosis of secondary adrenal insufficiency is the overnight metyrapone test (30 mg metyrapone/kg (maximum 3 g) with a snack at midnight). Metyrapone inhibits adrenal 11β-hydroxylase, i.e. the conversion of 11-deoxycortisol to cortisol. In normal subjects, HPA feedback activation will increase serum 11-deoxycortisol, while serum cortisol remains less

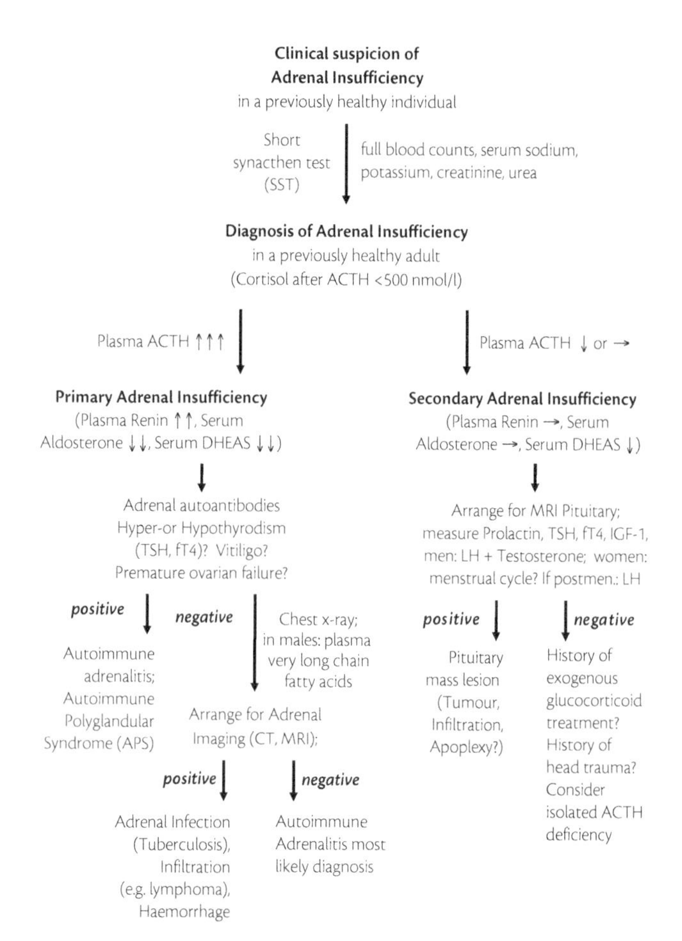

Fig. 5.9.4 Flowchart outlining the steps to be taken for the diagnostic management of adults with newly diagnosed adrenal insufficiency. DHEAS, dehydroepiandrosterone sulphate ester; IGF-1, insulin-like growth factor 1; LH, luteinizing hormone; TSH, thyroid-stimulating hormone.

than 230 nmol/l. In patients with secondary adrenal insufficiency, 11-deoxycortisol does not exceed 200 nmol/l at 8.00 hours after metyrapone. Shortcomings of the test are limited availability of reliable 11-deoxycortisol assays and of the drug itself, which cannot be obtained in all countries though it is readily available in the UK. As metyrapone may precipitate adrenal crisis in severe cortisol deficiency, a morning cortisol above 200 nmol/l should be documented prior to performing the test on an outpatient basis.

As both the ITT and the metapyrone test pose a significant burden to patients and physicians, there have been continuing efforts to replace these tests by more convenient tools. Sustained secondary adrenal insufficiency leads to adrenal atrophy and also to reduced adrenal ACTH receptor expression, as ACTH up-regulates its own receptor. Thus adrenal responsiveness to an acute exogenous ACTH challenge is impaired also in secondary adrenal insufficiency facilitating the use of the SST for the evaluation of HPA axis integrity (Fig. 5.9.4). Several studies have reported excellent agreement between peak cortisol values in SST and in ITT (13) and a recent study has convincingly demonstrated the long-term predictive accuracy of the SST (12). However, there is some evidence that some patients with secondary adrenal insufficiency will pass the SST while failing the ITT. The use of a higher cut-off value (600 nmol/l) for passing the SST may minimize the risk of overlooking secondary adrenal insufficiency but this is largely assay dependent as different radioimmunoassays will have different cut-offs. Our traditional cut-offs are certain to undergo changes in the imminent future with the introduction of more specific tandem mass spectrometry for the measurement of serum cortisol.

There are other tests that have been used in the diagnostic assessment of adrenal insufficiency but whose use is not recommended as a routine procedure. As the administration of 250 μg 1–24 ACTH represents a massive supraphysiological challenge, a low-dose corticotropin test (LDT) employing only 1 μg ACTH has been proposed as a more sensitive test for the diagnosis of secondary adrenal insufficiency. The LDT has been successfully used to monitor recovery of adrenal function after withdrawal of oral glucocorticoids and to detect subtle impairment of adrenal reserve during inhalative steroid therapy. However, the administration of 1 μg ACTH IV still results in ACTH levels above those required for maximum cortisol release. Accordingly, in normal subjects serum cortisol concentrations measured 30 min after the ACTH challenge do not differ between SST and LDT. Thus it is currently a matter of debate whether employing the LDT represents any advantage (16, 17), which would be further offset by handling problems due to the necessity of dilution from the commercially available 250 μg ACTH 1–24 ampoule and due to the potential binding of ACTH to the surface of injection devices.

CRH has been used to differentiate hypothalamic from pituitary disease in secondary adrenal insufficiency. However, CRH stimulation is not of great help in actually diagnosing secondary AI as individual responses to exogenous CRH are highly variable and cut-off values or even normal ranges are still not well defined.

Finally, a word of caution: none of the tests, including the ITT, will classify all patients correctly. Mild secondary adrenal insufficiency may pass as intact HPA axis and some healthy subjects may fail any single test by a small margin. Thus clinical judgement remains important. Persisting symptoms such as fatigue, myalgia, or reduced vitality should lead to reassessment.

Special diagnostic situations

Adrenal insufficiency after pituitary surgery

Screening for adrenal insufficiency by SST should not be performed immediately after pituitary surgery, but only 4 to 6 weeks later, as adrenal atrophy may develop only gradually after onset of ACTH deficiency. Until then, patients with a morning cortisol not excluding secondary adrenal insufficiency (<450 nmol/l at 3 days and <350 nmol/l at 7 days after surgery) should receive hydrocortisone replacement paused 24 h prior to scheduled adrenal function testing. The impairment of other hormonal axes after pituitary surgery increases the likelihood of ACTH deficiency, whereas isolated corticotropin deficiency is uncommon.

Adrenal insufficiency in critically ill patients

In critically ill patients the corticotropic axis is markedly activated (18, 19). Moreover, patients in intensive care units are less sensitive to dexamethasone suppression and achieve higher peak ACTH and cortisol concentrations after CRH. In addition, patients with critical illness show relatively low serum aldosterone levels with concurrently elevated plasma renin activity. Cortisol concentrations correlate with illness-severity scores and are highest in patients with the highest mortality. On the other hand, cytokine activation may induce relative secondary adrenal insufficiency in some patients with severe illness, thus putting them at risk of dying from adrenal crisis. Chronic inhibition of cortisol production by etomidate has been associated with increased mortality in intensive care unit patients. Unfortunately, no consensus exists how to diagnose adrenal insufficiency in critically ill patients. In patients with primary adrenal insufficiency or severe secondary adrenal insufficiency the SST will establish the diagnosis by demonstrating a low baseline cortisol (<165 nmol/l) not responding to corticotropin (peak cortisol <500 nmol/l). However, it has been suggested that 'relative' adrenal insufficiency may be present in a number of critically ill patients, characterized by a poor cortisol response (increment <248 nmol/l) to ACTH despite normal baseline cortisol. These patients often present with catecholamine-dependent hypodynamic shock responding to hydrocortisone administration. One study has reported decreased mortality in patients with septic shock and abnormal cortisol response in the SST (increment <248 nmol/l) after treatment with hydrocortisone (20) but a prospective study did not support this finding (21). At present it seems prudent to collect a random sample of serum cortisol and plasma ACTH in critically ill patients with suspected adrenal insufficiency followed by immediate hydrocortisone administration. Depending on the results of these hormone determinations (serum cortisol >700 nmol/l rules out adrenal insufficiency) hydrocortisone therapy is terminated or a more detailed evaluation employing the SST is performed.

Imaging requirements in adrenal insufficiency

If there is no coexisting autoimmune disease and adrenal and steroid autoantibodies are negative, imaging of the adrenals, preferably by CT, is warranted (Fig. 5.9.4). Tuberculosis should be considered, which is frequent in developing countries and therefore also in migrant populations. Chest radiography is helpful and imaging of the adrenals typically shows hyperplastic organs in the early phase and spotty calcifications in the late phase of tuberculous adrenalitis. Much rarer causes are bilateral infiltration by bilateral primary adrenal lymphoma, (predominantly lung cancer) metastases (22, 23), sarcoidosis, haemochromatosis, or amyloidosis. Bilateral adrenal haemorrhage is usually only seen during septic shock or in very rare instances in primary antiphospholipid syndrome (24). In male patients with isolated Addison's and negative autoantibodies, imaging should be preceded by measurement of plasma very long chain fatty acids to safely exclude X-linked adrenoleucodystrophy which affects 1 in 20 000 males (25). *ABCD1* gene mutations encoding for the peroxisomal ALD protein involved in cross-membrane transport manifest in 50% of cases in early childhood and primarily with CNS symptoms. However, the adrenomyoeloneuropathy variant, accounting for 35% of cases, can manifest with adrenal insufficiency prior to the development of spinal paraparesis during early adulthood (25).

If ACTH is inappropriately low in the presence of cortisol deficiency, imaging of the hypothalamic–pituitary region by MRI is the first diagnostic measure that should be arranged for, alongside an endocrine pituitary baseline profile (Fig. 5.9.4). Pituitary adenomas are most common, craniopharyngiomas are much rarer and may present at any age; very rare causes include meningioma, metastases, and infiltration by sarcoidosis, Langerhans' cell histiocytosis, or other granulomatous disease. Careful history taking should ask for previous head trauma (26, 27), surgery, radiotherapy, and for clinical indicators of pituitary apoplexy (28), i.e. the sudden onset of high-impact headache (29). The latter may occur spontaneously in larger pituitary adenomas or may result from sudden hypocirculation during surgery or as a consequence of complicated deliveries with significant blood loss, the classical cause of Sheehan's syndrome. Lymphocytic hypophysitis of autoimmune origin (30) commonly presents with panhypopititarism including diabetes insipidus and a pituitary mass effect. However, it may present with isolated ACTH deficiency, in some cases coinciding with autoimmune thyroid disease (31, 32).

Importantly, the most obvious should not be forgotten—suppression of the hypothalamic–pituitary axis by exogenous glucocorticoid treatment. This should always be excluded, considering not only oral steroid intake but also glucocorticoid inhalers, creams, or intra-articular injections.

Treatment of adrenal insufficiency

Glucocorticoid replacement

A patient with suspected acute adrenal insufficiency certainly needs immediate therapeutic attention, with signs and symptoms very suggestive of adrenal insufficiency including patchy hyperpigmentation of the oral mucosa and the presence of severe hypovolaemic hypotension. If peripheral veins are collapsed, a central line for IV fluid resuscitation may be required, administered at an initial rate of 1 l/h and with continuous cardiac monitoring. In addition, hydrocortisone replacement should be commenced by intravenous injection of 100 mg hydrocortisone followed by continuous infusion of 150 mg hydrocortisone in 5% glucose per 24 h. Mineralocorticoid replacement does not need to be added in the acute setting as long as the total daily hydrocortisone dose is greater than 50 mg as such a dose will ensure sufficient mineralocorticoid receptor activation by cortisol.

Chronic glucocorticoid replacement requires additional considerations. Physiological daily cortisol production rates vary between 5 and 10 mg/m^2 (33), which is equivalent to the oral administration of 15 to 25 mg hydrocortisone, i.e. cortisol. After oral ingestion cortisol produces highly variable peak concentrations within the supraphysiological range followed by a rapid decline to below 100 nmol/l 5 to 7 h after ingestion (Fig. 5.9.5). I usually recommend the administration of hydrocortisone in two to three divided doses, e.g. 15 mg in the morning upon awakening followed by 5 mg 6 h later, or 10 mg upon awakening followed by 5 mg 4 h and 8 h later. It is important to let the patient experiment with different timings to find the most suitable regimen for his individual needs.

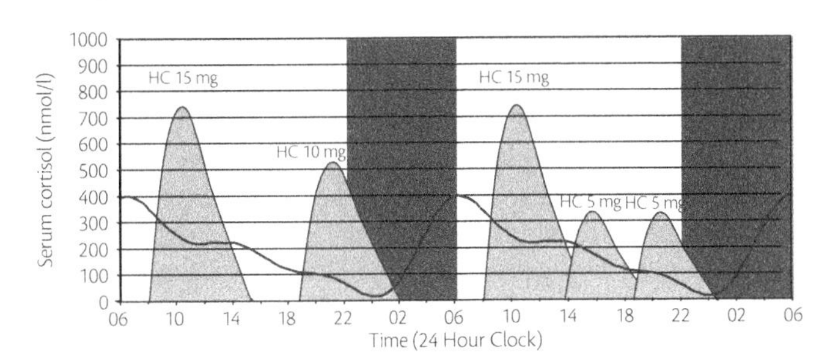

Fig. 5.9.5 Schematic graph depicting the physiological diurnal rhythm of cortisol secretion and typical mean serum cortisol concentrations observed after different doses of oral hydrocortisone (HC) in patients with adrenal insufficiency.

Importantly, patients who work shifts have to adjust the timing of the glucocorticoid doses to their working times and subsequent sleep–wake cycle. Whether a thrice daily glucocorticoid regimen should be preferred over twice daily administration is not clear as well-designed and appropriately powered studies are lacking. As Fig. 5.9.5 clearly illustrates, neither of the two regimens will be able to achieve cortisol availability similar to that of physiological diurnal secretion. Some groups advocate weight-related dosing (34) and this appears to generate a smoother pharmacokinetic profile but data demonstrating superiority of such a regimen are lacking. However, body surface area adjusted glucocorticoid dosing is commonly used for guiding glucocorticoid replacement in children.

The oral administration of currently available cortisol preparations is not able to mimic the physiological pattern of cortisol secretion, which follows a distinct circadian rhythm. Cortisol secretion begins to rise between 02.00 and 04.00 hours, peaks within an hour of waking and then declines gradually to low levels during the evening and nadir levels at and after midnight (35). There is evidence for a diurnal variability in glucocorticoid sensitivity. Plat *et al.* (36) have demonstrated that a more unfavourable metabolic response occurs to evening administration of hydrocortisone. Also, high levels of glucocorticoids may disrupt sleep, thus late evening hydrocortisone administration should be avoided; sleep disturbances contributing to increased fatigue are a common feature in chronic adrenal insufficiency (37, 38).The delivery of cortisol by intravenous infusion (39) or subcutaneous pump (40) can closely mirror diurnal secretion, but these administration modes are obviously not suited for routine delivery. Recently developed modified and delayed release hydrocortisone preparations mimicking physiological cortisol secretion represent a very promising therapeutic approach (41, 42).

Cortisone acetate requires intrahepatic activation to cortisol by 11β-hydroxysteroid dehydrogenase 1, which contributes to a higher pharmacokinetic variability compared to hydrocortisone; 25 mg cortisone acetate are equivalent to 15 mg hydrocortisone (43, 44). Long-acting glucocorticoids are also used for replacement, e.g. in 20% of respondents to the 2002 survey of the North American Addison Disease Foundation. Some countries do not have access to hydrocortisone or cortisone acetate and therefore have to resort to long-acting synthetic glucocorticoids. However, prednisolone and dexamethasone have considerably longer biological half-lives, likely to result in unfavourably high night-time glucocorticoid activity with potentially detrimental effects on insulin sensitivity and bone mineral density (45). In addition, available preparations offer limited options for dose titration. Therefore I generally recommend against the use of synthetic glucocorticoids for replacement therapy in adrenal insufficiency; the only exception are patients with concurrent insulin-dependent diabetes in whom prednisolone may help to avoid the peaks and troughs of hydrocortisone pharmacokinetics and thus also subsequent rapid changes in glucose control. For clinical purposes, I assume equipotency to 1 mg hydrocortisone for 1.6 mg cortisone acetate, 0.2 mg prednisolone, 0.25 mg prednisone, and 0.025 mg dexamethasone, respectively. While equipotency doses of hydrocortisone and cortisone acetate are based on pharmacokinetic studies (43, 44), suggested doses for synthetic steroids are based on estimates from older studies comparing the relative anti-inflammatory properties of various glucocorticoids.

Monitoring of glucocorticoid replacement is mainly based on clinical grounds as a reliable biomarker for glucocorticoid activity has yet to be identified (Table 5.9.4). Plasma ACTH cannot be used as a criterion for glucocorticoid dose adjustment. In primary adrenal insufficiency, ACTH is invariably high before the morning dose and rapidly declines with increasing cortisol levels after glucocorticoid ingestion (46, 47) (Fig. 5.9.6a). Aiming at ACTH levels within the normal range would therefore invariably result in over-replacement. In secondary adrenal insufficiency, plasma ACTH is anyway low and thus not informative. Urinary 24-h free cortisol excretion has been advocated for monitoring of replacement quality (48). However, after exogenous glucocorticoid administration, urinary cortisol excretion shows considerable interindividual variability. Also, following glucocorticoid absorption cortisol-binding globulin is rapidly saturated, resulting in transient but pronounced increases in renal cortisol excretion. Thus, one cannot refer to normal ranges for healthy subjects when judging urinary cortisol excretion during replacement therapy for adrenal insufficiency. Some authors have suggested regular measurements of serum cortisol day curves to monitor replacement therapy (48, 49). However, the efficacy of this approach is not supported by controlled studies and recent data indicate a poor correlation between clinical assessment and cortisol levels (50). Timed serum cortisol measurements can be of some value in selected patients, e.g. in case of suspected noncompliance or malabsorption; however, random serum cortisol measurements without information on the time of the hydrocortisone dose are not informative.

Thus, in the absence of objective parameters, the physician has to rely primarily on clinical judgment, carefully taking into account signs and symptoms potentially suggestive of glucocorticoid over- or under-replacement, recognizing their relative lack of specificity. Glucocorticoid under-replacement bears the risk of incipient crisis and significant impairment of well-being. Conversely, chronic over-replacement may lead to substantial morbidity including impaired glucose tolerance, obesity and osteoporosis. An increased incidence of osteoporosis has only been reported in patients receiving daily replacement doses of 30 mg hydrocortisone or higher (45, 51, 52) or 7.5 mg prednisone (45) whereas appropriate replacement doses of 20–25 mg hydrocortisone do not affect bone mineral density (50, 53). Therefore, bone mineral density measurements are not routinely required in patients with adrenal insufficiency receiving recommended glucocorticoid replacement doses.

Mineralocorticoid replacement

Patients with primary adrenal insufficiency require mineralocorticoid replacement, which usually consists of the oral administration of 9α-fludrocortisone; fluorination at the 9α position ensures selective binding to the MR and thus exclusive mineralocorticoid action. By contrast, cortisol binds with equal affinity to both the GR and MR. However, excessive MR binding of cortisol in the kidney is prevented by 11β-hydroxysteroid dehydrogenase type 2, which inactivates cortisol to cortisone. Oelkers has coined the term 'mineralocorticoid unit' (MCU), determining that 100 MCU are equivalent to 100 μg fludrocortisone and 40 mg hydrocortisone, respectively (54). By contrast, prednisolone exerts only reduced and dexamethasone no mineralocorticoid activity at all; therefore patients treated with synthetic glucocorticoids need particularly careful monitoring of their mineralocorticoid replacement.

Table 5.9.4 Treatment and monitoring in chronic adrenal insufficiency

Chronic adrenal insufficiency	
Glucocorticoid replacement	Primary adrenal insufficiency: 20–25 mg hydrocortisone per 24 h
	Secondary adrenal insufficiency: 15–20 mg hydrocortisone per 24 h; if borderline fail in cosyntropin test consider 10 mg or stress dose cover only
	Administer in 2–3 divided doses with two-thirds and half of the dose, respectively, administered immediately after awakening
	Monitoring: ◆ Check body weight, calculate body mass index ◆ Check for signs of underreplacement (weight loss, fatigue, nausea, myalgia, lack of energy) ◆ Check for signs of overreplacement (weight gain, central obesity, stretch marks, osteopenia/osteoporosis, impaired glucose tolerance, hypertension) ◆ Take a detailed account of stress-related glucocorticoid dose self-adjustments since last visit, potential adverse events including emergency treatment and/or hospitalization
Mineralocorticoid replacement	Only required in primary adrenal insufficiency
	Not required as long as hydrocortisone dose >50 mg per 24 h
	Start on 100 μg fludrocortisone (doses vary between 50 and 250 μg per 24 h) administered as a single dose in the morning immediately after waking up
	Monitoring: ◆ Blood pressure sitting and erect (postural drop ≥15 mm Hg indicative of underreplacement, high blood pressure may indicate overreplacement) ◆ Check for peripheral oedema (indicative of overreplacement) ◆ Check serum sodium and potassium ◆ Check plasma renin activity (at least every 2–3 years, upon clinical suspicion of over- and underreplacement and after significant changes in the hydrocortisone dose (40 mg hydrocortisone = 100 μg fludrocortisone)
Adrenal androgen replacement	Consider in patients with impaired well-being and mood despite apparently optimized glucocorticoid and mineralocorticoid replacement and in women with symptoms and signs of androgen deficiency (dry, itchy skin; reduced libido)
	DHEA 25–50 mg as a single morning dose
	If no perceived benefit after 6 months, consider stopping
	Monitoring: ◆ In women, serum testosterone and SHBG (to calculate free androgen index) ◆ In men and women on DHEA replacement, serum DHEAS and androstenedione levels ◆ Blood should be sampled at steady state, i.e. 12–24 h after the preceding DHEA dose
Additional monitoring requirements	Regular follow-up in specialist centre every 6–12 months
	In primary adrenal insufficiency of autoimmune origin (isolated Addison or autoimmune polyglandular syndrome) serum TSH every 12 months
	In female patients: check regularity of menstrual cycle, consider measurement of ovarian autoantibodies if family planning not finalized
	Check emergency bracelet/steroid card, update as required
	Check knowledge of 'sick day rules' and reinforce emergency guidelines involving partner/family members
	Consider prescription of a hydrocortisone emergency self-injection kit, in particular if delayed access to acute medical care is likely (rural areas, travel)
	Check if other medication includes drugs known to induce (e.g. rifampicin, mitotane, anticonvulsants such as phenytoin, carbamazepine, oxcarbazepine, phenobarbital, topiramate) or inhibit (e.g. antiretroviral agents) hepatic cortisol inactivation by CYP3A4, which may require glucocorticoid dose adjustment

DHEA, dehydroepiandrosterone; SHBG, sex hormon-binding hormone; TSH, thyroid-stimulating hormone.

In the newly diagnosed patient, mineralocorticoid replacement should be initiated at 100 μg once daily; optimized doses may vary between 50 and 250 μg. Children, in particular neonates and infants, have considerably higher mineralocorticoid dose requirements and often need additional salt supplementation. However, also amongst adults there is a good degree of interindividual variability. A high dietary salt intake may slightly reduce mineralocorticoid requirements. An important additional factor is temperature and humidity, e.g. individuals living in Mediterranean summer or tropical climates will require a 50% increase in fludrocortisone dose due to increased salt loss through perspiration. Monitoring (Table 5.9.4) includes supine and erect blood pressure and serum sodium and potassium; plasma renin activity should be checked regularly, aiming at the upper normal range (54). If essential hypertension develops, mineralocorticoid dose may be slightly reduced, accompanied by monitoring of serum sodium and potassium, but complete cessation of mineralocorticoid replacement should be avoided. It is important to recognize that plasma renin

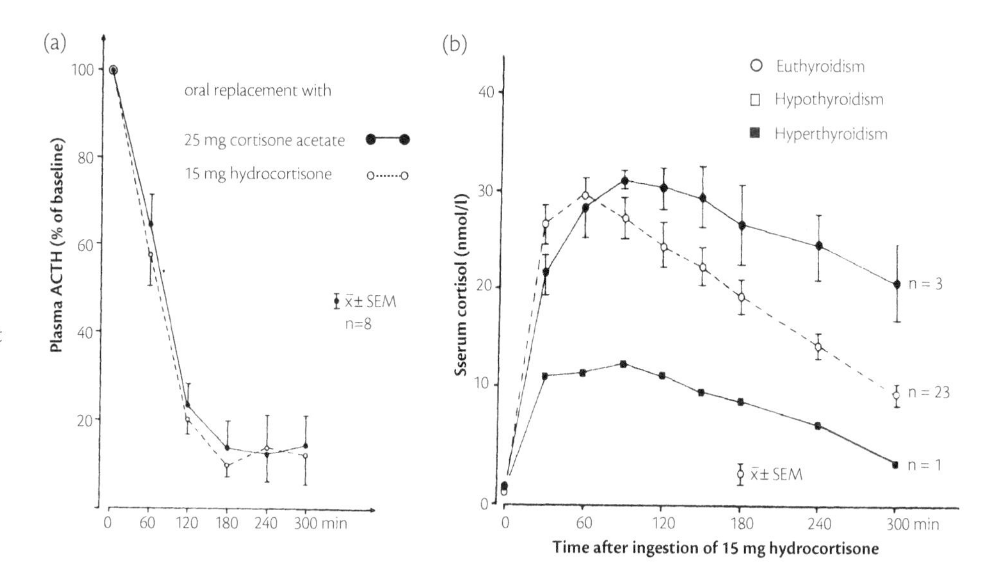

Fig. 5.9.6 (a) Plasma ACTH concentrations before and after administration of the hydrocortisone morning dose in patients with primary adrenal insufficiency (n = 8). (b) Serum cortisol and thyroid function. Serum cortisol concentrations after administration of 15 mg hydrocortisone orally in 27 patients with primary adrenal insufficiency. Patients with concurrent overt hypothyroidism (n = 3) or hyperthyroidism (n = 1) differ from euthyroid patients (n = 23), which has to be considered when choosing appropriate glucocorticoid replacement doses. Modified from Allolio *et al.*, *Akt Endokr Stoffw*, 1985: **6**: 35–39.

physiologically increases during pregnancy; therefore, monitoring in pregnancy should comprise blood pressure, serum sodium and potassium, and, if required, urinary sodium excretion. During the last term of pregnancy fludrocortisone dose may require adjustment, also due to increased progesterone levels exerting antimineralocorticoid activity (55).

Prevention of adrenal crisis

Risk of adrenal crisis is higher in primary adrenal insufficiency and several factors such as coincident APS or age have been suggested as additional modifiers (2, 56). Many crises are due to glucocorticoid dose reduction or lack of stress-related glucocorticoid dose adjustment by patients or general practitioners (2). A recent survey in 526 patients found that 42% of patients (47% in primary adrenal insufficiency, 35% in secondary adrenal insufficiency) had experienced at least one adrenal crisis during the course of their disease. Precipitating causes were mainly gastrointestinal infections and fever but also several other causes, including major pain, surgery, psychological distress, heat, and pregnancy. This was corroborated by data from a large patient survey (n = 841) (57) that also highlighted gastrointestinal infections as the single most important cause of crisis. Thus adrenal crises are a predictable and frequent, but still undermanaged event and crisis prevention is a key strategy that needs to be pursued.

All patients and their partners should receive regular crisis prevention training, including verification of steroid emergency card/bracelet and instruction on stress-related glucocorticoid dose adjustment (Table 5.9.4). Generally, hydrocortisone should be doubled during intercurrent illness, such as a respiratory infection with fever, until clinical recovery. Gastrointestinal infections, a frequent cause of crisis, may require parenteral hydrocortisone administration,. Preferably all patients, but at least patients travelling or living in areas with limited access to acute medical care should receive a hydrocortisone emergency self-injection kit (e.g. 100 mg for IM injection). For major surgery, trauma, delivery, and diseases requiring intensive care unit monitoring, patients should receive intravenous administration of 100–150 mg hydrocortisone per 24 h in 5% glucose or 25–50 mg hydrocortisone IM four times per day. Some authors have advocated lower doses (25–75 mg/24 h) for surgical stress (58). However, 60 years after the seminal observation that glucocorticoid replacement needs to be increased during periods of major stress (59) studies clarifying exact dose requirements are still outstanding.

DHEA replacement

The introduction of DHEA, the third major steroid produced by the adrenal gland, into the replacement regimen for adrenal insufficiency (60) represents a major advance, in particular for women who are invariably androgen deficient (60, 61). DHEA has been shown to significantly enhance well-being, mood, and subjective health status in women with primary and secondary adrenal insufficiency (60, 62–65) and also recently in children and adolescents with adrenal failure (66). Similar effects have been described for testosterone replacement in hypopituitarism (67), however, no study has yet directly compared DHEA to testosterone. In addition to acting as an androgen precursor, DHEA has neurosteroidal properties, exerting a primarily antidepressive effect, and also shows immunemodulatory properties (68). Of note, DHEA has been shown to exert beneficial effects on subjective health status and energy levels not only in women but also in men with primary adrenal insufficiency (63, 64) including significant beneficial effects on bone mineral density and truncal lean mass (63).

Currently, DHEA replacement is hampered by the lack of pharmaceutically controlled preparations, with questionable quality and content of several over-the-counter preparations (69). At present, DHEA should be reserved for patients with adrenal insufficiency suffering from significant impairment in well-being despite otherwise optimized replacement, in particular women with signs of androgen deficiency such as dry and itchy skin and loss of libido. DHEA should be taken as a single dose (25–50 mg) in the morning. Treatment monitoring (Table 5.9.4) should include blood sampling 24 h after the last preceding morning dose for measurement of serum DHEAS (in women also androstenedione, testosterone, sex hormone-binding hormone) aiming at the middle normal range for healthy young subjects. I usually start patients on 25 mg and increase to 50 mg after 2 to 4 weeks, advising them to halve the dose if androgenic skin side effects (greasy skin, spots) persist for more than a week. Obviously, transdermal testosterone represents an alternative androgen replacement tool in women with adrenal failure.

Special therapeutic situations impacting on corticosteroid replacement

Thyroid dysfunction

Hyperthyroidism results in increased cortisol metabolism and clearance and hypothyroidism the converse, principally due to an effect of thyroid hormone upon hepatic 11β-HSD1 and 5α/5β-reductases. Insulin-like growth factor 1 (IGF-1) increases cortisol clearance by inhibiting hepatic 11β-HSD1 (conversion of cortisone to cortisol). In patients with adrenal insufficiency and unresolved hyperthyroidism, glucocorticoid replacement should be doubled to tripled. To avoid adrenal crisis, thyroxine replacement for hypothyroidism should only be initiated after concomitant glucocorticoid deficiency has either been excluded or treated. Obviously overt endogenous hyperthyroidism will also increase hydrocortisone metabolism (Fig. 5.9.6b). Therefore, the initiation of glucocorticoid replacement in patients with newly diagnosed hypopituitarism should always precede the initiation of thyroxine replacement as the reverse might precipitate adrenal crisis.

Pregnancy

Pregnancy is physiologically associated with a gradual increase in CBG and during the last term of pregnancy also with an increase in free cortisol. In addition, serum progesterone increases, exerting antimineralocorticoid action. Therefore, during the third trimester, hydrocortisone replacement should be increased by 50%. Plasma renin activity cannot serve as a monitoring tool because it physiologically increases during pregnancy. Peripartal hydrocortisone replacement should follow the requirements for major surgery, i.e. 100 mg/24 h starting with labour until 48 h after delivery, followed by rapid tapering.

Concomitant drug therapy and interactions

When deciding on the glucocorticoid dose, it is important to consider concurrent medication, in particular drugs known to increase hepatic glucocorticoid metabolism by CYP3A4 induction, which results in increased 6β-hydroxylation and hence cortisol inactivation (2, 3). 6β-hydroxylation by CYP3A4 is normally a minor pathway but cortisol itself induces CYP3A4 so that 6β-hydroxycortisol excretion is markedly increased in patients with Cushing's syndrome. A multitude of drugs are known to induce CYP3A4 (Table 5.9.1), which require a two- to threefold increase in glucocorticoid dose. Conversely, the intake of drugs inhibiting CYP3A4 would require reduction of glucocorticoid replacement dose.

Of note, treatment of tuberculosis with rifampicin increases cortisol clearance but does not influence aldosterone clearance. Thus, glucocorticoid replacement should be doubled during rifampicin treatment. Mitotane (o,p′DDD, *ortho*, *para′*, dichlorodiphenyl-dichloroethane) decreases bioavailable glucocorticoid levels due to an increase in CBG and concurrently enhanced glucocorticoid metabolism following induction of CYP3A4. During chronic mitotane treatment, e.g. in adrenal carcinoma (70), usual glucocorticoid replacement doses should therefore be at least tripled.

Quality of life, disablement, and prognosis in adrenal insufficiency

Recent data demonstrate that current standard replacement fails to restore quality of life, which is significantly impaired in both patients with primary and secondary adrenal insufficiency (37, 71), with no apparent difference between prednisolone and hydrocortisone-treated patients (72). Predominant complaints are fatigue, lack of energy, depression, anxiety, and reduced ability to cope with daily demands; the degree of impairment is comparable to that observed in congestive heart failure and chronic haemodialysis patients (37, 71). Subjective health status is most reduced in younger patients but all age groups are significantly impaired (71), a persistent finding even if only analysing patients without any comorbidity (71) This also has a socioeconomic perspective as patients with Addison's disease have a two- to threefold higher likelihood of receiving disablement pensions (37, 71).

In addition, large cohort studies have demonstrated an increased mortality not only in patients with secondary adrenal insufficiency due to hypopituitarism (73) but also in primary adrenal insufficiency, i.e. Addison's disease (74, 75), a finding still valid when the influence of comorbidities is excluded. The causes underlying this increased mortality remain unclear, but we certainly need to consider the possible impact of current replacement regimens on the observed increase in mortality from cardiovascular and cerebrovascular disease and respiratory infections.

Conclusions

More than 150 years after Thomas Addison first described a disease characterized by salt wasting and hyperpigmentation as the result of adrenal gland destruction (1), adrenal insufficiency is no longer an invariably fatal condition. The landmark achievement of the synthesis of cortisone in the late 1940s and its introduction into therapy in the early 1950s quickly lead to widespread availability of life-saving glucocorticoid replacement therapy. However, while initial survival is routinely achieved nowadays, current replacement regimens may not be able to achieve normal quality of life. Future research has to uncover the causes underlying the increased mortality in adrenal insufficiency and should further explore the role of novel replacement modalities, such as DHEA and modified-release hydrocortisone.

References

1. Addison T. *On the Constitutional and Local Effects of Diseases of the Supra-Renal Capsules*. London: Warren and Son, 1855.
2. Arlt W, Allolio B. Adrenal insufficiency. *Lancet*, 2003; **361** (9372): 1881–93.
3. Bornstein SR. Predisposing factors for adrenal insufficiency. *N Engl J Med*, 2009; **360**: 2328–39.
4. Betterle C, Dal PC, Mantero F, Zanchetta R. Autoimmune adrenal insufficiency and autoimmune polyendocrine syndromes: autoantibodies, autoantigens, and their applicability in diagnosis and disease prediction. *Endocr Rev*, 2002; **23**: 327–64.
5. Ahonen P, Myllarniemi S, Sipila I, Perheentupa J. Clinical variation of autoimmune polyendocrinopathy-candidiasis-ectodermal dystrophy (APECED) in a series of 68 patients. *N Engl J Med*, 1990; **322**: 1829–36.
6. Finnish-German APECED Consortium. An autoimmune disease, APECED, caused by mutations in a novel gene featuring two PHD-type zinc-finger domains. *Nat Genet*, 1997; **17**: 399–403.
7. Nagamine K, Peterson P, Scott HS, Kudoh J, Minoshima S, Heino M, *et al*. Positional cloning of the APECED gene. *Nat Genet*, 1997; **17**: 393–8.
8. Mathis D, Benoist C. A decade of AIRE. *Nat Rev Immunol*, 2007; **7**: 645–50.
9. Kemp EH, Ajjan RA, Husebye ES, Peterson P, Uibo R, Imrie H, *et al*. A cytotoxic T lymphocyte antigen-4 (CTLA-4) gene polymorphism is associated with autoimmune Addison's disease in English patients. *Clin Endocrinol (Oxf)*, 1998; **49**: 609–13.

10. Skinningsrud B, Husebye ES, Gervin K, L vås K, Blomhoff A, Wolff AB, *et al.* Mutation screening of PTPN22: association of the 1858T-allele with Addison's disease. *Eur J Hum Genet*, 2008; **16**: 977–82.
11. Skinningsrud B, Husebye ES, Pearce SH, McDonald DO, Brandal K, Wolff AB, *et al.* Polymorphisms in CLEC16A and CIITA at 16p13 are associated with primary adrenal insufficiency. *J Clin Endocrinol Metab*, 2008; **93**: 3310–17.
12. Agha A, Tomlinson JW, Clark PM, Holder G, Stewart PM. The long-term predictive accuracy of the short synacthen (corticotropin) stimulation test for assessment of the hypothalamic-pituitary-adrenal axis. *J Clin Endocrinol Metab*, 2006; **91**: 43–7.
13. Stewart PM, Corrie J, Seckl JR, Edwards CR, Padfield PL. A rational approach for assessing the hypothalamo-pituitary-adrenal axis. *Lancet*, 1988; **1** (8596): 1208–10.
14. Clark PM, Neylon I, Raggatt PR, Sheppard MC, Stewart PM. Defining the normal cortisol response to the short Synacthen test: implications for the investigation of hypothalamic-pituitary disorders. *Clin Endocrinol (Oxf)*, 1998; **49**: 287–92.
15. Inder WJ, Hunt PJ. Glucocorticoid replacement in pituitary surgery: guidelines for perioperative assessment and management. *J Clin Endocrinol Metab*, 2002; **87**: 2745–50.
16. Kazlauskaite R, Evans AT, Villabona CV, Abdu TA, Ambrosi B, Atkinson AB, *et al.* Corticotropin tests for hypothalamic-pituitary-adrenal insufficiency: a metaanalysis. *J Clin Endocrinol Metab*, 2008; **93**: 4245–53.
17. Stewart PM, Clark PM. The low-dose corticotropin-stimulation test revisited: the less, the better?. *Nat Clin Pract Endocrinol Metab*, 2009; **5**: 68–9.
18. Cooper MS, Stewart PM. Corticosteroid insufficiency in acutely ill patients. *N Engl J Med*, 2003; **348**: 727–34.
19. Marik PE, Pastores SM, Annane D, Meduri GU, Sprung CL, Arlt W, *et al.* Recommendations for the diagnosis and management of corticosteroid insufficiency in critically ill adult patients: consensus statements from an international task force by the American College of Critical Care Medicine. *Crit Care Med*, 2008; **36**: 1937–49.
20. Annane D, Sebille V, Charpentier C, Bollaert PE, François B, Korach JM, *et al.* Effect of treatment with low doses of hydrocortisone and fludrocortisone on mortality in patients with septic shock. *JAMA*, 2002; **288**: 862–71.
21. Sprung CL, Annane D, Keh D, Moreno R, Singer M, Freivogel K, *et al.* Hydrocortisone therapy for patients with septic shock. *N Engl J Med*, 2008; **358**: 111–24.
22. Lutz A, Stojkovic M, Schmidt M, Arlt W, Allolio B, Reincke M. Adrenocortical function in patients with macrometastases of the adrenal gland. *Eur J Endocrinol*, 2000; **143**: 91–7.
23. Lam KY, Lo CY. Metastatic tumours of the adrenal glands: a 30-year experience in a teaching hospital. *Clin Endocrinol (Oxf)*, 2002; **56**: 95–101.
24. Presotto F, Fornasini F, Betterle C, Federspil G, Rossato M. Acute adrenal failure as the heralding symptom of primary antiphospholipid syndrome: report of a case and review of the literature. *Eur J Endocrinol*, 2005; **153**: 507–14.
25. Moser HW, Mahmood A, Raymond GV. X-linked adrenoleukodystrophy. *Nat Clin Pract Neurol*, 2007; **3**: 140–51.
26. Agha A, Rogers B, Sherlock M, O'Kelly P, Tormey W, Phillips J, *et al.* Anterior pituitary dysfunction in survivors of traumatic brain injury. *J Clin Endocrinol Metab*, 2004; **89**: 4929–36.
27. Giordano G, Aimaretti G, Ghigo E. Variations of pituitary function over time after brain injuries: the lesson from a prospective study. *Pituitary*, 2005; **8**: 227–31.
28. Chanson P, Lepeintre JF, Ducreux D. Management of pituitary apoplexy. *Expert Opin Pharmacother*, 2004; **5**: 1287–98.
29. Schwedt TJ, Matharu MS, Dodick DW. Thunderclap headache. *Lancet Neurol*, 2006; **5**: 621–31.
30. Caturegli P, Lupi I, Landek-Salgado M, Kimura H, Rose NR. Pituitary autoimmunity: 30 years later. *Autoimmun Rev*, 2008; **7**: 631–7.
31. Kasperlik-Zaluska AA, Czarnocka B, Czech W. Autoimmunity as the most frequent cause of idiopathic secondary adrenal insufficiency: report of 111 cases. *Autoimmunity*, 2003; **36**: 155–9.
32. Manetti L, Lupi I, Morselli LL, Albertini S, Cosottini M, Grasso L, *et al.* Prevalence and functional significance of antipituitary antibodies in patients with autoimmune and non-autoimmune thyroid diseases. *J Clin Endocrinol Metab*, 2007; **92**: 2176–81.
33. Esteban NV, Loughlin T, Yergey AL, Zawadzki JK, Booth JD, Winterer JC, *et al.* Daily cortisol production rate in man determined by stable isotope dilution/mass spectrometry. *J Clin Endocrinol Metab*, 1991; **72**: 39–45.
34. Mah PM, Jenkins RC, Rostami-Hodjegan A, Newell-Price J, Doane A, Ibbotson V, *et al.* Weight-related dosing, timing and monitoring hydrocortisone replacement therapy in patients with adrenal insufficiency. *Clin Endocrinol (Oxf)*, 2004; **61**: 367–75.
35. Krieger DT, Allen W, Rizzo F, Krieger HP. Characterization of the normal temporal pattern of plasma corticosteroid levels. *J Clin Endocrinol Metab*, 1971; **32**: 266–84.
36. Plat L, Leproult R, L'Hermite-Baleriaux M, Fery F, Mockel J, Polonsky KS, *et al.* Metabolic effects of short-term elevations of plasma cortisol are more pronounced in the evening than in the morning. *J Clin Endocrinol Metab*, 1999; **84**: 3082–92.
37. Lovas K, Loge JH, Husebye ES. Subjective health status in Norwegian patients with Addison's disease. *Clin Endocrinol (Oxf)*, 2002; **56**: 581–8.
38. Lovas K, Husebye ES, Holsten F, Bjorvatn B. Sleep disturbances in patients with Addison's disease. *Eur J Endocrinol*, 2003; **148**: 449–56.
39. Merza Z, Rostami-Hodjegan A, Memmott A, Doane A, Ibbotson V, Newell-Price J, *et al.* Circadian hydrocortisone infusions in patients with adrenal insufficiency and congenital adrenal hyperplasia. *Clin Endocrinol (Oxf)*, 2006; **65**: 45–50.
40. Lovas K, Husebye ES. Continuous subcutaneous hydrocortisone infusion in Addison's disease. *Eur J Endocrinol*, 2007; **157**: 109–12.
41. Newell-Price J, Whiteman M, Rostami-Hodjegan A, Darzy K, Shalet S, Tucker GT, *et al.* Modified-release hydrocortisone for circadian therapy: a proof-of-principle study in dexamethasone-suppressed normal volunteers. *Clin Endocrinol (Oxf)*, 2008; 68: 130–5.
42. Debono M, Ross R, Newell-Price J. Inadequacies of glucocorticoid replacement and improvements by physiological circadian therapy. *Eur J Endocrinol*, 2009; 160: 719–29.
43. Allolio B, Kaulen D, Deuss U, Hipp FX, Winkelmann W. Comparison between hydrocortisone and cortisone acetate as replacement therapy in adrenocortical insufficiency. *Akt Endokr Stoffw*, 1985; **6**: 35–9.
44. Kehlet H, Binder C, Blichert-Toft M. Glucocorticoid maintenance therapy following adrenalectomy: assessment of dosage and preparation. *Clin Endocrinol (Oxf)*, 1976; **5**: 37–41.
45. Jodar E, Valdepenas MP, Martinez G, Jara A, Hawkins F. Long-term follow-up of bone mineral density in Addison's disease. *Clin Endocrinol (Oxf)*, 2003; **58**: 617–20.
46. Feek CM, Ratcliffe JG, Seth J, Gray CE, Toft AD, Irvine WJ. Patterns of plasma cortisol and ACTH concentrations in patients with Addison's disease treated with conventional corticosteroid replacement. *Clin Endocrinol (Oxf)*, 1981; **14**: 451–8.
47. Scott RS, Donald RA, Espiner EA. Plasma ACTH and cortisol profiles in Addisonian patients receiving conventional substitution therapy. *Clin Endocrinol (Oxf)*, 1978; **9**: 571–6.
48. Howlett TA. An assessment of optimal hydrocortisone replacement therapy. *Clin Endocrinol (Oxf)*, 1997; **46**: 263–8.
49. Peacey SR, Guo CY, Robinson AM, Price A, Giles MA, Eastell R, *et al.* Glucocorticoid replacement therapy: are patients over treated and does it matter?. *Clin Endocrinol (Oxf)*, 1997; **46**: 255–61.
50. Arlt W, Rosenthal C, Hahner S, Allolio B. Quality of glucocorticoid replacement in adrenal insufficiency: clinical assessment vs. timed serum cortisol measurements. *Clin Endocrinol (Oxf)*, 2006; **64**: 384–9.
51. Zelissen PM, Croughs RJ, van Rijk PP, Raymakers JA. Effect of glucocorticoid replacement therapy on bone mineral density in patients with Addison disease. *Ann Intern Med*, 1994; **120**: 207–10.

52. Florkowski CM, Holmes SJ, Elliot JR, Donald RA, Espiner EA. Bone mineral density is reduced in female but not male subjects with Addison's disease. *N Z Med J*, 1994; **107**: 52–3.
53. Braatvedt GD, Joyce M, Evans M, Clearwater J, Reid IR. Bone mineral density in patients with treated Addison's disease. *Osteoporos Int*, 1999; **10**: 435–40.
54. Oelkers W, Diederich S, Bahr V. Diagnosis and therapy surveillance in Addison's disease: rapid adrenocorticotropin (ACTH) test and measurement of plasma ACTH, renin activity, and aldosterone. *J Clin Endocrinol Metab*, 1992; **75**: 259–64.
55. Ehrlich EN, Lindheimer MD. Effect of administered mineralocorticoids or ACTH in pregnant women. Attenuation of kaliuretic influence of mineralocorticoids during pregnancy. *J Clin Invest*, 1972; **51**: 1301–9.
56. Erichsen MM, Lovas K, Fougner KJ, Svartberg J, Hauge ER, ollerslev J, *et al.* Normal overall mortality rate in Addison's disease, but young patients are at risk of premature death. *Eur J Endocrinol*, 2009; **160**: 233–7.
57. White K, Arlt W. Adrenal crisis in treated Addison's disease: a predictable but under-managed event. *Eur J Endocrinol*, 2010; **162**: 115–20.
58. Glowniak JV, Loriaux DL. A double-blind study of perioperative steroid requirements in secondary adrenal insufficiency. *Surgery*, 1997; **121**: 123–9.
59. Nicholas JA, Burstein CL, Umberger CJ, Wilson PD. Management of adrenocortical insufficiency during surgery. *AMA Arch Surg*, 1955; **71**: 737–42.
60. Arlt W, Callies F, van Vlijmen JC, Koehler I, Reincke M, Bidlingmaier M, *et al.* Dehydroepiandrosterone replacement in women with adrenal insufficiency. *N Engl J Med*, 1999; **341**: 1013–20.
61. Miller KK, Sesmilo G, Schiller A, Schoenfeld D, Burton S, Klibanski A. Androgen deficiency in women with hypopituitarism. *J Clin Endocrinol Metab*, 2001; **86**: 561–7.
62. Brooke AM, Kalingag LA, Miraki-Moud F, Camacho-Hübner C, Maher KT, Walker DM, *et al.* Dehydroepiandrosterone improves psychological well-being in male and female hypopituitary patients on maintenance growth hormone replacement. *J Clin Endocrinol Metab*, 2006; **91**: 3773–9.
63. Gurnell EM, Hunt PJ, Curran SE, Conway CL, Pullenayegum EM, Huppert FA, *et al.* Long-term DHEA replacement in primary adrenal insufficiency: a randomized, controlled trial. *J Clin Endocrinol Metab*, 2008; **93**: 400–9.
64. Hunt PJ, Gurnell EM, Huppert FA, Richards C, Prevost AT, Wass JA, *et al.* Improvement in mood and fatigue after dehydroepiandrosterone replacement in Addison's disease in a randomized, double blind trial. *J Clin Endocrinol Metab*, 2000; **85**: 4650–6.
65. Johannsson G, Burman P, Wiren L, Engström BE, Nilsson AG, Ottosson M, *et al.* Low dose dehydroepiandrosterone affects behavior in hypopituitary androgen-deficient women: a placebo-controlled trial. *J Clin Endocrinol Metab*, 2002; **87**: 2046–52.
66. Binder G, Weber S, Ehrismann M, Zaiser N, Meisner C, Ranke MB, *et al.* Effects of dehydroepiandrosterone therapy on pubic hair growth and psychological well-being in adolescent girls and young women with central adrenal insufficiency: a double-blind, randomised, placebo-controlled phase III trial. *J Clin Endocrinol Metab*, 2009; 94 : 1182–90.
67. Miller KK, Biller BM, Beauregard C, Lipman JG, Jones J, Schoenfeld D, *et al.* Effects of testosterone replacement in androgen-deficient women with hypopituitarism: a randomized, double-blind, placebo-controlled study. *J Clin Endocrinol Metab*, 2006; **91**: 1683–90.
68. Arlt W. Androgen therapy in women. *Eur J Endocrinol*, 2006; **154**: 1–11.
69. Parasrampuria J, Schwartz K, Petesch R. Quality control of dehydroepiandrosterone dietary supplement products. *JAMA*, 1998; **280**: 1565.
70. Hahner S, Fassnacht M. Mitotane for adrenocortical carcinoma treatment. *Curr Opin Investig Drugs*, 2005; **6**: 386–94.
71. Hahner S, Loeffler M, Fassnacht M, Weismann D, Koschker AC, Quinkler M, *et al.* Impaired subjective health status in 256 patients with adrenal insufficiency on standard therapy based on cross-sectional analysis. *J Clin Endocrinol Metab*, 2007; **92**: 3912–22.
72. Bleicken B, Hahner S, Loeffler M, Ventz M, Allolio B, Quinkler M. Impaired subjective health status in chronic adrenal insufficiency: impact of different glucocorticoid replacement regimens. *Eur J Endocrinol*, 2008; **159**: 811–17.
73. Tomlinson JW, Holden N, Hills RK, Wheatley K, Clayton RN, Bates AS, *et al.* Association between premature mortality and hypopituitarism. West Midlands Prospective Hypopituitary Study Group. *Lancet*, 2001; **357**: 425–31.
74. Bergthorsdottir R, Leonsson-Zachrisson M, Oden A, Johannsson G. Premature mortality in patients with Addison's disease: a population-based study. *J Clin Endocrinol Metab*, 2006; **91**: 4849–53.
75. Bensing S, Brandt L, Tabaroj F, Sjöberg O, Nilsson B, Ekbom A, *et al.* Increased death risk and altered cancer incidence pattern in patients with isolated or combined autoimmune primary adrenocortical insufficiency. *Clin Endocrinol (Oxf)*, 2008; **69**: 697–704.

5.10

Familial glucocorticoid deficiency

Claire Hughes, Louise Metherell, Adrian J.L. Clark

Introduction

Familial glucocorticoid deficiency (FGD), also known as isolated glucocorticoid deficiency or hereditary unresponsiveness to ACTH, is a rare, genetically heterogeneous autosomal recessive disorder. It is characterized by resistance of the adrenal cortex to ACTH, resulting in adrenal failure with isolated glucocorticoid deficiency. Mineralocorticoid production by the adrenal gland remains near normal.

Patients with FGD usually present in early childhood with symptoms relating to cortisol deficiency, including hypoglycaemia, jaundice, recurrent infection, and failure to thrive. Patients are hyperpigmented due to grossly elevated ACTH levels.

FGD was first described in 1959 by Shepard *et al.* who reported two sisters as having Addison's disease without hypoaldosteronism (1). Subsequently, a number of patients were reported with an inherited form of adrenal insufficiency also without hypoaldosteronism (2–5). In contrast to Addison's disease (see Chapter 5.9), FGD is a genetic disorder resulting from mutations in genes encoding essential proteins involved in the early response to ACTH.

Aetiology and molecular genetics of FGD

Adenocorticotropic hormone

ACTH acts by binding to its specific cell-surface receptor, the ACTH receptor or melanocortin 2 receptor (MC2R) to induce adrenal steroidogenesis in all three zones of the adrenal cortex. The MC2R is the smallest member of the melanocortin receptor family, which includes five members, MC1R–MC5R. The melanocortin receptors are seven-transmembrane-domain G-protein-coupled receptors (GPCRs), which are involved in diverse functions including adrenal steroidogenesis, pigmentation, and weight and energy homoeostasis (6). The sole natural ligand for the MC2R is ACTH, in contrast to the other melanocortin receptors which show varying affinity to ACTH and α-, β-, and γ-melanocyte-stimulating hormone.

ACTH binding to the MC2R induces intracellular production of cAMP, one of the major actions of which is to stimulate cAMP-dependent protein kinase (protein kinase A). As a consequence of this stimulus, cholesterol ester is imported into the cell via the scavenger receptor B1 and hydrolysis of the ester by hormone-sensitive lipase occurs. Cholesterol is then taken up into the mitochondrion by a complex including the steroidogenic acute regulatory protein (StAR). Steroidogenic enzyme expression is stimulated via a number of mechanisms including activation of the cAMP response element binding protein, and ultimately results in an increased rate of cortisol synthesis.

FGD is characterized by ACTH resistance due to defects in the early events of ACTH action, leading to failure of cortisol synthesis. The resulting cortisol deficiency causes failure of the negative feedback loop to the pituitary and hypothalamus and grossly elevated ACTH levels. A number of autosomal recessive causes of FGD have been described and include FGD type 1, resulting from mutations in the MC2R, and FGD type 2, resulting from mutations in the melanocortin 2 receptor accessory protein (MRAP). A third subgroup of patients presenting with FGD have recently been shown to have mutations in StAR. A further 50% of patients with FGD have no identifiable mutation in MC2R, MRAP, or StAR.

FGD type 1

The *MC2R* gene (OMIM 607397) was first cloned in 1992 by Mountjoy *et al.* (7). Researchers were then able to identify point mutations in the *MC2R* in patients with FGD (8, 9). To date, more than 30 mutations in *MC2R* have been reported, including both homozygous and compound heterozygous defects. These mutations are distributed throughout the coding region and account for 25% of cases of FGD. A diagram detailing the position of all the known mutations is shown in Fig. 5.10.1. Interestingly, the majority of these are missense mutations. Nonsense mutations are uncommon and are usually compounded with a missense mutation on the other allele. This has led to the suggestion that homozygous nonsense mutations either lead to reduced survival *in utero* or are associated with a different phenotype (11).

The identification of homozygous mutations in affected individuals is highly suggestive but not definitive evidence of a causative role in the disease. Functional analysis of MC2R mutations has been problematic in view of difficulties expressing the receptor in transfected cells (12). However, since the discovery of MRAP (see below) it has been possible to show convincingly that mutations are associated with loss of receptor function. In the majority of cases the mutation results in a failure of the receptor to traffic to the cell surface, probably because the mutation leads to defective folding

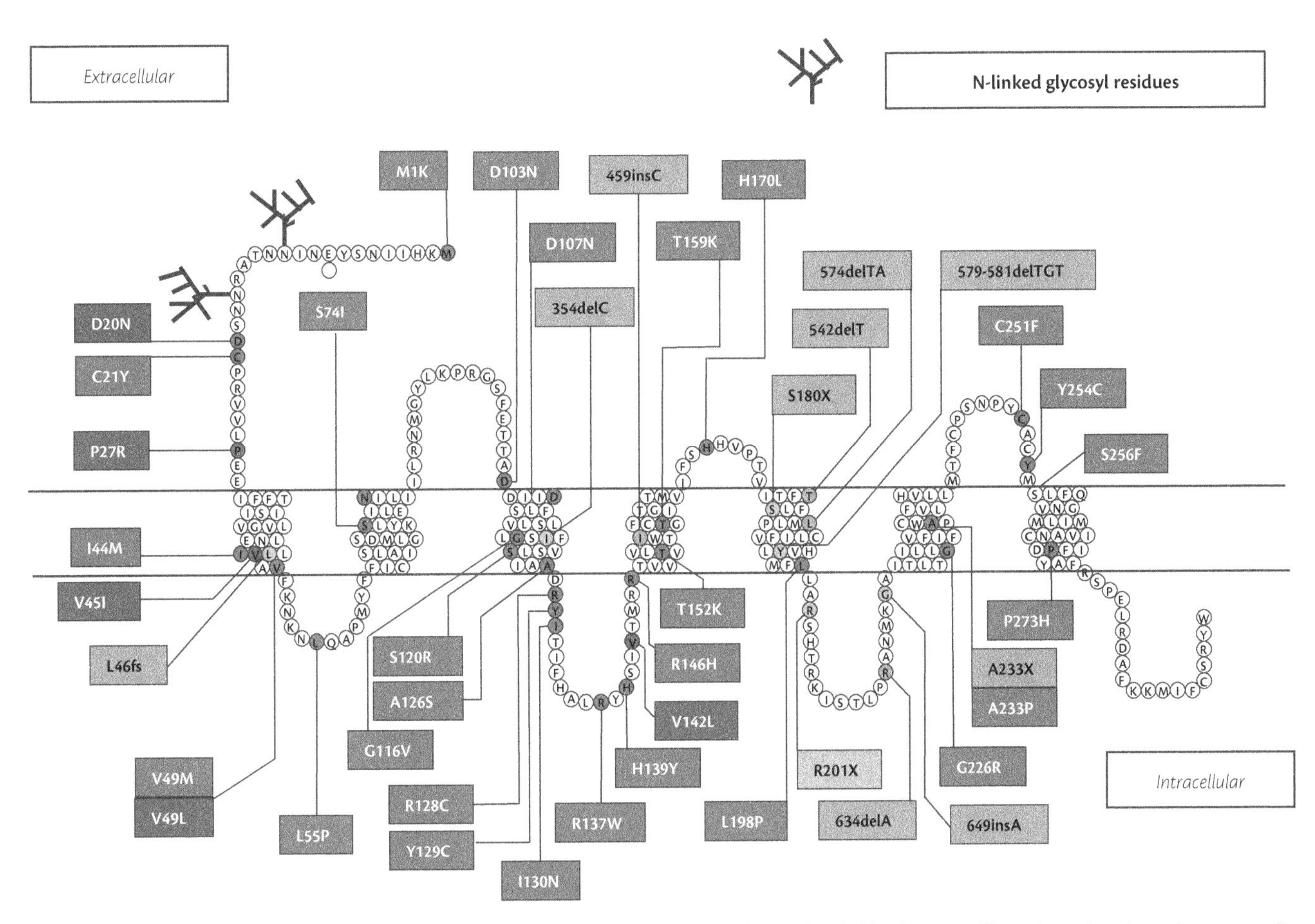

Fig. 5.10.1 Schematic diagram showing the locations of all MC2R mutations that are known to be associated with FGD type 1. Those shown in red are missense mutations, those in blue are probable benign polymorphisms, and those in green are nonsense or frameshift mutations. (Reprinted from Clark AJ, Metherell LA, Cheetham ME, Huebner A. Inherited ACTH insensitivity illuminates the mechanisms of ACTH action. *Trends Endocrinol Metab*, 2005; **16**: 451–7 (10) with permission.) (See also Plate 31)

of the receptor at the time of its synthesis (13). In a few cases, the mutant receptor is expressed at the cell surface, but the mutation interferes with ACTH binding or signal transduction (12). As is the case in many genetic disorders, there is a poor correlation between *in vitro* characterization of each mutant and clinical severity.

FGD type 2

MC2R is unable to form a functional ACTH-responsive receptor in nonadrenal cell lines due to lack of cell surface localization. This observation led to the hypothesis that a specific accessory factor, present in adrenal cells types, is required to facilitate trafficking of MC2R to the cell surface. Genetic studies were carried out using homozygosity mapping in consanguineous families affected with FGD. This identified a locus on chromosome 21q22.1. Further studies identified mutations in a candidate gene in this region, which showed high adrenal expression, and this gene was subsequently named the *MRAP* (OMIM 609196) (14).

MRAP is a small, single-transmembrane-domain protein. Alternative splicing gives rise to two protein isoforms—MRAPα of 19 kDa and MRAPβ of 11.5 kDa. Functional analysis of MRAP revealed that it was essential for normal MC2R function (15). MRAP forms a unique antiparallel homodimer, which directly interacts with the MC2R at the endoplasmic reticulum and is required for correct folding or trafficking of the receptor to the cell surface. Current evidence suggests that MRAP is also required at the plasma membrane for ACTH binding and signal transduction (15). These possible modes of action are summarized in Fig. 5.10.2. To date, nine *MRAP* mutations causing FGD have been reported, all of which result in either an absent or severely truncated protein (Fig. 5.10.3).

FGD type 3/nonclassical congenital lipoid adrenal hyperplasia

It was reported in 2002 (16) that in a small subset of patients with FGD the disease mapped to a locus on chromosome 8. This gene has recently been identified as the *STAR* gene (OMIM 600617) (17). StAR is a mitochondrial phosphoprotein that mediates the acute response to steroidogenic stimuli by increasing cholesterol transport from the outer to the inner mitochondrial membrane. Defects in StAR usually result in congenital lipoid adrenal hyperplasia (OMIM 201710) (CLAH), a severe form of congenital adrenal hyperplasia. Review of history, examination, and biochemical data in the individuals diagnosed with FGD confirmed they had isolated glucocorticoid deficiency with normal or near normal renin and aldosterone levels. However, some patients did have mild reproductive anomalies, including hypospadias and cryptorchidism which had not previously been connected to their adrenal failure. The mutations found in StAR in FGD appear to lead to only partial impairment of the cholesterol uptake function of this protein. Thus classical CLAH is caused by mutations that completely abolish any functioning

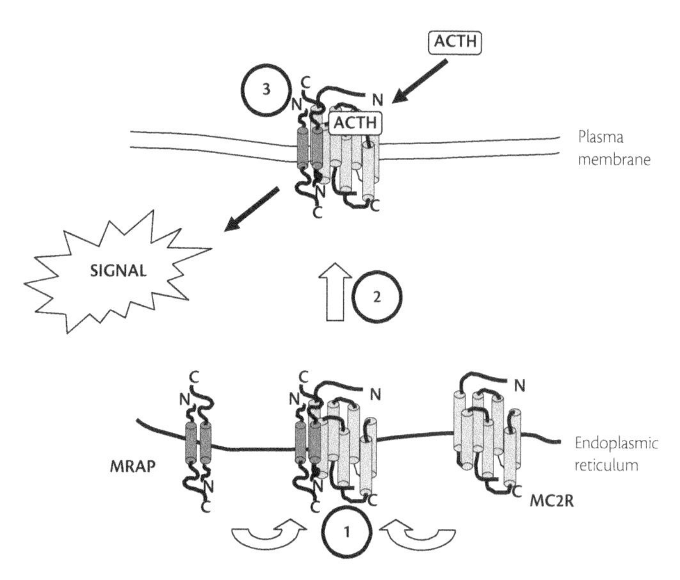

Fig. 5.10.2 Schematic diagram of the possible actions of melanocortin 2 receptor accessory protein (MRAP) in supporting melanocortin 2 receptor (MC2R) function. (1) MRAP exists as an antiparallel homodimer, and may have a chaperone-like function in assisting the correct folding of the MC2R in the endoplasmic reticulum. (2) MRAP may have an 'escort' function in assisting the trafficking of the correctly folded MC2R to the plasma membrane. (3) Finally, MRAP may form a trimeric structure with the MC2R at the cell surface and may be required for ACTH interaction and binding, or for generation of an intracellular signal.

StAR while mutations that allow the protein to retain some function are associated with a nonclassical CLAH or FGD (17).

There remain many FGD patients (*c.* 50%) without mutations in *MC2R*, *MRAP*, or *STAR* and who show no linkage to these loci. Ongoing research in this area is aimed at identifying new genes responsible for FGD.

Clinical presentation

Patients with FGD usually present during the neonatal period or early childhood with symptoms related to cortisol deficiency and ACTH excess. The most common presenting feature is hypoglycaemia. This may be overlooked in the postnatal period as it may respond to routine treatment, e.g. decreasing the time interval between feeds, and transient asymptomatic hypoglycaemia in healthy infants is relatively common. Symptoms secondary to hypoglycaemia include jitteriness, tremors, hypotonia, lethargy, apnoea, poor

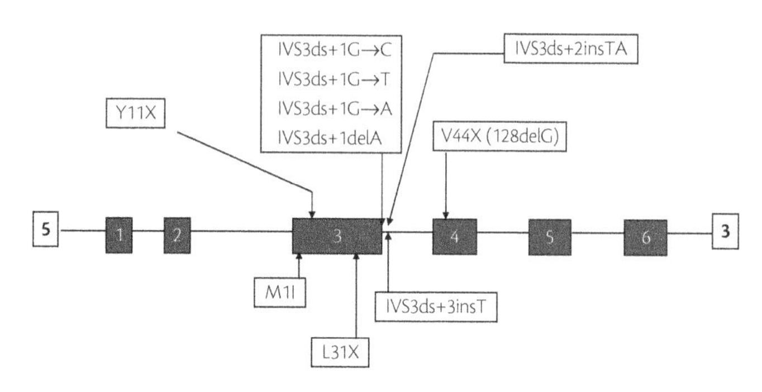

Fig. 5.10.3 Schematic diagram of human melanocortin 2 receptor accessory protein (MRAP) showing locations of all known mutations. Boxes represent exons; horizontal line representations.

feeding, and hypoglycaemic seizures. In a small number of patients, undiagnosed hypoglycaemia in infancy may have been sufficiently severe to cause serious long-term neurological sequelae.

Neonates may also present with jaundice, failure to thrive, and collapse. Transient neonatal hepatitis has been described in one case (18). There may be a history of unexplained neonatal or childhood death and as this is an autosomal recessive disorder there is frequently a history of consanguinity. Hyperpigmentation will usually develop by a few months of age due to the over-stimulation of MC1R by high circulating ACTH levels, and in some cases this is the presenting complaint. Older children may present with a variety of features including recurrent hypoglycaemia and lethargy, recurrent infections, and shock.

A feature that has been observed in patients with FGD type 1 is tall stature and discordant ossification (19, 20). The underlying mechanism is not clear and the limited data available suggests that the growth hormone–insulin-like growth factor (IGF-1) axis is normal. Hydrocortisone replacement appears to stop this excessive growth and bring the height back towards the midparental height (19). This suggests that either the cortisol deficiency itself or excessively high ACTH levels may have a causative role. Studies have shown a number of melanocortin receptors are expressed in bone and the cartilaginous growth plate and therefore ACTH at high concentrations may activate these receptors and stimulate growth (21). Alternatively, it has been reported that glucocorticoid inhibits the synthesis of IGF binding protein 5 (IGFBP-5) in the osteoblast (22). As bone growth is stimulated by IGFBP-5 it is conceivable that cortisol deficiency could result in a lack of inhibition and hence increased growth. Tall stature is not a recognized feature of FGD type 2 or other causes of adrenal failure, and it may be that the chronic exposure to high ACTH/low cortisol from birth is important. There is evidence that FGD type 2 presents at an earlier age than FGD type 1 (23) and thus the length of high ACTH/low cortisol exposure may be less.

ACTH is required for adrenal androgen synthesis and hence for adrenarche to occur normally in children. Children with FGD can have an absent adrenarche with delayed or absent pubic hair development associated with low or undetectable adrenal androgen levels. Normal pubertal development controlled by the hypothalamic–pituitary–gonadal axis is unaffected and fertility is normal.

Diagnosis

The hallmark of FGD is low or undetectable cortisol paired with high ACTH levels and normal electrolytes, renin, and aldosterone levels. ACTH levels are often extremely high—levels of above 200 pmol/l (normal range <18 pmol/l) are commonly found. A short ACTH stimulation test showing an impaired cortisol response (<550 nmol/l) may be necessary to confirm adrenal insufficiency.

The most important feature to distinguish FGD from other causes of adrenal insufficiency is the absence of mineralocorticoid deficiency. However, this is not always simple to ascertain for various reasons. Firstly, at presentation, children with FGD may be hypovolaemic, or pyrexial, and are usually stressed. Alternatively, they may be relatively water overloaded as a result of intravenous fluid replacement and because of reduced free water clearance associated with glucocorticoid deficiency. ACTH is normally an effective stimulus to aldosterone production and this action will be deficient in FGD. As a result, FGD patients frequently present with minor abnormalities of the renin–aldosterone axis. Furthermore, there is evidence that those rare patients with nonsense mutations of the *MC2R* in whom no MC2R function is possible often do have mild hyperreninaemia and/or partial aldosterone deficiency (24, 25). These investigations should nevertheless distinguish those patients with adrenal failure from other causes in whom there is overt aldosterone deficiency and compensatory elevated renin values. Usually, after introduction of appropriate hydrocortisone replacement renin and aldosterone normalize and fludrocortisone replacement is not required.

Adrenal imaging

MRI/CT scanning of the adrenal gland are not usually necessary to establish the diagnosis of FGD. In FGD the gland is usually small in size (26) in contrast to congenital adrenal hyperplasia or infiltrative disorders in which the adrenal is enlarged.

Histopathology

Some histopathology studies of adrenal glands are available from patients who died prior to diagnosis. These report the absence of fasciculata and/or reticularis cells with disorganization of granulosa cells (4, 5).

Differential diagnosis

Alternative diagnoses and their most likely distinguishing clinical and biochemical features that should be considered in patients potentially presenting with FGD are:

- congenital adrenal hyperplasia: disorders of sexual development, ambiguous genitalia, hypertension, elevated 17-hydroxyprogesterone, abnormal urinary steroid chromatography
- Addison's disease: age of onset, mineralocorticoid deficiency, positive adrenal autoantibodies, other autoimmune disease
- triple A syndrome: alacrima (demonstrated with the Schirmer test of tear production), achalasia, and various neurological defects
- adrenoleucodystrophy: progressive neurological manifestations, elevated very-long-chain fatty acids
- IMAGe syndrome: other dysmorphic features
- congenital adrenal hypoplasia: hypogonadism, delayed puberty, disorders of sexual development, mineralocorticoid deficiency
- autoimmune polyglandular syndromes: presence of other autoimmune deficiencies, positive adrenal autoantibodies
- lipoid congenital adrenal hyperplasia: disorders of sexual development, mineralocorticoid deficiency.

Treatment

The treatment is with physiological glucocorticoid replacement. This is usually given in the form of oral hydrocortisone 10–12 mg/m^2 per day in children and 20 mg/day in adults. The total daily dose is given in three divided doses throughout the day.

Glucocorticoid dosing must be increased during times of stress to two to three times the maintenance dose. It is vital to ensure the patient and their family have adequate education to understand when and how to increase hydrocortisone doses and emergency management with intramuscular hydrocortisone or hydrocortisone suppositories. Patients should also be given a Medic alert bracelet and 'steroid card'.

Patients should be monitored for symptoms and signs of excessive glucocorticoid replacement and the dose titrated to prevent overtreatment. In individuals with adequate replacement therapy, ACTH levels often remain elevated and therefore cutaneous pigmentation can persist. Attempting to suppress the ACTH levels must be avoided as it will lead to over treatment, iatrogenic Cushing's syndrome, and growth failure in children.

Summary

Primary adrenal failure in a child with a normal renin–angiotensin–aldosterone axis is highly suggestive of a diagnosis of FGD. Confirming the diagnosis with genetic analysis is now possible in approximately 50% of patients, this is important both in providing reassurance that mineralocorticoid replacement is unnecessary and for genetic counselling.

References

1. Shepard TH, Landing BH, Mason DG. Familial Addison's disease; case reports of two sisters with corticoid deficiency unassociated with hypoaldosteronism. *AMA J Dis Child*, 1959; **97**: 154–62.
2. Stempfel RS, Engel FL. A congenital, familial syndrome of adrenocortical insufficiency without hypoaldosteronism. *J Pediatr*, 1960; **57**: 443–51.
3. Migeon CJ, Kenny EM, Kowarski A, Snipes CA, Spaulding JS, Finkelstein JW, *et al*. The syndrome of congenital adrenocortical unresponsiveness to ACTH. Report of six cases. *Pediatr Res*, 1968; **2**: 501–13.
4. Kelch RP, Kaplan SL, Biglieri EG, Daniels GH, Epstein CJ, Grumbach MM. Hereditary adrenocortical unresponsiveness to adrenocorticotropic hormone. *J Pediatr*, 1972; **81**: 726–36.
5. Thistlethwaite D, Darling JA, Fraser R, Mason PA, Rees LH, Harkness RA. Familial glucocorticoid deficiency. Studies of diagnosis and pathogenesis. *Arch Dis Child*, 1975; **50**: 291–7.
6. Raffin-Sanson ML, de Keyzer Y, Bertagna X. Proopiomelanocortin, a polypeptide precursor with multiple functions: from physiology to pathological conditions. *Eur J Endocrinol*, 2003; **149**: 79–90.
7. Mountjoy KG, Robbins LS, Mortrud MT, Cone RD. The cloning of a family of genes that encode the melanocortin receptors. *Science*, 1992; **257**: 1248–51.
8. Clark AJ, McLoughlin L, Grossman A. Familial glucocorticoid deficiency associated with point mutation in the adrenocorticotropin receptor. *Lancet*, 1993; **341**: 461–2.
9. Tsigos C, Arai K, Hung W, Chrousos GP. Hereditary isolated glucocorticoid deficiency is associated with abnormalities of the adrenocorticotropin receptor gene. *J Clin Invest*, 1993; **92**: 2458–61.
10. Clark AJ, Metherell LA, Cheetham ME, Huebner A. Inherited ACTH insensitivity illuminates the mechanisms of ACTH action. *Trends Endocrinol Metab*, 2005; **16**: 451–7.
11. Clark JL, Metherell LA, Naville D, Begeot M, Huebner A. Genetics of ACTH insensitivity syndromes. *Ann Endocrinol (Paris)*, 2005; **66**: 247–9.
12. Elias LL, Huebner A, Pullinger GD, Mirtella A, Clark AJ. Functional characterization of naturally occurring mutations of the human adrenocorticotropin receptor: poor correlation of phenotype and genotype. *J Clin Endocrinol Metab*, 1999; **84**: 2766–70.
13. Chung TT, Webb TR, Chan LF, Cooray SN, Metherell LA, King PJ, *et al*. The majority of ACTH receptor (MC2R) mutations found in familial glucocorticoid deficiency type 1 lead to defective trafficking

of the receptor to the cell surface. *J Clin Endocrinol Metab*, 2008; 93: 4948–54.

14. Metherell LA, Chan LF, Clark AJ. The genetics of ACTH resistance syndromes. *Best Pract Res Clin Endocrinol Metab*, 2006; **20**: 547–60.
15. Metherell LA, Chapple JP, Cooray S, David A, Becker C, Rüschendorf F, *et al.* Mutations in MRAP, encoding a new interacting partner of the ACTH receptor, cause familial glucocorticoid deficiency type 2. *Nat Genet*, 2005; **37**: 166–70.
16. Genin E, Huebner A, Jaillard C, Faure A, Halaby G, Saka N, *et al.* Linkage of one gene for familial glucocorticoid deficiency type 2 (FGD2) to chromosome 8q and further evidence of heterogeneity. *Hum Genet*, 2002; **111**: 428–34.
17. Metherall LA, Naville D, Halaby G, Begeot M, Huebner A, Nurnberg G, *et al.* Nonclassic lipid congenital adrenal hyperplasia masquerading as familial glucocorticoid deficiency. *J Clin Endocrinol Metab*, 2009; **94**: 3865–71.
18. Lacy DE, Nathavitharana KA, Tarlow MJ. Neonatal hepatitis and congenital insensitivity to adrenocorticotropin (ACTH). *J Pediatr Gastroenterol Nutr*, 1993; **17**: 438–40.
19. Elias LL, Huebner A, Metherell LA, Canas A, Warne GL, Bitti ML, *et al.* Tall stature in familial glucocorticoid deficiency. *Clin Endocrinol (Oxf)*, 2000; **53**: 423–30.
20. Imamine H, Mizuno H, Sugiyama Y, Ohro Y, Sugiura T, Togari H. Possible relationship between elevated plasma ACTH and tall stature in familial glucocorticoid deficiency. *Tohoku J Exp Med*, 2005; **205**: 123–31.
21. Evans JF, Shen CL, Pollack S, Aloia JF, Yeh JK. Adrenocorticotropin evokes transient elevations in intracellular free calcium ($[Ca2+]_i$) and increases basal $[Ca2+]_i$ in resting chondrocytes through a phospholipase C-dependent mechanism. *Endocrinology*, 2005; **146**: 3123–32.
22. Gabbitas B, Pash JM, Delany AM, Canalis E. Cortisol inhibits the synthesis of insulin-like growth factor-binding protein-5 in bone cell cultures by transcriptional mechanisms. *J Biol Chem*, 1996; **271**: 9033–8.
23. Chung TT, Chan LF, Metherell LA, Clark AJL. Phenotypic characteristics of Familial Glucocorticoid Deficiency type 1 and 2. *Clin Endocrinol*, 2009; **72**: 589–94.
24. Lin L, Hindmarsh PC, Metherell LA, Alzyoud M, Al-Ali M, Brain CE, *et al.* Severe loss-of-function mutations in the adrenocorticotropin receptor (ACTHR, MC2R) can be found in patients diagnosed with salt-losing adrenal hypoplasia. *Clin Endocrinol (Oxf)*, 2007; **66**: 205–10.
25. Chan LF, Clark AJ, Metherell LA. Familial glucocorticoid deficiency: advances in the molecular understanding of ACTH action. *Horm Res*, 2008; **69**: 75–82.
26. Clark AJ, Weber A. Adrenocorticotropin insensitivity syndromes. *Endocr Rev*, 1998; **19**: 828–43.

5.11

Congenital adrenal hyperplasia

Nils Krone

Introduction

Congenital adrenal hyperplasia (CAH) represents a group of autosomal recessive disorders of steroidogenesis caused by defects in steroidogenic enzymes involved in glucocorticoid synthesis or in enzymes providing cofactors to steroidogenic enzymes (1, 2). Congenital lipoid adrenal hyperplasia (CLAH) caused by steroidogenic acute regulatory protein (StAR) deficiency is distinct in origin and presentation from the conventional variants of CAH, with the unique feature of lipid accumulation subsequently leading to destruction of adrenal function. This chapter will also mention aldosterone synthase deficiency, which is the only defect in adrenal steroidogenesis causing deficient mineralocorticoid biosynthesis without affecting glucocorticoid biosynthesis. The disorder cannot strictly be considered a CAH variant as it does not result in increased ACTH drive and thus not in adrenal hyperplasia.

Novel forms of CAH have emerged during recent years. These include P450 oxidoreductase deficiency (ORD), P450 side-chain cleavage (CYP11A1) deficiency, the nonclassic form of CLAH (StAR deficiency), and apparent cortisone reductase deficiency. All forms of congenital adrenal hyperplasia resemble a disease continuum spanning from mild nonclassic presentations to classic onset with severe signs and symptoms.

Normal physiology

The adrenal cortex consists of three zones: the outer zona glomerulosa is responsible for mineralocorticoid synthesis, the middle zona fasciculata for glucocorticoid synthesis, and the inner zona reticularis for synthesis of the adrenal androgen precursors dehydroepiandrosterone (DHEA) and androstenedione. All major enzymes involved in adrenal steroidogenesis are located either in the mitochondria or the endoplasmic reticulum. The function of mitochondrial (type I) cytochrome P450 (CYP) enzymes, such as P450 side-chain cleavage (CYP11A1), 11β-hydroxylase (CYP11B1), and aldosterone synthase (CYP11B2), depends on electron transfer facilitated by the proteins adrenodoxin and adrenodoxin reductase. Micrososomal (type II) CYP enzymes localized to the endoplasmic reticulum include 17α-hydroxylase (CYP17A1), 21-hydroxylase (CYP21A2), and P450 aromatase (CYP19A1). The function of CYP type II enzymes crucially depends on P450 oxidoreductase (POR) providing electrons required for monooxygenase reaction catalysed by the CYP enzyme.

Glucocorticoid synthesis is under negative feedback control of the hypothalamic–pituitary–adrenal (HPA) axis (see Chapter 5.9). The pituitary releases ACTH, which binds to its adrenal receptor (melanocortin receptor 2) and stimulates import of cholesterol into the mitochondrion by StAR. In parallel, transcription of genes encoding steroidogenic enzymes and their cofactor enzymes is increased. The rate-limiting step is the conversion of cholesterol into pregnenolone by CYP11A1, which is expressed in all three adrenocortical zones. The biosynthetic directionality of different steroid hormone pathways in the adrenal zones is facilitated by differential expression of steroidogenic enzymes and cofactors.

Glucocorticoids are mainly synthesized in the zona fasciculata, following the route from pregnenolone via progesterone, 17-hydroxyprogesterone (17OHP), or pregnenolone via 17-hydroxypregnenolone and 17OHP. 17-Hydroxyprogesterone is then 21-hydroxylated to 11-deoxycortisol and finally converted to cortisol.

Sex steroids are produced from pregnenolone by 17α-hydroxylation to 17OH-pregnenolone, which is converted by the 17,20-lyase activity of CYP17A1 into DHEA, the universal sex steroid precursor. Sufficient 17,20-lyase activity depends not only on POR but also on the availability of cytochrome b5, which facilitates close interaction between CYP17A1 and its electron donor POR. The conversion from 17OHP to androstenedione is negligible under normal physiological circumstances (Fig. 5.11.1). Androstenedione undergoes conversion to testosterone, which is facilitated by 17β-dehydrogenase type 3 (HSD17B3) in the gonad and also by 17β-dehydrogenase type 5 (AKR1C3) (3) in the adrenal cortex, albeit to a much lesser extent. High-volume production of androgens that bind and activate the androgen receptor, i.e. testosterone and 5α-dihydrotestoserone, and the conversion of androstenedione and testosterone to oestrogens, occurs in the gonad and in part in peripheral target tissues of sex steroid action but not in the adrenal.

Mineralocorticoid synthesis is mainly under the control of the renin–angiotensin–aldosterone system and a potassium feedback loop (see Chapter 5.9). The adrenal zona glomerulosa lacks 17α-hydroxylase activity and pregnenolone is subsequently converted into aldosterone in five enzymatic steps involving the endoplasmic HSD3B2 and CYP21A2 enzymes and mitochondrial CYP11B2 (Fig. 5.11.1). The latter facilitates the three final steps of mineralocorticoid biosynthesis providing 11β-hydroxylase, 18-hydroxylase, and 18-oxidase activities.

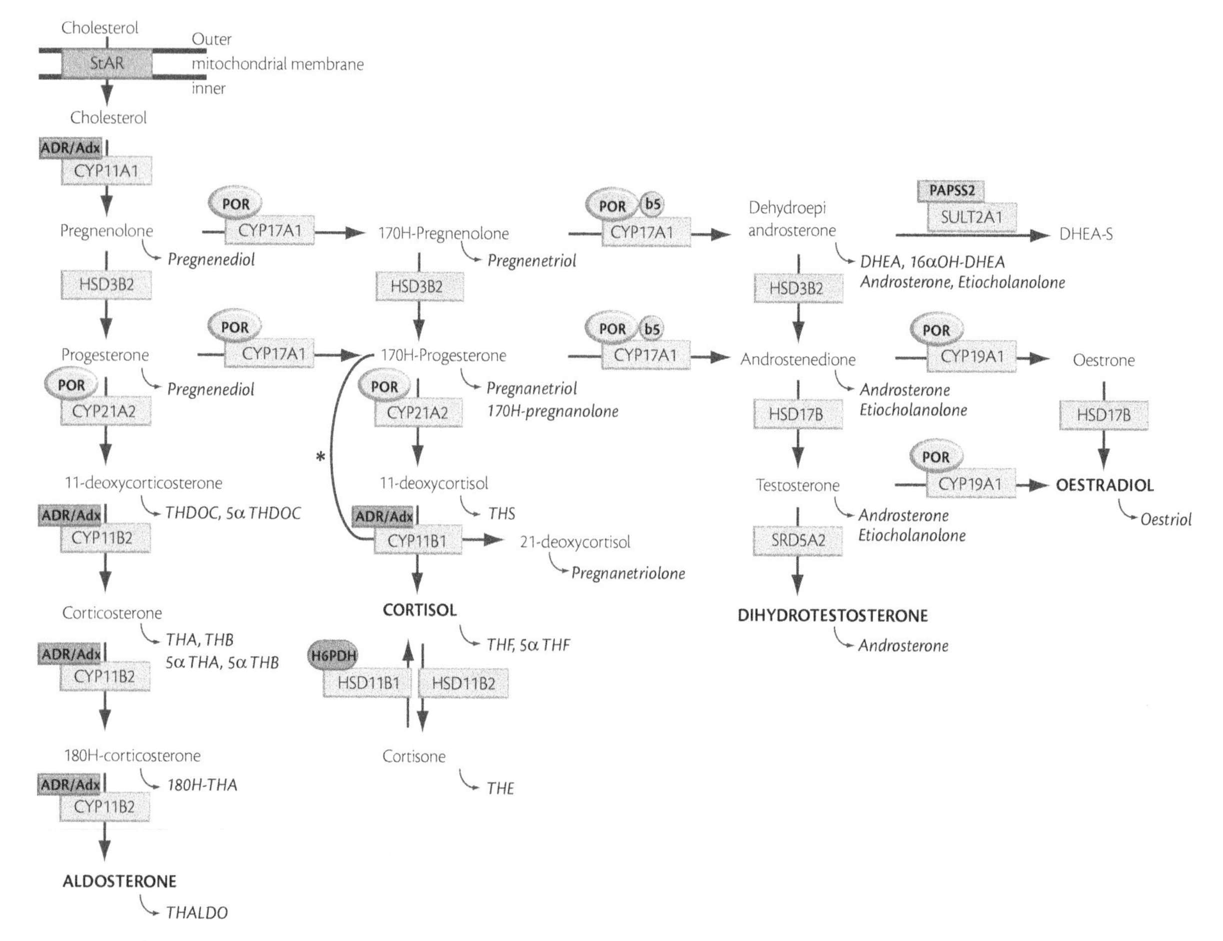

Fig. 5.11.1 Pathways of adrenal and gonadal steroid biosynthesis. Steroidogenic enzymes are marked with light grey boxes. Mitochondrial CYP type I enzymes requiring electron transfer via adrenodoxin reductase (ADR) and adrenodoxin (Adx) CYP11A1, CYP11B1, CYP11B2, are marked with a labelled box ADR/Adx. Microsomal CYP II enzymes receiving electrons from P450 oxidoreductase, CYP17A1, CYP21A2, CYP19A1, are marked by circled POR. The 17,20-lyase reaction catalysed by CYP17A1 requires in addition to POR also cytochrome b5, indicated by a circled b5. Hexose-6-phosphate dehydrogenase (H6PDH) is the cofactor to HSD11B1 and is given as an ellipse. Urinary steroid hormone metabolites are given in italics below the plasma hormones. The asterisk (*) indicates the pathognomonic 11-hydroxylation of 17OHP to 21-deoxycortisol in 21-hydroxylase deficiency. The conversion of androstenedione to testosterone is catalysed by HSD17B3 in the gonad and also, albeit to a much lesser extent, by AKR1C3 (HSD17B5) in the adrenal. The conversion of androgens to oestrogens takes place exclusively in the gonads. StAR, steroidogenic acute regulatory protein; CYP11A1, P450 side-chain cleavage enzyme; HSD3B2, 3β-hydroxysteroid dehydrogenase type 2; CYP17A1, 17α-hydroxylase; CYP21A2, 21-hydroxylase; CYP11B1, 11β-hydroxylase; CYP11B2, aldosterone synthase; HSD17B, 17β-hydroxysteroid dehydrogenase; CYP19A1, P450 aromatase; SRD5A2, 5α-reductase type 2; SULT2A1, sulphotransferase 2A1; PAPPS2, 3′-phosphoadenosine 5′-phosphosulfate synthase 2; PAPPS2, 3′-phosphoadenosine 5′-phosphosulfate synthase 2.

Different forms of congenital adrenal hyperplasia

The pathophysiology of the different forms of CAH is explained by the specific enzyme deficiency and their consequences on clinical phenotype expression. Table 5.11.1 provides a summary of the various forms.

21-Hydroxylase deficiency

Steroid 21-hydroxylase deficiency (21OHD) is caused by mutations in the *CYP21A2* gene encoding adrenal 21-hydroxylase. 21OHD ranks among the most common inborn errors and accounts for approximately 95% of all cases of CAH. The frequency of the classic form is about 1 in 10 000 to 15 000 livebirths. Nonclassic CAH, caused by milder mutations that do not completely disrupt enzymatic efficiency, is more frequent, with an incidence of about 1 in 500 to 1 in 1000. Glucocorticoid substitution therapy is available since the mid-20th century and the oldest surviving patients with classic CAH are now well within their fifties. Therefore, increasing awareness is necessary not only to address paediatric problems, but also to prevent and treat potential comorbidities during later life (1, 4, 5).

Pathophysiology

The most severe form due to completely absent 21-hydroxylase enzyme activity comprises mineralocorticoid deficiency, glucocorticoid deficiency, androgen excess (Fig. 5.11.1), and adrenomedullary dysfunction.

Aldosterone action is essential for sodium reabsorption and potassium excretion in the distal renal tubulus. In 21OHD, the deficient conversion of progesterone to 11-deoxycorticosterone results in a lack of aldosterone and its precursors (Fig. 5.11.1). This causes renal salt loss with subsequent severe hyponatraemia, hyperkalaemia, and metabolic acidosis. The clinical course in untreated patients includes dehydration, arterial hypotension, hypovolaemic shock, and finally death due to cardiovascular

Table 5.11.1 Differential diagnosis of congenital adrenal hyperplasia—clinical, biochemical, and genetic characteristics

	Deficiency									
Characteristic	**21-hydroxylase**		**11β-hydroxylase**	**17α-hydroxylase**	**3β-HSD type 2**	**P450 oxidoreductase**	**Lipoid adrenal hyperplasia**	**P450 side chain cleavage**	**Aldosterone synthase**	**Apparent cortisone reductase**
OMIM No.	+201910		#202010	#202110	+201810	#201750	*600617	*118485	*124080	*138090
Gene/protein	CYP21A2		CYP11B1	CYP17A1	HSD3B2	POR	StAR	CYP11A1	CYP11B2	H6PDH
alias	P450c21		P450c11	P450c17	3β-HSD	CPR, CYPOR		P450scc	P450aldo	
Subtype	Classic	Nonclassic								
Incidence	1: 10 000 to 15 000	1:500 to 1:1000	1: 100 000 to 1: 200 000	Rare	Rare	Unknown	Rare	Rare	Rare	Rare
DSD	46,XX	No	46,XX	46,XY	46,XY[a]	46,XX + 46,XY[c]	46,XX	46,XX	No	No
Primary affected organ	Adrenal	Adrenal	Adrenal	Adrenal, gonads	Adrenal, gonads	Adrenal, gonads, liver, all CYP type 2 expressing tissues	Adrenal, gonads	Adrenal, gonads	Adrenal	Liver, adrenal all H6PDH/HSD11B1 expressing tissues
Glucocorticoids	Reduced	Normal	Reduced	Reduced	Reduced	Reduced to normal, impaired stress response	Reduced	Reduced	Normal	Normal, but reduced tissue levels due to increased cortisol clearance
Mineralocorticoids	Reduced in SW	Normal	Increased, mainly precursors	Increased	Reduced often	Reduced to increased	Reduced	Reduced	Reduced	Normal
Sex hormones	Increased	Increased	Increased	Reduced	Reduced in males Increased in females[b]	Reduced	Reduced	Reduced	Normal	Increased
Increased marker metabolite										
Plasma	17OHP 21-deoxycortisol		DOC, S	Pregnenolone, Progesterone DOC, S	17OH-Pregnenolone, DHEA	Pregnenolone, progesterone, 17OHP			DOC, B 18OH-B	
Urine	Pregnanetriol, 17OHpregnanolone, pregnanetriolone		THDOC, THS	THDOC, THB, Pregnenediol, pregnanediol	Pregnantriol	Pregnenediol, pregnanediol pregnanetriol, 17OHpregnanolone				
PRA	Increased	Normal–mildly increased	Reduced	Reduced	Increased		Increased	Increased	Increased	Normal
Hypertension	No	No	Yes	Yes	No	No or mild	No	No	No	No
Plasma sodium	Reduced in SW	Normal	Increased	Increased	Reduced in SW	Normal	Reduced	Reduced	Reduced	Normal
Plasma potassium	Increased in SW	Normal	Reduced	Reduced	Increased in SW	Normal	Increased	Increased	Increased	Normal
Urinary salt loss	Yes	No	No	No	Yes	No	Yes	Yes	Yes	No
Skeletal malformation	No	No	No	No	No	Yes[d]	No	No	No	No

[a] Masculinization of the external genitalia in females at birth is rare and if present in most cases mild, signs of increased androgens usually present later.
[b] Steroid hormone conversion by 3β-HSD type 1 in peripheral tissues.
[c] DSD observed in both sexes as well as normal sex-specific sexual development reported.
[d] In majority of cases published thus far, but absence of skeletal malformations does not rule out P450 oxidoreducatase deficiency.
S,11-deoxycortisol; DOC, 11-deoxycorticosterone; B, corticosterone; THS, tetrahydrodeoxycortisol; THDOC, tetrahydrodeoxycorticosterone; PRA, plasma renin activity; SW, salt-wasting.

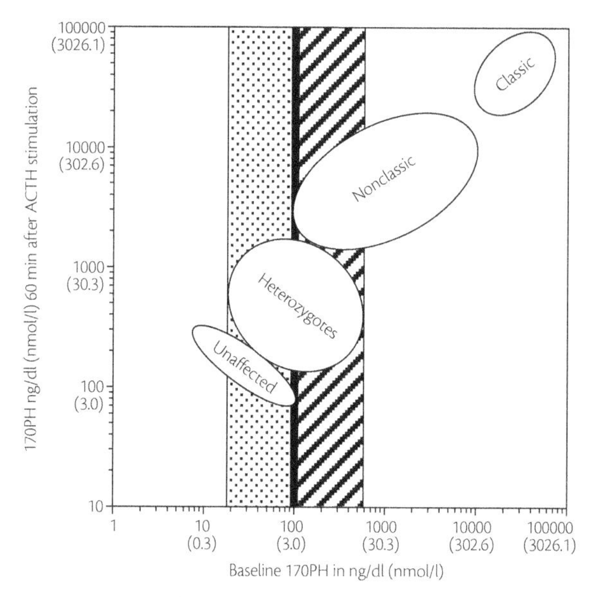

Fig. 5.11.2 Nomogram for comparing 17OHP concentrations before and 60 min after a 0.25 mg IV bolus of (1–1) ACTH in subjects with or without 21-hydroxylase deficiency. Dotted area indicated the overlap of basal 17OHP concentrations between unaffected individuals and heterozygous carriers. The striped area shows the overlap of basal 17OHP concentrations between heterozygous carriers and individuals with nonclassic CAH. SI units for 17OHP are given in brackets. It allows in the majority of cases for differentiation between heterozygous carriers, and patients with nonclassic CAH and classic CAH. (Adapted from New MI. Extensive clinical experience: nonclassical 21-hydroxylase deficiency. *J Clin Endocrinol Metab*, 2006; **91**: 4205–14. (6))

collapse. This so-called salt-wasting crisis usually develops in the second or third week of life.

Cortisol biosynthesis is impaired due to insufficient enzymatic conversion of 17OHP to 11-deoxycortisol (Fig. 5.11.1). The insufficient cortisol feedback to the hypothalamus and pituitary gland results in increased corticotropin-releasing hormone (CRH) and ACTH secretion leading to the pathological correlate of hyperplastic adrenal glands. Glucocorticoid deficiency results in hypoglycaemia due to impairment of gluconeogenesis, glycogenolysis, proteolysis, and lipolysis. Furthermore, glucocorticoid deficiency lowers myocardial contractility, cardiac output, and decreases the full pressor effects of catecholamines on the cardiovascular system, which can result in cardiovascular shock.

Impaired adrenomedullary development and function has been demonstrated in patients with CAH. Decreased adrenaline levels most likely contribute to the development of hypoglycaemia during intercurrent illness and the development of metabolic consequences such as hyperleptinaemia and hyperinsulinaemia. Adrenaline deficiency is associated with impaired blood glucose response to high-intensity exercise, and explains the failure of hydrocortisone to improve glucose levels during high-intensity exercise.

Accumulated steroid precursors are shunted in the sex hormone biosynthesis pathway resulting in androgen excess (Fig. 5.11.1). Prenatal androgen excess leads to virilization of the external genitalia in 46,XX individuals, i.e. 46,XX disordered sex development (DSD). However, affected patients have normal müllerian structures and thus normal internal female genital organs. The degree of external virilization is classified into five stages according to Prader, spanning a range from isolated mild clitoromegaly (Prader I) to complete labioscrotal fusion with the urethra traversing the penis-like enlarged clitoris (Prader V). External genitalia in affected male 46,XY individuals are normal, but sometimes may be hyperpigmented and slightly enlarged.

Clinical manifestation

A wide range of clinical manifestation of 21OHD exists and can be described as a disease continuum. Commonly, 21OHD is classified into classic (salt-wasting and simple-virilizing forms) and the milder nonclassic form. Disease severity correlates well with the underlying severity of the enzymatic defect. Disease classifications based only on the age of diagnosis is not helpful in clinical practice.

Classic 21-hydroxylase deficiency

The classic form comprises salt-wasting and simple-virilizing CAH variants with patients usually presenting during childhood. Cortisol deficiency is a characteristic feature. This results in adrenal stimulation and overproduction of steroid precursors that due to the enzymatic block in 21-hydroxylase are redirected towards adrenal androgen synthesis leading to androgen excess. About two-thirds of patients have additional clinically significant aldosterone deficiency and salt loss. Patients with salt-wasting CAH have complete or almost complete absence of 21-hydroxylase function. Patients with glucocorticoid deficiency without apparent mineralocorticoid deficiency are categorized as simple-virilizing CAH.

Almost all patients with classic CAH can be diagnosed by newborn screening within the first 2 weeks of life, before life-threatening salt loss manifests. In countries without implemented CAH newborn screening, girls with ambiguous genitalia are most likely diagnosed soon after birth before manifestation of salt loss. However, the diagnosis in boys with salt-wasting CAH is only established once the patient presents with salt loss. Salt-wasting often manifests with poor feeding, vomiting, failure to thrive, lethargy, and sepsis-like symptoms. The crisis can result in rapid deterioration and if diagnosis is not made in time will lead to a life-threatening situation and consequently death.

Male patients with simple-virilizing CAH, who escaped diagnosis during the neonatal period, commonly present at ages 2 to 7 years with signs of precocious pseudopuberty, including premature pubarche, acne, genitoscrotal hyperpigmentation, increased penile growth, growth acceleration, and advanced bone age. Most patients have a testicular volume in the prepubertal range. However, CAH should be ruled out during the baseline assessment of patients with larger testicular volumes as secondary central precocious puberty, triggered by high circulating androgens of adrenal origin, might have already developed.

Nonclassic 21-hydroxylase deficiency

The milder, nonclassic form is caused by partial impairment of 21-hydroxylase function and has an estimated incidence of 1:500 to 1 000 in the general population (1, 4, 6). Females are born with normal external genitalia. Most patients can produce sufficient amounts of mineralocorticoids and glucocorticoids, but to the expense of steroid precursor accumulation, leading to increased androgen production. Basal cortisol concentrations are generally normal, but response to 1–24ACTH is insufficient in a significant number of patients (7). Therefore, the need of glucocorticoid substitution has to be established in all patients with nonclassic CAH.

Signs and symptoms at presentation and the age at first presentation of this nonclassic form are highly variable. During childhood premature pubarche, i.e. early onset of pubic hair, and acceleration of growth and bone age are commonly observed signs. Mild clitoromegaly is infrequently found. In later life acne, hirsutism, oligomenorrhoea, sometimes even primary amenorrhoea, and infertility are frequent features. Nonclassic 21OHD is the most common specific cause in women presenting with androgen excess (8). The percentage of undiagnosed patients, in particular males, remains unknown and individuals are regularly diagnosed during family screening after the identification of an affected index patient.

Diagnosis

Neonatal period/infancy

The diagnosis of 21-hydroxylase deficiency has to be considered in all patients with genital ambiguity and/or salt-losing crisis. In case of any genital ambiguity, the karyotype analysis will provide essential information on DSD and guide towards diagnosis of the specific underlying CAH form (Table 5.11.1). The differential diagnosis between 21-hydroxylase deficiency and 11β-hydroxylase deficiency can already be established in the newborn screening using steroid hormone profiling by liquid chromatography–tandem mass spectrometry from filter paper (9). If such a method is unavailable, confirmation tests are similar to the diagnostic procedure for patients diagnosed within a clinical setting without CAH newborn screening (Table 5.11.2).

Randomly timed plasma 17OHP concentrations are significantly increased in classic 21OHD, but should be taken in the morning before 09,00 h to achieve maximal diagnostic value. Commonly, 17OHP concentrations in patients with salt-wasting CAH are higher than in nonsalt-losing patients. A short synacthen test is reserved to investigate borderline cases and is very useful to differentiate between nonclassic CAH and heterozygous carriers (Fig. 5.11.2). A highly specific marker for 21-hydroxylase deficiency is the metabolite 21-deoxycortisol, which is generated by 11-hydroxylation of 17OHP, which only occurs in the absence of 21-hydroxylase activity (Fig. 5.11.1). The analysis of a urine steroid profile is diagnostic with increased metabolites of 17OHP and 21-deoxycortisol. Plasma renin activity should be documented but in the first instance all affected children will be treated with glucocorticoids, mineralocorticoids, and sodium supplementation during the neonatal period and infancy.

Table 5.11.2 Initial diagnostic steps to establish the differential diagnosis of CAH in patients with ambiguous genitalia

Clinical question	Investigation
Chromosomal sex? 46,XX or 46,XY DSD?	FISH (X and Y specific probes), karyotype
Müllerian or wolffian structures?	Pelvic ultrasonography
Adrenal morphology? Enlarged?	Adrenal ultrasonography
Inborn error of steroidogenesis?	17OH-progesterone[a] Save plasma for: 11-deoxycortisol, 17OH-pregnenolone, DHEA, androstenedione, and testosterone
Salt loss?	U&Es, urinary electrolytes Plasma renin activity (aldosterone)
Differential diagnosis of inborn error of steroidogenesis/biochemical confirmation?	Urinary steroid metabolite profile (Gas chromatography/mass spectrometry)[b]

[a] Depending on local setting, only small blood sample volume required for steroid hormone profile by Liquid chromatography tandem/mass spectrometry including 17OHP, 11-deoxycortisol, 21-deoxycortisol, DHEA, androstenedione, testosterone.

[b] Spot urine is sufficient for the diagnosis of all forms except aldosterone synthase deficiency, which needs 24-h urine collection.

Childhood

In patients with simple-virilizing CAH with delayed diagnosis, plasma 17OHP and urine steroid analysis establish the diagnosis of 21OHD. The degree of 17OHP increase and of sex hormone excess can help to differentiate whether patients are suffering from classic or nonclassic CAH. Measurement of plasma renin activity is needed to assess if patients require additional mineralocorticoid replacement.

Nonclassic CAH

Early morning 17OHP concentrations below 2.5 nmol/l in children and below 6.0 nmol/l in women during the follicular phase make the diagnosis of nonclassic CAH unlikely. However, patients with nonclassic CAH may have normal random 17OHP concentrations. A short synacthen test with 17OHP measurements at baseline and after 60 min is the gold standard, and stimulated 17OHP concentrations above 45 nmol/l are diagnostic (Fig. 5.11.2). Cortisol levels should be included in the short synacthen test assessment to identify cases with impaired stress response that would require glucocorticoid cover, at least in increased stress situations such as intercurrent illness. Heterozygous carriers usually have circulating 17OHP levels below 30 nmol/l, but a diagnostic grey area exists for 17OHP concentrations between 30 and 45 nmol/l. Diagnostic sensitivity and specificity can be enhanced by including 21-deoxycortisol and 11-deoxycorticosterone in the measurements before and after ACTH stimulation, but is limited by availability of the tests.

The biochemical diagnosis of 21-hydroxylase deficiency should be confirmed by molecular genetic analysis of the 21-hydroxylase gene, *CYP21A2*. This provides information on severity of clinical disease expression, facilitates family screening, and aids possible subsequent discussions on future antenatal diagnosis, treatment, and family planning.

Molecular genetics of 21-hydroxylase deficiency

21-Hydroxylase (CYP21A2) gene and CYP21A2 gene locus

The 21-hydroxylase gene (*CYP21A2*, alias: *CYP21*, *CYP21B*) encodes a cytochrome P450 type II enzyme of 495 amino acids. *CYP21A2* and its nonfunctional pseudogene (*CYP21A1P*, alias: *CYP21P*, *CYP21A*) are located in the HLA region III on chromosome 6p21.3. Both genes consist of 10 exons sharing a high homology with a nucleotide identity of 98% at exon and of 96% at intron level. They are arranged in tandem repeat with the *C4A* and *C4B* genes encoding the fourth factor of the complement system (10).

CYP21A2 mutations and genotype–phenotype correlation

Complete gene deletions, large gene conversions, chimeric genes, single point mutations, and an 8-bp deletion account for the majority of *CYP21A2* mutations (1, 2). Microconversions or

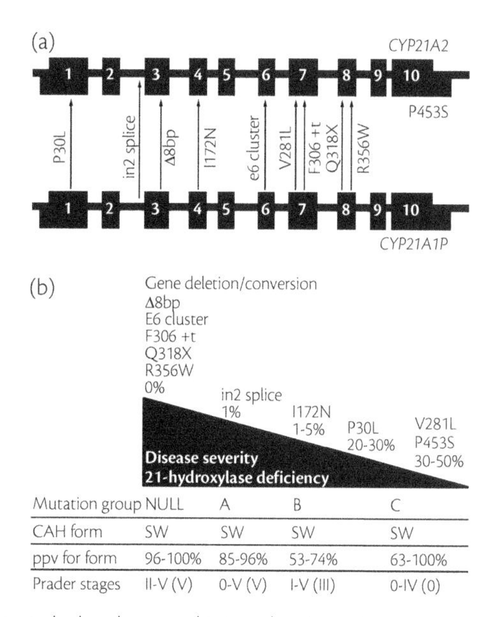

Fig. 5.11.3 21-hydroxylase gene (*CYP21A2*) and pseudogene (*CYP21A1P*). (a) Nine out of 10 common mutations are transferred by microconversions from the *CYP21A1P* gene into *CYP21A2*. In addition large gene deletions and chimeric genes between *CYP21A2* and *CYP21A1P* leading to nonfunctional product commonly occur. (b) Genotype–phenotype correlations in CAH due to 21-hydroxylase deficiency based on *in vitro* CYP21A2 activity. Mutation groups Null and A are associated with the salt-wasting (SW) form of 21OHD, group B with the simple virilizing (SV) form, and group C with the nonclassic (NC) form. Positive predictive values are usually higher with increasing severity of the mutation. The variability in the degree of virilization of the female external genitalia in the different mutation groups (grading according to Prader genital stages) is shown in the lower panel. Modal values are provided in parentheses.

apparent gene conversions transferring genetic material from the inactive *CYP21A1P* pseudogene into the active *CYP21A2* gene are the underlying cause for the eight most common point mutations and an 8-bp deletion in exon 3 (Fig. 5.11.3a). In most populations, pseudogene-derived mutations can be detected in similar frequencies. Novel or rare mutations account for about 3–5% of detected mutations in large cohorts. To date, over 90 additional rare pseudogene-independent mutations have been identified (http://www.hgmd.cf.ac.uk http://www.cypalleles.ki.se/cyp21.htm). The vast majority of these rare mutations have been identified in single families or small populations. Approximately 1% of *CYP21A2*-inactivating mutations arise *de novo*.

About 65–75% of CAH patients are compound heterozygous, i.e. they are affected, but carry different mutations on each chromosome. The clinical phenotype of CAH correlates well with the less severely mutated allele, and consequently with the allele encoding for the higher residual activity of 21-hydroxylase. This has major implications for genetic counselling in patients with nonclassic CAH. If a patient with nonclassic CAH is compound heterozygous for a mild and a severe mutation, the risk of having a child with classic CAH increases significantly to about 1 in 400 (1/50 × 1/2 × 1/4) assuming a heterozygous rate of 1/50 for classic mutations in the general population.

The correlation of genotype with the extent of glucocorticoid and mineralocorticoid deficiency is strong (Fig. 5.11.3b). However, divergence between genotype and phenotype occurs in some cases. Although a trend exists, the correlation between the genotype and the virilization phenotype assessed by Prader genital stages is less pronounced (Fig. 5.11.3b). This implies the importance of other factors modifying clinical androgen effects. This observed variability might be influenced by CAG repeat length of the androgen receptor modulating androgen action (11). Potential variations in the degree of recovery from glucocorticoid and mineralocorticoid deficiency during later life might be explained by significant 21-hydroxylase activity of the extra-adrenal enzymes CYP2C19 and CYP3A4 (12).

Treatment

Therapeutic management of CAH is challenging and treatment objectives differ with age. Generally, treatment includes glucocorticoid and mineralocorticoid replacement and also aims at the control of adrenal androgen excess. Therapeutic goals in affected children are the prevention of adrenal crisis and precocious pseudopuberty, and protection from long-term complications. Importantly, management in affected girls has to address the issue of genital corrective surgery and psychosexual development. In adults, long-term morbidity and infertility are in the focus.

Glucocorticoid treatment

Hydrocortisone is recommended for replacement therapy from the newborn period to adolescence (13). The average physiological cortisol secretion rate is about 8 mg/m^2 per day. Typical hydrocortisone doses are 10–15 mg/m^2 divided in three daily doses, with doses up to 25 mg/m^2 in infancy only seldom required. These doses are higher than those employed for replacement of adrenal insufficiency, because treatment also aims at normalization of ACTH-driven adrenal androgen excess. Cortisone acetate is not recommended as it requires activation to cortisol by 11β-hydroxysteroid dehydrogenase type 1, which leads to considerable interindividual variability in pharmacokinetics of cortisone acetate. The optimal timing for providing the highest dose of hydrocortisone remains unsolved with no endpoint data supporting either a circadian or reverse-circadian replacement strategy. Providing the highest dose in the evening has no or a minor effect on the ACTH surge occurring during the early morning hours. However, providing the highest dose in the morning, as done in the majority of paediatric endocrine centres in Europe, may also not suppress the ACTH surge sufficiently as hydrocortisone is usually given around 7 AM, thus 4–5 h after the surge (14). Ideally, the early glucocorticoid dose is given between 03.00 and 04.00 h, but this approach is rarely tolerated by patients and parents. Long-acting synthetic glucocorticoids, such as prednisone, prednisolone, and dexamethasone, are more likely to be associated with growth suppression and weight gain and should be avoided before final height is achieved.

At final height patients may be changed to treatment with longer-acting glucocorticoids, e.g. with prednisolone (2–4 mg/m^2 per day) and dexamethasone (0.25–0.375 mg/m^2 per day, seldom more than 0.5 mg total daily dose). Reassessment of mineralocorticoid deficiency is of paramount importance as prednisolone delivers reduced and dexamethasone exhibits virtually no mineralocorticoid activity. By contrast, hydrocortisone can mask mineralocorticoid deficiency by binding the mineralocorticoid receptor with similar affinity to aldosterone (0.1 mg fludrocortisone is equivalent to 40 mg hydrocortisone).

Table 5.11.3 Parameters used for therapy monitoring in steroid 21-hydroxylase deficiency

Parameters	Comment
Clinical	
Growth/ growth velocity/ BMI	
Pubertal status	
Virilization, hirsutism	
Striae	
Tiredness	
Hyperpigmentation	
Blood pressure	
Bone age	
Biochemistry[a]	
17-hydroxyprogesterone as: ◆ Single time point blood test ◆ Filter paper blood profile ◆ Salivary profile	Good indicator of glucocorticoid overtreatment if suppressed or in normal range
DHEA-S	Limited value for therapy monitoring
Androstenedione as: ◆ Single time point blood test ◆ Salivary profile	Good indicator of therapy quality with aim to achieve concentrations within the normal age- and sex-specific range
Testosterone	Aim to achieve concentrations within the normal age- and sex-specific range, differentiation between adrenal or gonadal origin not possible
Plasma renin activity/renin	Good indicator for appropriate mineralocorticoid replacement
Pregnanetriol, pregnanetriolone	Urine metabolites of 17-hydroxyprogesterone, not widely used
17-ketosteroids	Urine metabolites of 17-hydroxylated steroids including androgens, older and unspecific method, not widely used, largely obsolete

[a] Evidence for the superiority of either combination of parameters does not exist.
BMI, body mass index; DHEA-S, dehydroepiandrosterone sulphate.

Several monitoring strategies for corticosteroid therapy in CAH have been described, including clinical and biochemical markers (Table 5.11.3). Data on the superiority of either approach are not available. Similar to the situation in adrenal insufficiency (see Chapter 5.9) cortisol measurements are not useful to monitor quality of glucocorticoid substitution in adrenal insufficiency (15). Treatment of CAH should aim to normalize sex hormones. Commonly, the optimal glucocorticoid dose avoids suppression of 17OHP while maintaining sex hormone concentrations in the mid age- and sex-specific normal range.

Mineralocorticoid and sodium chloride replacement

Mineralocorticoid replacement is required in all patients with classic CAH, at least during infancy. Fludrocortisone doses during the first year of life are commonly 150 μg/m^2 per day and should be adjusted according to individual requirements. Total dose of 300 μg per day might be required (13). Sodium needs to be supplemented as milk feeds only provide maintenance sodium requirements. Sodium supplements up to 10 mmol/kg per day may be required at least in the first 6 months of life (16). Sodium supplementation may be discontinued when salt intake is sufficient via food. Sodium supplementation can be beneficial also in later life during episodes of increased sodium loss such as hot weather and intense exercise. Adequate mineralocorticoid replacement generally leads to hydrocortisone dose reduction. The need to continue this therapy should be reassessed after infancy or early childhood using plasma renin activity and blood pressure as reliable markers (13). The relative dose in relation to body surface decreases throughout life. After the first 2 years of life, fludrocortisone doses of 100 μg/m^2 per day are commonly sufficient. This requirement drops further with adolescents and adults are usually sufficiently supplemented with a total daily dose of 100 to 200 μg (50 to 100 μg/m^2 per day). Mineralocorticoid substitution is monitored by plasma renin, aiming at the upper normal reference range, and also by blood pressure measurements using age, sex, and height-adjusted references. A significant drop (>15 mmHg) in systolic blood pressure between seated and erect blood pressure recordings indicates postural hypotension suggestive of insufficient mineralocorticoid replacement.

Stress treatment

Adrenal crisis due to impaired cortisol response to stress is a serious threat in CAH. During febrile illness (>38.5 °C), trauma, and surgery the daily hydrocortisone dose should be doubled or tripled, with intravenous or intramuscular administration oral doses where appropriate. Fludrocortisone adjustment is commonly not required. However, extra sodium supplement may be necessary. Special attention should be paid towards glucose supply during severe illness as patients tend to hypoglycaemia due to impaired adrenomedullary function. Patients with diarrhoea and vomiting, who are unable to take their medication require IM hydrocortisone (100 mg/m^2 per dose, maximum 100 mg) and immediate review by a medical professional. Patients with severe illness or major surgery require IV hydrocortisone (Table 5.11.4). All CAH patients must carry a steroid emergency card or MedicAlert bracelet emphasizing the diagnosis 'adrenal insufficiency' in addition to CAH. Patients should have an emergency glucocorticoid injection kit and

Table 5.11.4 Intravenous glucocorticoids during critical illness or major surgery

Age		Bolus (single dose)	Maintenance
≤3 years	Hydrocortisone	25 mg IV	25–30 mg IV per day
>3 years and <12 years	Hydrocortisone	50 mg IV	50–60 mg IV per day
≥12 years	Hydrocortisone	100 mg IV	100 mg IV per day
Adults	Hydrocortisone	100 mg IV	100–200 mg IV per day

patients (and parents and partners) should undergo self-injection training.

Surgical management

Genital surgery should achieve a genital appearance compatible with gender, unobstructed urinary emptying without incontinence or infections, and good adult sexual and reproductive function (13). A one-stage surgical approach following the latest techniques of vaginoplasty, clitoral, and labial surgery has been recommended (13). Surgery is recommended to be timed at age 2 to 6 months. Surgical procedures between age 12 months and adolescence are usually not recommended in the absence of medical problems. Clitorectomy is absolutely contraindicated at any stage. Vaginal dilations are contraindicated until adolescence. It is important that female CAH patients remain under the follow-up of a specialized gynaecologist throughout adolescence and adulthood.

Prenatal treatment

Prenatal treatment is carried out with dexamethasone, which crosses the placenta and therefore can suppress the fetal HPA axis that drives androgen excess and virilization. However, prenatal treatment is controversial as the safety, including metabolic and psychointellectual long-term consequences of dexamethasone treatment, remains to be fully defined. Prenatal treatment has been shown to be effective to prevent severe genital virilization if started early enough, as major developments in fetal sexual differentiation take place between gestational weeks 4–10. Therefore, dexamethasone treatment needs to be established as soon as pregnancy is confirmed and ideally before the sixth and no later than the eighth week of gestation to achieve significant benefit in preventing 46,XX DSD. Counselling regarding prenatal dexamethasone therapy should be carried out ideally well before conception, involving an endocrinologist, fetal medicine specialist, and clinical geneticist. Patients should be included in ongoing multicentre studies with available protocols (17). The suggested dose is 20–25 μg/kg in three divided doses (total maximum dose 1.5 mg/day) (1). Maternal side effects resemble those of high-dose glucocorticoid treatment including oedema, striae, weight gain, mood fluctuations, and sleep disturbances. Arterial hypertension and impaired glucose tolerance seem not to be increased, but close monitoring for these complications should be carried out. Only one in eight children will benefit from prenatal dexamethasone treatment if the parents are heterozygous carriers, as the chance of carrying an affected girl is 12.5%. All other children are exposed to dexamethasone without benefit. The number of unnecessarily treated cases can be reduced to three out of eight using modern molecular genetic techniques. The fetal sex can be determined as early as week six of gestation by analysing free fetal DNA from maternal blood by using real time PCR approaches. Dexamethasone treatment can be stopped if the fetus is determined to be male. Otherwise, the fetal sex is established from a chorionic villous biopsy. If the fetal karyotype is 46,XX, *CYP21A2* mutation analysis is performed and subsequently dexamethasone treatment stopped in pregnancies with an unaffected female. In case of an affected female fetus, current recommendations suggest that dexamethasone treatment should be continued up until delivery.

Nonstandard therapies

Two main additional experimental pharmacological therapies in the paediatric setting have focussed on the improvement of final height. A promising approach within a study setting uses a combination of the antiandrogen flutamide to lower glucocorticoid doses (8 mg/m^2 per day) and the aromatase inhibitor testolactone to reduce oestrogen-mediated fusion of the growth plate. Final outcome data are unavailable, but 2-year follow-up data showed normal linear growth in children treated with this regimen. Another study, including 14 patients, achieved improvement of growth and final height with gonadotropin-releasing-hormone agonists used alone and in combination with growth hormone. Long-term safety and efficiency data are unavailable.

Bilateral adrenalectomy has been proposed as an alternative in severe CAH. However, the experience with bilateral adrenalectomy in CAH is limited. Long-term follow-up data indicated improved signs and symptoms of hyperandrogenism and less obesity after surgery. It has also been reported as a therapeutic approach to achieve successful pregnancies. However, this procedure bears also a number of risk, including surgical and anaesthetic complications and leaving the patients completely adrenal insufficient and thus exposing them to a higher risk of adrenal crisis. Currently, bilateral adrenalectomy for CAH has to be considered an experimental therapeutic strategy and its appropriateness needs to be carefully considered.

Psychosexual issues

Gender-related behaviour demonstrates shifts from female to male even in patients with the milder nonclassic CAH, becoming more obvious in the more severe CAH forms (18). Females with CAH have a more male-typical childhood play behaviour and more male-typical cognitive functioning during childhood than unaffected girls. The impact on adult life is unclear as adult women with CAH do not show a more male-typical cognitive pattern. Psychological health is not compromised and psychological adjustment is not significantly associated with genital virilization or age at genital surgery. Gender assignment is commonly not a problem even in heavily virilized 46,XX individuals. Importantly, most female CAH patients do not experience serious gender identity problems, such as gender dysphoria, reported in only 5% of 250 patients. Similar numbers have been observed in a series of 63 female CAH patients (18). Conversely, 90% of female CAH patients raised as males (n = 33) had a normal male gender identity (19).

Consequences of genital corrective surgery are of importance during adolescence and early adulthood. Inadequate vaginal reconstruction, which may be present in more than 50% of adult patients (20), and reduced clitoral sensitivity, impacts on sexual activity and sexual experience. This often has downstream effects on partner choice, steady relationships, marital status, and fertility (18). Although the surgical approach is continuously improving, physicians involved in the care of adult CAH patients will be confronted with the consequences of previous, now abandoned surgical techniques for several decades to follow. Another important mechanism resulting in sexual dysfunction in CAH patients is near complete suppression of sex hormones due to glucocorticoid overtreatment, with subsequently low libido.

Long-term prognosis in CAH

Growth and development

The final height outcome in many patients is not optimal. A meta-analysis, including 18 studies between 1977 and 2001, showed that the mean adult height in classic CAH was 10 cm (−1.4 standard deviation score (SDS)) below the population mean and −1.2 SDS calculated for target height. The pubertal growth spurt occurs earlier and is less pronounced than in the normal population. Hyperandrogenism and overexposure to glucocorticoids both contribute to the problem. Sex hormone excess leads to accelerated growth, early fusion of the epiphysis, and can also trigger secondary central precocious puberty, which further exacerbates the situation.

Glucocorticoid overexposure inhibits growth. Special attention should be drawn towards the infancy growth spurt during the first 2 years of life. This growth phase is characterized by the highest postnatal growth velocity and an impaired growth velocity during this time significantly impacts on final height outcome. Therefore, the lowest optimal dose for glucocorticoid substitution and sex hormone normalization has to be achieved as early in life as possible.

Metabolic consequences and cardiovascular risk

Obesity and increased fat mass is common amongst children and adolescents with CAH (21–23). Birth weight and length, serum leptin concentrations, or type of glucocorticoid and mineralocorticoid dose were not associated with obesity in 89 CAH patients (0.2–17.9 years). However, glucocorticoid dose, chronologic age, advanced bone age maturation, and parental obesity contributed to elevated body mass index (BMI)-SDS (22). CAH females older than 30 years had increased fat mass and higher insulin levels. However, clear evidence of cardiovascular risk factors could not be shown. Women with CAH have a significantly higher rate of gestational diabetes as a risk factor for the development of type 2 diabetes (24). Females with nonclassic CAH (25) and young adult CAH patients (26) have reduced insulin sensitivity. The risk of atherosclerosis might be increased; increased intima media thickness as a marker of atherosclerosis has been detected (26). The intima media thickness was independent of cardiovascular risk factors such as BMI, elevated blood pressure, or lipid profile changes (26).

Daytime systolic blood pressure in children and adolescents with CAH is elevated and the physiological nocturnal dip in blood pressure is absent (27). Elevated systolic blood pressure correlates with the degree of overweight and obesity. CAH patients with normal weight tend to suffer more frequently from diastolic hypotension (28). Older CAH patients had a higher standing diastolic blood pressure than younger patients, which was not observed in the control group (24). Data on mortality are unavailable.

Bone mineral density

Bone mineral density (BMD) is usually not grossly impaired if patients receive an appropriate glucocorticoid dose. Low BMD appears to be associated with glucocorticoid overtreatment. Androgen excess and subsequent aromatization can lead to enhanced bone density. A reduction of bone turnover markers in conjunction with normal BMD has been noticed by several groups (29, 30).

Fertility and pregnancy

Fertility prognosis has been improving over the recent years and is now less pessimistic than described in the first reports. Most adult males with CAH are fertile, but the impact on male fertility has possibly been underestimated.

Female fertility The fertility rate is the lowest in salt-wasting CAH patients, with markedly increasing fertility in patients with simple-virilizing and nonclassic CAH. The aetiology of decreased female fertility is multifactorial (Box 5.11.1). Optimization of fertility can often be achieved by close monitoring and adjustment of glucocorticoid replacement with the longer acting prednisolone. The situation may prove difficult because both over-replacement and under-replacement with glucocorticoids can result in anovulation. Even after achieving good control of 17-hydroxyprogesterone production, serum progesterone levels may remain elevated (31) thereby impairing follicle maturation and implantation of the fertilized egg. The successful use of adrenalectomy to achieve pregnancy has been reported in two patients (32).

Pregnancy in female CAH patients Prior to pregnancy, the carrier status of the male partner should be established. If the partner is not a carrier for CAH, the developing child will be an obligatory, clinically healthy carrier. If the partner of a CAH patient desiring pregnancy happens to be a heterozygous *CYP21A2* mutation carrier, the patient should be counselled with regard to the possibility of prenatal dexamethasone treatment. Recommendations for the management of women with adrenal insufficiency suggest that the glucocorticoid dose should be increased by 30–50% during the last trimester of pregnancy (33). Although it has been suggested that glucocorticoids have to be rarely adjusted during pregnancy (29), spontaneous miscarriage risk in untreated women with nonclassic CAH is significantly higher than in treated patients (34). Mineralocorticoid requirements may sometimes increase as well, due to the antimineralocorticoid properties of progesterone. Adjustment of the mineralocorticoid dose has to be performed according to postural blood pressure response, and serum sodium and potassium concentrations. Plasma renin activity is physiologically increased during pregnancy and therefore cannot serve as a monitoring tool. Delivery requires glucocorticoid coverage at doses recommended for major surgical stress, i.e. 100–200 mg/24 h, either per continuous intravenous infusion in a 5% glucose solution or per intramuscular injection (e.g. 50 mg four times per day), with rapid tapering after delivery if the clinical situation permits. Patients who underwent corrective surgery for ambiguous genitalia will more likely require a caesarean section.

Male fertility Two major issues are recognized to impact on male fertility (Box 5.11.1). Hypogonadotrophic hypogonadism is a consequence of increased aromatization of adrenal androgens, in particular androstenedione to oestrone. This results in suppression of pituitary luteinizing hormone and follicle-stimulating hormone secretion impacting on testicular androgen synthesis and spermatogenesis. The condition is reversible after optimization of glucocorticoid therapy.

Benign testicular adrenal rest tumours (TARTs) have been correlated with male infertility (35). Embryologically, testes and adrenal cortex both develop from the urogenital ridge. TARTs arise from adrenal cell nests within the testicular tissue that are subject to continuous ACTH stimulation. TART can result in Leydig cell failure and/or oligospermia. High-dose glucocorticoid treatment may reverse infertility. However, even high doses of steroids may not be sufficient to restore testicular function. Testes-sparing surgery may not reliably restore testicular function. TARTs have been detected in male patients as early as 7 years of age. Early treatment optimization to reduce these hyperplasic areas within the testes appears to be paramount to improve long-term fertility outcome. Of note, TARTs represent a benign entity that responds to glucocorticoid treatment in the early stages and should not be confused with testicular tumours. Treating physicians and urological surgeons need

Box 5.11.1 Causes of decreased fertility in congenital adrenal hyperplasia

Females

- Unsatisfactory intercourse due to inadequate vaginal introitus
- Decreased heterosexual activity
- Increased rate of homosexual orientation
- Poor adrenal suppression
- Ovulatory dysfunction due to polycystic ovaries
- Failure of implantation caused by increased follicular phase progesterone
- Amenorrhoea/oligomenorrhoea
- Insulin resistance, hyperandrogenism
- Reduced libido due to glucocorticoid overtreatment
- Gonadotrophin suppression due to glucocorticoid overtreatment
- Intrauterine androgen exposure—long-term effects on HPG axis?

Males

- Testicular adrenal rest tumours
- Hypogonadotrophic hypogonadism
- Adrenal androgen excess
- Glucocorticoid overtreatment

to be aware of this entity to avoid unnecessary gonadectomies based on the suspicion of seminoma.

11β-Hydroxylase deficiency

About 5–8% of CAH cases are due to 11β-hydroxylase deficiency (11OHD), which is equivalent to an incidence of 1 in 100 000 to 200 000 livebirths in nonconsanguineous populations (36). Steroid 11β-hydroxylase (CYP11B1) catalyses the final step in cortisol biosynthesis, the conversion of 11-deoxycortisol to cortisol (Fig. 5.11.1). It also catalyses the conversion of 11-deoxycorticosterone (DOC) to corticosterone, but is lacking noteworthy 18-hydroxylase and 18-oxidase activity (Fig. 5.11.1). Thus 11OHD results in decreased cortisol secretion and accumulation of the glucocorticoid precursor 11-deoxycortisol and the mineralocorticoid precursor DOC (Fig. 5.11.1). DOC activates the mineralocorticoid receptor and may lead to significant arterial hypertension. Accumulated precursors are shunted into the androgen synthesis pathway, leading to hyperandrogenism. Basal concentrations of 17OHP are commonly increased, but may be normal even during the first weeks of life (37).

Classic 11OHD results in virilization of the external genitalia in newborn females, and later on leads to precocious pseudopuberty combined with rapid somatic growth and bone age acceleration in both sexes. Nonclassic 11OHD is a rare condition (36, 38). Affected female patients are born with normal genitalia and present with signs of androgen excess during childhood. Alternatively, they may present as adults with hirsutism and oligomenorrhoea, though certainly only a small minority of women presenting with signs and symptoms suggestive of polycystic ovary syndrome suffer from nonclassic 11β-hydroxylase deficiency.

Steroid 11β-hydroxylase deficiency is caused by mutations in the 11β-hydroxylase gene (*CYP11B1*), which is localized on chromosome 8q21 approximately 40 kb from the highly homologous aldosterone synthase gene (*CYP11B2*) (39). *CYP11B1*-inactivating mutations have been shown to be distributed over the entire coding region consisting of nine exons. Although a cluster is reported in exons 2, 6, 7, and 8 (40, 41), real hot spots such as in 21OHD do not exist. A broad variety of mutations have been reported to cause either classic or nonclassic 11OHD (63).

Glucocorticoid replacement follows the same rules as in 21-hydroxylase deficiency. The blood pressure is often well controlled under glucocorticoid substitution. However, if no blood pressure control can be achieved, antihypertensive treatment should be commenced at an early stage and excessive glucocorticoid exposure should be avoided.

17α-Hydroxylase deficiency

Steroid 17α-hydroxylase deficiency (17OHD) is a rare form of CAH. It accounts for about 1% of all CAH cases and affects adrenal and gonadal steroid biosynthesis. The 17α-hydroxylase enzyme (CYP17A1) catalyses two different enzymatic reactions: firstly, the 17α-hydroxylation of pregnenolone and progesterone and, secondly, via its 17,20 lyase activity, the conversion of 17-hydroxypregenolone to DHEA and with lesser efficiency also that of 17OHP to androstenedione (Fig. 5.11.1). As a consequence, 17OHD results in both glucocorticoid deficiency and sex steroid deficiency. In addition, the mineralocorticoid precursors corticosterone and DOC accumulate (Fig. 5.11.1) Corticosterone has weaker glucocorticoid activity than cortisol, but corticosterone excess production generally prevents adrenal crisis in patients with 17OHD. Accumulation of corticosterone and DOC result in excess mineralocorticoid activity, causing severe hypokalaemic hypertension. Sex steroid deficiency caused by loss of 17,20 lyase activity results in 46,XY DSD presenting as undervirilization in male newborns and in primary amenorrhoea in 46,XX individuals. There is lack of pubertal development due to hypergonadotrophic hypogonadism in both sexes (42).

Due to the low incidence of adrenal crisis in untreated 17OHD, the diagnosis is often only established during adolescence or early adulthood following investigations for hypokalaemic hypertension or delayed pubertal development (42). This fact emphasizes the importance of blood pressure measurement as a clinical screening tool in all patients with delayed puberty. Typical biochemical findings include raised ACTH levels and suppressed plasma renin activity whilst serum aldosterone is decreased, with sex steroid deficiency further confirming the diagnosis (Table 5.11.1). Glucocorticoid replacement commonly normalizes plasma renin activity, aldosterone, blood pressure, and electrolyte disturbances. Doses are lower than required for treatment of 21OHD and 11OHD. Substitution of sex hormones is generally required.

A rare variant of 17OHD has been described, isolated 17,20 lyase deficiency with largely preserved 17α-hydroxylase activity. This manifests with impaired sex steroid biosynthesis only, without concurrent evidence of mineralocorticoid excess or glucocorticoid deficiency.

The *CYP17A1* gene consists of eight exons and is located on chromosome 10q24.3. A variety of different mutations have been described, without evidence of a hot spot. Mutations underlying the isolated 17,20 lyase deficiency variant are located within the area of the CYP17A1 molecule that is thought to interact with the cofactor cytochrome b5, thereby disrupting the electron transfer from POR to CYP17A1, specifically disrupting the conversion of 17OH-pregnenolone to DHEA (43, 44) (Fig. 5.11.1).

3β-Hydroxysteroid-dehydrogenase deficiency

Steroid 3β-hydroxysteroid-dehydrogenase type 2 (HSD3B2) deficiency represents a rare CAH variant and data on population-based incidence are lacking. HSD3B2, also termed Δ4/Δ5-isomerase, catalyses three key reactions in adrenal steroidogenesis: the conversion of the Δ5-steroids pregnenolone, 17OH-pregnenolone and DHEA to the Δ4-steroids progesterone, 17OHP and androstenedione, respectively (Fig. 5.11.1). Thereby HSD3B2 deficiency affects all three biosynthetic pathways (mineralocorticoids, glucocorticoids, sex steroids). The clinical spectrum shows a wide variety of disease expression, ranging from a severe salt-wasting form, with or without ambiguous genitalia in affected male neonates, to isolated premature pubarche in infants and children of both sexes and late-onset variant manifesting with hirsutism and menstrual irregularities. Patients with mild biochemical late-onset deficiency are commonly *HSD3B2* mutation negative. There is no strong correlation between salt-wasting and male undervirilization, primarily presenting with mostly perineoscrotal hypospadias and bifid scrotum. Female patients diagnosed during neonatal or infant life usually present with normal genitalia, though some cases of minor clitoromegaly have been reported. The diagnosis of HSD3B2 deficiency is often delayed in affected individuals without salt-wasting and with normal genitalia. Furthermore, HSD3B2-deficient patients are at risk to be misdiagnosed as suffering from of 21OHD (45).

The biochemical diagnosis of HSD3B2 deficiency is usually established by the elevated concentrations of Δ5-steroids, such as DHEA, 17OH-pregnenolone, and their metabolites, and a high ratio of Δ5 to Δ4 steroids or their respective urinary metabolites (45) (Fig. 5.11.1). Hormonal criteria have recently been refined for the diagnosis of HSD3B2 deficiency based on genotyping of the *HSD3B2* gene. 17OH-pregnenolone concentrations and 17OH-pregnenolone to cortisol ratios at baseline and after ACTH stimulations are of the highest discriminatory value in differentiating between patients affected by HSD3B2 deficiency and patients with milder biochemical abnormalities, who are negative for *HSD3B2* mutations (46, 47).

Two isoforms of 3β-hydroxysteroid dehydrogenase, 3β-HSD type 1 and 3β-HSD type 2, exist, which are encoded by the *HSD3B1* and *HSD3B2* genes, respectively. The *HSD3B2* gene is located on chromosome 1p13•1 and consists of four exons. 3β-HSD2 is mainly present in the adrenal and the gonad, while 3β-HSD1 is present in the placenta and almost ubiquitously in peripheral target tissues (45, 48). Both enzymes are NAD-dependant short chain dehydrogenases. HSD3B2 deficiency is caused by mutations in the *HSD3B2* gene. A reasonable degree of genotype–phenotype correlation with regard to mineralocorticoid deficiency exists, with major loss of function mutations resulting in the salt-wasting form and partial inactivating mutations allowing for some residual aldosterone synthesis capacity. However, the genotype cannot be used to predict the degree of male undervirilization (45).

P450 Oxidoreductase deficiency

ORD is the underlying cause of CAH presenting with apparent combined CYP17A1–CYP21A2 deficiency, which was first described in 1985 (49). However, the molecular pathology has only recently been elucidated as inactivating mutations in the electron donor enzyme POR which provides electrons to all microsomal CYP enzymes including CYP17A1 and CYP21A2 (50, 51). The incidence of ORD is unknown, but a considerable number of patients have been described since the molecular characterization of ORD.

The majority of ORD patients described have skeletal malformations (Box 5.11.2) resembling the Antley–Bixler syndrome phenotype with predominantly craniofacial malformations. Endocrine dysfunction is characterized by adrenal and gonadal insufficiency and disordered sexual development which may occur in affected individuals of both sexes (46,XX DSD and 46,XY DSD). An Antley–Bixler syndrome phenotype can also be caused by autosomal dominant mutations in the fibroblast growth factor receptor 2 gene (*FGFR2*), which does not manifest with abnormalities of steroid metabolism or ambiguous genitalia (52). Impairment of sterol biosynthesis, specifically of POR-dependent 14α-lanosterol demethylase (CYP51A1), may be causative for the development of skeletal malformation. This is supported by the finding that children born to mothers treated during pregnancy with the CYP51A1 inhibitor fluconazole show evidence of Antley–Bixler syndrome-like skeletal malformations.

Severe sexual ambiguity in ORD can be found in both sexes. Affected girls may present with significant virilization of the external genitalia. Affected boys can be undervirilized, with degrees varying from borderline micropenis to perineoscrotal hypospadias. Progressive postnatal virilization in affected girls does not occur and circulating sex hormone concentrations are invariably low or low normal in both sexes. Mothers pregnant with an affected child may present with virilization manifesting during midgestation and have often low oestriol concentrations. Generally, the androgen excess reverses after delivery (53).

Undervirilization in affected boys is easily conceivable based on the impairment of CYP17A1 function. The potential existence of an alternative 'backdoor' pathway towards prenatal androgen synthesis has been described, potentially explaining virilization in affected girls. Postnatally, the alternative pathway ceases and the

Box 5.11.2 Skeletal malformations in P450 oxidoreductase deficiency

- Craniofacial malformations
- Craniosynostosis
- Midface hypoplasia
- Low-set ears
- Pear-shaped nose
- Choanal atresia
- Digital malformations (e.g. arachnodactyly, clinodactyly)
- Radiohumeral synostosis
- Bowed femora, including neonatal fractures

conventional androgen pathway remains inefficient due to the POR mutations.

Pubertal development in ORD is not well studied yet. It appears to be dominated by the consequences of sex steroid deficiency (54). A common finding in females diagnosed in early adolescence are polycystic ovaries. Females may have large ovarian cysts that have a tendency to rupture and bilateral polycystic ovaries have even been reported in a 2-month old baby with ORD.

Typical biochemical findings include raised 17OHP, albeit not to the extent observed in 21-hydroxylase deficiency. In contrast to 21OHD, sex steroids are low and there is commonly no mineralocorticoid deficiency. The gold standard for diagnosis of ORD is GC/MS analysis of urinary steroid excretion. The metabolome is characterized by accumulation of pregnenolone and progesterone metabolites alongside low androgen metabolites and increased 17OHP metabolites, indicating pathognomonic combined CYP17A1–CYP21A2 deficiency (Fig. 5.11.1). Analysis of serum steroids may lead to misdiagnosis of patients because features of 17OHD and 21OHD are present in variable combinations (55). Prenatal biochemical diagnosis is possible as mothers pregnant with an affected child often present with low serum oestriol and a characteristic urinary steroid profile (2, 56). Recent data suggest that at least 50% of patients can be detected in newborn 17OHP screening (54).

Baseline glucocorticoid secretion is often sufficient, but the cortisol response to stress is usually impaired (54, 56). Affected patients without hydrocortisone replacement are at a high risk for developing a life-threatening adrenal crisis. Glucocorticoids are required in replacement doses only (commonly hydrocortisone 8–10 mg/m^2 per day) because of absent postnatal androgen excess. Mineralocorticoid production is generally uncompromised, plasma renin activity and serum aldosterone are generally normal. However, some patients show increased excretion of mineralocorticoid metabolites (51) and mild hypertension (50). The *POR* gene is located on chromosome 7q11.2. It consists of 15 translated exons spanning a region of approximately 32.9 kb and encodes for a protein of 680 amino acids. A variety of *POR*-inactivating mutations have been reported, including missense, frameshift, and splice site mutations (http://www.cypalleles.ki.se/por.htm). A287P is the most common mutation in Caucasians, while R457H is the most frequent founder mutation in the Japanese population. Although genotype–phenotype correlations are not fully established yet, certain patterns are evolving suggestive of genotype–phenotype correlations predicting the presence and severity of skeletal malformations as well as the correlation of karyotype and presence of genital ambiguity (54).

Steroid acute regulatory protein (StAR) deficiency—congenital lipoid adrenal hyperplasia

StAR mobilizes cholesterol from the outer mitochondrial membrane to the inner mitochondrial membrane (Fig. 5.11.1). StAR-independent cholesterol transport only occurs at a low rate. Therefore, a defect in StAR leads to almost no substrate provision for P450 side-chain cleavage and the production of all steroid hormones from adrenal and gonad is severely reduced. In contrast to the conventional CAH forms, the adrenals of individuals affected by CLAH show a characteristic accumulation of lipids, predominantly cholesterol esters (57). The most severe form presents with 46,XY DSD and combined adrenal insufficiency. Salt-wasting typically develops in the neonatal period or after a few weeks of life, but later onset also occurs. Females can show spontaneous pubertal development. Recently a milder form of StAR deficiency has been described with normally virilized 46,XY individuals, who presented with adrenal failure during early childhood (58). Treatment consists of glucocorticoid and mineralocorticoid replacement, and substitution of sex hormones in later life.

P450 Side chain cleavage deficiency

The deficiency of P450 side-chain cleavage (CYP11A1) enzyme is a rare inborn error of steroidogenesis. It presents clinically and biochemically with similar signs and symptoms as CLAH caused by StAR mutations. However, all patients with CYP11A1 deficiency had small or normal-sized adrenals (59). Depending on the impairment of CYP11A1 function a spectrum of clinical presentation ranging from 46,XY DSD with severe adrenal insufficiency in the newborn period over midshaft hypospadias and cryptorchidism and later manifestation of adrenal insufficiency during childhood (60). Concentrations of all steroid hormones are characteristically decreased as the first step in steroidogenesis, the conversion of cholesterol to pregnenolone is impaired. Treatment is similar to CLAH.

Aldosterone synthase deficiency

Aldosterone synthase (CYP11B2, corticosterone methyloxidase, CMO) deficiency (ASD) is a rare condition causing isolated mineralocorticoid deficiency (61). Patients present during the first days to weeks of life. Since patients are not glucocorticoid deficient and can synthesize DOC (and variable levels of corticosterone) the salt-wasting crisis is commonly less pronounced than in 21OHD. Two biochemical forms exist: ASD 1 (CMO I) has an increased ratio of corticosterone to 18OH-corticosterone and decreased 18OH-corticosterone to aldosterone ratio, whereas corticosterone to 18OH-corticosterone is decreased and 18OH-corticosterone to aldosterone is increased in ADS 2 (CMO II). Both forms are associated with mutations in the *CYP11B2* gene. The underlying molecular pathology defining these different forms is not fully understood. Patients with CYP11B2 deficiency generally respond well to fludrocortisone (start dose 150 μg/m^2 per day in neonates and infancy) and will also benefit from salt supplementation. Patients, who manifested with failure to thrive, generally show a good catch-up growth after initiation of treatment. Electrolytes often tend to normalize from age 3 to 4 years. Untreated patients are at significant risk of being growth retarded. Adults are generally asymptomatic, but are more susceptible to salt loss. The need for mineralocorticoid treatment in later life has to be established individually.

Apparent cortisone reductase deficiency

Apparent cortisone reductase deficiency is characterized by hyperandrogenism resulting in hirsutism, oligoamenorrhoea, and infertility in females and premature pseudopuberty in males. The condition is caused by mutations in the gene encoding hexose-6-dehydrogenase (62), which provides NADPH to 11β-hydroxysteroid dehydrogenase type 1 (HSD11B1). HSD11B1 activates inactive cortisone to cortisol within target tissues of glucocorticoid action, namely in the liver and adipose (Fig. 5.11.1). Defects in this system result in increased cortisol clearance leading to activation of the HPA axis and ACTH-mediated adrenal androgen excess.

References

1. White PC, Speiser PW. Congenital adrenal hyperplasia due to 21-hydroxylase deficiency. *Endocr Rev*, 2000; **21**: 245–91.
2. Krone N, Dhir V, Ivison HE, Arlt W. Congenital adrenal hyperplasia and P450 oxidoreductase deficiency. *Clin Endocrinol (Oxf)*, 2007; **66**: 162–72.
3. Nakamura Y, Hornsby PJ, Casson P, Morimoto R, Satoh F, Xing Y, *et al*. Type 5 17beta-hydroxysteroid dehydrogenase (AKR1C3) contributes to testosterone production in the adrenal reticularis. *J Clin Endocrinol Metab*, 2009; **94**: 2192–8.
4. Merke DP, Bornstein SR. Congenital adrenal hyperplasia. *Lancet*, 2005; **365**: 2125–36.
5. Arlt W, Krone N. Adult consequences of congenital adrenal hyperplasia. *Horm Res*,2007; **68** (Suppl. 5): 158–64.
6. New MI. Extensive clinical experience: nonclassical 21-hydroxylase deficiency. *J Clin Endocrinol Metab*, 2006; **91**: 4205–14.
7. Bidet M, Bellanne-Chantelot C, Galand-Portier M-B, Tardy V, Billaud L, Laborde K, *et al*. Clinical and molecular characterization of a cohort of 161 unrelated women with nonclassical congenital adrenal hyperplasia due to 21-hydroxylase deficiency and 330 family members. *J Clin Endocrinol Metab*, 2009; **94**: 1570–8.
8. Azziz R, Sanchez LA, Knochenhauer ES, Moran C, Lazenby J, Stephens KC, *et al*. Androgen excess in women: experience with over 1000 consecutive patients. *J Clin Endocrinol Metab*, 2004; **89**: 453–62.
9. Janzen N, Peter M, Sander S, Steuerwald U, Terhardt M, Holtkamp U, *et al*. Newborn screening for congenital adrenal hyperplasia: additional steroid profile using liquid chromatography-tandem mass spectrometry. *J Clin Endocrinol Metab*, 2007; **92**: 2581–9.
10. Krone N, Arlt W. Genetics of congenital adrenal hyperplasia. *Best Pract Res Endocrinol Metab*, 2009; **23**: 181–92.
11. Rocha RO, Billerbeck AE, Pinto EM, Melo KF, Lin CJ, Longui CA, *et al*. The degree of external genitalia virilization in girls with 21-hydroxylase deficiency appears to be influenced by the CAG repeats in the androgen receptor gene. *Clin Endocrinol (Oxf)* 2008; **68**: 226–32.
12. Gomes LG, Huang N, Agrawal V, Mendonca BB, Bachega TA, Miller WL. Extraadrenal 21-hydroxylation by CYP2C19 and CYP3A4: effect on 21-hydroxylase deficiency. *J Clin Endocrinol Metab*, 2009; **94**: 89–95.
13. Joint_LWPES/ESPE_CAH_Working_Group. Consensus statement on 21-hydroxylase deficiency from the Lawson Wilkins Pediatric Endocrine Society and the European Society for Paediatric Endocrinology. *J Clin Endocrinol Metab*, 2002; **87**: 4048–53.
14. Riepe FG, Krone N, Viemann M, Partsch CJ, Sippell WG. Management of congenital adrenal hyperplasia: results of the ESPE questionnaire. *Horm Res*, 2002; **58**: 196–205.
15. Arlt W, Rosenthal C, Hahner S, Allolio B. Quality of glucocorticoid replacement in adrenal insufficiency: clinical assessment vs. timed serum cortisol measurements. *Clin Endocrinol (Oxf)* 2006; **64**: 384–9.
16. Hindmarsh PC. Management of the child with congenital adrenal hyperplasia. *Best Pract Res Endocrinol Metab*, 2009; **23**: 193–208.
17. Lajic S, Nordenstrom A, Hirvikoski T. Long-term outcome of prenatal treatment of congenital adrenal hyperplasia. *Endocr Dev*, 2008; **13**: 82–98.
18. Meyer-Bahlburg HF, Dolezal C, Baker SW, Ehrhardt AA, New MI. Gender development in women with congenital adrenal hyperplasia as a function of disorder severity. *Arch Sex Behav*, 2006; **35**: 667–84.
19. Dessens AB, Slijper FM, Drop SL. Gender dysphoria and gender change in chromosomal females with congenital adrenal hyperplasia. *Arch Sex Behav*, 2005; **34**: 389–97.
20. Mulaikal RM, Migeon CJ, Rock JA. Fertility rates in female patients with congenital adrenal hyperplasia due to 21-hydroxylase deficiency. *New Engl J Med*, 1987; **316**: 178–82.
21. Cornean RE, Hindmarsh PC, Brook CG. Obesity in 21-hydroxylase deficient patients. *Arch Dis Child*, 1998; **78**: 261–3.
22. Volkl TM, Simm D, Beier C, Dorr HG. Obesity among children and adolescents with classic congenital adrenal hyperplasia due to 21-hydroxylase deficiency. *Pediatrics*, 2006; **117**: e98–105.
23. Stikkelbroeck NM, Oyen WJ, van der Wilt GJ, Hermus AR, Otten BJ. Normal bone mineral density and lean body mass, but increased fat mass, in young adult patients with congenital adrenal hyperplasia. *J Clin Endocrinol Metab*, 2003; **88**: 1036–42.
24. Falhammar H, Filipsson H, Holmdahl G, Janson P-O, Nordenskjold A, Hagenfeldt K, *et al*. Metabolic profile and body composition in adult women with congenital adrenal hyperplasia due to 21-hydroxylase deficiency. *J Clin Endocrinol Metab*, 2007; **92**: 110–6.
25. Speiser PW, Serrat J, New MI, Gertner JM. Insulin insensitivity in adrenal hyperplasia due to nonclassical steroid 21-hydroxylase deficiency. *J Clin Endocrinol Metab*, 1992; **75**: 1421–4.
26. Sartorato P, Zulian E, Benedini S, Mariniello B, Schiavi F, Bilora F, *et al*. Cardiovascular risk factors and ultrasound evaluation of intima-media thickness at common carotids, carotid bulbs, and femoral and abdominal aorta arteries in patients with classic congenital adrenal hyperplasia due to 21-hydroxylase deficiency. *J Clin Endocrinol Metab*, 2007; **92**: 1015–8.
27. Roche EF, Charmandari E, Dattani MT, Hindmarsh PC. Blood pressure in children and adolescents with congenital adrenal hyperplasia (21-hydroxylase deficiency): a preliminary report. *Clin Endocrinol*, 2003; **58**: 589–96.
28. Volkl TMK, Simm D, Dotsch J, Rascher W, Dorr HG. Altered 24-hour blood pressure profiles in children and adolescents with classical congenital adrenal hyperplasia due to 21-hydroxylase deficiency. *J Clin Endocrinol Metab*, 2006; **91**: 4888–95.
29. Ogilvie CM, Crouch NS, Rumsby G, Creighton SM, Liao L-M, Conway GS. Congenital adrenal hyperplasia in adults: a review of medical, surgical and psychological issues. *Clin Endocrinol*, 2006; **64**: 2–11.
30. Merke DP. Approach to the adult with congenital adrenal hyperplasia due to 21-hydroxylase deficiency. *J Clin Endocrinol Metab*, 2008; **93**: 653–60.
31. Holmes-Walker DJ, Conway GS, Honour JW, Rumsby G, Jacobs HS. Menstrual disturbance and hypersecretion of progesterone in women with congenital adrenal hyperplasia due to 21-hydroxylase deficiency, *Clin Endocrinol (Oxf)*, 1995; **43**: 291–6.
32. Ogilvie CM, Rumsby G, Kurzawinski T, Conway GS. Outcome of bilateral adrenalectomy in congenital adrenal hyperplasia: one unit's experience. *Eur J Endocrinol*, 2006; **154**: 405–8.
33. Arlt W, Allolio B. Adrenal insufficiency. *Lancet*, 2003; **361**: 1881–93.
34. Moran C, Azziz R, Weintrob N, Witchel SF, Rohmer V, Dewailly D, *et al*. Reproductive outcome of women with 21-hydroxylase-deficient nonclassic adrenal hyperplasia. *J Clin Endocrinol Metab*, 2006; **91**: 3451–6.
35. Claahsen-van der Grinten HL, Otten BJ, Stikkelbroeck MM, Sweep FC, Hermus AR. Testicular adrenal rest tumours in congenital adrenal hyperplasia. *Best Pract Res Endocrinol Metab*, 2009; **23**: 209–20.
36. White PC, Curnow KM, Pascoe L. Disorders of steroid 11β-hydroxylase isozymes. *Endocr Rev*, 1994; **15**: 421–38.
37. Peter M, Janzen N, Sander S, Korsch E, Riepe FG, Sander J. A case of 11β-hydroxylase deficiency detected in a newborn screening program by second-tier LC-MS/MS. *Horm Res*, 2008; **69**: 253–6.
38. Joehrer K, Geley S, Strasser-Wozak EM, Azziz R, Wollmann HA, Schmitt K, *et al*. CYP11B1 mutations causing non-classic adrenal hyperplasia due to 11 beta-hydroxylase deficiency. *Hum Mol Genet*, 1997; **6**: 1829–34.
39. Mornet E, Dupont J, Vitek A, White PC. Characterization of two genes encoding human steroid 11β-hydroxylase (P-450(11)β). *J Biol Chem*, 1989; **264**: 20961–7.
40. Curnow KM, Slutsker L, Vitek J, Cole T, Speiser PW, New MI, *et al*. Mutations in the CYP11B1 gene causing congenital adrenal hyperplasia and hypertension cluster in exons 6, 7, and 8. *Proc Natl Acad Sci U S A*, 1993; **90**: 4552–6.

41. Geley S, Kapelari K, Johrer K, Peter M, Glatzl J, Vierhapper H, *et al.* CYP11B1 mutations causing congenital adrenal hyperplasia due to 11 beta- hydroxylase deficiency. *J Clin Endocrinol Metab*, 1996; **81**: 2896–901.
42. Auchus RJ. The genetics, pathophysiology, and management of human deficiencies of P450c17. *Endocrinol Metab Clin North Am*, 2001; **30**: 101–19.
43. Geller DH, Auchus RJ, Mendonca BB, Miller WL. The genetic and functional basis of isolated 17,20/lyase deficiency. *Nat Genet*, 1997; **17**: 201–5.
44. Geller DH, Auchus RJ, Miller WL. P450c17 mutations R347H and R358Q selectively disrupt 17,20-lyase activity by disrupting interactions with P450 oxidoreductase and cytochrome b5. *Mol Endocrinol*, 1999; **13**: 167–75.
45. Simard J, Ricketts M-L, Gingras S, Soucy P, Feltus FA, Melner MH. Molecular biology of the 3β-hydroxysteroid dehydrogenase/Δ5-Δ4 isomerase gene family. *Endocr Rev*, 2005; **26**: 525–82.
46. Lutfallah C, Wang W, Mason JI, Chang YT, Haider A, Rich B, *et al.* Newly proposed hormonal criteria via genotypic proof for type II 3β-hydroxysteroid dehydrogenase deficiency. *J Clin Endocrinol Metab*, 2002; **87**: 2611–22.
47. Mermejo LM, Elias LLK, Marui S, Moreira AC, Mendonca BB, de Castro M. refining hormonal diagnosis of type II 3β-hydroxysteroid dehydrogenase deficiency in patients with premature pubarche and hirsutism based on HSD3B2 genotyping. *J Clin Endocrinol Metab*, 2005; **90**: 1287–93.
48. Payne AH, Hales DB. Overview of steroidogenic enzymes in the pathway from cholesterol to active steroid hormones. *Endocr Rev*, 2004; **25**: 947–70.
49. Peterson RE, Imperato-McGinley J, Gautier T, Shackleton C. Male pseudohermaphroditism due to multiple defects in steroid-biosynthetic microsomal mixed-function oxidases. A new variant of congenital adrenal hyperplasia. *N Engl J Med*, 1985; **313**: 1182–91.
50. Fluck CE, Tajima T, Pandey AV, Arlt W, Okuhara K, Verge CF, *et al.* Mutant P450 oxidoreductase causes disordered steroidogenesis with and without Antley-Bixler syndrome. *Nat Genet*, 2004; **36**: 228–30.
51. Arlt W, Walker EA, Draper N, Ivison HE, Ride JP, Hammer F, *et al.* Congenital adrenal hyperplasia caused by mutant P450 oxidoreductase and human androgen synthesis: analytical study. *Lancet*, 2004; **363**: 2128–35.
52. Fluck CE, Pandey AV, Huang N, Agrawal V, Miller WL. P450 oxidoreductase deficiency—a new form of congenital adrenal hyperplasia. *Endocr Devel* 2008; **13**: 67–81.
53. Shackleton C, Marcos J, Arlt W, Hauffa BP. Prenatal diagnosis of P450 oxidoreductase deficiency (ORD): a disorder causing low pregnancy estriol, maternal and fetal virilization, and the Antley-Bixler syndrome phenotype. *Am J Med Genet*, 2004; **129A**: 105–12.
54. Fukami M, Nishimura G, Homma K, Nagai T, Hanaki K, Uematsu A, *et al.* Cytochrome P450 oxidoreductase deficiency: identification and characterization of biallelic mutations and genotype-phenotype correlations in 35 Japanese patients. *J Clin Endocrinol Metab*, 2009; **94**: 1723–31.
55. Fukami M, Hasegawa T, Horikawa R, Ohashi T, Nishimura G, Homma K, *et al.* Cytochrome P450 oxidoreductase deficiency in three patients initially regarded as having 21-hydroxylase deficiency and/or aromatase deficiency: diagnostic value of urine steroid hormone analysis. *Pediatr Res*, 2006; **59**: 276–80.
56. Shackleton C, Malunowicz E. Apparent pregnene hydroxylation deficiency (APHD): seeking the parentage of an orphan metabolome. *Steroids*, 2003; **68**: 707–17.
57. Bose HS, Sugawara T, Strauss JF 3rd, Miller WL. The pathophysiology and genetics of congenital lipoid adrenal hyperplasia. International Congenital Lipoid Adrenal Hyperplasia Consortium. *N Engl J Med*, 1996; **335**: 1870–8.
58. Baker BY, Lin L, Kim CJ, Raza J, Smith CP, Miller WL, *et al.* Nonclassic congenital lipoid adrenal hyperplasia: a new disorder of the steroidogenic acute regulatory protein with very late presentation and normal male genitalia. *J Clin Endocrinol Metab*, 2006; **91**: 4781–5.
59. Kim CJ, Lin L, Huang N, Quigley CA, AvRuskin TW, Achermann JC, *et al.* Severe combined adrenal and gonadal deficiency caused by novel mutations in the cholesterol side chain cleavage enzyme, P450scc. *J Clin Endocrinol Metab*, 2008; **93**: 696–702.
60. Rubtsov P, Karmanov M, Sverdlova P, Spirin P, Tiulpakov A. A novel homozygous mutation in CYP11A1 gene is associated with late-onset adrenal insufficiency and hypospadias in a 46,XY patient. *J Clin Endocrinol Metab*, 2009; **94**: 936–9.
61. White PC. Aldosterone synthase deficiency and related disorders. *Mol Cell Endocrinol*, 2004; **217**: 81–7.
62. Lavery GG, Walker EA, Tiganescu A, Ride JP, Shackleton CH, Tomlinson JW, *et al.* Steroid biomarkers and genetic studies reveal inactivating mutations in hexose-6-phosphate dehydrogenase in patients with cortisone reductase deficiency. *J Clin Endocrinol Metab*, 2008; **93**: 3827–32.
63. Parajes S, Loidi L, Reisch N, Dhir V, Rose IT, Hampel R, *et al.* Functional consequences of seven novel mutations in the CYP11B1 gene: four mutations associated with nonclassic and three mutations causing classic 11{beta}-hydroxylase deficiency. *J Clin Endocrinol Metab*, 2010; **95**(2): 779–88.

PART 6

Neuroendocrine tumours and genetic disorders

6.1

Neuroendocrine tumours of the gastrointestinal tract: an appraisal of the past and perspectives for the future

Irvin M Modlin, Bjorn I Gustafsson, Mark Kidd

Introduction

Although Siegfried Oberndorfer is rightly credited with introducing the term karzinoide (carcinoma-like) in 1907, T. Langhans had in 1867 described a submucosal tumour that resembled poorly differentiated glandular tissue arranged in 'nests' with a rich, thick fibrous stroma (1). Thereafter in 1888, O. Lubarsch reported the post mortem identification of multiple ileal tumours, which he was reluctant to classify as 'carcinomas' due to a benign growth pattern appearance (2). In 1890, W.B. Ransom reported similar tumours at autopsy in the region of the ileocoecal valve with associated extensive hepatic tumours, but, in addition, emphasized the associated clinical symptoms, which included diarrhoea and wheezing (3). Nevertheless, despite these early descriptions, it remained for Oberndorfer to published his seminal paper *Carcinoid Tumours of the Small Intestine* in 1907 and recognize their unique nature; finally defining the lesions as a neoplasm distinct from carcinoma (Fig. 6.1.1) (4).

This manuscript was the first to describe and characterize the tumour that had previously been referred to as a 'benign carcinoma'. Histologically, the tumours consisted of small polymorphic cells with large nuclei and scant cytoplasm arranged in nests surrounded by dense, fibrous connective tissue composed of surrounding stroma with epithelial vascular growth adjacent to the tumour. Since the tumours appeared to have unique clinical characteristics incongruous with those evident in carcinomas, Oberndorfer labelled them as 'carcinoid-like' or 'karzinoide', mistakenly considering them to be 'benign' (4).

Although Oberndorfer's early contributions to the understanding of the biology of carcinoid tumours were prescient, his assertion that the tumours were of a benign nature subsequently proved to be incorrect. In 1929, 22 years after first publication, Oberndorfer revised his initial characterization of the benign behaviour of the tumour, confirming the possibility that 'karzinoide' might exhibit malignant features and metastasize (5).

Although considerable progress had been made in the elucidation of the pathological nature of this 'odd' tumour of the small intestine, there was a paucity of information available regarding the cellular basis of the lesions. In 1896, Heidenhain identified chromaffin cells in the gastric mucosa although he was unable to define their role (6). In 1897, Kulchitsky noted similar cells in the crypts of Lieberkuhn in the intestinal mucosa (7), as did others including, A. Nicolas (1891) (8) and H. Kull (1924) (9). In 1906, M.C. Ciaccio introduced the term 'enterochromaffin' (EC) in an attempt categorize them as a group of cells specifically located in the gut (10). In 1914, A. Gosset and P. Masson, using silver impregnation techniques, demonstrated the argentaffin-staining properties of carcinoid tumours and suggested that these neoplasms might arise from the enterochromaffin cells (Fig. 6.1.2) (11).

In 1931, A.J. Scholte, a Dutch pathologist, found an ileal carcinoid tumour in a 47-year-old male who had suffered from diarrhoea, cyanosis, cough, lower extremity oedema, and cutaneous telangiectasia before dying from cardiac failure and bronchopneumonia (12). Of particular note was Scholte's astute observation of hard thickening of the tricuspid valves and irregular endocardial thickening of the right atrium, probably representing the first documentation of carcinoid heart disease. The first clear descriptions of the carcinoid syndrome (flushing, diarrhoea, bronchospasm) and carcinoid heart disease, however, was published by Biörk and Thorson in the early 1950s (13, 14). In 1952, V. Erspamer identified the biogenic amine serotonin (5-hydroxy tryptamine (5-HT)) as a specific hormone of the enterochromaffin cell system and proposed its fundamental role as a 'gut hormone', and in 1953 Lembeck isolated 5-HT from a carcinoid tumour (15, 16). In 1938, F. Feyrter, formerly Professor of Pathology at the Medical Academy of Danzig, Poland and then in Graz, Austria, described the presence of argentaffin-positive and argyrophilic 'clear cells' ('Helle Zellen') throughout the gut and proposed the concept of a diffuse neuroendocrine system from which carcinoid tumours were derived (17). By 1948, A.B. Dawson had developed a technique by which enterochromaffin and enterochromaffin-like (ECL) cells of the gastrointestinal tract could be stained using silver nitrate (18). By the 1970s, electron microscopy could identify different secretory

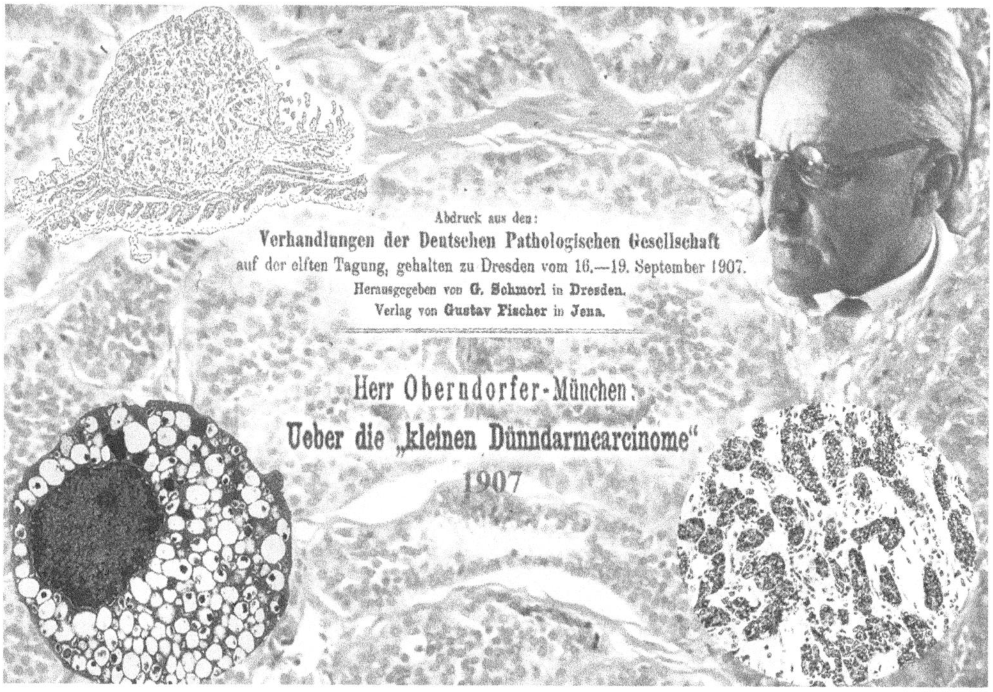

Fig. 6.1.1 Siegfried Oberndorfer (1876–1944) (top right) of the Pathological Institute at the University of Munich first presented his observations of multiple 'benign carcinomas' of the small intestine (top left, his original drawing of the morphology of the tumour) at the German Pathological Society meeting of 1907 in Dresden (centre). Current techniques of identification using immunohistochemical staining of tumour chromogranin positivity (bottom right) and electron micrographic appearance (bottom left) of the granule/ vesicle morphology of the enterochromaffin-like (ECL) cell.

granule structures and individual endocrine cells and their putative secretory products could be determined, and Pearse proposed the amine precursor uptake decarboxylation concept to link the diverse cell types (19–21). Similarly, the isolation and characterization of a variety of peptide hormones and amines enabled antibody production and the development of immunohistochemistry which further facilitated delineation of individual cell and tumour types by their biochemical secretory profile (Table 6.1.1) (22).

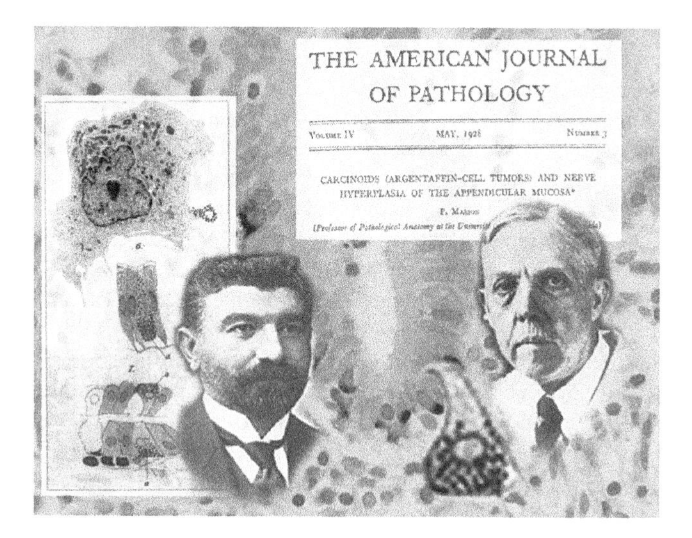

Fig. 6.1.2 Pierre Masson (1880–1959) (right) developed the eponymous trichrome stain (background), which became the standard in all pathology laboratories. The use of this technique in 1914 allowed him and Andre Gosset (1872–1944) (left) to demonstrate the argentaffin staining properties of carcinoid tumours (frontispiece, top right). They suggested that the Kulchitsky, or enterochromaffin (EC), cells in the gut (left, EM of an EC cell; bottom right, original drawing by Kulchitsky), which had been described in 1897 by Nikolai Kulchitsky, formed a diffuse endocrine organ. In 1928, they described these cells as being of neural origin, and proposed that they were the progenitors of neuroendocrine tumours of the gut (carcinoids).

Cell of origin, function, and tumour biology

Neuroendocrine tumours are derived from neuroendocrine cells in the gastrointestinal tract which themselves are derived from local tissue-specific stem cells, probably through a committed precursor cell (23). The mechanisms leading to tumourigenesis are, however, largely unknown.

Most endocrine tumours of the small and large intestines arise in a sporadic manner; others, notably (ECL) cell tumours of the stomach, are found associated with ECL cell hyperplasia, usually due to hypergastrinaemia, while gastrin-containing G-cell tumours and somatostatin-containing D-cell tumours of the duodenum are also associated with neuroendocrine cell hyperplasia related to a genetic defect such as multiple endocrine neoplasia type I (MEN 1), neurofibromatosis, von Hippel–Lindau, or tuberose sclerosis (24). Multifocal lesions are seen in approximately 30% of midgut neuroendocrine tumours (NETs) and comprise small intestinal enterochromaffin cell tumours (25). Most of these tumours develop as independent primary lesions, and only a minority are due to metastasis from a single primary (26). In both multiple jejunoileal enterochromaffin cell tumours and appendices containing enterochromaffin cell NETs, hyperplasia of neuroendocrine cells in the associated mucosa is evident (27, 28). Given the doctrine of multistage carcinogenesis, it is likely that the cell that accumulates the mutations necessary for development of NETs is a committed neuroendocrine progenitor, a cell not as yet defined in the human gastrointestinal tract. The mechanisms underlying the differentiation pathway of neuroendocrine cells remain poorly defined but transcription factors including Math1, Neurogenin 3, and beta2/ NeuroD are considered essential for final enteroendocrine cell specification (29).

Once differentiated, neuroendocrine cells occur throughout the length of the gut, constituting the largest group of hormone-producing cells in the body (30). At least 13 different gut neuroendocrine cells exist. Each produces an array of bioactive peptides/

Table 6.1.1 Gastrointestinal and pancreatic neuroendocrine cell types and secretory products

Cell type	Localization	Products
Delta (D)	Entire gastrointestinal tract	Somatostatin
Enterochromaffin	Entire gastrointestinal tract	Serotonin/substance P/guanylin/melatonin
Enterochromaffin-like (ECL)	Gastric fundus	Histamine
Gastrin (G)	Gastric antrum and duodenum	Gastrin
Ghrelin (Gr)	Entire gastrointestinal tract	Ghrelin
I	Duodenum	CCK
K	Duodenum/ jejunum	GIP
L	Small intestine	GLP-1, PYY, NPY
Motilin (M)	Duodenum	Motilin
Neurotensin (N)	Small intestine	Neurotensin
Secretin (S)	Duodenum	Secretin
Vasoactive intestinal peptide (VIP)	Entire gastrointestinal tract	VIP
X	Stomach: fundus and antrum	Amylin
Beta	Pancreas	Insulin
Alpha	Pancreas	Glucagon
Delta	Pancreas	Somatostatin
Pancreatic polypeptide (PP)	Pancreas	PP

CCK, cholecystokinin; GIP, gastric inhibitory peptide; GLP-1, glucagon-like peptide 1; PYY, polypeptide YY (tyrosine, tyrosine); NPY, neuropeptide Y (tyrosine); PP, pancreatic polypeptide.

amines, including serotonin (5-HT) from enterochromaffin cells, somatostatin from D cells, histamine (ECL cells), and gastrin (G cells) (Fig. 6.1.3).

The secretory products are stored in large dense-core and small synaptic-like vesicles, and proteins such as CgA A (CgA) and synaptophysin (in large dense-core and small synaptic-like vesicles, respectively) represent markers of neuroendocrine cells (31).

Secretory regulation

Secretion is regulated by G-protein coupled receptors, ion-gated receptors, and receptors with tyrosine kinase activity. Peptide hormones destined for regulated secretion are packaged into secretory granules (large dense-core secretory granules) which bud from the trans-Golgi network where prohormones and proneuropeptides are stored and processed prior to secretion in a regulated manner. CgA is a critical regulator of dense-core secretory granule biogenesis. Other granins (e.g. CgB) regulate proteolytic processing of peptide precursors and promote aggregation-mediated sorting into mature secretory granules, providing a mechanism whereby granules mature into regulatable exocytotic carriers. Secretagogue-evoked stimulation induces actin reorganization through sequential ordering of carrier proteins at the interface between granules and the plasma membrane. This calcium-dependent step is a prerequisite for regulated exocytosis and allows granule–membrane trafficking and release of neuroendocrine contents (Fig. 6.1.4) (32).

The apical part of the enterochromaffin cell often communicates with the gut through thin cytoplasmic extensions serving as mechano- and chemosensors, which project into the glandular lumen. The size, shape, and electron density of the secretory granules vary, representing important means to characterize and differentiate neuroendocrine cell types. As a general rule, different granules store individual peptide hormones; in some neuroendocrine cells, however, several different peptides or amines may be colocalized in the same granule (33).

ECL cells of the gastric fundus comprise a component of the gastric neuroendocrine cell system interacting with antral G cells. The latter secrete gastrin that activates the ECL cells to produce histamine, which drives the parietal cells of the fundus to produce acid. Loss of parietal cells (atrophic gastritis) or acid suppression culminates in increased gastrin secretion, ECL cell proliferation, and even neoplasia (gastric carcinoids) (34).

Enterochromaffin cells are the major small intestinal neuroendocrine cell type, secreting 5-HT, guanylin, and substance P in response to neurogenic and luminal, (mechanical and chemical) stimuli. Activating pathways include adenylyl cyclase, β-adrenoreceptors and PACAP-38, while somatostatin (acting via the $SSTR_2$ receptor), acetyl choline (muscarinic M_4 receptors), and γ-aminobutyric acid (GABA, via $GABA_A$ receptors) inhibit secretion (35). The effects of 5-HT, such as proliferation of epithelial cells and contraction of intestinal smooth muscle, are mediated via multiple 5-HT receptor

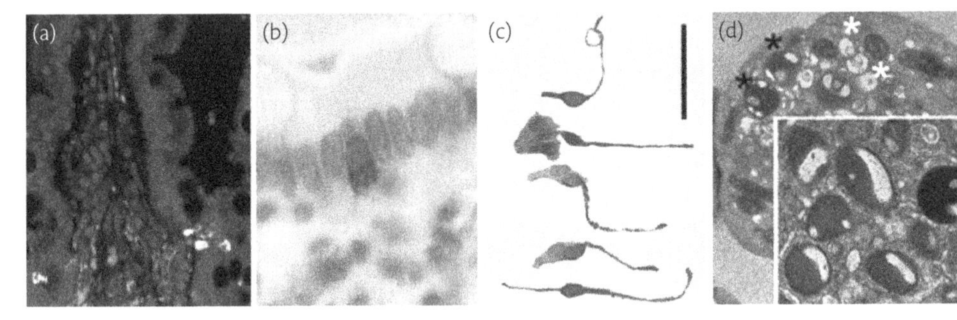

Fig. 6.1.3 Neuroendocrine cell morphology. (a) Confocal immunofluorescence micrograph of normal human intestine. Enterochromaffin cells (yellow fluorescence; colocalization of Cy5 (red-labelled), CgA, and Fluorescein isothiocyanate (FITC) (green-labelled) Tryptophan hydroxylase (TPH)) are located at the base of the crypt. (b) Serotonin immunostaining (brown) of an enterochromaffin cell demonstrating localization of serotonin in vesicles. (c) Microdissected rat rectal enterochromaffin cells immunostained with serotonin demonstrating lengthy dendritic-like basal extensions consistent with a neural and endocrine phenotype. (d) Electron micrograph (7200 × magnification) of rodent small intestinal enterochromaffin cells demonstrating a typical admixture of large dense granules and electroluscent (empty) vesicles (inset shows the characteristic dense content and pear or ovoid shape of the vesicles). (See also Plate 32)

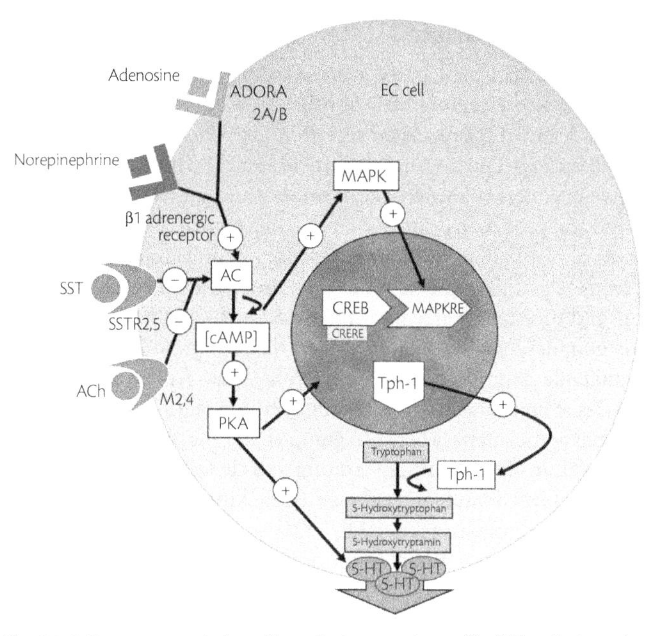

Fig. 6.1.4 Secretory regulation of intestinal enterochromaffin (EC) cells. Secretion is regulated by diverse hormonal (somatostatin (SST)) and neural agents (noradrenaline, acetylcholine (ACh), adenosine) through activation of adenylate cyclase (AC) and up-regulation of cellular cAMP. This activates MAPK and PKA to induce transcription of Tph-1 (through cAMP response element and MAPK response element) activation. Tph-1 catalyses 5-hydroxytryptophan which is then converted to its tryptamine derivate (5-HT) and then concentrated in vesicles prior to secretion. The later is mediated by PKA through activation of Ca^{2+} influx. Negative regulators (e.g. somatostatin and acetylcholine) inhibit secretion through inhibition of adenylate cyclase activity.

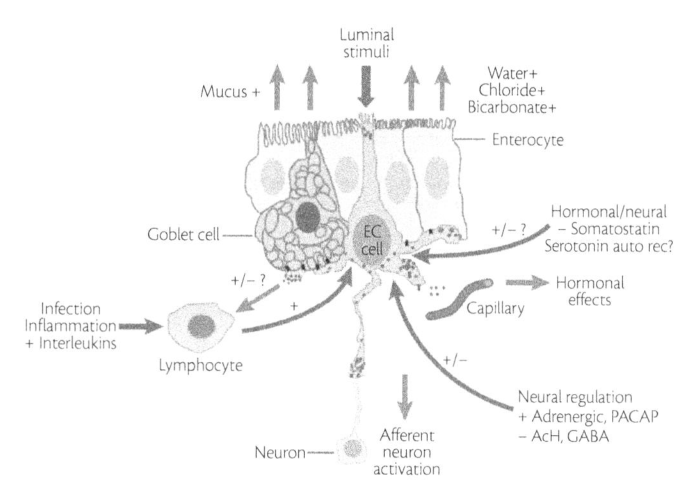

Fig. 6.1.5 Diagram of an intestinal enterochromaffin (EC) cell and its complex interactions in both local and systemic physiological events. Numerous activation pathways converge on this ubiquitous neuroendocrine cell and its activation has diverse physiological effects both locally and systemically. Local somatostatin is the key inhibitory regulator. AcH Acetyl choline; GABA, γ-aminobutyric acid; PACAP Pituitary adenylate cyclase-activating peptide.

subtypes (5-HT_{1-7}). Rapid inactivation of 5-HT is crucial to limit its actions; this is achieved by uptake into neighbouring enterocytes as well as reuptake into enterochromaffin cells (35, 36), followed by intracellular conversion of 5-HT to 5-hydroxyindoleacetic acid (5-HIAA) by monoamine oxidase (Fig. 6.1.5).

Proliferative regulation and neuroendocrine cell transformation

The proliferative regulation underlying the majority of neuroendocrine cells is largely unknown except for foregut/gastric ECL cells. For other cell types, difficulty in isolating the cells for investigation has led to a paucity of information regarding regulation of normal cell proliferation.

In the stomach, factors regulating normal and neoplastic ECL cells are well-defined. Gastrin produced by the antral G cells is the principal proliferative regulator of ECL cells in both humans and animals. In the Mastomys (*Praomys natalensis*), a sub-Saharan African muroid rodent phylogenetically related to the mouse (37), gastric NETs spontaneously develop in 20–50% by 2 years of age (38). Serum gastrin levels in these animals are normal (39) and the development of normogastrinaemic ECL cell tumours is probably due to a gastrin receptor mutant that shows ligand-independent activity (40). The Mastomys CCK2 receptor, when expressed in COS-7 cells, differs from human, canine, and rat receptor homologues in its ability to constitutively activate inositol phosphate formation (40). Functional characterization has revealed that three amino acids from the Mastomys transmembrane domain VI to the C-terminal end are sufficient to confer constitutive activity. Mutagenesis studies using a combination of ^{344}Leu, ^{353}Ile, and ^{407}Asp confer a level of comparable ligand-independent signalling when introduced into the human receptor (40).

Although multiple naturally occurring amino acid polymorphisms and/or mutations may result in an enhanced basal level of CCK2 receptor activity, endogenous gastrin, however, is required for ECL cell tumour development in the Mastomys (41) and in other rodent models, e.g. female hispid cotton rats (*Sigmodon hispidus*), which also spontaneously develops gastric carcinomas by about 10–16 months of age (42), an effect that can be accelerated by pharmacological acid suppression (43). Thus, drug-induced hypergastrinaemia consequent upon acid suppression, e.g. following oral ingestion of the histamine H_2 receptor blockers (loxtidine, cimetidine) or omeprazole (proton pump inhibitor (PPI) class of agents) significantly accelerates the development of ECL cell tumours (44).

In humans, low acid states, induced either by endogenous parietal cell destruction (autoimmune disease), or by exogenous pharmacotherapeutic agents such as H_2 receptor blockers or PPIs, result in G-cell hypersecretion and culminate in hypergastrinaemia. The association between low acid states and gastric neoplasia is well documented (45, 46). Similarly, the gastrin elevation noted in atrophic gastritis and the trophic effect of gastrin on ECL cells is consistent with the hypothesis that a low acid state with elevated plasma gastrin levels drives ECL proliferation (47). These gastrin-responsive lesions are termed Type I or Type II (if MEN 1 is associated). Normogastrinaemic lesions also develop; their aetiology is unknown (48). It is therefore likely that trophic regulatory agents (e.g. transforming growth factor (TGFβ), CCN2—discussed below) other than gastrin are involved in ECL cell tumourigenesis. Despite this, it appears that gastrin is the dominant effector (46, 49). The mechanisms by which gastrin-mediated growth regulation results in tumour formation is considered to be the end-result of a ligand-receptor activated signal transduction cascade (usually the MAP kinase pathway (50)) and induction of the activator protein-1 (AP-1) complex (a fos/jun-mer) transcription factor (51) which regulates genes necessary for cell cycle progression (e.g. cyclin genes) (52). Normal ECL cell proliferation is associated with activation of fos/jun transcription by the MAPK pathway (ERK1/2) following gastrin-mediated Ras activation (53). In these normal cells, gastrin activates the Ras-MAPK pathway and mediates cell growth via upstream activation of phosphatidyl inositol 3-kinase and the PKB/PKC pathways. In addition, there is evidence that gastrin also up-regulates epidermal growth factor (EGF)/TGFβ and the EGF receptor in neoplastic ECL cells (54). It is thus likely that perturbations in growth factor production and/or responsiveness are implicated in increased ECL cell proliferation, and ultimately NET neoplasia (54). Mechanisms by which gastrin mediates ECL tumourigenesis include a decrease in expression of the negative regulators (Jun D and Menin) of AP-1 which regulates cell cycle progression via cyclin D1 expression (44). Menin is interesting because foregut NETs have frequent deletions and mutations of this gene, which encodes a 610 amino acid protein. Menin mutations are responsible for most cases of MEN 1 and a small proportion of sporadic foregut and nongastrointestinal endocrine tumours. Menin is a predominantly nuclear protein but in dividing cells it interacts in the cytoplasm with several proteins involved in transcriptional regulation, genome stability, and cell division (55). Other factors that may be involved in gastric ECL cell proliferation include histamine. Blockade of the H1 receptor with the specific receptor antagonist, terfenadine, inhibited DNA synthesis in cultured tumour cells demonstrating that the H1 receptor has a significant influence on ECL cell proliferation (44). In addition, CCN2 or connective tissue growth factor, a prototypic member of the CCN family of proteins (56), is expressed in gastric rodent and human gastric NET cells, and functions as a proliferative agent during NET neoplasia through activation of the ERK1/2 pathway (57).

In contrast to ECL cells, there is, however, little information regarding proliferation in either normal or tumour neuroendocrine cells in the gastrointestinal tract. Small intestinal NETs, which do not express mutations of the menin gene are, however, characterized by a loss of responsiveness to TGFβ1-mediated growth inhibition that characterizes normal small intestinal enterochromaffin cell proliferation (Fig. 6.1.6) (58). Even less is known about hindgut NETs, except that they express TGFα and the EGF receptor (59).

Metastatic potential

Metastasis is present in 60–80% of small bowel and colonic NETs at diagnosis and overall approximately 35% of all NETs exhibit metastatic disease on presentation (60). The diversity in likelihood of metastasis probably reflects the heterogeneity of neuroendocrine cell types. Thus, gastric NETs whose aetiology is gastrin-dependent (i.e. the Type I or Type II tumours), very rarely metastasize (less than 10%) (61). In contrast, the normogastrinaemic tumours (Type III) have a high rate of metastasis (>50%) (61). This is reflected in tumours of the small intestine and colon which will almost all eventually metastasize (61). The biological reasons underlying the metastatic potential of these tumours is not known but probably reflects, at least in small intestinal NETs, a reconfiguration of the TGFβ signalling pathway that the cell uses to drive c-Myc transcription and pathways associated with metastasis (down-regulation of E-cadherin expression) (58).

Tumour-related fibrosis

A distinctive feature of the enterochromaffin tumours is their propensity to extensive mesenteric fibrosis and, occasionally, mesenteric ischaemia. Fibrosis may also involve the endocardium

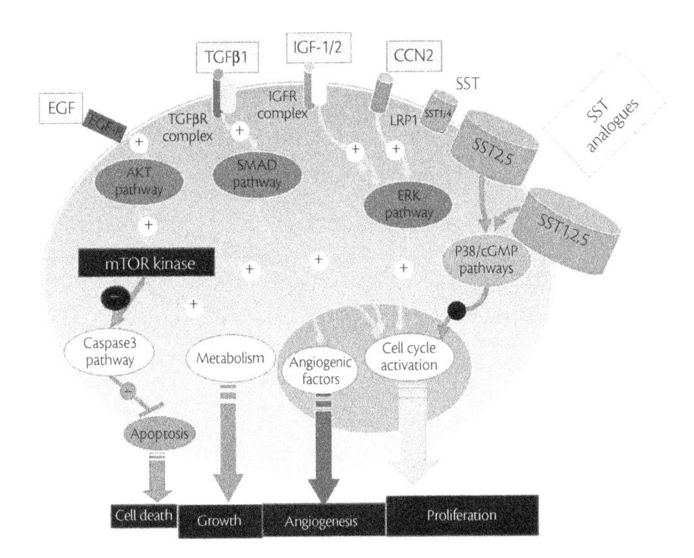

Fig. 6.1.6 Proliferative regulation of enterochromaffin (EC) cells. Proliferation is regulated by a number of different growth factors (e.g. transforming growth factor (TGFβ)) through activation of AKT/ERK/SMAD and mTOR pathways. Negative regulators include somatostatin (SST) which target cell cycle activators through the P38/cGMP pathways. Targeting mTOR kinase or somatostatin receptors are currently the most effective methods for inhibiting cell growth. EGF, epidermal growth factor; IGF1, insulin-like growth factor; CCN2 Connective tissue growth factor (CTGF); LRP1 low density lipoprotein receptor-related protein 1.

of the right heart as well as the tricuspid and pulmonary valves with impairment of cardiac function; 10–20% of patients with the carcinoid syndrome have heart disease at presentation and prior to the introduction of the somatostatin analogue class of pharmacotherapeutic agents as many as 50% of patients with serotonin-producing lesions developed cardiac manifestations (62).

Individuals that exhibit the most elevated levels of tachykinins/serotonin in plasma and 5-HIAA in the urine are prone to develop cardiac valve fibrosis, suggesting that one or more of these agents are involved in the development of fibrosis (63–65). Serotonin is a major agent involved in the pathogenic process and promotes proliferation of valvular subendocardial cells (66, 67), while hyperserotoninaemia induces cardiac fibrosis in rats (68). These effects can be prevented by terguride, an antagonist of the 5-HT2B receptor, indicating that the specific 5-HT2B receptor may be a therapeutic target in the development of NET-related fibrosis (69). Several other profibrotic agents, such as TGFβ1 and its downstream mediator, connective tissue growth factor, are also implicated in localized and cardiac fibrosis (Fig. 6.1.7) (70).

Unresolved issues and future perspectives

There remains a continuing uncertainty regarding the origins and differentiation of both normal and malignant neuroendocrine cells. In addition, the regulation of cell growth and secretion within neuroendocrine tumours, apart from gastric ECL cell NETs, remains largely obscure. This reflects a shortage of *in vitro* and animal models. The only natural model is the Mastomys rodent, which spontaneously generates gastric carcinoids whose development can be accelerated by the use of acid-suppressive medication (38). Other models include nude mice injected in the flank with either lung (NCI-H727) or pancreatic NET (BON) cell lines (71) or nude or athymic mice injected intrasplenically with BON cells (72, 73). In all instances, these represent xenografts of cell cultures and

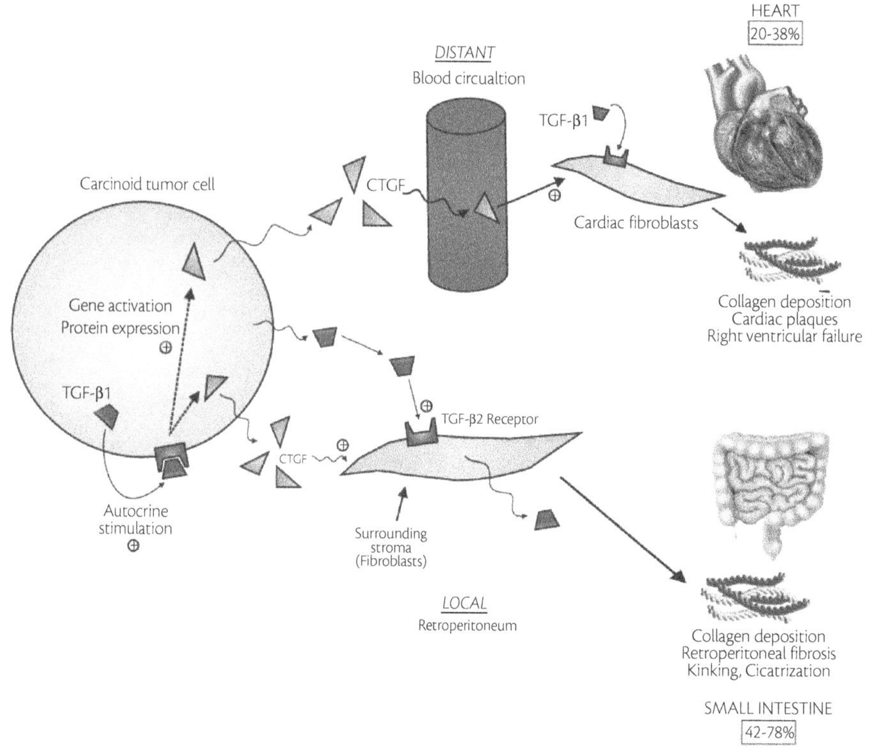

Fig. 6.1.7 Schematic model of putative mechanisms involved in fibrosis. TGFβ1, produced by carcinoid tumour cells, activates transcription and secretion of connective tissue growth factor (CTGF) which, either locally (peritoneal fibroblasts) or distantly (endomyocardial fibroblasts), activates collagen synthesis and deposition. Small intestinal NETs are associated (42–78%) with peritoneal fibrosis, bowel kinking, and cicatrization. In the heart (20–38%), fibrosis is associated with right-sided valvular plaques, endocardial fibrosis, and right ventricular failure. Other activators of fibrosis include TGFβ1 and may include nongrowth factors such as amines and tachykinins.

immune-compromised animals and are of uncertain biological relevance. As such, they may have limited correlation with disease pathogenesis and treatment although they may provide information on the efficacy of therapeutic agents.

These limitations underline the requirement for an improved understanding of the development of the diffuse neuroendocrine cell system, including enterochromaffin cells, to better understand the development of abnormalities in these cells. There is a need to develop validated NET cell lines and animal models to investigate the molecular mechanisms involved in the control of their growth and secretion, and fibrosis. This will be necessary to identify novel mechanisms and targets. An improvement in the molecular understanding of these tumours through the application of genomic, RNA interference, microRNA, proteomic, and small-molecule screen technologies should be a priority, while the establishment of national/ international clinical databases and biobanks of tumour, serum, and DNA for future collaborative clinical and translational studies of neuroendocrine tumour disease is an absolute necessity. The establishment of these facilities, as well as the development of a translational NET model, will enable improved early detection of NETs, a more accurate mechanism to anatomically localize tumours, better prediction of metastasis, and the development of targeted antisecretory and antiproliferative pharmacotherapy.

Histopathology/classification systems

Although the original term carcinoid sought to address a novel gut epithelial tumour of a relatively monotonous structure that was less aggressive than carcinoma, the utility of this definition has to a large extent been eclipsed by the advances in biology, biochemistry, and functional pathology. Currently, carcinoids should be regarded as gastroenteropancreatic neuroendocrine tumours and the early 20th century terminology (carcinoid), introduced by Oberndorfer, will probably fade into obsolescence. The understanding of carcinoids has evolved from a conglomeration of carcinoma-like lesions, mostly in the gut and lungs, to a diverse group of neuroendocrine lesions each defined by a specific cell of origin, secretory profile, and clinical presentation.

The recognition of carcinoids as endocrine-related tumours was first outlined by Gosset and Masson in 1914 (11), but it remained for Williams and Sandler in 1963 to classify carcinoid tumours on their putative embryological origin (foregut, midgut, or hindgut) (74). Thus, it was considered that foregut endocrine cells give rise to NETs in the respiratory tract, the stomach, the first part of the duodenum, and the pancreas. Midgut carcinoid tumours represent lesions of the bowel from the second part of the duodenum through to the ascending colon and appendix, and hindgut carcinoids constitute lesions of the transverse and descending colon and rectum. It subsequently became apparent that neuroendocrine tumours from different segments of the embryologic gut typically varied widely in the character of their bioactive products, diversity of symptoms and immunohistochemical profiles.

In recent years, standardizing the pathological reporting of gastroenteropancreatic neuroendocrine tumours has been attempted to further aid clinicians regarding the likely biology of individual tumours. The World Health Organization (WHO) classification has defined these tumours by degree of differentiation and the tumour site of origin (75). In this system, tumours are described as well-differentiated neuroendocrine tumours (benign behaviour or uncertain malignant potential), well-differentiated neuroendocrine carcinomas (low-grade malignancy), or poorly differentiated (usually small cell) neuroendocrine carcinomas of high-grade malignancy. The term 'carcinoid' applies to tumours classified as 'well-differentiated'. Size, angioinvasion, proliferative activity, histological differentiation, metastases, and hormonal activity (association with clinical syndromes or diseases) are also taken into consideration. Histochemical indicators of prognosis include the degree of expression of the proliferation protein Ki-67 and the p53 tumour suppressor protein (76, 77).

The European Neuroendocrine Tumour Society (ENETS) group and the Neuroendocrine Tumour Summit Consensus of 2009 have proposed to further refine this classification by including the Ki-67 scoring index and using a TNM classification system (Box 6.1.1; Tables 6.1.2 and 6.1.3) (78, 79). Some controversy exists, however, as to the utility of Ki-67 and its general application (80). The recent development and introduction of a minimal data set for pathologists will, however, add consistency and uniformity to the evaluation and classification of NETs (80).

Unsolved issues and future perspectives

Neither the WHO classification nor the newly proposed ENETS classification has so far been widely adopted. This lack of a defined and widely accepted classification and staging system has led to a lack of agreement on the minimum pathological investigations required to clearly define these tumours and to difficulties in comparing US data with that from European or Asian centres. Semantic issues continue to obfuscate the field, especially with regard to clinical trials, in which, as a result of the absence of a broadly accepted classification system, heterogeneous patient/ tumour populations have often been the norm. Standardization of pathology with incorporation of methods for minimum pathological diagnosis and classification is necessary to develop an easily adopted and well accepted classification system. The use of the TNM classification as proposed by ENETS and incorporation of the current WHO classification seems appealing, as does the recommendations of the recent 2009 NET Pathology Summit meeting (80).

Box 6.1.1 TNM classification of neuroendocrine tumours

T—primary tumour

- Tx: primary tumour cannot be assessed
- T0: no evidence of primary tumour
- T1: tumour limited to the pancreas with size <2 cm
- T2: tumour limited to the pancreas with size 2–4 cm
- T3: tumour limited to the pancreas with size >4 cm or invading duodenum or bile duct
- T4: tumour invading adjacent organs or the wall of large vessels

N—regional lymph nodes

- Nx: regional lymph nodes cannot be assessed
- No: no regional lymph node metastases
- N1: regional lymph node metastases

M—distant metastases

- Mx: distant metastases cannot be assessed
- M0: no distant metastases
- M1: distant metastases

Stage I: T1, N0, M0

Stage IIa: T2, N0, M0

Stage IIb: T3, N0, M0

Stage IIIa: T4, N0, M0

Stage IIIb: any T, N1, M0

Stage IV: any T, any M, M1

Table 6.1.2 Grading system

Grade	Mitotic count (10 HPF)[a]	Ki-67 index (%)[b]
G1	<2	≤2
G2	2–20	3–20
G3	>20	>20

[a] 10 HPF, high power field = 2 × 2 mm, at least 40 fields (at 40 × magnification) evaluated in areas of highest mitotic density.

[b] MIB1 antibody; % of 2000 tumour cells in areas of highest nuclear labelling.

Epidemiology

The Surveillance Epidemiology and End Results (SEER) database (1973–2006), containing 48 195 NETs (81), demonstrates that in the USA, NETs comprise 0.66% of all malignancies and the incidence is increasing at a rate of 3–10% per year depending on the subtype. Furthermore, NETs comprised 1.25% of all malignancies in 2004 compared to only 0.75% of all malignancies in 1994 (60, 81). Much of this increase probably reflects the introduction of more sensitive diagnostic tools (topographic and immunohistochemical) as well as an overall increased awareness among clinicians and pathologists. Nevertheless, over the last 30 years the incidence has increased approximately 740% (82, 83). The frequency (1.22%) of NETs in a large autopsy series also indicates that they have previously been underdiagnosed (84). In the USA, NETs occur most frequently in the gastrointestinal tract (66%) with the second most common location in the bronchopulmonary system (25%), followed by considerably less frequent locations such as the ovaries, testes, hepatobiliary, and pancreas (Fig. 6.1.8) (85).

In SEER, 1993–2006, African Americans exhibited a high overall NET incidence of 6.5/100 000 compared to 4.44/100 000 among Caucasians (Fig. 6.1.9). Rectal NETs were most common lesion (1.65/100 000, 27%) among African Americans, followed by small intestinal (1.42/100 000, 21%) and bronchopulmonary (1.20/100 000, 18%). Taking gender and ethnicity into consideration, the highest incidence rates of NET subtypes were small intestinal (1.83/100 000) and rectal NETs (1.81/100 000) in black males followed by bronchopulmonary NETs (1.51/100 000) in white females. Studies from Asian countries, although smaller, support

Table 6.1.3 Staging for gastrointestinal neuroendocrine tumours

Stage 0	Tis	N0	M0	Gastric only
Stage I	T1	N0	M0	All except colorectal
Stage Ia	T1a	N0	M0	Colorectal only
Stage Ib	T1b	N0	M0	Colorectal only
Stage IIa	T2	N0	M0	All
IIb	T3	N0	M0	All
Stage IIIa	T4	N0	M0	All
IIIb	Any T	N1	M0	All
Stage IV	Any T	Any N	M1	All

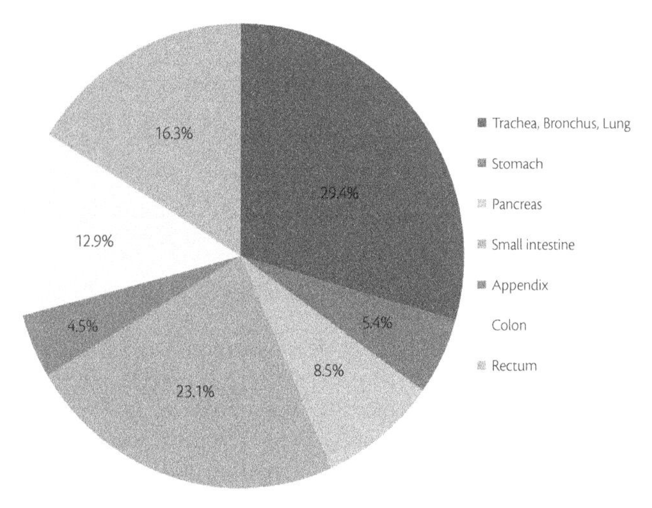

Fig. 6.1.8 Distribution of gastrointestinal and lung NETs. The majority of NETs occur in the gastrointestinal tract and constitute approximately 70% of all NETs. Within the gastrointestinal tract, approximately 40% occur in the small intestine (5202 tumours), 21% in the colon (2892), and 26% in the rectum (3657). A significant percentage occurs in the bronchopulmonary system (30%: 6606).

a genetic/racial variation in NET incidence and tumour localization. Among 228 Taiwanese NETs, 60.5% were rectal, 20.2% bronchopulmonary, 6% thymic, small intestine 4.8%, gastric 3.1%, ovarian 0.9%, and appendiceal only 0.4% (86). Similar results were evident in a recent Japanese study of 1027 NETs: 28.2% were foregut (respiratory tract, stomach, duodenum, biliary system, and pancreas), 5.2% midgut (small intestine, appendix, and proximal colon), and 66.0% hindgut (distal colon and rectum) (87). Among 10 804 NETs in the Niigata Registry the most frequent site was the respiratory system (19.8%), followed by the rectum (15.0%), jejunoileum (12.0%), stomach (11.4%), appendix (9.6%), and duodenum (8.3%) (88). Despite the relative rarity of the disease, the prevalence of gastrointestinal NETs is substantial given the often indolent nature of the disease process (89). As a matter of clinical practicality it is noteworthy that the prevalence of gastrointestinal NETs in the USA exceeds that of pancreatic, gastric, oesophageal, and hepatic cancer and is only exceeded by that of colon cancer (Fig. 6.1.10).

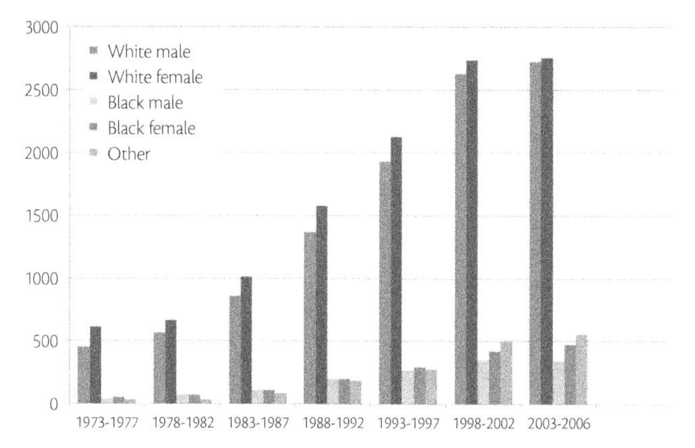

Fig. 6.1.9 Prevalence of NETs in Caucasian and African Americans in the USA. The prevalence of NETs is higher in Caucasians than in African Americans. However, normalization of the data based upon the National Census Data (2002) indicates that the incidence is approximately 1.5 times higher amongst the African American segment of the population (SEER 9 Registry, 1973–2006).

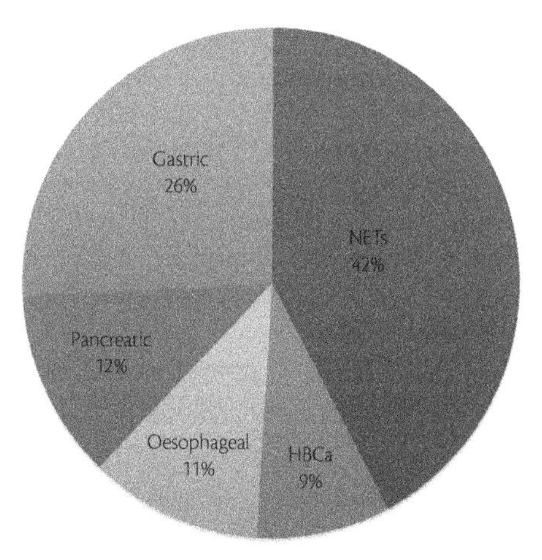

Fig. 6.1.10 Estimated prevalence of gastrointestinal adenocarcinomas and gastrointestinal NETs. NETs constitute approximately 42% of all gastrointestinal malignancies and are more prevalent than either gastric, pancreatic, oesophageal, or hepatobiliary carcinomas (HBCa). As such, NETs comprise a previously unrecognized and substantial burden for the health care system. (Adapted from Yao J, *et al.* One hundred years after 'carcinoid': epidemiology of and prognostic factors for neuroendocrine tumours in 35,825 cases in the United States. *J Clin Oncol*, 2008; **261**: 3063–72 (89).)

Unsolved issues and future perspectives

Even if the increase in incidence is in a great part due to the introduction of more sensitive diagnostic tools (topographic and immunohistochemical) as well as an overall increased awareness among physicians, it remains to be determined whether a true increase has occurred. It seems likely that a cell that senses the gut contents is susceptible to novel agents used to preserve, taste, or colour food. Similarly, there is a lack of understanding regarding genetic and environmental factors responsible for gender and racial differences in incidence which requires resolution. Large, validated clinical datasets are thus needed to determine whether the increased rate of diagnosis represents a true increased incidence of disease. Better mapping with both national and international registries, laboratories, and tumour banks is needed. Whatever the outcome, the increasing incidence has generated a substantial reappraisal of the prevalence and highlights the NET patient load that institutions need to consider in long-term planning.

Genetics

Several gene mutations and genetic disorders (e.g. MEN 1, von Hippel–Lindau disease, and neurofibromatosis 1) have been associated with NET disease (Fig. 6.1.11) and are discussed in detail in separate chapters in this book. Additionally, the neuroendocrine marker CgA is elevated approximately twofold in plasma in inflammatory bowel disease (90), and NET incidence is considerably higher (approximately 15 times) in Crohn's disease. Crohn's-associated NETs develop in areas not directly affected by Crohn's inflammation, suggesting that genetic or perhaps circulating proinflammatory mediators may account for the increased NET risk (91). There is also an increased association of adenocarcinoma with NETs (82, 92). A retrospective Swedish Cancer Registry analysis of 3055 cases of small bowel NETs indicated an increased risk of second malignancies: prostate cancer (increased 2.8 times), malignant melanoma (increased 6.3), and malignancies of endocrine organs (increased 2.3) (61).

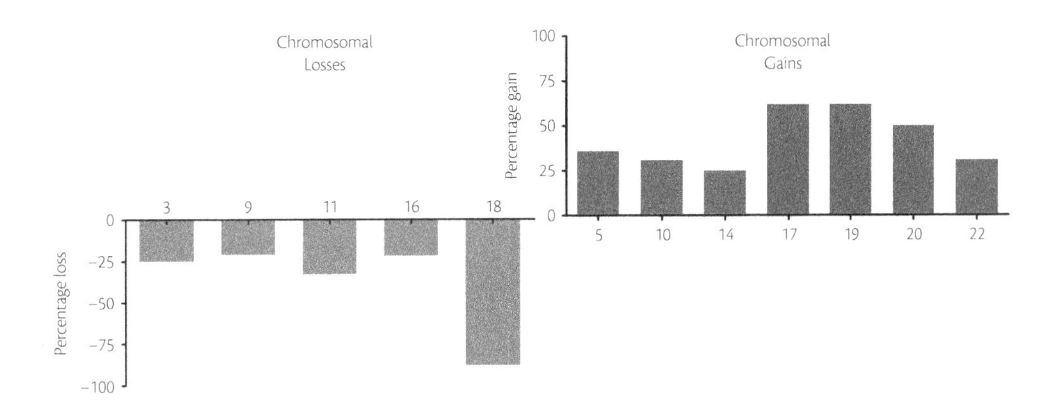

Fig. 6.1.11 Common chromosomal abnormalities in small intestine NETs. The commonest loss is on chromosome 18 (66%), while chromosomes 17 and 19 (approximately 60%) exhibit the most common gains. (Adapted from Zikusoka M, *et al.* The molecular genetics of gastroenteropancreatic neuroendocrine tumors. *Cancer*, 2005; **104**: 2292–309.)

Unsolved issues and future perspectives

There is a major paucity of information related to genetic abnormalities in NETs. In order to better define NET genetic abnormalities, identification of familial accumulations of NET disease require evaluation and, optimally, twin studies are needed. Resolution of this area of knowledge requires large-scale, well-organized biobanks of tumour, serum, and DNA.

Clinical diagnosis

NETs may present a considerable diagnostic and therapeutic challenge as their clinical presentation is protean, nonspecific, and usually late when metastases are already evident. The classical carcinoid syndrome is relatively uncommon (10–15%), typically consisting of diarrhoea, cutaneous flushing, bronchospasm, and right-sided heart failure (84). Biochemical tests including plasma serotonin and 24-h measurement of urinary 5-HIAA in 5-HT-producing lesions. The general gastrointestinal NET marker plasma CgA levels is sensitive (>90%) but nonspecific (elevated in other types of NETs, impaired kidney function, and during proton pump medication) and measurements often vary between laboratories (93). Plasma serotonin levels are often unreliable and difficult to quantify while 5-Hydroxyindoleacetic acid (5-HIAA) levels are cumbersome and insensitive. Topographic localization using CT, MRI, somatostatin receptor scintigraphy, whole body positron emission tomography (PET), or endoscopy/ultrasonography are all variously effective depending upon equipment availability and user skill. No modality alone is entirely secure and overall exhibit a sensitivity specificity of approximately 80–90% (94).

Unsolved issues and future perspectives

A key unmet need is the availability of a blood test for early diagnosis or surveillance. The recent demonstration of specific NET transcripts in plasma suggests that this strategy may enable early diagnosis and detection of such lesions and even provide a basis for prognostic determination and therapeutic recommendation (95) (Fig. 6.1.12). A major delay in diagnosis of 5–7 years remains characteristic of gastrointestinal NETs. Vague or nonspecific initial symptoms are typical, with extensive investigation by a primary care physician, endocrinologist, or gastroenterologist before the diagnosis is reached. This situation reflects the fact that many physicians lack experience with or have had education about neuroendocrine tumours as a result of inadequate attention to the subject (considered rare) both at medical schools and in training programmes. As a consequence, the clinical diagnosis is often not considered until the disease is advanced. Even once considered, identification of neuroendocrine tumours using imaging with radiolabelled octreotide scanning, which recognizes the somatostatin receptors expressed on the majority (>90%) these tumours, is not available at all institutions. Magnetic resonance imaging and multislice CT are the most sensitive of the widely available imaging modalities and are most effective when performed using protocols that have been optimized for the evaluation of NETs. The recent experience with Ga-68 DOTaTOC and the cost efficiency of such generators suggests that this technique may become the ideal anatomical imaging strategy of the near future (96). Some patients with gastrointestinal NETs have relatively slow-growing disease and may live for decades, whereas others have a rapidly progressive course. Determining the likely biological behaviour of the tumour is important for deciding who, how, and when to treat, but the choice of therapy is currently often empiric because the natural history of the disease is not well understood. There is thus a need for reliable diagnostic and prognostic tests and to identify molecular prognostic factors to recognize high-risk patients.

The general lack of multidisciplinary neuroendocrine tumour management teams further amplifies the issue of the current suboptimal clinical management of these tumours. The choice of imaging modality should depend on the clinical question being posed—this may vary from seeking to identify a small primary lesion responsible for a biochemically diagnosed syndrome to evaluating the extent and location of metastatic disease in the liver to plan cytoreductive surgery or embolic ablation. Selecting among diagnostic modalities and determining the optimal protocol for neuroendocrine tumour diagnosis ideally should reflect a multidisciplinary collaboration.

Therapy in brief

Despite the introduction of novel treatments including peptide receptor radionuclide therapy (PRRT) and enzyme inhibitors (tyrosine kinase inhibitors), primary surgical resection of the tumour and regional lymph nodes remains the only curative treatment available for gastrointestinal NETs. It is usually possible in approximately 20%, due to the delay in diagnosis and the presence of metastatic disease. Small, solitary, noninvasive (endosonographically proven) lesions in the stomach, duodenum, and rectum may be treated with endoscopic local resection (97, 98). Somatostatin analogues usually induce biochemical stabilization or effective biochemical response (approximately 85%) and manage clinical symptoms (approximately 80%) in patients with somatostatin receptor-positive tumours.

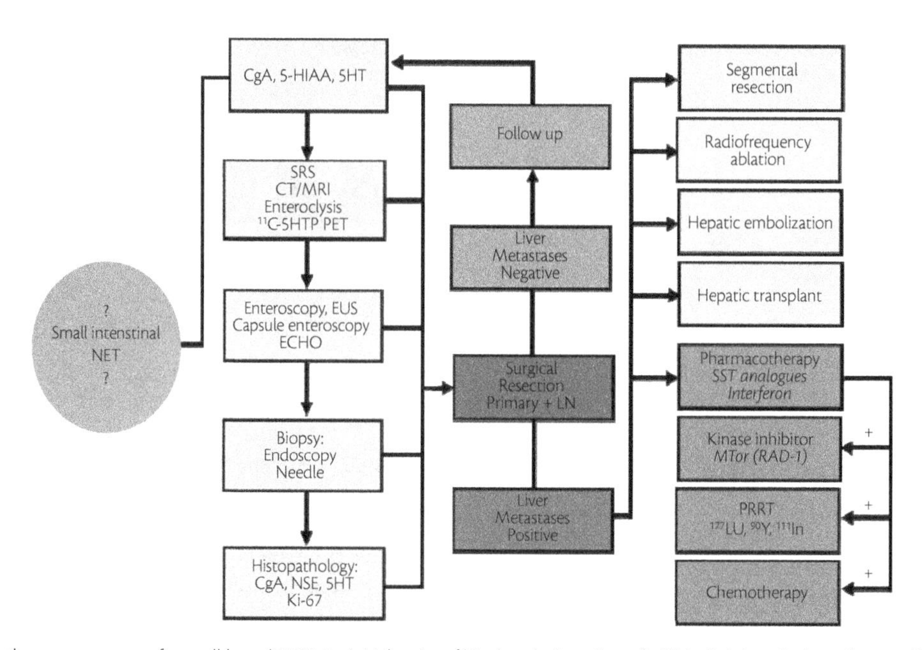

Fig. 6.1.12 Algorithm for the management of a small bowel NET. An initial series of biochemical studies, of which CgA has the broadest application, should be used to establish the presence of a NET. Subsequently, topographic studies are utilized to identify the location of the lesion and its metastases. Somatostatin receptor scintigraphy has special utility in that it establishes both the neuroendocrine nature of the lesion (somatostatin receptor expression) and as a whole body scan defines total tumour burden. Once disease extent is defined, surgical resection of the primary and ablation of hepatic metastases (when feasible) should be undertaken. All patients should receive a long acting somatostatin (SST) analogue to ameliorate symptomatology and inhibit tumour cell proliferation. If there is evidence of disease progression, the use of a novel kinase inhibitor or PRRT should be considered. Chemotherapy is only warranted for high-grade NETs with evidence of rapid progression. 5-HIAA, 5-hydroxyindoleacetic acid; 5-HT, 5-hydroxy tryptamine; ECHO, echocardiography; EUS, endoscopic ultrasonography; LN, lymph node; PET, positron emission tomography; PRRT, peptide receptor radionuclide therapy; SRS, somatostatin receptor scintigraphy.

More recently the PROMID and Radiant 001 studies have, respectively, indicated a positive effect of octreotide alone and the combination of octreotide and a mTOR kinase inhibitor on tumour progression and survival (99, 100). A diverse array of single-agent or multiagent chemotherapuetic regimes have been examined. Invariably they exhibit little, short-lasting, or no effect on NET response and in most circumstances the associated adverse events usually exceeds the efficacy of the agents (101). Novel agents, including inhibitors of the tyrosine kinase receptor family c-kit, platelet-derived growth factor receptors α and β, and epidermal growth factor receptor, have shown modest (approximately 10% tumour response rate) but nevertheless promising results (71, 102). The activity of the oral inhibitor of mTOR, everolimus (RAD001) in combination with octreotide LAR was recently studied in 60 patients with advanced low- to intermediate-grade neuroendocrine tumours (89). There were 13 (22%) with partial responses, 42 (70%) with stable disease, and five (8%) patients with progressive disease.

The recent introduction of PRRT using ^{111}Indium, ^{90}Yttrium or ^{177}Lutetium radionuclides linked to a somatostatin analogue has enabled SSTR-expressing tumour cells to be specifically targeted. At present, the most effective PRRT available for treatment of metastatic gastrointestinal NETs is ^{177}Lu bound to the somatostatin analogue, DOTA^{0}Tyr^{3}octreotate. ^{177}Lu-DOTA^{0}Tyr^{3}octreotate has a high affinity for the somatostatin 2 subtype and produces tumour responses in 35% and tumour stabilization in 80–90% of gastrointestinal NETs.

Unfortunately, most patients have multiple, bilateral liver metastases at diagnosis, and approximately 5–10% metastases are available for 'complete' resection (103). Liver transplantation may be an option in highly selected patients (104) but for the majority ablative techniques including hepatic arterial embolization or radio frequency ablation are effective in decreasing tumour load and reduce symptoms and prolong survival with a 5-year survival of up to 50% (105). The strategy of reducing liver tumour bulk to 10% followed by therapy with a somatostatin analogue in conjunction with everlimus warrants serious consideration.

Unsolved issues and perspectives for the future

Given the paucity of sufficiently powered randomized clinical trials using homogenous patient groups and adequate follow-up in this field, the correct treatment choice is challenging, even for clinicians who have considerable experience in the management of this disease. After an accurate diagnosis and evaluation of the site and extent of disease, the choice of therapy should also be highly individualized on the basis of current symptoms, pathological tumour type/grade, burden, and additional prognostic information. The patient's goals and expectations should also be considered in the context of the relative risks and the benefits of available treatments and their impact on quality of life. Choosing no treatment should also be a consideration.

Neuroendocrine cells exhibit a high density of cell surface receptors for somatostatin, an endogenous peptide that acts through paracrine pathways to inhibit secretion of neuropeptides. Initially, somatostatin analogues are usually highly effective at controlling many of the symptoms caused by excessive bioactive peptide or amine secretion; however, some patients develop a variable degree of resistance to these analogues. This may represent tachyphylaxis or increased tumour burden while in some instances it represents tumour transformation. Exploitation of the relative specificity and over-expression of somatostatin receptors in gastrointestinal NETs has led to the development of radionuclide therapy tagged to somatostatin analogues. Initial experience with PRRT appears promising (106), but, as for NET treatment in general, appropriate randomized clinical trials are lacking.

Few alternative therapies are available, and in many cases these are only marginally effective, and no specific targeted antineoplastic therapy exists. For disseminated disease, a new generation of drugs are currently being evaluated for efficacy in systemic disease; these include inhibitors of vascular endothelial growth factor, of receptor tyrosine kinases (e.g. sunitinib, sorafenib, and vatalanib), and of the mammalian target of rapamycin (e.g. temsirolimus and everolimus) (107–110). However, the clinical and/or radiological response rates in single-agent trials of these newer molecular targeted therapies are less than 20% (111), and their future use will probably depend on combination therapies. It is likely that the development of detailed molecular characterizations of individual tumours will facilitate identification of specific therapeutic agents and, in addition, enable use of the 'correct' drug for a specific tumour. Thus, many agents currently considered to exhibit suboptimal efficacy when utilized in the appropriate setting may well prove to be extremely effective. Apart from somatostatin and its analogues, all of the systemic chemotherapeutic agents under evaluation were developed for the treatment of non-neuroendocrine neoplasia and are only secondarily applied to gastrointestinal NETs. The key issue is the need to develop more specific therapies and this requires elucidation of NE cell biology as well as immortalized cell systems and animal tumour models.

The management and treatment of gastrointestinal NETs differ markedly from the treatment of the common malignancies in the expertise required for diagnosis, pathology, cytoreductive and curative neuroendocrine surgery, oncology, and interventional radiology and nuclear medicine. It is difficult at present not only to acquire but also to maintain this specialized expertise because of the limited number of patients most individual centres see annually. The limited number of patients also impedes the ability to carry out standardized studies and systematically assess new treatments. The need for specialized regional centres for the investigation and management of gastrointestinal NETs is therefore critical. These centres should participate in the establishment of a national clinical database and biobank of tumour, serum, and DNA for future collaborative clinical and translational studies of neuroendocrine tumour disease. Such centres would also make sufficiently powered randomized clinical trials using homogenous patient groups and adequate follow-up more feasible.

One of the characteristic features of NETs—particularly those of the ileum—is the development of fibrosis, both locally and at sites distant from the primary tumour. Fibrosis occurs as a result of the production of bioactive agents, such as serotonin and connective tissue growth factor, which have profibrotic effects (68, 112).

Table 6.1.4 Observed 5-year survival rates by grade and stage (SEER17: 1973–2006)

Grade	Localized (%)	Regional (%)	Distant (%)	Unknown (%)	All stages (%)
Grade I	83.52	76.95	44.90	58.51	72.19
Grade II	79.27	57.35	27.72	35.56	54.11
Grade III	43.45	27.97	4.39	14.69	18.57
Grade IV	49.44	25.18	5.11	22.29	20.40
Unknown	83.41	64.56	25.91	48.88	61.81
All grades	81.37	58.40	21.94	46.15	56.96

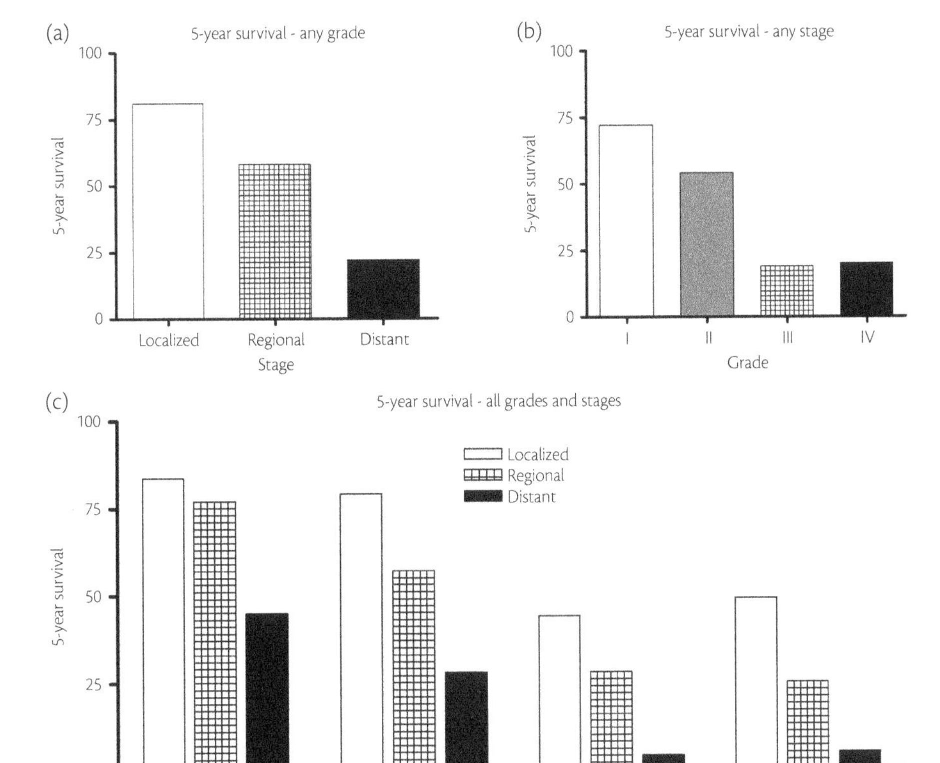

Fig. 6.1.13 Five-year survival by grade and stage. Localized, regional, and distant staged disease have decreasing survival (a), as do Grades I and II (irrespective of stage) (b). Interestingly, Grade III and IV tumours have similar survival irrespective of the stage (localized, regional, or distant). A breakdown of survival by stage and grade (c) emphasizes that a higher grade is generally associated with a lower survival. Conversely, however, Grade I tumours tend to have a higher survival rate except if the tumours have metastasized, when survival then drops to levels commensurate with Type III/IV tumours (i.e. <50% survival).

Cardiac fibrosis is particularly evident after metastasis to the liver and is associated with right-sided heart valve fibrosis and impairment of cardiac function. The frequency of carcinoid heart disease is as high as 20% at tumour diagnosis. Recent advances in its early detection (echocardiography) as well as aggressive surgical and medical management, have led to increased survival (64). The presence of extensive peritoneal fibrosis often renders surgical management difficult, and, if advanced, may culminate in an abdominal cocoon that is virtually untreatable. The precise mechanistic biological basis for the development of fibrosis remains obscure. Further clarification of the pathogenesis of carcinoid heart disease fibrosis is needed to facilitate the development of targeted antifibrotic therapeutic agents.

Prognosis

The 5-year survival rate for gastrointestinal NET disease in 1973–2005 ranged from 56.2 % for colon NETs to 87.6% for rectal NETs (Table 6.1.4, Fig. 6.1.13); disappointingly, the overall 5-year survival has not improved over this time period (81). The 5-year survival is highly dependent on tumour stage and grade and ranges from only 4.5% in undifferentiated NETs with distant spread to 83.4% in localize, well-differentiated NETs.

Unsolved issues and future perspectives

The understanding of the true natural history of gastroenteropancreatic neuroendocrine tumours is limited, especially regarding

Table 6.1.5 Summary of unsolved issues and future strategies

Issues	Barriers	Solutions
1. Limited understanding of cellular and molecular biology of neuroendocrine cells and mechanisms of tumourigenesis	Few investigators focused on neuroendocrine tumour pathogenesis Little opportunity for basic and clinical training in this field Paucity of relevant cell and animal models	Increase and earmark funding from government and charitable foundations for gastroenteropancreatic neuroendocrine tumours Develop novel *in vitro* and *in vivo* models
2. Paucity of specific targets for new therapies	Poor definition of specific molecular targets Paucity of high-quality clinical trials	Improve understanding of molecular pathogenesis Multicenter large clinical trials of homogenous patient groups Develop appropriate cell lines and animal models which can be used to assess possible new therapies
3. Shortage of *in vitro* and animal models to study disease pathogenesis and treatment	Few investigators focused on gastroenteropancreatic neuroendocrine disease Existing models have limited correlation with clinical states	Designate funding specifically for translational gastroenteropancreatic neuroendocrine model development Collaboration between basic and clinical scientists in gastroenteropancreatic neuroendocrine disease
4. No uniform pathological classification or staging system	Community pathologists unfamiliar with neuroendocrine tumours Reluctance for US pathologists to adopt WHO system without demonstration of clinical benefit Semantic problems of benign vs. malignant states in gastroenteropancreatic neuroendocrine tumours	Develop a consensus amongst US pathologists on classification and staging Prospectively validate WHO criteria Educate pathologists Referral for pathological 2nd opinions Develop minimal standards that are required for diagnosis and classification
5. Lack of molecular prognostic factors to identify high-risk patients and lack of an understanding of natural history of these tumours	Relative rarity of gastroenteropancreatic neuroendocrine tumours Heterogeneity of tumour types Long-term systematic studies of patients difficult Lack of a surveillance test for gastroenteropancreatic neuroendocrine tumours	Establish regional and national databases Develop long-term molecular-clinical correlative studies Fund research into biomarkers of gastroenteropancreatic neuroendocrine disease
6. Few centres offer the multidisciplinary expertise required for the diagnosis, staging, and management of gastroenteropancreatic neuroendocrine tumours	Numerous imaging options available Lack of widespread availability of sensitive and specific imaging Local resources and expertise variable Paucity of high-quality clinical trials	Development of regional multidiscipline centres of expertise with experienced and focused clinicians and radiologists Multicenter clinical trials of homogenous patient groups
7. Paucity of investigators in neuroendocrine tumour disease	Gastroenteropancreatic neuroendocrine tumours at the interface between disparate disciplines (oncology, endocrinology, surgery, gastroenterology) Underemphasized as a source of morbidity and mortality	Increase educational programmes Increase medical and public awareness of gastroenteropancreatic neuroendocrine tumours Increase funding for clinical and basic scientific research into this disease
8. Lack of understanding of the disease complications that lead to morbidity and mortality	Inexperience of many clinicians in gastroenteropancreatic neuroendocrine tumours Reliable diagnostic tests lacking	Develop regional centres of excellence with multidiscipline clinical teams Establish large prospective data bases, with well-defined patient groups

Adapted from Modlin IM, *et al.* Priorities for improving the management of gastroenteropancreatic neuroendocrine tumors. *J Natl Cancer Inst*, 2008; **100**: 1282–9.

survival; whereas most tumours grow relatively slowly, some exhibit highly aggressive behaviour that is clinically indistinguishable from adenocarcinoma. In addition, much of the published literature predates modern imaging methods and includes heterogeneous patient populations that have undergone a wide spectrum of therapies, often serially. Determining the likely biological behaviour of the tumour is critical to deciding who, how, and when to treat, but the choice of therapy is currently often empiric because the natural history of the specific disease entity is not well understood. The identification of NET molecular predictors of metastasis, invasion, and proliferation is a critical need in order to be able to determine specific treatment, define appropriate follow-up parameters, and improve survival.

Appropriate long-term therapy of NET patients requires a clear understanding of the natural history of these tumours, which at present is unavailable given the recent alterations in therapy (somatostatin analogue availability). Since few patients are systematically studied and followed in treatment centres that have an interest in all aspects of the disease, little is known of important natural history factors that might determine survival, including the development of secondary malignancies (15–20% in some series) (111, 113) or the effect of current therapeutic options in altering the natural history of disease.

Perspectives for the future

In contrast to the general assumption that gastrointestinal NETs are extremely rare and benign slow-growing tumours, it is evident that they are far more common than previously considered and have the highest prevalence of any gastrointestinal malignancy except colon cancer. Furthermore, in contradistinction to the notion that they are benign and indolent, they often exhibit a poor prognosis due to widespread metastatic disease and a low quality of life due to disabling symptoms. Although diagnostic modalities such as somatostatin receptor scintigraphy, PET, and the combination of nuclear imaging techniques with anatomical imaging are useful in accurate and early diagnosis, the critical lack is the absence of a plasma or genetic marker to identify early disease or predict and recognize micrometastasis. Apart from early diagnosis, delineation of the mechanistic and biological basis of NET biology is necessary to develop a rational and effective therapeutic approach using targeted agents. A major drawback to evaluating therapy is the absence of a universally acceptable pathology classification system and the ability to identify specific tumour types and thereby individualize therapy and define prognosis or time therapeutic intervention. Although treatment with somatostatin analogues very effectively palliates symptoms and delays disease progression, more effective and specific targeted therapies are needed to regulate NE cell proliferation. Peptide receptor radio therapies with somatostatin analogues or radiolabelled precursors of tumour amines and peptides have demonstrated therapeutic advantage but their efficacy remains modest. To date, other growth factor antagonists and antiangiogenic agents have demonstrated limited efficacy, although this may reflect an inability to identify the specific tumour for which they might be effective (114). Increased knowledge about NET cellular biology and their genetic characteristics is the key to the evolution of therapy. The primary goal is the need to develop a surveillance test and identify plasma markers that facilitate early diagnosis. The obvious therapeutic goal is based upon the identification of molecular targets in a particular tumour and the development of effective tumour-specific targeted therapeutic agents. Overall, there is a need to ensure that all NET patients are treated by multidisciplinary groups located within centres of excellence, or evaluated by such groups as part of a regional NET health network (Table 6.1.5).

References

1. Langhans T. Ueber einen drusenpolyp im ileum. *Virchows Arch Pathol Anat*, 1867; **38**: 550–60.
2. Lubarsch O. Ueber dem primaren Krebs des ileum nesbt bemerkungen uber das gleichzeitige vorkommenvon Krebs und tuberculose. *Virchows Arch Pathol Anat*, 1888; **111**: 280–317.
3. Ransom W. A case of primary carcinoma of the ileum. *Lancet*, 1890; **2**: 1020–3.
4. Oberndorfer S. Karzinoid tumouren des dunndarms. *Frankf Z Pathol*, 1907; **1**: 426–3.
5. Oberndorfer S. Karzinoide handbuch der speziellen. In: Henke F, Lubarsch O, eds. *Handbuch der Speziellen Pathologischen Anatomie und Histologie*. Berlin: Verlag von Julius Springer, 1928: 814–47.
6. Heidenhain R. Untersuchungen uber den bau der labdrusen. *Arch Mikr Anat*, 1870; **6**: 368.
7. Kulchitsky N. Zur Frage uber den Bau des Darmkanals. *Arch Mikr Anat*, 1897; 49: 7–35.
8. Nicolas A. Recherches sur l'epithelium de l'intestin grele. *Intern Monatsschr Anat Physiol*, 1891; 8: 1.
9. Kull H. Die chromaffinen Zellen des Verdauungstraktus. *Ztschr Mikr Anat Forsch*, 1924; **2**: 163.
10. Ciaccio M. Sur une nouvelle espece cellulaire dans les glandes de Lieberkuhn. *C R Seances Soc Biol Fil (Paris)*, 1906; **60**: 76–7.
11. Gosset A, Masson P. Tumeurs endocrines se l'appendice. *Prese Med*, 1914; **25**: 237–40.
12. Scholte A. Ein Fall von Angioma teleangieactaticum Cutis mit chronischer Endocarditis und malignem Dünndarmscarcinoid. *Beitrag Path Anat*, 1931; **86**: 440–3.
13. Biorck G, Axen O, Thorson A. Unusual cyanosis in a boy with congenital pulmonary stenosis and tricuspid insufficiency. Fatal outcome after angiocardiography. *Am Heart J*, 1952; **44**: 143–8.
14. Thorson A, Biorck G, Bjorkman G, Waldenstrom J. Malignant carcinoid of the small intestine with metastases to the liver, valvular disease of the right side of the heart (pulmonary stenosis and tricuspid regurgitation without septal defects), peripheral vasomotor symptoms, bronchoconstriction, and an unusual type of cyanosis; a clinical and pathologic syndrome. *Am Heart J*, 1954; **47**: 795–817.
15. Erspamer V, Asero B. Identification of enteramine, the specific hormone of the enterochromaffin cell system, as 5-hydroxytryptamine. *Nature*, 1952; **169**: 800–1.
16. Lembeck F. 5-Hydroxytryptamine in carcinoid tumour. *Nature*, 1953; **172**: 910–11.
17. Feyrter F. Zur Pathologie des Polysaccharidstoffwechsels im Epithel. II. Im Bronchialepithel und Alveolarepithel der menschlichen Lunge. *Virchows Arch*, 1957; **329**: 610–27.
18. Dawson A. Argentophile and argentaffin cells in gastric mucosa of rat. *Anat Rec*, 1948; **100**: 319–29.
19. Knowles F. Neuroendocrine correlations at the level of ultrastructure. *Arch Anat Microsc Morphol Exp*, 1965; **54**: 343–57.
20. Stachura J, Urban A, Bigaj M, Szczudrawa J, Wysocki A. Histochemical and ultrastructural observation of endocrine cells in pathological gastric mucosa. *Folia Histochemica Cytochemica (Krakow)*, 1978; **16**: 287–98.
21. Gould V, Chejfec G. Neuroendocrine carcinomas of the colon. Ultrastructural and biochemical evidence of their secretory function. *Am J Surg Pathol*, 1978; **2**: 31–8.

22. Wood S, Polak J, Bloom S. Gut hormone secreting tumours. *Scand J Gastroenterol*, 1983; (Suppl. 82): 165–70.
23. Wong WM, Wright NA. Cell proliferation in gastrointestinal mucosa. *J Clin Pathol*, 1999; **52**: 321–33.
24. Metz DC, Jensen RT. Gastrointestinal neuroendocrine tumours: pancreatic endocrine tumours. *Gastroenterology*, 2008; **135**: 1469–92.
25. Yantiss RK, Odze RD, Farraye FA, Rosenberg AE. Solitary versus multiple carcinoid tumours of the ileum: a clinical and pathologic review of 68 cases. *Am J Surg Pathol*, 2003; **27**: 811–17.
26. Hodges JR, Isaacson P, Wright R. Diffuse enterochromaffin-like (ECL) cell hyperplasia and multiple gastric carcinoids: a complication of pernicious anaemia. *Gut*, 1981; **22**: 237–41.
27. Moyana TN, Satkunam N. A comparative immunohistochemical study of jejunoileal and appendiceal carcinoids. Implications for histogenesis and pathogenesis. *Cancer*, 1992; **70**: 1081–8.
28. Slade MJ, Smith BM, Sinnett HD, Cross NC, Coombes RC. Quantitative polymerase chain reaction for the detection of micrometastases in patients with breast cancer. *J Clin Oncol*, 1999; **17**: 870–9.
29. Wang J, Cortina G, Wu SV, Tran R, Cho JH, Tsai MJ, *et al.* Mutant neurogenin-3 in congenital malabsorptive diarrhoea. *N Engl J Med*, 2006; **355**: 270–80.
30. Rehfeld JF. The new biology of gastrointestinal hormones. *Physiol Rev*, 1998; **78**: 1087–108.
31. Wiedenmann B, John M, Ahnert-Hilger G, Riecken EO. Molecular and cell biological aspects of neuroendocrine tumours of the gastroenteropancreatic system. *J Mol Med*, 1998; **76**: 637–47.
32. Bader MF, Doussau F, Chasserot-Golaz S, Vitale N, Gasman S. Coupling actin and membrane dynamics during calcium-regulated exocytosis: a role for Rho and ARF GTPases. *Biochim Biophys Acta*, 2004; **1742**: 37–49.
33. Bloom SR. *Gut Hormones*. Edinburgh: Churchill Livingstone, 1978.
34. Kidd M, Modlin IM, Tang LH. Gastrin and the enterochromaffin-like cell: an acid update. *Dig Surg*, 1998; **15**: 209–17.
35. Modlin IM, Kidd M, Pfragner R, Eick GN, Champaneria MC. The functional characterization of normal and neoplastic human enterochromaffin cells. *J Clin Endocrinol Metab*, 2006; **91**: 2340–8.
36. Takayanagi S, Hanai H, Kumagai J, Kaneko E. Serotonin uptake and its modulation in rat jejunal enterocyte preparation. *J Pharmacol Exp Ther*, 1995; **272**: 1151–9.
37. Jansa SA, Weksler M. Phylogeny of muroid rodents: relationships within and among major lineages as determined by IRBP gene sequences. *Mol Phylogenet Evol*, 2004; **31**: 256–76.
38. Modlin IM, Lawton GP, Tang LH, Geibel J, Abraham R, Darr U. The mastomys gastric carcinoid: aspects of enterochromaffin-like cell function. *Digestion*, 1994; **55** (Suppl. 3): 31–7.
39. Modlin IM, Esterline W, Kim H, Goldenring JR. Enterochromaffin-like cells and gastric argyrophil carcinoidosis. *Acta Oncol*, 1991; **30**: 493–8.
40. Schaffer K, McBride EW, Beinborn M, Kopin AS. Interspecies polymorphisms confer constitutive activity to the Mastomys cholecystokinin-B/gastrin receptor. *J Biol Chem*, 1998; **273**: 28779–84.
41. Bilchik AJ, Nilsson O, Modlin IM, Sussman J, Zucker KA, Adrian TE. H2-receptor blockade induces peptide YY and enteroglucagon-secreting gastric carcinoids in mastomys. *Surgery*, 1989; **106**: 1119–26; discussion 1026–7.
42. Kawase S, Ishikura H. Female-predominant occurrence of spontaneous gastric adenocarcinoma in cotton rats. *Lab Anim Sci*, 1995; **45**: 244–8.
43. Fossmark R, Martinsen TC, Bakkelund KE, Kawase S, Waldum HL. ECL-cell derived gastric cancer in male cotton rats dosed with the H2-blocker loxtidine. *Cancer Res*, 2004; **64**: 3687–93.
44. Kidd M, Hinoue T, Eick G, Lye KD, Mane SM, Wen Y, *et al.* Global expression analysis of ECL cells in Mastomys natalensis gastric mucosa identifies alterations in the AP-1 pathway induced by gastrin-mediated transformation. *Physiol Genomics*, 2004; **20**: 131–42.
45. McCloy RF, Arnold R, Bardhan KD, Cattan D, Klinkenberg-Knol E, Maton PN, *et al.* Pathophysiological effects of long-term acid suppression in man. *Dig Dis Sci*, 1995; **40**: 96S–120S.
46. Modlin IM, Lye KD, Kidd M. Carcinoid tumours of the stomach. *Surg Oncol*, 2003; **12**: 153–72.
47. Modlin IM, Goldenring JR, Lawton GP, Hunt R. Aspects of the theoretical basis and clinical relevance of low acid states. *Am J Gastroenterol*, 1994; **89**: 308–18.
48. Modlin I, Tang L. The gastric enterochromaffin-like cell: an enigmatic cellular link. *Gastroenterology*, 1996; **111**: 783–810.
49. Modlin IM, Kidd M, Latich I. Current status of gastrointestinal carcinoids. *Gastroenterology*, 2005; **128**: 1717–51.
50. Rozengurt E, Walsh JH. Gastrin, CCK, signalling, and cancer. *Ann Rev Physiol*, 2001; **63**: 49–76.
51. Chalmers CJ, Gilley R, March HN, Balmanno K, Cook SJ. The duration of ERK1/2 activity determines the activation of c-Fos and Fra-1 and the composition and quantitative transcriptional output of AP-1. *Cell Signal*, 2007; **19**: 695–704.
52. Treinies I, Paterson HF, Hooper S, Wilson R, Marshall CJ. Activated MEK stimulates expression of AP-1 components independently of phosphatidylinositol 3-kinase (PI3-kinase) but requires a PI3-kinase signal To stimulate DNA synthesis. *Mol Cell Biol*, 1999; **19**: 321–9.
53. Kinoshita Y, Nakata H, Kishi K, Kawanami C, Sawada M, Chiba T. Comparison of the signal transduction pathways activated by gastrin in enterochromaffin-like and parietal cells. *Gastroenterology*, 1998; **115**: 93–100.
54. Tang LH, Modlin IM, Lawton GP, Kidd M, Chinery R. The role of transforming growth factor alpha in the enterochromaffin-like cell tumour autonomy in an African rodent mastomys. *Gastroenterology*, 1996; **111**: 1212–23.
55. Thakker RV. Multiple endocrine neoplasia type 1. In: DeGroot LJ, Jamesson JL, eds. *Endocrinology*. 5th edn. Philadelphia: Elsevier Saunders, 2006: 3509–21.
56. Bradham DM, Igarashi A, Potter RL, Grotendorst GR. Connective tissue growth factor: a cysteine-rich mitogen secreted by human vascular endothelial cells is related to the SRC-induced immediate early gene product CEF-10. *J Cell Biol*, 1991; **114**: 1285–94.
57. Kidd M, Modlin IM, Eick GN, Camp RL, Mane SM. Role of CCN2/CTGF in the proliferation of Mastomys enterochromaffin-like cells and gastric carcinoid development. *Am J Physiol Gastrointest Liver Physiol*, 2007; **292**: G191–200.
58. Kidd M, Modlin IM, Pfragner R, Eick GN, Champaneria MC, Chan AK, *et al.* Small bowel carcinoid (enterochromaffin cell) neoplasia exhibits transforming growth factor-beta1-mediated regulatory abnormalities including up-regulation of C-Myc and MTA1. *Cancer*, 2007; **109**: 2420–31.
59. Lollgen RM, Hessman O, Szabo E, Westin G, Akerstrom G. Chromosome 18 deletions are common events in classical midgut carcinoid tumours. *Int J Cancer*, 2001; **92**: 812–15.
60. Modlin IM, Lye KD, Kidd M. A 5-decade analysis of 13,715 carcinoid tumours. *Cancer*, 2003; **97**: 934–59.
61. Modlin IM, Oberg K, Chung DC, Jensen RT, de Herder WW, Thakker RV, *et al.* Gastroenteropancreatic neuroendocrine tumours. *Lancet Oncol*, 2008; **9**: 61–72.
62. Gustafsson BI, Hauso O, Drozdov I, Kidd M, Modlin IM. Carcinoid heart disease. *Int J Cardiol*, 2008; 129: 318–24.
63. Lundin L, Norheim I, Landelius J, Oberg K, Theodorsson-Norheim E. Carcinoid heart disease: relationship of circulating vasoactive substances to ultrasound-detectable cardiac abnormalities. *Circulation*, 1988; **77**: 264–9.
64. Moller JE, Pellikka PA, Bernheim AM, Schaff HV, Rubin J, Connolly HM. Prognosis of carcinoid heart disease: analysis of 200 cases over two decades. *Circulation*, 2005; **112**: 3320–7.
65. Zuetenhorst JM, Bonfrer JM, Korse CM, Bakker R, van Tinteren H, Taal BG. Carcinoid heart disease: the role of urinary

5-hydroxyindoleacetic acid excretion and plasma levels of atrial natriuretic peptide, transforming growth factor-beta and fibroblast growth factor. *Cancer*, 2003; **97**: 1609–15.

66. Waldenstrom J, Ljungberg E. Studies on the functional circulatory influence from metastasizing carcinoid (argentaffine, enterochromaffine) tumours and their possible relation to enteramine production. I. Symptoms of cardinoidosis. *Acta Med Scand*, 1955; **152**: 293–309.
67. Rajamannan NM, Caplice N, Anthikad F, Sebo TJ, Orszulak TA, Edwards WD, *et al.* Cell proliferation in carcinoid valve disease: a mechanism for serotonin effects. *J Heart Valve Dis*, 2001; **10**: 827–31.
68. Gustafsson BI, Tommeras K, Nordrum I, Loennechen JP, Brunsvik A, Solligard E, *et al.* Long-term serotonin administration induces heart valve disease in rats. *Circulation*, 2005; **111**: 1517–22.
69. Hauso O, Gustafsson BI, Loennechen JP, Stunes AK, Nordrum I, Waldum HL. Long-term serotonin effects in the rat are prevented by terguride. *Regul Pept*, 2007; 143: 39–46.
70. Modlin IM, Shapiro MD, Kidd M. Carcinoid tumours and fibrosis: an association with no explanation. *Am J Gastroenterol*, 2004; **99**: 2466–78.
71. Moreno A, Akcakanat A, Munsell MF, Soni A, Yao JC, Meric-Bernstam F. Antitumour activity of rapamycin and octreotide as single agents or in combination in neuroendocrine tumours. *Endocr Relat Cancer*, 2008; **15**: 257–66.
72. Musunuru S, Carpenter JE, Sippel RS, Kunnimalaiyaan M, Chen H. A mouse model of carcinoid syndrome and heart disease. *J Surg Res*, 2005; **126**: 102–5.
73. Jackson LN, Chen LA, Larson SD, Silva SR, Rychahou PG, Boor PJ, *et al.* Development and characterization of a novel in vivo model of carcinoid syndrome. *Clin Cancer Res*, 2009; **15**: 2747–55.
74. Williams E, Sandler M. The classification of carcinoid tumours. *Lancet*, 1963; **1**: 238–9.
75. DeLellis RA, Lloyd RV, Heitz PU, Eng C. *World Health Organization Classification of Tumours, Pathology and Genetics of Tumours of Endocrine Organs.* Lyon: IARC Press, 2004.
76. Rorstad O. Prognostic indicators for carcinoid neuroendocrine tumours of the gastrointestinal tract. *J Surg Oncol*, 2005; **89**: 151–60.
77. Hotta K, Shimoda T, Nakanishi Y, Saito D. Usefulness of Ki-67 for predicting the metastatic potential of rectal carcinoids. *Pathol Int*, 2006; **56**: 591–6.
78. Ruszniewski P, Delle Fave G, Cadiot G, Komminoth P, Chung D, Kos-Kudla B, *et al.* Well-differentiated gastric tumours/carcinomas. *Neuroendocrinology*, 2006; **84**: 158–64.
79. Rindi G, Kloppel G, Couvelard A, Komminoth P, Korner M, Lopes JM, *et al.* TNM staging of midgut and hindgut (neuro) endocrine tumours: a consensus proposal including a grading system. *Virchows Arch*, 2007; **451**: 757–62.
80. Klimstra D, Modlin I, Adsay N, Chetty R, Deshpande V, Gonen M, *et al.* Pathologic reporting of neuroendocrine tumours: application of the delphic consensus process to the development of a minimum pathologic data set. *Am J Surg Pathol*, 2010; **34**: 300–13.
81. National Cancer Institute. *Surveillance Epidemiology and End Results (SEER) data base*, 1973–2004. Available at: http://seer.cancer.gov/. 2007 (accessed 16 June 2010).
82. Modlin IM, Oberg K, Chung DC, Jensen RT, de Herder WW, Thakker RV, *et al.* The current status of gastroenteropancreatic neuroendocrine tumours. *Lancet Oncol*, 2008; **9**: 61–72.
83. Modlin IM, Champaneria MC, Chan AK, Kidd M. A three-decade analysis of 3,911 small intestinal neuroendocrine tumours: the rapid pace of no progress. *Am J Gastroenterol*, 2007; **102**: 1464–73.
84. Berge T, Linell F. Carcinoid tumours. Frequency in a defined population during a 12-year period. *Acta Pathol Microbiol Scand A*, 1976; **84**: 322–30.
85. Gustafsson BI, Kidd M, Modlin IM. Neuroendocrine tumours of the diffuse neuroendocrine system. *Curr Opin Oncol*, 2008; **20**: 1–12.
86. Li AF, Hsu CY, Li A, Tai LC, Liang WY, Li WY, *et al.* A 35-year retrospective study of carcinoid tumours in Taiwan: differences in distribution with a high probability of associated second primary malignancies. *Cancer*, 2008; **112**: 274–83.
87. Onozato Y, Kakizaki S, Ishihara H, Iizuka H, Sohara N, Okamura S, *et al.* Endoscopic submucosal dissection for rectal tumours. *Endoscopy*, 2007; **39**: 423–7.
88. Soga J. Carcinoids and their variant endocrinomas. An analysis of 11842 reported cases. *J Exp Clin Cancer Res*, 2003; **22**: 517–30.
89. Yao J, Hassan M, Phan A, Dagohoy C, Leary C, Mares J, *et al.* One hundred years after 'carcinoid': epidemiology of and prognostic factors for neuroendocrine tumours in 35,825 cases in the United States. *J Clin Oncol*, 2008; **261**: 3063–72.
90. Sciola V, Massironi S, Conte D, Caprioli F, Ferrero S, Ciafardini C, *et al.* Plasma chromogranin A in patients with inflammatory bowel disease. *Inflamm Bowel Dis*, 2009; 15: 867–71.
91. West NE, Wise PE, Herline AJ, Muldoon RL, Chopp WV, Schwartz DA. Carcinoid tumours are 15 times more common in patients with Crohn's disease. *Inflamm Bowel Dis*, 2007; **13**: 1129–34.
92. Modlin I, Lye K, Kidd M. A five-decade analysis of 13,715 carcinoid tumours. *Cancer*, 2003; **97**: 934–59.
93. Sciarra A, Monti S, Gentile V, Salciccia S, Gomez AM, Pannunzi LP, *et al.* Chromogranin A expression in familial versus sporadic prostate cancer. *Urology*, 2005; **66**: 1010–14.
94. Modlin IM, Latich I, Zikusoka M, Kidd M, Eick G, Chan AK. Gastrointestinal carcinoids: the evolution of diagnostic strategies. *J Clin Gastroenterol*, 2006; **40**: 572–82.
95. Modlin IM, Gustafsson BI, Drozdov I, Nadler B, Pfragner R, Kidd M. Principal component analysis, hierarchical clustering, and decision tree assessment of plasma mRNA and hormone levels as an early detection strategy for small intestinal neuroendocrine (carcinoid) tumours. *Ann Surg Oncol*, 2009; **16**: 487–98.
96. Al-Nahhas A, Win Z, Szyszko T, Singh A, Nanni C, Fanti S, *et al.* Gallium-68 PET: a new frontier in receptor cancer imaging. *Anticancer Res*, 2007; **27**: 4087–94.
97. Itoi T, Sofuni A, Itokawa F, Tsuchiya T, Kurihara T, Moriyasu F. Endoscopic resection of carcinoid of the minor duodenal papilla. *World J Gastroenterol*, 2007; **13**: 3763–4.
98. Merg A, Wirtzfeld D, Wang J, Cheney R, Dunn KB, Rajput A. Viability of endoscopic and excisional treatment of early rectal carcinoids. *J Gastrointest Surg*, 2007; **11**: 893–7.
99. Yao JC, Phan AT, Chang DZ, Wolff RA, Hess K, Gupta S, *et al.* Efficacy of RAD001 (everolimus) and octreotide LAR in advanced low- to intermediate-grade neuroendocrine tumours: results of a phase II study. *J Clin Oncol*, 2008; **26**: 4311–18.
100. Arnold R, Muller H, Schade-Brittinger C, Rinke A, Klose K, Barth P, *et al.* Placebo-controlled, double-blind, prospective, randomized study of the effect of octreotide LAR in the control of tumour growth in patients with metastatic neuroendocrine midgut tumours: A report from the PROMID study group. *2009 Gastrointestinal Cancers Symposium.* American Society of Clinical Oncology, 2009: Abstract 121.
101. Bruns C, Lewis I, Briner U, Meno-Tetang G, Weckbecker G. SOM230: a novel somatostatin peptidomimetic with broad somatotropin release inhibiting factor (SRIF) receptor binding and a unique antisecretory profile. *Eur J Endocrinol*, 2002; **146**: 707–16.
102. Zhang J, Jia Z, Li Q, Wang L, Rashid A, Zhu Z, *et al.* Elevated expression of vascular endothelial growth factor correlates with increased angiogenesis and decreased progression-free survival among patients with low-grade neuroendocrine tumours. *Cancer*, 2007; **109**: 1478–86.
103. Akerstrom G, Hellman P. Surgery on neuroendocrine tumours. *Best Pract Res Clin Endocrinol Metab*, 2007; **21**: 87–109.
104. de Lecea L, Sutcliffe JG. The hypocretins and sleep. *FEBS J*, 2005; **272**: 5675–88.

105. Liapi E, Geschwind JF, Vossen JA, Buijs M, Georgiades CS, Bluemke DA, *et al.* Functional MRI evaluation of tumour response in patients with neuroendocrine hepatic metastasis treated with transcatheter arterial chemoembolization. *AJR Am J Roentgenol*, 2008; **190**: 67–73.
106. Forrer F, Valkema R, Kwekkeboom DJ, de Jong M, Krenning EP. Peptide receptor radionuclide therapy. *Best Pract Res Clin Endocrinol Metab*, 2007; **21**: 111–29.
107. Yao JC, Ng C, Hoff PM, Phan AT, Hess K, Chen H, *et al.* Improved progression free survival (PFS), and rapid, sustained decrease in tumour perfusion among patients with advanced carcinoid treated with bevacizumab. *Proc Am Soc Clin Oncol*, 2005; **23**: 309s.
108. Yao JC, Phan AT, Jacobs C, Mares JE, Meric-Bernstam F. Phase II study of RAD001 (everolimus) and depot octreotide (sandostatin LAR) in patients with advanced low grade neuroendocrine carcinoma (LGNET). 2006 American Society of Clinical Oncology Annual Meeting. *J Clin Oncol*, 2006; **24** (Suppl.): 4042.
109. Kulke M, Lenz HJ, Meropol N, Posey J, Ryan D, Picus J, *et al.* A phase 2 study to evaluate the efficacy and safety of SU11248 in patients (pts) with unresectable neuroendocrine tumours (NETs). *Proc Am Soc Clin Oncol*, 2005; **23**: 310S.
110. Duran I, Kortmansky J, Singh D, Hirte H, Kocha W, Goss G, *et al.* A Phase II clinical and pharmacodynamic study of temsirolimus in advanced neuroendocrine carcinomas. *Br J Cancer*, 2006; **95**: 1148–54.
111. Modlin IM, Kidd M, Latich I, Zikusoka MN, Shapiro MD. Current status of gastrointestinal carcinoids. *Gastroenterology*, 2005; **128**: 1717–51.
112. Kidd M, Modlin IM, Shapiro MD, Camp RL, Mane SM, Usinger W, *et al.* CTGF, intestinal stellate cells and carcinoid fibrogenesis. *World J Gastroenterol*, 2007; **13**: 5208–16.
113. Modlin I, Oberg K. *A Century of Advances in Neuroendocrine Tumour Biology and Treatment.* Hannover, Germany: Felsenstein CCCP, 2008.
114. Modlin IM, Latich I, Kidd M, Zikusoka M, Eick G. Therapeutic options for gastrointestinal carcinoids. *Clin Gastroenterol Hepatol*, 2006; **4**: 526–47.

6.2

Neuroendocrine tumour markers

R. Ramachandran, W. Dhillo

Introduction

Neuroendocrine cells occur either singly or in small groups in a variety of tissues and organs. Although morphologically and embryologically diverse, they are characterized by a number of unifying features. They have dense core secretory vesicles in the cytoplasm and hormone receptors on the cell membranes. There is evidence of prohormone activity within the cells and they synthesize, store, and secrete hormones. In addition, neuroendocrine cells possess an ability to take up and decarboxylate amine precursors.

Components of this diffuse endocrine system are particularly prominent in the gastrointestinal tract, pancreas, C cells of the thyroid, adrenal medulla, parathyroid tissue, respiratory tract, skin, and genitourinary system. Neuroendocrine tumours (NETs) are known to occur in all these tissues.

Historically, the diagnosis of NET was made on the basis of characteristic histological findings. The significantly worse prognosis in advanced disease and the availability of multiple therapeutic options have highlighted the need for robust tumour markers that can be used both for diagnosis and follow-up. Currently, a number of normal and abnormal forms of peptides, biogenic amines, and hormones, secreted by NETs, are routinely measured as markers of disease.

An ideal tumour marker would be one that is secreted exclusively by the tumour cells and is useful (1) for screening and differential diagnosis of NETs; (2) as a prognostic indicator; (3) as an estimate of tumour burden; and (4) as a surveillance tool. Although none of the currently available markers completely fits the paradigm for an ideal tumour marker, when measured in conjunction with each other, they are useful not only for making a diagnosis but also for monitoring response to therapy and in surveillance post-remission.

General neuroendocrine markers

NETs often express and secrete peptides that are common to most neuroendocrine cells and to cells that have undergone neuroendocrine differentiation.

Chromogranins

Neuroendocrine cells are characterized by the presence of electron-dense core secretory vesicles. Chromogranins (A, B, and C) form a major constituent of these granules (1) and are widely distributed in the neuroendocrine system. As a result, they are excellent tissue and serum markers for neuroendocrine tumours.

Chromogranin A

Chromogranin A (Cg A) was the first of the 'granins' to be identified and has the widest distribution (1, 2). It is quantitatively the major constituent of the secretory granules in the neuroendocrine cells and is expressed in the cells of the anterior pituitary, C cells of the thyroid, chief cells of the parathyroid, islet cells of the pancreas, and the chromaffin cells of the adrenal medulla. It is also widely distributed in the neuroendocrine cells of the bronchial and gastropancreatic systems and the skin.

The human form of Cg A is an acidic 439-amino acid protein, which is preceded by an 18-amino acid signal peptide. Both the N- and C-terminals are well conserved between species. The Cg A molecule contains a number of mono- and dibasic amino acid sites, thus implying fairly extensive and varied post-translational processing. This suggests that it may be a precursor to a number of other peptides. Although the function of Cg A has not yet been fully elucidated, it is often cosecreted with the neuroendocrine hormones and peptides and therefore thought to play a role in the processing, packaging, and secretion of neuropeptide precursors and hormones (3).

Most NETs are associated with increased circulating levels of Cg A. Even tumours that produce hormones with no identifiable clinical features or have lost the ability to synthesize peptides, continue to express Cg A (1). As a result, Cg A is routinely used as a marker for both diagnosis and monitoring of NETs. It is particularly useful (1) when existing cell specific markers (explained later in the chapter) are either unstable, rapidly fluctuating or inconvenient for clinical use; (2) to confirm the neuroendocrine origin of a tumour; and (3) as a general marker of disease when the neoplastic disease involves multiple neuroendocrine tissues, e.g. multiple endocrine neoplasia (1).

There are, however, some limitations to using Cg A as a tumour marker. Because of the wide distribution of Cg A-secreting cells, the basal circulating levels are much higher than most peptide hormones. Therefore, an increase in Cg A levels due to a tumour often goes undetected until it has reached a size capable of producing appreciably increased amounts of Cg A. Further, Cg A cannot differentiate between different subtypes of NET and it is not equally expressed in all NETs. Some only weakly express Cg A, e.g. small cell carcinoma of the lung (4). Concentrations are only minimally elevated in patients with insulinomas. Most patients with metastatic foregut and midgut carcinoids have increased (tumour burden-dependent) levels of Cg A. Gastrinomas may show increased levels of Cg A even in patients with very limited disease. This is probably because chronic hypergastrinaemia causes hyperplasia of the enterochromaffin cells (5).

A number of non-neoplastic conditions are associated with high Cg A levels. Patients on proton pump inhibitors (PPI) have raised Cg A levels. Renal and liver impairment also result in increased levels.

In spite of these shortcomings, the overall specificity and sensitivity of Cg A in NETs are 71.3% and 77.8%, respectively. It has a good negative predictive value of over 90% but the positive predictive value is poor, at around 50% or less depending on site of tumour (6).

Cg A undergoes post-translational changes before release. Tumours may, therefore, release different molecular forms of Cg A (7). As a result, a number of different forms of Cg A are released into circulation. Thus, levels measured are dependent on the antiserum used. Some assays measure only the whole Cg A, while others measure the whole Cg A plus fragments that contain the specific epitope to which the antisera was developed. Therefore reference ranges are assay specific. A lack of standardization between the various commercially available immunoassays makes comparison difficult. However, sequential measurement with the same assay can reliably be used to monitor disease progression in a patient.

Pancreastatin is a 49-amino acid (Cg A 240–288) peptide produced by dibasic cleavage of Cg A. Pancreastatin assays that use antisera raised to the midmolecule cross react strongly to Cg A and can be used to measure both pancreastatin and Cg A. Assays using antisera raised to the N- or C-terminals of pancreastatin are, however, specific for pancreastatin. Pancreastatin concentrations are shown to correlate well with extent of liver involvement. Specific pancreastatin assays may therefore be used to assess and monitor the extent liver involvement in patients with NET (8).

Chromogranin B

Chromogranin B (657 amino acid peptide) (Cg B) or GAWK (a partial sequence of Cg B 420–493) coexists with Cg A in the secretory granules and bears a strong homology to Cg A in the terminal regions. Like Cg A it is an acidic protein (9). The relative abundance of Cg A and Cg B is cell specific. Cg A is the dominant granin in the pancreatic endocrine tumours and in the serotonin-secreting tumours in the ileum and appendix. However, in rectal carcinoids, where Cg A is virtually absent, Cg B is the most abundant granin (10). Unlike Cg A, Cg B is unaffected by renal failure or use of PPI. It is, therefore, measured complementary to Cg A in some centres, and improves diagnostic sensitivity. Cg B assays are, however, associated with the same problems of standardization as the Cg A assays (10, 11). The combined measurement of Cg A and Cg B has a sensitivity of 89% for NETs (12). A polyclonal antiserum with cross reactivity to both Cg A and B has been developed by Eriksson *et al.* (13).

Chromogranins are best measured in plasma. Fasting samples are not required. Samples must be centrifuged, plasma aliquoted, and stored at −20 °C immediately after collection, to prevent degradation of the peptide. Patients on acid-suppressive therapy should be advised to come off treatment before Cg A is measured (see Summary).

Neuron-specific enolase

α–γ and γ–γ isomers of the glycolitic enzyme phosphopyruvate hydratase, 2-phospho-D-glycerate hydrolase, occur mainly in the neuronal and neuroectodermal tissue and are collectively known as neuron-specific enolase (NSE). NSE is expressed in a number of primary neuroendocrine tumours and in tumour with neuroendocrine differentiation (14, 15). It is specifically used in the diagnosis and follow-up of patients with neuroblastoma and small cell carcinoma of lung. This is particularly helpful as Cg A is poorly expressed in small cell lung carcinoma (16). Although the specificity of serum NSE in the diagnosis of neuroendocrine tumours is lower than that of Cg A, the combination of both markers has a higher sensitivity than both markers separately (17).

Other markers

Pancreatic polypeptide (PP) is a 36-amino acid peptide secreted by the normal pancreas. Levels increase in response to food. Although its function has not been fully elucidated, pancreatic polypeptide is known to slow gastric motility and is thought to play a role in the initiation of satiety (18). Its levels are increased in 74% of gastropancreatic tumours and roughly 50% of carcinoids. The term PPoma is used to describe tumours secreting particularly high levels of pancreatic polypeptide. Although no specific clinical symptoms have so far been attributed to elevated pancreatic polypeptide levels (7, 19), these tumours are sometimes associated with non-specific gastrointestinal symptoms. Due to a significant response to food, pancreatic polypeptideis best measured in plasma samples taken after an overnight fast. Samples must be centrifuged, plasma aliquoted, and stored at −20 °C immediately after collection, to prevent degradation of the peptide.

Tumours secreting somatostatin (stomatostatinoma) (20), ghrelin (21), and GLP-1 (GLPoma) (22) have been described. Due to significant changes in levels after food, all of these hormones are best measured in samples taken after an overnight fast. Samples must be centrifuged and plasma aliquoted, and stored at −20 °C immediately after collection, to prevent degradation of the peptide.

Neurotensin A and substance P are members of the tachykinin family and are expressed in midgut carcinoid cells. They act on lymphocytes and mast cell degranulation and cause vasodilatation and flushing and effect gastrointestinal motility. Levels of neurotensin A and its fragment neurotensin K are increased in 46% of patients with midgut carcinoids and serve as good prognostic markers. Levels correlate well with tumour burden and therapeutic response. Tachykinins can be measured in either plasma or serum. As tachykinins do not show a significant rise postprandially, fasting samples are not required (23).

Alpha subunit of the glycoprotein hormones and/or β-human chorionic gonadotropin (β-hGC) are elevated in about 25% of patients with neuroendocrine tumours such as carcinoids, islet cell tumours, medullary thyroid cancer, and small cell lung cancer. Locally invasive NETs are associated with higher prevalence of increased β-hCG and alpha subunit expression and circulating levels (24).

Carcinoembryonic antigen (CEA) is not specific to neuroendocrine tumours but is found to be elevated in some NETs such as medullary thyroid carcinoma. When used in conjunction with calcitonin, the specific marker for medullary thyroid carcinoma, CEA is a good prognostic marker as increased levels are associated with greater tumour aggressiveness and poorer prognosis (25).

Ki-67 is a proliferation antigen, which is expressed in G1, S, G2, and M phases of the mitotic cycle. Cells in G0 phase (resting phase) of the mitotic cycle do not express Ki-67. As a result, actively proliferating cells are seen to have a higher expression of Ki-67 on immunocytochemistry. Ki-67 proliferation index is a measure of its expression in the cell, based on the intensity of staining on immunocytochemistry. Nonfunctioning and metastatic NETs are seen to have a higher Ki-67 staining index. Increased expression of Ki-67 is associated with a poorer prognosis. Levels, however, cannot be measured in circulation, thus limiting the use of the marker to immunocytochemistry (26).

A number of other peptides, including adrenomedullin (27) and cocaine- and amphetamine- regulated transcript (CART) (12), have been proposed as candidate markers for NETs. The highest levels of adrenomedullin are found in neuroendocrine tumours of bronchial, midgut, and unknown origin. Levels seem to be predictive of progressive disease, suggesting a role for adrenomedullin as a prognostic marker. CART has been found to be a specific tumour marker in patients with a range of neuroendocrine tumours. Used in combination with Cg A, CART measurement has the potential to improve sensitivity in diagnosis and follow-up of neuroendocrine tumours, in particular progressive pancreatic neuroendocrine tumours.

Cell-specific markers

In addition to the markers mentioned above, neuroendocrine cells are often associated with the synthesis of specific hormones/peptides. Excessive production and/or release of hormones by tumours arising from these cells may result in clearly identifiable clinical syndromes (e.g. Zollinger–Ellison syndrome in patients with gastrinomas and recurrent hypoglycaemia in patients with insulinomas). Other NETs may present with unusual clinical symptoms as a result of ectopic secretion of hormones, such as growth hormone or ACTH. In such tumours (also known as functioning tumours), the specific hormone can be used as a marker for diagnosis, monitoring, and surveillance of disease. Some of these tumours and their markers are listed in Table 6.2.1. Each of these tumours is discussed in detail in elsewhere in this book.

Measurement of serum hormone concentrations can also be useful in the diagnosis of NETs in which the hormonal products produce a few nonspecific or no clinical symptoms. Hormones such as calcitonin, pancreatic polypeptide, and somatostatin and prohormones such as proopiomelanocortin (POMC) and calcitonin gene related peptide (CGRP) are examples of this.

Most peptides, hormones, and neuropeptides secreted by neuroendocrine cells are first synthesized as precursors or prohormones. In normal neuroendocrine cells they are then processed into mature hormones by sequence-specific and tissue-specific, post-translational modifications, including glycosylation, amidation, phophorylation, and sulphation. However, these processes are often defective in NETs. As a result, tumour cells may secrete a number of heterogeneous unprocessed or incorrectly/ incompletely processed forms of hormones/ peptides. A classic example is POMC, which is cleaved to ACTH and β-endorphin in an ordered manner in the normal pituitary. But in the presence of a tumour, high-molecular-weight forms of ACTH, as well as POMC, are secreted into the circulation. Other common examples of prohormones secreted by tumours include CGRP, progastrin, and proinsulin. Thus, the presence of incompletely or incorrectly processed prohormones is suggestive of the presence of a tumour.

Table 6.2.1 Cell specific markers for some of the neuroendocrine tumours

Tumour/syndrome	Marker (peptide(s)/hormone(s))
Gastrinoma	Gastrin (elevated fasting serum levels, off acid suppressive treatment)
Insulinoma	Insulin, proinsulin, and C-peptide (inappropriately elevated in the presence of hypoglycaemia: plasma glucose <2.2 mmol/l)
Glucagonoma	Glucagon (elevated fasting serum levels)
VIPoma	Vasoactive Intestinal polypeptide (elevated fasting serum levels)
Carcinoids	5-Hydroxyindoleacetic acid (5-HIAA) (elevated 24-h urinary) (elevated in midgut, occasionally in foregut, and rarely in hindgut carcinoids)
Phaeochromocytoma, carcinoids (occasionally)	Metanephrines (elevated plasma and 24-h urinary) Catecholamines (elevated plasma and 24-h urinary)
Hypercalcaemia	Parathyroid hormone (PTH) related peptide (elevated, in association with raised serum calcium and suppressed PTH)
Medullary thyroid carcinoma	Calcitonin (elevated plasma calcitonin)
Acromegaly	Growth hormone releasing hormone (elevated plasma levels due to ectopic secretion) Growth hormone (elevated plasma levels due to ectopic secretion) Insulin like growth factor (elevated plasma levels due to ectopic secretion)
Cushing's syndrome	Adrenocorticotropic hormone (elevated plasma levels due to ectopic secretion) Cortisol (elevated plasma levels due to high ACTH)

This fact has particular implications when validating assays for measuring hormones/ peptides as tumour markers. The antibody used must cross-react with as many forms of the hormone/ peptide as possible, in order to avoid false-negative results.

Dynamic function tests may sometimes improve the diagnostic sensitivity of hormone measurements. Common examples include the pentagastrin stimulation test for medullary thyroid carcinoma and 72-h fasting test for insulinomas.

Summary

Cg A is currently the best available NET marker. However, none of the currently available tumour markers are specific or sensitive enough to be used as a single definitive marker and, for most NETs, diagnosis by means of plasma level estimations of one hormone is not always clear cut. Therefore, two or more hormones are used for the diagnosis of most NET tumours.

Apart from the cell-specific hormones associated with functioning tumours, it is useful to monitor Cg A (+/– Cg B) as a marker of disease in almost all NETs. NSE is particularly useful in monitoring small cell carcinoma lung and neuroblastomas.

A panel of tumour markers is used to investigate both functioning and nonfunctioning gastropancreatic tumours. The markers most commonly measured include pancreatic polypeptide, somatostatin, Cg A, Cg B, VIP, gastrin, glucagon, and insulin. Of note, a number of these hormones (pancreatic polypeptide, somatostatin, VIP, gastrin, glucagon, and insulin) show a significant change in levels in response to food. Samples to measure these hormones must therefore be collected after an overnight fast.

Before collecting samples, it is always advisable to confirm sample requirements from the assaying laboratory, as requirements may sometimes differ. Guidelines offered by the supraregional assay service for gut hormone measurement in the UK (Imperial College Healthcare NHS Trust, London) suggest that all of these hormones, including Cg A and Cg B, are best measured in plasma samples collected in bottles containing ethylenediaminetetraacetic acid (EDTA) or LiHeparin (+ aprotinin). Neurotensin can only be measured in plasma samples collected in LiHeparin (+ aprotinin) bottles.

The peptides are prone to degradation. Samples must therefore be centrifuged, aliquoted, and frozen at −20 °C, immediately after collection. Both Cg A and gastrin levels are significantly affected by acid suppressive therapy. All patients must stop PPIs for 2 weeks, histamine-2 receptor blocker therapy for 3 days, and any other antacid therapy for 1 day before the measurement of Cg A or gastrin (28). Further details on sample requirements can be found on The Imperial Carcinoid and Neuroendocrine tumour service website (http://carcinoid.co.uk).

It is important to remember that, as with all other tumour markers, NET markers are only valuable when measured in the context of corroborative clinical and radiological findings.

It is hoped that future advances in microarrays and proteomics will lead to the discovery of more specific markers that will not only be more accurate diagnostic and prognostic indicators, but will also enable the use of highly effective, targeted, and individualized treatments for patients with NETs.

References

1. Nobels FR, Kwekkeboom DJ, Bouillon R, Lamberts SW. Chromogranin A: its clinical value as marker of neuroendocrine tumours. *Eur J Clin Invest*, 1998; **28**: 431–40.
2. Blaschko H, Comline RS, Schneider FH, Silver M, Smith AD. Secretion of a chromaffin granule protein, chromogranin, from the adrenal gland after splanchnic stimulation. *Nature*, 1967; **215**: 58–9.
3. Helle KB, Corti A, Metz-Boutigue MH, Tota B. The endocrine role for chromogranin A: a prohormone for peptides with regulatory properties. *Cell Mol Life Sci*, 2007; **64**: 2863–86.
4. Lloyd RV, Cano M, Rosa P, Hille A, Huttner WB. Distribution of chromogranin A and secretogranin I (chromogranin B) in neuroendocrine cells and tumors. *Am J Pathol*, 1988; **130**: 296–304.
5. Granberg D, Stridsberg M, Seensalu R, Eriksson B, Lundqvist G, Oberg K, *et al.* Plasma chromogranin A in patients with multiple endocrine neoplasia type 1. *J Clin Endocrinol Metab*, 1999; **84**: 2712–17.
6. Zatelli MC, Torta M, Leon A, Ambrosio MR, Gion M, Tomassetti P, *et al.* Chromogranin A as a marker of neuroendocrine neoplasia: an Italian Multicenter Study. *Endocr Relat Cancer*, 2007; **14**: 473–82.
7. de Herder WW. Biochemistry of neuroendocrine tumours. *Best Pract Res Clin Endocrinol Metab*, 2007; **21**: 33–41.
8. Ardill JES. Circulating markers for endocrine tumours of the gastroenteropancreatic tract. *Ann Clin Biochem*, 2008; **45**: 539–59.
9. Benedum UM, Lamouroux A, Konecki DS, Rosa P, Hille A, Baeuerle PA, *et al.* The primary structure of human secretogranin I (chromogranin B): comparison with chromogranin A reveals homologous terminal domains and a large intervening variable region. *EMBO J*, 1987; **6**: 1203–11.
10. Stridsberg M, Husebye E. Chromogranin A and chromogranin B are sensitive circulating markers for phaeochromocytoma. *Eur J Endocrinol*, 1997; **136**: 67–73.
11. Sekiya K, Ghatei MA, Salahuddin MJ, Bishop AE, Hamid QA, Ibayashi H, *et al.* Production of GAWK (chromogranin-B 420–493)-like immunoreactivity by endocrine tumors and its possible diagnostic value. *J Clin Invest*, 1989; **83**: 1834–42.
12. Bech P, Winstanley V, Murphy KG, Sam AH, Meeran K, Ghatei MA, *et al.* Elevated cocaine- and amphetamine-regulated transcript immunoreactivity in the circulation of patients with neuroendocrine malignancy. *J Clin Endocrinol Metab*, 2008; **93**: 1246–53.
13. Eriksson B, Arnberg H, Oberg K, Hellman U, Lundqvist G, Wernstedt C, *et al.* A polyclonal antiserum against chromogranin A and B—a new sensitive marker for neuroendocrine tumours. *Acta Endocrinol (Copenh)*, 1990; **122**: 145–55.
14. Gerbitz KD, Summer J, Schumacher I, Arnold H, Kraft A, Mross K. Enolase isoenzymes as tumour markers. *J Clin Chem Clin Biochem*, 1986; **24**: 1009–16.
15. Pahlman S, Esscher T, Bergvall P, Odelstad L. Purification and characterization of human neuron-specific enolase: radioimmunoassay development. *Tumour Biol*, 1984; **5**: 127–39.
16. Bajetta E, Catena L, Procopio G, Bichisao E, Ferrari L, Della Torre S, *et al.* Is the new WHO classification of neuroendocrine tumours useful for selecting an appropriate treatment? *Ann Oncol*, 2005; **16**: 1374–80.
17. Nobels FRE, Kwekkeboom DJ, Coopmans W, Schoenmakers CHH, Lindemans J, De Herder WW, *et al.* Chromogranin A as serum marker for neuroendocrine neoplasia: comparison with neuron-specific enolase and the α-subunit of glycoprotein hormones. *J Clin Endocrinol Metab*, 1997; **82**: 2622–8.
18. Gardiner JV, Jayasena CN, Bloom SR. Gut hormones: a weight off your mind. *J Neuroendocrinol*, 2008; **20**: 834–41.
19. Eriksson B, Arnberg H, Lindgren PG, Lorelius LE, Magnusson A, Lundqvist G, *et al.* Neuroendocrine pancreatic tumours: clinical presentation, biochemical and histopathological findings in 84 patients. *J Intern Med*, 1990; **228**: 103–13.
20. Garbrecht N, Anlauf M, Schmitt A, Henopp T, Sipos B, Raffel A, *et al.* Somatostatin-producing neuroendocrine tumors of the duodenum and pancreas: incidence, types, biological behavior, association with inherited syndromes, and functional activity. *Endocr Relat Cancer*, 2008; **15**: 229–41.
21. Tsolakis AV, Stridsberg M, Grimelius L, Portela-Gomes GM, Falkmer SE, Waldum HL, *et al.* Ghrelin immunoreactive cells in gastric endocrine tumors and their relation to plasma ghrelin concentration. *J Clin Gastroenterol*, 2008; **42**: 381–8.
22. Todd JF, Stanley SA, Roufosse CA, Bishop AE, Khoo B, Bloom SR, *et al.* A tumour that secretes glucagon-like peptide-1 and somatostatin in a patient with reactive hypoglycaemia and diabetes. *Lancet*, 2003; **361**: 228–30.
23. Turner GB, Johnston BT, McCance DR, McGinty A, Watson RGP, Patterson CC, *et al.* Circulating markers of prognosis and response to treatment in patients with midgut carcinoid tumours. *Gut*, 2006; **55**: 1586–91.
24. Grossmann M, Trautmann ME, Poertl S, Hoermann R, Berger P, Arnold R, *et al.* Alpha-subunit and human chorionic gonadotropin-beta immunoreactivity in patients with malignant endocrine gastroenteropancreatic tumours. *Eur J Clin Invest*, 1994; **24**: 131–6.
25. Machens A, Ukkat J, Hauptmann S, Dralle H. Abnormal carcinoembryonic antigen levels and medullary thyroid cancer progression: a multivariate analysis. *Arch Surg*, 2007; **142**: 289–93.
26. Vilar E, Salazar R, Perez-Garcia J, Cortes J, Oberg K, Tabernero J. Chemotherapy and role of the proliferation marker Ki-67 in digestive neuroendocrine tumors. *Endocr Relat Cancer*, 2007; **14**: 221–32.
27. Pavel ME, Hoppe S, Papadopoulos T, Linder V, Mohr B, Hahn EG, *et al.* Adrenomedullin is a novel marker of tumor progression in neuroendocrine carcinomas. *Horm Metab Res*, 2006; **38**: 112–18.
28. Dhillo W, Jayasena C, Lewis C, Martin N, Tang K, Meeran K, *et al.* Plasma gastrin measurement cannot be used to diagnose a gastrinoma in patients on either proton pump inhibitors or histamine type-2 receptor antagonists. *Ann Clin Biochem*, 2006; **43**: 153–5.

6.3

Neuroendocrine (carcinoid) tumours and the carcinoid syndrome

Rajaventhan Srirajaskanthan,
Martyn E. Caplin, Humphrey Hodgson

Introduction

Neuroendocrine tumours (NETs) are derived from cells of the diffuse neuroendocrine system, which are present in organs throughout the body. Originally, Pearse proposed that tumours develop from migration of cells from the neural crest; however, it is now thought that the tumour cells are derived from multipotent stem cells (1).

The term 'karzinoide' (meaning carcinoma like) was initially introduced by Siegfried Oberndorfer in 1907 (2). The term carcinoid tumour has historically been used; however, with advances in the understanding of the tumour biology, and the recent WHO classification, the term NET or endocrine tumour is considered more appropriate, and more details are given in the historical introduction in Chapter 6.1.

Incidence

The reported incidence is 2.5–5 cases per 100 000 population (3), however, due to their rather indolent nature the prevalence of these tumours is much higher—approximately 35 per 100 000 population in the USA (4). The incidence of different NETs has risen over the last three decades, with the greatest increased in bronchial NETs (5), which account for 10–30% of all NETs. This increase in incidence of NETs is partly due to improved diagnostic techniques, both radiological and endoscopic.

Aetiology

Most cases are sporadic; however, some occur as part of genetic syndromes, including multiple endocrine neoplasia 1 (MEN 1), MEN 2, von Hippel–Lindau syndrome and neurofibromatosis 1 (6). The incidence of MEN 1 in NETs varies dependent on the site, from very rare in midgut NETs but occurring in up to 25–40% of gastrinomas (7). Approximately one-third of individuals with MEN 1 develop gastric carcinoids.

Classification

NETs of the gastrointestinal tract have been classified according to their embryological origin into foregut (bronchial, stomach, pancreas, gall bladder, and duodenum), midgut (jejunum, ileum, appendix, and colon, up to ascending colon), and hindgut (transverse and remaining colon, rectum). It is becoming apparent that tumours within each region can have markedly different clinical behaviour and, therefore, a shift towards categorization of tumours purely by anatomical location is being introduced (8). Additional tumours considered to be neuroendocrine include: thymic carcinoids, medullary thyroid cancer, phaeochromocytomas, and paragangliomas.

Pathology

NETs can exhibit a diverse spectrum of pathology, from benign tumours to highly aggressive, poorly differentiated tumours (8). The WHO classification is used for describing tumours of gut and pancreas (9). Separate classifications systems are in use for bronchial, thymic, and thyroid NETs. The WHO classification for tumours is based on degree of differentiation and clinical behaviour; there are three types:

- well-differentiated endocrine tumours, with benign (1.1) or uncertain behaviour (1.2) at the time of diagnosis
- well-differentiated endocrine carcinomas with low-grade malignant behaviour
- poorly differentiated endocrine carcinomas, with high-grade malignant behaviour.

Bronchial carcinoid tumours are classified into four groups dependent on histological parameters, including mitotic activity and proliferation index. These groups are typical carcinoids, atypical carcinoids, large cell neuroendocrine carcinoma, and small cell lung carcinoma (10).

The European Neuroendocrine Tumour Society has proposed a TNM staging classification and this also includes a grading system of low, intermediate, or high-grade tumours dependent on their proliferation index, mitotic activity, and histological phenotype (11–13). Also, they stage tumours using the TMN classification. The classification so far has been published for GEP NETs but not other NETs. Further details are given in Chapter 6.1.

Clinical features

NETs can be separated into nonfunctioning and functioning tumours. The majority (approximately 60%) are nonfunctional tumours, i.e. with no symptoms attributable to secretion of metabolically active peptides. Functional tumours secrete substances that are metabolically active, which can lead to the development of specific clinical syndromes (Table 6.3.1). The most common functional syndrome is carcinoid syndrome, which is thought to be due to secretion of amines, kallikrein, and prostaglandins. Serotonin (5-hydroxytryptamine) is one of the main amines that is synthesized and secreted by these tumours.

Carcinoid syndrome

Carcinoid syndrome occurs in 20–30% of patients with midgut carcinoid tumours and approximately 5% of bronchial carcinoids (14). Other foregut tumours (e.g. pancreatic neuroendocrine tumours) can cause carcinoid syndrome although this is uncommon (1%). Hind gut tumours are generally nonfunctional and rarely cause carcinoid syndrome. Carcinoid syndrome is usually seen in patients with liver metastases (in 95% patients), but excess tachykinins, serotonin production from retroperitoneal metastases, or ovarian tumours can bypass the liver to cause the syndrome.

Table 6.3.1 The clinical features of neuroendocrine tumours

Site	Clinical features	Cell type	MEN 1
Pancreatic			
Insulinoma	Hypoglycaemia, Whipple's triad, clammy, sweating, weight gain	β-islet cell	5–10%
VIPoma	Werner–Morrison syndrome, watery diarrhoea	VIP	10%
Glucagonoma	Diabetes mellitus, necrolytic migratory erythyema		5–10%
Somatostatinoma	Gallstones, diabetes mellitus, steatorrhoea	D cells	5–10%
Gastrinoma	Zollinger—Ellison syndrome	G cells	25%
Nonfunctional	Symptoms related to mass effect		
Bronchial	Majority nonfunctional, 8% carcinoid syndrome, atypical flushing		
Midgut[a]	Majority nonfunctional, 40% develop carcinoid syndrome		
Hindgut[a]	Usually nonfunctional, however tumours may secrete somatostatin, other peptide, and occasionally carcinoid syndrome may occur		

[a] Midgut tumours arise from the jejunum to caecum and hindgut encompasses tumours from the ascending colon to rectum.

Normally, serotonin is synthesized from tryptophan, and is subsequently metabolized by monoamine oxidase to 5-hydroxyindoleacetic acid (5-HIAA), which is subsequently secreted in the urine in healthy individuals. Approximately 99% of tryptophan is used for the synthesis of nicotinic acid and less than 1% converted to 5-hydroxytryptamine (5-HT). However, in patients with carcinoid tumours there is a shift towards the production of 5-HT. The increased production of 5-HT and other products and their direct release into the systemic circulation, due to liver metastases, leads to the development of carcinoid syndrome (15).

Patients often describe having symptoms for many months prior to presentation. The two most common symptoms are diarrhoea and flushing, whilst wheeze occurs less commonly. Often diarrhoea is associated with crampy abdominal pain and urgency, and can occur during both day and night. Flushing is characteristically described as a sudden onset of pink to red discoloration involving the face and upper trunk. This usually lasts a few minutes and can occur intermittently throughout the day. Triggers leading to flushing and diarrhoea include stress, tyramine-containing foods (chocolate, bananas, walnuts) and alcohol. In patients with atypical flushing, which may last for several hours, telangiectasia and hypertrophy of the face may be seen. Wheeze is caused by bronchial constriction mediated via tachykinins and bradykinins. This is more common in those with bronchial carcinoid tumours.

A raised jugular venous pressure and features of right heart failure may be present in patients with carcinoid heart disease related to carcinoid syndrome. Right-sided cardiac murmurs of tricuspid regurgitation and pulmonary stenosis may be heard on cardiovascular examination (16).

Other hormone-related manifestations include morphoea (subcutaneous thickening of the lower limbs) and a pellagra-type rash if nicotinic acid deficiency has been induced. With severe, longstanding hepatomegaly or local infiltration, inferior vena cava obstruction, or even lymphangiectasia leading to ascites may occur.

The prognosis of patients with carcinoid syndrome varies widely and although some patients may have rapidly progressive disease, in others survival for decades may occur.

Diagnostic investigations

Diagnosis of NETs requires biochemical, topographical imaging, and, importantly, histological diagnosis. Efforts should be made to identify the primary tumour site, which can be difficult since some primary lesions are small and not detected by conventional cross-sectional imaging.

Biochemical tests

Patients with suspected NETs should undergo biochemical testing, including fasting gut hormones (glucagon, vasoactive intestinal peptide, somatostatin (SST), and gastrin), chromogranin A, and pancreatic polypeptide. In addition to specialized blood tests, routine lab tests including full blood count, urea and electrolytes, liver function tests, carcino-embryonic antigen, α-fetoprotein, β-human chorionic gonadotropin, Ca 19-9, and ESR should be performed. Urinary 5-HIAA assay should also be performed in all patients with suspected carcinoid syndrome (17). Table 6.3.2. shows the different biochemical tests that are used for diagnosis of NETs.

Histology

Histology remains the gold standard for diagnosing NETs. Specimens should be immunostained with a panel of antibodies to general neuroendocrine markers. These include chromogranin A, synaptophysin, and PGP9.5. In addition, the tumour should be stained with an antibody to the Ki-67 protein, since the Ki-67 proliferation index is of benefit in grading tumours (11).

The histological characteristics of NETs vary according to the degree of differentiation. Low-grade NETs originating from the gut were previously termed 'typical' carcinoids; these tumours had classic histological architecture of trabecular, or ribbon-like cell clusters, with little or no cellular pleomorphism and occasional mitoses. The higher grade and poorly differentiated tumours had increased mitotic activity and evidence of necrosis. The WHO classification gives clear parameters for categorizing NETs into the three main categories described earlier (9).

Imaging

Cross-sectional imaging is usually with contrast CT, including arterial phase enhancement, of the abdomen, chest, and pelvis. MRI is the most sensitive modality for liver metastases (18). Studies of CT in carcinoid tumours show an overall sensitivity of 80% in detecting lesions (19, 20). The sensitivity and specificity of CT and MRI alone are lower than the combination of ^{111}In-octreotide scan with CT or MRI (21).

Table 6.3.2 General biochemical plasma markers raised in neuroendocrine tumour-dependent on anatomical site

Type of tumour	Plasma marker	Urinary marker
Carcinoid	Chromogranin A Chromogranin B Neuron-specific enolase β-human chorionic gonadotropin Substance P Gherelin Neuropeptide K α fetoprotein	5-Hydroxyindoloacetic acid
Phaeochromocytoma	Chromogranin A Chromogranin B Neuron-specific enolase β-human chorionic gonadotropin Neuropeptide Y Metanephrins α fetoprotein	Catecholamines Vanillylmandelic acid Dopamine Homovanillic acid
Pancreatic NETs	Chromogranin A Chromogranin B Pancreatic polypeptide Neuron-specific enolase β-human chorionic gonadotropin α fetoprotein	

Nuclear medicine

Nuclear medicine imaging is important in staging of disease and determining suitability for therapy with SST analogues and peptide receptor. The two main nuclear medicine scans used in staging NETs are ^{111}In-octreotide and ^{123}I-metaiodobenzylguanidine (MIBG), with newer modalities, including PET scanning, being introduced.

There are five different SST receptor (SSTR) subtypes, all of which have strong affinity for SST (22). Octreotide is an SST analogue which has a strong affinity for SSTR-2 and to a lesser extent SSTR-5 receptors. NETs predominantly express SSTR-2. Synthetic radiolabelled SSTR analogues, such as ^{111}In-pentetreotide, enable SSTR scintigraphy to be performed (23).

SSTR scintigraphy is now established in localizing NET (24). Prospective studies have shown that inclusion of SSTR scintigraphy in the diagnostic work-up of patients alters management in up to 47% of cases (25). The sensitivity of SSTR scintigraphy for the detection of GEP NETs has been well studied. The sensitivity has been reported to be between 67 and 100%, with no significant difference in carcinoid tumours from foregut, midgut, or hindgut origin (26–28). With pancreatic NETs, sensitivity of SSTR scintigraphy is dependent on the type of functional tumour. Gastrinomas detection has a sensitivity between 56 and 80%, VIPoma is 60–70%, and insulinoma lower at 50% due to a lower expression of SSTR-2 (23). With phaeochromocytomas, SSTR scintigraphy is often negative and other imaging modalities, such as MIBG, should be used. Medullary thyroid cancer express SSTR-1 therefore may be negative on SSTR scintigraphy. False-positive scans can be seen in patients with chronic inflammation and granulomatous disease. SSTR scintigraphy detection is also affected by the size of NET and will often not detect lesions less than 1 cm (29).

MIBG has been used for two decades to visualize carcinoid tumours. The method was initially developed to detect phaeochromocytomas. MIBG shares the same method of uptake as noradrenaline and is not dependent on SSTR receptor expression. In phaeochromocytomas, MIBG has sensitivity of 87% and specificity of 99%; however, for carcinoid tumours it only has 50% sensitivity and specificity, whilst in pancreatic NETs uptake may be seen in less than 10% of cases (30). In general, ^{123}I-MIBG scintigraphy was shown to be less sensitive than ^{111}In-octreotide in identifying carcinoid tumours (30).

PET scanning in other malignancies is well established; however, its role for NETs is still evolving. [^{18}F]2-fluoro-2-deoxyglucose (FDG)-PET is only suitable for high-grade tumours and is of minimal use in low-grade tumours due to their slow glucose turnover. Experimental agents of interest include gallium-68 (Ga-68) DOTA-octreotide and Ga-68 DOTA-octreotate, 5-hydroxytryptophan (5-HTP) and 3,4-dihydroxyphenylalanine (DOPA). Studies with Ga-68 DOTA-octreotide had a greater sensitivity than conventional SSTR scintigraphy (31, 32) (Fig. 6.3.1).

Endoscopy

If the primary site has not been identified by conventional imaging, it is worthwhile performing endoscopy of the upper and lower gastrointestinal tract. In addition, if patients are known to have a primary lesion in the gastrointestinal tract endoscopy will allow visualization of the lesion and the option of histological diagnosis. For detection of gastric, pancreatic, and duodenal lesions, endoscopic

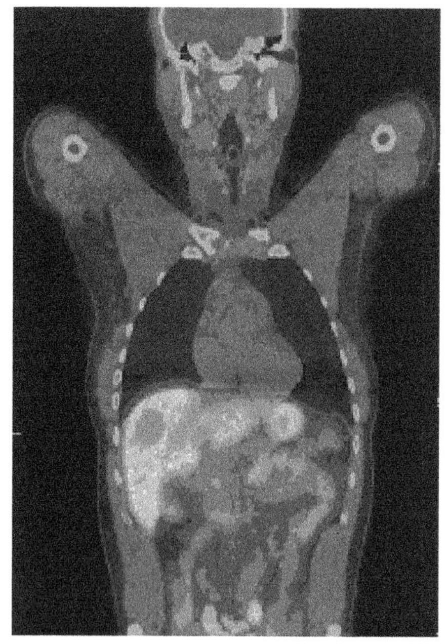

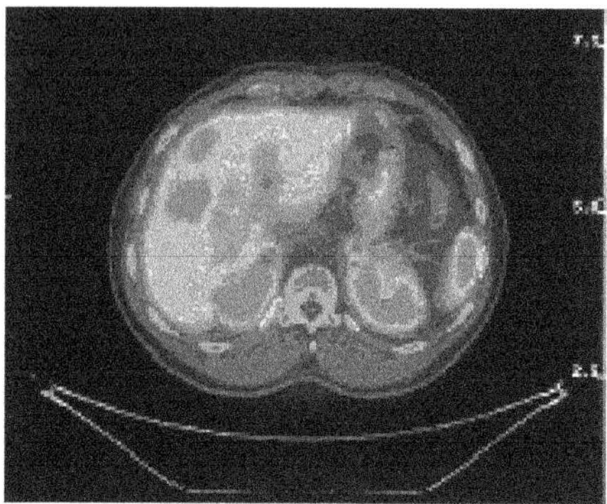

Fig. 6.3.1 Ga-68 DOTATATE PET images from patient with metastatic neuroendocrine tumour. Images show Ga-68 DOTATATE-avid liver metastases. (See also Plate 33)

ultrasonography is a sensitive method for staging disease and providing information regarding depth of invasion and potential resectability of the lesions. In addition, biopsies can be performed to provide histological diagnosis. Endoscopic ultrasonography has an accuracy of 90% in staging of rectal carcinoids (33).

Capsule endoscopy can be used to diagnose small bowel carcinoid tumours, and appears to be at least as good as enteroscopy for identifying lesions. Obviously, the drawback is the inability to obtain a histological diagnosis. In small case series there appears to be advantage of capsule endoscopy over conventional small bowel investigations using CT and barium follow-through (34). To exclude the possibility of obstruction, a barium follow-through should be performed prior to capsule endoscopy.

For bronchial NETs, which commonly arise in large to midsize airways, bronchoscopy is of use in assessing the lesion and obtaining histological diagnosis (5).

Management

Therapies for NETs incorporate those required for control of symptoms due to hormonal secretion from tumours, and also antiproliferative therapies. The management of NETs requires the use of a number of different therapies including: surgery, biotherapy, chemotherapy, peptide receptor targeted therapy, and tumour embolization. The best way to provide the most appropriate management plan for patients is through a multidisciplinary approach. Different therapies may be required at different clinical stages, and in patients with indolent disease and mild symptoms merely symptomatic relief may be all that is required for some years.

Surgery

Surgery is the only method of cure and therefore should be considered and undertaken in all patients where feasible. In patients with localized tumours resection of the primary lesion should be performed, especially with bronchial tumours which are often localized. Debulking surgery should be considered in cases where increasing hormonal symptoms are present that cannot be controlled using medical therapy.

Somatostatin analogues

SST is a small polypeptide hormone, which occurs naturally in the human body and binds with a high affinity to the five recognized SSTRs. Activation of SSTRs leads to activation of common signalling pathways, such as inhibition of adenyl cyclase and modulation of mitogen activated protein kinase through G-protein dependent mechanisms (35). The effect of SST on tumour growth may be through the suppression of the synthesis and secretion of growth factors and growth promoting hormones. SST also appears to inhibit angiogenesis and cell proliferation in *in vitro* models. Its antiangiogenic effect appears to be through inhibition of angiogenic factors such as vascular endothelial growth factor, insulin-like growth factor-1, and platelet-derived growth factor (36, 37).

Short-acting octreotide, which needs to be administered three times a day. Long-acting octreotide-LAR and Lanreotide Autogel have a 28 day duration of action (38). Both are equally effective at controlling symptoms related to carcinoid syndrome, with improvement seen in approximately 85% of cases (39). Biochemical markers, such as chromogranin A and urinary 5-HIAA, are found to decrease by at least 50% in 60–80% of cases following therapy (40). In a study performed by Garland *et al.*, of 27 patients with positive SSTR scintigraphy and commenced on octreotide-LAR, all had good symptom control initially; however, the majority of patients developed progressive disease and required further therapies for symptom control (41). Side effects include gastrointestinal disturbances, including pancreatic insufficiency which may require enzyme replacement therapy, gallstones, and glucose intolerance. Tolerance to SST analogues is a recognized phenomenon and there is a need for new biotherapy agents. Pasireotide, a new multiligand SST analogue, is currently being trialled. Recent studies have demonstrated that the majority of NETs coexpress dopamine and SSTRs, which has led to development of chimeric agents; these have shown promising results in NET cell lines (42, 43).

Interferon α

Interferon therapy has been used for symptomatic control in patients with NETs since 1982. It has been found to be beneficial in reducing symptoms of flushing and diarrhoea in patients with carcinoid syndrome in 50–60% of cases. Significant biochemical responses are reported in 40–50% of cases (44). Its mechanism is action is unclear though is thought to act through antisecretory and immunomodulatory functions. Its antitumour effect is not as pronounced as with SST analogues, with radiological evidence of tumour regression being less common. In a study of 111 patients treated with interferon-α, 15% demonstrated a greater than 50% reduction in tumour size (45).

Studies have shown that disease stabilization occurs in 40% of patients following combined therapy with SST analogues and interferon-α, which is similar to that of SST analogues alone (46). A randomized study with over 100 patients showed there was no significant survival benefit of SST analogues with interferon-α compared to SST analogues alone (47).

Chemotherapy

Chemotherapy has been widely used in the treatment of NETs for over three decades. Its precise role is not clearly defined; it is, however, often used as first-line therapy for unresectable, poorly differentiated NETs and pancreatic well-differentiated NETS, which are often chemosensitive. Studies have demonstrated wide variation in response rates with chemotherapy; this may, in part, be due to inclusion of different types and grades of NETs. The overall response rate for intestinal carcinoid is less than 30% (48–55).

Hepatic artery embolization

Metastases from NETs are often isolated to the liver and therefore embolization of the liver can result in necrosis of tumour tissue and consequent decrease in hormonal secretion. Embolization is commonly performed radiologically and can be performed with particles or chemoembolization. Contraindications to performing hepatic artery embolization include: portal vein thrombosis, liver failure, and biliary reconstruction.

Symptomatic response is seen in 40–80% of cases, with a biochemical response (56) for hepatic embolization of 7–75%, and 12–75% for hepatic chemoembolization (57). In the latter study (57), Gupta *et al.* demonstrated no additional benefit of chemotherapy to transarterial hepatic embolization in metastatic midgut tumours. Complications postprocedure include ileus, portal vein thrombosis, hepatic abscess, hepatic fistula, encephalopathy, and renal insufficiency.

Radionuclide peptide receptor therapy

The overexpression of SSTR-2 has allowed for the development of targeted peptide receptor therapy. The mechanism of action appears to be that the radiopeptide binds to the SSTR-2 receptor and is internalized by the cell, thereby delivering radioactivity for a long period of time, with beta emitting radionuclides irradiating neighbouring tumour cells. Contraindications include bone marrow suppression, renal impairment, liver failure, very poor performance status, and inability to self care. A number of studies have been published using peptide receptor radionuclide therapy; however, the criteria for objective response has varied in studies (Table 6.3.3). The two radiopeptides that are currently in use are Yttrium-90 and Lutetium-177. Unfortunately, there are no randomized studies of peptide–receptor radionuclide therapy, thus evaluation of their true benefit and optimal radionuclide is difficult.

Kwekkeboom *et al.* recently published the largest series to date of over 500 patients treated with Lu177-DOTATATE (58). Of these patients, response data was available in 310: 2% had complete response, 28% partial response, and 16% had minor response.

Table 6.3.3 Peptide receptor studies looking at different radiopeptides and response rates seen in neuroendocrine tumours

Authors	No.	Response (%)				
		CR	PR	MR	SD	PD
Y90-DOTATOC						
Otte *et al.* (59)	29	0	2 (7)	4 (14)	20 (69)	3 (10)
Waldherr *et al.* (60)	39	2 (55)	7 (18)	n/a	27 (69)	3 (8)
Bodei *et al.* (61)	29	1 (3)	7 (24)	n/a	14 (48)	7 (24)
Valkema *et al.* (62)	52	0	5 (10)	7 (13)	29 (56)	14 (26)
Y90-Lanreotide						
Virgolini *et al.* (63)	39	0	0	8 (20)	17 (44)	14 (36)
Y90-DOTATATE						
Baum *et al.* (64)	75	0	28 (37)	n/a	39 (52)	8 (11)
Lu177- DOTATATE						
Kwekkeboom *et al.* (58)	310	5 (2)	96 (28)	51 (16)	107 (35)	61 (20)

CR, complete response; PR, partial response; MR, minimal response; SD, stable disease; PD, progressive disease.

The median time to progression was 40 months and median overall survival from start of treatment was 46 months; median survival from diagnosis was 128 months. The overall survival for these patients seems much higher than historic controls, were survival was usually around 60 months.

Conclusion

The anatomical site and biology of NETs is important in determining management. With the wide variety of therapies and a number of trials underway, patients with NETs are best managed in a multidisciplinary team setting in a specialist centre. Further randomized control trials are needed to determine the optimal treatments for patients, which in view of the rarity of the cancers need to be performed in national and international studies.

References

1. Pearse AG. The diffuse neuroendocrine system and the APUD concept: related "endocrine" peptides in brain, intestine, pituitary, placenta, and anuran cutaneous glands. *Med Biol*, 1977; **55**: 115–25.
2. Oberndorfer S. Karzinoide tumoren des dunndarms. *Frankf Z Pathol*, 1907; **1**: 426–32.
3. Modlin IM, Lye KD, Kidd M. A 5-decade analysis of 13,715 carcinoid tumors. *Cancer*, 2003; **97**: 934–59.
4. Yao JC, Hassan M, Phan A, Dagohoy C, Leary C, Mares JE, *et al.* One hundred years after "carcinoid": epidemiology of and prognostic factors for neuroendocrine tumors in 35 825 cases in the United States. *J Clin Oncol*, 2008; **26**: 3063–72.
5. Gustafsson BI, Kidd M, Chan A, Malfertheiner MV, Modlin IM. Bronchopulmonary neuroendocrine tumors. *Cancer*, 2008; **113**: 5–21.
6. Modlin IM, Latich I, Zikusoka M, Kidd M, Eick G, Chan AK. Gastrointestinal carcinoids: the evolution of diagnostic strategies. *J Clin Gastroenterol*, 2006; **40**: 572–82.
7. Caplin ME, Buscombe JR, Hilson AJ, Jones AL, Watkinson AF, Burroughs AK. Carcinoid tumour. *Lancet*, 1998; **352**: 799–805.

8. Kloppel G, Rindi G, Anlauf M, Perren A, Komminoth P. Site-specific biology and pathology of gastroenteropancreatic neuroendocrine tumors. *Virchows Arch*, 2007; **451** (Suppl. 1): S9–27.
9. Kloppel G, Anlauf M. Epidemiology, tumour biology and histopathological classification of neuroendocrine tumours of the gastrointestinal tract. *Best Pract Res Clin Gastroenterol*, 2005; **19**: 507–17.
10. Skuladottir H, Hirsch FR, Hansen HH, Olsen JH. Pulmonary neuroendocrine tumors: incidence and prognosis of histological subtypes. A population-based study in Denmark. *Lung Cancer*, 2002; **37**: 127–35.
11. Ramage JK, Davies AH, Ardill J, Bax N, Caplin M, Grossman A, *et al.* Guidelines for the management of gastroenteropancreatic neuroendocrine (including carcinoid) tumours. *Gut*, 2005; **54** (Suppl. 4): 1–16.
12. Rindi G, de Herder WW, O'Toole D, Wiedenmann B. Consensus guidelines for the management of patients with digestive neuroendocrine tumors: why such guidelines and how we went about It. *Neuroendocrinology*, 2006; **84**: 155–7.
13. Rindi G, Kloppel G, Couvelard A, Komminoth P, Korner M, Lopes JM, *et al.* TNM staging of midgut and hindgut (neuro) endocrine tumors: a consensus proposal including a grading system. *Virchows Arch*, 2007; **451**: 757–62.
14. Kulke MH, Mayer RJ. Carcinoid tumors. *N Engl J Med*, 1999; **340**: 858–68.
15. Kaltsas G, Grossman AB. Clinical features of gastroenteropancreatic tumours. In: Caplin ME, Kvols L, eds. *Handbook of Neuroendocrine Tumours*. 1st edn. Bristol: BioScientifica, 2007: 53–82.
16. Bhattacharyya S, Davar J, Dreyfus G, Caplin ME. Carcinoid heart disease. *Circulation*, 2007; **116**: 2860–5.
17. Shah T, Srirajaskanthan R, Bhogal M, Toubanakis C, Meyer T, Noonan A, *et al.* Alpha-fetoprotein and human chorionic gonadotrophin-beta as prognostic markers in neuroendocrine tumour patients. *Br J Cancer*, 2008; **99**: 72–7.
18. Namasivayam S, Martin DR, Saini S. Imaging of liver metastases: MRI. *Cancer Imaging*, 2007; **7**: 2–9.
19. Chong S, Lee KS, Chung MJ, Han J, Kwon OJ, Kim TS. Neuroendocrine tumors of the lung: clinical, pathologic, and imaging findings. *Radiographics*, 2006; **26**: 41–57.
20. Rockall AG, Reznek RH. Imaging of neuroendocrine tumours (CT/MR/US). *Best Pract Res Clin Endocrinol Metab*, 2007; **21**: 43–68.
21. Plockinger U, Wiedenmann B. Treatment of gastroenteropancreatic neuroendocrine tumors. *Virchows Arch*, 2007; **451** (Suppl. 1): S71–80.
22. Patel YC. Somatostatin-receptor imaging for the detection of tumors. *N Engl J Med*, 1990; **323**: 1274–6.
23. Krenning EP, Bakker WH, Kooij PP, Breeman WA, Oei HY, de Jong M, *et al.* Somatostatin receptor scintigraphy with indium-111-DTPA-D-Phe-1-octreotide in man: metabolism, dosimetry and comparison with iodine-123-Tyr-3-octreotide. *J Nucl Med*, 1992; **33**: 652–8.
24. Kwekkeboom DJ, Krenning EP. Somatostatin receptor imaging. *Semin Nucl Med*, 2002; **32**: 84–91.
25. Termanini B, Gibril F, Reynolds JC, Doppman JL, Chen CC, Stewart CA, *et al.* Value of somatostatin receptor scintigraphy: a prospective study in gastrinoma of its effect on clinical management. *Gastroenterology*, 1997; **112**: 335–47.
26. Chiti A, Briganti V, Fanti S, Monetti N, Masi R, Bombardieri E. Results and potential of somatostatin receptor imaging in gastroenteropancreatic tract tumours. *Q J Nucl Med*, 2000; **44**: 42–9.
27. Schillaci O, Spanu A, Scopinaro F, Falchi A, Corleto V, Danieli R, *et al.* Somatostatin receptor scintigraphy with 111In-pentetreotide in non-functioning gastroenteropancreatic neuroendocrine tumors. *Int J Oncol*, 2003; **23**: 1687–95.
28. Schillaci O, Spanu A, Scopinaro F, Falchi A, Danieli R, Marongiu P, *et al.* Somatostatin receptor scintigraphy in liver metastasis detection from gastroenteropancreatic neuroendocrine tumors. *J Nucl Med*, 2003; **44**: 359–68.
29. Alexander HR, Fraker DL, Norton JA, Bartlett DL, Tio L, Benjamin SB, *et al.* Prospective study of somatostatin receptor scintigraphy and its effect on operative outcome in patients with Zollinger-Ellison syndrome. *Ann Surg*, 1998; **228**: 228–38.
30. Kaltsas GA, Mukherjee JJ, Grossman AB. The value of radiolabelled MIBG and octreotide in the diagnosis and management of neuroendocrine tumours. *Ann Oncol*, 2001; **12** (Suppl. 2): S47–50.
31. Buchmann I, Henze M, Engelbrecht S, Eisenhut M, Runz A, Schafer M, *et al.* Comparison of 68Ga-DOTATOC PET and 111In-DTPAOC (Octreoscan) SPECT in patients with neuroendocrine tumours. *Eur J Nucl Med Mol Imaging*, 2007; **34**: 1617–26.
32. Gabriel M, Decristoforo C, Kendler D, Dobrozemsky G, Heute D, Uprimny C, *et al.* 68Ga-DOTA-Tyr3-octreotide PET in neuroendocrine tumors: comparison with somatostatin receptor scintigraphy and CT. *J Nucl Med*, 2007; **48**: 508–18.
33. Yoshikane H, Tsukamoto Y, Niwa Y, Goto H, Hase S, Mizutani K, *et al.* Carcinoid tumors of the gastrointestinal tract: evaluation with endoscopic ultrasonography. *Gastrointest Endosc*, 1993; **39**: 375–83.
34. de Mascarenhas-Saraiva MN, da Silva Araujo Lopes LM. Small-bowel tumors diagnosed by wireless capsule endoscopy: report of five cases. *Endoscopy*, 2003; **35**: 865–8.
35. Grozinsky-Glasberg S, Shimon I, Korbonits M, Grossman AB. Somatostatin analogues in the control of neuroendocrine tumours: efficacy and mechanisms. *Endocr Relat Cancer*, 2008; **15**: 701–20.
36. Barrie R, Woltering EA, Hajarizadeh H, Mueller C, Ure T, Fletcher WS. Inhibition of angiogenesis by somatostatin and somatostatin-like compounds is structurally dependent. *J Surg Res*, 1993; **55**: 446–50.
37. Zatelli MC, Ambrosio MR, Bondanelli M, Uberti EC. Control of pituitary adenoma cell proliferation by somatostatin analogs, dopamine agonists and novel chimeric compounds. *Eur J Endocrinol*, 2007; **156** (Suppl. 1): S29–35.
38. Heron I, Thomas F, Dero M, Gancel A, Ruiz JM, Schatz B, *et al.* Pharmacokinetics and efficacy of a long-acting formulation of the new somatostatin analog BIM 23014 in patients with acromegaly. *J Clin Endocrinol Metab*, 1993; **76**: 721–7.
39. Oberg K, Kvols L, Caplin M, Delle FG, de Herder W, Rindi G, *et al.* Consensus report on the use of somatostatin analogs for the management of neuroendocrine tumors of the gastroenteropancreatic system. *Ann Oncol*, 2004; **15**: 966–73.
40. Kvols LK, Moertel CG, O'Connell MJ, Schutt AJ, Rubin J, Hahn RG. Treatment of the malignant carcinoid syndrome. Evaluation of a long-acting somatostatin analogue. *N Engl J Med*, 1986; **315**: 663–6.
41. Garland J, Buscombe JR, Bouvier C, Bouloux P, Chapman MH, Chow AC, *et al.* Sandostatin LAR (long-acting octreotide acetate) for malignant carcinoid syndrome: a 3-year experience. *Aliment Pharmacol Ther*, 2003; **17**: 437–44.
42. Kidd M, Drozdov I, Joseph R, Pfragner R, Culler M, Modlin I. Differential cytotoxicity of novel somatostatin and dopamine chimeric compounds on bronchopulmonary and small intestinal neuroendocrine tumor cell lines. *Cancer*, 2008; **113**: 690–700.
43. O'Toole D, Saveanu A, Couvelard A, Gunz G, Enjalbert A, Jaquet P, *et al.* The analysis of quantitative expression of somatostatin and dopamine receptors in gastro-entero-pancreatic tumours opens new therapeutic strategies. *Eur J Endocrinol*, 2006; **155**: 849–57.
44. Shah T, Caplin M. Endocrine tumours of the gastrointestinal tract. Biotherapy for metastatic endocrine tumours. *Best Pract Res Clin Gastroenterol*, 2005; **19**: 617–36.
45. Oberg K, Eriksson B. The role of interferons in the management of carcinoid tumours. *Br J Haematol*, 1991; **79** (Suppl. 1): 74–7.
46. Fazio N, de Braud F, Delle FG, Oberg K. Interferon-alpha and somatostatin analog in patients with gastroenteropancreatic neuroendocrine carcinoma: single agent or combination? *Ann Oncol*, 2007; **18**: 13–19.
47. Arnold R, Rinke A, Klose KJ, Muller HH, Wied M, Zamzow K, *et al.* Octreotide versus octreotide plus interferon-alpha in endocrine

gastroenteropancreatic tumors: a randomized trial. *Clin Gastroenterol Hepatol*, 2005; **3**: 761–71.

48. Eriksson B, Skogseid B, Lundqvist G, Wide L, Wilander E, Oberg K. Medical treatment and long-term survival in a prospective study of 84 patients with endocrine pancreatic tumors. *Cancer*, 1990; **65**: 1883–90.
49. Frame J, Kelsen D, Kemeny N, Cheng E, Niedzwiecki D, Heelan R, *et al.* A phase II trial of streptozotocin and adriamycin in advanced APUD tumors. *Am J Clin Oncol*, 1988; **11**: 490–5.
50. Kulke MH, Kim H, Clark JW, Enzinger PC, Lynch TJ, Morgan JA, *et al.* A Phase II trial of gemcitabine for metastatic neuroendocrine tumors. *Cancer*, 2004; **101**: 934–9.
51. Kulke MH, Stuart K, Enzinger PC, Ryan DP, Clark JW, Muzikansky A, *et al.* Phase II study of temozolomide and thalidomide in patients with metastatic neuroendocrine tumors. *J Clin Oncol*, 2006; **24**: 401–6.
52. Kunz PL, Kuo T, Kaiser JA, Norton JA, Longacre J, Ford JM, *et al.* A phase II study of capecitabine, oxaliplatin, and bevacizumab for metastatic or unresectable neuroendocrine tumors: Preliminary results. *J Clin Oncol*, 2008; **26**: abstract 15502.
53. Moertel CG, Hanley JA. Combination chemotherapy trials in metastatic carcinoid tumor and the malignant carcinoid syndrome. *Cancer Clin Trials*, 1979; **2**: 327–34.
54. Moertel CG, Kvols LK, O'Connell MJ, Rubin J. Treatment of neuroendocrine carcinomas with combined etoposide and cisplatin. Evidence of major therapeutic activity in the anaplastic variants of these neoplasms. *Cancer*, 1991; **68**: 227–32.
55. Moertel CG, Lefkopoulo M, Lipsitz S, Hahn RG, Klaassen D. Streptozocin-doxorubicin, streptozocin-fluorouracil or chlorozotocin in the treatment of advanced islet-cell carcinoma. *N Engl J Med*, 1992; **326**: 519–23.
56. Toumpanakis C, Meyer T, Caplin ME. Cytotoxic treatment including embolization/ chemoembolization for neuroendocrine tumours. *Best Pract Res Clin Endocrinol Metab*, 2007; **21**: 131–44.
57. Gupta S, Johnson MM, Murthy R, Ahrar K, Wallace MJ, Madoff DC, *et al.* Hepatic arterial embolization and chemoembolization for the treatment of patients with metastatic neuroendocrine tumors: variables affecting response rates and survival. *Cancer*, 2005; **104**: 1590–602.
58. Kwekkeboom DJ, de Herder WW, Kam BL, van Eijck CH, Van EM, Kooij PP, *et al.* Treatment with the radiolabeled somatostatin analog [177 Lu-DOTA 0,Tyr3]octreotate: toxicity, efficacy, and survival. *J Clin Oncol*, 2008; **26**: 2124–30.
59. Otte A, Herrmann R, Heppeler A, Behe M, Jermann E, Powell P, *et al.* Yttrium-90 DOTATOC: first clinical results. *Eur J Nucl Med*, 1999; **26**: 1439–47.
60. Waldherr C, Pless M, Maecke HR, Schumacher T, Crazzolara A, Nitzsche EU, *et al.* Tumor response and clinical benefit in neuroendocrine tumors after 7.4 GBq 90)Y-DOTATOC. *J Nucl Med*, 2002; **43**: 610–16.
61. Bodei L, Cremonesi M, Zoboli S, Grana C, Bartolomei M, Rocca P, *et al.* Receptor-mediated radionuclide therapy with 90Y-DOTATOC in association with amino acid infusion: a phase I study. *Eur J Nucl Med Mol Imaging*, 2003; **30**: 207–16.
62. Valkema R, Pauwels S, Kvols LK, Barone R, Jamar F, Bakker WH, *et al.* Survival and response after peptide receptor radionuclide therapy with [90Y-DOTA0,Tyr3]octreotide in patients with advanced gastroenteropancreatic neuroendocrine tumors. *Semin Nucl Med*, 2006; **36**: 147–56.
63. Virgolini I, Britton K, Buscombe J, Moncayo R, Paganelli G, Riva P. In- and Y-DOTA-lanreotide: results and implications of the MAURITIUS trial. *Semin Nucl Med*, 2002; **32**: 148–55.
64. Teunissen JJ, Kwekkeboom DJ, de Jong M, Esser JP, Valkema R, Krenning EP. Endocrine tumours of the gastrointestinal tract. Peptide receptor radionuclide therapy. *Best Pract Res Clin Gastroenterol*, 2005; **19**: 595–616.

6.4

Gastrinoma

Christos Toumpanakis, Martyn Caplin

Introduction

Gastrin is a gastrointestinal hormone, produced predominantly by the G cells of the gastric antrum and duodenum, although small amounts of gastrin have been isolated in the pituitary and some vagal nerve fibres. The biologically active forms of gastrin include carboxy-amidated gastrin-17 and carboxy-amidated gastrin-34, which bind mainly to the cholecystokinin (CCK)-2 receptor. The main role of amidated gastrin is the stimulation of gastric acid secretion by regulation of histamine release from the gastric enterochromaffin-like (ECL) cells, while it may also have a trophic effect on gastric mucosa. There is evidence that the precursor forms of gastrin, such as progastrin and glycine-extended gastrin, are also of biological importance, binding to a separate CCK-C receptor. These precursor may induce cellular and tumour growth and they are implicated in several cancers, such as colon and pancreatic adenocarcinomas.

Gastrinomas represent a group of functional pancreatic neuroendocrine tumours, characterized by autonomous release of gastrin by the tumour cells, which results in symptoms not only due to the tumour growth *per se*, but also to gastric acid hypersecretion.

In 1955, at the annual meeting of American Surgical Association, Robert M. Zollinger and Edwin H. Ellison presented a study entitled *Primary Peptic Ulcerations of the Jejunum Associated with Islet Cell Tumour of the Pancreas.* They proposed a new clinical syndrome of: (1) ulceration in unusual locations in the upper gastrointestinal tract or recurrent ulcerations; (2) gastric acid hyperseretion; and (3) non-β islet cell tumours of the pancreas. However, the potent gastric secretagogue for the Zollinger–Ellison syndrome was not identified until 1960, when Rodney Gregory and Hilda Tracy of the University of Liverpool discovered that the extract from the pancreas of a patient with Zollinger–Ellison syndrome was the hormone gastrin. Thus, these pancreatic tumours were termed 'gastrinomas'.

Epidemiology

The incidence of gastrinomas is 0.5–3/million population per year. There is a slight male predominance with an average age of diagnosis in the mid 40s, although patients may well have had symptoms for 5–6 years.

Genetics

Gastrinomas can either be sporadic or can be associated with multiple endocrine neoplasia type 1 (MEN 1) syndrome in 25% of cases. This syndrome should always be considered and excluded in every patient with gastrinoma, as it may have significant implications for patient management and also prognosis. MEN 1 is an autosomal dominant disorder which is passed to the offspring with high penetrance, and is discussed in Chapter 6.11. Approximately 23–29% of patients with gastrinomas associated with MEN 1 may develop gastric neuroendocrine (carcinoid) tumours type II.

Recently, it was found that *MEN1* mutations are also present in 37% of sporadic gastrinomas, which indicates that the *MEN1* gene may be involved in the pathogenesis of both familial and sporadic forms. Other genetic alterations associated with sporadic gastrinomas include those in the $p16^{INK4a}$ gene on chromosome 9p21 and in the *HER2/neu* gene. Mutations of the p53 gene are not common in gastrinomas.

Pathophysiology and molecular pathogenesis

Gastrinomas secrete mainly carboxy-amidated gastrin-17, which is associated with gastric acid hypersecretion and relevant clinical features. This autonomous hypergastrinaemia induces ECL cell hyperplasia, which may lead to the development of gastric neuroendocrine tumours. Apart from amidated gastrin, these tumours may also secrete precursor forms, progastrin and glycine-extended gastrin.

Gastrinomas overexpress various growth factor receptors (epidermal growth factor receptor (EGFR), insulin growth factor 1 receptor, and hepatocyte growth factor receptor) but among these only EGFR is known to correlate with angioinvasion. The activation of CCK-2 receptor by carboxy-amidated gastrin-17 initiates multiple signal transduction pathways, including activation of EGFR.

Clinicopathological features

Although gastrinomas were previously reported to be located predominantly in the pancreas, recent series have shown that the duodenum (especially the first and the second part) is the most common location for both sporadic and MEN 1-associated gastrinomas (50–88% and 70–100% of cases, respectively). In cases of pancreatic gastrinomas, the tumour is usually (70%) located in the pancreatic body/tail. At surgery, 70–85% of all gastrinomas are found in the so-called 'gastrinoma triangle'. The anatomy of this triangle is defined superiorly by the confluence of the cystic and common bile duct, inferiorly by the junction of the second and third portions of the duodenum, and medially by the junction of the neck and body of the pancreas. Rarely (10%), gastrinomas can be found in other abdominal (stomach, liver, bile duct, ovary) or extra-abdominal (heart, small lung cancer) sites.

At presentation, pancreatic gastrinomas are usually large lesions (mean size 3.8 cm), whereas the duodenal ones, especially those associated with MEN 1, are small (1–20 mm). The latter are usually multiple, while sporadic gastrinomas are predominantly (80%) solitary tumours.

Gastrinomas may metastasize to the liver, lymph nodes, and rarely to the bones as well. At presentation, the majority of patients have either localized (36%) or locally advanced disease with only lymph node metastases (29%). The development of metastases are independent of tumour size, as even small (<5 mm) duodenal gastrinomas may have a high malignant potential. However, liver metastases seem to be more common in pancreatic rather than duodenal gastrinomas (22–35% versus 0–10%, respectively).

Gastrinomas share histopathological features with the other gastroenteropancreatic neuroendocrine tumours (Fig. 6.4.1). In addition, they predominantly express gastrin (Fig. 6.4.2), and can produce other gastrointestinal peptides such as insulin. However, these additional peptides are either not released in the systemic circulation or they are released in small quantities and are thus not of any clinical significance. Other neuroendocrine tumours may express gastrin, but they are not considered to be gastrinomas if clinical and biochemical features are lacking.

According to the WHO for gastroenteropancreatic neuroendocrine tumours, gastrinomas are divided into: (1) well-differentiated endocrine tumours (benign or uncertain malignancy); (2) well-differentiated endocrine carcinomas with low-grade malignant behaviour; and (3) poorly differentiated endocrine carcinomas with high-grade malignant behaviour. Criteria for categorization of these tumours include general morphological description, mitotic rate (two or more mitoses/mm^2), proliferation index (as assessed by nuclear Ki-67 expression), tumour size, and evidence of invasion of blood vessels/nerves/adjacent organs. The majority of gastrinomas are well-differentiated endocrine carcinomas, with Ki-67: 2–10%.

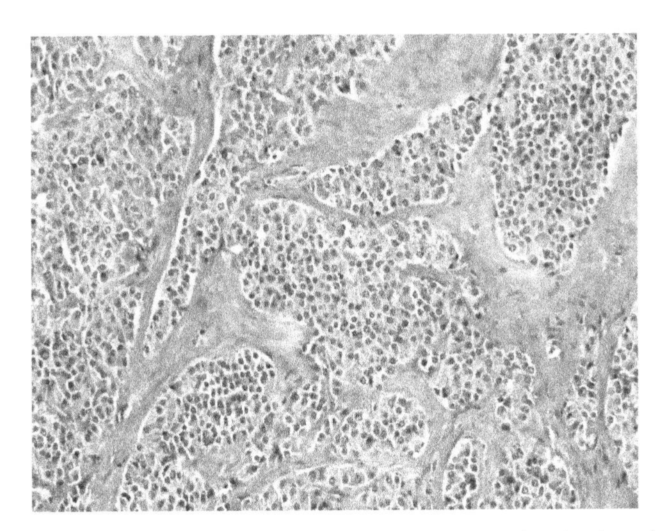

Fig. 6.4.1 Well-differentiated, low-grade pancreatic gastrinoma. (See also Plate 34)

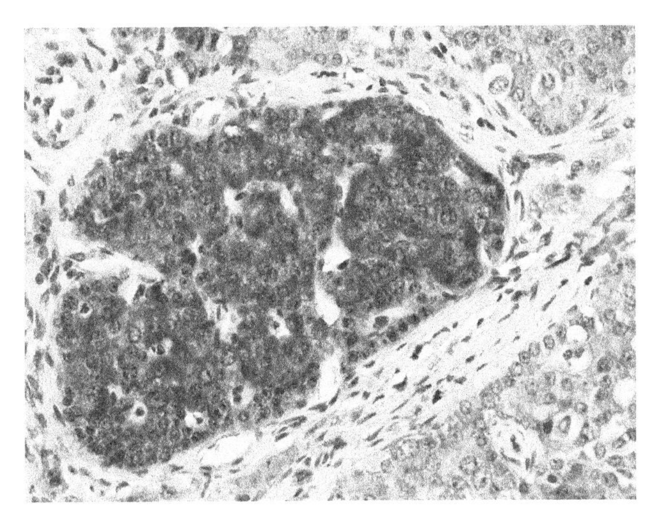

Fig. 6.4.2 Gastrin immunostaining in the same patient as in Fig. 6.4.1 with pancreatic gastrinoma. (See also Plate 35)

Recently, the European Neuroendocrine Tumour Society suggested the TNM system for staging of all gastroenteropancreatic neuroendocrine tumours, including gastrinomas, which also includes a grading system based on mitotic rate and proliferation index. The new TNM system as well as the grading system are summarized in Box 6.1.1 and Tables 6.1.2 and 6.1.3.

Diagnosis

Clinical presentation

Most of the symptoms in patients with gastrinomas are associated with gastric acid hypersecretion. The latter can lead to the development of peptic ulcers, erosive oesophagitis, and chronic diarrhoea. Symptoms associated with peptic ulcers and their complications (bleeding, perforation, pyloric stenosis) are the most common presenting clinical features in patients with gastrinoma (80%). Peptic ulcers in these patients are often multiple, located in unusual anatomic sites, and resistant to treatment. They are less associated with *Helicobacter pylori* infection compared to idiopathic peptic ulcers (24–48% versus >90%, respectively) and are not associated with nonsteroidals. Erosive oesophagitis, causing heartburn and potentially dysphagia, occurs in 50–60% of these patients. Finally, chronic diarrhoea is a result of inactivation of pancreatic enzymes (especially lipases), and damage of the intestinal mucosa, due to acid hypersecretion. Gastrinoma-related diarrhoea is usually watery, may be associated with malabsorption, and is the only diarrhoea that responds dramatically to proton pump inhibitors (PPIs). It occurs in 40–70% of patients with gastrinoma, and may be the only symptom in 20% of them.

Clinical suspicion for a gastrinoma associated with MEN 1 syndrome is raised when one or more of the above clinical features coexist with hyperparathyroidism or any other MEN 1-related endocrinopathies, and when there is a family history of MEN 1 syndrome. In patients with sporadic gastrinomas, the mean age at the onset of symptoms is 48–55 years, while patients with MEN 1 usually present at an earlier age (32–35 years). The frequency of most symptoms is similar in these two groups of patients, although it seems that diarrhoea is less common in MEN 1 patients. Up to 20% of gastrinoma patient may develop features of Cushing's syndrome, which is due to ectopic production of ACTH

Table 6.4.1 Clinical features indicating gastrinoma

Clinical feature	% of patients
Peptic ulcers resistant to treatment, multiple, located in unusual anatomic sites, less associated with *H. pylori*, and not associated with nonsteroidals.	80
Erosive oesophagitis causing heartburn and potentially dysphagia, resistant to treatment	50
Diarrhoea responding to proton pump inhibitors	40–70
The above features in combination with other endocrinopathies	20
The above features in combination with family history of neuroendocrine tumours	25

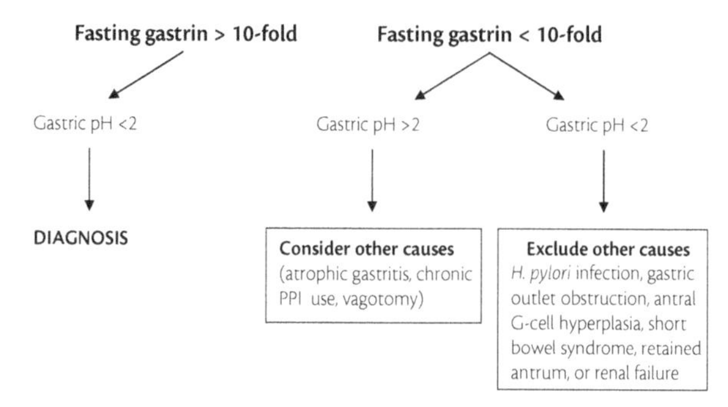

Fig. 6.4.3 Differential diagnosis of hypergastrinaemia. PPI, proton pump inhibitor.

and represents a poor prognostic sign. Suspicious clinical features that may indicate gastrinoma are summarized in Table 6.4.1.

Laboratory tests

The biochemical confirmation, following clinical suspicion, of a gastrinoma requires a significant elevation of fasting serum gastrin in combination with hyperchlorhydria. The presence of the latter is very important, as hypergastrinaemia alone can be a result of chronic hypochlorhydria/ achlorhydria, which is associated with chronic fundus atrophic gastritis, chronic PPI use, as well as vagotomy.

A fasting serum gastrin level of more than 10-fold the upper normal limit in the presence of gastric pH less than 2 or BAO more than 15 mmol/h is considered to be diagnostic of a gastrinoma. If possible, PPIs should be discontinued 2 weeks prior to serum gastrin estimation, while a discontinuation of histamine-2 receptor antagonists for only 48–72 h prior to the test seems to be adequate. Moderately elevated serum gastrin levels (<10-fold the upper normal limit) and hyperchlorhydria may occur in 66% of gastrinoma patients, but in this situation other clinical disorders need to be excluded, including *H. pylori* infection, gastric outlet obstruction, antral G-cell hyperplasia, short bowel syndrome, retained antrum, or renal failure. In this situation, a provocative test with IV administration of secretin is indicated. After an overnight fast, an IV bolus of secretin (2 U/kg) is given to the patient. A rise of serum gastrin concentration of 200 pg/ml, noted within 10 min of secretin administration, can establish the diagnosis of gastrinoma, whereas in the above mentioned nontumour-related causes the serum gastrin level remains flat. For the secretin provocative test, PPIs do not need to be stopped. A diagnostic algorithm for fasting serum gastrin levels is summarized in Fig. 6.4.3.

Another biochemical test that contributes to the diagnosis is the estimation of chromogranin-A (CgA). CgA is a general marker for neuroendocrine tumours and belongs to a family of water-soluble acidic glycoproteins, including at least three different members (CgA, CgB, CgC), which are stored in the secretory granules of neuroendocrine cells and released during exocytosis. CgA is found throughout the diffuse neuroendocrine system and is thought to be the best and most sensitive general marker for the diagnosis and follow-up of gastroenteropancreatic neuroendocrine tumours. Its levels may correlate with tumour progression or regression, while increases in CgA may precede radiographic evidence of progression. However, recent studies in patients with gastrinomas suggest that there is not always precise correlation between CgA levels and tumour burden, as in these patients CgA may also be produced by the ECL cells of the stomach in response to hypergastrinaemia.

As soon as the biochemical diagnosis of gastrinoma is established, it is important for all patients (even those without suspicious clinical features) to be screened for MEN 1 syndrome, with a baseline estimation of serum parathyroid hormone (PTH) levels, calcium levels (preferably ionized calcium or albumin-corrected calcium), as well as prolactin. In presence of suspicious clinical or biochemical data, a *MEN1*, germline mutation DNA test should be performed, and, if it is positive, genetic counselling is offered to all patients' kindreds after their first decade of life. Rarely, patients with gastrinoma may have hypercalcaemia with normal PTH levels, which may be a result of PTH-related peptide secreted by these tumours. Finally, in patients who develop clinical signs of Cushing's syndrome, appropriate investigations to exclude or confirm this should be performed.

Tumour localization

Precise localization of the primary tumour, as well as metastatic deposits, has a significant impact on the patient's management. Invasive and noninvasive localization studies are used in order to identify the primary lesion and determine the extent of resection when surgery is planned, and also to assess the tumour extent in patients with advanced disease.

Noninvasive techniques

Among the conventional radiological studies, transabdominal ultrasonography has the lowest sensitivity for detection of the primary site and hepatic metastases (20% and 45%, respectively), but its specificity may be greater than 90%. Spiral CT and MRI have better sensitivities for the primary lesion (35–55% and 40–65%, respectively) and for distant metastases (45–70% and 70–80%, respectively), with a specificity also above 90% (Fig. 6.4.4a,b).

Indium-111-diethylentriamine penta-acetic acid-octreotide (OctreoScan) is recognized as the gold standard and most sensitive modality for imaging of gastroenteropancreatic neuroendocrine tumours. It provides not only an accurate localization of the primary and metastatic lesions, but also may detect unsuspected lesions not shown by the previous conventional studies, which is crucial when surgery is planned. OctreoScan in combination with single photon emission CT is the most sensitive noninvasive test for detection of primary sites in patients with gastrinomas, with a

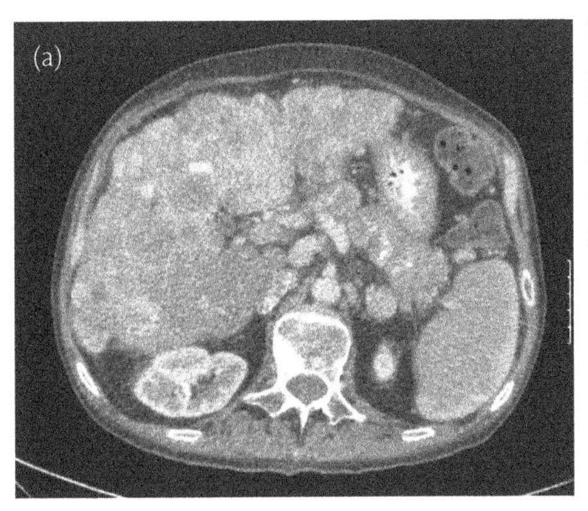

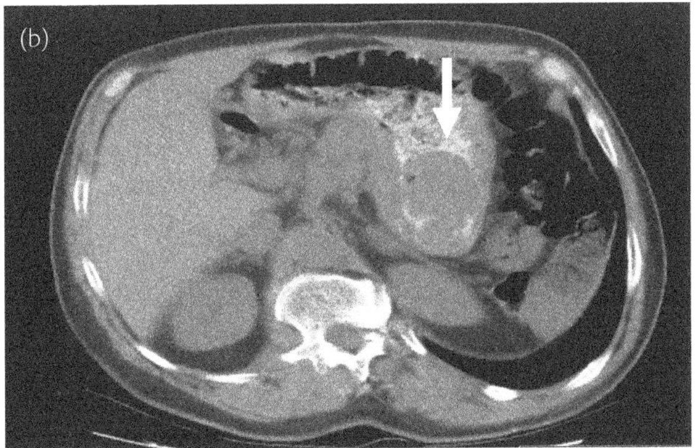

Fig. 6.4.4 (a) CT in metastatic sporadic gastrinoma. (b) CT in a patient with MEN 1 gastrinoma and type II gastric neuroendocrine tumour (arrow).

sensitivity of 70–85% and a specificity of 85%, while its sensitivity is above 90% for distant metastases (Fig. 6.4.5).

However, the diagnostic value of all conventional imaging studies, as well as OctreoScan, is limited when the size of the primary tumour is less than 1–2 cm. This is usually the case in gastrinomas associated with MEN 1, where the tumours are small (<1 cm), multiple, and located in the duodenum. Therefore, when the noninvasive techniques have failed to identify the primary tumour site, especially when surgery is planned, a variety of invasive localization studies can be performed.

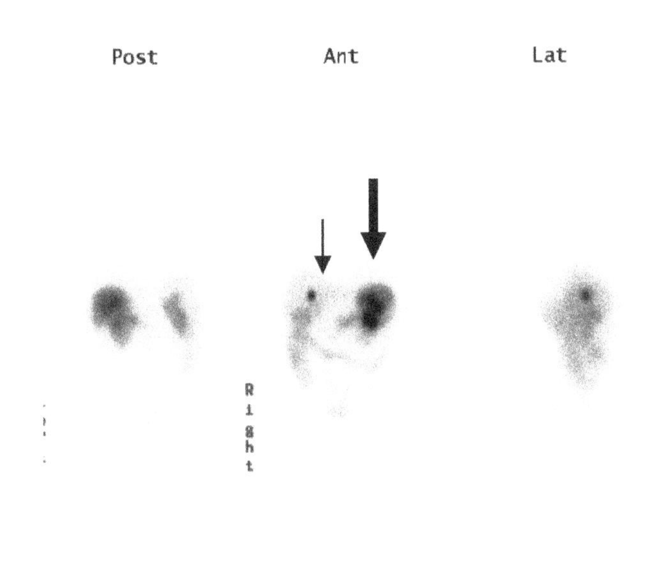

Fig. 6.4.5 OctreoScan in patient with metastatic MEN 1 gastrinoma. Solitary hepatic metastatic deposit (thin arrow), gastric neuroendocrine tumour (thick arrow).

Invasive techniques

Oesophagogastroduodenoscopy (OGD) needs to be performed in every patient with gastrinoma. OGD not only corroborates the clinical suspicion by demonstrating severe oesophagitis, peptic ulcers in uncommon locations, and prominent gastric folds, but also may reveal small duodenal gastrinomas, as well as gastric polyps, which may represent gastric neuroendocrine tumours type II in patients with MEN 1 gastrinomas (Fig. 6.4.6).

Endoscopic ultrasonography (EUS) should be considered in all patients who are due to have an operation and also in those with MEN 1 gastrinomas. In experienced hands, it has a sensitivity of 95% for pancreatic gastrinomas, while it also provides useful staging information. EUS can precisely estimate tumour size, distinguish a pancreatic tumour from a peripancreatic lymph node, and also enables histology samples via fine-needle aspiration. However, EUS has a lower sensitivity for duodenal gastrinomas (50%).

Angiography is less commonly used nowadays, and usually includes angiography with secretin stimulation and hepatic venous

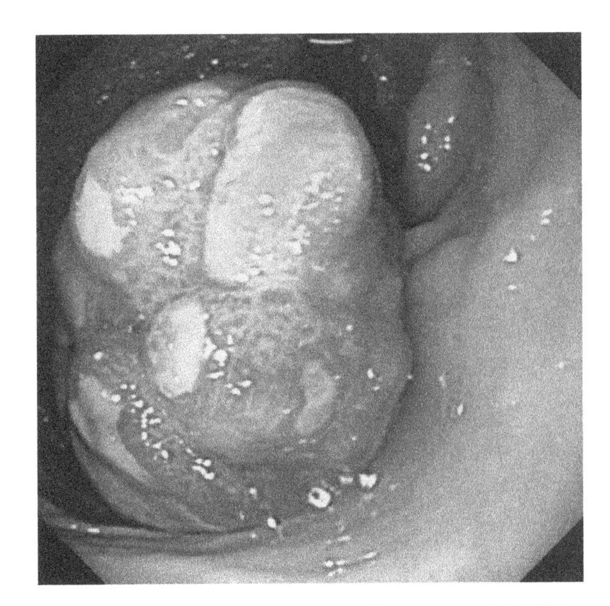

Fig. 6.4.6 Gastric neuroendocrine tumour type II in a patient with MEN 1 gastrinoma (same patient as in Fig. 6.4.4b).

sampling. During this test, small doses of secretin are injected into the splenic, hepatic, gastroduodenal, and then the superior mesenteric arteries, following a selective cannulation. Then, blood samples are taken from the right hepatic vein, at baseline, 20, 40, 60, and 120 s for gastrin estimation.

In patients, where all the above imaging techniques have failed to detect the primary lesion preoperatively, an intraoperative transillumination of the duodenum in combination with intraoperative ultrasonography should always be performed. These tests should always be followed by duodenotomy, which is able to detect up to 50% of duodenal tumours.

Management

Once the diagnosis of Zollinger–Ellison syndrome is established, and even before the completion of localization studies, it is important to start medical treatment in order to control gastric acid hypersecretion and prevent its complications.

Control of symptoms

In the early years, the treatment of choice was total gastrectomy. However, as soon as the antisecretory medications, initially H_2-receptor antagonists and subsequently PPIs, became widely available, an effective control of gastric acid secretion was achieved, and thus total gastrectomy is no longer necessary.

PPIs are superior to H_2-receptor antagonists in terms of effectiveness in gastric acid control and long-term action, and therefore they are considered as first-choice medical treatment for these patients. The initial dose is usually an equivalent dose to 60 mg/day of omeprazole in sporadic gastrinomas. Patients with MEN 1 gastrinomas and hypercalcaemia, patients with severe gastro-oesophageal reflux symptoms, as well as those with previous Bilroth-II resection may require higher initial doses (40–60 mg twice per day). The maintenance dose tends to be lower than the initial dose in 40–80% of patients. PPIs are considered as safe long-term treatment with patients being treated for more than 15 years with no significant adverse effects and no evidence of tachyphylaxis. It has been recommended, however, that long-term treatment with PPIs may be associated with vitamin B_{12} malabsorption, and thus vitamin B_{12} levels need to be monitored once a year. There may also be an increased predisposition to osteoporosis. Patients who cannot tolerate oral PPIs can be treated with high doses of H_2-receptor antagonists and the dose requirements tend to increase with time.

The use of somatostatin analogues (octreotide and lanreotide preparations) for antiacid control, although potentially effective, is not a first-line option and should be reserved for patients with difficult to control hyperacidity and those who develop gastric neuroendocrine tumours.

Gastric surgery (vagotomy, gastrectomy) for control of gastric acid hypersecretion is very rarely required in the era of antisecretory medications, and is only indicated in patients who cannot or will not take antisecretory medications. Parathyroidectomy in patients with MEN 1 gastrinomas and parathyroid adenomas is usually indicated at an early stage, as this results in a decrease in the basal acid output and fasting gastrin levels and therefore the required dosage of antisecretory medications as well.

Surgical therapy

Sporadic gastrinomas

The aim of surgery in sporadic gastrinomas patients is a long-term curative resection in order to decrease the risk of distant metastases, as well as to completely control the hormonal symptoms. Pancreatic head/body tumours may be enucleated, in combination with regional lymph node dissection (peripancreatic, periduodenal, and hepatoduodenal ligament), while duodenotomy is always required to detect small duodenal gastrinomas. Whipple's pancreaticoduodenectomy may be required for large gastrinomas. Tumours in the pancreatic tail may be enucleated, or for larger lesions a distal pancreatectomy is performed. The overall 15-year survival following a curative resection in sporadic gastrinoma patients is between 80 and 100%.

MEN 1 gastrinomas

The benefit of surgery in gastrinomas associated with MEN 1 syndrome is controversial. Tumours are usually small, multiple, and located in various sites in pancreas and duodenum. Surgical exploration, especially if the tumours have not been visualized in the preoperative imaging studies or their size is less than 2 cm, does not seem to be worth while, as the curative potential in these cases is low, metastases are usually regional, and the long-term prognosis is favourable. Surgical intervention should be considered when the tumour size is more than 2 cm. The concept of this approach is to reduce the possibility of subsequent liver metastases, although its efficacy remains controversial.

Management of advanced disease

All patients with advanced disease, consisting mainly of hepatic metastases, should have antitumour treatment in order to prolong the survival rates. Treatment options include invasive procedures or systemic medical treatment.

Invasive treatment

Cytoreductive surgery may be an option when hepatic metastases are confined to one lobe, and also in cases where more than 90% of disease can be removed surgically. Liver resection can also be combined with radiofrequency ablation at the same time for tumour lesions that cannot be resected. In patients with disease predominantly in the liver, transarterial hepatic embolization (TAE) or chemoembolization (TACE) may be considered, especially when a clinical or radiological progression is noted. TAE or TACE cannot be performed in patients with occluded portal vein and poor performance status. Finally, liver transplantation can be considered rarely in selective cases, mainly young patients with low-grade tumours, no significant comorbidities, and no evidence of extrahepatic disease.

Noninvasive treatment

In patients unsuitable for surgery, systemic medical treatment should be considered in order to control tumour growth and improve survival. Biological agents, such as somatostatin analogues and less commonly interferon, are considered as antitumour treatment in patients with low-grade tumour and slowly progressive disease. Disease stabilization can be achieved in up to 50% of these patients, whereas the objective response rate (decrease in tumour size >20%) with these medications is only 10%.

Cytotoxic chemotherapy, using combination regimens of streptozotocin, doxorubicin 5-fluorouracil, and cisplatin, may be an option in patients with disease progression despite treatment with biological agents, in patients with high-grade tumours. or in patients with distant metastases outside the liver. Objective responses and disease stabilization have been reported in 30–40% and 70% of patients, respectively.

Peptide receptor radionuclide therapy represent an alternative option to cytotoxic chemotherapy and can be considered in patients with avid tumour uptake in OctreoScan. The concept of this treatment is to transfer cytotoxic radiation directly to the tumour cells by using somatostatin analogues (octreotide or octreotate) radiolabelled with isotopes such as yttrium-90 or lutetium-177. Although, peptide receptor radionuclide therapy is still considered experimental, initial results from several studies have shown good efficacy and tolerability by the patients. Recently, molecular targeted therapies have been developed, for various types of neuroendocrine tumours including gastrinomas, with their efficacy and tolerability currently under evaluation in clinical trials.

Prognostic factors—survival

The 15-year survival rate in patients either sporadic or MEN 1 gastrinomas and localized disease (including lymph nodes metastasis) is more than 90%, whereas in those with hepatic metastases the 5-year survival is between 50 and 70%. Other poor prognostic factors include: short disease history; female gender; pancreatic primary location; primary tumour size more than 3 cm; absence of MEN 1 syndrome; extremely high serum gastrin levels; ectopic Cushing's syndrome; and presence of bone metastases. Histological features such as angioinvasion, perineural invasion, mitotic rate above 2/20 high power fields, and Ki-67 above 2% are associated with poor prognosis, as is the overexpression of EGFR and *HER2/neu* gene.

References

1. Zollinger RM, Ellison EH. Primary peptic ulcerations of the jejunum associated with islet cell tumours of the pancreas. *Ann Surg*, 1955; **142**: 709–23.
2. Caplin ME. Zollinger-Ellison syndrome. In: Modlin I, *From Gastrin to GERD A century of acid suppression*. Felsenstein: 2006.
3. Jensen RT. Gastrinomas: advances in diagnosis and management. *Neuroendocrinology*, 2004; **80** (Suppl. 1): 23–7.
4. Toumpanakis CG, Caplin ME. Molecular genetics of gastroenteropancreatic neuroendocrine tumors. *Am J Gastroenterol*, 2008; **103**: 729–32.
5. Ellison EC. Zollinger-Ellison syndrome: a personal perspective. *Am Surg*, 2008; **74**: 563–71.
6. Ramage JK, Davies AH, Ardill J, Bax N, Caplin M, Grossman A, *et al.* UKNETwork for Neuroendocrine Tumours. Guidelines for the management of gastroenteropancreatic neuroendocrine (including carcinoid) tumours. *Gut*, 2005; **54** (Suppl. 4): iv1–16.
7. Fendrich V, Langer P, Waldmann J, Bartsch DK, Rothmund M. Management of sporadic and multiple endocrine neoplasia type 1 gastrinomas. *Br J Surg*, 2007; **94**: 1331–41.
8. Alexakis N, Neoptolemos JP. Pancreatic neuroendocrine tumours. *Best Pract Res Clin Gastroenterol*, 2008; **22**: 183–205.
9. Shah T, Caplin M. Endocrine tumours of the gastrointestinal tract. Biotherapy for metastatic endocrine tumours. *Best Pract Res Clin Gastroenterol*, 2005; **19**: 617–36.
10. Jensen RT, Niederle B, Mitry E, Ramage JK, Steinmuller T, Lewington V, *et al.* Frascati Consensus Conference; European Neuroendocrine Tumor Society. Gastrinoma (duodenal and pancreatic). *Neuroendocrinology*, 2006; **84**: 173–82.
11. Forrer F, Valkema R, Kwekkeboom DJ, de Jong M, Krenning EP. Neuroendocrine tumors. Peptide receptor radionuclide therapy. *Best Pract Res Clin Endocrinol Metab*, 2007; **21**: 111–29.

6.5

Insulinoma and hypoglycaemia

Puja Mehta, Jeannie F. Todd

Insulinomas

Introduction

Hypoglycaemia is a clinical syndrome with diverse aetiology. Insulinomas, although rare, are the most common functioning pancreatic islet cell tumour and may be part of the multiple endocrine neoplasia type 1 (MEN 1) syndrome. Patients present with symptoms of neuroglycopenia and a catecholamine response. Diagnosis is confirmed by evidence of endogenous hyperinsulinaemic hypoglycaemia. Tumours are localized by ultrasonography, CT and/or intra-arterial calcium stimulation with venous sampling. Most tumours are benign and solitary, making surgical cure possible with complete resection. Medical options, including diazoxide or octreotide, are available for multifocal tumours.

Epidemiology

Insulinomas, although rare, are the most common hormone-producing neuroendocrine tumour of the gastrointestinal tract, with an estimated annual incidence of 0.5–1 per million of the population (similar to that of phaeochromocytomas). Insulinomas are four times more common in females. They can occur at any age, but present most commonly in middle age, with a median age at diagnosis of 47 years for sporadic cases and 23 years with MEN 1 (1). Most insulinomas are solitary (90%), benign (90%), small (65% diameter less than 1.5 cm), intrapancreatic (99%), and distributed equally throughout the pancreas. 16% are associated with MEN 1 and are often multiple, malignant in 25% of cases, and have a higher recurrence rate.

Clinical presentation

Hypoglycaemia is the hallmark of an insulinoma. Patients present with non-specific, episodic hypoglycaemic symptoms, which fall into two categories: neuroglycopenic or autonomic (catecholamine/neurogenic). Neuroglycopenia occurs when plasma glucose levels fall below 2.2 mmol/l and is due to central nervous system glucose deprivation. These symptoms include dizziness, confusion, fatigue, difficulty in speaking or concentrating, headache, changes in vision, seizures, and loss of consciousness. Autonomic catecholamine symptoms include sweating, hunger, paraesthesia, tremor, anxiety, palpitations, and nausea (2). These symptoms usually resolve with the ingestion of carbohydrate or injection of glucose. Patients with insulinomas are usually symptomatic in the morning, several hours after eating or post-exercise, and accommodate by eating regular, high-sugar snacks, usually resulting in weight gain. Diagnosis is usually delayed due to the non-specific presentation.

Diagnosis

The symptoms of hypoglycaemia are non-specific. Objective measurement of hypoglycaemia during a symptomatic period with relief following administration of glucose (Whipple's triad) (3) is strongly suggestive of endogenous hyperinsulinaemia. The combination of hypoglycaemic symptoms with biochemical hypoglycaemia (blood glucose less than 2.2 mmol/l), C-peptidaemia (above 300 pmol/l), and hyperinsulinaemia (above 30 pmol/l or 6 mU/l) is pathognomonic of an insulinoma. If the glucose level is normal, a hypoglycaemic disorder is excluded and no further investigation is necessary.

The 72-h fast

The 72-h fast is considered the gold standard (2) and involves a supervised, monitored fast. According to most reports 30% patients develop symptoms of hypoglycaemia within 12 h, 80% within 24 h, 90% in 48 h, and 100% at 72 h. Food is withheld, although the patient may consume water or non-caloric beverages. Intravenous access is established and blood is sampled for glucose, insulin, and C-peptide, as well as a serum and urine sample for a sulphonylurea screen at regular (4–6 h) intervals or more often if the patient is symptomatic. All these samples should be taken at the same time. Hypoglycaemia should only be reversed after laboratory confirmation or if the patient has a seizure or becomes unconscious. If the patient is asymptomatic, a short period of exercise (10–15 min) before the final sample may provoke hypoglycaemia.

True hypoglycaemia (glucose <2.2 mmol/l) must be demonstrated to interpret the results and allow consideration of an insulinoma (Table 6.5.1). Despite fasting, ketones and plasma β-hydroxybutyrate should be suppressed with an insulinoma, due to the antiketogenic hyperinsulinaemic status.

C-Peptide

Endogenous insulin is secreted as a proinsulin (a precursor prohormone), requiring post-translational proteolytic cleavage of a C-peptide for activity. Insulin and the C-peptide are thus secreted in equimolar amounts and the C-peptide acts as a surrogate marker of endogenous insulin production. Measurement of the C-peptide may act as a screening or confirmatory test. The C-peptide suppression test is not 100% reliable but can be completed in 2 h.

Table 6.5.1 Interpretation of prolonged supervised fast, when plasma glucose levels fall below 2.2 mmol/l

Insulin	C-peptide	Interpretation
↓ <3 mU/l	↓ <200 pmol/l	Normal response (or nonislet cell tumour if ↑ IGF 2)
↑	↓ /undetectable	Consider self-administration of insulin or autoimmune causes
↑ >3–6 mU/l	↑ 100–300 pmol/l	Further confirmatory tests required
↑↑ >6 mU/l	↑↑ >300 pmol/l	Insulinoma (sulphonylurea screen negative and C-peptide:insulin ratio high)

A patient with an insulinoma will fail to suppress endogenous insulin production after infusion of exogenous insulin, as demonstrated by a persistent, inappropriate C-peptidaemia. This test is mainly used when hypoglycaemic symptoms recur following successful surgical resection of insulinoma—distinguishing between recurrent hyperinsulinaemia and psychological aetiology. The test may also be useful when the 72-h fast is equivocal or weakly positive.

The most common cause of hypoglycaemia is exogenous administration of anti-diabetic medications (insulin or sulphonylureas) (4). This so-called 'factitious hypoglycaemia' is most commonly observed in female healthcare professionals. Commercially available insulin does not contain a C-peptide and therefore factitious hypoglycaemia is associated with elevated insulin levels and suppressed C-peptide. Insulin receptor stimulating antibodies are also associated with raised insulin and suppressed C-peptide levels.

Hypoglycaemia, elevated insulin and C-peptide levels are demonstrated with insulinomas and also sulphonylurea consumption and therefore measuring the sulphonylurea level is imperative for accurate diagnosis. Hypoglycaemia may also be due to ectopic insulin secretion from nonislet cell tumours. There is hypersecretion of insulin-like growth factor (IGF 2) with appropriate suppression of plasma insulin, C-peptide levels, and IGF 1 (5).

Stimulation tests

Insulinomas show an exaggerated response compared with normal β-cells to insulin secretagogues, for example tolbutamide, glucagon, and intravenous or oral glucose tolerance tests. These tests are rarely performed as the 72-h fast is so reliable.

Localization

Most insulinomas (>80%) are benign and solitary, making surgical cure possible with complete resection. Once a biochemical diagnosis of an insulinoma has been confirmed, preoperative localization and definition of the anatomy is necessary for optimal surgical outcome. However some believe that intraoperative exploration and ultrasonography may be more sensitive than preoperative localization. Virtually all insulinomas arise from within the pancreas and therefore localization techniques should be directed to this organ. A number of imaging modalities with varying degrees of invasiveness and sensitivity have been used for preoperative localization. Techniques employed include CT, ultrasonography (transabdominal and endoscopic), angiography, MRI, and selective intra-arterial injection of calcium with hepatic venous sampling.

Ultrasonography

Transabdominal ultrasonography is non-invasive, inexpensive, and readily available, but is heavily operator-dependent. This has a sensitivity of only 9–64% (6). Endoscopic ultrasonography (EUS) has a sensitivity of up to 94% (57–94%) (7). EUS may be useful in patients with MEN 1, who may have multiple intrapancreatic tumours not detectable by ultrasonography, CT, or other non-invasive techniques.

Computed tomography scan

A CT scan of the abdomen is usually performed, but may not detect an insulinoma as the tumours are often very small. Detection rates of approximately 20–40% have been regularly reported. Most malignant insulinomas may be detected and staged by CT scan (8). The advent of helical CT scanning has improved the detection of insulinomas compared with conventional CT. A recent study examined the sensitivity of abdominal CT in the detection of insulinoma in 32 patients between 1987 and 2000 (9). Diagnostic sensitivity was 94% for dual-phase thin-section multidetector CT, 57% for dual-phase multidetector CT without thin sections, and 29% for sequential CT (9). The combination of biphasic, thin-section, arterial phase, helical CT and EUS was shown to have a diagnostic sensitivity of 100%, but is subjective to false positives (9). MRI may allow localization of small insulinomas, where CT scanning has failed.

Selective intra-arterial calcium stimulation with hepatic venous sampling

Selective arteriography alone was formerly considered the gold-standard method, but has been superseded by selective arterial calcium stimulation with hepatic venous sampling. This has been proposed as the most sensitive preoperative localization technique. An angiogram is carried out by selective cannulation of the splenic (supplying the pancreatic body and tail), superior mesenteric (supplying the uncinate process) and gastroduodenal artery (supplying the head of the pancreas). Calcium gluconate, a potent β-cell secretagogue, is injected locally into each respective artery. Blood samples are taken from the right hepatic vein at 0, 30, 60, and 120 s post-injection to measure insulin. A twofold increase in insulin in the 30- and/or 60-s sample confirms the diagnosis (7). This technique has a reported sensitivity of over 90% (range 87.5–100%) in the localization of pancreatic insulinomas, but is invasive and not routinely available. It is therefore only considered when there is strong clinical suspicion of an insulinoma, but diagnosis with non-invasive tests has proved elusive (10). This technique also has the advantage that it confirms functionality of any lesion seen on cross-sectional imaging. Octreotide scanning is another method for preoperative localization but has low sensitivity in detecting insulinomas (30–40%).

Somatostatin receptor scintigraphy and PET scan

Insulinomas have a low density of somatostatin receptors thereby limiting the role of somatostatin receptor scintigraphy, which is useful in the detection of other neuroendocrine tumours such as gastrinomas. Newer techniques to preoperatively localize insulinomas include positron emission tomography (PET) scanning, although the sensitivity remains to be determined.

Management

Surgical management

As most insulinomas are benign, solitary adenomas surgical resection is the treatment of choice and offers a definitive cure, depending upon stage at presentation and limits of resection. After successful surgical removal, prognosis is good, with a 10-year survival of 88% (7). Surgery may be laparoscopic or open and may involve enucleation, resection, and metastatectomy. Enucleation is the preferred method of removal. Almost all insulinomas possess a pseudocapsule with a clear plane of dissection between the tumour and the surrounding soft pancreatic parenchyma. Enucleation is sufficient if the lesion is clearly localized before surgery, near or at the pancreatic surface, and easily defined intraoperatively (11). Histological confirmation of complete excision and the benign nature of the insulinoma are essential (11).

Resection is indicated when there is considerable ductal or vascular invasion, or where malignancy is suspected with a hard, infiltrating tumour and puckering of the surrounding soft tissue, distal dilatation of the pancreatic duct, or lymph node involvement. Splenic preservation is ideal to minimize postoperative complications. Histological analysis is important to confirm diagnosis and adequacy of resection.

Malignant insulinomas are managed with pancreatectomy and adjunctive treatment (such as hepatic artery embolization and/or chemotherapy). Hepatic metastases indicate a poor prognosis.

With advances in laparoscopic techniques, both laparoscopic enucleation and resection have been performed successfully (12). Although the conversion rate to open surgery is 14%, this most probably represents the learning curve for this procedure. Surgical treatment of insulinomas is effective and safe; reported success rates lie between 77 and 100% and mortality and morbidity rates are 2% and 26% respectively, including postoperative infection (particularly post-splenectomy) and pancreatic abscess, pseudocysts, and fistula formation. After resection, the risk of recurrence is greater in patients with MEN 1 (21% at 20 years) than those without MEN 1 (5% at 10 years and 7% at 20 years).

Medical management

Patients may be medically managed when awaiting surgery or medical therapies may be used alone for patients unsuitable for surgery (such as high anaesthetic risk or unresectable disease with metastases) or for patients with unsuccessful surgical outcomes (such as persistent symptoms post-resection or tumour non-localization in theatre). The aim of medical management is to prevent hypoglycaemia and to reduce tumour bulk in those with malignant tumours.

Dietary advice

Patients are encouraged to eat regular, small meals to avoid symptomatic hypoglycaemia. Complex carbohydrates for maintenance and high glycaemic index foods to relieve acute, symptomatic episodes are recommended. Guar gum has been shown to reduce insulin secretion in patients with insulinoma. Guar gum is an indigestible saccaride that delays gastric emptying and thus reduces the peak glucose load presented to the small intestine, which acts as a stimulus for insulin secretion. Guar gum thereby slows the rate of glucose absorption and has been used in patients with diabetes to improve postprandial glycaemic profiles.

Diazoxide

Diazoxide is an antihypertensive agent (potassium channel activator) with hyperglycaemic properties—stimulating extrapancreatic glycogenolysis and working directly on β cells to suppress insulin secretion. Significant side effects occur in 10–50% of patients, including oedema, weight gain, hirsutism, and hypokalaemia. Serious side effects, such as cardiomyopathy, myelosuppression, and cardiac arrhythmia, warrant close monitoring and cessation of therapy.

Calcium channel blockers

Verapamil has been used to treat hypoglycaemia from insulinoma and may be particularly useful for nesidioblastosis.

Somatostatin analogues

Somatostatin analogues, such as octreotide, have been used with variable success rates in palliation. This variability may due to the low expression of somatostatin receptors on insulinomas, which is in stark contrast to other gastrointestinal neuroendocrine tumours. Octreotide may improve hypoglycaemia by inhibition of insulin secretion by the tumour, or to a lesser extent may worsen it by suppressing counter-regulatory hormones such as glucagon or growth hormone. The potential for successful clinical improvement usually warrants a therapeutic trial.

Chemotherapy

Chemotherapy is usually ineffective in the treatment of insulinomas and carries the risk of considerable drug toxicity.

Hepatic artery embolization

The normal liver parenchyma is supplied predominantly from the portal vein, whereas hepatic metastases are supplied by the hepatic artery. Therefore hepatic metastases may be deprived of their blood supply by embolizing the hepatic artery, if the portal vein is patent.

Other causes of hypoglycaemia

Causes of hypoglycaemia

There are many causes of hypoglycaemia (Box 6.5.1) which may be due to inadequate glucose intake or increased utilization or losses. Iatrogenic causes are the most common. Hyperinsulinaemic hypoglycaemia may be due to β-cell stimulation which may be mitotic (insulinoma), iatrogenic (sulphonylurea), or autoimmune (stimulating antibodies).

Drugs

Drugs are the most common cause of hypoglycaemia.

Insulin

Hypoglycaemia is well-recognized side effect of insulin treatment and may account for 4% of deaths in patients with type 1 diabetes. Patients with type 1 diabetes may be vulnerable to iatrogenic hypoglycaemia due to 'hypoglycaemic unawareness' and impaired catecholamine responses to hypoglycaemia. Severe hypoglycaemia may be considered a barrier to improving and achieving strict glycaemic control in type 1 diabetes. Continuous subcutaneous insulin infusion (insulin pump therapy) is recommended by several national guidelines as a therapeutic option for people with type 1 diabetes who fail to achieve satisfactory glycaemic control on multiple dose insulin injections because of frequent severe hypoglycaemia.

Box 6.5.1 Causes of hypoglycaemia

Drugs
- Insulin
- Sulphonylureas
- Ethanol
- Salicylates
- Quinine
- Haloperidol
- Propranolol

Severe illness
- Sepsis
- Cardiac/renal/hepatic failure
- Starvation

Hormone deficiencies
- Cortisol
- Glucagon
- Catecholamine

Hyperinsulinaemia
- β-cell tumours (insulinoma)
- β-cell hyperplasia (nesidioblastosis)
- Autoimmune (insulin autoantibodies)
- β-cell stimulation
- Non-islet cell tumour (mesenchymal, epithelial, haematopoetic)

Reactive (post-prandial)
- In-born errors of metabolism, e.g. galactosaemia
- Postgastrectomy (dumping)

A recent meta-analysis showed that frequency of severe hypoglycaemia in type 1 diabetes was markedly reduced in trials during continuous subcutaneous insulin infusion compared with multiple dose insulin based on isophane and lente insulins (a mean 2.9-fold reduction for randomized controlled trials, 4.3-fold for before/after studies, and 4.2-fold for all studies), even though the mean level of glycaemia (measured by HbA_{1c}) was significantly less on insulin pump therapy (13). This is an important finding and counters the belief that an intensive insulin regimen is inherently associated with a high rate of severe hypoglycaemia and has an unfavourable risk:benefit ratio in those patients with severe hypoglycaemia (13).

Sulphonylurea

Sulphonylureas are insulin secretagogues and may cause hypoglycaemia and a biochemical picture indistinguishable from an insulinoma: hypoglycaemia with elevated plasma insulin and C-peptide levels. Demonstration of an elevated sulphonylurea level in the serum and/or plasma is therefore vital to exclude factitious hypoglycaemia.

Alcohol

Alcohol influences glucose metabolism in several ways. Ethanol inhibits gluconeogenesis (but has no effect on hepatic glycogenolysis) and the hormones that oppose insulin and enable a counter-regulatory response to hypoglycaemia—cortisol, growth hormone, and catecholamine. Glucagon secretion appears unaffected. In the malnourished or fasting state, patients may be glycogen depleted and gluconeogenesis is relied upon to maintain normoglycaemia. Therefore these subjects are vulnerable to hypoglycaemia, which is not normally seen in normal patients with adequate glucagon reserve and hepatic glycogenolysis.

Nesidioblastosis and islet cell hyperplasia

Hyperinsulinaemic hypoglycaemia in children and young adults is usually due to nesidioblastosis. The main histopathological characteristics of nesidioblastosis are hypertrophic β cells, which may be focal or diffuse. They are biochemically indistinguishable from insulinomas, but tend to abate when adolescence is reached. Children from consanguineous parents tend to have a more severe form of the disease, usually resistant to medical management, often requiring operative intervention. In other cases, medical management with diazoxide and/or octreotide is preferred. Surgery is only considered when medical options fail and should be restricted to removal of only 80% of the gland, which usually results in symptomatic improvement. Total pancreatectomy should be avoided, as common complications include endocrine (lifelong insulin-dependent diabetes) and exocrine dysfunction.

Non-islet cell tumour hypoglycaemia

Tumours may cause hypoglycaemia via three mechanisms. Firstly, they may cause hypersecretion of insulin (pancreatic insulinoma or ectopic insulin-secreting tumours). Secondly, tumours may cause infiltration or metastatic spread involving the liver and adrenal glands. Finally, with the case of non-islet cell tumour hypoglycaemia (NICTH), tumours may produce substances that interfere with normal glucose handling, such as insulin receptor antibodies (haematological malignancies including Hodgkin's lymphoma) and cytokines.

NICTH is a rare paraneoplastic phenomenon occurring in patients with tumours of mesenchymal, epithelial, and haematopoetic origin. Among mesenchymal tumours, the most common are fibrosarcomas, mesotheliomas, leiomyosarcomas, and hemangiopericytomas. The mesenchymal tumours are usually slow-growing, large (0.5–20 kg) and found in the thorax or retroperitoneal space. Epithelial tumours associated with NICTH include hepatomas, gastric, pancreatic exocrine, and lung carcinomas.

Insulin levels in NICTH are appropriately suppressed, eliminating its role in the pathogenesis. NICTH is associated with the secretion of incompletely processed precursors of IGF 2 by the tumour. This is not subject to regulation or inactivation by its binding protein, and circulates freely. IGF 2 fragments are therefore capable of activating the insulin receptor and inducing hypoglycaemia. Normally, serum IGF 2 is synthesized in the liver, where it is processed into a mature form which is secreted. In serum it forms a complex with an IGF-binding protein and with an acid-labile protein, such that it has little biological activity. It is excessive production of incompletely processed IFG 2, which circulate as smaller complexes with a greater capillary permeability, that is thought to increase IGF bioavailability. This aberrant IGF 2 is thought to be involved in the pathogenesis of NICTH as it interacts more readily with insulin receptors in the liver, muscle, and adipocytes, resulting in hypoglycaemia. This results in net increased peripheral glucose consumption and failure of hepatic compensatory mechanisms to increase glucose output. The incompletely processed IGF 2 binds not only to insulin receptors, but also to IGF 1 receptors in the pituitary gland and pancreas, leading to suppression of growth hormone and insulin secretion. The suppression of growth hormone secretion, in turn, causes a reduction in the serum concentrations of growth hormone-dependent proteins—IGF 1, IGF-binding protein 3, and acid-labile protein. This allows a greater percentage of free, unbound IGF 2 to circulate and exert hypoglycaemic effects. The diagnosis of NICTH is confirmed by demonstration of hypoglycaemia with low growth hormone, IGF 1, IGF 3, and insulin levels and a ratio of IGF 2: IGF 1 of greater than 10:1 (normally 3:1).

The metabolic derangements caused by NICTH are fully reversible after successful surgical removal of the tumour (complete or partial). Alleviating hypoglycaemia is a challenge; diazoxide, corticosteroids and growth hormone have been used with some success and immunosuppressants may be helpful when anti-insulin antibodies are implicated.

Autoimmune hypoglycaemia (insulin receptor antibodies)

Insulin receptor stimulating antibodies can cause hypoglycaemia. In these patients, insulin levels are high, and plasma glucose and C-peptide levels are low. Antibodies directed to insulin produce hypoglycaemia during the transition period from the post-prandial to post-absorptive state as insulin secreted in response to an earlier meal slowly dissociates from the antibodies. In these patients, total and free plasma insulin levels are inappropriately high, insulin secretion is appropriately suppressed, free plasma C-peptide levels and proinsulin levels are low, but total C-peptide and proinsulin levels are high because of cross-reactivity with antibody.

Hypoglycaemia caused by lymphoma may be caused by insulin receptor antibodies as suggested by reports where hypoglycaemia was associated with low or very low plasma IGF 2 levels or a normal IGF 2: IGF 1 ratio.

Organ failure

Hypoglycaemia is a common medical emergency. Among hospitalized patients, it is most common in those with diabetes mellitus, but it also occurs in patients with renal insufficiency, liver disease, malnutrition, congestive heart failure, sepsis, or cancer.

Liver failure

The liver is largely responsible for glycogenolysis and gluconeogenesis. Therefore hypoglycaemia rapidly ensues following hepatectomy. However there is a large reserve for hepatic glucose output and glucose levels fall severely only in cases of extensive liver damage and defective peripheral glucose production. Hypoglycaemia is unusual in conventional liver cirrhosis or hepatitis or metastatic hepatic deposits, but has been reported in cases of rapid and extensive hepatic damage, such as in fulminant viral or drug-induced hepatitis.

Cardiac failure

Hepatic congestion, anorexia, hepatic hypoxia, and impaired gluconeogenesis may be responsible for hypoglycaemia that may be associated with severe cardiac failure.

Sepsis

Sepsis may be associated with hypoglycaemia, associated with decreased hepatic glucose output and increased utilization. The use of intensive insulin therapy in patients with severe sepsis is unclear. A recent multicentre trial randomly assigned patients with severe sepsis to receive either intensive insulin therapy to maintain euglycaemia or conventional insulin therapy and either pentastarch (a low molecular weight hydroxyethyl starch) or modified Ringer's lactate for fluid resuscitation (14). This trial was stopped due to safety reasons; the rate of severe hypoglycaemia (glucose level ≤40 mg/dl (2.2 mmol/l)) was higher in the intensive therapy group than in the conventional therapy group (17.0 vs. 4.1%, $P < 0.001$), as was the rate of serious adverse events (10.9 vs. 5.2%, $P = 0.01$) (14). Fluid resuscitation with hydroxyethyl starch was harmful and associated with higher rates of acute renal failure and the need for renal replacement therapy, compared to Ringer's lactate (14).

Hormone deficiencies

Glucocorticoids have profound effects on hepatic glucose metabolism. Cortisol increases hepatic gluconeogenesis and prolonged cortisol excess enhances gluconeogenesis, increases hepatic glucose production, and decreases hepatic insulin sensitivity. Hypopituitarism in adults may be associated with hypoglycaemia when peripheral glucose consumption is increased (e.g. during exercise) or when glucose production is impaired (e.g. in alcohol excess). Young children are particularly vulnerable, with reduced gluconeogenesis, increased glucose utilization, reduced fat mobilization, and ketone body generation potentially contributing to susceptibility. Clinical hypoglycaemia may occur in children with growth hormone or cortisol deficiency, usually preceded by a prolonged fast (approximately 30 h) and relieved with administration of glucocorticoid. This suggests that defective gluconeogenesis may cause hypoglycaemia when glycogen stores are depleted. A recent study aimed to assess the response to fasting in children and adolescents with growth hormone and/or cortisol deficiency (15). Unrecognized overnight hypoglycaemia was uncommon in those on pituitary replacement, although blood glucose levels dropped quickly when treatment and meals were omitted (15). Patients with pituitary hormone deficiency were shown to have altered sympathetic activity, as evidenced by a compromised noradrenaline response (15).

Hypoglycaemia may occur when glucagon and catecholamines are deficient in the context of type 1 diabetes, but hypoglycaemia is generally not a feature of isolated catecholamine deficiency, resulting from bilateral adrenelectomy with replacement glucocorticoids or pharmacological catecholamine blockade. In the presence of intact catecholamine responses, glucagon deficiency would not be expected to cause hypoglycaemia.

Postprandial (reactive) hypoglycaemia

Postprandial reactive (late) dumping usually occurs within 4 h after eating, most commonly as sequel of gastroduodenal surgery (e.g. gastrectomy) and results from an exaggerated insulin and glucagon-like peptide-1 release in response to rapid transit of a carbohydrate load into the small intestine. Most patients can be treated with advice to eat small, frequent meals with slowly absorbed, complex carbohydrates. Octreotide may also be helpful in management.

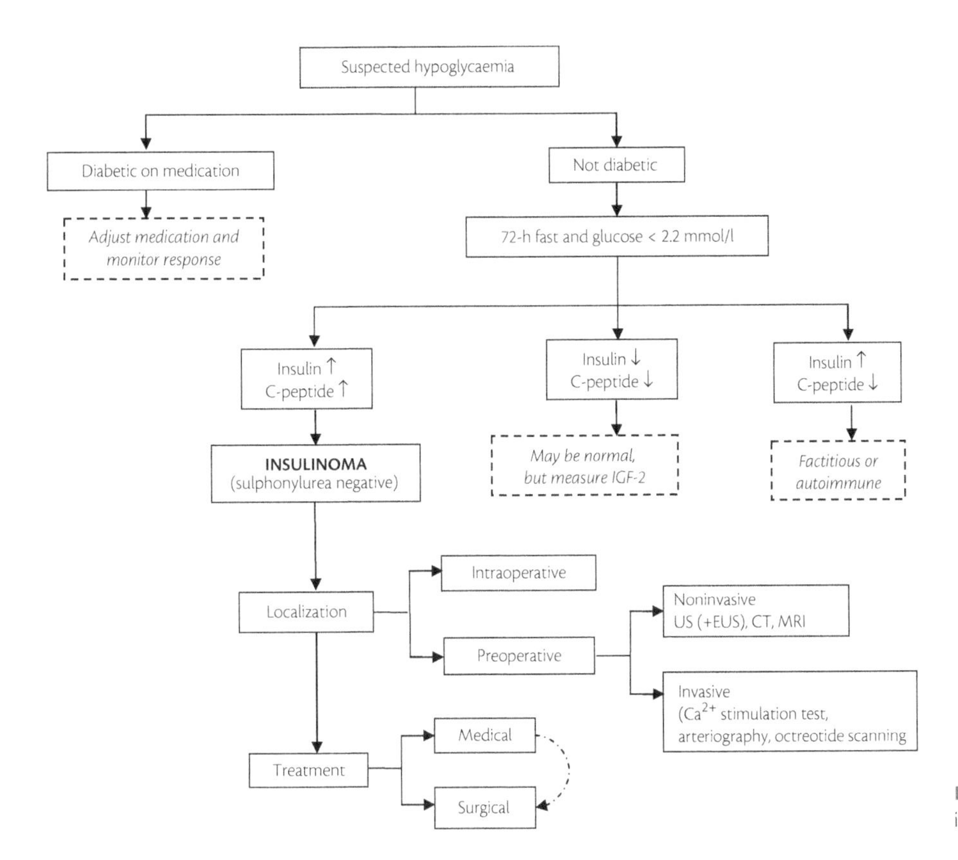

Fig. 6.5.1 Management algorithm for insulinomas.

Conclusions

Insulinomas are rare, but are the most common curable pancreatic tumours (Fig. 6.5.1). Most are small, benign, solitary, and intrapancreatic. Episodic neuroglycopenic symptoms predominate. Biochemical diagnosis is obtained with a supervised 72-h fast, demonstrating symptomatic hypoglycaemia with raised insulin and C-peptide levels in the absence of sulphonylureas in the plasma and urine. Preoperative localization is usually via helical CT with or without EUS and, particularly if the CT is normal, selective arterial calcium stimulation with hepatic venous sampling is usually successful for diagnostic confirmation. Surgical excision, particularly laparoscopic enucleation, is the treatment of choice with good chances of long-term cure.

References

1. Service FJ, McMahon MM, O'Brien PC, Ballard DJ. Functioning insulinoma incidence, recurrence, and long-term survival of patients: A 60-year study. *Mayo Clin Proc*, 1991; **66**: 711–19.
2. Service FJ. Hypoglycemic disorders. *N Engl J Med*, 1995; **332**: 1144–52.
3. Whipple AO, Frantz VK. Adenoma of islet cells with hyperinsulinism: A review. *Ann Surg*, 1935; **101**: 1299–335.
4. Marks V, Teale JD. Hypoglycemia: factitious and felonious. *Endocrinol Metab Clin North Am*, 1999; **28**: 579–601.
5. Teale JD, Marks V. Inappropriately elevated plasma insulin-like growth factor II in relation to suppressed insulin-like growth factor I in the diagnosis of non-islet cell tumour hypoglycaemia. *Clin Endocrinol (Oxf)*, 1990; **33**: 87–98.
6. Galiber AK, Reading CC, Charboneau JW, Sheedy PF 2nd, James EM, Gorman B, *et al.* Localization of pancreatic insulinoma: Comparison of pre- and intraoperative US with CT and angiography. *Radiology*, 1988; **166**: 405–8.
7. Tucker ON, Crotty PL, Conlon KC. The management of insulinoma. *Br J Surg*, 2006; **93**: 264–75.
8. Clark LR, Jaffe MH, Choyke PL, Grant EG, Zeman RK. Pancreatic imaging. *Radiol Clin North Am*, 1985; **23**: 489–501.
9. Gouya H, Vignaux O, Augui J, Dousset B, Palazzo L, Louvel A, *et al.* CT, endoscopic sonography, and a combined protocol for preoperative evaluation of pancreatic insulinomas. *AJR Am J Roentgenol*, 2003; **181**: 987–92.
10. Morganstein DL, Lewis DH, Jackson J, Isla A, Lynn J, Devendra D, *et al.* The role of arterial stimulation and simultaneous venous sampling in addition to cross-sectional imaging for localization of biochemically proven insulinomas. *Eur Radiol*, 2009; **19**: 2467–73.
11. Ramage JK, Davies AH, Ardill J, Bax N, Caplin M, Grossman A, *et al.* Guidelines for the management of gastroenteropancreatic neuroendocrine (including carcinoid) tumours. *Gut*, 2005; **54** (Suppl. 4): iv1–16.
12. Isla AM, Arbuckle JD, Kekis PB, Lim A, Jackson JE, Todd JF, *et al.* Laproscopic management of insulinomas. *Br J Surg*, 2009; **96**: 185–90.
13. Pickup JC, Sutton AJ. Severe hypoglycaemia and glycaemic control in type 1 diabetes: Meta-analysis of multiple daily insulin injections compared with continuous subcutaneous insulin infusion. *Diabet Med*, 2008; **25**: 765–74.
14. Brunkhorst FM, Engel C, Bloos F, Meier-Hellmann A, Ragaller M, Weiler N, *et al.* Intensive insulin therapy and pentastarch resuscitation in severe sepsis. *N Engl J Med*, 2008; **358**: 125–39.
15. Johnstone HC, McNally RJ, Cheetham TD. The impact of fasting and treatment omission on susceptibility to hypoglycaemia in children and adolescents with GH and cortisol insufficiency. *Clin Endocrinol (Oxf)*, 2008; **69**: 436–42.

6.6

Glucagonoma

G.M.K. Nijher, S.R. Bloom

Introduction

Glucagonomas are neuroendocrine tumours arising from the α cells of the islets of Langerhans, which result in excessive secretion of glucagon and peptides derived from preproglucagon. Post-translational modification of proglucagon is tissue specific and results in various glucagon peptides (1). It is the ratio of insulin to glucagon that controls the balance of gluconeogenesis and glycogenolysis in the liver. Glucagon stimulates hepatic gluconeogenesis and inhibits both glycolysis and glycogen synthesis. It increases production of free fatty acids from triglyceride breakdown by activating hormone-sensitive lipase; these undergo fatty oxidation in the liver via acetyl CoA, forming ketone bodies. The increase in free fatty acids from lipolysis inhibits hepatic lipogenesis. Glucagon also increases muscle proteolysis, resulting in an increase in amino acid supply to the liver.

Epidemiology

The incidence of glucagonomas is estimated to be only 1 per 20 million (2). The current data is either based upon single case reports or a few small series of cases. The majority of glucagonomas are sporadic, with only 3% associated with multiple endocrine neoplasia (MEN) (3). Table 6.6.1 illustrates the clinical features of 22 patients from the Hammersmith Hospital between 1970 and 1999. The median age of presentation is 64 years for sporadic tumours and 33 years for those associated with MEN. The earlier age of onset noted in those with glucagonomas associated with MEN may be due to the fact these patients may present with other disease-associated symptoms, e.g. hypercalcaemia of hyperparathyroidism . Alternatively, they may be detected through screening for neuroendocrine tumours.

Clinical features

The term glucagonoma syndrome was first used in 1974 with the description of a series of cases of glucagon-secreting pancreatic tumours associated with necrolytic migratory erythema, weight loss, diabetes mellitus, and stomatitis (4). Not all glucagonomas are symptomatic and they may be identified solely through screening of MEN patients. The nutrient deficiencies arising due to hyperglucagonoma and the secretion from the tumour of glucagon-like peptides 1 and 2, as well as cosecretion of other hormones such as pancreatic polypeptide, give rise to a spectrum of clinical features (5).

Necrolytic migratory erythema (NME)

This painful pruritic rash is a typical feature of the glucagonoma syndrome and one of the most common presenting signs, occurring in 72% of patients (6). Although characteristic for the glucagonoma syndrome, NME is not pathognomic (Fig. 6.6.1). The initial lesions of NME are erythematous plaques which may be associated with bullae. These lesions form erosions and crusts which eventually heal to leave central areas of hyperpigmentation and induration. The lesions demonstrate the koebner phenomenon, i.e. occurring at sites of trauma (4). Skin biopsy histology reveals necrolysis of the upper dermis and vacuolization of keratinocytes (7). The occurrence of NME does not correlate with metastases and has been noted in 60% of patients with benign glucagonoma.

The exact pathogenesis of NME remains unclear. There have been several postulated theories; the condition appears to be a multifactorial disease caused by a combination of zinc, amino acid, and fatty acid deficiencies (8). The glucagonoma syndrome shares a number of clinical features with vitamin B_2, B_3, B_6, and B_{12} deficiency. Indeed vitamin B deficiency may arise as a result of hyperglucagonaemia (5). There have been several cases of NME reported that were secondary to intravenous glucagon treatment, suggesting that NME is a direct consequence of glucagon action on the skin (9, 10). NME has also been associated with conditions other than glucagonoma, e.g. coeliac disease and cirrhosis; both of these conditions may have raised glucagon or glucagon-like peptides levels (6).

Diabetes mellitus

Diabetes mellitus is common in sporadic glucagonomas, occurring in 55% of patients at presentation and eventually developing in 75% of cases. Of these three-quarters require insulin therapy (11). Although rare, diabetic ketoacidosis has been reported (12).

Other clinical features

Weight loss or cachexia is a common presenting complaint, occurring in 72% of patients with metastases and 40% with local disease (6) Similar rates of 71% were noted in a review from the Mayo clinic of 21 patients with glucagonoma (11). Normocytic normochromic anaemia was noted in approximately a third of patients; and is probably the result of direct bone marrow suppression by glucagon (6). Diarrhoea occurs in approximately one-fifth of patients (6, 11); of these, 50% also have elevated gastrin and pancreatic polypeptide levels (6). Involvement of the mucous

Table 6.6.1 Presenting clinical features in 22 patients with glucagonoma at the Hammersmith Hospital (1970–1999)

Clinical feature	Sporadic cases[a] (%)	MEN 1 cases[a] (%)	Total (%)
Rash	14 (88)	1 (17)	15 (68)
Metastases	13 (81)	1 (17)	14 (64)
Diabetes mellitus	12 (75)	0	12 (55)
Cachexia	12 (75)	0	12 (55)
Anaemia	7 (44)	0	7 (32)
Cosecretion pancreatic polypeptide	7 (44)	0	7 (32)
Angular chelitis	6 (38)	0	6 (27)
Glossitis	5 (31)	0	5 (23)
Diarrhoea	4 (25)	0	4 (18)
Zollinger–Ellison syndrome	2 (13)	1 (17)	4 (18)
Psychiatric symptoms	3 (19)	0	3 (14)
Asymptomatic	0	3 (50)	3 (14)
Thrombosis	2 (13)	0	2 (9)
Cosecretion PTHrP	1 (6)	0	1 (9)
Hypoglycaemia cosecretion insulin	1 (6)	0	1 (5)

[a] Number of sporadic cases = 16, number of MEN 1 cases = 6.
PTHrP, parathyroid hormone-related protein; MEN 1, multiple endocrine neoplasia type 1.

membranes may lead to the development of stomatitis, glossitis, and chelitis in a third of cases (6). Psychiatric symptoms occur in 20% of patients and may vary from depression to paranoid delusions (6). Thromboembolism is a major source of morbidity and mortality in the glucagonoma syndrome and occurs in up to 11% of cases (6) and may account for up to 50% of deaths (13).

Metastases and site of primary tumour

Over 80% of patients with sporadic tumours have metastases at presentation (6, 11). Hepatic metastases usually involve both lobes of the liver and are multiple in two-thirds of cases; of the single hepatic metastases 75% occur in the right lobe (6). Of primary tumours, 41% are confined to the tail of the pancreas, 14% involve the head and body, 14% occur in the head alone, and 9% in the body alone (6). Sensitive imaging modalities and hepatic angiography may allow an increased detection of the primary tumour site (6).

Investigations

Biochemistry

Raised fasting plasma glucagon immunoreactivity is the basis for diagnosis. The reference range at the Hammersmith Clinical Chemistry Gut Hormone Laboratory is fasting plasma glucagon level below 50 pmol/l. False-positive results may occur due to other causes of a raised fasting plasma glucagon such as renal or hepatic failure, drugs, and prolonged fasting (14). Plasma glucagon levels may be elevated to various degrees ranging from only 1.5 to 150 times the upper limit of normal (6). Thus, if clinically supported, a marginally elevated plasma glucagon level may still be suspicious (15).

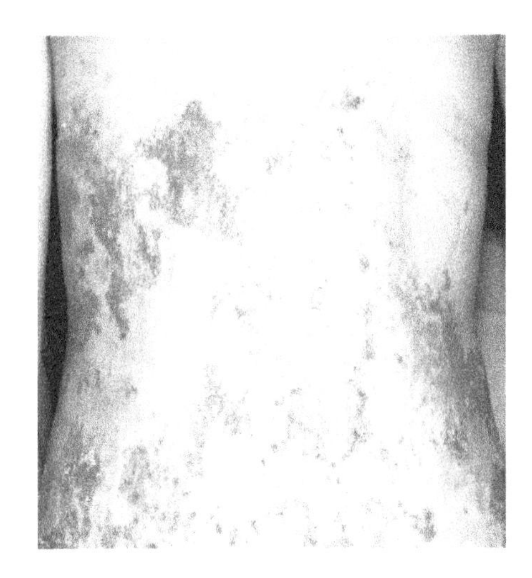

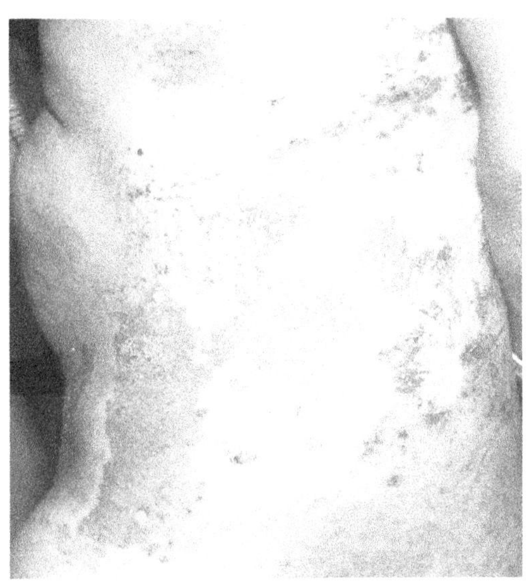

Fig. 6.6.1 Necrolytic migratory erythema on the back and trunk of patient with malignant glucagonoma. (See also Plate 36)

A raised fasting plasma gastrin level is noted in one-fifth of patients at presentation and may be associated with the Zollinger–Ellison syndrome (16). Plasma gastrin levels should be monitored regularly since they may rise up to 6 years after initial diagnosis. Other hormones may also be elevated, for example insulin, 5-hydroxyindoleacetic acid, human pancreatic polypeptide, chromogranin, and vasoactive intestinal peptide. It is therefore important an annual assessment of fasting gut hormone profile should be undertaken (6).

Biochemical investigations may reveal hypoproteinaemia, hypoalbuminaemia, and hypocholesterolaemia (13). Specific nutritional deficiencies, e.g. zinc deficiency, should be screened for (13), although plasma levels of trace elements may not reflect tissue levels (6).

Imaging

Contrast-enhanced CT and visceral angiography are the imaging modalities of choice and are more sensitive than abdominal ultrasound in tumour detection (17) (Fig. 6.6.2). The usefulness of MRI in tumour or metastases detection is as yet unclear (6).

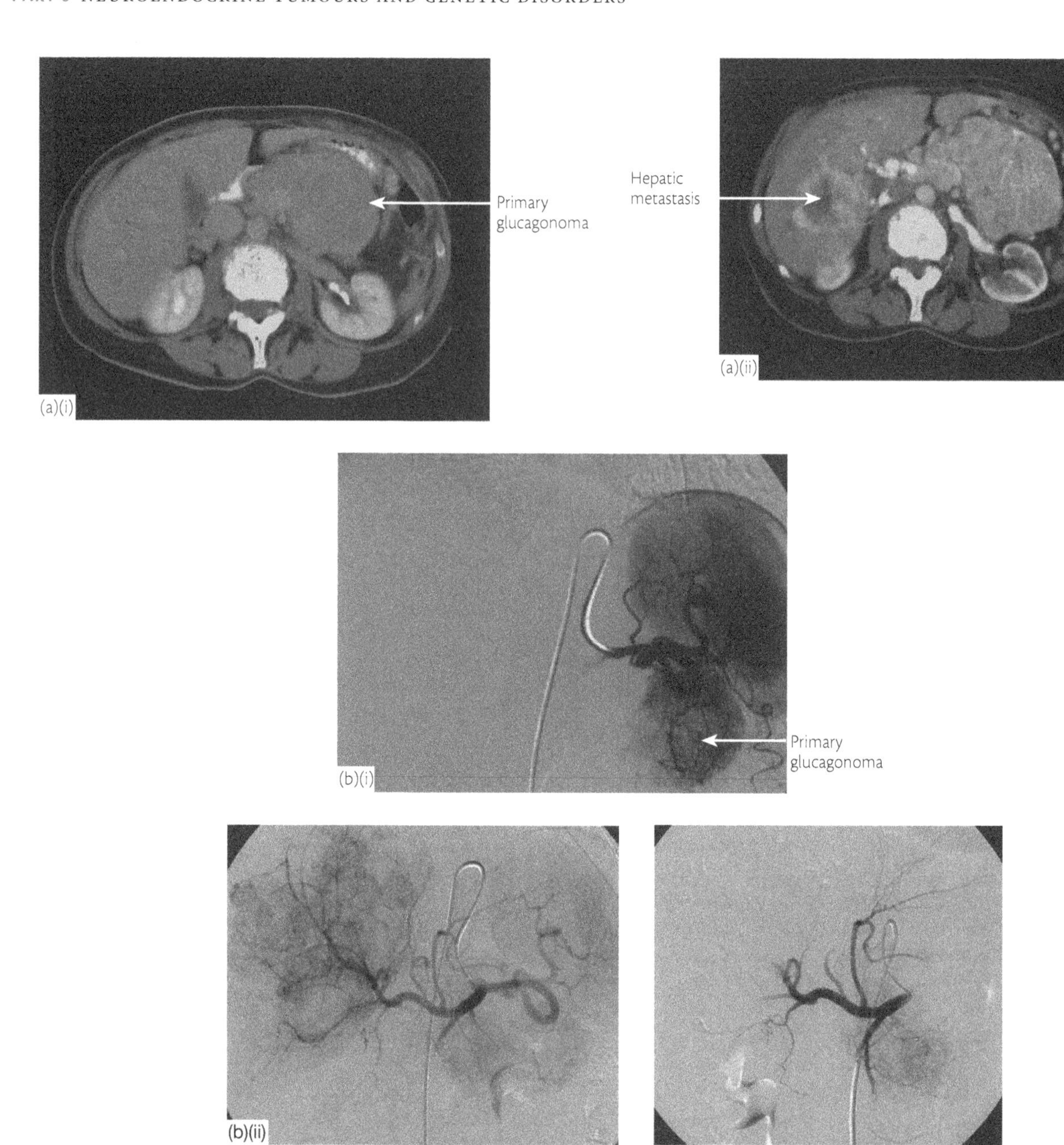

Fig. 6.6.2 (a) Abdominal CT scans showing (i) primary glucagonoma, (ii) progression of primary glucagonoma and hepatic metastases after 4 years. (b) (i) visceral angiogram showing cannulation of the splenic artery and vascular blush of primary glucagonoma, (ii) visceral angiogram showing cannulation of the hepatic artery and vascular blush of hepatic metastases, pre- and post-hepatic artery embolization.

Treatment

A multidisciplinary approach to treatment is required. Nutritional assessment, correction of any deficiencies and implementation of weight maintenance strategies is imperative. Where required, diabetic control should be optimized. Anticoagulation therapy should be instigated although there are currently no guidelines regarding which anticoagulant to use or the extent of anticoagulation required.

Surgical resection, either of the tumour itself or distal pancreatectomy and splenectomy in local disease, is the treatment of choice and offers 5-year survival rates of over 66% (6). However, 90% of patients have metastases at presentation and these commonly extend beyond lymph node metastases (6). Nevertheless, surgical resection or debulking of the tumour or distal pancreatectomy and splenectomy may offer good symptom relief (6). Unfortunately, symptoms return in a quarter of patients by 1 year, and 1-year survival rates are only 50% (6).

Hepatic artery embolization allows devascularization of hepatic metastases and symptomatic relief in 80% of patients; this may not correlate with a fall in plasma glucagon (18). Prior to the procedure, the patency of the portal vein must be established to ascertain whether there is adequate supply to the normal liver parenchyma. Complications of the procedure include massive peptide release, the effects of this may be minimized with the use of octreotide.

Vasodilating peptides and contrast load may lead to severe hypotension, thus optimal fluid balance must be maintained both pre- and postembolization. Additionally there are risks of infection in the necrotic tissue and of hepatic abscess formation (6).

Somatostatin analogues such as octreotide are the mainstay of medical therapy and provide rapid symptomatic relief, especially of NME (19), although they are less effective in control of weight loss and diabetes (20). Somatostatin inhibits growth hormone and other pituitary and pancreatic hormones. It has been demonstrated to both reduce plasma glucagon levels and shrink tumour size but its use was restricted by its very short plasma half-life. Octreotide is a somatostatin analogue with a longer plasma half-life of 2 h with intravenous administration. It is effective in reducing plasma glucagon levels, although tumour shrinkage or suppression of growth has not been demonstrated (21). Patients may require increasingly higher doses of octreotide after 6 months to control symptoms (6). Lanreotide is a longer-acting somatostatin analogue, which can be administered every 2 weeks, and has been shown to be effective (22) requires further evaluation in a larger number of cases. Patients should be monitored for symptoms of gall stone formation as cholestasis is noted in 50% of patients (6).

Chemotherapeutic agents such as streptozocin and 5-fluorouracil have been used in the treatment of glucagonoma. Streptozocin is a nitrosourea antibiotic with selective toxicity to pancreatic B cells, demonstrated in animals, and 5-fluorouracil inhibits DNA synthesis (6). Chemotherapy has a very limited role in management in those with symptoms persisting at 6 months and patients tend to survive for less than a year (6).

Prognosis

Patients with benign disease have a 85% survival rate at a mean follow-up of 4.7 years. Those with malignant disease treated with combination therapy have a 60% survival rate with a mean follow-up of 4.8 years.

References

1. Holst JJ. Enteroglucagon. *Annu Rev Physiol*, 1997; **59**: 257–71.
2. Kreijs GJ. Gastrointestinal endocrine tumours. *Am J Med*, 1987; **82** (Suppl. 5B): 1–3.
3. Wermers RA, Fatourechi V, Kvols LK. Clinical spectrum of hyperglucagonemia associated with malignant neuroendocrine tumors. *Mayo Clin Proc*, 1996; **71**: 1030–8.
4. Mallinson CN, Bloom SR, Warin AP. A glucagonoma syndrome. *Lancet*, 1979; **115**: 1429–32.
5. van Beek AP, de Haas ER, van Vloten WA, Lips CJM, Roijers JFM, Canninga-van Dijk M. The glucagonoma syndrome and necrolytic migratory erythema: a clinical review. *Eur J Endocrinol*, 2004; **151**: 531–7.
6. Frankton S, Bloom SR. Glucagonomas. *Baillieres Clin Gastroenterol*, 1996; **10**: 697–707.
7. Binnick AN, Spencer SK, Dennison WL Jr, Horton ES. Glucagonoma syndrome. Report of two cases and literature review. *Arch Dermatol*, 1977; **113**: 749–54.
8. Tierney EP, Badger J. Etiology and pathogenesis of necrolytic migratory erythema: review of the literature. *MedGenMed*, 2004; **6**: 4.
9. Mullans EA, Cohen PR. Iatrogenic necrolytic migratory erythema: a case report and review of the nonglucagonoma- associated necolytic migratory erythema. *J Am Acad Dermatol*, 1998; **38**: 866–73.
10. Wald M, Lawrence K, Luckner D, Seimann R, Mohnie K, Schober E. Glucagon therapy as a possible cause of erythema necrolyticum migrans in two neonates with persistent hypersinsulinaemic hypoglycaemia. *Eur J Pediatr*, 2002; **161**: 600–3.
11. Wermers RA, Fatourechi V, Wynne AG, Kvols LK, Lloyd RV. The glucagonoma syndrome. Clinical and pathologic features in 21 patients. *Medicine (Baltimore)*, 1996; **75**: 53–63.
12. Domen RE, Schaffer MB, Finke J, Sterin WK, Hurst CB. The glucagonoma syndrome: a report of a case. *Arch Intern Med*, 1980; **140**: 262–3.
13. Chastain MA. The glucagonoma syndrome: A review of its features and discussion of new perspectives. *Am J Med Sci*, 2001; **321**: 306–20.
14. Bloom SR, Polak JM. Glucagonoma syndrome. *Am J Med*, 1987; **82**: 25–36.
15. Edney JA, Hofmann S, Thompson JS, Kessinger A. Glucagonoma syndrome is an under diagnosed clinical entity. *Am J Surg*, 1990; **160**: 625–8.
16. White A, Tan K, Gray C, Roberts I, Ratcliffe JG. Multiple hormone secretion by a human pancreatic glucagonoma in culture. *Regul Pept*, 1985; **11**: 335–45.
17. Hammond PJ, Jackson JA, Bloom SR. Localization of pancreatic endocrine tumours. *Clin Endocrinol*, 1994; **40**: 3–14.
18. Ajani JA, Carraso CH, Charnsangavej C, Samaan NA, Levin B, Wallace S. Islet cell tumours metastatic to the liver. Effective palliation by sequential percutaneous artery embolization. *Ann Intern Med*, 1988; **108**: 340–4.
19. Anderson JV, Bloom SR. Neuroendocrine tumours of the gut: long term therapy with the somatostatin analogue SMS 201–995. *Scand J Gastroenterol*, 1986; **119** (Suppl.): 115–28.
20. Schmid R, Allescher HD, Schepp W, Hölscher A, Siewert R, Schusdziarra V, *et al.* Effect of stomatostatin in skin lesions and concentrations of plasma amino acids in a patient with glucagonoma syndrome. *Hepatogastroenterology*, 1988; **35**: 34–7.
21. Jockenhovel F, Lederbogen S, Olbricht T, Schmidt-Gayk H, Krenning EP, Lamberts SW, *et al.* The long acting somatostatin analogue octreotide alleviates symptoms by reducing post translational conversion of prepro-glucagon to glucagon in a patient with malignant glucagonoma, but does not prevent tumour growth. *Clin Investig*, 1994; **72**: 127–33.
22. Tomassetti P, Migliori M, Gullo L. Slow release lanreotide treatment in endocrine gastrointestinal tumours. *Am J Gastroenterol*, 1998; **93**: 1468–71.

6.7

VIPomas

Katie Wynne

Introduction

Vasoactive intestinal polypeptide (VIP) secreting tumours are rare neuroendocrine tumours. The associated syndrome was first described by Priest and Alexander in 1957. They reported a case that they thought to be a variant of the Zollinger–Ellison syndrome—a patient with an islet cell tumour associated with diarrhoea, peptic ulceration, and hypokalaemia (1). The following year, Verner and Morrison described a syndrome of profuse, refractory, watery diarrhoea with severe hypokalaemia and dehydration associated with a non-β-cell islet cell tumour (2). Historical terms for this syndrome have included 'pancreatic cholera' (as the diarrhoea is similar to the secretory diarrhoea observed in cholera) and the acronym WDHA (watery diarrhoea, hypokalaemia, and achlorhydria). However, these terms are inaccurate descriptions of a syndrome that can be associated with both extrapancreatic tumours and normal gastric acid secretion. In 1973, Bloom first connected the watery diarrhoea with an elevated plasma VIP level and an increased tumour content of VIP, suggesting the term 'VIPoma syndrome' (3). There followed a debate as to whether VIP was a marker for the syndrome or the causative agent for the diarrhoea. However, in 1983, Kane infused porcine VIP intravenously in healthy human subjects, achieving VIP levels similar to patients with VIPomas. Profuse watery diarrhoea developed within 4 h of infusion, providing evidence that VIP was indeed the mediator of the syndrome (4).

Epidemiology

VIPomas comprise approximately 2% of gastroenteropancreatic neuroendocrine tumours (5) with a reported annual incidence of 1 per 10 million individuals in the general population (6). Most cases present in the fifth decade and some series suggest an increased incidence in females (7–10). In adults, 80 to 90% of VIP-producing tumours originate in the pancreas (5). Reported extrapancreatic locations include the colon, bronchus, adrenals, liver, and sympathetic ganglia (11). Primary tumours are usually greater than 3 cm and solitary. The majority of these tumours are malignant (12) and over 70% of adult patients present with metastatic disease in lymph nodes, liver, or distant sites (9). Despite the severity of the clinical syndrome, symptoms may only present when the tumour reaches a certain size, which may account for the delay in diagnosis and advanced presentation (12). In children, VIP tumours most commonly occur along the autonomic chain and in the adrenal medulla as ganglioneuromas, ganglioblastomas, or neuroblastomas, which only occasionally metastasize.

It is estimated that 2% of VIPoma patients have multiple endocrine neoplasia syndrome type 1. However, VIPoma remains a rare feature of this syndrome with the incidence less than 1% (13). Other tumours, such as carcinoids, phaeochromocytomas, and bronchiogenic carcimonas, are also well recognized to occasionally produce VIP (7–10).

Pathophysiology

VIP is a 28-amino acid peptide, which normally functions as a neurotransmitter within enteric neurons and neurons of the brain, spinal cord, lung, urogenital system, and other endocrine organs. VIP has close structural homology to secretin and the two cloned VIP receptors (VIP1/VIP2 or VPAC1/VPAC2) are G-protein coupled receptors of the secretin family. The half-life of VIP is less than 1 min in circulation and plasma levels are usually low without prandial fluctuation. VIP is a potent vasodilator and physiological effects of VIP include smooth muscle relaxation (14), stimulation of pancreatic exocrine and gastrointestinal secretion (15), inhibition of gastric acid secretion (16), and modification of immune function and gastrointestinal blood flow (17).

Clinical and biochemical features

The VIPoma syndrome is caused by excessive VIP secretion from the tumour, although other substances can be cosecreted (18, 19). Watery diarrhoea occurs in nearly all patients (20) and is frequently produced in excess of 3 litres per day (9). The diarrhoea is secretory and typically persists despite 48 to 72 h of fasting. Diarrhoea is the results of the binding of VIP to high-affinity receptors on epithelial cells in all segments of the intestine, leading to secretion of Na^+, K^+, Cl^-, and HCO^{3-} as well as water into the lumen (7). This results in dehydration, severe hypokalaemia (often below 2.5 mmol/l), and hyperchloraemic metabolic acidosis. Diarrhoea-induced hypomagnesasaemia has occasionally been reported and may underlie the infrequent reports of tetany associated with VIPomas. High levels of circulating VIP are known to cause inhibition of gastric acid secretion, stimulation of bone resorption, increased hepatic glucose output, and vasodilation. These effects may clinically result in hypochlorhydria, hypercalcaemia, hyperglycaemia, or flushing (21). Common features are shown in Table 6.7.1.

Table 6.7.1 Features of the VIPoma syndrome

VIP action	Clinical/biochemical feature
Intestinal secretion of Na^+, Cl^-, and HCO^{3-}	Secretory diarrhoea Dehydration Weight loss Metabolic acidosis
Intestinal secretion of K^+ and hyperaldosteronism secondary to hypovolaemia	Hypokalaemia
Increased bone reabsorption Acidosis Tumour secretion of PTHrP Hyperparathyroidism secondary to MEN 1	Hypercalcaemia
Increased glycogenolysis	Hyperglycaemia
Vasodilation	Flushing

PTHrP, parathyroid hormone-related protein; MEN 1, multiple endocrine neoplasia type 1.

Diagnosis

The diagnosis of VIPoma syndrome can be established in a patient with otherwise unexplained secretory diarrhoea by demonstrating a raised fasting plasma VIP concentration with a localized source of VIP production (7–10). Secretory diarrhoea can be recognized by identifying a low osmotic gap as determined by faecal electrolyte measurement (22). The osmotic gap is calculated by subtracting twice the sum of the concentration of stool potassium and sodium from 290 mOsm/kg to account for unmeasured anions, i.e. measured osmolality = $290–2(Na^+ + K^+)$. An osmotic gap of less than 50 mOsm/kg suggests secretory diarrhoea. Other causes of secretory diarrhoea should be considered (23) and are listed in Box 6.7.1.

The VIPoma syndrome can be difficult to diagnose as other conditions may mimic its presentation, e.g. laxative abuse and Zollinger–Ellison syndrome. These can be differentiated using a careful history and by measurement of gastric pH, acid production, and circulating levels of gastrin and VIP. Fasting plasma VIP levels in healthy volunteers are generally low, whilst many patients with symptomatic VIPoma have levels more than three times the upper limit of normal (20). Chronic diarrhoea from other causes do not generally exhibit raised VIP levels (a rare exception being a carcinoid tumour cosecreting VIP). However, an elevation in plasma VIP can be found following a prolonged fast or in inflammatory bowel disease, small bowel resection, renal failure, or, uncommonly, in the normal population due to reduced clearance of non-bioactive high-molecular-weight VIP. A falsely low VIP level may be found if the hormone is allowed to undergo proteolytic enzymatic degradation prior to measurement. Samples of blood should be collected with the enzyme inhibitor aprotinin, the plasma rapidly separated, and frozen until assayed. It should be noted that patients with VIPoma syndrome may have normal VIP levels in early disease when symptoms are intermittent. Therefore repeated samples should be taken for evaluation of plasma VIP concentration during episodes of diarrhoea.

VIPomas may cosecrete additional peptides including pancreatic polypeptide, calcitonin, gastrin, neurotensin, gastric inhibitory peptide, serotonin, glucagon, insulin, somatostatin, growth hormone-release hormone, chromogranin A, chromogranin B GAWK fragment, and peptide histidine–methionine (PMH) (18, 19). PMH is a 27-amino acid peptide encoded by the same mRNA as VIP in humans. Therefore, PHM is invariably raised in the VIPoma syndrome and often to a greater extent than VIP itself as it has a longer circulating half-life. PMH further stimulates gastrointestinal secretion, although it is significantly less potent than VIP. The biochemical diagnosis of VIPoma should include measurement of general markers of neuroendocrine tumours such as chromogranin A and pancreatic peptide, as well as serum parathyroid hormone, calcium, and prolactin as a baseline screen for multiple endocrine neoplasia type 1 (24).

Box 6.7.1 Causes of secretory diarrhoea

- Infection
  - Cholera
  - *E. coli*
- Villous adenoma of the rectum
- Laxative abuse
- IgA deficiency
- Congenital
  - Dysautonomia
  - Chloridorrhoea
  - Structural enteric abnormalities
- Neuroendocrine tumours
  - VIPoma
  - Carcinoid
  - Gastrinoma (Zollinger–Ellison syndrome)
  - Medullary carcinoma of the thyroid
- Miscellaneous
  - Systemic mastocytosis
  - Basophilic leukaemia
- Idiopathic

VIPomas cannot be clearly distinguished from other pancreatic endocrine tumours by histological studies alone. Features are those of epithelial endocrine tumours with either solid, acinar, or trabelular cellular patterns with scant mitosis (25). VIP immunoreactivity is, however, strongly suggestive of a VIPoma, as this is found in less than 10% of other pancreatic endocrine tumours. Tissue examination should include immunohistological staining and histological classification according to the WHO system, which can be an important indicator of malignancy. However, the only method for confirming malignancy is the examination of local lymph nodes and metastatic sites such as the liver.

Localization

The optimal treatment for VIPoma is surgical resection and therefore the ability to localize a tumour is integral to a patient's subsequent management. As for other neuroendocrine tumours, standard imaging procedures include contrast-enhanced helical CT or MRI of the abdomen in combination with endoscopic ultrasonography or somatostatin receptor scintigraphy. The sensitivity of CT can approach 100% for most VIPomas, which are large at presentation (26). Furthermore, most pancreatic neuroendocrine tumours are highly vascular, making contrast-enhanced imaging able to identify up to 92% of lesions (27). MRI is particularly useful to differentiate smaller tumours, with reported sensitivity of 85% and specificity of 100% (28). If cross-sectional imaging is unable to identify the tumour, endoscopic ultrasonography has high sensitivity of up to 100% for detecting small pancreatic tumours, and may also demonstrate extrapancreatic lesions (27). VIPomas are somatostatin receptor positive in 80–90% of cases. Therefore somatostatin receptor scintigraphy is a useful functional scan which complements conventional imaging. Scintigraphy may also identify distant metastases to lymph nodes and rare cases of extra-abdominal spread to lung or bone (29). Positive scintigraphy may be predictive of the response to octreotide as the degree of VIP suppression is related to the number of high affinity receptors. Gallium-labelled somatostatin analogue positron emission tomography is also a promising method in the detection of small tumours or tumours bearing only a low density of somatostatin receptors (24).

Management

Supportive therapy

Initial therapeutic intervention in a patient with VIPoma should be focussed at correcting potentially life-threatening dehydration and electrolyte abnormalities. Patients are likely to require intensive fluid and potassium replacement (up to 350 mmol/day) in order to correct the substantial potassium deficit and prevent renal and cardiac dysfunction, which are common causes of death.

Surgery

Surgical resection is the treatment of choice for nonmetastatic islet cell tumours as half of tumours are resectable and 10% of those patients can be cured (30). In the remaining patients, distal pancreatectomy or tumour debulking can ameliorate symptoms for an extended period. Perioperative administration of a H_2 blocker or proton pump inhibitors is recommended in patients with VIPoma syndrome because of the possibility of rebound gastric acid hypersecretion following tumour removal. Postsurgery there may be profound circulatory changes as the VIP-induced vasodilatory drive is removed, leading to the possibility of circulatory overload. This is particularly problematic as preoperatively the gut is often dilated and contains large quantities of fluid that may be rapidly absorbed once the source of VIP is removed.

Pharmacotherapy

The somatostatin analogue, octreotide, is effective at suppressing hormone secretion in neuroendocrine tumours, especially glucagonomas and VIPomas. Symptomatic response occurs in 80 to 90% of patients within days of initiation, and it is therefore the treatment of choice to control diarrhoea in VIPoma syndrome (31, 32). The usual dose of subcutaneous octreotide is 50–100 μg 8 hourly, which can be increased by 50-μg increments up to 200 μg (and occasionally 500 μg) every 8 h (33). Titration should be by clinical response and symptomatic relief is not always accompanied by a reduction in circulating hormone levels. The improvement is mediated by both a direct inhibitory effect of hormone production of the tumour as well as indirect effects, such as the resorption of intestinal fluid and a reduction in bowel motility (34). Although there is some evidence that somatostatin analogues can reduce tumour burden in a minority of patients (32) this has not been clearly shown, but somatostatin therapy may be indicated as an antiproliferative treatment in selected cases base on positive scintigraphy (5).

One-third of patients experience nausea, abdominal discomfort, bloating, loose stools, and fat malabsorption during initial treatment with octreotide (34, 35). These effects on normal tissue usually subside within 2 weeks of initiation of therapy. Initially, diarrhoea can worsen due to steatorrhoea, which is secondary to suppression of pancreatic exocrine secretion; this responds to oral pancreatic enzyme supplements. Mild glucose intolerance rarely occurs due to transient inhibition of insulin secretion. Octreotide reduces postprandial gallbladder contractility and delays gallbladder emptying. One-quarter of patients develop asymptomatic cholesterol gallstones or sludge during the first 18 months of therapy (35). However, only 1% of patients develop symptoms during each year of treatment (34).

Somatostatin analogues can be considered for symptomatic control of the VIP syndrome in patients with unresectable or metastatic disease (12, 31). Treatment should be initiated with short-acting analogues, but once control is achieved the patient can be transferred to a long-acting analogue (e.g. octreotide acetate (Sandostatin-LAR) intramuscularly or Lanreotide autogel subcutaneously) every 4 weeks (36). The availability of long-acting monthly depot forms of octreotide avoids a frequent dosing regimen and improves quality of life in patients who may require pharmacological control over a longer period. The majority of patients have good sustained symptomatic response to octreotide-based therapy (37), but escape from symptomatic control can be seen quite frequently. In this instance an increase in the dose of pharmacotherapy may be temporarily effective. The loss of sensitivity of endocrine cancers to somatostatin analogues may occur due to the growth of tumour cells lacking somatostatin receptors (34).

Refractory disease

A number of different pharmacological agents have been reported to control the VIPoma syndrome with varying efficacy (7–10, 31). Prior to the use of somatostatin, glucocorticoids were often used as a first-line agent and patients have been reported to respond to combined glucocorticoid and octreotide therapy (31). α-interferons improve symptom control in up to 50% of patients with pancreatic islet cell tumours (37) and can be effective in VIPomas unresponsive to somatostatin analogues (38). It has also been reported to stabilize or regress tumours in a proportion of patients. The use of interferon is limited by side effects including fatigue, depression, and myelosuppression. Other potential agents, including angiotensin II and clonidine, may enhance sodium absorption in the jejunum, whereas indometacin, lithium carbonate, phenothiazines, propanolol, calcium channel blockers, and opiates may act by inhibition of intestinal secretion.

Metastatic disease

A wide range of treatment modalities are available for metastatic disease including hepatic resection and transplantation surgery, hepatic artery embolization, radiofrequency ablation, cryotherapy, intravenous chemotherapy, and peptide receptor radionuclide therapy.

Hepatic resection can be undertaken in patients with normal synthetic function and limited hepatic metastases if it is anticipated that 90% of the tumour burden can be removed (24). Although the majority of cases will not be cured by surgery, symptoms of hormone hypersecretion are effectively palliated and prolonged survival is often possible. Liver transplantation may be indicated for a small number of patients without extrahepatic metastases (39) in whom life-threatening hormonal symptoms persist despite maximal medical therapy and where standard surgery is not feasible (24).

Symptomatic liver metastases that are not amenable to surgery may respond to hepatic artery embolization. The goal of this palliative approach is to remove the blood supply to the metastases with only limited damage to normal hepatocytes, which derive most of their blood supply from the portal vein. This procedure can be repeated in metastatic disease with effective prolonged palliation (40). Fever, right upper quadrant pain, nausea, and vomiting are common sequelae postembolization. The possibility of infection must be excluded by regular cultures and, as the cystic artery is a branch of the hepatic artery, inadvertent gallbladder infarction is a possible complication of the procedure. The administration of broad-spectrum antibiotics and octreotide is recommended just prior to embolization and for several days afterwards in order to minimize the risk of infection and peptide release from necrotic tissue. Elevation of liver function tests, particularly liver transaminases, reflect unavoidable hepatic necrosis. However, massive necrosis or abscess formation is rare. Postprocedure hyperuricaemia can occasionally be clinically significant and allopurinol and urine alkalinization can be performed in addition to fluid hydration in order to reduce the risk of urate nephropathy (41).

Hepatic radiofrequency ablation, cryotherapy, or laser therapy can be used to treat hepatic lesions by a percutaneous or laparoscopic route or in combination with surgical debulking (42). This may not be as invasive as resection or embolization, but the technique is less well established and only applicable to limited disease—fewer than eight to ten metastases of less than 4–5 cm diameter (39).

Chemotherapy may be a useful therapeutic option in patients with metastatic and progressive neuroendocrine tumours (10, 31). A combination of streptozocin and doxorubicin has demonstrated response rates in the order of a third (43, 44), but few patients with VIPoma have been included in these series. The orally active agent temozolamide has also demonstrated antitumour activity in advanced neuroendocrine tumour disease (45). However, the relative benefits of these agents are uncertain and systemic chemotherapeutic agents have significant adverse effects with only modest success. An alternative approach is to deliver high doses of cytotoxic agent directly to the tumour in combination with hepatic embolization (chemoembolization). This technique can produce a transient partial remission (46).

Peptide receptor radionuclide therapy utilizes modified somatostatin analogues coupled with trivalent metal ions (indium, gallium, yttrium, lutetium, etc.) at a higher radioactivity than the radiolabelled somatostatin used for imaging. Limited experience is available in the treatment of VIPoma syndrome, but therapy with these agents are efficacious in other endocrine gastroenteropancreatic tumours (47, 48).

Prognosis

Insufficient data are available to provide accurate estimates of survival. However, in one study, the 5-year survival of patients with pancreatic VIPomas was reported as 68.5% (49). Patients with well-differentiated, small tumours and the absence of metastases have a more favourable prognosis (20, 30, 49).

References

1. Priest WM, Alexander MK. Isletcell tumour of the pancreas with peptic ulceration, diarrhoea, and hypokalaemia. *Lancet*, 1957; **273**: 1145–7.
2. Verner JV, Morrison AB. Islet cell tumor and a syndrome of refractory watery diarrhea and hypokalemia. *Am J Med*, 1958; **25**: 374–80.
3. Bloom SR, Polak JM, Pearse AG. Vasoactive intestinal peptide and watery-diarrhoea syndrome. *Lancet*, 1973; **2** (7819): 14–16.
4. Kane MG, O'Dorisio TM, Krejs GJ. Production of secretory diarrhea by intravenous infusion of vasoactive intestinal polypeptide. *N Engl J Med*, 1983; **309**: 1482–5.
5. O'Toole D, Salazar R, Falconi M, Kaltsas G, Couvelard A, De Herder WW, *et al.* Rare functioning pancreatic endocrine tumors. *Neuroendocrinology*, 2006; **84**: 189–95.
6. Friesen SR. Update on the diagnosis and treatment of rare neuroendocrine tumors. *Surg Clin North Am*, 1987; **67**: 379–93.
7. Bloom SR, Yiangou Y, Polak JM. Vasoactive intestinal peptide secreting tumors. Pathophysiological and clinical correlations. *Ann N Y Acad Sci*, 1988; **527**: 518–27.
8. Long RG, Bryant MG, Mitchell SJ, Adrian TE, Polak JM, Bloom SR. Clinicopathological study of pancreatic and ganglioneuroblastoma tumours secreting vasoactive intestinal polypeptide (vipomas). *BMJ (Clin Res Ed)*, 1981; **282**: 1767–71.
9. Mekhjian HS, O'Dorisio TM. VIPoma syndrome. *Semin Oncol*, 1987; **14**: 282–91.
10. Park SK, O'Dorisio MS, O'Dorisio TM. Vasoactive intestinal polypeptide-secreting tumours: biology and therapy. *Baillieres Clin Gastroenterol*, 1996; **10**: 673–96.
11. Ectors N. Pancreatic endocrine tumors: diagnostic pitfalls. *Hepatogastroenterology*, 1999; **46**: 679–90.
12. Peng SY, Li JT, Liu YB, Fang HQ, Wu YL, Peng CH, *et al.* Diagnosis and treatment of VIPoma in China: (case report and 31 cases review) diagnosis and treatment of VIPoma. *Pancreas*, 2004; **28**: 93–7.
13. Levy-Bohbot N, Merle C, Goudet P, Delemer B, Calender A, Jolly D, *et al.* Prevalence, characteristics and prognosis of MEN 1-associated glucagonomas, VIPomas, and somatostatinomas: study from the GTE (Groupe des Tumeurs Endocrines) registry. *Gastroenterol Clin Biol*, 2004; **28**: 1075–81.
14. Holst JJ, Fahrenkrug J, Knuhtsen S, Jensen SL, Poulsen SS, Nielsen OV. Vasoactive intestinal polypeptide (VIP) in the pig pancreas: role of VIPergic nerves in control of fluid and bicarbonate secretion. *Regul Pept*, 1984; **8**: 245–59.
15. Robberecht P, Conlon TP, Gardner JD. Interaction of porcine vasoactive intestinal peptide with dispersed pancreatic acinar cells from the guinea pig. Structural requirements for effects of vasoactive intestinal peptide and secretin on cellular adenosine 3':5'-monophosphate. *J Biol Chem*, 1976; **251**: 4635–9.
16. Barbezat GO, Grossman MI. Intestinal secretion: stimulation by peptides. *Science*, 1971; **174**: 422–4.
17. Fahrenkrug J. Transmitter role of vasoactive intestinal peptide. *Pharmacol Toxicol*, 1993; **72**: 354–63.
18. Meriney DK. Pathophysiology and management of VIPoma: a case study. *Oncol Nurs Forum*, 1996; **23**: 941–8.
19. Perry RR, Vinik AI. Clinical review 72: diagnosis and management of functioning islet cell tumors. *J Clin Endocrinol Metab*, 1995; **80**: 2273–8.
20. Nikou GC, Toubanakis C, Nikolaou P, Giannatou E, Safioleas M, Mallas E, *et al.* VIPomas: an update in diagnosis and management in a series of 11 patients. *Hepatogastroenterology*, 2005; **52**: 1259–65.

21. Rood RP, DeLellis RA, Dayal Y, Donowitz M. Pancreatic cholera syndrome due to a vasoactive intestinal polypeptide-producing tumor: further insights into the pathophysiology. *Gastroenterology*, 1988; **94**: 813–8.
22. Donowitz M, Kokke FT, Saidi R. Evaluation of patients with chronic diarrhea. *N Engl J Med*, 1995; **332**: 725–9.
23. American Gastroenterological Association. Medical position statement: guidelines for the evaluation and management of chronic diarrhea. *Gastroenterology*, 1999; **116**: 1461–3.
24. Kowalski J, Henze M, Schuhmacher J, Macke HR, Hofmann M, Haberkorn U. Evaluation of positron emission tomography imaging using [68Ga]-DOTA-D Phe(1)-Tyr(3)-Octreotide in comparison to [111In]-DTPAOC SPECT. First results in patients with neuroendocrine tumors. *Mol Imaging Biol*, 2003; **5**: 42–8.
25. Capella C, Polak JM, Buffa R, Tapia FJ, Heitz P, Usellini L, *et al.* Morphologic patterns and diagnostic criteria of VIP-producing endocrine tumors. A histologic, histochemical, ultrastructural, and biochemical study of 32 cases. *Cancer*, 1983; **52**: 1860–74.
26. King CM, Reznek RH, Dacie JE, Wass JA. Imaging islet cell tumours. *Clin Radiol*, 1994; **49**: 295–303.
27. Legmann P, Vignaux O, Dousset B, Baraza AJ, Palazzo L, Dumontier I, *et al.* Pancreatic tumors: comparison of dual-phase helical CT and endoscopic sonography. *AJR Am J Roentgenol*, 1998; **170**: 1315–22.
28. Thoeni RF, Mueller-Lisse UG, Chan R, Do NK, Shyn PB. Detection of small, functional islet cell tumors in the pancreas: selection of MR imaging sequences for optimal sensitivity. *Radiology*, 2000; **214**: 483–90.
29. Krenning EP, Kooij PP, Pauwels S, Breeman WA, Postema PT, De Herder WW, *et al.* Somatostatin receptor: scintigraphy and radionuclide therapy. *Digestion*, 1996; **57** (Suppl. 1): 57–61.
30. Thompson GB, van Heerden JA, Grant CS, Carney JA, Ilstrup DM. Islet cell carcinomas of the pancreas: a twenty-year experience. *Surgery*, 1988; **104**: 1011–7.
31. O'Dorisio TM, Mekhjian HS, Gaginella TS. Medical therapy of VIPomas. *Endocrinol Metab Clin North Am*, 1989; **18**: 545–56.
32. Kraenzlin ME, Ch'ng JL, Wood SM, Carr DH, Bloom SR. Long-term treatment of a VIPoma with somatostatin analogue resulting in remission of symptoms and possible shrinkage of metastases. *Gastroenterology*, 1985; **88**: 185–7.
33. Harris AG, O'Dorisio TM, Woltering EA, Anthony LB, Burton FR, Geller RB, *et al.* Consensus statement: octreotide dose titration in secretory diarrhea. Diarrhea Management Consensus Development Panel. *Dig Dis Sci*, 1995; **40**: 1464–73.
34. Lamberts SW, Van Der Lely AJ, De Herder WW, Hofland LJ. Octreotide. *N Engl J Med*, 1996; **334**: 246–54.
35. Newman CB, Melmed S, Snyder PJ, Young WF, Boyajy LD, Levy R, *et al.* Safety and efficacy of long-term octreotide therapy of acromegaly: results of a multicenter trial in 103 patients a clinical research center study. *J Clin Endocrinol Metab*, 1995; **80**: 2768–75.
36. Oberg K, Kvols L, Caplin M, Delle FG, de Herder W, Rindi G, *et al.* Consensus report on the use of somatostatin analogs for the management of neuroendocrine tumors of the gastroenteropancreatic system. *Ann Oncol*, 2004; **15**: 966–73.
37. Oberg K. Chemotherapy and biotherapy in the treatment of neuroendocrine tumours. *Ann Oncol*, 2001; **12** (Suppl. 2): S111–14.
38. Oberg K, Alm G, Lindstrom H, Lundqvist G. Successful treatment of therapy-resistant pancreatic cholera with human leucocyte interferon. *Lancet*, 1985; **1** (8431): 725–7.
39. Ahlman H, Friman S, Cahlin C, Nilsson O, Jansson S, Wangberg B, *et al.* Liver transplantation for treatment of metastatic neuroendocrine tumors. *Ann N Y Acad Sci*, 2004; **1014**: 265–9.
40. Ajani JA, Carrasco CH, Charnsangavej C, Samaan NA, Levin B, Wallace S. Islet cell tumors metastatic to the liver: effective palliation by sequential hepatic artery embolization. *Ann Intern Med*, 1988; **108**: 340–4.
41. Clouse ME, Lee RG. Management of the posthepatic artery embolization syndrome. *Radiology*, 1984; **152**: 238.
42. Moug SJ, Leen E, Horgan PG, Imrie CW. Radiofrequency ablation has a valuable therapeutic role in metastatic VIPoma. *Pancreatology*, 2006; **6**: 155–9.
43. Kouvaraki MA, Ajani JA, Hoff P, Wolff R, Evans DB, Lozano R, *et al.* Fluorouracil, doxorubicin, and streptozocin in the treatment of patients with locally advanced and metastatic pancreatic endocrine carcinomas. *J Clin Oncol*, 2004; **22**: 4762–71.
44. Delaunoit T, Ducreux M, Boige V, Dromain C, Sabourin JC, Duvillard P, *et al.* The doxorubicin-streptozotocin combination for the treatment of advanced well-differentiated pancreatic endocrine carcinoma; a judicious option? *Eur J Cancer*, 2004; **40**: 515–20.
45. Ekeblad S, Sundin A, Janson ET, Welin S, Granberg D, Kindmark H, *et al.* Temozolomide as monotherapy is effective in treatment of advanced malignant neuroendocrine tumors. *Clin Cancer Res*, 2007; **13**: 2986–91.
46. Valette PJ, Souquet JC. Pancreatic islet cell tumors metastatic to the liver: treatment by hepatic artery chemo-embolization. *Horm Res*, 1989; **32**: 77–9.
47. Kwekkeboom DJ, Teunissen JJ, Bakker WH, Kooij PP, De Herder WW, Feelders RA, *et al.* Radiolabeled somatostatin analog [177Lu-DOTA0,Tyr3]octreotate in patients with endocrine gastroenteropancreatic tumors. *J Clin Oncol*, 2005; **23**: 2754–62.
48. Forrer F, Valkema R, Kwekkeboom DJ, de Jong M, Krenning EP. Neuroendocrine tumors. Peptide receptor radionuclide therapy. *Best Pract Res Clin Endocrinol Metab*, 2007; **21**: 111–29.
49. Soga J, Yakuwa Y. Vipoma/ diarrheogenic syndrome: a statistical evaluation of 241 reported cases. *J Exp Clin Cancer Res*, 1998; **17**: 389–400.

6.8

Somatostatinoma

John A.H. Wass

Introduction

Somatostatin was isolated in 1973 by Paul Brazeau in Roger Guillemin's laboratory. It was found to have a widespread distribution, not only in the hypothalamus and brain but also in the gastrointestinal tract. Sixty-five per cent of the body's somatostatin is in the gut, mostly in the D cells of the gastric and intestinal epithelium. It is also present in the myometric and submucosal plexuses. The highest concentration is in the antrum of the stomach and there is a gradual decrease of concentrations down the gastrointestinal tract. Five per cent of the body's somatostatin is in the pancreas.

Infused somatostatin, which has a short half-life of 3 min, has a large number of actions on the pituitary gland, the endocrine and exocrine pancreas, gastrointestinal tract, other hormones, and on the nervous system (Box 6.8.1). Among its various actions of importance in the gastrointestinal tract is the inhibition of gastrin and cholecystokinin (CCK). In the pancreas, insulin and glucagon are inhibited. Nonendocrine actions include inhibition of gastric acid secretion, pancreatic exocrine function, gall bladder contraction, and intestinal motility. Intestinal absorption of nutrients, including glucose, triglycerides, and amino acids, is also inhibited (1).

Somatostatin exists in two main forms, as a 14-amino acid peptide (somatostatin 14) present mainly in the pancreas and the stomach, and as a 28-amino acid peptide present mainly in the intestine. Somatostatin 14 is the peptide present in enteric neurons.

Somatostatin receptors are present on many cell types, including the parietal cells of the stomach, G cells, D cells themselves, and cells of the exocrine and endocrine pancreas. A large number of tumours also have somatostatin receptors and these include pituitary adenomas, endocrine pancreatic tumours, carcinoid tumours, paragangliomas, phaeochromocytomas, small cell lung carcinomas, lymphomas, and meningiomas. Five different somatostatin receptors (SSTRs) have been cloned (SSTR1–SSTR5) and all are on different chromosomes. These have a varying affinity for somatostatin 14 and somatostatin 28 and a varying tissue distribution with SSTR2 and 5 being predominant in the pituitary (2).

Somatostatin can act either as an endocrine hormone or in a paracrine or autocrine way. It probably also has luminal effects in the gastrointestinal tract. Lastly, it can act as a neurotransmitter (3).

Somatostatinoma (4, 5)

Somatostatinomas are rare tumours with an estimated incidence of about 1 in 40 million. In total, over 200 have been described. They may be sporadic (90%) or familial (10%). Two main types exist: pancreatic somatostatinomas (56%), which are large tumours often associated with features of somatostatin excess; and duodenal tumours (44%), which are usually small and more amenable to surgical resection (6). They have also been described in the jejunum and cystic duct. The two types are compared in Table 6.8.1. They are infrequently associated with multiple endocrine neoplasia type 1 syndrome (7%), neurofibromatosis type 1, or Von Hippel–Lindau syndrome.

Pancreatic somatostatinoma

Somatostatinoma syndrome was first described in 1977 (8). Over 100 such cases have now been reported with features as in Box 6.8.2. The syndrome consists of cholelithiasis, the cause of which is multifactorial, including suppression of CCK production which results in impaired gallbladder contractility. High levels of somatostatin also inhibit bowel transit, which alters bowel flora, thus increasing bile acid reabsorption and this is associated with super saturated bile (9). Mild diabetes occurs and has often been present for many years before diagnosis. It is probably due to suppression of insulin secretion. Diarrhoea and steatorrhoea also occur and relate to the inhibition of pancreatic exocrine function. Hypochlorhydria relates to the inhibition of gastric acid secretion and gastrin. Anaemia, abdominal pain, and weight loss are also present and are nonspecific. They are probably related to the size of the tumour, which is usually large, and also to the fact that it is malignant. Those tumours are often diagnosed late and distant metastases may be present in lymph nodes, liver, or bone (55% are in the head of the pancreas).

Plasma and tissue levels of somatostatin are elevated and levels are higher in pancreatic as opposed to duodenal somatostatinomas. These somatostatin-secreting cells often also secrete ACTH, calcitonin, insulin, or some other peptides. This means that Cushing's syndrome, flushing, or hypoglycaemia (if there is cosecretion of insulin) may be present (10).

Box 6.8.1 Actions of exogenously administered somatostatin on endocrine and exocrine secretion

Endocrine secretion—inhibits the secretion of:

Pituitary

- Growth hormone
- Thyroid-stimulating hormone

Gastrointestinal tract

- Gastrin
- Cholecystokinin
- Secretin
- Vasoactive intestinal polypeptide
- Gastrin-inhibiting peptide
- Motilin
- Enteroglucagon
- Pancreatic polypeptide
- Insulin
- Glucagon
- Somatostatin

Other peptides

- Renin

Exocrine secretion—inhibition of:

- Gastric acid secretion
- Gastric emptying rate
- Pancreatic exocrine function: volume, electrolytes, and enzyme content
- Gall bladder contraction
- Intestinal motility
- Intestinal absorption of nutrients
- Splanchnic blood flow
- Renal water reabsorption
- Activity of some central nervous system neurons

Duodenal somatostatinoma

Duodenal somatostatinomas tend to be smaller and present earlier. The vast majority occur near the ampulla of Vater where they tend to cause obstructive biliary disease (NFI) (39%). Some are associated with neurofibromatosis type 1 and some are occasionally associated with phaeochromocytoma. Radiologically they can be difficult to diagnose. This may need endoscopic techniques. At presentation paraduodenal lymph nodes are involved because there is a high malignancy rate, although this is usually low grade. None of the duodenal somatostatinoma patients have developed the full-blown somatostatinoma syndrome but diabetes and gall stones have been noted in some cases.

Table 6.8.1 Comparison of pancreatic and extrapancreatic somatostatinomas (7)

Feature	Pancreatic	Extrapancreatic (duodenal)
Number of patients	81	81
Inhibitory syndrome (%)	18.5	2.5
von Recklinghausen's disease (%)	1.2	43.2
Large tumour (>20 mm) (%) (NFI)	85.5	41.4
Multisecretorary activity (%)	33.3	16.3
Metastatic rate and malignancy	No differences	
5-year survival	75.2% overall 59.9% with metastases 100% without metastases	

Box 6.8.2 Features of pancreatic somatostatinoma

- Hyperglycaemia 95%
- Cholelithiasis 68%, if inhibitory syndrome present
- Steatorrhoea 47%
- Hypochlorhydria
- Diarrhoea 60% with pancreatic; 11% with duodenal
- Abdominal pain 40%
- Weight loss 25%
- Anaemia 14%
- Elevated plasma and tissue somatostatin
- Histologically malignant, may be associated with ACTH, calcitonin and insulin secretion

Histologically these are psammomatous tumours. Treatment is with surgery if this is feasible, chemotherapy, and, if necessary, hepatic embolization. Somatostatin analogues may lower somatostatin levels and improve symptoms (such as diarrhoea) of both types of somatostatinoma if metastases are present.

References

1. Schultz A. Somatostatin: physiology and clinical application. *Clin Endocrinol Metabol*, 1994; **8**: 215–36.
2. Farooqi S, Bevan JS, Sheppard MC, Wass JAH. The therapeutic value of somatostatin and its analogues. *Pituitary*, 1999; **2**: 79–88.
3. Schonbrunn A. Somatostatin in endocrinology, De Groot LJ, Jameson JL, eds. Philadelphia: WB Saunders and Co., 2005: 427–77.
4. Nesi G, Marcucci T, Rubio CA, Brandi ML, Tonelli F. Somatostatinoma: Clinicopathological features of three cases and literature reviewed. *J Gastroenterol Hepatol*, 2008; **23**: 521–6.
5. Oberg K, Eriksson B. Endocrine tumours of the pancreas. *Best Pract Res Clin Gastroenterol*, 2005; **19**: 753–81.
6. Krejs GJ, Orci L, Conlon JM, Ravazzola M, Davis GR, Raskin P, Collins SM, *et al.* Somatostatinoma syndrome. Biochemical, morphological and clinical features. *N Engl J Med*, 1979; **301**: 285–92.
7. Soga J, Yakuwa Y. Somatostatinoma/inhibitory syndrome: a statistical evaluation of 173 reported cases as compared to other pancreatic endocrinomas. *J Exp Clin Cancer Res*, 1999; **18**: 13–22.

8. Ganda OP, Weir GC, Soeldner JS, Legg MA, Chick WL, Patel YC, Ebeid AM, *et al*. 'Somatostatinoma'; the somatostatin containing tumour of the endocrine pancreas. *N Engl J Med*, 1977; **296**: 963–7.
9. Dowling RH, Hussaini SH, Murphy GM, Besser GM, Wass JAH. Gallstones during octreotide therapy. *Clin Exp Metabol*, 1992; **41**: 22–33.
10. Wright J, Abolfathr A, Penman E, Marks V. Pancreatic somatostatinoma presenting with hypoglycaemia. *Clin Endocrinol*, 1980; **12**: 603–8.

6.9

Imaging neuroendocrine tumours of the gastrointestinal tract

James E. Jackson, Mary E. Roddie

Introduction

Gastroenteropancreatic (GEP) tumours are best divided into two distinct groups when discussing their radiological imaging. First are the functioning insulinomas and gastrinomas, which are often small at presentation; imaging of these lesions is usually aimed at localization of the primary tumour (and exclusion of metastatic disease) with a view to surgical excision. Second are the nonfunctioning neoplasms and the functioning tumours—carcinoids being the most common—which secrete a variety of other hormones including glucagon, vasoactive intestinal polypeptide, 5-hydroxytryptamine, somatostatin, serotonin, and pancreatic polypeptide. These are often large at presentation and are, therefore, obvious on cross-sectional imaging studies or have already metastasized; the role of the radiologist in this group is usually that of documenting the extent of disease to guide operative or nonoperative therapy. These two groups will be discussed separately.

Insulinomas and gastrinomas

Insulinomas

These tumours are rare with a reported incidence of 4 to 6 per million but are usually associated with severe symptoms due to recurrent hypoglycaemia and weight gain. More than 90% are benign, solitary, intrapancreatic neoplasms and are, therefore, amenable to cure by surgical excision (1) (see Chapter 6.5). Because of the potent effects of their hormonal output they are, however, often less than 1 cm in diameter at the time of presentation and for this reason may be very difficult to localize preoperatively. The necessity for preoperative imaging of insulinomas has been debated as it is universally recognized that an experienced surgeon using direct palpation of the pancreas together with intraoperative ultrasonography will be able to localize the tumour in close to 100% of cases. Most surgeons agree, however, that preoperative localization is helpful in that it will often reduce the duration of surgery and will, in some cases, decrease the extent of pancreatic resection, thereby improving morbidity and mortality rates. Furthermore, laparoscopic resection of insulinomas has become increasingly popular in recent years and precise tumour localization is essential when this technique is to be used as patient positioning on the operating table and the surgical approach will vary depending upon the site of the neoplasm (2–5). Many investigations are used to help in their preoperative detection, including transabdominal ultrasonography, endoscopic ultrasonography (EUS), CT, MRI, somatostatin receptor scintigraphy (SRS), angiography, and venous sampling, and the reported results for successful localization using each of these modalities vary considerably between centres.

Multidetector computed tomography (MDCT) and MRI provide the mainstay of noninvasive investigation but, despite the advances that have occurred in both of these modalities since the first edition of this book, there will still be a significant number of patients in whom a tumour will not be visualized. EUS and angiography combined with arterial stimulation venous sampling (ASVS) are invasive investigations but remain the most sensitive modalities for the detection of insulinomas.

So-called adult idiopathic nesidioblastosis is an extremely rare condition in which there is diffuse β-cell hyperplasia and resultant hyperinsulinaemic hypoglycaemia. None of the different imaging modalities discussed below will allow a preoperative diagnosis, which can only be made by biopsy.

Transabdominal ultrasonography

Transabdominal ultrasonography is often the first imaging investigation in an individual who has a biochemical diagnosis of an insulinoma. It will, however, only be useful in demonstrating the tumour in fewer than half the patients, largely related to the problems associated with imaging the whole of the pancreas in many individuals due to the presence of overlying bowel gas and this is one of the major limitations of this technique. Tumours are usually seen as rounded areas of lower reflectivity than the surrounding pancreatic parenchyma and may be buried within the gland or lie more superficially and, thereby, cause some contour deformity.

Contrast ultrasonography

Contrast ultrasonography involves the intravenous injection of a 'microbubble' agent that allows the assessment of tissue perfusion.

Small intrapancreatic tumours, which are not visible on conventional transabdominal ultrasonography, may become apparent when such an agent is used because of their increased vascularity with respect to the surrounding pancreatic parenchyma. These agents are being used increasingly during EUS (see below) to help differentiate neuroendocrine tumours from other pancreatic neoplasms. Contrast ultrasonography may also prove useful in the detection of hepatic metastases as small deposits that are not visible on other imaging modalities may be demonstrated.

Endoscopic ultrasonography (6–8)

EUS is increasingly being reported as the most sensitive investigation for the localization of insulinomas with detection rates in several series of over 90%. As with any 'interventional' technique, the results, in terms of successful localization, depend upon the experience of the operator and considerable expertise is required to image the pancreas completely.

Unlike transabdominal ultrasonography, the entire pancreas can be imaged in the majority of individuals although the tip of the pancreatic tail at the splenic hilum may remain a blindspot. The body and tail of the pancreas are imaged through the gastric wall and the pancreatic head via the duodenum. As the EUS probe is placed in almost direct contact with the pancreas, high-frequency transducers (7.5–20 MHz) are used with a resulting increase in resolution when compared with the lower-frequency probes required for transabdominal imaging; tumours as small as 5 mm may, therefore, be detected. Neoplasms are usually seen as focal areas of decreased echogenicity when compared with the surrounding normal pancreatic parenchyma although lesions may occasionally be of increased reflectivity. Most of these tumours will be markedly hypervascular on colour Doppler ultrasonography and tumour conspicuity may be further enhanced by using intravenous 'bubble' contrast medium.

Computed tomography (5, 9, 10)

The emergence of MDCT has had a profound effect on pancreatic imaging; exquisite images can be obtained during a single breath hold at any phase of contrast medium enhancement and the volume of axial data that is acquired can be instantly viewed in any plane. Insulinomas are highly vascular tumours and will enhance avidly during arterial phase images; a typical lesion will, therefore, be seen as a focal area of increased density when compared with the surrounding normal pancreas. A meticulous scanning technique is essential if optimal images are to be obtained, including the use of a negative oral contrast medium (e.g. water) within the stomach and duodenum and data acquisition during both arterial and portal venous phase studies as the enhancement of a few neoplasms will be delayed (Fig. 6.9.1).

Reports of the studies should include a description of the size and position of any visualized tumour and its relationship to the pancreatic duct and to normal visceral vessels to help determine whether surgical resection is likely to be possible by simple enucleation or whether a formal pancreatic resection will be necessary.

Despite the undoubted improvement in image quality that has occurred with MDCT there is surprisingly, as yet, no published evidence that this has increased the detection of insulinomas; a recent series documenting the results from two tertiary referral centres (5) quoted the accuracy of CT as being only 64%, which is similar to that at the current authors' institution.

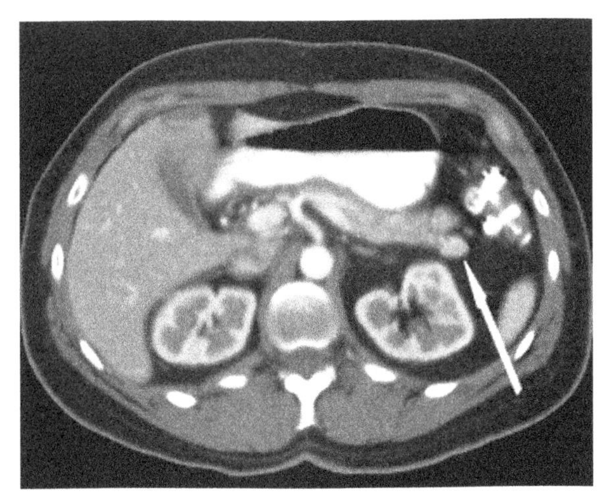

Fig. 6.9.1 Insulinoma. Contrast-enhanced CT demonstrates a well-defined vascular tumour nodule protruding from the posterior aspect of the pancreatic tail consistent with a neuroendocrine tumour subsequently confirmed at surgery.

Magnetic resonance imaging (11)

There has been great interest in recent years in the use of MRI for the localization of insulinomas, particularly since the development of rapid imaging sequences allowing breath-holding scanning. Once again a meticulous scanning technique, including bowel paralysis, is important and intravenous enhancement with gadolinium may be required. Tumours are usually of low signal intensity on T1-weighted images, especially if fat suppression sequences are used, and will show enhancement following intravenous contrast medium. On T2-weighted images, tumours are more likely to be hyper- or isointense when compared with the normal surrounding hepatic parenchyma.

The reported sensitivity for the detection of primary pancreatic insulinomas varies considerably from as low as 20% to one report approaching 100%; a figure of between 50% and 70% is probably reasonable. It is important to recognize, however, that MRI will not infrequently demonstrate tumours that have not been localized on MDCT. This is especially true in patients with multiple endocrine neoplasia type 1 (MEN 1) in whom multiple pancreatic neoplasms, both functioning and nonfunctioning, may be present and individuals with this condition and biochemical evidence of a functioning insulinoma should always undergo both MDCT and MRI before considering surgery (Fig. 6.9.2).

Radionuclide imaging

Radiolabelled somatostatin analogues

A variety of tumours, both neuroendocrine and non-neuroendocrine, contain somatostatin receptors and these are often expressed in particularly high density in well-differentiated gastroenteropancreatic tumours. SRS with ^{111}In-DTPA-octreotide has, therefore, proved to be highly sensitive in localizing and documenting the extent of disease in the majority of these neoplasms. As a result, it is justifiably considered the first-choice imaging modality for most gastroenteropancreatic tumours (see below). The one exception is insulinomas; these tumours have a lower incidence of somatostatin receptors in general and of the subtype 2 in particular. This, taken together with the small size of these neoplasms at the time of symptom onset, means that SRS is rarely helpful in the localization of these tumours.

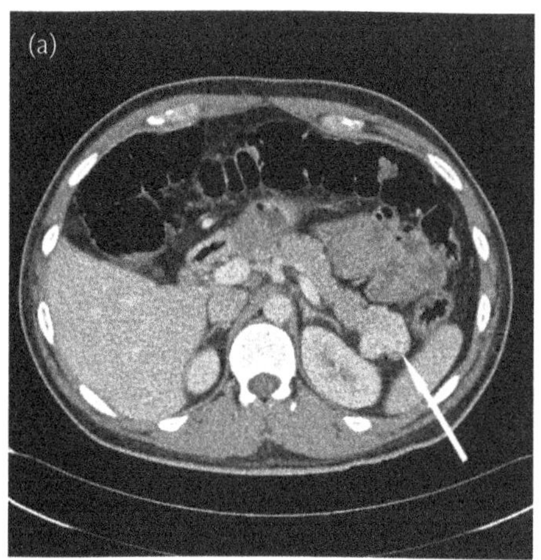

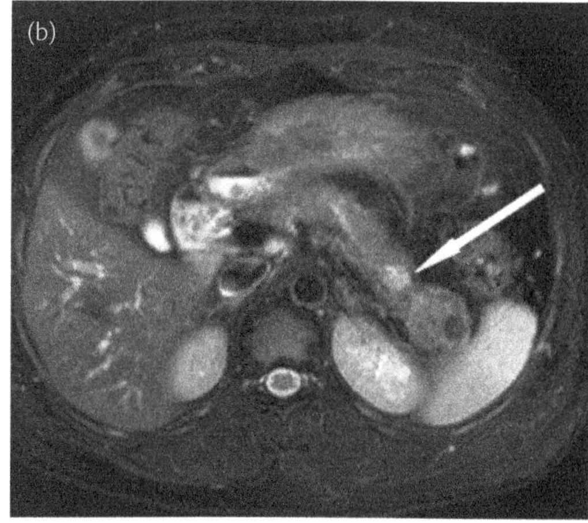

Fig. 6.9.2 Patient with multiple endocrine neoplasia type 1 and hyperinsulinaemic hypoglycaemia. (a) Contrast enhanced CT demonstrates a large enhancing tumour mass involving the pancreatic tail consistent with a neuroendocrine tumour. No other intrapancreatic tumours were demonstrated on CT. (b) T2-weighted MRI demonstrates a second tumour in the pancreatic body. Three additional pancreatic tumours (not shown) were identified on MRI in the pancreatic head, neck, and body. Subsequent angiography and arterial stimulation venous sampling documented that the large lesion in the tail was the dominant source of insulin and this lesion was subsequently resected.

Positron emission tomography (PET) combined with CT (PET-CT)

PET using ([^{18}F]2-fluoro-2-deoxy-D-glucose (FDG)) has become a powerful functional imaging modality in general oncology but has not, as yet, shown any advantages over other imaging techniques in the investigation of pancreatic neuroendocrine tumours and, in particular, insulinomas. Gallium-68-PET imaging has shown greater promise than FDG in the documentation of disease extent for both low and high-grade gastroenteropancreatic tumours. It plays little or no role, however, in the localization of insulinomas.

Angiography

Visceral angiography was for many years considered to be the most sensitive investigation for the detection of insulinomas but this has been questioned by a number of authors more recently since the improvements that have occurred in the cross-sectional imaging techniques discussed above. There can be little doubt that angiography should not precede the noninvasive investigations of transabdominal ultrasonography, CT, and MRI but it remains a highly sensitive investigation for the precise localization of this tumour. It also has the advantage over other imaging modalities, including EUS, in that it can very usefully be combined with arterial stimulation venous sampling (see below) to confirm that a visualized angiographic abnormality is due to a functioning neuroendocrine tumour. This is important in any individual as incidental nonfunctioning pancreatic tumours or pseudotumours may be present but is especially important in the context of multiple endocrine neoplasia; patients with this condition may have multiple pancreatic tumours and confirmation of function from one or more of these lesions and not from others may be essential when planning therapy.

A selective coeliac axis arteriogram using a digital subtraction technique should be performed initially as this will usually demonstrate most of the pancreas; it is not unusual for the insulinoma to be identified on this first run. A meticulous technique is absolutely essential; bowel movement must be completely abolished by the liberal use of appropriate antiperistaltic agents and complete immobility of the patient during breath-holding must be obtained. Selective splenic arteriograms in frontal and left anterior oblique projections and common hepatic, gastroduodenal, and superior mesenteric angiograms are subsequently performed. In many instances, the dorsal pancreatic and inferior pancreaticoduodenal arteries will also require catheterization in order to interrogate further a possible angiographic abnormality.

An insulinoma is seen as a well-defined, round or oval vascular blush that is of increased density when compared with the surrounding normal pancreatic parenchyma. It is usually visualized in the early arterial phase and persists for a variable length of time into the venous phase of the run. Early and prominent venous return from the tumour is common (Fig. 6.9.3).

Like many of the other investigations already discussed, the sensitivity reported for angiography for the detection of insulinomas varies considerably, from as low as 27% to over 90%. In the current authors' series of patients, angiography localizes over 95% of these tumours.

Arterial stimulation venous sampling (12–14)

The localization of an insulinoma by ASVS relies upon a detectable rise in insulin in hepatic venous samples after the selective injection of calcium gluconate in turn into the arteries supplying different portions of the pancreas. The splenic, gastroduodenal, superior mesenteric, and proper hepatic (i.e. beyond the origin of the gastroduodenal) arteries are those vessels most commonly studied during this technique; an appropriate rise in the level of insulin in the hepatic vein (sampled through a second catheter introduced via a femoral venous approach) will localize the insulinoma to the pancreatic body/tail, anterosuperior portion of the pancreatic head, and posteroinferior portion of the pancreatic head, respectively. A rise in insulin after injection into the proper hepatic artery suggests the presence of hepatic metastases. Depending upon the results of the selective angiogram performed immediately prior to ASVS, further injections may be made into other vessels supplying an area of angiographic abnormality, e.g. the inferior pancreaticoduodenal or dorsal pancreatic arteries. Published data confirm that this technique is a very useful addition to selective angiography with a sensitivity of close to 100%. It only localizes the tumour to a region of the pancreas rather than to a specific site if the

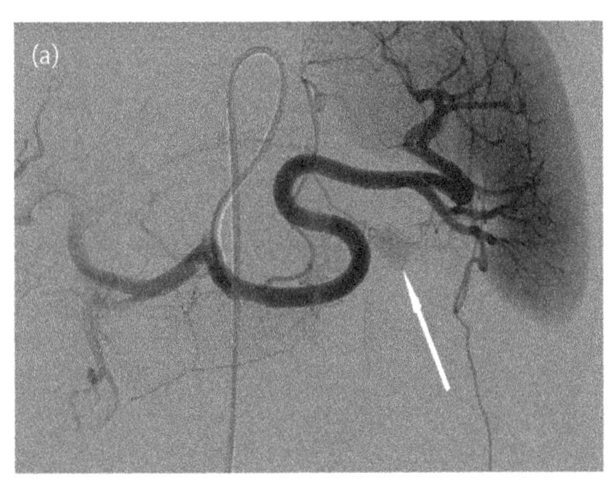

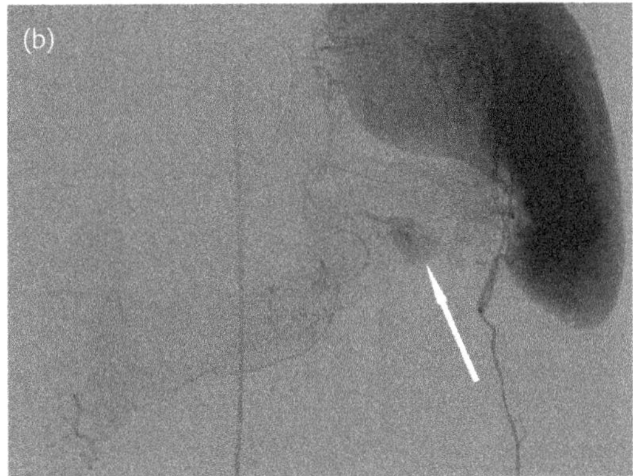

Fig. 6.9.3 Woman with biochemical diagnosis of insulinoma; CT, MRI, and endoscopic ultrasonography all negative. (a) Arterial phase image from selective splenic artery angiogram demonstrates an 8 mm diameter, well-defined vascular tumour in the pancreatic tail. (b) Early venous phase image from the same study demonstrates prominent venous drainage from the tumour nodule. Arterial stimulation venous sampling confirmed that this lesion secreted insulin and it was subsequently successfully resected laparoscopically.

angiogram does not demonstrate a tumour blush. However, it has the advantage of being able to confirm that a visualized angiographic abnormality is a functioning tumour.

Transhepatic portal venous sampling

This invasive investigation involves the direct percutaneous transhepatic puncture of the right portal vein and the selective catheterization via this route of the portal venous tributaries. Venous samples are then obtained from the splenic, pancreatic, pancreaticoduodenal, and superior mesenteric veins, the site of each sample being recorded on a 'map' of the portal venous system. Tumour localization is based upon demonstrating a rise in hormone concentration for a specific region of the pancreas. Although the reported sensitivity of this technique is high at approximately 84%, complications, which mainly relate to the transhepatic portal vein catheterization, are not infrequent with a reported incidence of approximately 10% and a mortality rate of 0.7%. For these reasons, together with the development of the less-invasive technique of ASVS, described above, this investigation is no longer necessary for the preoperative localization of pancreatic neuroendocrine tumours.

Gastrinomas

Unlike insulinomas 60% of gastrinomas are multicentric or have metastasized at the time of diagnosis and 40% are extrapancreatic, most commonly within the duodenum (see Chapter 6.4); they are similar to insulinomas, however, in that many are small (less than 1 cm in diameter) at the time of diagnosis. Ninety per cent of these neoplasms occur within what is termed the 'gastrinoma triangle', an area bounded by the junction of the neck and body of the pancreas medially, the junction of the second and third parts of the duodenum inferiorly, and the junction of the cystic and common bile ducts superiorly. Tumours within the duodenum are often less than 5 mm in diameter and are notoriously difficult to localize preoperatively despite the large number of different investigations available. It should be remembered that one-third of gastrinoma patients will have MEN 1 (see Chapter 6.11) and such individuals are more likely to have multiple duodenal gastrinomas. While many of the comments made above regarding the role of the numerous imaging modalities available for the localization of insulinomas also apply to gastrinomas, there are some important differences which will be discussed below.

Ultrasonography

Transabdominal ultrasonography is even less likely to detect a primary gastrinoma than an insulinoma because of the proportion of these tumours that are located in an extrahepatic location. It may, however, demonstrate hepatic or lymph node metastases. Primary tumours may be hypo-, iso-, or hyperechoic with respect to the surrounding normal pancreatic parenchyma whereas hepatic metastases are normally of increased echogenicity when compared with adjacent liver.

Contrast ultrasonography

See comments above regarding localization of insulinomas.

Endoscopic ultrasonography

EUS has been reported as being a highly sensitive technique (about 80%) for the demonstration of both pancreatic and extrapancreatic tumours although small duodenal tumours may be difficult to visualize. It has been suggested that EUS may be useful in excluding an intrapancreatic primary so that subsequent localization techniques can be aimed at finding an extrapancreatic neoplasm. Tumours may be hypo-, iso-, or hyperechoic with respect to normal pancreatic parenchyma. As discussed above, contrast Doppler ultrasonography may be helpful.

Computed tomography

As one might expect, CT is poor at localizing small primary tumours, especially those within the duodenum. A reported sensitivity of approximately 30% is quoted. Hepatic metastases are usually easily identified, although this is a less-sensitive technique for their detection than MRI or SRS, and are seen as low attenuation lesions on precontrast scans and high attenuation lesions on 'arterial phase' contrast enhanced images. As is the case with any neuroendocrine tumour, the extent of hepatic metastatic disease can easily be under-reported, or missed altogether, if scans are performed at a portal venous or 'equilibrium' phase of contrast enhancement when the normal liver and hepatic tumours are likely to be of similar attenuation.

Magnetic resonance imaging

Like transabdominal ultrasonography and CT, the role of MRI is principally for the demonstration or exclusion of hepatic metastases, although intrapancreatic tumours or lymph node metastases may be demonstrated. Primary gastrinomas are typically of increased signal intensity on T2-weighted scans when compared with normal pancreas and show ring enhancement with central low signal following intravenous gadolinium. MRI has a greater sensitivity than both ultrasonography and CT for hepatic metastases, although small hepatic haemangiomas may occasionally cause diagnostic confusion.

Radionuclide imaging

Somatostatin receptor scintigraphy

Unlike insulinomas the majority of gastrinomas contain a high density of somatostatin receptors and this form of imaging has been reported as being extremely useful for the localization of primary tumours and, more particularly, for the demonstration of distant spread to regional lymph nodes or the liver. It will often identify deposits previously unrecognized on other imaging modalities. There is, therefore, a good argument in favour of performing this investigation first and only proceeding to other imaging studies if the SRS is negative and surgery is being contemplated. Single photon emission computed tomography (SPECT) images should be performed in all cases as this considerably improves the sensitivity of the investigation. Small duodenal tumours remain difficult lesions to identify using this technique and although SRS is the most sensitive preoperative imaging study for extrahepatic gastrinomas and should, therefore, replace other 'conventional' investigations, it may still miss one-third of all lesions found at surgery. Negative results of SRS should not, therefore, be used to decide operability. Over 90% of gastrinoma hepatic metastases are identified by SRS and this investigation has been shown to be accurate at distinguishing between small metastatic deposits and hepatic haemangiomas. SRS clearly also has an important role in follow-up after surgery and in the evaluation of the response to medical therapy.

PET and PET-CT (15–20)

Like insulinomas, most gastrinomas have a low proliferation rate and PET is generally unhelpful. Those tumours with an aggressive clinical behaviour, however, are usually less well differentiated and may as a result be negative on SRS but show intense FDG uptake because of a higher proliferative activity (Fig. 6.9.4). In such cases FDG-PET is of prognostic significance. Gallium68-DOTATATE and DOTATOC have recently been shown to be of greater value than FDG in the documentation of disease extent in poorly differentiated gastroenteropancreatic tumours and may also have a role in the imaging of better differentiated neoplasms. These diagnostic radiopharmaceuticals also have a therapeutic application as they may be labelled with yttrium or lutetium to allow targeted radionuclide therapy of somatostatin receptor-positive gastroenteropancreatic tumours which are inoperable and/or metastatic.

Angiography

The technique of visceral angiography is similar to that used for the localization of pancreatic insulinomas although selective catheterization of the gastroduodenal and inferior pancreaticoduodenal arteries is more frequently required in order to try to visualize duodenal primaries. These tumours tend to be less intensely vascular than insulinomas and their differentiation from normally enhancing pancreatic parenchyma may, therefore, be more difficult. Patients with Zollinger–Ellision syndrome usually have marked thickening of gastric and duodenal walls and these will sometimes produce focal blushes, which may be confused with hypervascular tumours. The use of oblique projections will, however, usually allow differentiation between a mucosal fold and a gastrinoma. Hepatic metastases are usually well demonstrated.

The reported sensitivity of angiography for the localization of gastrinomas varies considerably but is less than that for insulinomas; in the best hands it may approach 70% but figures as low as 30–40% are not uncommon. Like insulinomas, however, the results may be improved by the use of arterial stimulation venous sampling.

Arterial stimulation venous sampling (21, 22)

The technique of ASVS is identical to that used for insulinomas. Secretin used to be the 'provocative agent' of choice but calcium gluconate is now more commonly used as it has been shown to work just as well. When injected into the vessel supplying a gastrinoma, both of these secretagogues will produce a significant rise in gastrin concentration in the hepatic vein of at least 25% at 20 s or 50% at 30 s after administration; a similar rise does not occur when the injection is made into a vessel supplying normal territory (Fig. 6.9.5).

There are relatively few data available regarding the usefulness of this technique for localizing primary gastrinomas but a few small

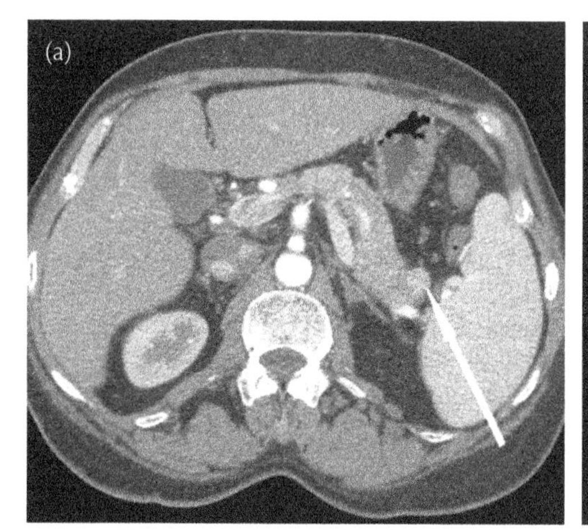

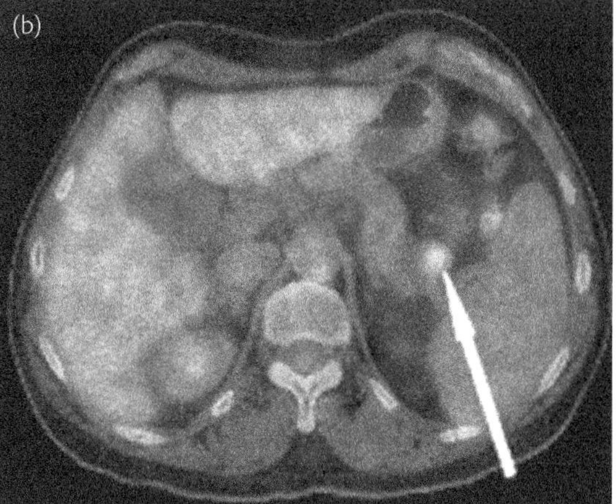

Fig. 6.9.4 Man with Zollinger–Ellison syndrome. (a) Contrast-enhanced CT documents a single enhancing tumour in the pancreatic tail. (b) Fused FDG-PET/CT image demonstrates localization of the radiopharmaceutical to the tumour. No other lesions were identified on this study and only this single tumour was found at subsequent surgery. (See also Plate 37)

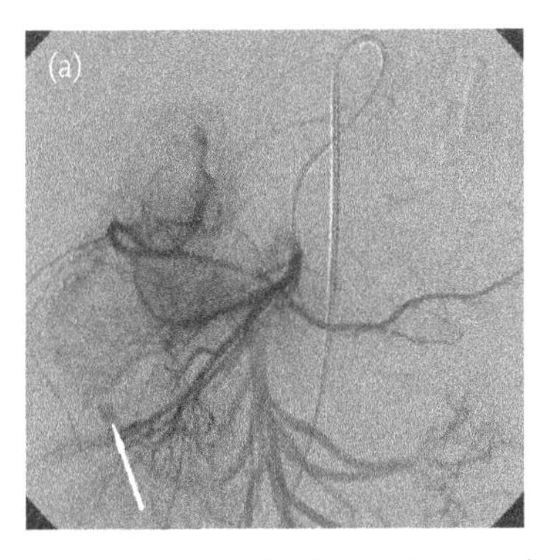

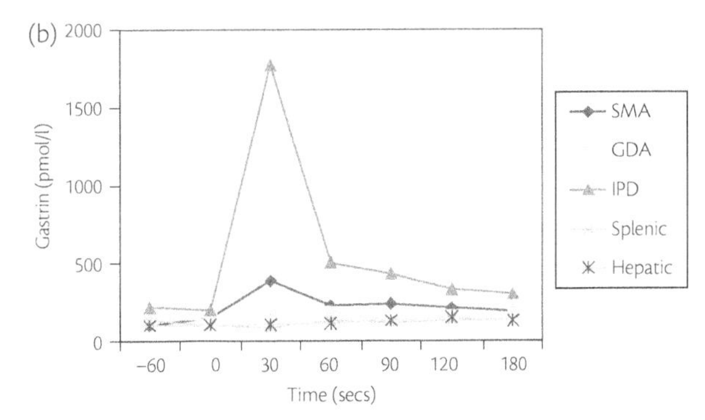

Fig. 6.9.5 Man with biochemical evidence of Zollinger–Ellison syndrome. (a) Arterial phase image from selective inferior pancreaticoduodenal artery angiogram demonstrates round vascular blush in the distal second part of the duodenum consistent with an intramural gastrinoma. (b) Graph of gastrin concentration within the hepatic vein after injection of calcium gluconate into the superior mesenteric artery (SMA), gastroduodenal artery (GDA), splenic artery, proper hepatic artery, and inferior pancreaticoduodenal (IPD) artery demonstrates the large rise in gastrin which occurred after injection into the IPD. A much smaller rise occurred after injection into the SMA due to the fact that the IPD arises from this vessel. The duodenal tumour was subsequently removed surgically.

series report high sensitivities, between 80 and 100%. Whether this 'localization' to a region of the pancreas or duodenum is associated with a significant improvement in disease-free survival, however, is difficult to determine. The technique has also been evaluated to see if it is able to reliably detect hepatic metastases but was shown to have a low sensitivity of only 41% but high specificity (a positive result was only seen in 2% of patients without liver deposits).

Transhepatic portal venous sampling

There is good evidence that the technique of ASVS is more sensitive than transhepatic portal venous sampling, and this invasive investigation is, therefore, no longer necessary (see comments above under localization of insulinomas).

Other functioning and nonfunctioning neuroendocrine tumours

Pancreatic tumours

The majority of these tumours are large at presentation and their demonstration by transabdominal ultrasonography and/or CT is rarely a problem (Fig. 6.9.6). Their malignant potential is high and many have metastasized at the time of diagnosis and imaging is primarily aimed, therefore, at either excluding or confirming the presence of hepatic metastases or other extrapancreatic spread. Primary tumours are usually of inhomogeneous soft-tissue density on CT and may contain areas of cystic degeneration or calcification; the latter is frequently seen in glucagonomas. They are commonly highly vascular and will, therefore, show marked contrast enhancement, which may be inhomogeneous due to areas of necrosis, on arterial phase scans.

Most of these neoplasms express somatostatin receptors and scintigraphy using ^{111}In-DTPA-octreotide has, until recently, been the best method for evaluating the presence and extent of metastatic disease. Gallium68-DOTATATE or DOTATOC PET imaging combined with CT is now, however, considered by many to be the most useful modality for these tumours (20).

Extrapancreatic tumours

Midgut carcinoids are the commonest extrapancreatic neuroendocrine tumours (see Chapter 6.3). These are most frequently located in the appendix where they have a low malignant potential and are usually an incidental finding following appendicectomy. Ileal carcinoids will metastasize in 30–60% of individuals and in an even greater proportion when over 2 cm in diameter. Metastatic disease to the liver results in the carcinoid syndrome and will be the reason for presentation in approximately two-thirds of patients, with the remainder developing symptoms due to local effects of the primary tumour, in particular, intestinal obstruction. The role of the imaging in this group of patients depends, therefore, upon the mode of presentation. Small bowel obstructive symptoms or chronic gastrointestinal blood loss may be investigated by a number of different imaging modalities and a specific diagnosis of a carcinoid tumour can often be made due to the frequent presence of a surrounding desmoplastic reaction. The most useful investigations are: CT, which may show a soft-tissue mass containing some calcification associated with marked stranding of the adjacent mesentery commonly associated with mesenteric venous and arterial occlusions and subsequent collaterals, small bowel dilatation, and bowel wall thickening (Fig. 6.9.7c, d); the small bowel enema (conventional barium, CT, or MRI), which will typically demonstrate small bowel dilatation and angulation with thickening of the valvulae conniventes with or without an associated mass lesion; and angiography, which may demonstrate a vascular blush with associated 'corkscrewing', narrowing, and occlusion of the adjacent mesenteric arteries and veins.

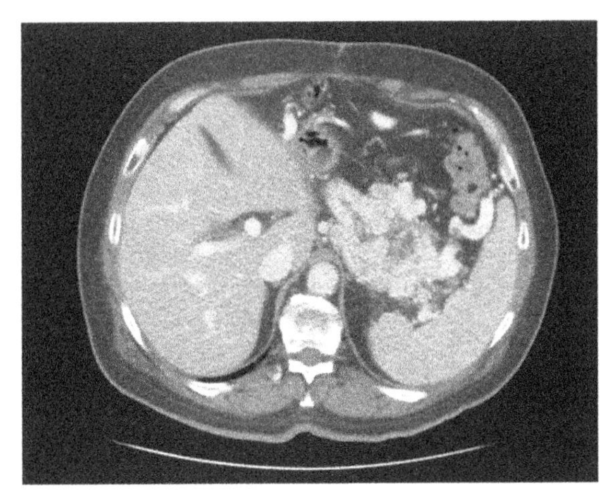

Fig. 6.9.6 Inoperable non-functioning neuroendocrine tumour. Contrast enhanced MDCT demonstrates a large vascular neoplasm containing central areas of low attenuation consistent with necrosis replacing the body and tail of the pancreas associated with splenic venous occlusion and resultant large varices.

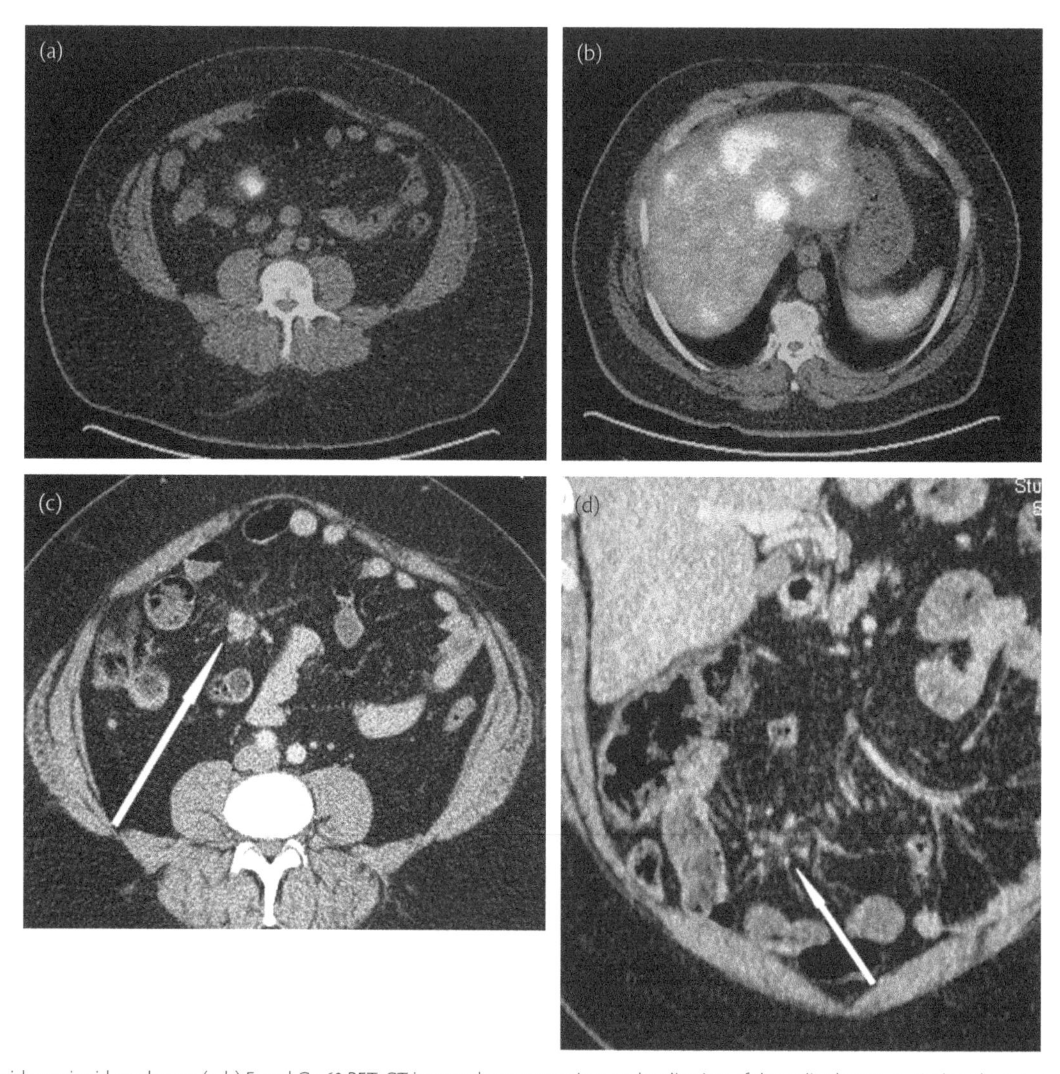

Fig. 6.9.7 Man with carcinoid syndrome. (a, b) Fused Ga-68 PET-CT images demonstrate intense localization of the radiopharmaceutical to the primary tumour and liver metastases. (c, d) Multidetector CT images in axial and coronal planes demonstrate the primary tumour and the surrounding mesenteric stranding due to the desmoplastic reaction which typically surrounds these neoplasms. (See also Plate 38)

In patients with carcinoid syndrome, imaging is primarily aimed at confirming the presence and extent of hepatic, and extrahepatic, metastases. Approximately 85% of carcinoid tumours express somatostatin receptors and scintigraphy with ^{111}In-pentetreotide is a reliable investigation for staging of disease. PET-CT imaging with Ga68-DOTATATE or DOTATOC may also be helpful (Fig. 6.9.7a,b), not only to demonstrate the full extent of disease but also, in some cases, to determine whether there is any role for targeted radionuclide therapy using yttrium- or lutetium-labelled radiopharmaceuticals. As previously mentioned, both of these agents may be useful for the palliative treatment of any metastatic somatostatin receptor-positive gastroenteropancreatic tumour.

References

1. Nikfarjam M, Warshaw AL, Axelrod L, Deshpande V, Thayer SP, Ferrone CR, *et al.* Improved contemporary surgical management of insulinomas: a 25-year experience at the Massachusetts General Hospital. *Ann Surg*, 2008; **247**: 165–73.
2. Ayav A, Bresler L, Brunaud L, Boissel P, SFCL, AFCE. Laparoscopic approach for solitary insulinoma: a multicentre study. *Langenbecks Arch Surg*, 2005; **390**: 134–40.
3. Fernandez-Cruz L, Blanco L, Cosa R, Rendon H. Is laparoscopic resection adequate in patients with neuroendocrine pancreatic tumours? *World J Surg*, 2008; **32**: 904–17.
4. Isla A, Arbuckle JD, Kekis PB, Lim A, Jackson JE, Todd JF, *et al.* Laparoscopic management of insulinomas. *Br J Surg*, 2009; **96**: 185–90.
5. Roland CL, Lo Cy, Miller BS, Holt S, Nwariaku FE. Surgical approach and perioperative complications determine short-term outcomes in patients with insulinoma: results of a bi-institutional study. *Ann Surg Oncol*, 2008; **15**: 3532–7.
6. Alsohaibani F, Bigam D, Kneteman N, Shapiro AM, Sandha GS. The impact of preoperative endoscopic ultrasound on the surgical management of pancreatic neuroendocrine tumours. *Can J Gastroenterol*, 2008; **22**: 817–20.
7. Chatzipantelis P, Salla C, Konstantinou P, Karoumpalis I, Sakellariou S, Doumani I. Endoscopic ultrasound-guided fine-needle aspiration cytology of pancreatic neuroendocrine tumors: a study of 48 cases. *Cancer*, 2008; **114**: 255–62.
8. Patel KK, Kim MK. Neuroendocrine tumors of the pancreas: endoscopic diagnosis. *Curr Opin Gastroenterol*, 2008; **24**: 638–42.
9. Rappeport ED, Hansen CP, Kjaer A, Knigge U. Multidetector computed tomography and neuroendocrine pancreaticoduodenal tumors. *Acta Radiol*, 2006; **47**: 248–56.

10. Rockall AG, Reznek RH. Imaging of neuroendocrine tumours (CT/MR/US). *Best Pract Res Clin Endocrinol Metab*, 2007; **21**: 43–68.
11. Zanello A, Nicoletti R, Brambilla P, Boccuni R, Di Carlo V, Staudacher C, *et al.* Magnetic resonance with manganese-DPDP (mangafodipir) of focal solid pancreatic lesions. *Radiol Med*, 2004; **108**: 194–207.
12. O'Shea D, Rohrer-Theurs AW, Lynn JA, Jackson JE, Bloom SR. Localization of insulinomas by selective intra arterial calcium injection. *J Clin Endocrinol Metabol*, 1996; **81**: 1623–7.
13. Jackson JE. Angiography and arterial stimulation venous sampling in the localization of pancreatic islet cell tumours. *Best Pract Res Clin Endocrinol Metabol,* 2005: **19** 229–39.
14. Kenney B, Tormey CA, Qin L, Sosa JA, Jain D, Neto A. Adult nesidioblastosis. Clinicopathological correlation between pre-operative selective arterial calcium stimulation studies and post-operative pathologic findings. *JOP*, 2008; **9**: 504–11.
15. Kayani I, Bomanji JB, Groves A, Conway G, Gacinovic S, Win T, *et al.* Functional imaging of neuroendocrine tumours with combined PET/CT using 68Ga-DOTATATE (DOTA-DPhe1, Tyr3-octreotate) and 18F-FDG. *Cancer*, 2008; **112**: 2447–55.
16. Khan MU, Khan S, El-Refaie S, Win Z, Rubello D, Al-Nahhas A. Clinical indications for Gallium-68 positron emission tomography imaging. *Eur J Surg Oncol*, 2009; **35**: 561–7.
17. Khan S, Lloyd C, Szyszko T, Win Z, Rubello D, Al-Nahhas A. PET imaging in endocrine tumours. *Minerva Endocrinol*, 2008; **33**: 41–52.
18. Lopci E, Nanni C, Rampin L, Rubello D, Fanti S. Clinical applications of 68Ga-DOTANOC in neuroendocrine tumours. *Minerva Endocrinol*, 2008; **33**: 277–81.
19. Basu S, Kumar R, Rubello D, Fanti S, Alavi A. PET imaging in neuroendocrine tumors: current status and future prospects. *Minerva Endocrinol*, 2008; **33**: 257–75.
20. Buchmann I, Henze M, Engelbrecht S, Eisenhut M, Runz A, Schäfer M, *et al.* Comparison of 68Ga-DOTATOC PET and 111In-DTPAOC (Octreoscan) SPECT in patients with neuroendocrine tumours. *Eur J Nucl Med Mol Imaging*, 2007; **34**: 1617–26.
21. Turner JJ, Wren AM, Jackson JE, Thakker RV, Meeran K. Localization of gastrinomas by selective intra-arterial calcium injection. *Clin Endocrinol (Oxf)*, 2002; **57**: 821–5.
22. Dhillo WS, Jayasena CN, Jackson JE, Lynn JA, Bloom SR, Meeran K, *et al.* Localization of gastrinomas by selective intra-arterial calcium injection in patients on proton pump inhibitor or H2 receptor antagonist therapy. *Eur J Gastroenterol Hepatol*, 2005; **17**: 429–33.

6.10

Systemic mastocytosis

Tomás Ahern, Donal O'Shea

Introduction

Mastocytosis is a heterogeneous group of rare disorders characterized by the abnormal growth and accumulation of mast cells in one or more organs. Mast cells are myeloid lineage cells that express the CD117 (KIT), CD45, and FcεRI cell surface markers. Patients with mastocytosis often present with abdominal cramps and diarrhoea and episodes of flushing, lightheadedness, and headache, which may prompt investigation for a neuroendocrine cause.

Cutaneous manifestations are common to all forms of mastocytosis. The majority of cases of mastocytosis are relatively benign, although some forms are associated with significant early death. The clinical course of mastocytosis is variable and can include shifting between the different forms.

Epidemiology

Mastocytosis is a rare condition with an unknown incidence or prevalence. It occurs equally in both sexes. Cutaneous mastocytosis first manifests before the age of 15 years in approximately two-thirds of patients (1); 85% of these cases manifest during the first 2 years of life (1–4). Systemic mastocytosis, on the other hand, is usually diagnosed after puberty (3).

Prognosis

Cutaneous lesions regress in 10–15% of patients with indolent systemic mastocytosis although repeated bone marrow examinations show persistence of disease (5). A minority progress to more aggressive forms of disease (6, 7). The prognosis of mastocytosis associated with other haematological disease is similar to that of the associated disease (8). Death usually occurs within 48 months of the diagnosis of aggressive systemic mastocytosis and within 18 months of the diagnosis of mast cell leukaemia (6, 9, 10).

Causes

The fundamental cause of mastocytosis is unknown. Germline and somatically acquired constitutively activating mutations of c-*kit*, the gene encoding KIT (CD117), are clearly associated with most forms of mastocytosis (11). Whether these mutations are necessary to cause mast cell transformation remains unclear—they do not occur in all cases of mastocytosis (12).

Pathogenesis

The complications and features of mastocytosis result from organ infiltration with mast cells and/or release of mast cell mediators. Mast cell mediators include histamine, serotonin, heparin, proteases, lipid mediators, cytokines, chemokines, and growth factors.

Complications

Organ infiltration can lead to lytic bone lesions, bone fractures, bone marrow suppression, portal hypertension, hypersplenism, and malabsorption (13). It is likely that mediator release contributes to increased bone fracture risk.

Features

The cutaneous lesions of mastocytosis represent collections of mast cells and usually involve the extremities, trunk, and abdomen with sparing of the palms, soles, and scalp. They vary in colour from yellow tan to reddish brown and generally take the form of macules or papules although occasionally they take the form of plaques or nodules (Fig. 6.10.1). The lesions commonly exhibit the classical urticarial reaction (wheal and erythema) when rubbed or scratched. This reaction, and the commonly associated itch, is due to mast cell degranulation and the release of mediators.

Telangiectasia macularis eruptiva perstans accounts for less than 1% of cases of maculopapular cutaneous mastocytosis and is distinguishable by the presence of generalized, red, telangiectatic macules with a tan brown background colour. Diffuse cutaneous mastocytosis is characterized by widespread, confluent areas of skin that are red-yellow-brown in colour and are of increased thickness due to infiltration with mast cells. This condition may be associated with bullous, sometimes haemorrhagic, eruptions and with flushing due to the release of mediators from the enormous mast cell load. Mastocytomas are similar in quality to the typical cutaneous lesions although they tend to be larger and may be associated with bullae (14).

Symptoms of noncutaneous organ infiltration by mast cells include poorly localized bone and joint pain. Gastrointestinal symptoms occur in about 50% of cases and include diarrhoea, steatorrhoea, and abdominal cramps (15). Hepatomegaly, splenomegaly, and/or palpable lymph nodes are common. Ascites, due to portal hypertension, occurs in more severe forms of the disease.

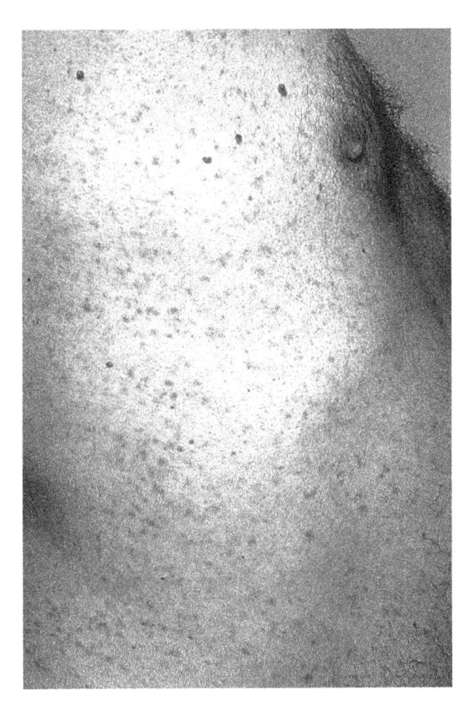

Fig. 6.10.1 Urticaria pigmentosa. We are grateful to Dr C. Bunker for providing this figure. (See also Plate 39)

Symptoms of mediator release occur with variable frequency and intensity and may take the form of discrete attacks. Histamine-mediated symptoms include pruritis, urticaria, angioedema, flushing, wheeze, and dyspepsia. Release of histamine, leukotrienes, prostaglandins, and cytokines are all thought to contribute to increased vasopermeability and vasodilation, which can lead to flushing, lightheadedness, and syncope, and may be life-threatening (13). It is likely that these mediators are also responsible for the increased susceptibility to anaphylaxis during allergic reactions. Recognized triggers of mast cell degranulation include temperature change, exercise, alcohol, insect or animal bites, infection, nonsteroidal anti-inflammatory drugs, opiates, radiocontrast material, anaesthetic agents, and invasive procedures.

Diagnosis and classification

The *Year 2000 Working Conference on Mastocytosis* published diagnostic and classification systems in 2001 (16) (Boxes 6.10.1 and 6.10.2). The diagnosis of a cutaneous manifestation requires the presence of typical skin lesions and identification of typical mast cell infiltrates within these lesions by microscopic examination.

The presence of B or C findings, as given in Box 6.10.3, allows classification of those diagnosed with systemic mastocytosis. Those with indolent systemic mastocytosis have neither evidence of high mast cell burden nor evidence of impaired organ function, whereas the presence of B findings confers a diagnosis of smouldering systemic mastocytosis, and any C finding confers a diagnosis of aggressive systemic mastocytosis.

Mast cell leukaemia is characterized by increased numbers of mast cells (>20% of cells), with blast-like morphology in bone marrow aspirates. Mast cell sarcoma is a unifocal tumour that consists of atypical mast cells and shows a destructive growth which is not associated with systemic involvement. Mastocytoma is a localized benign tumour composed of mature mast cells in either skin or extracutaneous organs (most commonly lung).

Box 6.10.1 Diagnostic criteria for systemic mastocytosis

Major criteria

Detection of multifocal dense infiltrates of mast cells (>15 cells aggregating) by tryptase immunohistochemistry or another stain in sections of:

1 Bone marrow, and/or

2 Other extracutaneous organ(s)

Minor criteria

1 Detection of either:

a. Greater than 25% mast cells with spindle-shaped morphology in aggregates in extracutaneous organ(s) sections, or

b. Greater than 25% mast cells with atypical morphology in aggregates in bone marrow aspirates

2 Detection of a c-*kit* point mutation at codon 816 in an extracutaneous organ

3 Coexpression of KIT (CD 117) and either CD2, CD25, or both on mast cells in bone marrow or blood

4 Serum total tryptase concentration >20 ng/ml (not valid in case of an) associated haematological non-mast cell disease (AHNMD)

A diagnosis requires the fulfilment of either 1 major and 1 minor criteria or 3 minor criteria.

Consensus proposal derived from the *Year 2000 Working Conference on Mastocytosis* (16).

Investigations

Blood tests

A full blood count, liver blood tests, and a serum tryptase level are all useful in the initial evaluation of the patient with mastocytosis.

Urine testing

Establishment of elevated levels of mast-cell mediators in a 24-h urine collection is supportive, but not diagnostic, of mastocytosis (17). Measurable urine histamine and prostaglandin metabolites include *N*-methylhistamine, *N*-methylimidazoleacetic acid, and 11-β-prostaglandin F_2.

Skin biopsy

A 3-mm punch biopsy that is fixed in formalin and stained with Giemsa is usually sufficient for microscopic examination. Mast cell infiltrates are typically perivascular and located in the papillary and upper dermis.

Bone marrow biopsy and aspirate

Bone marrow examination enables both diagnosis of systemic mastocytosis and detection of a possible associated haematological

Box 6.10.2 Classification and variants of mastocytosis

- Cutaneous mastocytosis
  - Urticaria pigmentosa/ maculopapular cutaneous mastocytosis
  - Diffuse cutaneous mastocytosis
  - Mastocytoma of the skin
- Indolent systemic mastocytosis
  - Classical indolent systemic mastocytosis
  - (Isolated) bone marrow mastocytosis
  - Smouldering systemic mastocytosis
- Systemic mastocytosis with an associated clonal haematological non-mast cell lineage disease (AHNMD)
  - Systemic mastocytosis–myelodysplastic syndrome
  - Systemic mastocytosis–myeloproliferative disorder
  - Systemic mastocytosis–chronic eosinophilic leukaemia
  - Systemic mastocytosis–acute myeloid leukaemia
  - Systemic mastocytosis–non-Hodgkin lymphoma
- Aggressive systemic mastocytosis
- Mast cell leukaemia
  - Classical mast cell leukaemia
  - Aleukaemic variant of mast cell leukaemia
- Mast cell sarcoma
- Extracutaneous mastocytoma

Consensus proposal derived from the *Year 2000 Working Conference on Mastocytosis* (16).

Box 6.10.3 B and C findings in systemic mastocytosis

B findings: evidence of high mast cell burden

1 Detection of either:

a. Greater than 30% mast cells in aggregates in bone marrow sections, or

b. Elevated serum tryptase level (>200 ng/ml)

2 Dysmyelopoiesis

3 Organomegaly:

a. Palpable hepatomegaly

b. Palpable splenomegaly

c. Palpable lymph nodes, or

d. Visceral lymph nodes >2 cm on imaging

C findings: evidence of impaired organ function

1 Bone marrow: cytopenia(s), any of:

a. Absolute neutrophil count <1000/μl

b. Haemoglobin <10 g/dl

c. Platelet count <100 000/μl

2 Liver: hepatomegaly with portal hypertension or ascites

3 Spleen: splenomegaly with hypersplenism

4 Gastrointestinal tract: malabsorption with hypoalbuminaemia and weight loss

5 Skeleton: large osteolyses, severe osteoporosis, and/or pathological fractures

Consensus proposal derived from the *Year 2000 Working Conference on Mastocytosis*(16).

disease. Although it is not usually necessary for children with cutaneous manifestations of mastocytosis, it should be performed on almost all adults who develop these manifestations (18). Other indications for bone marrow examination include unexplained other features of mastocytosis if a baseline serum tryptase concentration is measured at greater than 20 ng/ml.

The bone marrow biopsy should be immunohistochemically stained with antibodies to tryptase, KIT, and/or CD25 prior to microscopic examination (19). The multifocal dense mast cell aggregates are frequently located in perivascular and/or paratrabecular areas. The bone marrow aspirate should be submitted for flow cytometric analysis of mast cells and/or genetic analysis for c-*kit* mutations.

Imaging

Plain bone radiographs and/or whole body radionuclide bone scans may be useful in the diagnosis of bony lesions in those with mastocytosis and musculoskeletal symptoms. Abdominal CT cross-sectional imaging may be useful in those with gastrointestinal symptoms, palpable organomegaly, or palpable lymphadenopathy.

Treatments

There is no cure for mastocytosis and treatment is largely based on amelioration of symptoms. The mainstay of therapy is avoidance of recognized triggers of mast cell degranulation.

Cutaneous manifestations of mastocytosis

Psoralen ultraviolet A therapy and glucocorticoid therapy can be considered for the treatment of severe mastocytosis cutaneous lesions (20).

Inhibition of mast cell mediator action

By inhibiting mediator release from mast cells, cromolyn sodium can ameliorate pruritis, whealing, flushing, diarrhoea, and disorders of cognitive function (21). Ketotifen, another mast cell stabilizer, may be of use in patients with prominent pruritis and whealing (22). Histamine receptor antagonists are used to control flushing, pruritis, urticaria, and gastrointestinal cramping (H_1 antagonists) as well as oversecretion of gastric acid (H_2 antagonists) (23). Montelukast, the leukotriene receptor antagonist, has been reported to bring about significant amelioration of skin vesicles and wheeze in one paediatric case of systemic mastocytosis (24). Patients with an history of anaphylaxis should carry adrenaline filled syringes and be prepared to self-medicate to abort attacks (25). Oral glucocorticoid therapy can be considered for those with severe skin disease (bullous lesions) or those with refractory symptoms related to mediator release. Similarly, splenectomy has been performed for those with extreme hypersplenism.

Antiresorptive agents

Bone pain and increased fracture risk are commonly treated with calcium, vitamin D, and bisphosphonate therapy.

Immunomodulatory and cytoreductive agents

Those with more severe forms of mastocytosis generally require more aggressive therapy. Interferon-α2b, frequently combined with oral glucocorticoid therapy, brings about a partial response rate in one-third of patients and a minor response rate in another one-third (26). This, however, is associated with a 35% incidence of depression and only 65% of patients are able to tolerate at least 6 months of therapy. Cladribine, the purine nucleoside analogue, has been used in small numbers of patients with systemic mastocytosis and has been reported to bring about decreases in symptom severity and serum tryptase levels in 70 to 90% of subjects (27). Its use is limited by bone marrow toxicity. The chemotherapeutic approach and bone marrow transplantation has been generally found not to be successful—mast cell infiltration persists (9, 28).

Tyrosine kinase inhibitors

Imatinib has proved effective in the treatment of other haematological disorders that are associated with constitutive tyrosine kinase activity: chronic myelogenous leukaemia, gastrointestinal stromal cell tumours, and the myeloproliferative hypereosinophilic syndrome (29).

The majority of patients with systemic mastocytosis, however, are refractory to imatinib therapy (30). This appears to be due to resistance conferred by mutations at the 816 codon of c-*kit*; mutations at this site disrupt the enzymatic cleft of KIT, to which imatinib binds (31). In the uncommon patients who carry mutations of platelet-derived growth factor receptor or who carry mutations of c-*kit* which code for nonenzymatic cleft portions of KIT, however, imatinib has brought about dramatic and complete responses.

Dasatinib and PKC412 are two tyrosine kinase inhibitors that have been shown to have activity against human mast cell leukaemia cell lines that harbour imatinib-resistant mutations. They have shown promise in preclinical studies and clinical trials are currently underway to investigate their effect in the treatment of systemic mastocytosis (32, 33).

References

1. Kettelhut BV, Metcalfe DD. Pediatric mastocytosis. *J Invest Dermatol*, 1991; **96**: 15S–18S.
2. Azana JM, Torrelo A, Mediero IG, Zambrano A. Urticaria pigmentosa: a review of 67 pediatric cases. *Pediatr Dermatol*, 1994; **11**: 102–6.
3. Middelkamp Hup MA, Heide R, Tank B, Mulder PG, Orange AP. Comparison of mastocytosis with onset in children and adults. *J Eur Acad Dermatol Venereol*, 2002; **16**: 115–20.
4. Caplan RM. The natural course of urticaria pigmentosa. Analysis and follow-up of 112 cases. *Arch Dermatol*, 1963; **87**: 146–57.
5. Brockow K, Scott LM, Worobec AS, Kirshenbaum A, Akin C, Huber MM, *et al.* Regression of urticaria pigmentosa in adult patients with systemic mastocytosis: correlation with clinical patterns of disease. *Arch Dermatol*, 2002; **138**: 785–90.
6. Lawrence JB, Friedman BS, Travis WD, Chincilli VM, Metcalfe DD, Gralnick HR. Hematologic manifestations of systemic mast cell disease: a prospective study of laboratory and morphologic features and their relation to prognosis. *Am J Med*, 1991; **91**: 612–24.
7. Travis WD, Li CY, Bergstralh EJ, Yam LT, Swee RG. Systemic mast cell disease. Analysis of 58 cases and literature review. *Medicine (Baltimore)*, 1998; **67**: 345–68.
8. Travis WD, Li CY, Yam LT, Bergstralh EJ, Swee RG. Significance of systemic mast cell disease with associated hematologic disorders. *Cancer*, 1988; **62**: 965–72.
9. Nakamura R, Chakrabarti S, Akin C, Robyn J, Bahceci E, Greene A, *et al.* A pilot study of nonmyeloablative allogeneic hematopoietic stem cell transplant for advanced systemic mastocytosis. *Bone Marrow Transplant*, 2006; **37**: 353–8.
10. Pardanani A, Baek JY, Li CY, Butterfield JH, Tefferi A. Systemic mast cell disease without associated hematologic disorder: a combined retrospective and prospective study. *Mayo Clin Proc*, 2002; **77**: 1169–75.
11. Nagata H, Worobec AS, Oh CK, Chowdhury BA, Tannenbaum S, Suzuki Y, *et al.* Identification of a point mutation in the catalytic domain of the protooncogene c-kit in peripheral blood mononuclear cells of patients who have mastocytosis with an associated hematologic disorder. *Proc Natl Acad Sci USA*, 1995; **92**: 10560–4.
12. Valent P, Akin C, Sperr WR, Mayerhofer M, Fodinger M, Fritsche-Polanz R, *et al.* Mastocytosis: pathology, genetics, and current options for therapy. *Leuk Lymphoma*, 2005; **46**: 35–48.
13. Horan RF, Austen KF. Systemic mastocytosis: retrospective of a decade's clinical experience at the Brigham and Women's hospital. *J Invest Dermatol*, 1991; **96**: 5S–13S.
14. Chargin L, Sachs PM. Urticaria pigmentoasa appearing as a solitary nodular lesion. *AMA Arch Derm Syphilol*, 1954; **63**: 345–55.
15. Cherner JA, Jensen RT, Dubois A, O'Dorisio TM, Gardner JD, Metcalfe DD. Gastrointestinal dysfunction in systemic mastocytosis. A prospective study. *Gastroenterology*, 1988; **95**: 657–67.
16. Valent P, Horny HP, Escribano L, Longley BJ, Li CY, Schwartz LB, *et al.* Diagnostic criteria and classification of mastocytosis: a consensus proposal. *Leuk Res*, 2001; **25**: 603–25.
17. Keyzer JJ, de Monchy JG, van Doormaal JJ, van Voorst Vader PC. Improved diagnosis of mastocytosis by measurement of urinary histamine metabolites. *N Engl J Med*, 1983; **309**: 1603–5.
18. Czarnetzki BM, Kolde G, Schoemann A, Urbanitz S, Urbanitz D. Bone marrow findings in adult patients with urticaria pigmentosa. *J Am Acad Dermatol*, 1988; **18**: 45–51.
19. Miettinen M, Lasota J. KIT (CD117): a review on expression in normal and neoplastic tissues, and mutations and their clinicopathologic correlation. *Appl Immunohistochem Mol Morphol*, 2005; **13**: 205–20.
20. Czarnetzki MB, Rosenbach T, Kolde G, Frosch PJ. Phototherapy of urticaria pigmentosa: clinical response and changes of cutaneous reactivity, histamine and chemotactic leukotrienes. *Arch Dermatol Res*, 1985; **277**: 105–13.
21. Soter NA, Austen KF, Wasserman SI. Oral disodium cromoglycate in the treatment of systemic mastocytosis. *N Engl J Med*, 1979; **301**: 465–9.
22. Czarnetzki BM. A double-blind cross-over study of the effect of ketotifen in urticaria pigmentosa. *Dermatologica*, 1983; **166**: 44–7.
23. Frieri M, Alling DW, Metcalfe DD. Comparison of the therapeutic efficacy of cromolyn sodium with that of combined chlorpheniramine and cimetidine in systemic mastocytosis. Results of a double-blind clinical trial. *Am J Med*, 1985; **78**: 9–14.
24. Tolar J, Tope WD, Neglia JP. Leukotriene-receptor inhibition for the treatment of systemic mastocytosis. *N Engl J Med*, 2004; **350**: 735–6.
25. Turk J, Oates JA, Roberts LJ 2nd. Intervention with epinephrine in hypotension associated with mastocytosis. *J Allergy Clin Immunol*, 1983; **71**: 189–92.
26. Casassus P, Caillat-Vigneron N, Martin A, Simon J, Gallais V, Beaudry P, *et al.* Treatment of adult systemic mastocytosis with interferon-alpha: results of a multicentre phase II trial on 20 patients. *Br J Haematol*, 2002; **119**: 1090–7.

27. Kluin-Nelemans HC, Oldhoff JM, Van Doormaal JJ, Van't Wout JW, Verhoef G, Gerrits WB, *et al.* Cladribine therapy for systemic mastocytosis. *Blood*, 2003; **102**: 4270–6.
28. Hennessy B, Giles F, Cortes J, O'Brien S, Ferrajoli A, Ossa G, *et al.* Management of patients with systemic mastocytosis: review of M.D. Anderson Cancer Center experience. *Am J Hematol*, 2004; **77**: 209–14.
29. Demetri GD, von Mehren M, Blanke CD, Van den Abbeele AD, Eisenberg B, Roberts PJ, *et al.* Efficacy and safety of imatinib mesylate in advance gastrointestinal stromal tumors. *N Engl J Med*, 2002; **347**: 472–80.
30. Musto P, Falcone A, Sanpaolo G, Bodenizza C, Carella AM. Inefficacy of imatinib-mesylate in sporadic, aggressive systemic mastocytosis. *Leuk Res*, 2004; **28**: 421–2.
31. Ma Y, Zeng S, Metcalfe DD, Akin C, Dimitrijevic S, Butterfield JH, *et al.* The c-kit mutation causing human mastocytosis is resistant to sti571 and other kit kinase inhibitors; kinases with enzymatic site mutation show different inhibitor sensitivity profiles than wild-type kinases and those with regulatory-type mutation. *Blood*, 2002; **99**: 1741–4.
32. Shah NP, Lee FY, Luo R, Jiang Y, Donker M, Akin C. Dasatinib (BMS-354825) inhibits KITD816V, an imatinib-resistant activating mutation that triggers neoplastic growth in most patients with systemic mastocytosis. *Blood*, 2006; **108**: 286–91.
33. Gotlib J, Berube C, Growney JD, Chen C, George TI, Williams C, *et al.* Activity of the tyrosine kinase inhibitor PKC412 in a patient with mast cell leukaemia with the D816V KIT mutation. *Blood*, 2005; **106**: 2865–70.

6.11

Multiple endocrine neoplasia type 1

R.V. Thakker

Introduction

Multiple endocrine neoplasia (1, 2) is characterized by the occurrence of tumours involving two or more endocrine glands within a single patient. The disorder has previously been referred to as multiple endocrine adenopathy (MEA) or the pluriglandular syndrome. However, glandular hyperplasia and malignancy may also occur in some patients and the term multiple endocrine neoplasia (MEN) is now preferred. There are two major forms of multiple endocrine neoplasia, referred to as type 1 and type 2, and each form is characterized by the development of tumours within specific endocrine glands (Table 6.11.1). Thus, the combined occurrence of tumours of the parathyroid glands, the pancreatic islet cells, and the anterior pituitary is characteristic of multiple endocrine neoplasia type 1 (MEN 1), which is also referred to as Wermer's syndrome. However, in multiple endocrine neoplasia type 2 (MEN 2), which is also called Sipple's syndrome, medullary thyroid carcinoma (MTC) occurs in association with phaeochromocytoma, and three clinical variants, referred to as MEN 2a, MEN 2b and MTC-only, are recognized (Table 6.11.1). Although MEN 1 and MEN 2 usually occur as distinct and separate syndromes as outlined above, some patients occasionally may develop tumours that are associated with both MEN 1 and MEN 2. For example, patients suffering from islet cell tumours of the pancreas and phaeochromocytomas or from acromegaly and phaeochromocytoma have been described, and these patients may represent 'overlap' syndromes. All these forms of MEN may either be inherited as autosomal dominant syndromes or they may occur sporadically, i.e. without a family history. However, this distinction between sporadic and familial cases may sometimes be difficult as in some sporadic cases the family history may be absent because the parent with the disease may have died before developing symptoms. In this chapter, the main clinical features and molecular genetics of the MEN 1 syndrome will be discussed.

Clinical features of MEN 1

Parathyroid, pancreatic, and pituitary tumours constitute the major components of MEN 1 (Fig. 6.11.1). In addition to these tumours adrenal cortical, carcinoid, facial angiofibromas, collagenomas, and lipomatous tumours may also occur in some patients (2, 3).

Parathyroid tumours

Primary hyperparathyroidism is the most common feature of MEN 1 and occurs in more than 95% of all MEN 1 patients (1, 3). Patients may present with asymptomatic hypercalcaemia, or nephrolithiasis, or osteitis fibrosa cystica, or vague symptoms associated with hypercalcaemia, for example polyuria, polydipsia, constipation, malaise, or occasionally with peptic ulcers. Biochemical investigations reveal hypercalcaemia, usually in association with raised circulating parathyroid hormone concentrations. The hypercalcaemia is usually mild, and severe hypercalcaemia resulting in crisis or parathyroid carcinoma are rare occurrences. Additional differences in the primary hyperparathyroidism of MEN 1 patients from that in non-MEN 1 patients include an earlier age of onset (20 to 25 years versus 55 years), and an equal male:female ratio (1:1 versus 1:3). Primary hyperparathyroidism in MEN 1 patients is unusual before the age of 15 years, and the age of conversion from being unaffected to affected has been observed to be between 20 and 21 years in some individuals (3). No effective medical treatment for primary hyperparathyroidism is generally available and surgical removal of the abnormally overactive parathyroids is the definitive treatment. However, all four parathyroid glands are usually affected with multiple adenomas or hyperplasia, although this histological distinction may be difficult, and total parathyroidectomy has been proposed as the definitive treatment for primary hyperparathyroidism in MEN 1, with the resultant lifelong hypocalcaemia being treated with oral calcitriol (1,25 dihydroxyvitamin D_3). It is recommended that such total parathyroidectomy should be reserved for the symptomatic hypercalcaemic patient with MEN 1, and that the asymptomatic hypercalcaemic MEN 1 patient should not have parathyroid surgery but have regular assessments for the onset of symptoms and complications, when total parathyroidectomy should be undertaken.

Pancreatic tumours

The incidence of pancreatic islet cell tumours in MEN 1 patients varies from 30 to 80% in different series (1, 3). The majority of these tumours produce excessive amounts of hormone, for example gastrin, insulin, glucagon, or vasoactive intestinal polypeptide (VIP), and are associated with distinct clinical syndromes.

Table 6.11.1 The multiple endocrine neoplasia (MEN) syndromes, their characteristic tumours and associated biochemical abnormalities

Type	Tumours	Biochemical features
MEN 1	Parathyroids	Hypercalcaemia and ↑
	Pancreatic islets	
	Gastrinoma	↑ Gastrin and ↑ basal gastric acid output
	Insulinoma	Hypoglycaemia and ↑ insulin
	Glucagonoma	Glucose intolerance and ↑ glucagon
	VIPoma	↑ VIP and WDHA
	PPoma	↑ PP
	Pituitary (anterior)	
	Prolactinoma	Hyperprolactinaemia
	GH-secreting	↑ GH ↑ IGF1
	ACTH-secreting	Hypercortisolaemia and ↑ ATCH
	Nonfunctioning	Nil or α subunit
	Associated tumours:	
	Adrenal cortical	Hypercortisolaemia or primary hyperaldosteronism
	Carcinoid	↑ 5-HIAA
	Lipoma	Nil
MEN 2a	Medullary thyroid carcinoma	Hypercalcitoninaemia[a]
	Phaeochromocytoma	↑ Catecholamines
	Parathyroid	Hypercalcaemia and ↑
MEN 2b	Medullary thyroid carcinoma	Hypercalcitoninaemia
	Phaeochromocytoma	↑ Catecholamines
	Associated abnormalities:	
	Mucosal neuromas	
	Marfanoid habitus	
	Medullated corneal nerve fibres	
	Megacolon	

Autosomal dominant inheritance of the MEN syndromes has been established.

[a] In some patients, basal serum calcitonin concentrations may be normal, but may show an abnormal rise at 1 min and 5 min after stimulation with pentagastrin, 0.5 µg/kg.

↑, increased; PTH, parathyroid hormone; VIP, vasoactive intestinal peptide; WDHA, watery diarrhoea, hypokalaemia, and achlorhydria; PP, pancreatic polypeptide; GH, growth hormone; IGF1, insulin like growth factor1; ACTH, adrenocorticotrophic hormone; 5-HIAA, 5-hydroxyindoleacetic acid.

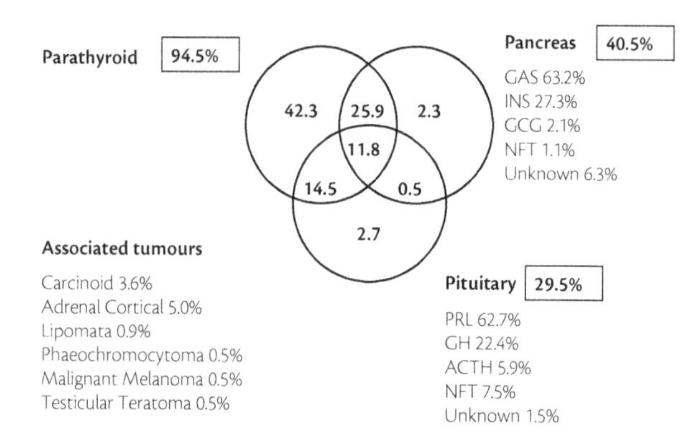

Fig. 6.11.1 Schematic representation of the distribution of 384 MEN 1 tumours in 220 MEN 1 patients. The proportions of patients in whom parathyroid, pancreatic, or pituitary tumours occurred are shown in the respective boxes, e.g. 94.5% of patients had a parathyroid tumour. The Venn diagram indicates the proportions of patients with each combination of tumours, e.g. 37.7% (25.9% + 11.8%) of patients had both a parathyroid and pancreatic tumour, whereas 2.3% of patients had a pancreatic tumour only. In addition to these tumours observed in one series, multiple facial angiofibromas have been observed in 88% of 32 patients, and collagenomas in 72% of patients. The hormones secreted by each of these tumours are indicated: GAS, gastrin; INS, insulin; GCG, glucagon; NFT, nonfunctioning tumours; PRL, prolactin; GH, growth hormone; ACTH, adrenocorticotrophic hormone. Parathyroid tumours represent the most common form of MEN 1 tumours and occur in approximately 95% of patients, with pancreatic islet cell tumours occurring in approximately 40% of patients, and anterior pituitary tumours occurring in approximately 30% of patients. (Reproduced with permission from Trump D, Farren B, Wooding C, Pang JT, Besser GM, Buchanan KD, *et al.* Clinical studies of multiple endocrine neoplasia type 1 (MEN1) in 220 patients. *Q J Med*, 1996; **89**: 653–69 (3).)

Gastrinoma

These gastrin-secreting tumours represent over 50% of all pancreatic islet cell tumours in MEN 1 and approximately 20% of patients with gastrinomas will have MEN 1. Gastrinomas are the major cause of morbidity and mortality in MEN 1 patients. This is due to the recurrent, severe multiple peptic ulcers which may perforate. This association of recurrent peptic ulceration, marked gastric acid production, and non-β-islet cell tumours of the pancreas is referred to as the Zollinger–Ellison syndrome. Additional prominent clinical features of this syndrome include diarrhoea and steatorrhoea. The diagnosis is established by demonstration of a raised fasting serum gastrin concentration in association with an increased basal gastric acid secretion (4). Medical treatment of MEN 1 patients with the Zollinger–Ellison syndrome is directed to reducing basal acid output to less than 10 mmol/l, and this may be achieved by the parietal cell H^+-K^+-ATPase inhibitor, e.g. omeprazole. The ideal treatment for a nonmetastatic gastrinoma is surgical excision of the gastrinoma. However, in patients with MEN 1 the gastrinomas are frequently multiple or extrapancreatic and the role of surgery has been controversial (5). For example, in one study (5), only 16% of MEN 1 patients were free of disease immediately after surgery, and at 5 years this had declined to 6%; the respective outcomes in non-MEN 1 patients were better at 45 and 40%. The treatment of disseminated gastrinomas is difficult and hormonal therapy with human somatostatin analogues, e.g. Octreotide chemotherapy with streptozotocin and 5-fluoroaracil, hepatic artery embolization, and removal of all resectable tumour have all occasionally been successful (1).

Insulinoma

These β-islet cell tumours secreting insulin represent one-third of all pancreatic tumours in MEN 1 patients (1, 3). Insulinomas also occur in association with gastrinomas in 10% of MEN 1 patients, and the two tumours may arise at different times. Insulinomas occur more often in MEN 1 patients who are below the age of 40 years, and many of these arise in individuals before the age of 20 years (3), whereas in non-MEN 1 patients insulinomas generally occur in those above the age of 40 years. Insulinomas may be the

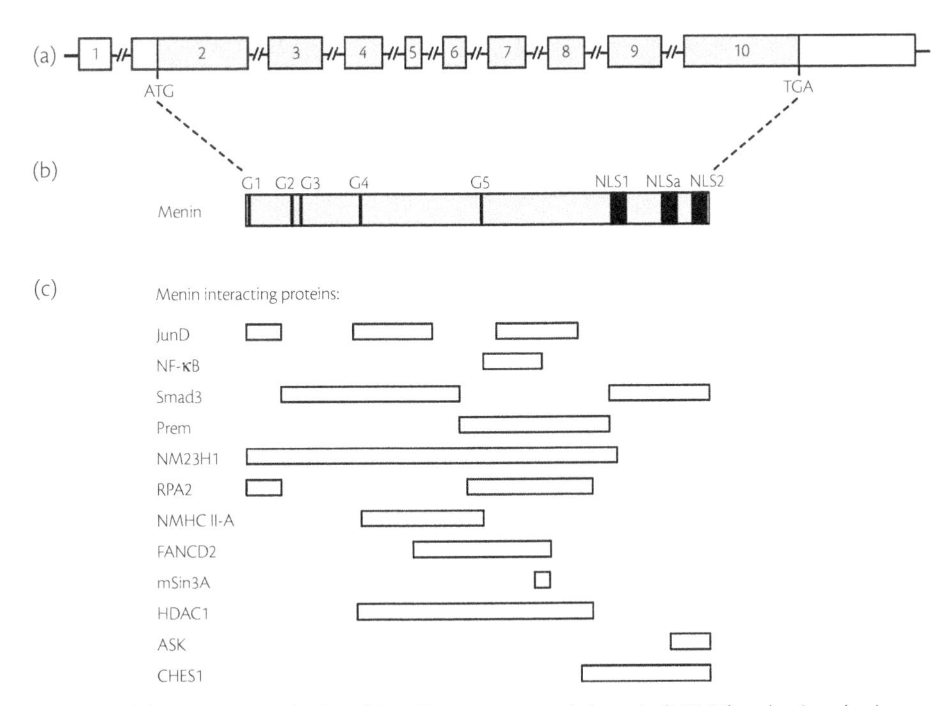

Fig. 6.11.2 Schematic representation of the genomic organization of the *MEN1* gene, its encoded protein (MENIN), and regions that interact with other proteins. (a) The human *MEN1* gene consists of 10 exons that span more than 9 kb of genomic DNA and encodes a 610-amino acid protein. The 1.83 kb coding region (indicated by shaded region) is organized into nine exons (exons 2–10) and eight introns (indicated by a line but not to scale). The sizes of the exons (boxes) range from 41 to 1297 bp, and that of the introns range from 80 to 1564 bp. The start (ATG) and stop (TGA) codons in exons 2 and 10, respectively, are indicated. Exon 1, the 5′ part of exon 2, and the 3′ part of exon 10 are untranslated (indicated by open boxes). The promoter region is located within a few 100 bp upstream of exon 2. (b) MENIN has three nuclear localization signals (NLSs) at codons 479–497 (NLS1), 546–572 (NLSa), and 588–608 (NLS2), indicated by closed boxes, and five putative guanosine triphosphatase (GTPase) sites (G1–G5) indicated by closed bars. (c) MENIN regions that have been implicated in the binding to different interacting proteins are indicated by open boxes. These are JunD (codons 1–40, 139–242, 323–428); nuclear factor-kappa B (NF-κB) (codons 305–381); Smad3 (codons 40–278, 477–610); placenta and embryonic expression, Pem (codons 278–476); NM23H1 (codons 1–486); a subunit of replication protein A (RPA2) (codons 1–40, 286–448); NMHC II-A (codons 154–306); FANCD2 (codons 219–395); mSin3A (codons 371–387); HDAC1 (codons 145–450); ASK (codons 558–610), and CHES1 (codons 428–610). The regions of MENIN that interact with GFAP, vimentin, Smad 1/5, Runx2, MLL-histone methyltransferase complex, and oestrogen receptor-α remain to be determined. (Reproduced with permission from Lemos M, Thakker RV. Multiple endocrine neoplasia type 1 (MEN1): analysis of 1336 mutations reported in the first decade following identification of the gene. *Hum Mutat*, 2008; **29**: 22–32 (16).)

first manifestation of MEN 1 in 10% of patients and approximately 4% of patients presenting with insulinoma will have MEN 1. Patients with an insulinoma present with hypoglycaemic symptoms, which develop after a fast or exertion and improve after glucose intake. Biochemical investigations reveal raised plasma insulin concentrations in association with hypoglycaemia. Circulating concentrations of C-peptide and proinsulin, which are also raised, may be useful in establishing the diagnosis, as may an insulin suppression test. Medical treatment, which consists of frequent carbohydrate feeds and diazoxide, may be useful in the short-term, with surgery being the definitive treatment. Most insulinomas are multiple and small and preoperative localization with computed tomography scanning, coeliac axis angiography, and preoperative percutaneous transhepatic portal venous sampling is difficult and success rates have varied. Surgical treatment, which ranges from enucleation of a single tumour to a distal pancreatectomy or partial pancreatectomy, has been curative in some patients. Chemotherapy, which consists of streptozotocin or octreotide, is used for metastatic disease.

Glucagonoma

These α-islet cell, glucagon-secreting pancreatic tumours occur in less than 3% of MEN 1 patients (1, 3). The characteristic clinical manifestations of a skin rash (necrolytic migratory erythyema), weight loss, anaemia, and stomatitis may be absent and the presence of the tumour is indicated only by glucose intolerance and hyperglucagonaemia. The tail of the pancreas is the most frequent site for glucagonomas and surgical removal of these is the treatment of choice. However, treatment may be difficult as 50% of patients have metastases at the time of diagnosis. Medical treatment of these with somatostatin analogues, or with streptozotocin has been successful in some patients.

VIPoma

Patients with VIPomas, which are VIP-secreting pancreatic tumours, develop watery diarrhoea, hypokalaemia, and achlorhydria, referred to as the WDHA syndrome. This clinical syndrome has also been referred to as the Verner–Morrison syndrome or the VIPoma syndrome. VIPomas have been reported in only a few MEN 1 patients and the diagnosis is established by documenting a markedly raised plasma VIP concentration (1). Surgical management of VIPomas, which are mostly located in the tail of the pancreas, has been curative. However, in patients with unresectable tumour, treatment with somatostatin analogues, streptozotocin, corticosteroids, indomethicin, metoclopramide, and lithium carbonate has proved beneficial.

PPoma

These tumours, which secrete pancreatic polypeptide (PP) are found in a large number of patients with MEN 1 (1, 6). No pathological sequelae of excessive pancreatic polypeptide secretion are apparent and the clinical significance of pancreatic polypeptide is unknown, although the use of serum pancreatic polypeptide measurements has been suggested for the detection of pancreatic tumours in MEN 1 patients.

Pituitary tumours

The incidence of pituitary tumours in MEN 1 patients varies from 15 to 90% in different series (1, 3). Approximately 60% of MEN 1 associated pituitary tumours secrete prolactin, less than 25% secrete growth hormone, 5% secrete ACTH, and the remainder appear to be nonfunctioning. Prolactinomas may be the first manifestation of MEN 1 in less than 10% of patients and somatotrophinomas occur more often in patients over the age of 40 years (3). Less than 3% of patients with anterior pituitary tumours will have MEN 1. The clinical manifestations depend upon the size of the pituitary tumour and its product of secretion. Enlarging pituitary tumours may compress adjacent structures such as the optic chiasm or normal pituitary tissue and cause bitemporal hemianopia or hypopituitarism, respectively. The tumour size and extension are radiologically assessed by CT scanning and MRI. Treatment of pituitary tumours in MEN 1 patients is similar to that in non-MEN 1 patients and consists of medical therapy or selective hypophysectomy by the transphenoidal approach if feasible, with radiotherapy being reserved for residual unresectable tumour.

Associated tumours

Patients with MEN 1 may have tumours involving glands other than the parathyroids, pancreas, and pituitary. Thus carcinoid, adrenal cortical, facial angiofibromas, collagenomas, thyroid, and lipomatous tumours have been described in association with MEN 1 (1, 3).

Carcinoid tumours

Carcinoid tumours, which occur in more than 3% of patients with MEN 1, may be inherited as an autosomal dominant trait in association with MEN 1. The carcinoid tumour may be located in the bronchi, the gastrointestinal tract, the pancreas, or the thymus (7). Bronchial carcinoids in MEN 1 patients predominantly occur in women (M:F = 1:4) whereas thymic carcinoids predominantly occur in men, with cigarette smokers having a higher risk of developing tumours. Most patients are asymptomatic and do not suffer from the flushing attacks and dyspnoea associated with the carcinoid syndrome, which usually develops after the tumour has metastasized to the liver. Somatostatin analogues have been successfully used to treat symptoms and may in some patients result in regression of gastric carcinoids (8).

Adrenal cortical tumours

The incidence of asymptomatic adrenal cortical tumours in MEN 1 patients has been reported to be as high as 40% (9). The majority of these tumours are nonfunctioning. However, functioning adrenal cortical tumours in MEN 1 patients have been documented to cause hypercortisolaemia and Cushing's syndrome, and primary hyperaldosteronism, as in Conn's syndrome (1, 3).

Lipomas

Lipomas may occur in more than 33% of patients (2, 10), and frequently they are multiple. In addition, pleural or retroperitoneal lipomas may also occur in patients with MEN 1.

Thyroid tumours

Thyroid tumours consisting of adenomas, colloid goitres, and carcinomas have been reported to occur in over 25% of MEN 1 patients (1, 2). However, the prevalence of thyroid disorders in the general population is high and it has been suggested that the association of thyroid abnormalities in MEN 1 patients may be incidental and not significant.

Facial angiofibromas and collagenomas

Multiple facial angiofibromas, which are similar to those observed in patients with tuberous sclerosis, have been observed in 88% of MEN 1 patients (2, 10) and collagenomas have been reported in over 70% of MEN 1 patients (2, 10).

Genetics

The gene causing MEN 1 was localized to chromosome 11q13 by genetic mapping studies that investigated MEN 1 associated tumours for loss of heterozygosity (LOH) and by segregation studies in MEN 1 families (11, 12). The results of these studies, which were consistent with Knudson's model for tumour development (13), indicated that the *MEN1* gene represented a putative tumour suppressor gene. Further genetic mapping studies defined a less than 300-Kb region as the minimal critical segment that contained the *MEN1* gene and characterization of genes from this region led to the identification, in 1997, of the *MEN1* gene (14, 15), which consists of 10 exons with a 1830-bp coding region (Fig. 6.11.2) that encodes a novel 610-amino acid protein, referred to as 'MENIN' (14). Over 1100 germline and over 200 somatic mutations of the *MEN1* gene have been identified, and the majority (>70%) of these are inactivating, and are consistent with its role as a tumour suppressor gene (16). These mutations are diverse in their types and approximately 25% are nonsense mutations, approximately 40% are frameshift deletions or insertions, approximately 5% are in-frame deletions or insertions, approximately 10% are splice site mutations, approximately 20% are missense mutations, and less than 1% are whole or partial gene deletions. More than 10% of the *MEN1* mutations arise *de novo* and may be transmitted to subsequent generations (16–18). It is also important to note that between 5% and 10% of MEN 1 patients may not harbour mutations in the coding region of the *MEN1* gene (16), and that these individuals may have mutations in the promoter or untranslated regions, which remain to be investigated. The mutations are not only diverse in their types but are also scattered throughout the 1830-bp coding region of the *MEN1* gene with no evidence for clustering as observed in MEN 2 (see Chapter 6.12). Correlations between the *MEN1* mutations and the clinical manifestations of the disorder appear to be absent (16). Tumours from MEN 1 patients and non-MEN 1 patients have been observed to harbour the germ line mutation together with a somatic LOH involving chromosome 11q13, as expected from Knudson's model and the proposed role of the *MEN1* gene as a tumour suppressor (16). MENIN has been shown to have three nuclear localization sites (NLSs) and to be located predominantly in the nucleus (16, 19).

Studies of protein–protein interactions have revealed that MENIN interacts with several proteins involved in transcriptional regulation, genome stability, cell division, and proliferation (Fig. 6.11.2) (16). Thus, in transcriptional regulation, MENIN has been shown to interact with: the activating protein-1 transcription factor JunD and to suppress Jun-mediated transcriptional activation members (e.g. p50, p52, and p65) of the NF-κB family of transcriptional regulators to repress NF-κB-mediated transcriptional activation; members of the Smad family, Smad3 and the Smad 1/5 complex, which are involved in the transforming growth factor-β (TGFβ) and the bone morphogenetic protein-2 (BMP-2) signalling pathways, respectively; Runx2, also called cbfa1, which is a common target of TGFβ and BMP-2 in differentiating osteoblasts; and the mouse placental embryonic (*Pem*) expression gene, which encodes a homeobox-containing protein. Additional studies have shown that the interaction of MENIN with JunD may be mediated by a histone deacetylase-dependent mechanism, via recruitment of an mSin3A-histone deacetylase complex to repress JunD transcriptional activity. Recently, the forkhead transcription factor CHES1 has been shown to be a component of this transcriptional repressor complex and to interact with MENIN in an S-phase checkpoint pathway related to DNA damage response. MENIN uncouples ELK-1, JunD, and c-Jun phosphorylation from mitogen-activated protein kinase (MAPK) activation and suppresses insulin-induced c-Jun-mediated transactivation in CHO-1R cells (16).

A wider role in transcription regulation has also been suggested, as MENIN has been shown to be an integral component of histone methyltransferase complexes that contain members from the mixed-lineage leukaemia (MLL) and trithorax protein family. These can methylate the lysine 4 residue of histone H3 (H3K4) and H3K4 trimethylation is linked to activation of transcription. MENIN, as a component of this MLL complex, regulates the expression of genes such as the *Hox* homeobox genes and the genes for cyclin-dependent kinase inhibitors, p27 and p18. MENIN has been shown to directly interact with the nuclear receptor for oestrogen (ERα) and to act as a coactivator for ERα–mediated transcription, linking the activated oestrogen receptor to histone H3K4 trimethylation. MENIN has also been shown to bind to a broad range of gene promoters, independently of the histone methyltransferase complex, suggesting that MENIN functions as a general transcriptional regulator that helps maintain stable gene expression, perhaps by cooperating with other, currently unknown, proteins. MENIN also directly binds to doubled-stranded DNA and this is mediated by the positively charged residues in the NLSs in the carboxyl terminus of MENIN. The NLSs appear to be necessary for MENIN to repress the expression of the insulin-like growth factor binding protein-2 (IGFBP-2) gene by binding to the IGFBP-2 promoter. In addition, each of the NLSs has also been reported to be involved in MENIN-mediated induction of caspase 8 expression. The NLSs may therefore have roles in controlling gene transcription as well as targeting MENIN into the nucleus (16).

A role for MENIN in controlling genome stability (16) has been proposed because of its interactions with: a subunit of replication protein (RPA2), which is a heterotrimeric protein required for DNA replication, recombination, and repair; and the FANCD2 protein, which is involved in DNA repair and mutations of which result in the inherited cancer-prone syndrome of Fanconi's anaemia. MENIN also has a role in regulating cell division as it interacts with: the nonmuscle myosin II-A heavy chain (NMHC II-A), which participates in mediating alterations in cytokinesis and cell shape during cell division and the glial fibrillary acidic protein (GFAP) and vimentin, which are involved in the intermediate filament network. MENIN also has a role in cell cycle control as it interacts with: the tumour metastases suppressor NM23H1/nucleoside diphosphate kinase, which induces guanosine triphosphatase activity and the activator of S-phase kinase (ASK), which is a component of the Cdc7/ASK kinase complex that is crucial for cell proliferation. Indeed, MENIN has been shown to completely repress ASK-induced cell proliferation.

The functional role of MENIN as a tumour suppressor also has been investigated, and studies in human fibroblasts have revealed that MENIN acts as a repressor of telomerase activity via hTERT (a protein component of telomerase) (16). Furthermore, overexpression of MENIN in the human endocrine pancreatic tumour cell line (BON1) resulted in an inhibition of cell growth which was accompanied by up-regulation of JunD expression but down-regulation of delta-like protein 1/preadipocyte factor-1, proliferating cell nuclear antigen, and QM/Jif-1, which is a negative regulator of c-Jun. These findings of growth suppression by MENIN were observed in other cell types. Thus, expression of MENIN in the RAS-transformed NIH3T3 cells partially suppressed the RAS-mediated tumour phenotype *in vitro* and *in vivo*. Overexpression of MENIN in CHO-IR cells also suppressed insulin-induced activating protein-1 transactivation, and this was accompanied by an inhibition of c-Fos induction at the transcriptional level. Furthermore, MENIN re-expression in *Men1*-deficient mouse Leydig tumour cell lines induced cell cycle arrest and apoptosis. In contrast, depletion of MENIN in human fibroblasts resulted in their immortalization. Thus, MENIN appears to have a large number of functions through interactions with proteins, and these mediate alterations in cell proliferation.

Acknowledgements

I am grateful to the Medical Research Council (MRC), UK, for support and to Mrs Tracey Walker for expert secretarial assistance.

References

1. Thakker RV. Multiple endocrine neoplasia type 1 (MEN1). In: DeGroot LJ, Besser GK, Burger HG, Jameson JL, Loriaux DL, Marshall JC, *et al*, eds. *Endocrinology*. Philadelphia: W. B. Saunders, 1995: 2815–31.
2. Marx SJ. Multiple endocrine neoplasia type 1. In: Vogelstein B, Kinzler KW, eds. *Genetic Basis of Human Cancer*. New York: McGraw Hill, 1998: 489–506.
3. Trump D, Farren B, Wooding C, Pang JT, Besser GM, Buchanan KD, *et al*. Clinical studies of multiple endocrine neoplasia type 1 (MEN1) in 220 patients. *Q J Med*, 1996; **89**: 653–69.
4. Wolfe MM, Jensen RT. Zollinger-Ellison syndrome. Current concepts in diagnosis and management. *N Engl J Med*, 1987; **317**: 1200–9.
5. Norton JA, Fraker DL, Alexander R, *et al*. Surgery to cure the Zollinger-Ellison syndrome. *N Engl J Med*, 1999; **341**: 635–44.
6. Skogseid B, Oberg K, Benson L, Lindgren PS, Lörelius LE, Lundquist G, *et al*. A standardized meal stimulation test of the endocrine pancreas for early detection of pancreatic endocrine tumours in Multiple endocrine Neoplasia Type 1 syndrome: Five years experience. *J Clin Endocrinol Metabol*, 1987; **64**: 1233–40.
7. Teh BT, Zedenius J, Kytola S, Skogseid B, Trotter J, Choplin H, *et al*. Thymic carcinoids in multiple endocrine neoplasia type 1. *Ann Surg*, 1998; **228**: 99–105.

8. Tomassetti P, Migliori M, Caletti GC, Fusaroli P, Corinaldesi R, Gullo L. Treatment of type II gastric carcinoid tumours with somatostatin analogues. *N Engl J Med*, 2000; **343**: 551–4.
9. Skogseid B, Larsson C, Lindgren PG, Kvanta E, Rastad J, Theodorsson E, *et al.* Clinical and genetic features of adrenocortical lesions in multiple endocrine neoplasia type 1. *J Clin Endocrinol Metabol*, 1992; **75**: 76–81.
10. Darling TN, Skarulis MC, Steinberg SM, Marx SJ, Spiegel AM, Turner M. Multiple facial angiofibromas and collagenomas in patients with multiple endocrine neoplasia type 1. *Arch Dermatol*, 1997; **133**: 853–61.
11. Larsson C, Skogseid B, Oberg K, Nakamura Y, Nordenskjold MC. Multiple endocrine neoplasia type I gene maps to chromosome 11 and is lost in insulinoma. *Nature*, 1988; **332**: 85–7.
12. Thakker RV. The molecular genetics of the multiple endocrine neoplasia syndromes. *Clin Endocrinol*, 1993; **39**: 1–14.
13. Knudson AG. Antioncogenes and human cancer. *Proc Natl Acad Sci U S A*, 1993; **90**: 10914–21.
14. Chandrasekharappa SC, Guru SC, Manickam P, Olufemi S-E, Collins FS, Emmert-Buck MR, *et al.* Positional cloning of the gene for multiple endocrine neoplasia-type 1. *Science*, 1997; **276**: 404–7.
15. The European Consortium on MEN1. Identification of the multiple endocrine neoplasia type 1 (MEN1) gene. *Hum Mol Genet*, 1997; **6**: 1177–83.
16. Lemos M, Thakker RV. Multiple endocrine neoplasia type 1 (MEN1): analysis of 1336 mutations reported in the first decade following identification of the gene. *Hum Mutat*, 2008; **29**: 22–32.
17. Agarwal SK, Kester MB, Deblenko LV, Heppner C, Emmert-Buck MR, Skarulis MC, *et al.* Germline mutations of the MEN1 gene in familial multiple endocrine neoplasia type 1 and related states. *Hum Mol Genet*, 1997; **6**: 1169–75.
18. Bassett JHD, Forbes SA, Pannett AAJ, Lloyd SE, Christie PT, Wooding C, *et al.* Characterisation of mutations in patients with multiple endocrine neoplasia type 1 (MEN1). *Am J Hum Genet*, 1998; **62**: 232–44.
19. Guru SC, Goldsmith PK, Burns AL, Marx SJ, Spiegel AM, Collins FS, *et al.* MENIN, the product of the *MEN1* gene, is a nuclear protein. *Proc Natl Acad Sci U S A*, 1998; **95**: 1630–4.

6.12

Multiple endocrine neoplasia type 2

Niamh M. Martin, Karim Meeran, Stephen R. Bloom

Introduction

Multiple endocrine neoplasia type 2 (MEN 2) is a rare cancer susceptibility syndrome which has at least three distinct variants: MEN 2A, MEN 2B, and familial medullary thyroid carcinoma (FMTC). The syndrome was first described by John Sipple in 1961 (1). The features of MEN 2A and its clinical variants are outlined in Box 6.12.1. Medullary thyroid carcinoma (MTC) is seen in all variants of MEN 2A and is frequently the earliest neoplastic manifestation, reflecting its earlier and overall higher penetrance. MEN 2 is due to the autosomal dominant inheritance of a germline missense mutation in the 'hotspot' regions of the rearranged during transfection (*RET*) (OMIM 164761) proto-oncogene (2, 3). MEN 2 has an estimated prevalence of 1:30000, with MEN 2A accounting for more than 75% of cases. The introduction of *RET* screening in family members of affected individuals has significantly altered the clinical outcome of MEN 2, by allowing prophylactic surgery for MTC, and screening enabling early intervention for phaeochromocytoma (4, 5). Prior to the availability of genetic screening, more that half of MEN 2 affected individuals died before or during the fifth decade from metastatic MTC or cardiovascular complications from an underlying phaeochromocytoma.

Clinical variants of MEN 2

MEN 2A is characterized by MTC, unilateral or bilateral phaeochromocytoma, and primary hyperparathyroidism, due to parathyroid cell hyperplasia or adenomas. Rare variants include MEN 2A with cutaneous lichen amyloidosis, a pruritic cutaneous rash over the upper back, and MEN 2A associated with Hirschsprung's disease, characterized by the absence of autonomic ganglion cells within the distal colonic parasympathetic plexus. In FMTC, MTC is the only clinical manifestation and this diagnosis requires more than 10 carriers in the kindred, multiple carriers or affected members over the age of 50 years, and an adequate medical history, especially in family members (4). These strict criteria attempt to prevent incorrect diagnosis of FMTC rather than MEN 2A and hence avoid the potentially catastrophic effects of failing to screen for a phaeochromocytoma. MEN 2B is the most aggressive MEN 2 variant and is characterized by MTC and phaeochromocytomas, but not primary hyperparathyroidism. Affected individuals may exhibit mucosal neuromas (lips, tongue, gastrointestinal tract) and skeletal abnormalities including a marfanoid habitus and kyphoscoliosis. In contrast to patients with Marfan's syndrome, MEN 2B patients do not exhibit lens or aortic abnormalities.

Molecular genetics

The *RET* gene is situated on the pericentromeric region of chromosome 10 and has 20 exons. It encodes for the transmembrane RET receptor tyrosine kinase, expressed by cells derived from the neural crest. This receptor comprises an extracellular region which includes four cadherin-like domains, a calcium-binding site and a cysteine-rich domain, a transmembrane region, and an intracellular component containing at least two tyrosine kinase domains (Fig. 6.12.1). The extracellular domain is important for receptor dimerization and cross-phosphorylation whereas the intracellular tyrosine kinase domains affect adenosine triphosphate binding. Several functional ligands of RET have been identified, including glial cell line-derived neurotrophic factor (GDNF). These ligands, in association with the extracellular protein GDNF receptor α-1 (GFRα-1), bind to the extracellular RET receptor domain, inducing a homodimerization of RET molecules and a specific activation of the intracellular tyrosine kinase domain.

Whereas *RET* mutations associated with nonsyndromic Hirschprung's disease arise from loss of function mutations, *RET* gain of function mutations in tyrosine signalling are associated with MEN 2 (6). The exact sequence of molecular events directing the transition from normal to hyperplasia to tumour is unclear. Oncogenic activation of the RET receptor due to germline mutations of *RET* are likely to initiate events as an inherited 'first hit', resulting in C cell and adrenal medullary hyperplasia. Progression to MTC and phaeochromocytoma requires second somatic 'hits' in activated C cells and adrenal medullary cells. The higher penetrance of MTC compared to phaeochromocytoma or parathyroid hyperplasia/ adenoma within MEN 2 suggests increased susceptibility of C-cell *RET* activation compared to adrenal medullary or parathyroid cells (7).

Genotype–phenotype correlation

Unlike MEN 1, strong genotype–phenotype correlations exist within MEN 2 such that there are clear associations between mutations at specific codons and MEN 2 subtypes (4). Mutations

Box 6.12.1 Clinical features of MEN 2 with estimated prevalence in parentheses

- **MEN 2A** (75% of all MEN 2 cases)
  - MTC (99%)
  - Phaeochromocytoma (>50%)
  - Parathyroid hyperplasia/adenoma (15–30%)
  - MEN 2A with cutaneous lichen amyloidosis
  - MEN 2A/FMTC with Hirschsprung's disease
- **FMTC** (20% of all MEN 2 cases)
  - MTC is sole manifestation
- **MEN 2B** (5% of all MEN 2 cases)
  - MTC (100%)
  - Phaeochromocytoma (40–50%)
  - Intestinal ganglioneuromatosis and mucosal neuromas (40%)
  - Marfanoid habitus

MTC, medullary thyroid carcinoma; FMTC, familial medullary thyroid carcinoma.

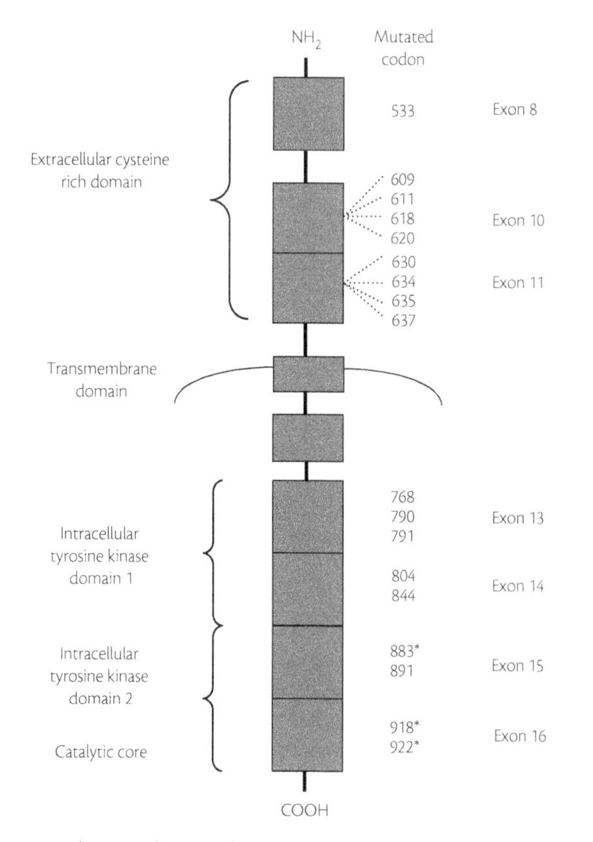

Fig. 6.12.1 Schematic diagram of RET tyrosine kinase receptor. *RET* mutations at codons marked with an asterisk are associated with the most aggressive forms of medullary thyroid carcinoma and a prophylactic thyroidectomy at 6–12 months of age is recommended.

clustered in the cysteine-rich extracellular domain (codons 609, 611, 618, 620, 630, and 634) are the primary causative factor in approximately 98% of cases of MEN 2A. Since these highly conserved cysteines are important for receptor dimerization, mutations result in ligand-independent dimerization and activation of the RET receptor complex (7). Mutations in the intracellular tyrosine kinase domain (codons 768, 790, and 804) are less common, traditionally associated with FMTC, and rarely associated with other MEN 2A-related tumours (5). Ninety-five per cent of MEN 2B cases involve a single point mutation leading to the substitution of methionine 918 for a threonine altering the substrate recognition pocket of the catalytic core of the receptor. Reports of the MEN 2A variant associated with cutaneous lichen amyloidosis all describe mutations in codon 634. MEN 2A-Hirschprung disease variants are associated with mutations in codons 609, 618, and 620 (6).

Clinical management of medullary thyroid cancer in MEN 2

MTC arises from the parafollicular C cells of the thyroid. These neuroendocrine cells are derived from the neural crest and secrete calcitonin. Most patients with MTC have sporadic (nonfamilial) disease and 25–30% of cases of MTC are associated with MEN 2. In patients with MEN 2, MTC is usually bilateral and multifocal and C-cell hyperplasia represents the premalignant precursor of MTC. The aggressiveness of MEN 2-associated MTC depends on the variant of MTC, with MEN 2B being associated with the most aggressive forms. This variability reflects the underlying mutated *RET* codon. Presentation of MTC may be with a neck mass, or symptoms from distant metastases in association with elevated calcitonin (diarrhoea, flushing, weight loss, or bone pain). Circulating calcitonin concentrations, either basal or stimulated following pentagastrin administration, may be used as a tumour marker to detect MTC or to monitor disease progression or recurrence following surgery. However, biochemical screening for diagnosis of MTC in MEN 2 by measuring basal or stimulated calcitonin is largely obsolete due to the widespread availability and high diagnostic accuracy of genetic screening for *RET* mutations (4). Cross-sectional imaging of MTC using CT or MRI may be useful when planning surgery and metastatic disease can be detected using radioisotopes including ^{131}I-metaiodobenzylguanidine (MIBG) and pentavalent ^{99m}Tc-dimercaptosiuccininc acid (8).

Surgery represents prevention or cure in MTC and timing of prophylactic thyroidectomy is dictated by the underlying *RET* mutation. The major prognostic factor is tumour stage at presentation and, hence, early surgical intervention before cervical lymph node metastases appear is necessary to improve survival. Predictive genetic testing of members of MEN 2 families has enabled presymptomatic individuals at risk of developing MTC to be identified and a prophylactic thyroidectomy to be performed. *RET* mutations have been categorized as highest, high, and least risk in terms of guiding appropriate timing of thyroidectomy (4, 5). Patients with the highest risk mutations (codons 883, 918, or 922) should have a total thyroidectomy with central compartment node dissection performed between 6 and 12 months of age. In those with high-risk *RET* mutations, in codons 609, 611, 618, 620, 630, and 634, prophylactic thyroidectomy should be performed by age 5 years. The least risk is associated with *RET* codon mutations 768, 790, 791, 804, and 891, where surgery should be performed between age 5 and 10 years. MTC is not radiosensitive and standard chemotherapy regimens are of limited benefit. A recent development is targeted oncoprotein-specific therapy in the form of tyrosine kinase inhibitors and clinical trials are underway to ascertain their efficacy (9).

Clinical management of phaeochromocytoma in MEN 2

Phaeochromocytomas occur in approximately 50% of MEN 2A or 2B patients. These are usually benign, but are bilateral in up to 80% of cases and invariably arise from the adrenal medulla. In 25% of cases, phaeochromocytoma is the first clinical manifestation of MEN 2, compared to MTC in 40%. The highest risk of developing phaeochromocytoma is associated with *RET* mutations in codons 634 or 918 (10). Although certain *RET* mutations are not associated with phaeochromocytomas, these data describe only a small number of patients (11) and therefore, periodic biochemical screening of all *RET* mutation carriers for phaeochromocytoma should be performed from age 5–10 years.

Screening should take the form of urine or plasma metanephrine or catecholamine measurements. Following confirmation of the diagnosis biochemically, localization of the tumour can be carried out using cross-sectional imaging and MIBG scintigraphy (8). Surgical removal is the mainstay of treatment and the first-line choice is a laparoscopic approach if the tumour(s) is amenable to this technique. Some centres advocate the use of cortical sparing adrenalectomy for bilateral disease to reduce the increased mortality associated with bilateral adrenalectomy, which results from adrenal cortical insufficiency. Regular screening postoperatively should be undertaken to assess for recurrence or the development of a contralateral phaeochromocytoma in unilateral disease. Patients should be prepared for surgery using α-blockade, initially using intravenous phenoxybenzamine, and subsequent β-blockade if there are concerns regarding tachycardia. Prior to thyroidectomy, biochemical screening for phaeochromocytoma should be performed to prevent an intraoperative hypertensive crisis secondary to an undiagnosed phaeochromocytoma.

Clinical management of primary hyperparathyroidism in MEN 2

Primary hyperparathyroidism is a feature in approximately 30% of patients with MEN 2 and results from hyperplasia of the parathyroid glands. Adenomas may develop on a background of hyperplasia. Compared to MEN 1, parathyroid disease in MEN 2A is usually milder and has a later onset. Diagnosis is made by demonstrating hypercalcaemia in the context of an inappropriately normal or elevated parathyroid hormone level. In view of multigland involvement, a common surgical approach is removal of three and a half parathyroid glands.

RET mutation testing for MEN 2 carrier determination

In view of the clear associations between specific *RET* mutations and the potential risk for local and distant metastases from MTC at an early age, *RET* mutation testing allows guidance regarding timing of prophylactic thyroidectomy (4, 12) (see above, Clinical Management of Medullary Thyroid Cancer in MEN 2). *RET* mutational analysis should be initially performed in a family member known to have MEN 2 to determine the specific *RET* mutation for that family. Ninety-eight per cent of MEN 2 index cases have an identifiable *RET* mutation. Therefore, following the likely identification of the *RET* mutation in the index case, all members of that family of unknown *RET* status should be subsequently definitively genotyped. RET genotyping requires only a small volume of blood and can therefore be performed at birth or shortly after.

Approximately 98% *RET* mutations predisposing to MEN 2A and of 80% of FMTC are confined to exons 10 and 11. The majority of MEN 2B cases are associated with mutations in exon 16. However, as genetic analysis has become more common place in screening for *RET* mutations, cases of FMTC–MEN 2A have also been described associated with mutations in exons 8, 13, 14, and 15. Therefore, if a *RET* mutation in a family is unknown, it is important that if exons 10, 11, and 16 are negative, sequencing of exons 8, 13, 14, and 15 should be performed.

Conclusion

Since the discovery more than a decade ago that germline mutations in the *RET* proto-oncogene are associated with MEN 2, the subsequent introduction of genetic screening for *RET* mutations has had a significant impact on the clinical outcome of MEN 2. The clear genotype–phenotype relationship which exists in MEN 2 has enabled the risk stratification of *RET* mutation carriers following genetic screening. This, in turn, has allowed early intervention and potential cure in MTC by guiding prophylactic thyroidectomy and regular screening for development of phaeochromocytoma, once both major causes of death in these individuals. It is hoped that the future will see targeted molecular therapies to improve outcome in those previously unscreened individuals who are diagnosed with disease manifestations of MEN 2.

References

1. Sipple JH. The association of phaeochromocytoma with carcinoma of the thyroid gland. *Am J Med*, 1961; **31**: 163–6.
2. Donis-Keller H, Dou S, Chi D, Carlson KM, Toshima K, Lairmore TC, *et al.* Mutations in the RET proto-oncogene are associated with MEN 2A and FMTC. *Hum Mol Genet*, 1993; **2**: 851–6.
3. Mulligan LM, Kwok JB, Healey CS, Elsdon MJ, Eng C, Gardner E, *et al.* Germ-line mutations of the RET proto-oncogene in multiple endocrine neoplasia type 2A. *Nature*, 1993; **363**: 458–60.
4. Brandi ML, Gagel RF, Angeli A, Bilezikian JP, Beck-Peccoz P, Bordi C, *et al.* Guidelines for diagnosis and therapy of MEN type 1 and type 2. *J Clin Endocrinol Metab*, 2001; **86**: 5658–71.
5. Machens A, Dralle H. Genotype-phenotype based surgical concept of hereditary medullary thyroid carcinoma. *World J Surg*, 2007; **31**: 957–68.
6. Moore SW, Zaahl MG. Multiple endocrine neoplasia syndromes, children, Hirschsprung's disease and RET. *Pediatr Surg Int*, 2008; **24**: 521–30.
7. Machens A, Dralle H. Multiple endocrine neoplasia type 2 and the RET protooncogene: from bedside to bench to bedside. *Mol Cell Endocrinol*, 2006; **247**: 34–40.
8. Scarsbrook AF, Thakker RV, Wass JA, Gleeson FV, Phillips RR. Multiple endocrine neoplasia: spectrum of radiologic appearances and discussion of a multitechnique imaging approach. *Radiographics*, 2006; **26**: 433–51.
9. Lewis CE, Yeh MW. Inherited endocrinopathies: an update. *Mol Genet Metab*, 2008; **94**: 271–82.
10. Machens A, Brauckhoff M, Holzhausen HJ, Thanh PN, Lehnert H, Dralle H. Codon-specific development of pheochromocytoma in multiple endocrine neoplasia type 2. *J Clin Endocrinol Metab*, 2005; **90**: 3999–4003.
11. Jimenez C, Gagel RF. Genetic testing in endocrinology: lessons learned from experience with multiple endocrine neoplasia type 2 (MEN2). *Growth Horm IGF Res*, 2004; **14** (Suppl. A): S150–7.
12. Marini F, Falchetti A, Del Monte F, Carbonell Sala S, Tognarini I, Luzi E, *et al.* Multiple endocrine neoplasia type 2. *Orphanet J Rare Dis*, 2006; **1**: 45.

6.13

von Hippel–Lindau disease and succinate dehydrogenase subunit (*SDHB*, *SDHC*, and *SDHD*) genes

Eamonn R. Maher

Introduction

This chapter considers the clinical and molecular features of von Hippel–Lindau (VHL) disease (OMIM 193300) and mutations in succinate dehydrogenase subunit genes (*SDHB* (OMIM 115310), *SDHC* (OMIM 605373), and *SDHD* (OMIM 168000)). Both disorders are important causes of phaeochromocytoma and, in addition to having overlapping clinical phenotypes, also share some similarities in mechanisms of tumourigenesis.

von Hippel–Lindau disease

VHL is a dominantly inherited familial cancer syndrome with multisystem involvement. The most frequent features are retinal and central nervous system haemangioblastomas, renal cell carcinoma (RCC), and renal, pancreatic, and epididymal cysts (1). The most important endocrine complications are phaeochromocytoma and pancreatic islet cell tumours.

Clinical features and management of VHL disease

The earliest features of VHL disease are usually retinal or central nervous system haemangioblastomas (CHB) (Table 6.13.1 and Fig. 6.13.1) (4). However there is marked phenotypic variability. Thus phaeochromocytoma or RCC can be the presenting feature (5). In such cases the detection of subclinical haemangioblastomas (e.g. retinal by ophthalmological screening, or cerebellar by brain MRI) or the detection of visceral cysts and tumours by abdominal imaging can aid diagnosis. If there is a positive family history, a clinical diagnosis of VHL disease can be made in an at risk individual by the identification of a single retinal or cerebellar haemangioblastoma, RCC, or phaeochromocytoma (6). In isolated cases conventional diagnostic criteria require the presence two or more retinal or cerebellar haemangioblastomas or a single haemangioblastoma and a visceral tumour. However, in many cases molecular genetic testing can allow a diagnosis of VHL disease to be made in patients who do not satisfy clinical diagnostic criteria (7). When a mutation has been identified in a family, other relatives can be tested to determine their mutation status and hence their need for surveillance.

Endocrine tumours

There are marked interfamilial differences in phaeochromocytoma frequency in VHL disease. Thus in some families phaeochromocytoma is the most common manifestation, but in others it is rare. These differences reflect genotype–phenotype correlations and the high risk of phaeochromocytoma associated with certain *VHL* missense mutations. Large deletions, protein truncating mutations, and missense mutations that disrupt protein stability are associated with a high risk of retinal angioma, CHB, and RCC but a low risk of phaeochromocytoma (type 1 VHL phenotype) whereas missense mutations affecting amino acids on the VHL protein (pVHL) surface predominate in VHL patients with phaeochromocytoma (8, 9, 11). However not all phaeochromocytoma-associated missense mutations are equivalent. Most cause a high risk of retinal angioma, CHB, RCC, *and* phaeochromocytoma (type 2B VHL disease), but rare missense mutations may cause type 2A (haemangioblastomas and phaeochromocytoma but rarely RCC) or type 2C (phaeochromocytoma only) phenotypes (3, 5, 10, 11).

The clinical presentation of phaeochromocytoma in VHL disease is similar to that in sporadic cases except that there is a higher frequency of bilateral or multiple tumours and, on average, an earlier onset (mean approximately 30 years) in VHL disease. As with sporadic tumours, phaeochromocytomas in VHL disease may be extra-adrenal and, in about 5% of cases, malignant. Early detection of phaeochromocytoma in VHL disease facilitates management and so screening for phaeochromocytoma should be offered to all VHL patients and at-risk individuals irrespective of whether there is a family history of phaeochromocytoma. However, the presence of a positive family history or a missense mutation known to be associated with a high risk of phaeochromocytoma indicate a need for enhanced phaeochromocytoma surveillance. Patients with apparently nonsyndromic familial or bilateral phaeochromocytoma, or phaeochromocytoma at a young age may have a germline

Table 6.13.1 Clinical frequencies and mean ages at diagnosis of the major complications of von Hippel–Lindau disease (3)

Lesion	Prevalence n = 52	Mean age at diagnosis[a]
Retinal angioma	89 (59%)	25.4 ± 12.7 years (Range: 4–68 years)
Cerebellar haemangioblastoma	89 (59%)	29.0 ± 10.0 years (Range: 13–61 years)
Spinal cord haemangioblastoma	20 (13%)	33.9 ± 12.6 years (Range: 11–60 years)
Renal cell carcinoma	43 (28%)	44.0 ± 10.9 years (Range: from 16 years)
Phaeochromocytoma	11 (7%)	20.2 ± 7.6 years (Range: 12–36 years)

[a]Includes both symptomatic and presymptomatic diagnoses.

VHL gene mutation (4, 12) and should be offered *VHL* mutation analysis. In such cases the nature of the *VHL* mutation identified will indicate the risk of other types of VHL related tumours (e.g. whether a type 2A, 2B, or 2C associated mutation).

The most frequent pancreatic feature of VHL disease is multiple cystadenomas, which rarely cause clinical disease. However, pancreatic tumours, most commonly nonsecretary islet cell tumours, occur in a minority (5–10%) of cases. These tumours are often asymptomatic and are detected by routine abdominal imaging. Initial experience of pancreatic tumours in VHL disease suggested a high frequency of malignancy, but more recent studies have suggested that surgery may be delayed for small tumours (13). Although there is a clinical impression that there are interfamilial differences in pancreatic tumour incidence and that the risk of pancreatic islet cell tumours and phaeochromocytomas may be correlated, the genotype–phenotype correlations reported for pancreatic tumours are less clear than for phaeochromocytoma.

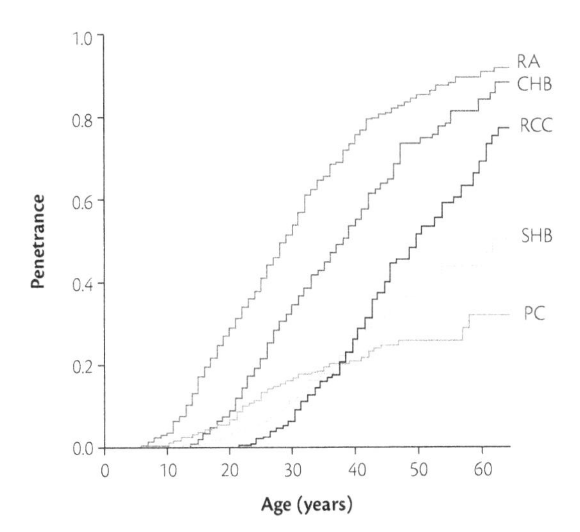

Fig. 6.13.1 Age-related risks for the five major manifestations of von Hippel–Lindau disease. RA, retinal angioma; CHB, cerebellar haemangioblastoma; SHB, spinal haemangioblastoma; RCC, renal cell carcinoma; PC, phaeochromocytoma. (Reprinted with permission from Ong KR, Woodward ER, Killick P, Lim C, Macdonald F, Maher ER. Genotype–phenotype correlations in von Hippel–Lindau disease. *Hum Mutat*, 2007; **28**: 143–9 (2).)

Nonendocrine tumours

Retinal and central nervous system haemangioblastomas are benign vascular tumours consisting of endothelial lined vascular channels and surrounding stromal cells and pericytes. Although benign, they are frequently cystic and neurological symptoms result from compression of the adjacent structures and/or raised intracranial pressure. Cerebellar involvement is most frequent and these usually respond well to surgery. However, both retinal and CHB are frequently multiple. Surgery for brainstem and spinal haemangioblastomas can be hazardous and CNS lesions remain an important cause of morbidity and mortality. Although the natural history of retinal lesions is to enlarge and cause retinal detachment and haemorrhage resulting in blindness, most small haemangioblastomas respond to laser- or cryotherapy so early detection is important (see below).

The lifetime risk of RCC in most cases of VHL disease (types 1 and 2B) is high (>70%) (4, 11). VHL disease is characterized not only by a high risk of RCC but also by an earlier age at onset (mean age 44 years for symptomatic lesions but as early as 16 years for early tumours detected by renal imaging) and a high risk of bilateral and multicentric tumours. Microscopically, VHL kidneys may contain numerous, small tumours and the risk of recurrence (from new primary tumours) after local excision for RCC is very high. However, a nephron-sparing approach is considered the optimal management for RCC in VHL disease in most centres. Thus, renal tumours detected at an early presymptomatic stage by routine surveillance are followed until 3 cm in size when nephron sparing resection is performed and other small lesions are also excised. The aim of this conservative approach to surgery is to delay dialysis for as long as possible. Although there is a high rate of reoperation for new primary tumours with this approach, the risk of metastatic spread appears small.

Endolymphatic sac tumours have also been recognized as a complication of VHL disease (3). These papillary adenocarcinomas may be asymptomatic or cause patients to present with symptoms such as tinnitus or deafness.

Molecular genetics of VHL disease

The *VHL* tumour suppressor gene was isolated in 1993 and encodes a 213-amino acid protein (pVHL) which is widely expressed in human tissues (7). A wide variety of germline *VHL* gene mutations have been identified, including large deletions, protein truncating mutations, and missense amino acid substitutions (11). Tumours from VHL patients show inactivation (by loss, mutation, or methylation) of the wild-type allele so that the mechanism of tumourigenesis appears similar to that of a classical tumour suppressor gene such as the retinoblastoma gene (14). However, an added complexity in VHL disease is the existence of intricate genotype–phenotype correlations, which suggested that the *VHL* gene product (pVHL) had multiple and tissue-specific functions (see above).

Although pVHL has been implicated in multiple signalling pathways, the signature pVHL function is the ability to regulate expression of the hypoxia-inducible transcription factors HIF-1 and HIF-2 (15, 16). Thus pVHL is the recognition component of an E3 ubiquitin ligase complex that, in normoxic cells, binds to hydroxylated prolines on the HIF-1 and HIF-2 α subunits, resulting in ubiquitylation and proteosomal degradation of the subunits (Fig. 6.13.2). Oxygen is an essential cofactor of the prolyl hydroxylation

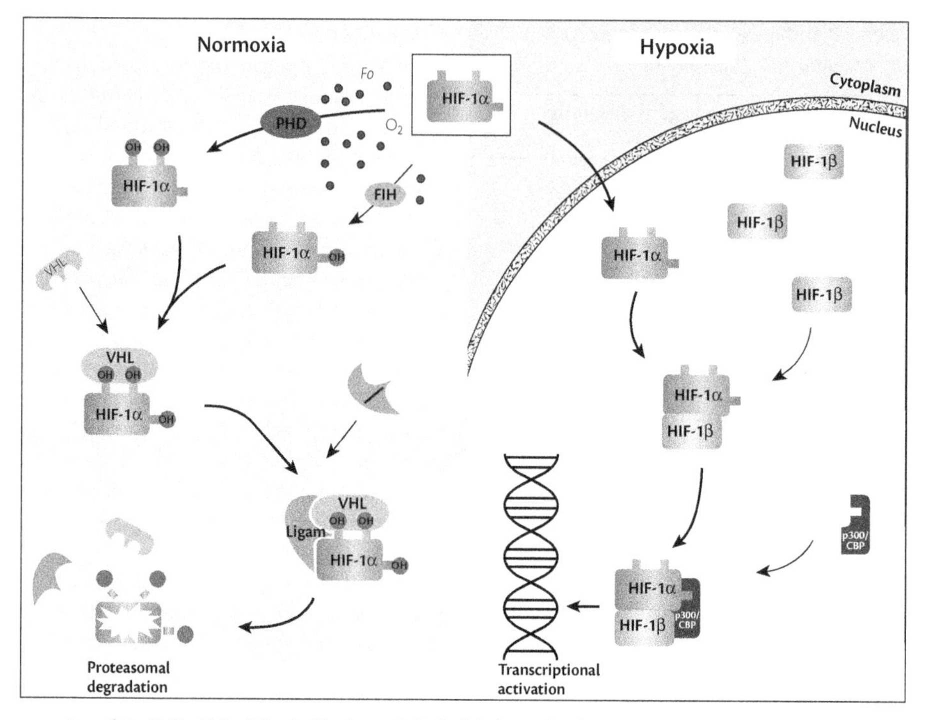

Fig. 6.13.2 Schematic representation of the PHD–VHL–HIF axis. The hypoxia-inducible factor (HIF)-α subunit is synthesized continuously but is rapidly destroyed in the presence of oxygen and iron. Oxygen- and iron-dependent prolyl hydroxylase domain (PHD) enzymes hydroxylate specific proline residues in HIF-α, increasing its affinity for the von Hippel–Lindau tumour suppressor protein (VHL). The binding of VHL to hydroxylated HIF-α then targets HIF-α for destruction by a multiprotein ubiquitin ligase (denoted 'ligase') that mediates proteasomal degradation of HIF-α subunits. Under hypoxic conditions, the hydroxylation of HIF-α by PHDs inhibited, proteasomal degradation is slowed. HIF-α accumulates and dimerizes with HIF-β and regulates hypoxia-responsive genes. If the vHL protein is mutated and unable to bind HIF-α then proteasomal degradation does not occur and HIF-α and HIF-β can dimerize and activate gene expression. Similarly if succinate dehydrogenase function is compromised, the PHDs are inhibited and a pseudohypoxic state ensues. (Reprinted with permission from Smith TG, Robbins PA, Ratcliffe PJ. The human side of hypoxia-inducible factor. *Br J Haematol*, 2008; **141**: 325–34.)

enzymes that regulate the ability of pVHL to bind to HIF-α subunits (16). In hypoxic conditions, pVHL is unable to bind to HIF-α subunits and HIF-1 and HIF-2 transcription factors are stabilized and cause activation of hypoxic-response genes, promoting angiogenesis, alterations in cell metabolism, and proliferation. Targets of HIF-2 are thought to be particularly implicated in the pathogenesis of RCC (17). Although many VHL mutations that are associated with phaeochromocytoma lead to dysregulation of HIF pathways, a second VHL-regulated pathway has been implicated in the pathogenesis of phaeochromocytoma in VHL disease. Thus pVHL has been implicated in a developmental apoptotic pathway that is normally activated when nerve growth factor becomes limiting for neuronal progenitor cells and results in developmental culling of the sympathetic neuronal (thought to be the phaeochromocytoma precursor cells) in late fetal life. Germline *VHL*– mutations associated with phaeochromocytoma are thought to impair this developmental apoptosis pathway and so predispose to phaeochromocytoma (17).

Surveillance in VHL disease

The ascertainment, diagnosis and surveillance of patients and relatives at risk of VHL disease is essential to prevent morbidity and mortality. The multisystem nature of the disease can lead to inconsistent and uncoordinated follow-up and it is important that a process is established to coordinate the multidisciplinary surveillance required. Following the diagnosis of VHL disease in an individual, all at-risk relatives should be contacted and informed of the need for investigation. Surveillance should commence in childhood (Box 6.13.1) and continue until there is no evidence of VHL disease at an advanced age (penetrance is almost complete by age 65 years). However, in most families it is possible to determine the need for surveillance by molecular genetic testing. Lifelong surveillance is indicated in affected individuals and asymptomatic gene carriers, whilst noncarriers can be reassured and discharged. The introduction of systematic surveillance protocols for following up affected and at-risk members of VHL kindreds has led to the early diagnosis of VHL tumours with a reduction in morbidity.

Succinate dehydrogenase subunit (*SDHB, SDHC*, and *SDHD*) genes

Succinate dehydrogenase is a heterotetrameric protein consisting of A, B, C, and D subunits located on the inner mitochondrial membrane (18). Succinate dehydrogenase has a critical role in cellular energy metabolism through its dual role in the Krebs citric acid cycle and as part of the respiratory chain (mitochondrial complex 2). The SDH-B subunit (also known as iron-sulphur protein), contains three iron-sulphur clusters ([2Fe-2S], [4Fe-4S], and [3Fe-4S]), is part of the hydrophilic catalytic domain, and binds to the A subunit, which contains a covalently attached flavin adenine dinucleotide cofactor and the substrate binding site. The B subunit also binds to the two hydrophobic membrane anchor subunits, C and D. The SDH-C and -D subunits attach the complex to the mitochondrial inner membrane and also contain the ubiquinone

Box 6.13.1 Birmingham surveillance protocol for von Hippel–Lindau disease in asymptomatic affected patients and at-risk relatives

Affected patient:

- Annual physical examination, and direct and indirect ophthalmoscopy
- MRI brain scan every 3 years to age 50 years and every 5 years thereafter
- Annual abdominal MRI (or ultrasonography if MRI is unavailable) for renal, adrenal, and pancreatic masses
- Annual 24-h urine collection for catecholamines and vanillylmandelic acid (VMA)

At-risk relative:

- Annual physical examination, and direct and indirect ophthalmoscopy from age 5 years until age 60 years
- MRI brain scan every 3 years to from age 15 to 40 years and then every 5 years until age 60 years
- Annual renal MRI or ultrasonography from age 16 years to age 65 years
- Annual 24-h urine collection for catecholamines and VMAs

binding site to which the electrons are transferred from the SDH-B subunit iron-sulphur clusters within the B subunit.

Germline mutations in the gene encoding the D subunit of succinate hydrogenase were first found to be associated with familial head and neck paragangliomas (HNPGL) and then phaeochromocytoma (19, 20). Thereafter, germline mutations in the B subunit gene (*SDHB*) were also demonstrated to cause susceptibility to HNPGL and adrenal and extra-adrenal phaeochromocytoma (21). Germline *SDHB* and *SDHD* mutations are now recognized as a major cause of phaeochromocytoma susceptibility. Mutations in SDHA have been associated rarely with neoplasia (but can cause an autosomal recessive juvenile encephalopathy (22)) and *SDHC* mutations are an infrequent cause of HNPGL and a rare cause of phaeochromocytoma (23). With increasing availability and application of molecular testing for *SDHB* and *SDHD* mutations the phenotype has been expanded to include renal and thyroid tumours and gastrointestinal stromal cell tumours. Furthermore, *SDHB* mutations have been associated with a high risk of malignant phaeochromocytoma (24).

Clinical features of germline *SDHB*, *SDHC*, and *SDHD* mutations

There is considerable overlap between the clinical features associated with mutations in the three genes that encode the B, C, and D subunits of succinate dehydrogenase, but there are also some important differences with respect to inheritance pattern and risks of individual tumours.

SDHB *mutations* Although germline mutations in *SDHB*, *SDHC*, and *SDHD* mutations can each be associated with the development of phaeochromocytoma and HNPGL, *SDHB* mutations are particularly associated with phaeochromocytoma and *SDHD* and *SDHC* with HNPGL. Thus in molecular genetic studies of population-based cohorts of phaeochromocytoma and HNPGL patients, the frequency of *SDHB* mutations is higher in the former group and *SDHD* in the latter (24–26). Mean age of phaeochromocytoma in *SDHB* mutation carriers is younger than in sporadic cases and similar to that in VHL disease. In contrast to sporadic and VHL-associated phaeochromocytomas, many phaeochromocytomas in *SDHB* mutation carriers occur at extra-adrenal sites (such tumours are also known as 'paragangliomas'). Furthermore, there is a high frequency of malignancy in *SDHB*-associated phaeochromocytomas such that germline *SDHB* mutations may be detected in 30–50% of patients with malignant phaeochromocytoma. Patients with germline *SDHB* mutations are at risk for RCC. although the lifetime of approximately 15% is much less than in VHL disease. Familial or bilateral RCC without a personal or family history of phaeochromocytoma or HNPGL can be the presenting feature of germline *SDHB* mutations (27). Germline mutations in *SDHB* (and *SDHC* and *SDHD*) may also present with phaeochromocytoma and gastrointestinal stromal tumours (Carney–Stratakis syndrome) (28).

SDHC *mutations* Patients with germline *SDHC* mutations are less common than those with *SDHB* and *SDHD* mutations. Germline *SDHC* mutation carriers most commonly present with HNPGL (which tend to be unifocal) and only occasionally with phaeochromocytoma.

SDHD *mutations* Germline *SDHD* mutations were first characterized in patients with familial HNPGL and subsequently in familial phaeochromocytoma (19, 20). HNPGL in *SDHD* mutation carriers are often bilateral and multifocal. On average, the risk of HNPGL is higher in *SDHD* mutation carriers than in *SDHB* mutation carriers, whereas the reverse is true for phaeochromocytoma (Fig. 6.13.3). Nevertheless, germline *SDHD* mutations are an important cause of phaeochromocytoma susceptibility. The risk of malignancy is highest, but not confined to, *SDHB* mutations. The unusual inheritance pattern of *SDHD*-associated tumours may often lead to the possibility of familial disease being overlooked. Thus both *SDHB* and *SDHC* mutations cause dominantly inherited disease (so the risk of a child inheriting the mutation from an affected parent is 1 in 2) although age-dependent penetrance is apparent and incomplete penetrance is common. However, *SDHD* mutations display an unusual pattern of inheritance. Thus although the risk of a child inheriting the mutation from an affected parent is 1 in 2, the risk of a child who inherits a mutation becoming clinically affected is dependent on which parent has transmitted the mutation (19). Thus children who inherit a mutation from their father have a high risk of tumours but children who inherit the mutation from their mother are almost always unaffected. This parent of origin effect on disease expression is reminiscent of genomic imprinting, but the *SDHD* gene has not been demonstrated to be imprinted.

Molecular genetics of germline *SDHB*, *SDHC*, and *SDHD* mutations

More than 200 different germline *SDHB*, *SDHC*, and *SDHD* mutations have been described (see the LOVD database (http://chromium.liacs.nl/LOVD2/SDH/home.php)). These mutations represent a wide variety of mutation types (e.g. missense, frameshift, splice-site and exonic deletions) and are loss of function mutations. As with any relatively recently described gene, the pathogenic significance of rare variants may be difficult to assess.

Tumours from individuals with *SDHB/C/D* subunit mutations demonstrate loss of the wild-type allele, as seen in VHL disease

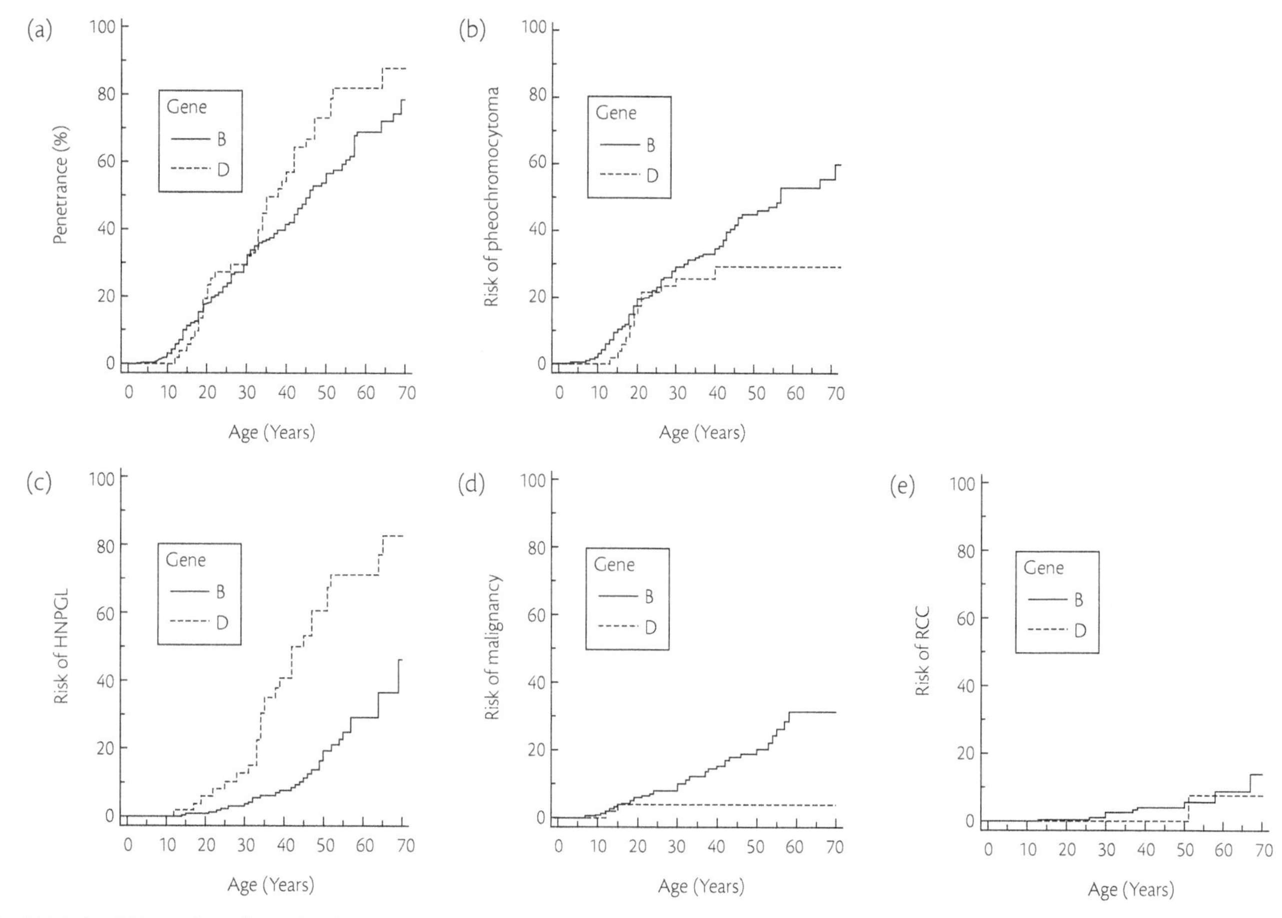

Fig. 6.13.3 (a–c) Comparison of age-related penetrances in *SDHB* and *SDHD* mutation carriers. (a) Head and neck paraganglioma or phaeochromocytoma; (b) phaeochromocytoma only; (c) head and neck paraganglioma only; (d) malignant phaeochromocytoma; (e) penetrance of renal tumours in *SDHB* mutation carriers. (Reprinted with permission from Ricketts C, *et al. Human Mutation*, 2010; **31**: 41–51.)

and other classic tumour suppressor genes. Several mechanisms have been implicated in the development of *SDHB/C/D*-related phaeochromocytomas. Thus inactivation of *SDHB/D* can result in a pseudohypoxic state (similar to that seen in VHL tumours) (29) and activation of HIF pathways with SDH inactivation has been linked to accumulation of succinate and resulting inhibition of prolyl hydroxylase enzymes that are necessary for proteosomal degradation of HIF-α subunits (Fig. 6.13.2) (30). Also, animal models of SDH inactivation suggest that reactive oxygen species may be increased and these might also provoke a pseudohypoxic state (31). As in VHL disease (see above), germline *SDHB/D* mutations have also been reported to predispose to a failure of normal developmental apoptosis of sympathetic neuronal cells, leading to persistence of 'phaeochromocytoma precursor cells' (17).

Surveillance

Unlike VHL disease, there is relatively little experience of the utility of surveillance in *SDHB/C/D* gene carriers. However, anecdotal evidence suggests that surveillance of asymptomatic gene carriers can lead to early tumour detection. As experience with surveillance programmes increases, a consensus should emerge as to the optimum methodologies and frequency of surveillance. However, currently no such consensus exists and the protocol proposed in Box 6.13.2 is provided as an example of a programme used in one centre.

The role of genetic testing in phaeochromocytoma

Up to a third of patients with phaeochromocytoma will have an underlying genetic cause. In some cases this will have been suspected because of a family or personal history of other features of a known phaeochromocytoma susceptibility syndrome (e.g. VHL

Box 6.13.2 Example of a surveillance protocol for asymptomatic *SDHB/SDHD* mutation carriers

Proven *SDHB* mutation carrier:

- Annual 24-h urine for catecholamines and VMA measurements from age 5 years
- Annual abdominal MRI scans from age 7 years (abdominal and thoracic every 3 years)
- MRI neck age 20 years and every 3 years thereafter

Proven *SDHD* mutation carrier (paternally transmitted):

- Annual 24-h urine for catecholamines and VMA measurements from age 5 years
- Two-yearly abdominal MRI scans from age 7 years (abdominal and thoracic every 5 years)
- MRI neck age 20 years and every 1–2 years thereafter

disease, multiple endocrine neoplasia type 2, neurofibromatosis type 1 (von Recklinghausen's disease)). However genetic testing of apparently sporadic, nonsyndromic cases can reveal a germline mutation in 12–25% of cases (24, 26). Although this observation led to suggestions that all patients with phaeochromocytoma might be offered mutation analysis of *RET, SDHB, SDHD,* and *VHL* the detection rate for mutations in older patients with sporadic, non-syndromic adrenal phaeochromocytomas is very low. Hence mutation analysis in sporadic patients with a single phaeochromocytoma should be prioritized for those with: (1) features of a known inherited phaeochromocytoma syndrome (e.g. RCC, HNPGL, medullary thyroid cancer, etc.); (2) malignant tumours (*SDHB*); (c) extra-adrenal phaeochromocytoma (*SDHB, SDHD*); or (3) age at diagnosis less than 40 years (*VHL, SDHB, SDHD*).

References

1. Maher ER, Kaelin WG. von Hippel-Lindau disease. *Medicine*, 1997; **76**: 381–91.
2. Ong KR, Woodward ER, Killick P, Lim C, Macdonald F, Maher ER. Genotype-phenotype correlations in von Hippel-Lindau disease. *Hum Mutat*, 2007; **28**: 143–9.
3. Prowse A, Webster A, Richards F, Richard F, Olschwang S, Resche F, *et al.* Somatic inactivation of the VHL gene in von Hippel-Lindau disease tumors. *Am J Hum Genet*, 1997; **60**: 765–71.
4. Maher ER, Yates JRW, Harries R, Benjamin C, Harris R, Moore AT, *et al.* Clinical features and natural history of von Hippel-Lindau disease. *QJMed*, 1990; **77**: 1151–63.
5. Woodward ER, Eng C, McMahon R, Voutilainen R, Affara NA, Ponder BAJ, *et al.* Genetic predisposition to phaeochromocytoma: analysis of candidate genes GDNF, RET and VHL. *Hum Mol Genet*, 1997; **7**: 1051–6.
6. Melmon K, Rosen S. Lindau's disease. *Am J Med*, 1964; **36**: 595–617.
7. Latif F, Tory K, Gnarra J, Yao M, Duh FM, Orcutt ML, *et al.* Identification of the von Hippel-Lindau disease tumour suppressor gene. *Science*, 1993; **260**: 1317–20.
8. Crossey PA, Richards FM, Foster K, Green JS, Prowse A, Latif F, *et al.* Identification of intragenic mutations in the von Hippel-Lindau disease tumour suppressor gene and correlation with disease phenotype. *Hum Mol Genet*, 1994; **3**: 1303–8.
9. Maher ER, Webster AR, Richards FM, Green JS, Crossey PA, Payne SJ, *et al.* Phenotypic expression in von Hippel-Lindau disease: correlations with germline *VHL* gene mutations. *J Med Genet*, 1996; **33**: 328–32.
10. Brauch H, Kishida T, Glavac D, Chen F, Pausch, F, Hofler H, *et al.* von Hippel-Lindau disease with phaeochromocytoma in the Black Forest region in Germany: Evidence for a founder effect. *Hum Genet*, 1995; **95**: 551–6.
11. Neumann HP, Bausch B, McWhinney SR, Bender BU, Gimm O, Franke G, *et al*; Freiburg-Warsaw-Columbus Pheochromocytoma Study Group. Germ-line mutationsin nonsyndromic pheochromocytoma. *N Engl J Med*, 2002; **346**: 1459–66.
12. Blansfield JA, Choyke L, Morita SY, Choyke PL, Pingpank JF, Alexander HR, *et al.* Clinical, genetic and radiographic analysis of 108 patients with von Hippel-Lindau disease (VHL) manifested by pancreatic neuroendocrine neoplasms (PNETs). *Surgery*, 2007; **142**: 814–8.
13. Manski TJ, Heffner DK, Glenn GM, Patronas NJ, Pikus AT, Katz D, *et al.* Endolymphatic sac tumors—a source of morbid hearing loss in von Hippel-Lindau disease. *JAMA*, 1997; **277**: 1461–6.
14. Clifford SC, Cockman ME, Smallwood AC, Mole DR, Woodward ER, Maxwell PH, *et al.* Contrasting effects on HIF-1alpha regulation by disease-causing pVHL mutations correlate with patterns of tumourigenesis in vonHippel-Lindau disease. *Hum Mol Genet*, 2001; **10**: 1029–38.
15. Maxwell P, Wiesener M, Chang G-W, Clifford SC, Vaux E, Cockman M, *et al.* The tumour suppressor protein VHL targets hypoxia-inducible factors for oxygen-dependent proteolysis. *Nature*, 1999; **399**: 271–5.
16. Kaelin WG Jr. The von Hippel-Lindau tumour suppressor protein: O2 sensing and cancer. *Nat Rev Cancer*, 2008; **8**: 865–73.
17. Lee S, Nakamura E, Yang H, Wei W, Linggi MS, Sajan MP, *et al.* Neuronal apoptosis linked to EglN3 prolyl hydroxylase and familial pheochromocytoma genes: developmental culling and cancer. *Cancer Cell*, 2005; **8**: 155–67.
18. Sun F, Huo X, Zhai Y, Wang A, Xu J, Su D, *et al.* Crystal structure of mitochondrial respiratory membrane protein complex II. *Cell*, 2005; **121**: 1043–57.
19. Baysal BE, Ferrell RE, Willett-Brozick JE, Lawrence EC, Myssiorek D, Bosch A, *et al.* Mutations in SDHD, a mitochondrial complex II gene, in hereditary paraganglioma. *Science*, 2000; **287**: 848–51.
20. Astuti D, Douglas F, Lennard TW, Aligianis IA, Woodward ER, Evans DG, *et al.* Germline SDHD mutation in familial phaeochromocytoma. *Lancet*, 2001; **357**: 1181–2.
21. Astuti D, Latif F, Dallol A, Dahia PL, Douglas F, George E, *et al.* Gene mutations in the succinate dehydrogenase subunit SDHB cause susceptibility to familial pheochromocytoma and to familial paraganglioma. *Am J Hum Genet*, 2001; **69**: 49–54.
22. Bourgeron T, Rustin P, Chretien D, Birch-Machin M, Bourgeois M, Viegas-Pequignot E, *et al.* Mutation of a nuclear succinate dehydrogenase gene results in mitochondrial respiratory chain deficiency. *Nat Genet*, 1995; **11**: 144–9.
23. Baysal BE. Clinical and molecular progress in hereditary paraganglioma. *J Med Genet*, 2008; **45**: 689–94.
24. Gimenez-Roqueplo AP, Favier J, Rustin P, Rieubland C, Crespin M, Nau V, *et al*; COMETE Network. Mutations in the SDHB gene are associated with extra-adrenal and/or malignant phaeochromocytomas. *Cancer Res*, 2003; **63**: 5615–21.
25. Baysal BE, Willett-Brozick JE, Lawrence EC, Drovdlic CM, Savul SA, McLeod DR, *et al.* Prevalence of SDHB, SDHC, and SDHD germline mutations in clinic patients with head and neck paragangliomas. *J Med Genet*, 2002; **39**: 178–83.
26. Neumann HP, Bausch B, McWhinney SR, Bender BU, Gimm O, Franke G, *et al.* The Freiburg-Warsaw-Columbus Pheochromocytoma Study Group. Germ-line mutations in nonsyndromic pheochromocytoma. *N Engl J Med*, 2002; **346**: 1459–66.
27. Ricketts C, Woodward ER, Killick P, Morris MR, Astuti D, Latif F, *et al.* Germline SDHB mutations and familial renal cell carcinoma. *J Natl Cancer Inst*, 2008; **100**: 1260–2.
28. Stratakis CA, Carney JA. The triad of paragangliomas, gastric stromal tumours and pulmonary chondromas (Carney triad), and the dyad of paragangliomas and gastric stromal sarcomas (Carney-Stratakis syndrome): molecular genetics and clinical implications. *J Intern Med*, 2009; **266**: 43–52.
29. Pollard PJ, El-Bahrawy M, Poulsom R, Elia G, Killick P, Kelly G, *et al.* Expression of HIF-1alpha, HIF-2alpha (EPAS1), and their target genes in paraganglioma and pheochromocytoma with VHL and SDH mutations. *J Clin Endocrinol Metab*, 2006; **91**: 4593–8.
30. Selak MA, Armour SM, MacKenzie ED, Boulahbel H, Watson DG, Mansfield KD, *et al.* Succinate links TCA cycle dysfunction to oncogenesis by inhibiting HIF-alpha prolyl hydroxylase. *Cancer Cell*, 2005; **7**: 77–85.
31. Szeto SS, Reinke SN, Sykes BD, Lemire BD. Ubiquinone-binding site mutations in the Saccharomyces cerevisiae succinate dehydrogenase generate superoxide and lead to the accumulation of succinate. *J Biol Chem*, 2007; **282**: 27518–26.

6.14

Neurofibromatosis

George Tharakan

Introduction

Neurofibromatosis 1 and 2 have historically been grouped together. However they represent two distinct diseases separated both genetically and clinically. Both diseases are discussed in this chapter with the emphasis on neurofibromatosis 1 (NF 1), which has more endocrine manifestations.

Neurofibromatosis 1

Clinical descriptions of NF 1 have been documented since AD 1000 (1). Its eponymous name honours a German pathologist, von Recklinghausen. It is a neurocutaneous condition that is hereditary but 50% of cases are accounted by sporadic mutations (2). The diagnostic criteria and clinical features are described in Table 6.14.1 and Boxes 6.14.1, 6.14.2, and 6.14.3.

Genetic/molecular basis of neurofibromatosis 1

Neurofibromatosis 1 occurs due to a defect in a single gene known as *NF1* (OMIM 166220) located on chromosome 17q11.2(3). It is a large gene containing 60 exons or 350 kilobase pairs. It is inherited in an autosomal dominant pattern. Hence each NF 1 patient has a 50% chance of having an affected offspring. However, predicting the clinical picture is complicated because although there is 100% penetrance with features being present by the age of 5 there is variable expression.

Somatic mutations are common, occurring in 1 in 10 000 births and representing 50% of new cases. Mutations that occur early in embryogenesis produce a clinical picture that is indistinguishable from the inherited form but mutations that occur later produce a localized form of the disease. *NF1* is a tumour suppressor gene and hence tumour genesis requires a second hit to occur prior to disease being present.

The *NF1* product is a 2818-amino acid protein known as neurofibromin. This cytoplasmic protein is mostly expressed in neurological tissue. It contains a GTPase activating protein (GAP) domain that is important in the Ras pathway. GAP inhibits signal transduction by dephosphorylating the Ras protein. Loss of neurofibromin function results in uncontrolled Ras signalling, which is involved in the differentiation of Schwann cells. This explains a possible mechanism for neurofibroma development. The signalling pathway involves mTOR, which is a target of the drug rapamycin. This implies a potential pharmacological intervention in the growth of neurofibromas (4).

General management of neurofibromatosis 1

The manifestations of neurofibromatosis are varied (Table 6.14.1). Recent guidelines recommend that the two main principles of management be age-specific monitoring and patient education. Whilst the presence of unidentified bright objects on an MRI of the brain can be used as a diagnostic tool in young children this will invariably require general anaesthetic. Subsequently, baseline imaging to identify asymptomatic tumours is not advocated. Assessment in a specialist NF clinic should be conducted annually with opportunities for the patient with concerns to seek specialist advice if needed.

Consultations with young children should include assessment of learning and behavioural issues. The initial appointment should also include visual assessment to exclude an optic glioma. Adolescents may require psychological support. Adults will need, at a minimum, annual blood pressure measurement. All patients should be made aware of the complications of the disease and information on support groups, such as the Neurofibromatosis Association, should be made available.

Management of specific endocrine problems

Phaeochromocytoma

Phaeochromocytoma occurs in 0.1–5.7% of patients with neurofibromatosis. The European-American Phaeochromocytoma study group's database demonstrates no significant difference in the characteristics between patients with sporadic phaeochromocytomas and those with associated neurofibromatosis. Twelve per cent of phaeochromocytomas associated with NF 1 are malignant (5).

Consideration of phaeochromocytoma should occur in NF 1 patients who are hypertensive (an alternative diagnosis being renal hypertension). The hypertension can be episodic or sustained. Other symptoms included flushing, palpitations, and headache. Management remains the same as for sporadic phaeochromocytomas.

Carcinoid

Carcinoid (enterochromaffin cell) tumours have been associated with NF 1 in case reports since 1970. The incidence is less than 1% but has an unusual predisposition to being located in the periampullary region, which is very rare for sporadic tumours. A quarter of all periampullary carcinoid have occurred in association with neurofibromatosis (6).

Common presenting features are of obstructive jaundice and abdominal pain. The presence of carcinoid syndrome is rare.

Table 6.14.1 Clinical features of neurofibromatosis 1

Clinical features and complications of NF 1	Frequency
Dermatological	
Café-au-lait spots	>99%
Axillary and inguinal freckling	>60%
Juvenile xanthogranuloma	<1%
Neurological	
Peripheral neurofibroma	100%
Plexiform neurofibroma	30%
Malignant peripheral sheath tumours	7–12%
Gliomas	1%
Spinal neurofibromatosis	1–2%
Epilepsy	5%
Endocrine	
Phaeochromocytoma	<1%
Carcinoid	<1%
Precocious puberty	1–2%
Psychology	
Moderate to severe learning difficulties	3%
Behavioural problems	30%
Visual–spatial problems	50%
Vascular	
Renal artery stenosis	1–2%
Intercranial artery stenosis	<1%
Growth	
Macrocephaly	30%
Short stature	25%
Skeletal	
Scoliosis	10%
Pseudoarthrosis	2%
Sphenoid wing dysplasia	>1%
Localized overgrowth	<1%
Ophthalmic	
Lisch nodules	>90%
Orbital and eyelid plexiform neurofibromas	3%

The tumours metastasize early and so aggressive management with surgery is recommended (7).

Growth

Impaired growth in NF 1 is well documented. Studies have identified that the mean adult height of NF 1 patients to correspond to the 25th percentile of the general population. Analysis of growth velocity charts have demonstrated that growth occurs normally in children until the onset of puberty. The subsequent decreased growth is currently debated with possible causes being decreased growth hormone, inadequate nutrition due to the requirement of large tumours/ neurofibromas, and psychosocial issues (8).

Box 6.14.1 Diagnostic criteria for neurofibromatosis 1, based on 1988 NIH development conference

Two of the following seven required:

- Six or more café-au-lait macules (>0.5 cm prepuberty, >1.5 cm postpuberty)
- Two or more cutaneous/subcutaneous neurofibromas or one plexiform neurofibroma
- Freckling found in axilla/groin
- Optic pathway glioma
- Two or more lisch nodules on slit lamp examination
- Bony dysplasia
- First-degree relative with neurofibromatosis 1

Puberty

Both delayed puberty and precocious puberty have been reported in NF 1. The incidence of precocious puberty with the NF 1 population has been reported as between 2.4 and 3%. There is a strong association with optic glioma pathways. Precocious puberty can occur in the absence of an optic pathway glioma at a prevalence thought to be similar to the general population. Treatment of precocious puberty is with gonadotrophin releasing hormone agonists and is essential when puberty starts before the age of 6 years in girls and 7 years in boys. Delayed puberty occurs at a higher incidence than precocious puberty, at a rate of 16% in the NF 1 population (8).

Genetic counselling

The difficulties of genetic counselling in respect to NF 1 lie in its variable expression. Although it has classical mendelian autosomal dominance and 100% penetration, the severity and expression vary within families.

The United Kingdom Neurofibromatosis Association Clinical Advisory Board has recommended that the parents of any 'new' diagnosis of neurofibromatosis should be examined for any cutaneous stigmata or lisch nodules. This is to identify parents that have segmental/ mosaic forms of the disease as these patients will

Box 6.14.2 Diagnostic criteria for neurofibromatosis 2, based on 1987 NIH development conference

1. Bilateral eight nerve masses seen by appropriate imaging (for example CT or MRI)
2. A first-degree relative with neurofibromatosis 2 AND unilateral eighth nerve mass OR at least two of:
   - Neurofibroma
   - Meningioma
   - Glioma
   - Schwannoma
   - Juvenile posterior subcapsular lenticular opacity

Box 6.14.3 Diagnostic criteria for neurofibromatosis 2 (Manchester criteria)

- Bilateral vestibular schwannomas
- First-degree relative with NF 2 and unilateral vestibular schwannoma or any two of meningioma, schwannoma, glioma, neurofibroma, or posterior subcapsular opacities
- Unilateral vestibular schwannoma and any two of meningioma, schwannoma, glioma, neurofibroma, or posterior subcapsular opacities
- Multiple meningiomas (two or more), and unilateral vestibular schwannoma or any two of schwannoma, glioma, neurofibroma, or cataract

have had gamete mutations and so carry the 50% chance of having affected offspring. If no clinical features are present, the risk of the parent having an affected offspring is reduced to less than 1%.

Prenatal testing is possible via amniocentesis or chorionic villous sampling but interpretation remains difficult as it does not predict expression of disease. A more clinically applicable option for couples wishing to avoid therapeutic intervention is preimplantation genetic diagnosis. This can occur via a single cell removed from a 3-day-old embryo (9).

Neurofibromatosis 2

Neurofibromatosis 2 (NF 2) is genetically and clinically distinct from NF 1. It has a much lower incidence of 1 in 40 000 (10).

Genetic/molecular basis of neurofibromatosis 2

While also an autosomal dominant condition with 100% penetrance, it is due to a single gene defect on chromosome 22q12. The *NF2* (OMIM 101000) gene known as Merlin or Schwannomin encodes a 595-amino acid protein (11). It is also a tumour suppressor gene, requiring loss of both genes (the first an inherited genetic defect and the second a somatic mutation) for clinical expression. However, unlike neurofibromin, Merlin is widely expressed.

The molecular mechanism by which Merlin acts as a tumour suppressor gene remains to be confirmed. However, at present it is proposed that Merlin is associated with other ERM proteins that are thought to be involved in intercellular contact and signalling. Merlin promotes the suppression of mitogenic signalling. Loss of Merlin subsequently results in unregulated cell proliferation (12).

Diagnostic features

There are at least four sets of criteria for the diagnosis of NF 2; the first to be established was the NIH criteria, created in 1987. These were later revised in 1991 to be more sensitive as improved neuroimaging and genetic analysis revealed that the original criteria were too restrictive. However, the most sensitive criteria to date were established by the Manchester group, which do not require any family history of the condition (13).

Clinical features

The characteristic tumours of NF 2 are vestibular schwannomas. These present with reduced hearing (60% of patients), which initially is usually unilateral. Other symptoms include tinnitus, dizziness, and imbalance. Visual problems are common in NF 2 patients. The most common cause for this is posterior subcapsular opacities (60–80% of patients). Optic nerve sheath meningiomas and retinal hamartomas may also cause reduced visual acuity. Other clinical features include mononeuropathies (most commonly affecting the VIIth cranial nerve) and skin tumours (most commonly schwannomas).

Management

A consensus statement written by the United Kingdom Neurofibromatosis Association recommends that NF 2 patients are managed in specialist centres. A multidisciplinary team is advocated, which should include a neurosurgeon (with experience in managing vestibular schwannomas and auditory rehabilitation), otolaryngologist, neurologist/ geneticist, nurse, and audiologist. In contrast to NF 1, baseline scans are advocated. These should include an MRI scan of the brain, auditory canals, and spine. Scanning should be initiated at the age of 10 years and continue every 2 years for patients below the age of 20 years and then every 3 years provided that the patient is asymptomatic. Annual audiological tests should complement scanning although tumour growth may occur in the absence of hearing deficit. In addition to imaging, genetic testing and counselling should be available to all NF 2 patients and their families. Should imaging detect a vestibular schwannoma, current treatment modalities that should be made available to the patient include surgery and radiotherapy (14).

References

1. Zanca A, Zanca A. Antique illustrations of neurofibromatosis. *Int J Dermatol*, 1980; **19**: 55–8.
2. Huson SM, Harper PS, Compston DA. Von Recklinghausen neurofibromatosis. A clinical and population study in south-east Wales. *Brain*, 1988; **111**: 1355–81.
3. Wallace MR, Marchuk DA, Andersen LB, Letcher R, Odeh HM, Saulino AM, *et al.* Type 1 neurofibromatosis gene: identification of a large transcript disrupted in three NF1 patients. *Science*, 1990; **249**: 181–6.
4. Ferner RE. Neurofibromatosis 1. *Eur J Hum Genet*, 2007; **15**: 131–8.
5. Bausch B, Borozdin W, Neumann HP. Clinical and genetic characteristics of patients with neurofibromatosis type 1 and pheochromocytoma. *N Engl J Med*, 2006; **354**: 2729–31.
6. Makhlouf HR, Burke AP, Sobin LH. Carcinoid tumors of the ampulla of Vater: a comparison with duodenal carcinoid tumors. *Cancer*, 1999; **85**: 1241–9.
7. Zyromski NJ, Kendrick ML, Nagorney DM, Grant CS, Donohue JH, Farnell MB, *et al.* Duodenal carcinoid tumors: how aggressive should we be? *J Gastrointest Surg*, 2001; **5**: 588–93.
8. Virdis R, Street ME, Bandello MA, Tripodi C, Donadio A, Villani AR, *et al.* Growth and pubertal disorders in neurofibromatosis type 1. *J Pediatr Endocrinol Metab*, 2003; **16** (Suppl. 2): 289–92.
9. Radtke HB, Sebold CD, Allison C, Haidle JL, Schneider G. Neurofibromatosis type 1 in genetic counseling practice: recommendations of the National Society of Genetic Counselors. *J Genet Couns*, 2007; **16**: 387–407.
10. Evans DG, Huson SM, Donnai D, Neary W, Blair V, Newton V, *et al.* A genetic study of type 2 neurofibromatosis in the United Kingdom. II. Guidelines for genetic counselling. *J Med Genet*, 1992; **29**: 847–52.
11. Trofatter JA, MacCollin MM, Rutter JL, Murrell JR, Duyao MP, Parry DM, *et al.* A novel moesin-, ezrin-, radixin-like gene is a candidate for the neurofibromatosis 2 tumor suppressor. *Cell*, 1993; **72**: 791–800.

12. Okada T, You L, Giancotti FG. Shedding light on Merlin's wizardry. *Trends Cell Biol*, 2007; **17**: 222–9.
13. Baser ME, Friedman JM, Wallace AJ, Ramsden RT, Joe H, Evans DG. Evaluation of clinical diagnostic criteria for neurofibromatosis 2. *Neurology*, 2002; **59**: 1759–65.
14. Evans DG, Baser ME, O'Reilly B, Rowe J, Gleeson M, Saeed S, *et al.* Management of the patient and family with neurofibromatosis 2: a consensus conference statement. *Br J Neurosurg*, 2005; **19**: 5–12.

6.15

Carney's complex

Constantine A. Stratakis

Introduction

Carney's complex (CNC) is an autosomal dominant disorder, which was described in 1985 as 'the complex of myxomas, spotty pigmentation, and endocrine overactivity' in 40 patients (1). Since then, more than 500 index cases have been reported, resulting in better definition of the disease and the establishment of diagnostic criteria (2, 3). As implied from the initial description, CNC is not only a multiple neoplasia syndrome, but also causes a variety of pigmented lesions of the skin and mucosae. (4) Several patients described in earlier years under the acronyms NAME (nevi, atrial myxomas, and ephelides) and LAMB (lentigines, atrial myxomas, and blue nevi) probably had CNC (5, 6). Thus, lentigines, blue nevi, café-au-lait spots, and cutaneous tumours, such as myxomas, fibromas, and others, are major features of the disease (4, 7–10).

The clinical characteristics of CNC have been reviewed and are presented in Box 6.15.1 (2, 9). A definite diagnosis of CNC is given if two or more major manifestations are present (4, 9, 11, 12). A number of related manifestations may accompany or suggest the presence of CNC but are not considered diagnostic of the disease (Box 6.15.1). Cutaneous manifestations constitute three of the major disease manifestations: (1) spotty skin pigmentation with a typical distribution (lips, conjunctiva, and inner or outer canthi, genital mucosa); (2) cutaneous or mucosal myxoma; and (3) blue nevi (multiple) or epithelioid blue nevus. Suggestive or associated with CNC findings but not diagnostic are: (1) intense freckling (without darkly pigmented spots or typical distribution); (2) multiple blue nevi of common type; (3) café-au-lait spots or other 'birthmarks'; and (4) multiple skin tags or other skin lesions, including lipomas and angiofibromas.

The relationship between the cutaneous and noncutaneous manifestations of CNC appears to be an essential clue to the molecular aetiology of the disease. According to the latest reports, more than half of CNC patients present with both characteristic dermatological and endocrine signs; however, a significant number of patients present with skin lesions that are only 'suggestive' and not characteristic of CNC (9). A recent classification based on both dermatological and endocrine markers has subgrouped CNC patients as: multisymptomatic (with extensive endocrine and skin signs); intermediate (with few dermatological and endocrine manifestations); and, paucisymptomatic (with isolated primary pigmented nodular adrenocortical disease (PPNAD) alone and no cutaneous signs) (9).

Skin manifestations in CNC

Skin lesions are consistently reported in the majority of the CNC patients (above 80%), the most common being lentigines (in 70–75% of cases). Other pigmented lesions, most frequently blue nevi and café-au-lait spots, with or without lentigines, are seen in approximately 50% of CNC patients. The effort to systemize the knowledge on the cutaneous lesions in CNC patients is driven by their high diagnostic value—presented early in life and easily recognizable, the skin manifestations are an early sign that directs dermatologists' attention towards underlying endocrine or other pathology. In an attempt to outline the most specific and sensitive skin abnormalities in CNC, several research groups have published exhaustive analyses that add to an improved diagnostic and preventive approach (9, 10, 13). The major challenge appears to be in distinguishing the disease-associated prominent lesions from the more common non-CNC-specific, age- or sun-related skin alterations.

Characteristic CNC pigmented skin lesions are shown in Fig. 6.15.1. Lentigo is a hamartomatous melanocytic lesion, clinically similar but histologically different from freckles (14). Morphologically, lentigines are flat, poorly circumscribed, brown-to-black macules, usually less than 0.5 cm in diameter, but these may differ in different ethnic groups. In African-Americans, for example, lentigines may be slightly raised, dark papules, similar to nevi (14). In contrast to the common freckles, on histological examination lentigines show basal cell layer hyperpigmentation associated with an increased number of melanocytes (hyperplasia), the majority of which appear hypertrophic. This distinguishes them from freckles (ephelides), which present with a regular number of melanocytes and are pigmented as a result of melanin disposition in the surrounding keratinocytes.

Lentiginosis is one of the manifestations of CNC that can occur early; lentigines usually acquire their typical intensity and distribution during the peripubertal period (9, 10, 15). They typically involve the centrofacial area, including the vermilion border of the lips, and the conjunctiva, especially the lacrimal caruncle and the conjunctival semilunar fold; intraoral pigmented spots have also been reported (16). In contrast to age-related skin lesions, CNC-associated lentigines tend to fade after the fourth decade of life, but may be detectable as late as the eighth decade (9, 15).

The next very common skin manifestation in CNC is a lesion known as blue nevus, which is infrequent in the general population. Blue nevi can be seen as small (usually <5 mm), blue to black-coloured marks with a circular or star-shaped appearance.

Box 6.15.1 Diagnostic criteria for Carney's complex

Major diagnostic criteria for Carney's complex

1. Spotty skin pigmentation with typical distribution (lips, conjunctiva and inner or outer canthi, vaginal and penile mucosal)
2. Myxoma[a] (cutaneous and mucosal)
3. Cardiac myxoma[a]
4. Breast myxomatosis[a] or fat-suppressed magnetic resonance imaging findings suggestive of this diagnosis
5. Primary pigmented nodular adrenocortical disease[a] or paradoxical positive response of urinary glucocorticosteroid excretion to dexamethasone administration during Liddle's test[b]
6. Acromegaly due to growth hormone-producing adenoma[a]
7. Large-cell calcifying Sertoli cell tumour[a] or characteristic calcification on testicular ultrasound
8. Thyroid carcinoma[a] or multiple, hypoechoic nodules on thyroid ultrasound in a young patient
9. Psammomatous melanotic schwannomas[a]
10. Blue naevus, epithelioid blue naevus[a]
11. Breast ductal adenoma[a]
12. Osteochondromyxoma[a]

Supplementary criteria

1. Affected first-degree relative
2. Inactivating mutation of the *PRKAR1A* gene

Findings suggestive of or possibly associated with Carney's complex, but not diagnostic for the disease

1. Intense freckling (without darkly pigmented spots or typical distribution)
2. Blue naevus, common type (if multiple)
3. Café-au-lait spots or other birthmarks
4. Elevated insulin-like growth factor -1 levels, abnormal glucose tolerance test, or paradoxical growth hormone response to thyrotropin-releasing hormone testing in the absence of clinical acromegaly
5. Cardiomyopathy
6. Pilonidal sinus
7. History of Cushing's syndrome, acromegaly, or sudden death in extended family
8. Multiple skin tags or other skin lesions; lipomas
9. Colonic polyps (usually in association with acromegaly)
10. Hyperprolactinaemia (usually mild and almost always combined with clinical or subclinical acromegaly)
11. Single, benign thyroid nodule in a young patient; multiple thyroid nodules in an older patient (detected on ultrasonography)
12. Family history of carcinoma, in particular of the thyroid, colon, pancreas, and ovary; other multiple benign or malignant tumours

[a] After histological confirmation.
[b] It has been shown that patients with primary pigmented nodular adrenocortical disease exhibit a paradoxical increase in cortisol secretion in response to Liddle's test (administration of dexamethasone at doses of 2 mg/d for 2 days followed by 8 mg/d for 2 days); this abnormal cortisol response is now used as a criterion for the diagnosis of the disease.

Their distribution is variable; most often they occur on the face, trunk, and limbs, and less frequently on the hands or feet.

An interesting subtype of blue nevus, which is exceedingly rare as a sporadic lesion in the general population but is sometimes seen in patients with CNC, is the epithelioid blue nevus (17). Epithelioid blue nevus usually presents with intensive pigmentation and poorly circumscribed proliferative regions containing two cell types: heavily pigmented globular and fusiform cells; and lightly pigmented, polygonal spindle melanocytes with a single prominent nucleolus. In contrast to blue nevi, epithelioid blue nevi display no dermal fibrosis (18). After comprehensive comparative analysis, and based on the fact the epithelioid blue nevi have also been reported in patients with none of the other features of CNC, epithelioid blue nevi are not considered pathognomonic for CNC but simply associated with the disease (9, 18).

Blue nevi and lentigines in CNC are often accompanied by café-au-lait spots, which are otherwise rarely present as an isolated skin manifestation of CNC. Like lentigines, café-au-lait spots can be present at birth. In general, café-au-lait spots in CNC are less intensely pigmented than those seen in McCune–Albright syndrome and they are more similar to those seen in the neurofibromatosis syndromes.

The third most common skin manifestation of CNC—cutaneous myxoma—is reported in between 30 and 55% of the studied patients (4, 9, 10). Cutaneous myxomas rarely exceed 1 cm in diameter and often affect the eyelids, ears, and nipples, but may also be seen on other areas of the face, ears, trunk, and perineum. They usually appear as asymptomatic, sessile, small, opalescent, or dark pink papules and large, finger-like, pedunculated lesions. They are typically diagnosed early in life, most often during the teenage years (mean age, 18 years). In the majority of patients (>70%) cutaneous myxomas show multiple appearance and a tendency to recur. The frequency of myxoma may be underestimated because of the sometimes difficult clinical diagnosis; therefore histological examination is strongly recommended when in doubt. Histopathologically, myxomas are characterized by a location in the dermis or, occasionally, more superficially in the subcutaneous tissues, sharp circumscription (sometimes encapsulation), relative hypocellularity with abundant myxoid stroma, prominent capillaries, lobulation (larger lesions), and occasional presence of an epithelial component. It is estimated that approximately 80% of CNC patients with life-threatening cardiac myxoma present with cutaneous myxoma earlier in life; therefore, cutaneous myxoma

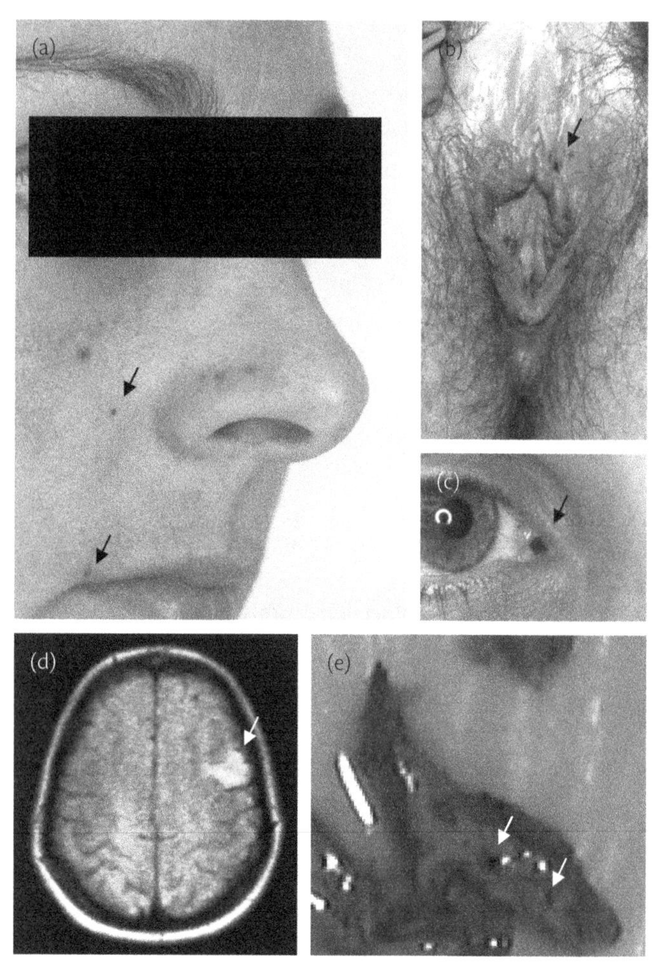

Fig. 6.15.1 A patient with Carney's complex (CAR47.01) with the germline IVS2+1 G>A *PRKAR1A* mutation. (a) Since childhood the patient had freckling on the vermillion border of the upper lip (lower arrow) and blue nevi on the face (upper arrow) and elsewhere. (b) Extensive genital pigmented nevi and lentigines (arrow). (c) Pigmentation of the inner canthus that is pathognomonic for Carney's complex. (d) The patient first presented with a stroke (arrow) and right-sided paralysis due to dislodged right atrial cardiac myxoma. (e) She developed Cushing's syndrome due to primary pigmented nodular adrenocortical disease, which is characterized by the many brown micronodules (arrows) present throughout the adrenal cortex. (See also Plate 40)

can serve as good marker for the disease with high prognostic significance (4, 9, 10).

Other CNC-related skin abnormalities include melanocytic and atypical nevi, and the so-called Spitz nevus. Occasionally, depigmented lesions can be present at birth or, more often, develop in early childhood. These manifestations, although usually not considered specific, may be suggestive for the disease or may accompany other CNC signs of importance for the diagnosis.

Molecular genetics

Most cases of CNC are caused by inactivating mutations in the gene encoding one of the subunits of the protein kinase A (PKA) tetrameric enzyme, namely regulatory subunit type 1 α (*PRKAR1A*), located at 17q22–24 (4). Although a second locus (2p16) has been implicated, sequencing of the region in the linked families did not reveal alterations in other coding sequences (19).

PRKAR1A extends to a total genomic length of approximately 21 kb and consists of 11 exons, encoding a total of 381 amino acids, with a dimerization/ docking domain, and two cAMP binding domains, A and B. Since the identification of *PRKAR1A* mutations in CNC, more than 100 disease-causing pathogenic sequence changes have been reported; they are spread over the entire coding sequence of the gene, without a notable preference for a region or exon. Structurally, the vast majority of the mutations consist of base substitutions, small deletions, and insertions or combined rearrangements, involving up to 15 bp (4); although rare, large *PRKAR1A* deletions have been reported (20).

Mutations in *PRKAR1A* are seen in more than 70% of the patients with classical CNC and, in the majority of these cases, they lead to complete inactivation of one of the *PRKAR1A* alleles as a result of premature stop codon generation and subsequent nonsense-mediated mRNA decay (NMD) (4, 10). In its inactive form, PKA is a tetramer composed of two regulatory and two catalytic subunits (21). The decreased cellular concentration of regulatory subunits results in a balance shift between the formation and the disassembly of the PKA tetramer, towards the release of the catalytic subunits. The free catalytic subunits, which are active serine–threonine kinases, further phosphorylate a series of targets that regulate downstream effectors and transcription of specific genes, mediating cell growth and differentiation (22). Thus, functionally, the mechanism by which *PRKAR1A* haploinsufficiency causes CNC is through excess cellular cAMP signalling in affected tissues (23). CNC lesions frequently show loss-of-heterozygosity, suggesting a tumour-suppressor function for PRKAR1A (4, 3).

Although significantly less frequent, mutations that escape NMD and lead to the expression of an abnormal, defective PRKAR1A protein have been reported (20, 24, 25). These expressed mutations may lead to a characteristic phenotype that reflects the location and the type of the genetic change. Examples include a germline in-frame deletion of exon 3 which results in severe expression of the majority of the CNC manifestations—a phenotype illustrating the importance of exon 3 in linking the dimerization/docking and the first cAMP binding domain (20). In contrast, another in-frame variant—a splice-site deletion that eliminates exon 7—is seen associated mostly with lentiginosis and the adrenal component of CNC, PPNAD. Just as lentiginosis is the most common nonendocrine CNC manifestation, PPNAD is the most frequently observed endocrine tumour of the disease. Thus, the presence of only two features of CNC, the most common ones, with this splice-site variant is consistent with the anticipation of a milder phenotype associated with certain splice mutations, due to their incomplete penetrance at the mRNA level, (i.e. not all DNA molecules harbouring the splice variant result in mRNA species lacking exon 7) (24–26).

Apart from the above mentioned, expressed mutant PRKAR1A isoforms, several other expressed isoforms that result from single amino acid substitutions have been reported (25, 26). Detailed *in vitro* analysis of their effects on protein function have revealed important PRKAR1A domain features (26, 27). The six naturally occurring missense substitutions examined by this study (Ser9Asn, Arg74Cys, Arg146Ser, Asp183Tyr, Ala213Asp, Gly289Trp) are spread over all the functional domains of the protein. Although, as mentioned before, the low number of individuals affected by each of these mutations prevented detailed phenotype–genotype analysis, these studies support the previous suggestion that the alteration of

PRKAR1A function alone (and not only its complete loss) is sufficient to increase PKA activity, leading to CNC.

Until recently, no genotype–phenotype correlations had been found for the different stop codon mutations, which are expected to uniformly lead to lack of the *PRKAR1A* mutant allele's protein product in cells. This was because most of the mutations were identified in single patients only and only two (c.491–492delTG/p. Val164fsX4, and c.709(−7–2) del6(TTTTTA)) had been seen in more than three kindreds (4, 24). The first study to explore all *PRKAR1A* mutations found to date against all CNC phenotypes was recently completed; 353 individuals, 258 of whom (73%) were positive for a *PRKAR1A* mutation, were studied (10). Several features that distinguish *PRKAR1A* mutation carriers from mutation-negative CNC patients were identified; the former presented more frequently and earlier in life with pigmented skin lesions, myxomas, thyroid, and gonadal tumours. In addition, essential correlations between certain genetic defects and the severity and type of CNC manifestations were found. Bertherat *et al.* (10) outlined subgroups of patients; the first group presented with isolated PPNAD, in some cases accompanied with lentiginosis. In this group the following tendencies were observed: (1) patients diagnosed before 8 years of age were rarely carriers of *PRKAR1A* mutations; and (2) most of the patients with isolated PPNAD and the presence of *PRKAR1A* mutation were carriers of either the c.709(−7–2) del6(TTTTTA) mutation ($p < 0.0001$) or the c.1A>G/p.Met1Val substitution affecting the initiation codon of the protein. These observations were in line with previously published reports (4, 24) and both mutations are rather rare. Although the molecular mechanism of the Met1Val substitution is not completely clear, it is the only mutation that alters the protein initiation site, and may, in theory, result in alternative initiation (28); c.709(−7–2) del6(TTTTTA) is a splice variant that is expected to result in an exon skip, frame shift, and premature stop codon generation. However, since it does not affect the two immediate nucleotides on either site of the splice junction, it is expected to lead to splicing in less than 100% of the molecules that harbour it, and thus, presumably, to lead to a milder phenotype. The fact that a milder phenotype involves only the adrenal and skin is suggestive of their high sensitivity to changes in PKA activity.

The second group of CNC patients that was suggested to have a particular genotype–phenotype correlation comprised individuals with myxomas (affecting all locations—skin, heart, and breast), PMS, thyroid tumours, and large-cell calcifying Sertoli cell tumours (LCCSCT). In these patients, *PRKAR1A* mutations were seen substantially more often. Related to this is the recognition that certain tumours present at a significantly younger age in *PRKAR1A* mutation carriers: cardiac myxomas ($p = 0.02$), thyroid tumours ($p = 0.03$), and LCCSCTs ($p = 0.04$) (10). Another finding in these patients was that mutations that escaped NMD and led to an alternate, usually shorter, protein were associated with an overall higher total number of CNC manifestations ($p = 0.04$).

In terms of pigmented skin lesions in CNC, two important correlations have been observed: (1) lentigines (as well as PMS, acromegaly, and cardiac myxomas), were seen significantly more often in CNC patients with exonic *PRKAR1A* mutations, compared to those with intronic ones ($p = 0.04$); and (2) lentigines (as well as cardiac myxoma and thyroid tumours) were significantly associated with the hot spot c.491–492delTG mutation compared to all other *PRKAR1A* defects ($p = 0.03$). These data add greatly to the understanding of the molecular mechanisms of the involvement of *PRKAR1A* in endocrine and other tumourigenesis and, thus, for genetic counselling and prognosis in CNC families.

Interestingly, a 2.3-Mb deletion in chromosome band 17q24.2–q24.3, which involved *PRKAR1A* together with another 13 genes, resulted in a number of clinical features, including posterior laryngeal cleft, growth restriction, microcephaly, and moderate mental retardation. The only CNC manifestation was numerous freckles and lentigines at a young age (29); the authors called the observed phenotype 'CNC plus'.

To date, the molecular causes underlying the formation of pigmented skin lesions in CNC are not fully understood. A possible mechanism involves the PKA-mediated activation of pathways downstream of the melanocortin receptors (MCRs), which form a subfamily of the G protein-coupled receptors (GPCRs) and regulate a wide variety of processes, including skin pigmentation (30–32). The melanocortin 1 receptor (MC1R) is expressed preferentially in epidermal melanocytes and is known to be the key regulator of mammalian pigmentation (31, 33). MC1R is stimulated by the proopiomelanocortin-derived melanocyte-stimulating hormone and ACTH and, in turn, activates the rate-limiting enzyme in melanin synthesis, tyrosinase. As a GPCR, MC1R is positively coupled with adenylate cyclase, and its actions are mainly mediated by PKA, in coordination with other signalling molecules involving protein kinase C (PKC) and MAPKs (34–36).

Relationship to other syndromes

CNC shares clinical features and molecular pathways with several other familial lentiginosis syndromes, such as McCune–Albright syndrome (OMIM #174800), Peutz–Jeghers (OMIM #175200), LEOPARD (OMIM #151100), Noonan's (OMIM #163950), Cowden's disease (OMIM #158350), and Bannayan–Ruvalcaba–Riley syndrome (OMIM #153480). In all of these conditions skin lesions accompany underlying endocrine and/or other abnormalities, which, as in CNC, are considered an important diagnostic sign.

Probably the closest, at least in terms of a molecular pathway link, to CNC is McCune–Albright syndrome. Patients with this condition have characteristic lesions that affect predominantly three systems: the skin, the endocrine system, and the skeleton. The café-au-lait spots in McCune–Albright syndrome patients are similar to those observed in CNC, but tend to be more intensely pigmented. McCune–Albright syndrome is caused by postzygotic, activating, somatic mutations of *GNAS*, located on 20q13, which encodes the adenylate cyclase-stimulating G α protein (Gsa) of the heterotrimeric G protein (37). G proteins couple hormone receptors to adenylyl cyclase and are therefore required for hormone-stimulated cAMP synthesis. Because of the somatic nature of the genetic defect, the presentation of the disease is mosaic and the level of clinical involvement of any tissue is highly variable. The mutations in *GNAS* are always missense substitutions at the critical sites for the GTPase inactivation (amino acid positions Arg201 and Gln227), and, in contrast to *PRKAR1A* defects, lead to constant protein activation and prolonged cAMP production.

We have reported another endocrine lesion that is associated with increased tissue levels of cAMP, isolated micronodular adrenocortical hyperplasia (iMAD). In these patients, inactivating mutations in the genes encoding phosphodiesterases types 11A (*PDE11A*) and 8B (*PDE8B*) have been reported (38–40). iMAD patients were initially considered CNC patients, but it soon became clear that iMAD is not the same as PPNAD (41).

Peutz–Jeghers syndrome, another autosomal dominant familial lentiginosis syndrome, is characterized by melanocytic macules of the lips, buccal mucosa, and digits, multiple gastrointestinal hamartomatous polyps, and an increased risk of various neoplasms. The lentigines observed in patients with Peutz–Jeghers syndrome shows similar density and distribution to the ones in CNC. Peutz–Jeghers syndrome has been elucidated at the molecular level (42, 43); the disease was first mapped to chromosome 19p13.3 and, soon after, the gene encoding the serine–threonine kinase 11 (*STK11* also known as *LKB1*) was found to be mutated in most patients (44–49). The proposed mechanism of the disease is through elimination of the kinase activity of the STK11/LKB1 tumour suppressor protein.

LEOPARD is an acronym for the manifestations of the syndrome comprising: multiple lentigines, electrocardiographic conduction abnormalities, ocular hypertelorism, pulmonic stenosis, abnormal genitalia, retardation of growth, and sensorineural deafness (50). LEOPARD is allelic to Noonan's syndrome; both diseases are linked to mutations in *PTPN11* (12q24), the gene encoding the nonreceptor tyrosine phosphatase Shp-2 (51, 52). The protein encoded by this gene is a member of the protein tyrosine phosphatase family, proteins that are known to regulate a variety of cellular processes including cell growth, differentiation, mitotic cycle, and oncogenic transformation.

Cowden's disease and Bannayan–Ruvalcaba–Riley syndrome share clinical characteristics, including mucocutaneous lesions, hamartomatous polyps of the gastrointestinal tract, and increased risk of developing neoplasms. Both conditions are caused by mutations in the *PTEN* gene (53–55). *PTEN* is located on 10q23.31 and encodes phosphatidylinositol-3, 4, 5-trisphosphate 3-phosphatase. The gene was recognized as a tumour suppressor gene and has been found to be mutated in a number of tumours (56). It contains a tensin-like domain as well as a catalytic domain similar to that of the dual-specificity protein tyrosine phosphatases. Unlike most of the protein tyrosine phosphatases, PTEN preferentially dephosphorylates phosphoinositide substrates. It negatively regulates intracellular levels of phosphatidylinositol-3, 4, 5-trisphosphate in cells and its tumour suppressor effect is expressed by inhibition of the AKT/PKB signalling pathway.

The overlapping clinical manifestations of these syndromes, which are caused by distinct molecular defects, suggest crosstalk between the involved pathways. Indeed, PRKAR1A inactivation leads to phosphorylation of mTOR and ERK1/2 (57, 58), LKB1 is phosphorylated by PKA (59), and PTEN expression is positively regulated by transcription factor Egr-1 in a PKA-dependent manner (60).

Acknowledgements

Studies on CNC and related syndromes have been supported by the Eunice Kennedy Shriver National Institute of Child Health & Human Development, NIH, intramural project Z01-HD-000642–04 (to Dr C. A. Stratakis).

References

1. Carney JA, Gordon H, Carpenter PC, Shenoy BV, Go VL. The complex of myxomas, spotty pigmentation, and endocrine overactivity. *Medicine (Baltimore)*, 1985; **64**: 270–83.
2. Boikos SA, Stratakis CA. Carney complex: pathology and molecular genetics. *Neuroendocrinology*, 2006; **83**: 189–99.
3. Boikos SA, Stratakis CA. Carney complex: the first 20 years. *Curr Opin Oncol*, 2007; **19**: 24–9.
4. Stratakis CA, Kirschner LS, Carney JA. Clinical and molecular features of the Carney complex: diagnostic criteria and recommendations for patient evaluation. *J Clin Endocrinol Metab*, 2001; **86**: 4041–6.
5. Atherton DJ, Pitcher DW, Wells RS, Macdonald DM. A syndrome of various cutaneous pigmented lesions, myxoid neurofibromata and atrial myxoma: the NAME syndrome. *Br J Dermatol*, 1980; **103**: 421–9.
6. Rhodes AR, Silverman RA, Harrist TJ, Perez-Atayde AR. Mucocutaneous lentigines, cardiomucocutaneous myxomas, and multiple blue nevi: the "LAMB" syndrome. *J Am Acad Dermatol*, 1984; **10**: 72–82.
7. Carney JA, Headington JT, Su WP. Cutaneous myxomas. A major component of the complex of myxomas, spotty pigmentation, and endocrine overactivity. *Arch Dermatol*, 1986; **122**: 790–8.
8. Jabbour SA, Davidovici BB, Wolf R. Rare syndromes. *Clin Dermatol*, 2006; **24**: 299–316.
9. Mateus C, Palangie A, Franck N, Groussin L, Bertagna X, Avril MF, *et al.* Heterogeneity of skin manifestations in patients with Carney complex. *J Am Acad Dermatol*, 2008; **59**: 801–10.
10. Bertherat J, Horvath A, Groussin L, Grabar S, Boikos S, Cazabat L, *et al.* Mutations in regulatory subunit type 1A of cyclic AMP-dependent protein kinase (PRKAR1A): phenotype analysis in 353 patients and 80 different genotypes. *J Clin Endocrinol Metab*, 2009; **94**: 2085–91.
11. Bertherat J. Carney complex (CNC). *Orphanet J Rare Dis*, 2006; **1**: 21.
12. Sandrini F, Stratakis CA. Clinical and molecular genetics of Carney complex. *Mol Genet Metab*, 2003; **78**: 83–92.
13. Bauer AJ, Stratakis CA. The lentiginoses: cutaneous markers of systemic disease and a window to new aspects of tumourigenesis. *J Med Genet*, 2005; **42**: 801–10.
14. Stratakis CA. Genetics of Peutz-Jeghers syndrome, Carney complex and other familial lentiginoses. *Horm Res*, 2000; **54**: 334–43.
15. Young WF JR, Carney JA, Musa BU, Wulffraat NM, Lens JW, Drexhage HA. Familial Cushing's syndrome due to primary pigmented nodular adrenocortical disease. Reinvestigation 50 years later. *N Engl J Med*, 1989; **321**: 1659–64.
16. Carney JA. Carney complex: the complex of myxomas, spotty pigmentation, endocrine overactivity, and schwannomas. *Semin Dermatol*, 1995; **14**: 90–8.
17. Zembowicz A, Carney JA, Mihm MC. Pigmented epithelioid melanocytoma: a low-grade melanocytic tumor with metastatic potential indistinguishable from animal-type melanoma and epithelioid blue nevus. *Am J Surg Pathol*, 2004; **28**: 31–40.
18. Carney JA, Ferreiro JA. The epithelioid blue nevus. A multicentric familial tumor with important associations, including cardiac myxoma and psammomatous melanotic schwannoma. *Am J Surg Pathol*, 1996; **20**: 259–72.
19. Stratakis CA, Carney JA, Lin JP, Papanicolaou DA, Karl M, Kastner DL, *et al.* Carney complex, a familial multiple neoplasia and lentiginosis syndrome. *J Clin Invest*, 1996; **97**: 699–705.
20. Horvath A, Bossis I, Giatzakis C, Levine E, Weinberg F, Meoli E, *et al.* Large deletions of the PRKAR1A gene in Carney complex. *Clin Cancer Res*, 2008; **14**: 388–95.
21. Tasken K, Skalhegg BS, Tasken KA, Solberg R, Knutsen HK, Levy FO, *et al.* Structure, function, and regulation of human cAMP-dependent protein kinases. *Adv Second Messenger Phosphoprotein Res*, 1997; **31**: 191–204.

22. Shabb JB. Physiological substrates of cAMP-dependent protein kinase. *Chem Rev*, 2001; **101**: 2381–411.
23. Robinson-White A, Meoli E, Stergiopoulos S, Horvath A, Boikos S, Bossis I, *et al.* PRKAR1A Mutations and protein kinase A interactions with other signaling pathways in the adrenal cortex. *J Clin Endocrinol Metab*, 2006; **91**: 2380–8.
24. Groussin L, Horvath A, Jullian E, Boikos S, Rene-Corail F, Lefebvre H, *et al.* A PRKAR1A mutation associated with primary pigmented nodular adrenocortical disease in 12 kindreds. *J Clin Endocrinol Metab*, 2006; **91**: 1943–9.
25. Veugelers M, Wilkes D, Burton K, Mcdermott DA, Song Y, Goldstein MM, *et al.* Comparative PRKAR1A genotype-phenotype analyses in humans with Carney complex and prkar1a haploinsufficient mice. *Proc Natl Acad Sci U S A*, 2004; **101**: 14222–7.
26. Greene EL, Horvath AD, Nesterova M, Giatzakis C, Bossis I, Stratakis CA. In vitro functional studies of naturally occurring pathogenic PRKAR1A mutations that are not subject to nonsense mRNA decay. *Hum Mutat*, 2008; **29**: 633–9.
27. Horvath A, Giatzakis C, Tsang K, Greene E, Osorio P, Boikos S, *et al.* A cAMP-specific phosphodiesterase (PDE8B) that is mutated in adrenal hyperplasia is expressed widely in human and mouse tissues: a novel PDE8B isoform in human adrenal cortex. *Eur J Hum Genet*, 2008; **16**: 1245–53.
28. Kirschner LS, Sandrini F, Monbo J, Lin JP, Carney JA, Stratakis CA. Genetic heterogeneity and spectrum of mutations of the PRKAR1A gene in patients with the carney complex. *Hum Mol Genet*, 2000; **9**: 3037–46.
29. Blyth M, Huang S, Maloney V, Crolla JA, Temple KI. A 2.3Mb deletion of 17q24.2-q24.3 associated with 'Carney Complex plus'. *Eur J Med Genet*, 2008; **51**: 672–8.
30. Butler AA, Cone RD. The melanocortin receptors: lessons from knockout models. *Neuropeptides*, 2005; **36**: 77–84.
31. Abdel-Malek ZA. Melanocortin receptors: their functions and regulation by physiological agonists and antagonists. *Cell Mol Life Sci*, 2001; **58**: 434–41.
32. Gantz I, Fong TM. The melanocortin system. *Am J Physiol Endocrinol Metab*, 2003; **284**: E468–74.
33. Kadekaro AL, Kanto H, Kavanagh R, Abdel-Malek ZA. Significance of the melanocortin 1 receptor in regulating human melanocyte pigmentation, proliferation, and survival. *Ann N Y Acad Sci*, 2003; **994**: 359–65.
34. Busca R, Ballotti R. Cyclic AMP a key messenger in the regulation of skin pigmentation. *Pigment Cell Res*, 2000; **13**: 60–9.
35. Tsatmali M, Ancans J, Yukitake J, Thody AJ. Skin POMC peptides: their actions at the human MC-1 receptor and roles in the tanning response. *Pigment Cell Res*, 2000; **13** (Suppl. 8): 125–9.
36. Busca R, Abbe P, Mantoux F, Aberdam E, Peyssonnaux C, Eychene A, *et al.* Ras mediates the cAMP-dependent activation of extracellular signal-regulated kinases (ERKs) in melanocytes. *EMBO J*, 2000; **19**: 2900–10.
37. Weinstein LS, Shenker A, Gejman PV, Merino MJ, Friedman E, Spiegel AM. Activating mutations of the stimulatory G protein in the McCune-Albright syndrome. *N Engl J Med*, 1991; **325**: 1688–95.
38. Horvath A, Giatzakis C, Robinson-White A, Boikos S, Levine E, Griffin K, *et al.* Adrenal hyperplasia and adenomas are associated with inhibition of phosphodiesterase 11A in carriers of PDE11A sequence variants that are frequent in the population. *Cancer Res*, 2006; **66**: 11571–5.
39. Horvath A, Boikos S, Giatzakis C, Robinson-White A, Groussin L, Griffin KJ, *et al.* A genome-wide scan identifies mutations in the gene encoding phosphodiesterase 11A4 (PDE11A) in individuals with adrenocortical hyperplasia. *Nat Genet*, 2006; **38**: 794–800.
40. Horvath A, Mericq V, Stratakis CA. Mutation in PDE8B, a cyclic AMP-specific phosphodiesterase in adrenal hyperplasia. *N Engl J Med*, 2008; **358**: 750–2.
41. Gunther DF, Bourdeau I, Matyakhina L, Cassarino D, Kleiner DE, Griffin K, *et al.* Cyclical Cushing syndrome presenting in infancy: an early form of primary pigmented nodular adrenocortical disease, or a new entity?. *J Clin Endocrinol Metab*, 2004; **89**: 3173–82.
42. Hemminki A, Markie D, Tomlinson I, Avizienyte E, Roth S, Loukola A *et al.* A serine/threonine kinase gene defective in Peutz-Jeghers syndrome. *Nature*, 1998; **391**: 184–7.
43. Jenne DE, Reimann H, Nezu J, Friedel W, Loff S, Jeschke R, *et al.* Peutz-Jeghers syndrome is caused by mutations in a novel serine threonine kinase. *Nat Genet*, 1998; **18**: 38–43.
44. Westerman AM, Entius MM, Boor PP, Koole R, De Baar E, Offerhaus GJ, *et al.* Novel mutations in the LKB1/STK11 gene in Dutch Peutz-Jeghers families. *Hum Mutat*, 1999; **13**: 476–81.
45. Wang ZJ, Churchman M, Avizienyte E, Mckeown C, Davies S, Evans DG, *et al.* Germline mutations of the LKB1 (STK11) gene in Peutz-Jeghers patients. *J Med Genet*, 1999; **36**: 365–8.
46. Resta N, Simone C, Mareni C, Montera M, Gentile M, Susca F, *et al.* STK11 mutations in Peutz-Jeghers syndrome and sporadic colon cancer. *Cancer Res*, 1998; **58**: 4799–801.
47. Jiang CY, Esufali S, Berk T, Gallinger S, Cohen Z, Tobi M, *et al.* STK11/LKB1 germline mutations are not identified in most Peutz-Jeghers syndrome patients. *Clin Genet*, 1999; **56**: 136–41.
48. Ylikorkala A, Avizienyte E, Tomlinson IP, Tiainen M, Roth S, Loukola A, *et al.* Mutations and impaired function of LKB1 in familial and non-familial Peutz-Jeghers syndrome and a sporadic testicular cancer. *Hum Mol Genet*, 1999; **8**: 45–51.
49. Boardman LA, Couch FJ, Burgart LJ, Schwartz D, Berry R, Mcdonnell SK, *et al.* Genetic heterogeneity in Peutz-Jeghers syndrome. *Hum Mutat*, 2000; **16**: 23–30.
50. Gorlin RJ, Anderson RC, Blaw M. Multiple lentigenes syndrome. *Am J Dis Child*, 1969; **117**: 652–62.
51. Jamieson CR, Van Der Burgt I, Brady AF, Van Reen M, Elsawi MM, Hol F, *et al.* Mapping a gene for Noonan syndrome to the long arm of chromosome 12. *Nat Genet*, 1994; **8**: 357–60.
52. Van Der Burgt I, Berends E, Lommen E, Van Beersum S, Hamel B, Mariman E. Clinical and molecular studies in a large Dutch family with Noonan syndrome. *Am J Med Genet*, 1994; **53**: 187–91.
53. Nelen MR, Padberg GW, Peeters EA, Lin AY, Van Den Helm B, Frants RR, *et al.* Localization of the gene for Cowden disease to chromosome 10q22–23. *Nat Genet*, 1996; **13**: 114–6.
54. Liaw D, Marsh DJ, Li J, Dahia PL, Wang SI, Zheng Z, *et al.* Germline mutations of the PTEN gene in Cowden disease, an inherited breast and thyroid cancer syndrome. *Nat Genet*, 1997; **16**: 64–7.
55. Marsh DJ, Dahia PL, Zheng Z, Liaw D, Parsons R, Gorlin RJ, Eng C. Germline mutations in PTEN are present in Bannayan-Zonana syndrome. *Nat Genet*, 1997; **16**: 333–4.
56. Yin Y, Shen WH. PTEN: a new guardian of the genome. *Oncogene*, 2008; **27**: 5443–53.
57. Robinson-White A, Hundley TR, Shiferaw M, Bertherat J, Sandrini F, Stratakis CA. Protein kinase-A activity in PRKAR1A-mutant cells, and regulation of mitogen-activated protein kinases ERK1/2. *Hum Mol Genet*, 2003; **12**: 1475–84.
58. Mavrakis M, Lippincott-Schwartz J, Stratakis CA, Bossis I. Depletion of type IA regulatory subunit (RIalpha) of protein kinase A (PKA) in mammalian cells and tissues activates mTOR and causes autophagic deficiency. *Hum Mol Genet*, 2006; **15**: 2962–71.
59. Collins SP, Reoma JL, Gamm DM, Uhler MD. LKB1, a novel serine/threonine protein kinase and potential tumour suppressor, is phosphorylated by cAMP-dependent protein kinase (PKA) and prenylated in vivo. *Biochem J*, 2000; **345**: 673–80.
60. Fernandez S, Garcia-Garcia M, Torres-Aleman I. Modulation by insulin-like growth factor I of the phosphatase PTEN in astrocytes. *Biochim Biophys Acta*, 2008; **1783**: 803–12.

6.16

Molecular and clinical characteristics of the McCune–Albright syndrome

Steven A. Lietman, Michael A. Levine

Introduction

Heterotrimeric guanine nucleotide-binding proteins (G proteins) couple extracellular receptor proteins to intracellular effector enzymes and ion channels. The observation that alterations in G protein-coupled signalling pathways can impact cellular function and proliferation, and cause human disease, has stimulated investigation into the molecular and pharmacological regulation of G protein expression and action. The most well characterized models for altered G protein expression defects have been based on naturally occurring mutations in *GNAS*, a complex gene at 20q13 which encodes the α subunit of Gs, the G protein that stimulates adenylyl cyclase. Somatic mutations in *GNAS* (OMIM 139320) that activate $G\alpha_s$ are present in a subset of endocrine tumours and in patients with the McCune–Albright syndrome (OMIM 174800), a sporadic disorder characterized by increased hormone production and/or cellular proliferation of many tissues. By contrast, germline mutations of the *GNAS* gene that decrease expression or function of $G\alpha_s$ are present in subjects with Albright's hereditary osteodystrophy (AHO), a heritable disorder associated with a constellation of developmental defects and, in many patients, reduced responsiveness to multiple hormones that signal through receptors that require $G\alpha_s$ to activate adenylyl cyclase *EC 4.6.1.1* (i.e. pseudohypoparathyroidism type 1a (OMIM 103580)). McCune–Albright syndrome (MAS) and AHO represent contrasting gain of function and loss of function mutations in the *GNAS* gene, respectively. Clinical and biochemical analyses of subjects with these syndromes have extended our understanding of the developmental and functional consequences of dysfunctional G protein action, and have provided unexpected insights into the importance of cAMP as a regulator of the growth and/or function of many tissues. This chapter will focus on the clinical implications of activating mutations of *GNAS* as the basis for MAS.

G protein structure and signalling

G proteins share a common heterotrimeric structure, consisting of an α subunit and a tightly coupled βγ dimer. The α subunit interacts with detector and effector molecules, binds GTP, and possesses intrinsic GTPase activity (1). There are 16 genes in mammals that encode some 20 different α chains. The α subunits associate with a smaller group of β (at least five) and γ (more than 12) subunits (2). Combinatorial specificity in the associations between various G protein subunits provides the potential for enormous diversity, and may allow distinct heterotrimers to interact selectively with only a limited number of G protein-coupled receptors and effector proteins.

G protein-coupled signalling is regulated by a mechanism in which the binding and hydrolysis of GTP acts a molecular timing switch (Fig. 6.16.1). In the basal (inactive) state, G proteins exist in the heterotrimeric form with GDP bound to the α chain. The interaction of a ligand-bound receptor with a G protein facilitates the release of tightly bound GDP and the subsequent binding of cytosolic GTP. The binding of GTP to the α chain induces conformational changes that facilitate the dissociation of the α-GTP chain from the βγ dimer and the receptor. The free α-GTP chain assumes an active conformation in which a new surface is formed which enables the α chain to interact with target enzymes and ion channels with 20- to 100-fold higher affinity than in the GDP bound state. The βγ dimers also participate in downstream signalling events through interaction with an ever-widening array of targets, including certain forms of adenylyl cyclase and phospholipase C, potassium channels, and G protein-coupled receptor kinases.

G protein signalling is terminated by the hydrolysis of α-GTP to α-GDP by an intrinsic GTPase. The GTPase reaction is a high-energy transition state which requires association of the γ-phosphorus atom with the oxygen of a water molecule. To catalyse this reaction, the γ-phosphate of GTP must be stabilized so that a straight line, perpendicular to the plane of the γ-phosphate, connects the water, the γ-phosphorus, and the oxygen molecule leaving the β-phosphate. In $G\alpha_s$ amino acids arginine^{201} and glutamine^{227} function as 'fingers' to position the γ-phosphate of GTP. With hydrolysis of GTP to GDP, the α-GDP chain reassociates with the βγ dimer and the heterotrimeric G protein is capable of participating in another cycle of receptor-activated signalling (Fig. 6.16.1).

The GTPase of the Gα chain is a molecular timer that controls the duration, and thereby the intensity, of the signalling event.

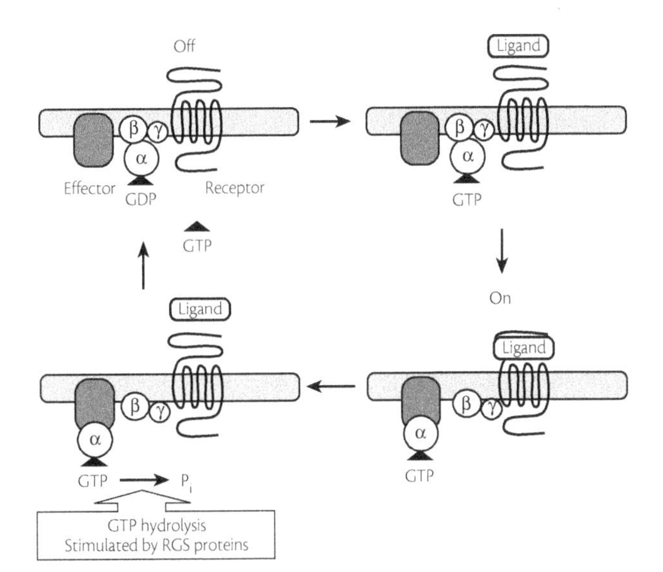

Fig. 6.16.1 The cycle of hormone-dependent GTP binding and hydrolysis that regulates heterotrimeric G protein signal transduction. In the nonstimulated, basal (Off) state, GDP is tightly bound to the α chain of the heterotrimeric G protein. Binding of an agonist (Ligand) to its receptor (depicted with seven transmembrane-spanning domains) induces a conformational change in the receptor, and enables it to activate the G protein. The G protein now releases GDP and binds GTP present in the cytosol. The binding of GTP to the α chain leads to dissociation of the α-GTP from the βγ dimer, and each of these molecules is now free to regulate downstream effector proteins. The hydrolysis of GTP to GDP by the intrinsic GTPase of the α chain promotes reassociation of α-GDP with βγ and the inactive state is restored. The heterotrimeric G protein is ready for another cycle of hormone-induced activation.

Different G protein α have distinctive rates of GTP hydrolysis, and changes in GTPase activity can have profound consequences on signalling. Several factors, termed 'GTPase activating proteins' (GAPs) (3), can interact directly with specific α chains to accelerate the slow intrinsic rate of GTP hydrolysis. One important class of GAPs is represented by the evolutionarily conserved superfamily of proteins, termed 'regulators of G protein signalling', that can stimulate a 40-fold increase in the catalytic rate of GTP hydrolysis, and thus can markedly accelerate the termination of G protein signalling. On the other hand, inhibition of intrinsic GTPase by modification or replacement of key amino acid residues (e.g. arginine[201] or glutamine[227] in $G\alpha_s$) can delay termination of the signal transduction process, and cause persistent and excessive signalling. For example, exotoxins secreted by *Vibrio cholerae* and some strains of *E. coli* catalyse the addition of an ADP-ribose moiety to the side chain of arginine[201] in $G\alpha_s$. This covalent modification markedly reduces GTP hydrolysis and maintains $G\alpha_s$ in its active GTP-bound form, thus resulting in persistent stimulation of adenylyl cyclase (4). The subsequent accumulation of cAMP in intestinal epithelial cells stimulates secretion of salt and water into the intestine and produces, in part, the watery diarrhoea associated with cholera.

Activating mutations of the *GNAS* gene induce cellular proliferation

Activity of adenylyl cyclase is under dual regulatory control through receptors that interact with either G_s to stimulate adenylyl cyclase or with G_i to inhibit adenylyl cyclase. Increased intracellular cAMP stimulates proliferation of many cell types, and can increase synthesis and secretion of endogenous hormones and neurotransmitters. Both germline and somatic mutations in *GNAS* that lead to a gain of function in $G\alpha_s$ produce constitutive (i.e. hormone independent) activation of adenylyl cyclase (5, 6). Vallar, *et al.* (7) initially described a subset of human growth hormone-secreting pituitary tumours in which basal adenylyl cyclase activity *in vitro* was very high and failed to increase further with addition of growth hormone releasing hormone. Subsequent studies showed that these somatotropic tumours contained unusual forms of $G\alpha_s$ that lacked GTPase activity. Loss of GTPase results from somatic mutations in *GNAS* that replace either arginine[201] or glutamine[227] and thereby convert *GNAS* into the *gsp* oncogene. Arginine[201] corresponds to the site of choleragen modification of $G\alpha_s$ (described above), whereas glutamine[227] in $G\alpha_s$ corresponds to the cognate amino acid Gln[61] in the low-molecular-weight GTP-binding protein $p21^{ras}$. Naturally occurring Gln[61] mutations convert $p21^{ras}$ into an oncogene that plays a role in the development of a variety of human tumours (8). Replacement of either arginine[201] or glutamine[227] in $G\alpha_s$ enables the protein to remain in the active, GTP-bound state, and the consequent increase in cAMP leads to cellular proliferation and excessive hormone secretion (9, 10). Such activating mutations occur in approximately 40% of somatotropic tumours (Box 6.16.1). In addition to growth hormone-secreting pituitary tumours, *gsp* mutations are also present in a small number of ACTH-secreting pituitary tumours (11, 12), a subset of thyroid neoplasms, and testicular and ovarian stromal Leydig tumours (13), but are rare in other endocrine tumours (Box 6.16.1). Moreover, *gsp* mutations have been described in ovarian cysts that cause isosexual gonadotropin-independent precocious puberty (14, 15), in intramuscular myxomas (16), and in isolated fibrous dysplasia of the bone (17).

Molecular basis for the McCune–Albright syndrome

In 1937, McCune and Bruch (18) and Albright and associates (19) independently described a sporadic syndrome characterized by the clinical triad of polyostotic fibrous dysplasia, café-au-lait skin lesions, and endocrine hyperfunction, now known as McCune–Albright syndrome (MAS) (Fig. 6.16.2). Despite excessive activity of endocrine tissues, serum levels of the relevant regulatory or tropic hormones were either normal or decreased, suggesting autonomous function. Based on the observation that the cutaneous hyperpigmentation in MAS typically follows the developmental lines of Blaschko, Happle proposed that the underlying genetic abnormality might be a dominantly acting somatic mutation that occurs early in development, leading to a mosaic pattern of distribution of mutant cells (20). Similarly, a lack of documented heritability of MAS has been interpreted as evidence that germline transmission of the mutation would be lethal (20).

The molecular basis for MAS is a somatic mutation in exon 8 of *GNAS* which replaces the residue arginine at position 201, generally by histidine or cysteine (21, 22) but occasionally by serine, glycine, or leucine (23–29). Although missense mutations that replace the nearby glutamine at position 227 have been identified in solitary endocrine tumours, they have not been described in patients with MAS.

Consistent with a postzygotic somatic mutation, cells containing the *gsp* mutation are not present in all tissues of patients with MAS.

Table 6.16.1 Clinical manifestations of McCune–Albright syndrome

Clinical manifestations	% of all patients affected	% of males affected	% of females affected	Age at diagnosis, years (range)	Comments
Fibrous dysplasia	98	96	98	7.7 (0–52)	Polyostotic more common than monostotic
Café-au-lait lesions	85	92	82	7.7 (0–52)	Variable size and number of lesions, irregular border ('coast of Maine')
Precocious puberty	52	15	70	4.9 (0.3–9)	Common initial manifestation
Acromegaly/gigantism	27	38	21	14.8 (0.2–42)	65% with adenoma on MRI/ CT
Hyperprolactinaemia	15	17	13	16.0 (0.2–42)	55% of acromegalic patients with ↑ PRL
Hyperthyroidism	19	13	22	14.4 (0.5–37)	Euthyroid goitre is common
Hypercortisolism	6	8	5	4.4 (0.2–17)	All primary adrenal
Myxomas	5	6	5	34 (17–50)	Extremity myxomas
Osteosarcoma	2	2	3	36 (34–37)	At sites of fibrous dysplasia, not related to prior radiation therapy
Rickets/ osteomalacia	3	2	3	27.3 (8–52)	Responsive to phosphorus plus calcitriol
Cardiac abnormalities	11	15	9	(0.1–66)	Arrhythmias and CHF reported
Hepatic abnormalities	10	11	10	1.9 (0.3–4)	Neonatal icterus is most common

Clinical data compiled from approximately 190 cases of MAS reported in the literature and summarized in (50, 51). Evaluations include clinical and biochemical data; other rarely described manifestations include metabolic acidosis, nephrocalcinosis, mental retardation, thymic and splenic hyperplasia, and colonic polyps.
CHF, congestive heart failure; PRL, prolactin.

Rather, cells containing a mutant *GNAS* gene are distributed in a mosaic pattern, with the greatest number of *gsp*-containing cells present in the most abnormal areas of affected tissues (Fig. 6.16.3) (21, 22, 24, 30, 31). In some cases, *gsp* alleles may be present in only some cell types within tissues that are derived from different embryological precursors. For example, a 3-year-old male MAS patient with macro-orchidism but no precocious puberty was reported to have an Arg201His *gsp* allele present only in Sertoli cells, resulting in isolated Sertoli cell hyperfunction, evidenced by increased AMH expression and cell hyperplasia leading to prepubertal macro-orchidism. There were no signs of Leydig cell activation, and no evidence of excess androgen action (32, 33). The different early embryologic origin of precursors contributing to Sertoli and Leydig cell lineages may underlie the differential distribution of the mutated *GNAS* gene.

Box 6.16.1 Clinical syndromes associated with activating mutations of *GNAS*

Missense mutations of *GNAS* at Arg^{201} and Gln^{227} which cause constitutive activation of AC and the cAMP signalling cascade have been identified in patients with McCune–Albright syndrome and subsets of a variety of endocrine tumours.

- McCune–Albright syndrome (100%)
- Pituitary adenomas (4–50%)
  - Growth hormone-secreting adenomas (35–40%)
  - ACTH-secreting adenomas (4–9%)
  - Clinically nonfunctioning adenomas (rare)
- Thyroid neoplasms (3–70%)
  - Hyperfunctioning and nonfunctioning follicular adenomas
- Papillary and follicular carcinomas
- Parathyroid neoplasms (<5%)
  - Parathyroid adenomas
- Adrenocortical disorders (<5%)
  - Aldosterone-producing adenomas
  - Adrenal hyperplasia
  - Phaeochromocytoma
- Leydig cell and ovarian neoplasms (66%)

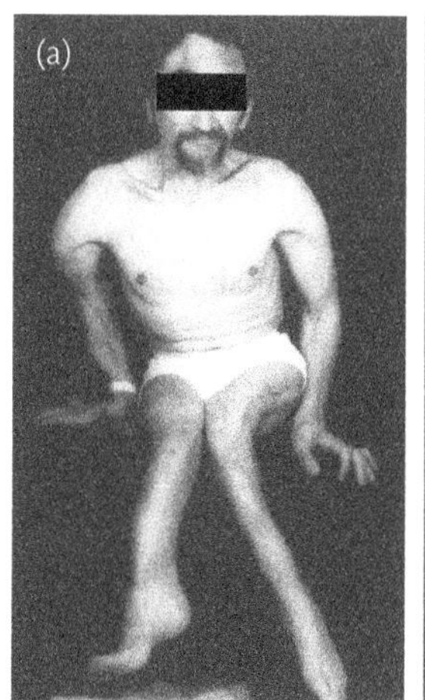

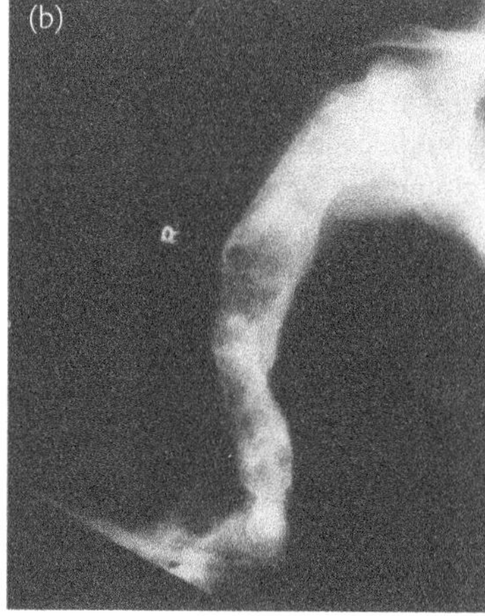

Fig. 6.16.2 Patient with McCune–Albright syndrome. (a) This patient demonstrates the complete clinical triad of McCune–Albright syndrome, with café-au-lait, polyostotic fibrous dysplasia, and excessive endocrine function (hyperthyroidism). The fibrous dysplasia has affected his skull and long bones and led to progressive and debilitating deformity. (b) The classic features of fibrous dysplasia are illustrated in this radiograph of his right upper extremity, which reveals expansile, lytic lesions with a 'ground glass' pattern and a scalloped border secondary to endosteal erosion.

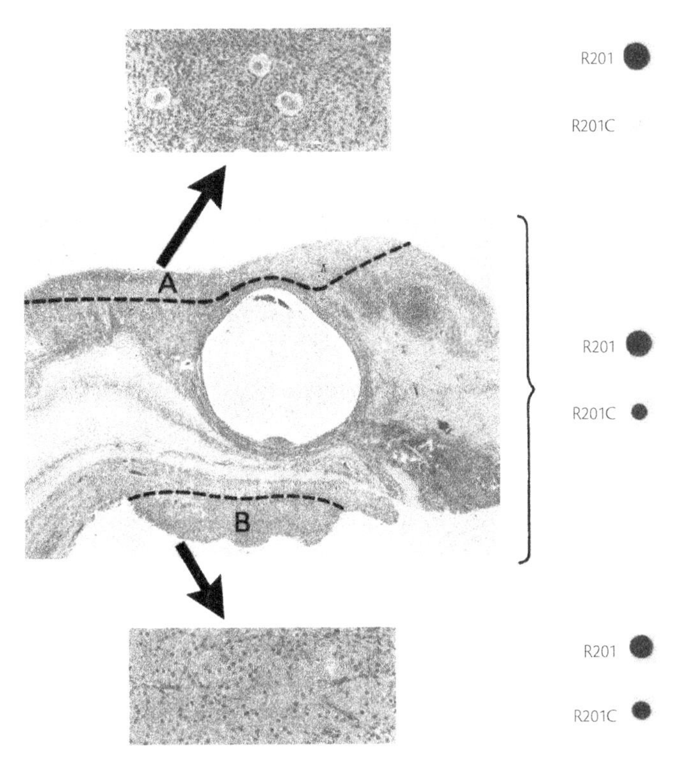

Fig. 6.16.3 Correlation of the abundance of mutant alleles with the pathological abnormalities in ovarian tissue from a young girl with McCune–Albright syndrome and precocious puberty. A cross-section from a paraffin-embedded section of ovary from a patient (patient 1 in (22)) with McCune–Albright syndrome is shown in the centre (× 50). The two outlined areas, shown at × 120, were dissected and analysed independently; area A shows ovarian cortex containing primordial follicles, and area B shows follicular cyst lining containing stimulated luteinized theca. On the right are blots showing the results of allele-specific oligonucleotide hybridization of DNA with wild type (R201) or mutant (R201C) radioactively labelled primers after PCR amplification; DNA was isolated from total ovary (centre) or specific regions as shown. (From Weinstein LS, Shenker A, Gejman PV, Merino MJ, Friedman E, Spiegel AM. Activating mutations of the stimulatory G protein in the McCune-Albright syndrome. *N Engl J Med*, 1991; **325**: 1688–95 (22).)

The variable involvement of different tissues in patients with MAS, as well as the clinical heterogeneity among affected patients, is assumed to be a result of several unique features. First, the number of tissues in which the *gsp* is present, and the proportion and distribution of affected cells in a tissue, will be determined by the timing of the mutational event. Thus, mutations that arise early in embryogenesis are likely to affect several cell lineages and produce a more severe phenotype than mutational events that occur later. For example, acquisition of a *gsp* mutation months or even years after birth could explain the development of a solitary endocrine tumour or a single fibrous dysplasia lesion in some patients.

Second, epigenetic and/or microenvironmental factors that regulate *GNAS* expression can influence the MAS phenotype. For example, stochastic effects, such as allelic imbalance, may favour expression of the mutant allele in some tissues (34), thus exaggerating the effect of a *gsp* mutation. Even more importantly, tissue-specific imprinting of *GNAS* can exert a discrete effect on expression of *gsp* alleles. *GNAS* transcripts that encode $G\alpha_s$ are preferentially expressed from the maternal allele in some cells (e.g. renal proximal tubule cells, thyroid follicular cells, and pituitary somatotrophs) (35, 36). In those cells in which $G\alpha_s$ is expressed predominately, if not exclusively, from the maternal allele, it is more likely that somatic mutations of the maternal allele will have pathophysiological consequences. This is the case for sporadic growth hormone-secreting pituitary adenomas as well as patients with MAS who have growth hormone-secreting pituitary adenomas, where activating mutations of $G\alpha_s$ almost always occur on the maternal allele (37, 38). By contrast, the parental origin of a *gsp* allele will be far less important in cells and tissues where both $G\alpha_s$ alleles are expressed (e.g. bone lesions of fibrous dysplasia).

Additional transcripts are generated by *GNAS* using alternative first exons that are spliced to exons 2–13, but the effect of these proteins on the MAS phenotype remains uncertain. Exon 1A is located approximately 2.5 kb upstream of exon 1. Transcripts beginning with exon 1A are expressed only from the paternal allele, and are probably untranslated (39). Further upstream are two additional alternative first exons; one encodes the N-terminus of the $XL\alpha_s$ protein, which is expressed only from paternal alleles. $XL\alpha_s$ shares C-terminal sequences with $G\alpha_s$, and functions in G protein-coupled signal transduction (40). Although *gsp* mutations in $XL\alpha_s$ can affect signal transduction *in vitro* (41, 42), a role for *gsp* mutations in $XL\alpha_s$ in human disease has yet to be defined. The other alternative first exon is approximately 52 kb upstream of exon 1 and is expressed exclusively from the maternal allele. This exon contains the entire coding sequence for the neurosecretory protein NESP55 (43), a chromogranin-like protein that is present in secretory granules and shares no protein homology with $G\alpha_s$. Thus, activating mutations in exon 8 of *GNAS* would not be present in NESP55.

Third, the clinical and endocrinological features of MAS will be influenced by the particular effects of cAMP in a specific cell type. A *gsp* oncogene will produce the most significant consequences in those tissues in which cAMP stimulates cellular proliferation and/or hormone secretion rather than differentiation. Cyclic AMP is not mitogenic in all cell types, and in some cell types cAMP can actually inhibit growth. Moreover, even in cells in which cAMP is a strong growth stimulator, changes in the expression of other genes (44) or induction of counter-regulatory responses (such as increased cAMP phosphodiesterase activity (45–49)) could mitigate or even reverse the effects of the *gsp* oncogene.

Clinical manifestations of McCune–Albright syndrome

Comprehensive reviews of the clinical spectrum of MAS have extended our appreciation of this unusual disorder (50–54) (Table 6.16.1). The mean age at the time of clinical diagnosis of MAS is 5.7 years, with a range of 0.7 to 11 years. Almost all patients who ultimately manifest the complete clinical triad of pigmented skin lesions, excessive endocrine function, and fibrous dysplasia will have evidence of café-au-lait skin lesions at birth. There is a 50% likelihood of precocious puberty in females by age 4 years, and a 50% likelihood of bone lesions by age 8 years.

Fibrous dysplasia

Fibrous dysplasia of the skeleton occurs in nearly all (98%) patients with MAS, and the proportion of patients with MAS is likely to be less than 5% of all individuals with fibrous dysplasia. Although fibrous dysplasia is usually monostotic (70%), patients with MAS are more likely to have multiple fibrous dysplasia lesions (polyostotic, two-thirds of patients) than a solitary fibrous dysplasia lesion (monostotic, one-third of patients). Fibrous dysplasia typically develops during the first decade of life (Table 6.16.1), and fractures are seen to peak at age 6–10 years (55). Fibrous dysplasia seems to progress over time in most patients, with an increase in both the extent and number of bone lesions. The femur and pelvis are most commonly involved, and the shepherd's crook deformity of the femur is a pathognomonic lesion. Spinal involvement, with progressive scoliosis, is apparently more common than originally thought (56, 57). Most affected patients will experience at least one fracture (peak age 7–12 years) and many patients will have multiple fractures. Radiographs of affected bones reveal expansile, lytic lesions with a 'ground glass' pattern and a scalloped cortical bone border secondary to endosteal erosion (Fig. 6.16.2). Craniofacial involvement occurs in many patients, and should be evaluated with both CT and MRI in order to demonstrate the extent of disease, and potential compressive complications of polyostotic fibrous dysplasia (PFD) (58). The marrow cavity, which usually has a cellular fatty tissue, is replaced by fibro-osseous tissue. Bone histology discloses three primary, but distinct, histological patterns, defined as Chinese writing type, sclerotic/pagetoid type, and sclerotic/hypercellular type, which are characteristically associated with the axial/appendicular skeleton, cranial bones, or gnathic bones, respectively (59).

The basis for the unusual cellular changes in fibrous dysplasia is poorly understood. Recent evidence indicates that the fibrotic areas consist of an excess of preosteogenic cells, whereas the bone formed *de novo* within fibrotic areas is produced by mature but abnormal osteoblasts (60). It is likely that at least some of the phenotypic changes in affected osteogenic cells result from cAMP-induced increases in protein kinase A and CREB pathways that induces overexpression of interleukin-6 and the c-fos proto-oncogene (27, 61, 62). Fos overexpression in transgenic mice results in bone lesions reminiscent of fibrous dysplasia (63). The mosaic distribution of lesions in fibrous dysplasia may also play an important pathogenic role, as close contact between transplanted normal bone cells and osteogenic cells containing the *gsp* mutation is necessary to reproduce the fibrous dysplasia lesion in mice (64).

Sarcomatous degeneration (e.g. osteosarcoma, fibrosarcoma, and chondrosarcoma, in descending order of frequency) occurs as a rare complication of fibrous dysplasia in MAS patients (mean age of 36 years) (65). F-18 fluorodeoxyglucose positron emission tomography may be a useful technique to identify early malignant transformation of fibrous dysplasia lesions (58, 66).

No treatment for fibrous dysplasia is entirely satisfactory. Most, but not all, studies have demonstrated that bisphosphonates can relieve bone pain, decrease bone resorption, and improve the radiological appearance (e.g. filling of lytic lesions and/or thickening of cortices) of bone lesions in about 50% of patients. Bone mineral density in affected sites is also significantly increased after treatment with pamidronate, a potent second-generation bisphosphonate which is administered intravenously (67, 68). In a series of nine patients on long-term pamidronate treatment who became resistant to this medication, a switch to intravenous zoledronic acid did not produce any substantial improvement (69).

Café-au-lait skin lesions

Patients with MAS typically have one or more pigmented macules, termed café-au-lait lesions, that have irregular borders (coast of Maine) (Fig. 6.16.4). By contrast, café-au-lait skin lesions that occur in patients with neurofibromatosis (von Recklinghausen's syndrome) have a smooth border (coast of California) (Fig. 6.16.5). The distribution of skin lesions in MAS is also characteristic (Fig. 6.16.4), consisting of an S-shaped pattern on the chest, a V-shaped pattern on the back, and a linear distribution on the extremities, which conforms to the embryological lines of ectodermal migration (i.e. lines of Blashko) and reflects the dorsoventral outgrowth of two populations of cells (20). Lesions rarely extend beyond the midline and in most patients the skin lesions tend to be on the same side of the body as the skeletal lesions. They occur most commonly on the buttocks and lumbosacral regions.

Endocrine abnormalities

Autonomous endocrine function is common in MAS (Table 6.16.1). Precocious puberty is the most common endocrine disorder in MAS, and has been reported in over 60% of patients. Precocious puberty is a common initial manifestation of MAS in girls, and characteristically presents as thelarche and/or vaginal bleeding in a girl under 5 years of age (50). Vaginal bleeding may occur in the absence of significant breast development or pubarche. Some young girls will have seemingly regular menses and progressive pubertal development, including rapid advancement of bone age, whereas others will have irregular or intermittent bleeding that is associated with relatively normal rates of growth. The production of oestrogen appears related to the growth and involution of small ovarian cysts, and is typically not associated with follicular maturation or ovulation. Ovarian activity can undergo a spontaneous remission in some cases. Large, benign ovarian cysts

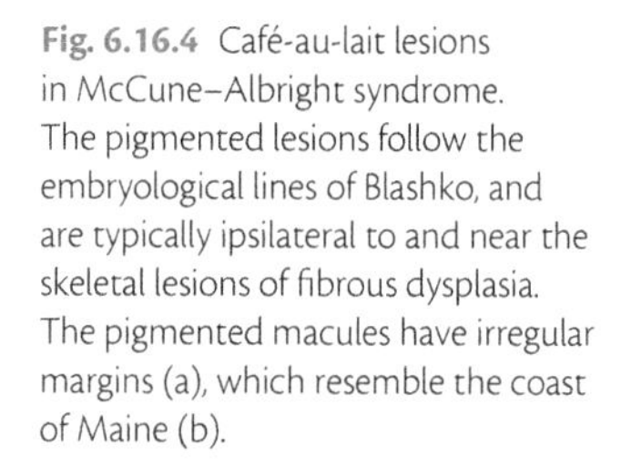
Fig. 6.16.4 Café-au-lait lesions in McCune–Albright syndrome. The pigmented lesions follow the embryological lines of Blashko, and are typically ipsilateral to and near the skeletal lesions of fibrous dysplasia. The pigmented macules have irregular margins (a), which resemble the coast of Maine (b).

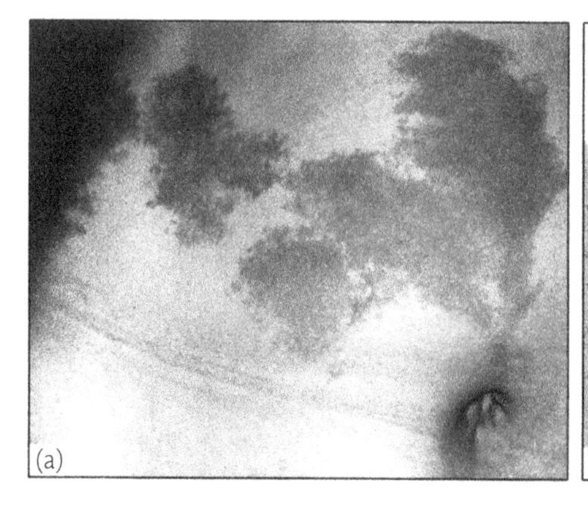

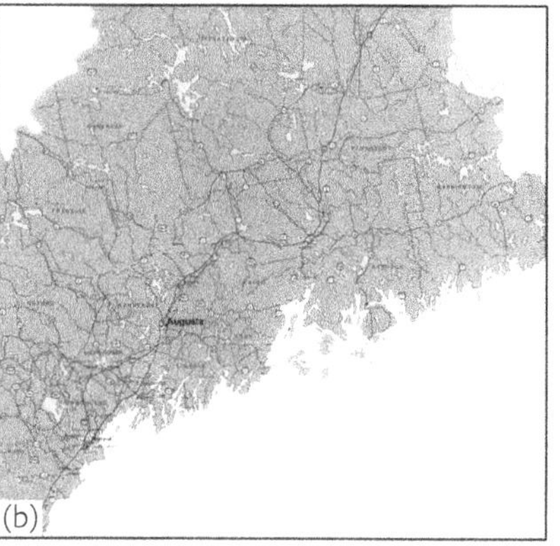

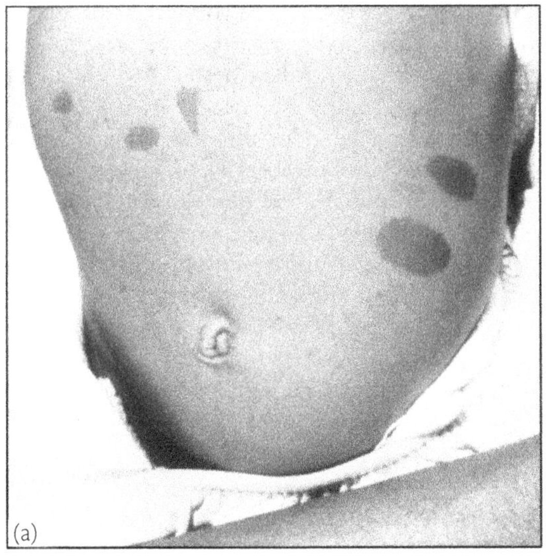

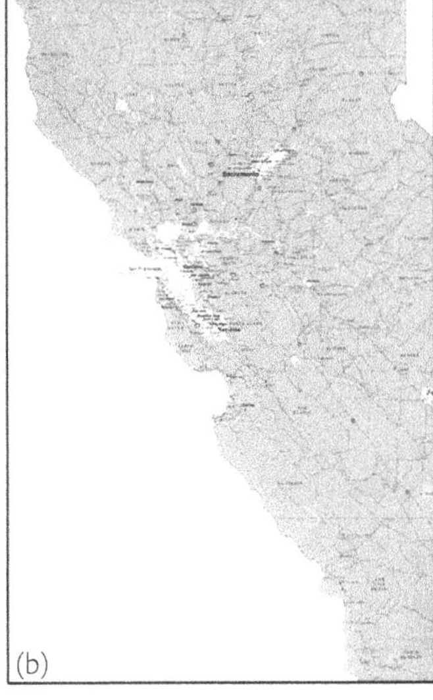

Fig. 6.16.5 Café-au-lait lesions in neurofibromatosis. The pigmented macules have smooth margins (a), which resemble the coast of California (b).

may also occur (14, 15), and surgical excision may result in regression of secondary sexual characteristics until the onset of normal pubertal development. Patients typically have low or suppressed levels of serum luteinizing hormone and follicle-stimulating hormone, which fail to increase significantly after administration of gonadotropin-releasing hormone (GnRH), a characteristic of gonadotropin-independent precocious puberty (i.e. precocious 'pseudopuberty'). Testing may be normal during intervals of apparent ovarian inactivity, however. Given the episodic nature of oestrogen production, and the poor performance characteristic of many clinical assays for oestradiol, serum concentrations of this steroid are often not elevated. Of interest, after several years of excessive sex steroid exposure some girls experience a transition to central precocious puberty, particularly those whose bone age is 11 years or greater (70–72). As adults, women with a past history of gonadotropin-independent precocious puberty may have irregular menses and reduced fertility due to continued autonomous production of oestrogen (73, 74).

Treatment of precocious puberty in girls with MAS is problematic. Therapy with GnRH analogues and superagonists is not effective unless there has been a progression to central precocious puberty (71). Treatment with aromatase inhibitors (70, 75) has been successful for short periods of time, but long-term therapy has generally been disappointing (75, 76). The efficacy of compounds with antioestrogenic activity, such as the selective oestrogen receptor modulators, tamoxifen or raloxifene, appears promising (77).

Precocious pseudopuberty also occurs in boys with MAS, but it is much less common than in young girls. Testicular biopsy reveals variable degrees of seminiferous tube development and Leydig cell hyperplasia. Testicular enlargement is generally bilateral but can be unilateral (78). Although testicular enlargement is usually associated with excessive production of testosterone and precocious puberty, occasionally the enlargement is limited to autonomous hyperfunction of Sertoli cells with no activation of Leydig cells (32). Treatment is similar to that for familial male precocious puberty due to activating mutations of the luteinizing hormone receptor (i.e. testitoxicosis) (79), and consists of the combination of an aromatase inhibitor plus an androgen receptor blocker (78, 80). In those cases where gonadotropin-independent precocious puberty leads to early activation of central puberty, the addition of a GnRH analogue may be required to arrest further pubertal development (81, 82).

Growth hormone excess is common in MAS, and may produce either gigantism or acromegaly (49, 83). The biochemical behaviour of growth hormone-producing pituitary tumours in patients with MAS appears indistinguishable from that of sporadic tumours with and without *gsp* mutations. Growth hormone secretion is stimulated by TRH, growth hormone releasing hormone, and sleep, and is incompletely suppressed by glucose administration. However, only 65% of MAS patients with growth hormone excess have radiographic evidence of a pituitary tumour, a much lower incidence than in sporadic cases of acromegaly (99%) (50). In addition, hyperprolactinaemia occurs in over 50% of MAS patients with elevated growth hormone levels, a frequency that is somewhat greater than occurs in patients with sporadic pituitary tumours (40%) (50).

Medical therapy with bromocriptine has been shown to reduce tumour size and hormonal secretion in many, but not all, patients (12, 44). Other medical treatments, such as long-acting octreotide and pegvisomant (84–86), appear more promising.

Hyperthyroidism and/or autonomous thyroid nodules have been identified in approximately 33% of MAS patients who underwent thyroid evaluation (50, 51, 87, 88). Radioactive iodine ablation or surgery has been used to treat thyroid nodules. The degree of hyperthyroidism is variable, and serum concentrations of TSH are typically low and thyroid stimulating immunoglobulins are undetectable. The thyroid gland will often appear normal by physical exam, but nodules are nearly always detectable by sonography.

Patients with MAS occasionally develop autonomous function of the adrenal gland and primary hypercortisolism at a young age (mean age of 4.4 years) (50). Adrenal gland histopathology reveals either nodular hyperplasia or solitary adenoma (89).

Other features

Recent analyses have documented the occurrence of additional nonendocrine features in patients with MAS that extend the clinical spectrum of the disorder. These include hypophosphataemia, hepatobiliary disease, and cardiac disease. Hypophosphataemia and/or decreased renal tubular reabsorption of phosphate occurs in over 50% of subjects with MAS, and may lead to the development of rickets or osteomalacia (90), A similar syndrome of hypophosphataemic rickets has been described in patients with fibrous dysplasia who lack other features of MAS, as well as in other patients who have various mesenchymal tumours (91), and appears due to secretion of circulating phosphaturic factors termed 'phosphatonins' (92, 93). FGF23 is the best characterized of the phosphatonins, and is produced by the abnormal osteogenic precursors present in fibrous dysplasia lesions. The concentration of circulating FGF23 correlates with the extent of fibrous dysplasia throughout the skeleton (94, 95). An alternative explanation for hypophosphataemia in patients with MAS is the presence of the *gsp* oncogene in the proximal renal tubule, where it induces increased cAMP production and an intrinsic defect in reabsorption of phosphate (96).

While neonatal jaundice in patients with MAS typical resolves, liver function enzymes typically remain mildly elevated. Liver histology varies from near normal to discrete portal fibrosis to giant cell hepatitis (97). Liver disease is due to the presence of the gsp mutation in hepatic tissue (30, 88, 97), and the degree of histological abnormality correlates with the relative amount of abnormal $G\alpha_s$ protein and adenylyl cyclase activation (30). Another unusual manifestation of MAS is cardiac disease (88). Cardiac involvement in patients with MAS most commonly manifests as tachycardia and/or hypertension (88). Affected cardiac tissue contains cells with the *gsp* mutation (88), and it is likely that elevated levels of cAMP account directly for the abnormal cardiac function.

Diagnosis

The diagnosis of MAS remains a clinical exercise, and is straightforward when all three cardinal features are present. However, many patients with MAS lack some features at the time of initial presentation, which makes it desirable to have a molecular test that can confirm the diagnosis. The mosaic distribution of cells bearing the *GNAS* mutation, and the variable number of affected cells in a tissue, makes it technically difficult to detect mutant *GNAS* alleles even in affected tissues, as they may represent only a small proportion of the *GNAS* alleles present in a DNA sample. Detection of a *gsp* mutant in DNA samples can be greatly enhanced by protocols that enrich the relative abundance of mutant alleles as PCR targets and thereby facilitate selective amplification. These techniques have relied upon either multiple rounds of PCR and restriction endonuclease digestion of wild type amplicons (25) or inclusion of a peptide nucleic acid (PNA) in the PCR to block amplification of wild-type *GNAS* targets (98, 99). The sensitivity of nested PCR and PNA-clamping appear comparable, but the nested PCR method requires more time and expense than PNA clamping (100). A recent improvement over standard PNA clamping uses a labelled PNA hybridization probe and fluorescence resonance energy transfer to allow for the direct and rapid quantification of *gsp* alleles with a sensitivity that allows detection in tissues that contain as few as 5% mutant cells (101). While analysis of DNA from lesional tissue affords greatest sensitivity, it is neither practical nor expedient to biopsy affected tissue(s) in all patients. Both nested PCR and PNA-clamping have been used to detect *gsp* mutations in peripheral blood samples (100, 102).

The detection of a *gsp* mutation in circulating cells from a patient with fibrous dysplasia or an isolated endocrinopathy (e.g. growth hormone-producing pituitary tumour, ovarian cysts) does not necessarily imply that the patient has MAS, however. Even with molecular demonstration of a *gsp* mutation, additional studies and clinical interpretation will be needed to distinguish between MAS and an isolated lesion.

On the other hand, identification of a *gsp* mutation can distinguish between fibrous dysplasia and similar lesion such as osteofibrous dysplasia (103), and may assist in distinguishing between atypical forms of MAS and Carney's complex (OMIM 160980) (104–107) or Mazabraud's syndrome (108, 109). These molecular techniques will require additional refinement and further development, however, before they can be considered as standard diagnostic tests, and at the present time no molecular technique is offered as a test for MAS in a commercial reference laboratory.

Conclusion

The diagnosis of MAS remains a clinical one, and requires a careful integration of physical findings, biochemical evaluation, and radiological examination. The disorder can present as a form fruste, and identification of a specific *GNAS* mutation in DNA from affected tissues and in many cases peripheral blood cells may one day confirm a clinical diagnosis of MAS. Finally, the genetic basis for MAS, mosaicism of a somatic *gsp* mutation, provides new insights into the role of imprinting as a modulator of human disease.

Acknowledgements

This work was supported in part by United States Public Health Service Grant R01 DK34281 from the NIDDK and grant RR00055 from NCRR to the Johns Hopkins General Clinical Research Center.

References

1. Bohm A, Gaudet R, Sigler PB. Structural aspects of heterotrimeric G-protein signaling. *Curr Opin Biotechnol*, 1997; **8**: 480–7.
2. Clapham DE, Neer EJ. G protein beta gamma subunits. *Annu Rev Pharmacol Toxicol*, 1997; **37**: 167–203.
3. Ross EM, Wang J, Tu Y, Biddlecome GH. Guanosine triphosphatase-activating proteins for heterotrimeric G- proteins. *Adv Pharmacol*, 1998; **42**: 458–61.
4. Kahn RA, Gilman AG. ADP-ribosylation of Gs promotes the dissociation of its alpha and beta subunits. *J Biol Chem*, 1984; **259**: 6235–40.
5. Farfel Z, Bourne HR, Iiri T. The expanding spectrum of G protein diseases. *N Engl J Med*, 1999; **340**: 1012–20.
6. Spiegel AM. The molecular basis of disorders caused by defects in G proteins. *Horm Res*, 1997; **47**: 89–96.
7. Vallar L, Spada A, Giannattasio G. Altered Gs and adenylate cyclase activity in human GH- secreting pituitary adenomas. *Nature*, 1987; **330**: 566–8.
8. Conti CJ. Mutations of genes of the ras family in human and experimental tumors. *Prog Clin Biol Res*, 1992; **376**: 357–78.
9. Landis CA, Masters SB, Spada A, Pace AM, Bourne HR, Vallar L. GTPase inhibiting mutations activate the alpha chain of Gs and stimulate adenylyl cyclase in human pituitary tumours. *Nature*, 1989; **340**: 692–6.
10. Lyons J, Landis CA, Griffith H, Vallar L, Grunewald K, Feichtinger H, *et al.* Two G protein oncogenes in human endocrine tumors. *Science*, 1990; **249**: 655–9.
11. Spada A, Lania A, Ballare E. G protein abnormalities in pituitary adenomas. *Mol Cell Endocrinol*, 1998; **142**: 1–14.

12. Barlier A, Gunz G, Zamora AJ, Morange-Ramos I, Figarella-Branger D, Dufour H, *et al.* Pronostic and therapeutic consequences of Gs alpha mutations in somatotroph adenomas. *J Clin Endocrinol Metab*, 1998; **83**: 1604–10.
13. Fragoso MC, Latronico AC, Carvalho FM, Zerbini MC, Marcondes JA, Araujo LM, *et al.* Activating mutation of the stimulatory G protein (gsp) as a putative cause of ovarian and testicular human stromal Leydig cell tumors. *J Clin Endocrinol Metab*, 1998; **83**: 2074–8.
14. Pienkowski C, Lumbroso S, Bieth E, Sultan C, Rochiccioli P, Tauber M. Recurrent ovarian cyst and mutation of the Gs alpha gene in ovarian cyst fluid cells: what is the link with McCune-Albright syndrome? *Acta Paediatr*, 1997; **86**: 1019–21.
15. Rodriguez-Macias KA, Thibaud E, Houang M, Duflos C, Beldjord C, Rappaport R. Follow up of precocious pseudopuberty associated with isolated ovarian follicular cysts. *Arch Dis Child*, 1999; **81**: 53–6.
16. Okamoto S, Hisaoka M, Ushijima M, Nakahara S, Toyoshima S, Hashimoto H. Activating Gs(alpha) mutation in intramuscular myxomas with and without fibrous dysplasia of bone. *Virchows Arch*, 2000; **437**: 133–7.
17. Alman BA, Greel DA, Wolfe HJ. Activating mutations of Gs protein in monostotic fibrous lesions of bone. *J Orthop Res*, 1996; **14**: 311–5.
18. McCune DJ, Bruch H. Osteodystrophia fibrosa. *Am J Dis Child*, 1937; **54**: 806–48.
19. Albright F, Butler AM, Hampton AO, Smith P. Syndrome characterized by osteitis fibrosa disseminata, areas of pigmentation and endocrine dysfunction, with precocious puberty in females. *N Engl J Med*, 1937; **216**: 727–41.
20. Happle R. The McCune-Albright syndrome: A lethal gene surviving by mosaicism. *Clin Genet*, 1986; **29**: 321–4.
21. Schwindinger WF, Francomano CA, Levine MA. Identification of a mutation in the gene encoding the alpha subunit of the stimulatory G protein of adenylyl cyclase in McCune-Albright syndrome. *Proc Natl Acad Sci U S A*, 1992; **89**: 5152–6.
22. Weinstein LS, Shenker A, Gejman PV, Merino MJ, Friedman E, Spiegel AM. Activating mutations of the stimulatory G protein in the McCune- Albright syndrome. *N Engl J Med*, 1991; **325**: 1688–95.
23. Dotsch J, Kiess W, Hanze J, Repp R, Ludecke D, Blum WF, *et al.* Gs alpha mutation at codon 201 in pituitary adenoma causing gigantism in a 6-year-old boy with McCune-Albright syndrome. *J Clin Endocrinol Metab*, 1996; **81**: 3839–42.
24. Tinschert S, Gerl H, Gewies A, Jung HP, Nurnberg P. McCune-Albright syndrome: clinical and molecular evidence of mosaicism in an unusual giant patient. *Am J Med Genet*, 1999; **83**: 100–8.
25. Candeliere GA, Roughley PJ, Glorieux FH. Polymerase chain reaction-based technique for the selective enrichment and analysis of mosaic arg201 mutations in G alpha s from patients with fibrous dysplasia of bone. *Bone*, 1997; **21**: 201–6.
26. Riminucci M, Fisher LW, Majolagbe A, Corsi A, Lala R, de Sanctis C, *et al.* A Novel GNAS1 Mutation, R201G, in McCune-Albright Syndrome. *J Bone Miner Res*, 1999; **14**: 1987–9.
27. Candeliere GA, Glorieux FH, Prud'homme J, St-Arnaud R. Increased expression of the c-fos proto-oncogene in bone from patients with fibrous dysplasia. *N Engl J Med*, 1995; **332**: 1546–51.
28. Lumbroso S, Paris F, Sultan C. Activating Gsalpha mutations: analysis of 113 patients with signs of McCune-Albright syndrome—a European Collaborative Study. *J Clin Endocrinol Metab*, 2004; **89**: 2107–13.
29. Malchoff C, Reardon G, MacGillivray DC, Yamase H, Rogol AD, Malchoff DM. An unusual presentation of McCune-Albright syndrome confirmed by an activating mutation of the Gsα-subunit from a bone lesion. *J Clin Endocrinol Metab*, 1994; **78**: 803–6.
30. Schwindinger WF, Yang SQ, Miskovsky EP, Diehl AM, Levine MA. An activating Gsα mutation in McCune-Albright syndrome increases hepatic adenylyl cyclase activity. *The Endocrine Society Program and Abstracts*. Bethesda: Endocrine Society Press, 1993; 517.
31. Gorelov VN, Gyenes M, Neser F, Roher HD, Goretzki PE. Distribution of Gs-alpha activating mutations in human thyroid tumors measured by subcloning. *J Cancer Res Clin Oncol*, 1996; **122**: 453–7.
32. Coutant R, Lumbroso S, Rey R, Lahlou N, Venara M, Rouleau S, *et al.* Macroorchidism due to autonomous hyperfunction of Sertoli cells and G(s)alpha gene mutation: an unusual expression of McCune-Albright syndrome in a prepubertal boy. *J Clin Endocrinol Metab*, 2001; **86**: 1778–81.
33. Rey RA, Venara M, Coutant R, Trabut JB, Rouleau S, Lahlou N, *et al.* Unexpected mosaicism of R201H-GNAS1 mutant-bearing cells in the testes underlie macro-orchidism without sexual precocity in McCune-Albright syndrome. *Hum Mol Genet*, 2006; **15**: 3538–43.
34. Michienzi S, Cherman N, Holmbeck K, Funari A, Collins MT, Bianco P, *et al.* GNAS transcripts in skeletal progenitors: evidence for random asymmetric allelic expression of Gs alpha. *Hum Mol Genet*, 2007; **16**: 1921–30.
35. Germain-Lee EL, Ding CL, Deng Z, Crane JK, Saji M, Ringel MD, *et al.* Paternal imprinting of Galpha(s) in the human thyroid as the basis of TSH resistance in pseudohypoparathyroidism type 1a. *Biochem Biophys Res Commun*, 2002; **296**: 62–72.
36. Liu J, Erlichman B, Weinstein LS. The stimulatory G protein alpha-subunit Gs alpha is imprinted in human thyroid glands: implications for thyroid function in pseudohypoparathyroidism types 1A and 1B. *J Clin Endocrinol Metab*, 2003; **88**: 4336–41.
37. Mantovani G, Bondioni S, Locatelli M, Pedroni C, Lania AG, Ferrante E, *et al.* Biallelic expression of the Gsalpha gene in human bone and adipose tissue. *J Clin Endocrinol Metab*, 2004; **89**: 6316–9.
38. Hayward BE, Barlier A, Korbonits M, Grossman AB, Jacquet P, Enjalbert A, *et al.* Imprinting of the G(s)alpha gene GNAS1 in the pathogenesis of acromegaly. *J Clin Invest*, 2001; **107**: R31–6.
39. Swaroop A, Agarwal N, Gruen JR, Bick D, Weissman SM. Differential expression of novel Gsα signal transduction protein cDNA species. *Nucleic Acids Res*, 1991; **17**: 4725–9.
40. Kehlenbach RH, Matthey J, Huttner WB. XLαs is a new type of G protein. *Nature*, 1994; **372**: 804–8.
41. Linglart A, Mahon MJ, Kerachian MA, Berlach DM, Hendy GN, Juppner H, *et al.* Coding GNAS mutations leading to hormone resistance impair in vitro agonist- and cholera toxin-induced adenosine cyclic 3′,5′-monophosphate formation mediated by human XLalphas. *Endocrinology*, 2006; **147**: 2253–62.
42. Aydin C, Aytan N, Mahon MJ, Tawfeek HA, Kowall NW, Dedeoglu A, *et al.* Extralarge XL(alpha)s (XXL(alpha)s), a variant of stimulatory G protein alpha-subunit (Gs(alpha)), is a distinct, membrane-anchored GNAS product that can mimic Gs(alpha). *Endocrinology*, 2009; **150**: 3567–75.
43. Hayward BE, Moran V, Strain L, Bonthron DT. Bidirectional imprinting of a single gene: GNAS1 encodes maternally, paternally, and biallelically derived proteins. *Proc Natl Acad Sci U S A*, 1998; **95**: 15475–80.
44. Barlier A, Pellegrini-Bouiller I, Gunz G, Zamora AJ, Jaquet P, Enjalbert A. Impact of gsp oncogene on the expression of genes coding for Gsalpha, Pit-1, Gi2alpha, and somatostatin receptor 2 in human somatotroph adenomas: involvement in octreotide sensitivity. *J Clin Endocrinol Metab*, 1999; **84**: 2759–65.
45. Nemoz G, Sette C, Hess M, Muca C, Vallar L, Conti M. Activation of cyclic nucleotide phosphodiesterases in FRTL-5 thyroid cells expressing consitutitively active Gs alpha. *Mol Endocrinol*, 1995; **9**: 1279–87.
46. Lania A, Persani L, Ballare E, Mantovani S, Losa M, Spada A. Constitutively active Gs alpha is associated with an increased phosphodiesterase activity in human growth hormone-secreting adenomas. *J Clin Endocrinol Metab*, 1998; **83**: 1624–8.
47. Wogensen L, Ma Y-H, Grodsky GM, Robertson RP, Burton F, Sutcliffe JG, *et al.* Functional effects of transgenic expression of cholera toxin in pancreatic beta-cells. *Mol Cell Endocrinol*, 1993; **98**: 33–42.

48. Ma YH, Landis C, Tchao N, Wang J, Rodd G, Hanahan D, Bourne HR, *et al.* Constitutively active stimulatory G-protein alpha s in beta- cells of transgenic mice causes counterregulation of the increased adenosine 3',5'-monophosphate and insulin secretion. *Endocrinology*, 1994; **134**: 42–7.
49. Ham J, Ivan M, Wynford-Thomas D, Scanlon MF. GH3 cells expressing constitutively active Gs alpha (Q227L) show enhanced hormone secretion and proliferation. *Mol Cell Endocrinol*, 1997; **127**: 41–7.
50. Ringel MD, Schwindinger WF, Levine MA. Clinical implications of genetic defects in G proteins. The molecular basis of McCune-Albright syndrome and Albright hereditary osteodystrophy. *Medicine*, 1996; **75**: 171–84.
51. de Sanctis C, Lala R, Matarazzo P, Balsamo A, Bergamaschi R, Cappa M, *et al.* McCune-Albright syndrome: a longitudinal clinical study of 32 patients. *J Pediatr Endocrinol Metab*, 1999; **12**: 817–26.
52. Diaz A, Danon M, Crawford J. McCune-Albright syndrome and disorders due to activating mutations of GNAS1. *J Pediatr Endocrinol Metab*, 2007; **20**: 853–80.
53. Zacharin M. The spectrum of McCune Albright syndrome. *Pediatr Endocrinol Rev*, 2007; 4 (Suppl. 4): 412–8.
54. Volkl TM, Dorr HG. McCune-Albright syndrome: clinical picture and natural history in children and adolescents. *J Pediatr Endocrinol Metab*, 2006; 19 (Suppl. 2): 551–9.
55. Leet AI, Chebli C, Kushner H, Chen CC, Kelly MH, Brillante BA, *et al.* Fracture incidence in polyostotic fibrous dysplasia and the McCune-Albright syndrome. *J Bone Miner Res*, 2004; **19**: 571–7.
56. Leet AI, Magur E, Lee JS, Wientroub S, Robey PG, Collins MT. Fibrous dysplasia in the spine: prevalence of lesions and association with scoliosis. *J Bone Joint Surg Am*, 2004; 86-A: 531–7.
57. Mancini F, Corsi A, De Maio F, Riminucci M, Ippolito E. Scoliosis and spine involvement in fibrous dysplasia of bone. *Eur Spine J*, 2009; **18**: 196–202.
58. Bulakbasi N, Bozlar U, Karademir I, Kocaoglu M, Somuncu I. CT and MRI in the evaluation of craniospinal involvement with polyostotic fibrous dysplasia in McCune-Albright syndrome. *Diagn Interv Radiol*, 2008; **14**: 177–81.
59. Riminucci M, Liu B, Corsi A, Shenker A, Spiegel AM, Robey PG, *et al.* The histopathology of fibrous dysplasia of bone in patients with activating mutations of the Gs alpha gene: site-specific patterns and recurrent histological hallmarks. *J Pathol*, 1999; **187**: 249–58.
60. Riminucci M, Robey PG, Bianco P. The pathology of fibrous dysplasia and the McCune-Albright syndrome. *Pediatr Endocrinol Rev*, 2007; 4 (Suppl. 4): 401–11.
61. Shenker A, Weinstein LS, Sweet DE, Spiegel AM. An activating Gsα mutation is present in fibrous dysplasia of bone in McCune-Albright syndrome. *J Clin Endocrinol Metab*, 1994; **79**: 750–5.
62. Riminucci M, Fisher LW, Shenker A, Spiegel AM, Bianco P, Gehron RP. Fibrous dysplasia of bone in the McCune-Albright syndrome: abnormalities in bone formation. *Am J Pathol*, 1997; **151**: 1587–600.
63. Ruther U, Garber C, Komitowski D, Muller R, Wagner EF. Deregulated c-fos expression interferes with normal bone development in transgenic mice. *Nature*, 1987; **325**: 412–6.
64. Bianco P, Kuznetsov SA, Riminucci M, Fisher LW, Spiegel AM, Robey PG. Reproduction of human fibrous dysplasia of bone in immunocompromised mice by transplanted mosaics of normal and Gsalpha-mutated skeletal progenitor cells. *J Clin Invest*, 1998; **101**: 1737–44.
65. Ruggieri P, Sim FH, Bond JR, Unni KK. Osteosarcoma in a patient with polyostotic fibrous dysplasia and Albright's syndrome. *Orthopedics*, 1995; **18**: 71–5.
66. Berrebi O, Steiner C, Keller A, Rougemont AL, Ratib O. F-18 fluorodeoxyglucose (FDG) PET in the diagnosis of malignant transformation of fibrous dysplasia in the pelvic bones. *Clin Nucl Med*, 2008; **33**: 469–71.
67. Mandrioli S, Carinci F, Dallera V, Calura G. [Fibrous dysplasia. The clinico-therapeutic picture and new data on its etiology. A review of the literature]. *Minerva Stomatol*, 1998; **47**: 37–44.
68. Pfeilschifter J, Ziegler R. [Effect of pamidronate on clinical symptoms and bone metabolism in fibrous dysplasia and McCune-Albright syndrome]. *Med Klin*, 1998; **93**: 352–9.
69. Chapurlat RD. Medical therapy in adults with fibrous dysplasia of bone. *J Bone Miner Res*, 2006; 21 (Suppl. 2): P114–9.
70. Feuillan PP, Jones J, Cutler GBJ. Long-term testolactone therapy for precocious puberty in girls with the McCune-Albright syndrome. *J Clin Endocrinol Metab*, 1993; **77**: 647–51.
71. Schmidt H, Kiess W. Secondary central precocious puberty in a girl with McCune-Albright syndrome responds to treatment with GnRH analogue. *J Pediatr Endocrinol Metab*, 1998; **11**: 77–81.
72. Boepple PA, Frisch LS, Wierman ME, Hoffman WH, Crowley WFJ. The natural history of autonomous gonadal function, adrenarche, and central puberty in gonadotropin-independent precocious puberty. *J Clin Endocrinol Metab*, 1992; **75**: 1550–5.
73. Lala R, Andreo M, Pucci A, Matarazzo P. Persistent hyperestrogenism after precocious puberty in young females with McCune-Albright syndrome. *Pediatr Endocrinol Rev*, 2007; 4 (Suppl. 4): 423–8.
74. Chanson P, Salenave S, Orcel P. McCune-Albright syndrome in adulthood. *Pediatr Endocrinol Rev*, 2007; 4 (Suppl. 4): 453–62.
75. Feuillan P, Calis K, Hill S, Shawker T, Robey PG, Collins MT. Letrozole treatment of precocious puberty in girls with the McCune-Albright syndrome: a pilot study. *J Clin Endocrinol Metab*, 2007; **92**: 2100–6.
76. Mieszczak J, Lowe ES, Plourde P, Eugster EA. The aromatase inhibitor anastrozole is ineffective in the treatment of precocious puberty in girls with McCune-Albright syndrome. *J Clin Endocrinol Metab*, 2008; **93**: 2751–4.
77. Eugster EA, Rubin SD, Reiter EO, Plourde P, Jou HC, Pescovitz OH, McCune-Albright Study Group. Tamoxifen treatment for precocious puberty in McCune-Albright syndrome: a multicenter trial. *J Pediatr*, 2003; **143**: 60–6.
78. Arrigo T, Pirazzoli P, de Sanctis L, Leone O, Wasniewska M, Messina MF, *et al.* McCune-Albright syndrome in a boy may present with a monolateral macroorchidism as an early and isolated clinical manifestation. *Horm Res*, 2006; **65**: 114–9.
79. DiMeglio LA, Pescovitz OH. Disorders of puberty: inactivating and activating molecular mutations. *J Pediatr*, 1997; **131**: S8–12.
80. Mieszczak J, Eugster EA. Treatment of precocious puberty in McCune-Albright syndrome. *Pediatr Endocrinol Rev*, 2007; 4 (Suppl. 4): 419–22.
81. Leschek EW, Cutler GBJ. Familial male precocious puberty. *Curr Ther Endocrinol Metab*, 1997; **6**: 343–5.
82. Leschek EW, Jones J, Barnes KM, Hill SC, Cutler GBJ. Six-year results of spironolactone and testolactone treatment of familial male-limited precocious puberty with addition of deslorelin after central puberty onset. *J Clin Endocrinol Metab*, 1999; **84**: 175–8.
83. Lee PA, Van Dop C, Migeon CJ. McCune-Albright syndrome. Long-term follow-up. *JAMA*, 1986; **256**: 2980–4.
84. Akintoye SO, Kelly MH, Brillante B, Cherman N, Turner S, Butman JA, *et al.* Pegvisomant for the treatment of gsp-mediated growth hormone excess in patients with McCune-Albright syndrome. *J Clin Endocrinol Metab*, 2006; **91**: 2960–6.
85. Tajima T, Tsubaki J, Ishizu K, Jo W, Ishi N, Fujieda K. Case study of a 15-year-old boy with McCune-Albright syndrome combined with pituitary gigantism: effect of octreotide-long acting release (LAR) and cabergoline therapy. *Endocr J*, 2008; **55**: 595–9.
86. Almeida JP, Albuquerque LA, Ferraz CL, Mota I, Gondim J, Ferraz TM. McCune-Albright syndrome and acromegaly: hormonal control with use of cabergoline and long-acting somatostatin—case report. *Arq Bras Endocrinol Metabol*, 2009; **53**: 102–6.

87. Mastorakos G, Mitsiades NS, Doufas AG, Koutras DA. Hyperthyroidism in McCune-Albright syndrome with a review of thyroid abnormalities sixty years after the first report. *Thyroid*, 1997; **7**: 433–9.
88. Shenker A, Weinstein LS, Moran A, Pescovitz OH, Charest NJ, Boney CM, *et al.* Severe endocrine and nonendocrine manifestations of the McCune- Albright syndrome associated with activating mutations of stimulatory G protein GS. *J Pediatr*, 1993; **123**: 509–18.
89. Mauras N, Blizzard RM. The McCune-Albright syndrome. *Acta Endocrinol Suppl (Copenh)*, 1986; **279**: 207–17.
90. Lala R, Matarazzo P, Andreo M, Defilippi C, de Sanctis C. Impact of endocrine hyperfunction and phosphate wasting on bone in McCune-Albright syndrome. *J Pediatr Endocrinol Metab*, 2002; 15 (Suppl. 3): 913–20.
91. Drezner MK, Murray JF, Michael FH, Sylvia C, Steven RG, Frederick SK. Tumor-induced osteomalacia. In: Favus MJ, Christakos S, Robey PG, *et al.*, eds. *Primer on the Metabolic Bone Diseases and Disorders of Mineral Metabolism*. 4th edn. Philadelphia: Lippincott Williams & Wilkins, 1999: 331–7.
92. Econs MJ, Drezner MK. Tumor-induced osteomalacia—unveiling a new hormone. *N Engl J Med*, 1994; **330**: 1679–81.
93. Kumar R. Phosphatonin—a new phosphaturetic hormone? (lessons from tumour- induced osteomalacia and X-linked hypophosphataemia). *Nephrol Dial Transplant*, 1997; **12**: 11–3.
94. Imel EA, Econs MJ. Fibrous dysplasia, phosphate wasting and fibroblast growth factor 23. *Pediatr Endocrinol Rev*, 2007; 4 (Suppl. 4): 434–9.
95. Riminucci M, Collins MT, Fedarko NS, Cherman N, Corsi A, White KE, *et al.* FGF-23 in fibrous dysplasia of bone and its relationship to renal phosphate wasting. *J Clin Invest*, 2003; **112**: 683–92.
96. Zung A, Chalew SA, Schwindinger WF, Levine MA, Phillip M, Jara A, *et al.* Urinary cyclic adenosine 3',5'-monophosphate response in McCune- Albright syndrome: clinical evidence for altered renal adenylate cyclase activity. *J Clin Endocrinol Metab*, 1995; **80**: 3576–81.
97. Silva ES, Lumbroso S, Medina M, Gillerot Y, Sultan C, Sokal EM. Demonstration of McCune-Albright mutations in the liver of children with high gammaGT progressive cholestasis. *J Hepatol*, 2000; **32**: 154–8.
98. Bianco P, Riminucci M, Majolagbe A, Kuznetsov SA, Collins MT, Mankani MH, *et al.* Mutations of the GNAS1 gene, stromal cell dysfunction, and osteomalacic changes in non-McCune-Albright fibrous dysplasia of bone. *J Bone Miner Res*, 2000; **15**: 120–8.
99. Lietman SA, Ding C, Levine MA. A highly sensitive polymerase chain reaction method detects activating mutations of the GNAS gene in peripheral blood cells in McCune-Albright syndrome or isolated fibrous dysplasia. *J Bone Joint Surg Am*, 2005; 87: 2489–94.
100. Lietman SA, Schwindinger WF, Levine MA. Genetic and molecular aspects of McCune-Albright syndrome. *Pediatr Endocrinol Rev*, 2007; 4 (Suppl. 4): 380–5.
101. Karadag A, Riminucci M, Bianco P, Cherman N, Kuznetsov SA, Nguyen N, *et al.* A novel technique based on a PNA hybridization probe and FRET principle for quantification of mutant genotype in fibrous dysplasia/McCune-Albright syndrome. *Nucleic Acids Res*, 2004; 32: e63.
102. Kalfa N, Philibert P, Audran F, Ecochard A, Hannon T, Lumbroso S, *et al.* Searching for somatic mutations in McCune-Albright syndrome: a comparative study of the peptidic nucleic acid versus the nested PCR method based on 148 DNA samples. *Eur J Endocrinol*, 2006; 155: 839–43.
103. Sakamoto A, Oda Y, Iwamoto Y, Tsuneyoshi M. A comparative study of fibrous dysplasia and osteofibrous dysplasia with regard to Gsalpha mutation at the Arg201 codon: polymerase chain reaction-restriction fragment length polymorphism analysis of paraffin-embedded tissues. *J Mol Diagn*, 2000; 2: 67–72.
104. Libe R, Mantovani G, Bondioni S, Lania AG, Pedroni C, Beck-Peccoz P, *et al.* Mutational analysis of PRKAR1A and Gs(alpha) in sporadic adrenocortical tumors. *Exp Clin Endocrinol Diabetes*, 2005; 113: 248–51.
105. Horvath A, Stratakis CA. Clinical and molecular genetics of acromegaly: MEN1, Carney complex, McCune-Albright syndrome, familial acromegaly and genetic defects in sporadic tumors. *Rev Endocr Metab Disord*, 2008; 9: 1–11.
106. DeMarco L, Stratakis CA, Boson WL, Jakbovitz O, Carson E, Andrade LM, *et al.* Sporadic cardiac myxomas and tumors from patients with Carney complex are not associated with activating mutations of the Gs alpha gene. *Hum Genet*, 1996; 98: 185–8.
107. Mantovani G, Corbetta S, Bondioni S, Menicanti L, Rubino B, Peverelli E, *et al.* Analysis of GNAS and PRKAR1A gene mutations in human cardiac myxomas not associated with multiple endocrine disorders. *J Endocrinol Invest*, 2009; **32**: 501–4.
108. Tagliafico A, Succio G, Martinoli C, Serafini G. Clinical overlap between Mazabraud and McCune-Albright syndromes. *J Ultrasound Med*, 2009; 28: 397–9.
109. Zoccali C, Teori G, Prencipe U, Erba F. Mazabraud's syndrome: a new case and review of the literature. *Int Orthop*, 2009; 33: 605–10.

6.17

Cowden's syndrome

Charis Eng

Introduction

Cowden's syndrome (OMIM 158350), named after Rachel Cowden, is an autosomal dominant inherited cancer syndrome characterized by multiple hamartomas involving organ systems derived from all three germ cell layers and a risk of breast and thyroid cancers (1, 2). Endocrinologists may make the diagnosis of Cowden's syndrome when they are presented with these patients' endocrine lesions, chief of which are multinodular goitre, thyroid adenomas, and epithelial thyroid cancer. The Cowden's syndrome susceptibility gene, *PTEN*, is located on chromosome sub-band 10q23.3 (3, 4).

Epidemiology

Cowden's syndrome has not been well recognized; as of 1993, there were approximately 160 reported cases in the world literature. From an informal population-based study, the estimated gene frequency is one in a million. Multiple case reports have appeared after the identification of the gene in 1997, resulting in incidence estimates of 1:300 000. Because of the variable, protean, and often subtle external manifestations of Cowden's syndrome, many cases remain undiagnosed. Despite the apparent rarity, the syndrome is worthy of note from both scientific and clinical viewpoints. Because Cowden's syndrome is probably underdiagnosed, a true count of the fraction of isolated cases (defined as no obvious family history) and familial cases (defined as two or more related affected individuals) cannot be performed. From the literature and the experience of both major US Cowden's syndrome centres, most cases are isolated. As a broad estimate, perhaps 10–50% of cases are familial.

Aetiology and pathogenesis

Genetics

Inheritance patterns in families with Cowden's syndrome implicate an autosomal dominant pattern. Expression is variable and true penetrance is unknown. Based on the only population-based clinical epidemiology study to date, some believe that the penetrance is 90% after the age of 20 years (3). The precise penetrance will be clarified after further study of the susceptibility gene within families and affected individuals. Cowden's syndrome was mapped to 10q22–23, without genetic heterogeneity (3). Further germline and somatic genetic analysis helped place the putative gene between the markers D10S215 and D10S541, a region of less than 1 cM (3, 5).

PTEN

A candidate tumour suppressor gene *PTEN/MMAC1/TEP1* was located precisely in the Cowden's syndrome critical interval (3, 6). The gene comprises 1209 coding bp in nine exons and predicted to result in a 403-amino acid protein (6, 7). The protein has a tyrosine phosphatase domain and homology to tensin and auxilin (6, 7). Hence, this new gene was dubbed *PTEN* for *p*hosphatase and *ten*sin homologue deleted on chromosome *ten*. *In vitro*, PTEN has been shown to act as a dual specificity phosphatase, meaning it is both a lipid phosphatase and a protein phosphatase as well as a tyrosine phosphatase and serine–threonine phosphatase (8–11). Subsequent *in vivo* work in mouse models has suggested that PTEN plays a role in the PI3Kinase/Akt cell survival/apoptosis pathway (12–14). Because of its homology to the focal adhesion molecules tensin and auxilin, it was hypothesized that PTEN may also play a role in cell migration and focal adhesion. When PTEN was overexpressed in NIH 3T3 cells, it appeared that cell migration was inhibited while antisense PTEN enhanced migration (15). Evidence for PTEN interaction with focal adhesions kinases (FAK) was given when integrin-mediated cell spreading and focal adhesion formation were down-regulated by wild-type but not mutant PTEN; PTEN must interact with FAK to reduce its tyrosine phosphorylation (15). This leads to the hypothesis that PTEN functions as a phosphatase by negatively regulating cell interactions with the extracellular matrix. Although the genetic evidence that points to PTEN as a tumour suppressor—broad spectrum of mutations scattered throughout the gene, truncating mutations, and location of the gene in a region of loss of heterozygosity (see below)—is strong, functional demonstration was still required. When functional wild-type PTEN was transfected into a series of glioma cell lines which carry endogenous *PTEN* mutations or are PTEN null, growth suppression was observed (16–18). Multiple *in vitro* studies where wild-type and mutant PTEN were overexpressed in a broad variety of cancer cell lines, including those of the breast, thyroid, and prostate, demonstrate that PTEN-phosphatase- and PI3K-dependent G1 cell cycle arrest and/or apoptosis result in growth suppression (19–25). This is *in vitro* functional evidence that PTEN acts as a tumour suppressor.

PTEN is the Cowden's syndrome gene

The spectrum of tumour cell lines with *PTEN* mutations, its putative function as suggested by structural motifs, and its location within 10q23.3 all argued strongly that *PTEN* was an ideal candidate for the Cowden's syndrome susceptibility gene. Therefore, to determine if germline *PTEN* mutations could be aetiological for Cowden's syndrome, five families, with a high prior probability of having mutations, were chosen for initial analysis (3, 4). Two families had nonsense mutations, Arg233Xaa and Glu157Xaa, while two unrelated families shared an identical missense mutation, Gly129Glu, which is a nonconservative amino acid alteration occurring in one of the conserved glycines of the phosphatase signature motif (see above). No unaffected family member carried these mutations. In each family, the family-specific germline *PTEN* mutation segregated with disease but not in unaffected family members nor normal controls. Given these data, *PTEN* was most likely the susceptibility gene for Cowden's syndrome. Further support that *PTEN* is indeed the susceptibility gene came when multiple other groups confirmed that germline mutations in *PTEN* are associated with Cowden's syndrome.

PTEN mutation spectrum and genotype–phenotype correlations in Cowden's syndrome

In the single largest series of Cowden's syndrome cases ascertained under the strict operational diagnostic criteria of the International Cowden Consortium (3, 26), 37 unrelated families were examined for frequency and spectrum of germline intragenic *PTEN* mutations (27). Of these, 30 (81%) had germline mutations. The 30 mutations were scattered along the length of the gene. Forty-three per cent of all mutations were found in exon 5, which encodes the phosphatase core motif, although exon 5 only represents 20% of the entire coding sequence.

An exploratory genotype–phenotype association analysis was performed in these 37 Cowden's syndrome families. Two potential associations were noted. The first is the association between the presence of detectable germline mutation in *PTEN* and the presence of malignant breast disease. The second is the association between the presence of missense mutation and/or position of mutation within the phosphatase core motif and the development of multiorgan disease. Because most missense mutations occur within the core motif, it is unclear whether the nature and/or position of the mutation is significant. One could imagine that while missense mutations could disrupt phosphatase activity, the ability to bind substrate is maintained. In this scenario, substrates are sequestered but not dephosphorylated. Conceivably, this could lead to multiorgan involvement. Obviously, given the relatively small numbers, a second larger independent cohort needs to be accrued for genotype–phenotype analyses. If proven true, these preliminary associations might be helpful in tailoring medical management with regard to surveillance. It is also suspected that with a larger series, other associations might be found as well.

Another 10% of Cowden's syndrome individuals not found to have intragenic mutations have germline mutations in the promoter of *PTEN* (28). These promoter mutations result in decreased transcription of *PTEN* as well as decreased translation of *PTEN* due to altered RNA secondary structure (28, 29). Based on small numbers, it would appear that women with germline promoter mutations are at further increased risk of developing breast cancer than those with intragenic mutations.

PTEN is also the Bannayan–Riley–Ruvalcaba gene

Bannayan–Riley–Ruvalcaba syndrome (BRRS) (OMIM 153480) is a rare autosomal dominant disorder characterized by macrocephaly, lipomatoses, hamartomas, hemangiomas, and speckled penis (30). Unlike Cowden's syndrome, however, malignancies have not previously been rigorously shown to be components of BRRS and onset is usually at birth or shortly thereafter. Because of sharing of some, but not all, features of BRRS and Cowden's syndrome, it was postulated that BRR and Cowden's syndrome might be allelic. Initially, two of two BRRS families were shown to have germline *PTEN* mutations (31). Multiple *PTEN* mutations have now been described in both familial and isolated cases of BRRS, such that approximately 60% of BRRS individuals have been found to harbour intragenic *PTEN* mutations (26, 32). Amongst those without intragenic mutations, another 10% have been found to harbour large deletions encompassing or including *PTEN* (28). Since identical mutations (e.g. Arg233Xaa) have been found in Cowden's syndrome as well as BRRS individuals, genetic and nongenetic modifiers must play a role in helping dictate the ultimate phenotype. Overall, the mutational spectrum of Cowden's syndrome cases appears to favour the 5′ two-thirds of *PTEN* while that of BRRS the 3′ two-thirds of the gene (26).

Concept of the *PTEN* hamartoma-tumour syndrome (PHTS)

In addition to Cowden's syndrome and BRRS, germline *PTEN* mutations were found in variable subsets of several seemingly unrelated clinical syndromes. For example, up to 20% of individuals with Proteus syndrome have germline *PTEN* mutations (33). Approximately 10–20% of individuals with autism spectrum disorder and macrocephaly harbour germline *PTEN* mutations (34–37). Single cases of VATER and megalencephaly and hemimegencephaly have been reported to carry germline *PTEN* mutations as well (38, 39). The concept of PHTS to encompass any clinical disorder with germline *PTEN* mutation was proposed because it is clinically useful (32). Finding a germline *PTEN* mutation should trigger cancer risk management and genetic counselling similar to those used for Cowden's syndrome.

PTEN mutation-negative Cowden's syndrome

Approximately 15% of classic Cowden's syndrome and perhaps 90% of Cowden's syndrome-like individuals, defined as having features of Cowden's syndrome but not meeting the diagnostic criteria, remain without detectable *PTEN* mutations. Recently, a subset of such individuals were found to carry germline variants in *SDHB* and *SDHD*, encoding the B and D subunits of mitochondrial succinate dehydrogenase (40). In this pilot series, Cowden's syndrome or Cowden's syndrome-like individuals carrying a germline *SDHB/D* variant had higher frequencies of developing breast, thyroid, and renal cancers than even those with germline *PTEN* mutations.

Pathology

Like other inherited cancer syndromes, multifocality and bilateral involvement is the rule. Hamartomas are the hallmark of Cowden's syndrome. These are classic hamartomas in general and are benign tumours comprising all the elements of a particular organ but in a disorganized fashion. Of note, the hamartomatous polyps found in this syndrome are different in histomorphology from Peutz–Jeghers polyps, which have a distinct appearance. However, caution must be taken when the polyp histology is not read by a dedicated gastrointestinal pathologist as histological diagnoses are often incorrect when compared to genetic classification (41).

With regard to the individual cancers, even of the breast and thyroid, as of 2009, there has yet to be a systematic study published. Recently, however, one study has attempted to look at benign and malignant breast pathology in Cowden's syndrome patients. Although these are preliminary studies, without true matched controls, it is, to date, the only study to examine breast pathology in a series of Cowden's syndrome cases. Breast histopathology from 59 cases belonging to 19 Cowden's syndrome women was systematically analysed (42). Thirty-five specimens had some form of malignant pathology. Of these, 31 (90%) had ductal adenocarcinoma, one tubular carcinoma, and one lobular carcinoma *in situ*. Sixteen of the 31 had both invasive and *in situ* (DCIS) components of ductal carcinoma, while 12 had DCIS only and two only invasive adenocarcinoma.

Benign thyroid pathology is more common in Cowden's syndrome than malignant. Multinodular goitre and thyroid adenomas are often noted. Follicular thyroid carcinomas are much more common than papillary histology in PHTS although *SDHB/D*-related thyroid carcinomas are more likely to be papillary (2, 40). No systematic studies on thyroid pathology in Cowden's syndrome have been performed.

Clinical aspects

Diagnostic criteria

Cowden's syndrome usually presents by the late 20s. It has variable expression and, probably, an age-related penetrance. As with most syndromes prior to gene identification, the precise penetrance is unknown. By the third decade, 99% of affected individuals would have developed the mucocutaneous stigmata although any of the features could be present already (Boxes 6.17.1 and 6.17.2). It is believed that the penetrance is less than 10% under the age of 20 years. The most commonly reported manifestations are mucocutaneous lesions, thyroid abnormalities, fibrocystic disease, and carcinoma of the breast, gastrointestinal hamartomas, multiple, early onset uterine leiomyoma, macrocephaly (specifically, megencephaly), and developmental delay (Box 6.17.1) (2, 43). Pathognomonic mucocutaneous lesions are trichilemmomas and papillomatous papules (Box 6.17.2). Because of the lack of uniform diagnostic criteria for Cowden's syndrome prior to 1995, a group of individuals, the International Cowden Consortium (2, 3), interested in systematically studying this syndrome arrived at a set of consensus operational diagnostic criteria (Box 6.17.2). Subsequently, when virtually all adult-onset presentations of Lhermitte–Duclos disease (LDD; dysplastic gangliocytoma of the cerebellum) were shown to have *PTEN* mutations, LDD was made a pathognomonic diagnostic criterion as well (44).

The two most commonly recognized cancers in Cowden's syndrome are carcinoma of the breast and thyroid. By contrast, in the general population, lifetime risks for breast and thyroid cancers are approximately 11% (in women) and 1%, respectively. In women with Cowden's syndrome, lifetime risk estimates for the development of breast cancer range from 25 to 50% (43, 45). The mean age at diagnosis is probably 10 years earlier than breast cancer occurring in the general population. Although Rachel Cowden died of breast cancer at the age of 31 (46) and the earliest recorded age at diagnosis of breast cancer is 14, the great majority of breast cancers are diagnosed after the age of 30–35 (range 14–65).

Box 6.17.1 Common manifestations of Cowden's syndrome

- Mucocutaneous lesions (90–100%)
  - Trichilemmomas
  - Acral keratoses
  - Verucoid or papillomatous papules
- Thyroid abnormalities (50–67%)
  - Goitre
  - Adenoma
  - Cancer (3–10%)
- Breast lesions
  - Fibroadenomas/fibrocystic disease (76% of affected females)
  - Adenocarcinoma (25–50% of affected females)
- Gastrointestinal lesions (40%)
  - Hamartomatous polyps
- Macrocephaly (38%)
- Genitourinary abnormalities (44% of females)
  - Uterine leiomyoma (multiple, early onset)

The lifetime risk for epithelial thyroid cancer can be as high as 10% in males and females with Cowden's syndrome. Because of small numbers, it is unclear if the age of onset is earlier than that of the general population. Histologically, the thyroid cancer is predominantly follicular carcinoma although papillary histology has also been observed. Medullary thyroid carcinoma has yet to be observed in patients with Cowden's syndrome.

Benign tumours are also very common in Cowden's syndrome. Apart from those of the skin, benign tumours or disorders of breast and thyroid are the most frequently noted and probably represent true component features of this syndrome (Box 6.17.1). Fibroadenomas and fibrocystic disease of the breast are common signs in Cowden's syndrome, as are follicular adenomas and multinodular goitre of the thyroid. Exponents of this field believe that endometrial carcinoma could be an important component tumour of Cowden's syndrome as well. Other tumours that are seen in Cowden's syndrome include renal cell carcinoma, malignant melanoma, and glial tumours. Whether each of these tumours is a true component of Cowden's syndrome or whether some are coincidental findings is as yet unknown.

Role of endocrinologists in Cowden's syndrome

There are several ways in which Cowden's syndrome patients can come to the attention of endocrinologists or endocrine surgeons. Sometimes, an individual with known Cowden's syndrome is referred for management of their endocrine problems, chief of which are multinodular goitre, thyroid adenomas, and epithelial thyroid carcinomas. More commonly, such patients are not previously diagnosed and seek endocrinological attention because of abnormal thyroid function or a thyroid mass. Over two-thirds of

Box 6.17.2 International Cowden Syndrome Consortium operational criteria for the diagnosis of Cowden's syndrome (Version 1996)*

- Pathognomonic criteria
  Mucocutanous lesions:
  - Trichilemmomas, facial
  - Acral keratoses
  - Papillomatous papules
  - Mucosal lesions
- Major criteria
  - Breast carcinoma
  - Thyroid carcinoma, especially follicular thyroid
  - Macrocephaly (Megalencephaly) (greater than 97%)
  - Lhermitte–Duclos disease (LDD)
- Minor criteria
  - Other thyroid lesions (e.g. adenoma or multinodular goitre)
  - Mental retardation (e.g. IQ less than 75)
  - Gastrointestinal hamartomas
  - Fibrocystic disease of the breast
  - Lipomas
  - Fibromas
  - Genitourinary tumours (e.g. uterine fibroids) or malformation
- Operational diagnosis in an individual
  Mucocutanous lesions alone if:
  - There are 6 or more facial papules, of which 3 or more must be trichilemmoma, or
  - Cutaneous facial papules and oral mucosal papillomatosis, or
  - Oral mucosal papillomatosis and acral keratoses, or
  - Palmo plantar keratoses, 6 or more
- 2 major criteria but one must include macrocephaly or LDD
- 1 major and 3 minor criteria
- 4 minor criteria
- Operational diagnosis in a family where one individual is diagnostic for Cowden's syndrome
  - The pathognomonic criteria
  - Any one major criterion with or without minor criteria
  - Two minor criteria

*Operational diagnostic criteria are reviewed and revised on a continuous basis as new clinical information becomes available.

Cowden's syndrome patients have thyroid problems, which may occur at any age. However, finding multifocal lesions, especially in young individuals, should raise suspicion. Endocrinologists and endocrine surgeons should be especially mindful of the differential diagnosis of Cowden's syndrome should they see patients with these thyroid lesions. A careful history and physical examination, as well as a meticulous family history to look for other component symptoms and signs of Cowden's syndrome, are warranted.

Rarely, Cowden's syndrome individuals present with an uncommon feature of Cowden's syndrome, for example, hyperparathyroidism or parathyroid adenomas. When these occur together with 'a thyroid cancer', the initial diagnosis that endocrinologists might think of is multiple endocrine neoplasia type 2 (MEN 2) (see Chapter 6.12) (2, 47). However, it would be prudent to pursue the histology of the thyroid cancer as this might turn out to be a Cowden's syndrome patient and not a MEN 2 case. Even more unusual, Cowden's syndrome can present with ganglioneuromas of the gut and are referred to the endocrinologist as MEN 2B. However, in general, MEN 2B and Cowden's syndrome, are clinically and genetically distinct (2, 47). A few MEN 2B cases can present with apparently isolated intestinal ganglioneuromatosis without the other classic stigmata of MEN 2B, yet all were found to have the MEN 2B-defining germline *RET* mutation Met918Thr and all developed medullary thyroid carcinoma (48).

Implications for molecular diagnosis and predictive testing

With the identification of *PTEN* as the susceptibility gene for Cowden's syndrome and the original linkage studies indicating no genetic heterogeneity, it is theoretically possible to perform direct mutation analysis of *PTEN* for molecular diagnosis of Cowden's syndrome. Direct mutation analysis has advantages over linkage analysis as it can be performed even if only one individual is available. However, since the discovery of *PTEN*'s involvement in Cowden's syndrome was relatively recent, the actual proportion of isolated and familial cases who carry germline *PTEN* mutations is unknown. If a germline *PTEN* mutation was detected in a previously undiagnosed individual or an individual with an unclear clinical presentation, then the diagnosis becomes obvious. If, however, no germline *PTEN* mutation was found in such an individual, then the result should be considered nondiagnostic. While *SDHB/D* are novel susceptibility alleles, these should be considered experimental until a validation series is achieved.

If a family-specific mutation is already known, then screening for that particular mutation in as yet unaffected family members would yield results which are 100% accurate, barring administrative error. If a family-specific mutation cannot be identified in a family that clearly fits the International Cowden Consortium operational diagnostic criteria for Cowden's syndrome, then predictive testing based on direct mutation analysis is not possible. However, in the rare instances where the family is large and many affected members are available, then linkage analysis using makers within and closely flanking *PTEN* (D10S579, D10S1765, D10S2491/S2492, and D10S541) might be considered.

Interestingly, families or individuals with only breast and thyroid cancers or a Cowden's syndrome-like phenotype that does not fulfil the diagnostic criteria of the International Cowden Consortium have a low frequency of germline *PTEN* mutation, approximately 2%. Having endometrial carcinoma might increase the likelihood for finding an occult germline *PTEN* mutation.

Although initially believed to be a locus for juvenile polyposis syndrome (OMIM 174900) (49), *PTEN* has been excluded (50). Further, the first susceptibility gene for juvenile polyposis syndrome has been identified as *SMAD4/DPC4* on 18q21.1 and a second susceptibility gene is *BMPR1A* on 10q22 (51–53). Interestingly, germline deletions encompassing *BMPR1A* and *PTEN* seem to be peculiar to the so-called juvenile polyposis of infancy, clinically defined as juvenile polyposis presenting before the age of 6 years old (54).

Genetic counselling and medical management

The key to proper genetic counselling in Cowden's syndrome is recognition of the syndrome. Families with Cowden's syndrome should be counselled as for any autosomal dominant trait with high penetrance. What is unclear, however, is the variability of expression between and within families. We suspect that there are Cowden's syndrome families who have nothing but trichilemmomas and, therefore, never come to medical attention.

The two most serious and established, component tumours in Cowden's syndrome are breast cancer and epithelial thyroid cancer. Patients with Cowden's syndrome or those who are at risk for Cowden's syndrome should undergo surveillance for these two cancers. Beginning in their teens, these individuals should undergo annual physical examinations paying particular attention to the thyroid examination. Beginning in their mid 20s, women with Cowden's syndrome or those at risk for it should be encouraged to perform monthly breast self-examinations and to have careful breast examinations during their annual physicals. The value of annual imaging studies is unclear since there are no objective data available. We usually recommend annual mammography and/or breast ultrasonography performed by skilled individuals in women at risk, beginning at age 30 or 5 years earlier than the earliest breast cancer case in the family, whichever is younger. Some women with Cowden's syndrome develop severe, sometimes disfiguring, fibroadenomas of the breasts well before age 30. This situation should be treated individually. For example, if the fibroadenomas cause pain or if they make breast cancer surveillance impossible, then some have advocated prophylactic mastectomies.

Whether other tumours are true components of Cowden's syndrome is unknown. It is believed, however, that endometrial carcinomas and possibly, skin cancers, might be true features of Cowden's syndrome as well. For now, therefore, surveillance for other organs should follow the American Cancer Society guidelines, although proponents of Cowden's syndrome will advise routine skin and uterine surveillance as well.

The key to successful management of Cowden's syndrome patients and their families is a multidisciplinary team. There should always be a primary care provider, who orchestrates the care of such patients, some of whom will need the care of surgeons, gynaecologists, dermatologists, oncologists, and geneticists at some point.

Approximately 65% of all BRRS cases will have germline *PTEN* mutations (2, 28, 32). Since clinical epidemiological studies on already small numbers of BRRS suggest no formal association with cancer, it becomes difficult to interpret how finding such a mutation in a BRRS patient would alter medical management. If one were to extrapolate from the Cowden's syndrome–*PTEN* data, then it might be conservative to suggest that all BRRS patients and all other PHTS patients be followed for cancer development similar to that practised for Cowden's syndrome.

Acknowledgements

I am grateful to my collaborators and members of my laboratory, past and present, especially Debbie J. Marsh, PhD and Xiao-Ping Zhou, MD, PhD, for contributing to the work described in this chapter. I am deeply appreciative of Kathy Schneider, MPH, CGC for her superb coordination of the PTEN Study during its infancy, and for her continued friendship and support. My laboratory has been and is supported by the American Cancer Society, the Breast Cancer Research Foundation, the Department of Defence USARMC Breast Cancer Research Programme, the Susan G. Komen Breast Cancer Foundation, and the National Cancer Institute. CE is a Doris Duke Distinguished Clinical Scientist Awardee, an American Cancer Society Clinical Research Professor, and the Sondra J. and Stephen R. Hardis Chair of Cancer Genomic Medicine at the Cleveland Clinic.

References

1. Zbuk K, Stein J, Eng C. *PTEN Hamartoma Tumor Syndrome (PHTS): GeneReviews at GeneTests: Medical Genetics Information Resource [database online]*. Seattle: University of Washington, copyright 1997–2006. 2006:
2. Zbuk K, Eng C. Cancer phenomics: RET and PTEN as illustrative models. *Nat Rev Cancer*, 2007; **7**: 35–45.
3. Nelen MR, Padberg GW, Peeters EAJ, Lin AY, van den Helm B, Frants RR, *et al*. Localization of the gene for Cowden disease to 10q22–23. *Nat Genet*, 1996; **13**: 114–16.
4. Liaw D, Marsh DJ, Li J, Dahia PLM, Wang SI, Zheng Z, *et al*. Germline mutations of the *PTEN* gene in Cowden disease, an inherited breast and thyroid cancer syndrome. *Nat Genet*, 1997; **16**: 64–7.
5. Dahia PLM, Marsh DJ, Zheng Z, Zedenius J, Komminoth P, Frisk T, *et al*. Somatic deletions and mutations in the Cowden disease gene, *PTEN*, in sporadic thyroid tumors. *Cancer Res*, 1997; **57**: 4710–13.
6. Li J, Yen C, Liaw D, Podsypanina K, Bose S, Wang S, *et al*. *PTEN*, a putative protein tyrosine phosphatase gene mutated in human brain, breast and prostate cancer. *Science*, 1997; **275**: 1943–7.
7. Li D-M, Sun H. TEP1, encoded by a candidate tumor suppressor locus, is a novel protein tyrosine phosphatase regulated by transforming growth factor B. *Cancer Res*, 1997; **57**: 2124–9.
8. Maehama T, Dixon JE. The tumor suppressor, PTEN/MMAC1, dephosphorylates the lipid second messenger phosphoinositol 3,4,5-triphosphate. *J Biol Chem*, 1998; **273**: 13375–8.
9. Myers MP, Stolarov J, Eng C, Li J, Wang SI, Wigler MH, *et al*. PTEN, the tumor suppressor from human chromosome 10q23, is a dual specificity phosphatase. *Proc Natl Acad Sci U S A*, 1997; **94**: 9052–7.
10. Myers MP, Tonks NK. PTEN: Sometimes taking it off can be better than putting it on. *Am J Hum Genet*, 1997; **61**: 1234–8.
11. Myers MP, Pass I, Batty IH, van der Kaay J, Storalov JP, Hemmings BA, *et al*. The lipid phosphatase activity of PTEN is critical for its tumor suppressor function. *Proc Natl Acad Sci U S A*, 1998; **95**: 13513–18.
12. Suzuki A, de la Pompa JL, Stambolic V, Elia AJ, Sasaki T, del Barco Barrantes I, *et al*. High cancer susceptibility and embryonic lethality associated with mutation of the *PTEN* tumor suppressor gene in mice. *Curr Biol*, 1998; **8**: 1169–78.
13. Stambolic V, Suzuki A, de la Pompa JL, Brothers GM, Mirtsos C, Sasaki T, *et al*. Negative regulation of PKB/Akt-dependent cell survival by the tumor suppressor PTEN. *Cell*, 1998; **95**: 1–20.
14. Dahia PLM, Aguiar RCT, Alberta J, Kum J, Caron S, Sills H, *et al*. PTEN is inversely correlated with the cell survival factor PKB/Akt and is inactivated by diverse mechanisms in haematologic malignancies. *Hum Mol Genet*, 1999; **8**: 185–93.

15. Tamura M, Gu J, Danen EHJ, Takino T, Miyamoto S, Yamada KM. PTEN interactions with focal adhesion kinase and suppression of the extracellular matrix-dependent phosphotidyinositol 3-kinase/Akt cell survival pathway. *J Biol Chem*, 1999; **274**: 20693–703.
16. Furnari FB, Lin H, Huang H-JS, Cavanee WK. Growth suppression of glioma cells by PTEN requires a functional catalytic domain. *Proc Natl Acad Sci U S A*, 1997; **94**: 12479–84.
17. Cheney IW, Johnson DE, Vaillancourt M-T, Avanzini J, Morimoto A, Demers GW, *et al.* Suppression of tumorigenicity of glioblastoma cells by adenovirus-mediated *MMAC1/PTEN* gene transfer. *Cancer Res*, 1998; **58**: 2331–4.
18. Li DM, Sun H. PTEN/MMAC1/TEP1 suppresses the tumorigenecity and induces G1 cell cycle arrest in human glioblastoma cells. *Proc Natl Acad Sci U S A*, 1998; **95**: 15406–11.
19. Weng L-P, Smith WM, Dahia PLM, Ziebold U, Gil E, Lees JA, *et al.* PTEN suppresses breast cancer cell growth by phosphatase function-dependent G1 arrest followed by apoptosis. *Cancer Res*, 1999; **59**: 5808–14.
20. Weng LP, Brown JL, Baker KM, Ostrowski MC, Eng C. PTEN blocks insulin-mediated Ets-2 phosphorylation through MAP kinase, independent of the phosphoinositide-3-kinase pathway. *Hum Mol Genet*, 2002; **11**: 1687–96.
21. Weng LP, Brown JL, Eng C. PTEN induces apoptosis and cell cycle arrest through phosphoinositol-3-kinase/Akt-dependent and independent pathways. *Hum Mol Genet*, 2001; **10**: 237–42.
22. Weng LP, Brown JL, Eng C. PTEN coordinates G1 arrest by down regulating cyclin D1 via its protein phosphatase activity and up regulating p27 via its lipid phosphatase activity. *Hum Mol Genet*, 2001; **10**: 599–604.
23. Weng LP, Gimm O, Kum JB, Smith WM, Zhou XP, Wynford-Thomas D, *et al.* Transient ectopic expression of *PTEN* in thyroid cancer cell lines induces cell cycle arrest and cell type-dependent cell death. *Hum Mol Genet*, 2001; **10**: 251–8.
24. Weng LP, Smith WM, Brown JL, Eng C. PTEN inhibits insulin-stimulated MEK/MAPK activation and cell growth by blocking IRS-1 phosphorylation and IRS-1/Grb-2/Sos complex formation in a breast cancer model. *Hum Mol Genet*, 2001; **10**: 605–16.
25. Davies MA, Kim SJ, Parikh NU, Dong Z, Bucana CD, Gallick GE. Adenoviral-mediated expression of MMAC/PTEN inhibits proliferation and metastasis of human prostate cancer cells. *Clin Cancer Res*, 2002; **8**: 1904–14.
26. Eng C. *PTEN*: One gene, many syndromes. *Hum Mutat*, 2003; **22**: 183–98.
27. Marsh DJ, Coulon V, Lunetta KL, Rocca-Serra P, Dahia PLM, Zheng Z, *et al.* Mutation spectrum and genotype-phenotype analyses in Cowden disease and Bannayan-Zonana syndrome, two hamartoma syndromes with germline *PTEN* mutation. *Hum Mol Genet*, 1998; **7**: 507–15.
28. Zhou XP, Waite KA, Pilarski R, Hampel H, Fernandez MJ, Bos C, *et al.* Germline *PTEN* promoter mutations and deletions in Cowden/Bannayan-Riley-Ruvalcaba syndrome result in aberrant PTEN protein and dysregulation of the phosphoinositol-3-kinase/Akt pathway. *Am J Hum Genet*, 2003; **73**: 404–11.
29. Teresi RE, Planchon SM, Waite KA, Eng C. Regulation of the *PTEN* promoter by statins and SREBP. *Hum Mol Genet*, 2008; **17**: 919–28.
30. Gorlin RJ, Cohen MM, Condon LM, Burke BA. Bannayan-Riley-Ruvalcaba syndrome. *Am J Med Genet*, 1992; **44**: 307–14.
31. Marsh DJ, Dahia PLM, Zheng Z, Liaw D, Parsons R, Gorlin RJ, *et al.* Germline mutations in *PTEN* are present in Bannayan-Zonana syndrome. *Nature Genet*, 1997; **16**: 333–4.
32. Marsh DJ, Kum JB, Lunetta KL, Bennett MJ, Gorlin RJ, Ahmed SF, *et al.* *PTEN* mutation spectrum and genotype-phenotype correlations in Bannayan-Riley-Ruvalcaba syndrome suggest a single entity with Cowden syndrome. *Hum Mol Genet*, 1999; **8**: 1461–72.
33. Zhou XP, Hampel H, Thiele H, Gorlin RJ, Hennekam R, Parisi M, *et al.* Association of germline mutation in the *PTEN* tumour suppressor gene and a subset of Proteus sand Proteus-like syndromes. *Lancet*, 2001; **358**: 210–11.
34. Butler MG, Dasouki MJ, Zhou XP, Talebizadeh Z, Brown M, Takahashi TN, *et al.* Subset of individuals with autism spectrum disorders and macrocephaly associated with germline mutations in the PTEN tumour suppressor gene. *J Med Genet*, 2005; **42**: 318–21.
35. Herman GE, Butter E, Enrile B, Pastore M, Prior TW, Sommer A. Increasing knowledge of germline PTEN mutations: two additional patients with autism and macrocephaly. *Am J Med Genet A*, 2007; **143**: 589–93.
36. Herman GE, Henninger N, Ratliff-Schaub K, Pastore M, FitzGerald S, McBride KL. Genetic testing in autism: how much is enough? *Genet Med*, 2007; **9**: 268–74.
37. Varga EA, Pastore M, Prior T, Herman GE, McBride KL. The prevalence of PTEN mutations in a clinical pediatric cohort with autism spectrum disorders, developmental delay and macrocephaly. *Genet Med*, 2009; **11**: 111–17.
38. Reardon W, Zhou XP, Eng C. A novel germline mutation of the *PTEN* gene in a patient with macrocephaly, ventricular dilatation and features of VATER association. *J Med Genet*, 2001; **38**: 820–3.
39. Merks JHM, de Vries LS, Zhou XP, Nikkels P, Barth PG, Eng C, *et al.* Cowden/Bannayan-Riley-Ruvalcaba syndrome: variability of an entity. *J Med Genet*, 2003; **40**.
40. Ni Y, Zbuk KM, Sadler T, Patocs A, Lobo G, Edelman E, *et al.* Germline mutations and variants in the succinate dehydrogenase genes in Cowden and Cowden-like syndromes. *Am J Hum Genet*, 2008; **83**: 261–8.
41. Sweet K, Willis J, Zhou XP, Gallione C, Sawada T, Alhopuro P, *et al.* Molecular classification of patients with unexplained hamartomatous and hyperplastic polyposis. *JAMA*, 2005; **294**: 2465–73.
42. Schrager CA, Schneider D, Gruener AC, Tsou HC, Peacocke M. Clinical and pathological features of breast disease in Cowden's syndrome: an underrecognised syndrome with an increased risk of breast cancer. *Hum Pathol*, 1997; **29**: 47–53.
43. Hanssen AMN, Fryns JP. Cowden syndrome. *J Med Genet*, 1995; **32**: 117–19.
44. Zhou XP, Marsh DJ, Morrison CD, Maxwell M, Reifenberger G, Eng C. Germline and somatic PTEN mutations and decreased expression of PTEN protein and dysfunction of the PI3K/Akt pathway in Lhermitte-Duclos disease. *Am J Hum Genet*, 2003; **73**: 1191–8.
45. Starink TM, van der Veen JPW, Arwert F, de Waal LP, de Lange GG, Gille JJP, *et al.* The cowden syndrome: a clinical and genetic study in 21 patients. *Clin Genet*, 1986; **29**: 222–33.
46. Lloyd KM, Denis M. Cowden's disease: a possible new symptom complex with multiple system involvement. *Ann Intern Med*, 1963; **58**: 136–42.
47. Eng C. The *RET* proto-oncogene in multiple endocrine neoplasia type 2 and Hirschsprung disease. *N Engl J Med*, 1996; **335**: 943–51.
48. Gordon CM, Majzoub JA, Marsh DJ, Mulliken JB, Ponder BAJ, Robinson BG, *et al.* Four cases of mucosal neuroma syndrome: MEN 2B or not 2B. *J Clin Endocrinol Metab*, 1998; **83**: 17–20.
49. Olschwang S, Serova-Sinilnikova OM, Lenoir GM, Thomas G. *PTEN* germline mutations in juvenile polyposis coli. *Nat Genet*, 1998; **18**: 12–14.
50. Eng C, Peacocke M. *PTEN* and inherited hamartoma-cancer syndromes. *Nat Genet*, 1998; **19**: 223.
51. Howe JR, Roth S, Ringold JC, Summers RW, Jarvinen HJ, Sistonen P, *et al.* Mutations in the *SMAD4/DPC4* gene in juvenile polyposis. *Science*, 1998; **280**: 1086–8.
52. Howe JR, Blair JA, Sayed MG, Anderson ME, Mitros FA, Petersen GM, *et al.* Germline mutations of *BMPR1A* in juvenile polyposis. *Nat Genet*, 2001; **28**: 184–7.
53. Eng C. News and views: to be or not to BMP. *Nat Genet*, 2001; **28**: 105–7.
54. Delnatte C, Sanlaville D, Mougenot JF, Houdayer C, Vermeesch J, de Blois MC, *et al.* Contiguous gene deletion within chromosome arm 10q is associated with juvenile polyposis of infancy reflecting cooperation between the *BMPRIA* and *PTEN* tumor suppressor genes. *Am J Hum Genet*, 2006; **78**: 1066–74.

Index

Note:
Major discussions of topics are indicated by page numbers in **bold.** Page numbers in *italics* refer to tables.

O

Q

S

U

Y

Z